D1241428

Yen and Jaffe's
REPRODUCTIVE ENDOCRINOLOGY

Yen and Jaffe's

REPRODUCTIVE ENDOCRINOLOGY

Physiology, Pathophysiology, and Clinical Management

6TH EDITION

Jerome F. Strauss III, MD, PhD
Executive Vice President for Medical Affairs, VCU Health System
Dean, School of Medicine and Professor of Obstetrics and Gynecology
Virginia Commonwealth University
Richmond, Virginia

Robert L. Barbieri, MD
Kate Macy Ladd Professor, Department of Obstetrics, Gynecology and Reproductive Biology
Harvard Medical School
Chair, Department of Obstetrics and Gynecology
Brigham and Women's Hospital
Boston, Massachusetts

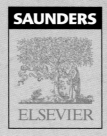

SAUNDERS

ELSEVIER

SAUNDERS
ELSEVIER

1600 John F. Kennedy Blvd.
Ste 1800
Philadelphia, PA 19103-2899

Notice

Knowledge and best practice in this field are constantly changing. As new research and experience broaden our knowledge, changes in practice, treatment, and drug therapy may become necessary or appropriate. Readers are advised to check the most current information provided (i) on procedures featured or (ii) by the manufacturer of each product to be administered, to verify the recommended dose or formula, the method and duration of administration, and contraindications. It is the responsibility of the practitioner, relying on his or her own experience and knowledge of the patient, to make diagnoses, to determine dosages and the best treatment for each individual patient, and to take all appropriate safety precautions. To the fullest extent of the law, neither the Publisher nor the Editors assume any liability for any injury and/or damage to persons or property arising out or related to any use of the material contained in this book.

Library of Congress Cataloging-in-Publication Data
Yen and Jaffe's reproductive endocrinology / [edited by] Jerome F.
Strauss, Robert L. Barbieri.—6th ed.
   p. ; cm.
Includes bibliographical references and index.
ISBN 978-1-4160-4907-4
  1. Human reproduction—Endocrine aspects. 2. Endocrine gynecology.
3. Generative organs—Diseases—Endocrine aspects. I. Strauss, Jerome F.
(Jerome Frank) II. Barbieri, Robert L. III. Yen, Samuel S. C.
Reproductive endocrinology. IV. Title: Reproductive endocrinology.
[DNLM: 1. Reproduction—physiology. 2. Endocrine Glands—physiology.
3. Endocrine System Diseases—physiopathology. WQ 205 Y4467 2009]
QP252.Y46 2009
612.6—dc22

2008037592

Acquisitions Editor: Stefanie Jewell-Thomas
Developmental Editor: Colleen McGonigal
Project Manager: Mary Stermel
Marketing Manager: Courtney Ingram
Design Direction: Ellen Zanolle
Multi-Media Producer: Adrienne Simon

Printed in China

Last digit is the print number: 9 8 7 6 5 4 3 2 1

Remembrance

Samuel S. C. Yen, MD, DSc
1927–2006

In 2006, endocrinology in general, and reproductive endocrinology in particular, lost a giant in clinical and translational reproductive endocrinologic research, Samuel S. C. Yen. He was insightful and a visionary and demanded excellence from his trainees, but no more so than from himself. He was arguably the leading clinical reproductive neuroendocrinologist of his time.

He and I coedited the first four editions of this textbook, which has since been translated from English into five languages—including a pirated version from China. The genesis of our textbook was crystallized during our time at the magnificent, idyllic Rockefeller Foundation retreat, the Villa Serbelloni, at the nexus of the three legs of Lake Como in Italy. It was there, surrounded by scholars from a panoply of disciplines and countries (Sam and I were the only physicians in the group), that we had the time and freedom to finalize the chapters. We mutually selected the authors, most of whom were outstanding investigators and clinicians in the areas about which they wrote (albeit not all as expeditiously as we had hoped).

Fortunately, our first editor, John Hanley, was a true scholar who shared our passion for quality and excellence. Our original publisher, W. B. Saunders, shared that same passion.

Sam continued his insistence on excellence for each edition, and he cajoled several of our authors until they did the same.

Sam's chapters on neuroendocrine regulation of the brain and of the hypothalamic-pituitary-ovarian axis are classic. His extensive and productive collaboration with his very close friend, the Nobel Laureate Roger Guillemin, who characterized many of the hypothalamic secretagogues that Sam used in his clinical studies, enabled him to base many of his comments in the textbook on his own laboratory's studies.

Sam was hard-driving, yet charming, as demanding of himself and our authors as he was of the myriad investigators with whom he worked and trained. His was a rich, full, productive, and creative life. He was a unique and colorful individual.

His like comes along very rarely.

Robert B. Jaffe, MD
University of California, San Francisco
2008

Contributors

Valerie A. Arboleda
Department of Human Genetics, David Geffen School of
Medicine at UCLA, Los Angeles, California
16: *Disorders of Sex Development*

Mario Ascoli, PhD
Professor, Department of Pharmacology, Carver College
of Medicine, The University of Iowa, Iowa City, Iowa
2: *The Gonadotropin Hormones and Their Receptors*

Richard J. Auchus, MD, PhD
The Charles A. and Elizabeth Ann Sanders Chair in
Translational Research, Professor of Internal Medicine,
Division of Endocrinology and Metabolism, University
of Texas Southwestern Medical Center, Dallas, Texas
23: *Endocrine Disturbances Affecting Reproduction*

Robert L. Barbieri, MD
Kate Macy Ladd Professor, Department of Obstetrics,
Gynecology and Reproductive Biology, Harvard
Medical School; Chair, Department of Obstetrics and
Gynecology Brigham and Women's Hospital, Boston,
Massachusetts
10: *The Breast;* **21:** *Female Infertility*

Kurt Barnhart, MD, MSCE
Director, Women's Health Clinical Research Center,
Assistant Dean, Clinical Trial Operations, University
of Pennsylvania School of Medicine, Philadelphia,
Pennsylvania
34: *Contraception*

Breton F. Barrier, MD
Assistant Professor, Department of Obstetrics,
Gynecology and Women's Health, University of
Missouri, Columbia, Columbia, Missouri
13: *Reproductive Immunology and Its Disorders*

Enrico Carmina, MD
Professor of Endocrinology, Department of
Clinical Medicine, University of Palermo,
Palermo, Italy
32: *Evaluation of Hormonal Status*

Alice Y. Chang, MD, MS
Assistant Professor, Department of Internal Medicine,
Division of Endocrinology and Metabolism,
University of Texas Southwestern Medical Center,
Dallas, Texas
23: *Endocrine Disturbances Affecting Reproduction*

R. Jeffrey Chang, MD
Professor and Division Director, University of California
School of Medicine, San Diego, California
20: *Polycystic Ovary Syndrome and Hyperandrogenic
States*

Charles Chapron, MD
Professor and Chair, Obstetrics and Gynecology II,
Université Descartes GHU Cochin-St. Vincent
de Paul, Paris, France
33: *Pelvic Imaging in Reproductive Endocrinology*

John A. Cidlowski, PhD
Chief, Laboratory of Signal Transduction, Head,
Molecular Endocrinology Group, National Institute
of Environmental Health Science, National
Institutes of Health, Research Triangle Park,
North Carolina
5: *Steroid Hormone Action*

Donald K. Clifton, PhD
Professor of Obstetrics and Gynecology, University of
Washington, Seattle, Washington
1: *Neuroendocrinology of Reproduction*

Anick De Vos, PhD
Clinical Embryologist, Centre for Reproductive
    Medicine, Universitair Ziekenhuis Brussel, Brussels,
    Belgium
30: Gamete and Embryo Manipulation

Dominique de Ziegler, MD
Professor and Head, Reproductive Endocrine and
    Infertility, Obstetrics and Gynecology II, Université
    Descartes GHU Cochin-St. Vincent de Paul, Paris,
    France
33: Pelvic Imaging in Reproductive Endocrinology

William S. Evans, MD
Professor, Departments of Medicine and Obstetrics and
    Gynecology, University of Virginia, Charlottesville,
    Virginia
*19: Physiologic and Pathophysiologic Alterations of the
    Neuroendocrine Components of the Reproductive Axis*

Bart C. J. M. Fauser, MD, PhD
Professor of Reproductive Medicine; Chair, University
    Medical Center Utrecht, Utrecht, The Netherlands
*28: Medical Approaches to Ovarian Stimulation for
    Infertility*

Garret A. FitzGerald, MD
Robert L. McNeil, Jr., Professor in Translational Medicine
    and Therapeutics, Department of Pharmacology,
    University of Pennsylvania School of Medicine,
    Philadelphia, Pennsylvania
*6: Prostaglandins and Other Lipid Mediators in
    Reproductive Medicine*

Timothée Fraisse, MD, MSc
Joint Division Reproductive Endocrine and Infertility,
    University Hospitals Geneva and Lausanne, Geneva
    and Lausanne, Switzerland
33: Pelvic Imaging in Reproductive Endocrinology

Colin D. Funk, PhD
Professor, Departments of Physiology and Biochemistry,
    Queen's University, Kingston, Canada
*6: Prostaglandins and Other Lipid Mediators in
    Reproductive Medicine*

Antonio R. Gargiulo, MD
Assistant Professor, Department of Obstetrics,
    Gynecology and Reproductive Biology, Harvard
    Medical School; Associate Reproductive
    Endocrinologist, Department of Obstetrics,
    Gynecology and Reproductive Biology,
    Brigham and Women's Hospital, Boston,
    Massachusetts
13: Reproductive Immunology and Its Disorders

Janet E. Hall, MD
Professor of Medicine, Harvard Medical School;
    Reproductive Endocrine Unit, Massachusetts
    General Hospital, Boston, Massachusetts
7: Neuroendocrine Control of the Menstrual Cycle

Kristin D. Helm, MD
Fellow, Division of Endocrinology and Metabolism,
    South Shore Hospital, South Weymouth,
    Massachusetts
*19: Physiologic and Pathophysiologic Alterations of the
    Neuroendocrine Components of the Reproductive Axis*

Mark D. Hornstein, MD
Associate Professor of Obstetrics, Gynecology and
    Reproductive Biology, Harvard Medical School;
    Director, Division of Reproductive Endocrinology and
    Infertility; Director, Center for Reproductive Medicine,
    Brigham and Women's Hospital, Boston, Massachusetts
29: Assisted Reproduction

Dan I. Lebovic, MD, MA
Director, Division of Reproductive Endocrinology and
    Infertility, Department of Obstetrics and Gynecology,
    University of Wisconsin School of Medicine, Madison,
    Wisconsin
24: Endometriosis

Charles Lee, PhD, FACMG
Director of Cytogenetics, Harvard Cancer Center;
    Associate Professor, Harvard Medical School; Associate
    Faculty Member, MIT Broad Institute; Clinical
    Cytogeneticist, Brigham and Women's Hospital,
    Boston, Massachusetts
31: Cytogenetics in Reproduction

Bruce A. Lessey, MD, PhD
Greenville Professor, University of South Carolina
    School of Medicine; Vice Chair, Research and Division
    Director, Reproductive Endocrinology and Infertility,
    Greenville Hospital System, Greenville, South Carolina
*9: The Structure, Function, and Evaluation of the Female
    Reproductive Tract*

Peter Y. Liu, MBBS, FRACP, PhD
Associate Professor and Head, Endocrinology and
    Metabolism, Woolcock Institute of Medical Research
    and ANZAC Research Institute, University of Sydney,
    Sydney, Australia; Associate Professor and Consultant,
    Concord Hospital, Concord, Australia
*12: The Hypothalamo-Pituitary Unit, Testes, and Male
    Accessory Organs*

Rogerio A. Lobo, MD
Professor, Columbia University College of Physicians and
    Surgeons; Attending Physician, New York Presbyterian
    Hospital; Director, REI Fellowship Program, New
    York, New York
*14: Menopause and Aging; 32: Evaluation of Hormonal
    Status*

Nicholas S. Macklon, MB, ChB, MD,
Professor and Chair, Department of Reproductive
    Medicine and Gynaecology, University Medical Centre
    Utrecht, Utrecht, The Netherlands
*28: Medical Approaches to Ovarian Stimulation for
    Infertility*

Sam Mesiano, PhD
Assistant Professor, Department of Reproductive Biology,
   Case Western Reserve University; Assistant Professor,
   Department of Obstetrics and Gynecology, University
   Hospitals Case Medical Center, Cleveland, Ohio
*11: The Endocrinology of Human Pregnancy and
Fetoplacental Neuroendocrine Development*

Anne Elodie Millischer-Belaïche, MD
Obstetrics and Gynecology II, Université Descartes GHU
   Cochin-St. Vincent de Paul, Paris, France
33: Pelvic Imaging in Reproductive Endocrinology

Mark E. Molitch, MD
Professor of Medicine, Division of Endocrinology,
   Metabolism, and Molecular Medicine, Department
   of Medicine, Northwestern University Feinberg
   School of Medicine; Attending Physician,
   Northwestern Memorial Hospital, Chicago,
   Illinois
3: Prolactin in Human Reproduction

Cynthia C. Morton, PhD
William Lambert Richardson Professor of Obstetrics,
   Gynecology and Reproductive Biology, Brigham and
   Women's Hospital, Boston, Massachusetts
31: Cytogenetics in Reproduction

Ralf M. Nass, MD
Research Assistant Professor, Department of Medicine,
   University of Virginia School of Medicine, University
   of Virginia Health System, Charlottesville, Virginia
*19: Physiologic and Pathophysiologic Alterations
of the Neuroendocrine Components of the Reproductive
Axis*

Errol R. Norwitz, MD, PhD
Professor, Yale University School of Medicine;
   Co-Director, Division of Maternal-Fetal Medicine;
   Director, Maternal-Fetal Medicine Fellowship Program;
   Director, Obstetrics and Gynecology Residency
   Program, Department of Obstetrics, Gynecology
   and Reproductive Sciences, Yale-New Haven Hospital,
   New Haven, Connecticut
26: Endocrine Diseases of Pregnancy

Tony M. Plant, PhD
Professor, Departments of Cell Biology and Physiology
   and Obstetrics, Gynecology and Reproductive
   Sciences, University of Pittsburgh School of Medicine,
   Pittsburgh, Pennsylvania
17: Puberty: Gonadarche and Adrenarche

Staci Pollack, MD
Assistant Professor of Obstetrics and Gynecology
   and Women's Health, Associate Reproductive
   Endocrinology and Infertility Fellowship Director,
   Albert Einstein College of Medicine, New York,
   New York
18: Nutrition and the Pubertal Transition

Alex J. Polotsky, MD, MSc
Assistant Professor of Obstetrics and Gynecology
   and Women's Health, Albert Einstein College
   of Medicine; Attending Physician, Montefiore
   Medical Center, New York, New York
18: Nutrition and the Pubertal Transition

David Puett, PhD
Regents Professor of Biochemistry and Molecular Biology,
   University of Georgia, Athens, Georgia
2: The Gonadotropin Hormones and Their Receptors

Catherine Racowsky, PhD
Associate Professor of Obstetrics, Gynecology and
   Reproductive Biology, Harvard Medical School;
   Director, Assisted Reproductive Technology
   Laboratory, Brigham and Women's Hospital,
   Boston, Massachusetts
29: Assisted Reproduction

Turk Rhen, PhD
Assistant Professor of Biology, University of North
   Dakota, Grand Forks, North Dakota
5: Steroid Hormone Action

Jessica Rieder, MD, MS
Assistant Professor, Department of Pediatrics,
   Division of Adolescent Medicine, Albert Einstein
   College of Medicine; Attending Physician,
   Department of Pediatrics, Division of Adolescent
   Medicine, Children's Hospital at Montefiore,
   New York, New York
18: Nutrition and the Pubertal Transition

Richard J. Santen, MD
Professor of Medicine, University of Virginia Health
   Sciences System, Charlottesville, Virginia
27: Breast Cancer

Nanette Santoro, MD
Professor and Director, Division of Reproductive
   Endocrinology, Department of Obstetrics and
   Gynecology and Women's Health, Albert Einstein
   College of Medicine/Montefiore Medical Center,
   New York, New York
18: Nutrition and the Pubertal Transition

Courtney A. Schreiber, MD, MPH
Assistant Professor of Obstetrics and Gynecology,
   University of Pennsylvania, Philadelphia,
   Pennsylvania
34: Contraception

Danny J. Schust, MD
Associate Professor of Obstetrics, Gynecology and
   Women's Health; Chief, Division of Reproductive
   Endocrinolgy and Infertility, Department of Obstetrics,
   Gynecology and Women's Health, University of
   Missouri, Columbia, Missouri
13: Reproductive Immunology and Its Disorders

Peter J. Snyder, MD
Professor of Medicine, University of Pennsylvania, Philadelphia, Pennsylvania
15: Male Reproductive Aging

Wen-Chao Song, PhD
Professor, Department of Pharmacology, Institute for Translational Medicine and Therapeutics, University of Pennsylvania School of Medicine, Philadelphia, Pennsylvania
6: Prostaglandins and Other Lipid Mediators in Reproductive Medicine

Robert A. Steiner, PhD
Professor, Departments of Obstetrics and Gynecology and Physiology and Biophysics, University of Washington, Seattle, Washington
1: Neuroendocrinology of Reproduction

Elizabeth A. Stewart, MD
Professor, Department of Obstetrics and Gynecology, Mayo Clinic College of Medicine; Senior Associate Consultant, Mayo Clinic, Rochester, Minnesota
25: Benign Uterine Disorders

Jerome F. Strauss III, MD, PhD
Executive Vice President for Medical Affairs, VCU Health System; Dean, School of Medicine and Professor of Obstetrics and Gynecology, Virginia Commonwealth University, Richmond, Virginia
4: The Synthesis and Metabolism of Steroid Hormones; 8: The Ovarian Life Cycle; 9: The Structure, Function, and Evaluation of the Female Reproductive Tract

Robert N. Taylor, MD, PhD
Willaford Leach-Armand Hendee Professor and Vice Chair for Research, Department of Gynecology and Obstetrics, Emory University School of Medicine, Atlanta, Georgia
24: Endometriosis

Stephen F. Thung, MD, MSCI
Assistant Professor, Department of Obstetrics, Gynecology and Reproductive Sciences, Yale University School of Medicine; Director, Yale Maternal-Fetal Medicine Practice; Director, Yale Diabetes during Pregnancy Program, New Haven, Connecticut
26: Endocrine Diseases of Pregnancy

Paul J. Turek, MD, FACS, FRSM
Former Professor and Endowed Chair in Urologic Education, Department of Urology, Obstetrics, Gynecology and Reproductive Sciences, University of San Fransiscco; Director, The Turek Clinic, San Francisco, California
22: Male Infertility

André Van Steirteghem, MD, PhD
Emeritus Professor, Faculty of Medicine, Vrije Universiteit Brussel; Honorary Consultant, Centre for Reproductive Medicine, Universitair Ziekenhuis Brussel, Brussels, Belgium
30: Gamete and Embryo Manipulation

Johannes D. Veldhuis, MD
Professor of Medicine and Clinical Investigator, Mayo Clinic College of Medicine; Consultant, Division of Endocrinology, Diabetes, Metabolism, Nutrition, Department of Internal Medicine, Mayo Clinic, Rochester, Minnesota
12: The Hypothalamo-Pituitary Unit, Testes, and Male Accessory Organs

Eric Vilain, MD, PhD
Professor of Human Genetics, Pediatrics, and Urology; Chief, Medical Genetics, Department of Pediatrics, David Geffen School of Medicine at UCLA, Los Angeles, California
16: Disorders of Sex Development

Carmen J. Williams, MD, PhD
Clinical Investigator, Laboratory of Reproductive and Developmental Toxicology, National Institute of Environmental Health Sciences, Research Triangle Park, North Carolina
8: The Ovarian Life Cycle

Selma Feldman Witchel, MD
Associate Professor, Department of Pediatrics, University of Pittsburgh School of Medicine; Associate Professor, Division of Endocrinology, Children's Hospital of Pittsburgh, Pittsburgh, Pennsylvania
17: Puberty: Gonadarche and Adrenarche

Preface

The year 2008 marked the 30th anniversary of the clinical success of in vitro fertilization and embryo transfer, a technology that has revolutionized the treatment of infertility. This landmark event came about through the marriage of reproductive biology, endocrinology, and gynecology, in what was at the time a new model of translational science. Today, the field of reproductive endocrinology continues to be broad-based with contributions from the fields of developmental and reproductive biology, neuroscience, genetics and genomics, endocrinology, gynecology, obstetrics, andrology, pediatrics, pathology and laboratory medicine, and diagnostic imaging, among others. The multiple disciplines and their respective perspectives have brought forth what can arguably be considered the greatest medical advance in the past century: the capacity of humans to master the process of reproduction. The 6th edition of *Yen and Jaffe's Reproductive Endocrinology* has been expanded to reflect the position of our field as the nexus of basic and clinical research, and as a source of innovation that shapes the scientific foundations of physiology and medicine. The editors thank the chapter authors, both old and new, for delivering the insightful synthesis of their topics. In many instances, advances in research and clinical practice have resulted in substantial changes in scope and direction that necessitated critical appraisal of information offered in the 5th edition.

Since the previous edition of this text, we lost Samuel S. C. Yen, one of the founders of contemporary reproductive endocrinology and one half of the brilliant team that birthed this text. As noted in the remembrance, his legacy is profound, and the editors once again acknowledge his transformative influence on the field.

Jerome F. Strauss III, MD, PhD
Richmond, Virginia

Robert L. Barbieri, MD
Boston, Massachusetts

Contents

PART II

Pathophysiology and Therapy

PART III

Reproductive Technologies

PART I

Endocrinology of Reproduction

CHAPTER 1

Neuroendocrinology of Reproduction

Donald K. Clifton and Robert A. Steiner

Historical Perspective[1]

ENDOCRINOLOGY TAKES FLIGHT

In 1849, A. A. Berthold conducted the first known experiment in endocrinology—long before the word *endocrinology* was invented. He castrated roosters and showed that after the surgery, the animals lost the ability to crow, their combs drooped, and they stopped chasing hens. Berthold went on to show that if he transplanted testes from other roosters into the castrated animals, the newly transplanted organs would survive and the roosters became sexually rejuvenated—crowing, strutting, and mounting the hens, as they did before castration. Berthold observed that the transplanted testes became revascularized and thus revitalized—despite having no obvious regeneration of nerve supply to the organ. Berthold deduced correctly that without the action of nerves, the testes must release blood-borne substances that are transported to distant target sites in the body and thus support the secondary sex characteristics of the rooster and its behavior.

THE ANTERIOR PITUITARY AND NEUROHYPOPHYSIS

The thought that the pituitary gland serves some physiologic function can be traced to the first century AD, when Galen postulated that the pituitary was a sump for wastes distilled from the brain—an idea that was also championed by the Belgian physician and anatomist Andreas Vesalius in the middle of the 16th century. However, the true physiologic significance of the pituitary traces its roots to the late 19th and early 20th century with early attempts of physiologists to perform hypophysectomies and study the outcome on survival, growth, and reproduction. The

work of Harvey Cushing, Bernard Aschner, and others established that the pituitary was indeed important and that experimental manipulations or tumors of the pituitary were associated with disorders of growth, metabolism, adrenal function, and reproduction. Also in the 19th century, Ramón y Cajal described a neural tract that led from the brain to the neural lobe of the pituitary, and in the mid 1920s, it was recognized that the supraoptic and paraventricular nuclei in the hypothalamus were the origins of this neural tract. Cushing observed that the anterior lobe of the pituitary was highly vascularized, and he postulated that this organ was anatomically and physiologically distinct from the pars intermedia, which he incorrectly thought was part of the "neural lobe." Confusion about the anatomy of the pituitary persisted until the mid 1930s, when G. B. Wislocki and L. S. King finally got it right.

ANTERIOR PITUITARY AS A SOURCE FOR GONADOTROPINS

The turn of the 20th century brought with it the first clue that the gonads were somehow physiologically linked to the pituitary gland. In 1905, Fichera reported that castration produced a gross enlargement of the pituitary gland and the appearance of large vacuolated cells—"castration cells." In 1926, working independently, Philip Smith and Bernard Zondek showed that daily injections of fresh pituitary glands into immature mice and rats would induce precocious puberty in recipient animals. In 1927, Smith and E. T. Engle showed that hypophysectomy would prevent sexual maturation, thus establishing a critical role for the pituitary in reproduction. In the early 1930s, Zondek also proposed that the pituitary produced two "gonadotropic" hormones, which he termed *Prolan A* (FSH) and *Prolan B* (LH), and shortly thereafter, H. L. Fevold and

3

F. L. Hisaw, working at the University of Wisconsin, successfully isolated and purified these two hormones, which came to be known as *luteinizing hormone* (LH) and *follicle-stimulating hormone* (FSH).

PROLACTIN AND LACTATION

In the late 1920s, the idea that the pituitary gland plays some role in lactation grew from observations that daily injections of extracts from the anterior pituitary would stimulate mammary gland development in rabbits. In the early 1930s, Oscar Riddle conducted experiments in pigeons and ring doves, showing that secretion of crop milk in birds was stimulated by the same hormone that induced milk secretion in mammals, and Riddle named this hormone *prolactin*. A spate of experimental work over the next several decades would establish that prolactin has complicated effects on the reproductive axis in mammals—acting as a luteotropic factor in some species, but inhibiting FSH secretion (and thus estrous cyclicity) in others. The isolation of prolactin from growth hormone would not come until 1962, when R. W. Bates and his colleagues finally separated these closely related molecules and thus helped to explain 30 years of confusing experimental results involving studies of "pituitary extracts" on growth, reproduction, and lactation.

THE HYPOTHALAMIC–PITUITARY–GONADAL (HPG) AXIS

As early as 1901, Alfred Frohlich had described a clinical syndrome termed *urogenital dystrophy*, which was associated with damage to the pituitary gland and basal forebrain, but for the next 40 years, it remained controversial whether the condition was caused by damage to either the hypothalamus or the pituitary. Nevertheless, by 1930, it had become clear that experimental manipulations of the anterior pituitary gland (e.g., hypophysectomy) could influence gonadal function and likewise that alterations in gonadal function (i.e., castration) would influence the cellular architecture of the pituitary. These observations led Dorothy Price and Carl Moore to postulate that there was a reciprocal relationship between the pituitary and gonads, such that pituitary hormones stimulate gonadal function, whereas gonadal hormones inhibit "gonadotropin" secretion—a concept that has come to be known as *gonadal steroid negative feedback*. The idea that the brain might also be involved in this process was presaged by studies in the late 1920s of coitally induced ovulation in rabbits, but Walter Holweg and Karl Junkmann were the first to argue that the brain serves as an intermediary target for gonadal hormones, and then in turn controls the activity of the anterior pituitary. Later in the 1930s, F. H. Marshall, G. W. Harris, and others went on to show that stimulation of the brain and hypothalamus, in particular, could induce ovulation in the rabbit. In the early 1940s, Frederick Dey, working at Northwestern University, showed that discrete lesions placed in the hypothalamus could induce either constant estrus or diestrus in the rat. This work established the idea that different areas of the hypothalamus coordinate particular aspects of reproductive

cyclicity. By the late 1940s, experiments conducted by J. W. Everett, C. H. Sawyer, and J. E. Markee clearly showed in the rat and rabbit that ovulation could be either blocked or induced by drugs that act on the central nervous system, thus reinforcing the idea that the brain plays a central role in the events that trigger ovulation. Although it had also become evident that communication between the brain and the pituitary was essential for pituitary function, the anatomic basis for this communication (later discovered to be the pituitary portal vessels) remained unappreciated for many years. In fact, it remained dogmatic that the brain–pituitary connection must be "neural," notwithstanding the anatomic observations of A. T. Rasmussen, who had reported finding very few nerve fibers in the anterior pituitary.

In the early 1930s, G. T. Popa and U. Fielding reported finding blood vessels that connected the basal forebrain to the anterior pituitary gland. However, they incorrectly deduced that blood flowed from the pituitary to the brain—not the other way around. In 1935, using microscopy, B. Houssay visualized the blood vessels along the pituitary stalk in the toad and observed blood flowing from the brain to the pituitary. One year later, G. B. Wislocki and L. S. King performed careful histologic studies of the median eminence and pituitary and described a dense capillary bed that drained blood from the median eminence, which collected into the large portal vessels along the infundibular stalk, and in turn fed a secondary capillary bed in the pars distalis (anterior pituitary). This came to be known as the *hypothalamo-hypophysial portal system*.

The notion that there is a humoral (instead of neural) connection between the hypothalamus and the anterior pituitary was seeded by the early observations of J. C. Hinsey and J. E. Markee in the rabbit, showing that coitally induced ovulation persists in rabbits with severed cervical sympathetic nerves. They deduced that some substances must somehow diffuse from the posterior lobe (neurohypophysis) into the anterior pituitary to control its function. The exact method by which the brain communicates with the pituitary remained controversial (and unproven) until an elegant series of investigations by J. D. Green, G. W. Harris, and D. Jacobsohn provided compelling evidence that humeral agents must be released by the brain into the hypophysial portal system, which then spews "hypophysiotropic factors" into the anterior pituitary to regulate its function. However, it still was not clear precisely how the brain could control all aspects of pituitary function—i.e., the secretion not only of the gonadotropins, but also of growth hormone, prolactin, thyroid-stimulating hormone (TSH), and adrenocorticotropic hormone (ACTH). Although it had been postulated by J. D. Green, G. W. Harris, and S. M. McCann that the brain produces separate excitatory and inhibitory factors that regulate the various pituitary hormones, proof of the existence of such factors (e.g., thyrotropin-releasing hormone [TRH], somatostatin, gonadotropin-releasing hormone [GnRH], corticotropin-releasing hormone [CRH]) was not forthcoming until the final isolation, characterization, and purification of these "hypophysiotropic hormones" in the early 1970s by R. Guillemin, A. Schally, and their coworkers, for which they received the Nobel Prize in 1977.

PRIMATES ARE PHYSIOLOGICALLY UNIQUE[2]

Until the early 1970s, the foundation of modern reproductive neuroendocrinology had been built on studies of *infra* primate species—most notably, the rabbit, rat, mouse, and sheep. Classical studies in these nonprimate species established basic principles that apply to *all mammals*—such as the negative feedback regulation of gonadotropin secretion by sex steroids and the stimulatory action of GnRH on pituitary gonadotropes. However, there are fundamental aspects of the neuroendocrine regulation of reproduction that are dramatically different among species and several that are unique to higher primates, such as Old World monkeys, the great apes, and humans. These include the cellular and molecular mechanisms that govern the onset of puberty, the circuitry that triggers the preovulatory surge of gonadotropins, and circadian inputs to GnRH neurons. The neuroendocrine mechanisms that control these processes are different in higher primates compared with rodent and ovine species. Thus, caution must be exercised when making generalizations and drawing inferences based on work performed in certain laboratory animals because the data may or may not apply to humans. This fact has implications that extend beyond physiology into the realms of pathophysiology and the translational relevance of the various models of disorders of reproduction.

Neuroendocrine Anatomy[3]

NEURONS AND GLIA

The brain has two predominant cell types—neurons, which constitute approximately 10% of the brain, and glia, which make up the other 90%. Neurons represent a highly differentiated and phenotypically diverse array of excitable cells that receive, transduce, and relay information through action potentials and the release of neurotransmitters and neuromodulators at synaptic junctions. Glia comprise several general types of non-neuronal cells, the most numerous of which are astrocytes. Astrocytes can respond to neurotransmitters, neuromodulators, and hormones, and they may provide substrates and signals to neurons and thus regulate their activity and metabolism (e.g., insulin-like growth factor-1, transforming growth factor α and β). Changes in the activity of astrocytes have been linked to the mechanisms that control the onset of puberty. Astrocytes have highly motile processes that may cover nerve terminals (and thus restrict secretion) or retract to expose nerve terminals and allow unrestricted neurosecretion. Pituicytes are modified glial cells that reside in the neural lobe of the pituitary, and their movable processes either ensheath or expose nerve terminals that release oxytocin or vasopressin. Oligodendrocytes are cells that form the myelin sheaths around axons, allowing neurons to conduct action potentials rapidly across long distances without decrement. Ependymal cells are epithelial cells (often ciliated), which line the third ventricle. The end feet processes of these cells govern exchange between the parenchyma of the brain and the fluid-filled ventricular cavities of the brain.

NEUROTRANSMITTERS, NEUROMODULATORS, AND THEIR RECEPTORS

Communication in the brain is mediated through synaptic transmission involving three classes of neurotransmitters—amino acids, biogenic amines, and neuropeptides. Examples of amino acid transmitters include acetylcholine (excitatory), glutamate and aspartate (excitatory), glycine (inhibitory), and γ-aminobutyric acid (GABA), which is predominantly inhibitory but may also be excitatory. The biogenic amines include the catecholamines (e.g., norepinephrine, epinephrine, dopamine) and the indoleamine serotonin. There are many neuropeptides that act as neurotransmitters, neuromodulators, or hypophysiolotropic factors in the brain. These include proopiomelanocortin (POMC) and its derivatives, including α-melanocyte-stimulating hormone and β-endorphin); neuropeptide Y (NPY); growth hormone–releasing hormone (GHRH); TRH; CRH; somatostatin; vasoactive intestinal peptide (VIP); vasopressin; oxytocin; cholecystokinin; peptide PYY; neurotensin; angiotensin II; galanin-like peptide (GALP); kisspeptin (and other RF amides, including gonadotropin-inhibitory peptide); galanin; neurokinin B; dynorphin; enkephalin; GnRH; and others. In some cases, the function of these neurotransmitters is clear—e.g., GnRH stimulates the release of the gonadotropins—but in other (most) cases, the physiologic function of a particular factor either is unknown or is complex and diverse (e.g., NPY, which has functions in feeding behavior and reproduction, but is likely to play other physiologic roles as well). These various neurotransmitters have multiple receptors and cellular mechanisms of action (e.g., five receptor subtypes for NPY), which adds layers of complexity to their divergent and diverse functions.

HYPOTHALAMIC NEUROANATOMY AND LIMBIC INPUTS

The hypothalamus is part of the diencephalon. It lies rostral to the midbrain and caudal to the forebrain. The hypothalamus is bounded dorsally by the thalamus, posteriorly by the mammillary bodies, and anteriorly by the lamina terminalis and optic chiasm, and the third ventricle splits the hypothalamus bilaterally (Figs. 1-1 and 1-2). The hypothalamus receives rich input from the autonomic areas and reticular nuclei of the brain stem, particularly the catecholaminergic cell groups (many of which have neuropeptides as cotransmitters, such as galanin and NPY). The hypothalamus also receives dense innervation from the limbic areas of the forebrain, including the hippocampus, amygdala, septum, and orbitofrontal cortex.

The hypothalamus serves as the primary site for the integration and regulation of many important physiologic processes. These include homeostatic control of temperature, metabolism, and body weight, aspects of cardiovascular function, physiologic adaptation to stress, regulation of growth, reproduction (including sexual behavior), and lactation. Although the regulation of these complex processes depends on the circuitry of the hypothalamus (and its afferent inputs), the control of these systems cannot be defined on the basis of strict anatomic criteria.

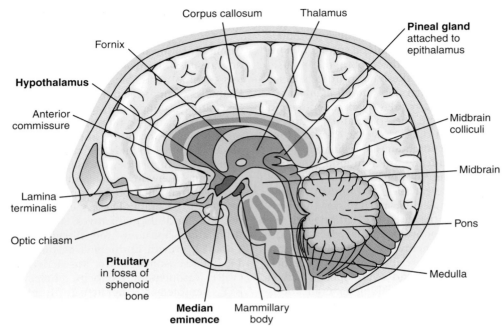

Figure 1-1. *Saggital section of the human brain, including the pituitary and pineal glands. (Adapted from Johnson MH, Everitt BJ. Essential Reproduction, ed 5. Blackwell Science, 2000, Fig. 6.1.)*

The hypothalamus comprises distinct nuclei (collections of cell bodies), including the supraoptic, paraventricular, suprachiasmatic, ventro- and dorsomedial, and arcuate nuclei. The suprachiasmatic nucleus (SCN; Fig. 1-3) is the site of the brain's circadian "clock." Cells in the SCN receive input from the retinohypothalamic pathway, through which the

brain keeps track of the diurnal rhythm of light and dark and controls rhythmic cycles of activity and hormone secretion (e.g., sleep–wake and CRH/ACTH/cortisol rhythms). Subgroups of neurons in the SCN that express VIP and arginine vasopressin project to different parts of the hypothalamus to coordinate diverse physiologic functions, including activity

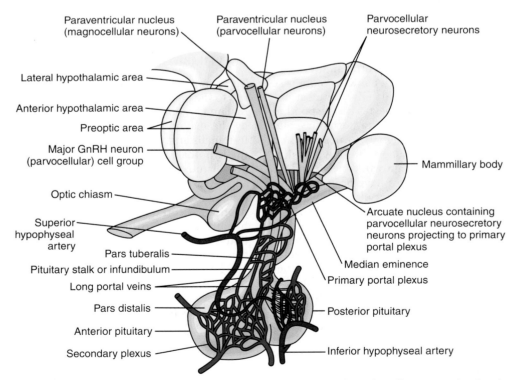

Figure 1-2. *Schematic, three-dimensional view of the human hypothalamus, pituitary, and portal capillary system showing the approximate locations of the major nuclei. GnRH, gonadotropin-releasing hormone. (Adapted from Johnson MH, Everitt BJ. Essential Reproduction. Oxford, Blackwell Science, 2000, Fig. 6.2.)*

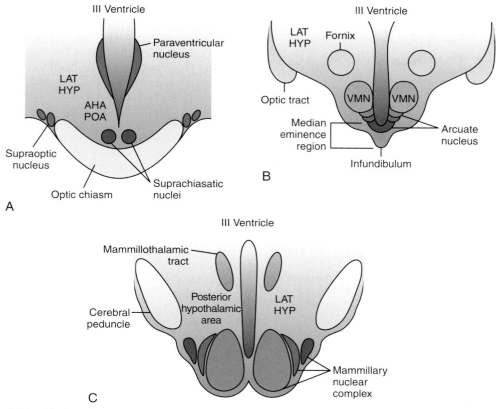

Figure 1-3. *Rostral (**A**), mid (**B**), and caudal (**C**) coronal sections of the human hypothalamus. AHA, anterior hypothalamic area; LAT HYP, lateral hypothalamus; POA, preoptic area; VMN, ventromedial nucleus. (Adapted from Johnson MH, Everitt BJ. Essential Reproduction, ed 5. Blackwell Science, 2000, Fig. 6.3.)*

rhythms and the preovulatory GnRH/LH surge (at least in rodent and ruminant species). Neurons in the SCN express genes that display endogenous rhythmicity, approximating a 24-hour period—hence, the term *circadian*, with components *circa* ("about") and *dian* ("day"). The *clock* and *per* genes, among many others expressed by cells in the SCN, generate pacemaker activity, which may be entrained by external cues (e.g., light or activity) to help the body keep track of time. Cells in the SCN express estrogen receptor α (ERα) and are believed to be involved in the neuroendocrine regulation of gonadotropin secretion, at least in rodent and ruminant species, where the evidence is most compelling.[4-6]

The arcuate nucleus (ARC; see Figs. 1-2 to 1-5) is the nodal point for the regulation of many complex physiologic functions.[7-9] The ARC comprises many phenotypically distinct groups of neurons—including cells that produce pro-opiomelanocortin (POMC) and its derivatives (e.g., β-endorphin and the melanocortin α-melanocyte–stimulating hormone, α-MSH), NPY, GHRH, kisspeptin, GALP, and dopamine. Most, if not all, neurons in the ARC express two or more neuropeptides. For example, NPY-expressing cells also express agouti-related peptide (AgRP). POMC neurons coexpress cocaine- and amphetamine-regulated transcript (CART). GHRH neurons coexpress galanin, and kisspeptin neurons coexpress both dynorphin and neurokinin B. Dopamine-containing neurons are concentrated in the tuberoinfundibular track within the ARC, and these cells play a critical role in the neuroendocrine regulation of prolactin secretion. Certain neurons whose cell bodies reside in

the ARC project to other areas within the hypothalamus, including the preoptic area and paraventricular nucleus (e.g., NPY neurons project to the paraventricular nucleus).

Together, the lateral hypothalamus, dorsomedial nucleus (DMN), ventromedial nucleus (VMN), and parvocellular region of the paraventricular nucleus (PVN) exert regulatory control over feeding, body weight, and activity rhythms.[10] In experimental animals (e.g., rats and cats) lesions of the VMN stimulate appetite and cause obesity, whereas stimulation of the VMN reduces feeding and body weight subsequently declines as a result. The VMN may also play a role in sexual behavior, particularly in females. The lateral hypothalamus comprises other unique cell groups, including neurons that produce orexins (also known as *hypocretins*), which have profound effects on sleep–wake cycles, feeding, and reward-seeking behavior, and can influence GnRH secretion. Neurons in the parvocellular region of the PVN produce TRH and CRH, which regulate the hypothalamic–pituitary–thyroid and hypothalamic–pituitary–adrenal axes, respectively, but both of these neuropeptides also play a critical role in the control of feeding and metabolism. CRH has been implicated in the stress-induced inhibition of GnRH secretion—perhaps through its interaction with β-endorphin–producing neurons in the ARC.

Just rostral to the formal boundaries of the hypothalamus lies the medial preoptic area, which contains many GnRH neurons that project (along with GnRH neurons in the ARC) to the median eminence. (In the primate, GnRH

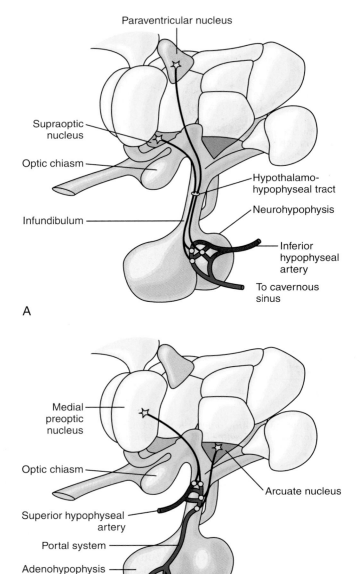

Figure 1-4. *Schematic illustration of the neurosecretory systems in the human that regulate reproduction. A, The locations of oxytocin cell bodies, which reside in the hypothalamus, and their fibers, which project to the neurohypophysis. B, The primary locations of gonadotropin-releasing hormone (GnRH) cell bodies in the human hypothalamus and their axons, which terminate near portal capillaries in the median eminence. (Adapted from Johnson MH, Everitt BJ. Essential Reproduction, ed 5. Blackwell Science, 2000, Fig. 6.4.)*

in the midbrain raphe and provide dense innervation of the hypothalamus, particularly the mammillary complex, periventricular nucleus, ARC, and SCN. The hypothalamus also receives descending input from several sources. These include projections from the basal forebrain, olfactory tubercle, piriform cortex, amygdala, and hippocampus.

Hypophysiotropic neurons whose cell bodies reside within the hypothalamus send their projections to the median eminence, where their secretory products enter the portal vasculature and thus regulate anterior pituitary function. In the context of reproduction, GnRH neurons, with cell bodies in the preoptic area and ARC, send projections into the external zone of the median eminence. From nerve terminals in the median eminence, GnRH is secreted into the fenestrated capillaries and transported to the anterior pituitary (see Figs. 1-4B and 1-5). Kisspeptin neurons (whose cell bodies are in the ARC and rostral hypothalamus) interact with GnRH neurons by projecting directly to GnRH cell bodies, but may also send axoaxonal projections into the zona internal of the median eminence and thereby influence GnRH secretion by several different mechanisms (see Fig. 1-5). Magnocellular neurons in the PVN and supraoptic nucleus (SON) send long axons into the neurohypophysis, where they release vasopressin and oxytocin into the vasculature (see Fig. 1-4A).

THE HYPOTHALAMUS AS A TARGET FOR HORMONE ACTION

The hypothalamus is packed with cells that are direct targets for the action of sex steroids—including many cells that express the ERα estrogen receptor β (ERβ), the progesterone receptor (PR), and the androgen receptor (AR)—all expressed abundantly in various hypothalamic nuclei and the entire periventricular region of the diencephalon. Many specific populations of neurons in the hypothalamus have been shown to express ERα, ERβ, and AR, including kisspeptin neurons in the ARC and AVPV. These observations underscore the idea that the hypothalamus is a prime target for the action of sex steroids, which control GnRH and gonadotropin secretion and exert a profound effect on sexual behavior in both the male and female.[11,12]

The hypothalamus is also a prime target for the action of important metabolic hormones that influence reproduction. For example, the insulin receptor is expressed abundantly in the ARC, by or near NPY and POMC neurons. The hypothalamus is also a target for the action of leptin, which has profound effects on the neuroendocrine reproductive axis. POMC, GALP, and kisspeptin neurons all express the leptin receptor, showing that these populations of cells in the ARC are direct targets for the action of this satiety factor and may serve as a cellular link coupling metabolism and reproduction.[13,14]

THE NEUROHYPOPHYSIS AND MAGNOCELLULAR NEUROSECRETORY SYSTEM

Axons of the magnocellular ("large cell") neurons in the supraoptic and paraventricular nuclei project directly to the neural (or posterior) lobe of the pituitary gland, sometimes

neurons are widely dispersed in the anterior hypothalamus, medial preoptic area, and ARC, whereas in rodent species, GnRH cell bodies are restricted to the rostral hypothalamus and medial preoptic area [Figs. 1-4B and 1-5]).

The hypothalamus receives input from many regions of the brain. Ascending noradrenergic projections arise from the medulla and pons and innervate many nuclear groups within the hypothalamus, including the medial preoptic area and ARC (see Fig. 1-5). Serotonin projections originate

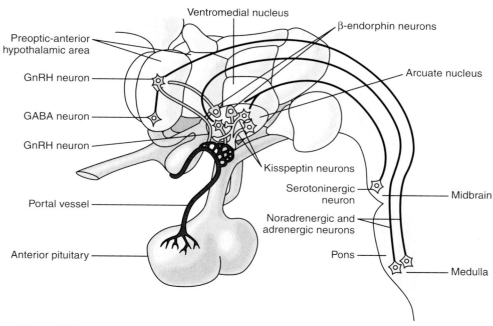

Figure 1-5. *Diagram of some of the neurotransmitter systems that are believed to play a role in regulating gonadotropin-releasing hormone (GnRH) secretion. GABA, γ-aminobutyric acid. (Adapted from Johnson MH, Everitt BJ. Essential Reproduction, ed 5. Blackwell Science, 2000, Fig. 6.18.)*

called the *neurohypophysis* (see Fig. 1-4A). The hormones secreted by the neurohypophysis—oxytocin and arginine vasopressin (AVP)—are synthesized in cell bodies that reside in the PVN and SON. Oxytocin and vasopressin are both cyclic nonapeptides (containing nine amino acids), and their structure differs by only two amino acids at positions 3 and 8 (Fig. 1-6B). These neuropeptides are packaged together in association with a binding protein called *neurophysin,* derived from the precursor proteins of oxytocin and AVP. Neurophysins aid the transport of oxytocin and AVP down the long axons leading to the posterior pituitary. Oxytocin and vasopressin and their neurophysins are cosynthesized, co-packaged in granules, and cosecreted along with neurophysin (Fig. 1-6A). (Some neurons in the SON and PVN produce predominantly one or the other peptide.) Galanin and dynorphin are coexpressed with AVP in many magnocellular neurons. Oxytocin neurons also coexpress other neuropeptides, including galanin, CRH, TRH, and cholecystokinin.

In addition to axonal projections to the neurohypophysis, the magnocellular neurons of the SON and PVN also project to the median eminence, where their nerve terminals release AVP and oxytocin into the hypophysial–portal vasculature. The concentrations of AVP and oxytocin are 50-fold higher in the portal circulation than in the peripheral plasma, suggesting that these neuropeptides play a role in the control of anterior pituitary function, particularly with respect to ACTH secretion.

Afferent Inputs Controlling Oxytocin and Vasopressin Secretion

The magnocellular neurons of the SON and PVN receive afferent input from a variety of sources, including cholinergic, noradrenergic, and peptidergic pathways.

Acetylcholine stimulates AVP secretion through nicotinic receptors, and tobacco derivatives induce antidiuresis by activating AVP neurons. Noradrenergic projections from the brain stem (locus coeruleus) influence the secretion of AVP and oxytocin by acting through α- and β-adrenergic receptors. The firing rate of magnocellular neurons is reduced by α-adrenergic antagonists and stimulated by β-adrenergic antagonists (e.g., propranolol). Agents such as propranolol are sometimes used to facilitate milk let-down, and the stress-induced inhibition of the milk let-down reflex in nursing mothers is likely mediated by activation of β-adrenergic receptors. AVP and oxytocin neurons also receive input from endogenous opioid pathways projecting from the ARC and the nucleus tractus solitarius, whose activities may influence the secretion of AVP and oxytocin under stress. Furthermore, dynorphin may act directly on nerve terminals in the neurohypophysis (through κ receptors) to attenuate oxytocin secretion, contributing to the stress-induced inhibition of milk let-down. Estradiol induces the expression of oxytocin, most remarkably during pregnancy.

Functional Significance and Regulation of AVP and Oxytocin Secretion

Arginine vasopressin plays a critical role in the regulation of plasma volume, blood pressure, and osmolality. AVP is a powerful vasoconstrictor (acting through V1R vasopressin receptor) and an antidiuretic hormone, acting on the kidney through V2R. The synthesis and secretion of AVP from the magnocellular neurons in the SON and PVN are regulated within a narrow range by changes in osmolality, intravascular tone (reflected by baroreceptors

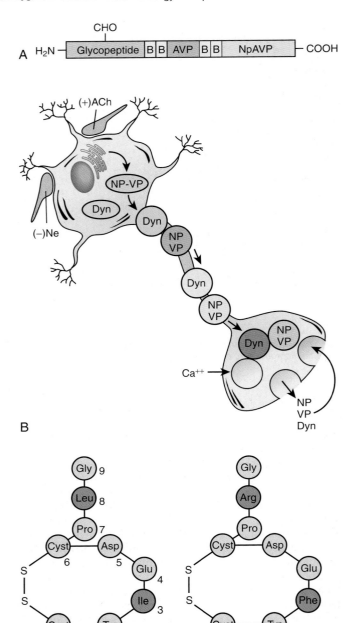

Figure 1-6. *Synthesis, secretion, and structure of oxytocin and arginine vasopressin (AVP). **A,** The basic structure of propressophysin, from which AVP and AVP-associated neurophysin (Np-AVP) are cleaved. Oxytocin is derived from a similar prohormone called prooxyphysin. **B,** The packaging and secretion of AVP. Propressophysin is packaged in secretory granules, where it is cleaved into AVP (VP) and Np-AVP (NP). Dynorphin (Dyn) is also synthesized in the soma of AVP neurons (but not oxytocin neurons) and packaged into granules. Granules are transported down the axons to terminals (arrows), from which they are released—a process that is calcium-dependent. The activity of oxytocin and vasopressin neurons is regulated, in part, by acetylcholine (ACh) and norepinephrine (NE). **C,** The structures and amino acid compositions of oxytocin and AVP.*

in the great vessels that project to the hypothalamus), and angiotensin II, which work in concert to maintain homeostasis. Inadequate or inappropriate AVP secretion may result in hyper- or hyponatremia and excess loss (diabetes insipidus) or retention of body water.

In 1906, oxytocin was the first hormone linked directly to reproduction, when Sir Henry Dale established that extracts of the neurophysis could induce uterine contractility, and oxytocin was the first peptide hormone to be synthesized—for which du Vigneaud received the Nobel prize in 1955. Oxytocin plays key roles in various aspects of reproduction, including lactation, parturition, and sexual, maternal, and partnership behaviors. Oxytocin triggers milk ejection by acting on the myoepithelial cells lining the alveoli of the breast, to expel milk into the ducts. Suckling triggers milk let-down by a neuroendocrine reflex (Fig. 1-7). Stimulation of the nipple during suckling activates sensory nerves that project to the dorsal horn of the spinal cord. From there, second-order neurons project through the anterolateral columns to the brain stem reticular formation, through the medial forebrain bundle, and on to the magnocellular neurons of the PVN and SON.[15]

Oxytocin also plays an important role in parturition. Although oxytocin does not appear to be involved in the initiation of labor in humans, it stimulates myometrial contractions in the late stages of labor and induces hemostasis after delivery. The primary stimulus for the release of oxytocin during labor is believed to be vaginal distention, which is called the *Fergusson reflex*. Estrogen induces the expression of oxytocin receptors in the myometrial and decidual tissues in pregnant women near term, enhancing the sensitivity of the uterus to oxytocin late in pregnancy. Oxytocin may facilitate expulsion of the fetus by stimulating prostaglandin secretion, and of course, labor is often facilitated in obstetric settings by the appropriate administration of oxytocin (Pitocin).

Some evidence gleaned from studies in rodents suggests that a "central oxytocin system," which is activated in parallel to the magnocellular/peripheral oxytocinergic pathway during and subsequent to parturition, plays a role in stimulating maternal behavior. Whether this applies to primate species, including humans, is unknown.

THE CIRCUMVENTRICULAR ORGANS

The circumventricular organs are specialized anatomic features of the brain that are adjacent to the ventricular system and lie outside of the blood–brain barrier. These organs have fenestrated ("windowed") capillaries that permit the transport of relatively large, charged molecules into (and out of) the brain, sometimes by direct and specific transport mechanisms. There are five of these specialized regions of the brain—the median eminence, the pineal gland, the organum vasculosum at the lamina terminalis (OVLT), the subfornical organ, and the subcommissural organ. The ARC lies in close proximity to the median eminence, and the dense plexus of fenestrated capillaries in this region exposes the neurons in the ARC to molecules that would otherwise be blocked from access in other regions of the brain by the blood–brain barrier.[16]

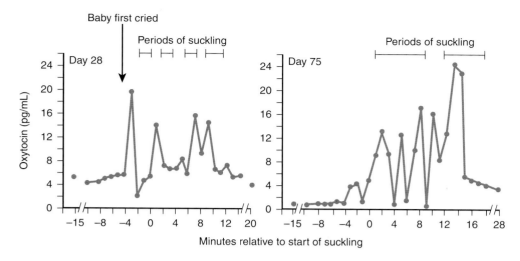

Figure 1-7. *Pulsatile release of oxytocin before and during suckling at 28 and 75 days postpartum. (Adapted from McNeilly AS, Robinson IC, Houston MJ, Howie PW. Release of oxytocin and prolactin in response to suckling. Br Med J 286:257-259, 1983.)*

THE PINEAL GLAND AND MELATONIN

The pineal gland is appended by a stalk to the habenular region of the epithalamus, just above the midbrain colliculi in the roof of the diencephalons. The pineal gland contains pineal cells (or pinealocytes), glial cells, and dense nerve terminals, which arise from the superior cervical ganglia (SCG) and lie in the perivascular space near the pinealocytes. In the human, there is no evidence that the pineal gland plays a significant role in the neuroendocrine regulation of reproduction during either puberty or adulthood. However, in seasonally breeding animals, such as sheep and hamsters, the pineal gland plays a critical role in determining day length and thus gating reproduction as a function of season. In these animals, the presence of environmental light is transmitted to the SCN (via the retinohypothalamic tract). This signal is then relayed from the SCN to the PVN, from the PVN to the SCG, and from the SCG to the pineal gland, where it regulates the secretion of melatonin, produced by the pineal cells.

GnRH–Gonadotropin Axis

GnRH

GnRH and the neurons that secrete it are critical components of the reproductive system. The loss of GnRH leads to hypogonadotropic hypogonadism, a condition in which the reproductive system is completely shut down. Although there may be other brain-derived factors that can influence pituitary gonadotropin secretion, the primary way the brain stimulates and controls the release of gonadotropins from the pituitary is by regulating the secretion of GnRH into the portal system. Thus GnRH neurons are often referred to as the *motor neurons* and the *final common pathway* of the reproductive neuroendocrine system.

FORMS OF GnRH AND ITS RECEPTOR

Since the isolation of GnRH from the hypothalami of pigs and sheep by Andrew Schally and Roger Guillemin, more than 20 additional isoforms have been identified in a variety of species.[17] The originally isolated form of

GnRH appears to be present in most vertebrate species, and to distinguish it from the other forms, is referred to as GnRH I. Another common form of GnRH was first found in chickens and is referred to as GnRH II. With a few exceptions (most notably, mice and rats), nearly all animals that have been studied express both GnRH I and GnRH II. GnRH I and GnRH II are encoded by separate genes, are located in different regions of the brain and periphery, and are believed to perform different physiologic functions. Although the role of GnRH I in the regulation of pituitary gonadotropin secretion has been clearly understood since its discovery, the function of GnRH II remains uncertain. GnRH II has been implicated in the regulation of feeding and in mediating the effects of food restriction on reproductive behavior; however, it is likely to have other roles unrelated to reproduction. In this chapter, we focus on GnRH I, and we refer to it simply as GnRH.

Like the GnRH peptide, there are two main types of GnRH receptors.[18] Both GnRH I and GnRH II bind to type 1 and type 2 GnRH receptors, but the affinity of the type 1 receptor is much greater for GnRH 1, and likewise, the type 2 receptor has a much greater affinity for GnRH II. In addition, in most species, both receptor types are expressed in various brain regions and peripheral tissues. However, in the human, transcripts of the type 2 receptor contain a premature stop codon, casting doubt on the functionality of the human type 2 GnRH receptor. Only the type 1 GnRH receptor is expressed in the mammalian pituitary, and is thus directly involved in the regulation of gonadotropin secretion.

GnRH NEURONS

Morphology

The morphologic features of GnRH neurons are peculiar in many ways. The cell bodies are usually ovoid, tapering on each end into single neurites. These neurites appear to contain all of the organelles of the cell body, except for the nucleus, making it difficult to determine where the cell body ends and the neurite begins.[19] In fact, neither neurite appears to contain the components associated with an axon hillock. GnRH neurites do contain both small, electron-translucent vesicles and larger, electron-dense vesicles. The fact that only some of the larger vesicles are immunopositive for GnRH in rats suggests that these neurons synthesize and secrete other neurotransmitters/neuromodulators in addition to GnRH. GnRH neurites do occasionally bifurcate, but usually not until they are a considerable distance from the cell body.

GnRH neurons are classified as either smooth or spiny. The spines on GnRH neurons are believed to be sites of excitatory synaptic input.[20] However, smooth GnRH neurons have been reported to have roughly the same number of synaptic contacts as the spiny ones.[21] Spiny GnRH neurons appear to be more common in rats, where they are uniformly distributed along with the smooth type. In the monkey, spiny GnRH neurons are relatively more abundant in the medial basal hypothalamus than in the preoptic area. The physiologic significance of the two different morphologic phenotypes associated with GnRH neurons is unclear. Spiny cells contain more Golgi apparatus and mitochondria, whereas smooth cells contain more and larger nucleoli. Thus, it has been suggested that smooth cells are more involved in gene transcription, whereas spiny cells are more invested in peptide processing and packaging, but that conjecture remains untested. It is also unknown whether these cells transform from one phenotype to the other, depending on their state, or whether they represent two separate populations of neurons with unique physiologic functions. Nevertheless, the relative frequency of the two phenotypes has been reported to depend on the reproductive state of the animal. The ratio of spiny to smooth GnRH neurons increases during postnatal development and decreases after gonadectomy in both the rat and the monkey.[22]

Neuroanatomy

It has been estimated that the brain of adult mammals contains between 800 and 2000 GnRH neurons.[23] These neurons are mostly found scattered along a continuum from the olfactory bulbs to the medial basal hypothalamus (MBH), spread out more laterally as they progress toward the more caudal regions. The exact distribution is somewhat species-specific. In the rat and mouse, most of the GnRH neurons are found in the medial septum (MS), the diagonal band of Broca (DBB), and the mPOA. Notably, they are not found in the ARC, an area believed to play an important role in the regulation of gonadotropin secretion. In the primate and some other mammals, the distribution is shifted more caudally, with fewer cells in the MS/DBB/mPOA region, more cells in the MBH (including the ARC or its analog in the primate, the infundibular nucleus), and some cells located as far caudal as the mammillary complex.

Most of the GnRH neurons in the brain send projections to the median eminence. In the rat, these projections follow one of two pathways. The first pathway runs caudally near the midline, along the floor of the third ventricle. The second swings out laterally, follows the medial forebrain bundle caudally, and then curves back medially into the median eminence. In mammals with GnRH neurons in the ARC, those cells send their fibers directly into the median eminence. All of the GnRH projections to the median eminence terminate in the vicinity of portal capillaries in the external

zone. However, very few of the GnRH neuronal terminals make direct contact with the portal vasculature. Although the percentage making direct contact varies, depending on the reproductive state of the animal, most of the terminals remain physically isolated from the portal capillaries by the basal processes of specialized ependymal cells called *tanycytes*.[24,25] In humans and some other mammals, some of the GnRH fibers that enter the median eminence have been reported to continue into the posterior pituitary.[26]

Besides the median eminence, GnRH neurons also project to the other circumventricular organs in the brain. These specialized areas, like the median eminence, contain fenestrated capillaries and therefore are outside the blood–brain barrier. The principal circumventricular target of GnRH projections is the OVLT. This structure is located at the rostral tip of the third ventricle and is believed to contain receptors for circulating signals, such as those for osmolarity, cytokines, angiotensin II, and relaxin.[27,28] The physiologic significance of GnRH fibers in this region is unclear. It is possible that some circulating factors access and modulate GnRH neurons via the OVLT. However, it is also possible that substances released from GnRH neurons into the OVLT act as signals that are conveyed in the cerebrospinal fluid or blood to distal targets.

In addition to projecting to areas outside the blood–brain barrier, GnRH fibers terminate in a number of areas within the brain, where GnRH may act as a neurotransmitter/neuromodulator. These areas include the amygdala, hippocampus, habenula, neocortex, and periaqueductal gray. GnRH projections to some of these sites are likely to be involved in mediating the effects of GnRH on reproductive behavior,[29] but the physiologic functions of GnRH projections to the other areas are a matter of speculation.

One other known target of GnRH fibers is other GnRH neurons throughout their rostral–caudal distribution. GnRH synaptic contacts on both the cell bodies and neurites of GnRH neurons have been reported.[30,31] Thus, even though GnRH neurons are not densely clustered in one region, they still maintain contact with each other. These interconnections may provide the framework whereby ensembles of individual GnRH cells maintain synchronous activity.

Development

The development of the GnRH neurosecretory system has been the subject of intense investigation, primarily in the mouse. Originally, GnRH neurons in the forebrain were believed to arise from multiple precursor sites because they are scattered across areas that originate in different parts of the neuroepithelium. However, when studied carefully, the spaciotemporal appearance of GnRH neurons throughout the forebrain suggests the possibility that they originate in nasal regions and migrate into the forebrain.[32-34] In the mouse, cells containing GnRH peptide are first seen within the nasal placode on embryonic day 11 (E11). Two days later (E13), fewer cells are found in the nasal placode. At this time, most of the cells are seen in the vicinity of the cribriform plate and a few are located in the rostral preoptic area. Late on E14, only a few cells can be found in the nasal placode, whereas at the same time, cells begin to appear in the caudal preoptic area and rostral hypothalamus (Fig. 1-8). By E16, cells have

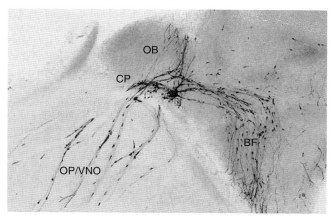

Figure 1-8. Saggital section from an E15 mouse brain stained for gonadotropin-releasing hormone (GnRH) and preipherin, showing the migratory route of GnRH neurons from the olfactory placode/vomeronasal region (OP/VNO), across the cribriform plate (CP), past the olfactory bulb (OB), and into the basal forebrain (BF). (Adapted from Wierman ME, Pawlowski JE, Allen MP, et al. Molecular mechanisms of gonadotropin-releasing hormone neuronal migration. Trends Endocrinol Metab 2004;15:96-102.)

begun to show up in their most caudal positions in the hypothalamus, and by birth, the final distribution of GnRH neurons in the mouse has been established.

Initial evidence that the observed temporal changes in the distribution of GnRH neurons are caused by a rostral to caudal migration of cells originating in the nasal placode came from the results of thymidine injection experiments.[32,33] When radiolabeled thymidine is injected, it becomes incorporated into the DNA of cells that are dividing at the time. By injecting thymidine into animals at various times during development and examining the brains of those animals for the presence of radiolabeled thymidine in GnRH neurons, one can estimate the time of the final division. In the mouse, most cells are labeled by injections occurring on or before day 10, a time at which GnRH neurons are found only in the nasal placode.[34] More recently, the rostral to caudal movement of GnRH neurons has been visualized directly either in embryonic nasal explant cultures[35] or by examining slices from the heads of transgenic mice that express green fluorescent protein under the control of the GnRH promoter.[36]

The mechanisms that guide and propel the GnRH neurons along their way to their final locations inside the forebrain are still being identified. However, it is clear that axons that form part of the vomeronasal nerve (VNN) play an important role.[23,37] These axons arise in the vomeronasal organ and project primarily to the accessory olfactory bulb. On reaching the cribriform plate, the nerve defasciculates and a subset of fibers branches off, heading through the forebrain ventrally and caudally toward the median eminence. Evidence suggests that netrin-1 binding to DCC (deleted in colorectal cancer, the netrin-1 receptor) helps to guide the caudally projecting VNN fibers, because these fibers end up in the cortex instead of the hypothalamus in *DCC* knockout mice.[38]

While traveling through the nasal region, GnRH cells are always found in the axon fascicles of the VNN.[39] Presumably, some set of cell adhesion molecules is responsible for the movement of GnRH cells along VNN axons. One of the first molecules with cell adhesion-like properties to be associated

with GnRH neuronal migration was anosmin-1, the product of the *KAL1* gene. Mutations of the *KAL1* gene lead to the anosmia and hypogonadotropic hypogonadism that accompany Kallmann's syndrome. Those deficiencies appear to be caused by a failure of olfactory fibers and GnRH neurons to reach the forebrain.[40] Neural cell adhesion molecule (N-CAM) is also expressed in olfactory regions during embryonic development, and has been the subject of considerable interest with respect to GnRH migration. However, N-CAM is not expressed in GnRH neurons of the mouse, and manipulations that interfere with N-CAM function, although disruptive, do not prevent GnRH migration.[23] In addition to cell adhesion molecules, a chemokine known as SDF-1 is expressed in the nasal compartment, starting on E10 in the mouse.[41] The expression of SDF-1 forms a gradient across the caudal half of the nasal region, with the highest concentration at the junction with the cribriform plate. Embryonic GnRH cells express the SDF-1 receptor CXCR4, and the migration of GnRH cells through the nasal compartment is severely retarded in CXCR4 mice, suggesting that SDF-1 acts as an important signaling molecule directing the early migration of GnRH cells. Prokinecticin 2, a secreted protein, may function as a chemo-attractant since mutations in the *PROK2* gene (as well as its receptor gene, *PROKR2*) cause Kallmann syndrome. Another potentially important protein called *nasal embryonic LH-releasing hormone factor* (NELF) has been identified through the use of a subtractive screen comparing the messenger ribonucleic acid expressed in migrating and nonmigrating GnRH cells.[42] NELF is expressed in both VNN axons and GnRH cells in nasal regions, and NELF antisense probes interfere with axonal outgrowth and GnRH neuronal migration in explant cultures.[42] The movement of GnRH cells across the nasal compartment appears to be a complex process, and the role that NELF plays in that process warrants further investigation.

When they arrive at the cribriform plate, GnRH cells appear to pause for a while before plunging into the forebrain. Associated with the pause is an increase in the expression of glutamate decarboxylase (GAD) in neurons whose axons terminate in the vicinity of the cribriform plate.[43] GAD is the enzyme that produces GABA, and GABA, along with GABA agonists, has been shown to inhibit GnRH neuronal migration both in vitro and in vivo.[36,44,45] These observations implicate increased GABAergic activity in delaying the entry of GnRH neurons into the forebrain. Even less is known about the mechanisms involved in the migration of GnRH neurons after they traverse the cribriform plate and enter the brain. NELF does not appear to be a factor because the branch of the VNN that projects to the hypothalamus does not express NELF.[42] Nevertheless, GnRH neurons appear to continue to travel in association with the caudal VNN pathway. In *DCC* knockout mice, in which the VNN turns toward the cortex instead of toward the hypothalamus, GnRH neurons end up in the cortex as well.[38] Both GABA and N-methyl-D-aspartate receptors have been implicated along this pathway, but their role remains unclear.[45,46]

Molecular Phenotypes

Although all of the GnRH neurons in the rostral forebrain share a common site of origin, they end up in a variety of locations, participating in the positive and negative feedback regulation of gonadotropin secretion and possibly influencing reproductive behaviors. Thus, it would be reasonable to expect their molecular phenotypes to reflect their diverse physiologic roles. The majority of these cells project to the median eminence, reflecting their role as the output drivers of the reproductive neuroendocrine system. As such, the receptor molecules that sense the neural and hormonal input signals, along with the neurotransmitters and neurohormones that comprise the output signals of the cell, play major roles in the function of GnRH neurons.

Based on the results of immunohistochemical studies, early reports suggested that GnRH neurons expressed only a few different kinds of receptors. More recently, the use of molecular biology-based techniques, such as double-label in situ hybridization and single-cell reverse transcription polymerase chain reaction, along with electrophysiologic recordings from single cells, have provided evidence that GnRH neurons express a much wider variety of receptors than previously believed (see Herbison[47] for a catalog). Among them are receptors for classic neurotransmitters that have long been believed to play an important role in the regulation of GnRH secretion, including norepinephrine (NE), glutamate, and GABA.[47] Conspicuously absent from that list, however, is solid evidence for the expression of cholinergic, dopaminergic, and serotoninergic receptors, suggesting that either the expression of those receptors is too low to be detected or the effects of those neurotransmitters on GnRH secretion are mediated by intervening neurons.

GnRH neurons also express a number of receptors for neuropeptides that are believed to regulate GnRH secretion. These include (among others) receptors for NPY, galanin, neurotensin, VIP, kisspeptin, and GnRH. The ligands for those receptors have all been shown to either stimulate or inhibit the release of gonadotropin secretion when injected into the brain.[47] It is worthwhile to note that even though pharmacologic disruptions of neuropeptide signaling to receptors expressed in GnRH neurons usually have dramatic effects on gonadotropin secretion, targeted deletions of the respective neuropeptides generally have no detectable effect on fertility.[48-50] For example, the administration of galantide (a galanin antagonist) on the afternoon of proestrus completely blocks the preovulatory LH surge[51]; however, galanin knockout mice are fertile.[49] The one exception is kisspeptin and its receptor KISS1R (formerly GPR54). Animals and people with mutations that block KISS1R function exhibit hypogonadotropic hypogonadism because of inadequate GnRH secretion.[52-54] These observations suggest that most neurotransmitter/receptor interactions on GnRH neurons are modulatory, but kisspeptin/KISS1R signaling is mandatory for even the most basic reproductive functions.

Because metabolic and reproductive hormones regulate GnRH release, it seems reasonable to expect GnRH neurons to express receptors for hormones such as insulin, leptin, estrogen, progesterone, and testosterone. Although the expression of some of these receptors has been found in transformed GnRH cell lines,[55-58] with few exceptions, investigators have been unable to obtain evidence for their expression within GnRH neurons in vivo. One notable exception is estrogen receptor beta (ERβ), which has been shown to be expressed in GnRH neurons of female rats.[59,60]

The disparity of receptor expression between transformed cell lines and GnRH neurons in vivo raises a cautionary flag with regard to naively assuming that results obtained through the use of those cell lines can be directly applied to GnRH neurons in their native environment. Nevertheless, in most cases, it appears that information about circulating hormone concentrations reaches GnRH cells via intermediary neurons that express the appropriate receptors.

Although neurotransmitter and endocrine receptor molecules mediate the input signals that regulate GnRH neuronal activity, there are several neuropeptides expressed in GnRH neurons that are candidates for output signals. The most important of these is GnRH itself, without which pituitary gonadotropin secretion is essentially shut down.[61] Accompanying GnRH in nerve terminals and released with it is GnRH-associated peptide (GAP).[62] GAP is the peptide left over after GnRH is cleaved from proGnRH. GAP appears to have a mild stimulatory effect on gonadotropin secretion in some species,[63,64] and under some conditions, it inhibits prolactin secretion.[65,66] However, beyond these tenuous effects, the physiologic significance (if any) of the release of GAP from GnRH neurons remains obscure. Delta sleep-inducing peptide (DSIP) is an even more mysterious neuropeptide that is contained in GnRH neurons.[67] DSIP was named for its ability to induce slow-wave (delta) sleep when infused intraventricularly. This peptide is colocalized with GnRH within axon terminals in the median eminence,[68,69] and it also induces LH when injected in vivo, apparently by stimulating the release of GnRH.[70,71] Outside of these very basic observations, nothing more is known about the possible function of DSIP contained in GnRH neurons. Recently, another neuropeptide known as *orphanin FQ* (OFQ), which is a member of the endogenous opioid family, was reported to be expressed in essentially all GnRH neurons in sheep, regardless of their location.[72] Because it inhibits LH secretion when infused into the third ventricle of either luteal-phase or ovariectomized animals, it has been suggested that OFQ in GnRH neurons acts in an autoregulatory loop to control the activity of those neurons[72]; however, acceptance of that hypothesis awaits evidence that GnRH neurons express OFQ receptors.

The most thoroughly studied neuropeptide expressed in GnRH neurons is galanin. The expression of galanin in GnRH neurons and its regulation is species-specific. In the rat, not all GnRH neurons contain galanin, but galanin is found in the GnRH neurons of a much larger percentage of females compared with males.[73] In female rats, galanin gene expression in GnRH neurons is regulated by estrogen, with galanin expression being very low in ovariectomized animals, moderate during diestrus, and highest at the time of the proestrus LH surge.[74] This effect of estrogen in the rat is probably mediated by neurons that synapse on GnRH neurons because it can be blocked by pharmacologic agents that inhibit neuronal activity and the LH surge.[75] In the mouse, the percentage of cells containing galanin is also sexually dimorphic and dependent on the animal's endocrine state, but it is not as clearly dependent on estrogen as in the rat.[76] In the sheep, all GnRH neurons in both sexes contain galanin, independent of reproductive state,[77] whereas none of the GnRH neurons in the macaque appear to express galanin.[78] Because galanin (1) induces the release of GnRH from the median eminence,[79] (2) is released into the portal system,[80] and (3) enhances GnRH-stimulated release of LH from the pituitary,[80] galanin in GnRH neurons is believed to facilitate the ability of those neurons to evoke LH secretion, particularly during the generation of an LH surge. The fact that galantide, a galanin antagonist, blocks the LH surge in rats supports that conjecture. However, the importance of galanin has been called into question by the observation that LH levels are not lower in galanin knockout mice, and those mice have an apparently normal reproductive phenotype.[49]

Electrophysiology

Because GnRH neurons are few in number and are scattered throughout the forebrain, until recently, recording from GnRH neurons was a very tedious process. However, through the use of transgenic animals that express green fluorescent protein (GFP) under the control of the GnRH promoter, it has been possible to record from visually identified GFP-labeled GnRH cells in forebrain slices from both mice and rats.[81,82] So far, no special electrophysiologic characteristics of GnRH neurons have been identified that would mark them as uniquely different from other hypothalamic neurons.[47] They appear to contain voltage-dependent sodium channels, voltage-activated calcium channels, and a variety of potassium channels. They have also been found to exhibit a variety of firing patterns, including completely inactive, constant, and phasic. GFP-labeled GnRH cells in forebrain slices are now beginning to provide important information about the receptor mechanisms by which neurotransmitters act directly on GnRH neurons.[47]

THE PORTAL SYSTEM

The hypothalamic–hypophysial portal system is the conduit that connects the brain to the anterior pituitary. The portal system is made up of two capillary beds, one in the median eminence and the other in the anterior pituitary. The portal capillary bed in the median eminence is fed from the superior hypophysial arteries, and is divided into an external and an internal plexus.[83] The capillaries of the external plexus form a hexagonal, chicken wire–like mesh embedded in the external surface of the median eminence (Fig. 1-9). The interior of each hexagonal unit is filled with axon terminals and glial tissue, including tanycyte processes. The internal plexus consists of capillary loops that emanate from the external plexus and rise into the upper regions of the internal zone. Blood coming from the capillary plexus of the median eminence is carried into a capillary bed in the anterior pituitary by long portal veins. From the anterior pituitary capillary bed, portal blood drains into the cavernous and posterior intercavernous sinuses. The capillaries and veins of the portal system are fenestrated; thus, molecules that are normally blocked by the blood–brain barrier can readily pass into and out of the portal circulation. Although in their original description of the portal system, Popa and Fielding speculated that the portal system delivered pituitary hormones to the brain,[84] observations in living animals have shown that portal blood generally flows from the median eminence to the anterior pituitary,[85] delivering hypothalamic hormones, such as GnRH, to the secretory cells they control.

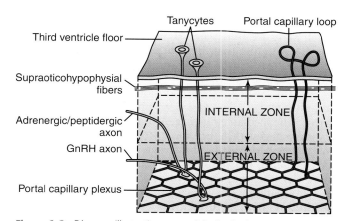

Figure 1-9. *Diagram illustrating some of the basic elements and nomenclature of the median eminence. GnRH, gonadotropin-releasing hormone.*

THE MEDIAN EMINENCE

The brain's regulation of the reproductive system culminates in the median eminence, where GnRH, along with other releasing and inhibiting factors, are released into the portal system to be delivered to gonadotropes and lactotropes in the anterior pituitary. The median eminence, which resides at the base of the third ventricle, consists of two main layers: the internal zone and the external zone (see Fig. 1-9). The internal zone abuts against the ventral floor of the third ventricle, which is lined with specialized ependymal cells known as *tanycytes*.[83] Tanycytes are bipolar, with a short apical process that extends into the ventricular surface and a long basal process.[86] In the median eminence, the basal processes of tanycytes extend through the internal zone and into the external zone, where they terminate in the perivascular space of fenestrated capillaries. The internal zone also contains portal capillary loops and fibers of the supraopticohypophysial tract, which originates in the magnocellular neurons of the supraoptic and periventricular nuclei and terminates in the posterior pituitary. The external zone receives fibers from parvocellular neurons throughout the forebrain. Among other neuroactive substances, these fibers comprise the hypothalamic hormones that regulate secretion of pituitary hormones, including GnRH. Capillaries of the hypophysial portal system are also located in the external zone.

The tanycytes in the median eminence have attracted a considerable amount of attention. The third ventricle contains two types of tanycytes, α and β.[86] The apical processes of α tanycytes protrude into a region of the third ventricle just dorsal to the lateral recess, and their basal processes extend into the ARC. The apical processes of β tanycytes are embedded in the lateral recess and floor of the third ventricle. The β tanycytes are further divided into two subtypes. The β1 tanycytes line the lateral recesses of the third ventricle, and their basal processes form tight junctions with each other, creating a barrier between the ARC and the median eminence. The β2 tanycytes line the floor of the third ventricle, forming an effective barrier between the third ventricle and the median eminence. Their basal processes project to the portal capillaries and into the neuropil that fills the hexagonal units of the external capillary plexus. The tanycytic projections into the external zone are innervated by aminergic and peptidergic fibers, suggesting that they are actively regulated by neurotransmitters/neuromodulators,[86] and at least some of them contain ERα.[87]

Based on their location and morphologic features, several physiologic roles have been proposed for the β tanycytes in the median eminence. Although their morphologic features suggest that they form a conduit for transporting substances between the third ventricle and the portal system, evidence that this might be the case is limited.[83] A more clear-cut role for the β tanycytes is to form a tight barrier separating the median eminence from the ARC and the third ventricle. A further role for isolation has been suggested by the observation that tanycytes ensheath GnRH terminals, separating them from the portal capillaries. Because the degree of isolation appears to depend on the endocrine state of the animal,[88] it has been suggested that the retraction and extension of tanycytic processes modulates the ability of GnRH to reach the portal capillaries. More recent work in the rat has provided evidence that during the preovulatory LH surge, GnRH terminals sprout philopodia that reach out toward the portal capillaries, while tanycytes pull the basal lamina, along with the pericapillary space, toward the terminals.[25] Working together, these processes most likely serve to modulate the efficacy of GnRH release.

THE PITUITARY

Anatomy

The pituitary (hypophysis) is divided into two distinctly different lobes (see Fig. 1-2). The posterior lobe (neurohypophysis, or neural lobe) is an extension of nervous tissue from the hypothalamus/median eminence, primarily containing nerve terminals, glial pituicytes, and capillaries. The nerve terminals derive from magnocellular neurons in the supraoptic and paraventricular nuclei (SON and PVN, respectively) and thus contain oxytocin and vasopressin. The anterior lobe (adenohypophysis, or anterior pituitary) is made of glandular epithelial tissue that is closely applied to the neurohypophysis. The anterior pituitary has been further divided into the pars tuberalis, which is located immediately under the median eminence and adjacent to the infundibular stalk, and the pars distalis, which is distal to the pars tuberalis, adjacent to the neural lobe. In most species, but not humans or birds, there is a third division, called the *intermediate lobe* (pars intermedia) that is interposed between the neural lobe and the pars distalis.

The pars distalis is the largest and best understood division of the anterior lobe. It is predominantly composed of secretory epithelial cells and capillaries. The capillaries are fenestrated, allowing the secreted products of the epithelial cells to freely enter the general circulation. The fenestrations also allow hormones from outside the pituitary (e.g., GnRH from the hypothalamus and inhibin from the gonads) to reach the secretory cells and hormones from the endothelial cells to act on other secretory cells in the same region of the pituitary. The secretory cells synthesize and release the six major anterior pituitary hormones: growth hormone, ACTH, TSH, prolactin, LH, and FSH. Each hormone is produced by its own endocrine cell type, except for LH and FSH, which are produced by a common type. Growth hormone, ACTH, TSH, and prolactin are synthesized by somatotropes, corticotropes, thyrotropes, and lactotropes, respectively, whereas LH and FSH are synthesized by gonadotropes. These various epithelial cell types are not innervated and are scattered throughout the pars distalis, interspersed with folliculostellate cells, dendritic cells, and resident macrophages.[83]

Most of the secretory epithelial cells of the pars tuberalis are of a type that is not found in other regions of the pituitary. These cells (referred to as *PT cells*) line the hypophysial portal vessels, and presumably, they release their secretory products into those vessels. They express the α glycoprotein subunit (αGSU) that is shared by TSH, FSH, and LH, and in some cases, may also express the β-TSH subunit. More recently, PT cells have been shown to express a peptide called *tuberalin* that stimulates the release of prolactin from lactotropes.[89] PT cells express melatonin receptors; this and other evidence suggest that those cells are involved in the seasonal regulation of pituitary hormones, especially prolactin.[90] In humans, who do not undergo seasonal changes in prolactin secretion, the expression of melatonin receptors in the pars tuberalis is questionable.[83] Besides PT cells, the other secretory endothelial cells in the pars tuberalis are, for the most part, gonadotropes that have migrated into that region from the pars distalis.

The epithelial cells of the pars intermedia contain both α- and β-melanocyte–stimulating hormone (α-MSH), along with other products of the *POMC* gene. Unlike epithelial cells in other parts of the anterior pituitary, those in the pars intermedia are innervated by nerve fibers, some of which contain dopamine and GABA.[83] The pars intermedia also contains a capillary bed that connects to the capillary bed in the pars distalis via portal veins. Furthermore, the extracellular space of the pars intermedia communicates with the extracellular space of the neural lobe.[83] This means that secretory products of the pars intermedia can easily reach and act on elements in both the posterior pituitary and the pars distalis. It also means that the secretory cells in the pars intermedia can be regulated by (1) hypothalamic hormones, (2) anterior lobe hormones, and (3) posterior lobe hormones.

Development

The anterior pituitary arises from the anterior neural ridge, which consists of ectodermal tissue and abuts the anterior tip of the neural plate. The posterior pituitary (and hypothalamus) develops from the portion of the neural plate that is adjacent to the neural ridge. The development of the pituitary itself begins with an invagination of the roof of the oral cavity called *Rathke's pouch* that eventually becomes the anterior pituitary. At nearly the same time, the ventral diencephalon begins to produce an outgrowth called the *infundibulum* that is destined to form the posterior pituitary. A number of signaling molecules and transcription factors that play important roles in the formation of the pituitary have been identified.[91] Those will not be discussed here in detail; however, our current knowledge of the steps involved in the terminal differentiation of gonadotropes and lactotropes in mice will be summarized.

Differentiation of lactotropes begins at approximately E10, when the expression of a paired-like homeodomain transcription factor called Prop-1 commences. Prop-1 expression is required for the activation on E13.5 of Pit-1 expression. Pit-1 is a POU domain-containing transcription factor that is essential for the development of lactotropes, somatotropes, and thyrotropes; those cell types are completely absent in both *Prop-1* and *Pit-1* knockouts. The expression of GATA-2, a transcription factor that binds to GATA DNA sequences, appears to play a role in differentiating thyrotropes from somatotropes and lactotropes. Furthermore, the interaction of the transcriptional corepressor N-CoR with Pit-1 forms a corepressor complex that inhibits the expression of growth hormone in lactotropes. Thus, a lack of GATA-2 expression and the expression of N-CoR appear to contribute to the final lactotrope phenotype.

Gonadotropes are the last cells to reach their final state, but their differentiation commences at approximately E13.5, when those cells begin to express steroidogenic factor-1 (SF-1). SF-1 is a zinc finger nuclear receptor that regulates a variety of reproductive genes, including those that encode αGSU, LHβ, FSHβ, and the GnRH receptor. GATA-2 also plays a role in gonadotrope differentiation by repressing the expression of Pit-1. However, neither SF-1 nor GATA-2 appears to be absolutely essential for gonadotrope development. Other transcription factors that appear to be active (but not essential) in the differentiation of gonadotropes include Egr-1 and Otx-1.

GONADOTROPINS

Gonadotropins are glycoprotein hormones that consist of a 92–amino acid α subunit (αGSU) and an approximately 120–amino acid β subunit. The α subunit is common to LH, FSH, and TSH (which is also a glycoprotein), and the β subunit confers specificity to the hormone. Both subunits have a cystine knot motif, which consists of three loops that are attached to each other with disulfide bonds. The α–β heterodimer is held together by disulfide bonds as well. For most mammalian species, each subunit has one or two binding sites at which oligosaccharide structures are attached. Each oligosaccharide contains a variety of carbohydrate moieties. Although the function of the carbohydrates is not completely understood, it is clear that they affect both the rate of degradation in the circulation and the specific activities of the hormones. Deglycosylated gonadotropins bind to their receptors with higher affinity but lower specific activity compared with the native forms of the hormones.

Gonadotropin synthesis and secretion is regulated by a variety of endocrine and paracrine factors that originate in the brain, gonads, and pituitary. GnRH is the primary signal the brain uses to regulate gonadotropin production and release. The GnRH receptor (GnRHR) is a G protein–coupled receptor. The binding of GnRH to GnRHR activates the $G_{q/11}$ α subunit, leading to the release of intracellular Ca^{2+} and the activation of protein kinase C pathways that lead to the expression and secretion of gonadotropins.[92] GnRH also regulates the efficacy of GnRHR signaling in gonadotropes. Constant exposure to elevated levels of GnRH leads to a desensitization of the signaling pathway. GnRH is normally released in discrete pulses that lead to optimal stimulation of gonadotropins. The effect of pulse frequency on LH and FSH expression and release has been extensively investigated.[93] Low pulse frequencies favor the synthesis and secretion of FSH, whereas higher frequencies tend to favor those of LH. However, the molecular mechanisms responsible for these effects remain a matter of speculation.

The gonads control pituitary gonadotropins principally through gonadal steroids (estrogens, androgens, and progestogens) and inhibin. Although most of the effects of gonadal steroids on gonadotropins are believed to be mediated by the brain through the release of GnRH, steroids also act directly on gonadotropes. Within gonadotropes, gonadal steroids control gonadotropins both by regulating GnRHR expression and signaling and by directly regulating the production of gonadotropins. The effects of estradiol and progesterone can be inhibitory or stimulatory, depending on sex, timing, species, and hormonal milieu, whereas the effects of testosterone are mainly inhibitory. Inhibin is a dimmer consisting of α and β subunits. There are two forms of the β subunit, $β_A$ and $β_B$. Inhibin is secreted into the circulation by both the ovary and the testis. The primary site of action for circulating inhibin is the pituitary, where it specifically inhibits the expression of the FSHβ subunit[94]; inhibin has little or no effect on the release of GnRH from the brain.

Two additional peptide hormones are known to regulate gonadotropin production and secretion. Activin, a hormone formed by the dimerization of two inhibin β subunits, was originally isolated from gonadal tissue, but does not appear to be released from the gonads into the circulation in significant quantities. However, both activin A (containing two $β_A$ subunits) and activin B (containing two $β_B$ subunits) have potent stimulatory effects on FSHβ expression in gonadotropes and increase GnRHR synthesis in rat pituitary cells.[92] Because activin A is produced in the pituitary, it is believed to work in a paracrine fashion to regulate FSH. Furthermore, activin B is synthesized exclusively in gonadotropes, suggesting an autocrine role for that hormone.[95] Another peptide hormone that is produced in the pituitary and regulates gonadotropins is follistatin. Follistatin is a potent inhibitor of FSHβ expression and secretion, and this effect is additive with the inhibitory effects of inhibin. The expression of follistatin in gonadotropes is stimulated by activin and GnRH, and is inhibited by inhibin and testosterone.[92] In addition, follistatin has been reported to inhibit its own expression,[96] suggesting that its presence in gonadotropes is under autoregulatory negative feedback control. The regulation of follistatin by GnRH is dependent on GnRH pulse frequency.[97] High-frequency GnRH pulses increase the expression of follistatin, thus providing a possible mechanism whereby GnRH pulse frequency differentially regulates the expression and release of LH and FSH.

PROLACTIN

Prolactin is a monomeric protein consisting of approximately 200 amino acids. Its structure is very similar to that of growth hormone, but prolactin is encoded by its own unique gene. Like growth hormone, prolactin is believed to comprise a number of α-helix bundles. The mature hormone contains one small loop on each end and a large loop in the middle. The loops are held together by disulfide bridges. The two small loops do not affect biologic activity, but the large central loop is absolutely necessary for prolactin to activate its receptor. Sometimes prolactin is glycolsylated or phosphorylated. The reasons for glycosylation and phosphorylation are not clear, although both of those processes tend to reduce the specific activity of prolactin.[98]

In mammals, prolactin is secreted spontaneously from lactotropes, so there is little need for a prolactin-releasing hormone. Nevertheless, a number of factors found in portal blood have been shown to stimulate prolactin release, including VIP, TRH, oxytocin, and galanin.[99] The principal prolactin-inhibiting factor appears to be dopamine, released from tuberoinfundibular dopamine neurons. The pituitary expresses type 2 and type 4 dopamine receptors, both of which incorporate $G_{i/o}$ α subunits. When dopamine binds to these receptors, the $G_{i/o}$ α subunit disassociates, inhibiting adenylate cyclase and the production of cyclic adenosine monophosphate, which subsequently leads to a suppression of prolactin gene expression. At the same time, the G βγ subunit activates potassium channels, causing hyperpolarization of the membrane, reducing Ca^{+2} influx, and inhibiting the secretion of prolactin. Estrogen is another important factor regulating prolactin secretion. Estrogen acts directly on lactotropes to induce prolactin gene expression. Estrogen does not appear to directly stimulate the release of prolactin, but the increased synthesis leads to increased release.[98]

Temporal Patterns of GnRH/LH Secretion

Successful reproduction depends on a complex interplay of biologic rhythms in which the reproductive neuroendocrine system is intimately involved. These include ultradian rhythms with periods of minutes to hours, diurnal and circadian rhythms that recur daily, reproductive cycle rhythms that range from a few days to several months, and annual rhythms that repeat yearly. These rhythms are generated by different mechanisms, and they play different roles in the regulation of the reproductive system.

ULTRADIAN RHYTHMS

Before sensitive methods for measuring hormones became available, hormone release was believed to be basically tonic, changing only as necessary to meet physiologic demands. With the advent of the radioimmunoassay, it became possible to measure hormone levels in small blood samples, paving the way for assessing the minute-to-minute changes in hormone secretion in individual animals. It soon became apparent that most pituitary hormones are secreted episodically, with episodes occurring many times each day (Fig. 1-10). LH is released in discrete bursts that occur at intervals ranging from 15 minutes to several hours. This mode of hormone release is referred to as *pulsatile*, or *episodic*, and is the result of short bursts of GnRH released into the portal system, with each burst causing a rapid rise in pituitary LH secretion. Between the bursts of GnRH, LH release is low, and blood LH concentrations decline asymptotically toward basal levels as LH is cleared from the circulation. Although GnRH pulses stimulate both LH and FSH secretion, blood concentrations of FSH are not as clearly pulsatile as LH concentrations because the FSH response to GnRH is slower and more prolonged compared with the LH response, and FSH is cleared from the circulation more slowly than LH. The amplitude and frequency of the pulses depends on the species and the endocrine environment. In gonadectomized rats, LH pulses occur every 15 to 30 minutes,[100] whereas in sheep and both human and nonhuman primates, they occur about once an hour,[101-103] and thus, they have been referred to as *circhoral* (*circa* = approximately; *horal* = hourly).

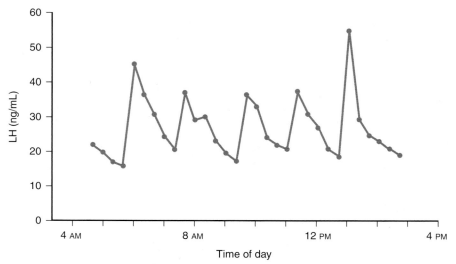

Figure 1-10. Luteinizing hormone (LH) pulses during the early follicular phase of the menstrual cycle in a normal woman. (Adapted from Soules MR, Steiner RA, Clifton DK, et al. Progesterone modulation of pulsatile luteinizing hormone secretion in normal women. J Clin Endocrinol Metab 58:378-383, 1984.)

The existence of pulsatile LH secretion has been known for a long time; nevertheless, the mechanisms responsible for its generation are still a matter of debate and investigation. One important aspect of pulsatile LH secretion that has become clear is that it is the result of the episodic release of GnRH into the portal system. Through the measurement of GnRH in samples collected from the median eminence with push-pull cannulae, or taken directly from pituitary stalk blood, GnRH has been shown to be released in discrete pulses that correlate with pulsatile LH secretion in monkeys, rats, and sheep.[104-106] Furthermore, a one-to-one correspondence between bursts of electrical activity in hypothalamic neurons and the pulsatile release of LH into the circulation has been shown in ovariectomized monkeys (Fig. 1-11).[107] These observations indicate that a GnRH pulse–generating mechanism resides within the brain and drives episodic LH secretion. If this explanation is accurate, are GnRH neurons driven by neural inputs from an external pulse generator, or are they intrinsically rhythmic? Evidence from in vitro experiments suggests that the latter may be the case. Cultures containing only GT1 cells appear to release GnRH in an episodic manner,[108] suggesting that their activity is intrinsically rhythmic. Similarly, cultures of embryonic olfactory placodes from monkeys, rats, and sheep release rhythmic pulses of GnRH into the medium.[109-111] Nevertheless, it should be noted that olfactory placodes contain other types of cells besides GnRH neurons that might be capable of generating pulsatile GnRH release. If GnRH neurons are intrinsically rhythmic, then there must be some mechanism that synchronizes their activity, so they act in concert to effect pulsatile LH release. Presumably, GnRH neurons can interact with each other through synaptic interconnections that have been shown to exist in both rats and monkeys.[30,31] Either GnRH or galanin, both of which are expressed in GnRH neurons, could be active at those synapses because GnRH neurons have been shown to express receptors for both of those peptides.[47]

Despite the evidence that intrinsic rhythmicity of GnRH neurons plays an important role in the generation of GnRH pulses, there are observations that are difficult to reconcile with that model. Possibly the most difficult is the observation that mice in which the receptor for kisspeptin (KISS1R) is knocked out have very low levels of LH, even when castrated.[112] If GnRH neurons were intrinsically pulsatile, the removal of external inputs would not be expected to abolish those pulses. In fact, it is quite possible that episodic kisspeptin activity drives GnRH pulses. Earlier reports implicated a role for the ARC in GnRH pulse generation of the rat,[113,114] and the ARC of the rat contains a large population of kisspeptin neurons that are believed to control GnRH secretion in both males and females.[115] These observations are consistent with a model in which kisspeptin neurons play a critical role in the generation and delivery of a pulsatile signal that drives GnRH neurons. Thus, even though several decades have passed since pulsatile GnRH secretion was first discovered, we still cannot say for sure how GnRH pulses are generated. However, there is hope that, through the use of molecular tools that are now becoming available, we will be able to answer that important question in the near future.

Why is GnRH released in discrete pulses? Several reasons have been identified, and there may be some others that have not yet been discovered. First, it appears that the pituitary is able to respond only transiently to stimulation by GnRH. When GnRH is infused at a constant rate into animals with hypothalamic lesions that block endogenous GnRH secretion, gonadotropin levels are initially stimulated, but within hours, they begin to decline and continue to recede to baseline levels, even while GnRH continues to be administered (Fig. 1-12).[116] Although the mechanisms are not completely understood, the pituitary loses its ability to respond to GnRH after long-term exposure. This desensitization of the pituitary to GnRH has allowed physicians to use long-acting GnRH analogs to provide long-term blockade of gonadotropin secretion. Second, modulation of pulse frequency provides a mechanism for differential regulation of the synthesis and release of two hormones (LH and FSH) from the same cells (gonadotropes) by the same stimulus (GnRH). Higher-frequency GnRH pulses tend to favor the synthesis and release of LH over FSH, whereas lower frequencies favor FSH over LH.[117,118] However, FSH levels decline throughout the luteal phase of the menstrual cycle—a time when GnRH pulse frequency is at its lowest—and they begin to rise at the transition between the luteal and the follicular phase—a time when GnRH pulse frequency is rapidly accelerating.[119] Except for the preovulatory LH surge, average LH levels remain relatively constant throughout the luteal and follicular phases. These observations call into question the importance of GnRH pulse frequency in the differential regulation of LH and FSH secretion. Third, the frequency of GnRH/LH pulses has been shown to affect follicular development in the primate. In monkeys with hypothalamic lesions, low pulse frequencies, similar to those found during the luteal phase, do not produce follicular development, whereas higher-frequency (similar to those occurring during the follicular phase) pulses do.[120] Thus, the perimenstrual transition from low-frequency to high-frequency pulses likely plays a role in promoting the development of follicles for the subsequent cycle.

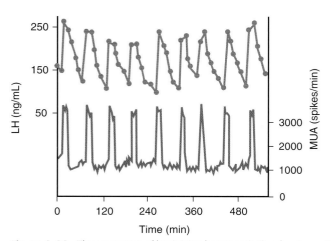

Figure 1-11. *The occurrence of luteinizing hormone (LH) pulses (green) is associated with the firing of neurons (as measured by multiple unit activity [MUA] [purple]) in the hypothalamus of an ovariectomized monkey (Adapted from Knobil E. The electrophysiology of the GnRH pulse generator in the rhesus monkey. J Steroid Biochem 33:669-671, 1989.)*

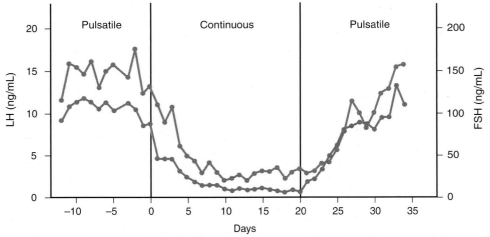

Figure 1-12. *The effects of exogenous gonadotropin-releasing hormone (GnRH) infusions on circulating gonadotropin levels in a monkey that has a hypothalamic lesion that prevents endogenous GnRH release. Pulsatile GnRH infusions lead to elevated luteinizing hormone (LH) (green) and follicle-stimulating hormone (FSH) (purple) levels, but the pituitary becomes refractory when the same amount of GnRH is infused continuously, causing gonadotropin levels to drop dramatically. (Adapted from Belchetz PE, Plant TM, Nakai Y, et al. Hypophysial responses to continuous and intermittent delivery of hypopthalamic gonadotropin-releasing hormone. Science 202:631-633, 1978.)*

DIURNAL/CIRCADIAN RHYTHMS

The term *diurnal* is used to refer to rhythms that cycle once daily. *Circadian rhythms* are diurnal rhythms based on endogenous, cyclic events that occur approximately once each day. To be classified as circadian, a diurnal rhythm must be synchronized to environmental cues, but not driven by them. This means that the rhythm should persist for a period of approximately 24 hours in the absence of any environmental cues and should use environmental cues, when they are available, to synchronize itself to the time of day. A number of organs throughout the body display intrinsic circadian rhythmicity, but most of these are synchronized to a "master clock" that resides in the SCN. The molecular circuitry that generates circadian activity has been described in considerable detail and involves complex feedback interactions among genes and transcription factors, including *Clock, Bmal1, per,* and *cry* genes.[121] The clock in the SCN is synchronized to the time of day by light-induced signals from the retina that are conveyed in fibers that traverse the optic nerve, branch off in the optic chiasm, and terminate in the SCN (the retinohypothalamic tract). Its location in the hypothalamus provides the circadian oscillator in the SCN with easy access to the neural circuits that regulate reproduction.

Diurnal rhythms have been associated with both the basal and surge modes of gonadotropin secretion, depending on a number of factors, including species, sex, and age. For example, during puberty in boys, LH levels are lower during the day and higher at night.[122] A diurnal rhythm in circulating testosterone accompanies this LH rhythm. Underlying the rhythm is a rhythm in LH pulse amplitude, and to a lesser extent, pulse frequency.[123] This is not a true circadian rhythm, however, because it occurs in association with sleep, not time of day. In young men, mean LH levels do not show a significant diurnal rhythm, although the pulse pattern of LH secretion does undergo circadian variations, with lower pulse frequency and higher pulse amplitude at night.[124] Accompanying these changes in LH

pulse patterns is a significant diurnal rhythm in mean testosterone levels (Fig. 1-13). As men age, the amplitude of these rhythms declines.[124] Similar observations have been made in women with respect to LH and estradiol secretion over puberty and during the follicular phase of the menstrual cycle (Fig. 1-14).[125] The mechanisms that generate these rhythms and their physiologic importance—if any—are still unknown.

A definite circadian rhythm associated with the reproductive neuroendocrine system that has clear physiologic significance is the occurrence of the preovulatory LH surge in many species, especially rodents. For example, the LH surge in the rat is dependent on two factors: (1) circulating

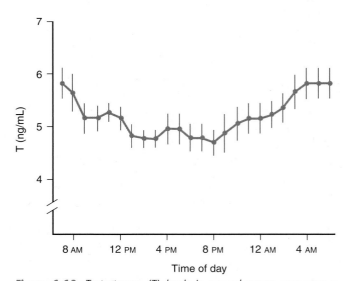

Figure 1-13. *Testosterone (T) levels in normal young men over a 24-hour period. (Adapted from Tenover JS, Matsumoto AM, Clifton DK, Bremner WJ. Age-related alterations in the circadian rhythms of pulsatile luteinizing hormone and testosterone secretion in healthy men. J Gerontol 43:M163-M169, 1988.)*

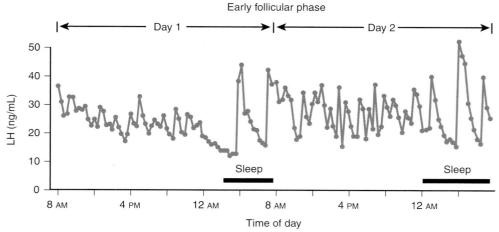

Figure 1-14. *Variation of luteinizing hormone (LH) pulse amplitude and frequency over two 24-hour periods during the early follicular phase of the menstrual cycle in a normal woman. Day 2 occurred 68 days after Day 1. (From Soules MR, Steiner RA, Cohen NL, et al. Nocturnal slowing of pulsatile luteinizing hormone secretion in women during the follicular phase of the menstrual cycle. J Clin Endocrinol Metab 61:43-49, 1985.)*

gonadal steroid levels and (2) time of day. In the adult female rat, the preovulatory LH surge occurs on the afternoon of proestrus. Proestrus is the only time during the estrous cycle in which high levels of ovarian steroids are present, and the afternoon is the only time of day when high levels of ovarian steroids can cause an LH surge to occur. Female rats that are ovariectomized and treated with high levels of estradiol undergo daily LH surges that occur at the same time every afternoon.[126] The surge is synchronized to the environmental light cycle and occurs several hours before the onset of the dark period, which is the time when rats become active. This timing results in ovulation at a time when copulation is most likely to take place. Although the timing of the LH surge has not been studied extensively in humans, based on blood samples collected at 4-hour intervals, the surge has been reported to commence between 4 AM and 8 AM most of the time.[127] However, the physiologic significance of LH surges in humans that are closely associated with the time of day is called into question by the observation that intercourse that takes place as much as 2 days before ovulation is almost as likely to result in conception as intercourse that happens on the day of ovulation.[128]

REPRODUCTIVE CYCLE RHYTHMS

Among mammals, full-fledged reproductive cycles are mainly restricted to females. Although the regional development of gametes is a temporal process that can span a period of several months, neuroendocrine activity in the male is relatively static, allowing the male to successfully mate whenever the female is ready. In contrast, cyclic reproductive activity is a critical component of female fertility and encompasses a sequence of ovarian events that intimately involve the reproductive neuroendocrine system. The relative contribution of each component of the reproductive system toward the timing of the female reproductive cycle has not been completely defined and probably depends on the species. However, it is clear that the first half of the cycle is determined by the length of time required to recruit and develop mature follicles, which may

depend on the circulating levels of LH that are maintained by hypothalamic GnRH release. For the most part, the hypothalamus decides when it is time to induce ovulation by monitoring circulating estrogen levels and generating an LH surge. The last half of the reproductive cycle is determined by the lifespan of the corpus luteum, which may be as long as 6 months in some canines or as little as less than 1 day in some rodents, where the life of the corpus luteum is essentially over before it even begins.

ANNUAL RHYTHMS

Yearly rhythms in reproductive activity are characteristic of animals that live in climates where the weather undergoes dramatic seasonal changes. Allowing conception to occur only at a time of the year when it is likely that a viable offspring will be produced helps to preserve the life of the mother and prevents the wasting of precious energy resources associated with reproductive failure. Animals whose reproduction is regulated by the time of year are referred to as *seasonal breeders*. The effects of season can affect both male and female reproductive functions, depending on the species. A considerable amount of progress has been made toward understanding the general framework whereby the time of year controls the reproductive system, yet many details remain unclear.

In general, the time of year is sensed by measuring the length of the daylight period. Short daylight periods are associated with winter and long daylight periods with summer, whereas daylight periods that are growing longer are associated with spring and those growing shorter with fall. Day length information originates in the eye and is conveyed through the retinohypothalamic tract to the SCN. From the SCN, the signal is relayed through the PVN, down through the spinal cord to the superior cervical ganglion, and then via sympathetic fibers to the pineal gland. This sympathetic input regulates the synthesis of melatonin and its release into both a capillary bed located in and around the pineal and the cerebrospinal fluid. Melatonin thus acts as an endocrine signal to inform systems both inside and outside the brain about day length based on the length of time it is secreted during the night.

Although the primary effect of melatonin on the reproductive system is believed to occur upstream of GnRH neurons, the anatomic sites of its action in the brain appear to be species-dependent.[129] Two sites that seem to be common among most mammals are the pars tuberalis of the anterior pituitary and the SCN. Although the pars tuberalis may have some role in regulating gonadotropin secretion, this region has been associated primarily with seasonal prolactin secretion, at least in sheep.[130] Besides the SCN, the premammillary hypothalamic area in sheep and the medial basal hypothalamus in Syrian hamsters, along with the nucleus reunions of the thalamus and the paraventricular nucleus of the thalamus in Siberian hamsters, are also sites of melatonin action that are believed to be involved in the seasonal regulation of gonadotropin secretion.[129,131] The cellular and molecular mechanisms that decode the melatonin signal at these sites to provide time-of-year information remain poorly understood, but theoretical frameworks for these processes have been proposed.[132,133]

Feedback Regulation of GnRH and Gonadotropins

Gonadal steroids play a critical role in the regulation of gonadotropin secretion. These hormones transmit information about the status of the gonad to the reproductive neuroendocrine system in the brain. The reproductive neuroendocrine system processes this information and adjusts gonadotropin secretion to meet the gonad's needs and ensure that successful reproduction occurs. The transmission of information from the gonad to the brain is referred to as *feedback regulation*. Depending on the sex of the individual and the stage of the reproductive cycle, the feedback signal can either inhibit (negative feedback) or stimulate (positive feedback) GnRH secretion, and subsequently the secretion of gonadotropins. Gonadal steroids also feed back on the pituitary to modulate its response to GnRH, thus complementing the effects of the hormones that are mediated by the brain.

STEROID RECEPTORS

Steroid receptors mediate the negative and positive feedback effects of gonadal steroids. In the female, estradiol levels reflect the status of developing follicles, and progesterone levels indicate the occurrence of ovulation and provide information about the status of the corpus luteum. The primary mechanism by which estradiol acts is through nuclear estrogen receptors that regulate gene transcription within the target cell. Two forms of nuclear ER have been identified (ERα and ERβ), each of which appears to have distinct functions.[134] Evidence suggests that estrogen can also act through nongenomic receptors, and one of these, GPR30, has recently been identified. GPR30 is a G protein–coupled receptor that, when activated by estrogen, mobilizes calcium and activates phosphatidylinositol 3,4,5-triphosphate synthesis.[135] Progesterone,

like estradiol, acts through two different forms of nuclear receptor (PR-A and PR-B). Unlike ERs, the same gene encodes PR-A and PR-B, with PR-A being a truncated form of PR-B. The expression of these two isoforms is differentially regulated, and they appear to have different functions.[136] In the male, testosterone is the primary circulating gonadal steroid, and many effects of testosterone are mediated by nuclear ARs. However, testosterone is also aromatized to estradiol both peripherally and centrally, and thus it can act through the various ERs as well.

The sex steroid receptors ER, PR, and AR are differentially expressed in distinct areas throughout the forebrain and brain stem.[137-139] Because gonadal steroids perform many functions within the CNS, it is likely that only a small subset of the cells in the brain that express gonadal steroid receptors are directly involved in the regulation of gonadotropin secretion. Areas known to play an important role in the regulation of gonadotropin secretion, such as the mPOA, AVPV, and ARC, have been shown to express one or more forms of each of the gonadal steroid receptors.

NEGATIVE FEEDBACK

In the gonad-intact adult animal, gonadotropin secretion is under constant inhibition by circulating gonadal steroids. After gonadectomy, gonadotropin levels rise dramatically over a period of several weeks. The initial response to gonad removal depends somewhat on species and sex. In the male rat, circulating LH levels rise abruptly within 24 hours after castration, whereas in the female rat, ovariectomy results in little change for the first week, after which LH levels begin to rise more rapidly.[140] In women, the initial response depends on the phase of the menstrual cycle in which ovariectomy is performed. When ovariectomy occurs in the follicular phase, LH increases severalfold within 24 hours, but when ovariectomy is performed in the luteal phase, it takes several days for LH levels to begin to rise.[141] Immediately after gonadectomy in the male monkey, LH can be maintained at gonad-intact levels with the administration of physiologic levels of either estradiol or testosterone.[142] However, evidence in male monkeys suggests that after the negative feedback system has not been exposed to testosterone for a long time, physiologic levels of testosterone become incapable of suppressing LH secretion.[142] In contrast with estradiol and testosterone, progesterone by itself does not exert negative feedback inhibition of LH secretion in most species,[143,144] but does appear to enhance the ability of low levels of estradiol to suppress LH secretion.[144,145]

In addition to their ability to regulate mean circulating levels of gonadotropins, gonadal steroids modulate both the amplitude and the frequency of LH pulses. LH pulse frequency is generally highest in the absence of gonadal steroids. In ovariectomized rats, estradiol slows the frequency of LH pulses by approximately 50% and leads to a small decrease in pulse amplitude.[144] The effects of estradiol on LH pulses in sheep depend on the time of year. When ewes are in anestrus (i.e., not breeding), estradiol dramatically reduces LH pulse frequency, but during the breeding season, estradiol either has no effect or increases

LH pulse frequency and inhibits pulse amplitude.[146] In the human and monkey, LH pulse frequency during the follicular phase of the menstrual cycle is similar to that seen in the complete absence of ovarian estrogen secretion.[102,103,147] These observations have led to the conclusion that estradiol has no effect on pulse frequency in the primate. However, carefully controlled studies have shown that physiologic levels of estradiol either slow or completely block LH pulses in ovariectomized monkeys.[148] This apparent discrepancy may be due to an increased sensitivity to estradiol after ovariectomy,[149] coupled with the fact that, during the follicular phase of the menstrual cycle, there is a dynamic interplay between estradiol and LH that does not exist in ovariectomized animals given constant levels of estradiol. The effects of progesterone on pulsatile LH secretion are, for the most part, subtle and dependent on species and endocrine status. However, progesterone appears to be responsible for the decreased frequency and increased amplitude of LH pulses that occur during the luteal phase of the menstrual cycle.[150]

In males, gonadectomy generally leads to a rapid increase in LH pulse frequency. This occurs within 24 hours in the rat and 48 hours in the monkey, and in those two species, an increase in pulse amplitude occurs at the same time.[151,152] The temporal effects of castration on LH pulse parameters have not been reported in humans, but hypogonadal men have higher-frequency and higher-amplitude pulses compared with eugonadal men.[153] As might be expected, differences in LH pulse characteristics between males with and without functional testes are caused, at least in part, by differences in circulating testosterone. Testosterone replacement reduces LH pulse frequency to near-intact levels; however, replacement with physiologic levels of testosterone, by itself, does not appear to be capable of reducing LH pulse amplitude to that found in males with functional testes.[152-154] This suggests that other factors from the testis are involved in regulating LH pulse amplitude. One of these factors is probably inhibin, because inhibin antibodies have been shown to increase LH pulse amplitude in intact rams without altering LH pulse frequency.[155] It is likely that testosterone exerts at least some of its effects on LH pulses by acting through an AR that is expressed in the brain and pituitary. Nevertheless, testosterone can also be aromatized to estradiol and thus act through ERs. That aromatization and ER play a role in the regulation of pulsatile LH secretion is suggested by the observations that (1) a centrally administered aromatase inhibitor increased LH pulse frequency in intact rams[156] and (2) a peripherally administered aromatase inhibitor increased both LH pulse frequency and amplitude in normal men.[157]

Gonadal steroids can regulate LH pulse characteristics by acting on the brain, the pituitary, or both. Because pulses of LH reflect pulses of GnRH that drive the output of LH from gonadotropes, steroid effects on pulse frequency are generally interpreted as the result of steroid action on the brain. However, changes in LH pulse amplitude could result either from altered GnRH pulse amplitude or from changes in the response of gonadotropes to GnRH stimulation. Several approaches have been used to distinguish between these two possibilities. One is to

test for changes in pituitary sensitivity by administering exogenous GnRH pulses and measuring the LH response. This testing is fairly easy to perform, but the results can be confounded by interference from endogenous GnRH secretion. To avoid problems with interference, some investigators have surgically disrupted the connection between the hypothalamus and the pituitary. The second approach is to directly measure the release of GnRH in the median eminence/portal system/pituitary through the use of push-pull perfusion, microdialysis, or sampling directly from portal blood. These techniques can be technically demanding, and interpretation of the results can be complicated by the relatively small samples that can be collected. To appreciate the difficulties associated with some of these techniques, consider the fact that there have been at least seven articles describing the effects of castration on GnRH pulses in conscious male rats through the use of push-pull perfusion or microdialysis in the median eminence or pituitary. Three of them report that castration increases GnRH pulse amplitude, one reports no effect, and two report a decrease in pulse amplitude.[158]

A clearer picture of how gonadal steroids regulate LH pulse amplitude has emerged for sheep and monkeys. In male sheep, LH pulse amplitude remains relatively constant for several weeks after castration and then gradually declines. GnRH pulse amplitude, as measured by the collection of portal blood samples in conscious rams, roughly parallels that of GnRH, suggesting that castration has little effect on pituitary sensitivity.[159] That conclusion is also supported by the observation that testosterone does not alter the pituitary response to GnRH when administered to castrated male sheep in which endogenous GnRH has been blocked.[160] In the male monkey, direct measurements of GnRH in portal blood have not been performed; however, based on measurements made in monkeys with lesions that block endogenous GnRH secretion, pituitary sensitivity is only slightly increased by castration and is unaltered by testosterone treatment.[161] Because LH pulse amplitude increases dramatically with castration and decreases to intact levels after testosterone administration, it appears that testosterone suppresses GnRH pulse amplitude in male monkeys. In men, it is not ethically possible to perform hypothalamic–pituitary disconnections. Nevertheless, the results from GnRH injections into normal men have led to conclusions that are similar to those derived from studies in sheep and monkeys. The inhibitory effect of testosterone on LH pulse amplitude in men appears to be due to a suppression of GnRH pulse amplitude and is not caused by a change in pituitary sensitivity to GnRH.[162]

Unlike testosterone in the male, estradiol appears to modulate LH pulse amplitude by changing pituitary sensitivity to GnRH, in addition to regulating GnRH pulse amplitude. For example, the response of the pituitary to GnRH decreases dramatically immediately after the administration of estradiol to ovariectomized monkeys in which endogenous GnRH secretion has been blocked by hypothalamic lesions.[163] Similar observations have been made in female sheep.[164] Furthermore, measurement of GnRH levels in the portal blood of ovariectomized ewes has shown that GnRH pulse amplitude is also suppressed by estradiol administration.[165] In both the monkey and the sheep, the reduction of pituitary sensitivity to GnRH after estradiol administration is transient; within several hours (in sheep) or days (in monkeys), the response of the pituitary to GnRH increases dramatically above pretreatment levels. This enhancement of pituitary sensitivity is associated with the positive feedback effect of estradiol.

POSITIVE FEEDBACK

One critically important function of the reproductive neuroendocrine system in the female is to monitor the progress of developing follicles so that it can induce ovulation by generating an LH surge at the right time. The primary ovarian signal indicating follicular maturation is estradiol. Although low levels of estradiol produce negative feedback inhibition of LH secretion, elevated levels of estradiol trigger a large but transient release of LH known as the *preovulatory LH surge*. Because under these circumstances increasing gonadal steroid levels lead to increased LH release, this phenomenon is often referred to as *positive feedback*. The relationship between estradiol levels and the LH surge has been most carefully described in the monkey. By adjusting the number of estradiol-filled capsules administered to monkeys on day 3 of the menstrual cycle, Karsch and colleagues found that, to generate unambiguous LH surges, circulating estradiol levels had to be elevated to more than 100 pg/mL.[166] Estradiol levels of 100 to 200 pg/mL were capable of generating an LH surge, but only if they remained elevated for at least 42 hours. However, circulating estradiol levels of approximately 1500 pg/mL were able to induce an LH surge after only a 24-hour period of exposure. Thus, both the strength of the estradiol signal and its duration play a role in determining if and when the preovulatory LH surge in the monkey will occur. Such strength–duration relationships are probably present in other species, including humans, although similar studies in those species have not been reported. Nevertheless, it is unlikely that the duration of exposure is an important factor in the generation of preovulatory LH surges in rodents because their reproductive cycle is so short. In the rodent, another condition, in addition to elevated estradiol levels, must be satisfied before an LH surge can be generated. As mentioned earlier, the LH surge in rats and mice can occur only at a certain time of day. If a surge is delayed, it will occur exactly 24 hours later.[167] Furthermore, if levels that are high enough to trigger an LH surge are maintained for several days in ovariectomized rats, LH surges are generated at the same time on consecutive days.[126] The generation of multiple LH surges under continuous exposure to estradiol has not been documented in primates.

Progesterone by itself is unable to induce an LH surge, but in combination with estradiol, it can have either stimulatory or inhibitory effects on the generation of LH surges in humans, monkeys, and rats, depending on the relative timing of its administration. When administered before or at the same time that estradiol is given, progesterone blocks the LH surge that would have been generated by estradiol alone.[168-170] However, if progesterone is administered after estradiol but before the LH surge, it causes the surge to occur earlier than it normally would.[168,171,172] Similar effects of exogenous progesterone on the spontaneous LH surge

have been found in females during regular reproductive cycles.[173-175]

The generation of an LH surge involves the action of estradiol at both the brain and the pituitary. During the LH surge, there is an increase in the amount of GnRH released into the hypophysial portal system, which has been verified by direct measurements in sheep and rats,[176,177] and by indirect measurements in monkeys.[178] At the same time, high levels of circulating estradiol increase the pituitary response to GnRH.[62,179] In fact, the importance of changes in pituitary sensitivity, at least in the monkey, are highlighted by the observation that normal menstrual cycles, including preovulatory LH surges, can be produced by administering constant-amplitude pulses of GnRH once per hour to animals in which endogenous GnRH secretion has been blocked by hypothalamic lesions.[180] Thus, even though GnRH release normally increases at the time of the surge in the monkey, that increase does not appear to be essential for the production of a surge. In other species, increased GnRH secretion from the brain appears to play a more important role. In rats, a wide variety of evidence indicates that a GnRH surge emanating from the brain is critical for the generation of an LH surge. For example, brain lesions and deafferentations that spare basal GnRH support of the pituitary effectively block the LH surge.[181,182] Furthermore, estradiol implanted into the medial preoptic area is as effective as systemic estradiol in inducing LH surges, without elevating pituitary estradiol to the levels seen just before the preovulatory LH surge, whereas estradiol implanted in the mediobasal hypothalamus, which results in very high pituitary estradiol levels, does not lead to the generation of an LH surge.[183] Evidence for the importance of increased GnRH secretion in the generation of LH surges has also been found in sheep.[184]

A MODEL OF NEGATIVE AND POSITIVE FEEDBACK REGULATION OF GnRH BY KISSPEPTINS

The fact that GnRH plays a critical role in the feedback regulation of gonadotropin secretion has been known for many years. Nevertheless, the neural mechanisms by which steroids control GnRH release are, for the most part, still unclear. Much of our understanding of how feedback control of GnRH operates comes from work in rats, and more recently, mice. It is now generally accepted that GnRH neurons in rats do not express gonadal steroid receptors, except ERβ.[47] It is unlikely that ERβ plays an important role in gonadal feedback because animals that lack a functional *ERβ* gene exhibit both negative and positive feedback responses to estradiol, whereas these functions are lacking in ERα knockouts.[185,186] These observations suggest that steroids regulate the activity of GnRH neurons indirectly by acting through other neurons. Although the identity of those neurons remains a mystery, candidates would include neurons that exhibit a number of specific characteristics. First, they would express one or more gonadal steroid receptors. Second, gonadal steroids would regulate their activity. Third, they would express one or more neurotransmitters that are known to control GnRH secretion. Fourth, they would make either direct or indirect connections to GnRH neurons. Fifth, disruption of those neurons would interrupt feedback regulation of GnRH secretion. Among the numerous neurons and neurotransmitters that have been implicated in the regulation of LH/GnRH secretion over the years, a newcomer, kisspeptin, stands out as a potentially important mediator of both the negative and positive feedback effects of gonadal steroids.

As mentioned earlier, kisspeptin is a potent stimulator of GnRH release and *Kiss1* (the gene that encodes kisspeptin) is expressed primarily in the ARC in males and in both the AVPV and ARC in females.[115] Furthermore, the majority of GnRH neurons express kisspeptin receptors (KISS1R),[187] suggesting that *Kiss1* neurons in one or both of those areas project to GnRH neurons. In the rat, the ARC has long been associated with negative feedback regulation of gonadotropin secretion. Virtually all of the *Kiss1*-expressing neurons in the ARC of the female express ERα, and most of those in the male express ERα and AR.[188,189] Estrogen inhibits *Kiss1* expression in the ARC and testosterone does the same in males, as would be expected if *Kiss1* neurons were to mediate gonadal steroid negative feedback. Finally, animals in which the kisspeptin/KISS1R signaling pathway has been disrupted (i.e., KISS1R knockout mice) do not undergo negative feedback regulation.[112] In fact, those animals appear to lack basal LH secretion, suggesting that inhibition of tonic kisspeptin stimulation is the mode by which gonadal steroids inhibit GnRH secretion. Taken together, these observations strongly support the idea that kisspeptins acting through KISS1R play an important role in negative feedback regulation of GnRH/LH secretion by gonadal steroids.

In addition to a possible negative feedback role in the ARC, it is likely that *Kiss1* neurons in the AVPV are involved in the positive feedback of estradiol on LH secretion in the female, based on several lines of evidence. First, AVPV is known to be an essential part of the neural circuit that generates LH surges in the rat.[47] Second, only female rodents are capable of generating LH surges, and only female rodents have large numbers of *Kiss1* neurons in the AVPV.[190] Third, estradiol induces the expression of *Kiss1* messenger ribonucleic acid in the AVPV.[189] Fourth, in the AVPV, *Kiss1* neurons are activated during LH surges, as indicated by increased expression of Fos.[191] Fifth, *Kiss1* neurons in the AVPV project directly to GnRH neurons.[192] Sixth, kisspeptin antiserum blocks the proestrous LH surge in rats.[193] However, despite this strong evidence that kisspeptins normally play an important role in generating LH surges, it appears that they are not absolutely essential. KISS1R knockout mice, which lack a functional kisspeptin/KISS1R signaling pathway, have been shown to be capable of producing an LH surge in response to exogenous estradiol. This observation suggests that alternative surge mechanisms exist in animals that chronically lack a functional kisspeptin signaling system.

Figure 1-15 summarizes the model for kisspeptin/KISS1R-mediated negative and positive feedback regulation of GnRH/LH in female rodents. In the male and during most of the estrous cycle in females, gonadal steroid feedback inhibits the activity of *Kiss1* neurons in the ARC, maintaining the proper basal gonadotropin stimulation of

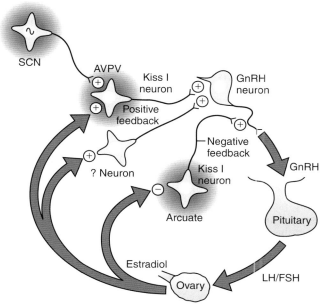

Figure 1-15. *Simplified model of kisspeptin-mediated positive and negative feedback regulation of gonadotropin-releasing hormone (GnRH)/gonadotropin secretion. Negative feedback: Kiss1 neurons in the arcuate nucleus express estrogen receptor α (ERα) and are inhibited by circulating estradiol. These neurons project to GnRH neurons, stimulating GnRH activity. In the absence of estradiol, Kiss1 neurons are highly active, leading to elevated GnRH/gonadotropin secretion. When estradiol levels rise, Kiss1 activity decreases, leading to a reduction in GnRH activity and gonadotropin secretion. Positive feedback: Kiss1 neurons in the anteroventral periventricular nucleus (AVPV) also express ERα, but they are stimulated by estradiol. They may also receive inputs from the suprachiasmatic nucleus (SCN), which relay time-of-day information and project to GnRH neurons. When estradiol levels are high and it is the right time of day, Kiss1 neurons in the AVPV become active, leading to the activation of GnRH neurons and a surge release of LH. Observations in KISS1R knockout animals suggest that other neuronal circuits (labeled "? Neuron" in the figure) may also be involved in the positive feedback generation of GnRH/gonadotropin luteinizing hormone (LH) surges. FSH, follicle-stimulating hormone.*

the developing gamete. When the gonads are removed, *Kiss1* neurons in the ARC are no longer inhibited by gonadal steroids; thus, their activity increases, leading to an increase in the release of GnRH and gonadotropins. The AVPV does not play an important role in the male, but it does in the female. For most of the estrous cycle, estrogen levels are too low to activate *Kiss1* neurons in the AVPV, but rising levels of estrogen associated with follicular maturation induce the expression of *Kiss1* in the AVPV, preparing the *Kiss1* neurons for activation. On the afternoon of proestrus, when those neurons are ready, they are activated by a daily signal that comes from the SCN. Although it is simplistic, this model is strikingly consistent with our understanding of how feedback works and it provides a solid framework on which subsequent investigations can be planned. Some important issues that need to be addressed include determining whether *Kiss1* neurons are involved in the generation of pulsatile GnRH secretion, learning how progesterone feedback affects the kisspeptin/KISS1R system, and investigating the interactions of kisspeptins with other neurotransmitter systems known to influence GnRH release. In addition, although this model is mostly consistent with results obtained in the monkey and sheep, details need to be studied and confirmed in other species.

Metabolism, Stress, and Reproduction[194]

METABOLIC STRESSES THAT INFLUENCE REPRODUCTION

Caloric Restriction

Reproduction is energetically taxing. Darwin wrote extensively about the effect of nutrition on fertility in sheep and other animals, observing that ewes feeding on lush lowland pastures were more fertile (and more likely to bear twins) than those grazing on sparse high ground. Indeed, the phenomenon of seasonal breeding—which is characteristic of most nonequatorial mammals—reflects the effect of seasonal food availability on reproductive success. Metabolic fuels are required for the intracellular oxidation of glucose and fatty acids to produce adenosine triphosphate, but in the longer term, there must be adequate stored fuels (i.e., fat) to address the caloric demands of mating (consider the rutting elk), pregnancy, and lactation. The energy burden of reproduction rests more heavily on females than on males, and thus the effect of caloric restriction (and limited fat reserves) is greater in females. Caloric restriction leads to a classic metabolic profile, with gradually diminishing plasma levels of insulin, leptin, and other metabolic hormones, along with changes in blood levels of metabolic fuels (i.e., glucose, amino acids, fatty acids). One of the most astonishing features of the effect of diet on reproduction is how rapidly the body responds—often within just days (Fig. 1-16).[195,196] However, despite having a reasonably clear understanding of what happens to the body with food restriction, we do not know precisely how this information leads to alterations in the activity of the brain–pituitary–gonadal axis.

The effect of diet (restricted or ample) is also reflected in the age of puberty onset. This is the case in all mammals, including humans. In the early 1960s, Gordon Kennedy established that the timing of puberty in rats was dependent on body weight (and thus diet). This work presaged the classic epidemiologic studies of Rose Frisch and her colleagues in the 1970s in humans, showing that the age of menarche was more closely associated (and predicted) by body weight than by chronologic age. During the 18th century, in Western Europe, the average age of puberty onset (as reflected by menarche) was close to 18 years, whereas today, it stands at approximately 12.5 years. It is presumed that the decline in the age of puberty (in girls and boys) reflects improved nutrition of Western societies that resulted from improved socioeconomic conditions. This in turn is associated with an increase in the rate of growth and a constellation of metabolic events that somehow contribute to the acceleration of pubertal maturation. Although "body weight," "body fat," and "rate of growth" have all been variously associated with the timing of pubertal maturation, it has become clear that these are associated (not causal) variables—such as foot size.

Studies over the next several decades led to the conclusion that neither body weight nor fat itself is the proximate trigger for puberty, but rather, a complex derivative of growth (e.g., some combination of metabolic hormones or fuels) reports to the brain about the status of metabolic reserves—and thus acts permissively to allow sexual maturation to proceed when conditions are ripe. The corollary to this phenomenon is found in clinical syndromes, such as anorexia nervosa, where inadequate caloric intake either delays puberty or causes secondary amenorrhea and a regression to the prepubertal reproductive state. Although the advantage of having caloric reserves (i.e., fat) act as a gate to either permit or restrict reproductive activity makes good sense, it is less clear precisely how this happens at a cellular and molecular level. No doubt, the brain is the final arbiter that determines whether the individual's metabolic state is sufficient to permit reproduction to proceed, but exactly how the brain accomplishes this feat remains poorly understood.

Exercise

Exercise, especially in females, has a similar metabolic effect on reproduction as caloric restriction (and lactation). The metabolic profile associated with intense exercise—a state of negative energy balance—closely resembles that of fasting, particularly when the individual has minimal fat reserves. Severe exercise can delay the onset of puberty and inhibit reproductive function in adults. The mechanisms

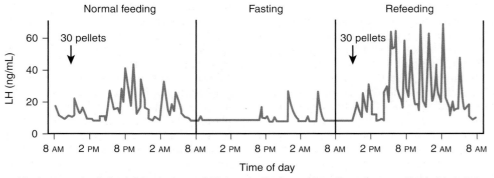

Figure 1-16. *Effects of fasting on pulsatile luteinizing hormone (LH) secretion in the monkey. (From Cameron JL, Nosbisch C. Suppression of pulsatile luteinizing hormone and testosterone secretion during short term food restriction in the adult male rhesus monkey* [Macaca mulatta]. *Endocrinology 128:1532-1540, 1991.)*

that drive this inhibition are not well understood; however, everything points to common denominators with fasting and dietary restriction, because at least under experimental circumstances, exercise-induced amenorrhea can be reversed by exogenously administering GnRH or simply replenishing the calorie deficit (Fig 1-17).[196] Ideas about how the brain keeps tab of exercise have included suggestions that endogenous opioid peptides, such as β-endorphin (derived from the *POMC* gene), may play a role in shutting down the reproductive axis as a result of intense exercise; however, studies in humans would appear to negate this idea.

Lactation

Lactation, like exercise, presents a tremendous energetic drain. Although many animals, including humans, build fat reserves during pregnancy, these reserves are inadequate to meet the metabolic demands of nursing without enormous maternal hyperphagia and reduced energy expenditures. During this period of high energy demand, it would be disadvantageous for the animal (and the species) if it were to expend energy to become pregnant again, and with a few notable exceptions, postpartum lactation represents a period of infertility. In many animals, including humans, lactational infertility reflects an inhibition of folliculogenesis and ovulation, attributable to low circulating levels of gonadotropins (mostly LH)—although in other cases, such as kangaroos, animals may become

pregnant, with the blastocyst remaining in suspended animation. Lactational infertility is associated with reduced GnRH (and hence LH) secretion. Although negative energy balance contributes the lion's share to reduced GnRH/LH secretion during lactation (analogous to dietary restriction and exercise), the suckling stimulus itself (and activation of neural pathways leading from the breast to the hypothalamus) plays a direct inhibitory role in suppressing GnRH secretion. Thus, fasting, exercise, and lactation share similar features—association with diminished activity of the brain–pituitary–ovarian axis, a metabolic profile of low circulating levels of insulin and leptin, and changes in other metabolic hormones and fuels. Although it is known that the brain is responsible for garnering the physiologic response to the metabolic challenges of lactation and suckling, we are still not sure precisely how this happens.[197]

CIRCULATING METABOLIC SIGNALS THAT LINK NUTRITION, GROWTH, AND REPRODUCTION

Negative energy balance leads to predictable changes in circulating levels of metabolic hormones and fuels, and one could imagine that such changes might act on the brain to inhibit GnRH secretion during metabolic stress (e.g., fasting). There is compelling evidence to indicate that insulin is one critical signal to the neuroendocrine reproductive axis. Plasma levels of insulin increase and decrease as

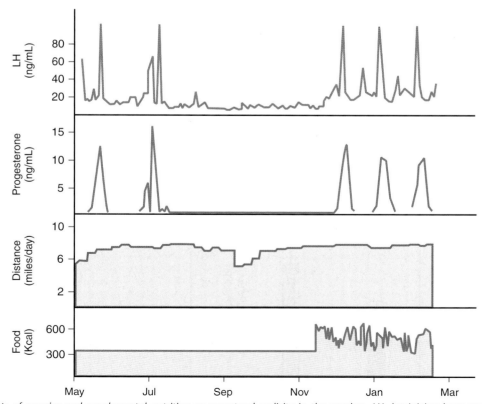

Figure 1-17. *Effects of exercise and supplemental nutrition on menstrual cyclicity in the monkey. LH, luteinizing hormone. (From Williams NI, Caston-Balderrama AL, Helmreich DL, et al. Longitudinal changes in reproductive hormones and menstrual cyclicity in cynomolgus monkeys during strenuous exercise training: Abrupt transition to exercise-induced amenorrhea. Endocrinology 142:2381-2389, 2001.)*

an immediate function of plasma levels of glucose; however, insulin levels change in rough proportion to body weight—or more precisely—body adiposity. Insulin acts directly on the brain as a satiety factor to regulate body weight and energy expenditure. Thus, it seems plausible to think that the insulin signal could also be borrowed by the neuroendocrine reproductive axis to gate its operation as a function of body fat reserves. Diabetic animals, including humans (lacking insulin or appropriate responsiveness), often have impaired reproductive function, which can, under some circumstances, be reversed by appropriate insulin treatment. Moreover, animals bearing brain-specific, genetically targeted deletions of the insulin receptor have impaired reproductive function, underscoring the prerequisite role of insulin in reproduction. Although insulin has direct effects on hypothalamic neurons, particularly in the ARC, its effects on GnRH and LH secretion are controversial and complicated by the difficulty in isolating its direct action from that of other metabolic hormones and fuels. Insulin is necessary for proper reproductive function, but alone, it is insufficient to account for the complex effects of metabolism on reproduction. There is also strong evidence to suggest that metabolic fuels, such as glucose fatty acids, have profound effects on GnRH and LH secretion—at least in a permissive sense. Blockade of glucose metabolism in experimental animals produces an immediate and profound inhibitory effect on reproductive function, including behavior; however, because glucose is an absolute prerequisite for all neuronal function, it is perhaps not surprising that glucoprivation inhibits GnRH and LH secretion.

Leptin is an adipocyte-derived hormone that circulates in proportion to fat reserves. Leptin is believed to act on the brain as a satiety hormone, and the absence of leptin (with nutritional deprivation) increases appetite, feeding, and body weight. Animals, including humans, with disabling mutations in the leptin or leptin receptor genes are obese and have severely impaired reproductive function, suggesting that leptin may be necessary for initiating and supporting reproductive function (as well as regulating body weight). Moreover, administering exogenous leptin to leptin-deficient *ob/ob* mice can activate their reproductive function (Fig. 1-18).[198] Leptin acts directly on neurons in the hypothalamus that produce POMC, NPY, GALP, and kisspeptin—all of which have been implicated in the regulation of GnRH and LH secretion. The exogenous administration of leptin can partially reverse the diet-induced delay of puberty in the rat and mouse, and under some circumstances, leptin can stimulate LH secretion in primate species. On the other hand, leptin's putative role in the neuroendocrine regulation of GnRH/gonadotropin secretion is confounded by several contradictory observations. First, people with certain lipodystrophies and profoundly low circulating levels of leptin do not always have reproductive abnormalities. Second, despite the fact that leptin-deficient ob/ob female mice have low levels of gonadotopins and reproductive failure, male ob/ob mice that are crossed into a BALB/cJ background are fertile. This suggests that leptin interacts with other factors that must be present at some level to influence GnRH and LH secretion to support normal spermatogenesis and sexual behavior. Thus, the preponderance of evidence suggests that leptin plays a permissive role in gonadotropin secretion—but by itself, leptin is not the Holy Grail linking metabolism and reproduction.

The thyroid gland synthesizes and secretes thyroid hormones (TH), predominantly thyroxine (T_4), which is metabolized in peripheral tissue to the more biologically active triiodothyronine (T_3). T_3 stimulates metabolism in many target cells in the body, by acting through TH receptors, which are members of the nuclear hormone receptor superfamily. Alterations in diet—particularly negative energy balance—can produce changes in circulating levels of thyroid hormones, which decline with food restriction and

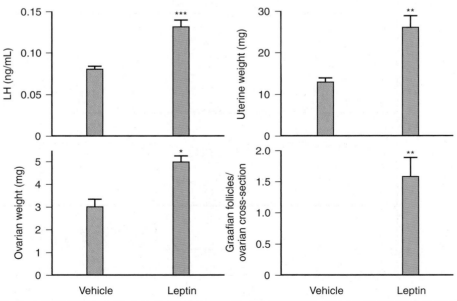

Figure 1-18. *Effects of leptin administration on the reproductive axis of leptin-deficient* ob/ob *mice. LH, luteinizing hormone. *P < 0.01; **P < 0.001; ***P < 0.0001. (Adapted from Barash IA, Cheung CC, Weigle DS, et al. Leptin is a metabolic signal to the reproductive system. Endocrinology 137:3144-3147, 1996.)*

thus reduce the basal metabolic rate. Either a deficiency or an excess of thyroid hormones can have adverse consequences on the reproductive axis. Hypothyroidism often causes hypogonadotropic hypogonadism, but occasionally can be associated with sexual precocity in boys and girls. Hyperthyroidism is also linked to impaired reproductive function, including delayed puberty and hypogonadotropic hypogonadism. TH receptors are found in the brain, and are expressed by GnRH neurons. However, TH receptors are widely distributed in the reproductive system, including the gonads, and it is likely that TH has direct effects on the activity of many cell types in the HPG axis. Although departures from normal circulating levels of TH can affect reproductive function, it seems likely that TH is likely just one of many metabolic signals that influence the HPG axis during swings in food availability.

Other metabolic hormones, such as growth hormone, insulin-like growth factor-1 (IGF-1), cholecystokinin, glucagon-like peptide-1, and ghrelin, have been shown to influence the reproductive axis by acting on the brain—at least under some experimental circumstances. However, the physiologic role—if any—of these other factors in specifically linking metabolism to reproduction remains to be established. Vagal afferents may relay information about metabolic status (or at least meal size) from the gut to the brain, and manipulations of the vagus have been shown to influence LH secretion. Thus, blood-borne factors produced by fat, the endocrine pancreas, and the gastrointestinal tract, as well as neuronal afferents from the gut, may all serve some physiologic role in coupling metabolic status to reproductive function, by acting somewhere in the brain to regulate GnRH secretion.

CENTRAL PATHWAYS THAT INTEGRATE METABOLISM AND REPRODUCTION

Metabolic hormones, such as leptin and insulin, act on the brain to regulate feeding and energy metabolism. These hormones (and fuels, such as fatty acids) are believed to serve as satiety factors to reflect fuel status and thereby serve as one limb of the control system to regulate fuel homeostasis and body weight. They accomplish this task by acting on specific target cells in the brain that act as a complex neural circuit that coordinates energy regulation, metabolism, and feeding behavior. These same hormones are believed to provide signals to the neuroendocrine reproductive axis, allowing reproduction to proceed when fuel reserves are adequate, but inhibiting reproduction if reserves are too low to support the energy demands of reproduction. It has become clear during the last several decades that none of these groups of target cells is likely to be the final common pathway through which metabolic information is conveyed to the neuroendocrine reproductive axis. Instead, it would appear that an ensemble of target cells and neuropeptides acts in concert to integrate and coordinate this complex task and that, in the congenital absence of one of these peptides (or its receptor), the system has proved to be resilient and well compensated by redundancy.

Neurons that produce POMC-derived peptides (i.e., the melanocortin α-melanocyte–stimulating hormone,

α-MSH, and the endogenous opioid, β-endorphin) are targets for the actions of leptin, insulin, and metabolic fuels, and these peptides exert profound effects on feeding and metabolism. Cellular levels of POMC mRNA are reduced in states of negative energy balance and up-regulated by overfeeding. POMC neurons in the ARC are direct targets for the action of leptin (and insulin), which increases firing rate and induces Fos expression in these cells. The melanocortin receptors, MC3-R and MC4-R, and their principal ligand, α-MSH, an anorexigenic peptide, have been unequivocally implicated in the regulation of metabolism and body weight. However, any role for the central melanocortin system in the neuroendocrine regulation of reproduction remains to be established—particularly in view of the fact that reproduction continues unabated, even in the chronic absence of melanocortin signaling. On the other hand, β-endorphin would appear to play a vital role in the control of GnRH and gonadotropin secretion. Exogenous administration of β-endorphin (or morphine) inhibits GnRH and LH secretion, whereas opiate receptor antagonists, such as naloxone, stimulate GnRH and gonadotropin secretion. β-Endorphin–containing neurons appear to make direct synaptic contact with GnRH neurons, and GnRH neurons are hyperpolarized by opiate receptor agonists. Nevertheless, there is no clear evidence that GnRH neurons express any of the classic opiate receptors, so it remains uncertain how endogenous opioid peptides exert their effects on GnRH neurons. Endogenous opioids are plausible candidates for mediating some of the stress-induced effects on reproduction. In the case of metabolic stress, the inhibitory effects of food restriction can be attenuated (or reversed) in fasted rats, lactating animals, and women with anorexia nervosa, by the administration of opiate receptor antagonists; however, this does not appear to be universally the case because nalaxone does not increase LH secretion in some other experimental models (fasted monkeys).

Neuropeptide Y is an orexigenic peptide that has been a central focus for elucidating the neuroendocrine regulation of body weight and metabolism. Central injections of NPY evoke an astonishing increase in appetite and feeding—even in satiated animals. NPY-expressing neurons are found in many places in the brain—but most conspicuously for energy regulation and reproduction—in the ARC and brain stem. The synthesis and secretion of NPY in the ARC is profoundly influenced by energy status. Fasting and other states of negative energy balance, as well as leptin and insulin deficiency (e.g., lactation and exercise), stimulate the production of NPY, whereas states of energy repletion are associated with reduced expression of NPY.

NPY is also believed to play a central role in the neuroendocrine regulation of GnRH and gonadotropin secretion. GnRH neurons receive direct synaptic input from NPY-containing neurons, whose cell bodies reside in the ARC and brain stem. GnRH neurons express one or more of the six NPY receptor subtypes (likely Y5 and possibly Y1), setting the anatomic framework for NPY regulating GnRH secretion. Studies of the effect of NPY on GnRH and LH secretion show a complicated picture. In normal intact animals (or gonadectomized animals that are treated with sex steroids), central injections of NPY exert a stimulatory effect on GnRH and LH secretion, whereas in animals that are castrated, NPY inhibits GnRH/LH secretion. This bimodal, steroid-dependent action of NPY on GnRH/LH is not unusual because other neurotransmitters exert steroid-dependent effects on gonadotropin secretion (e.g., norepinephrine and orexins). Adding to this complexity is the observation that continuous central infusions of NPY given to normal intact animals delays sexual maturation in prepubertal animals and disrupts estrous cyclicity in adults—reminiscent of the fact that leptin-deficient *ob/ob* mice, which express extraordinarily high levels of NPY in the ARC, have profoundly disturbed reproductive function; moreover, targeted deletions of the Y4 receptor rescue fertility in the *ob/ob* mouse, implying that excessive NPY-Y4 signaling is responsible for inhibiting reproduction when the body perceives a state of depleted energy reserves (i.e., in the *ob/ob* mouse). Notwithstanding, mice with null mutations in the *NPY* gene appear to have relatively normal reproductive function, which would argue that whatever role NPY plays in reproduction represents only one of many inputs and part of a highly redundant network.

Galanin-like peptide is a neuropeptide, distantly related to galanin, but coded by a separate gene on a different chromosome. GALP is expressed discretely in the ARC of the hypothalamus. GALP neurons are targets for regulation by leptin and insulin, and GALP neurons express the leptin receptor.[199] The expression of GALP is reduced in physiologic states when circulating levels of leptin and insulin are low (e.g., in diabetic and leptin-deficient animals), and leptin and insulin can stimulate the expression of GALP. These observations suggest that GALP may serve an important role in the regulation of metabolism and body weight. Moreover, GALP has been implicated in the regulation of GnRH and gonadotropin secretion. GALP (administered intracerebroventricularly into the brain) can stimulate GnRH and LH secretion and can induce precocious puberty in experimental animals. GALP-containing fibers are found in close proximity to GnRH cell bodies and fibers, and intracerebroventricular injection of GALP induces Fos expression in GnRH neurons. GALP can also reverse the deleterious effects of diabetes on reproduction and sexual behavior in the rat, and antiserum to GALP can block leptin's stimulatory effect on gonadotropin secretion. Thus, GALP neurons are poised to serve as important cellular motifs that integrate metabolism and reproduction. The only caveat to this story is the fact that mice bearing null mutations in the *GALP* gene apparently have normal reproductive function—perhaps a testimony to the redundancy of the circuits that serve this role.

CRH-expressing neurons that control the release of ACTH from the pituitary provide the central target for feedback control of ACTH by glucocorticoids, such as cortisol (in humans) and corticosterone (in rodent species). The hypothalamic–pituitary–adrenal axis plays a critical regulatory role in the body's response and adaptation to stress—stresses of many kinds, including trauma, metabolic stress (e.g., fasting), environmental stress (e.g., temperature extremes), and psychological stress, and it would make sense that reproduction would be inhibited and delayed under circumstances that might compromise an individual's viability. CRH-expressing neurons are found in the parvicellular region of the PVN, which receives and processes information about metabolism, fuel status, and sympathetic tone. CRH (administered intracerebroventricularly) acts as a catabolic molecule, decreasing feeding and reducing body weight. Leptin and other metabolic hormones stimulate CRH secretion, which is believed to mediate at least part of the inhibitory effects of leptin on feeding behavior and body weight. Central injections of CRH inhibit the HPG axis in many experimental animal models, including the rat and monkey—perhaps by acting directly on GnRH neurons or acting indirectly by stimulating β-endorphin, which in turn inhibits GnRH.[200] However, the fasting-induced inhibition of gonadotropin secretion persists in the *CRH* knockout, which would imply that other factors besides CRH play a critical role in mediating the effects of metabolic stress on the reproductive axis.

Orexins (also known as hypocretins) are produced by neurons whose cell bodies reside in the lateral hypothalamus, and these neuropeptides (orexin-A/hypocretin-1 and orexin-B/hypocretin-2) have been implicated in the neuroendocrine regulation of feeding behavior and the control of sleep–wake cycles, although the nature of their involvement in body weight regulation is a matter of some controversy. Orexins are also known to influence GnRH and LH secretion. Centrally administered orexins stimulate LH secretion. Orexin-containing fibers are found in close apposition to GnRH neurons, which express orexin receptor-1. Moreover, orexin antibodies block the LH surge in rats. These observations suggest that orexins and their receptors could serve as a molecular link between metabolism and reproduction; however, this remains unproven.

Melanin-concentrating hormone (MCH) is a neuropeptide that is also expressed in the lateral hypothalamus. These neurons are targets are for regulation by metabolic hormones, including leptin, which inhibits MCH expression. Central infusions of MCH stimulate feeding, and transgenic mice that overexpress MCH overeat and become obese. MCH also stimulates GnRH and LH secretion, and MCH-containing fibers are found in close approximation to GnRH neurons. Thus, MCH, like orexins, could conceivably be part of the hypothalamic circuitry that integrates metabolism and reproduction.

Kiss1 neurons express the leptin receptor, and the expression of *Kiss1* mRNA is regulated (induced) by leptin. Animals made diabetic with streptozotocin (i.e., insulin deficient) have profoundly reduced expression of *Kiss1* in the hypothalamus. This pharmacologically induced form of type 1 diabetes is associated with reduced circulating levels of gonadotropins and sex steroids, and chronic infusions of kisspeptin can rescue reproductive function in these diabetic animals. Thus, it would appear that *Kiss1* neurons may be involved in coupling the response of the neuroendocrine reproductive axis to metabolic disorders, such as diabetes.[201,202]

In addition to neuropeptides, classic neurotransmitters have also been implicated in the integration of metabolism and reproduction. These include catecholaminergic neurons producing NE, whose cell bodies reside in the brain stem and send projections to the hypothalamus via the ascending noradrenergic pathway. Considerable evidence suggests that NE neurons play an important—if only permissive—role in the regulation of GnRH secretion, and they are key players in the regulation of fuel metabolism. Neurons that produce GABA make direct synaptic contact with GnRH neurons, and it is clear that GABA plays a key role in the regulation of GnRH secretion. Changes in circulating levels of leptin alter GABAergic drive to GnRH neurons, and GABA neurons are believed to integrate input from NPY and endogenous opioid peptides to reflect metabolic status and thus gate the activity of GnRH neurons.[203,204]

Sexual Differentiation of the Brain[205]

NEURONAL CIRCUITRY

The brain is sexually differentiated—in all mammals, including humans. In 1971, Raisman and Field reported that female rats have more dendritic spines in the preoptic area (POA) than males do.[206] A few years later, Roger Gorski and his colleagues showed that male rats have a larger number of neuronal cells in a subregion of the POA than do females, and this area became known as the *sexually dimorphic nucleus of the POA* (SDN-POA). Many other nuclei in the brain of the rodent are sexually differentiated on the basis of size and presumably function. These include the vomeronasal organ, the medial amygdala, the bed nucleus of the stria terminalis, the AVPV, the SON, the SCN, the locus ceruleus, and the spinal nucleus of the bulbocavernosus (in the spinal cord). There is less consensus on which and to what degree various structures in the human brain are sexually differentiated. In 1982, Delacoste-Utamsing and Holloway reported that a portion of the corpus callosum, the splenium, is more bulbous in men than in women,[207] although this finding has been controversial. Notwithstanding, other areas of the human brain have been reported (by other groups) to be sexually dimorphic, including the central division of the bed nucleus of the stria terminalis, the human homolog of the rat SDN-POA, and the relative asymmetry and lateralization of the cerebral hemispheres.[208-211] Recent studies with functional magnetic resonance imaging have also showed sexual differentiation of activation patterns in the amygdala.[212] The gross structures of the brain and the cellular architecture are sexually differentiated, and females have more projections from the AVPV to the medial POA and a greater degree of dendritic arborizations of dopamine neurons in the ARC than do males—including the extent of dendritic aborization, the pattern of synaptic contacts, and the morphologic features of astrocytes .[213-215]

The intensity and distribution of the classic and amino acid neurotransmitter systems and many of their receptor types in the brain show remarkable differences between the sexes, beginning even in early development. For example, the expression of glutamate, GABA, glutamic acid decarboxylase (the rate-liming enzyme for GABA synthesis), and GABA A receptors is more abundant in certain regions of the forebrain, such as the ventromedial nucleus, amygdala, and hippocampus, in male than in female rats. This

sex difference becomes apparent during the first few days of postnatal life in many areas of the brain—but persists into adulthood only in some nuclei (e.g., AVPV).[204,213,216-218] It has been postulated that GABA plays an important role in mediating the effects of sex steroids during the neonatal critical period, where GABA influences differential neuronal survival and synaptogenesis between the sexes and sex-specific activity of GABA circuits may contribute to differences in the control of GnRH secretion between the sexes. The expression of indole- and catecholamines is also sexually differentiated. Serotonin expression is generally higher in the brain of adult female rats compared with males.[219,220] The expression of dopamine in the AVPV, as reflected by tyrosine hydroxylase, is higher in female compared with male rats, whereas the expression of NE in the POA is greater in males.[220] Moreover, in virtually all of these cases, the pattern of expression of these transmitters and receptors is influenced by the prevailing sex steroid milieu during development (at least in rodent species, where it has been most comprehensively studied).

Most neuropeptide systems are also sexually differentiated—at least in certain brain regions. For example, male rats have greater numbers of enkephalin neurons in the AVPV and medial preoptic area than do females. Males show greater expression of vasopressin (in the bed nucleus stria terminalis and SCN) and GHRH (in the ARC) than do females,[220-225] whereas females show more expression of neurotensin and *Kiss1*/kisspeptin in the AVPV.[190] As is the case with the classic neurotransmitters, the adult pattern of expression of these neuropeptides appears to be strongly influenced by the sex steroid environment present during the neonatal critical period. In humans, the expression of somatostatin and VIP is sexually differentiated in the bed nucleus of the stria terminalis (Fig. 1-19) and in CRH neurons, whose cell bodies reside in the hypothalamic paraventricular nucleus.[226,227] The differential expression of these neuropeptides can be related (by inference) to sex differences in the neuroendocrine regulation of pituitary function (e.g., growth hormone or gonadotropin secretion) or behaviors (e.g., sexual behavior, aggression, exploration); however, in many cases, the physiologic significance of sex differences in the pattern and degree of neurotransmitter expression is unknown. The mechanisms through which sex steroids permanently alter the expression of neurotransmitter systems are believed to involve regulation of apoptosis (programmed cell death), neuronal migration, neurite outgrowth, synaptogenesis, and astrocyte morphology.

SEXUAL DIFFERENTIATION OF THE GnRH/LH SURGE MECHANISM

The neuroendocrine mechanisms that control the preovulatory GnRH/LH surge are sexually differentiated—at least in rodent and ovine species. The initial observation can be traced back to the work of C. A. Pfeiffer, who in 1936 published the results of ingenious experiments in rats. He transplanted ovarian tissue from rats to the anterior chamber of the eye, where he could observe follicular development and cyclic ovulation. He found that only if the ovaries were implanted into normal adult females—not

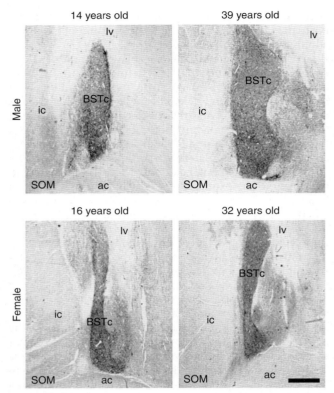

Figure 1-19. Sexual differentiation of somatostatin expression (visualized by immunocytochemistry) in the bed nucleus of the stria terminalis (BSTc) in the human. Scale bar = 1 mm. ac, anterior commissure; ic, internal capsule; lv, lateral ventricle; SOM, somatostatin. (Adapted from Chung WC, De Vries GJ, Swaab DF. Sexual differentiation of the bed nucleus of the stria terminalis in humans may extend into adulthood. J Neurosci 22:1027-1033, 2002.)

males—would they show cyclic function. However, if males were castrated at birth (before their so-called critical period), then allowed to develop to adulthood, these adult males were capable of supporting cyclic ovarian function after receiving transplants. On the other hand, if females were given testicular implants as neonates, then allowed to mature, these "androgenized" females were incapable of supporting ovarian cyclicity. These experiments laid the foundation for subsequent research showing that the pituitary itself was not sexually differentiated in its capacity to produce a preovulatory LH surge. Rather, the brain is sexually differentiated and holds the capacity to generate the neurosecretory events that trigger an LH surge in females, but lacks this capacity in males—in rodent and other nonprimate species, including sheep. Moreover, the capacity of the brain to produce an LH surge is determined early in development. In rodents, this ability becomes manifest as a function of the endocrine milieu during the critical period of neonatal development, which is usually from the time of birth (or shortly before) extending through the first 7 to 10 days of postnatal life. Recent evidence suggests that the critical period may even extend to the peripubertal period, where the effects of testosterone (or its relative absence) may become manifest as sexually differentiated behaviors in the adult. In primates—including Old World monkeys, the great apes, and humans—the GnRH/LH surge mechanism is not sexually differentiated—at least grossly. Adult males, like females, retain the capacity to elicit an LH surge in response to an estrogen challenge, and indeed, castrated adult male monkeys can even support cyclic ovarian function in transplanted ovaries!

ROLE OF HORMONES, CHROMOSOMES, AND GENES IN SEXUAL DIFFERENTIATION OF THE BRAIN AND BEHAVIOR

In the normal male, the *Sry* gene present on the Y chromosome acts as a molecular switch that initiates the cascade of events leading to the development of the testis in the fetus. In the male, this process leads to the production of testosterone, which in turn causes the brain (and other parts of the body) to develop along phenotypic male lines. In the female—who is unexposed to the androgenic products of the testis, and under the influence of other genes whose expression is altered in the absence of *Sry*—the brain develops to become phenotypically female. Among its effects in the male, testosterone permanently thwarts the brain's capacity to generate a GnRH/LH surge. However, in the normal female, the GnRH/LH surge mechanism develops unimpeded because of a lack of testosterone during the neonatal period. The effects of testosterone on the brain are believed to reflect predominantly the action of estradiol, which is converted from androgen by the cytochrome P450 enzyme, aromatase. Estradiol then acts on target cells in the brain through ERα and ERβ to masculinize and defeminize its circuitry. Other aspects of sexual differentiation of the brain (such as male sexual behavior and aggression) may be attributable to the complementary action of either testosterone itself or one of its androgenic metabolites, such as dihydrotestosterone, which acts through the AR to permanently alter pathways in the limbic system of the brain. In the male primate, the brain is also exposed to testosterone during development—at least three times. The first exposure occurs in fetal life, when sexual differentiation of the genital structures occurs. A second exposure occurs during the neonatal period (between 2 weeks and 8 months after birth), and the brain is re-exposed to testosterone during the awakening of the reproductive system at the time of puberty. Despite the fact that the GnRH/LH surge mechanism is not sexually differentiated in the primate, other aspects of brain function and behavior are clearly sexually differentiated.

Many behaviors in the adult animal are sexually differentiated. This concept applies to all mammals—including humans. In rats, sexually differentiated behaviors include behavior with sexual encounters, orientation toward the opposite sex, locomotion, aggression, exploratory behavior, spatial perception, and many social behaviors. The notion that behavior might be influenced by the steroidal milieu during development had its origins in a classic study by Phoenix and associates, in 1959, who showed that, in the male guinea pig, testosterone acts during a narrow window of fetal development to permanently "organize" the ability of the brain to express stereotypical sexual behavior in adulthood. Moreover, female guinea pigs that are artificially exposed to testosterone during

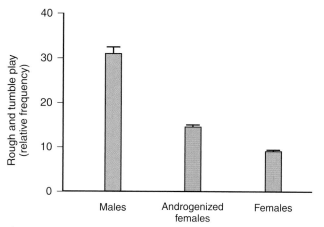

Figure 1-20. *Sexual differentiation of play behavior in normal juvenile monkeys and the effects of intrauterine exposure to testosterone on play behavior in juvenile genetic female monkeys. (Adapted from Young WC, Goy RW, Phoenix CH. Hormones and Sexual Behavior. Science 143:212-218, 1964.)*

this same critical period develop phenotypically male patterns of behavior that are permanently etched into the brain.[228] This principle was shown to apply to primates by Young and colleagues and Eaton and associates, who demonstrated that prepubertal monkeys show sexually differentiated behaviors (e.g., mounting and rough and tumble play), which are influenced by exposure to testosterone during fetal life (Fig. 1-20).[229,230] Likewise, many behaviors in humans are sexually differentiated, and although social conditioning plays a significant role in shaping adult behaviors, so too does biology. Differences between male and female humans in their exposure to the effects of sex steroids during fetal, neonatal, and peripubertal life influence—if not determine—many complex behaviors.

Although exposure to sex steroids occurs during critical periods of development (predominantly prenatally in humans), it has become clear that hormones (most notably, testosterone or its relative absence) are not the only factors influencing the development of the brain and behavior. The sex chromosomes themselves and presumably differences in the pattern of expression of genes coded by the sex chromosomes (besides *Sry*) have a direct effect on the developing brain.[231-234]

SEXUAL DIFFERENTIATION OF GENDER IDENTITY

The role of hormones and genes in influencing gender identity has been the subject of intense discussion and controversy. There have been several serious reports on the differences in brain structures and the pattern of gene expression that appear to be associated with gender identity, sexual orientation, and transsexualism.[231-237] However, debate about study design and interpretation of this work adds a strong measure of caution—and perhaps doubt—about the strength and validity of any conclusions.[238-240]

The complete reference list can be found on the companion Expert Consult Web site at www.expertconsultbook.com.

Suggested Readings

Everett J. Pituitary and hypothalamus: Perspectives and overview. *In* Neill J (ed). Knobil and Neill's Physiology of Reproduction, vol 1. Oxford, Elsevier, 2006, pp 1289-1307.

Gooren L. The biology of human psychosexual differentiation. Horm Behav 50:589-601, 2006.

Herbison A. Physiology of the gonadotropin-releasing hormone neuronal network. *In* Neill J (ed). Knobil and Neill's Physiology of Reproduction, vol 1. Oxford, Elsevier, 2006, pp 1415-1482.

Karsch F. Central actions of ovarian steroids in the feedback regulation of pulsatile secretion of luteinizing hormone. Annu Rev Physiol 49:365-382, 1987.

Krasnow S, Steiner R. Physiological mechanisms integrating metabolism and reproduction. *In* Neill J (ed). Knobil and Neill's Physiology of Reproduction, vol 2. Oxford, Elsevier, 2006, pp 2553-2625.

Page RB. Anatomy of the hypothalamo-hypophysial complex. *In* Neill J (ed). Knobil and Neill's Physiology of Reproduction, vol 2. Oxford, Elsevier, 2006, pp 1309-1413.

Popa S, Clifton D, Steiner R. The role of kisspeptins and GPR54 in the neuroendocrine regulation of reproduction. Annu Rev Physiol 70:213-238, 2008.

Simerly R. Wired for reproduction: Organization and development of sexually dimorphic circuits in the mammalian forebrain. Annu Rev Neurosci 25:507-536, 2002.

Wilson CA, Davies DC. The control of sexual differentiation of the reproductive system and brain. Reproduction 133:331-359, 2007.

Wray S. Development of gonadotropin-releasing hormone-1 neurons. Front Neuroendocrinol 23:292-316, 2002.

CHAPTER 2

The Gonadotropin Hormones and Their Receptors

Mario Ascoli and David Puett

The regulation of gonadal functions, namely gametogenesis and steroidogenesis, is mediated by the hypothalamic decapeptide gonadotropin-releasing hormone (GnRH) and the two pituitary gonadotropins luteinizing hormone (LH) and follicle-stimulating hormone (FSH), which are biosynthesized in and secreted by gonadotropes. Along with placental-derived human chorionic gonadotropin (hCG), these three gonadotropins regulate male and female reproductive endocrinology, including androgen, estrogen, and progesterone production, follicle and sperm maturation, ovulation, and maintenance of early pregnancy.

Structurally, the three gonadodotropins (as well as the related thyroid-stimulating hormone [TSH]) exist as heterodimers, sharing a common α subunit and homologous hormone-specific β subunits. Highly elongated molecules with the two subunits, intertwined and having similar conformations, the gonadotropins are members of the larger cystine knot–containing growth factor family that includes transforming growth factor β, activin, and others.

The three gonadotropins act via two G-protein–coupled receptors (GPCRs). The gonadotropin receptors (as well as the TSH receptor [TSHR] and several others) are characterized by the presence of a large extracellular domain composed of leucine-rich repeats (LRRs). This large extracellular domain is responsible for the recognition and high-affinity binding of the appropriate hormones. The LH receptor (LHR) recognizes both LH and hCG, and the FSH receptor (FSHR) is specific for FSH. The LHR is expressed in Leydig, theca, granulosa, and luteal cells, whereas the FSHR is expressed in granulosa and Sertoli cells. Expression of the gonadotropin receptors (especially the LHR) in many nongonadal tissues has also been reported, but these findings are still controversial and the physiologic significance, if any, of the extragonadal expression of the gonadotropin receptors is

debatable. This chapter focuses on the three gonadotropins and their two receptors.

Gonadotropins

GONADOTROPIC PROTEINS

Amino Acid Sequences and Three-Dimensional Structures

The three gonadotropins (LH, hCG, and FSH) and TSH comprise the better characterized members of a family of complex proteins known as the *glycoprotein hormones*.[1] They are noncovalently bound heterodimers composed of a common α subunit and distinct β subunits. The common α gonadotropin subunit (α-GSU), encoded by the *CGH* gene, contains 92 amino acid residues, and LHβ, FSHβ, and hCGβ are, respectively, 121, 110, and 145 amino acid residues in length. The additional length of hCGβ is due to a carboxy-terminal extension arising from a frameshift mutation in an ancestral LHβ gene, resulting in a read-through into an untranslated region of LHβ and an extension of the open reading frame.[2-4] This extension is known as the *carboxy-terminal peptide* (CTP). The amino acid sequences of the human (h) subunits are shown in Figure 2-1. It can be seen that the α and β subunits are relatively rich in Cys residues and that considerable homology exists in the β subunits.

Crystal structures are available for deglycosylated hCG[5,6]; glycosylated, antibody-bound hCG[7]; a partially deglycosylated hFSH obtained by replacement of Thr26 with Ala to eliminate a site of N-glycosylation[8]; and a partially deglycosylated complex of a single-chain hFSH bound to a large N-terminal fragment (residues 1-268) of the hFSHR ectodomain (ECD).[9-11] In hCG, electron densities were obtained for amino acid residues 5 to 89 of

```
hFSHβ   1  - - - - - - NSCELTNI T I A I EKEECRFC I S I NTTWCAGYCYTRDLVYKDPARPK I QKTCTFKEL VYETVRVPVCAH68
hLHβ    1  SREPLRPWCHP I NATLAVEKEGCPVC I TVNTT I CAGYCPTMMRVLQAVL PPLPQVVCTYRDVRFES I RLPGCPR74
hCGβ    1  SKEPLRPRCRP I NATLAVEKEGCPVC I TVNTT I CAGYCPTMTRVLQGVL PALPQVVCNYRDVRFES I RLPGCPR74


hFSHβ  69 HADSLYTYPVATQCHCGKCDSDSTDCTVRGLGPSYCSFGEMKE- - - - - - - - - - - - - - - EMKE- - - - - - - - - - 111
hLHβ   75 GVDPVVSFPVALSCRCGPCRRSTSDCGGPKDHPLTCDHP- - - - - - - - - - - - - - - - - - - - QLSG- - - - - LLFL 121
hCGβ   75 GVNPVVSYAVALSCQCALCRRSTTDCGGPKDHPLTCDDPRFQDSSSSKAPPPSLPSPSRLPGPSDTP I LPQ 145


α   1  APDVQDCPECTLQENPFFSQPGAPILQCMGCCFSRAYPTPLRSKKTMLVQKNVTSESTCCVAKSYNRVTVMG 74
   75  KVENHTACHCSTCYYHKS                                                          92
```

Figure 2-1. *Amino acid sequences of human α gonadotropin subunit (α-GSU), luteinizing hormone (LH)β, chorionic gonadotropin (CG)β, and follicle-stimulating hormone (FSH)β. Amino acid sequences were obtained from the Ensembl web site (http://www.ensembl.org/index.html), and the β subunits are aligned to maximize homology. Identical, highly conserved, and semiconserved residues among the three β subunits are highlighted by the* blue, green, *and* yellow *boxes, respectively. All cysteines participate in disulfide bond formation in the native proteins. hCG, human chorionic gonadotropin; hFSH, human follicle-stimulating hormone; hLH, human luteinizing hormone. (Copyright © 1999–2008 The European Bioinformatics Institute and Genome Research Limited, and others. All rights reserved.)*

α-GSU and 2 to 111 of deglycosylated hCG. The remaining residues in the two subunits could not be identified, presumably because of their flexible nature. Another structure of an antibody–hCG complex also enabled visualization of hCGβ residues 2 to 111; in addition, the three C-terminal amino acid residues (90-92) in α-GSU were determined in the complex. In FSH, electron densities were measured for amino acid residues 5-90 in α-GSU and 3-108 in the β subunit. Figure 2-2 shows the crystal structures of hCG and hFSH.

The conformations of hCG and hFSH are quite similar, each being highly elongated molecules with the two

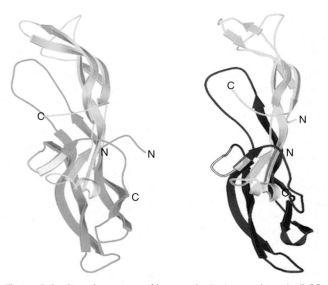

Figure 2-2. *Crystal structures of human chorionic gonadotropin (hCG; left) and human follicle-stimulating hormone (hFSH; right). The structures[5-8] show that the two subunits are highly elongated and intertwined (hCGα, yellow; hCGβ, green; and hFSH, blue), forming a relatively large contact surface area. As discussed in the text, there are several interesting features associated with the structures: each subunit contains a cystine knot motif; the β subunit wraps around a portion of the α subunit, forming what is termed a* seatbelt *(shown in* white*); although having little sequence homology, the two subunits adopt similar folding patterns; hCG and hFSH form very similar structures, but the respective subunits of each exhibit subtle differences in their conformations. C, C-terminus; N, N-terminus.*

subunits intertwined in a slightly twisted manner. Despite the absence of any striking sequence homology, the two subunits in both heterodimers have similar folds, characterized by three major loops, and each subunit contains a cystine knot motif, consisting of three disulfides located in the core of each subunit. The α and β subunits contain, in addition to the three disulfides in the cystine knot, two and three disulfides, respectively. In both hCG and hFSH, the two subunits are associated in a head-to-tail arrangement. Although there are no structures available for LH and TSH, the similarities of the hCG and FSH structures engender confidence that the overall conformations of LH and TSH will be closely related to the known structures.

There are subtle, but perhaps important differences in the common α-GSU in hCG and hFSH. Larger differences were found between hCGβ and hFSHβ, particularly in the C-terminal region of the seatbelt, an important region of the β subunit that wraps around a portion of α-GSU. The seatbelt contains the amino acid residue sequence between Cys90 and Cys110 in hCG and the sequence between Cys84 and Cys104 in hFSH. Within each seatbelt is a determinant loop (Cys93 to Cys100 in hCGβ and Cys87 to Cys94 in FSHβ) originally proposed to provide receptor specificity to the hormones.[12] The determinant loops of hCG and hFSH are similar in conformation, but the loop is shifted several angstroms at its C-terminal portion in hFSHβ because of conformational differences of loop 2 of α-GSU and loops 1 and 3 of hFSHβ. Asp93 of hFSHβ and the equivalent Asp99 of hCGβ, essential residues for receptor binding, are in similar conformations in the two hormones, but Asp88, Asp90, and Asp93 of hFSHβ form a negatively charged region on one side of the determinant loop; in hCGβ, Arg94 and Arg95 point to the opposite side of the loop. The C-terminal portions of the seatbelts in hCGβ and hFSHβ exhibit distinct conformations.

Solution structures have been obtained for deglycosylated human α-GSU[13,14] using nuclear magnetic resonance (NMR) spectroscopy. The overall ensemble of structures determined for α-GSU is similar to that obtained in the crystal structures of hCG and hFSH, although there are some differences. Similar to the crystal structures of the heterodimers, amino acid residues 1 to 10 and 85 to 92 are disordered; moreover, residues 33 to 57 and the conformations of Val76 and Glu77 are less ordered in free α-GSU structure when there is no stabilization by the β subunit. NMR and circular dichroism spectroscopy have shown that the CTP of hCGβ is unordered,[15,16] consistent with the inability to detect this region in crystallographic studies of heterodimeric hCG.

With crystal structures available for FSH[8] and an FSH–FSHR ECD complex (discussed elsewhere in this review),[9,10] it is possible to delineate the conformational changes of the free heterodimer and that bound to receptor. The unbound form of the hormone is more flexible than the bound form. It is the C-terminal region of the α-GSU, however, that undergoes the greatest change in conformation. When bound to receptor, the C-terminal region rotates nearly 180 degrees, placing it more than 20 Å from its position in unbound FSH. The two C-terminal residues in α-GSU are unordered in the crystal structure of FSH, but in the complex with receptor, they are fully ordered.

Glycosylation

The human subunits contain N-linked glycans: two on α-GSU at Asn52 and Asn78, two on CGβ (Asn13 and Asn30), two on FSHβ (Asn7 and Asn24), and one on LHβ at Asn30. In addition, hCGβ contains four mucin-type O-linked glycans at serines 121, 127, 132, and 138, located on the CTP (Fig. 2-3). The carbohydrate moieties appear to be important in subunit assembly and stabilization, secretion, and circulatory half-life. Although earlier studies suggested a role for N-linked glycan at Asn52 on α-GSU in receptor activation, more recent evidence

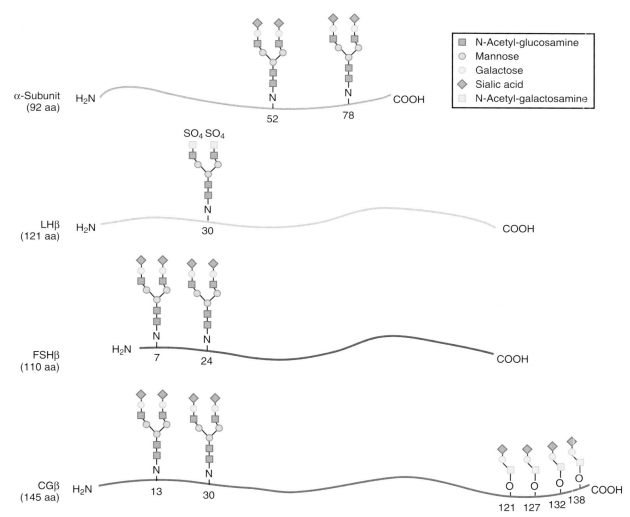

Figure 2-3. *Location and typical structures of the N-linked and O-linked glycans on the gonadotropins. The sites of glycosylation on each of the gonadotropin subunits and representative structures of the various N-linked glycans on human luteinizing hormone (hLH), human chorionic gonadotropin (hCG), and human follicle-stimulating hormone (hFSH). As discussed in the text, scores of different structures have been identified, often with fucose present; moreover, some sites are devoid of glycosylation in various gonadotropin preparations. A representative structure of type 1 O-linked glycans on the carboxy-terminal peptide of hCGβ is shown; type 2 structures have been reported as well, and some sites show no glycosylation in various gonadotropin preparations.* Blue squares, *GlcNAc;* yellow squares, *GalNAc;* green circles, *mannose;* yellow circles, *galactose;* purple diamonds, *sialic acid.*

indicates that the glycan acts more as a conformational or stabilizing determinant of the protein.[17,18] At another N-linked site on α-GSU, Asn78, NMR spectroscopy was used to identify interaction of the glycan with the protein.[19] Moreover, there is growing evidence that the particular type of glycosylation may influence biologic activity.[20-24] As one example, there are reports that hyperglycosylated hCG directly influences implantation of the embryo, an effect not observed with hCG produced later in pregnancy.[25,26]

The biantennary N-linked glycans on hFSH and hCG terminate in sialic acid (and, to a lesser extent, sulfate), although the number of such moieties varies from zero to two, accounting in large part for the microheterogeneity of these glycoprotein hormones. In LH, the biantennary N-linked structures tend to terminate mainly in sulfate. These are but generalizations because, for example, hFSH also contains triantennary and tetraantennary N-linked glycans,[27] and some hFSHβ subunits lack N-linked structures completely.[28] Also, fucose is often found in the glycoprotein hormones. Earlier studies identified the major glycoforms of some of the glycoprotein hormones, but more recent studies using mass spectrometry have focused on the microheterogeneity at individual sites.[29-34] As recently summarized, nearly 50 different N-linked and O-linked glycans have been reported in hCGα and β preparations.[31,33,35] In one study on hCG, eight glycoforms were detected on hCGα, none of which contained fucose, and hCGβ had nine distinct N-linked glycans and five different O-linked glycans.[31] Focusing on pregnancy urinary hCGβ, others reported interesting differences between the two N-linked glycans.[33] In this study, the glycans at Asn13 and Asn30 contained mainly biantennary structures, with lesser amounts of no glycan (approximately 4% at Asn13 and <1% at Asn30) and monoantennary and tetraantennary (0% to 1%) glycans. Fucose was present on fewer than 30% of the N-linked glycans at Asn13, but on most of the Asn30 N-linked glycans. Analysis of the O-glycans showed that Ser121 had primarily core-2 (biantennary) structures, whereas Ser138 was predominantly core-1 (monoantennary); in some cases, there was no glycosylation at these two sites. Analyzed together, Ser127 and Ser132 exhibited mainly core-1 structures.[36] Site-specific differences were found in a comparison of glycan structures on human and equine FSH.[32] The major gonadotropin N-linked and C-linked glycans are shown in Figure 2-3.

Folding, Assembly, and Secretion

Extensive studies have been performed on the folding characteristics and assembly of the α and β subunits of hCG. Based on the similarities of the amino acid sequences of the various β subunits, it is anticipated that similar folding patterns will hold for the other hormones as well. Several special features of the hCG and FSH structures[5-8] pose challenging problems in elucidating folding patterns: as discussed earlier, each subunit contains a cystine knot motif consisting of six cysteines forming three disulfides; in addition to the cystine knot motif, other disulfides are present in each subunit; and a 20–amino acid residue region of the β subunit, denoted as the *seatbelt,* wraps around and latches a portion of the α subunit.

Investigations into the kinetic folding pathways of the hCG subunits led to the interesting suggestion that disulfide exchange occurs during the maturation process and that subunit association occurred before the completion of protein folding and disulfide formation.[37-44] Moreover, it was posited that subunit association occurred before the seatbelt was latched by closure of Cys26 and Cys110. In contrast to these reports, a different mechanism in which subunit assembly involved closure of the seatbelt latch, followed by threading of α loop 2, has been proposed.[45-49] Others have also studied the folding patterns of hCG and reported that subunit association occurred between an almost completely folded α subunit and an immature β subunit.[50-53] Interestingly, the presence of the α subunit was found to reduce the maturation of the β subunit, and in contrast to an earlier report,[37] this group did not support the proposition that four of the six disulfides had formed in hCGβ before association with the α subunit.

In addition to the heterodimeric nature of the hormones, homodimers have also been found for LHβ,[54,55] consistent with molecular modeling results,[56] and for the α subunit.[52,53,57] Whether these homodimeric forms of the glycoprotein hormones have any associated bioactivity remains to be shown, although it has been reported that the free α subunit potentiates progesterone-mediated decidualization.[58]

Other Heterodimeric Glycoproteins Related to Gonadotropins

A search of the human genome showed two proteins similar to the glycoprotein hormone subunits A2 and B5.[59] Heterodimers can be formed between A2 and B5, and the complex is capable of stimulating the TSHR. This heterodimer was named *thyrostimulin* and is postulated to act in a paracrine manner in the pituitary, which also contains TSHR.[60] Thus, the human genome is known to contain the four canonical glycoprotein hormones, LH, CG, FSH, and TSH, and possibly a fifth, thyrostimulin.

STRUCTURE–FUNCTION STUDIES

Amino Acid Mutations

As discussed later, a limited number of naturally occurring mutations have been identified in the α and β subunits of the glycoprotein hormones. In contrast, there is a wealth of information available from site-directed mutagenesis followed by biologic characterization of the mutant hormones. Few mutants have been described in which there was a significant increase in bioactivity; most mutations either have no effect or are loss-of-function mutations, disrupting folding, subunit assembly, or receptor binding/activation. Gain-of-function mutations in hCG were obtained by replacing single or multiple amino acid residues at the N-terminal region of the α subunit with Lys.[61] A twofold increase in the potency of hCG was obtained with a single replacement of Phe with Thr at position 18 of α-GSU.[62] Of great interest would be the development of potent receptor antagonists, but the structure–function studies reported have suggested only one possibility. Mutant forms of α-GSU missing the N-linked oligosaccharide at Asn52 are capable of associating with the hCGβ or FSHβ subunit, giving a heterodimer that binds to the cognate receptor, but has diminished signaling efficacy.[63-65] Although still controversial, it appears that the role of N-linked glycosylation at Asn52 is to stabilize the active conformation of the heterodimer by formation of a hydrogen bond with a Tyr on the β subunit.[8] Mutations in the central region of α-GSU[66-68] and at the C-terminus[69,70] yielded mutants that associated with the β subunits of hCG and hFSH, but displayed compromised functionality in receptor binding.

A large number of β subunit mutations have been prepared and characterized.[71-79] As with mutations in α, many interfere with folding, subunit assembly, or receptor binding. The data, overall, are consistent with the structures of hCG and FSH. Unlike α-GSU mutants, however, there have been no reports of β mutants that retain the ability to form heterodimers and bind to a receptor, yet do not signal. Of great interest, however, was the report that single-chain hCGβ–hCGβ homodimers bind to LHR with an affinity about three times lower than that of wild-type hCG; this engineered homodimer does not elicit a biologic response and blocks hCG binding to LHR.[80] Mutation data collected on the β subunit have, by and large, confirmed a role for residues in the central portion and determinant loops in receptor binding.

The many mutations made and characterized in the two subunits of the various glycoprotein hormones are, in general, supported by the structural data available for hCG, FSH, and the FSH–FSHR ECD complex. Combining the results from the mutagenesis and structural biology of the hormones and receptor (using the FSH–FSHR ECD structure as prototypical of all members of this class) permits a better understanding of specific site function in the glycoprotein hormones.

Protein Engineering

Protein engineering has been used to produce a variety of subunit deletion derivatives, single-chain hormones, and chimeric hormones yielding interesting results. As mentioned earlier, C-terminal deletion mutants of the α subunit result in large N-terminal fragments that retain the ability to bind to the β subunit, but the resulting heterodimers exhibit minimal, if any, receptor-binding capability. Deletion mutants at the N- and C-termini of hCGβ have been reported by several groups,[71,72,75,81] and the shortest form that retains minimal functionality in subunit assembly and subsequent receptor binding and activation is a fragment consisting of residues 8 to 100.[75]

A number of glycoprotein hormone chimeras have been designed and characterized, providing useful information on specific amino acid residues involved in receptor binding and activation.[82-90] In general, these results emphasize the role of the β subunit seatbelt region in receptor binding, although different portions are important in receptor specificity.

A novel approach to the study of gonadotropin structure–function relationships involved the design of single-chain hormones (i.e., fusion proteins of the α and β subunits). The first reports of a yoked or tethered hCG showed that the single-chain gonadotropin, in the configuration N-hCGβ-α-C, was bioactive.[91,92] Later, different fusion proteins with different linkers were expressed and characterized, in many cases, with interesting mutations in one or both subunits.[93-106] From these studies, it was concluded that the N-α-hCGβ-C configuration was also bioactive and, quite surprisingly, that each disulfide of the subunits could be eliminated without a loss of activity.[107-109] Extending the approach of covalently linking the two subunits, others designed and expressed disulfide-linked heterodimers.[95,96,110-112] These results further substantiated the possibility that α-Asn52 contributed to heterodimer stability and was not involved directly in signal transduction,[17] and also led to suggestions that the C-terminus of the α-GSU is not required for LHR binding. This latter finding is consistent with the observation that the five C-terminal residues can be removed from α-GSU without a loss of LHR binding. As discussed earlier, N-hCGβ-hCGβ-C acts as a receptor antagonist, the first such β-designed analog with potential clinical applications.[80] These selected results, along with others not covered here, indicate that single-chain glycoprotein hormones exhibit some properties distinct from those in heterodimers. The increased stability of the single-chain proteins and the dual activities, bioactive LH/hCG-like and FSH-like, make them attractive candidates for clinical use.

The approach of converting glycoprotein hormones to single chains has been extended to produce fusion proteins with dual and triple activities. For example, a three-domain fusion protein of the form N-FSHβ-hCGβ-α-C exhibited both LH and FSH activities.[113-115] Interestingly, the bifunctional gonadotropin is secreted from cells as two species, one with LHR and the other with FSHR activities.[116] A four-domain fusion protein, N-TSHβ-FSHβ-hCGβ-α-C, although secreted inefficiently, was found to exhibit three distinct bioactivities in both cellular and whole animal studies.[117,118] These results raise intriguing questions about subunit association and conformation as manifested in receptor binding and activation. A provocative finding was based on a bifunctional, triple-domain fusion protein of the form N-FSHβ-hCGβ-α-C.[109] These investigators showed that disruption of heterodimer formation by mutation of either Cys10 to Cys60 or Cys32 to Cys84 did not eliminate bioactivity, and thus concluded that αβ contacts are not required for receptor binding and activation. The use of single-chain gonadotropins, particularly in the N-α-β-C configuration, also raises interesting questions about the role of the C-terminal region of α-GSU in FSH, where the structure of the FSH–FSHR ECD complex shows a large movement of α-GSU in the receptor complex compared with the heterodimer.[9,10]

The concept of single-chain gonadotropins was extended to produce fusion proteins of hCG and LHR (i.e., covalent attachment of a single-chain hCG to LHR), which when expressed, led to constitutive receptor activation in transfected cells and transgenic mice.[100,101,119-121] This model was also used to show that the individual subunits are devoid of bioactivity.[122]

GONADOTROPIN SUBUNIT GENES AND TRANSCRIPTS

Gonadotropin Subunit Genes

The three gonadotropins, LH, CG, and FSH, are encoded by one gene each for the common α subunit and the β subunits of LH and FSH; in contrast, the CGβ subunit, expressed in primates and equids, is encoded by six genes.[123,124] It has been suggested that the glycoprotein hormone α and β subunits diverged from a common ancestral gene more than 900 million years ago,[125] with the β gene undergoing duplications and mutations to yield the current family. In humans, the gene encoding the common α subunit is on chromosome 6, that for *FSHB* is on chromosome 11, and those for *LHB* and *CGB* are on chromosome 19 (www.ensembl.org). The gene for human α is 9.4 kb and contains four exons and three introns; that for *FSHB* is 4.2 kb, with three exons and two introns; that for *LHB* is 1.1 kb, with three exons and two introns; and those for *CGB* are variable in length.

The seven genes for LHβ and CGβ exist in a large cluster spanning approximately 52 kbp, and it is believed that CGβ arose from a duplication of the gene encoding LHβ.[3,123,124,126,127] The six genes encoding the β subunit of CG (i.e., *CGB*, *CGB1*, *CGB2*, *CGB5*, *CGB7*, and *CGB8*) exist as tandem and inverted repeats.[124] The genes for CGβ have been analyzed in detail,[128-130] extending and, in many cases, complementing earlier work.[131,132] Four of the CGβ genes, *CGβ*, *CGβ5*, *CGβ7*, and *CGβ8*, exhibit 97% to 99% sequence identity with one another, whereas their identity with LHβ is 92% to 93%. These gene similarities lead to protein amino acid sequences that are 98% to 100% identical for the four CGβ genes and 85% identical with LHβ. Interestingly, the identity of the four similar CGβ genes is approximately 85% with the CGβ1 and CGβ2 genes, but there is no similarity between the predicted amino acid sequences of the CGβ1 and CGβ2 proteins and those of LHβ and the four related CGβ genes.[129] These differences arise from the use of an alternative exon 1 and a shifted open reading frame in CGβ1 and CGβ2.[130,131] The genes for *CGB*, *CGB5*, *CGB7*, and *CGβ8* encode proteins with a carboxy-terminal extension, the CTP, that appears to have arisen from the LHβ gene by frameshift mutations, leading to a read-through into a previously untranslated region, thus extending the reading frame.[2,3,127] The CTP contains mucin-type O-glycans, resulting in properties of hCG not found in LH.[4]

Multiple response elements are located in the 5' flanking region of the α subunit gene. In the pituitary, for example, there are elements responsive to sex steroids, GnRH, steroidogenic factor 1 (SF-1), and others, whereas the placenta requires cyclic AMP (cAMP) response elements and another domain that binds various transcription factors.[133-141] The *LHβ* and *FSHβ* genes have regulatory elements that are responsive to sex steroids, GnRH, SF-1, and others; moreover, *LHβ* and *FSHβ* require Egr-1 and activin-mediated response elements.[141]

Response elements for CGβ include cAMP response elements, AP-2, and others.[141-143]

Gonadotropin Subunit Transcripts

The available evidence indicates single transcripts for the gonadotropin genes, with the exception of the human FSHβ gene, for which four messenger RNA (mRNA) species have been described, arising from alternate splicing and the use of two polyadenylation sites.[144] The CGβ family is interesting in that all six genes appear to be expressed, giving transcripts of varying lengths. Original reports suggested that CGβ5 is expressed more frequently by the placenta,[131,132] with a transcript approximately 1000 nucleotides long, whereas, in contrast, CGβ8 was predominant.[128] Although expressed in the placenta,[131,142,145] pituitary,[146] testis,[147] and breast cancer,[148] no proteins have yet been identified for the CGβ1 and CGβ2 genes. The predicted sizes of CGβ1 and CGβ2 are smaller than that of hCGβ; this observation, coupled with the distinct amino acid sequences predicted, suggests that these proteins, if biosynthesized, may have quite different functions than those of hCG. Using transgenic mice expressing a 36-kb cosmid insert that contained the six CGβ genes, transcripts of CGβ1 and CGβ2 genes were found to be present in brain at levels comparable to those of the other four CGβ genes.[149] The LHβ mRNA is 700 nucleotides in length, and depending on the species, the gene for α encodes an mRNA species of some 730 to 800 nucleotides.

Naturally Occurring Mutations in α, *LHB*, and *FSHB*

The only mutation reported in the α gene is that from a human carcinoma.[150] This mutation led to a replacement of Glu56 to Ala, resulting in a mutant form of α-GSU that does not associate with LHβ. The highly conserved nature of the α subunit throughout evolution and the absence of any known mutations in somatic cells argue strongly for the importance of the majority of the amino acid residues in the structure and function of this common subunit.

In contrast, there are several reports of mutations in the genes encoding the β subunits, resulting in loss-of-function and thus hypogonadism.[151-158] The first report of a mutation in *LHB* was that of a missense mutation in a male presenting with delayed puberty and hypogonadism.[159] This mutant led to a replacement of Gln54 with Arg; although subunit assembly could occur, the heterodimer was unable to bind to LHR. Other studies showed that LHβ and hCGβ subunits with Gln54 replacements formed heterodimers with α-GSU, but these heterodimers exhibited reduced binding to LHR.[76,79] Another missense mutation reported in *LHB* was that of Gly36 to Asp, reported in a male with delayed puberty and infertility.[160] Gly36 is part of the CAGYC sequence in LHβ that is critical to the formation of the disulfide knot; presumably, an Asp at this position prevents at least one of the disulfides from forming.

An unusual mutation in *LHB* was recently reported.[161] This mutation, a G-C substitution at the +1 position of intron 2 (a 5' splice-donor site) leads to a hypothetical aberrant protein with a 79–amino acid residue insert beginning after Met41 and a frameshift in exon 3, thus removing the essential seatbelt loop of β and important cysteines. The offspring of consanguineous parents (second cousins) who were heterozygous for this heretofore unreported mutation were analyzed. Three siblings, two 46,XY and one 46,XX, were homozygous for the mutation, and three other siblings were heterozygous. Two did not harbor the mutation, and three more either were deceased or were not evaluated. The three homozygous siblings presented with hypogonadism and infertility, and interestingly, the sister underwent normal pubertal development and menarche at age 13 years; the three heterozygous siblings were fertile. Analysis of serum hormone concentrations of the three siblings homozygous for the LHβ gene mutation showed undetectable levels of LH and high levels of free α-GSU; the two males had elevated FSH and low testosterone levels, whereas the female had FSH, estradiol, and progesterone values in the normal range, albeit on the low end of normal for the sex steroids.

Several mutations have been described in exon 3 of *FSHB* that lead to an absence of pubertal development, amenorrhea, and of course, infertility in females and azoospermia in males. The first report was of a 27-year-old woman presenting with the described symptoms and undetectable serum FSH, both before and after administration of GnRH.[162] She was found to be homozygous for a two–base-pair deletion at codon 61 of *FSHB*, which caused a frameshift, namely an alteration of codons 61 to 86, and premature termination of the β subunit. A similar mutation was found in an 18-year-old man who was evaluated for delayed puberty.[163]

Other reports identified a compound heterozygous mutation at codon 51, leading to a Cys51 to Gly replacement and a two–base-pair deletion at codon 61.[152,153,164] A missense mutation was found in a 28-year-old man who presented with infertility and was found to have Cys82 replaced with Arg.[165] One case of hypoglycosylation was reported for FSH, resulting in a hormone with diminished activity.[166]

Overall, the observed phenotypes associated with the naturally occurring mutations in *LHB* and *FSHB* are consistent with the known structures and actions of the gonadotropins, although fertility in men is not totally dependent on FSH as it is in women.

Polymorphisms in *LHB*, *CGB*, and *FSHB*

A fairly well-characterized polymorphism in *Lhβ* appears in variable frequencies in ethnic groups throughout the world and results from two single-nucleotide polymorphisms (SNPs) leading to replacements of Trp8 with Arg and Ile15 with Thr.[167-173] There is, however, no association of this polymorphism with infertility or cancer,[157,167,174-178] although biopotencies are increased in vitro and decreased in vivo, perhaps because of aberrant glycosylation.[179] Individuals harboring this double polymorphism appear to exhibit low, if detectable, levels of immunoreactive LH, but this results from the use of antibodies that do not recognize the altered LH. The Thr15 mutant has an additional site of glycosylation, but Arg8 may be responsible for most of the altered properties.

Another *LHB* variant is a replacement of Gly102 in LHβ with Ser,[177,180-183] resulting in reduced LH biopotency in vitro.[184] The frequency of this polymorphism, however, seems to be quite low.[174,181]

An unusual polymorphic variant of *LHB* involves an Ala to Thr replacement three residues before the signal peptide cleavage site.[185] Using in vitro assays, it was found, rather surprisingly, that the mature protein from the variant appears less potent than wild-type LH in cAMP production, but more potent in inositol phosphate production. The SNP-related alteration may interfere with proper processing of the β subunit, although studies have not addressed this possibility.

A polymorphism has been reported in exon 3 of *CGB5*, resulting in a Val79 replacement with Met.[186] This SNP results in a β subunit deficient in folding and interaction with the α subunit. The frequency and physiologic consequences of this polymorphic variant are unknown; one sampling of just under 600 samples from four European groups did not detect a single case.[187] Other polymorphic variants have been detected, but these were silent or located in intron regions.[188]

A very limited number of polymorphic variants of FSHB have been reported.[157,164,188] There has not, however, been a detailed study correlating FSH function with particular SNPs, some being silent.[164]

REGULATION OF EXPRESSION AND SECRETION OF GONADOTROPINS

Transcriptional Regulation

The neurocrine reproductive axis, composed of the hypothalamus, anterior pituitary, and gonads, is now known to be regulated, apparently in large part, by kisspeptin, a product of *Kiss-1*, acting via the G-protein–coupled receptor GPR54, which is located on GnRH neurons.[189-191] Indeed, many of the feedback actions of sex steroids may be mediated by this recently discovered system. GnRH pulses regulate transcription of *α-GSU*, *LHB*, and *FSHB* through several signaling pathways (e.g., protein kinase C, mitogen-activated protein kinase, calcium influx, and calcium-calmodulin kinase). The GnRH-provoked activation of some of these pathways is greatly influenced by pulse frequency and magnitude.[192] The three pituitary genes are differentially responsive to GnRH frequencies: *α-GSU* is preferentially transcribed at high GnRH pulse frequencies, *LHB* at intermediate frequencies, and *FSHB* at lower frequencies. Sex steroid–mediated regulation of the gonadotropin genes may result from direct effects on the hypothalamus and pituitary, although recent evidence suggests a critical role of the kisspeptin–GPR54 system in sex steroid action.

A number of promoter–regulatory elements have been described that regulate expression of the gonadotropin genes in pituitary.[193-196] Regulatory elements on *CGA* include, most importantly, the cAMP response elements (CREs),[197] as well as numerous others in the 5'-flanking region, including the GnRH responsive unit and pituitary homeobox 1 (Pitx1) response elements. Fewer regulatory elements have been characterized on the *LHB* gene, but the early growth response protein 1 (Egr-1), the orphan nuclear receptor (SF-1), and Pitx1 have been relatively well characterized and are known to be involved in GnRH regulation.[193,196] Recent studies have shown an important role for β-catenin in the GnRH regulation of *LHB* expression.[198] β-Catenin first binds to SF-1 and then the complex interacts with Egr-1 to give maximal response to GnRH. The *FSHB* gene also contains regulatory elements for transcription factors, such as SF-1 and Pitx1, in addition to nuclear factor Y (NFY), Ptx2, activator protein-1 (AP-1), and Smads.[196] Moreover, activin and the bone morphogenic proteins regulate the *FSHB* gene. Activin regulation of *FSHB* expression has been shown to involve the Smads and the TALE homeodomain proteins, Pbx-1 and Prep-1.[199]

Regulatory elements of *CGA* in the trophoblast layer of the placental villous, containing syncytiotrophoblast and cytotrophoblast, include two adjoining CREs that act synergistically, as well as Ets2 sites. It has been proposed that association of CRE-binding protein (CREB) and Ets-2, augmented by protein kinase A, regulates *CGA* expression and coordinates expression with *hCGB*. An upstream regulatory element (URE) on *CGA* contains binding sites for several transcription factors, and a second control element, α-ACT, binds a GATA factor and AP-2γ. The *hCGB5* promoter binds both CREB and Ets-2, and there is a suggestion of an AP-1 site as well.[200-202]

Post-Translational Regulation (Glycosylation)

It is now well established that the glycosylation patterns of at least some of the glycoprotein hormones change during various physiologic states.[20,21] Examples include a shift in the structures of hCG N-linked oligosaccharides in the differentiation of cytotrophoblasts to syncyciotrophoblasts,[25,203-207] changes in LH and FSH N-linked glycosylation during the menstrual cycle,[206,208] and alterations in FSH N-linked glycans during adolescence in boys.[21,24] Indeed, a portion of FSH contains a nonglycosylated β subunit.[28,30]

The circulatory half-life of the sulfated gonadotropins, notably LH, is invariably less than that of the sialic acid–containing hormones. This arises from a hepatic receptor that recognizes the terminal N-acetyl galactosamine-sulfate, rapidly removing it from circulation.[209]

Various laboratories have shown that the carbohydrate moieties of hCG produced in early pregnancy (i.e., from cytotrophoblasts) and in gestational trophoblastic diseases differ from those on hCG secreted by syncytiotrophoblast.[210] It has been suggested that the hyperglycosylated hCG in early pregnancy has autocrine functions in addition to the canonical physiologic function of "rescuing" the corpus luteum.[25,26,211] There are also data suggesting that the hCG produced by cytotrophoblasts and choriocarcinoma have distinct carbohydrate moieties.[212] The N-linked oligosaccharides on hCG from invasive moles and testicular cancer are characterized by both biantennary and triantennary structures and often more heavily fucosylated glycans, whereas the four O-linked units tend to have more core-2 type structures.[33]

Samples from patients with choriocarcinoma, testicular cancer, and invasive moles showed interesting differences in their glycans. Triantennary N-linked glycans increase in choriocarcinoma[210] at Asn30, but not at Asn13,[33] whereas the reported increase in monoantennary N-linked glycans was observed at both Asn13 and Asn30.[33] The status of hCG fucosylation in pregnancy and in patients with cancer has been investigated by several groups,[36,210,213,214] with some conflicting results. In malignancies, fucosylation was recently reported to increase at Asn13, but not at Asn30.[33]

Although a daunting task, elucidation of the nature of the heterogeneity in the glycoprotein hormone subunits, particularly their alterations in different physiologic and pathophysiologic states, can be used for diagnostic purposes and may also offer additional evidence of specific roles for the various glycans. Whereas mass spectrometry is the method of choice for glycan identification (e.g., in patient samples), it has been shown that lectins can be used in a surface plasmon resonance–based sandwich assay to distinguish pregnancy hCG from that produced by malignant gestational trophoblastic neoplasias and male germ cell tumors.[207]

Regulation of Secretion

Luteinizing hormone is stored in dense core granules, under the control of the pulsatile secretogogue, GnRH, with regulated secretion occurring from the basolateral surface.[141] In contrast, hCG is not stored in granules, but rather is secreted constitutively into the maternal circulation at the apical side of trophoblasts.[215] The differential sorting determinant (e.g., for the very similar hormones LH and hCG) was found to reside in the CTP O-glycans.[216-218] As with LH, GnRH activates transcription of the α and FSHβ genes, with secretion of the translated and processed glycoprotein believed to be, in large part, via a constitutive route.[141] The various glycoprotein hormones are trafficked from the endoplasmic reticulum to the cis-Golgi and undergo glycosylation as they traverse the Golgi, reaching the trans-Golgi, to yield the mature hormones. A variety of glycosyltransferases are responsible for N- and O-glycan biosynthesis; notably, sulfation in the pituitary requires N-acetylgalactosamine transferase and sulfotransferase, both of which are missing in the placenta.[27,219-221]

Expression in Physiologic and Pathophysiologic Conditions

The accepted physiologic action of hCG is to maintain functionality of the corpus luteum, particularly during the first trimester of pregnancy. It has also been suggested that hCG can promote angiogenesis by influencing the expression of the potent vascular endothelial growth factor.[222] In addition, hCG is located in the pituitary,[223] but its physiologic significance is unknown. As with pituitary hCG, there are reports of small amounts of glycoprotein hormone synthesis in various nonpituitary and nonplacental tissues, but specific functions have not been ascribed to these ectopically produced hormones. For example, testis and prostate produce hCGα, hCGβ, and intact hCG, with the α subunit being expressed in excess.[57] Interestingly, seminal plasma contains the highest known concentration of the free α subunit. In general, the low concentrations of heterodimeric hCG would argue for an autocrine or paracrine role if indeed there is any physiologic function associated with expression in these other sites. The major forms of circulating LH and hCG have been delineated, along with their patterns in normal physiologic conditions and various disorders.[206]

There is ample evidence supporting ectopic production in a variety of disorders. It is well known that hCG is expressed in malignant forms of gestational trophoblastic disease (e.g., invasive moles and choriocarcinoma)[207,211,224-226] and in testicular cancer.[227] In men and women, hCGβ, and only occasionally intact hCG, is expressed in a variety of other malignancies, including breast, bladder, colorectal, gynecologic, head and neck, hematologic, lung, neuroendocrine, oral/facial, pancreatic, and prostate cancer.[228,229] It has been reported that free α subunit could be detected in breast and prostate cancer, and the level of expression correlated with the amount of estrogen receptor-α.[230,231]

In an analysis of human α, *LHB*, and *hCGB* gene expression in breast cancer, studies showed that most normal tissues expressed only *CGB7*, whereas *CGB3*, *CGB5*, and *CGB8* were expressed in trophoblastic tissues and correlated with the malignant transformation of breast cancer and other nontrophoblastic malignancies.[148,232] Human α, *LHB*, *CGB1*, *CGB2*, and *CGB7* were not, however, upregulated in breast cancer.

DIAGNOSTIC AND THERAPEUTIC APPLICATIONS OF GONADOTROPINS

Immunoassay-based measurements of the serum concentrations of pituitary-derived gonadotropins have been used extensively to monitor functionality of the hypothalamic–pituitary–gonadal axis, and measurements of urinary concentrations of hCG are widely used for pregnancy determinations and management, as well as monitoring trophoblastic malignancies. In addition, studies have shown that hyperglycosylated hCG can be used to detect Down syndrome pregnancies,[233,234] particularly when coupled with the other serum markers α-fetoprotein and estradiol.[235] Immunocytochemistry is also commonly used in evaluating expression of hCGβ in suspected tumor tissue sections. It has been recognized for decades, however, that multiple forms of the glycoproteins exist, giving rise to microheterogeneity and macroheterogeneity.[236] For example, considering hCG, assays must be capable of distinguishing the following: intact or heterodimeric hormone, nicked hCG, heterodimeric hormone with bond cleavages in the hCGβ 43 to 48 region, free α and β subunits, nicked hCGβ core fragment (i.e., free β subunit with bond cleavages in the 43 to 48 region), and hCGβ core fragment, consisting of two disulfide-linked fragments, 6 to 40 connected to 55 to 92.[237] Hyperglycosylated hCG can present with a similar number of derivatives. Several reviews, workshop proceedings, and reports have addressed this issue and

the challenges of obtaining and using appropriate standards.[25,212,226,236-239] The preparation and adoption of universal standards, coupled with complete characterization and disclosure of antibody specificities, will greatly facilitate standardization of glycoprotein hormone immunoassays.

Although immunoreactivity is the primary technique for determining hormone concentrations in body fluids, it is often necessary to measure bioactivity. The earlier cumbersome in vivo assays for the glycoprotein hormones have, by and large, been replaced with radioreceptor and signaling assays in transfected cells. Such measurements provide quantitative data on hormone–receptor binding and the efficacy of signal transduction, but they give no information on circulatory half-life and thus in vivo potency. For this, animal and human studies are obviously required.

Therapeutically, the gonadotropins are used in the treatment of infertility. The longer circulatory half-life of hCG, attributed to the β subunit CTP, has been used most effectively in producing long-acting analogs of FSH and TSH with a CTP engineered to the β C-terminus.[240-244] Another approach that has proven successful in extending the half-life of FSH is an engineered extension at the α N-terminus with two sites of N-glycosylation.[245] The resulting analog was glycosylated as judged by mobility on sodium dodecyl sulfate polyacrylamide gel electrophoresis (SDS-PAGE) and exhibited increased circulatory half-life and in vivo potency.

Recently, a number of reports have appeared suggesting that hCG, in particular, could be used therapeutically in the treatment of cancer. A recent phase I clinical trial has shown that administration of hCG to postmenopausal patients with breast cancer led to a reduction in the proliferative index (Ki-67) and the levels of estrogen and progesterone receptors.[246] In contrast, female transgenic mice overexpressing hCG or LH exhibit multiple sites of tumorigenesis.[247-251] A conjugate of the lytic peptide hecate (a 23–amino acid residue peptide, similar to bee venom mellitin, that disrupts cell membranes) to a 15–amino acid residue peptide from hCGβ (residues 81-95) was found to kill cultured prostate and ovarian cancer cells and reduce the tumor xenografts in nude mice.[252-255] In a transgenic mouse model, it was found that the hecate–hCGβ 15–amino acid residue peptide reduced malignant Leydig and granulosa cell tumors via necrosis or necrosis-like cell death.[256] Although it is surprising that such a short hCGβ peptide is capable of LHR binding, the results are quite dramatic and may lead to specific therapies for LHR-positive tumors.

Early studies found that some crude preparations of hCG, as well as hCGβ-derived peptides, were effective in inhibiting the growth of Kaposi's sarcoma tumors,[257] but later studies showed the effects to arise from a factor that copurifies with hCG and induces cell death via apoptosis.[258] Others have reported that recombinant hCG was only transiently effective in inhibiting the growth of xenografts in nude mice, whereas a fairly pure preparation of hCG was more effective.[259] Despite the controversy in this area, the identification of bioactive proteins and peptides is promising for clinical applications.

A possible role of LH in the etiology and progression of Alzheimer disease has been postulated.[260-262] Of interest was the observation that LH modulates the processing of the amyloid-β precursor protein, yielding deposition of amyloid-β peptide.

The purported extragonadal actions of the gonadotropins remain controversial, but this is an area that will surely be investigated more thoroughly in view of the enormous clinical implications.

Gonadotropin Receptors

GONADOTROPIN RECEPTOR PROTEINS

Amino Acid Sequences and Three-Dimensional Structures

The fully processed hLHR and hFSHR are 675 and 678 amino acid residues long, respectively (www.ensembl.org). By convention, the amino acid residues of the hLHR and hFSHR have been numbered from the initiator methionine of their precursor sequences, which were obtained by virtual translation of the open reading frames of the cognate complementary DNA (cDNA).[263-266] Algorithms that predict the most likely site of cleavage of signal peptides predict signal peptides of the hLHR that are 24 residues long and peptides of the hFSHR that are 17 residues long. Therefore, the N-terminus of the mature hLHR and hFSHR are predicted to be Leu25 and Cys18, respectively. An alignment of the amino acid sequences of the hLHR and hFSHR is presented in Figure 2-4.

When grouped with the TSH receptor, the gonadotropin receptors form the glycoprotein hormone receptor family. One can readily recognize three distinct domains in this family of receptors, a large N-terminal domain that contains approximately 300 residues and is predicted to be extracellular, a serpentine region containing seven transmembrane segments connected by three extracellular loops and three intracellular loops, and a C-terminal tail that is predicted to be located intracellularly (see Fig. 2-4). The presence of seven transmembrane segments is, of course, indicative of the fact that the gonadotropin receptors are members of the superfamily of GPCRs. The GPCR superfamily can be readily divided into several major subfamilies, and the glycoprotein hormone receptors belong to the rhodopsin/β₂-adrenergic receptor–like subfamily of GPCRs.[267-269]

The amino acid sequences of the ECDs of the gonadotropin receptors are 46% identical, and this region is of particular interest because it is responsible for the recognition and high-affinity binding of the hormones to their cognate receptors.[270] It can be divided into three subregions: an N-terminal cysteine-rich region, a region composed of several copies of a structural motif rich in leucine and other hydrophobic residues (the LRR), and a C-terminal cysteine-rich region also known as the *hinge region* (see Fig. 2-4).

The recently determined crystal structure of a large portion of the ECD of the hFSHR (Fig. 2-5B) complexed with a single-chain hFSH analog[10] has provided much-needed insight into the three-dimensional structure of this important receptor region and its involvement in ligand binding. The nine LRRs predicted from the primary structure form nine parallel β sheets, as expected, but an additional β sheet is composed of residues in the N-terminal cysteine-rich region. The first seven β sheets form a fairly flat structure, but the last three have a horseshoe-like curvature that gives the ECD the overall shape of a slightly curved tube (see Fig. 2-5A). The individual LRRs are irregular in length and conformation, but they each have a β strand. These β strands collectively form the concave surface and a coiled structure, and these collectively form the outer surface of the LRR domain (see Fig. 2-5A). FSH is bound to the concave surface of the ECD of the FSHR like two hands clasping each other, with the receptor wrapping itself around the middle section of the hormone (see Fig. 2-5A). All 10 β strands (as well as additional structures) of the LRRs of the hFSHR are in contact with the hormone, and many of these contacting amino acid residues of the hFSHR are conserved between the other two glycoprotein hormone receptors (see Fig. 2-5A and B). The contact surface area between the hormone and the receptor is large and highly charged.

As expected, both hormone subunits participate in receptor binding. Important points of receptor contact for the hormone involve the C-terminal portions of the α and β subunits as well as the α and β L2 loops (see Fig. 2-5C and D). A comparison of the crystal structure of free hFSH[8] with that of the complexed hormone[10] showed that the structures of the free and bound hFSH are quite similar, but the hormone is more rigid when bound to the receptor. The most obvious change in the hormone is on the C-terminus of FSHα, which becomes buried at the receptor interface, where it forms contacts with receptor residues that are highly conserved among the three glycoprotein hormone receptors.[10]

The crystal structure of a large region of the TSHR ECD in complex with a TSHR autoantibody was also solved recently.[271] Although the number of LRRs is different between the TSHR and the FSHR, the overall structure of the ECD of the TSHR is very similar to that of the ECD of the FSHR.[271] Interestingly, the TSHR surface that binds the autoantibody is remarkably similar to the surface of the FSHR that binds FSH.[271]

The crystal structure also showed that the complex of FSH with the FSHR is a dimer, a finding that was confirmed by several other methods.[10] Dimerization involves the outer surface of LRRs 2 to 4 in the FSHR. The finding that one residue (Tyr110, highlighted in yellow in Fig. 2-4) that is fully conserved in the glycoprotein hormone receptors contributes most of the intermolecular contacts in the dimer suggests that dimerization of the other glycoprotein hormone receptors is also likely. The crystal structure of the TSHR in complex with a TSHR antibody did not show any dimers, however.[271]

Because the hinge region is missing from the two ECD crystal structures, nothing is known about its contribution to the overall conformation of the ECD or the receptors. The finding that residues 1 to 268 of the hFSHR (the fragment used for the crystal structure) bind hFSH with high affinity suggests that the hinge region of the hFSHR is not involved in binding. Likewise, a number of laboratory-designed and

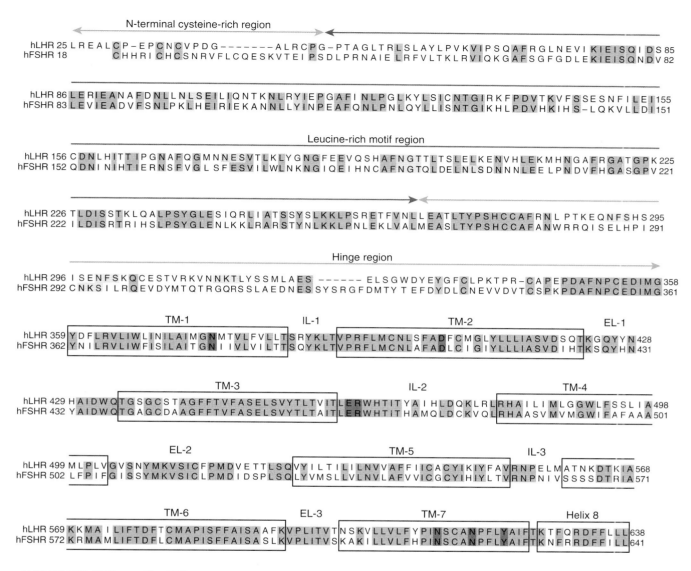

Figure 2-4. Amino acid sequence alignment of the human luteinizing hormone receptor (hLHR) and human follicle-stimulating hormone receptor (hFSHR). Amino acid sequences were obtained from a public Web site (www.ensembl.org/index.html). The boundaries of the three distinct regions of the extracellular domain discussed in the text (N-terminal cysteine-rich region, leucine-rich motif region, and hinge region) are marked with green, red, and green arrows, respectively. The seven transmembrane (TM) helices and the putative cytoplasmic helix 8 are delineated by black boxes and labeled TM-1 through TM-7 and helix 8, respectively. The three extracellular (EL) and four intracellular (IL) loops that connect the transmembrane regions are labeled EL-1 through EL-3 and IL-1 through IL-4, respectively. Identical residues between the two receptors are shown with gray boxes. The consensus sequences for N-linked glycosylation are shown with blue boxes. The tyrosine that participates in dimer formation for the FSHR and is conserved in the hLHR is shown in yellow. The conserved tyrosines that may be sulfated are shown in pink. The conserved cysteines that are believed to be palmitoylated are shown with the green box. Residues that are highly conserved among the rhodopsin/β2-adrenergic family of G-protein–coupled receptors are shown in red. (Copyright © 1999-2008 The European Bioinformatics Institute and Genome Research Limited, and others. All rights reserved.)

naturally occurring mutations of the LHR show that the hinge region of the hLHR is not necessary for the high-affinity binding of hLH or hCG.[270] Nevertheless, the high degree of conservation of some hinge region residues in the glycoprotein hormone receptor family (see Fig. 2-4) suggests that this region plays an important role in other aspects of receptor function, such as activation (discussed later in this section). A highly conserved Tyr present in this region (highlighted in pink in Fig. 2-4) was shown to be sulfated in

the cell surface TSHR, and mutation of this Tyr impairs TSH binding and activation.[272] Sulfation of the equivalent Tyr in the LHR or FSHR has not been shown, but mutations of this residue in the gonadotropin receptors also impair hormone binding and activation.[272]

The serpentine domain of the LHR is characterized by the canonical GPCR structure containing seven transmembrane (TM) segments joined by three alternating intracellular and extracellular loops (see Fig. 2-4). The

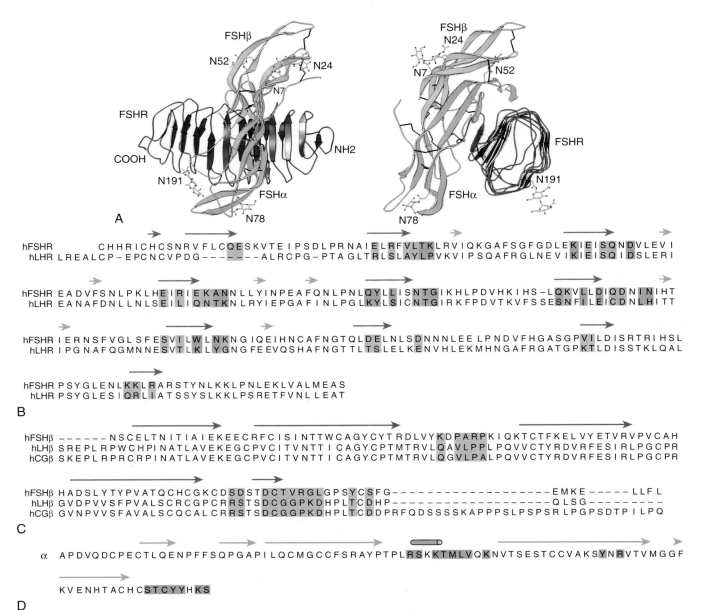

Figure 2-5. *Interactions between the gonadotropin receptors and their cognate hormones.* ***A,*** *Ribbon diagrams of two views of the human follicle-stimulating hormone (hFSH)/follicle-stimulating hormone receptor (FSHR) ectodomain (ECD) rotated 90° around the vertical axis. The α and β chains of FSH are shown in* green *and* blue, *respectively, and the ECD of the FSHR is shown in* red. *Disulfides are shown in* black, *and the N-linked carbohydrates (of the hormone and the receptor) present in the crystal structure are shown in* yellow. ***B*** *to **D,*** *Sequence alignments and secondary structure of portions of the ECD of the two gonadotropin receptors **(B),** the β-subunits of the three gonadotropins **(C),** and the common α subunit **(D).*** Arrows *designate β strands and* cylinders *designate α helices. For the receptor ectodomains **(B),** β strands located on the concave face of the FSHR ectodomain are shown in* red, *and those located in the convex face are shown in* beige. *The FSHR ectodomain residues shown in* green, blue, *or* pink *are buried at the receptor–ligand interface by the α subunit, the β subunit, or both, respectively. The residues in FSHβ shown in* blue ***(C)*** *and those shown in* green *on FSHα **(D)** are buried at the receptor interface. hCG, human chorionic gonadotropin; hLH, human luteinizing hormone; LHR, luteinizing hormone receptor. (Modified from Fan QR, Hendrickson WA. Structure of human follicle-stimulating hormone in complex with its receptor. Nature 433:269-277, 2005. © The Nature Publishing Group [2005].)*

amino acid sequences of this region of the hLHR and hFSHR are 72% identical (see Fig. 2-4). A three-dimensional structure of the transmembrane domain of the gonadotropin receptors is lacking, but models based on the crystal structure of rhodopsin[273] have been built.[274,275] The boundaries of the seven α-helical TM segments predicted for the hLHR and hFSHR based on the rhodopsin structure

are shown in Figure 2-4. Serpentine domain residues that are highly conserved among the rhodopsin/β₂-adrenergic receptor–like subfamily of GPCRs are also highlighted in red in Figure 2-4. All agree that activation of the gonadotropin receptors involves conformational changes in this region,[270,274-276] but little is known about the nature of these changes and how they are brought about (see "Models for Activation of Gonadotropin Receptors"). Two recent publications showed that the LHR and TSHR can be activated by a family of low–molecular-weight compounds that appear to interact with the TM region rather than the ECD.[277,278] These are now being used as lead compounds for the generation of low–molecular-weight agonists of the LHR that may be useful in the treatment of infertility.

Surprisingly, the intracellular domains of the gonadotropin receptors are the most divergent of the three domains (approximately 27% identity; see Fig. 2-4). An intracellular cysteine residue present in the juxtamembrane region of the C-terminal tail of the rhodopsin/β_2-adrenergic receptor–like subfamily of GPCRs is, however, among the most highly conserved residues of this subfamily of GPCRs, and all members of this subfamily examined to date have been shown to be palmitoylated at this site. This cysteine is directed toward the C-terminal end of a cytoplasmic helical segment of rhodopsin that is referred to as "helix 8,"[273] and the palmitate present at this highly conserved position is believed to be embedded in the membrane. Thus, the amino acid residues present between the cytoplasmic end of TM helix 7 and these conserved cysteines are believed to form a fourth intracellular α-helical loop for this subfamily of GPCRs. The LHR is unusual in that it has two adjacent cysteines in this position (see Fig. 2-4). Although the palmitoylation of the hLHR has not been studied, the mature form of the rat (r) LHR expressed in 293 cells has been shown to be palmitoylated at both of these residues.[279-281] Mutation of the palmitoylation sites of the rLHR had no effect on hCG binding or hCG-stimulated signal transduction,[279,280] but it was reported to affect the postendocytotic trafficking of the receptor.[280,282] It is likely that the equivalent cysteine in the hFSHR is also palmitoylated, but this has not been experimentally addressed.

Some residues in the intracellular regions of the gonadotropin receptors are phosphorylated in response to hormone binding. The location of the phosphorylated residues and the functional significance of phosphorylation are discussed elsewhere (see section "Post-Translational Regulation").

Glycosylation

The ectodomains of the hLHR and hFSHR have six and three consensus sites for N-linked glycosylation, respectively (see Fig. 2-4). Although it is clear that the hLHR and hFSHR contain N-linked glycans, studies determining whether all potential sites for carbohydrate attachment are used have not been performed with the human receptors. This question has only been addressed for the recombinant rLHR and FSHR expressed in heterologus cell lines as well as the endogenous porcine LHR. In the porcine LHR, the site equivalent to Asp299 in the hLHR does not appear to be glycosylated, but the other five sites are.[283] One study done with the rLHR expressed in mammalian cells concluded that all potential glycosylation sites are glycosylated,[284] whereas another study done with the rLHR expressed in insect cells concluded that the site equivalent to Asp299 in the hLHR was not glycosylated.[285] A single study done with the recombinant rFSHR expressed

in mammalian cells concluded that the site equivalent to Asp199 in the hFSHR is not glycosylated.[286]

The FSHR/FSHR complex used in the crystallography studies is partially deglycosylated; therefore, full carbohydrate structures are not available. It is clear, however, that carbohydrate residues are present in all four potential glycosylation sites of the hormone (αAsp52, αAsp78, βAsp7, and βAsp24) as well at the first potential glycosylation site of the receptor (Asp191). It is also clear that these are not part of the hormone/receptor interface (see Fig. 2-4). Similarly, the potential glycosylation sites of the TSHR are located on the surface of the TSHR that is not involved in antibody-binding autoantibodies.[271] These data are consistent with the findings that glycosylation of the gonadotropins or the receptors is not required for the formation of the hormone receptor complex.

Folding, Maturation, and Transport to the Plasma Membrane

Mammalian cells expressing the recombinant hLHR show several distinct glycoprotein species with molecular masses (estimated from SDS gels) ranging from 65 to 240 kDa.[270] The mature LHR present at the cell surface has been identified as an 85- to 95-kDa protein, whereas a 65- to 75-kDa band has been identified as an immature precursor that is located in the endoplasmic reticulum.[270] The higher–molecular-weight bands, ranging from 165 to 240 kDa, are oligomers of the immature or mature receptors.[270,287] Precursor, mature, and oligomerized forms of the hFSHR can also be detected in transfected cells, but there is more variation in the reported molecular weights of these products. Estimates of the molecular mass of the mature cell surface that FSHR forms range from 74 to 89 kDa, whereas estimates of the molecular mass of the immature intracellular precursors range from 67 to 82 kDa.[286,288-290] Higher–molecular-weight forms of the FSHR (approximately 170 kDa) have also been identified and appear to be oligomers of the immature intracellular precursor.[290]

Two different studies using the hLHR and the rLHR, along with site-directed mutagenesis, removal of carbohydrate moieties by glycosidase treatment, or pharmacologic inhibition of carbohydrate attachment, suggest that the nonglycosylated LHR can be properly folded, expressed at the cell surface (albeit at reduced levels), and bound to hormone. It can also transduce signals.[284,291] A similar series of studies done with the rFSHR suggests that one of the two carbohydrate moieties present in this receptor (discussed earlier) is required for the proper folding of the nascent receptor into the conformation that can bind FSH with high affinity.[286] Interestingly, the intracellular precursor of the LHR can bind LH and hCG with high affinity,[292,293] but the intracellular precursor of the FSHR cannot bind FSH.[294]

Many of the studies on the sizes and nature of the different forms of gonadotropin receptors have been done by immunologic detection of the epitope-tagged receptors expressed in heterologous cell lines. Immunologic detection of the endogenous gonadotropin receptors expressed in the testes or ovaries has been much more difficult because they are expressed at low densities and because of the nature of the gonadotropin receptor antibodies available. With monoclonal or polyclonal antibodies that have been rigorously validated, the mature and immature forms of the LHR and FSHR described earlier can be immunologically detected in target tissues.[288,295-298]

OTHER RECEPTORS RELATED TO GONADOTROPIN RECEPTORS

The homologous nature of the four glycoprotein hormones (LH, CG, FSH, and TSH) forecasted the homology of their receptors, and the cloning of the cDNAs for these receptors as well as the two recently identified crystal structures clearly fulfilled this prediction.[10,270,271,299,300] The LHR, FSHR, and TSHR defined a subfamily of GPCRs that is characterized by the presence of a large N-terminal ECD containing several LRRs (discussed earlier). This glycoprotein hormone receptor family, which has been renamed the *leucine-rich repeat-containing G-protein–coupled receptor (LGR) family*, has been expanded to include five additional receptors designated LGR4-8[301] and has been further subdivided into three subfamilies. Subfamily A is composed of the three glycoprotein hormone receptors. Subfamily B includes three orphan receptors (LGR4, LGR5, and LGR6), and subfamily C is composed of LGR7 and LGR8, which are receptors for relaxin and relaxin-like hormones.[301-303] The extracellular domains of the LGRs of subfamilies B and C have more LRRs than those of subfamily A, and those of subfamily C also have an N-terminal cysteine rich-motif related to that found in the LDL receptor.[301-303] The hinge region is also subtype-specific.[301]

GONADOTROPIN RECEPTOR GENES AND TRANSCRIPTS

Genes

The human lutropin and follitropin receptors are encoded by single genes located approximately 200 Kb apart on the short arm of chromosome 2 (*LHCGR* and *FSHR*; www.ensembl.org). This region of chromosome 2 is largely devoid of other coding genes.

Lhcgr is approximately 70 Kb in length and is composed of 11 exons, whereas *Fshr* is approximately 190 Kb long and is composed of 10 exons. The transmembrane and C-terminal domains of the receptors are encoded by exon 10 for *Fshr* and by exon 11 for *Lhcgr*. These exons also code for the C-terminal end of the hinge region of the ECD of each receptor. The N-terminal cysteine-rich region, all of the LRRs, and the N-terminal end of the hinge region of the ECD arise from the splicing of the remaining exons.

The 5′ flanking regions of *Lhcgr* and *Fshr* are rich in GC, and the proximal promoters of both genes are devoid of TATA boxes.[304,305] The cis- and trans-acting elements that control the transcription of mouse, rat, and human *Lhcgr* have been examined in some detail.[304] The core promoter of *Lhcgr* in these three species lies within the first 200 bp upstream of the transcriptional start site. This region of rat or human *Lhcgr* has four or five transcription start sites, respectively, as well as two Sp1 sites and one ERE half-site direct repeat (DR). The Sp1 sites bind Sp1/Sp3 proteins or other unidentified proteins, and they

are important for basal transcription. The DR site binds the orphan receptors ER2 and ER3, which inhibit transcription, or testicular receptor 4 (TR4), which stimulates transcription.[306-308] An upstream initiator-like inhibitory element capable of interacting with transcription factor II-I lies approximately at position −300,[309] with one or more (depending on the species) GATA elements in the −1000 to −2000 region.[304] GATA-4 binds to the single GATA element present in the mouse *Lhcgr* promoter and stimulates transcription.[310]

In initial studies, transgenic mice harboring reporter genes driven by approximately 7, approximately 2, or approximately 0.2 kb of the 5′-flanking sequence of the mouse *Lhcgr* expressed the transgene in adult Leydig cells, but not in fetal Leydig cells or ovarian cells.[311] More recent studies have shown that transgenic mice harboring reporter genes driven by 2 to 4 kb of the 5′-flanking sequence of the rat *Lhcgr* express the transgene in the gonads, adrenal glands, kidneys, and several areas of the peripheral and central nervous systems.[298,312]

Studies of the transcriptional control of *Fshr* have been done mostly with the rat gene.[305,313-318] The minimal promoter of rat *Fshr* contains approximately 200 bp upstream of the translation start site.[305] This region has two transcription start sites located within 100 bp upstream of the translation start site.[319] Several elements important for transcription and present in this region include GATA, E2F, and AP1 sites and an E box.[305] Among these, the E box and its binding proteins (upstream stimulatory factors 1 [Usf1] and 2 [Usf2]) are particularly important for expression of *Fshr* in the ovary, but not in the testes.[305] Other transcription factors, such as SF-1, as well as several distal regions of the promoter that are evolutionary conserved,[317,318,320] also contribute to the transcriptional regulation of *FSHR*.[305]

Transcripts

There is controversial evidence regarding the number and nature of multiple FSHR transcripts.[321,322] Most of the studies on this issue have been done in sheep and mouse models, and as many as four different transcripts, arising from alternative splicing and presumably translated into functional proteins with distinct signaling properties, have been reported.[323] Multiple transcripts of the LHR have been identified and arise from alternative splicing or from the use of two different polyadenylation domains present in the 3′ flanking region of *Lhcgr*.[304] Although the presence of these transcripts raises intriguing questions about their possible physiologic roles, it is important to point out that, for the most part, data showing the presence of proteins arising from such transcripts are lacking.

Naturally Occurring Mutations of *Lhcgr* and *Fshr*

A number of naturally occurring mutations of *Lhcgr* and *Fshr* associated with human reproductive disorders have also been reported. These are also shown in Figures 2-6 and 2-7 and have been extensively reviewed.[157,270,300,324-326]

Naturally occurring loss-of-function or inactivating mutations of the hLHR occur throughout the polypeptide

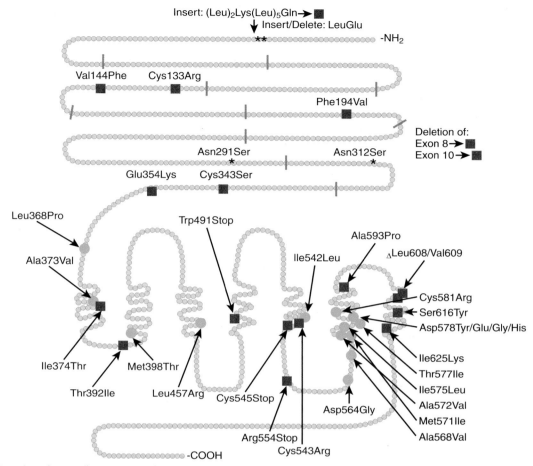

Figure 2-6. *Location of naturally occurring polymorphisms, loss-of-function mutations, and gain-of-function mutations of the human luteinizing hormone receptor (hLHR). Polymorphisms are shown with asterisks, loss-of-function mutations are shown with red squares, and gain-of-function mutations are shown with green dots. The sequences coded for by the different exons are demarcated by vertical blue bars. (From Themmen APN. An update of the pathophysiology of human gonadotrophin subunit and receptor gene mutations and polymorphisms. Reproduction 130:263-274, 2005. © Society for Reproduction and Fertility [2005]. Reproduced by permission.)*

chain, as shown in Figure 2-6. These are all germline mutations, and a phenotype is obvious only in individuals who are homozygotes or compound heterozygotes. The most severe phenotype in 46XY individuals is complete absence of Leydig cells (Leydig cell hypoplasia) and pseudohermaphroditism. Other milder phenotypes in 46XY individuals include hypospadias and micropenis.[324,325] In women, inactivating mutations of the hLHR are associated with low estrogen production and anovulatory disorders.[324,325]

Loss-of-function mutations of the hLHR can take many forms, including single–amino acid mutations, nonsense mutations that result in truncated receptors, small insertions or deletions, and large insertions or deletions. Some of these mutations prevent hormone binding per se, but all of them impair the maturation or transport of the hLHR precursor so that the expression of the mature hLHR at the cell surface is completely lost or at least partially reduced.[270] Therefore, the phenotype of these individuals is mostly due to a net loss of cell surface hLHR rather than to the expression of a receptor that binds hormone but cannot become activated.

The phenotype associated with the exon 10 deletion deserves special mention. This mutation was initially found in a 46XY individual who did not undergo puberty in spite of normal sex differentiation.[327] When expressed in a heterologous cell line, an hLHR construct lacking the amino acids encoded by exon 10 (residues 290-316 in the hinge region of the ECD; see Fig. 2-4) is transported properly to the cell surface and binds hLH and hCG with high affinity.[328] Interestingly, cells expressing this mutant receptor respond to hCG normally, but their sensitivity to hLH was reduced approximately 40-fold.[328] Therefore, the residues encoded by exon 10 of the hLHR do not participate in hormone binding, but appear to be involved in receptor activation by hLH, but not by hCG.

The LHR of the marmoset monkey provides an interesting evolutionary parallel to the hLHR variant lacking exon 10. The marmoset pituitary does not express LHβ,[329] and exon 10 of the marmoset monkey *Lhcgr* is spliced out of the mature mRNA[330]; yet, this receptor can bind hCG with a high affinity and respond to the bound hCG.[330] A recent study has begun to identify regulatory elements of *Lhcgr* that influence the usage of exon 10.[331]

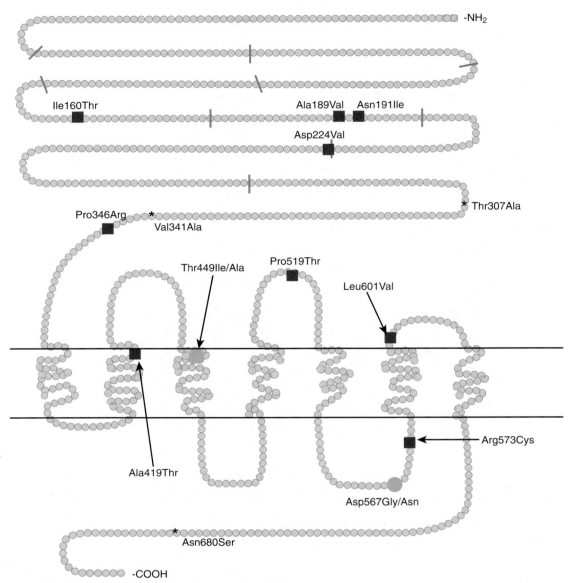

Figure 2-7. *Location of the naturally occurring polymorphisms, loss-of-function mutations, and gain-of-function mutations of the human follicle-stimulating hormone receptor (hFSHR). Polymorphisms are shown with asterisks, loss-of-function mutations are shown with red squares, and gain-of-function mutations are shown with green dots. The sequences coded for by the different exons are shown with vertical blue bars (From Themmen APN. An update of the pathophysiology of human gonadotrophin subunit and receptor gene mutations and polymorphisms. Reproduction 130:263-274, 2005. © Society for Reproduction and Fertility [2005]. Reproduced by permission.)*

In contrast to the heterogeneous location of the naturally occurring loss-of-function mutations of the hLHR, all naturally occurring gain-of-function mutations reported to date are localized to exon 11, which codes for the transmembrane and intracellular regions of the hLHR (see Fig. 2-6).[157,270,300,324-326] All of these are single-point mutations, and many of them cluster to transmembrane helix 6 and intracellular loop 3 (see Fig. 2-6). Four of these mutations are associated with a single residue (Asp578), which is found mutated to Gly, Glu, Tyr, and His (see Fig. 2-6). Although the restricted location of these mutations is in agreement with the perceived importance of the serpentine region of the hLHR in signal transduction, their restricted location may also be a function of the methods used to

search for mutations. Because earlier efforts to find activating mutations of the hLHR were restricted to this region of the gene, it is possible that further studies will show the presence of activating mutations of the hLHR elsewhere. Such a finding can indeed be forecasted by the recent demonstration that certain laboratory-designed mutations of the hinge region of the hLHR can also induce constitutive activation.[332,333] In addition, naturally occurring activating mutations have been recently identified in the hinge region of the ECD of the structurally related TSHR.[334-336]

Gain-of-function mutations of the hLHR are found in heterozygous boys with familial male limited precocious puberty, but there is no phenotype in female carriers.[157,270,324-326] All of these mutations are also germline, with the exception of the Asp578His mutation, which has only been found as a somatic mutation in the Leydig cells of several unrelated boys with precocious puberty and Leydig cell adenomas.[337-339]

When expressed in heterologous cell types, these gain-of-function hLHR mutants show variable levels of constitutive (i.e., hormone-independent) activity, and the addition of LH or hCG to cells expressing these mutants may or may not result in additional activation.[157,270,324-326]

Naturally occurring mutations of *Fshr* are fewer in number, but can be similarly classified (see Fig. 2-7). The most severe phenotype in homozygous females harboring inactivating mutations, such as Ala189Val and Pro419Thr, is hypergonadotropic hypogonadism, arrest of follicular maturation beyond the primary stage and complete lack of responsiveness to hFSH. Less severe phenotypes are observed in individuals who are homozygous or compound heterozygous, and they include secondary amenorrhea, gonadotropin resistance, and follicular development up to the antral stage.[157,325] The phenotype in homozygous males is not nearly as obvious. Sperm quality is reduced, but fertility is maintained.[157,325] The functional properties of many of these hFSHR mutants have been studied by expressing the mutants in heterologous cell lines. As in the case of the hLHR, many of these mutations impair the transport of the hFSHR to the plasma membrane, thus inducing a complete lack of hFSH binding and therefore responsiveness.[157,325] At least one of them, however (the mutation of Ala419 to Thr in TM helix 2), impairs signal transduction while having little or no effect on hFSH binding or the proper trafficking of the hFSHR to the plasma membrane.[340]

Four activating mutations of *Fshr* have been described. These are two mutations of two residues of exon 10, as shown in Figure 2-7. The Asp567Gly mutation in intracellular loop 3 was identified in a hypophysectomized male with undetectable gonadotropins who responded to testosterone treatment with normal spermatogenesis.[341] The activating nature of this mutation is not readily apparent, however, when the mutant receptor is expressed in heterologous cells.[341] The Asp567An, Thr449Ile, and Thr449Ala mutations (see Fig. 2-7) were initially discovered in women with recurrent spontaneous ovarian hyperstimulation syndrome.[342-344] When these mutants are expressed in heterologous cell types, they display a weak but detectable level of constitutive activity; they also display increased sensitivity to hCG and to TSH, while maintaining normal sensitivity to hFSH.[300] This latter change in binding specificity is responsible for the ovarian hyperstimulation experienced by women harboring these mutations. In this context, it is worth mentioning that one naturally occurring mutation of the TSHR ECD that renders it more sensitive to hCG was found in two women who experienced hyperthyroidism during pregnancy.[345]

Polymorphisms of *Lhcgr* and *Fshr*

Hundreds of SNPs of *Lhcgr* and *Fshr* have been identified, but many of them are intronic (http://SNPper.chip.org).

Three SNPs of *Lhcgr* occur in exons. A six-nucleotide in-frame insertion/deletion between codons 18 and 19 of exon 1 results in the expression of two hLHR variants that differ by the presence or absence of a LeuGln pair near the the C-terminus of the signal peptide (see Fig. 2-6).[346-348] The functional implications of the presence or absence of this insertion are unclear. One group reported no effect on hormone binding or responsiveness,[346] whereas another reported that the LeuGln insertion enhances receptor expression and sensitivity to hCG.[349] The variant of the LHR containing the LeuGln insertion is associated with adverse outcomes in women with breast cancer.[349,350] Two additional frequent SNPs in exon 10 of the hLHR gene code for either Asn or Ser in codons 291 and 312 in the hinge region of the ECD of the hLHR (see Fig. 2-6). The presence of Asn or Ser at either of these positions does not appear to change the expression or function of the hLHR.[351] This is interesting because codon 291 is a glycosylation site when Asn is present in this position.[350]

Only five of the *Fshr* SNPs are exonic. They are all located in exon 10, but only four cause a coding change (Ala307Thr, Arg524Ser, Ala665Thr, and Ser680Asn). The most common and best studied are Ala307Thr and Ser680Asn (see Fig. 2-7). These are in linkage disequilibrium, and the most common allelic variants, Thr307/Asn680 and Ala307/Ser680, are almost equally distributed among white populations.[157] Several studies have reported that women carrying the Ser-680 *Fshr* allele who are injected with FSH during in vitro fertilization treatment are less sensitive to FSH. In addition, studies of women with normal menstrual cycles indicate that the Ser680 allele leads to higher FSH serum levels and a prolonged cycle.[157,352] The presence of the Ala307 and Ser680 polymorphism carriers may affect the susceptibility of women to specific subtypes of ovarian cancer.[353] Interestingly, studies of the Ser680 or Asn680 hFSHR expressed in heterologous cell types have not shown any differences in the functional properties of these receptors.[354,355]

REGULATION OF THE EXPRESSION OF GONADOTROPIN RECEPTORS

Transcriptional Regulation

In addition to directing the basal expression of *Lhcgr* and *Fshr*, transcriptional regulation of these genes is involved in the hormonal regulation of receptor expression in the ovary and perhaps the testes as well. For example, the increase in LHR that occurs during the growth and differentiation of granulosa cells is accompanied by an increase in LHR mRNA that is mediated, at least in part, by an increase in the transcription of *Lhcgr*.[356-359] An exhaustive review of the hormonal regulation of the transcription of *Lhcgr* and *Fshr* is, however, beyond the scope of this chapter. Several recent reviews have addressed this important but complex area.[270,304,305,315,320,360-362] A summary of the regulatory elements and the transcription factors that modulate basal expression of *Lhcgr* and *Fhsr* was presented earlier.

Post-Transcriptional Regulation

Post-transcriptional regulation is also an important aspect of the regulation of the LHR mRNA and the LHR during the preovulatory LH surge.[356,362-366] This important level of regulation seems to be mediated by mevalonate kinase, an enzyme that is involved in cholesterol metabolism that is also an LHR mRNA-binding protein.[367-371] LH-induced activation of steroidogenesis and subsequent depletion of cholesterol trigger an increase in the transcription of genes that participate in cholesterol biosynthesis, including mevalonate kinase. The increased levels of this protein may thus serve the dual role of enhancing cholesterol synthesis (an enzymatic function) and decreasing the levels of LHR mRNA by virtue of its ability to bind LHR mRNA and enhance its degradation.[366,372]

Post-Translational Regulation

There are two levels of post-translational regulation of gonadotropin receptors. The first has been documented only with the LHR, and it occurs at the level of processing, maturation, and transport of the intracellular LHR precursor to the mature cell surface LHR.

During development, several rat tissues, such as the gonads, adrenal glands, and kidneys, seem to express only the immature form of the LHR, whereas others, such as nervous tissues, express both the mature and immature forms.[298,312] Interestingly, rodent gonads appear to express the mature LHR only after birth,[312] suggesting that the developing rat gonads are insensitive to the actions of LH. This finding is consistent with the phenotype of the LHR knockout mice, which displays arrested gonadal development only after birth.[373,374] The expression of the mature LHR in rat tissues also seems to be under hormonal control, as indicated by the finding that the mature LHR becomes detectable in the female adrenal glands and kidneys during pregnancy.[312] Direct actions of gonadotropins on the kidneys are controversial, but expression of functional LHR that mediates direct actions on LH/CG in the pregnant adrenal gland has been well documented (discussed later).

Coexpression of splice variants of the LHR may also regulate the expression of the LHR and FSHR by forming intracellular oligomers that prevent the proper processing of the intracellular LHR precursor.[375,376] For example, LHR transcripts lacking exon 9 are prevalent in normal human ovaries, but the resulting protein is not able to bind hCG or to be adequately processed to be expressed at the cell surface.[377,378] When coexpressed with the wild-type hLHR or hFSHR in heterologous cell lines, however, the mutant lacking exon 9 appeared to associate with the immature forms of these receptors and decrease their cell surface expression.[377,378]

The second level of post-translational regulation involves phosphorylation and regulated degradation of the mature gonadotropin receptors. This has been shown for both the LHR and the FSHR, but most of these experiments have been done in heterologous cell types, and their physiologic significance is still debated.

Like many other GPCRs studied to date,[379-382] the mature forms of the LHR[383-386] and FSHR[387-391] have been shown to be phosphorylated in transfected cells exposed to the appropriate hormone. The kinases involved are likely to be members of the GPCR kinase family.[381,384,387,391] The agonist-induced phosphorylation of the hLHR and rLHR occur on several serine residues present in the

C-terminal tail.[384-386,392,393] The phosphorylation of the FSHR has been studied only using the rat receptor. The rFSHR becomes phosphorylated on serine and threonine residues,[390] but the location of these phosphorylation sites is controversial. One laboratory has mapped the phosphorylation sites to the first and third intracellular loops,[388,389] whereas another laboratory reported that phosphorylation of the FSHR occurs in the C-terminal tail.[391]

Phosphorylation of GPCRs is an important event for binding arrestins, a family of GPCR-binding proteins that are involved in signaling, internalization, and desensitization.[380,381,394,395] The phosphorylation of the hLHR appears to be largely dispensable for arrestin binding and internalization, however.[384,396-398] In contrast, phosphorylation of the rFSHR appears to be needed for arrestin binding and internalization.[391,397,399-401]

Hormone-induced internalization of gonadotropin receptors is an important process because, depending on the fate of the internalized receptor, it can serve the function of preserving or preventing hormonal responsiveness. Interestingly, after hormone-induced internalization, the complex formed by hCG and the rodent or porcine LHR is largely routed to an intracellular degradation pathway[402-406] that is ultimately responsible for the degradation of hCG and a net loss of cell surface LHR and hormonal responsiveness.[407-410] The fate of the internalized hLHR is different, however, in that a substantial portion of the hCG–hLHR complex is routed to a recycling rather than a degradation pathway.[410-413] Cells expressing the hLHR recycle most of the internalized hormone and receptor; thus, the loss of hormonal responsiveness induced by gonadotropins is not as pronounced in cells expressing the hLHR as in those expressing the rLHR.[410] One would predict then that LH/CG responsiveness in humans would be largely preserved on prolonged activation of the LHR, whereas LH responsiveness in rodents would be largely lost on prolonged activation of the LHR. In contrast to the difference in the fates of the internalized hLHR and rFSHR, the internalized hFSHR and rFSHR are both routed mostly to a recycling pathway.[414] Cells expressing these receptors recycle most of the internalized FSH and FSH; consequently, the loss of hormonal responsiveness induced by FSH is relatively minor.[410]

Several amino acids present in the extreme C-terminus of the hLHR and one cellular protein that is important for recycling of the hLHR have been identified.[412,413,415] Amino acids of the FSHR that are important for recycling are also located in the extreme C-terminal tail.[414]

EXPRESSION OF GONADOTROPIN RECEPTORS IN EXTRAGONADAL TISSUES

For many years, the LHR and FSHR were believed to localize strictly to gonadal cells. In the testes, the LHR and FSHR are believed to be restricted to Leydig and Sertoli cells, respectively. In the ovary, expression of the LHR occurs in theca, interstitial, and granulosa cells, whereas the FSHR is localized to granulosa cells. Certainly, the main physiologic roles of the gonadotropin receptors can be attributed to their actions in the ovaries and testes, as shown by the phenotypes of individuals harboring activating or inactivating mutations of *Lhcgr* and *Fshr* (discussed earlier) and by the phenotypes of mice with targeted inactivation of *Lhcgr*[373,374] or *Fshr*.[416,417] There is a large and growing body of literature, however, suggesting that functional gonadotropin receptors, particularly the LHR, may be present in extragonadal tissues.[418-422]

The suggestion of extragonadal LHR expression has been based in many cases on the detection of fragments of LHR mRNA. Attempts to detect immunoreactive LHR protein often result in the identification of one or more proteins that do not match the expected molecular weight of the authentic gonadal LHR (discussed earlier). A comparison of the actions of LH/CG in isolated cells or tissues from wild-type and LHR-null mice would go a long way toward shedding light on this controversy, but curiously, this has not been done often. In a recent study of the potential angiogenic activity of hCG, it was shown that the proangiogenic effect of hCG was clearly ameliorated in blood vessels isolated from LHR-null mice.[423] This finding clearly shows that a functional, classic LHR is expressed in blood vessels.

Some of the clearest evidence of extragonadal expression of a functional LHR comes from studies done on a woman who had pregnancy-dependent Cushing's syndrome and had this syndrome again after menopause.[424] After menopause, there was clear evidence that this patient's cortisol levels were controlled by LH because suppression of the hypothalamic–pituitary axis with leuprolide controlled the hypercortisolism.[424] Clinical findings in a number of other cases also seem to be explained by the inappropriate expression of the LHR in the adrenal cortex or in adrenocortical tumors.[425] Lastly, ectopic expression of functional LHR in the adrenal cortex appears to be a common finding in transgenic or knockout mouse models with elevated levels of gonadotropins,[426-429] and expression of the mature LHR can be readily documented in the adrenal glands of pregnant rats.[312]

Studies of potential extragonadal expression of the FSHR are much more limited. A recent study suggesting that FSH has direct actions in bone because of the expression of the FSHR in osteoclasts[430] has generated a substantial amount of controversy, but remains unresolved.[431,432] There is also some evidence of the expression of the FSHR in the prostate.[433]

In spite of this newly emerging information, the phenotypes of genetically engineered mice with exaggerated or absent gonadotropin action, as well as the phenotypes of men or women harboring activating or inactivating mutations of these gonadotropin receptors (discussed earlier), appear to be explained entirely by the classic actions of LH and FSH in gonadal tissues.[249,422,434] Nonetheless, the controversy about extragonadal actions of these hormones is far from over.[435,436]

MODELS FOR ACTIVATION OF GONADOTROPIN RECEPTORS

Because there is a physical separation between the region of the gonadotropin receptors that binds the hormones (ECD) and the region involved in receptor activation (TM domain), there are at least three models that one may consider as being responsible for receptor activation.[270,299,300]

Model 1

Portions of the hormones bound to the ECD interact with either the hinge or the serpentine region to induce an active conformation in the serpentine region.

The specificity of binding is clearly dictated by the amino acid sequences of the ECD of the receptors and of the β subunit of the hormone. One can envision the activation step as being common to all glycoprotein hormone receptors and mediated by specific interactions of conserved amino acids present in the common α subunit of the four glycoprotein hormones and conserved amino acids present in the serpentine region of the three glycoprotein hormone receptors. This model is supported by the finding that certain mutations of the gonadotropins or their receptors can impair receptor activation without affecting hormone binding[270] and by the three-dimensional structure of FSH bound to the ECD of the FSHR.[10] This structure shows that some portions of the hormone do not interact with the ECD and thus are free to interact with other portions of the receptor.[10] Although not proven, this structure also suggests that the tips of FSHα in the complex are oriented toward the membrane.[10]

Model 2

The binding of gonadotropins to the ECD allows the ECD to directly interact with and activate the serpentine region.

This model is similar to model 1, except that the ECDs, instead of the bound hormones, are the activators of the serpentine region. This model is supported by the finding that discrete mutations of the ECDs can impair signal transduction without affecting hormone binding,[270] and it suggests that, in the inactive state, the ECDs are not as tightly associated with the serpentine region as in the activated state. This suggestion is supported by the observation that some mutations of the transmembrane domains of the LHR, FSHR, or TSHR influence the affinity or specificity of hormone binding to the ECD.[300,344,437]

Model 3

The ECD may hold the serpentine domain in an inactive state, and hormone binding to the ECD activates the serpentine domain by relaxing this interaction.

This model is supported by the finding that discrete mutations of the hinge region of the glycoprotein hormone receptors can induce constitutive activation[332,333] and predicts that expression of receptor variants lacking the ECD would display constitutive signaling. Gonadotropin receptor variants lacking the ECDs are, however, either inactive or not fully active.[270,299,300]

Regardless of which model is correct, it appears likely that dimerization of the gonadotropin receptors is an important component of the process of activation. As mentioned earlier, the complex of the ECD of the FSHR with FSH is a dimer, and several other laboratories have shown agonist-dependent or constitutive homo- and heterodimerization of the LHR and FSHR.[287,438-440]

SIGNALING PATHWAYS ACTIVATED BY GONADOTROPIN RECEPTORS

Although most investigators agree that the effects of gonadotropins on the differentiated function of their target cells are mediated mostly (if not entirely) by the activation of the Gs/adenylyl cyclase/cAMP/protein kinase A pathway, it is abundantly clear that this is not the only pathway activated by these receptors. Additional pathways are activated, as discussed later, and these may be involved in other gonadotropin-dependent events, such as the proliferation or differentiation of target cells.

The LHR was one of the first GPCRs shown to independently activate two G-protein–dependent signaling pathways, adenylyl cyclase and phospholipase C.[441,442] This observation was initially made in heterologoous cells expressing the recombinant mouse LHR, but it has now been extensively reproduced by a number of investigators using a variety of cell lines transfected with either the rodent or human LHR.[270] The FSHR also activates both of these cascades when expressed in heterologous cell types.[388-390] In general, however, the gonadotropin receptor–mediated activation of phospholipase C is detectable only when cells expressing a high density of receptors are exposed to high concentrations of gonadotropins.[385,386,388-390,392,443-446] This has led to the suggestion that the LHR-induced activation of this signaling pathway is important only in females during the preovulatory LH surge or during pregnancy,[441] and some recent studies conducted in granulosa cells expressing different densities of the LHR or FSHR support this idea.[447,448] Because maternal hCG is also important in the development of the normal male phenotype, it is also possible that exposure of the male fetus to the high levels of maternal hCG may result in stimulation of the phospholipase C cascade in fetal Leydig cells.

All investigators agree that the gonadotropin receptor–induced activation of adenylyl cyclase occurs through $G\alpha_s$.[449-452] In addition, the LHR has been reported to activate members of the other three families of G proteins,[449-452] but little is known about the gonadal cell effectors that are sensitive to the activation of these G proteins. There is also no agreement on the identity of the G protein or G protein subunits that mediate the effects of the LHR on phospholipase C activation. Some investigators have concluded that LHR-induced activation of phospholipase C is mediated by the β/γ subunits liberated by the activation of G_i and possibly G_s,[449,453] whereas others have concluded that it is mediated by $G\alpha_{q/11}$.[441,442,452]

The classification of naturally occurring mutants of the hLHR as gain- or loss-of-function mutants (discussed earlier) and the effect of laboratory-designed mutations on the activation of the LHR were initially based on measurements of cAMP accumulation as an index of receptor activation. More recent experiments have compared the effects of a given LHR mutation (naturally occurring or laboratory-designed) on the cAMP and inositol phosphate responses. This issue is particularly important in view of the initial proposal stating that constitutive activity toward the inositol phosphate pathway may be restricted to naturally occurring somatic gain-of-function mutations of the LHR that are associated with Leydig cell adenomas.[337] This proposal arose from the finding that the single gain-of-function mutation of the hLHR associated with Leydig cell adenomas (Asp578His; see Fig. 2-6) showed constitutive activity toward the cAMP and inositol phosphate responses, whereas a similar gain-of-function mutation of the hLHR associated with Leydig cell hyperplasia (Asp578Tyr, see Fig. 2-6) showed constitutive activity only toward the cAMP response.[337] Subsequent experiments generated an extensive comparison of the functional properties of two germline hLHR constitutively activating mutants (CAMs) associated with Leydig cell hyperplasia, hLHR-Leu457Arg and hLHR-Asp578Tyr,[454-457] with the functional properties of the single somatic hLHR CAM (hLHR-Asp578His) associated with Leydig cell adenomas. These experiments showed that the G proteins and signaling pathways activated by constitutively active mutants of the hLHR associated with Leydig cell hyperplasia or tumors are identical and are the same as those activated by the agonist-engaged hLHR-wild type.[384,396,446,452] The reasons why the Asp578His mutation is uniquely associated with Leydig cell adenomas remain a mystery.

The ERK1/2 cascade, a signaling pathway that figures prominently in cell proliferation, is also under the control of gonadotropins in the ovary and testes.[458-468] The mechanisms by which this pathway is activated also seem to involve the activation of the Gs/adenylyl cyclase, but other, less characterized modes of activation seem to be involved as well.[464,466]

More recently, gonadotropin receptors have been shown to activate certain tyrosine kinases, such as members of the Src and ErB receptor families.[460,464,466,469-476] The molecular bases of the activation of these pathways are not well understood, and they could be downstream of the Gs/adenylyl cyclase signaling cascade,[473,474] or they could be independently stimulated through G-protein–dependent or -independent pathways.[464,466,469] The EGF network, which involves several EGF-like growth factors and several ErB receptors, has now been shown to mediate the ovulatory response.[471-475]

Lastly, a number of other cAMP-dependent and -independent signaling cascades that are stimulated by gonadotropins in the ovaries and testes have been recently reviewed.[360,458,468,477,478]

ACKNOWLEDGMENTS: It is a pleasure to thank Geneva DeMars, Diana Hartle, and Susan Brunn Puett for their capable assistance. We also thank Dr. Michael Tiemeyer for his assistance with Figure 2-3, Drs. Wayne Hendrickson and Qin Fan for providing Figures 2-5A and B, and Drs. Axel Themmen and Ilpo Huhtaniemi for providing us with editable versions of Figures 2-6 and 2-7. Research in the authors' laboratories on gonadotropins and their receptors was funded by NIH grants CA40629 and HD28962 to MA and DK33973 and DK69711 to DP.

The complete reference list can be found on the companion Expert Consult Web site at www.expertconsultbook.com.

Suggested Readings

Ahtiainen P, Rulli S, Pakarainen T, et al. Phenotypic characterization of mice with exaggerated and missing LH/hCG action. Mol Cell Endocrinol 260-262:255-263, 2007.

Ascoli M. Potential Leydig cell mitogenic signals generated by the wild-type and constitutively active mutants of the lutropin/choriogonadotropin receptor. Mol Cell Endocrinol 260-262:244-248, 2007.

Ascoli M, Fanelli F, Segaloff DL. The lutropin/choriogonadotropin receptor: a 2002 perspective. Endocr Rev 23:141-174, 2002.

Boime I, Garcia-Campayo V, Hsueh AJW. The glycoprotein hormones and their receptors. In Strauss III J, Barbieri RL (eds). Reproductive Endocrinology: Physiology, Pathophysiology, and Clinica Management. Philadelphia, Saunders, 2004,pp 75-92.

Conti M, Hsieh M, Park JY, et al. Role of the EGF network in ovarian follicles. Mol Endocrinol 20:715-723, 2005.

Costagliola S, Urizar E, Mendive F, et al. Specificity and promiscuity of gonadotropin receptors. Reproduction 130:275-281, 2005.

Fan QR, Hendrickson WA. Structure of human follicle-stimulating hormone in complex with its receptor. Nature 433:269-277, 2005.

Hearn MTW, Gomme PT. Molecular architecture and biorecognition processes of the cystine knot protein superfamily: Part I. The glycoprotein hormones. J Mol Recog 13:223-278, 2000.

Hunzicker-Dunn M, Maizels ET. FSH signaling pathways in immature granulosa cells that regulate target gene expression: branching out from protein kinase A. Cell Signal 18:1351-1359, 2006.

Lapthorn AJ, Harris DC, Littlejohn A, et al. Crystal-structure of human chorionic-gonadotropin. Nature 369:455-461, 1994.

Latronico AC, Segaloff DL. Insights learned from L457(3.43)R, an activating mutant of the human lutropin receptor. Mol Cell Endocrinol 260-262:287-293, 2007.

Puett D, Wu CB, Narayan P. The tie that binds: design of biologically active single-chain human chorionic gonadotropins and a gonadotropin-receptor complex using protein engineering. Biol Reprod 58:1337-1342, 1998.

Tegoni M, Spinelli S, Verhoeyen M, et al. Crystal structure of a ternary complex between human chorionic gonadotropin (hCG) and two Fv fragments specific for the alpha and beta-subunits. J Mol Biol 289:1375-1385, 1999.

Themmen APN. An update of the pathophysiology of human gonadotrophin subunit and receptor gene mutations and polymorphisms. Reproduction 130:263-274, 2005.

Wu H, Lustbader JW, Liu Y, et al. Structure of human chorionic-gonadotropin at 2.6-Angstrom resolution from MAD analysis of the selenomethionyl protein. Structure 2:545-558, 1994.

CHAPTER 3

Prolactin in Human Reproduction

Mark E. Molitch

Prolactin (PRL), a hormone with roles in reproduction, lactation, and metabolism, is made by the pituitary lactotrophs which, in the normal human pituitary, comprise approximately 15% to 25% of the total number of cells, are similar in number in both sexes, and do not change significantly with age.[1] During gestation and subsequent lactation, there is considerable lactotroph hyperplasia because of the stimulatory effect of the hormonal milieu of pregnancy.[2,3] The hyperplastic process involutes within several months after delivery, although breast-feeding retards this process.[3] This stimulatory effect of pregnancy on the lactotrophs also holds true for prolactinomas, explaining why very significant tumor enlargement may occur during pregnancy. As described later in this chapter, the proliferation of lactotrophs and the increase in PRL secretion is due, at least in part, to autocrine and paracrine mechanisms playing out within the pituitary gland. This chapter reviews the physiology of PRL and the pathophysiology of hyperprolactinemic states and their diagnosis and management.

Anatomy and Physiology

LACTOTROPH MORPHOLOGY AND ONTOGENY

During embryologic development, the ectodermal primordial cells of the anterior and intermediate lobes of the pituitary make contact with the neuroectoderm of the floor of the diencephalon. Inductive interactions between these tissues occur that are necessary for their subsequent interdependent development.[4,5] There are a number of homeodomain transcription factors that are sequentially expressed in the developing hypothalamus and pituitary that lead to the final determination of the five mature pituitary cell types and the functional integration of the hypothalamic–pituitary system.[4-6]

The POU homeodomain transcription factor Pit-1 is necessary for the activation of the *PRL,* growth hormone *(GH),* and thyroid-stimulating hormone *(TSH)* genes as well as being necessary for the differentiation and proliferation of these cell lineages. Point mutations in the POU homeodomain of the *Pit-1* gene have been found to be the cause of the syndrome of combined GH, PRL, and TSH deficiencies found in humans, with absence of somatotroph, lactotroph, and thyrotroph cells.[4-6] A second paired-like homeodomain factor, known as Prophet of Pit-1 (Prop-1), has also been found to be necessary for the expression of Pit-1, and mutations of the *Prop-1* gene cause variable deficiencies of GH, PRL, TSH, luteinizing hormone (LH), and follicle-stimulating hormone (FSH).[4-6] Mutations in the *Lhx4* and *Hesx1* genes cause combined pituitary hormone deficiencies as well as other brain developmental defects.[5,6] Lactotrophs and somatorophs are believed to arise from a common progenitor, the mammosomatotroph, under the regulation of these and other transcription factors during embryologic development, but it is possible that some lactotrophs arise directly from a common pituitary progenitor cell without passing through this mammosomatotroph step.[7]

PROLACTIN GENE STRUCTURE AND REGULATION

The *PRL* gene in the human is located on chromosome 6.[8] The human *PRL* gene is approximately 10 kb long from the 5′ transcription initiation site to the poly(A) addition site at the 3′ end; it consists of five exons separated by four large introns.[9,10] In the 5′ flanking region, there are specific regions responsible for tissue-specific Pit-1 transcription activation. The transcription enhancement of the *PRL* gene by Pit-1 can be modified by other factors, such as thyrotropin-releasing hormone (TRH), epidermal growth factor (EGF), cyclic adenosine monophosphate (cAMP),[11-13] glucocorticoids,[14] and estrogens.[15] Other areas of the 5′ flanking region have also been found to be involved in the suppression of *PRL* gene transcription by thyroid hormone and stimulation by estrogen.[15-19] Estrogen also increases PRL by modulating the inhibitory effect of dopamine (DA) on *PRL* gene transcription.[20,21]

A number of factors affecting PRL secretion, including TRH and DA, act through the phosphoinositide-signaling pathways, with resultant release of calcium from the endoplasmic reticulum and an activation of membrane calcium channels.[22] Increases in intracellular calcium result in activation of protein kinase C, which phosphorylates downstream effector proteins.

A second transduction pathway involving membrane phospholipids is the arachidonate pathway. In vitro stimulation of membrane-bound phospholipase A_2 by TRH, angiotensin II, neurotensin, and other direct stimulators releases PRL and arachidonic acid from pituitary cells.[23,24] This stimulated release of arachidonic acid is blocked by inhibitors of phospholipase A_2[23] and by DA.[25] Arachidonic acid increases PRL release primarily by an increase in calcium influx, not through mobilization of intracellular calcium stores.[26]

In addition to effects on protein kinase C, calcium also binds to topoisomerase II, which then interacts with specific DNA binding sites, and to calmodulin. In turn, calmodulin then binds to a number of different intracellular enzymes.[27] TRH appears to cause rapid release of PRL via activation of protein kinase C and calcium store mobilization, but not calcium channel–mediated transport, and its effects on *PRL* gene transcription and PRL synthesis involve all three processes.[27]

Dopamine, the primary PRL inhibitory factor (PIF), acts through the D_2 DA receptor, partly by inhibiting adenyl cyclase and decreasing intracellular cAMP.[28] DA inhibits the PRL release induced by activation of calcium channels and by mobilization of intracellular calcium stores.[29] Conversely, the calcium channel blockers nimodipine, verapamil, and diltiazem antagonize the inhibitory effect of DA in vitro.[30] However, administration of the calcium channel blocker verapamil to humans causes an *increase* in serum PRL levels[31,32] and does *not* inhibit the TRH-induced increase in PRL.[32] This effect was shown to be due to a decrease in tuberoinfundibular generation of DA.[33] Dihydropyridine and benzothiazepine calcium channel blockers have no effect on PRL levels in humans,[33] and it is likely that the effect of verapamil is via action at N-type calcium channels present in neuronal tissues.[33]

Vasoactive intestinal peptide (VIP) stimulates PRL release primarily through stimulation of adenyl cyclase and the production of intracellular cAMP.[34,35]

HORMONE BIOSYNTHESIS

The mature PRL messenger RNA (mRNA) formed after nuclear processing of the original heteronuclear RNA is only approximately 1 kb long and codes for a 227–amino acid sequence that includes an initial 28–amino acid signal peptide and the 199–amino acid structural peptide.[9,10]

There is considerable heterogeneity in the final PRL product, depending on variations in the extent of post-translational modifications (which include cleavage, polymerization, glycosylation, phosphorylation, and degradation). Approximately 80% to 90% of PRL extractable from pituitaries and in serum is monomeric, 8% to 20% is dimeric (molecular mass, 45-50 kDa) and 1% to 5% is polymeric.[36,37] These higher–molecular-weight polymers have decreased binding to receptors and show decreased bioactivity in a variety of receptor assays,[36,37] but have normal bioactivity in the Nb_2 lymphoma cell bioassay.[37] Some of the cleavage products of PRL have been found to have antiangiogenic function, but their physiologic significance is not clear.[38]

Several patients described as having elevated basal serum PRL levels but normal reproductive function were found to have elevated proportions of polymeric PRL. This "macroprolactinemia" presumably resulted in less PRL bioactivity.[39-42] In other cases, the higher–molecular-weight moieties consist of monomeric PRL bound to immunoglobulin[43]; however, in many such reported cases, the proportion of monomeric PRL in the blood is still elevated (see "Clinical Testing of Hyperprolactinemic Patients").

DECIDUAL PROLACTIN

Prolactin levels in maternal blood increase throughout gestation and are of pituitary origin.[44,45] However, PRL concentrations in amniotic fluid are 10- to 100-fold higher than either maternal or fetal blood levels.[44] Cultured human chorion and decidual cells synthesize and release a PRL into the amniotic fluid that is identical to pituitary PRL in structure and bioactivity.[46-49] Decidual PRL mRNA is indistinguishable from pituitary PRL mRNA, except for four silent nucleotide differences, and the decidual *PRL* gene is approximately 150 nucleotides longer in the 5′ untranslated region.[50-52]

The regulation of decidual PRL production differs from that of pituitary PRL. DA agonists[53] and antagonists[54] given to the mother respectively decrease and increase maternal serum PRL levels, but have no effect on amniotic fluid PRL levels. Decidual PRL production is increased by progesterone and progesterone plus estrogen (but not estrogen alone),[51,55] insulin, insulin-like growth factor 1 (IGF-1), and relaxin.[51,56,57] The function of decidual PRL remains obscure, although there is some evidence that it may contribute to the osmoregulation of the amniotic fluid, fetal lung maturation, and uterine contractility and modulation of the uterine immune system.[58] Recent evidence suggests that decidual PRL may silence the expression of genes detrimental to pregnancy.[59] Interestingly, in some animal species, a large number of PRL-related genes in trophoblastic tissue have evolved whose products involve the coordination of maternal, extraembryonic, and fetal tissues, including immunologic activity.[60]

MEASUREMENT OF PROLACTIN

With conventional radioimmunoassays (RIAs), there is considerable variation in different laboratories in the measurement of PRL levels, and normal values need to be established for each laboratory.[61] Over the last decade, two-site immunoradiometric assays (IRMA) and chemi-luminometric assays (ICMA) have come into wide use because of improved sensitivity and precision and short incubation periods.

Hook Effect

In patients with large prolactinomas, very high PRL levels may saturate the antibodies in two-site assays, preventing the formation of the PRL–antibody sandwich. As a result, labeled antibody is lost and a falsely low PRL value may be reported.[62,63] St-Jean and colleagues noted this high-end "hook effect" in 5.6% of 69 patients believed to have clinically nonfunctioning adenomas.[62] Therefore, in patients with large macroadenomas, PRL assessments should always be performed in both undiluted and 1:100 diluted serum to exclude the hook effect when two-site assays are used.

Macroprolactin

Normally, more than 90% of PRL is present in serum as the 23-kDa monomer and less than 10% is in higher–molecular-weight forms (discussed earlier in section "Hormone Biosynthesis"). These large-molecular forms are referred to as *macroprolactin* and are usually composed of PRL bound to immunoglobulin (IgG), but sometimes it is in the form of oligomers.[64-66] The gold standard method of measurement is to put a serum sample on a gel chromatography sizing column.[65-67] However, another more easily done method is to add polyethylene glycol (PEG) to the serum; the higher–molecular-weight forms precipitate and the monomeric form is left in the supernatant.[64-68] However, this method is very assay-dependent.[69]

Some investigators have stated that in a patient with hyperprolactinemia, if the amount of PRL left after PEG precipitation is less than 50% or 40%, then the hyperprolactinemia is caused by macroprolactin.[68] However, others have suggested that, because some macroprolactin is present in normal serum or some monomer is precipitated with PEG, the "normal" range should be recalculated from normal samples after PEG treatment; therefore, hyperprolactinemia can be attributed to macroprolactin only when the level of nonprecipitated PRL is within the normal range.[70] It is clear that in many studies, even when the amount of nonprecipitated PRL is less than 40% of the total, the level is still above the normal range.

An important issue is the bioactivity of the macroprolactin because it is implied that it is of no biologic significance. In most series of patients with macroprolactin, there tend to be fewer symptoms in those whose hyperprolactinemia has been attributed to macroprolactin than in those with true hyperprolactinemia.[67-71] When macroprolactin is put into the rat Nb2 lymphoma cell culture system, a standard in vitro prolactin bioassay system, macroprolactin tends to have the same bioassayable activity as monomeric PRL.[72] However, when bioassays are used in which the human PRL receptor was stably transfected and expressed in murine Ba/F-3 cells or human embryonic kidney-derived 293 (HEK-293) cells, the bioactivity of macroprolactin was shown to be decreased.[73,74]

In studies in which patients with hyperprolactinemia believed to be due (often in retrospect) to macroprolactin have been treated with DA agonists, galactorrhea, when present, has generally disappeared, but oligo/amenorrhea has been variably responsive.[67,68,70,71] Long-term follow-up studies of patients diagnosed with macroprolactinemia shows considerable instability of levels (up to fivefold).[67]

In clinical practice, if a patient has relatively typical symptoms, such as galactorrhea, amenorrhea, or impotence, and is found to have mild hyperprolactinemia, the usual exclusions should be looked for (medication history, hypothyroidism, elevated creatinine, pregnancy—discussed in section "Pathologic States of Prolactin Secretion"), and then the patient should have a magnetic resonance imaging scan, primarily to exclude a large lesion, such as a craniopharyngioma or clinically nonfunctioning adenoma. If the patient has equivocal symptoms (such as headaches or decreased libido) but has normal menses and no galactorrhea and is found to have mild hyperprolactinemia, assessment for macroprolactin using PEG would seem reasonable. The decision that the hyperprolactinemia is due to macroprolactin then would consist of finding an abnormal amount of PEG-precipitable PRL as well as an absolute level or monomer that is within the normal range. Only in such a patient would an MRI scan not be indicated, but such patients should continue to be followed carefully.

HORMONE SECRETION PATTERNS

Episodic Secretion

Prolactin is secreted episodically. There are 13 to 14 peaks per day in young subjects, with a peak duration lasting 67 to 76 minutes, a mean peak amplitude of 3 to 4 ng/mL, and an interpulse interval of 93 to 95 minutes.[75,76] Disinhibition seen with hypothalamic tumors causes an increase in basal PRL levels due to an increase in pulse amplitude, not pulse frequency.[77] There is an increase in the amplitude of the PRL secretory pulses that begins approximately 60 to 90 minutes after the onset of sleep; the secretory pulses increase with non–rapid eye movement (REM) sleep and fall before the next period of REM sleep.[78] An increase in circulating PRL levels of 50% to 100% occurs within 30 minutes of meals[79] due to the amino acids generated from the protein component of the meals, with phenylalanine, tyrosine, and glutamic acid being the most potent.[80]

Changes in Prolactin with Age

Prolactin levels are elevated almost 10-fold in infants after delivery due to the stimulatory effect of maternal estrogen, but then they gradually decrease so that levels are normal by 3 months of age.[81] PRL levels then rise modestly during puberty to adult levels.[81] PRL levels in women gradually fall by approximately 50% over the first 18 months after menopause, but this decrease is considerably less in women treated with estrogen replacement therapy[82] (although some studies have shown no change in PRL levels with hormone replacement therapy[83]). In hyperprolactinemic women, estrogen replacement therapy causes no change in PRL levels.[84] In men, mean serum PRL concentrations are approximately 50% lower in older men compared with younger men.[85]

Changes in Prolactin Levels during the Menstrual Cycle

Some, but not all, subjects have higher PRL levels at mid-cycle and lower levels in the follicular phase.[44,61,86-89] Some studies have shown that PRL and LH secretion are often synchronous in the luteal phase and that very small doses of gonadotropin-releasing hormone (GnRH) can cause the secretion of both PRL and LH at this time.[90]

Changes in Prolactin Levels during Pregnancy

Basal PRL levels gradually increase throughout the course of pregnancy.[44,45] This has generally been attributed to the stimulatory effect of the hormonal milieu of pregnancy (primarily estrogenic), causing lactotroph hyperplasia.[2,3] By term, PRL levels may be increased 10-fold to more than 200 ng/mL,[44,45,81] preparing the breast for lactation.

Changes in Prolactin Levels with Postpartum Lactation

Within the first 4 to 6 weeks postpartum, basal PRL levels remain elevated in lactating women and each suckling episode triggers a rapid release of pituitary PRL.[44,91] Over the next 4 to 12 weeks, basal PRL levels gradually decrease to normal, whereas the PRL increase that occurs with each suckling episode is gradually extinguished.[44,91] The decreases in basal and stimulated PRL levels between 3 and 6 months postpartum are largely the result of decreased breast-feeding as formula is introduced into the baby's diet. If intense nursing behavior is maintained, basal PRL levels remain elevated and postpartum amenorrhea persists.[92] High-intensity lactation–induced failure to ovulate and menstruate has long been used as a method of contraception in a number of developing countries.[92]

Breast stimulation may cause an increase in PRL levels in some healthy women who are not breast-feeding; such increases have not been found in men,[91,93] except for one study showing PRL increases in men after breast stimulation by their wives.[93]

Changes in Prolactin Secretion with Stress

Prolactin is one of the pituitary hormones released by stress, along with adrenocorticotropic hormone (ACTH) and GH. The stress-induced increase in PRL in humans generally results in a doubling or tripling of PRL levels and lasts less than 1 hour.[94] However, prolonged critical illness does *not* cause a sustained elevation of PRL; rather, there is a reduction in the pulsatile secretion with an overall lowering of levels.[95] Acute exercise has also been regarded as a form of stress and results in an acute, transient increase in PRL levels.[94] Although chronic, high-level exercise, such as occurs in runners training for a marathon, is often associated with menstrual disturbances, it is not associated with sustained hyperprolactinemia.[96]

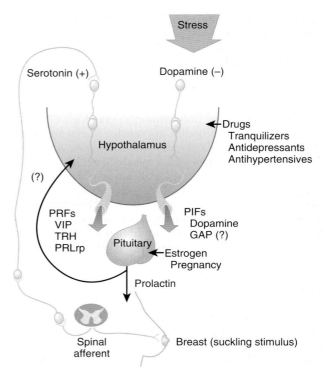

Figure 3-1. Regulation of prolactin (PRL) secretion. PRL release is stimulated by a number of PRL-releasing factors (PRFs), including vasoactive intestinal peptide (VIP), thyrotropin-releasing hormone (TRH), and PRL-releasing peptide (PRLrp), and is inhibited by PRL-inhibiting factors (PIFs), predominantly dopamine, but possibly also by the 56–amino acid peptide portion of the precursor to gonadotropin-releasing hormone (GnRH), known as GnRH-associated peptide (GAP). Estrogens and the hormonal milieu of pregnancy are also stimulatory to PRL production. The primary target organ for PRL is the breast. Suckling activates neural afferent pathways to the hypothalamus, where appropriate increases in PRFs or decreases in PIFs effect PRL release in the puerperium. Within the hypothalamus, serotoninergic pathways are stimulatory and dopaminergic pathways are inhibitory to PRL release. (Reproduced from Molitch ME. Disorders of prolactin secretion. Endocrinol Metab Clin North Am 2001;30, 585-610, with permission.)

Neuroendocrine Regulation

The hypothalamus exerts a predominantly inhibitory influence on PRL secretion through one or more PIFs that reach the pituitary via the hypothalamic–pituitary portal vessels (Fig. 3-1). There are PRL-releasing factors (PRFs) as well. Disruption of the pituitary stalk leads to a moderate increase in PRL secretion in addition to decreased secretion of the other pituitary hormones.

PROLACTIN INHIBITORY FACTORS

Dopamine

Dopamine is the predominant physiologic PIF. The concentration of DA found in the pituitary stalk plasma (approximately 6 ng/mL) is sufficient to decrease PRL levels and is 5- to 10-fold higher than levels found in peripheral plasma.[97] Stimuli that result in an acute release of PRL usually also result in an acute decline in portal vessel DA levels.[98-100] In most physiologic circumstances that cause a rise in PRL, such as lactation, there is likely to be a fall in DA along with a simultaneous rise in PRFs (such as VIP).[101]

Experiments in mice in which the DA D_2 receptor or DA transporter has been "knocked out" (KO) with inactivating mutations have confirmed the results of earlier studies that used pharmacologic methods or lesioning. DA D_2 receptor-KO mice have lactotroph hyperplasia with scattered multifocal prolactinomas and sustained hyperprolactinemia.[102-104] DA action within the synapse terminates as a result of DA reuptake by the DA-secreting neurons via the DA transporter. In contrast to the findings with the DA receptor-KO mice, DA transporter-KO mice have increased dopaminergic tone and lactotroph hypoplasia.[105] Although such mice have normal circulating levels of PRL, these levels cannot increase in response to various stimuli and the mice are therefore unable to lactate.[105]

In humans, infusion of DA causes a rapid suppression of basal and stimulated PRL levels.[106,107] Studies of low-dose DA infusions in humans have shown that DA blood concentrations similar to those found in rat and monkey hypothalamic–pituitary portal blood[97,108] are able to suppress PRL secretion.[109,110] Blockade of endogenous DA receptors by a variety of drugs causes a rise in PRL.[111,112]

The axons responsible for the release of DA into the median eminence originate in the dorsal portion of the arcuate nucleus and the inferior portion of the ventromedial nucleus of the hypothalamus. These axons terminate in the median eminence, a pathway known as the *tuberoinfundibular DA (TIDA) pathway*.[113,114] The DA that traverses the TIDA pathway binds to the D_2 DA receptors on the lactotroph cell membrane.[114]

The inhibitory action of DA on PRL secretion is partially blocked by estrogen administration. This is largely because of the direct action of estrogen on the estrogen response element of the *PRL* gene, as previously mentioned. Judd and coworkers found that infusions of DA into women during the early follicular phase (when estrogen levels are low) resulted in a greater suppression of PRL than infusions of the same dose administered during the late follicular or periovulatory phase (when estrogen levels are higher).[115]

Other Inhibitory Factors

Whether DA alone can account for all of the PIF activity of the hypothalamus has long been a question. Inhibitory activity has been shown by GnRH-associated protein (GAP), a peptide in the carboxyterminal region of the precursor to GnRH,[116] and by γ-aminobutyric acid (GABA)[117,118] in various experimental studies, but their physiologic importance in the human remains unknown.

PROLACTIN-RELEASING FACTORS

Thyrotropin-Releasing Hormone

Thyrotropin-releasing hormone causes a rapid release of PRL from pituitary cell cultures[119] and humans after intravenous injection.[120] The smallest dose of TRH that releases TSH also releases PRL in humans.[121] However,

immunoneutralization of endogenous TRH with TRH antisera only causes suppression of basal PRL levels in rats in some studies[122] but not in others[123,124]; mice with targeted disruption of the *TRH* gene (TRH-KO) become hypothyroid, but have normal PRL levels.[125] Suckling causes an increase in PRL but not in TSH.[126] On the other hand, in hypothyroidism, basal TSH and PRL levels are elevated,[127] with both being normalized by thyroxine treatment.[127,128] Conversely, in hyperthyroidism, PRL levels are not low basally, but the PRL response to TRH is markedly blunted and returns to normal with correction of the hyperthyroidism.[127,128] These conflicting data support a role for TRH as a physiologic PRF, albeit not the primary one or even one of major physiologic importance.

Vasoactive Intestinal Peptide and Peptide Histidine Methionine

Vasoactive intestinal peptide stimulates PRL synthesis and release from pituitary cell preparations and humans in vivo.[129-133] VIP neuronal perikarya are present in the paraventricular nucleus, with axons terminating in the external zone of the median eminence.[134] Passive immunoneutralization with anti-VIP antisera in rats partially inhibits the PRL responses to suckling, ether-induced stress,[135,136] and estrogen.[137] This same type of VIP immunoneutralization in DA receptor-blocked rats suppresses PRL pulsatile secretion.[138] Similar results for suckling have been obtained with a VIP antagonist.[139]

Within the VIP precursor is another similarly sized peptide known as *peptide histidine methionine* (PHM).[140] PHM and VIP colocalize in the hypothalamus and median eminence.[141] PHM given to humans has caused a PRL increment in some experiments,[141] but not in others.[133]

Complicating the role of VIP as a PRF is the finding that VIP is actually synthesized by anterior pituitary tissue.[142] Antisera to VIP inhibit basal PRL secretion from dispersed pituitary cells in vitro,[143,144] suggesting a local "autocrine" role for VIP in PRL regulation within the pituitary. The precise physiologic roles of VIP versus PHM and hypothalamic VIP versus pituitary VIP are still not clear.

Serotonin

Serotonin and its precursor, 5-hydroxytryptophan, cause a release of PRL in rats, whether injected systemically[145] or into the third ventricle.[146] A variety of experiments using blockers of serotonin synthesis, receptors, or reuptake by nerve terminals have shown that serotonin mediates, in part, the PRL elevations associated with suckling and proestrus.[147-149] In humans, infusion of the serotonin precursor, 5-hydroxytryptophan, results in a prompt increase in PRL levels.[150,151] Nocturnal PRL secretion is inhibited by cyproheptadine.[152] Fenfluramine, a serotonin-releasing agent, caused a fourfold rise in PRL in humans that could be partially blocked by cyproheptadine.[153] Fluoxetine, a serotonin reuptake inhibitor, also increases PRL levels modestly (with levels remaining within the normal range).[154] Although it is possible that serotonin is a direct secretagog for PRL, either through transport from the hypothalamus by the portal vessels or through an autocrine action within the pituitary, its role in this regard is still uncertain. Serotonin likely mediates, in part, the nocturnal surge of PRL; it may well participate in the suckling-induced rise in PRL through the ascending serotoninergic pathways from the dorsal raphe nucleus by causing VIP release.

Other Neuroactive Peptides and Neurotransmitters

Opioid Peptides. In rats, various opioid peptides cause the release of PRL.[155,156] Studies using specific agonists and antagonists have shown that the μ receptor is the predominant one involved in PRL release.[157,158] Most evidence suggests that the opioid peptides do not have a direct effect on the pituitary[156] and that they stimulate PRL release by inhibiting DA turnover and release by the TIDA pathway.[159,160] In humans, morphine and morphine analogs increase PRL release acutely[161] and chronically.[162] However, blockade of the μ receptor with naloxone has minimal to no effect on PRL levels, either basally or with stimulation by hypoglycemia, exercise, sleep, TRH, or physical stress.[163,164]

In contrast to these findings, two groups have reported an increase in PRL levels in response to naloxone given in the late follicular and midluteal phases of the menstrual cycle.[165,166] The interpretation of these changes is not straightforward, but overall, it appears that the endogenous opioid pathways play, at most, only a minor role in the regulation of PRL secretion.

Growth Hormone–Releasing Hormone. A number of studies have found GH-releasing hormone (GHRH) to have PRL-releasing properties. The initial clue to this action of GHRH came when patients with acromegaly due to GHRH-secreting tumors were found to be hyperprolactinemic and their PRL levels fell in parallel with GH after tumor excision.[167] GHRH has also been reported to release PRL in vivo in healthy humans,[168] and long-term therapy with GHRH in children with GH neurosecretory dysfunction results in a sustained elevation of PRL levels.[169] Although large amounts of GHRH clearly can release PRL, the physiologic significance of these observations remains unknown.

Posterior Pituitary, Oxytocin, and Vasopressin. Studies in animals have shown that oxytocin, in levels found in the hypothalamic–pituitary portal vessels, can stimulate PRL release when added to the incubation medium of pituitary cells or when given intravenously; however, it lowers PRL levels when directly injected into the third ventricle.[170] Studies in which endogenous oxytocin was eliminated by passive immunization with oxytocin antisera or by administration of oxytocin antagonists show a reduction and a delay in the suckling-induced PRL surges.[170] Very limited studies in humans suggest that oxytocin administered intravenously has no effect on basal PRL levels and causes only a minimal increase in TRH-stimulated PRL levels.[171]

To date, there are no studies of the effects of vasopressin on PRL secretion in humans. Whether there are other PRFs in the posterior pituitary in addition to oxytocin, vasopressin, and their respective neurophysins has been a matter of controversy.

Gonadotropin-Releasing Hormone. Gonadotropin-releasing hormone releases PRL from rat pituitary cells in vitro.[172] GnRH has been found to cause a release of PRL in anovulatory women[173,174] and in women with anorexia nervosa who were gaining weight.[175] In 24% to 78% of normal women, there is a PRL response to GnRH; this response is dependent on the phase of the menstrual cycle, with the highest number of subjects responding in the periovulatory phase.[176]

Postmenopausal women also have a PRL response to GnRH that is augmented with estrogen supplementation.[177] There is no PRL release in response to GnRH in healthy, eugonadal men, but such a release does occur in transsexual men who receive high doses of estrogen.[178] Analysis of PRL and LH secretory pulses in women shows a high degree of concordance.[90] This cosecretion of LH and PRL suggests that the response to GnRH is physiologic and is evidence against a physiologic role for the inhibitory effect of cosecreted GAP.

Prolactin-Releasing Peptide. Hinuma and colleagues discovered a 31–amino acid peptide capable of releasing PRL that has been termed *prolactin-releasing peptide* (PrRP); the discovery came while the investigators were looking for endogenous ligands for an orphan receptor (termed *HGR3*) present in the human pituitary.[179] In pituitary cell preparations, PrRP released PRL with a potency equal to that of TRH.[179] However, although PrRP is found in neuronal perikarya in the paraventricular and supraoptic nuclei, PrRP-immunoreactive nerve fibers are found only in the internal zone of the median eminence and not the external zone,[180] casting uncertainty on the physiologic significance of this peptide with respect to PRL secretion. In subsequent studies, PrRP has been shown to affect the hypothalamic–pituitary–adrenal axis stress response and feeding behavior.[181]

Other Neuroactive Peptides and Neurotransmitters. There is evidence that several other neuropeptides and neurotransmitters affect PRL secretion in a variety of experimental paradigms in animals, including angiotensin, neurotensin, substance P, cholecystokinin, bombesin, secretin, gastrin, galanin, endothelin, somatostatin, relaxin, melatonin, basic fibroblast-growth factor, bradykinin, calcitonin, calcitonin gene-related peptide, histamine, norepinephrine, and acetylcholine. However, their physiologic significance, especially in humans, is unknown.

PROLACTIN SHORT-LOOP FEEDBACK

Experiments conducted in rats suggest that PRL is able to feed back negatively on its own secretion (*short-loop feedback* or *autofeedback*).[182] Most evidence suggests that such feedback occurs via augmentation of hypothalamic TIDA turnover.[183] Direct confirmation of the importance of short-loop feedback in rodents comes from recent studies using mice with targeted disruption of the *PRL* gene

(*PRL* gene-KO mice). Mice with the *PRL* KO have no pituitary PRL and have markedly decreased DA in TIDA neurons, along with hyperplasia of lactotrophs that do not make PRL.[184-186] Direct evidence for such PRL short-loop feedback in the human has not been shown. However, it has been suggested that altered regulation of gonadotropin and TSH secretion in hyperprolactinemic patients may constitute indirect evidence of PRL-induced augmentation of TIDA activity.[187]

Prolactin Action

Prolactin has a great diversity of actions in many species of animals, including osmoregulation, growth and developmental effects, metabolic effects, actions on ectodermal and integumentary structures, and actions related to reproduction.[188] Its primary physiologic action in humans, however, is the preparation of the breast for lactation in the postpartum period.[189] Elevated levels of PRL affect many tissues, and PRL receptors are found in many tissues.

PROLACTIN RECEPTORS

The *PRL receptor* is a member of the class 1 cytokine receptor family. The human PRL receptor gene has 10 exons, with exons 3 to 10 encoding the full length of the long form of the receptor.[190] A hydrophobic region of the receptor (amino acids 211-234) corresponds to the single-transmembrane–spanning region of the receptor.[191] Two isoforms of the PRL receptor result from alternative splicing and differ in the length and composition of the cytoplasmic tail, being referred to as the *long* and *intermediate* forms; the short form found in the mouse is not present in humans.[192]

Prolactin binds to its receptor with high affinity, the dissociation constant (K_d) being 10^{-10} mol/L.[192] Half-saturation of the receptor occurs at a hormone concentration of 7 ng/mL.[192] PRL binding causes dimerization of the receptor, a necessary step for signaling.[192]

Prolactin receptors are widely distributed throughout the body, being present in the breast, pituitary, liver, kidney tubules, adrenal cortex, prostate, ovary, testes, seminal vesicles, epididymis, intestine, skin, pancreatic islets, lymphocytes, lung, myocardium, and brain.[192] PRL release caused by suckling increases PRL receptor levels in the breast and liver, resulting in much greater PRL-binding activity in lactating animals than in those not lactating.[192] Signal transduction of the activated, dimerized receptor involves the JAK-STAT pathway.[192] Activation of the mitogen-activated protein kinase cascade has also been reported after receptor activation, but whether this involves JAK 2 is unknown.[192]

The physiologic roles of PRL in most of the tissues in which receptors are present are not known. Although some have suggested that PRL may play a role in the development of breast and other cancers, this has not been firmly established. Future research with PRL receptor antagonists acting at the tissue level may allow a more clear delineation of additional physiologic and pathologic functions of PRL.[193]

PROLACTIN EFFECTS ON THE BREAST

Prolactin, GH, cortisol, insulin, estrogen, progesterone, and thyroxine all contribute to breast development. The high concentrations of estrogen and progesterone produced by the placenta, coupled with the estrogen-induced high concentration of circulating PRL and the high concentrations of placental lactogen, cause development of the lobular alveolar tissue during pregnancy.[189] Once the breast is fully developed and hormonally primed, PRL stimulates the production of milk proteins and other components.[189] Before term, the high estrogen levels suppress the effects of the high PRL levels on milk production, but the rapid decrease in estrogen levels after delivery allows milk production to proceed.[194] Bromocriptine-induced suppression of this physiologic hyperprolactinemia in the puerperium causes a rapid cessation of milk production.[195] The key role of PRL in milk formation has been shown by the finding that mice with either the *PRL* gene KO[184] or the PRL receptor KO[196] are unable to lactate.

Galactorrhea

The persistence of galactorrhea for more than 1 year after normal delivery and cessation of breast-feeding or its occurrence in the absence of pregnancy generally is taken as a definition of inappropriate lactation. The incidence of galactorrhea in healthy women has been reported as 1% to 45% in subjects tested.[197,198] This variability probably is the result of differences in the techniques used to express milk from the breast and the way in which nonmilky secretions are classified.

Inappropriate lactation may be an important clue to the presence of pituitary–hypothalamic disease, especially if accompanied by amenorrhea. Combined data from 14 published series suggest that 27.9% of galactorrheic women with normal menses have elevated PRL levels.[199] More recent experience, however, suggests that galactorrhea may be present in approximately 5% to 10% of normally menstruating women and that basal PRL levels are normal in more than 90% of these women. Decreasing PRL levels will almost always lead to a marked decrease or abolition of lactation, regardless of whether PRL levels are initially elevated.

PROLACTIN EFFECTS ON GONADOTROPIN SECRETION

The effects of PRL levels in the normal range on gonadotropin secretion are not known. However, *PRL* gene-KO and PRL receptor-KO female mice are sterile and have disordered estrous cycles.[184,196] Females with the PRL receptor KO had fewer primary follicles, fewer eggs ovulated, fewer eggs fertilized, poorer progression of those eggs that were fertilized to the blastocyst stage, and uteruses that were refractory to implantation by the blastocyst.[196] Furthermore, they had decreased estradiol and progesterone levels.[200]

In healthy women treated with short-term bromocriptine to lower PRL levels to approximately 5 ng/mL, there was no change in the pulsatile secretion of LH and FSH,

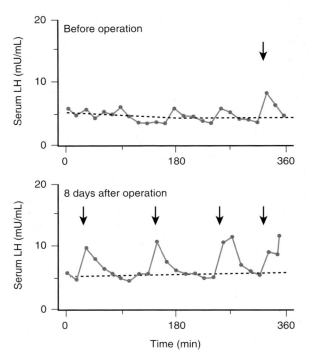

Figure 3-2. *Pre- and postoperative serum luteinizing hormone (LH) concentrations after selective resection of a prolactinoma. The start of an LH pulse is indicated by an* arrow. *(Reproduced by copyright permission from the Endocrine Society from Stevenaert A, Beckers A, Vandalem JL, et al. Early normalization of luteinizing hormone pulsatility after successful transsphenoidal surgery in women with microprolactinomas. J Clin Endocrinol Metab 1986;62:1044-1047.)*

but estradiol levels were higher the last 3 days of the follicular cycle. Progesterone levels were lower during the luteal phase.[201]

Hyperprolactinemia has a number of effects on various steps in the reproductive axis. Hyperprolactinemia has been found in most studies to suppress LH pulsatile secretion (Fig. 3-2) by decreasing pulse amplitude and frequency.[202-204] With menopause in humans, hyperprolactinemia can prevent the expected rise in gonadotropins[205]; normalization of PRL levels with bromocriptine results in elevation of gonadotropin levels and hot flashes.[205]

Hyperprolactinemia inhibits pulsatile gonadotropin secretion by a number of mechanisms. It had been postulated that the pulsatile gonadotropin secretion was directed by the hypothalamic GnRH pulse generator and that alteration of pulsatile secretion necessarily means a direct hypothalamic action of PRL. Consistent with that notion, PRL inhibits GnRH release from hypothalamic neuron cell lines through an action on PRL receptors expressed by these cells.[206] Measurement of portal vessel GnRH levels in rats showed a marked inhibitory effect of hyperprolactinemia in one study,[207] but not in another.[208]

The pituitary gonadotroph response to GnRH in hyperprolactinemia has generally been found to be decreased in rats[208,209]; in contrast, the response may be normal, increased, or decreased in humans.[210,211] The number of GnRH receptors on gonadotroph cells in hyperprolactinemic rats

is reduced,[212] even when endogenous GnRH is replaced with intra-arterial pulses of GnRH.[205,213] In addition to these effects, hyperprolactinemia in women has been associated with loss of positive estrogen feedback on gonadotropin secretion.[214]

PROLACTIN EFFECTS ON THE OVARY

Prolactin is trophic to corpus luteum function in rats, giving rise to the name *luteotrophic hormone*.[215] The role of PRL in normal ovarian function in humans is not as well established, however. McNatty and coworkers showed that low physiologic concentrations of PRL are necessary for progesterone synthesis by human granulosa cells, but that high concentrations are inhibitory in vitro.[216] Other studies suggest that PRL can activate the expression of type 2 β-hydroxysteroid dehydrogenase, the final enzymatic step in progesterone biosynthesis.[217] Del Pozo and coworkers found no effect on luteal function in women treated with bromocriptine to lower normal PRL levels[218]; others, however, have found that such a decrease in PRL resulted in lowered progesterone levels and short luteal phases.[203,219,220] On the other hand, short luteal phases have also been reported in hyperprolactinemic women.[221]

In humans, plasma PRL levels greater than 100 ng/mL have been found to cause an increase of antral fluid PRL levels and reductions in antral fluid FSH and estradiol levels and a decrease in the number of granulosa cells.[222] Perfusion studies of human ovaries in vitro show a direct suppressive effect of PRL on progesterone and estrogen secretion.[223] PRL can inhibit estrogen formation by antagonizing the stimulatory effects of FSH on aromatase activity[224]; direct inhibition of aromatase synthesis has also been shown.[225]

In early studies, PRL levels were found to be elevated in 19% to 50% of women with a polycystic ovary (PCO).[226,227] Bromocriptine treatment of hyperprolactinemic patients with a PCO usually resulted in a reduction of testosterone and LH levels and often a resumption of ovulatory cycles. One hypothesis suggests that the increased estrogen levels found in PCO stimulate increased PRL secretion,[227] but the association between PCO and hyperprolactinemia has been questioned.[228]

When amenorrhea or oligo/amenorrhea is associated with galactorrhea, it usually is a manifestation of hyperprolactinemia. In combined series totaling 471 patients with galactorrhea/amenorrhea, 75.4% were found to have hyperprolactinemia.[199] Although the amenorrhea caused by hyperprolactinemia usually is secondary, it may be primary if the disorder begins before the usual age of puberty.[229,230] In two studies of 33 patients evaluated for primary amenorrhea and low gonadotropin levels, 9 (27%) were found to have hyperprolactinemia.[229,230] In patients with primary amenorrhea due to hyperprolactinemia, failure to develop normal secondary sexual characteristics may be the presenting problem. Galactorrhea is variable in this setting because the breast may not have been exposed to appropriate priming with estrogen and progesterone. Young women with hyperprolactinemia and primary amenorrhea tend to have macroadenomas more commonly than those with secondary amenorrhea; the reason for this difference remains uncertain.

Hyperprolactinemia has been found in many women with a short luteal phase, as noted previously. A short luteal phase is likely to be the first evidence of interference in the normal cycle by hyperprolactinemia.[231] In the initial period of shortened luteal phase, progesterone levels are subnormal, suggesting deficient corpus luteum function.

Infertility also may be a presenting symptom of patients with hyperprolactinemia and is invariable when gonadotropin levels are suppressed with anovulation. In women (367 women combined from multiple studies) studied for infertility, one third were found to have hyperprolactinemia.[199] Most of the women had amenorrhea and galactorrhea as well, but in one series of 113 cases of infertility, 5 of the 22 hyperprolactinemic women had neither amenorrhea nor galactorrhea.[232] PRL excess may be important in this type of patient, as suggested by the finding that treatment of similar patients with bromocriptine restored fertility.[232] In some of these women, transient hyperprolactinemia lasting for 1 to 2 days during the cycle can be documented; this subset usually responded to bromocriptine, experiencing increased progesterone during the luteal phase and improved fertility.[233]

Reduced libido and orgasmic dysfunction are found in most hyperprolactinemic amenorrheic women when such complaints are specifically elicited.[210] Reduction of PRL levels to normal restores normal libido and sexual function in most of these women.[234]

PROLACTIN EFFECTS ON THE TESTES

The role of PRL in normal testicular function is not well understood. Half of the male rats with PRL receptor-KO mutations were fully fertile, but the remainder were either completely or partially infertile, despite normal sexual behavior and normal spermatogenesis (as determined by histologic evaluation of the testes).[196] Male mice with the *PRL* gene KO were fully fertile and had normal plasma testosterone levels and normal testosterone release from the testes, despite decreased plasma LH levels and LH and FSH secretion from the pituitary in vitro and decreased weights of the seminal vesicles and ventral prostate.[235]

In studies of healthy men, bromocriptine-induced suppression of normal PRL levels for 8 weeks resulted in suppression of basal and human chorionic gonadotropin (hCG)-stimulated testosterone levels.[236] This finding implies a physiologic role for PRL in normal testosterone production in humans. PRL is present in human semen in very high concentrations,[237] and PRL has been shown to stimulate adenyl cyclase, fructose use, glycolysis, and glucose oxidation in human spermatozoa.[238]

Chronic hyperprolactinemia results in impotence and decreased libido in more than 90% of cases.[239-247] Galactorrhea in men has been reported in 10% to 20% of cases and is virtually pathognomonic of a prolactinoma.[239-246,248] As previously noted, there is a decrease in the pulsatile secretion of LH and FSH in hyperprolactinemic men, and testosterone levels are low or are in the lower part of the normal range.[239-248] With normalization of PRL levels with cabergoline, testosterone levels normalize in

approximately two thirds of men and erectile function normalizes in 60%.[249]

The testosterone response to stimulation with hCG has been reported to be both decreased[243,250] and normal[239,251]; in those with decreased responses, there is improvement in the response when PRL levels are lowered with bromocriptine.[243] If there is sufficient normal pituitary tissue, reduction of elevated PRL levels to normal usually results in a return of normal testosterone levels.[244-246,252,253] Although some studies in rats have suggested that drug-induced elevated PRL levels cause a partial block of the enzyme 5α reductase, resulting in a decrease in dihydrotestosterone levels, this has not been found in studies in men with prolactinomas.[250] Carter and colleagues noted that testosterone therapy in hyperprolactinemic men does not always correct the impotence until PRL levels are brought down to normal.[239] Whether this is due to a decrease in dihydrotestosterone levels has not been verified directly.

Sperm count and motility are decreased, with an increase in abnormal forms, in hyperprolactinemic men.[249,251] Histologic studies show abnormal seminiferous tubule walls and altered Sertoli cell ultrastructure.[254] Results of semen analysis do not always return to normal, despite normalization of testosterone and PRL levels.[249,252]

A number of surveys have attempted to assess the frequency of hyperprolactinemia among men with complaints of impotence or infertility. Between 2% and 25% of men with impotence have been found to be hyperprolactinemic in various series.[232,243,245,255-258] However, only 1% to 5% of infertile men have been found to be hyperprolactinemic.[259-261] Although these frequencies are relatively low, the modest cost of measuring PRL is justified, given that hyperprolactinemia is, in general, easily treatable.

PROLACTIN EFFECTS ON THE ADRENAL CORTEX

Although PRL receptors are found on cells of the adrenal cortex, the physiologic role of PRL in adrenal steroidogenesis is unknown. Plasma dehydroepiandrosterone (DHEA) and DHEA sulfate (DHEAS) levels have been found to be mildly elevated in approximately 50% of women with hyperprolactinemia in most,[262-264] but not all, studies.[265-267] In most of these studies, however, the investigators did not try to correlate the androgen levels with the presence of hirsutism or other indices of hyperandrogenism. The abnormal androgen levels return to normal with correction of the hyperprolactinemia by bromocriptine.[232]

PROLACTIN EFFECTS ON BONES

Prolactin may have a physiologic role in calcium and bone metabolism. The PRL receptor-KO mouse has a decrease in bone formation rate and bone mineral density in association with increased parathyroid hormone levels, but also has decreased estradiol and progesterone levels.[200] Thus, it is difficult to know how much of the abnormal bone metabolism is attributable to the inability to respond to PRL as opposed to estrogen deficiency.

Hyperprolactinemic women have decreased bone mineral density,[268-270] but whether this effect is mediated by estrogen deficiency[268] or is a direct effect of the hyperprolactinemia[269,270] has been debated. Correction of the hyperprolactinemia results in an increase in bone mass.[271,272] Studies of hyperprolactinemic women who were not amenorrheic and hypoestrogenemic have shown that their bone mineral density is normal,[273,274] confirming the initial hypothesis that estrogen deficiency mediates the bone mineral loss. A similar, androgen-dependent loss of bone mineral is found in hyperprolactinemic men and is reversible with reversal of the hypoandrogenic state.[275]

PROLACTIN EFFECTS ON THE IMMUNE SYSTEM

Prolactin is produced by T and B lymphocytes, but its synthesis is under control of an alternative upstream promoter.[276] In animal studies, lowering of normal PRL levels by bromocriptine or anti-PRL antibodies results in impaired lymphocyte proliferation and macrophage-activating factor production,[277] but in *PRL* gene-KO and PRL receptor-KO mice, PRL has not been found to be essential for normal immune function.[278,279] Conversely, in rat models of systemic lupus erythematosus, PRL levels are elevated and bromocriptine causes improvement in a variety of autoimmune parameters.[280-282]

Studies in humans have been conflicting. Some studies of patients with hyperprolactinemia have shown increased rates of autoantibodies (including antithyroid, anti–double-stranded DNA, anti-Ro, anticardiolipin, and antinuclear antibodies), without clinical evidence of disease.[283-285] Conversely, elevated levels of PRL have been found in patients with systemic lupus erythematosus, rheumatoid arthritis, psoriatic arthritis, multiple sclerosis, Reiter's syndrome, Sjögren's syndrome, and uveitis.[285-288] In some studies, conventional immunosuppressive treatment of these disorders resulted in a lowering of PRL levels, and conversely, treatment with bromocriptine resulted in clinical improvement in the autoimmune condition (see Chuang and Molitch for a detailed review).[289] Although PRL appears to have an immunomodulatory function, the relationship of pituitary versus lymphocytic PRL to these autoimmune conditions in humans is still uncertain, and some aspects of treatment remain to be established.

PATHOLOGIC STATES OF PROLACTIN SECRETION

Hypoprolactinemia

Prolactin deficiency may occur in the setting of panhypopituitarism, generally as a result of pituitary infarction or after pituitary surgery. When the cause of the hypopituitarism is hypothalamic or stalk dysfunction, PRL levels generally rise due to disinhibition of PRL secretion (discussed in section "Hypothalamic-Pituitary Stalk Disease"). However, when the pituitary tissue is actually destroyed, as in Sheehan's peripartum necrosis, PRL levels are usually low.[290] The finding of low PRL levels after surgery for a pituitary tumor usually is indicative of very severe hypopituitarism.[291] Idiopathic PRL deficiency has been described in only a single human.[292] Clinically, hypoprolactinemia manifests as an inability to lactate postpartum.

Hyperprolactinemia

The differential diagnosis of sustained hyperprolactinemia encompasses a spectrum of pharmacologic and pathologic entities (Box 3-1). This section discusses those causes of hyperprolactinemia other than prolactinomas.

BOX 3-1

Etiologies of Hyperprolactinemia

Pituitary Disease
Prolactinomas
Acromegaly
Empty sella syndrome
Lymphocytic hypophysitis
Cushing's disease

Hypothalamic Disease
Craniopharyngiomas
Meningiomas
Dysgerminomas
Nonsecreting pituitary adenomas
Other tumors
Sarcoidosis
Eosinophilic granuloma
Neuraxis irradiation
Vascular
Pituitary stalk section

Medications
Phenothiazines
Haloperidol
Risperidone
Monoamine oxidase inhibitors
Reserpine
Methyldopa
Metoclopramide
Tricyclic antidepressants
Cocaine
Verapamil

Neurogenic
Chest wall lesions
Spinal cord lesions
Breast stimulation

Other
Pregnancy
Hypothyroidism
Chronic renal failure
Cirrhosis
Pseudocyesis
Adrenal insufficiency
Ectopic

Idiopathic

Medications

Psychoactive Medications. The antipsychotic agents (phenothiazines and butyrophenones) are DA receptor blockers and uniformly result in elevated PRL levels, generally no higher than 100 ng/mL, but some patients have been reported with levels as high as 365 ng/mL.[111,112] PRL levels usually fall to normal within 48 to 96 hours of discontinuation of antipsychotic drug therapy.[293] Combined serotonin/dopamine receptor antagonists, such as risperidone and molindone, cause similar elevations of PRL.[294] However, many of the newer atypical antipsychotic agents, such as quetiapine, olanzapine, and aripiprazole, do not cause hyperprolactinemia, and when feasible, hyperprolactinemic patients may be switched to these drugs.[294-297]

Tricyclic antidepressants cause modest hyperprolactinemia in approximately 25% of patients.[298] Long-term use of monoamine oxidase inhibitors may also cause a minimal elevation of PRL levels.[299] The mechanisms by which these drugs cause increased PRL levels are not certain, and they likely facilitate several possible stimulatory pathways. Serotonin reuptake inhibitors, by increasing synaptic serotonin levels, very rarely cause hyperprolactinemia.[154,294,300,301] Other antidepressants, including nefazodone, bupropion, venlafaxine, trazodone, and lithium, do not cause hyperprolactinemia.[294] Chronic opiate abuse is associated with mild hyperprolactinemia and menstrual dysfunction.[294] Cocaine abuse has also been associated with chronic, mild hyperprolactinemia.[302]

Antihypertensive Drugs. Alpha-methyldopa causes moderate hyperprolactinemia by inhibiting the enzyme L-aromatic amino acid decarboxylase (which is responsible for converting L-dopa to DA) and by acting as a false neurotransmitter to decrease DA synthesis. Short-term and long-term verapamil therapy has been found to increase basal PRL secretion and the PRL response to TRH[31-33,303-305]; patients have been described with galactorrhea associated with sustained hyperprolactinemia as a result of verapamil therapy.[303,304] In a survey of patients taking verapamil in an outpatient clinic, PRL levels were found to be elevated in 8.5% of patients.[305] Verapamil blocks the hypothalamic generation of DA.[33] Other calcium channel blockers, such as the dihydropyridines and benzothiazepines, have no action on PRL secretion, implying that the action of the phenylakylamine, verapamil, likely is acting on the neuronal N-type calcium channel.[33]

Protease Inhibitors. Although one report showed that some HIV-positive patients treated with protease inhibitors had galactorrhea and hyperprolactinemia,[306] a second report implied that the elevations of PRL seen in some patients can largely be attributed to other medications and to stress.[307] The mechanism and frequency of this effect are unknown.

Stress

As previously mentioned, physical stress (such as physical discomfort, exercise, and hypoglycemia) causes an acute, transient rise in PRL levels (discussed earlier). Chronic hyperprolactinemia as a result of prolonged physical stress has not been reported, and chronic illness generally suppresses PRL levels. Psychological stress may cause minimal increases of PRL, but chronic hyperprolactinemia has not been reported with any chronic psychiatric state except pseudocyesis; in this condition, PRL levels fall with psychotherapy.[308]

Renal Disease

Hyperprolactinemia occurs in 73% to 91% of women and 25% to 57% of men with end-stage renal disease.[309,310] The hyperprolactinemia is due to decreased PRL clearance as well as autonomous production and bromocriptine results in suppression of PRL levels.[309] Approximately one fourth of individuals with renal insufficiency not requiring dialysis (serum creatinine, 2 to 12 ng/mL) have PRL levels of 25 to 100 ng/mL.[310] When such patients take medications known to alter hypothalamic regulation of PRL (such as methyldopa or metoclopramide), PRL levels may rise to more than 2000 ng/mL.[310] Correction of the renal failure with transplantation causes a return of PRL levels to normal.[310]

Cirrhosis

Basal PRL levels are elevated in patients with alcoholic cirrhosis in frequencies varying from 16% to 100%,[311-313] and in patients with nonalcoholic cirrhosis, they range from 5% to 13%.[311] In one study, 50% of patients with hepatic encephalopathy were found to be hyperprolactinemic.[314] An underlying defect in hypothalamic DA generation has been hypothesized as the cause of the hyperprolactinemia in these encephalopathic patients.

Hypothyroidism

Primary hypothyroidism is associated with a modest increase in the level of PRL in 40% of patients, but levels greater than 25 ng/mL are reached in only 10%.[315] The mechanisms involved probably include increased TRH production, increased sensitivity of lactotrophs to TRH, and possibly increased pituitary VIP generation. Therapy with L-thyroxine will cause the PRL levels to return to normal and can even result in a regression of pituitary size (which was due to thyrotroph hyperplasia).[316]

Adrenal Insufficiency

Glucocorticoids have a suppressive effect on *PRL* gene transcription and PRL release. Rare cases of hyperprolactinemia have been reported in patients with adrenal insufficiency whose PRL levels return to normal with glucocorticoid replacement.[317,318]

Neurogenic Stimulation

Sexual breast stimulation and suckling cause a reflex release of PRL that is mediated by afferent neural pathways going through the spinal cord. Chest wall and cervical cord lesions have been reported to result in elevated PRL levels and galactorrhea through stimulation of these afferent neural pathways.[319] Similar chronic elevations of PRL have been reported after mastectomy, nipple piercing, thoracotomy, and chronic spinal cord injuries.[320,321]

Ectopic Prolactin Secretion

Ectopic production of PRL is exceedingly rare[322]; however, there have been reported cases of symptomatic hyperprolactinemia due to well-documented PRL production from renal cell carcinoma,[323] gonadoblastoma,[324] and ectopic pituitary tissue in two ovarian teratomas.[325,326] Given the great frequency of prolactinomas, "idiopathic hyperprolactinemia," and other causes of hyperprolactinemia, a search for an ectopic source of PRL secretion is not warranted unless some other tumor is found coincidentally.

Hypothalamic–Pituitary Stalk Disease

Hyperprolactinemia caused by lesions of the hypothalamus and the pituitary stalk is due to disturbance of the neuroendocrine mechanisms that control PRL secretion.[327] From hypothalamic lesion work in animals, it has been assumed that this PRL elevation is due to disinhibition of the tonic PIF (DA) acting at the level of the pituitary lactotrophs. However, many of these patients have normal TSH and ACTH function, implying that there still is significant transmission of hypothalamic-releasing factors to the pituitary.

Generally, patients with total stalk section (in whom the increase in PRL is due solely to DA deficiency) have lower PRL levels than those with partial stalk–hypothalamic dysfunction who have DA plus continued PRF activity. In a recent series of 226 patients with clinically nonfunctioning pituitary adenomas, 99% had serum PRL levels less than 84 ng/mL.[328] However, a number of cases have been reported in the literature of PRL levels between 104 and 219 ng/mL.[327,329-331]

Idiopathic Hyperprolactinemia

When no specific cause for hyperprolactinemia is found, it is designated as *idiopathic*. In many such cases, small prolactinomas may be present that are too small to be detected by current radiologic techniques. In other cases, hyperprolactinemia may be attributed to presumed hypothalamic regulatory dysfunction, but no dysfunction specific to idiopathic hyperprolactinemia has been definitively elucidated. Long-term follow-up of such patients has found that in approximately one third, PRL levels return to normal; in 10% to 15%, there is a rise in PRL levels to greater than 50% over baseline; and in the remaining patients, prolactin levels remain stable.[332,333] Over a 2- to 6-year follow-up of 199 patients, only 23 were found to have evidence of microadenomas, and none had macroadenomas.[332-336]

CLINICAL TESTING OF HYPERPROLACTINEMIC PATIENTS

Because PRL is secreted episodically and some PRL levels during the day may be above the upper limit of normal established for a given laboratory, the finding of minimally elevated

levels in blood requires confirmation in several samples. As indicated in the previous section, there are a number of conditions that may cause moderate PRL elevations of less than 250 ng/mL. A careful history and physical examination, screening blood chemistries, thyroid function tests, and a pregnancy test will exclude virtually all causes except for hypothalamic–pituitary disease.[337] In cases with less certain symptoms, macroprolactinemia should be looked for (discussed earlier in section "Macroprolactinemia").

When there is no obvious cause of hyperprolactinemia from the routine screening, a radiologic evaluation of the hypothalamic–pituitary area is mandatory to evaluate for a mass lesion.[337] This includes patients with even mild PRL elevations. Currently, such an evaluation is generally done using magnetic resonance imaging with gadolinium enhancement or computed tomography (CT) with intravenous contrast enhancement. For prolactinomas, there is a fairly good correlation between PRL level and tumor size.[338] Patients with microprolactinomas rarely have PRL levels of more than 250 mg/dL.[338] It should be emphasized here that it is very important to distinguish between a large nonsecreting tumor causing modest PRL elevations (usually < 250 ng/mL) from a PRL-secreting macroadenoma (PRL level usually > 250 ng/mL), because the therapy may be quite different. It is important to have serum tested at 1:100 dilution in patients with large macroadenomas to exclude the "hook effect." Stimulation and suppression tests give nonspecific results with regard to the differential diagnosis of hyperprolactinemia and provide no more information than measurement of basal PRL levels.[337,339]

Prolactinoma

CLASSIFICATION AND EPIDEMIOLOGY

Prolactinomas are generally classified clinically by size: microadenomas are less than 10 mm in diameter; macroadenomas are greater than 10 mm in diameter; and macroadenomas have extrasellar extension. The direction and the degree of extrasellar extension are of obvious clinical importance. Serum PRL levels usually parallel tumor size.

Prolactinomas are the most common of the secreting pituitary adenomas, occurring with an incidence of 6 to 10 cases per million and a prevalence of 60 to 100 cases per million.[340] However, a recent series from Belgium reported a prevalence approximately 10 times higher.[341] Prolactinomas occur more commonly in women, in whom they generally are microadenomas, whereas those in men generally are macroadenomas (discussed later in the chapter).

NATURAL HISTORY OF PROLACTINOMAS

Autopsy Studies

Pituitary adenomas have been found at autopsy in approximately 11% of subjects not suspected of having pituitary disease while alive.[342] In the studies in which PRL immunohistochemistry was performed, 40% stained positively for PRL.[342] In these postmortem studies, all but three of the tumors (99.97%) were less than 10 mm in diameter; however, there are a number of clinical reports of incidentally found macroadenomas.[342]

Natural History of Untreated Prolactinomas

Six studies have been published in which patients with microadenomas were observed for long periods without treatment. In these studies, women who had prolactinomas documented by sella tomography or CT who refused surgery or medical treatment were followed for a period of up to 8 years.[343-348] Of the 139 women observed, there was evidence of tumor growth by these methods in only 9 (6.5%). In retrospect, we now know the high false-positive and false-negative rates associated with polytomography.

One potential stimulus to the growth of a microadenoma was hypothesized to be the use of oral contraceptives. However, careful case–control studies using normal or amenorrheic control subjects and long-term epidemiologic surveys have not shown such a relationship.[349] In other studies, estrogens were administered for 2 to 4 years to women with microadenomas and idiopathic hyperprolactinemia, resulting in no tumor enlargement in any patients.[350-352] However, individual patients with enlargement of tumors during estrogen therapy have been reported,[353] so hyperprolactinemic patients treated with estrogens should be followed carefully with periodic monitoring of PRL levels.

Many other potential factors have been investigated to determine why some tumors grow to become macroadenomas and why some macroadenomas are extremely large and invasive. Histologically, invasive prolactinomas have a high Ki-67 (MIB-1) labeling index, which reflects increased cell proliferation.[354] Altered expression of adhesion molecules, matrix metaloproteinases, and extracellular matrix components have also been found.[354] An increase in angiogenesis has also been found in these large tumors.[355]

PATHOGENESIS OF PROLACTINOMAS

A primary defect in hypothalamic regulation of PRL secretion, such as a defect in dopaminergic tone, had earlier been hypothesized to either cause or facilitate the growth of prolactinomas.[356] However, most information now favors the hypothesis that prolactinomas arise de novo as intrinsic disorders of the pituitary due to a single-cell mutation with monoclonal cell proliferation and that most changes in hypothalamic function in patients with tumors are secondary to the tumors.[357,358]

A large number of potential mutations that could be pathogenetic for prolactinomas in humans have been investigated (Box 3-2). Mutations causing loss of function in the DA D_2 receptor or gain of function of the TRH receptor have been looked for without succes.[359-361] Evaluation of prolactinomas for mutations in the G proteins coupling the D_2 receptor to adenyl cyclase and the TRH receptor to its intracellular activating pathways have also been unsuccessful,[362,363] although prolactinomas resistant to bromocriptine may have decreased levels of the $G_{i2}\alpha$ protein that couples the D_2 receptor to adenyl cyclase.[362] As noted later, bromocriptine-resistant prolactinomas also have a decrease in the short D_2 receptor isoform, resulting in decreased inhibition of adenyl cyclase.[364] Thus, these alterations in D_2 isoforms and $G_{i2}\alpha$ may play a role in the

pathogenesis of DA-resistant prolactinomas, but those tumors comprise only 8% to 15% of prolactinomas.[362]

Many other studies have examined prolactinomas for putative oncogenes and tumor suppressor genes. No amplifications or rearrangements have been found for the putative oncogenes *Pit-1, Prop-1, N-ras, H-ras, K-ras, myc II, N-myc, c-myc, myb, blc1, h-SF1, p16, p27, p53, sea, nm23,* or *c-fos,* or for the *menin* tumor suppressor gene.[357,358,365] Investigations are ongoing regarding the transforming heparin-binding secretory transforming (*hst*) gene, which encodes the fibroblast growth factor 4[366] and pituitary tumor transforming gene 1 (*PTTG1*),[367-369] but their roles in the pathogenesis of prolactinomas and the stimulation of their growth still remain unclear.

PROLACTINOMAS IN MULTIPLE ENDOCRINE NEOPLASIA TYPE I

Prolactinomas occur in approximately 20% of patients with multiple endocrine neoplasia type I (MEN-I).[370] The MEN-I (*MENIN*) gene is believed to function as a constitutive tumor suppressor gene, so an inactivating mutation results in tumor development. As noted previously, similar mutations have not been found in sporadic prolactinomas.

BOX 3-2

Potential Sites for Mutations That Could Be Implicated in Prolactinoma Tumorigenesis

Oncogenes
Release and Inhibitory Hypophysiotropic Factor Receptors
Releasing factor (thyrotropin-releasing hormone, vasoactive intestinal peptide, other prolactin-peptide–releasing factors) receptors (activating mutations)
Inhibitory factor (dopamine) receptors (inactivating mutations)
Signal Transduction Mechanisms
G-proteins
Adenylyl cyclase/cyclic adenosine monophosphate/cyclic adenosine monophosphate response element–binding protein
Protein kinase C
Transcription Factors
Pit-1
Prop-1
Other
Heparin-binding secretory transforming gene *(hst)*
Pituitary tumor transforming gene *(PTTG)*
Ras, myc, myb, fos, jun
Cyclins
Tumor Suppressor Genes
Menin
Other (p53, p21, p16, p27Rb, nm23)

From Molitch ME. Prolactinoma. *In* Melmed S (ed). The Pituitary, 2nd ed. Malden, Mass, Blackwell 2002, pp 455-495.

The fact that prolactinomas develop in only a subset of patients with MEN-1 suggests that there may be a secondary modifying gene at a different locus that acts with the *MENIN* gene to produce prolactinomas.[370] There is evidence that the prolactinomas in patients with MEN-1 may be more aggressive and more resistant to treatment than sporadic prolactinomas.[371,372]

When patients with apparently sporadic prolactinomas were screened for hypercalcemia, 14.3% in one series were found to have hyperparathyroidism, of whom one third were found to have gastrinomas on screening for pancreatic tumors.[373] This figure is higher than the 2% to 3% reported previously.[374,375] However, even a figure of 2% suggests that obtaining a careful family history and measuring calcium levels are useful in the evaluation of all cases of prolactinoma. Familial cases of prolactinomas without MEN-I have also been reported.[376]

Pathology

Prolactinomas can invade local tissues and may have varying histologic features, but they cannot be considered truly malignant unless metastases distant from the original tumor can be shown. Fortunately, true malignant prolactinomas are exceedingly rare, and just over 40 have been reported.[377,378]

Prolactin-secreting tumors may also secrete other hormones. The most common combination is PRL plus GH, and approximately 25% to 40% of GH-secreting tumors have been found to make PRL. One particular variant of these PRL/GH-secreting tumors is the *acidophil stem cell adenoma.* These tumors have irregular, elongated cells, with irregular nuclei, and may have oncytic changes with very large mitochondria. In contrast to the other tumors secreting both hormones, patients with these tumors have more marked elevations of PRL than of GH, and they usually present with menstrual abnormalities, galactorrhea, decreased libido, or impotence. They may have little in the way of acromegalic features.[342,379] These tumors are usually macroadenomas at the time of presentation and generally have had a relatively short course.[379] Other hormone combinations include PRL and ACTH, PRL and TSH, and PRL and FSH.[380] Interestingly, these plurihormonal tumors are generally monoclonal in origin,[381] as are most pure prolactinomas (discussed earlier in the chapter).

Local Mass Effects

Local mass effects may well cause symptoms in patients with macroadenomas, depending on the size and extent of extrasellar extension. The frequency of such symptoms is much lower than in patients with nonsecreting tumors because patients with prolactinomas usually present with symptoms of reproductive or sexual dysfunction (discussed later in the chapter). Visual field defects due to chiasmal compression depend on the amount of suprasellar extension. Because of the great variation in how these tumors grow superiorly with respect to the location of the chiasm, visual field defects can range from the classic complete bitemporal hemianopsia, to small partial quadrantic defects, to scotomas.[382] There are no specific types of visual field defects peculiar to prolactinomas compared with other types of tumors.

Ophthalmoplegias are relatively uncommon and are due to invasion of the cavernous sinus, with entrapment of cranial nerves III, IV, V_1, V_2, and VI. In some patients, a cavernous sinus syndrome may develop, consisting of ophthalmoplegia and pain or hyperesthesia in the distribution of V_1.[383] The carotid artery may be encased within the tumor, but narrowing of the artery is not seen. Shrinkage of these very large, invasive tumors with DA agonists can be quite dramatic and satisfying,[383-385] because surgery rarely is curative and is potentially fraught with complications.[386,387]

Extensive invasion of the floor of the skull, with massive destruction of bone, may occur, but rarely causes problems with entrapping cranial nerves or compressing vital brain structures.[385-389] Extrasellar extension in other directions may rarely cause temporal lobe epilepsy and hydrocephalus.[386] These large, invasive tumors are uncommon but not rare, and should be differentiated from true carcinomas; the finding of metastases distant from the primary tumor is necessary for the latter diagnosis. Histologically, these invasive tumors have no specific features to differentiate them from noninvasive prolactinomas.[386] Many of these patients respond quite well to DA agonists, with tumors occasionally shrinking to the point where they are undetectable on MRI and PRL levels are normal.[383,384,386-389] Rarely, these tumors function as a "cork" at the base of the skull so that cerebrospinal fluid (CSF) leaks may occur with substantial tumor shrinkage.[387] Surgery is necessary to repair such leaks to avoid the risk of meningitis.[387]

Surgery for large macroadenomas is never curative and may be dangerous.[385,387] However, for some tumors that do not respond to medication, surgical debulking and irradiation may be necessary (discussed later in the chapter).[386]

Local mass effects may also cause hypopituitarism because of direct pituitary compression or hypothalamic/stalk dysfunction. The larger the tumor, the more likely there is to be one or more hormonal deficits.[253,386,388,389] All patients with macroadenomas need to be evaluated for possible deficits in pituitary function.[337]

Clinical Manifestations

The clinical manifestations of hyperprolactinemia were discussed earlier in section "Prolactin Action." The frequencies with which various clinical manifestations occur in patients with prolactinomas vary depending on referral patterns.

Women. In older series, almost all premenopausal women presented because of symptoms of galactorrhea, amenorrhea, or infertility. In a summary of 21 series of 1621 women with prolactinomas who underwent transsphenoidal surgery, the frequency of oligoamenorrhea was 92.9% and of galactorrhea was 84.7%.[390]

Although secondary amenorrhea is more common, primary amenorrhea may also occur. Presentation because of severe headaches or visual field disturbance due to large tumors is uncommon in women because they usually initially seek medical attention for menstrual dysfunction or galactorrhea (which generally occur even with minimal PRL elevations and long before the tumors have grown large).[391] Postmenopausal women with prolactinomas usually present with mass effects from large tumors,[383] although other patients simply have a history of "premature" menopause.[392]

Men. Men with prolactinomas often seek medical attention because of symptoms related to the size of the tumor, not because of impotence, loss of libido, or infertility.[393] Prostate volume is reduced when men are hyperprolactinemic, presumably due to their low testosterone levels; prostate size returns to normal when PRL levels are normalized.[394] In a summary of 16 series comprising 444 men with prolactinomas (not all of whom went to surgery), 77.9% were impotent, 36.6% had visual field defects, 33.8% had partial or complete hypopituitarism, 29.1% complained of headaches, and 10.9% had galactorrhea.[390] Thus, approximately one third of men had symptoms due to tumor size. Radiologic investigation shows a macroadenoma in 80% to 90% of cases in most studies.[390,393]

There has been much speculation about the possible reason why a considerably greater proportion of men have macroadenomas compared with women. One hypothesis suggests that men tend to ignore symptoms of sexual dysfunction longer than do women, writing off impotence and decrease in libido to aging.[395] Thus, the prolonged course without therapy permits tumors to grow large. This line of reasoning ignores the data from women regarding the rather uncommon occurrence of progression of size of microadenomas. This observation would point to a more fundamental biologic difference in the growth of prolactinomas between the sexes. The difference is unlikely to be due to the differences in target organ sex hormones (i.e., estrogens and testosterone), because estrogens tend to be strongly growth-promoting. It is not known whether there are tumor growth factors that might have a differential effect on prolactinoma growth in the different sexes. Immunohistochemical studies of tumors using the Ki-67 (MIB-1) antibody, which correlates with tumor growth, showed no difference between the sexes when corrected for tumor size.[396] Further examination of these issues may yield important information about the pathophysiology of these tumors.

Children and Adolescents. Children and adolescents may present with growth arrest, pubertal delay, or primary amenorrhea, in addition to the more standard presentations of galactorrhea, oligo/amenorrhea, and mass effects, such as headaches or visual disturbances.[397-401] Low bone mineral density is also commonly seen.[402] In contrast to adults, there is a disproportionately large number of patients who have macroadenomas (64%), even allowing for possible selection bias because of reporting from neurosurgical units. Hypopituitarism may be present in those with macroadenomas.[393] Furthermore, the percentage of children and adolescents resistant to DA agonists may be higher than in adults; Colao and coworkers reported that PRL levels were normalized in only 10 of 26 children and adolescents taking bromocriptine, 5 of 15 taking quinagolide, and 15 of 20 taking cabergoline.[401] The reasons

for the high percentage of large macroadenomas and the relative resistance to DA agonists are not known, but it is tempting to speculate that these peculiarities may be linked.

Treatment

The indications for therapy in patients with prolactinomas may be divided into two categories: effects of tumor size and effects of hyperprolactinemia. In 93% of patients, microprolactinomas do not enlarge over a 4- to 6-year period of observation. Thus, the simple argument that therapy is indicated for a microadenoma to prevent it from growing is fallacious. On the other hand, if a documented adenoma exists, it needs to be followed closely to determine if it is growing. It is very unlikely for a prolactinoma to grow significantly with no increase in serum PRL levels, although this phenomenon has been reported.[403] Therefore, after an initial MRI showing a microadenoma, most patients can just be followed with serial PRL measurements. If PRL levels rise or if the patient has symptoms of mass effects, such as headaches, then repeat scanning is indicated. Certainly, a microadenoma that is documented to be growing demands therapy for the size change alone because it may be one of the 7% that will grow to be a macroadenoma.

Macroadenomas have already shown their propensity for growth. Therefore, observation alone is inappropriate unless there are specific contraindications to therapy. Local or diffuse invasion and compression of adjacent structures, such as the stalk or optic chiasm, are additional indications for therapy.

Other indications for therapy are relative and are due to the hyperprolactinemia itself. These include decreased libido, menstrual dysfunction, galactorrhea, infertility, hirsutism, impotence, and premature osteoporosis. If a woman with a microadenoma has normal menses and libido and is not bothered by the galactorrhea, there is no specific reason for therapy. On the other hand, therapy clearly is indicated for a woman with amenorrhea and anovulation who wishes to become pregnant. However, if such a woman does *not* wish to become pregnant, then therapy to prevent osteoporosis or improve libido clearly is only relatively indicated.

The ability to follow a patient closely with PRL measurements, CT or MRI scans, and estimations of bone mineral density, coupled with rather precise estimates of the efficacy of various modes of therapy, allows a highly individualized way of following patients and choosing the proper timing and mode of therapy.

Surgery

Transsphenoidal surgical success rates are highly dependent on the experience and skill of the surgeon as well as the size of the tumor. An analysis of the surgical results from 50 published series shows that normalization of PRL levels was achieved in 1596 of 2137 (74.7%) microadenomas and 755 of 2226 (33.9%) macroadenomas.[393] Clearly, for the macroadenomas, the success rate in large part was dependent on the size of tumors chosen for surgery. In many series, the object was, appropriately, debulking of a very large tumor rather than cure, and in other series, very large tumors were not operated on.

From the series, compiled recurrence rates for microadenomas (147/809 = 18.2%) and macroadenomas (106/465 = 22.8%) were similar.[393] It should be stressed here that for virtually all of these recurrences, the recurrence is that of hyperprolactinemia and not documented radiologic evidence of tumor regrowth. With recurrence of the hyperprolactinemia, there usually is also a recurrence of sexual/reproductive dysfunction that usually is an indication for medical therapy to reduce PRL levels. Based on the cure and recurrence rates cited earlier, the ultimate long-term surgical cure rates, using a normal PRL level as the criterion, are 61.1% for microadenomas and 26.2% for macroadenomas.

In an analysis of 84 patients with macroadenomas (36 were prolactinomas), Nelson and colleagues found that of those with normal preoperative pituitary function, only 78% retained normal function postoperatively.[404] One third with some pituitary deficits before surgery improved, and one third with such deficits had worsened pituitary function after surgery; none of the patients in the panhypopituitary group improved after surgery.[404]

Complications from transsphenoidal surgery for microadenomas are infrequent, with a mortality rate of at most 0.6%, a major morbidity rate of approximately 3.4% (visual loss, stroke/vascular injury, meningitis/abscess, oculomotor palsy), and CSF rhinorrhea occurring in 1.9%.[393,405-407] The mortality rate for transsphenoidal surgery for all types of secreting and nonsecreting macroadenomas ranges from 0.2% to 1.2%, the major morbidity rate is approximately 6.5% (visual loss, stroke/vascular injury, meningitis/abscess, and oculomotor palsy), and the rate of CSF rhinorrhea is approximately 3%.[393,405-407] Transient diabetes insipidus is quite common with transsphenoidal surgery for both micro- and macroadenomas, and permanent diabetes insipidus occurs in approximately 1% of patients who undergo surgery for macroadenomas.[405-407] Although visual field defects and reduction in visual acuity can be improved in 74% of patients whose macroadenomas abut the optic chiasm,[408] a small number of patients with normal visual fields may have a reduction of vision after surgery due to herniation of the chiasm into an empty sella, direct injury or devascularization of the optic apparatus, fracture of the orbit, postoperative hematoma, or cerebral vasospasm.[409] In general, complication rates fall with increasing experience of the neurosurgeon.[406,407]

In recent years, endoscopic endonasal transsphenoidal surgery has evolved into a commonly used technique. This method gives a superior panoramic view, with a shorter operating time and a lower local complication rate. However, surgical remission rates are no better with this newer approach.[410,411]

Radiation Therapy

Because of the excellent therapeutic responses to transsphenoidal surgery and medical therapy (described in the next section), radiation therapy is generally not considered a primary mode of treatment for prolactinomas. Just over 250 patients have been reported who had been treated with conventional radiation therapy alone, in combination with bromocriptine, or after failure of surgical cure.[393] Approximately 35% of patients can achieve normal PRL levels after surgery plus irradiation, usually between 5 and 15 years after irradiation.[393]

The major adverse effect of radiation therapy is hypopituitarism. This complication occurs with frequencies as high as 93%.[393,412] Additional complications that occur months to years after radiation therapy for pituitary adenomas include second malignancies, cerebrovascular accidents, optic nerve damage, radiation brain necrosis, neurologic dysfunction, and soft tissue reactions. Second malignancies have been reported to be significantly increased 15 to 20 years after the primary irradiation.[413-415] Radiation-induced optic atrophy occurs in 2% to 5% of patients and is due to ischemic damage to the optic apparatus.[416] Radiation therapy–induced encephalopathy is rare, but can be devastating and occurs only with high doses.[417]

A new form of radiation therapy used increasingly in recent years, which allows the precise delivery of a single, necrotizing dose to the tumor with little radiation to surrounding tissue, is referred to as "stereotactic" radiation therapy (Gamma Knife and linear accelerator).[418] Cranial nerves in the cavernous sinus are relatively radioresistant, but the optic nerves, chiasm, and tracts are radiosensitive,[419] so this type of treatment appears to be advantageous for postoperative tumor residing in the cavernous sinus. Data extending out to only 2 to 3 years on almost 300 patients suggest that this technique may be more effective at reducing hormone levels and tumor size in a shorter period with fewer complications than conventional radiation therapy.[393] However, only one study reported using stereotactic radiation therapy as primary therapy without DA agonist, finding that only 16 of 77 (21%) patients achieved normal PRL levels.[420] Although it is hoped that many of the complications from brain irradiation will be less frequent with focused radiation therapy compared with conventional radiation therapy, preliminary data suggest that the frequency of hypopituitarism will likely be the same.[421]

Thus, with radiation therapy, only small numbers of patients reach normal levels of PRL and then only after many years. Radiation therapy seems best reserved as adjunctive therapy for those patients with enlarging lesions who have not responded to either medical or surgical treatment, and the newer technique of focused radiation therapy would appear to offer advantages of efficacy, rapid effect, and possibly fewer adverse effects, especially for residual tumor in the cavernous sinus.

Medical Therapy

Bromocriptine. Bromocriptine was the first D_2 DA receptor agonist to be used for the treatment of hyperprolactinemia. Because of its short half-life, it usually must be taken two or three times daily. Bromocriptine is successful in normalizing PRL levels or causing return of ovulatory menses in 80% to 90% of patients.[422,423] When PRL levels and return of menses were studied in the same patients, it was found that substantially reducing PRL levels to slightly

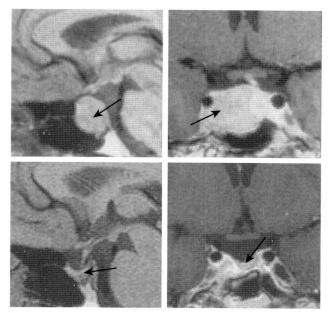

Figure 3-3. Magnetic resonance imaging scans of a patient with a macroadenoma before (top row) and during (bottom row) bromocriptine treatment. Left column, Sagittal view, Right column, Coronal view. Note the marked decrease in tumor size (arrows).

elevated levels was often enough to restore ovulation and menses, despite the fact that normal PRL levels were achieved in only 70% to 80% of treated patients.

There is little intraindividual variability in the absorption and peak blood levels achieved, but there is considerable interindividual variability.[424] There is also considerable variability in the PRL-lowering effects of a given dose of bromocriptine that does not correlate with serum bromocriptine levels, implying differences in sensitivity to the drug.[425] Decreased response to bromocriptine in vivo has been shown to correspond to decreased numbers of DA receptors on lactotroph cell membranes and decreased inhibition of adenyl cyclase when the same tumors are studied in vitro after surgery.[426]

In vitro studies have shown that bromocriptine decreases not only PRL synthesis but also DNA synthesis, cell multiplication, and tumor growth.[427] The initial report that bromocriptine was able to reduce tumor size in humans was by Corenblum and coworkers.[428] An analysis of tumor size response to bromocriptine from 24 different series of patients (totaling 302 patients) with macroadenomas showed that 76.8% had some tumor size decrease in response to bromocriptine, with periods of observation ranging from 6 weeks to more than 10 years (Fig. 3-3).[390] In 10 studies with 112 patients in whom the change in tumor size was quantified, 45 (40.2%) had a greater than 50% reduction in tumor size, 32 (28.6%) had a 25% to 50% reduction in tumor size, 14 (12.5%) had a less than 25% reduction, and 21 (18.7%) had no evidence of any reduction in tumor size.[390] In 15 patients with microadenomas, Bonneville and colleagues found that 6 tumors disappeared completely, 5 decreased approximately 50% in volume, and 4 remained unchanged with treatment of 3 to 12 months.[429]

The time course of tumor size reduction is variable. Some patients may experience an extremely rapid decrease in tumor size, with significant changes in visual fields being noted within 24 to 72 hours and significant changes noted on MRI within 2 weeks.[430] In others, little change may be noted at 6 weeks, but scanning again at 6 months may show significant changes.[390,431] In many patients, progressive tumor size reduction can be noted over several years.[390,431,432]

Visual field improvement occurs in 80% to 90% of patients with defects.[253,390,431,433] The visual field improvement generally parallels and often precedes the changes seen on MRI.[253,433] It is often difficult to determine before treatment whether visual defects are temporary or permanent, and only the response to therapy provides a final answer. These studies with medical therapy are reassuring in that a relatively slow chiasmal decompression over several weeks provides excellent restoration of visual fields and immediate surgical decompression is not necessary. Usually, when there is no significant change in visual fields despite significant evidence of tumor reduction on scan, subsequent surgery also does not improve these fields.[434] Reduction in tumor size may also be accompanied by improved pituitary function.[253,435] When the prolactinoma is present prepubertally, improved pituitary function allows resumption of normal growth and pubertal development.[436]

The extent of tumor size reduction does not correlate with basal PRL levels, nadir PRL levels achieved, the percentage of decrease in PRL levels, or whether PRL levels reached normal. Some patients have excellent reduction in PRL levels into the normal range, but only modest changes in tumor size; others may have persistent, mild hyperprolactinemia (although suppressed > 88% from basal values), with almost complete disappearance of tumor.[253] A reduction in PRL levels always precedes any detectable change in tumor size; therefore, patients whose PRL levels do not respond to therapy have no reduction in tumor size. Once maximum tumor size reduction is achieved, the dose of bromocriptine can often be substantially reduced, gradually.[437]

Rarely, the prolactinoma serves as a "cork," and tumor size reduction with bromocriptine may cause CSF rhinorrhea.[387,438] Fibrosis has been reported in some tumors, with marked shrinkage that may hinder later surgical cure of macroadenomas.[439,440] For most patients, however, continued DA agonist treatment is preferable to late surgery. Prolonged bromocriptine treatment for up to 10 years appears to be well tolerated,[435,441-446] and the dose can often be reduced considerably.[437]

With discontinuation of short-term (several weeks to months) treatment, macroadenomas can reexpand within 2 weeks.[447] However, more than 90% of tumors treated for several years that show good size reduction remain reduced in size when the drug is discontinued, although PRL levels may increase to above normal and require treatment.[393,441,443,445] In a study of 69 patients with macroadenomas and 62 with microadenomas, Passos and colleagues found that 16% of patients with macroadenomas and 21% with microadenomas maintained normal PRL levels after stopping a median of 47 months of therapy.[448] In two more recent studies, approximately 50% of patients with micro-adenomas maintained normal PRL levels after stopping therapy.[446,449]

Therapy discontinuation must be done very cautiously, if at all, in patients with very large tumors who have excellent tumor size reduction. The best approach is probably to reduce the dose gradually, following PRL levels, discontinuing the drug only if there are no increases in PRL levels or tumor size on low doses.

The most common adverse effects are nausea and sometimes vomiting; these are usually transient, but may recur with each dose increase. Orthostatic hypotension usually is only a problem when initiating therapy, and it rarely recurs with dose increases. Dose-limiting nausea and vomiting occurs in 5% to 10% of patients, and digital vasospasm, nasal congestion, and depression occur in rare patients when doses less than 7.5 mg/day are used.[422]

Side effects can be minimized by starting with one daily 1.25-mg dose taken with a snack at bedtime. The dose can then be gradually increased to 2.5 mg twice daily with meals over 7 to 10 days. PRL levels should be checked after 1 to 2 months; most patients who respond to this therapy will do so within this period. Doses higher than 7.5 mg/day are usually not necessary, except in some patients with very large tumors.

One other notable side effect is a psychotic reaction. Turner and coworkers noted psychotic reactions in 8 of 600 patients receiving either bromocriptine or lisuride for hyperprolactinemia or acromegaly.[450] Symptoms included auditory hallucinations, delusional ideas, and changes in mood. Rare reports of exacerbation of preexisting schizophrenia also exist; therefore, the drug should be given cautiously to such patients.[451] Psychotic reactions usually resolve within 72 hours of stopping the drug. It should be noted that phenothiazines given to such patients may also blunt the action of bromocriptine on prolactinomas.[253]

One concerning problem is the tumor that initially shrinks in response to a DA agonist, but then enlarges. This is usually due to noncompliance, which is further worsened by the tendency for the patient and physician to resume the full dose instead of gradually restarting the drug. This tends to make side effects worse, further exacerbating the noncompliance. However, several case reports of tumor enlargement in compliant patients have been reported.[452-455] Pelligrini and colleagues have shown markedly fewer DA binding sites in tumors that grew during bromocriptine treatment compared with those that shrank or remained unchanged in response to therapy.[455]

In other studies, Caccavelli and coworkers have shown that resistant cells express a decreased proportion of the shorter DA D_2 receptor isoform that is coupled to phospholipase C more efficiently than the long DA D_2 receptor isoform.[456] Prolactinomas that are resistant to bromocriptine are often sensitive to cabergoline.[457,458]

Although extremely rare, tumors that continue to enlarge while being treated with DA agonists may turn out to be carcinomas. A rare case of an adenoma transforming to a sarcoma during bromocriptine therapy has also been reported.[459]

An alternative method of giving bromocriptine has been found to be successful in some cases. Vermesh and colleagues reported that similar reductions in PRL levels are achieved with oral and intravaginal administration of oral bromocriptine tablets.[460] However, the drug effect lasts for up to 24 hours with a single dose, and gastrointestinal side effects were much less with the intravaginal route. Katz and coworkers reported that a macroadenoma in a woman who was unable to tolerate oral bromocriptine responded well, with tumor shrinkage, to intravaginal bromocriptine.[461] Many women have now been treated with intravaginal bromocriptine with similar results, although some have local irritation at the site of tablet placement. Thus, the gastrointestinal side effects appear to be caused by local effects rather than being mediated centrally.

Pergolide. Another DA agonist that has been shown to have efficacy in the treatment of prolactinomas is pergolide, which had been approved by the U.S. Food and Drug Administration for the treatment of Parkinson's disease. Several studies have shown comparability to bromocriptine with respect to tolerance and efficacy, including tumor size reduction.[462-464] However, pergolide was withdrawn from the U.S. market in 2007 because of an association with cardiac valvular lesions similar to those seen in patients with carcinoid syndrome. These associations were seen only when the drug was used in the high doses needed to treat Parkinson's disease.[465,466] No such lesions were seen in patients treated with bromocriptine.[465,466] No cardiac valvular lesions have been reported in patients treated with the lower doses used for prolactinomas.

Quinagolide. Quinagolide (CV 205-502) is a nonergot DA that can be given once daily, with similar tolerance and efficacy to bromocriptine and pergolide.[390,467] Approximately 50% of patients who have tumors that are resistant to bromocriptine respond to quinagolide.[390,467-469] Although side effects are similar, some patients appear to tolerate quinagolide better than bromocriptine.[390,467-469] In studies in which 105 patients were assessed for tumor size reduction in a semiquantitative way, 50 (48.1%) experienced greater than 50% tumor size reduction, 21 (20.2%) experienced a 25% to 50% size reduction, 18 (17.3%) experienced less than 25% reduction, and 15 (14.4%) had no change in tumor size.[390] Quinagolide is not approved for use in the United States.

Cabergoline. Cabergoline is different from the other DA agonists in that it has a very long half-life and can be given orally once or twice weekly. The long duration of action stems from its slow elimination from pituitary tissue,[470] its high-affinity binding to pituitary DA receptors,[471] and extensive enterohepatic recycling.[472] After oral administration, PRL-lowering effects are initially detectable at 3 hours, then gradually increase so that there is a plateau of effect between 48 and 120 hours[472,473]; with weekly doses, there is a sustained reduction of PRL.[474]

Several studies have shown that cabergoline is generally more effective than bromocriptine in lowering PRL levels and has substantially fewer side effects.[473-478] In a prospective, double-blind comparison study of 459 women (279 microadenomas, 3 macroadenomas, 167 idiopathic hyperprolactinemia, 10 other), of women treated with cabergoline, 83% achieved normoprolactinemia, 72% achieved ovulatory cycles, and 3% discontinued the medication because of adverse effects. Of women treated with bromocriptine, 59% achieved normoprolactinemia, 52% achieved ovulatory cycles, and 12% stopped the drug because of adverse effects.[477] In other studies, cabergoline treatment of men caused a rapid improvement of sperm number and quality.[478] Rare patients experience dose-limiting nausea and vomiting with cabergoline, and they may be treated with intravaginal cabergoline as well.[479]

Several studies have assessed the effect of cabergoline on macroadenoma size.[474-476,480-486] A total of 130 patients in these series had their tumor size assessed in a semiquantitative way in studies ranging from 3 to 24 months of treatment. Of these 130 patients, 33 (25.4%) experienced greater than 50% tumor size reduction, 61 (46.9%) had 25% to 50% reduction, 8 (6.9%) had less than 25% reduction, and 28 (21.5%) had no change in tumor size. In many of these studies, many of the patients had been previously treated with other DA agonists, changing therapy because of intolerance or resistance, and this may color the findings. In a comparison of groups of patients, Colao and colleagues found that 25 of 26 (96%) patients who had never received previous DA agonists had tumor shrinkage of greater than 50%, whereas 13 of 19 (68%) who had been intolerant of previous use of bromocriptine, 21 of 33 (64%) who had tumors resistant to bromocriptine, and 14 of 20 (70%) who had been responsive to bromocriptine had similar reductions.[487] Thus, in the drug-naive patient, cabergoline clearly seems to be the most efficacious in reducing PRL levels to normal and decreasing tumor size, and has the least adverse effects. Visual defects tend to improve with the decreases in tumor size with cabergoline, similar to what has been seen with bromocriptine.[488]

In patients who have had normalization of their PRL levels for several years, cabergoline may be withdrawn gradually to see if hyperprolactinemia recurs. Colao and coworkers reported that after cabergoline withdrawal, of 105 normoprolactinemic patients with microadenomas, hyperprolactinemia recurred in 40% of those with tumors visible on MRI scan, but in only 24% of those without visible tumors, and of 70 normoprolactinemic patients with macroadenomas, hyperprolactinemia recurred in 58 of those with tumors still visible on MRI scan, but in only 26% of those without visible tumors.[489] In a similar study of 67 patients with microadenomas, Biswas and colleagues found that only 31% remained free of recurrence of hyperprolactinemia.[449]

Some patients have giant prolactinomas that are very resistant even to cabergoline, and these patients may require very high doses. The dose of cabergoline can be gradually increased, as long as there is a stepwise fall in PRL with each stepwise increase in cabergoline dose and the patient is not experiencing side effects.[457,458] An additional approach involves adding an aromatase inhibitor to reduce testosterone-to-estrogen conversion in men.[490] In rare cases, the alkylating agent, temozolomide, has been found to be effective in reducing tumor size and PRL levels in an invasive giant prolactinoma that was not malignant.[491,492] This drug has also been used successfully in some cases of the very rare PRL-secreting pituitary carcinomas.[493,494]

Cardiac valvular lesions similar to those seen in patients treated with pergolide have also been found in patients treated with cabergoline. As with pergolide, these associations were seen only when it was used in the high doses needed for Parkinson's disease.[465,466] No cardiac valvular lesions have been reported in patients treated with the lower doses generally used for treatment of prolactinomas. In patients with resistant tumors who are receiving much greater than usual doses, echocardiographic monitoring may be prudent.

Conclusions about Treatment

Microadenomas. The risk of progression of microadenoma to macroadenoma is less than 7%, so the patient who is unconcerned with fertility has no pressing need for therapy. On the other hand, long-term hypogonadism due to hyperprolactinemia may be associated with premature osteoporosis in both sexes; treatment reverses the increased rate of bone loss. For the woman with continued menses and no hypoestrogenemia, the risk of osteoporosis is not increased. For the correction of gonadal function with prevention of osteoporosis and restoration of libido, most patients should be treated unless they have normal estrogen and testosterone function.

If fertility is not an issue, then estrogen replacement therapy or a DA agonist could be tried. Because of its efficacy in reducing PRL levels, its favorable adverse effect profile, and once- or twice-weekly dosing, cabergoline appears to be the initial drug of choice for most patients with prolactinomas. If fertility is the primary reason to restore ovulation, then bromocriptine may be better because of its more established safety profile (discussed in section "Effects of Dopamine Agonists on the Developing Fetus").

The cost of treatment and the necessity of taking medications for many years make some patients choose transsphenoidal surgery as their primary option. Surgery may also be preferable for the 5% of patients who either cannot tolerate or do not respond to DA agonists. Initial surgical cure rates for microadenomas appear to be in the range of 65% to 85%, with a later recurrence rate for hyperprolactinemia of approximately 20% (thus, the ultimate cure rate is in the 60% range). Radiation therapy has a very restricted role in patients with microadenomas, being limited to those who do not respond to DA agonists and who are not cured by surgery.

Macroadenomas. Because of their excellent results and the rather poor results of surgery in most patients, DA agonists are recommended as initial therapy for patients with PRL-secreting macroadenomas. Surgery can be performed later in patients whose tumor responses to such medications are not optimal. Even if this subsequent surgery is necessary for tumor debulking, it rarely is curative and a DA agonist is usually necessary for treatment of the hyperprolactinemia. Because of its better tolerability and generally better efficacy, cabergoline is the DA agonist of choice. Radiation therapy again has a very limited role, being used for those who have no response to DA agonists and those whose tumor was documented to grow during treatment with DA agonists, after incomplete surgical removal. Stereotactic radiation therapy appears to be the best form of radiation therapy at this point, although long-term complications have not yet been assessed fully.

When DA agonist therapy is stopped, the prolactinoma may return to its original size, often within days to weeks. However, most studies with longer-term treatment have found reexpansion in fewer than 10% of patients in whom DA agonists were withdrawn, despite recurrence of hyperprolactinemia in 80% to 85% of those treated with bromocriptine. Considerably lower rates of recurrence of hyperprolactinemia have been found in those discontinuing cabergoline. This potential return to pretherapy size dictates extreme caution when withdrawing DA agonist therapy, because rapid tumor expansion may produce far more clinical symptoms than slow tumor enlargement. Often, however, the dose can be gradually tapered once maximal size reduction has occurred, and in suitable cases, the treatment can be stopped entirely if no reexpansion occurs.

The anatomic response of tumors to DA agonist treatment must be monitored carefully by CT or MRI scan and by visual field examination to detect tumors that do not respond, including the very rare carcinomas and cases of tumor reenlargement.

Pregnancy in Women with Prolactinomas

Hyperprolactinemia is usually associated with anovulation and infertility; correction of the hyperprolactinemia with DA agonists restores ovulation in approximately 90% of cases. When a woman harbors a prolactinoma as the cause of the hyperprolactinemia, two major issues arise when ovulation and fertility are restored: the effects of the DA agonist on early fetal development, and the effect of the pregnancy itself on the prolactinoma.

EFFECTS OF DOPAMINE AGONISTS ON THE DEVELOPING FETUS

As a general principle, it is advised that fetal exposure to medications be limited to as short a period as possible. Most advise that mechanical contraception be used after institution of DA agonist therapy until the first two to three cycles have occurred, so that an intermenstrual interval can be established. In this way, a woman will know when she has missed a menstrual period, a pregnancy test can be performed quickly, and the DA agonist can be stopped. Thus, the drug will have been given for only approximately 3 to 4 weeks of the gestation.

When used in this fashion, bromocriptine has not been found to cause any increase in spontaneous abortions, ectopic pregnancies, trophoblastic disease, multiple pregnancies, or congenital malformations (Table 3-1).[495,496] Long-term follow-up studies of 64 children between the ages of 6 months and 9 years whose mothers took bromocriptine in this fashion have shown no ill effects.[497] Experience with the use of bromocriptine throughout gestation, however, is limited to just over 100 women; no abnormalities were noted in the infants, except for one with an undescended testicle and one with a talipes deformity.[495,498-500]

Pergolide has been shown to cross the placenta in mice,[501] and limited data suggest that there is an unacceptable risk of congenital malformations.[502,503] Initially, no detrimental effects on pregnancy or fetal development in women who became pregnant during treatment with quinagolide were found.[504] However, a review of 176 pregnancies reported 24 spontaneous abortions, 1 ectopic pregnancy, 1 stillbirth, and 9 fetal malformations.[505] Therefore, neither pergolide nor quinagolide can be recommended if pregnancy is desired.

TABLE 3-1
Effect of Bromocriptine on Pregnancies

	Bromocriptine		Normal Population (%)
	n	%	
Pregnancies	6239	100	100
Spontaneous abortions	620	9.9	10-15
Terminations	75	1.25	
Ectopic pregnancies	31	0.5	0.5-1
Hydatidiform moles	11	0.2	0.05-0.7
Deliveries (known duration)	4139	100	100
At term (>38 wk)	3620	87.5	85
Preterm (<38 wk)	519	12.5	15
Deliveries (known outcome)	5120	100	100
Single births	5031	9.3	8.7
Multiple births	89	1.7	1.3
Infants (known details)	5213	100	100
Normal infants	5030	96.5	95
Infants with malformations	93	1.8	3-4
Infants with perinatal disorders	90	1.7	>2

Data from Krupp P, Monka C, Richter K. The safety aspects of infertility treatments. Program of the Second World Congress of Gynecology and Obstetrics, Rio De Janeiro, October 1988.

Cabergoline has been shown to cross the placenta in animal studies, but such data are lacking in humans. Data on exposure of the fetus during the first several weeks of pregnancy have been reported in just over 350 cases, and such use has not shown an increased percentage of spontaneous abortion, premature delivery, multiple pregnancy, or congenital abnormalities.[506-510] Available data from 107 children whose mothers had taken cabergoline in the first few weeks of gestation and who were followed for 1 to 72 months showed normal physical and mental development.[506]

In conclusion, with respect to using a DA agonist to facilitate ovulation and fertility, bromocriptine has the largest safety database and has a proven safety record for pregnancy. Although the database for cabergoline use in pregnancy is much smaller, it does not appear that cabergoline exerts any deleterious effects on pregnant women, and the incidence of malformation in their offspring is not greater than in the general population. The safety databases for pergolide and quinagolide are quite limited, but they raise concerns, so these drugs should not be used when fertility is desired. The effects of transsphenoidal surgery during gestation are not known specifically, but they would not be expected to be significantly different from the effects of other types of surgery,[511] unless hypopituitarism should ensue.

EFFECT OF PREGNANCY ON PROLACTINOMA SIZE

Estrogens have a marked stimulatory effect on PRL synthesis and secretion, and the hormonal milieu of pregnancy can stimulate lactotroph cell hyperplasia.[2,3] Those autopsy studies showing lactotroph cell hyperplasia during pregnancy have now been corroborated in vivo; MRI scans show a gradual increase in pituitary volume over the course of gestation, beginning by the second month and peaking during the first week postpartum. In some cases, a final height of almost 12 mm is reached.[512]

The stimulatory effect of the hormonal milieu of pregnancy may also result in significant prolactinoma enlargement during gestation (Fig. 3-4). Tumor enlargement may also occur because the DA agonist that had caused the tumor to shrink has now been discontinued. Data have been compiled from five studies that analyzed the risk of symptomatic tumor enlargement in pregnant women with prolactinomas, divided according to tumor size (Table 3-2).[510,513-516] For women with microadenomas, only 12 of 457 pregnancies (2.6%) were complicated by symptoms of tumor enlargement (headaches or visual disturbances). Surgical intervention was not required in a single case, and medical therapy with reinstitution of bromocriptine resolved the symptoms in the five patients in whom it was tried. In 45 of 142 pregnancies (31%) in women who had not undergone previous surgery or radiation therapy for their macroprolactinomas, there were similar symptoms of tumor enlargement. Of these 45, surgical intervention was undertaken in 12 and medical therapy in 17, leading to resolution of symptoms. In addition, 140 women with macroadenomas were identified who had undergone surgery or radiation before pregnancy; their risk of tumor enlargement was low (5%).

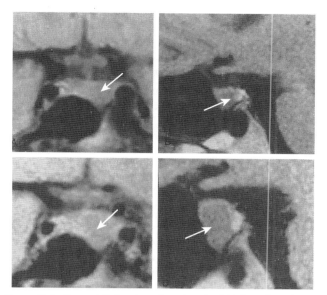

Figure 3-4. Coronal (left column) and sagittal (right column) magnetic resonance imaging scans of an intrasellar prolactin-secreting macroadenoma in a woman before conception (top row) and at 7 months of gestation (bottom row). Note the marked tumor (arrows) enlargement at the latter point, at which time the patient was complaining of headaches. (From Molitch ME. Medical treatment of prolactinomas. Endocrinol Metab Clin North Am 1999;28:143-169,with permission.)

RECOMMENDATIONS FOR MANAGEMENT DURING PREGNANCY

Because of its well-established safety record and the relative paucity of data with cabergoline, bromocriptine is favored by some clinicians for women wishing to become pregnant. However, there really are no data to show that cabergoline is not safe, and it is also commonly used in this setting. A patient with a microadenoma or a small intrasellar macroadenoma treated only with a DA agonist should be carefully followed throughout gestation. PRL levels do not always rise during pregnancy in women with prolactinomas, as they do in healthy women. PRL levels also may not rise with tumor enlargement.[517] Therefore, periodic checking of PRL levels is of no benefit. Because of the low incidence of tumor enlargement, routine periodic visual field testing is not cost-effective. Visual field testing and scanning are performed only in patients who become symptomatic. In the patient with tumor enlargement who does not respond to reinstitution of a DA agonist, surgery or early delivery may be required.

In a woman with a larger macroadenoma that may have suprasellar extension, there is approximately a 30% risk of clinically serious tumor enlargement during pregnancy

TABLE 3-2

Effect of Pregnancy on Prolactinomas

Tumor Type	Previous Therapy	Number of Patients	Symptomatic Enlargement
Microadenomas	No	457	12 (2.6%)
Macroadenomas	No	142	45 (31%)
Macroadenomas	Yes	140	7 (5%)

when only a DA agonist is used. There is no clear-cut answer as to the best therapeutic approach, so this must be a highly individualized decision that the patient has to make after a clear, documented discussion of the various therapeutic alternatives.

One approach is to perform a prepregnancy transsphenoidal surgical debulking of the tumor. This should greatly reduce the risk of serious tumor enlargement, but cases with massive tumor expansion during pregnancy after such surgery have been reported.[518] After surgical debulking, bromocriptine or cabergoline would be required to restore normal PRL levels and allow ovulation.

A second approach would be to treat the patient with bromocriptine or cabergoline to allow ovulation and then stop the drugs once pregnancy has been achieved, as in a woman with a microadenoma.

A third approach, that of giving bromocriptine continuously throughout gestation, has been advocated.[500] At this point, however, data on the effects of continuous bromocriptine therapy on the developing fetus are still quite meager, and such therapy cannot be recommended without reservation. There are no data documenting the safety of giving cabergoline throughout pregnancy. Should pregnancy at an advanced stage be discovered in a woman taking bromocriptine or cabergoline, the data that exist are reassuring and would not justify therapeutic abortion.

For patients with macroadenomas treated with DA agonists alone or after surgery, careful follow-up with visual field testing every 1 to 3 months is warranted. Repeat scanning (without gadolinium) is reserved for patients with symptoms of tumor enlargement, evidence of a developing visual field defect, or both. Repeat scanning after delivery to detect asymptomatic tumor enlargement may be useful as well.

Should symptomatic tumor enlargement occur with any of these approaches, reinstitution of a DA agonist is probably less harmful to the mother and child than surgery. There have been a number of cases reported where such reinstitution of bromocriptine has worked quite satisfactorily, causing rapid tumor size reduction with no adverse effects on the infant.[514] Similarly, one case has been reported with the successful reinstitution of cabergoline.[519] Any type of surgery during pregnancy results in a 1.5-fold increase in fetal loss in the first trimester and a 5-fold increase in fetal loss in the second trimester, although there is no risk of congenital malformations from such surgery.[511] Thus, DA agonist reinstitution would appear to be preferable to surgical decompression. However, such medical therapy must be very closely monitored, and transsphenoidal surgery or delivery (if the pregnancy is far enough advanced) should be performed is there is no response to the DA agonist and if vision progressively worsens.

There is no evidence that breast-feeding stimulates tumor growth.[520,521] For women who wish to breast-feed, DA agonists must be withheld until such time as the woman wishes to stop, unless pregnancy-induced tumor growth required treatment.

Interestingly, postpartum PRL levels are often lower than they were prepartum, with some patients achieving normalization of PRL without any therapy; the mechanism for this is not known.[521] However, in many patients, it may be reasonable to observe patients for a few months to determine their PRL and ovulatory status after delivery and cessation of breast-feeding, rather than automatically resuming treatment with DA agonists.

The complete reference list can be found on the companion Expert Consult Web site at www.expertconsultbook.com.

Suggested Readings

Bracero N, Zacur HA. Polycystic ovary syndrome and hyperprolactinemia. Obstet Gynecol Clin North Am 28:77-84, 2001.

Bronstein MD. Prolactinomas and pregnancy. Pituitary 8:31-38, 2005.

Casaneuva FF, Molitch ME, Schlechte JA, et al. Guidelines of the Pituitary Society for the diagnosis and management of prolactinomas. Clin Endocrinol 65:265-273, 2006.

Ciccarelli A, Daly AF, Beckers A. The epidemiology of prolactinomas. Pituitary 8:3-6, 2005.

Colao A, DiSarno A, Cappabianca P, et al. Withdrawal of long-term cabergoline therapy for tumoral and nontumoral hyperprolactinemia. N Engl J Med 349:2023-2033, 2003.

Colao A, Vitale G, Cappabianca P, et al. Outcome of cabergoline treatment in men with prolactinoma: effects of a 24-month treatment on prolactin levels, tumor mass, recovery of pituitary function, and semen analysis. J Clin Endocrinol Metab 89:1704-1711, 2004.

Donangelo I, Melmed S. Pathophysiology of pituitary adenomas. J Endocrinol Invest 28(11 Suppl Int):100-105, 2005.

Gillam MP, Molitch ME, Lombardi G, et al. Advances in the treatment of prolactinomas. Endocrine Rev 27:485-534, 2006.

Healy M-L, Smith TP, McKenna TJ. Diagnosis, misdiagnosis and management of hyperprolactinemia. Expert Rev Endocrinol Metab 1:123-132, 2006.

Karavitaki N, Thanabalasingham G, Shore HCA, et al. Do the limits of serum prolactin in disconnection hyperprolactinaemia need re-definition? A study of 226 patients with histologically verified non-functioning pituitary macroadenoma. Clin Endocrinol 65:524-529, 2006.

Molitch ME. Medication-induced hyperprolactinemia. Mayo Clin Proc 80:1050-1057, 2005.

Molitch ME. Pharmacologic resistance in prolactinoma patients. Pituitary 8:43-52, 2005.

Shrivastava RK, Arginteanu MS, King WA, et al. Giant prolactinomas: clinical management and long-term follow up. J Neurosurg 97:299-306, 2002.

CHAPTER 4

The Synthesis and Metabolism of Steroid Hormones

Jerome F. Strauss III

Steroid hormones are derived from cholesterol, a relatively abundant structural component of plasma membranes and other organelles. They belong to an ancient family of signaling molecules with diverse functions, including central roles in the regulation of female and male reproductive processes. These hormones are generated by seemingly subtle modifications of the four fused rings of the sterol skeleton and side chain. This chapter reviews the general features of the synthesis and metabolism of steroid hormones, the ways in which these processes are controlled physiologically, and the ways in which these processes can be modified by pharmacologic intervention.

Steroid Hormone Structure and Nomenclature

Steroid hormones are lipids that share a cyclopentanoperhydrophenanthrene backbone. Each carbon in this fused-ring structure is assigned a number identifier, and each ring, a letter (Fig. 4-1). The naturally occurring steroid hormones are named according to the saturated ring structures of the parent compound: *cholestanes,* of which cholesterol (5-cholesten-3β-ol) is a representative, have 27 carbons; *pregnanes* have 21 carbons (e.g., 4-pregnen-3-20-dione, also known by its trivial name, *progesterone*); *androstanes* have 19 carbons (e.g., 17β-hydroxy-4-androsten-3-one, or *testosterone*); and *estranes* have 18 carbons (e.g., 1,2,5(10)-estratriene-17β-ol, or *estradiol*). *Gonanes* contain 17 carbons (the cyclopentanoperhydrophenanthrene backbone), represented by synthetic progestins (e.g., desogestrel, norgestimate, gestodene). The backbone name is not synonymous with

biologic activity because glucocorticoids, mineralocorticoids, and progestins are all members of the pregnane family, and potent progestins and androgens containing 18 carbons (19-nortestosterone derivatives) are members of the estrane family.

The locations of substituents in the steroid backbone are indicated by the carbon number to which they are attached. Substituents at several positions have a significant effect on metabolism and biologic activity of steroid hormones, including carbons 3, 7, 11, and 17. Atoms attached to asymmetric centers are, by convention, given the designation α if they project below the plane of the ring structure (in figures of structures, a dashed line indicates the α configuration). The designation β (a solid line or filled triangle) is given to atoms that project above the plane. Hormone receptors distinguish between stereoisomers. In the case of estrogen receptors, 17β-estradiol is active, but 17α-estradiol is essentially inert. In the case of androgen receptors, testosterone with a 17β-hydroxyl function is active, but epitestosterone with a 17α-hydroxyl group has little activity.

Different enzymes catalyze the oxidation or reduction of α and β hydroxyl groups and reduce the Δ4 double bond in the steroid A ring to form 5α or 5β molecules. Such 5α-reduced steroids can be active (e.g., 5α-dihydrotestosterone) or inactive (e.g., 5α-dihydroprogesterone) with respect to steroid hormone receptor function, whereas the 5β-reduced steroids are not capable of activating steroid hormone receptors. The naturally occurring steroid hormones are rarely referred to in the medical literature by their systematic names, which designate the parent structure and the number, location, and (if appropriate) orientation of substituents; instead, the trivial names are preferred.

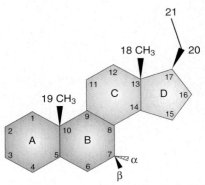

Figure 4-1. *The steroid nucleus. Rings are identified with capital letters and carbon atoms are numbered. Substituents and hydrogens are shown projecting above (β) or below (α) the plane of the steroid nucleus.*

Organization of Steroidogenic Organs and Cells

The steroidogenic machinery is compartmentalized at the organ, cellular, and subcellular levels, which has important implications for the control of steroid hormone production.[1,2] Steroid synthesis involves a series of sequential modifications of cholesterol that result in the clipping of the side chain; alterations in olefinic bonds; and the addition of hydroxyl functions, proceeding invariably (although some have argued that shortcuts do exist) from cholesterol through the pregnane, androstane, and finally, estrane families.

Specific cell types can accomplish several of these sequential steps, but rarely can they generate an estrogen from cholesterol. Indeed, the requirement for cooperative efforts by two different tissues or cell types is a characteristic of estrogen biosynthesis. This joint effort enables the modulation of estrogen production by factors that independently influence the cells involved in precursor synthesis, in addition to the cell type in which the final step, aromatization, occurs.

This cooperation is exemplified by estradiol synthesis in the ovarian follicle, where luteinizing hormone (LH) acts on the theca cells to stimulate production of androgen precursors and follicle-stimulating hormone (FSH) acts on granulosa cells to stimulate aromatization of these androgens into estrogens.

Placental estrogen synthesis likewise requires precursors from another tissue, the fetal adrenal gland that is under the control of fetal pituitary adrenocorticotropic hormone (ACTH). The sulfated dehydroepiandrosterone secreted from the fetal zone of the adrenal cortex has negligible androgenic activity in the fetus and increased solubility in plasma, so it can be efficiently transported to the placenta, where cleavage of the sulfate group, followed by aromatization, takes place in the syncytiotrophoblast. Cooperative interaction among different cell types is also important in regulating the production of steroid hormones in the brain and hormone production in endometriosis and endometrial cancers.

Another example of compartmentalization of the steroidogenic machinery at the organ level is the adrenal cortex, which has histologically and functionally distinct zones that determine the relative production rates of mineralocorticoids, glucocorticoids, and adrenal androgens.[3,4] The zona glomerulosa synthesizes mineralocorticoids; the zona fasciculata, glucocorticoids; and the zona reticularis and fetal zone of the fetal adrenal cortex produce androgens. One major functional distinction between the zona glomerulosa and the zonae fasciculata and reticularis is that aldosterone synthase is exclusively expressed in the zona glomerulosa, but 17α-hydroxylase is not; however, 17α-hydroxylase is abundant in the zonae fasciculata and reticularis. The zona reticularis expresses lower levels of type 2 3β-hydroxysteroid dehydrogenase and higher levels of cytochrome b_5 and sulfotransferase, a constellation that favors synthesis of dehydroepiandrosterone sulfate.

Acquisition, Storage, and Trafficking of Cholesterol

Steroidogenic cells have ultrastructural features that enhance their ability to obtain and store substrate cholesterol (Fig. 4-2).[2,5] Unlike protein hormone–producing cells, steroid-producing cells do not store prefabricated hormone; they synthesize hormones on demand from cholesterol that has been acquired from the plasma, synthesized de novo, or stored as esters in lipid droplets.

The plasma membrane has the highest content of free cholesterol, which is derived from lipoproteins and de novo sterol synthesis. This sterol pool is not static, but instead regularly cycles through the cell and back to the plasma membrane. During this cycling process, sterols can be diverted for use in steroid hormone synthesis.

Numerous microvilli project from the plasma membrane on which lipoprotein-gathering receptors of the low-density lipoprotein (LDL) receptor family are located (e.g., LDL receptors; LDL receptor–related protein, very–low-density (VLDL) lipoprotein receptors). These receptors mediate lipoprotein uptake by an endocytic mechanism that delivers the lipoproteins to the lysosomes where the apolipoproteins are degraded. The lipoprotein cholesterol esters are then hydrolyzed by acid lipase to release free cholesterol. Severe acid lipase deficiency (Wolman's disease) is associated with lysosomal accumulation of cholesterol esters and triglycerides, which can lead to damage of steroidogenic cells. Stimulation of steroidogenic cells by trophic hormones increases the number of LDL receptors and also accelerates the rate of LDL internalization and degradation.[6]

High-density lipoproteins (HDL) can also provide cholesterol for hormone synthesis.[7] Receptors for HDL (scavenger receptor type B, class 1 [abbreviated SR-B1] and its orthologs) are located in closely apposed microvilli that form "microvillar channels" in which HDL particles are lodged.[8,9] Hepatic lipase or endothelial cell–derived lipases that cleave HDL-associated phospholipids may facilitate uptake of the HDL sterols by altering the phospholipid-to-sterol ratio of the particles. SR-B1 expression is upregulated in response to trophic stimulation of steroidogenic glands, facilitating the usage of HDL-delivered substrate.

The process by which cholesterol is accumulated by the "HDL pathway" differs from that of the "LDL pathway":

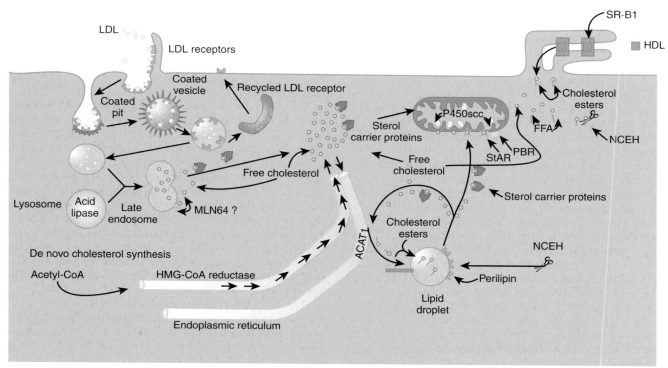

Figure 4-2. *The acquisition, storage, and trafficking of cholesterol in steroidogenic cells. ACAT1, acetyl-coenzyme A:cholesterol acyltransferase-1; FFA, free fatty acid; HDL, high-density lipoprotein; HMG-COA, 3-hydroxy-3-methyl-glutaryl-coenzyme A; LDL, low-density lipoprotein; MLN64, also known as StarD3; NCEH, neutral pH cholesterol ester hydrolase; PBR, peripheral benzodiazepine receptor; SR-B1 scavenger receptor type B; StAR, steroidogenic acute regulatory protein.*

HDL cholesterol esters are selectively internalized by SR-B1, leaving the apolipoproteins on the cell surface. The internalized HDL cholesterol esters are cleaved, presumably by a cytosolic, neutral pH optimum sterol esterase, thereby releasing free cholesterol.[5]

De novo synthesis of cholesterol, a process that involves at least 17 enzymes, takes place primarily in the abundant smooth endoplasmic reticulum (SER).[10] Steroidogenic cells have up to 10-fold more SER by volume than rough endoplasmic reticulum. In certain cells, the SER takes on unique forms, exemplified by the whorls found in testicular Leydig cells. Enzymes involved in steroid formation and metabolism are also embedded in the SER. Trophic hormones that stimulate steroidogenesis generally increase both cellular cholesterol synthesis and lipoprotein uptake. Of note, biosynthetic intermediates between lanosterol and cholesterol stimulate oocyte maturation in some in vitro assays. These 4,4-dimethyl sterols, referred to as *meiosis-activating sterols*, contain 29 carbons and are found in the testis and follicular fluid in low micromolar concentrations. However, their physiologic role in gamete maturation is the subject of current debate (see Chapter 8).

The quantitative importance of circulating cholesterol carried by LDL, HDL, and other lipoproteins as a hormone precursor (as opposed to de novo cholesterol synthesis) is demonstrated by the fact that radiolabeled plasma cholesterol in humans is almost fully equilibrated with the steroidogenic pool of cholesterol.[5] Additional evidence for an important role of lipoprotein cholesterol in steroidogenesis comes from the study of hypobetalipoproteinemia,

a disorder in which there is virtually no circulating LDL.[11,12] This rare metabolic disease is associated with reduced adrenocortical steroid production and diminished progesterone levels in the luteal phase and in pregnancy, although the lower levels of progesterone elaborated are still sufficient to achieve a term pregnancy.

Conversely, the commonly used statins (which inhibit 3-hydroxy-3-methylglutaryl coenzyme A reductase, the rate-limiting enzyme in de novo cholesterol synthesis) do not impair adrenal, testicular, or luteal steroidogenesis in adult humans despite the lowering of plasma LDL levels.[13,14] However, individuals with familial hypercholesterolemia due to inactivating mutations in the LDL receptor have only modest impairment of steroidogenic gland function, reflecting the capacity of alternative sterol uptake mechanisms to compensate for LDL receptor deficiency.

Smith-Lemli-Opitz syndrome, an autosomal recessive disease, offers interesting insight into the relationship of plasma cholesterol and de novo sterol synthesis for the supply of precursors for steroidogenesis.[15] The disease is caused by inactivating mutations in an enzyme involved in the terminal steps of cholesterol synthesis, 3β-hydroxysteroid Δ^7-reductase. As a result, cholesterol levels are quite low and 7-dehydrocholesterol levels are elevated. Adrenal insufficiency has been reported in affected individuals,[16,17] and hypospadias or ambiguous genitalia is a frequent finding in affected male neonates, reflecting diminished fetal testicular testosterone synthesis. Estrogen production during pregnancy is also reduced, resulting from impaired fetal adrenal hormone production. Thus, severely reduced plasma cholesterol levels are associated with impaired steroidogenesis, which is further compromised by the defect in de novo sterol synthesis. Interestingly, B-ring unsaturated equine-like steroids (1,3,5[10], 7-estratetrenes) are produced from the 7-dehydrocholesterol that accumulates, showing that the steroidogenic enzymes do not have an absolute requirement for cholesterol as a starting material.[18] Desmosterolosis, a rare autosomal recessive disease caused by mutations in the 3β-hydroxysterol Δ^{24} reductase, is also associated with ambiguous genitalia in affected males, presumably as a result of impaired fetal testicular testosterone synthesis.[15]

Cytoplasmic lipid droplets represent another major depot of substrate in steroidogenic cells: as much as 80% of the total cholesterol content of steroidogenic cells can be found esterified in these droplets.[2] The sterol esters are synthesized in the endoplasmic reticulum from cholesterol acquired from lipoproteins or de novo synthesis by acyl-coenzyme A:cholesterol acyltransferase-1 (ACAT1), encoded by one of two related ACAT genes.[19] The esters generated by ACAT accumulate within the endoplasmic reticulum membranes and subsequently bud off as lipid droplets (see Fig. 4-2). Targeted deletion of the *Acat 1* gene in mice resulted in a marked reduction of sterol esters in the adrenal glands, without impairment of basal or ACTH-stimulated glucocorticoid production. This finding shows that transit through the sterol ester pool is not part of an obligatory itinerary for steroidogenic cholesterol.

The limiting membranes of the nascent lipid droplets undergo modification in phospholipid and protein composition, including the collection of perilipins on the droplet surface.[20] Perilipins protect the droplet contents from hydrolysis in the basal state. They also serve as scaffolds, anchoring lipases and intermediate filaments to the lipid droplet surface. Perilipins, which are phosphorylated by protein kinase A, work via phosphorylation-dependent and phosphorylation-independent mechanisms to promote the mobilization of lipid stores when cells are stimulated by trophic hormones.

The sterol esters in lipid droplets are hydrolyzed by a hormone-sensitive lipase known as *neutral cholesterol ester hydrolase* because of its neutral pH optimum for hydrolytic activity (see Fig. 4-2).[21,22] Protein kinase A activates this enzyme by phosphorylation of serine residues, promoting binding of the sterol esterase to lipid droplets. This enzyme's role in steroidogenesis was suggested by the reduced production of stimulated (but not basal) corticosterone associated with an accumulation of lipid droplets in the adrenal cortex of mice deficient in the hormone-sensitive lipase. The male mice were infertile due to a defect in spermatogenesis that appeared to be unrelated to abnormalities in steroidogenesis, implicating sterol ester hydrolysis in Sertoli or male germ cell function.

The size and number of lipid droplets change as the ester pool expands or contracts.[2] The quantity of sterol ester stored is determined by the availability of cholesterol to the cell through de novo synthesis, through accumulation of lipoprotein-carried cholesterol, and by the steroidogenic activity of the cell. Trophic stimulation promotes cholesterol ester hydrolysis and diverts cholesterol into the steroidogenic pool away from ACAT, preventing re-esterification and resulting in a net depletion of cholesterol from the lipid droplets. Conversely, pharmacologic blockade of steroid hormone synthesis (e.g., aminoglutethimide) or defects in cholesterol use for steroidogenesis (e.g., congenital lipoid adrenal hyperplasia) increase sterol ester storage by increasing the amount of cholesterol available to ACAT.

The exact intracellular itinerary of lipoprotein-derived cholesterol (or free cholesterol from the plasma membrane, or free cholesterol released from lipid droplets) remains to be elucidated. In particular, much is still unknown about the ways in which sterol is presented to the mitochondria, where the first committed step in steroidogenesis takes place. It is likely that sterol distribution to and from organelles occurs through a dynamic vesicular–tubular late endosomal compartment, as well as through the assistance of lipid transfer proteins.[23] The lipid transfer proteins involved in this process may include *sterol carrier protein-2* and cytosolic proteins with a structure resembling the *steroidogenic acute regulatory protein (StAR),* including StarD3 (also known as MLN64), StarD4, and StarD5 (see Fig. 4-2).

The mitochondria of steroidogenic cells are frequently found in close association with cytoplasmic lipid droplets, which may facilitate movement of substrate from these depots to the mitochondria.[1,2] The mitochondria generally have tubulovesicular cristae, in contrast to the lamellar cristae that are characteristic of mitochondria in other cells. The inner mitochondrial membranes contain the cholesterol side-chain cleavage system needed for generation of pregnenolone, the first committed enzymatic step in steroidogenesis. The hydrophobic cholesterol substrate must move from the mitochondrial outer membrane across the aqueous intermembranous space to reach the inner membrane. This translocation process is the major rate-limiting step in steroidogenesis.

Indeed, the capacity to produce large amounts of steroid hormone in rapid response to trophic stimulation requires the action of StAR, which greatly enhances the flux of substrate to the side-chain cleavage system (see Fig. 4-2). The cholesterol side-chain cleavage system is closely juxtaposed to downstream enzymes in the steroidogenic pathway on the endoplasmic reticulum, allowing for efficient metabolism of pregnenolone.[24]

Overview of Steroidogenesis

The manufacture of steroid hormones involves the action of several classes of enzymes, primarily, the cytochromes P450, which are hemeprotein mixed-function oxidases (named because of their distinct absorption peak at 450 nm in the Soret region when reduced in the presence of carbon monoxide), as well as hydroxysteroid dehydrogenases and reductases.

Cytochrome P450s catalyze the major alterations in the sterol framework, cleavage of the side chain, hydroxylations, and aromatization. These hemeproteins, measuring approximately 55 kDa, require molecular oxygen and a source of reducing equivalents (i.e., electrons) to complete a catalytic cycle. Each member of the steroidogenic cytochrome P450 family of genes is designated "CYP," followed by a unique identifying number that usually refers to the carbon atom at which the enzyme acts.

The hydroxysteroid dehydrogenases reduce ketone groups or oxidize hydroxyl functions, employing pyridine nucleotide cofactors, usually with a stereospecific substrate preference and reaction direction. In addition to being involved in hormone biosynthesis in steroidogenic cells, this family of enzymes works with the reductases, steroid sulfotransferases, and steroid sulfatase to regulate the level of bioactive hormone in target tissues. The hydroxysteroid dehydrogenases are key determinants of the cellular response to endogenous steroid hormones as well as steroidal drugs (e.g., tibolone).

The reductases, using nicotinamide adenine dinucleotide phosphate (NADPH) as a cofactor, produce saturated ring A steroids from Δ^4-steroids (again, with stereospecificity). Table 4-1 lists the key steroidogenic enzymes by class and the respective gene designation. Figure 4-3 outlines the pathways of steroid hormone synthesis, indicating where specific enzymes act.

KEY PROTEINS IN THE BIOSYNTHESIS AND CATABOLISM OF STEROID HORMONES

StAR: The Principal Regulator of Gonadal and Adrenal Steroidogenesis

Translocation of cholesterol from the outer mitochondrial membranes to the relatively sterol-poor inner membranes is the critical step in steroidogenesis.[25] This sterol translocation process occurs at modest rates in the absence of specific effectors. It is markedly enhanced by StAR, a protein with a short biologic half-life. The following evidence supports the notion that StAR is the key mediator of substrate flux to the side-chain cleavage system:

1. Expression of StAR is directly correlated with steroidogenesis.
2. Cotransfection of StAR and the cholesterol side-chain cleavage system into cells that are not normally steroidogenic results in substantial pregnenolone synthesis above that produced by cells transfected with the cholesterol side-chain cleavage enzyme system alone.
3. Mutations that inactivate StAR cause congenital lipoid adrenal hyperplasia, a rare autosomal recessive disorder in which the synthesis of all adrenal and gonadal steroid hormones is severely impaired before the cholesterol side-chain cleavage step. This impairment leads to the accumulation of cholesterol ester–laden droplets in the adrenal cortex and testicular Leydig cells.
4. Targeted deletion of the murine *Star* gene results in a phenotype in nullizygous mice that mimics human congenital lipoid adrenal hyperplasia.

Human StAR is synthesized as a 285–amino acid protein. The N-terminus of StAR is characteristic of proteins synthesized in the cytoplasm and then imported into mitochondria, with the first 26 amino acid residues predicted to form an amphipathic helix. Newly synthesized StAR preprotein (37 kDa) is rapidly imported into mitochondria and processed to the mature 30-kDa form. The preprotein

has a very short half-life (minutes), but the mature form is longer-lived (hours).

Drugs that collapse the mitochondrial proton gradient inhibit StAR import, and agents that block mitochondrial matrix metalloendoproteinases prevent the cleavage of the StAR N-terminal mitochondrial targeting sequence from the imported protein. StAR contains two consensus sequences for cyclic AMP (cAMP)-dependent protein kinase phosphorylation at serine 57 and serine 195. Phosphorylation is one mechanism by which preexisting or newly synthesized StAR can be rapidly activated. Incorporation of ^{32}P into StAR is correlated with steroidogenesis in cultured cells, and serine 195 of human StAR must be phosphorylated for maximal steroidogenic activity in model systems.

Tissues that express StAR at high levels carry out trophic hormone–regulated mitochondrial sterol hydroxylations through the intermediacy of cAMP.[25,26] StAR messenger RNA (mRNA) and protein are not present in the human placenta, an observation that is consistent with the fact that pregnancies hosting a fetus affected with congenital lipoid adrenal hyperplasia go to term.[27] Although estrogen production is impaired in these pregnancies as a result of diminished fetal adrenal androgen production, placental progesterone synthesis is not significantly affected, indicating that the trophoblast cholesterol side-chain cleavage reaction is independent of StAR.

The abundance of StAR protein in steroidogenic cells is determined primarily by the rate of *STAR* gene transcription, although translational mechanisms may also contribute. In differentiated cells, the *STAR* gene is activated by the cAMP signal transduction cascade within 15 to 30 minutes. In differentiating cells (e.g., luteinizing granulosa cells), the induction of StAR transcription takes hours and requires ongoing protein synthesis.

Originally, StAR was believed to stimulate cholesterol movement from the outer to the inner mitochondrial membrane as it was imported into the mitochondria. The importation process was proposed to create contact sites between the two membranes, allowing cholesterol to flow down a chemical gradient. However, a StAR protein lacking the N-terminal 62 amino acids (N-62 StAR), which contain the mitochondrial targeting sequence, was found to be as effective as wild-type StAR in stimulating steroidogenesis. Other StAR constructs engineered for prolonged tethering to the surface of the mitochondria were very active in stimulating pregnenolone production, suggesting that the residency time of the protein on the mitochondrial surface determines the duration of the steroidogenic stimulus.[28] Recombinant human N-62 StAR in nanomolar concentrations enhanced pregnenolone production by isolated ovarian mitochondria in a dose- and time-dependent fashion, with significant increases in steroid production observed within minutes. Collectively, these findings strongly suggest that StAR acts on the outer mitochondrial membrane to promote cholesterol translocation. This perspective implies that import of the protein into the mitochondrial matrix, rather than being the *trigger* to steroid production, is actually the "off" mechanism because it removes StAR from its site of action (Fig. 4-4). This model explains three key points:

TABLE 4-1

Key Human Steroidogenic Proteins and Their Genes

Protein	Gene	Chromosomal Locus	Substrates*	Major Activities	Known Deficiency States
StAR	STAR	8p11.2	Cholesterol flux within mitochondria	Sterol delivery to P450scc	Congenital lipoid adrenal hyperplasia
P450scc	CYP11A1	15q23-q24	Cholesterol Hydroxysterols	Cholesterol side chain cleavage	Side chain cleavage enzyme deficiency
P450c17	CYP17	10q24.3	Preg, 170H-Preg Prog, [170H-Prog] DHEA	17α-Hydroxylase 1 6α-Hydroxylase 17,20-Lyase	17α-Hydroxylase deficiency Isolated 17,20-lyase deficiency
P450c21	CYP21B	6p21.1	Prog, 170H-Prog	21-Hydroxylase	21-Hydroxylase deficiency
P450c11β	CYP11B1	8q21-q22	11-Deoxycortisol	11-Hydroxylase	11-Hydroxylase deficiency
P450c11AS	CYP11B2	8q21-q22	Corticosterone 11-DOC 18OH-Corticosterone	11-Hydroxylase 18-Hydroxylase 18-Oxidase	CMO I deficiency CMO II deficiency
P450arom	CYP19	15q21.1	Androstenedione	19-Hydroxylase	Aromatase deficiency
P450 oxido reductase	POR	7q11.2	Androgens/corticoids Testosterone	17α-hydroxylase/17-20 lyase and 21-hydrxylase Aromatization	Combined partial 17α-hydroxylase/17-20 desmolase and 21-hydroxylase deficiencies
3β-HSDl	HSD3B1	1p13	Preg, 170H-Preg DHEA, Adiol	3β-Dehydrogenase Δ^{5,4}-Isomerase	
3β-HSD2	HSD3B2	1p13	Preg, 170H-Preg DHEA, Adiol	3β-Dehydrogenase Δ^{5–4}-Isomerase	3β-HSD deficiency
17β-HSD1	HSD17B1	17q21	Estrone, [DHEA]	17β-Ketosteroid reductase	
17β-HSD2	HSD17B2	16q24	Estradiol, testosterone DHT, 20α-OH-prog	17β-Hydroxysteroid dehydrogenase 20α-Hydroxysteroid dehydrogenase	
17β-HSD3	HSD17B3	9q22	Androstenedione	17β-Ketosteroid reductase	Male 17-ketosteroid reductase deficiency
17β-HSD4	HSD17B4	5q2.3	Estradiol, Adiol, 3-hydroxyacyl-CoA	17β-Hydroxysteroid dehydrogenase	D-hydroxy-acyl-CoA dehydrogenase deficiency
17β-HSD5	HSD17B5	10p14-15	Androstenedione, DHT, 3α-Asdiol 3α-Androstanediol Asone, Asdione	17β-Ketosteroid reductase 3α-Hydroxysteroid dehydrogenase	
5α-Reductase type 1	SRD5A1	5p15	Testosterone, C21 steroids	5α-Reductase	
5α-Reductase type 2	SRD5A2	2p23	Testosterone, C21 steroids	5α-Reductase	5α-Reductase deficiency
11β-HSDI	HSD11B1	1q32.2	Cortisol, cortisone, corticosterone, 11-dehydro-corticosterone	11β-Ketosteroid reductase	
11β-HSDII	HSD11B2	16p22	Cortisol, cortisterone	11β-Hydroxysteroid dehydrogenase	Syndrome of apparent mineralocorticoid excess
Estrogen sulfo-transferase	STE	4q13.1	Estradiol, estrone	Sulfonation	
Hydroxysteroid sulfotransferase	SULT2A1	19q13.4	DHEA, Preg	Sulfonation	
Steroid sulfatase	STS	Xp23.3	DHEA sulfate Cholesterol sulfate	Sulfatase	Sulfatase deficiency

*Bracketed compounds are minor substrates.

Adiol, Δ^5,3β-androstanediol; 3α-Asdiol, 3α-androstanedione; 11-DOC, 11-deoxycorticosterone; Asdione, androstanedione; Asone, androsterone; COA, coenzyme A; CMO, corticosterone methyl oxidase; DHEA, dehydroepiandrosterone; DHT, dihydrotestosterone; HSD, hydroxysteroid dehydrogenase; Preg, pregnenolone; Prog, progesterone.

1. Why continuous synthesis of StAR is needed to sustain steroidogenesis at high levels
2. How the steroidogenic response is efficiently terminated
3. Why inhibitors of protein synthesis (e.g., cycloheximides) rapidly and reversibly block cAMP stimulated steroidogenesis

The findings of the previously described experiments are most consistent with the idea that StAR enhances desorption of cholesterol from the sterol-rich outer mitochondrial membrane to the relatively sterol-poor inner membranes. The desorption process may involve a pH-dependent conformational change (molten globule transition). Even though StAR contains a hydrophobic pocket that binds cholesterol, sterol binding is not required for steroidogenic activity.[29]

The molecule or structure (protonated phospholipids?) on the mitochondrial outer membrane that StAR acts on has not yet been identified. It could be a lipid configuration or a protein. One protein candidate is the peripheral-type benzodiazepine receptor (PBR), an outer mitochondrial membrane protein that also binds cholesterol.[30] Suppression of PBR expression blocks steroidogenesis in cultured cells, even in the presence of StAR, suggesting that PBR is required for StAR action and that it may serve as a pore through which cholesterol could flow to the inner mitochondrial membrane in the presence of StAR. However, high-affinity binding of StAR to PBR has not been demonstrated, and the nature of StAR–PBR interaction remains to be elucidated.

Mutations in the *STAR* gene cause congenital lipoid adrenal hyperplasia, a rare autosomal recessive disease. Exceptions occur in Japan and Korea, however, where the mutation accounts for at least 5% of all cases of congenital adrenal hyperplasia.[27,28] The pathophysiology of the disease entails a two-step process in which impaired use of cholesterol for steroidogenesis leads to accumulation of sterol esters in lipid droplets. These droplets ultimately compress cellular organelles, causing damage through the formation of lipid peroxides. This damage occurs prominently in the adrenal cortex and Leydig cells.

Mutations found in the StAR gene, which is composed of seven exons and is located on band 8p11.2, include frameshifts caused by deletions or insertions, splicing errors, and nonsense and missense mutations. All of these mutations lead to the absence of StAR protein or the production of functionally inactive protein. Several nonsense mutations were shown to result in C-terminus truncations of StAR. One of these mutations, Q258X, results in the

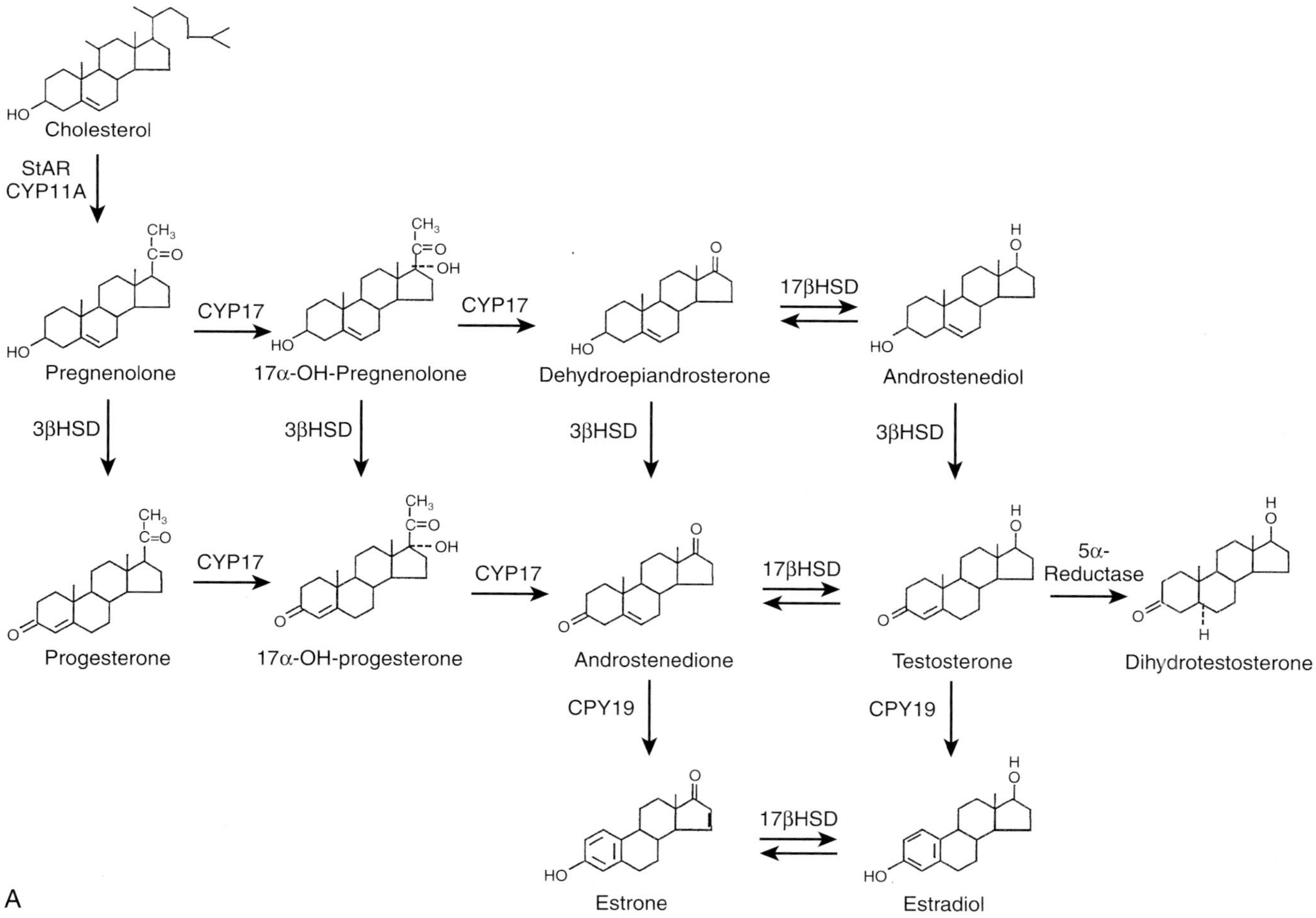

Figure 4-3. *A, Biosynthetic pathway for sex steroid hormones.*

Continued

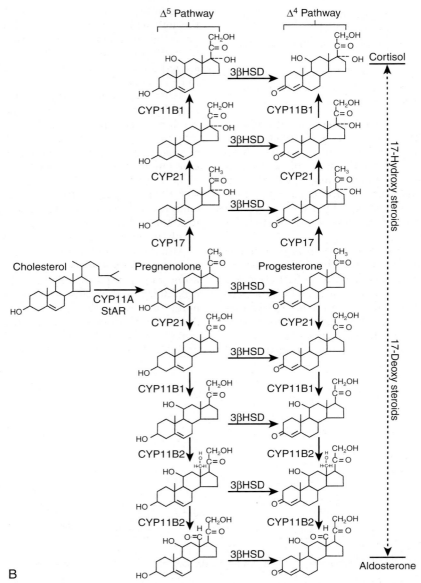

Figure 4-3, cont'd *B, Biosynthetic pathway for adrenal steroid hormones. Note that the 3β-hydroxysteroid dehydrogenase in the gonads and adrenal cortex is the type 2 enzyme, whereas the type 1 enzyme is responsible for this activity in the placenta. Note also that the 17β-hydroxysteroid dehydrogenases involved in the reduction and oxidation of steroids are different enzymes, as described in the text. CYP, cytochrome P; HSD, hydroxysteroid dehydrogenase; StAR, steroidogenic acute regulatory protein.*

deletion of the final 28 amino acids of the StAR protein and accounts for 80% of the known mutant alleles in the affected Japanese population. Known point mutations that produce amino acid substitutions occur in exons 5 to 7 of the gene, the exons that encode the C-terminus.

Although affected XY subjects are pseudohermaphrodites because of an inability to generate sufficient fetal testicular testosterone to masculinize the external genitalia, one should note that XX subjects have normal external genitalia, develop female secondary sexual characteristics, and experience menarche. They are, however, anovulatory and unable to produce large amounts of estradiol and progesterone in a cyclic fashion. The fact that some ovarian estradiol synthesis occurs reflects the existence of StAR-independent substrate movement to the cholesterol side-chain cleavage system.

Other START Domain Proteins

When StAR was discovered, it was believed to be a unique molecule. It is now evident that a family of proteins exists sharing a domain that is similar to the C-terminus of StAR, the *StAR-related lipid transfer (START) domain proteins.*[31,32] The absence of StAR from the human placenta, an organ that produces a significant amount of pregnenolone, documented the existence of StAR-independent steroidogenesis, but raised the possibility that another protein, possibly MLN64, also known as "StarD3," might subserve

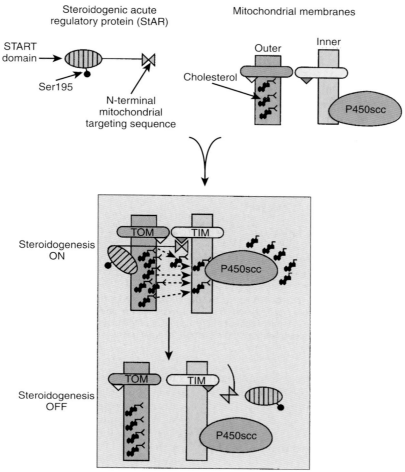

Figure 4-4. *Structure of steroidogenic acute regulatory protein (StAR) and model for its mechanism of action on intramitochondrial cholesterol translocation. TIM, inner mitochondrial membrane translocator; TOM, outer mitochondrial membrane protein translocator.*

the function of StAR in the placenta. Other cytosolic StAR domain proteins could be involved in the movement of cholesterol to the mitochondria as sterol carrier proteins, although their specific roles in sterol trafficking remain to be elucidated (see Fig. 4-2).

STEROIDOGENIC ENZYMES

The Cholesterol Side-Chain Cleavage Enzyme (P450scc Encoded by *CYP11A1*)

Cholesterol side-chain cleavage is catalyzed by cytochrome P450scc and its associated electron transport system, consisting of a flavoprotein reductase (ferredoxin or adrenodoxin reductase) and an iron sulfoprotein (ferredoxin or adrenodoxin), which shuttles electrons to cytochrome P450scc.[33,34] The side-chain cleavage reaction involves three catalytic cycles: the first two lead to the introduction of hydroxyl groups at positions C-22 and C-20, and the third results in scission of the side chain between these carbons (Fig. 4-5). Each catalytic cycle requires one molecule of NADPH and one molecule of oxygen so that the formation of one mole of the cleavage products (pregnenolone and isocroapraldehyde) uses three moles of NADPH and three moles of oxygen.

The slowest step of the reaction is the binding of cholesterol to the hydrophobic pocket of P450scc, where the heme resides. The sterol substrate remains bound to a single active site on cytochrome P450scc for all three cycles because of the tight binding of the reaction intermediates. The dissociation constant (K_d) for binding of cholesterol, a measure of the enzyme's affinity for its substrate, is approximately 5000 nM, whereas the K_d for the binding of the intermediate product 22-hydroxycholesterol is 4.9 nM; the K_d for 20,22-dihydroxycholesterol is 81 nM. However, the estimated K_d for pregnenolone, the end product, is 2900 nM, which permits its dissociation from the enzyme at the end of the reaction.

Reducing equivalents are shuttled to cytochrome P450scc by ferredoxin in cycles of reduction and oxidation, facilitated by differential affinities of the proteins, depending on their state of oxidation or reduction.[34] Ferredoxin forms a 1:1 complex with ferredoxin reductase, which catalyzes reduction of the iron-sulfur protein. The reduced ferredoxin then dissociates and forms a 1:1 complex with cytochrome P450scc and is subsequently oxidized when it donates its electrons to P450scc. Oxidized ferredoxin returns to ferredoxin reductase for electron recharging. This recharging is facilitated by the fact that

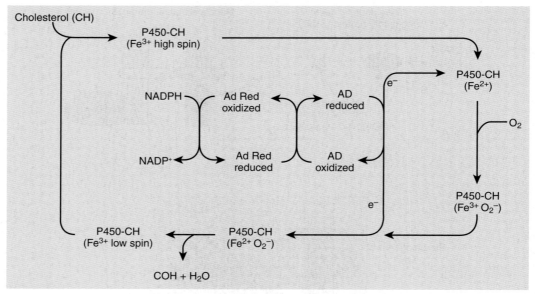

Figure 4-5. *Catalytic cycle for P450scc. Cholesterol (CH) binds to P450scc. Reducing equivalents are shuttled to P450scc by adrenodoxin (AD), which receives electrons from adrenodoxin reductase (Ad Red), which oxidizes nicotinamide adenine dinucleotide phosphate (NADPH). P450scc goes through three sequential catalytic cycles to convert 1 mole of cholesterol to 1 mole of pregnenolone and isocaproic acid, using 3 moles of NADPH and molecular oxygen. The P450scc heme iron undergoes oxidation and reduction, changing its spin state. NADP, nicotinamide adenine dinucleotide.*

ferredoxin reductase has a greater affinity for oxidized over reduced ferredoxin. The binding of cholesterol to cytochrome P450scc increases its affinity for reduced ferredoxin, which enhances the shuttle of electrons to substrate-loaded enzyme.

The rate of formation of pregnenolone is determined by the following factors:

1. The delivery of cholesterol to the mitochondria
2. The access of cholesterol to the inner mitochondrial membranes, which is regulated by StAR
3. The quantity of cholesterol side-chain cleavage enzyme, and secondarily, its flavoprotein and iron-sulfur protein electron transport chain
4. The catalytic activity of P450scc, which can be influenced by post-translational modification

Acute alterations in steroidogenesis generally result from changes in the delivery of cholesterol to P450scc, whereas long-term alterations involve changes in the quantity of enzyme proteins as well as cholesterol delivery.

The 20 kb *CYP11A1* gene, whose expression is regulated by a cAMP-mediated signal transduction cascade, is located on chromosome 15q23-q24. The gene consists of nine exons, an organization shared by the other mitochondrial steroidogenic P450 enzymes, 11β-hydroxylase and aldosterone synthase.

Mutations in the *CYP11A1* gene that result in diminished cholesterol side-chain cleavage activity have been reported in association with adrenal insufficiency and complete XY sex reversal.[35-37] One mutation in a heterozygous individual, an in-frame insertion of Gly and Asp between codons 271 and 272, resulted in an enzyme with no catalytic activity. It was suggested that the impaired flux through the side-chain cleavage system due to haploinsufficiency caused cholesterol accumulation

similar to what is seen in congenital lipoid adrenal hyperplasia, damaging the adrenal cortex and Leydig cells and causing the resultant clinical phenotype. A second XY subject with complete sex reversal and adrenal insufficiency was homozygous for a A359V mutation had P450scc activity that was 11% of normal. A female subject with adrenal insufficiency who was a compound heterozygote for two missense mutations has been described. One mutation (Arg353Trp) reduced cholesterol side-chain cleavage activity by greater than 90%, whereas the other created an alternative splice-donor site. The most interesting P450scc mutation was discovered in an XY subject, born prematurely with complete sex reversal and severe adrenal failure, with a homozygous single-nucleotide deletion leading to a premature termination codon at codon 288. This mutation is predicted to delete the C-terminal 242 amino acids, which are highly conserved regions of the P450scc enzyme, including the heme-binding site, and thus to result in a nonfunctional protein. Notably, the affected individual's parents were heterozygous for the mutation.

The discovery of mutations causing severe P450scc deficiency in humans challenges the notion that absence of P450scc activity in the fetus would be incompatible with pregnancy, raising the possibility of compensatory mechanisms to supply sufficient progesterone to sustain pregnancy to fetal viability.

17α-Hydroxylase/17,20-Lyase (P450c17)

P450c17 is a microsomal enzyme that catalyzes two reactions: hydroxylation of pregnenolone and progesterone at carbon 17, and conversion of pregnenolone into C19 steroids (in the case of the human enzyme, progesterone is also converted, but to a lesser extent).[38] The 17α-hydroxylation reaction requires one pair of electrons and

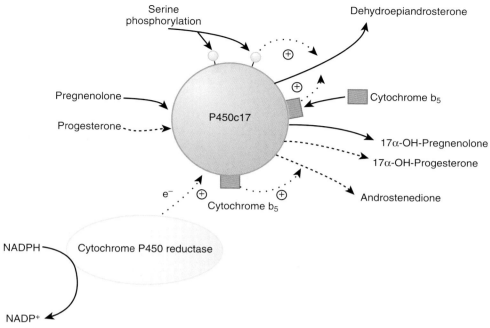

Figure 4-6. *Factors modulating 17α-hydroxylase and 17,20-lyase activities of P450c17. Phosphorylation of serine/threonine residues and cytochrome b5 stimulate (designated by* plus symbol*) lyase activity, with pregnenolone being the preferred substrate for the lyase reaction. Dephosphorylation of the serine/threonine residues by protein phosphatase 2A reduces lyase activity. Flow of reducing equivalents (e⁻, electrons) from cytochrome P450 reductase stimulates both 17α-hydroxylase and lyase activities. NADP, nicotinamide adenine dinucleotide; NADPH, nicotinamide adenine dinucleotide phosphate.*

molecular oxygen, whereas the lyase reaction requires a second electron pair and molecular oxygen. The reducing equivalents are transferred to the P450c17 heme iron from NADPH by NADPH cytochrome P450 reductase.[39] The hydroxylase and lyase reactions are both believed to proceed through a ferryl oxene mechanism, with the substrate bound in the enzyme in the catalytic pocket in the same orientation.[38] P450c17 also catalyzes 16α-hydroxylation of progesterone and dehydroepiandrosterone.

Several factors determine whether substrates undergo 17α-hydroxylation or subsequent scission of the 17,20 bond, including:

1. The nature of the substrate
2. Allosteric effectors
3. Post-translational modification of P450c17
4. Possibly the flux of reducing equivalents (Fig. 4-6)

Collectively, these factors determine the nature of the products produced by the enzyme, which, in the gonads and zona reticularis, favor androgens through augmentation of lyase activity. In contrast, the 17α-hydroxylation required for glucocorticoid and mineralocorticoid synthesis is favored in the zona fasciculata and glomerulosa.

Human P450c17 preferentially uses Δ^5 substrates for 17,20 bond cleavage. Cytochrome b_5, acting as an allosteric effector and not in an electron transport role (because the apo b_5 protein is also effective), increases 17,20-lyase activity.[40] Cytochrome b_5 also increases the use of 17α-hydroxyprogesterone as a substrate for androstenedione synthesis. The distribution and regulation of cytochrome b_5 expression in the adrenal cortex, being greatest in the adult zona reticularis, supports a role for this protein in the regulation of lyase activity. A second cytochrome b_5

gene (type 2 cytochrome b_5), found in human testis and expressed in the adrenals, also increases lyase activity. Its role relative to type 1 cytochrome b_5 protein in modulating 17,20-lyase activity remains to be determined.

The importance to steroidogenesis of P450 oxidoreductase, an 82-kDa membrane-associated protein encoded by a 32-kb gene on chromosome 7q11.2, is illustrated by the phenotype of individuals with P450 oxidoreductase deficiency, a newly described form of congenital adrenal hyperplasia.[40] The autosomal recessive disorder results in a steroid profile suggestive of combined 21-hydroxylase and 17-hydroxylase/17-20 desmolase deficiency, which presents as a range of phenotypes, including ambiguous genitalia, adrenal insufficiency, and Antley-Bixler skeletal malformation syndrome.

Phosphorylation of P450c17 at serine and threonine residues by a yet-to-be-identified protein kinase appears to be necessary for maximal 17,20-lyase activity.[41] The phosphorylated P450c17 protein is evidently a substrate for protein phosphatase 2A (PP2A). Inhibitors of PP2A enhance lyase activity in cultured adrenal tumor cells.

Adrenarche, the increased production of adrenal androgens in the absence of increased production of cortisol or levels of ACTH, may result from enhanced P450c17 lyase activity due to increased expression of cytochrome b_5 or the state of P450c17 phosphorylation. The availability of electrons to P450c17 has been proposed to influence the relative ratio of 17,20-lyase activity to 17α-hydroxylase activity. However, increasing the ratio of P450-oxidoreductase to P450c17 augments the formation of both 17α-hydroxylated products and the lyase reaction, making this an unlikely mechanism by which lyase-to-hydroxylase activity is differentially regulated.

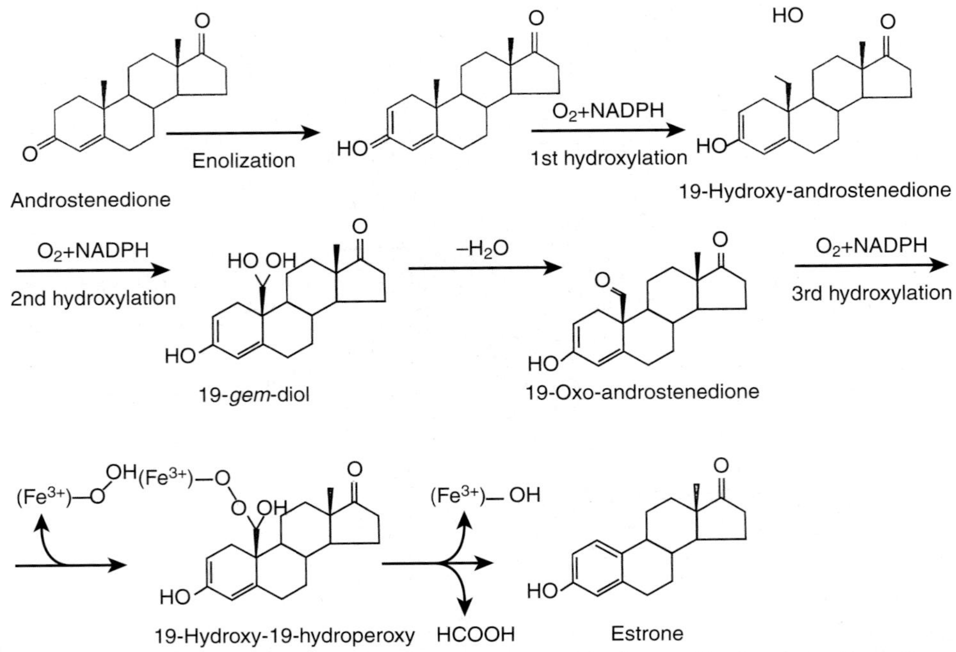

Figure 4-7. *The catalytic mechanism of aromatase. NADPH, nicotinamide adenine dinucleotide phosphate. (From Strauss JF III, Penning TM. Synthesis of the sex steroid hormones: molecular and structural biology with application to clinical practice. In Fauser BCJM, Rutherford AJ, Strauss JF III, et al [eds]. Molecular Biology in Reproductive Medicine. New York, Parthenon 1999, pp 201-232.)*

A P450c17-independent mechanism for conversion of pregnenolone into dehydroepiandrosterone in glial tumor cell homogenates promoted by $FeSO_4$ has been described. This conversion presumably originates from the fragmentation of tertiary hydroperoxides, which are probably derived from pregnenolone molecules oxygenated at carbons 17 and 20.[42] The significance of this pathway to the formation of C19 steroids in the brain or other tissues is unknown.

The *CYP17* gene, located on band 10q24.3, is divided into eight exons. Mutations in this gene cause separate or combined deficiency states for each activity of P450c17. Those with combined deficiency have marked diminution in production of C19 and C18 steroids, low levels of cortisol in association with hypertension, and hypokalemia resulting from increased production of 11-deoxycorticosterone.

The most common mutation causing combined 17α-hydroxylase and lyase deficiency is a 4-bp insertion that leads to an altered C-terminus sequence. Other mutations involving deletions in the C-terminus also result in complete loss of activity, indicating a critical role for this domain. Selective 17,20-lyase deficiency is rare; it results from point mutations that permit pregnenolone or progesterone to be bound and undergo 17α-hydroxylation but prohibit receipt or usage of a second pair of electrons to support the 17,20-lyase reaction.[43,44]

Aromatase (P450arom)

Aromatase, a microsomal enzyme, catalyzes three sequential hydroxylations of a C19 substrate by using 3 moles of NADPH and 3 moles of molecular oxygen to produce C18 steroids with a phenolic A ring (Fig. 4-7). The first hydroxylation yields a C19 hydroxyl derivative, which is converted in a second hydroxylation to a gem diol that

collapses to yield a C19 aldehyde. The final hydroxylation involves the formation of a 19-hydroxy-19-hydroperoxide intermediate that results in the elimination of the C19 methyl group as formic acid and concurrent aromatization. This sequence of reactions takes place at a single active site on the enzyme, with reducing equivalents transferred to P450arom by NADPH cytochrome P450 reductase.

The aromatase protein is encoded by a single large gene, *CYP19*, on band 15q21.1; this gene gives rise to cell-specific transcripts from different promoters (Fig. 4-8).[45-47] The promoter driving ovarian aromatase expression lies adjacent to the exon encoding the translation start site (promoter II). In granulosa cells, FSH stimulates transcription of the genes encoding both aromatase and the NADPH P450 reductase, which provides its reducing equivalents. A separate promoter lying approximately 100 kb upstream from the start of translation controls placental *CYP19* transcription. Expression of aromatase in adipose tissue, skin, and brain is driven from other promoters. Cytokines (including interleukin-11, interleukin-6, oncostatin-M, and leukemia-inhibiting factor) increase P450arom expression in adipose tissue in the presence of glucocorticoids. The cytokines increase aromatase gene transcription driven by the I.4 promoter through a JAK-STAT signaling cascade.

A number of cases of aromatase deficiency have been described.[46] Pregnancies in which the fetus is affected with aromatase deficiency are characterized by low maternal urinary estrogen excretion, maternal virilization, and pseudohermaphroditism in affected genetic females. Maternal and fetal virilization in the absence of placental aromatase activity highlights the importance and efficiency of the placenta in converting maternal and fetal androgens into estrogens.

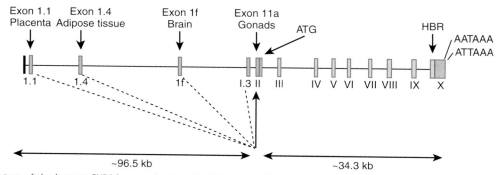

Figure 4-8. *Structure of the human* CYP19 *gene showing the 10 exons indicated by Roman numerals and the different tissue-specific promoters. The P450arom heme-binding region (HBR) and polyadenylation signals in exon 10 are indicated. ATG, methionine codon. (Modified from Kamat A, Hinshelwood MM, Murry BA, et al. Mechanisms in tissue-specific regulation of estrogen biosynthesis in humans. Trends Endocrinol Metab 13: 122, 2002.)*

Among the mutations identified in the *CYP19* gene are an 87-bp insertion at the splice junction between exon 6 and intron 6, causing the addition of 29 in-frame amino acid residues, with the other mutations being mainly missense or nonsense mutations in exons 4, 9, and 10. The mutant protein with the 29 in-frame amino acid residues displayed less than 3% of "wild-type" aromatase activity. Expression of the mutant complementary DNA confirmed that the protein had only a trace of aromatase activity. Compound heterozygous mutations in coding sequences found in patients with aromatase deficiency have also been shown to have minimal activity when expressed, documenting the effect of missense mutations. When aromatase activity has been measured in placenta from offspring with *CYP19* mutations, activities have been markedly reduced to 21% of control values.

Mice deficient in aromatase have been created by gene targeting.[47] The aromatase-deficient (ArKO) mice show many of the features of human aromatase deficiency and the consequential lack of estrogens, including a profound bone phenotype with reductions in all indices of bone mineralization.

Elevated aromatase activity in adipose tissue is associated with gynecomastia in prepubertal boys. Feminization of males and females caused by an autosomal dominant syndrome of aromatase excess in peripheral tissues has been reported, in which transcripts were found to originate near the gonadal promoter.[48-50]

Inappropriate expression of aromatase in neoplastic and non-neoplastic tissue has also been found. In these pathologic conditions, exemplified by breast cancer, there appears to be a shift in promoter use to favor the stronger gonadal (promoter IIa or I.3) over the weaker adipose tissue promoter (promoter I.4). This shift allows for activation of a cAMP-dependent signaling pathway, accounting for excessive aromatase expression and the resulting increase in estrogen synthesis.[49]

11β-Hydroxylases (P450c11β and P450c11AS)

The human genome contains two genes located on band 8q24.3 that encode related mitochondrial enzymes involved in 11β-hydroxylation and aldosterone synthesis, respectively, P450011β, encoded by *CYP11B1*, and

P450c11AS (also referred to as "P450aldo," "P450c18," or "P450cmo"), encoded by *CYP11B2*. These two genes are located 40 kb apart; each gene contains nine exons, and the encoded proteins differ in only 33 amino acid residues. Both enzymes display 11β-hydroxylase activities, but P450c11AS can also carry out the two oxygenation steps at carbon 18 required for the production of aldosterone. They require molecular oxygen and reducing equivalents shuttled by the adrenodoxin reductase–adrenodoxin system for catalysis.

CYP11B1, a gene whose transcription is stimulated by ACTH-triggered cAMP signaling pathways, is expressed in the zonae fasciculata and reticularis of the adrenal cortex. In contrast, *CYP11B2* expression is restricted to the zona glomerulosa; transcription of this gene is activated by protein kinase C signaling pathways that are turned on by angiotensin II.

Mutations in the *CYP11B1* gene cause 11β-hydroxylase deficiency, whereas mutations in *CYP11B2* cause 18-hydroxylase or corticosterone methyl oxidase I deficiency and 18-oxidase or corticosterone methyl oxidase II deficiency.[51,52] Accounting for 5% to 8% of cases of congenital adrenal hyperplasia, 11β-hydroxylase deficiency is characterized by high levels of deoxycorticosterone and 11-deoxycortisol. Unequal crossover of the adjacent *CYP11B1* and *CYP11B2* genes creates a third hybrid gene, in which the cAMP-regulated promoter of the *CYP11B1* gene drives expression of a chimeric protein with aldosterone synthase activity. This activity leads to glucocorticoid suppressible aldosteronism.

21-Hydroxylase (P450c21 Encoded by *CYP21B*)

P450c21 is an adrenal microsomal enzyme that catalyzes the 21-hydroxylation of progesterone and 17α-hydroxyprogesterone in the pathway of mineralocorticoid and glucocorticoid biosynthesis. The Michaelis constant (K_m) for 17α-hydroxyprogesterone (1.2 μM) is lower than that for progesterone (2.8 μM), and the apparent maximum velocity (V_{max}) for the former substrate is twice that for progesterone. The enzyme requires 1 mole of molecular oxygen and reducing equivalents (generated from NADPH through NADPH P450 reductase) to accomplish

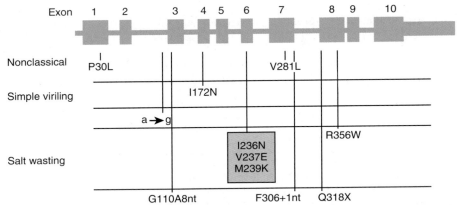

Figure 4-9. *Structure of the* CYP21B *gene and mutations causing 21-hydroxylase deficiency. (Modified from White PC, Speiser PW. Congenital adrenal hyperplasia due to 21-hydroxylase deficiency. Endocr Rev 21:245, 2000.)*

the hydroxylation of carbon 21. As noted previously, mutations inactivating P450 oxidoreductase cause a partial deficiency in 21-hydroxylase activity, as well as a partial deficiency in 17α-hydroxylase/17-20 lyase activity.[40] The primary regulator of *CYP21B* expression in the zona fasciculata is ACTH by way of a cAMP-mediated signal transduction cascade.

The *CYP21B* gene is adjacent to a pseudogene (*CYP21A*), separated by the complement *C4B* gene. These genes are embedded in the human leukocyte antigen region on band 6p21.1. The fairly frequent unequal crossovers and gene conversions make 21-hydroxylase deficiency one of the most common autosomal recessive metabolic diseases, occurring in 1:10,000 to 1:15,000 births.[53] Unequal crossover, with the complete loss of the *C4B* gene and a net deletion of *CYP21B1,* along with gene conversion events in which mutations in the pseudogene are introduced into the expressed gene, result in reduced 21-hydroxylase enzyme levels or impaired catalytic activity (Fig. 4-9).

Large-scale deletions/gene conversions may extend into the adjacent gene encoding tenascin-X, which when mutated in both alleles, causes a form of Ehlers-Danlos syndrome.[54] The clinical signs and symptoms of congenital adrenal hyperplasia caused by 21-hydroxylase deficiency reflect deficits in cortisol (because of inability to convert 17α-hydroxyprogesterone into 11-deoxycortisol) and aldosterone (because of inability to convert progesterone into deoxycorticosterone). Another contributing factor is the accumulation of adrenal androgens that results from elevated ACTH levels, due to the absence of cortisol-negative feedback on the hypothalamic–corticotrophic axis.

The clinical phenotypes are, however, variable and dependent on the severity of the 21-hydroxylase deficiency. The non–salt-wasting, salt-wasting, and nonclassic forms are associated with certain mutations that affect the amount of residual 21-hydroxylase activity, with the salt-wasting form being characteristic of severe enzyme deficiency (deletions and large conversions). The simple virilizing (non–salt-wasting) form is associated with mutations that substantially reduce activity (e.g., Ile172Asp), and the nonclassic (or *late-onset*) form is caused by

mutations that do not severely impair the level of expression or activity of P450c21 (e.g., Val28Leu, Pro30Leu).

Hydroxysteroid Dehydrogenases

Hydroxysteroid dehydrogenases (HSDs) or oxidoreductases catalyze the interconversion of alcohol and carbonyl functions in a position- and stereospecific manner on the steroid nucleus and side chain, using oxidized (+) or reduced (H) nicotinamide adenine dinucleotide (NADCH) or nicotinamide adenine dinucleotide phosphate (NADPCH) NAD(H) or NADP(H) as cofactors. In some instances, HSDs display bifunctionality (e.g., they oxidize or reduce 17β and 20α oxy functions), such as the type 2 17β-HSD.[55]

Multiple isoforms of HSDs exist, and coupled with their tissue-specific expression, account for the ability of specific enzymes to act predominantly as reductases (ketone reduction) or dehydrogenases (alcohol oxidation). In steroidogenic tissues, HSDs catalyze the final steps in progestin, androgen, and estrogen biosynthesis. In steroid target tissues, HSDs can regulate the occupancy of steroid hormone receptors by converting active steroid hormones into inactive metabolites or relatively inactive steroids to molecules with greater binding activity. The enzymes are members of the short chain dehydrogenase reductase or aldo-keto superfamilies. The nomenclature for these enzymes has recently been revised to reflect the membership of many of the hydroxysteroid dehydrogenases in the aldo-keto reductase superfamily (www.med.upenn.edu/akr/).

This is best exemplified by the human type 2 11β-HSD, which controls mineralocorticoid activity in the kidney by converting cortisol (which has high affinity for both the glucocorticoid and mineralocorticoid receptors) to cortisone (which does not bind to the mineralocorticoid receptor).[56] Thus, the specificity of mineralocorticoid receptor activation is not determined by the receptor, but by activity of the HSD that removes the more abundant potential mineralocorticoid receptor ligand, leaving aldosterone as the controlling activator (Fig. 4-10). Because of their tissue-specific roles in controlling the bioavailability of steroids, HSDs are interesting targets for pharmacologic manipulation.

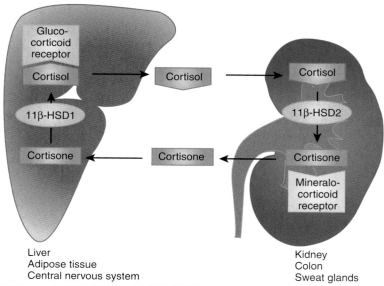

Figure 4-10. *The roles of 11β-HSD types 1 (11β-HSD1) and 2 (11β-HSD2) in controlling levels of bioactive glucocorticoids. 11β-HSD1 reduces inactive cortisone into cortisol in liver and other tissues, whereas 11β-HSD2 oxidizes cortisol to cortisone. Cortisone cannot activate the mineralocorticoid receptor, thus allowing aldosterone (a steroid that is less abundant than cortisol) to specifically regulate the mineralocorticoid receptor. (Modified from Seckl J, Walker B. 11β-Hydroxysteroid dehydrogenase type I-A tissue-specific amplifier of glucocorticoid action. Endocrinology 142:1371, 2001.)*

3β-Hydroxysteroid Dehydrogenase/Δ^{5-4} Isomerases

The 3β-HSD/Δ^{5-4} isomerases are membrane-bound enzymes localized to the endoplasmic reticulum and mitochondria that use nicotinamide adenine dinucleotide (NAD+) as a cofactor. These enzymes catalyze dehydrogenation of the 3β-hydroxyl group and the subsequent isomerization of the Δ^{5} olefinic bond to yield a Δ^{4} three-ketone structure. They convert pregnenolone into progesterone, 17α-hydroxypregnenolone into 17α-hydroxyprogesterone, and dehydroepiandrosterone into androstenedione.[57]

The dehydrogenase and isomerase reactions are believed to be performed at a single bifunctional catalytic site that adopts different conformations for each activity. The 3β-hydroxysteroid dehydrogenase step is rate-limiting in the overall reaction sequence, and the NADH formed in this reaction is believed to alter the enzyme conformation to promote the isomerase reaction.

There are two different human 3β-HSD genes, each consisting of four exons and lying 100 kb apart on band 1p13.1. The human genome also contains five unprocessed pseudogenes closely related to *HSD3B1* and *HSD3B2* on band 1p13.1, with two of them lying between the expressed genes. The type 1 gene (HSD3B1), identified first, is expressed primarily in the human placenta, skin, and adipose tissue. The type 2 gene (*HSD3B2*), identified subsequently, encodes the primary 3β-HSD expressed in the gonads and adrenal cortex.

The DNA sequences of the exons of the two genes are very similar, and the encoded proteins differ in only 23 amino acid residues. The type 1 enzyme has a lower K_{m} for substrate than the type 2 enzyme (<1 μM vs 1–4 μM), which facilitates metabolism of lower concentrations of Δ^{5} substrate. Electron microscope cytochemistry has localized type 2 3β-HSD activity to the perimitochondrial endoplasmic reticulum and in subcellular fractions containing StAR and P450scc. Some types of type 1 3β-HSD in the placenta are also localized to mitochondria. Thus, 3β-HSDs are closely associated with mitochondria and are positioned to act on pregnenolone produced by the cholesterol side-chain cleavage system.

Because most steroidogenic cells have a large capacity to generate progesterone when presented with exogenous pregnenolone, 3β-HSD is not believed to be a rate-determining enzyme. However, mutations resulting in deficiency in type 2 3β-HSD activity cause a form of congenital adrenal hyperplasia characterized by impaired adrenal and gonadal steroidogenesis with accumulation of $\Delta 5$ steroids in the circulation.[58]

In its severest form, 3β-HSD deficiency is associated with salt wasting because of insufficient mineralocorticoid production. Kinetic analysis of mutant proteins associated with the salt-wasting and non–salt-wasting forms of the disease in cell homogenates showed a 4- to 40-fold reduction in catalytic efficiency for the conversion of pregnenolone into progesterone. The salt-wasting form of the disease is associated with frameshift mutations resulting in protein truncation and a variety of missense mutations that affect affinity for cofactor and protein stability. The greater instability of the mutant proteins found in subjects with salt-wasting disease compared with those proteins found in the non–salt-wasting form appears to account, in part, for the different clinical phenotypes.

A so-called attenuated, or late-onset, form of 3β-HSD deficiency, diagnosed by steroid measurements, has been described in the literature. However, no mutations have yet been found in the gene encoding 3β-HSD type 1 or 2 in subjects with this clinical diagnosis. Although mutations in the distal promoter that might alter enzyme expression

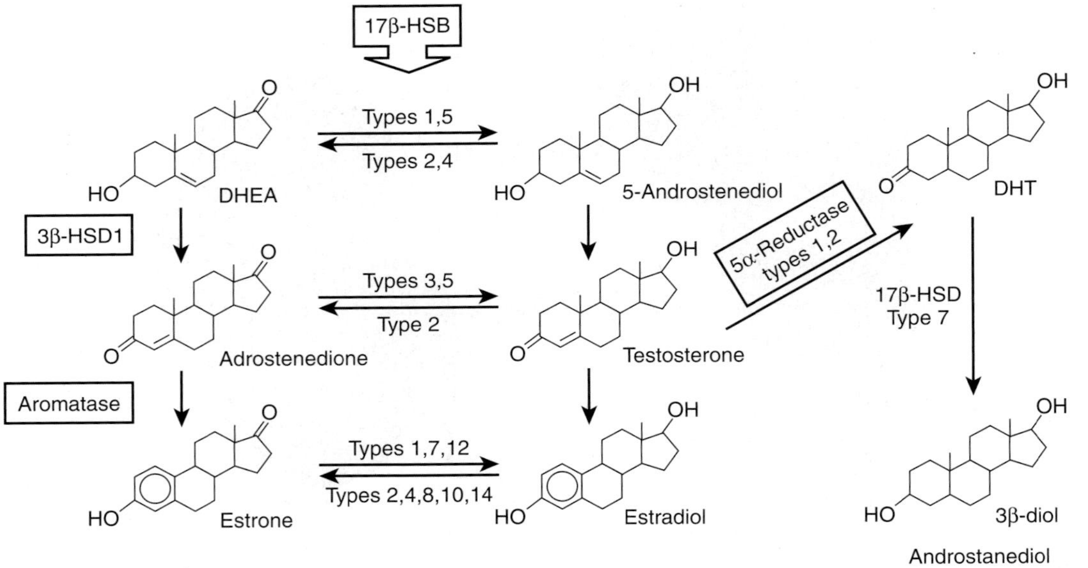

Figure 4-11. *The family of 17β-HSDs and their role in androgen and estrogen synthesis and metabolism. DHT, dihydrotestosterone. (Modified from Luu-The V. Analysis and characteristics of multiple types of human 17β-hydroxysteroid dehydrogenase. Steroid Biochem Mol Biol 76:143, 2001.)*

cannot be ruled out, the apparent reduced 3β-HSD activity could also be the result of alterations in the membrane environment that affect catalytic activity. The reduced activity could also be the result of post-translational modifications to the enzyme that diminish its function.

Mutations in *HSD3B1* have not been detected, although several sequence variants that are evidently without functional significance have been described. Because the type 1 enzyme is the primary 3β-HSD in the placenta, it is possible that mutations that inactivate the type 1 gene would lead to miscarriage as a result of insufficient placental progesterone production.

11β-Hydroxysteroid Dehydrogenases: Key Regulators of the Activity of Glucocorticoids

The biologic activity of cortisol in target tissues is controlled by the action of two different 11β-hydroxysteroid dehydrogenases that are members of the short-chain alcohol dehydrogenase family (see Fig. 4-10). These enzymes catalyze the interconversion of active glucocorticoids and their inert 11-keto metabolites.[59-61] The type 2 enzyme is a microsomal protein that has reversible oxidoreductase activity in vitro, but preferentially catalyzes the reduction of the 11-keto group, using NADPH as a cofactor in vivo. This enzyme is expressed in the liver, lung, adipose tissue, brain, vascular tissue, and gonads, where it regenerates cortisol from abundant 11-ketosteroids. In the case of the placenta, the activity ensures transport of biologically active cortisol to the fetus in the first half of pregnancy.

Targeted deletion of the type 1 enzyme in mice results in animals with lower blood glucose levels in response to overfeeding and stress, impaired activation of gluconeogenesis, and blunted sensitivity to natural glucocorticoids. This finding substantiates a role for the type 1 enzyme in the amplification of cortisol and corticosterone action.

The type 2 enzyme, also microsomal, has a higher affinity for its substrate than the type 1 enzyme and catalyzes

the oxidation of cortisol with NAD+ as a cofactor. It shares only modest amino acid sequence identity (21%) with the type 1 enzyme. Type 2 11β-HSD is highly expressed in the kidney, colon, salivary glands, and placenta, all tissues that respond to aldosterone, or in the case of the placenta, tissues that act to separate the maternal and fetal endocrine systems (which is important in the third trimester). By converting cortisol and corticosterone to 11-keto compounds, type 2 11β-hydroxysteroid dehydrogenase protects the renal mineralocorticoid receptors (which cannot distinguish cortisol or corticosterone from aldosterone) from inappropriate activation by the glucocorticoids.

Mutations that inactivate the type 2 enzyme produce a syndrome of apparent mineralocorticoid excess in humans, which is mimicked in the mice deficient in type 2 11βHSD that display hypertension, hypokalemia, and renal structural abnormalities.[59] Glycyrrhizic acid, a component of licorice, and its metabolite carbenoxolone, are competitive inhibitors of the type 2 enzyme, but also cause reduced expression of the type 2 enzyme mRNA when administered in vivo. As a result, a drug-induced syndrome of apparent mineralocorticoid excess is produced.[60]

17β-Hydroxysteroid Dehydrogenases: Multiple Enzymes with Specific Synthetic and Catabolic Roles

The adrenals, gonads, and placenta reduce 17-ketosteroids into 17β-hydroxysteroids (which have greater biologic potency), whereas target tissues usually oxidize 17β-hydroxysteroids, inactivating them.[61-63] In humans, these metabolic processes are mediated by at least seven of the known mammalian 17β-HSDs, designated types 1 through 14, according to the chronologic order in which they were identified (Fig. 4-11). They are all members of the short-chain dehydrogenase–reductase family of enzymes, except the type 5 enzyme, which is an aldo-keto reductase. They have different cofactor and substrate specificities, subcellular locations, and tissue-specific patterns of expression. The structures of the genes encoding 14 of the known 17β-hydroxysteroid dehydrogenases differ, and their nucleotide sequence homology is low. They can be grouped into enzymes that catalyze NAD+-dependent oxidation (types 2, 4, 6, 8, 9, 10, 11, and 14) and those that catalyze NADPH-dependent reduction (types 1, 3, 5, and 7). Because of the broad substrate specificities of these enzymes, the primary role of several of them lies in basic metabolic pathways unrelated to steroid metabolism, and deficiencies of these enzymes cause metabolic disease.

The type 1 enzyme is often referred to as the "estrogenic" 17β-HSD because it catalyzes the final step in estrogen biosynthesis by preferentially reducing the weak estrogen estrone to yield the potent estrogen 17β-estradiol. The enzyme is a cytoplasmic member of the short-chain dehydrogenase–reductase enzyme family that uses either NADH or NADPH as a cofactor. Type 1 17β-HSD has 100-fold higher affinity for C18 steroids than for C19 steroids.

The type 1 enzyme also shows modest 20α-HSD activity. The 6.2-kb structural gene encoding the type 1 enzyme in six exons is located on bands 17q11-12 in tandem with a highly homologous pseudogene. The structural gene gives rise to a major transcript of 1.3 kb and a minor transcript of 2.2 kb, which are abundant in granulosa cells of the ovary and the placental syncytiotrophoblast. It is also expressed at higher levels in breast cancer cells relative to the type 2 enzyme described later, which converts estradiol to the less potent estrogen estrone. The crystal structure of the type 1 enzyme has been determined to a resolution of 2.2 Å with and without bound substrates, providing a molecular framework for the design of specific inhibitors.

The type 2 17β-HSD is a microsomal enzyme that contains an N-terminal signal sequence, targeting it to endoplasmic reticulum, and a C-terminal endoplasmic reticulum retention motif. It inactivates hormones and preferentially oxidizes testosterone to yield androstenedione, and it also oxidizes estradiol into estrone using NAD+ as its cofactor. The type 2 enzyme also has the ability to convert 20α-hydroxyprogesterone into progesterone.

The gene encoding the type 2 enzyme is located on band 16q24, contains five exons, and gives rise to a 1.5-kb mRNA transcript. It is expressed in liver, secretory endometrium, and the fetal capillary endothelial cells of the placenta, as well as the endothelial cells of the larger vessels. This expression pattern is consistent with its role of inactivating testosterone and estradiol. Type 2 enzyme in the fetal capillary endothelium protects the fetal compartment from estradiol formed in the syncytiotrophoblast and from testosterone that escaped aromatization. Its expression in the secretory endometrium permits the conversion of estradiol to estrone, whereas 20α-hydroxyprogesterone is converted back into progesterone, resulting in progestational dominance. In normal breast tissue, type 2 17β-HSD expression predominates over type 1 enzyme expression.

The type 3 enzyme is referred to as the "androgenic" 17β-HSD because it catalyzes the final step in androgen biosynthesis in the Leydig cells, reducing androstenedione to testosterone using NADPH as cofactor.[63] It also can reduce estrone to estradiol and is microsomal in location. The type 3 enzyme is not expressed in the ovary, requiring androgen-producing cells of the ovary to employ

another enzyme, probably the type 5 17β-HSD, to synthesize testosterone. The type 3 gene is 60 kb in length and is located on band 9q22. It comprises 11 exons and gives rise to a 1.3-kb mRNA transcript.

In the absence of type 3 17β-HSD activity, the testes produce large amounts of androstenedione; deficiency of type 3 17β-HSD results in male pseudohermaphroditism, with 10-to 15-fold elevations in the ratio of blood androstenedione to testosterone. Females with mutations in the HSD17B3 gene are asymptomatic. Molecular analysis of the type 3 17β-HSD gene in affected individuals has shown mutations that affect splicing, amino acid replacements in exons 9 and 10, and a small deletion leading to a frameshift. Many of the missense mutations result in proteins that are devoid of catalytic activity when expressed in eukaryotic cells.

The type 4 17β-HSD is a peroxisomal protein expressed in the liver, breast, and uterus, and in granulosa, Leydig, and Sertoli cells. It serves a catabolic role by oxidizing 17β-estradiol and androgens, using NAD+ as cofactor. This 80-kDa enzyme is bifunctional, having 17β-HSD activity and participating in β-oxidation of fatty acids. Mutations in the 17BHSD4 gene cause peroxisomal D-hydroxy-acyl-coenzyme A dehydrogenase deficiency, a fatal form of Zellweger syndrome.

The type 5 enzyme, mapped to bands 10p15-14, is a member of the aldo-keto reductase family that produces testosterone from androstenedione. It appears to be the "androgenic" 17β-HSD of the ovarian theca cells.[64,65] Type 5 17β-HSD is also expressed in prostate, mammary gland, and Leydig cells.

The human type 7 17β-HSD produces active estrogens and inactivates androgens: it transforms estrone into estradiol and has 3-keto reductase activity, converting dihydrotestosterone into 3α-dihydrotestosterone. The protein is derived from a 1.5-kb transcript expressed in the ovary, breast, placenta, testes, prostate, and liver cells, and is encoded by a 21.8-kb gene located on band 10p11.2.

The type 8 17β-HSD, also known as Ke 6, is a microsomal protein that converts 17β-estradiol into estrone and is thus a hormone-inactivating enzyme. Relatively little is known about its expression in humans compared with the other 17β-HSDs, although type 8 17β-HSD mRNA has been found to be constitutively expressed in the primate uterus.

The type 10 enzyme, encoded by a gene on Xp11.22, oxidizes estrogens and also plays a role in beta oxidation of fatty acids, and mutations in the enzyme cause 2-methyl-3-hydroxybutyryl-CoA dehydrogenase deficiency.

20α-Hydroxysteroid Dehydrogenases: Regulators of Progestational Potency

Some 20α-HSDs are members of the aldo-keto reductase family of enzymes that reduce progesterone to yield the inactive steroid 20α-hydroxyprogesterone. They are cytosolic monomeric proteins with a molecular weight of approximately 34 kDa, exemplified by genes expressed in human keratinocytes and cells of the liver, prostate, testis, adrenal gland, brain, uterus, and mammary gland. These enzymes prefer NADPH to NADH as a cofactor.[66] As noted previously, some enzymes of the short-chain dehydrogenase–reductase family have 20α-HSD activity, including the type 1 and type 2 17β-HSDs. The type 2 17β-HSD preferentially oxidizes 20α-hydroxyprogesterone into progesterone.

Reductases

The reductases are membrane-associated enzymes that reduce the Δ5-4 double bond in steroid hormones by catalyzing direct hydride transfer from NADPH to the carbon 5 position of the steroid substrate. They produce either 5α or 5β-dihydrosteroids.

5α-Reductase Types 1 and 2. Two different human 5α-reductases sharing 50% similarity in amino acid sequence and a molecular weight of approximately 29 kDa have been identified.[67,68] The genes for type 1 and 2 5α-reductases each have five exons; the substrate-binding domain of the 5α-reductases is encoded by exon 1, and the cofactor-binding domain is encoded by exons 4 and 5. The type 2 5α-reductase gene, SRA5A2, is located on band 2p23, whereas the type 1 5α-reductase gene, SRA5A1, is located on band 5p15, with a pseudogene on Xq24-qter.

Type 2 5α-reductase is predominantly expressed in male genital structures (including genital skin and prostate), where it reduces testosterone to yield the more potent androgen, 5α-dihydrotestosterone. The type 1 enzyme, which catalyzes a similar reaction on both C21 and C19 steroid hormones, is expressed in the liver, kidneys, skin, and brain. Although this enzyme can also make 5α-dihydrotestosterone, its tissue distribution suggests that its predominant function is to inactivate steroid hormones.

The type 2 enzyme has an acidic pH optimum and a K_m for testosterone in the nanomolar range, whereas the type 1 enzyme has a broad alkaline pH optimum and a lower affinity for its substrates in the micromolar range. The type 2 enzyme can also be distinguished from the type 1 enzyme by its selective inhibition by finasteride, with an inhibition constant (K_i) equal to 3 nM.

Inactivating mutations in SRD5A2 cause male pseudohermaphrodism. The enzyme defect is characterized by abnormal testosterone-to-5α-dihydrotestosterone ratios. Affected males have varying degrees of abnormal development of the external genitalia, ranging from mild hypospadias to severe defects in which the external genitalia are essentially female. Wolffian ducts develop normally in response to adequate levels of testosterone.

Females carrying mutations in the SRD5A2 gene have a normal phenotype and normal menstrual cycles. They have a low incidence of hirsutism and acne, and like males with the disease, have low ratios of 5α- to 5β-dihydrosteroid metabolites in the urine. The infrequency of acne in both affected males and females, the rarity of hirsutism in affected females, the absence of male pattern baldness, and the finding of an atrophied prostate in affected males indicates that type 2 5α-reductase plays an important role in androgen metabolism in skin and in the androgen-dependent growth of the prostate.

Among the mutations reported are deletions that inactivate the type 2 enzyme and missense mutations that impair enzyme activity by affecting substrate or cofactor binding. A SRD5A2 variant (Ala49Thr) that has increased catalytic activity has been linked to an increased risk of prostate cancer.

Mutations have not been described in the human SRA5A1 gene. However, targeted deletion of the murine counterpart results in a female phenotype of reduced fecundity and a parturition defect caused by failed cervical ripening. This defect can be reversed by administration of 5α-androstanediol.[69,70]

5β-Reductases. The only known human 5β-reductase (SRD5B1) is a member of the aldo-keto reductase superfamily (AKR1D1), related to the HSDs of the same family.[71] This enzyme is involved in steroid hormone inactivation in the liver. Its reaction mechanism is similar to that described for 5α-reductase, except that an A/B cis-fused ring product is formed. The enzyme efficiently catalyzes the NADPH-dependent reduction of the Δ5-4 double bond in C27, C21, and C19 steroids to yield the 5β-dihydrosteroids with a distinct preference for C27 steroids.

In keeping with this observation, mutations in the SRD5B1 (AKR1D1) gene on bands 7q32-q33 that encodes this enzyme result in abnormal bile acid synthesis, along with a marked reduction in the primary bile acids and 5β-reduced steroid metabolites.

Sulfotransferases

A family of enzymes introduce the sulfonate (SO_3^-) anion from an activated donor, 3′-phosphoadenosine-5′-phosphosulfate, to a steroid hydroxyl acceptor, inactivating the hormone.[72] The major enzymes carrying out this reaction include estrogen sulfotransferase (SULT1E1, encoded by the STE gene on band 4q13.1), an enzyme that sulfonates the 3-hydroxyl function of phenolic steroids, and the hydroxysteroid sulfotransferases, encoded by the closely linked SULT2A1 and SULT2B1 genes on band 19q13.4.[72,73]

The SULT2A1 enzyme, also known as *dehydroepiandrosterone sulfotransferase,* has a broader substrate range than the products of the SULT2B1 gene, including the 3α-, 3β-, and 17β-hydroxy functions of steroid hormones. SULT2A1 enzyme is expressed at high levels in the fetal zone of the adrenal cortex, as well as in the zona reticularis after adrenarche, and in the liver, gut, and testes.[4] This enzyme is developmentally regulated in the adrenal cortex, with expression increasing between ages 5 and 13 years in association with adrenarche. The GATA6 transcription factor, which is known to increase transcription of other genes involved in androgen biosynthesis, also activates expression of the SULT2A1 gene.

The SULT2B1 gene gives rise to two protein isoforms through alternative splicing. The SULT2B1a isoform sulfonates pregnenolone, whereas the SULT2B1b isoform preferentially sulfonates cholesterol. They both sulfonate dihydrotestosterone. Unlike the SULT2A1 gene that is expressed in a limited number of tissues, SULTB1 isoforms are present in a variety of hormone-producing and hormone-responsive tissues, including the placenta, ovary, uterus, and prostate.[73] Phenol sulfotransferases can also act on steroid hormones.

Estrogen sulfotransferase (SULT1E) is expressed in many tissues, including the adrenal gland, liver, kidneys, muscle, fat, and uterus. In the endometrium, progesterone increases its activity, contributing to the inactivation of estradiol in the secretory phase. The importance of estrogen sulfotransferase in modulating local levels of bioactive estrogens has been shown in mice with targeted deletions of the gene.[74] Males with estrogen sulfotransferase deficiency have Leydig cell hyperplasia and become infertile with age, due to elevated testicular levels of estrogen. Such elevations are a consequence of the inability to inactivate these hormones by sulfonation. Adipose tissue mass also increases. Hydroxylated metabolites of polychlorinated biphenyls are potent inhibitors of estrogen sulfotransferase, with IC_{50} values in the picomolar range.[75] The blockade of estradiol inactivation by this compound may account for the reported "estrogenic" activity of polychlorinated biphenyls.

Steroid Sulfatase

The sulfonate function on steroids is cleaved by steroid sulfatase, an enzyme encoded by the *STS* gene on human Xp22.3. The syncytiotrophoblast is enriched in this enzyme, which plays a key role in placental estrogen synthesis by liberating sulfonated androgen precursors produced in the fetal compartment before their aromatization in the trophoblast. The enzyme is also expressed in skin, where it metabolizes cholesterol sulfate and sulfated estrogens.

Sulfatase deficiency is associated with marked impairment of placental estrogen synthesis during pregnancy and ichthyosis developing after birth.[76-78] It occurs mostly in males because of the X chromosome location of the sulfatase gene, at a frequency of 1:2000 to 1:6000 liveborn males. The majority of subjects with steroid sulfatase deficiency have a deletion of the entire gene that results from recombination of repetitive elements that flank the locus. The large deletions of the *STS* gene occur in association with mutations in the adjacent Kallmann's syndrome gene. Partial deletions in the *STS* gene causing enzyme deficiency have also been described.

Characteristically, in pregnancies hosting an affected fetus, maternal plasma estriol and urinary estriol excretion are quite low, approximately 5% of the levels found in normal pregnancies. Excretion of estrone and estradiol are also reduced, at approximately 15% of normal. Maternal serum 16α-hydroxydehydroepiandrosterone levels are elevated, and intravenous administration of dehydroepiandrosterone sulfate to the mother does not lead to an increase in estrogen excretion, whereas administration of dehydroepiandrosterone does.

Steroid sulfatase is expressed in estrogen target tissues, including endometrium, bone, and breast. Increased sulfatase expression may also contribute to greater bioavailability of estradiol in certain tumors, including breast cancers.

UDP-Glucuronosyl Transferases

Glucuronidation, catalyzed by a family of UDP-glucuronosyl transferases, is part of the metabolic clearance mechanism for steroid hormones by the liver and extrahepatic tissues.[80-82] There are two families of UDP-glucuronosyl transferases, UGT1 and UGT2. UGT1 enzymes are encoded by a single gene that gives rise to alternatively spliced products capable of acting on estrogens; in contrast, the UGT2 enzymes are products of separate genes subdivided into two families, UGT2A and UGT2B. UGT2A is expressed in olfactory epithelium, and UGT2B is expressed in the liver, kidney, breast, lung, and prostate. At least seven members of the UGT2B family have been identified with different steroid substrate specificities. UGT2B7 glucuronidates estrogens, catechol estrogens, and androstane-3α-17β-diol; UGT2B15 and UGT2B17 glucuronidate the latter steroid with similar activity, but with less activity than UGT2B7; UGT2B4 acts on 5α-reduced androgens and catechol estrogens, but with lower activity than UTG2B7, UGT2B15, and UGT2B17.

Interesting Steroid Hormone Metabolic Pathways

There are several metabolic fates of steroid hormones that have a significant effect on the activity and distribution of the molecules. Among these fates are esterification to long-chain fatty acids, formation of catechol estrogens, and the 7α-hydroxylation of androgens. Equine steroidogenic tissues also have a novel pathway for biosynthesis of estrogens, resulting in a phenolic A ring and an unsaturated B ring. The equine estrogens are of interest because of their extensive use in hormone replacement therapy.

SYNTHESIS OF EQUINE ESTROGENS

The pregnant mare produces estradiol and estrone, but also B-ring unsaturated estrogens (equilin [with an 8,9 olefinic bond], equilenin [with a phenolic B ring], 17α-dihydroequilin, 17α-dihydroequilenin, 17β-dihydroequilin, and 17β-dihydroiequilenin) by a mechanism that is yet to be fully understood (Fig. 4-12).[83]

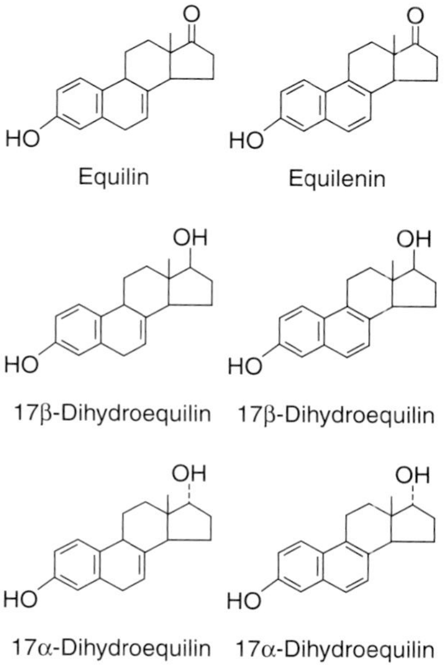

Figure 4-12. *Structures of equine estrogens.*

These B-ring unsaturated compounds are potent estrogens in vivo. Although 7-dehydrocholesterol can be converted into B-ring unsaturated estrogens (as occurs in Smith-Lemli-Opitz syndrome), the biosynthesis of these compounds in the pregnant mare occurs by a pathway not requiring the synthesis of squalene or cholesterol, and thus does not involve 7-dehydrocholesterol. Evidently, they are derived from a C25 sesterterpene pathway that coexists with the normal biosynthetic route of "standard" estrogens from a cholesterol precursor.

CATECHOL ESTROGENS

Catechol estrogens are generated by the actions of genes encoded by *CYP1A1* and *CYP1A2* (which catalyze 2-hydroxylation of estrogens), and *CYP1B1*, which is an estrogen 4-hydroxylase.[84-86] Peroxidative reactions can also generate catechol estrogens. Although the catechol estrogens are short-lived in vivo and are postulated to have physiologic functions as locally generated signaling molecules, they also yield potent genotoxic molecules implicated in carcinogenesis. The 4-hydroxyestrogens can be oxidized to quinone intermediates that react with purine bases of DNA, resulting in depurinating adducts that generate highly mutagenic apurinic sites (Fig. 4-13). Quinones derived from the 2-hydroxyestrogens produce stable DNA adducts and are presumed to be less genotoxic.

Metabolism of catechol estrogens may also generate oxygen free radicals. Catechol estrogens are methylated by catechol-*O*-methyltransferase, resulting in a catecholamine-like substance. The methylated catechol estrogens have a reduced genotoxic potential, but may act on catecholamine receptors.

Contrasting with its potential role in genotoxicity, 2-methoxyestradiol has been found to have antiangiogenic and antitumor activity; 2-methoxyestradiol inhibits expression of the hypoxia-inducible factor-1α (HIF-1α)

pro-angiogenic transcription factor that interacts with hypoxia response elements.

STEROID FATTY ACID ESTERS

Steroids esterified to long-chain fatty acids are present in blood, are bound to lipoproteins, or are found in tissue, particularly steroidogenic glands and fat.[89] These hydrophobic molecules may serve as a depot form of steroid, but they also have unique biochemical attributes. Estradiol 17-esters are produced in blood by the action of lecithin-cholesterol acyl transferase and in tissues by ACAT. The fatty acid esters of estradiol have pronounced antioxidant activity. Fatty acid esters of other steroids, including pregnenolone, testosterone, dehydroepiandrosterone, and glucocorticoids, have also been described.

STEROID 7α-HYDROXYLATION

Substituents on carbon 7 of the steroid nucleus can have a significant effect on activity. A cytochrome P450 encoded by the *CYP7B* gene catalyzes 7α-hydroxylation of steroid hormones and oxysterols. The 7α-hydroxylation of dehydroepiandrosterone produces a molecule with enhanced immunostimulatory activity, a property demonstrable in animal bioassays.[88]

Regulation of Expression of the Steroidogenic Machinery

The regulation of expression of genes encoding proteins involved in steroidogenesis in the ovary, testes, and adrenal cortex shares a number of similarities with respect to the involvement of *cis* elements and transcription factors. *Steroidogenic factor 1* (SF-1), an orphan nuclear receptor also known as "Ad4BP" and by the new family member

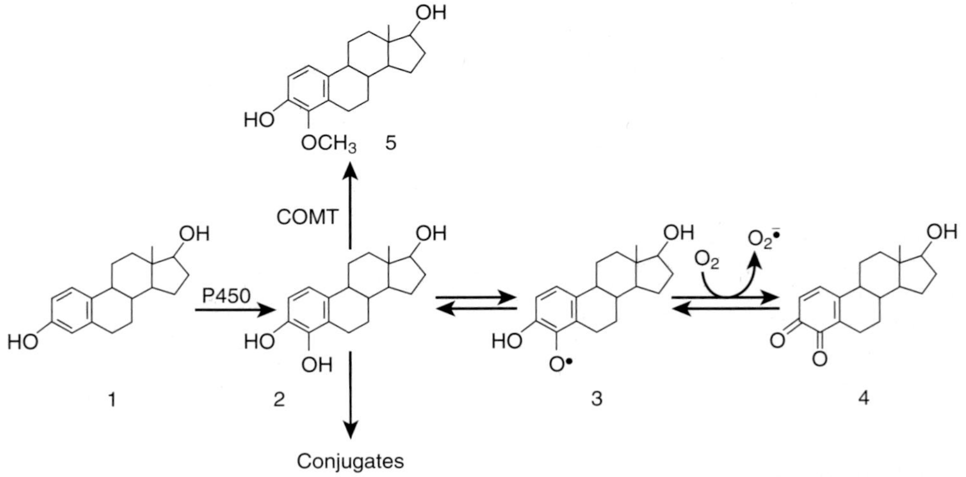

Figure 4-13. Metabolism of estradiol (1) by P450 enzymes, including P4501B1 to 4-hydroxyestradiol (2). Metabolic cycling between 4-hydroxyestradiol and estradiol 3,4-quinone (4) can be catalyzed by P4501A1 for the oxidation step and cytochrome P450 reductase for the reduction step. The semiquinone intermediate (3) is a free radical that can react with molecular oxygen to form superoxide radical and quinone. 4-Hydroxyestradiol can be converted to 4-methoxyestradiol (5) by catechol-O-methyltransferase (COMT). (From Liehr JG. Catecholestrogens in the induction of tumors in the kidney of the Syrian hamster. In Goldstein DS, Eisenhofer G, McCarty R [eds]. Advances in Pharmacology: Catecholamines. Bridging Basic Science with Clinical Medicine, vol 42. San Diego, Academic Press, 1998, pp 824-828.)

designation "NR5A1," is essential for development of steroidogenic glands. Most of the genes encoding key proteins involved in steroidogenesis (e.g., *SRB1, STAR, CYP11A1, CYP11B2, CYP17, CYP19, CYP21*) contain one or more SF-1 response elements in their proximal promoters. These elements are important for basal as well as stimulated expression of these genes, generally by a cAMP-mediated signal transduction pathway. Transactivation by SF-1 can be modified by phosphorylation, providing a link between this transcription factor and intracellular kinases that transduce signals from plasma membrane receptors.[89]

The importance of SF-1 to the regulation of steroidogenic tissues was documented by gene targeting. Mice deficient in SF-1 lacked adrenal glands and gonads, and males were consequently sex-reversed. Haploinsufficiency of SF-1 in the mouse resulted in an impaired adrenal steroidogenic response to stress, although basal steroidogenesis was not affected due to compensatory hypertrophy.[90] A human case of SF-1 haploinsufficiency has been reported in which there was primary adrenal failure and XY sex reversal.[91] However, recent reports indicate that heterozygous mutations can be found in patients with 46,XY partial gonadal dysgenesis and underandrogenization, but normal adrenal function. Among the SF-1 mutations reported are missense mutations within the DNA-binding region (C33S, R84H), a nonsense mutation (Y138X), a frameshift mutation (1277dupT) predicted to disrupt RNA stability or protein function, and a duplication and missense mutation. Functional studies of the missense mutants (C33S, R84H) and of one nonsense mutant (Y138X) showed impaired activation of SF-1–responsive target genes.[92]

Although SF-1 is clearly an important regulator of embryologic development of steroidogenic glands and control of transcription of proteins comprising the steroidogenic machinery, other transcription factors participate in the latter process. A related transcription factor, liver receptor homologue-1 (SF-2 or NR5A2) recognizes the same canonical DNA motif to which SF-1 binds and may share functions with SF-1 in certain tissues, including the adrenal cortex, testis, and ovary.[93] Both SF-1 ad LRH-1 have been crystallized and found to contain phospholipid-binding pockets, with phosphatidyl inositols being the presumed ligands. These observations suggest that phospholipids may be regulatory molecules controlling expression of genes involved in steroidogenesis.[94]

The tissue-specific regulation of genes expressed in multiple steroidogenic glands (e.g., CYP17) requires the action of other transcription factors working either independently or in concert with SF-1 in a combinatorial fashion. In addition, the activity of SF-1 is regulated by transcription factors that either bind to SF-1 response elements and prevent activation of transcription (chicken ovalbumin upstream promoter-transcription factor [COUP-TF]) or bind to SF-1 and block its ability to transactivate promoters (DAX-1, also known as "NR0B1").[95] Interestingly, expression of the latter gene is up-regulated by SF-1, so there is a complex control mechanism in place for modulating these antagonistic molecules.

Other transcription factors that are known to be important for the expression of genes involved in steroidogenesis include GATA4 and GATA6, members of the GATA family of transcription factors originally identified as being central to hematopoiesis and endoderm development, and the orphan nuclear receptor liver X receptor (LXRα).[96,97]

It is notable that the human placenta is an outlier in many respects in terms of the regulation of steroidogenesis.[98-100] First, the placenta does not express certain genes that are pivotal to gonadal and adrenal steroid hormone synthesis, including *SF1/NR5A1, STAR, HSD3B2,* and *CYP17*. Moreover, HSD3B1 replaces the type 2 3β-HSD enzyme in the placenta, and a START domain protein, MLN64 (which is not subject to acute regulation), may subserve StAR's role in cholesterol movement to the placental side-chain cleavage system.

Unlike the gonads and adrenal cortex, the placenta's capacity to produce progestins is believed to be largely determined by levels of adrenodoxin reductase (which governs the availability of reducing equivalents) and P450scc.[99] In addition, *CYP19* transcription in the placenta is driven by a different promoter than that used by the gonads.[45] Thus, placental steroidogenesis is controlled in a distinctly different way than gonadal and adrenal steroid production. The mechanism is more tonic, with steroidogenic capacity determined primarily by differentiation of trophoblast cells and growth of the placenta as opposed to tight regulation by trophic hormones.

Examples of Extraglandular Steroidogenesis

Although steroid hormone synthesis traditionally has been studied in the classic steroidogenic glands (ovaries, testes, adrenal cortex, and placenta), it is now evident that production of bioactive steroids, albeit at much lower levels, occurs at extraglandular sites, such as the brain, vascular tree, and adipose tissue. Synthesis also occurs in pathologic conditions affecting the endometrium (endometriosis and endometrial cancers)[101] and breast (breast cancer).[102] The latter are discussed in detail in Chapters 25 and 27.

SYNTHESIS OF NEUROSTEROIDS

The notion that steroid hormones could be synthesized in the central nervous system evolved from the discovery of appreciable levels of pregnenolone and dehydroepiandrosterone (DHEA) and their fatty acid esters in the brains of animals, even after gonadectomy or adrenalectomy.[102,103] It was subsequently shown that enzymes required for steroid hormone synthesis were expressed in the brain, spinal cord, and peripheral nervous system at the mRNA and protein levels. Included in this category are StAR, P450scc, P450c17, 3β-HSD, aromatase, 17β-HSD types 1 and 2, 5α-reductase, 3α-HSD, 11β-HSD, P450c11β, and aldosterone synthase (P450c11AS). An alternative enzymatic process has also been proposed for conversion of C21 steroids into C19 steroids in the brain through a P450c17-independent chemical reaction.[42]

The enzymes and their associated activities are distributed in different brain regions and cell types, including glia (astrocytes and oligodendrocytes) and neurons. They probably can act on circulating "prohormones" as well as participate in the de novo synthesis of steroids. The expression of the steroidogenic enzymes in the brain is developmentally regulated, although little is known about the mechanisms that control expression.

The known neurosteroids may act via the classic nuclear hormone receptors, but there is also good evidence that nonclassic signaling pathways are involved, including actions on gamma-aminobutyric acid (GABA)$_A$, N-methyl-D-aspartic acid (NMDA), alpha-amino-3-hydroxy-5-methyl-4-isoxazolepropionic acid (AMPA), glycine, serotonin, Sigma type 1, nicotinic acetylcholine, and oxytocin receptors. The actions of neurosteroids on these receptors have been implicated in stress responses, anxiolysis, seizure disorders, memory, unipolar and postpartum depression, and protection against neuronal injury. The evidence supporting these notions has mostly been derived from in vitro studies and animal studies. However, pharmacologic evidence from human studies based on synthetic neurosteroids (e.g., the short-acting anesthetic alphaxolone) substantiates the concepts derived from animal experimentation.

STEROID HORMONE METABOLISM IN SKIN

Skin makes a contribution to testosterone production in women by metabolizing prohormones, such as dehydroepiandrosterone sulfate and androstenedione into testosterone.[104] The *HSD3B1, 17BHSD3*, and type 1 and 2 5α-reductase genes are expressed in skin, allowing for local formation of androgens that can activate the androgen receptors present in the stroma, sebocytes, and dermal papillae.

Secretion, Production, and Metabolic Clearance Rates of Steroid Hormones

The concentration of a steroid in the circulation is determined by the rate at which it is secreted from glands, the rate of metabolism of precursor or prehormones into the steroid, and the rate at which it is extracted by tissues and metabolized. The *secretion rate* of a steroid refers to the total secretion of the compound from a gland per unit time.

Secretion rates have been assessed by sampling the venous effluent from a gland over time and subtracting out the arterial or peripheral venous hormone concentration. Although seemingly simple in concept, this procedure is quite challenging in practice. Much of the difficulty originates from the potential of the catheterization process to disturb gland function (e.g., endocrine changes resulting from the stress of the procedure) and the possibility of dilution or contamination from blood draining other glands. For example, the role of the postmenopausal ovary in androgen production has been challenged because of potential contamination of adrenal venous blood in ovarian venous samples.[105]

The *metabolic clearance rate* of a steroid is defined as the volume of blood that has been completely cleared of the hormone per unit time. The *whole-body metabolic clearance rate* is usually measured, reflecting the sum of clearance rates for each tissue or organ. Experimentally, this measurement is accomplished by infusion of an isotopically labeled steroid at a constant rate.[106] At equilibrium, the concentration of the infused steroid in peripheral venous blood is constant, and the rate of clearance from the blood equals the rate of entry. The metabolic clearance rate is calculated by dividing the infusion rate by the concentration of the steroid isotope in peripheral blood, giving the metabolic clearance rate in milliliters per day or liters per day.

Most of the circulating steroids are removed from blood by the liver. Hepatic blood flow in humans is approximately 1500 L/day, so metabolic clearance rates exceeding this level generally reflect extraction of steroids by other organs in addition to the liver. The lung, with its high rate of blood flow, is another potentially important site of C21 and C19 steroid metabolism.[107,108]

The uptake of steroids into the liver as well as other organs is highly influenced by their affinity for plasma steroid–binding proteins and albumin. Binding of steroid hormones to sex hormone–binding globulin (SHBG) and corticosteroid-binding globulin (CBG) reduces peripheral metabolism.[109,110] The binding of free steroids to albumin is of relatively low affinity; consequently, metabolic clearance rates of albumin-bound unconjugated steroids are relatively high compared with those of hormones, such as testosterone and cortisol, which bind, respectively, to SHBG and CBG with high affinity.[110-112] Sulfoconjugated steroids are an exception because they bind tightly to albumin, and as a result, are cleared very slowly from the blood. Consequently, concentrations of sulfated steroids in blood are usually several-fold higher than their respective unconjugated forms. In contrast, steroid glucuronates are weakly bound to albumin and are rapidly cleared.

The *production rate* of a steroid hormone refers to entry into the blood of the compound from all possible sources, including secretion from glands and conversion of prohormones into the steroid of interest.[113] At steady state, the amount of hormone entering into the blood from all sources will be equal to the rate at which it is being cleared (metabolic clearance rate) multiplied by blood concentration (production rate = metabolic clearance rate × concentration). If there is little contribution of prohormone metabolism to the circulating pool of steroid, then the production rate will approximate the secretion rate.

The fraction of prohormone that is metabolized into the steroid of interest, known as the *rho (ρ) value*, can be estimated by infusing an isotope of the prohormone at a constant rate until equilibrium is reached, then determining the blood concentrations of the unconjugated prohormone isotope and the isotopic product.[113] The amount of prohormone entering into the circulation can be calculated using the ρ value and by the production rate.

Table 4-2 shows the secretion, production, and metabolic clearance rates of the major steroids, and Table 4-3 provides the ρ values of selected sex steroid hormones. Note that there are some differences in these values between sexes and in the favored direction of interconversion,

TABLE 4-2

Blood Production Rates, Secretion Rates, Metabolic Clearance Rates, and Normal Serum Concentration of Sex Steroid Hormones

Steroid Hormone	Reproductive Phase	MCR (L/day)	PR (mg/day)	SR (mg/day)	Reference Values
Men				Testes	
Androstenedione		2200	2.8	1.6	2.8-7.3 nmol/L
Testosterone		950	6.5	6.2	6.9-34.7 nmol/L
Estrone		2050	0.15	0.11	37-250 nmol/L
Estradiol		1600	0.06	0.05	<37-210 pmol/L
Estrone sulfate		167	0.08	Insignificant	600-2500 pmo/L
Women				Ovary	
Androstenedione		2000	3.2	2.8	3.1-12.2 nmol/L
Testosterone		500	0.19	0.06	0.7-2.8 nmol/L
Estrone	Follicular	2200	0.11	0.08	110-400 pmol/L
	Luteal	2200	0.26	0.15	310-660 pmol/L
	Postmenopausal	1610	0.04	Insignificant	22-230 pmol/L
Estradiol	Follicular	1200	0.09	0.08	<37-360 pmol/L
	Luteal	1200	0.25	0.24	699-1250 pmol/L
	Postmenopausal	910	0.006	Insignificant	<37-140 pmol/L
Estrone sulfate	Follicular	146	0.1	Insignificant	700-3600 pmol/L
	Luteal	146	0.18	Insignificant	1100-7300 pmol/L
Progesterone	Follicular	2100	2	1.7	0.3-3 nmol/L
	Luteal	2100	25	24	19-45 nmol/L

MCR, metabolic clearance rate; PR, production rate; SR, secretion rate

which reflects the integrated activities of the different 17β-hydroxysteroid dehydrogenases that selectively oxidize or reduce androgens and estrogens.

Plasma Steroid Hormone–Binding Proteins

As noted previously, steroid hormones are present in blood, either free or associated with proteins.[110-112] Greater than 97% of the circulating fractions of testosterone, estradiol, cortisol, and progesterone are bound by plasma proteins of hepatic origin. SHBG and albumin bind testosterone and estradiol, whereas CBG and albumin bind cortisol and progesterone. Testosterone has a greater affinity for SHBG than does estradiol; 65% and 78% of circulating testosterone is bound to SHBG in men and women, respectively, whereas only 30% and 58% of estradiol in men

and women, respectively, is associated with SHBG. The remainder is mostly bound to albumin. Genome-wide linkage scans suggest that variation in plasma SHBG levels is influenced by several genes with different loci in different ethnic groups.[114]

The protein-bound steroid hormone is generally considered a reservoir, restrained from free diffusion into cells, where it can act and can be metabolized. This notion is substantiated by the discovery of variants in the SHBG gene that include a missense mutation (Pro156Leu) that causes abnormal glycosylation and impaired secretion. Women with this variant display symptoms of hyperandrogenemia, reflecting a greater proportion of bioavailable testosterone.[115]

A pentanucleotide TAAAA repeat in the 5′-untranslated region of the *SHBG* gene and a D327N polymorphism have been associated with serum SHBG concentrations in hirsute women. Individuals carrying the major allele of the D327N polymorphism were also found to have lower SHBG concentrations.[116]

Although SHBG is generally believed to reduce the entry of sex steroids into target tissues, it has been argued that the steroid bound to binding globulins may be selectively accumulated by some cell types by receptors, and that target tissues also synthesize SHBG that acts locally to facilitate signal transduction by way of a cAMP mechanism.[117,118] A role for receptor-mediated endocytosis of steroids bound to SHBG during development is suggested from the phenotype of mice lacking megalin, a member of the LDL receptor family. These mice show steroid hormone insensitivity indicative of cell type–specific endocytic pathways for uptake of protein-bound androgens and estrogens.[119]

TABLE 4-3

Mean ρ Values for Interconversion of Key Sex Steroid Hormones

Interconversion			ρ Values Female	Male
Androstenedione	→	Testosterone	0.03	0.052
Testosterone	→	Androstenedione	0.122	0.076
Androstenedione	→	Estrone	0.007	0.0114
Testosterone	→	Estradiol	0.0014	0.0033
Estrone	→	Estradiol	0.041	0.05
Estradiol	→	Estrone	0.176	0.156

TABLE 4-4

Factors Influencing the Binding Capacity of Sex Hormone-Binding Globulin and Cortisol-Binding Globulin

Factors and Endocrine Status	Binding Capacity	
	SHBG	CBG
Exogenous estrogen	↑	↑
Pregnancy	↑	↑
Exogenous androgens	↓	↓
Anabolic steroids	↓	NC
Synthetic progestins (androgenic properties)	↓	NC
Thyroid hormone (hyperthyroidism)	↑	↓
Prolactin (hyperprolactinemia)	↓	NC
Growth hormone (acromegaly)	↓	NC
Old age (men)	↑	NC
Postmenopausal	↓	↓
Obesity	↓	NC
Hyperinsulinemia	↓	↓

CBG, Cortisol-binding globulin; NC, no change; SHBG, Sex hormone-binding globulin.

Because of the importance of plasma steroid–binding proteins in influencing the amount of bioavailable hormone, any genetic or physiologic variation or pharmacologically induced change in the production of these proteins by the liver can have a significant effect on steroid hormone action and metabolism. The clinical evaluation of subjects with suspected disorders of hormone production or action may require an assessment of the level of binding protein or a measurement of the bioavailable or free fraction of hormone to clarify the basis for the clinical presentation. For example, the suppression of SHBG production by insulin contributes to the hyperandrogenemia associated with polycystic ovary syndrome, which frequently accompanies obesity and insulin resistance.[120] Table 4-4 summarizes changes in SHBG-and CBG-binding capacity under different physiologic and pathophysiologic conditions, as well as the influence of certain pharmacologic agents.

Inhibitors of Steroidogenic Enzymes

The inhibition of steroidogenic enzymes has been shown to be an effective strategy for terminating pregnancy and treating disorders of excessive hormone production (including Cushing's syndrome, steroid hormone–secreting malignancies, and hormone-dependent cancers of the prostate and breast). Inhibitors of aromatase may also have use in the induction of ovulation. The inhibitors include steroid-based and non–steroid-based molecules that act as competitive inhibitors or mechanism-based enzyme poisons (Fig. 4-14).

Endocrine-disrupting chemicals, often believed to act through direct effects on steroid hormone receptors, are now known to interefere with steroidogenic enzymes and enzymes involved in steroid metabolism. These actions may alter endogenous steroid hormone production and catabolism and lead indirectly to altered responses of hormone-responsive target tissues.[121]

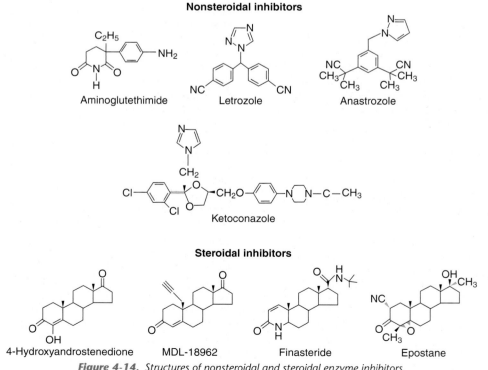

Figure 4-14. *Structures of nonsteroidal and steroidal enzyme inhibitors.*

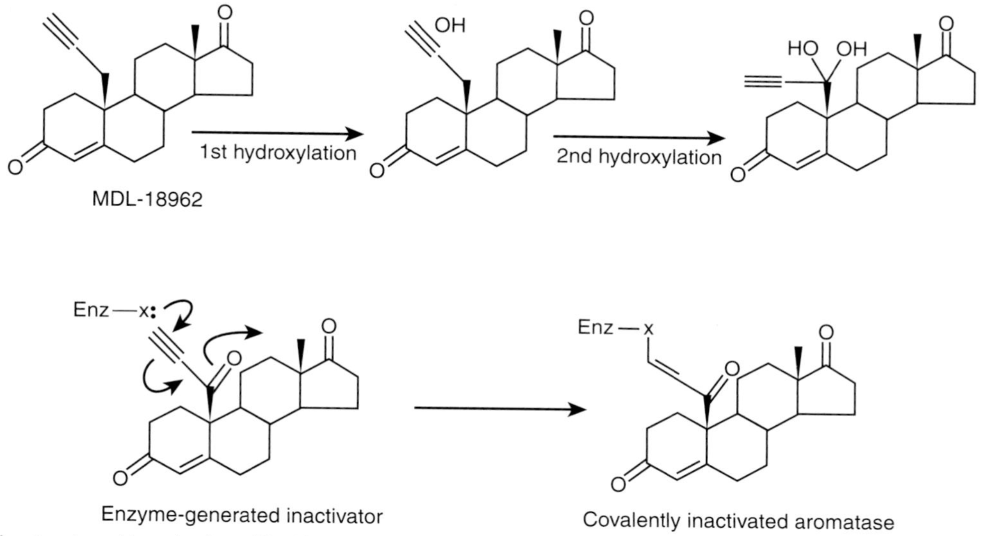

Figure 4-15. *Mechanism-based inactivation of P450arom by MDL-18962. The acetylenic steroid substrate MDL-18962 is activated by the first two aromatase hydroxylation steps to produce an acetylenic ketone. This enzyme-generated inactivator covalently links to the aromatase enzyme. (From Strauss JF III, Penning TM. Synthesis of the sex steroid hormones: molecular and structural biology with application to clinical practice. In Fauser BCJM, Rutherford AJ, Strauss IF III, et al [eds]. Molecular Biology in Reproductive Medicine. New York, Parthenon, 1999, pp 201-232.)*

INHIBITORS OF P450scc

Aminoglutethimide, a drug originally introduced as an antiepileptic, is a nonsteroidal competitive inhibitor of P450scc and P450arom.[122] The free amine of the drug (essential to the drug's inhibitory activity) interacts with the P450 heme to prevent reduction of Fe^{3+}, which is an obligatory step in the P450 catalytic mechanism.

P450c17 INHIBITORS

Ketoconazole, an antifungal agent that blocks P450s involved in ergosterol biosynthesis, is an effective inhibitor of the 17,20-lyase activity and blocks androgen biosynthesis.[123] Other compounds that are used in experimental systems to block 17α-hydroxylase/17,20-lyase activity are too toxic for clinical application. However, there is significant interest in developing new inhibitors that are specific for P450c17 and less toxic, and several new compounds are in development, including abiraterone and VN/124-1.[124]

P450c11 INHIBITORS

Metyrapone, an 11β-hydroxylase inhibitor, reduces cortisol production, with a concomitant increase in 11-deoxycortisol. It is used in diagnostic testing of the hypothalamic–pituitary–adrenal axis and has also been used to treat Cushing's syndrome, but its utility in this regard is limited by side effects.[125]

AROMATASE INHIBITORS

Two major classes of aromatase inhibitors have been developed, the nonsteroidal imidazole and triazole analogs based on ketoconazole, and the steroidal mechanism-based inactivators.[124] The first class of compounds is relatively nonspecific because they can inhibit other steroidogenic

P450s. Two triazole compounds that are reversible competitive inhibitors of P450arom are in clinical use (letrozole [Femara] and anastrozole [Arimidex]). These drugs bind to the iron atom of the heme protein and exclude the substrate from the catalytic pocket.

The steroidal mechanism–based inhibitors include 4-hydroxyandrostenedione (formestane) and 6-methyl-androsta-1,4-diene-3,17-dione (exemestane) (Fig. 4-15). They are innocuous by themselves, but are activated by the catalytic mechanism of P450arom to produce electrophilic species, which then covalently modify the active site. Inactivation requires both NADPH and oxygen. Inhibition by these drugs is long-lasting because new aromatase must be synthesized to overcome the inactivation event. The mechanism-based inhibitors are selective because they only inactivate the target enzyme. In the case of 4-hydroxyandrostenedione, the ultimate electrophilic species responsible for enzyme inactivation is unknown.

5α-REDUCTASE INHIBITORS

The 4-azasteroids represented by finasteride were developed as selective inhibitors of type 2 5α-reductase to prevent the formation of the potent androgen 5α-dihydrotestosterone.[126] These inhibitors contain a heterocyclic A ring with a nitrogen substitution at C4. The potent competitive inhibition of the type 2 enzyme ($K_i = 3$ nM) seen with finasteride was originally attributed to the ability of this compound to produce a mimetic of the enolate transition state. It is now evident that finasteride acts as a mechanism-based inactivator of 5α-reductase to form an isocitrate dehydrogenase (NADP+)–dihydrofinasteride bisubstrate analog with a K_i equal to 10^{-13} M (Fig. 4-16).

Other steroidal-based inhibitors include steroid acrylates, which contain a carboxylic acid substituent at C3.

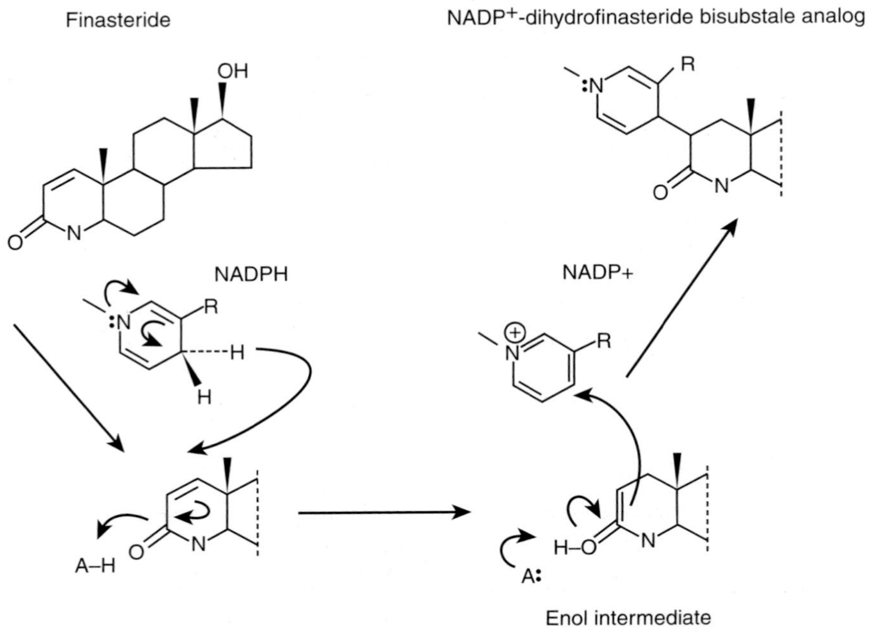

Figure 4-16. *Inhibition of 5α-Reductase type 2 by finasteride. Finasteride is reduced by 5-reductase via an enol intermediate, which then reacts with NADP+ to produce a NADP+–dihydrofinasteride bisubstrate analog, which is a potent enzyme inhibitor. NADP, nicotinamide adenine dinucleotide phosphate. (From Strauss JF III, Penning TM. Synthesis of the sex steroid hormones: molecular and structural biology with application to clinical practice. In Fauser BCJM, Rutherford AJ, Strauss JF III, et al [eds]. Molecular Biology in Reproductive Medicine. New York, Parthenon, 1999, pp 201-232.)*

The carboxylate moiety again mimics the enolate transition state. Interestingly, these compounds are potent noncompetitive inhibitors because they form an abortive enzyme—NADP+—acrylate complex. Dual-enzyme 5α-reductase inhibitors (e.g., GI198745) that are under development can suppress dihydrotestosterone production by 99% 24 hours after oral administration.

3β-HYDROXYSTEROID DEHYDROGENASE/Δ⁵⁻⁴ ISOMERASE INHIBITORS

Compounds originally developed to target 3β-HSD were derivatives of 2α-cyanoketone (2α-cyano-4,4,17α-trimethylandrost-5-en-17β-ol-3-one).[127] The subsequently developed compounds trilostane and epostane are relatively specific competitive inhibitors for blocking steroidogenesis in the adrenal cortex and placenta, respectively.[128]

OTHER ENZYME TARGETS

Inhibition of 17β-HSD type 1 and steroid sulfatase[129,130] is an approach to the reduction of bioavailable estradiol levels. Tibolone, a drug used in hormone replacement therapy, has the interesting property of inhibiting sulfatase activity in breast cancer cells, but not in bone cells, a tissue-selective pattern of action that could reduce estradiol bioavailability in breast, but not in bone.[130] The basis of this tissue-selective action of tibolone has not been elucidated. As noted previously, hydroxylated metabolites of polychlorinated biphenyls are potent inhibitors of estrogen sulfotransferase and thus increase the bioavailability of estradiol.[131]

The complete reference list can be found on the companion Expert Consult Web site at www.expertconsultbook.com.

Suggested Readings

Auchus RJ, Miller WL. Human 17α-hydroxylase/17,20-lyase. *In* Mason JI (ed). Genetics of Steroid Biosynthesis and Function, London, Taylor & Francis, 2002p 259-286.

Baird DT, Horton R, Longcope C, et al. Steroid dynamics under steady-state conditions. Recent Prog Horm Res 25:611, 1969.

Bose HS, Sugawara T, Strauss JF III, et al. The pathophysiology and genetics of congenital lipoid adrenal hyperplasia. N Engl J Med 335:1870, 1996.

Bruno RD, Njar VC. Targeting cytochrome P450 enzymes: a new approach in anti-cancer drug development. Bioorg Med Chem 15:5047, 2007.

Miller WL. Steroidogenic acute regulatory protein (StAR), a novel mitochondrial cholesterol transporter. Biochim Biophys Acta 1771:663, 2007.

Moeller G, Adamski J. Multifunctionality of human 17beta-hydroxysteroid dehydrogenases. Mol Cell Endocrinol 248:47, 2006.

Payne AH, Hales DB. Overview of steroidogenic enzymes in the pathway from cholesterol to active steroid hormones. Endocr Rev 25:947, 2004.

Penning TM. Molecular endocrinology of hydroxysteroid dehydrogenases. Endocr Rev 18:281, 1997.

Sanderson. The steroid hormone biosynthesis pathway as a target for endocrine-disrupting chemicals. Toxicol Sci 94:3, 2006.

Simard J, Ricketts M-L, Gingras S, et al. Molecular biology of the 3ß-hydroxysteroid dehydrogenase/δ5-δ4 isomerase gene family. Endocr Rev 226:525, 2005.

Simpson E, Clyne C, Rubin C. Aromatase: a brief overview. Annu Rev Physiol 64:93, 2002.

Tuckey RC. Progesterone synthesis by the human placenta. Placenta 26:273, 2005.

White PC. Steroid 11β-hydroxylase deficiency and related disorders. Endocrinol Metab Clin North Am 30:61, 2001.

White PC, Speiser PW. Congenital adrenal hyperplasia due to 21-hydroxylase deficiency. Endocr Rev 21:245, 2000.

CHAPTER 5

Steroid Hormone Action

Turk Rhen and John A. Cidlowski

Steroid Hormone Receptors Act as Ligand-dependent Transcription Factors or Repressors

Steroids are small, lipophilic hormones synthesized from a common precursor molecule, cholesterol, within the adrenal glands or the gonads (see Chapter 4). The adrenal cortex is the primary source of circulating mineralocorticoids and glucocorticoids, while the gonads are the main source of circulating active sex steroids called *estrogens, progestins*, and *androgens*. Despite their shared molecular origin and basic structural similarities, mineralocorticoids, glucocorticoids, estrogens, progestins, and androgens are distinct classes of steroid hormones that interact with specific, high-affinity receptors to exert their biologic effects. These hormones control diverse physiologic and cellular processes and affect virtually every aspect of vertebrate biology, from sexual differentiation, growth, and reproduction to immunity, brain function, and behavior. Consequently, a clear and complete understanding of the basic mechanisms of steroid hormone action is of critical importance for reproductive health and general well-being. Also of significance are the unique mechanisms that lead to hormone-specific effects and function and to differences in hormone responsiveness between species.

This chapter reviews what is known about the mechanisms of steroid action. Briefly, the classic mode of action of steroid hormones is to enter cells, interact with cognate receptors, and stimulate or inhibit transcription of target genes (Fig. 5-1).[1] Hormone-dependent changes in receptor conformation ultimately influence transactivation and transrepression of gene expression by (1) disrupting interactions with molecular chaperones that keep the receptor in an inactive state; (2) promoting the formation of receptor dimers; (3) promoting interactions with specific DNA sequences in the promoter of target genes; and (4) facilitating recruitment of coactivator or corepressor proteins that alter chromatin structure and contact the basal transcription machinery. To fully understand the commonalities of steroid hormone action and appreciate the specificity of signaling by different classes of steroids, it is important to understand the evolution of receptors (mineralocorticoid [MR], glucocorticoid [GR], estrogen [ER], progestin [PR], and androgen [AR]) from a common ancestral protein. Next is a discussion of hormone-dependent activation and repression of gene expression and the physiologic roles played by each of these receptors. This is followed by a discussion of general factors that influence steroid hormone action. Finally, the chapter examines more recent work, which has begun to elucidate alternative modes of action for steroid hormones and their receptors. Such mechanisms include interactions with other transcription factors and nongenomic effects mediated by second messenger signaling pathways.

Evolution of Steroid Hormone Receptor Structure and Function

Steroid receptors belong to a larger family of structurally and evolutionarily related proteins called *nuclear receptors*.[2-4] A recent bioinformatics analysis of the human genome has identified 49 genes for nuclear receptors, which appears to represent the total number of paralogs found in humans.[5] Paralogs are related genes found within a single genome that evolved by gene duplication. Although a complete review of the nuclear receptor family of transcription factors is beyond the scope of this chapter, a brief discussion is in order. All nuclear receptors, including steroid receptors, exhibit a modular structure composed of distinct domains (Fig. 5-2). In general, these receptors contain a variable amino-terminal region (A/B), a highly conserved DNA-binding region (C), a highly variable hinge region (D), and a moderately conserved hormone or ligand-binding domain

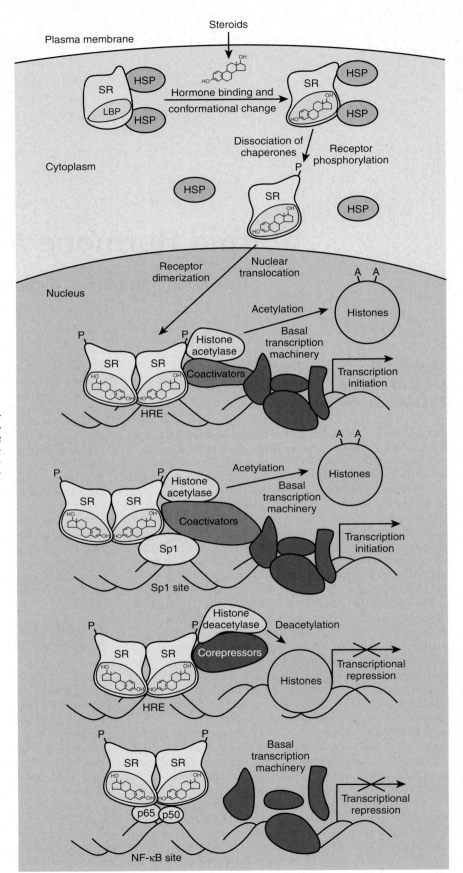

Figure 5-1. *General mechanism of action for cytoplasmic steroid receptors as described in the text. The two subunits of nuclear factor kappa B are p50 and p65. A, acetyl group; HSP, heat shock protein; HRE, hormone response element; LBP, ligand-binding pocket; NF, nuclear factor; P, phosphate group; SR, steroid receptor.*

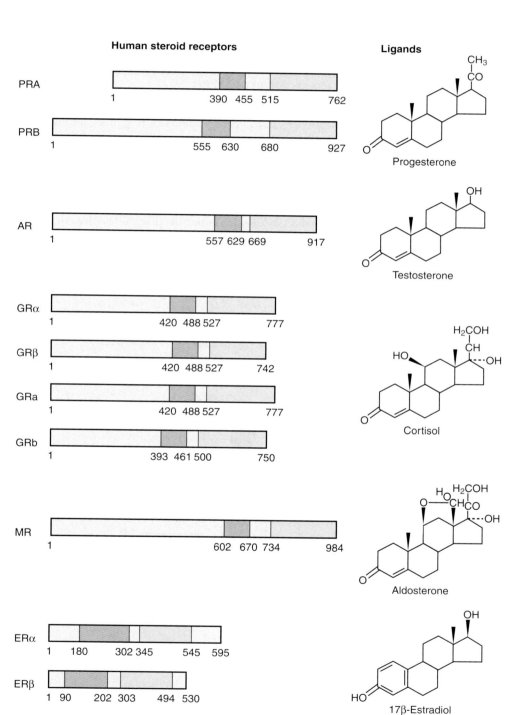

Figure 5-2. Schematic diagram of the primary structure of a generic steroid receptor and its functional domains. Region A/B contains transactivation function 1 domain (AF1). Region C contains the DNA-binding domain. Region D is the hinge region. Region E contains the ligand-binding domain. Region F contains the transactivation function 2 (AF2) domain. The primary structure of human steroid receptors, their isoforms, and their physiologic ligands. AR, androgen receptor; ER, estrogen receptor; GR, glucocorticoid receptor; MR, mineralocorticoid receptor; PRA, progestin receptor isoform A; PRB progestin receptor receptor isoform B.

(E). The primary structure of each human steroid receptor is shown, along with its physiologic ligand, in Figure 5-2. Some receptors also contain a carboxy-terminal F domain. Specific regions within the DNA-binding (C) and ligand-binding (E) domains play an important part in receptor dimerization, which is critical because most nuclear receptors are only transcriptionally active as homo- or heterodimers. In addition, nuclear receptors have one or two regions called *activation function 1 and 2* (AF1 and AF2) that are required to transactivate gene expression. Whereas AF1 activity is usually ligand-independent and located in the A/B domain, AF2 is found in the ligand-binding domain and is predominantly regulated by hormone binding.

Some nuclear receptors have defined natural ligands, such as steroid hormones, thyroid hormones, retinoids, or vitamin D, but others have no identified ligand and are called *orphan receptors*. The finding that diverse compounds act as ligands for nuclear receptors and that some receptors have no apparent ligand led to the hypothesis that ancestral nuclear receptors were constitutive transcription factors that independently evolved the ability to bind ligand.[6,7] However, it is also possible that ancestral receptors were ligand-dependent transcription factors that evolved specificity for different ligands by gene duplication, mutation, and functional divergence. Evidence favors the latter hypothesis for the evolution of ligand binding in the steroid receptor family. In fact, the primary, secondary, and tertiary structures of the ligand-binding domain of different steroid receptors are highly similar.[8-11] Moreover, detailed sequence, structural, and functional analyses strongly support the hypothesis that the ancestral steroid receptor bound estrogens. Specificity for other steroids evolved by serial and parallel duplications of the ancestral gene, mutation of nucleotides coding for specific amino acids, and structural and functional divergence of the paralogs.[12-14] Finally, steroid hormone receptors are nuclear receptors unique to the chordate lineage, indicating that they originated when the first chordates evolved.

GENE DUPLICATION OF ANCESTRAL STEROID HORMONE RECEPTORS

Sequence and phylogenetic analysis of 73 steroid receptor sequences from jawed vertebrates (e.g., fish, amphibians, reptiles, birds, and mammals) and a jawless fish (the sea lamprey) indicate that there were two serial duplications of an ancestral steroid receptor before the divergence of these lineages approximately 450 million years ago.[13] Maximum likelihood reconstructions of the ancestral amino acid sequence indicate that the first steroid receptor was probably an ER-like molecule (Fig. 5-3). After this gene was duplicated, one copy was constrained by natural selection and retained its function as an "estrogen receptor," whereas the other copy evolved specificity for 3-ketosteroid–like ligands (see Fig. 5-3). Duplication of the latter gene then produced a corticoid receptor–like protein

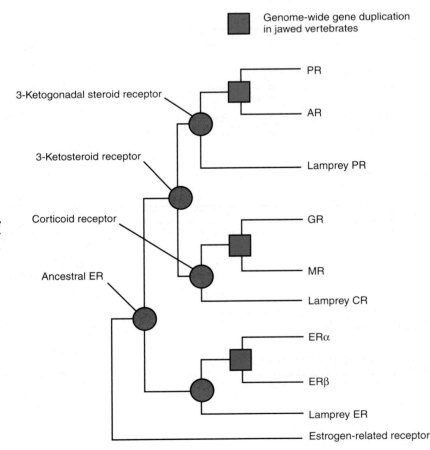

Figure 5-3. *Phylogeny of the steroid receptor gene family. AR, androgen receptor; CR, corticoid receptor; ER, estrogen receptor; GR, glucocorticoid receptor; MR, mineralocorticoid receptor; PR progestin receptor.*

and a receiver for 3-ketogonadal steroid–like molecules (e.g., androgens, progestins, or both). Whereas these three steroid receptors (i.e., the ER, corticoid, and 3-ketogonadal steroid receptors) are present in the sea lamprey, six steroid receptors are present in fish and tetrapods, suggesting a genome-wide duplication in the last common ancestor of jawed vertebrates (indicated by blue boxes in Fig. 5-3). This final duplication then led to the evolution of the true androgen and progesterone receptors from the ancestral 3-ketogonadal steroid receptor, glucocorticoid and mineralocorticoid receptors from the ancestral corticoid receptor, and ERα and ERβ from the ancestral estrogen receptor. The number of paralogs for other gene families, such as the *Hox* genes, supports the hypothesis that many genes were duplicated in parallel in the ancestor of jawed vertebrates.

STRUCTURAL AND FUNCTIONAL DIVERGENCE OF STEROID HORMONE RECEPTORS

Experiments deleting large regions of different steroid receptors have clearly shown that domain C is responsible for DNA binding and that domain E is responsible for ligand binding (see Fig. 5-2). Further studies swapping the entire ligand-binding domain among different receptors show that this region determines specificity for particular classes of steroid hormone. Nevertheless, crystal structures of various steroid hormone receptors show that all ligand-binding domains fold into a highly homologous three-layered structure with a small ligand-binding pocket in the center. This pocket is composed of roughly 30 amino acids that are in close proximity or direct contact with hormones bound to their cognate receptors. In agreement with structural studies, experiments using site-directed mutagenesis indicate that relatively specific, but minor, changes in amino acids within the ligand-binding pocket can lead to dramatic changes in the hormone-binding specificity of steroid receptors. For example, a cysteine residue at position 891 in the human PR is conserved at the corresponding position in the GR and MR and appears to be critical for contacting the C20 keto

group found in progestins, glucocorticoids, and mineralocorticoids.[13,15] Mutation of the corresponding threonine to cysteine in the AR changes its affinity for androgens and makes the receptor transactivate gene expression in the presence of progesterone and corticoids.[16] Based on structure–function studies of this sort and phylogenetic analyses, Thornton[13] proposed a series of relatively minor amino acid changes that may account for broad changes in hormone specificity during the evolution of steroid receptors.

Similar studies of the DNA-binding domain have defined the structural basis for interactions between steroid receptors and particular DNA sequences.[17,18] For instance, mutation of just three residues in the DNA-binding domain of the GR or ER to the corresponding residues in the other receptor changes the binding specificity for DNA sequences called *glucocorticoid-responsive* elements and *estrogen-responsive* elements. These three amino acids reside in a five-residue motif called the *P box*, which is found in the first of two zinc fingers (Fig. 5-4). The first finger interacts with the major groove of DNA, whereas the second is involved in receptor dimerization. Although the DNA-binding domain is very highly conserved among nuclear receptors, the three residues just discussed are variable among different receptors, which may in part account for receptor-specific regulation of distinct sets of genes. These examples illustrate that site-directed mutagenesis and fine-scale comparison of amino acid sequences among receptors, in the context of the tertiary structure of the DNA- and ligand-binding domains, can lead to testable hypotheses about the evolution of signaling and regulation of gene expression by different classes of steroids.[19]

Activation and Repression of Gene Expression

Given this background on the evolution of different steroid receptors, we will now focus on the general function of these receptors and the activation and repression of gene expression by each class of steroid hormone. Steroid receptors have taken on more or less distinct physiologic roles during evolution. ERα, ERβ, PR, and AR are primarily involved in sexual differentiation and reproduction. Estrogens and progestins are essential for normal female development and reproduction. Androgens are involved in various aspects of male reproductive physiology and development. Although androgens, estrogens, and progestins are sex-typical hormones, they are not sex-limited, and they play a physiologic role in both sexes. In contrast, GR and MR principally regulate nonreproductive traits. Glucocorticoids are considered stress hormones that control the function of many tissues, whereas mineralocorticoids play a more restricted role in regulating electrolyte balance and a few other traits. Despite the general separation of these functions, each class of steroid can also modulate the action of other steroids. Cross-talk among steroid hormones is therefore an important subject that will be addressed subsequently.

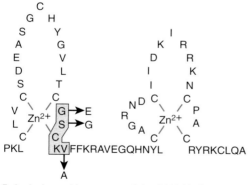

Figure 5-4. *Amino acid sequence of the DNA-binding domain of human glucocorticoid receptor showing two zinc fingers and the P box, which is outlined. The three mutant residues that change glucocorticoid receptor binding specificity from glucocorticoid-responsive element and estrogen-responsive element are indicated by the* **arrows.**

TABLE 5-1

Tissue-Specific Patterns of ERα and ERβ mRNA Expression in the Rat

Tissue	Receptor*	
	ERα	ERβ
Epididymis	+++	+
Prostate	+	+++
Testis	+++	+
Pituitary	++	+
Ovary	+++	+++
Uterus	+++	++
Bladder	+	++
Lung	0	+
Liver	+	0
Kidney	++	0
Thymus	+	+
Adrenal	++	0
Olfactory lobe	0	+
Cerebellum	0	+
Brain stem	0	+
Spinal cord	0	+
Heart	+	0

*Relative levels of expression are indicated by the number of plus signs: 0, not detected; +, low; ++, medium; +++, high.
From Kuiper GGJM, Carlsson B, Grandien K, et al. 1997. Comparison of the ligand binding specificity and transcript tissue distribution of estrogen receptors α and β. Endocrinology 138:863-870,1997.

TABLE 5-2

Binding Affinity of Various Ligands for ERα and ERβ Relative to Binding Affinity of E2

Ligand	Relative Binding Affinity*	
	ERα	ERβ
E2	100	100
Diethylstilbestrol	468	295
Hexestrol	302	234
Dienestrol	223	404
Estrone	60	37
17α-Estradiol	58	11
Moxestrol	43	5
Estriol	14	21
4-OH-Estradiol	13	7
2-OH-Estradiol	7	11
Estrone-3-sulfate	<1	<1
4-OH-Tamoxifen	178	339
ICI-164384	85	166
Nafoxidine	44	16
Clomifene	25	12
Tamoxifen	7	6
Coumestrol	94	185
Genestein	5	36
Bisphenol A	0.05	0.33
Methoxychlor	0.01	0.13

*Relative binding affinity is the ratio of concentrations of E2 and competitor required to displace 50% of specific radioligand binding. Relative binding affinity was set to 100% for E2.
From Kuiper GGJM, Carlsson B, Grandien K, et al. 1997. Comparison of the ligand binding specificity and transcript tissue distribution of estrogen receptors α and β. Endocrinology 138:863-870,1997.

ESTROGEN RECEPTOR

The biologic effects of estrogens were believed to be mediated by a single receptor (i.e., ERα) until the cloning of a second receptor (i.e., ERβ): ERα and ERβ are products of different genes.[20] It has subsequently been shown that these two receptors play distinctive roles in estrogen signaling and that the genes encoding ERα and ERβ are differentially expressed in different tissues (Table 5-1).[21,22] Although both ERα and ERβ are required for normal ovarian function, the phenotypes of ERα and ERβ knockout mice are dissimilar. The ERα knockout mouse is anovulatory and accumulates cystic follicles. The ERβ knockout mouse contains ovaries that appear normal histologically, but still display impaired ovulation. Based on the available evidence, it appears that ERα bears much of the load for mediating the effects of estrogen in other tissues. For instance, only ERα is required for estrogen effects on growth and differentiation of the uterus. Studies using knockout mice also showed that estrogens regulate mammary gland development exclusively via ERα. Female reproductive behavior is also severely impaired in ERα knockout mice. Whereas ERα knockout males are infertile, ERβ knockout males reproduce normally. Studies conducted in vitro further demonstrate unique roles for ERα and ERβ, even though both receptors bind natural estrogens with similar affinity (Table 5-2).[21] Based on these studies, it is generally believed that many of the functional differences between the receptors arise from their unique amino terminal (A/B) domains.

A number of estrogen-regulated genes have been identified in the uterus. Lactoferrin is induced by estrogen, but the function of this gene in the uterus is currently unknown.[23] Estrogens induce insulin-like growth factor 1 (IGF-1) and down-regulate IGF binding protein 3 and IGF binding protein 5. Given the repression of IGF binding proteins that sequester IGF-1, the net effect of these changes is to increase IGF-1 signaling and the proliferation of uterine epithelial cells. The epithelium of the female reproductive tract is also coated by glycoproteins such as mucin 1 (Muc-1) that play a role in blastocyst attachment and provide a barrier against uterine infections.[24] Muc-1 protein and messenger RNA (mRNA) expression is induced by estrogens.[25]

In addition to their normal role in regulating uterine function, estrogens are a risk factor for the initiation and progression of breast cancer. Moreover, ER antagonists slow or stop the growth of breast cancer by blocking estrogen-regulated gene expression. Part of these effects may be mediated by vascular endothelial growth factor (VEGF) because tumor growth is generally dependent on angiogenesis and a steady blood supply. Estrogen increases the expression of VEGF in breast cancer cells.[26] Interestingly, this effect on VEGF can be suppressed by direct interactions between ER and the wild-type breast cancer susceptibility gene BRCA1. Mutations that inactivate *BRCA1* confer increased risk for breast cancer, perhaps due to a loss of the ability to antagonize estrogen action.

Somatic mutations and genetic polymorphisms in the human ER itself are also associated with various disease states. An adult male without functional ERα (i.e., the mutation produces a premature stop codon) had decreased bone mineral density, signs of increased bone turnover, and incomplete closure of bone epiphyses, indicating that estrogens and ERs play an important role in bone growth and homeostasis in humans.[27] This finding is in general accord with studies of male ERα knockout mice, which have decreased bone mineral density. ER genetic polymorphisms have also been associated with increased risk of osteoporosis in humans, although the mechanisms responsible for these associations are not clear (reviewed in Gennari et al.[28]). A number of ER mutations have been detected in breast cancer.[29] For example, deletion of exon 5 within the ligand-binding domain generated a receptor that was constitutively active in the absence of estrogens. Deletion of exon 7 within the ligand-binding domain produced a receptor that displayed dominant negative activity and prevented the function of wild-type ER when expressed in the same cells. Additional mutations include base pair insertions and deletions and alternative splice variants that result in deletion of other exons. Although many of these mutations clearly alter signaling through the ER and influence responsiveness to anti-estrogen therapy, it is not known whether the mutations occurred before or after the development of malignancy.

PROGESTERONE RECEPTOR

Like estrogens, progestins have broad effects, including the establishment and maintenance of pregnancy, regulation of mammary gland development, control of ovulation, and regulation of female reproductive behavior. Interestingly, the PR has two isoforms, "PRA" and "PRB," which are derived from the same gene. PRA and PRB are identical except for an additional 164 amino acids at the amino-terminal end of PRB due to an alternative translation initiation site. Female mice with a targeted disruption of the PR gene (i.e., both A and B isoforms are inactive) are unresponsive to progesterone, strongly indicating that the pleiotropic effects of progestins are mediated by the PR.[30] In contrast to females, male mice that lack a functional PR appear normal and are able to reproduce as well as wild-type males. Analyses of PRA and PRB activity using transient transfection assays have shown that the two isoforms have distinct transcriptional activities. Whereas PRB is a transcriptional activator in most promoter contexts and cell types, PRA appears to have promoter and cell-specific effects on progestin target genes. It is also important that PRA can inhibit PRB action in contexts where PRA alone is inactive.

The specific role of each PR isoform in different tissues in vivo remains to be fully elucidated, but it is becoming clear that PRA and PRB have distinct functions.[31] PRA is required for normal ovarian and uterine function, but is dispensable in the mammary gland. However, transgenic mice carrying an extra copy of PRA have abnormal morphologic development of mammary glands.[32] These results suggest that overexpression of PRA and an increased ratio of PRA:PRB can have important physiologic consequences. Although the ratio of PRA:PRB changes during development and as a function of reproductive stage in different tissues,[33,34] it remains to be determined whether these changes influence progesterone signaling. Specific ablation of PRB shows that this isoform is not required in the ovary or uterus, but is required for normal development of mammary glands. A third PR isoform, "PRC," has also been cloned and appears to result from translation initiation at a downstream methionine.[35] Although PRC lacks the first zinc finger in the DNA-binding domain, it modulates the transcriptional activity of PRA and PRB on a reporter gene.

In accord with the finding that PRB is necessary for full differentiation and branching of the mammary ducts, progesterone has also been shown to regulate a number of genes that may be involved in breast cancer.[36] The PROGINS allele of PR is characterized by an Alu insertion in intron G, which is linked to additional mutations in exons 4 and 5. Interestingly, there is epidemiologic evidence that individuals carrying the PROGINS allele have reduced risk of breast cancer.[37] The functional consequence of these mutations is to increase the stability and transcriptional activity of the receptor in vitro. Conversely, PROGINS was found at a higher frequency in patients with ovarian cancer than in control individuals.[38] Subsequent work confirmed the association of this polymorphism with increased risk of ovarian cancer, but only in women who had not used oral contraceptives.[39] In the uterus, progesterone up-regulates expression of regulators of cell cycle progression, growth factors, and their receptors, but represses cell cycle arrest proteins.[40] Localized suppression of the immune system during gestation of the semi-allogenic embryo is another essential role played by progesterone and PR. Part of this effect may be mediated by down-regulation of RANTES (regulated on activation, normal T cell expressed and secreted) in endometrial stromal cells.[41] Although the PR also inhibits uterine inflammation in the nonpregnant uterus, the genes mediating this effect are unknown. Osteopontin is yet another gene induced by progesterone in the uterus; it codes for a glycoprotein constituent of the extracellular matrix that is believed to bind integrin receptors.[42] Progesterone repression of oxytocin receptor gene expression is also important because oxytocin plays a central role in uterine physiology and parturition.[43]

ANDROGEN RECEPTOR

Androgens produced by the testes during and after the sex-determining period coordinate the development and differentiation of many sexually dimorphic tissues by specifically activating the AR.[44] Only one isoform of the AR has been recognized to date. Leydig cells in the embryonic testes produce testosterone, which directs development of the male external genitalia, vas deferens, and related structures from the wolffian ducts. Evidence indicates that the early surge in testosterone also directs male-typical patterns of neural development and behavior that are expressed later in life. In the absence of androgens and in AR knockout mice, the wolffian ducts regress and female external genitalia develop.[45] Likewise, mutations in the human AR can lead to complete androgen insensitivity and development of female genitalia or partial androgen insensitivity and ambiguous genitalia. Given the readily observed phenotype, a large number of AR mutations have been described.[46,47] For example, it was suggested that a mutation substituting proline for histidine at residue 689 alters the conformation of the second helix in the ligand-binding domain. This mutation greatly reduces affinity of the AR for dihydrotestosterone and abolishes its ability to transactivate androgen-responsive elements.[48] A serine-to-proline mutation at residue 865 in helix 10/11 also causes complete androgen insensitivity by eliminating androgen-binding and androgen-dependent transactivation.[49] It is interesting to note that different mutations at a given residue can generate different phenotypes. Substitution of threonine for methionine at residue 807 produces partial androgen insensitivity and ambiguous genitalia by reducing but not completely blocking androgen binding to AR. In contrast, arginine or valine substitutions at the same site totally abrogate androgen binding and produce complete androgen insensitivity syndrome.[50]

Androgens are secreted at low levels in immature males, but are again produced at high levels later in development (i.e., at puberty and in sexually mature males). At this point, androgens govern the development of secondary sexual characteristics, activate male reproductive and aggressive behavior, and allow spermatogenesis. Meiosis in germ cells begins at puberty in males and is continuous thereafter. The rate of programmed cell death (or apoptosis) in germ cells during spermatogenesis has a large influence on sperm output and male fertility. Androgens play an important role as a survival factor because testosterone withdrawal from mature males increases germ cell apoptosis.[51] Expression of *Bax* is elevated in germ cells after testosterone withdrawal.[52] *Bax* is a well-known proapoptotic gene that could be involved in germ cell death. Evidence suggests that the Fas pathway may also play a role in germ cell apoptosis: Fas ligand and Fas receptor are expressed at elevated levels in dying germ cells. Androgens regulate prostate development and differentiation in the embryo and the adult and are believed to be a risk factor for prostate cancer in humans. Treatment of prostate cells with dihydrotestoterone induces changes in cell morphology and regulates a large number of genes.[53] Genes induced by dihydrotestoterone in prostate cells are involved in small molecule transport, membrane signal transduction, intracellular signal transduction, and metabolism. Other important aspects of AR function relate to physiologic differences in signaling by different androgens.[54] In particular, dihydrotestosterone is a more potent androgen than testosterone. Studies conducted in vivo and in vitro indicate that AR has higher affinity for dihydrotestosterone than does testosterone, which leads to greater stabilization of the receptor and more efficient signaling. Local conversion of testosterone to dihydrotestosterone to enhance androgen action is discussed in another section of this chapter.

GLUCOCORTICOID RECEPTOR

Glucocorticoids are often referred to as *stress hormones* because they are synthesized and secreted in response to pain and emotional trauma, caloric restriction, agonistic social encounters, and general anxiety. Mice homozygous for a null mutation in the GR (i.e., GR knockouts) die around the time of birth, indicating that the GR and glucocorticoids are essential for life.[55] In humans, there are at least four GR isoforms produced from a single gene. Whereas GRα and GRβ are produced by alternative splicing at the 3′ end of GR mRNA, GRA and GRB are produced by alternative translation initiation at the 5′ end of GR mRNA.[56] Glucocorticoids alter the physiology of numerous tissues throughout the body during periods of acute stress. For example, the inhibitory effects of stress on reproduction are mediated by glucocorticoids at all levels of the hypothalamic–pituitary–gonadal axis. These hormones also influence brain function and behavior. Glucocorticoids mobilize energy stores by inducing the degradation of proteins to free amino acids in muscle, lipolysis in adipose tissue, and gluconeogenesis in the liver. Glucocorticoids play a role in the immune and vascular systems, where they induce programmed cell death in lymphocytes and block inflammatory responses. Although these changes are adaptive in the short term, chronic stress accompanied by prolonged glucocorticoid secretion is pathologic.

In addition to mediating stress responses, glucocorticoids play an essential part in normal physiology. For example, glucocorticoids regulate the expression of numerous genes involved in energy homeostasis. Induction of the gene for phosphoenolpyruvate carboxykinase (*PEPCK*), the rate-limiting enzyme in gluconeogenesis, has recently been elucidated.[57,58] Glucocorticoids were shown to up-regulate the transcriptional coactivator peroxisome proliferator-activated receptor gamma coactivator 1 (PGC-1) in the liver. This protein then serves as an essential GR coactivator that increases transcription from the *PEPCK* promoter. Full induction of *PEPCK* expression involves PGC-1 coactivation of the liver-enriched transcription factor hepatocyte nuclear factor 4α. It has been reported that glucocorticoids also increase pyruvate dehydrogenase kinase 4 levels.[59] This kinase catalyzes phosphorylation and inactivation of the pyruvate dehydrogenase complex (PDC). In turn, PDC inactivation promotes gluconeogenesis by conserving three-carbon substrates. Glucocorticoids regulate the expression of genes related to other physiologic processes. The well-known anti-inflammatory effects of glucocorticoids are mediated in part by induction of the gene for inhibitor of nuclear factor kappa B alpha (IκBα), which keeps the proinflammatory transcription factor nuclear factor kappa B (NF-κB) in an inactive state in the cytoplasm.

MINERALOCORTICOID RECEPTOR

Aldosterone, the major circulating mineralocorticoid, specifically binds to and activates the MR. In contrast, cortisol (or corticosterone in rodents) binds to and activates both the MR and GR. To prevent inappropriate MR activation by glucocorticoids, 11β-hydroxysteroid dehydrogenase converts cortisol (or corticosterone) to inactive metabolites in cells containing MR (discussed in detail in Chapter 4). One critical function of aldosterone is to regulate electrolyte balance and blood pressure. Aldosterone's primary target tissue is the distal tubule of the kidney, where it promotes the retention of Na+ and the elimination of K+ during urine formation. Retention of Na+ leads to absorption of water from the distal tubules, an increase in blood volume, and maintenance of blood pressure. Mineralocorticoid insufficiency causes death by Na+ and water loss, a fall in blood volume, and circulatory shock. Accordingly, MR knockout mice also die of sodium and water loss.[60] On the other hand, mineralocorticoid excess contributes to hypertension and pathologies associated with high blood pressure. Additional targets of aldosterone include the heart, brain, smooth muscle, endothelial cells, and adipose tissue. Less is known about the cellular and molecular mechanisms involved in mineralocorticoid effects on these tissues.

Recent work has identified several mineralocorticoid-induced genes involved in Na+ resorption in tight epithelia.[61,62] Aldosterone, for example, increases mRNA levels of serum- and glucocorticoid-regulated kinase (Sgk) within 1 hour and increases Sgk protein levels within 2 hours. An increase in Sgk activity appears to activate the phosphatidylinositol-3-OH kinase (PI3K) pathway, which in turn stabilizes the epithelial Na+ channel (ENaC) in the open state and increases the number of ENaCs in the apical membrane. These changes have a corresponding effect on the amiloride-sensitive Na+ current. It is important to note that aldosterone induces the α subunit of ENaC and the α_1 subunit of Na+/K+-ATPase by the classic transcriptional mechanism attributed to steroid hormones. Pumping of Na+ from the serosal membrane of epithelial cells by Na+/K+-ATPase generates the electrochemical gradient necessary for Na+ resorption at the apical membrane. Aldosterone also induces the expression of the Na+/H+ transporter and numerous other genes that may play a role in electrolyte balance. The role of genes repressed by aldosterone, however, remains unclear.[62] Given this background on the function of different steroid receptors and a few genes regulated by these receptors, we will now focus on commonalities of steroid hormone action that were most likely present in the ancestral steroid receptor.

General Factors That Influence Steroid Hormone Action

Although numerous factors affect signaling by steroid hormones in vivo, this chapter focuses on some of the more important and well-characterized regulatory mechanisms. Foremost among the factors determining whether a cell responds to circulating steroid hormones is the intracellular availability of a given steroid and its receptor. Intracellular enzymes metabolize active steroids to inactive forms or vice versa, providing preemptory control over steroid hormone action (see Chapter 4). The number of receptors within a cell also determines its responsiveness to hormone, with regulation of receptor expression at all conceivable levels from transcription to protein degradation. When sufficient hormone and receptor are present in a cell, the ligand binds and activates the monomeric

receptor (see Fig. 5-1). The ligand-bound receptor undergoes a conformational change, dissociates from regulatory heat shock proteins, and is phosphorylated. Cytoplasmic receptors translocate to the nucleus, where they bind as homodimers to specific DNA sequences called *hormone-responsive elements*. The MR, GR, PR, and AR are predominantly cytoplasmic in the absence of ligand. In contrast, ERα and ERβ are localized in the nucleus in the absence of ligand and do not require nuclear translocation for their transcriptional activity. Within the nucleus, the ligand–receptor complex interacts with coactivator and corepressor proteins that remodel chromatin or contact the basal transcription machinery, thereby increasing or decreasing the probability of initiation of transcription. Although we discuss basic regulatory mechanisms at each step in the dynamic process just outlined, the reader is referred to primary research and review articles that treat each mechanism in greater detail.

HORMONE AVAILABILITY

Intracellular enzymes can activate or inactivate steroid hormones to produce tissue-specific or even cell-specific patterns of hormone responsiveness. Aromatase P450, which converts androgens to estrogens, is expressed in the gonads, brain, adipose tissue, skin, and placenta.[63] Estrogen concentration in plasma varies in a cyclic manner during the menstrual or estrous cycle in most female mammals. Whereas estrogen levels at the nadir of the cycle are usually below the concentration necessary for activation of the ER, estrogen levels at the peak of the cycle generally activate the ER. Consequently, synthesis and secretion of estrogens from the ovary into the general circulation is the main mechanism controlling estrogen action in females. In contrast, males have plasma levels of estrogens that are below the concentration necessary for activation of intracellular ER. Nevertheless, males still require estrogen for normal reproductive function and behavior, as demonstrated by ERα knockout mice.[64,65] Expression of male copulatory behavior in a variety of vertebrates therefore depends on the local conversion of testosterone to 17β-estradiol by aromatase and the activation of ER within the medial preoptic area of the brain.[66,67]

Similarly, localized expression of 5α-reductase plays a crucial role in regulating androgen action.[68] Testosterone is converted to dihydrotestosterone by 5α-reductase in a variety of androgen-sensitive tissues. This reaction is particularly important because dihydrotestosterone binds to the AR with higher affinity than does testosterone and because dihydrotestosterone is essential for full virilization of the external genitalia during male development. Interestingly, female knockout mice for type 1 5α-reductase show significant impairment of parturition, suggesting that androgens also play an important role in female reproductive physiology.[69] In general accord with this finding, female knockout mice for AR have smaller litter sizes than wild-type littermates.[45]

In yet another example of steroid-metabolizing enzymes regulating steroid hormone action, two isoforms of 11β-hydroxysteroid dehydrogenase (11β-HSD) oppose each other's action and regulate local levels of active and inactive glucocorticoids (see Chapter 4).[70] Whereas 11β-HSD type 1 is a reductase that converts weak glucocorticoids (i.e., cortisone and 11-deoxycorticosterone) into potent glucocorticoids (i.e., cortisol and corticosterone), 11β-HSD type 2 is a dehydrogenase that catalyzes the reverse reaction to inactivate the more potent glucocorticoids. Clinical and experimental evidence suggests that the relative activity of these enzymes in particular tissues may play an important role in normal glucocorticoid physiology and pathophysiology. These examples illustrate how local biosynthesis or inactivation of steroid hormones can facilitate or inhibit steroid hormone action in a tissue- or cell-specific manner.

RECEPTOR EXPRESSION

All other factors being equal, the level of expression of steroid receptors is a major factor regulating steroid hormone action. Whereas certain cells or tissues are insensitive to steroid hormones because they lack the appropriate receptors, other cells and tissues express large numbers of receptors and are exquisitely sensitive to low concentrations of hormones. In addition, hormone responsiveness is often modulated by up- or down-regulation of steroid receptors. One of the best-characterized mechanisms of sensitization is induction of PR gene expression by estrogens. During the ovarian cycle in the rat, 17β-estradiol concentrations slowly rise as ovulation approaches, and four hours before ovulation, progesterone concentrations surge.[71] These changes in hormone levels lead to biochemical changes in neurons of the ventromedial hypothalamus that facilitate the display of female sexual behavior. In particular, 17β-estradiol activates the ER and increases transcription of the PR gene. The increased abundance of PR mRNA is translated into PR protein, which thereby sensitizes the ventromedial hypothalamus to the subsequent surge in progesterone.[71,72] Essentially the same pattern and mechanism of PR induction by estrogens occurs in stromal cells of the uterus, priming these cells for decidualization in response to progesterone and the implanting blastocyst.[73] Another uterine cell type, the luminal epithelium, displays the opposite pattern of PR expression during the reproductive cycle.[74] Uterine epithelial cells express PR constitutively and rapidly down-regulate PR in response to estrogens. However, the mechanism responsible for this decrease in PR protein is currently unknown. It is also unclear whether PR down-regulation leads to hormone desensitization in these cells.

Receptor expression can be regulated by changes in mRNA stability. The preovulatory surge in luteinizing hormone (LH) decreases levels of ERβ mRNA in granulosa cells of rat preovulatory follicles.[75] This decrease in ERβ mRNA is due to a decrease in the half-life of the message from approximately 18 to 5 hours, rather than a decrease in transcription of the ERβ gene. Moreover, the LH-induced decline in steady-state levels of ERβ mRNA is mimicked by forskolin and the protein kinase C (PKC) activator phorbol myristoyl acetate (PMA), indicating that LH signaling occurs through generation of cyclic AMP (cAMP). The stability of ERα mRNA is also regulated in MCF-7 breast cancer cells. In these cells, 17β-estradiol decreases the half-life of ERα mRNA from 4 hours to 40 minutes by increasing the ribonuclease activity associated with polyribosomes.[76] In contrast, 17β-estradiol up-regulates ERα mRNA in the endometrium by selectively increasing message half-life from 9 to 24 hours.[77] These studies demonstrate hormone- and tissue-specific effects on the stability of steroid receptor mRNA.

Another well-established mechanism for steroid receptor regulation occurs at the protein level. Treatment with a given steroid generally results in a time-dependent decrease in the level of its cognate receptor in a process called *homologous down-regulation*. Accordingly, a decrease in receptor levels usually results in desensitization to subsequent treatment with the same steroid. Receptor degradation occurs by targeting of the receptor into the ubiquitin–proteasome pathway. Although this mechanism has been implicated in down-regulation of ER, GR, AR, and PR, the role of the proteasome in MR down-regulation has not been studied. The effects of proteasome inhibition on steroid hormone action clearly need further study because there are paradoxical effects on receptor levels and receptor function. Whereas GR accumulation by proteasome inhibition leads to increased transcriptional activity of the receptor, proteasome inhibition of ER and PR degradation results in a decrease in hormone-induced transcription.[78,79] In sum, regulation of steroid receptor expression occurs at multiple levels from gene transcription to mRNA stability to degradation of the mature protein (Fig. 5-5).

HORMONE BINDING AND CHANGES IN RECEPTOR CONFORMATION

Various lines of evidence show that ligand-induced changes in steroid receptor conformation play a central role in transduction of the hormonal signal into a transcriptional response. Early studies, for example, found that trypsin digestion produced different patterns of cleavage for inactive and active (i.e., ligand-bound) receptors: it was reasoned that binding of ligand to receptor caused conformational changes that either concealed or revealed trypsin cleavage sites. Other experiments found that protein–protein interactions between steroid receptors and heat shock proteins were disrupted by the addition of ligand. This result could also be explained by ligand-induced conformational changes that disturb putative contact sites between these proteins. Release of molecular chaperones is critical for receptor activation. Recent work verified inferences about receptor conformation by directly examining the crystal structure of the ligand-binding domain of the AR, ER, PR, and GR, either alone or in complex with ligand.[11,80-82] In particular, these studies showed that the ligand-binding domain is composed of 12 alpha helixes and 4 beta strands folded into a three-layered sandwich (Fig. 5-6). It was also shown that steroid hormones bind within a hydrophobic pocket in the core of the ligand-binding domain and that there are substantial structural differences between ligand-free and ligand-bound receptors.

One of these structural differences provides a basis for the ligand-induced increase in AF-2 activity. The C-terminal helix 12 moves like a trap door to close behind the ligand as it enters the hormone-binding pocket. The

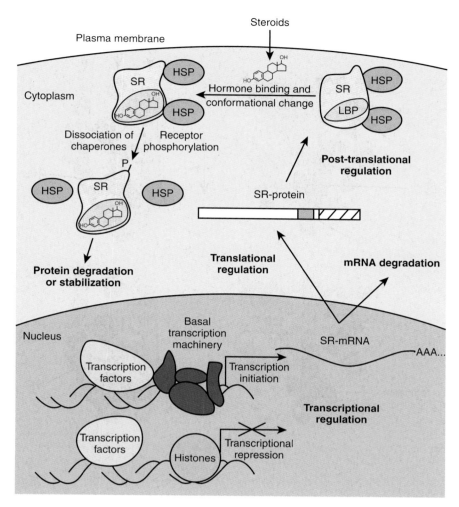

Figure 5-5. *Schematic diagram showing levels of regulation of steroid receptor expression. AAA, polyadenylated mRNA tail; HSP, heat shock protein; LBP, ligand-binding pocket; mRNA, messenger RNA; SR, steroid receptor.*

new position of helix 12, which contains AF-2, allows the receptor to interact with proteins called *coactivators* that are required for ligand-dependent transcription (see Fig. 5-6). Although hormone antagonists bind the same site as agonists, they induce a different receptor conformation (see Fig. 5-6). In general, antagonists have a bulky side chain that sticks out of the ligand-binding pocket and prevents movement of helix 12 into a position favorable for coactivator recruitment. Conformational changes are also important for a number of other aspects of steroid hormone action, including cooperativity for hormone binding and receptor dimerization. *Cooperativity* simply means that binding of hormone to a monomeric receptor facilitates binding of hormone to a second receptor, presumably through receptor dimerization.

Steroids have been found to have opposing effects in different tissues in postmenopausal women undergoing hormone replacement therapy (i.e., reduced risk of colorectal cancer and hip fractures, but increased risk of coronary heart disease, pulmonary embolism, stroke, and breast cancer).[83] The finding that combined estrogen–progestin therapy can have beneficial effects in some tissues and harmful effects in others highlights the importance of designing new ligands that dissociate these effects. Selective

ER modulators (SERMs) are compounds that have been developed to retain the beneficial effects of estrogens while eliminating unwanted side effects. Raloxifene and tamoxifen are two of the best-characterized ligands in this regard, having been crystalized in complex with ERα.[84-86] Raloxifene acts as an estrogen agonist in bone by increasing bone mineral density and decreasing the risk of vertebral fractures in women with osteoporosis. In contrast, raloxifene acts as an estrogen antagonist in the breast and uterus. Tamoxifen, on the other hand, antagonizes estrogen action in the breast, but acts as an agonist in the uterus. Tamoxifen is therefore an effective treatment for breast cancer, but it increases the risk of endometrial cancer.

It has been hypothesized that differences in receptor conformation induced by different SERMs are responsible for the tissue-specific effects of these compounds. For example, raloxifene and tamoxifen may elicit different interactions between a particular ER subtype (i.e., ERα) and tissue-specific coactivators and corepressors. Alternatively, a given SERM could have opposing effects on different ER subtypes (i.e., ERα versus ERβ), which are differentially expressed in estrogen-responsive tissues. The compound tetrahydrocannabinol is just such a ligand, activating ERα by allowing interaction with the coactivator GR-interacting

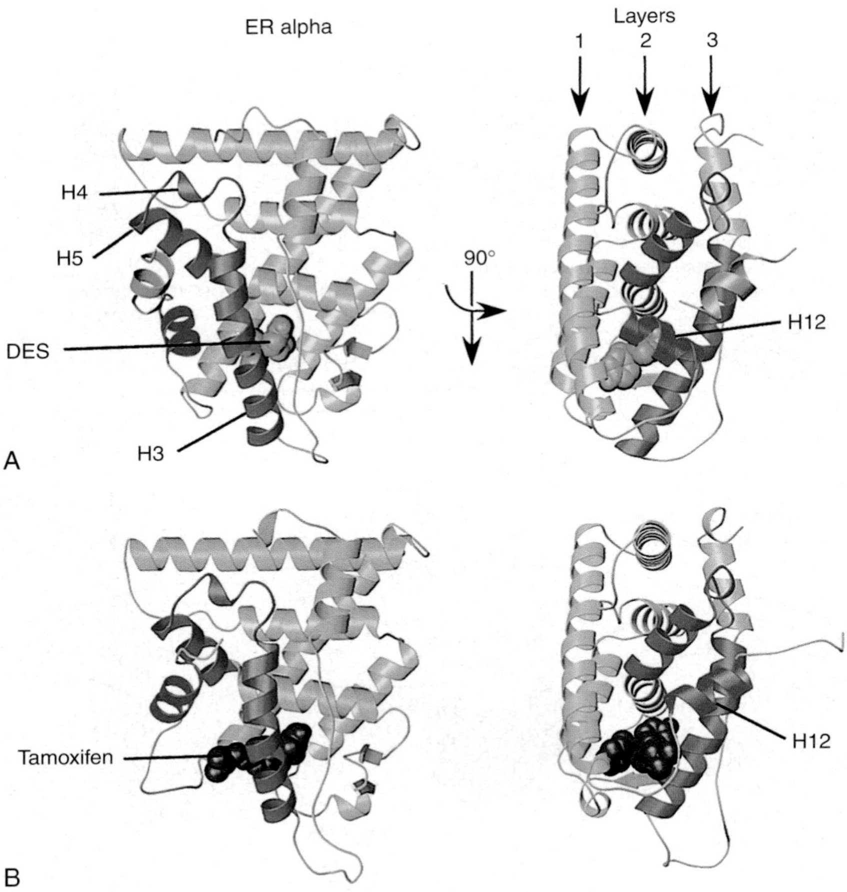

Figure 5-6. A, *Structure of the ERα ligand-binding domain (LBD) bound to diethylstilbestrol (DES; green) and interacting with a peptide from the GR-interacting protein (GRIP1) nuclear receptor box II (orange).* **B,** *Structure of the ERα LBD bound to tamoxifen (red). Note that the position of helix 12 differs between the receptor bound to agonist (DES) and antagonist (tamoxifen). H, helix. (From Shiau AK, Barstad PM, Loria L, et al. The structural basis of estrogen receptor/coactivator recognition and the antagonism of this interaction by tamoxifen. Cell 95:927-937, 1998, with permission from Elsevier).*

protein 1 (GRIP1) or transcriptional intermediary factor 2 (TIF2) and inhibiting ERβ by preventing interaction with the same coactivator.[82] Progress is also being made with selective progesterone receptor and AR modulators.[87,88] Although such compounds hold much promise, there is still a tremendous amount of research to be done. Ultimately, it will be essential to examine structural changes induced by a variety of ligands, ranging from pure and partial agonists to full antagonists as well as selective steroid modulators, to determine whether they work by similar or different mechanisms (i.e., by altering the position of helix 12 or changing cooperativity in hormone binding and receptor dimerization). The structure of an entire steroid receptor, rather than that of isolated domains, is also needed to fully understand steroid hormone action.

RECEPTOR PHOSPHORYLATION

Steroid receptors are proteins modified by phosphorylation at multiple sites. These modifications have distinct effects on the function of different receptors, often in a cell- or promoter-specific manner. Studies mapping phosphorylation sites have shown that steroid receptors are generally phosphorylated at specific serine residues adjacent to proline residues, although particular threonine and tyrosine residues can also be phosphorylated. Although some residues appear to be basally phosphorylated, others are modified in response to ligand binding or activation of other signaling pathways; these include cyclin-dependent kinases, mitogen-activated protein (MAP) kinases, and stress-activated kinases. For example, GR is basally phosphorylated in the S phase and hyperphosphorylated at the G2/M phase during the cell cycle, implicating cyclin-dependent kinases.[89] It is interesting to note that GR can be phosphorylated in response to glucocorticoid treatment during the S phase, but not the G2/M phase. This pattern of GR phosphorylation is correlated with the ability of glucocorticoids to activate gene expression at different stages of the cell cycle. The phosphorylation status of the mouse GR has been shown to have a promoter-specific effect in transient transfection assays.[90] Mutation of phosphorylation sites reduced transcriptional activity on a minimal promoter containing simple glucocorticoid response elements, but not on the more complex mouse mammary tumor virus promoter.

Mutation of just one serine at position 118 of the ER reduced transcriptional activity by as much as 75%, but this effect was also cell- and promoter-specific.[91] This particular residue can be phosphorylated by MAP kinase in vitro. Additional studies have shown that in vivo activation of MAP kinase by growth factors leads to phosphorylation of serine 118 and potentiation of transcription via recruitment of a specific coactivator to AF1.[92] Phosphorylation of ER at other sites has been reported to alter receptor dimerization and DNA binding.[91] A role for phosphorylation has been shown for other steroid receptors as well. For instance, a phosphoserine at position 650 in the hinge region of the AR appears to be required for full transcriptional activity of this receptor.[93] Cross-talk between the PR and the neurotransmitter dopamine plays a physiologic role in the control of sexual behavior in female mice: PR and sexual receptivity can be activated by dopamine in the absence of progesterone.[94] Like the ER, the PR can be phosphorylated in a ligand-independent manner at serine 294 by activation of MAP kinases.[95] Phosphorylation at this residue targets the PR for degradation by the proteasome, but paradoxically enhances transcriptional activity of the receptor.[96] In summary, various kinases can phosphorylate steroid receptors via ligand-dependent and ligand-independent mechanisms. In turn, receptor phosphorylation can alter steroid hormone action. Given the general importance of these modifications, it is somewhat surprising that protein phosphatases have not been more widely studied for their effects on steroid hormone action.

INTERACTION WITH DNA

Steroid receptors enhance or repress gene transcription by forming homodimers that interact with specific DNA sequences in the promoter of target genes.[97] The core motif for hormone response elements consists of two six–base-pair sequences arranged as a palindrome with a three–base-pair spacer (i.e., the consensus estrogen-responsive element is AGGTCAnnnTGACCT, where *n* can be any nucleotide). One receptor in each homodimer contacts each half site. As described earlier, three amino acids in the DNA-binding domain are responsible for specific interactions between the ER and the consensus estrogen-responsive element versus the GR and the consensus glucocorticoid-responsive element (i.e., GGTACAnnnTGTTCT). However, hormone-specific patterns of gene regulation cannot be totally explained by this mechanism because the GR, MR, AR, and PR have similar consensus response elements, as determined by in vitro studies.

One explanation for specific regulation of gene expression by glucocorticoids, mineralocorticoids, androgens, and progestins is that natural hormone response elements diverge significantly from the glucocorticoid-response element consensus sequence described earlier. Although nucleotide variants generally lower the affinity of steroid receptors for the hormone response element, they increase binding specificity. In fact, a study of many different hormone response elements in vitro indicates that receptors discriminate among nucleotides in the spacer region and in the sequences flanking the six–base-pair motifs that directly interact with the receptor.[18] In other words, each steroid receptor responds in a unique way to different hormone response elements. Studies analyzing ERα and ERβ activity on different natural estrogen response elements support the hypothesis that steroid receptors interact with DNA in an allosteric manner.[98,99] In turn, DNA-induced variation in receptor structure can influence the recruitment of coactivators to the receptor. Studies of hormone response elements from androgen-sensitive genes suggest another mechanism for steroid receptor specificity; the AR

binds direct repeats of the six–base-pair motif, rather than the inverted palindrome typical of other steroid receptors.[100] Additional studies have shown that the distance of the hormone response element from the promoter influences transcriptional activity of steroid receptors.[101] In short, steroid receptor–DNA interactions contribute significantly to the specificity of steroid hormone action, as well as to variation in hormone responsiveness among genes.

INTERACTION WITH COACTIVATORS AND COREPRESSORS

Within the last decade, it has become clear that the ability of steroid receptors to induce or inhibit gene transcription depends on interactions with proteins called *coactivators* and *corepressors*.[4,102] Steroid receptor recruitment of these proteins serves as a molecular switch regulating chromatin organization at target genes. Coactivators such as CREB-binding protein and p300 have intrinsic histone acetylase activity. Covalent attachment of acetyl groups to specific lysine residues modifies nucleosome function and increases the access of basal transcription factors to promoters (see Fig. 5-1).

Conversely, low levels of histone acetylation are associated with tightly wound nucleosomes and gene repression (see Fig. 5-1). Nuclear receptor corepressor (NCoR) is a protein that interacts with some but not all nuclear receptors to repress transcription. In the case of antagonist-bound ER and PR, NCoR is recruited along with proteins, such as HDAC3, that have histone deacetylase activity.

The discovery of additional coregulatory proteins with enzymatic activity expands on the relatively simple model of transcriptional regulation by histone acetylation and deacetylation. These proteins have diverse functions, including methylation, demethylation, phosphorylation, dephosphorylation, poly(ADP-ribosylation), ubiquitination, and sumoylation of steroid receptors, coactivators, corepressors, and histones.[103,104] Overall, the transition between transcriptional repression and activation of a given gene by steroids appears to result from highly dynamic and context-dependent interactions among these cofactors.

The kinetics of ER-dependent recruitment of coregulatory proteins to promoters has been examined in detail for two estrogen-responsive genes.[105-107] The general picture emerging from these studies is that different cofactors are brought to and then released from the promoter in a specific order. Another important observation was that cofactor recruitment and release was cyclical, suggesting that recruitment of a particular cofactor is required for the subsequent recruitment of another cofactor and so on, until the final coregulatory complex is assembled. The final steps in this cycle are formation of the preinitiation complex and transcription by RNA polymerase. Repetition of this cycle suggests that steroid-dependent transcription within a cell would occur in waves and could be rapidly modulated by reversible covalent modifications of coregulatory proteins at each step during cofactor exchange.

Although some coactivators only enhance transcription on chromatin templates, others are able to augment steroid receptor transcriptional activity on naked DNA.[102] These proteins act as molecular bridges spanning the

DNA-bound receptor and the basal transcription machinery, thereby stabilizing the preinitiation complex and facilitating transcription initiation. Steroid receptor coactivator 1 (SRC-1) and GRIP1 are two such proteins among a growing family of related nuclear receptor coactivators. These proteins contain multiple leucine-X-X-leucine-leucine (LXXLL, where X indicates any amino acid) motifs that are required for specific interactions with AF2 of different steroid receptors. For example, whereas the second LXXLL motif of GRIP1 interacts with the ER and is required to potentiate transcription, the third LXXLL motif of GRIP1 interacts with the GR to potentiate transcription.[11]

Although different coactivators may contribute to receptor-specific patterns of gene expression, there is a certain degree of functional overlap among members of the coactivator family. Recent studies have identified a host of other coactivator proteins (i.e., DRIP, TRAP, and Brg1) that presumably add to the complexity and specificity of steroid hormone action.[102,108]

INTERACTION WITH OTHER TRANSCRIPTION FACTORS

Steroid receptors can interact with other transcription factors to facilitate or inhibit their activity. Interestingly, these effects are mediated by direct protein–protein interactions and do not require the DNA-binding domain of steroid receptors. A well-characterized example is the mutually antagonistic interaction between GR and NF-κB. These transcription factors are involved in the regulation of many proinflammatory genes, with glucocorticoids inhibiting gene expression and activators of NF-κB enhancing gene expression.[109] It appears that the GR hinders the transcriptional activity of NF-κB by multiple mechanisms, including direct and indirect interactions with NF-κB. There is some indication that GR–NF-κB interactions can prevent NF-κB from binding κB-responsive elements. In other cases, the GR does not block DNA binding, but interacts with the transactivation domain of the p65 subunit of NF-κB (see Fig. 5-1). The GR thereby disrupts NF-κB interactions with the basal transcription machinery. Another hypothesis is that the GR competes for a limited number of coactivators that are required to form a bridge between NF-κB and the basal transcription machinery. Additional studies are required to clarify the relative importance of these mechanisms and whether they contribute to cell- or tissue-specific patterns of glucocorticoid antagonism of NF-κB signaling.

Interactions also occur between steroid receptors and the transcription factor AP-1 (Jun:Fos heterodimers). Whereas glucocorticoids and the GR generally antagonize AP-1 activity, estrogens and the ER can stimulate transcription via interactions with AP-1.[110,111] The mechanism responsible for the opposing effects of glucocorticoids and estrogens is currently unknown, but there is some evidence from transient transfection studies that antagonism between glucocorticoids and estrogens may be mediated by interactions at AP-1–responsive sites.[112] There are two distinct pathways for interaction between the ER and AP-1.[110] In the first, AP-1 stimulates transcription by recruiting CBP/p300 and p160 coactivators, such as GRIP1. The estrogen–ER complex then interacts with GRIP1 by the same AF1 and AF2 contacts as it does at estrogen-responsive elements. In a second pathway, estrogen antagonists bound to ER enhance the activity of AP-1 without physically interacting in the AP-1 complex. The antagonist–ER complex is believed to recruit corepressor proteins, such as N-CoR, away from the AP-1 complex, thus relieving repression.

The ligand-bound ER can also interact with the C-terminal DNA-binding domain of the transcription factor Sp1. However, this interaction is independent of the DNA-binding domain of ER because DNA-binding–deficient forms of the ER can stimulate transcription via consensus GC-rich Sp1-binding sites. Taken together, these results indicate that protein–protein interactions are critical for cross-talk between ER and Sp1.[113] In yet another example of cross-talk, signal transducer and activator of transcription 5 (STAT5) and the GR synergistically activate the beta-casein gene.[114] Although steroid receptors interact with numerous transcription factors to enhance or inhibit gene expression in artificial systems, additional work is required to establish the physiologic relevance of these mechanisms in whole organisms.

Nongenomic Actions of Steroids

Some effects of steroid hormones are entirely independent of their classic genomic action and are also independent of interactions with other transcription factors.[115] In general, these "nongenomic" effects occur rapidly and sometimes before those required for transcriptional activation. It is interesting to note that estrogen can have rapid, nongenomic effects, even though the ER is primarily nuclear in its localization. Roughly 2% of the cellular ER, however, is located at or near the plasma membrane and has been implicated in nongenomic signaling by estrogens.[116,117] Moreover, these early steroid effects cannot be blocked by inhibitors of transcription, such as actinomycin D, or inhibitors of translation, such as cycloheximide. Although rapid, nongenomic actions of steroids have been recognized for decades, the mechanisms responsible for these effects have only recently begun to be elucidated.[118] In this section, we will review a few examples of nongenomic actions for each class of steroid hormone. This area of research is currently the most exciting and dynamic in the study of steroid hormone action.

SIGNALING VIA SECOND MESSENGER CASCADES

Skepticism surrounded many of the early studies of nongenomic effects because pharmacologic doses of steroids were used. One of the first studies with physiologically relevant steroid levels showed that intravenous injection of 17β-estradiol produced a rapid increase in uterine cAMP in the presence of an inhibitor of transcription.[119] Subsequent work by others repeated these observations and extended them to show that estrogen-induced generation of cAMP could indirectly stimulate transcription via a cAMP response element.[120] Studies in breast cancer cells have shown that the G-protein–coupled receptor, GPR30, is required for activation of adenylate cyclase by estrogen antagonists.[121] Interestingly, estrogen antagonists could activate GPR30 in cells that lacked the classic ER. However, it is unclear whether the same mechanism is responsible for the rapid effects of estrogen agonists on cAMP levels in the uterus.

Estrogens have also been shown to activate phosphatidylinositol-3-OH kinase in an ER-dependent manner and to modulate cardiovascular function.[122] The ER binds in a ligand-dependent manner to the p85alpha regulatory subunit of PI3K, thereby increasing its activity. Activation of PI3K leads to the activation of protein kinase B (Akt), which directly phosphorylates and activates endothelial nitric oxide synthase (eNOS). Activated eNOS generates NO, causes vasodilation, and decreases vascular leukocyte accumulation. Estrogen-induced inhibition of leukocyte accumulation protects against ischemia–reperfusion injury. Inhibitors of PI3K and eNOS blocked the protective effect of estrogen. Much like the indirect activation of transcription via cAMP, estrogen can activate transcription indirectly by activating the PI3K/Akt pathway.[123] Hafezi-Moghadam and coworkers.[124] showed a similar pattern of activation of eNOS by ligand-activated GR. Briefly, dexamethasone stimulated PI3-kinase and Akt, thereby activating eNOS. NO-dependent vasorelaxation led to decreased inflammation and reduced myocardial infarct size after ischemia–reperfusion injury in the mouse heart.

Glucocorticoids have rapid behavioral effects in a variety of vertebrates.[125] Sexual behavior is inhibited in less than 10 minutes by corticosterone in the roughskin newt. In contrast, glucocorticoids enhance lordosis within 5 minutes in female rats. Although the mechanisms involved have not been clearly defined, it appears that glucocorticoids influence neuronal signaling through the N-methyl-D-aspartic acid (NMDA) receptor. Corticosterone decreases female preference for male odors in mice. When coadministered with corticosterone, NMDA antagonists blocked this effect.[126] Preincubation of rat hippocampal neurons with glucocorticoids for just 10 minutes prolonged the NMDA-induced rise in intracellular Ca^{2+}.[127] Studies in rats have shown that extracellular aspartate and glutamate (excitatory neurotransmitters) levels increase in the hippocampus shortly after corticosterone administration.[128]

Mineralocorticoids also produce rapid, nongenomic effects that are not blocked by inhibitors of transcription or translation. For example, aldosterone administered at physiologically relevant concentrations (i.e., approximately 0.1 nM) activates the Na+/H+ transporter and increases intracellular pH in renal cells within 3 to 20 minutes.[129] In addition to this rapid effect on transporter activity, aldosterone induces transcription of the Na+/H+ transporter gene by the classic mode of steroid hormone action.[130] Nongenomic and genomic mechanisms of aldosterone action may therefore play important roles in acute and long-term electrolyte balance, respectively. Aldosterone also produces rapid effects on Na+/H+ transporter activity in other cell types, including human mononuclear leukocytes, endothelial cells, and vascular smooth muscle cells. Glucocorticoids were generally unable to activate the Na+/H+ transporter, indicating that the effect is specific for mineralocorticoids. A diacylglycerol-dependent mechanism involving PKC has been implicated in aldosterone activation of the Na+/H+ transporter in some, but not all studies.[131] Intracellular levels of IP3 and calcium are rapidly elevated after mineralocorticoid treatment in colon cells. Whereas low calcium in the medium prevented the increase in intracellular calcium, depletion of intracellular calcium stores by pretreatment with thapsigargin had no effect. Thus, calcium appears to enter from outside the cell in response to aldosterone, rather than being released from intracellular stores. Nevertheless, the MR does not appear to be required for rapid, nongenomic effects on calcium levels, thus implicating a nonclassic receptor that has yet to be identified.[132]

Progesterone stimulates motility, Ca^{2+} influx, and the acrosome reaction in spermatozoa.[118,133] These effects are most likely nongenomic because they occur within a few seconds to minutes and because mature sperm have highly condensed chromatin that is transcriptionally inactive.[134] Given that progesterone is found in follicular fluid, in oviductal fluid, and in the extracellular matrix of oocytes around the time of fertilization, progesterone may play a physiologic role in the acrosome reaction. In any case, progesterone induces a rapid Ca^{2+} influx in sperm that is blocked by Ca^{2+} chelators or La^{3+}. Thapsigargin, which elicits a rise in cytoplasmic Ca^{2+} by releasing intracellular stores, also triggers the acrosome reaction. Interestingly, PKC appears to be involved in mediating progesterone-induced increase in Ca^{2+}.[135] In conjunction with these changes, progesterone activates phospholipase C, causes rapid hydrolosis of phosphatidylinositol 4,5-biphosphate, and stimulates the synthesis and secretion of platelet-activating factor, which can itself induce the acrosome reaction. There is also evidence that progesterone may activate a distinct membrane receptor that interacts with and activates a gamma-aminobutyric acid GABA(A) receptor/chloride channel. In turn, this channel modulates the acrosome reaction.[133]

Androgens and estrogens rapidly activate the MAP kinase (i.e., Src/Shc/ERK) pathway and block programmed cell death (apoptosis) in a variety of cell types.[136] Androgen action on this signaling pathway is mediated by the classic AR and results from an interaction between the ligand-binding domain and Src homology domain 3 of the protein tyrosine kinase Src. Androgen activation of this pathway is dependent on a conformational change in Src and its subsequent interaction with Shc, which links receptor tyrosine kinases with intracellular signaling proteins. Further studies show that Shc is required for phosphorylation and activation of ERK1/2 in response to androgens. Although the events downstream of ERK 1/2 have not been elucidated, evidence is accumulating that the MAP kinase pathways play an important role in cell survival.[137] Estrogens activate the same MAP kinase pathway, but via interaction between ER and the SH2 domain of Src.[136] Based on these results, it was proposed that cross-talk between androgens and estrogens in vivo may be mediated in part by AR and ER interactions with Src. Another important finding from that study was that nongenomic and genomic effects mediated by the classic ER can be dissociated using synthetic ligands. Estren did not activate a reporter gene containing estrogen responsive element (EREs), but

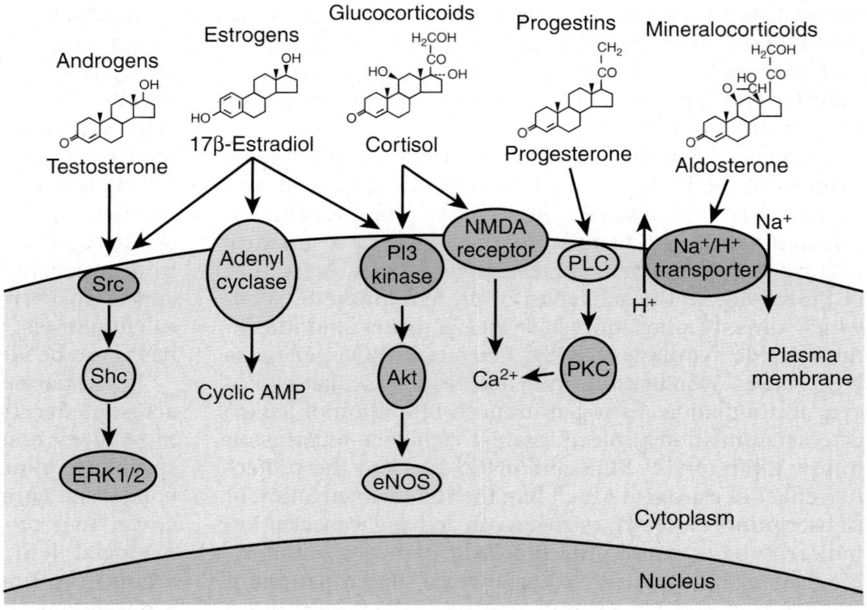

Figure 5-7. *Schematic diagram showing representative nongenomic effects of steroids. Akt, protein kinase B; eNOS, endothelial nitric oxide synthase; ERK, extracellular signal-regulated kinase; PI3, phosphoinositide 3-kinase; PKC, protein kinase C; PLC, phospholipase C; Shc, Src homology 2 domain; Src, sarcoma-inducing proto-oncogene.*

was able to protect against apoptosis. Conversely, pryazole activated a reporter gene containing EREs, but was unable to protect against apoptosis.

Summary

In conclusion, multiple interactions between steroid hormones and other signaling molecules increase the complexity of steroid hormone action. It has become widely accepted in recent years that physiologically relevant levels of steroids can activate second messenger pathways independently of their classic effects on gene expression (Fig. 5-7). In turn, these second messengers can significantly alter cell, organ, and whole animal physiology. It is important to note that steroid-dependent activation of nonclassic pathways can also lead to changes in gene transcription.[120,123] Steroid hormones can therefore have strictly nongenomic effects, genomic effects that are indirectly mediated by second messenger pathways, and genomic effects mediated by steroid receptors that act as ligand-gated transcription factors. Inhibitory and synergistic cross-talk with other transcription factors is another important mode of action for steroid receptors. It has also been shown that steroid receptors can be activated by various factors (e.g., MAP kinases, dopamine) in a ligand-independent manner. As basic mechanisms of steroid hormone action are further

elucidated, we will be able to address questions of critical importance for the treatment of disease and for maintenance of general health and well-being. For example, it will be critical to determine whether different mechanisms of steroid hormone action are independent of each other or whether inhibition or activation of one mechanism always affects other mechanisms. It is imperative to obtain such information if we hope to correct abnormal physiologic and cellular processes without disrupting normal processes.

The complete reference list can be found on the companion Expert Consult Web site at www.expertconsultbook.com.

Suggested Readings

Boonyaratanakornkit V, Edwards DP. Receptor mechanisms of rapid extranuclear signalling initiated by steroid hormones. Essays Biochem 40:105-120, 2004.

Heemers HV, Tindall DJ. Androgen receptor (AR) coregulators: a diversity of functions converging on and regulating the AR transcriptional complex. Endocr Rev 28:778-808, 2007.

Lonard DM, Lanz RB. O'Malley BW. Nuclear receptor coregulators and human disease. Endocr Rev 28:575-587, 2007.

Pike AC. Lessons learnt from structural studies of the oestrogen receptor. Best Pract Res Clin Endocrinol Metab 20:1-14, 2006.

Weigel NL, Moore NL. Kinases and protein phosphorylation as regulators of steroid hormone action. Nucl Recept Signal 5:e005, 2007.

Zhou J, Cidlowski JA. The human glucocorticoid receptor: one gene, multiple proteins and diverse responses. Steroids 70:407-417, 2005.

CHAPTER 6

Prostaglandins and Other Lipid Mediators in Reproductive Medicine

Colin D. Funk, Wen-Chao Song, and Garret A. FitzGerald

The study of prostaglandins had its beginning in reproductive biology. In the 1930s, von Euler first characterized the presence in semen of active substances that induced uterine contractility.[1] The active elements were named *prostaglandins,* based on the erroneous belief that they were produced by the prostate gland. We now know that the copious quantities of prostaglandins in semen are actually produced by the seminal vesicle gland and that prostaglandin biosynthesis is not limited to the accessory glands of the male reproductive system.

Discovery of the widespread occurrence of prostaglandins, their broad range of biologic activities, chemical structures, and biosynthetic pathways, and determination of their relevance to the mechanism of action of nonsteroidal anti-inflammatory drugs (NSAIDs) and aspirin have engaged the interest of generations of reproductive endocrinologists. The general relevance of the field to diverse aspects of biology has prompted an era of intense and broad-based research that few other fields have experienced.[2] The Nobel Prize was awarded to Bergström, Samuelsson, and Vane in 1982 for elucidating the structure and biosynthesis of prostaglandins and for revealing the mechanism of action of NSAIDs.[3]

Today, prostaglandins and related lipid mediators are collectively referred to as *eicosanoids.* Eicosanoids (from *eicosa,* a Greek root meaning "20") are derived enzymatically from 20-carbon polyunsaturated fatty acids, principally arachidonic acid in mammalian species. They are produced by almost all cells in the body in response to hormonal stimulation or mechanical trauma. They evoke a wide array of biologic actions in diverse tissues (including

the reproductive system) at extremely low concentrations. Tissue specificity in eicosanoid action is afforded by selective expression of biosynthetic enzymes and membrane receptors (and also nuclear receptors) for eicosanoids. They are generally believed to be short-lived because they are susceptible to spontaneous or metabolic inactivation. They are believed to act as paracrine or autocrine modulators of cellular function.

In this chapter, we first summarize the salient features of eicosanoid biosynthesis and pharmacology, and then we review the current understanding of their actions in the reproductive system. We also introduce at the end of the chapter other noneicosanoid lipid mediators that are now gaining recognition in reproductive medicine. For a more detailed and comprehensive review of the earlier literature on eicosanoids in reproduction, readers are urged to consult the corresponding chapter in a previous edition of this book.[4]

Biosynthesis of Eicosanoids

NOMENCLATURE

The term *eicosanoid* refers to both prostaglandins and thromboxanes (products of the cyclooxygenase pathway, abbreviated as PG and TX, respectively) and leukotrienes (products of the 5-lipoxygenase pathway, abbreviated as LT). All PGs have a hairpin configuration and contain a cyclopentane ring with two side chains oriented in *trans* positions relative to the cyclopentenone ring. Each group of prostaglandins is allocated a letter (e.g., A, E, F), which denotes particular functional groups at carbons 9 and 11 of the ring structure.

The degree of unsaturation of the side chains is indicated by the subscript numeral after the letter; thus, PGE_1, PGE_2, and PGE_3 have one, two, and three double bonds, respectively. In the case of $PGF_{2\alpha}$, the subscript α denotes the stereochemistry of the 9-hydroxyl group in the cyclopentane ring.

A similar system is used for nomenclature of TXs that have oxygen-bridged six-member rings in place of the five-member ring seen in PGs. All LTs have three conjugated double bonds, and the subscript numeral (e.g., the 4 in LTA_4 and LTC_4) denotes the total number of double bonds in the molecule. LTA_4 is an unstable epoxide and serves as a parent molecule in the biosynthesis of LTB_4 (hydrolysis product), LTC_4, LTD_4, and LTE_4 (peptide derivatives).

RELEASE OF ARACHIDONIC ACID FROM PHOSPHOLIPID STORES

Eicosanoids are not stored, but rather are synthesized de novo when cells are activated by hormonal or mechanical stimuli. The first obligatory (and often rate-limiting) step in eicosanoid biosynthesis is the release of arachidonic acid from membrane phospholipid stores (Fig. 6-1).[5,6] This process is exquisitely regulated by a host of enzymes, particularly several types of phospholipase A_2 (PLA_2),[7] and it appears to be coordinated with the induction of downstream eicosanoid biosynthetic enzymes.[6,8-10]

Recent studies suggest that at least three types of PLA_2 are involved in arachidonic acid release during different stages of cell activation.[6] Under basal conditions, the Ca^{2+}-independent PLA_2 ($iPLA_2$) is the dominant phospholipase involved in the liberation of arachidonic acid and other polyunsaturated fatty acids from membrane phospholipids.[6] The phospholipase $iPLA_2$ is primarily involved in membrane remodeling and usually does not cause significant eicosanoid production, because its activity in arachidonic acid release is balanced by acylase enzymes. However, the activity of $iPLA_2$ may become significant when acylase enzymes are down-regulated. For example, mice heterozygous for acyl-coenzyme A synthetase 4 deficiency accumulated high levels of uterine PGs, had abnormal uterus polycysts, and displayed reduced fertility.[11]

When cells are activated, such as by receptor ligation or calcium ionophore stimulation, intracellular calcium levels rise and the Ca^{2+}-dependent cytosolic PLA_2 ($cPLA_2$) becomes involved.[6] The activity of $cPLA_2$ far exceeds that of acylase enzymes, and as a result, there is rapid accumulation of free arachidonic acid to be acted on by either constitutive or inducible eicosanoid-synthesizing enzymes.

Under certain situations of sustained cell activation, secreted PLA_2 ($sPLA_2$) family members may also participate, further increasing the supply of free arachidonic acid to meet the need of eicosanoid-synthesizing enzymes. Clearly, $cPLA_2$ plays a key role among these enzymes because cells lacking $cPLA_2$ are generally devoid of eicosanoid biosynthesis.[7]

PATHWAYS OF EICOSANOID BIOSYNTHESIS

After its release from membrane phospholipid stores, arachidonic acid is transformed enzymatically to various eicosanoids through multiple pathways (Fig. 6-2). One pathway is initiated by the enzyme PG H synthase (PGHS, also known as *cyclooxygenase* [COX])[12] and results in the production of PGs, TX (TxA_2), and prostacyclin (PGI_2). These cyclooxygenase-derived products are sometimes also referred to as *prostanoids*.

The initial cyclized fatty acid derivative formed in this reaction is PG G_2 (PGG_2). The peroxide moiety at the 15-carbon position of PGG_2 is subsequently reduced to an alcohol group to form PGH_2 as a result of the inherent peroxidase activity of PGHS (see Fig. 6-2). Both PGG_2 and PGH_2 are unstable intermediates with very short half-lives.

The conversion of PGH_2 to individual PGs is relatively tissue-specific, depending on the local expression of specific PG-synthesizing enzymes.[12,13] For example, TxA_2 is synthesized in platelets and macrophages, whereas PGI_2 is the dominant COX product of macrovascular endothelial cells.[2,13]

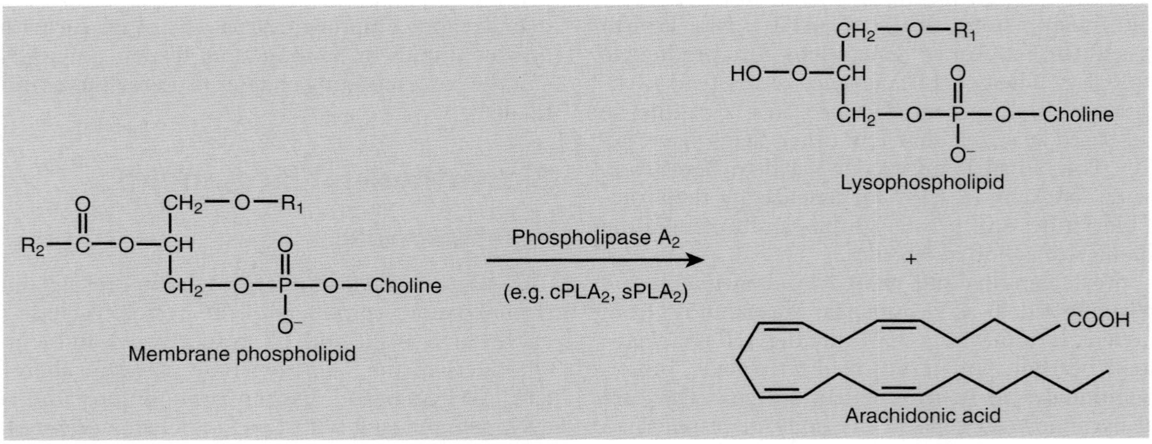

Figure 6-1. Release of free arachidonic acid from membrane phospholipid stores is the first step in eicosanoid biosynthesis. Arachidonic acid (R_2-COOH), located at the sn-2 position of phospholipids (phosphatidylcholine, phosphatidylethanolamine, and phospatidylinositol) is mainly cleaved by phospholipase A_2 enzymes when cells are activated. R_1 is often a C16 or C18 saturated or monounsaturated fatty acid in acyl linkage.

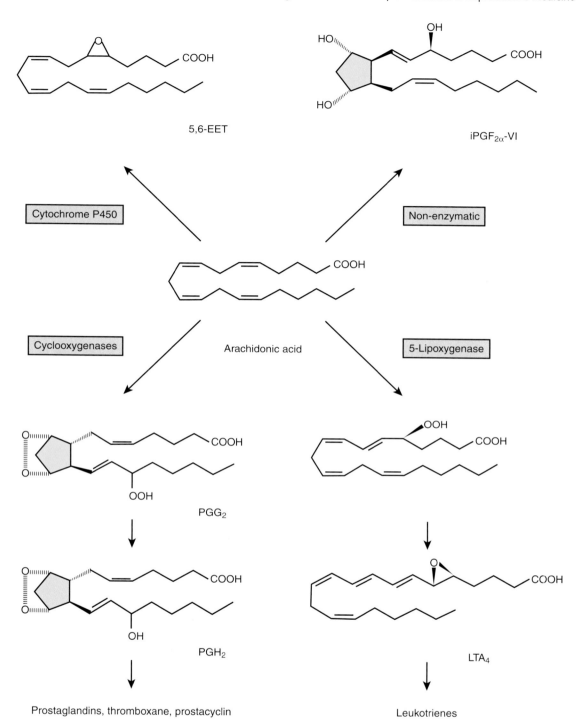

Figure 6-2. *Major pathways of eicosanoid biosynthesis from arachidonic acid. Arachidonic acid is converted by two forms of cyclooxygenase (formally known as* prostaglandin H synthase) *to PGH$_2$ and then to prostaglandins, thromboxane, and prostacyclin; by lipoxygenases to leukotrienes (depicted) and other products, such as hydroxy-eicosatetraenoic acids (HETEs) (not shown); by cytochrome P450 enzymes to epoxy-eicosatrienoic acids (EETs; 5,6-EET is shown as an example). Arachidonic acid can also be converted nonenzymatically to isoprostanes through free radical–catalyzed peroxidation and cyclization (there are 64 potential isomers of isoprostanes[22,23]; the structure of isoprostane isomer VI of prostaglandin F2 alpha (iPGF$_{2\alpha}$-VI) is shown as an example). In contrast to the enzymatic pathways, formation of isoprostanes can occur on phospholipids, and release of free arachidonic acid is not a prerequisite.[24]*

The second major pathway of arachidonic acid metabolism is initiated by lipoxygenases. Like cyclooxygenase, lipoxygenases (LOX) are also dioxygenases that catalyze the insertion of molecular oxygen into arachidonic acid to form a hydroperoxy derivative.[14] The insertion of molecular oxygen can occur at several carbon positions (e.g., 5, 12, and 15) along the fatty acid chain. These determine the specificity of the enzymes, hence, the origin of names such as *5-lipoxygenase* and *12-lipoxygenase*.[14] The enzyme 5-lipoxygenase is of particular importance because its product, 5-hydroperoxy-eicosatetraenoic acid (5-HPETE), serves as a precursor for the LT family of eicosanoids, which are involved in host defense and immediate-type hypersensitivity reactions.[2,15]

Other important eicosanoids formed from the lipoxygenase pathway include lipoxins, which are mostly produced by the interaction of neutrophils with other cells in the vascular compartment. They are believed to play a role in the resolution of inflammatory responses.[16]

Arachidonic acid can also be metabolized by an additional pathway, through the activity of cytochrome P450 enzymes.[17] Unlike the cyclooxygenases or lipoxygenases, cytochrome P450 enzymes catalyze the mono oxygenation (insertion of one atom of oxygen from O_2) of arachidonic acid, with hydroxy or epoxy derivatives of arachidonic acid as their major products.[17] Cytochrome P450 products modulate nephron ion transit and renovascular tone.[17-19] Some cytochrome P450–derived epoxy metabolites of arachidonic acid are elevated in women with pregnancy-induced hypertension,[20] and others may have anti-inflammatory activities.[21]

Lastly, peroxidation of arachidonic acid and cyclization to PG-like compounds called *isoprostanes* can also occur nonenzymatically by free radical–catalyzed reactions.[22,23] In contrast to the enzyme-produced eicosanoids, isoprostanes can be formed in situ on phospholipids and then released by phospholipases.[24] Isoprostanes may serve as incidental ligands for eicosanoid receptors under certain conditions.[23,25]

More importantly in the clinical setting, urine and plasma isoprostane levels have proven to be reliable markers of lipid peroxidation and oxidant stress in vivo.[22,23] For example, elevated levels of urinary isoprostanes were detected in women with android obesity[26] and in individuals with alcohol-induced liver injury.[27] Both conditions are associated with increased oxidant stress and inflammation, as determined by other independent markers.

MAJOR PRODUCTS OF THE CYCLOOXYGENASE PATHWAY: PROSTAGLANDINS, THROMBOXANES, AND PROSTACYCLIN

The first PGs whose chemical structures were deduced were PGE_2 and $PGF_{2\alpha}$ (which partitioned, respectively, into the *ether* [E] and *fosfat* [F; Swedish for *phosphate*] buffer phases, during the initial organic solvent extraction experiments). The discoveries of TxA_2 and PGI_2 occurred much later, partly because these compounds have extremely short half-lives (seconds to minutes), in solutions of neutral pH or under physiologic conditions.

As discussed previously, the formation of individual PGs in the cyclooxygenase pathway starts with the formation of PGH_2 by PGHS enzymes (see Fig. 6-2). Two COX enzymes, encoded by separate genes, have been identified in vertebrates.[12,28] One COX enzyme (COX-1) is constitutively expressed, whereas the other (COX-2) is inducible by cytokines, growth factors, and hormones. This categorization as constitutive COX-1 and inducible COX-2 is useful, but is not always the case (i.e., COX-2 is constitutively expressed in some organs, such as the kidney glomerulus[29]).

The subsequent conversion of PGH_2 to individual prostanoids is tissue-specific and is catalyzed by the corresponding isomerases and synthases (Fig. 6-3).[13] For example, TxA_2 synthase is expressed in platelets and macrophages, PGI_2 synthase is found in endothelial cells, and $PGF_{2\alpha}$ synthase is abundant in the uterus.[2]

There are at least two types of glutathione-dependent PGE_2 synthases.[8-10,30] One PGE_2 synthase, cPGES, is a constitutively expressed cytosolic enzyme functionally coupled to COX-1; the other is a microsomal and inducible enzyme, mPGES-1, which appears to be coupled to COX-2.[8-10,30] Another enzyme, mPGES-2, found in bovine endometrium and other sites, is less well characterized, and its role in PGE_2 synthesis is unclear.[31]

Two points relating to prostanoid synthesis must be mentioned. First, the various synthesizing enzymes all use the endoperoxide intermediate PGH_2 as a common substrate, but they are not always related phylogenetically. For example, PGF synthase belongs to the aldo-keto reductase (AKR) superfamily of enzymes, whereas both TxA_2 and PGI_2 synthases are heme-containing proteins, belonging to the cytochrome P450 superfamily of enzymes.[32]

Second, in addition to derivation from the endoperoxide PGH_2, one class of PGs can also be derived from another class of PGs. For example, $PGF_{2\alpha}$ can also be synthesized from PGE_2 by PGE_2 9-keto reductase; PGA_2 and PGJ_2, which contain an α, β-unsaturated ketone, can be formed from PGE_2 and PGD_2 by slow and spontaneous dehydration in vitro in biologic fluids containing serum albumin.[33]

MAJOR PRODUCTS OF THE 5-LIPOXYGENASE PATHWAY: THE LEUKOTRIENES

Products of the 5-lipoxygenase pathway with well-defined biologic activities are mainly produced by inflammatory cells.[2,34] The activation and biochemical cascade of the 5-lipoxygenase (5-LOX) pathway in leukocytes is particularly well understood, because it gives rise to the potent LT family of lipid mediators that have chemotactic or smooth muscle–contracting properties.[2]

Biosynthesis of LTs is initiated by the formation of 5-HPETE from arachidonic acid by 5-LOX in a Ca^{2+}-dependent process that involves translocation of both 5-LOX and $cPLA_2$ to the nuclear envelope.[2,35,36] The activity of 5-LOX also requires the cooperation of an accessory protein, 5-lipoxygenase–activating protein (FLAP), in intact cells.[37]

Some 5-HPETE molecules can escape from the active site of the 5-LOX enzyme and are ultimately reduced by cellular peroxidases to the corresponding 5-hydroxy derivative of arachidonic acid (5-HETE). Other 5-HPETE molecules may be further converted to the labile epoxide known as *leukotriene A4* (LTA_4) by a secondary dehydrase activity contained in 5-LOX (Fig. 6-4).[34] LTA_4 undergoes one of several potential transformation routes, depending on the cellular context.

Hydrolytic attack of LTA_4 by LTA_4 hydrolase produces LTB_4,[38] a potent chemotactic agent for neutrophils. The conjugation of LTA_4 with glutathione is catalyzed by LTC_4 synthase, thereby forming LTC_4 at the nuclear envelope.[39]

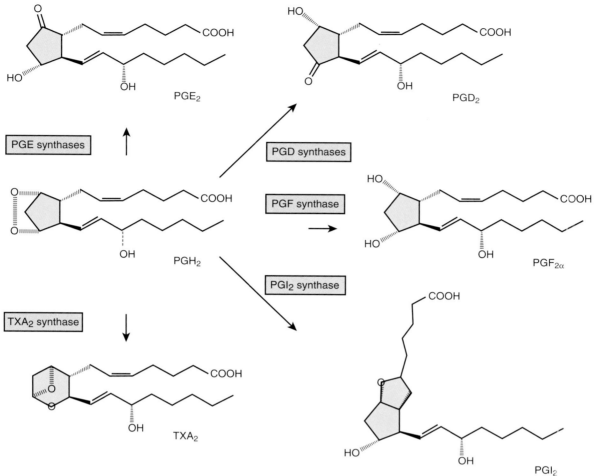

Figure 6-3. *Biosynthesis and structures of prostanoids from prostaglandin (PG) H$_2$ (PGH$_2$). Formation of PGE$_2$ is catalyzed by PGE synthases, of which at least three have been identified.[8-10,30,31] Formation of PGD$_2$ is catalyzed by at least three different PGD$_2$ synthases.[192] Formation of PGF$_{2\alpha}$ is catalyzed by PGF synthase, a member of the aldo-keto reductase family of enzymes. Thromboxane A$_2$ (TxA$_2$) and PGI$_2$ are formed by TxA$_2$ synthase and PGI$_2$ synthase, respectively. Both enzymes are cytochrome P450 enzymes associated with microsomal membranes.*

Sequential cleavage of the peptide moiety of LTC$_4$ by extracellular peptidases produces LTD$_4$ and LTE$_4$ (see Fig. 6-4).

The three cysteinyl LTs, LTC$_4$, LTD$_4$, and LTE$_4$, are the major constituents of the *slow-reacting substance of anaphylaxis* released from antigen-sensitized guinea pig lungs that produced slow and sustained smooth muscle contraction of intestinal smooth muscle strips, observed more than 60 years ago.[34] LTA$_4$ can also serve as a precursor for the transcellular biosynthesis of lipoxins.[40] A number of biologic activities, particularly in the resolution of the inflammatory response, have been proposed for lipoxins.[16]

Lipoxygenases with catalytic oxygenase specificity at different carbon positions of arachidonic acid, such as 12-LOX and 15-LOX, produce the corresponding HETEs as their main end products.[14] The physiologic role of these enzymes and their specific products has proven to be elusive—although the murine 15-LOX homologue, which produces both 12-and 15-LOX products, has been implicated in atherogenesis.[41,42] Interestingly, the HPETE product of this enzyme is involved in the initiation and propagation of low-density lipoprotein oxidation, a process known to contribute to the accumulation of fat-laden macrophages in atherosclerotic lesions.[41,42] Products of the same enzyme may also regulate local interleukin-12 production by macrophages in atherosclerotic lesions.[43]

TRANSPORT AND METABOLISM OF EICOSANOIDS

Although eicosanoids are lipid compounds, they do not permeate the cell membrane freely. One PG transporter (PGT)—a member of the organic anion transporter polypeptide family—has been identified and is found in a limited range of cells, where it is subject to humoral and physical stimuli.[44] PGT mediates the cellular uptake of most prostanoids, but not PGI$_2$.[44] Vascular expression of PGT appears to be responsible for clearing most classes of PGs when these compounds are infused into an animal and enter the pulmonary circulation.[44] On the other hand, multidrug-resistance protein 4 (MRP4) functions as a PG efflux transporter.[45] In the LT pathway, newly synthesized LTC$_4$ is transported outside of the cells by transporters such as multidrug-resistance protein 1 (MRP1).[46]

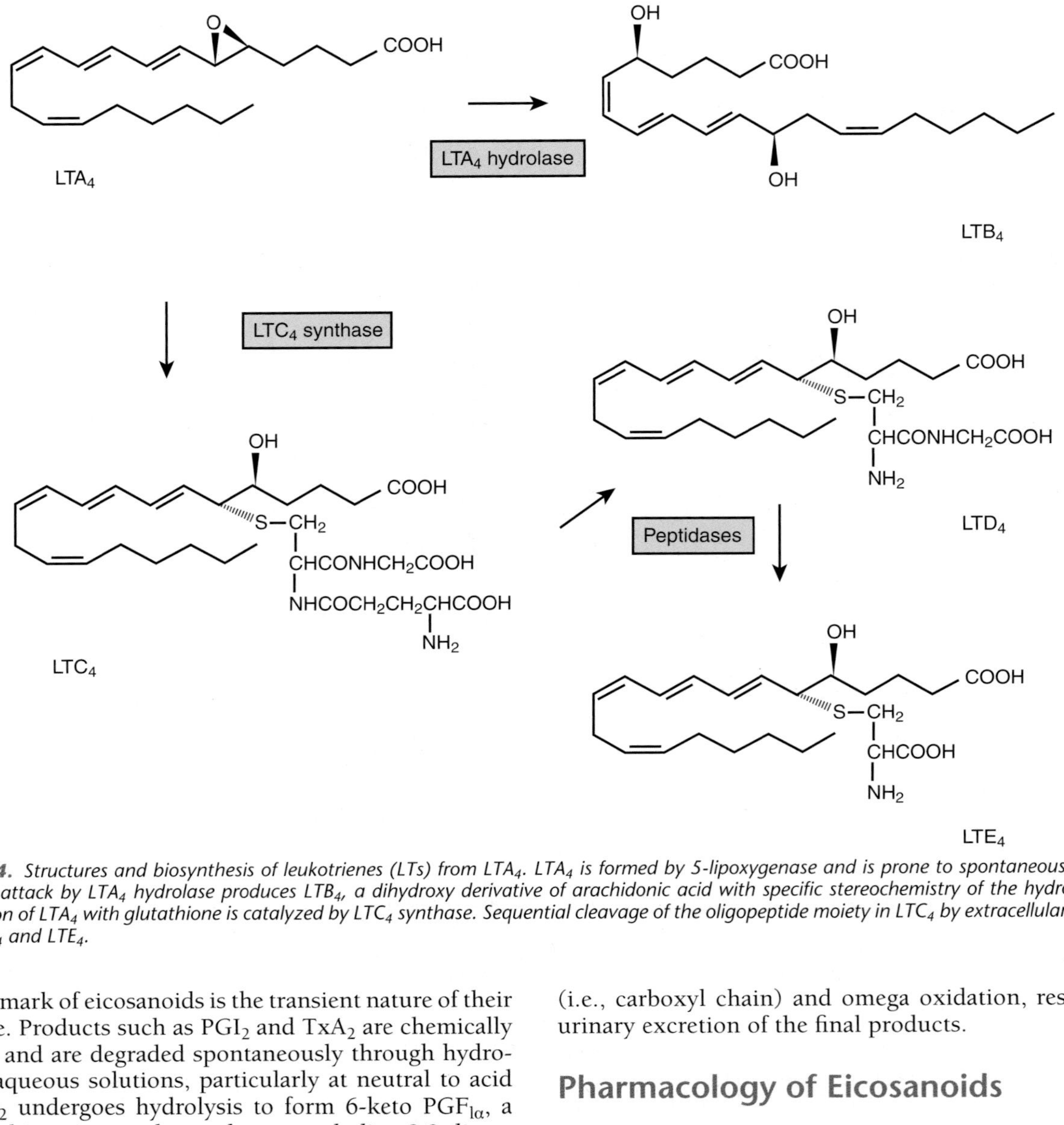

Figure 6-4. *Structures and biosynthesis of leukotrienes (LTs) from LTA₄. LTA₄ is formed by 5-lipoxygenase and is prone to spontaneous hydrolysis. Hydrolytic attack by LTA₄ hydrolase produces LTB₄, a dihydroxy derivative of arachidonic acid with specific stereochemistry of the hydroxy groups. Conjugation of LTA₄ with glutathione is catalyzed by LTC₄ synthase. Sequential cleavage of the oligopeptide moiety in LTC₄ by extracellular peptidases yields LTD₄ and LTE₄.*

A hallmark of eicosanoids is the transient nature of their existence. Products such as PGI_2 and TxA_2 are chemically unstable and are degraded spontaneously through hydrolysis in aqueous solutions, particularly at neutral to acid pH. PGI_2 undergoes hydrolysis to form 6-keto $PGF_{1\alpha}$, a stable and inactive product, whose metabolite, 2,3-dinor-6-keto-$PGF_{1\alpha}$, has been used as a surrogate marker for systemic PGI_2 biosynthesis in vivo. Similarly, TxA_2 rapidly undergoes facile hydrolysis to form the inactive product TxB_2, which is subject to beta oxidation. Plasma or urinary TxB_2 metabolites have served as useful indices of TxA_2 formation in vivo.

The most important catabolic step for PGs is the conversion of the 15-hydroxy group to a 15-keto group by a NAD(+)-dependent 15-hydroxyprostaglandin dehydrogenase (15-OH-PGDH).[47] 15-OH-PGDH is a cytosolic protein with highest concentrations in the lungs, the placenta, the spleen, and the kidney cortex.[47] Both PGE_2 and $PGF_{2\alpha}$ are excellent substrates for 15-OH-PGDH.[47]

The second notable step in the degradation of PGs is reduction of the double bond at position 13 by $\Delta^{13,14}$-PG reductase, which is highly specific for 15-keto PGs; this enzyme has a tissue distribution similar to that of 15-OH-PGDH.[48] The metabolites then undergo both beta

(i.e., carboxyl chain) and omega oxidation, resulting in urinary excretion of the final products.

Pharmacology of Eicosanoids

COX-1, COX-2, TRADITONAL NSAIDS, AND SELECTIVE COX-2 INHIBITORS

A major advance in the field of eicosanoid research during the last decade has been the discovery of the COX-2 enzyme and its physiologic and pharmacologic characterization.[49] COX-2 expression is readily inducible by cytokines, growth factors, and hormonal stimulation.[12] The two enzymes, within a given species, share a 60% to 65% sequence identity in their primary structures.[12]

Both enzymes are membrane-anchored proteins, localizing primarily to the luminal surface of the endoplasmic reticulum and the nuclear envelope.[12] The crystal structures of COX-1 and COX-2 are remarkably similar, as are their catalytic mechanisms and kinetics. However, two subtle structural and biochemical differences have been noted between the two isozymes. First, the active site of COX-2 is larger and more accommodating than COX-1; this property has been exploited by the pharmaceutical industry for the

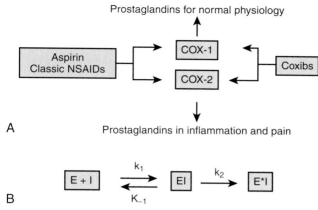

A Prostaglandins for normal physiology

Aspirin Classic NSAIDs → COX-1, COX-2 ← Coxibs

Prostaglandins in inflammation and pain

B

$$E + I \underset{K_{-1}}{\overset{k_1}{\rightleftharpoons}} EI \overset{k_2}{\longrightarrow} E*I$$

*Figure 6-5. Mechanism of action of aspirin, traditional nonsteroidal anti-inflammatory drugs (NSAIDs), and coxibs. **A**, Aspirin and traditional NSAIDs inhibit both COX-1 and COX-2, whereas coxibs preferentially inhibit COX-2. **B**, All COX enzyme (E) inhibitors (I) exhibit one of three kinetic models of inhibition: (1) rapid, reversible binding to form EI (e.g., ibuprofen); (2) rapid, lower-affinity reversible binding, followed by time-dependent, higher-affinity, slowly reversible binding (e.g., flurbiprofen and coxibs); (3) rapid, reversible binding, followed by covalent modification (acetylation) of a serine residue in COX (aspirin). The mechanism for the time-dependent inhibition is not well understood, but may involve conformational change of the enzyme (E*I). Coxibs confer their selectivity for COX-2 by causing time-dependent inhibition of COX-2, but not COX-1 enzymes.*

TABLE 6-1

Summary of Eicosanoid Receptor Types and Properties

Receptor	Cognate Ligand	Property*	Intracellular Signaling
IP	PGI_2	Relaxing	↑ cAMP
TP	TXA_2	Contractile	↑ Ca^{2+}
FP	$PGF_{2\alpha}$	Contractile	↑ Ca^{2+}
DP1	PGD_2	Relaxing	↑ cAMP
DP2 (CRTH2)	PGD_2	Chemoattractant	↑ Ca^{2+}
EP1	PGE_2	Contractile	↑ Ca^{2+}
EP2	PGE_2	Relaxing	↑ cAMP
EP3	PGE_2	Inhibitory	↓ cAMP
EP4	PGE_2	Relaxing	↑ cAMP
BLT1	LTB_4	Leukocyte Restricted	↑ Ca^{2+} ↓ cAMP
BLT2	LTB_4	Widely distributed	↑ Ca^{2+} ↓ cAMP
CysLT1	LTD_4	Lung SMC, macrophages	↑ Ca^{2+}
CysLT2	LTC_4, LTD_4	Spleen, Purkinje fibers, etc.	↑ Ca^{2+}

*Smooth muscle activities.
cAMP, cyclic AMP; SMC, smooth muscle cells.

purpose of developing selective COX-2–specific NSAIDs. Second, the gross kinetics (e.g., K_m, V_{max}) for COX-1 and COX-2 are similar, but COX-2 competes more efficiently with COX-1 in intact cells when the release of arachidonic acid is limiting.[6,28] Thus, when COX-1 and COX-2 are both present in the same cells, catalysis of arachidonic acid (provided exogenously or through activation of cellular lipases) is favored by COX-2.[6] COX-1 appears to function independently only when COX-2 is absent or inhibited.[6,28,50]

Researchers have proposed that this difference in sensitivity to arachidonic acid concentration is related to the sensitivity of their heme groups to lipid peroxide–catalyzed oxidation, and thus activation of the cyclooxygenase enzymes.[51] The concentration of lipid peroxide required to activate COX-1 is 10 times more than that required to activate COX-2 in the presence of low concentrations of arachidonic acid.[51]

Aspirin and traditional NSAIDs (e.g., indomethacin) function as nonselective inhibitors of both COX-1 and COX-2,[12] and their mechanisms of action had been extensively investigated, even before the discovery of COX-2. Long-term use of aspirin and traditional NSAIDs in managing inflammatory disorders is associated with significant adverse effects, such as impaired kidney function and gastrointestinal bleeding (Fig. 6-5).[2,12,28,49] COX-2 may be primarily responsible for producing PGs that contribute to the inflammatory process, a suggestion that offers a rationale for developing more specific inhibitors targeted at COX-2.

According to this paradigm, COX-1 is responsible for synthesizing the "housekeeping" PGs; these PGs are required for maintaining normal physiologic processes such as mucosal protection in the stomach and normal kidney function. Thus, the adverse effects associated with traditional NSAID use would result from their inhibition of the COX-1 enzyme, whereas their anti-inflammatory efficacy would be attributable to coincidental inhibition of COX-2 (see Fig. 6-5). This principle has formed the basis for the development and marketing of the selective COX-2 inhibitors known as the coxibs (e.g., celecoxib, rofecoxib, and valdecoxib) for treating the arthritides[2,52]; however, a designation of COX-1 and COX-2 as "good" and "bad" enzymes is an oversimplification.

Recent studies have identified both COX-1 and COX-2 genes and enzymes in such diverse species as human, chicken, and zebrafish.[12,53] This finding suggests that both enzymes have fundamental physiologic roles to play. Indeed, both COX-1 and COX-2 gene–disrupted mice display multiple developmental and physiologic defects, including abnormalities in steps of reproduction.[54-57] Also, the administration of the selective COX-2 inhibitor celecoxib in human subjects unexpectedly suppressed systemic prostacyclin biosynthesis.[58] This discovery further supports the notion that, in some settings, COX-2 may be constitutively expressed and active, participating in normal physiologic processes.

EICOSANOID RECEPTORS

The last decade has also seen an explosion of knowledge regarding the expression, structure, signaling pathways, and physiologic functions of eicosanoid receptors.[59,60] The existence of membrane receptors for eicosanoids was supported by pharmacologic evidence[61] and was consistent with the notion that eicosanoids are locally released paracrine mediators acting on self and neighboring cells.

The first eicosanoid receptor to be cloned was the human TX receptor in 1991.[62] There are now a total of 13 distinct eicosanoid receptors cloned and characterized, 9 for cyclooxygenase-derived prostanoids and 4 for LTs (Table 6-1).[2,59,60] All 13 eicosanoid receptors characterized so far are rhodopsin-like, seven transmembrane domain–containing, G-protein–coupled receptors.[59,60] The nine G-protein–coupled prostanoid receptors, conserved in mammals from mouse to human, are the TX receptor (TP), the prostacyclin receptor (IP), the $PGF_{2\alpha}$ receptor (FP), two PGD receptors (DP_1 and DP_2), and four PGE_2 receptors (EP1, EP2, EP3, and EP4). These receptors are encoded by different genes. In addition, there are several splice variants for the EP3, FP, and TP receptors, which differ only in their C-terminal tails[59,63-65] (Fig. 6-6).

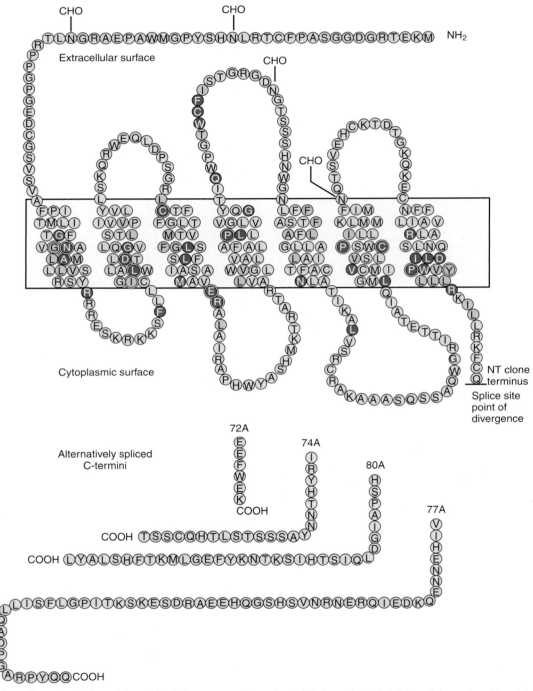

Figure 6-6. *Schematic representation of five rabbit EP3 receptor splice variants differing only in their intracellular carboxyl termini. The carboxyl-variable tails range from 56–amino acid residues for clone 77A to none for the NT (no-tail) clone. Conserved residues in the EP3 receptor are also identified after EP3 receptor sequences from various species are aligned with those of other prostanoid receptors. Conserved residues are indicated by* yellow circles, *and invariant residues are indicated by* red circles. *Residues with* bulls-eye symbols *are conserved across the entire superfamily of G-protein–coupled receptors; those without this inset are unique to the prostanoid receptors. The amino acid sequences of each splice variant are represented by a one-letter amino acid code. (From Breyer RM, Bagdassarian CK, Myers SA, et al. Prostanoid receptors: subtypes and signaling. Annu Rev Pharmacol Toxicol 41:661-690, 2001, with permission.)*

The second PGD receptor, DP2 (also known as CRTH2),[66] induces intracellular calcium mobilization and is a chemoattractant receptor for type 2 T-helper cells.[66] DP2 has also been demonstrated on human eosinophils where both PGD_2 and 15-deoxy-PGJ_2 (a degradation product of PGD_2) serve as activation ligands at nanomolar concentrations.[67,68]

The remaining eight prostanoid receptors fall into three categories according to their functional properties and the secondary messenger systems to which they couple. IP, DP1, EP2, and EP4 are smooth muscle–"relaxing" receptors that signal predominantly through a G_s-mediated increase in intracellular cyclic AMP (cAMP). The FP, TP, and EP1 receptors form the "contractile" subgroup and transduce their signals through a G_q-mediated increase of intracellular calcium. The EP3 receptor is regarded as an "inhibitory" receptor because it is coupled to G_i and causes inhibition of intracellular cAMP.

Several aspects of prostanoid receptor biology and pharmacology require comment. First, the existence of four subtypes of PGE_2 receptors is quite remarkable because all other prostanoids (except PGD_2) each have only a single receptor. Sequence-based phylogenetic tree analysis of the prostanoid receptors showed that the four PGE_2 receptors were the first to evolve because homology among these subtypes is less than that among receptors of different classes of prostanoids.[59,60] Thus, the four PGE_2 receptors must have evolved to play distinctive physiologic functions, and other prostanoid receptors are likely derived from functionally related PGE_2 receptor subtypes through gene duplication.[60]

Second, although there is high ligand selectivity for each of the prostanoid receptors, cross-activation by prostanoids other than the cognate ligand may occur; coupling to alternative downstream signaling pathways at different concentrations of the same ligand may also take place.[60] For example, at high concentrations, PGD_2 can activate the FP receptor.[59] Although PGI_2 analogs activate IP and cause a rise in intracellular cAMP in a dose-dependent manner, higher concentrations have been shown to couple IP to phospholipase C and calcium mobilization.[69]

Third, the multiplicity in prostanoid receptor subtypes and signaling pathways, coupled with their differential tissue expression, explains why the same PG at different concentrations or in different tissues can sometimes produce opposing effects.

Among the four membrane LT receptors characterized to date, two are receptors for LTB_4 (BLT1 and BLT2) and two are for the cysteinyl LTs (CysLTl and CysLT2). The high-affinity ligand-binding BLT1 is primarily expressed on leukocytes,[70] whereas BLT2 has a wider tissue distribution and binds LTB_4 with lower affinity.[71] Both of these receptors signal through intracellular calcium mobilization, as well as through inhibition of adenylyl cyclase.

However, a BLT1-mediated decrease in adenylyl cyclase activity, but not calcium mobilization, is sensitive to pertussis toxin inhibition.[70] In contrast, pertussis toxin treatment partially inhibited a BLT2-induced calcium increase, but had no effect on BLT2-mediated adenylyl cyclase inhibition.[71] Thus, BLT1 and BLT2 appear to use different assortments or ratios of G-proteins for downstream signaling.[71]

The existence of distinct cysteinyl LT receptors has been supported by pharmacologic evidence.[72] CysLT1 has been the primary target for the development of anti-LT drugs for asthma symptom management. Molecular characterization of CysLTl confirmed it to be a G-protein–coupled receptor, with LTD_4 as its preferred endogenous ligand.[73] CysLTl is expressed on lung smooth muscle cells and tissue macrophages, and activation of the receptor results in an elevation of intracellular calcium.[73]

CysLT2, originally defined by pharmacologic methods in trachea and pulmonary vein preparations, is expressed in the spleen, in Purkinje fibers of the heart, and in the adrenal gland.[74] Both LTD_4 and LTC_4 are equipotent agonists for this receptor, which also causes intracellular calcium increase when activated.[74] Recent studies indicate that a third subtype of CysLT receptor exists.[75] Further studies will be required to evaluate its function in mediating LT signaling.

Apart from activating plasma membrane receptors, there is considerable interest in the putative functions of eicosanoids as ligand for nuclear receptors, specifically members of the peroxisomal proliferator–activated receptor (PPAR) family. However, unlike the well-accepted functions of the membrane receptors, the involvement and in vivo significance of nuclear receptors in eicosanoid signaling remains an evolving concept.[2,60,76] Several prostanoids in the PGA and PGD series have been shown to be ligands for PPARα or PPARδ in receptor activation and functional assays (e.g., promotion of fibroblast differentiation to adipocytes); dehydration products of these prostanoids (such as 15-deoxy-$\Delta^{12,14}$-PGJ_2) and products of lipoxygenase pathways, such as 8(S)-HETE and LTB_4, have similar activities.[77-80]

More recently, PGI_2 formed from COX-2 has been proposed to act as a natural ligand for PPARδ to mediate processes ranging from colorectal carcinogenesis,[81] to apoptosis,[82] to embryo implantation.[83] However, most of these studies used nonphysiologic concentrations of eicosanoids or relied on indirect evidence (e.g., the use of synthetic PGI_2 analogs, co-localizations of COX-2, PGI_2 synthase, and PPARδ).[57,83] Whether eicosanoids can indeed signal through nuclear receptors under physiologic settings remains an open question.

Eicosanoids and Reproduction

The role of eicosanoids in reproductive processes is one of the most intensely investigated of their biologic functions. In fact, the uterine-contracting property of PGs led to their discovery. The activity of PGs in stimulating uterine contractility and inducing cervical ripening rendered them and their synthetic analogs attractive candidates as abortifacients in the first or second trimester of pregnancy. For example, misoprostol, a PGE_1 analog, has been used, alone or in combination with mifepristone, for first-, second-, and third-trimester abortions.[84-86]

Traditional NSAIDs, via their capacity to inhibit eicosanoid biosynthesis, block ovulation in several mammalian species,[87] and PGE_2 and $PGF_{2\alpha}$ are well known as effective luteolytic agents within the veterinary community.[88,89] PGs were believed to be involved in maintaining ductus

TABLE 6-2

Physiologic Roles and Therapeutics of Eicosanoids in Reproduction

Function	COX Enzyme	Eicosanoids	Receptor	Therapeutics
Ovulation	COX-2	PGE_2	EP2	
Luteolysis		$PGF_{2\alpha}$	FP	
Fertilization	COX-2			
Implantation	COX-2	PGI_2	PPAR	
Decidualization	COX-2	PGI_2	PPAR	
Dysmenorrhea	COX-2	$PGE_2/PGF_{2\alpha}/PGI_2$		NSAIDs/coxibs
Ductus arteriosus remodeling	COX-2	PGE_2	EP4	
Preeclampsia		PGI_2/TxA_2		Aspirin?
Cervical ripening				PGE analogs
Preterm labor	COX-2	$PGE_2/PGF_{2\alpha}$		NSAIDs/coxibs
Labor	COX-1	$PGF_{2\alpha}$	FP	
Erectile dysfunction				PGE_1

COX, cyclooxygenase; NSAIDs, nonsteroidal anti-inflammatory drugs.

arteriosus (DA) patency during fetal life, and in anecdotal reports, NSAID use during pregnancy was associated with increased risk of premature DA closure and fetal demise.[90,91] Recent advances in eicosanoid pathway molecular biology have significantly improved our understanding of the role PGs play in reproduction. Much of the new knowledge has emerged from studies using knockout mice. Table 6-2 summarizes the major reproductive steps where eicosanoids are known to play a physiologic role or have been shown to have therapeutic relevance.

GONADOTROPIN RELEASE

Prostaglandins have been shown to modulate the secretion of luteinizing hormone (LH) and, to some extent, follicle-stimulating hormone (FSH).[92] This is believed to occur through modulation of hypothalamic LH-releasing hormone (LHRH), because PGE_2 stimulates the release of LHRH in vivo,[93] but does not directly affect the release of LH from the pituitary.[92-93] Furthermore, immortalized neurons contain transcripts of both COX-1 and COX-2.[94] PGE_2 may also regulate the LHRH pulse generator.[92,94-95]

However, studies of COX-deficient mice have shown that the hypothalamic content of LHRH in COX-1-deficient and COX-2-deficient mice is comparable to that of wild-type mice.[96] This observation suggests that neither COX-1 nor COX-2 plays an indispensable role in LHRH production. Additionally, the potential effect of COX enzyme deficiency on the pulsatility of LHRH release during the estrous cycle remains to be evaluated.

In contrast to hypothalamic LHRH, pituitary FSH content was significantly elevated in both COX-1– and COX-2–deficient mice.[96] There was also a tendency for increased pituitary LH content in the COX-deficient mice, although the increase was less pronounced.[96] The mechanism for the increase in pituitary FSH content in the COX-deficient mice is not clear. Nevertheless, serum gonadotropin and steroid levels in COX-1– and COX-2–deficient mice were unchanged compared with wild-type mice.[96]

Furthermore, COX-1– and COX-2–deficient mice exhibited estrous cycles and normal mating behavior. Thus, one can conclude that neither COX-1 nor COX-2 is indispensable in the regulation of the neuroendocrine axis. The reproductive abnormalities observed in COX-deficient mice[54-57] must have resulted from defects in peripheral reproductive organs.

OVULATION

Although an essential role for PGs in ovarian function was established many years ago,[87] the intricacies of their mechanism of action began to be delineated only recently (see Chapter 8). A series of elegant studies established that induction of an antigenically distinct form of COX in the preovulatory follicles of the rat ovary (later to be confirmed as COX-2) was an obligatory downstream event in the LH surge–induced ovulation process.[97-100]

In contrast to the COX-1 enzyme, which was constitutively expressed in thecal cells and corpora lutea, LH-induced COX-2 enzyme was present in granulosa cells of the rat preovulatory follicles.[97-100] This observation was later extended to other mammalian species, including the cow and mare.[101] Interestingly, the time required for COX-2 induction in preovulatory follicles after the LH surge differed considerably in various species (2 to 4 hours in the rat, 18 hours in the cow, and 30 hours in the mare), yet induction of COX-2 expression always occurred approximately 10 hours before ovulation in each of these mammals.[101]

LH surge–induced COX-2 expression in the granulosa cells of macaques, a primate species, has also been established recently using reverse transcriptase–polymerase chain reaction and immunocytochemistry methods.[102] Furthermore, follicular administration of indomethacin in the rhesus monkey was demonstrated to significantly, although not completely, inhibit oocyte release from the ovary.[103]

Thus, in primate, rodent, and domesticated animal species, the induction of COX-2 seems to serve as an "alarm" signal for ovulation.[101,104] Ovulation, initiated by the LH surge that leads to a cascade of proteolytic events that culminate in follicle rupture and release of the ovum, has often been compared to an inflammatory response.[105] In this regard, it is perhaps fitting that COX-2, rather than COX-1, should be implicated in this process.

The predominant role of COX-2 in the ovulation process was subsequently ratified by studies using COX-1– and COX-2–deficient mice. Mice lacking the COX-2 enzyme had multiple reproductive failures, including ovulation defects, whereas COX-1–deficient mice had impaired parturition, but ovulated normally.[57,96] Biochemical studies showed that exogenous gonadotropins (pregnant mare serum gonadotropin [PMSG] and human chorionic gonadotropin [hCG]) stimulated a fourfold increase in ovarian PGE_2 levels in wild-type and COX-1–deficient mice 8 hours after hormonal challenge; COX-2–deficient mice showed no such increase.[96]

Examination at the cellular level showed that the primary defect responsible for failed ovulation in COX-2–deficient mice was impaired expansion of the cumulus oophorus. This impairment possibly originated from an alteration in the proteoglycan contents of the cumulus oophorus and follicular wall.[96] Whether COX-2 deficiency might also have affected the activation of proteolytic enzymes that participate in the breakdown of the follicular wall is not yet known. Indomethacin treatment, however, did cause oocyte retention but did not prevent follicular rupture in the rhesus monkey ovary.[103]

The critical role of COX-2 in ovulation has also been corroborated by pharmacologic studies using coxibs as selective inhibitors of this enzyme in wild-type animals. Administration of celecoxib to mice[106] and NS-398 to rats[107] decreased, but did not abolish, ovulation in the treated animals. NS-398 also reduced PGE_2 synthesis in isolated LH-stimulated rat preovulatory follicles in vitro.

The degree of inhibition of PGE_2 synthesis by NS-398 in this assay was similar to that achieved by indomethacin, supporting the conclusion that COX-2 mediated the previously observed ovulation blockade by traditional NSAIDs.[87] Finally, delayed follicular rupture in humans by the selective COX-2 inhibitor rofecoxib was observed in a recent randomized double-blind study,[108] supporting a link between NSAID use and reversible female infertility originating from ovulation interference.[108-109]

Several lines of evidence suggest that PGE_2 is the principal COX-2 product that mediates the ovulation process. First, ovarian PGE_2 production is increased in response to the LH surge. Second, application of exogenous PGE_2 to gonadotropin-primed, COX-2–deficient mice corrected the anovulatory phenotype.[96] Administration of $PGF_{2\alpha}$ in the same experiment also slightly improved the ovulation outcome, but this was most likely attributable to cross-activation of PGE receptors by $PGF_{2\alpha}$[59] because no ovulatory abnormality was detected in FP-deficient mice.[110]

Third, a moderate reduction in the ovulation rate has been detected in two independently generated EP2-deficient mouse lines,[111-112] but no apparent ovulation defect has been seen in other prostanoid receptor–mutant mice.[59] EP2-deficient mice had severely compromised fertility, which was attributed partially to an ovulation defect and predominantly to fertilization failure.[111-112]

A role for EP2 in ovulation and fertilization is supported by its specific expression in the cumulus cells of the preovulatory follicles, where it is up-regulated in response

to gonadotropin stimulation.[112] The impaired fertilization of EP2-deficient mouse eggs was shown to result from abortive cumulus expansion in the oviduct,[112] a phenomenon also observed in the preovulatory follicles of COX-2–deficient mice.[96] These studies suggested that EP2 may be essential for the late-stage events of ovulation by inducing ordered cumulus expansion after ovulation to ensure successful fertilization; however, it is relevant but not indispensable for follicular rupture and ova release.

Contrary to these initial findings, another follow-up study of adult COX-2–deficient and EP2-deficient mice concluded that the ovulatory process, *not* follicular growth, oocyte maturation, or fertilization, is primarily affected by these deficiencies.[113] This study also showed that severely compromised ovulation, seen in adult COX-2–deficient and EP2-deficient mice, was not manifested in immature (3-week-old) mice with those same deficiencies. This finding suggests that the process of ovulation may be more dependent on PGs in adult mice.[113]

If EP2 is the receptor subtype physiologically responsible for initiating PGE_2-induced ovulation in follicles, then the incomplete penetration of the ovulation phenotype in EP2-deficient mice could indicate compensatory responses from other EP receptor subtypes in this process. In addition to EP2, EP4 messenger RNA (mRNA) has also been detected in the mouse ovary,[59] but its cellular localization has not been determined.

CORPUS LUTEUM FUNCTION AND LUTEOLYSIS

Ovarian PGE_2 levels were slightly suppressed in both COX-1–and COX-2–mutant mice 24 hours after hormonal stimulation.[96] This discovery suggested that, whereas COX-2–derived PGs are responsible for ovulation, both isozymes may contribute to PG production during formation of the corpora lutea. However, neither COX isoform is indispensable for granulosa cell development or corpora lutea formation, because ovarian morphology and steroid hormone production in COX-deficient mice were similar to those of wild-type mice 24 to 30 hours after gonadotropin stimulation.[96] There was also no apparent difference in estrous cyclicity between wild-type, COX-1-deficient, and COX-2–deficient mice.[96]

The role of $PGF_{2\alpha}$ as a physiologic luteolysin has been well established in many nonprimate mammalian species that depend on the presence of the uterus for corpus luteum regression. Indeed, this finding proved to be a major breakthrough in the livestock industry, where $PGF_{2\alpha}$ and its synthetic analogs are now routinely used to regulate the breeding of domesticated animals.

Although FP is expressed in the corpora lutea of mice during a normal estrous cycle,[114] no change was found in the estrous cycle or in the number of corpora lutea in homozygous FP-deficient mice.[110] On the other hand, FP-deficient pregnant mice showed a parturition defect due to lack of luteolysis before the onset of labor.[110] Thus, $PGF_{2\alpha}$ acts as a luteolysin in pregnant mice, but not in nonpregnant, normally cycling female mice.

The involvement of PGs in the luteolysis of primate species is not as well defined (see Chapter 8). Unlike in other mammals, the primate corpus luteum undergoes luteolysis in the absence of the uterus. There is, however, evidence to suggest that locally produced PGs in the ovary may act as mediators to promote luteolysis. For example, $PGF_{2\alpha}$ is produced by the human corpus luteum, and specific receptors for $PGF_{2\alpha}$ are located in human luteal tissue.[115] High doses of $PGF_{2\alpha}$ injected directly into human corpus luteum in vivo also caused premature regression of the corpus luteum and shortening of cycle length.[116]

On the other hand, results from PG synthesis–inhibitor experiments in the rhesus monkey have been equivocal.[117,118] Also, it is not known whether PG levels change significantly in the primate ovary or corpus luteum during the luteal phase.[119] Thus, although there is considerable evidence that PGs of ovarian or luteal origin may participate in the induction of corpus luteum regression in primates, further studies will be required to conclusively resolve this question.[119]

FERTILIZATION, IMPLANTATION, AND DECIDUALIZATION

The importance of the role of PGs in oocyte maturation and fertilization is further supported by the phenotype of COX-2–deficient mice (see Chapter 8).[57] In addition to an ovulation defect, the few ovulated eggs from COX-2–deficient female mice recovered after PMSG and hCG challenge were totally incapable of being fertilized.[57] In accordance with this observation, immunostaining detected COX-2 enzyme in wild-type mouse cumulus cells enclosing ovulated eggs.[57] Thus, local COX-2–derived PGE_2 in the cumulus cells may function as an autocrine factor to activate an EP receptor and induce cumulus cell expansion necessary for successful fertilization.

Also, COX-2 but *not* COX-1 has been found to be essential for embryo implantation and uterine decidualization,[57] although a critical role for COX-2 in implantation per se was not confirmed in a more recent study, as described later.[120] Because COX-2–deficient mice are defective in ovulation and fertilization, the implantation and decidualization processes in these animals could be investigated only by embryo transfer (from wild-type mice) and by a procedure involving intraluminal infusion of oil to induce artificial decidualization.[57,83,120]

Initial published studies showed that 50% of the transferred embryos were successfully implanted in the uteri of wild-type mice at day 5 after pseudopregnancy, but fewer than 2% of the embryos implanted in the uteri of COX-2–deficient mice were successfully transferred.[57] Likewise, induction of artificial decidualization in wild-type mice caused a 16-fold increase in uterine wet weight, but did not produce any appreciable weight gain in COX-2–deficient mouse uteri.[57] The failure of implantation and decidualization in COX-2–deficient mice is not secondary to steroid hormone insufficiency from ovarian dysfunction, because supplementation of progesterone and estradiol did not rescue the phenotype.[57]

A specific role for COX-2 (but not COX-1) in these processes is also supported by the dynamic regulation of COX-2 expression in mouse uterus. Although COX-2 is normally expressed minimally in the uterus, it was robustly induced at 2 hours after artificial decidualization and its expression returned to basal levels within 8 hours. COX-1, in contrast, is constitutively expressed in the mouse uterus and barely changes its expression during decidualization.[57]

It should be noted that a critical role for COX-2 in implantation was disputed in a separate study conducted by Cheng and Stewart.[120] Their investigation into the role of COX-2 in embryo implantation and uterine decidualization concluded that COX-2 has a role in mediating the initial uterine decidual response, but is *not* essential for embryo implantation, sustained decidual growth, or embryo development throughout the remainder of pregnancy.[120]

In addition, PGI_2 is believed to be the eicosanoid that mediates COX-2–dependent embryo implantation and uterine decidualization.[57,83] Furthermore, researchers have proposed that the effect of PGI_2 in these processes is mediated by the nuclear receptor PPARδ. PGI_2 has been reported to be the most abundant prostanoid formed at implantation and decidualization sites, and PGI_2 synthase transcript is also present and up-regulated at the implantation sites between day 5 and day 8 of pregnancy.[57,83]

The finding in earlier studies that two PGI_2 analogs (carbaprostacyclin [cPGI] and iloprost) activated PPARδ[121] and the finding that IP-deficient mice had normal fertility[122] led to the hypothesis that endogenous PGI_2 mediates embryo implantation and decidualization through PPARδ.[57,83] The coordinated uterine expression of PPARδ and COX-2 during decidualization supports this contention. The hypothesis was also supported by the finding that PGI_2 agonists such as cPGI and iloprost (as well as a classic PPARδ-selective agonist, L-165,041) restored implantation and decidualization in COX-2–deficient mice.[57,83] Moreover, in a recent study, PPARδ was found to be essential for spontaneous and preimplantation PGI_2-stimulated embryo development and blastocyst hatching.[123] The implantation of cultured embryos was enhanced by PPARδ activation.

Nevertheless, many questions remain to be answered about the validity of this hypothesis. First, varied phenotypes of PPARδ-deficient mice have been reported.[124] Second, cPGI and iloprost have been shown to activate PPARδ,[57,83,121] but one cannot assume with certainty that endogenous PGI_2 will do the same. Indeed, cicaprost, another PGI_2 agonist for membrane IP, was not an activator of PPARδ,[121] suggesting that caution should be exercised when extrapolating data from PGI_2 analogs. Third, it is possible that implantation and decidualization could be mediated by COX-2 and PPARδ as separate and redundant pathways. To further muddy the waters, recent work suggests that IP receptors play an important role in preimplantation embryo development and mediate the embryo's response to exogenous PGI_2.[125] Clearly, more research is needed on this topic, and even though PGI_2-deficient mice (lacking PGI_2 synthase) have been developed, there have been no reports of the reproductive function in these mice to shed new light on this subject.

Even if the PGI_2-PPARδ hypothesis is accepted at face value, the mechanism and downstream events of this signaling pathway in the uterus remain to be established. No specific defect in the expression of implantation-related genes or steroid responsiveness has been found in the uterus of COX-2–deficient mice.[57] The direct causes of impaired implantation and decidualization failure in these animals are still unknown. Clearly, however, other eicosanoids are needed for the implanted embryos to develop to term. Thus, administration of cPGI was shown to improve implantation and decidualization in COX-2–deficient mice, but the subsequent growth of the implanted embryos in these mice was not comparable to that implanted in the wild-type mice.[57,83] Interestingly, coadministration of cPGI with PGE_2 markedly improved embryonic and decidual growth in COX-2–deficient mice.[83]

MENSTRUATION AND DYSMENORRHEA

Abnormal PG biosynthesis is involved in the pathogenesis of human dysmenorrhea, a gynecologic disorder that is defined as the occurrence of pain associated with menstruation (for a more detailed discussion of this topic, please see Chapter 25). Elevated levels of $PGF_{2\alpha}$ and PGE_2 occur in the endometrium and menstrual fluid of women who have dysmenorrhea, with an elevated ratio of $PGF_{2\alpha}$ to PGE_2.

Markedly increased PGI_2 levels have also been detected in endometriosis tissue. This elevation is considered to cause hyperalgesia and to contribute significantly to dysmenorrhea in endometriosis.[126] Furthermore, intrauterine administration of $PGF_{2\alpha}$ induces uterine contractility and dysmenorrhea-like pain.[4]

Cumulative data of clinical trials have indicated that 80% of patients with significant primary dysmenorrhea experience adequate pain relief with the use of NSAIDs.[127] Both celecoxib and valdecoxib, two COX-2–selective inhibitors, have been used for the treatment of primary dysmenorrhea.[128] Clinical studies confirmed valdecoxib to be both effective and well tolerated for the treatment of primary dysmenorrhea.[129] However, valdecoxib was removed from clinical use in 2005 because of an association with elevated risk of Stevens-Johnson syndrome and cardiovascular hazard, whereas celecoxib remains in use.

PARTURITION AND NSAID USE IN PRETERM LABOR

There has been a great deal of interest in the role that PGs play in term and preterm labor (see Chapters 11 and 26). Aspirin-like drugs were shown to delay parturition in humans more than 30 years ago,[130] and NSAIDs are also well known to be effective agents in attenuating the progression of term and preterm labor in various animal species.[131,132] PGE_2 and $PGF_{2\alpha}$, produced by both maternal and fetal tissues during pregnancy,[133] stimulate uterine contractions in vitro and in vivo; they also promote the coordinated inflammatory response that results in dilation and thinning of the cervix.[133] Studies with COX-1– and prostanoid receptor–deficient mice have provided additional insight into the role and mechanism of action of PGs in the process of parturition and preterm labor.

Although FP-deficient female mice grew and developed normally and became pregnant as expected, they did not deliver fetuses normally at term.[110] This complication was due entirely to impaired parturition. Fetuses could be rescued from FP-deficient mothers by cesarean operation before or at the expected term and survive normally. Uterine induction of the oxytocin receptor at term, an event believed to trigger parturition, did not occur in the FP-deficient mouse uterus.[110]

Additionally, FP-deficient mice did not experience a decline in maternal plasma progesterone level close to term; this decline usually occurs before parturition in mammals. It was quite revealing, however, that ovariectomy just before term completely normalized the parturition defect in FP-deficient mice.[110] Thus, ovariectomy of gravid FP-deficient mice decreased plasma progesterone levels, induced uterine oxytocin receptor expression, and initiated the onset of labor within 24 hours.[110] These observations suggest that $PGF_{2\alpha}$ induces labor through its luteolytic action in the ovary in rodents; its uterotonic action in the myometrium apparently is not essential for parturition.

A similar parturition defect was characterized in COX-1–deficient mice, and administration of $PGF_{2\alpha}$ was sufficient to correct this defect.[134] Thus, COX-1 is essential for the normal onset and progression of term labor and cannot be compensated for by unimpaired COX-2 activity. Remarkably, ovarian $PGF_{2\alpha}$ levels could be blocked by 85% in a COX-1 knockdown mouse model, and residual PG was still sufficient to promote timely luteolysis for initiation of labor.[135] There is still uncertainty regarding the contribution of fetal $PGF_{2\alpha}$ to this process. In one experiment involving reciprocal blastocyst transfers between wild-type and COX-1–deficient mice, maternal COX-1 expression was found to be both sufficient and necessary for the normal onset of labor.[134]

However, in another study, COX-1–deficient females carrying wild-type fetuses delivered their pups on schedule and with normal survival rates,[136] suggesting that maternally derived $PGF_{2\alpha}$ is dispensable. The idea that fetal $PGF_{2\alpha}$ contributes to parturition is also supported by another study by Cook and coworkers who found that increased mouse placental $PGF_{2\alpha}$ biosynthesis, catalyzed at least in part by up-regulated COX-2, is associated with uterine activation and the timing of birth.[137]

It is notable that studies of FP-deficient mice suggested that the primary target of $PGF_{2\alpha}$ action with regard to parturition is the corpus luteum, yet COX-1 mRNA levels in the ovary were quite low and relatively unchanged during pregnancy.[110] This contrasted with a 40-fold induction of COX-1 in the uterus in late gestation.[110] In addition, PGF synthase and a $PGF_{2\alpha}$-metabolizing enzyme, 15-OH-PGDH, were also time-dependently regulated in the pregnant mouse uterus, with a dramatic increase in PGFS and a decrease in 15-OH-PGDH toward late gestation.[138] Thus, primarily uterine-derived $PGF_{2\alpha}$ apparently activates ovarian FP and determines the timing of labor.

The lack of a parturition phenotype in PG receptor–deficient mice other than FP knockout mice suggests that PGs are less important in promoting cervical ripening and myometrial contraction in the mouse. This hypothesis is supported by the finding that the luteolytic effect alone of $PGF_{2\alpha}$ made its function indispensable for murine parturition. This role contrasts greatly with what is believed to occur in human labor. Various PGs are produced in the human uterine cervix, and their increased production is associated with cervical ripening.[139] Receptor sites for EP and FP are also present in the cervix, and a topically applied PG product, containing either dinoprostone or misoprostol, is the most popular means to soften and dilate the cervix in human labor induction.[140]

Local administration of PGs to the cervix in pregnant women results in clinical, histologic, and biochemical changes that are consistent with those observed during physiologic cervical ripening. The mechanism of action of PGs in human cervical ripening is not known, but may include induction of major degrading enzymes and alterations in the expression of genes encoding proteins that modify proteoglycan function. The lack of a phenotype in COX and PG receptor knockout mice in cervical ripening and uterotonic responses may indicate a species difference, or it may suggest compensation in these tissues between the two COX enzymes.

Although COX-1 is involved in term labor, COX-2 induction is likely to be primarily responsible for PG-mediated preterm labor. COX-2, but not COX-1, is induced during inflammation-mediated preterm labor elicited by lipopolysaccharide (LPS) administration.[141] In a murine model, the COX-2–selective inhibitor SC-236 was found to be more effective than the COX-1–selective inhibitor SC-560 in stopping LPS-prompted preterm labor and increasing uterine PG synthesis.[141] Furthermore, COX-1–deficient mice, which showed delay in the onset of term labor, exhibited no delay in the onset of preterm labor after LPS treatment.[141]

Although it is likely that COX-2–derived $PGF_{2\alpha}$ acted as a luteolysin in the mouse model of LPS-induced preterm labor, it is not known whether the uterotonic effect of $PGF_{2\alpha}$ and other COX-2–derived PGs may also have played a role in this setting. The latter possibility may be particularly relevant to human preterm labor, because indomethacin, an inhibitor of both COX-1 and COX-2, has been used successfully in treating human preterm labor, both when given systemically and when delivered locally through the vaginal route.[142-144]

The clinical utility of indomethacin as a tocolytic agent, however, is tempered by concerns over fetal and neonatal complications, such as constriction of the ductus arteriosus.[144] The adverse effects associated with indomethacin use in preterm labor have been mainly linked to inhibition of COX-2 based on mouse studies using selective COX-1 and COX-2 inhibitors.[145] COX-1–selective inhibitors, should they be developed clinically, would be expected to produce fewer adverse effects than traditional NSAIDs when used as tocolytic agents.[145] Studies in animals and pregnant women comparing indomethacin and coxibs produced mixed results when fetal ductus blood flow was used as a measure of potential adverse effects.[146-148]

DUCTUS ARTERIOSUS REMODELING

As mentioned earlier in the chapter, one of the complications of using NSAIDs such as indomethacin to treat preterm labor is the induction of premature closure of the fetal DA.[90,149] The DA is a large fetal vessel that shunts deoxygenated blood away from the pulmonary circulation to the descending aorta and to the umbilicoplacental circulation, where oxygenation takes place. In neonates, rapid remodeling of the DA leads to its closure after adaptation of spontaneous breathing in newborn infants. Although patency of the DA in utero is essential for proper fetal growth and development, failure of the DA to close after birth, called *patent DA*, compromises postnatal health by causing circulatory complications such as pulmonary hypertension and congestive heart failure.[149]

Prostaglandins are intimately involved in DA function and its perinatal remodeling, and details of their mechanism of action are beginning to emerge. The finding that indomethacin administration induced premature DA closure in fetuses[90,149] suggested that fetal PGs are essential for maintaining DA patency. However, mice lacking both COX-1 and COX-2 die postnatally with patent DA,[136,150] indicating that fetal-derived PGs are not necessary for maintaining DA patency in utero. Such PGs *do*, however, play an indispensable role in DA remodeling after birth.

How does one reconcile this phenotype with the results of pharmacologic inhibition studies? Researchers have proposed that PGE_2 in the fetal circulation (supplied in part by the placenta) maintains dilation of the DA in utero, and that COX-2 in the DA produces constrictor PGs that are important for DA contraction after birth.[150] Thus, indomethacin-induced premature DA closure in fetuses may have reflected inhibition of dilatory PGE_2 synthesis in the placenta without sufficient inhibition of ductal COX-2 to attenuate DA contraction. Although COX-1 deficiency alone did not affect perinatal DA remodeling, it was found to exacerbate the phenotype of patent DA on the background of COX-2 deficiency.[150]

In other studies, mice deficient in the dilatory receptor EP4[151,152] or the PGE_2-metabolizing enzyme 15-OH-PGDH[153] also failed to survive postnatally due to patent DA. EP4 expression in DA and 15-OH-PGDH expression in the fetal lung increase dramatically just before birth, supporting the conclusion that these proteins play an important role in perinatal DA remodeling.

The phenotypes of EP4-deficient and 15-OH-PGDH–deficient mice, together with the results of pharmacologic studies, support alternative models for the DA remodeling process.[152-154] Signals through EP4 have two essential roles in DA patency and remodeling, namely, vascular dilation and intimal cushion formation (ICF). The vascular smooth muscle–relaxing ability of PGE_2 acting via EP4 maintains patency during fetal life. When PGE_2 levels plummet at birth due to rapid and efficient metabolism by late gestation–induced 15-OH-PGDH activity, the vasodilatory role is curtailed and functional DA closure is triggered rapidly by an increase in oxygen tension. ICF occludes the vascular lumen and results in permanent closure after birth. ICF within the DA is a result of an increase in vascular smooth muscle cell migration and proliferation and the production of hyaluronic acid (HA) under the endothelial layer, along with decreased elastin fiber assembly. PGE_2 via EP4 signaling during late gestation controls a gene, *HAS2*, that regulates HA synthesis and ICF.[154]

PREGNANCY-INDUCED HYPERTENSION AND PREECLAMPSIA

The possible involvement of PGs in pregnancy-induced hypertension (PIH) and preeclampsia and the potential therapeutic efficacy of low-dose aspirin in their prophylactic treatment have received considerable attention. PIH and preeclampsia occur in 10% of pregnancies and are recognized as important, prevalent sources of risk to both mother and fetus (see Chapter 26).

Although the exact cause of the disease is unknown, dysregulated production of PGI_2 and TxA_2 has been postulated as one of many potential etiologic factors.[155] Decreased urinary and blood PGI_2 metabolites are found to precede the development of PIH,[156] and increased TxA_2 metabolite excretion occurs in patients with severe preeclampsia.[157,158]

An altered ratio of PGI_2 to TxA_2 may cause vasoconstriction of small arteries, activation of platelets, and uteroplacental insufficiency—clinical outcomes that are associated with PIH and preeclampsia. In a murine model of enhanced TxA_2 activity, transgenic overexpression of TP in the vasculature resulted in intrauterine growth retardation that was rescued by timed suppression of TxA_2 synthesis with indomethacin.[159]

Many clinical trials have been conducted to evaluate the use of low-dose aspirin in the prevention of preeclampsia. Although some randomized studies indicated a beneficial effect for women at increased risk, most large-scale clinical trials did not establish a positive effect of low-dose aspirin use on reducing the incidence of preeclampsia or on improving perinatal outcomes in pregnant women at high risk for preeclampsia.[160-162]

In some studies, neither maternal serum TxB_2 concentrations at enrollment nor their subsequent reduction by low-dose aspirin intake were correlated with adverse pregnancy outcomes.[163-164] Thus, aspirin trials may have failed because an increase in TX production is not the initial anomaly. Future interventions should make correcting prostacyclin deficiency a major part of the strategy to balance the abnormal vasoconstrictor–vasodilator eicosanoid ratio present in preeclampsia. Other issues that potentially could have confounded the outcome of these clinical trials include wrong inclusion criteria, late initiation of treatment, low patient compliance, and ill-defined end points.[160]

EICOSANOIDS IN MALE REPRODUCTION

Although PGs are critically involved in multiple steps of female reproduction, as previously discussed, their physiologic role in male reproduction is not well understood—although it appears to be less remarkable, based on gene knockout studies. No discernible male reproductive phenotype has been noted in any of the COX-deficient or prostanoid receptor–deficient mice.[54-55,59]

On the other hand, a number of studies have described androgen-dependent regulation and distinctive tissue distribution patterns of COX-1 and COX-2 enzymes, as well as PG-synthesizing enzymes, in the male reproductive tracts of rodents and humans.[165-169] Specific functions have also been documented for COX-2–derived PGD_2 and PGE_2 in mediating cytokine production in Leydig cells and in regulating apoptosis in the rat epididymis.[170-171] Although they are not definitive, such studies do suggest that PGs may be synthesized and functional in a regulated manner in the male reproductive organs, even though their physiologic roles in these sites are not indispensable.

In the future, a better understanding of the eicosanoid network in the male reproductive system may lead to new PG-based therapies or provide mechanistic insight about existing therapies. For example, highly specific expression of COX-2 has been found in the distal end of the rat vas deferens.[165] Because the distal vas comprises an extensive submucosal venous plexus connected to the penile corpora cavernosa, PGs from the vas may play a role in erection.[165] In this context, it is notable that intracavernosal injection of PGE_1 has been used clinically as an effective therapy for erectile dysfunction in man.[172-173]

OTHER LIPID MEDIATORS: LYSOPHOSPHATIDIC ACID AND SPHINGOSINE-1-PHOSPHATE

Besides eicosanoids, other lipid mediators have been implicated in reproductive function, in particular, lysophosphatidic acid (LPA) and sphingosine-1-phosphate (S1P). First, we briefly examine the features, synthesis, and signal transduction of LPA, and then we turn our attention to S1P.

The lipid mediator LPA is a lipid-signaling molecule as well as an intermediate in the de novo biosynthetic pathway of phospholipids, consisting of a glycerol backbone, a phosphate head group, and a long-chain fatty acid (usually oleic acid or palmitic acid), most commonly in acyl linkage (see Fig. 6-1).[174] LPA generation is complex, proceeding by at least two pathways: conversion from lysophospholipids or via phosphatidic acid. Several phospholipase activities are necessary, including phospholipase A_1 (PLA_1)/PLA_2 plus lysophospholipase D (lysoPLD) and phospholipase D (PLD). Additional extracellular phospholipases, such as secretory PLA_2 ($sPLA_2$-IIA), membrane-associated PA-selective PLA_1 (mPA-PLA_1), and lecithin–cholesterol acyltransferase (LCAT), can also be involved.[175] LPA signaling is mediated primarily by at least five members of the G-protein–coupled receptor family, currently referred to as LPA_1, LPA_2, LPA_3, LPA_4, and LPA_5.[176]

The lipid mediator S1P is a bioactive sphingolipid derived from the abundant phospholipid sphingomyelin. Sphingomyelinases generate ceramide, which is cleaved by ceramidases to sphingosine, followed by phosphorylation by sphingosine kinase to S1P (Fig. 6-7).[177] The initial mode of signaling for S1P was believed to be intracellular.[178] However, in 1992, S1P was postulated to act extracellularly via a putative transmembrane receptor.[179] We now know that there are five S1P receptors, also members of the GPCR family, referred to as $S1P_1$, $S1P_2$, $S1P_3$, $S1P_4$, and $S1P_5$.[180] S1P stimulation of these receptors elicits a battery of downstream effects, including inhibition of cAMP and activation of mitogen-activated protein kinases, phospholipase C, and PI3 kinase to evoke a broad range of cellular activities.[180]

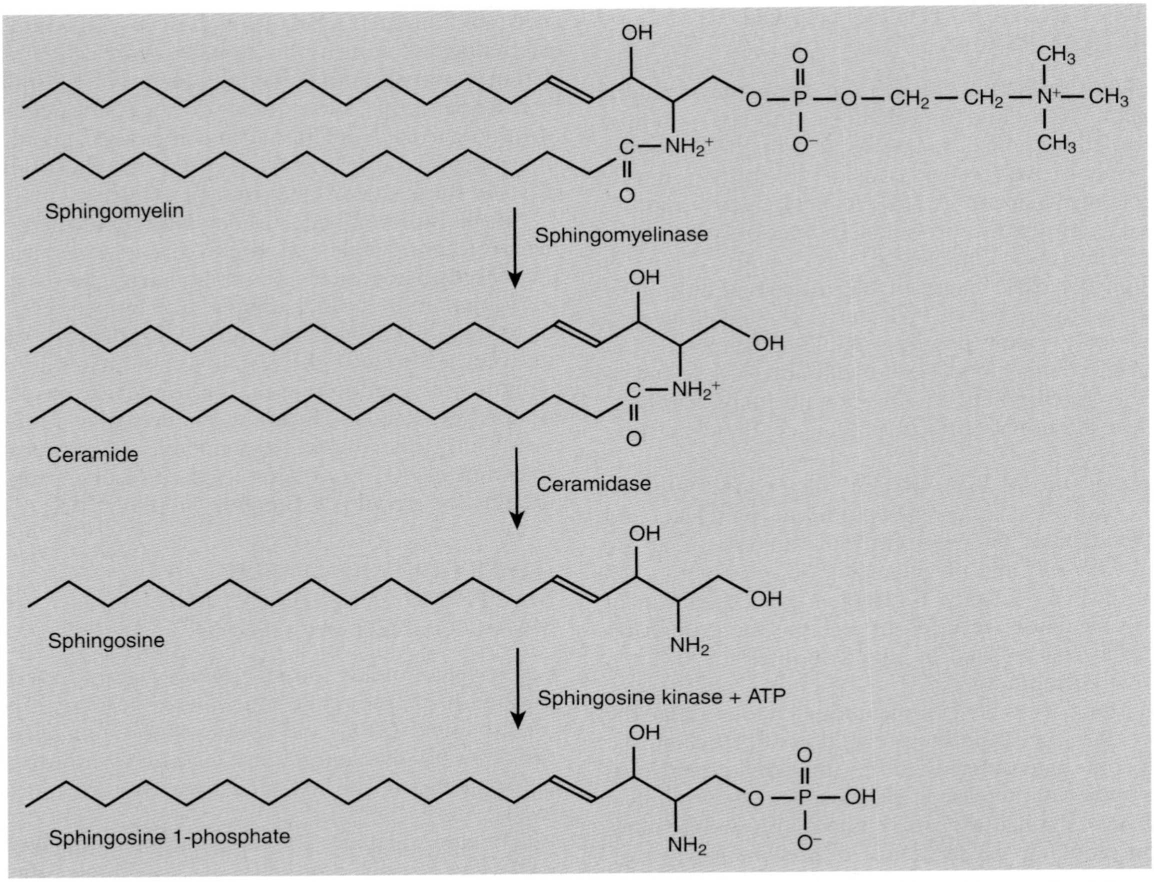

Figure 6-7. *Structures and biosynthesis of a representative sphingosine-1-phosphate (S1P) lipid mediator from sphingomyelin. Sphingomyelinase removes the phosphorylcholine head group to yield ceramide. Ceramidase cleaves the amide bond removing one aliphatic chain to generate sphingosine. In the presence of ATP, sphingosine kinase will phosphorylate sphingosine to generate S1P.*

LPA AND S1P IN REPRODUCTIVE FUNCTION

The effect of LPA on the female reproductive system was recognized as early as 1980, when a series of LPA molecules with variable fatty acyl side chain lengths and degrees of saturation were shown to stimulate rat uterine smooth muscle contraction.[181] To date, three of the LPA receptor genes have been disrupted in mice, with only one (LPA$_3$, also known as *Edg7*) showing a female reproductive phenotype.[182] LPA$_3$ mRNA has been detected in oviduct, placenta, and uterus, but not in ovary and oocytes. Its expression is highest early in pregnancy, at approximately embryonic day 3.5 (E3.5) in mice, and it is regulated positively by progesterone and negatively by estrogen.[182,183] LPA$_3$-deficient females produce small litters and show a prolongation of pregnancy by approximately 1.5 days (normal gestation, 19.5 days).[182] The mice show no obvious defects in ovulation, ovum transport, or blastocyst development. However, the defects were related to delayed implantation and altered crowding or positioning of embryos, which led to delayed embryonic development and death, accounting for the reduced litter size. The observed phenotypes were the result of maternal LPA$_3$ signaling and were not due to embryo LPA$_3$ signaling.[182] Strikingly, the phenotypes were similar to those seen with cPLA$_2$ female knockout mice and rodents treated with indomethacin.[184-186] Remarkably,

LPA$_3$-deficient female uteri had markedly reduced COX-2 expression and PGE$_2$/PGI$_2$ levels at E3.5, thus linking LPA signaling to PG biosynthesis and fertility control.[182] Overall, this particular study raises speculation that therapeutic manipulation of LPA$_3$ signaling could influence the low implantation rate that is a major drawback during infertility treatments using assisted reproductive technologies.

Clues to the roles of S1P in reproductive function have come from various sources. Based on expression studies of the five receptor subtypes that bind S1P, it is known that only three (S1P$_1$, S1P$_2$, and S1P$_3$) show widespread distribution in mice, with evidence in gonadal tissues and in the uterus during decidualization (E4.5-7.5).[180,187] S1P$_1$ and S1P$_2$ colocalize with COX-2 at the maternal/fetal interface throughout pregnancy, suggesting a link between sphingolipid and PG signaling and indicating that S1P coordinates uterine mesometrial angiogenesis during implantation.[187]

Because S1P$_1$-deficient mice die in midembryogenesis as a result of complications of vasculogenesis, it has not been possible to decipher a role for this particular signaling pathway in reproductive function.[180] Both S1P$_2$- and S1P$_3$-null mice show no obvious phenotypes, with the exception of slightly smaller litter sizes.[180] Therefore, the specific roles of each S1P receptor subtype in implantation still require more study.

A role for S1P in the preservation of female fertility is now being recognized.[188] Programmed cell death (apoptosis) is an established paradigm in the mammalian female germline. Ceramide generated by membrane cleavage of sphingomyelin by sphingomyelinase or via de novo biosynthesis by ceramide synthase is translocated from cumulus cells to adjacent oocytes to induce germ cell apoptosis.[189] This is prevented by S1P, a ceramide metabolite within the same pathway or by acid sphingomyelinase (ASM) deficiency. The therapeutic management of infertility by S1P in premature menopause and in female patients with cancer appears promising, but awaits further study.[188]

Sphingolipids also seem to play a role in male germ cell apoptosis.[190,191] Ceramide induces an early apoptotic pathway event in male germ cells that is partially suppressed by S1P. However, although maintenance of normal sphingomyelin levels in testes and normal sperm motility are dependent on ASM, testicular ceramide production and the ability of germ cells to undergo apoptosis do not require ASM.

Summary

Prostaglandins and other lipid mediators are involved in many steps of the human reproductive process. Detailed understanding of their mechanisms of action in these steps has been greatly facilitated by the characterization of two COX enzymes, individual PG, LPA, and S1P receptors, and by the engineering of COX, PG, and LPA receptor gene–disrupted animal models. These studies have shown some distinct roles played by each of the two COX enzymes and by specific PG and LPA receptor pathways in mammalian reproduction.

Despite the tremendous progress made so far, much remains to be learned, particularly with regard to the molecular events downstream of PG, LPA, and S1P receptor activation in each of the reproductive steps where PGs, LPA, and S1P were found to be essential. Another challenge is to integrate the findings in animal models into the study of PGs, LPA, and S1P in human reproductive endocrinology. Continued interest and research in the field may lead to new PG-based and other lipid mediator therapies for reproductive disorders (such as endometriosis and preterm labor) and the reduction of adverse effects of NSAID use in women of reproductive age.

The complete reference list can be found on the companion Expert Consult Web site at www.expertconsultbook.com.

Suggested Readings

Funk CD. Prostaglandins and leukotrienes: advances in eicosanoid biology. Science 294:1871-1875, 2001.

Gross GA, Imamura T, Luedke C, et al. Opposing actions of prostaglandins and oxytocin determine the onset of murine labor. Proc Natl Acad Sci U S A 95:11875-11879, 1998.

Narumiya S, FitzGerald GA. Genetic and pharmacological analysis of prostanoid receptor function. J Clin Invest 108:25-30, 2001.

Reese J, Paria BC, Brown N, et al. Coordinated regulation of fetal and maternal prostaglandins directs successful birth and postnatal adaptation in the mouse. Proc Natl Acad Sci U S A 97:9759-9764, 2000.

Reese J, Zhao X, Ma WG, et al. Comparative analysis of pharmacologic and/or genetic disruption of cyclooxygenase-1 and cyclooxygenase-2 function in female reproduction in mice. Endocrinology 142:3198-3206, 2001.

Richards JS, Russell DL, Ochsner S, et al. Ovulation: new dimensions and new regulators of the inflammatory-like response. Annu Rev Physiol 64:69-92, 2002.

Sugimoto Y, Yamasaki A, Segi E, et al. Failure of parturition in mice lacking the prostaglandin F receptor. Science 277:681-683, 1997.

Tilly JL. Commuting the death sentence: how oocytes strive to survive. Nat Rev Mol Cell Biol 2:838-848, 2001.

Vermillion ST, Landen CN. Prostaglandin inhibitors as tocolytic agents. Semin Perinatol 25:256-262, 2001.

CHAPTER 7

Neuroendocrine Control of the Menstrual Cycle

Janet E. Hall

The Reproductive Axis

Normal reproductive function in women involves repetitive cycles of follicle development, ovulation, and preparation of the endometrium for implantation should conception occur in that cycle. This pattern of regular ovulatory cycles is achieved through precise functional and temporal integration of stimulatory and inhibitory signals from the hypothalamus, pituitary, and ovary (Fig. 7-1). The reproductive system functions in a classic endocrine mode initiated by pulsatile secretion of gonadotropin-releasing hormone (GnRH) from the hypothalamus into the pituitary portal venous system. GnRH regulates the synthesis and subsequent release of follicle-stimulating hormone (FSH) and luteinizing hormone (LH) from the anterior pituitary into the circulation. FSH and LH stimulate ovarian follicular development, ovulation, and corpus luteum formation and the coordinated secretion of estradiol, progesterone, inhibin A, and inhibin B. A key component of this system is the modulatory effect of ovarian steroids and inhibins on gonadotropin secretion, acting either directly at the pituitary level or through alterations in the amplitude or frequency of GnRH secretion. Negative feedback restraint of FSH secretion is critical to the development of the single mature oocyte that characterizes human reproductive cycles. In addition to negative feedback controls, the menstrual cycle is unique among endocrine systems in its dependence on positive feedback. Estrogen positive feedback induces the preovulatory LH surge that is essential for ovulation.

Neuroendocrine Components of the Reproductive Axis

GONADOTROPIN-RELEASING HORMONES

Luteinizing hormone–releasing hormone (LHRH) was isolated, characterized, and synthesized in 1971.[1] It was expected that separate releasing hormones for LH and FSH would be discovered. However, subsequent studies provided evidence that both LH and FSH are secreted in response to LHRH, resulting in the common use of the term *gonadotropin-releasing hormone* (GnRH) for the decapeptide originally referred to as "LHRH." It is now known that *GnRH* is located on chromosome 8p and works through its own receptor, which is encoded on chromosome 4.

Neurons for GnRH differentiate in the olfactory placode, cross the cribriform plate into the forebrain, and migrate to the medial basal hypothalamus, where they establish connections with the pituitary portal system in the median eminence as part of the hypothalamic tuberoinfundibular system. The initial leg of this migratory journey occurs along the scaffold of the olfactory, vomeronasal, and terminal nerves. Studies in knockout models and in patients with hypogonadotropic hypogonadism due to abnormalities in GnRH secretion, some of whom have concomitant disruption of the olfactory system (Kallmann syndrome), have begun to provide critical insights into the complex developmental regulation of GnRH neurons.[2] Adhesion molecules, such as anosmin-1, which is encoded on the *KAL1* gene, fibroblast growth factor

Throughout this chapter, LH and FSH are expressed in IU/L of the 2nd International Reference Preparation (IRP) of human menopausal gonadotropins (hMG). To convert to the clinically used pituitary standards, LH IU [pit] = (LH IU [hMG] − 0.32) × 0.41 and FSH IU [pit] = (FSH IU [hMG] − 0.25) × 0.57.

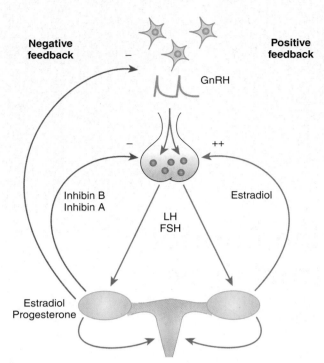

Figure 7-1. *Neuroendocrine control of reproduction requires the pulsatile secretion of gonadotropin-releasing hormone (GnRH) released into the pituitary portal system to stimulate the synthesis and secretion of luteinizing hormone (LH) and follicle-stimulating hormone (FSH) from the gonadotropes. The gonadotropins, in turn, stimulate follicular development and secretion of gonadal steroids and peptides whose negative feedback effects on the hypothalamus and pituitary restrain gonadotropin secretion. At midcycle, rising levels of estradiol are responsible for the positive feedback that generates the preovulatory gonadotropin surge.*

receptor 1 (*FGFR1*), and specific ligands for this receptor, such as *FGF8*,[3] as well other factors, such as prokineticin 2 (*PROK2*) and its receptor (*PROKR2*), appear to play a role in GnRH neuronal development and migration in the human.[2] There are approximately 7000 GnRH neurons responsible for gonadotropin regulation in the human.[4] Unlike neurons secreting other hypothalamic-releasing factors, GnRH neurons do not exist in a clearly defined nucleus, but are scattered throughout the medial basal hypothalamus.

There is now evidence that mammals, including humans, simultaneously express more than one molecular form of GnRH (Table 7-1).[5] *GnRH II* is located on chromosome 20p13 and works through its own receptor,

TABLE 7-1
Amino Acid Sequences of Mammalian GnRH, GnRH II, and GnRH III

GnRH (1) (Mammal)	pGLu- His- Trp- Ser- **Tyr- Gly- Leu-** Arg- Pro- Gly- NH2
GnRH II (Chicken I)	pGLu- His- Trp- Ser- **His- Gly- Trp-** Tyr- Pro- Gly- NH2
GnRH III (Lamprey III)	pGLu- His- Trp- Ser- **His** -Asp- Trp- Lys- Pro- Gly- NH2

Amino acids that differ between GnRH forms are bolded.

which is encoded on chromosome 1. GnRH II is widely expressed both within and outside the brain. It likely plays a role in reproductive behavior in lower animal species. It is a potent stimulator of LH and FSH in vitro and in vivo in animal models, but its role in the human is unknown. GnRH III has been identified in the human brain by immunohistochemistry and high-performance liquid chromatography, it has a hypothalamic distribution similar to that of GnRH, and it may act through the GnRH receptor. Although there is some evidence in lower animal species that GnRH III may have preferential FSH-releasing properties,[6] a GnRH III consensus sequence has not been found in the human genome,[5] and thus, its role in the human is unclear.

PULSATILE SECRETION OF GnRH

A prominent feature of the reproductive system is the absolute requirement for pulsatile secretion of GnRH into the pituitary portal system for normal gonadotropin secretion. The now classic studies of Knobil and colleagues in hypothalamic-lesioned monkeys receiving GnRH first showed that intermittent stimulation of the pituitary results in secretion of LH and FSH, whereas constant GnRH stimulation is associated with suppression of gonadotropin levels.[7] Isolated GnRH neurons exhibit an intrinsic pulsatility,[8] but there is also a significant body of research indicating that external influences modify and coordinate the secretion of GnRH, influencing both the amplitude and the frequency of pulsatile GnRH secretion.

Neuromodulators of GnRH Secretion

Although a number of neurotransmitters are involved in the control of GnRH secretion in animal species, only a few have been shown to have an effect in the human.[9] Although there is evidence for a stimulatory role of the α adrenergic system in a number of animal models, it is much less likely that it plays a role in control of the human menstrual cycle. The role of the dopaminergic system remains controversial, but several studies have documented an increase in LH pulse frequency in response to a dopamine antagonist in women with hypothalamic amenorrhea.[10,11] There is substantial evidence for the involvement of endorphins in transducing the negative feedback effects of progesterone on pulsatile GnRH secretion.[12,13] Recent evidence has excluded a role of the endorphin system in the hypothalamic negative feedback actions of estradiol, although it may play an inhibitory role in the GnRH network that contributes to the dynamics of individual GnRH pulses. On the other hand, there is evidence that γ-aminobutyric acid (GABA) may well be involved in mediating estrogen negative feedback on GnRH secretion.[9]

Although knockout models suggest that there is considerable redundancy in the systems that ultimately control GnRH secretion, an emerging body of evidence indicates a central role for the newly discovered kisspeptin/GPR54 pathway in the control of GnRH secretion. Kisspeptin is a powerful stimulant of gonadotropin secretion, and the kisspeptin/GPR54 pathway system has been implicated in the onset of puberty and in estrogen feedback.[14-16]

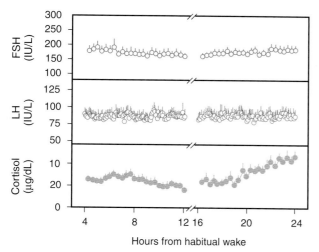

Figure 7-2. *Absence of circadian changes in luteinizing hormone (LH) and follicle-stimulating hormone (FSH) in normal women. Frequent blood sampling studies in young postmenopausal women (n = 11) under conditions of a constant routine of light, food intake, position, temperature, and persistent waking indicate the presence of a robust cortisol rhythm, but no circadian rhythm of FSH or LH. LH and FSH are expressed in IU/L of the 2nd IRP hMG. To convert to pituitary units, LH IU [pit] = (LH IU [hMG] − 0.32) × 0.41, and FSH IU [pit] = (FSH IU [hMG] − 0.25) × 0.57. (Adapted from Lavoie HB, Marsh EE, Hall JE. Absence of apparent circadian rhythms of gonadotropins and free α subunit in postmenopausal women: evidence for distinct regulation relative to other hormonal rhythms. J Biol Rhythms 21[1]:58-67, 2006.)*

Sleep and Circadian Effects on GnRH Secretion in Women

Endocrine systems are profoundly influenced by both sleep and endogenous circadian rhythms, which persist in the absence of sleep or other environmental cues. Diurnal (day/night) rhythms of LH and gonadal steroids have been

well described in men and women, and there is some evidence that the LH surge occurs most commonly at night in women.[17] Studies in which sleep and other environmental cues were controlled have not shown an endogenous circadian rhythm of LH or FSH in young postmenopausal women (Fig. 7-2), despite the presence of robust circadian rhythms of cortisol and thyroid-stimulating hormone.[18] In contrast, there is now considerable evidence that sleep directly affects the pulsatile secretion of LH and presumably that of GnRH, although the underlying mechanism is unknown. Studies that have been designed to separate the effects of sleep from time of day indicate that puberty in boys and girls is characterized by a specific stimulatory effect of sleep on pulsatile LH secretion.[19] In contrast, with maturation of the reproductive system and the onset of ovulatory menstrual cycles, there is a notable slowing of pulsatile LH secretion at night in the early follicular phase of the cycle.[20,21] Interestingly, sleep reversal studies in women[22] have shown not only that the early follicular–phase nighttime slowing of LH pulses is due to sleep rather than to time of day, but also that within sleep, brief periods of wakefulness are associated with the onset of LH pulses (Fig. 7-3).

GONADOTROPIN-PRODUCING CELLS OF THE PITUITARY

Synthesis of LH and FSH occurs in gonadotropes that comprise 7% to 15% of the cells in the pituitary. Immunohistochemical studies in the rat indicate that approximately 70% of gonadotropes stain for both LH and FSH, whereas the remainder are monohormonal, with approximately equal numbers of cells staining for each. Interestingly, this distribution is altered in different physiologic settings.[23]

The process of biosynthesis and secretion of intact gonadotropins involves translation of βLH, βFSH, and the common gonadotropin α-subunit, post-translational

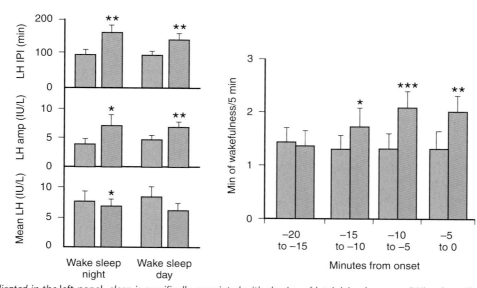

Figure 7-3. *As indicated in the left panel, sleep is specifically associated with slowing of luteinizing hormone (LH) pulses. The LH interpulse interval (IPI) is longer and the amplitude is higher in normal women during sleep (blue bars) than when awake (purple bars), whether sleep occurs at night or during the day. As indicated in the right panel, wakefulness is more likely in the 5 to 10 minutes before the onset of an LH pulse (blue bars) than in a similar time frame indexed to a random LH point that is not associated with an LH pulse (gray bars). (From Hall JE, Sullivan JP, Richardson GS. Brief wake episodes modulate sleep-inhibited luteinizing hormone secretion in the early follicular phase. J Clin Endocrinol Metab 90[4]:2050-2055, 2005.)*

TABLE 7-2

The Half-Life of Luteinizing Hormone (LH), but Not Follicle-Stimulating Hormone (FAS), Is Influenced by the Gonadal Steroid Milieu

	LH		FAS	
	Baseline (IU/L) Mean ± SEM	$T_{1/2}$ (min) Mean ± SEM	Baseline (pg/mL) Mean ± SEM	$T_{1/2}$ (min) Mean ± SEM
Postmenopausal	62 ± 3	139 ± 35	774 ± 45	51 ± 26
EFP, LFP, ELP	10 ± 1	57 ± 28	266 ± 44	41 ± 12
MCS	56 ± 11	78 ± 20	627 ± 122	41 ± 19

EFP, early follicular phase; ELP, early luteal phase; LFP, late follicular phase; MCS, midcycle surge.
Reproduced from Sharpless JL, Supko JG, Martin KA, et al. Disappearance of endogenous luteinizing hormone is prolonged in postmenopausal women. J Clin Endocrinol Metab 84(2):688-694, 1999, with permission.

modification and folding, a combination of the β and α subunits, and finally, hormone packaging and secretion. LH, FSH, and uncombined or free α subunit (FAS) are all secreted in response to GnRH stimulation of the gonadotrope.

Multiple isoforms of LH and FSH, differing in their carbohydrate structure and charge, coexist in both pituitary and serum. More basic forms of both LH and FSH yield a greater in vitro potency, but a shorter half-life in the circulation, whereas the opposite is true for less basic forms.[24] The greater number of sialic acid residues on FSH prolongs its half-life,[25] whereas the greater number of sulfonated N-acetyl-galactosamine (GalNAc) asparagine-linked oligosaccharides on LH is associated with more rapid clearance due to binding to a specific hepatic receptor.[26] Sulfonation and sialylation of LH and FSH vary across the menstrual cycle and in the absence of gonadal steroids; postmenopausal women have a greater preponderance of sialylated forms of both LH and FSH.[27] Consistent with these changes, the disappearance of LH after GnRH receptor blockade with a potent GnRH antagonist is significantly prolonged in postmenopausal women compared with women in the follicular phase and at the midcycle surge, whereas the disappearance of FAS is unaffected by the absence of gonadal function (Table 7-2).[28]

There is also evidence that gonadotropin secretion is modulated by a factor or factors related to obesity. Serum levels of LH are inversely related to body mass index in normal women and in women with polycystic ovarian syndrome.[29] Recent studies have indicated that the inhibitory effect of obesity on LH secretion in PCOS is not mediated at the hypothalamus, but is associated with a decrease in both the pituitary response to GnRH and the half-life of endogenous, but not exogenous, LH.[30,31] The latter finding is consistent with the increase in sulfonated isoforms of LH and FSH as a function of increasing BMI in women with PCOS.[27]

Differential Control of LH and FSH Secretion

Although secreted from a common cell type within the gonadotrope, LH and FSH have markedly different functions in the control of ovarian physiology. These differences in function are reflected in their different patterns of secretion during normal reproductive cycles. The divergent control of LH and FSH is achieved through a combination of differential control of the synthesis and secretion of LH and FSH by GnRH, the preferential control of FSH synthesis by the activin/follistatin system, and differential feedback by ovarian steroids and the inhibins. Understanding the control of LH and FSH secretion is critical to our understanding of the dynamics of the menstrual cycle.

GONADOTROPIN-RELEASING HORMONE

Along with LH, FSH is secreted in response to acute stimulation by GnRH, but the relative role of GnRH in the overall control of FSH synthesis is much less than for LH. Blockade of the GnRH receptor using a specific GnRH receptor antagonist results in 90% inhibition of LH secretion, but only 40% to 60% inhibition of FSH.[32]

Synthesis and secretion of LH and FSH are differentially controlled by the amplitude and frequency of GnRH stimulation.[33,34] Although LH secretion is highly responsive to increases in the dose of GnRH, this is not the case for FSH. A physiologic frequency of GnRH results in synthesis and secretion of all three gonadotropin subunits. However, increases or decreases from the physiologic frequency have differential effects on LH and FSH (Table 7-3). Slow frequencies of GnRH stimulation favor the synthesis and secretion of FSH in vitro and are

TABLE 7-3

Differential Effects of Gonadotropin-Releasing Hormones (GnRH) Pulse Frequency on Luteinizing Hormone (LH) and Follicle-Stimulating Hormone (FSH)

	LH	FSH
Increased Frequency		
In vitro mRNA	↑	→
GnRH-deficient men/women		
Mean	↑	→↓
Amplitude	↓	
Decreased Frequency		
In vitro mRNA	↓	↑
GnRH-deficient men/women		
Mean	↓	→↑
Amplitude	↑	

mRNA, messenger RNA.

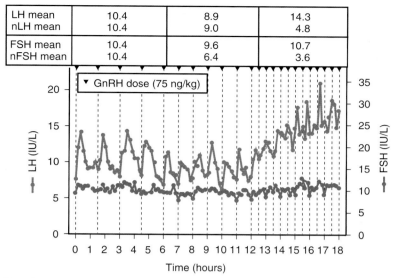

LH mean	10.4	8.9	14.3
nLH mean	10.4	9.0	4.8
FSH mean	10.4	9.6	10.7
nFSH mean	10.4	6.4	3.6

Figure 7-4. *The differential effect of increasing gonadotropin-releasing hormone (GnRH) pulse frequency on luteinizing hormone (LH) and follicle-stimulating hormone (FSH) as shown in a GnRH-deficient woman receiving intravenous pulsatile GnRH. After 7 days of administration of pulsatile GnRH at a dose of 75 ng/kg and a frequency of every 90 minutes, blood was sampled for 6 hours. The frequency was then increased to every 60 minutes for 6 hours and every 30 minutes for 6 hours, with evidence of an increase in LH but not FSH. The mean LH and FSH are given for each frequency as indicated. The means, normalized for the overall amount of GnRH administered, suggest that faster frequencies are associated with early stages of pituitary desensitization. LH and FSH are expressed in IU/L of the 2nd IRP hMG. To convert to pituitary units, LH IU [pit] = (LH IU [hMG] − 0.32) × 0.41, and FSH IU [pit] = (FSH IU [hMG] − 0.25) × 0.57. (From Hall JE, Taylor AE, Hayes FJ, Crowley WF Jr. Insights into hypothalamic-pituitary dysfunction in polycystic ovary syndrome. J Endocrinol Invest 21[9]:602-611, 1998.)*

associated with an increase in FSH in vivo in settings in which gonadal feedback is low.[35] In GnRH-deficient men and women, an increase in the frequency of GnRH stimulation results in an increase in mean levels of LH, with no appreciable change in FSH (Fig. 7-4),[36,37] effects that have implications for the pathophysiology of PCOS, in which the frequency of GnRH is consistently increased.[30] The direct effect of GnRH pulse frequency on GnRH receptor number[38] and the downstream effects of modulation of receptor number appear to underlie the frequency modulation of LH and FSH secretion.

In contrast to the effects of GnRH pulse frequency on the synthesis and mean levels of LH, studies in GnRH-deficient men and women have shown that the amplitude of pulsatile LH secretion is inversely related to GnRH pulse frequency.[39,40] Thus, slower GnRH pulse frequencies are associated with a higher LH amplitude in response to GnRH, whereas faster frequencies are associated with a decrease in the amplitude response to GnRH. The decrease in LH amplitude seen with pulse frequencies that are faster than those encountered in physiologic settings[36,37] may be the earliest sign of the pituitary desensitization that is well recognized in association with continuous infusions of GnRH or the use of a GnRH agonist.

AUTOCRINE/PARACRINE REGULATION OF GONADOTROPINS: ACTIVIN, INHIBIN, AND FOLLISTATIN

Activins, inhibins, and follistatins were first discovered as gonadal factors with preferential actions on FSH secretion from pituitary gonadotropes.[41] The inhibins, named for their inhibitory control of FSH, are composed of one of two inhibin/activin β subunits and a closely related α subunit

to form inhibin A or inhibin B. In contrast, the activins, which stimulate the synthesis and secretion of FSH, are composed of two inhibin/activin β subunits. There is evidence that activin is secreted by gonadotropes and other pituitary cell populations, and like other members of the TGF-β superfamily of growth and differentiation factors, activins exert most of there effects by autocrine or paracrine mechanisms. Activins sequentially interact with one of the two known type II activin receptors, ActRII or ActRIIB, and the type I receptor, activin receptor–like kinase (ALK) 4. The expression of *FSHβ* is extremely sensitive to the stimulatory action of activins, which work in concert with and are permissive for the actions of GnRH through promotion of transcription of both FSHβ and the GnRH receptor gene (*GNRHR*).[42]

The inhibins act as specific antagonists of the FSH stimulatory actions of activin by binding to betaglycan and sequestering the type II activin receptors. Although inhibin is made in the pituitary, circulating inhibin plays a far greater role in the negative control of FSH. In addition, Bone morphogenetic protein (BMP)-6 and BMP-7 are capable of modulating FSH synthesis in gonadotropes, suggesting that other systems may also be involved in the control of FSH.[43]

Follistatin is a monomeric protein that is distinct from the activin/inhibin family and acts as a virtually irreversible binding protein by complexing with activin and masking the binding sites on activin for the type I and type II receptors.[41] The follistatin 288 isoform (FS288) has a high affinity for cell surface proteoglycans and is presumed to act within the pituitary.[43] Follistatin is synthesized in many tissues in the body, including the pituitary, where its synthesis in pituitary folliculostellate cells and gonadotropes is controlled by activin and GnRH and may be additionally modulated by gonadal steroids. Activin synthesis does not appear to vary during reproductive cycles. However, specific changes in follistatin have been noted during the rat estrous cycle, suggesting that the effects of activin on FSH may be modulated through changes in follistatin.[43] Follistatin is increased in the presence of fast frequencies of GnRH stimulation and decreased with slower frequencies,[44] compatible with a role for the activin/follistatin system in transducing the effects of GnRH pulse frequency on FSH. Thus, whereas GnRH appears to be sufficient for control of LH synthesis and secretion, the activin/inhibin/follistatin system and perhaps BMPs play a significant role in conjunction with GnRH in the regulation of FSH synthesis and secretion.

OVARIAN FEEDBACK ON THE HYPOTHALAMUS AND PITUITARY

Negative Feedback

Estrogen. It is well known that low doses of estrogen inhibit gonadotropin secretion. Increased gonadotropin levels in patients with aromatase deficiency provide the most specific evidence of estrogen negative feedback on the control of both LH and FSH in men and women,[45] although this is supported by the marked increase in LH and FSH levels in postmenopausal and ovariectomized women.[46] The loss of gonadal feedback in ovariectomized rats is associated with an increase in LH and FSH secretion, increased expression of LHβ, FSHβ, and α messenger RNA (mRNA), an increase in the number of cells expressing LHβ, an increase in cell size, and an increase in the amount of expression per cell. These changes are reversed by administration of low doses of estradiol,[47] which has also been shown to reverse the increases in gonadotropin secretion in the ovariectomized sheep and monkey.

The majority of evidence suggests that negative feedback of estrogen on pituitary gonadotropin secretion is secondary to changes in GnRH.[9,48] Studies in which GnRH secretion has been measured using a push–pull hypothalamic perifusion technique in the rat and cannulation of the pituitary portal circulation in the sheep and monkey indicate that GnRH is increased after ovariectomy and decreased with estrogen replacement. Estradiol administration is associated with a decrease in GnRH expression in rat hypothalamic tissue slices and in a GnRH neuronal cell line. Both indirect and direct mechanisms for estrogen regulation of hypothalamic GnRH neurons have been proposed. Studies in estrogen receptor (ER) knockout animals support an important role of ERα in mediating estrogen negative feedback, although both forms of the receptor have been found in the hypothalamus.[48] Estrogen-receptive GABA neurons within the preoptic area may play a role in mediating the negative feedback effects of estrogen on GnRH secretion, whereas a role for β endorphin has been excluded.[9] In addition, there is compelling evidence of a role of kisspeptin in estrogen negative feedback in rodents.[16]

The mechanisms underlying estrogen negative feedback have generally been investigated in postmenopausal or ovariectomized women. The quantity of GnRH, estimated in vivo using submaximal GnRH antagonist administration, is higher in postmenopausal compared with premenopausal women,[49] consistent with the increase in GnRH mRNA that has been shown in postmenopausal women studied at autopsy.[50] Because the quantity of GnRH returned to follicular phase levels with administration of low levels of estradiol, the increase in GnRH in the absence of gonadal feedback can be attributed to loss of estrogen.[49] Neuroimaging studies have provided evidence of decreased metabolic activity in the medial basal hypothalamus in association with brief exposure to relatively low doses of estradiol.[51] Estradiol administration does not decrease GnRH pulse frequency in the majority of studies in postmenopausal women, and thus, the negative feedback effect of estradiol on the hypothalamus is likely to be mediated through changes in GnRH pulse amplitude.[46] These results in women are similar to those in which GnRH was measured directly in pituitary portal blood in ovariectomized sheep and monkeys and showed a decrease in GnRH pulse amplitude, but not frequency, in response to estradiol administration.[52,53] Autopsy studies in women are consistent with a role for neurons expressing kisspeptin, neurokinin B, substance P, dynorphin, and ERα in mediating the negative feedback of estrogen in the medial basal hypothalamus.[54]

Although these studies show a significant hypothalamic effect of estrogen negative feedback, they do not rule out a pituitary site of action. This remains a controversial question. Both ERα and ERβ are present on gonadotropes.[48] In cultured pituitary cells, estradiol transiently reduces the LH response to GnRH,[55] and administration of estradiol to hypothalamic-lesioned monkeys receiving pulsatile GnRH decreased LH secretion.[56] However, in studies in GnRH-deficient women, estradiol administration reduced the FSH, but not the LH response to pulsatile GnRH,[57] whereas ER blockade in GnRH-deficient women receiving pulsatile GnRH had no effect on either FSH or LH.[58]

Progesterone. Progesterone has a profound effect on gonadotropin secretion that operates at a hypothalamic level through slowing of the frequency of pulsatile GnRH secretion,[59,60] although estrogen priming appears to be essential for its effect,[61] likely through up-regulation of progesterone receptors in the hypothalamus.[62] In postmenopausal women receiving low doses of estradiol, addition of progesterone uniformly suppresses GnRH pulse frequency using either LH or FAS as markers of GnRH secretion.[63-65] In addition, administration of progesterone decreases the overall amount of GnRH secretion.[49] It is likely that progesterone exerts its effects on GnRH secretion through both direct and indirect mechanisms,[9,66] and there is ample evidence that the β-endorphin system plays a critical role in mediating the effects of progesterone on GnRH pulse frequency.

Inhibin. Evidence for a nonsteroidal gonadal factor with feedback effects on the pituitary dates to the early 1900s, but it was not until the mid-1980s that inhibin was isolated and subsequently found to be part of a family of peptides that includes inhibin A, inhibin B, activin, and the functionally related protein follistatin.[43] Inhibin B is present in the circulation in men, whereas both inhibin A[67-69] and inhibin B[70-75] are detected in the serum and follicular fluid in women during their reproductive years. Further studies have determined that inhibin B is produced by granulosa cells in the ovary[76] and by Sertoli cells in the testis,[77,78] whereas inhibin A is produced by granulosa cells and by the luteinized granulosa cells of the corpus luteum.[76,79] Inhibin subunits are expressed in a variety of tissues, including the adrenal. However, the only significant source of circulating dimeric inhibins is the gonads, and there is compelling evidence that its principal mechanism of action in suppressing pituitary FSH secretion is an endocrine action.

Activin acts as a local growth and differentiation factor in a variety of tissues, including the pituitary and ovary.[43] Although activin has been measured in serum, circulating activin is irreversibly bound by the circulating isoform of follistatin, FS315.[80] As yet, no mechanisms have been identified within tissues that would alter neutralization by follistatin; therefore, it is almost certain that activin acts in an autocrine/paracrine fashion rather than in an endocrine fashion.

Positive Feedback

Estrogen. In addition to inhibition of gonadotropin secretion, estrogen exerts a stimulatory effect to generate the preovulatory LH surge. This positive feedback effect is seen in multiple animal species[48] and in women, and it is dependent on both the degree of estrogen exposure and its duration.[81,82] What is less clear is how estrogen can exert both inhibitory and stimulatory effects on LH secretion and whether the stimulatory effects are mediated at the pituitary or the hypothalamus. There is ample evidence that high levels of estrogen augment the pituitary response to GnRH, increase GnRH receptor number, affect the function of ion channels in the plasma membrane, and regulate both gene expression and second messenger systems within gonadotropes.[38,83,84] Studies in the LβT2 pituitary cell indicate that activin may also play a role in stimulating GnRH receptors on pituitary gonadotropes.[42] In addition, there is evidence that progesterone may have a direct pituitary effect because low doses of progesterone augment the LH pulse amplitude in response to pulsatile GnRH replacement in GnRH-deficient women.[85] Finally, neuropeptide Y secretion from the median eminence is increased at the time of the preovulatory surge in the rat and may contribute to pituitary sensitization through changes in the affinity of the GnRH receptor for its ligand.[86]

In the rat and the sheep, there is evidence of an increase in GnRH secretion associated with the preovulatory surge,[87] and in rodents, this increase in GnRH secretion requires specific circadian signals.[88] In contrast, an increase in GnRH is not required for generation of the surge in normal women, although there is a requirement for ongoing secretion of GnRH (see "Midcycle Surge"). Thus, GnRH appears to play a permissive rather than an obligatory role in generation of the preovulatory LH surge in normal women, as it does in the monkey.[87]

The Normal Menstrual Cycle

CLINICAL CHARACTERISTICS

By convention, the first day of menses is designated day 1 and marks the onset of the follicular phase of the menstrual cycle. The follicular phase encompasses the period of recruitment of multiple follicles and emergence and growth of the dominant follicle (Fig. 7-5). During the follicular

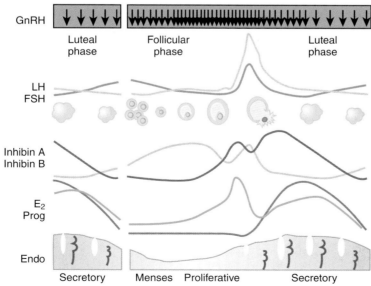

Figure 7-5. *The hormonal, follicular, and endometrial dynamics of the normal menstrual cycle from the late luteal phase, through menses and the beginning of a new cycle of follicle development, ovulation, and corpus luteum function, as indicated. With the support of the changing frequency of pulsatile gonadotropin-releasing hormone (GnRH) secretion, the integrated actions of follicle-stimulating hormone (FSH; green) and luteinizing hormone (LH; light blue) are responsible for (1) follicular development with secretion of estradiol (E₂; light green), inhibin B (pink) and inhibin A (blue), (2) the preovulatory surge and ovulation; and (3) secretion of progesterone (Prog; purple), estradiol, and inhibin A from the corpus luteum. Secretion of estradiol and progesterone result in proliferative and secretory changes in the endometrium (Endo), preparing it for implantation should conception occur. In the absence of conception, endometrial shedding follows the decline in hormone secretion secondary to demise of the corpus luteum.*

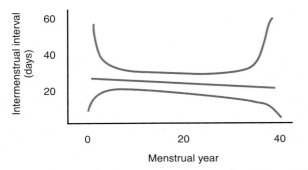

Figure 7-6. *Median menstrual cycle lengths* (purple line) *from menarche (menstrual year 0) until menopause. The* green lines *indicate the 95% confidence limits. (From Treloar AE, Boynton RE, Behn BG, Brown BW. Variation of the human menstrual cycle through reproductive life. Int J Fertil 12[1 Pt 2]:77-126, 1967.)*

phase, rising levels of estradiol are associated with endometrial proliferation. The luteal phase, which begins on the day after the LH surge, is characterized by formation of the corpus luteum, secretion of progesterone, and a coordinated series of changes in the endometrium as it first prepares for implantation and then loses its blood supply and sloughs with decline of the corpus luteum in the absence of pregnancy.

The classic studies of Treloar and coworkers[89] indicate that the median menstrual cycle length is 28 days, with a normal range between 25 and 35 days (Fig 7-6). For the majority of reproductive life, there is little cycle-to-cycle variability, although the intermenstrual interval declines between the ages of 36 and 40 years. Both immediately after menarche and preceding menopause there is a significant degree of variability in the intermenstrual interval between

and within individuals. Fluctuations in the length of the follicular phase are primarily responsible for the variations in cycle length both between women and as a function of normal aging in an individual woman. Luteal phase duration is more constant, lasting 10 to 16 days in 95% of cycles. During the follicular phase, the progressive increase in diameter of the largest follicle as assessed by ultrasound is highly predictable at approximately 2 mm/day until ovulation (Fig 7-7). The accompanying increase in estradiol is associated with a progressive increase in the thickness of the endometrium, whereas the effects of the luteal phase on the endometrium result in increased echogenicity (see Fig. 7-7).

GnRH DYNAMICS AND PITUITARY RESPONSIVENESS

Secretion of GnRH can be measured directly in animal species, and studies have indicated that, under physiologic circumstances, peripheral LH secretion occurs concomitantly with secretion of GnRH measured in pituitary portal blood.[90-92] LH has therefore been used as a marker of GnRH pulse frequency in the human, based on these studies and two additional lines of evidence. The first is that pulsatile secretion of LH is absent in patients with congenital isolated GnRH deficiency and can be restored with pulsatile administration of GnRH.[93] The second is that pulsatile secretion of LH in normal subjects is reversibly abolished by administration of a specific GnRH antagonist.[32] Thus, the occurrence of LH pulses can be taken as evidence of the occurrence of a preceding stimulatory GnRH pulse, and LH pulse frequency can be used as a peripheral monitor of the frequency of pulsatile GnRH secretion. Although the glycoprotein FAS

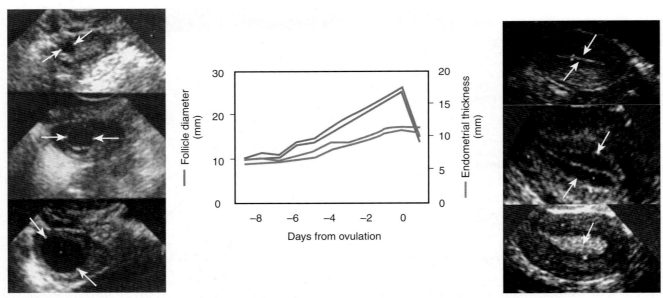

Figure 7-7. *Follicular development is associated with a progressive increase in the diameter of the dominant follicle* (arrows), *as seen on ultrasound* (left panels, top *to* bottom), *and an increase in endometrial thickness (between* arrows) *during the follicular phase* (right top *and* middle panels). *Follicle diameter* (blue lines *represent ±1 SEM) and endometrial thickness* (brown lines *represent ±1 SEM) derived from studies in 42 women with normal menstrual cycles are shown in relation to the day of ovulation, which is indicated as 0. The appearance of the endometrium* (single arrow) *is markedly different in the luteal phase, showing increased echogenicity* (right bottom panel). *(From Adams JM, Hall JE. Increase in the size of the dominant follicle and endometrial thickness as measured by ultrasound during the follicular phase in 42 normal women. Personal communication, 2003.)*

is secreted from both the gonadotrope and the thyrotrope under the control of GnRH and TRH, the pulsatile component of FAS secretion is entirely under the control of GnRH in euthyroid women.[94] Thus, FAS can also be used as a surrogate marker of GnRH pulse frequency. Because its clearance is faster than that of intact LH, it is a preferable marker when GnRH pulse frequency is rapid. The amplitude of the LH or FAS response to GnRH may depend on either the amplitude of the GnRH signal or pituitary responsiveness to GnRH, and other techniques must therefore be used to assess the amplitude of GnRH secretion.

Results of frequent sampling studies (every 5 or 10 minutes for up to 48 hours) have shown marked variations in the frequency and amplitude of LH pulses across the normal menstrual cycle (Fig. 7-8) and their precise regulation in relation to the preovulatory LH surge.[93-96]

FOLLICULAR PHASE

In the early follicular phase (days −14 to −9 from the LH surge), the mean interpulse interval of GnRH is approximately 90 to 100 minutes.[20,96] The early follicular phase of established reproductive cycles is characterized by a marked slowing of GnRH pulse frequency during sleep[22] (see Figs. 7-3 and 7-8), which may serve the function of maintaining FSH synthesis during this critical period of follicle recruitment.

In the midfollicular phase, GnRH pulse frequency increases and the interpulse interval shortens to approximately 60 minutes. LH pulse amplitude is markedly attenuated in the midfollicular phase. This may be due in part to the increase in frequency and its effect on gonadotrope responsiveness and is also likely to reflect the negative feedback of estradiol secreted from developing follicles on the amplitude of GnRH pulses.

The circhoral frequency of GnRH secretion is maintained through the late follicular phase as LH pulse amplitude begins to increase due to the stimulatory effects of rising levels of estradiol on gonadotrope responsiveness to GnRH.

MIDCYCLE SURGE

In response to the exponential increase in estradiol secretion in the late follicular phase, LH levels increase 10-fold over a period of 2 to 3 days, whereas FSH levels increase fourfold (see Fig. 7-8). This midcycle surge of LH is absolutely required for final maturation of the oocyte and initiation of follicular rupture, which generally occurs 36 hours after the surge. The gonadotropin surge is therefore a critical component of normal reproductive cycles. However, the mechanisms responsible for this dramatic increase in gonadotropin secretion are incompletely understood and appear to be species-specific. The classic studies of Wang and coworkers showed that the responses of LH and FSH to exogenous GnRH administration are markedly influenced by the stage of the menstrual cycle, with an exaggerated increase in

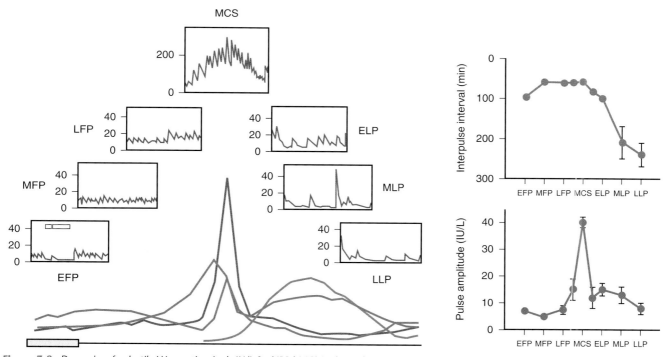

Figure 7-8. *Dynamics of pulsatile LH secretion (red; IU/L 2nd IRP hMG) in the early, mid-, and late follicular phases (EFP, MFP, LFP), during the midcycle surge (MCS), and in the early, mid-, and late luteal phases (ELP, MLP, LLP) presented in relation to the pattern of LH (red), FSH (teal), estradiol (green) and progesterone (brown) across the normal menstrual cycle. The* open rectangles *in the EFP denote sleep. Menses in indicated by the* blue rectangle. *The dynamic changes in the interpulse interval and amplitude of pulsatile LH secretion in relation to the phases of the menstrual cycle are indicated in the* right panel. *(From Hall JE, Martin KA, Taylor AE. Body weight and gonadotropin secretion in normal women and women with reproductive abnormalities. In Hansel W, Bray GA, Ryan DH [eds]. Nutrition and Reproduction, vol 8. Pennington Center Nutrition Series. Baton Rouge, Louisiana State University Press, 1998, pp 378-393; Hall JE. Neuroendocrine physiology of the early and late menopause. Endocrinol Metab Clin North Am 33[4]:637-659, 2004.)*

secretion of both gonadotropins at the time of the mid-cycle surge.[97]

The pattern of estrogen exposure is critical to positive feedback. Exogenous administration of estradiol to normal women in the early follicular phase[81,82] or to postmenopausal women[51] induces an increase in both basal and GnRH-stimulated LH release that is both dose- and time-dependent. There is further evidence that the surge occurs in response to the increase in estradiol rather than the drop in estradiol that frequently accompanies the onset of the surge. In other words, the surge results from estrogen positive feedback rather than removal of estrogen negative feedback.

Other evidence indicates that a small increase in progesterone augments this surge. Secretion of progesterone is typically associated with the luteal phase; however, the earliest increase in progesterone is evident in normal women before the LH surge. Blockade of progesterone receptors by mifepristone delays the surge by up to 3 days, despite continued growth of the dominant follicle and rising levels of estradiol.[98] In studies in normal women in whom a graduated estrogen infusion was initiated in the early follicular phase, it has now been demonstrated that progesterone does not influence the height of the surge, but decreases the variability in its timing relative to the onset of the infusion.[82] Although an LH surge can be generated in response to recreation of normal preovulatory estradiol and progesterone levels, the amplitude of the surge is less that in normal women. This suggests that there may also be other ovarian factors required for generation of a normal surge amplitude. One possibility is inhibin A, which increases dramatically before the LH surge in normal cycles[69,74] and has been shown to

increase GnRHR number and LH secretion in an ovine pituitary cell culture system.[99] Finally, it has long been speculated that gonadotropin surge–inhibiting factor (GnSAF) contributes to the LH surge. GnSAF is a nonsteroidal factor whose activity is highest in small follicles and decreases with development of the dominant follicle.[100]

A key question is whether estrogen positive feedback in women is mediated at the hypothalamus, the pituitary, or both. There is increasing evidence that the mechanisms underlying this critical process may be species-specific. As reviewed earlier in the chapter, there is compelling evidence from a variety of animal and in vitro studies that estradiol acts directly at the pituitary to increase gonadotrope sensitivity to GnRH.[38,83,84] In lower animal species, there is also evidence that hypothalamic mechanisms play a critical role in generating the preovulatory surge, although studies in sheep indicate that the amplitude of the GnRH surge exceeds that needed to generate the LH surge.[87] Additional studies have indicated that in both the rat and sheep the sites of estrogen negative and positive feedback within the hypothalamus may well be distinct.[9]

Studies in GnRH-deficient women receiving exogenous GnRH replacement provide the most compelling evidence for the importance of pituitary sensitization to GnRH in the generation of the midcycle surge in women. When GnRH is administered at a dose and frequency that mimic GnRH pulse frequency in the normal menstrual cycle with development of a single dominant follicle, an abrupt increase in LH and FAS pulse amplitude is observed in the absence of any change in the dose or frequency of GnRH (Fig. 7-9) and a normal LH surge is achieved (Fig. 7-10). These studies

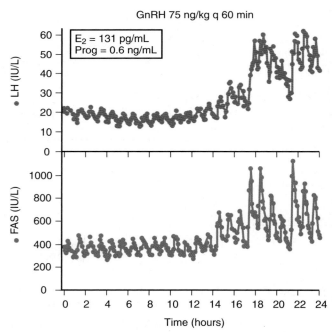

Figure 7-9. *Luteinizing hormone (LH) and free α subunit (FAS) sampled every 5 minutes in a gonadotropin-releasing hormone (GnRH)-deficient woman receiving pulsatile GnRH intravenously, showing the abrupt increase in LH and FAS pulse amplitude and mean levels associated with estrogen positive feedback in the absence of any change in the dose or frequency of GnRH. E₂, estradiol; Prog, progesterone. LH is expressed in IU/L of the 2nd IRP hMG. To convert to pituitary units, LH IU [pit] = (LH IU [hMG] – 0.32) × 0.41.*

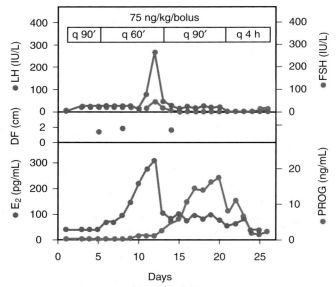

Figure 7-10. *Administration of intravenous pulsatile gonadotropin-releasing hormone (GnRH) to a GnRH-deficient woman at a physiologic frequency with follicular development, ovulation, and normal luteal phase function. Note that the LH surge is generated in association with an increase in follicle size and estradiol (E₂), but in the absence of an increase in the dose or frequency of pulsatile GnRH administration. LH and FSH are expressed in IU/L of the 2nd IRP hMG. To convert to pituitary units, LH IU [pit] = (LH IU [hMG] – 0.32) × 0.41, and FSH IU [pit] = (FSH IU [hMG] – 0.25) × 0.57. (From Hall JE, Martin KA, Whitney HA, et al. Potential for fertility with replacement of hypothalamic gonadotropin-releasing hormone in long term female survivors of cranial tumors. J Clin Endocrinol Metab 79[4]:1166-1172, 1994.)*

indicate that positive feedback can be achieved in women through pituitary mechanisms alone, with no increase in hypothalamic input.

Further studies indicate that this mechanism is also how gonadotropin surges are achieved in normal women. At the onset of both spontaneous and steroid-induced LH surges, complete GnRH receptor blockade results in termination of the surge,[101-103] indicating that ongoing GnRH secretion is essential for generation of the gonadotropin surge. However, neither the frequency nor the overall amount of GnRH is increased in association with the onset of the gonadotropin surge in normal women.[94,101] Studies in normal women in which blood samples were drawn every 5 minutes for up to 36 hours indicate a striking increase in LH and FAS pulse amplitude from the late follicular phase to the early and midportions of the surge, with no change in pulse frequency during the same period (see Fig. 7-8).[94] To address the question of whether generation of the surge in women is associated with an increase in the amplitude of GnRH secreted with each bolus, submaximal GnRH receptor blockade was used to provide a semiquantitative estimate of the overall amount of endogenous GnRH secreted.[101] Results of these studies provide no evidence for an increase in the overall amount of GnRH secreted; in fact, they suggest that the amount of GnRH at the surge is less than in the early and late follicular phases. Consistent with this finding, further studies have shown that in GnRH-deficient women, the replacement dose of GnRH can be reduced by two thirds in the late follicular phase from that required for development of a single dominant follicle without compromising the timing or height of the midcycle surge or the subsequent luteal phase (Fig 7-11).[104]

Taken together, these studies indicate that GnRH is absolutely required for generation of the midcycle surge in normal women; however, there is no evidence for an increase in either the amplitude or the frequency of GnRH secretion. Consistent with this conclusion, neuroimaging studies in postmenopausal women, in whom a gonadotropin surge was induced by administration of a graded estradiol infusion, show a marked increase in metabolic activity at the pituitary, but not the hypothalamus, in association with estrogen positive feedback on LH.[51]

The termination of the LH surge is associated with a dramatic decrease in pulse amplitude, accompanied by a decrease in pulse frequency to approximately every 70 minutes[94] (see Fig. 7-8). The decline in pulse frequency that accompanies the termination of the surge is due, at least in part, to the hypothalamic effects of progesterone on the GnRH pulse generator. Although a decrease in GnRH pulse frequency may contribute, the mechanisms responsible for termination of the surge remain poorly understood.[87] In normal cycles, the preovulatory increase in estradiol is followed by a rapid decline before estradiol increases again in the luteal phase. However, studies in the sheep indicate that termination of the surge is not dependent on this transient decrease in estradiol. Studies in the sheep also indicate that termination of the surge is not due to desensitization of the pituitary to GnRH.

LUTEAL PHASE

Slowing of pulsatile GnRH secretion begins during the termination of the midcycle surge and continues through the early, mid, and late luteal phases (see Fig. 7-8). In the late luteal phase, interpulse intervals of as long as 4 to 8 hours are observed. This slowing of the GnRH pulse generator is due to the effect of progesterone,[105] but is not expressed without the additional presence of estradiol.[61]

In the luteal phase, LH pulses are significantly higher than in the follicular phase. The known inverse relationship between LH responsiveness to GnRH and GnRH pulse frequency[39,40] suggests that this increase in LH pulse amplitude is secondary to progesterone-induced slowing of GnRH pulse frequency. However, there is additional evidence from studies in GnRH-deficient women, in whom it is possible to control the dose of GnRH administered, that progesterone may act directly at the pituitary to increase LH responsiveness to GnRH.[85]

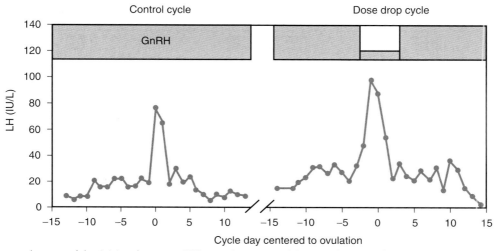

Figure 7-11. A normal surge of luteinizing hormone (LH) can be recreated in gonadotropin-releasing hormone (GnRH)-deficient women when the dose of exogenous GnRH is reduced from 75 ng/kg to 25 ng/kg before the onset of the LH surge. LH is expressed in IU/L of the 2nd IRP hMG. To convert to pituitary units, LH IU [pit] = (LH IU [hMG] − 0.32) × 0.41. (From Martin KA, Welt CK, Taylor AE, et al. Is GnRH reduced at the midcycle surge in the human? Evidence from a GnRH-deficient model. Neuroendocrinology 67[6]:363-369, 1998.)

LUTEAL–FOLLICULAR TRANSITION

The luteal–follicular transition is characterized by declining function of the corpus luteum and declining levels of progesterone, estradiol, and inhibin A. Release from negative feedback permits FSH to rise, an increase that begins before menses and is critical for recruitment of a new cohort of follicles into the developing pool (see Fig. 7-5). Maintenance of midluteal phase levels of estradiol prevents this increase in FSH.[106,107] Thus, it has been proposed that release from estrogen negative feedback is the key factor in the luteal–follicular rise in FSH and that other factors, such as the decline in inhibin A secretion from the corpus luteum, may not play a role. However, studies using tamoxifen to block the ER in normal cycles suggest that inhibin A also plays a role in restraining FSH secretion during the normal luteal phase.[58]

The LH/GnRH pulse frequency increases before the onset of menses (Fig. 7-12).[95] LH pulse frequency is inversely related to progesterone levels,[95] and administration of midluteal phase levels of progesterone in conjunction with estradiol prevents the normal luteal–follicular increase in GnRH pulse frequency in normal women.[61] There is convincing evidence that the increase in GnRH pulse frequency that occurs between the luteal and follicular phases facilitates the increase in FSH secretion. In normal women, the increase in FSH was significantly correlated with LH pulse frequency, whereas the inverse relationship between FSH and estradiol was not significant.[95] In GnRH-deficient women receiving pulsatile GnRH at a physiologic frequency to recreate normal cycle dynamics, there is a partial increase in FSH associated with release from the negative feedback effects of estradiol and possibly inhibin A.[72] However, an increase in GnRH pulse frequency from the luteal phase frequency of every 4 hours to the follicular phase frequency of every 90 minutes is essential to recreate the normal intercycle rise in FSH (Fig. 7-13).

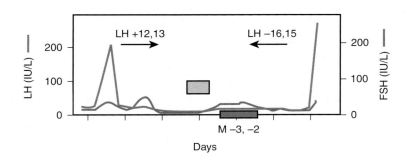

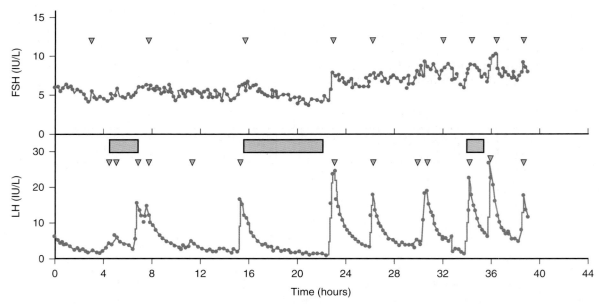

Figure 7-12. *Luteinizing hormone (LH) and follicle-stimulating hormone (FSH) in a subject studied during the luteal–follicular transition. The timing of the frequent sampling in relation to the hormonal dynamics of the preceding and subsequent LH surge and menses (green rectangle) is indicated in the light blue box in the upper panel. This study was conducted beginning 3 days before menses (M −3, −2) and indicates the rise in FSH that begins before menses and is associated with an increase in the frequency of pulsatile LH secretion. In this panel, the light blue rectangles indicate sleep and the inverted triangles indicate pulses. LH and FSH are expressed in IU/L of the 2nd IRP hMG. To convert to pituitary units, LH IU [pit] = (LH IU [hMG] − 0.32) × 0.41, and FSH IU [pit] = (FSH IU [hMG] − 0.25) × 0.57. (From Hall JE, Schoenfeld DA, Martin KA, Crowley WF Jr. Hypothalamic gonadotropin-releasing hormone secretion and follicle-stimulating hormone dynamics during the luteal-follicular transition. J Clin Endocrinol Metab 74[3]:600-607, 1992.)*

Thus, the slow frequency of GnRH secretion in the luteal phase is hypothesized to increase FSH synthesis, either directly or through a decrease in follistatin and a concomitant increase in activin signaling. However, FSH secretion is inhibited by estradiol and possibly inhibin A. With the demise of the corpus luteum, estradiol and inhibin A levels fall, as do those of progesterone. FSH is allowed to increase with release from negative feedback and is further stimulated by the increase in GnRH pulse frequency to its physiologic frequency.

There is now evidence that the progressive increase in GnRH pulse frequency from the early to the midfollicular phase represents a gradual loss of the restraining effects of low levels of progesterone on the GnRH pulse generator.[108] Because the early follicular phase is characterized by sleep-related inhibition of pulsatile LH secretion, it is intriguing to speculate that a similar prolonged effect of progesterone is also involved in sensitizing the hypothalamus to the inhibitory effects of sleep during this cycle phase. The possibility that sleep-related slowing of GnRH pulse frequency in the early follicular phase may play an important role in maintaining synthesis of FSH at this critical time is suggested by the association of menstrual cycle abnormalities with altered sleep–wake cycles in women exposed to transmeridian travel or rotating shifts.[109,110]

SECRETION OF INHIBIN A AND INHIBIN B

The pattern of inhibin A secretion is characterized by a periovulatory increase and maximal levels in the luteal phase (see Fig. 7-5).[67,68,74] In contrast, inhibin B is at its nadir in the luteal phase, begins to rise during the luteal–follicular transition to attain its highest levels in the early and midfollicular phases, and declines in the late follicular phase, followed by a brief periovulatory increase (see Fig. 7-5).[69,73] The differential patterns of inhibin B and inhibin A in serum across the menstrual cycle suggest different sources and differential control of these two inhibin forms in normal reproductive cycles. Interestingly, their relationship to the secretion of the gonadotropins and estradiol does not easily confirm the anticipated endocrine role for either inhibin in the control of FSH. Inhibin B and FSH levels are positively rather than negatively related, particularly during the luteal–follicular transition, whereas the potential negative feedback effects of inhibin A on FSH could just as easily be accounted for by estradiol, whose levels change in parallel to those of inhibin A.

Sources of Inhibin A and Inhibin B

The peak in inhibin A in the luteal phase and its decline with luteolysis are consistent with production by the corpus luteum, as expected from the high levels of βA inhibin subunit expression in the corpus luteum.[76] During folliculogenesis, peak levels of inhibin A are attained in the preovulatory period and inhibin A is correlated with the size of the dominant follicle in normal cycles,[68,69] as is estradiol. Inhibin A is primarily the product of granulosa cells; however, there is some evidence for theca cell production in the mature follicle.[76] Studies of βA inhibin subunit expression[76] and measurement of dimeric inhibin A in follicular fluid[111] are consistent in indicating maximal levels in the preovulatory follicle. However, it is now appreciated that inhibin A is synthesized and secreted at earlier stages

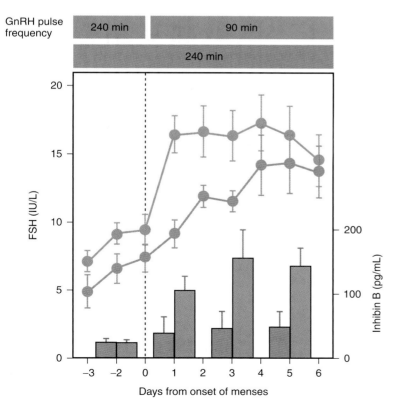

Figure 7-13. *The increased frequency of pulsatile gonadotropin-releasing hormone (GnRH) during the luteal–follicular transition facilitates the secretion of follicle-stimulating hormone (FSH), as indicated in this study in GnRH-deficient women. The normal rise in FSH in relation to menses is attenuated when the frequency of intravenous GnRH (75 ng/kg) remains at the luteal phase frequency of every 240 minutes (green circles) compared with the usual increase to every 90 minutes at the time of menses (purple circles). The bars indicate that the follicular phase increase in inhibin B is also attenuated in association with a persistently slow frequency of GnRH replacement (green) compared with the physiologic frequency of every 90 minutes (purple) secondary to an inadequate rise in FSH. FSH is expressed in IU/L of the 2nd IRP hMG. To convert to pituitary units, FSH IU [pit] = (FSH IU [hMG] − 0.25) × 0.57. (From Welt CK, Martin KA, Taylor AE, et al. Frequency modulation of follicle-stimulating hormone [FSH] during the luteal-follicular transition: evidence for FSH control of inhibin B in normal women. J Clin Endocrinol Metab 82[8]:2645-2652, 1997.)*

of follicular development than previously suggested by serum levels.[112]

In contrast to inhibin A, the pattern of inhibin B in serum suggests that it is primarily secreted from small antral follicles. A correlation of inhibin B levels with the size of the dominant follicle is remarkably absent in women undergoing spontaneous ovulatory cycles,[69] suggesting that inhibin B is not regulated in relation to dominant follicle growth. These data are consistent with studies showing that inhibin B levels in follicular fluid do not change as a function of follicle size or maturity.[111] They are also consistent with earlier studies showing that expression of βB inhibin subunit mRNA is highest in early antral follicles, with lower levels in the dominant follicle and no evidence of βB subunit expression in the corpus luteum.[76] The latter studies have also shown that inhibin B synthesis is confined to the granulosa cells and is absent in theca cells.

Regulation of Inhibin A and Inhibin B by Gonadotropins

Studies have shown an increase in inhibin B secretion in conjunction with early follicular development stimulated by physiologic levels of FSH. This was initially suggested by the relationship between the rise in FSH during the luteal–follicular transition and the concomitant increase

in inhibin B (see Fig. 7-5). In GnRH-deficient women, replacement of pulsatile GnRH at the slower luteal phase frequency of every 4 hours compared with the early follicular phase frequency of every 90 minutes was associated not only with failure of FSH to rise normally during the luteal-follicular transition, but also with the absence of both follicular growth and any increase in secretion of inhibin B (see Fig 7-13).[72] This study demonstrated the remarkable sensitivity of serum inhibin B levels to changes in FSH stimulation within the physiologic range during the earliest stages of follicular development.

In studies designed to examine the time course of the response to specific and physiologic gonadotropin stimulation, recombinant human LH (rhLH) or FSH (rhFSH) was administered to women after down-regulation of endogenous GnRH secretion with a potent GnRH agonist.[112] The rhLH (150 IU) alone had no effect on follicle growth or hormone secretion when administered daily for up to 7 days, consistent with failure to observe LH receptors in small antral follicles. However, daily subcutaneous administration of 150 IU rhFSH resulted in normal early follicular phase levels of FSH and an increase in inhibin B secretion that preceded that of estradiol and inhibin A (Fig 7-14). One interpretation of these findings is that FSH directly stimulates inhibin B secretion from granulosa cells. However, administration of FSH at this stage of development also results in the recruitment of a cohort of

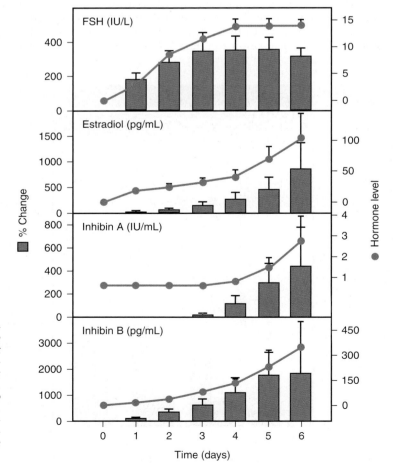

Figure 7-14. Hormone response to recombinant human follicle-stimulating hormone (rhFSH; 150 IU daily) for 6 days in normal women after gonadotropin-releasing hormone agonist down-regulation of endogenous gonadotropin secretion. Hormone responses are presented as percent change (left axis; green bars) or as absolute levels (right axis, purple circles). FSH is expressed in IU/L of the 2nd IRP hMG. To convert to pituitary units, FSH IU [pit] = (FSH IU [hMG] − 0.25) × 0.57. (From Welt CK, Smith ZA, Pauler DK, Hall JE. Differential regulation of inhibin A and inhibin B by luteinizing hormone, follicle-stimulating hormone, and stage of follicle development. J Clin Endocrinol Metab 86[6]:2531-2537, 2001.)

follicles into the growing pool and a dramatic stimulation of granulosa cell numbers.

To determine whether the increase in inhibin B observed in vivo in the early stages of folliculogenesis results from direct stimulation of granulosa cell secretion or from an increase in granulosa cell numbers, studies were conducted with preantral and small antral follicles obtained from ovaries at the time of oophorectomy for nonovarian indications.[113] Results of these studies indicated that inhibin B is constitutively secreted from preantral follicles and that FSH stimulates the secretion of inhibin A, but not secretion of inhibin B. Taken together, these studies show that inhibin B is constitutively secreted from granulosa cells and that the increase in inhibin B observed in vivo in response to FSH results from an increased number of granulosa cells rather than from direct stimulation of secretion by FSH. At later stages of follicular development, both LH and FSH stimulate secretion of inhibin A and estradiol from the dominant follicle, but have no effect on inhibin B.[112]

Evidence for an Endocrine Role of Inhibin A or Inhibin B

Although an endocrine role of either inhibin A or inhibin B cannot be implied from their relationship to FSH during the normal menstrual cycle, several lines of evidence support such a role in the negative feedback regulation of FSH. Inhibin was initially discovered based on its ability to inhibit FSH secretion in pituitary culture.[114] In addition, FSH levels decrease in response to administration of pharmacologic doses of inhibin A in the follicular and luteal phases in the rhesus monkey,[115,116] but α inhibin immunoneutralization did not decrease FSH when administered in the luteal phase of the macaque.[117]

The most compelling line of evidence that inhibin regulates FSH secretion under normal physiologic circumstances in women is the failure of physiologic levels of gonadal steroids to restore FSH levels to normal in postmenopausal women. The model of reproductive aging has been used by a number of investigators to refine this evidence. FSH levels increase with age, before increases in LH or decreases in estradiol,[118-120] and a number of studies have shown an inverse relationship between increasing FSH and decreasing inhibin B[119-122] in association with reproductive aging.

Reproductive aging is associated with a decline in fertility that begins in the third decade, but accelerates rapidly after age 35 years. A gradual decrease in the pool of ovarian follicles that first accelerates around the same age would appear to underlie this decline in fertility.[123] It is also at age 35 years that an increase in follicular phase FSH is first seen. In women 35 years or older with regular ovulatory cycles and follicular phase FSH levels within the normal range, there is a small, but significant increase in FSH in the early follicular phase only. These women also have decreased inhibin B levels across the entire follicular phase and estradiol levels that do not differ in the early follicular phase, but increase in the mid and late follicular phases.[69] In the luteal phase, inhibin B, inhibin A, and progesterone are lower in the older cycling women, whereas estradiol

levels are preserved. Thus, the very earliest decrease in inhibin B occurs at a time that is marked by the beginning of the more rapid follicular depletion that heralds the menopause, suggesting that lower inhibin B levels reflect a decrease in available follicle number with aging. This change in inhibin B is associated with higher levels of FSH in the absence of alterations in estradiol, providing evidence of an endocrine role of inhibin B in the control of FSH secretion in women of reproductive age. Studies conducted at later stages in the process of reproductive aging have uniformly confirmed increased FSH in conjunction with normal to higher levels of estradiol and lower levels of inhibin B and further support the negative feedback role of inhibin B in the control of FSH. Although a decrease in inhibin A may occur slightly later in reproductive aging, it precedes the decline in estradiol levels.[124]

Although studies of reproductive aging provide evidence of a negative feedback role of inhibin B on FSH secretion in normal women, these studies have not clarified the role of inhibin A or inhibin B relative to that of estradiol in the dynamic control of FSH during normal reproductive cycles. A key question is whether inhibin A or inhibin B contributes to the midfollicular decrease in FSH that is critical to the monofollicular development that characterizes reproductive cycles in normal women. The tools to determine the role of inhibin directly by either administration or blockade are not available. However, it is possible to investigate the estrogen component of FSH negative feedback and thereby infer the physiologic role of inhibin. Studies in which estradiol levels were maintained by estradiol administration during the luteal–follicular transition have been interpreted to suggest that inhibin A is not involved in the negative feedback control of FSH in the luteal phase.[106,107] An alternative approach is to block estrogen negative feedback. The use of tamoxifen to block the ER permitted evaluation of the relative role of estradiol and the inhibins in negative feedback on FSH.[58] Results suggest that the low levels of estradiol in the early follicular phase do contribute to negative feedback on FSH, as attested to by a prompt increase in early follicular phase FSH levels. However, these studies also suggest that inhibin B may be more important in restraining FSH in the mid and late follicular phases, as shown by a decrease in FSH to control levels in the late follicular phase. An increase in FSH in response to ER blockade was not seen in GnRH-deficient women receiving pulsatile GnRH replacement, suggesting that the negative feedback of estradiol on FSH secretion in normal women is mediated entirely at the hypothalamic level in the early follicular phase.

Taken together, these studies suggest that estradiol plays a critical role in FSH negative feedback in the luteal phase and during the luteal–follicular transition, whereas inhibin may play an increasingly important role as the follicular phase progresses. However, the failure of FSH to increase to menopausal levels in the luteal phase suggests additional restraint by inhibin A.

The control of FSH is dependent not only on inhibin and estradiol, but also on the activin/follistatin system. During the normal menstrual cycle, total activin A levels are highest at midcycle and during the luteal–follicular transition.[125] However, there is no change in activin A in follicular fluid as a function of follicular development,[111] no change in free activin across the menstrual cycle,[126] and no difference in activin B between the follicular and luteal phases.[127] Taken together, these data suggest that activin does not play an endocrine role in the control of FSH secretion.

The complete reference list can be found on the companion Expert Consult Web site at www.expertconsultbook.com.

Suggested Readings

Conn PM, Crowley WF Jr. Gonadotropin-releasing hormone and its analogs. Annu Rev Med 45:391-405, 1994.

Couse JF, Korach KS. Estrogen receptor null mice: what have we learned and where will they lead us? Endocr Rev 20(3):358-417, 1999.

Crowley WF, Pitteloud N, Seminara S. New genes controlling human reproduction and how you find them. Trans Am Clin Climatol Assoc 119:29-38, 2008.

Hall JE. Neuroendocrine physiology of the early and late menopause. Endocrinol Metab Clin North Am 33(4):637-659, 2004.

Herbison AE. Multimodal influence of estrogen upon gonadotropin-releasing hormone neurons. Endocr Rev 19(3):302-330, 1998.

Kaiser UB. Molecular mechanisms of the regulation of gonadotropin gene expression by gonadotropin-releasing hormone. Mol Cells 8(6):647-656, 1998.

Karsch FJ, Bowen JM, Caraty A, et al. Gonadotropin-releasing hormone requirements for ovulation. Biol Reprod 56(2):303-309, 1997.

Neill JD. GnRH and GnRH receptor genes in the human genome. Endocrinology 143(3):737-743, 2002.

Seminara SB. Kisspeptin in reproduction. Semin Reprod Med 25(5):337-343, 2007.

Welt C, Sidis Y, Keutmann H, Schneyer A. Activins, inhibins, and follistatins: from endocrinology to signaling. A paradigm for the new millennium. Exp Biol Med (Maywood) 227(9):724-752, 2002.

CHAPTER 8

The Ovarian Life Cycle

Jerome F. Strauss III and Carmen J. Williams

The ovary is a dynamic organ that undergoes some of the most dramatic changes in structure and function of any adult human tissue. The follicle, the major endocrine and reproductive compartment of the ovary, is a nonrenewable structure whose health and numbers determine both reproductive potential and reproductive life span (Fig. 8-1). The cells of the follicular compartment interact in a highly integrated manner to secrete sex steroids that prepare the reproductive tract for conception, program pituitary responses to promote follicular maturation, entrain an ovulatory surge of luteinizing hormone (LH) when follicular maturation is completed, and maintain the corpus luteum. Although many follicles initiate development, only a few (<1%) make the complete journey to ovulation. The factors that govern the seemingly profligate expenditure of the fixed complement of follicles remain largely obscure.

The follicle is the residence of the oocyte, which in its mature state is one of the largest cells and among the rarest in the body. The oocyte is both totipotent and highly specialized in that it is capable of undergoing meiosis and fertilization, with the resulting formation of a new human being. Remarkably, these attributes can be suspended for years, only becoming operative when a lengthy process of maturation has been completed.

Germ Cells and Ovarian Morphogenesis

The mammalian germ cell lineage is established early in development. Primordial germ cells originate in the proximal region of the epiblast, close to the extraembryonic endoderm, when a small number of cells emerge under the influence of inductive signals delivered by members of the transforming growth factor-β (TGF-β) superfamily, including bone morphogenetic protein (BMP)-2, BMP-4, and BMP-8B.[1-4] Loss of any of these signals prevents the appearance of all or most of the primordial germ cells. The primordial germ cell precursors must express SMAD1, SMAD5, and SMAD8, which are phosphoprotein downstream mediators of BMP signaling. The absence of SMAD1, SMAD4, and SMAD5 results in a marked reduction in the founder cells of the germ cell lineage.[5-6] The BMP–Smad gene dosage is critical, and distortion of the ratios impairs germ cell development.

Primordial germ cells are identifiable in the endoderm of the yolk sac as early as the end of the third week of gestation by their large size and clear cytoplasm, which contains fewer organelles than the endoderm cells.[7-8] The expression of Fragilis/Iftm3 and Blimp1/Prdm1 marks the emergence of primordial germ cells, which then express Dppa3 (also known as Stella), marking the founder primordial germ cells.[9-11] Other markers of primordial germ cells include tissue-nonspecific alkaline phosphatase[12] and Pou5f1 (also known as Oct4), a transcription factor present in embryonic stem cells and primordial germ cells.[13-14]

Once specified, primordial germ cells enter a period of migration and proliferation. In the human, they migrate from the yolk sac epithelium to the hindgut by approximately 4 weeks postfertilization, then migrate through the dorsal mesentery, finally reaching the genital ridge by approximately 6 weeks postfertilization. The cells change during this migration from a "resting" morphology, taking on an irregular shape, with protrusions and pseudopodia required for active amoeboid movement.[15] Primordial germ cell proliferation is characterized by incomplete cytokinesis, resulting in clusters of cells known as "oocyte nests" that form a network as a result of cytoplasmic continuity via intracellular bridges.[16-19]

Studies in the mouse have identified genes required for primordial germ cell proliferation and migration. The c-kit receptor tyrosine kinase and its ligand (kit ligand, or stem cell factor) are required for primordial germ cell survival and migration.[20-21] Expression of integrin β1 on the primordial germ cell surface is also required for successful

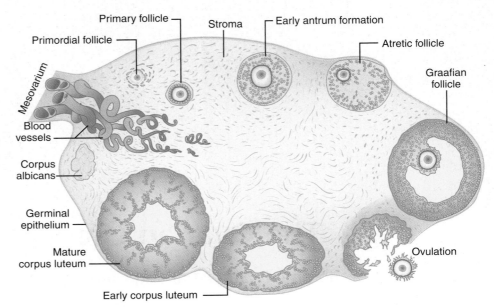

Figure 8-1. The follicular cycle of the human ovary. (Modified from Ham AW, Leeson TS. Histology, 4th ed. Philadelphia, JB Lippincott, 1961.)

migration to the genital ridge.[22] Genes involved in primordial germ cell proliferation include *TIAR1*, which encodes the RNA-binding protein TIAR23, and *Pog* (proliferation of germ cells), the gene responsible for the mouse "germ cell–deficient" mutation that likely encodes a DNA-binding protein.[23-24] In addition, leukemia inhibitory factor (LIF) and related cytokines appear to be responsible, in part, for primordial germ cell proliferation.[25]

Germ cells are unable to persist outside the genital ridge. Conversely, germ cells play an indispensable role in the induction of gonadal development. In the absence of germ cells, pregranulosa cells are not maintained and an inert streak gonad containing only stromal cells results, as occurs in humans with Turner syndrome and in mice homozygous for mutations in the White-spotting (*W*) or Steel (*Sl*) loci.

Germ cells that arrive at the genital ridge are referred to as *oogonia*. A critical step in mammalian germ cell development, the modification of genomic imprinting, occurs at this time. In mammals, there is an absolute requirement for the inheritance of a chromosomal complement from both the mother and the father.[26-28] The basis for this requirement is that specific genes must be expressed from *one* allele, not both, for successful development.[29-31] This task is accomplished by a tightly orchestrated set of modifications of the maternal and paternal chromatin that include methylation of CpG sequences of specific "imprinted" genes, depending on the parent of origin; the result is differential transcriptional regulation.[31-36] The erasure of imprints is required in preparation for switching the inherited maternal and paternal imprinted patterns to reflect the sex of the progeny. In the case of oogonia, both maternal and paternal imprints are erased, and maternal imprints are later established during oogenesis in the fetal ovary and during oocyte growth (Fig. 8-2).[34,37-38]

By 6 to 7 weeks of intrauterine life, the oogonia population has expanded by mitosis to reach some 10,000 cells, and it reaches approximately 600,000 cells by 8 weeks of intrauterine life. However, from this juncture, the oogonial endowment is influenced by three concurrent processes: mitosis, meiosis, and oogonial atresia. As a result of the combined effect of these processes, the number of germ cells peaks at 6 to 7 million by 20 weeks of gestation. Between weeks 8 and 13 of fetal life, some of the oogonia enter the prophase of the first meiotic division. The entry into meiosis is triggered by retinoic acid, produced by mesonephros. This change marks the conversion to primary oocytes, well before actual follicle formation. Meiosis, if correctly executed, appears to provide temporary protection from oogonial atresia, thereby allowing the germ cells to invest themselves with granulosa cells and to form primordial follicles. Oogonia that persist beyond the seventh month of gestation without entering meiosis undergo apoptotic cell death[39]; consequently, oogonia are usually not present at birth.

At midgestation, when the ovarian germ cell endowment is at its apex, two thirds of the total germ cells are intrameiotic primary oocytes; the remaining one third are oogonia. One reason for the subsequent decline in germ cell numbers is the declining rate of oogonial mitosis, a process that ends by approximately 7 months of intrauterine life. The reduction in germ cells is also the result of an increasing rate of oogonial atresia, which peaks at about month 5 of gestation, followed by follicular atresia, which begins around the sixth month of gestation.[40] Apoptosis is believed to be triggered by either a deficiency in survival factors, such as kit ligand, LIF, or basic fibroblast growth factor, or by death-inducing factors, such as Fas ligand, TGF-β, and activin. The relentless and irreversible attrition from midgestation onward progressively diminishes the gonadal germ cell complement, leaving approximately 700,000 primordial follicles in the ovaries at birth.[41] This number decreases further to approximately 300,000 by the onset of puberty; of these follicles, only 400 to 500 will ovulate in the course of a reproductive life span (Fig. 8-3). Although there is good evidence that embryonic stem cells

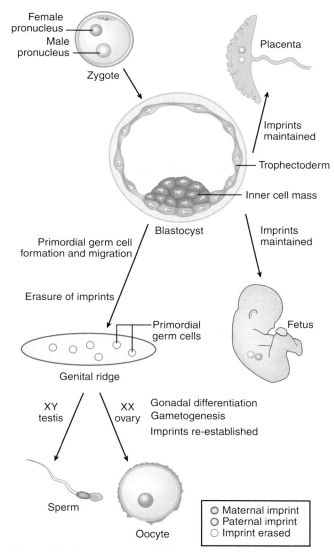

Figure 8-2. *Erasure and reestablishment of genetic imprints during development (Adapted from Surani MA. Reprogramming of genome function through epigenetic inheritance. Nature 414:122-128, 2001.)*

can give rise to oocyte-like cells and follicle-like structures in culture, the notion that germ cells and follicles can arise in vivo in the mammalian ovary during postnatal life from stem cells and contribute to the ovarian reserve has been rejected by most serious investigators.[42-43]

The oocyte persists in prophase of the first meiotic division until just before ovulation, when meiosis is resumed and the first polar body is formed and extruded. Although the exact cellular mechanisms responsible for this meiotic arrest remain uncertain, a granulosa cell–derived meiosis inhibitor is generally presumed to be responsible. This hypothesis is based on the observation that denuded (granulosa-free) oocytes are capable of spontaneously completing meiotic maturation in vitro.

Primordial follicles in the human ovary (30 to 60 μm in diameter) are composed of a late diplotene primary oocyte (9 to 25 μm in diameter) surrounded by a single layer of flattened granulosa cells (Figs. 8-4 and 8-5).[44] Follicles at

this stage of development are not believed to be influenced by gonadotropins. Primary follicles (>60 μm in diameter) are characterized by a primary oocyte surrounded by a single layer of cuboidal granulosa cells. Secondary follicles (<120 μm) consist of a primary oocyte surrounded by several layers of cuboidal granulosa cells (<600 cells), as shown in Figure 8-4.

GENES INVOLVED IN OVARIAN DEVELOPMENT AND FOLLICLE FORMATION IN MICE

Many of the genes governing the development of the human ovary remain to be identified and their specific functions described. However, a number of the murine genes involved in the early stages of gonadal development have been discovered through the study of spontaneous and induced mutations. Among these genes are the transcription factors *Lim1*, *Lhx9*, *Emx2*, *Wt1*, and *Sf1* (also known as *Nr5a1*) (Table 8-1).[45] The genital ridge is absent or does not develop normally in mice homozygous for null mutations in these genes. In addition, nullizygous mice have other abnormalities because some of these genes regulate renal or adrenal development. As noted previously, mice homozygous for null mutations of the *Bmp4* and *Blimp1/Prdm1* genes do not generate primordial germ cells, and heterozygous mutants have a reduced number of primordial germ cells.[1,10-11] Mice nullizygous for *Bmp8b* and the downstream BMP signaling molecules *Smad1* and *Smad5* also have defects in primordial germ cell development. Homozygous mutations in the gene that encodes the kit ligand (also known as *stem cell factor* or *mast cell growth factor*) result in streak gonads. Mice with the White-spotted (*W*) mutation, which disrupts the tyrosine kinase kit receptor, have a similar ovarian phenotype.

Mice homozygous for a null mutation in the X-linked zinc finger gene *Zfx* have a reduced number of oocytes, resulting in a diminished reproductive life span. Mutations in the *Atm* gene, the murine homologue of the human ataxia-telangiectasia gene, disrupt gametogenesis at the leptotene stage of meiosis, and consequently result in sterility. Inactivation of the *Wnt4* gene alters the expression of steroidogenic enzymes in the ovary, resulting in increased testosterone synthesis and wolffian duct masculinization.[46]

GENETICS OF HUMAN OVARIAN DEVELOPMENT

Normal ovarian development requires the activity of autosomal genes and the presence of two functional X chromosomes. X chromosome inactivation is random in germ cells before their entry into the genital ridge, when the silenced X chromosome is then reactivated. Although the requirement for two X chromosomes for ovarian development has long been recognized, the essential X-linked genes and their functions are largely unknown.[47] Cytogenetic studies showed that terminal deletions from Xp11 to Xp22.1 are associated with primary amenorrhea, and deletions from Xq13 to Xq27 usually coincide with primary amenorrhea or premature ovarian dysfunction.[48] The latter stretch of

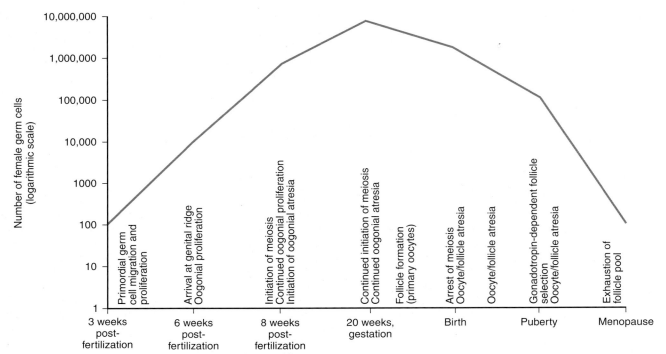

Figure 8-3. *Changes in oocyte numbers during fetal and postnatal life. The total number of oocytes is a reflection of the balance between active proliferation and oocyte/follicle atresia.*

the X chromosome is considered to be the critical region for normal ovarian function. Based on the study of interstitial deletions and breakpoints, this critical region has been subdivided into two domains encompassing Xq13-21 and Xq23-Xq27.[49] Deletions in these critical regions may cause

premature ovarian failure because of haploinsufficiency. Although translocations associated with premature ovarian failure might, on the surface, be thought to cause the phenotype because of the disruption of a critical X chromosome gene, definitive evidence for a key role of disrupted

Figure 8-4. *Ovarian follicles. A, Primordial follicles. Primary oocytes are surrounded by a single layer of flattened granulosa cells. B, Secondary follicle. The oocyte is surrounded by the early zona pellucida and several layers of cuboidal granulosa cells. C, Antral follicle. The oocyte is surrounded by a fully formed zona pellucida and many layers of granulosa cells. A Call-Exner body (arrow) is seen in the granulosa cell layer. Follicular fluid has accumulated, forming an antrum, and the theca interna layer is visible. D, Graafian follicle. The oocyte is surrounded by a fully formed zona pellucida and several layers of cumulus cells. Follicular fluid has accumulated, forming a large antrum. The mural granulosa cells and the theca interna layer are well defined. a, antrum; c, cumulus cells; g, granulosa cells; o, oocyte; t, theca interna; z, zona pellucida. (A originally published in Baca M, Zamboni L. The fine structure of the human follicular oocyte. J Ultrastruct Res 19:354, 1967; B to D adapted from Kurman RJ. Blaustein's Pathology of the Female Genital Tract, 3rd ed. New York, Springer-Verlag,1989.)*

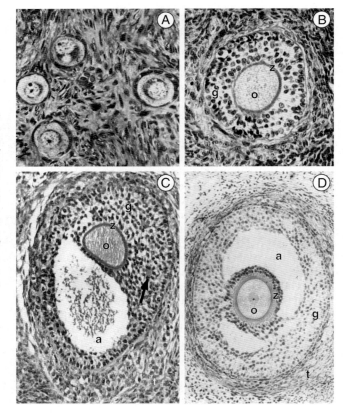

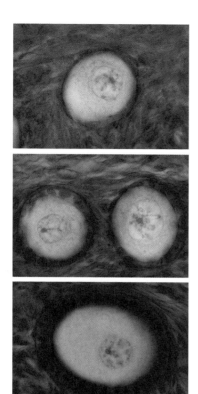

Figure 8-5. *Changes in the structure of primordial follicles with initiation of growth. The change in morphology of the cumulus cells from flat to cuboidal represents the earliest morphologic feature of this process. (From Westergaard CG, Byskov AG, Andersen CY. Morphometric characteristics of the primordial to primary follicle transition in the human ovary in relation to age. Hum Reprod 22[8]:2225-2231, 2007.)*

loci, as described later, is frequently lacking. Alternatively, these translocations may interfere with ovarian function as a result of aberrations in chromosome dynamics in general or position effects on flanking genes.[48-51]

Among candidate genes for ovarian failure is the fragile X syndrome gene *(FMR1)* on Xq27.3, which encodes an RNA-binding protein and is clearly linked to premature ovarian failure. "Premutations" in *FMR1,* consisting of increases in the number of CGG repeats in the 5' untranslated region that result in reduced translation of FMR1 messenger RNA (mRNA), are associated with premature ovarian failure, but the underlying mechanism of ovarian dysfunction is yet to be determined.[52] In the future, genetic screening for FMR1 alleles associated with reduced follicular content may identify women who should reproduce at an early age. The *FMR2* gene, located at Xq28, is another candidate. One report, which has yet to be replicated, suggests a high incidence of premature ovarian failure in women with microdeletions in *FMR2* (FRAXE fragile site–associated mental retardation).

The human homologue of *Drosophila* diaphanous 2 *(DIAPH2)* on Xq22 encodes a protein involved in cytokinesis that, when mutated, causes sterility in flies. A family affected by human premature ovarian failure associated with a translocation that disrupted the *DIAPH2* gene has been described. However, the relevance of this gene to premature ovarian failure has yet to be determined. *XPNPEP2,* a gene located at Xp25 that encodes a membrane-bound form of aminopeptidase P, was disrupted by a translocation associated with secondary amenorrhea. Again, the pathophysiologic role of this gene product in premature ovarian failure has not been established. Another gene, *POF1B,* also requires further study to identify its role, if any, in premature ovarian failure.

TABLE 8-1

Genes Involved in the Development of the Ovary

Gene	Protein Type	Role
Wt1	Transcription factor	Genital ridge formation[300]
Sf1 (Nr5a1)	Transcription factor	Genital ridge formation[301-302]
Lim1	Transcription factor	Genital ridge formation[303]
Lhx9	Transcription factor	Genital ridge formation[42]
Emx2	Transcription factor	Genital ridge formation[304]
Bmp4	Extracellular growth factor	Primordial germ cell development[1, 305]
Bmp8B	Extracellular growth factor	Primordial germ cell development[2]
Smad1	Transcription regulator	Primordial germ cell development[6]
Smad5	Transcription regulator	Primordial germ cell development[5]
Dazl	Translation regulator	Primordial germ cell development
TIAR	RNA-binding protein	Primordial germ cell development[23]
Pog	Unknown	Primordial germ cell proliferation[24]
Integrin β1	Integrin beta subunit	Primordial germ cell migration[22]
Steel (kit ligand)	Transmembrane growth factor	Primordial germ cell migration, follicle formation and growth[306]
W (c-kit receptor)	Tyrosine kinase receptor	Primordial germ cell migration, follicle formation and growth[307-308]
Figla	Transcription factor	Primordial follicle formation, follicle growth[55]
Foxo3	Transcription factor	Follicle growth
Nobox	Transcription factor	Follicle growth
Gdf-9	Growth factor	Follicle growth[62]
Bmp-15	Growth factor	Follicle growth[309]
Zfx	Transcription factor	Oocyte proliferation/survival[310]
Atm	Cell cycle kinase	Meiosis[311]
Wnt4	Secreted ligand	Steroidogenic enzyme expression[43]

Genes lying on the short arm of the X chromosome that may have a role in human ovarian function include *BMP15*, which lies on Xp11.2. It is a candidate gene for ovarian failure, based on its involvement in follicular arrest in the Inverdale and Hanna sheep (described in the section "Factors Initiating Follicle Growth"). Although two sisters with a normal karyotype with hypergonadotropic ovarian failure were found to be heterozygous for a nonconservative amino acid substitution in the pro region of *BMP15* (Y235C) and other *BMP15* variants have been reported in women with premature ovarian failure, there is no definitive evidence that these putative *BMP15* mutations lead to premature ovarian failure in women.[53-54] The zinc finger gene *ZFX*, on Xp22.1, which is important in ovarian development in the mouse because heterozygous and homozygous mutations are associated with a reduced germ cell number, is another candidate gene for ovarian failure, but little is known with respect to human ovarian biology.

Autosomal genes associated with abnormal ovarian differentiation or premature ovarian failure in humans include mutations in the follicle-stimulating hormone (FSH) receptor gene; the ataxia-telangiectasia gene (*ATM*), which is implicated in DNA repair and cell cycle control; the homeobox gene *NOBOX;* and the forkhead transcription factor *FOXL2*.[55] Mutations in the latter gene cause blepharophimosis–ptosis–epicanthus inversus syndrome (BPES), the type 1 form of which is associated with premature ovarian failure.[56-57] Genitourinary malformations, including sex reversal and streak gonads, are characteristic of syndromes associated with heterozygous mutations in the *WT1* gene. Heterozygous mutation in the *SF1* (*NR5A1*) gene also results in sex reversal. Rare genetic variants or mutations in the *GDF9* gene have been associated with premature ovarian failure, although definitive evidence of their causal role is lacking.[58-59] Polymorphisms in the gene encoding the inhibin α subunit (*INHA* 769G>A, A257T) have also been reported by some to be associated with premature ovarian failure, but others dispute this claim.[60-61] Mutations in the catalytic subunit of the mitochondrial DNA polymerase gamma (*POLG*) segregate with premature ovarian failure and progressive external ophthalmoplegia.[62]

The Follicle and Its Surroundings

THE OOCYTE

Oocyte-Specific Genes

The growing oocyte expresses a number of genes that are essential for successful follicular development, fertilization, and preimplantation development. Mouse knockout studies have identified several germ cell–specific transcription factors essential for folliculogenesis, including FIGLA (factor in the germline alpha), SOHLH1 (spermatogenesis- and oogenesis-specific basic helix-loop-helix 1), LXH8 (LIM homeobox 8), and NOBOX (newborn ovary homeobox). FIGLA, SOHLH1, and LXH8 appear to be required for the formation of primordial follicles from naked primordial oocytes, whereas NOBOX is involved in the transition of primordial to primary follicles. DAZLA (deleted in azoospermia-like autosomal), CPEB1 (cytoplasmic

polyadenylation element binding protein 1), and YBX2 (also known as MSY2) are DNA- or RNA-binding proteins involved in regulating mRNA translation within the oocyte. [63-64]

Oocyte growth is accompanied by formation of the *zona pellucida*, an extracellular matrix surrounding the oocyte.[63-66] The zona pellucida protects the developing germ cell in the follicle, the ovulated egg in the oviduct, and the cleavage-stage embryo. It also serves as the initial site of contact with sperm, and after fertilization, it becomes a barrier that discourages polyspermy. Three genes have been characterized that encode ZP1 (ZPA), ZP2 (ZPB), and ZP3 (ZPC), which are the main sulphated glycoproteins of the zona. A polymer of ZP2 and ZP3 proteins forms filaments that are interconnected by ZP1, a minor component of the zona pellucida. FIGLA regulates the coordinated expression of these genes during the oocyte growth phase. Humans and rats have a fourth ZP-1 like subunit (ZP4), which is not expressed in mice.[67]

In the mouse, ZP3 was believed for many years to be the primary sperm receptor, with ZP2 being a secondary receptor. However, recent compelling evidence indicates that this "ligand-receptor" model of sperm–ZP3 interaction may not be correct, and suggests that, instead, sperm specifically recognize and bind, not to ZP3 alone, but to the three-dimensional matrix formed by all three zona proteins.[68] Indeed, in the human, it is evident that components beyond ZP3 are required for sperm binding to the zona. After fertilization, small diffusible components, including cortical granule proteases, are released from the egg. These components cause modifications of the ZP, including cleavage of ZP2, that prevent additional sperm from binding the ZP and comprise the ZP to block polyspermy.

Mice lacking ZP1 form structurally abnormal zonae and have reduced fecundity. In mice lacking ZP2, a thin zona forms that is not retained in preovulatory follicles. The antral-stage follicle number is substantially reduced, few eggs are ovulated, and no two-cell–stage embryos can be found in mated animals. Moreover, blastocysts derived from in vitro fertilized oocytes from females lacking ZP2 do not undergo normal development. Mice lacking ZP3 form no zona pellucida despite the expression of the other zona proteins. Few eggs are ovulated, and the females are sterile. As in the ZP2 mutant, in vitro fertilized eggs from ZP3-deficient mice do not develop beyond the blastocyst stage.

Several oocyte-specific "maternal effect" genes have been identified in mouse models that are expressed in the oocyte, but are only required during preimplantation embryo development. These include *Nalp5* (NACHT, leucine-rich repeat and PYD-containing 5; also known as *MATER*), a 125-kD, leucine-rich cytoplasmic protein of unknown function encoded by a gene transcribed in the growing oocyte.[69] Although *Nalp5* transcripts are degraded during meiotic maturation, the protein remains until the blastocyst stage. NALP5 protein is required for development of embryos beyond the two-cell stage, as evidenced by female mice lacking the protein that produce no offspring because of this early block in development.[70] Three other mouse oocyte-specific genes were recently found to be maternal effect genes. *Zar1* (zygote arrest 1) is a cytoplasmic protein required for the transition from fertilized egg to cleaving embryo by an unknown mechanism. *Npm2*

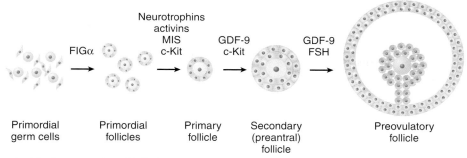

Neurotrophins
activins
MIS
FIGα   c-Kit   GDF-9   GDF-9
                          c-Kit   FSH

Primordial   Primordial   Primary   Secondary   Preovulatory
germ cells   follicles   follicle   (preantral)   follicle
                                                     follicle

Figure 8-6. *Factors involved in the progression of folliculogenesis and oogenesis. Communication between oocytes and their associated somatic cells is established with primordial follicle formation. Granulosa cells proliferate during the ensuing stages of folliculogenesis. Oocyte–granulosa cell communication mediated by secreted paracrine factors and gap junctions is essential for the developmental progression of follicles, female gametogenesis, and embryonic development after fertilization. Several factors (described in the text) function to promote or inhibit specific stages in this progression. FSH, follicle-stimulating hormone; FIG, factor in the germline; GDF, growth differentiation factor; MIS, müllerian inhibitory substance. (Adapted from Matzuk MM, Burns KH, Viveiros MM, Eppig JJ. Intercellular communication in the mammalian ovary: oocytes carry the conversation. Science 296:2178-2180, 2002.)*

(nucleoplasmin 2) is a nuclear protein generated before oocyte maturation that affects heterochromatin organization and histone deacetylation. In the absence of *Npm2*, ovulation and fertilization occur normally, but there is a complete failure of preimplantation embryo development. *Dppa3 (Stella)*, in addition to its role in primordial germ cell specification, is a maternal effect gene required for normal preimplantation embryo development.

Oocyte-Derived Factors and the Control of Follicular Growth and Differentiation

The concept that the oocyte plays an important role in follicular function and is far more than a passive inhabitant of the follicle emerged from two realizations: (1) that follicular survival depends on the presence of viable germ cells and (2) that removal of the oocyte from an antral follicle is followed by luteinization, indicating that the oocyte produces factors that restrain the terminal differentiation of granulosa cells.[71-72] Additional support for this concept was derived from experiments in which midsized oocytes from mouse secondary follicles were transferred by a grafting procedure into primordial follicles. This transfer resulted in a doubling of the rate of development of the primordial follicular cells in the presence of the secondary follicle oocyte.[73]

The effects of the oocyte on follicular growth are mediated in part by recently identified factors that are selectively or specifically produced by the oocyte. These factors, growth differentiation factor (GDF)-9 and BMP-15, influence granulosa and theca cell function (Fig. 8-6). The importance of GDF-9 and BMP-15 has been established through genetic manipulation of mice and the discovery of spontaneous mutations in the gene encoding BMP-15, which affects follicular dynamics in sheep.[74-76]

THE GRANULOSA CELLS

The granulosa cells are believed to originate from ovarian surface epithelial mesothelium or possibly from the rete ovarii.[77] The cohort of granulosa cells that surrounds each oocyte has an oligoclonal origin, with three to five parent cells giving rise to the full complement of granulosa cells in a mature follicle.[78] Granulosa cells receive no direct blood supply, and because a basal lamina separates them from the vascularized theca interna, there is a relative blood–follicle barrier that restricts the entry of leukocytes and high–molecular-weight substances (such as low-density lipoproteins). The absence of a blood supply also necessitates intimate intercellular contact between neighboring granulosa cells and the oocyte.

Granulosa Cell–Granulosa Cell and Granulosa Cell–Oocyte Communication via Gap Junctions

Granulosa cells are interconnected by an extensive network of gap junctions, and this network effectively couples them into an integrated and functional syncytium. These specialized cell junctions are important for metabolic exchange and transport of small molecules between neighboring cells. Moreover, granulosa cells extend cytoplasmic processes through the zona pellucida to form gap junctions with the plasma membrane of the oocyte (Fig. 8-7). Cyclic AMP (cAMP), produced by granulosa cells, may be one of the factors passed into the oocyte via gap junctions to maintain oocytes in a state of maturational arrest.

Gap junctions are composed of hexameric arrays of proteins called *connexins*. Connexin-37 and connexin-43 are two of the important follicular connexins. Connexin-37 is reported to be the predominant connexin in the oocyte, whereas connexin-43 predominates in the granulosa cells. As a result, communication between granulosa cells and the oocyte occurs through heterologous gap junctions, whereas gap junctional communication between granulosa cells is via homologous complexes.[79] FSH induces connexin-43 expression in granulosa cells, whereas the ovulatory surge of LH suppresses connexin-43 mRNA expression and causes post-translational modifications that lead to the loss of connexin-43 protein and the subsequent uncoupling of the gap junction network between granulosa cells and between granulosa cells and the oocyte.

The importance of connexins to follicular function was shown in the ovarian phenotype of connexin-37 and connexin-43 knockout mice.[80-81] In connexin-37–deficient mice, created by targeting the *Gja4* gene, follicle growth is arrested at the preantral stage; oocyte growth, although it

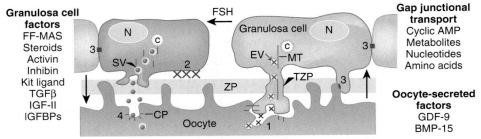

Figure 8-7. *Model proposing regulated delivery of paracrine factors at the oocyte–granulosa cell interface. Four (1-4) communication modalities are described: (1) Localized uptake of oocyte factors (x), such as GDF9, by endocytosis at stabilized attachment sites of transzonal projections (TZPs) at the oolemma; vectorial transport of endocytic vesicles (EVs) to the granulosa cell body occurs along microtubules (MTs) in preparation for intracellular processing and release of factors after transcytosis. (2) Granulosa–zona pellucida anchoring is required for TZP orientation. Contact sites may play a signaling role for oocytes and granulosa cells, and changes in adhesion would occur in response to changes in the composition of the zona pellucida. (3) Gap junctions allow for direct intercellular communication between granulosa cells, or between oocyte microvilli and granulosa cell TZPs. (4) A pathway is used for delivery of granulosa cell–derived factors (blue dots) packaged in secretory vesides (SVs) that are subsequently endocytosed by receptor-mediated endocytosis at the oocyte surface through coated pits (CPs). Note that remodeling of the microtubule cytoskeleton (MT) in response to granulosa cell stimulation by FSH would lead to TZP retraction and thus modulating of either the delivery of granulosa cell factors to the oocyte (left arrow) or uptake of oocyte-secreted factors (x) by granulosa cells (right arrow). BMP, bone morphogenetic protein; c, centrosome; FF-MAS, follicular fluid meiosis–activating substance; FSH, follicle-stimulating hormone; GDF, growth differentiation factor; IGF, insulin-like growth factor; IGFBP, IGF-binding protein; N, nucleus; TGF, transforming growth factor; ZP, zona pellucida. (Adapted from Albertini DF, Combelles CMH, Benecchi E, Carabatsos MJ. Cellular basis for paracrine regulation of ovarian follicle development. Reproduction 121:647-653, 2001.)*

commences, is also subsequently arrested before meiotic competence is achieved, resulting in loss of oocytes and formation of luteinized structures. Connexin-43–deficient mice, created by targeting the *Gja1* gene, have an ovarian phenotype characterized by diminished germ cell number and impaired growth of follicles beyond the primary stage.

Granulosa Cell Steroidogenic Activity

The primary steroid hormone produced by the preovulatory granulosa cells is estradiol. The synthesis of this hormone requires a collaborative relationship with adjacent theca cells, which produce the immediate precursors for the aromatization reaction. The control of this process is under the direction of LH, acting on thecal elements, and FSH, acting on the granulosa compartment (Fig. 8-8). The two cell–two gonadotropin model is a formidable example of the integrated function of the different cellular components of the follicle.

Granulosa Phenotypic Heterogeneity

Granulosa cells display different phenotypes within the follicle, depending on their location.[82-85] The mural granulosa cells, antral granulosa cells, and cumulus granulosa cells each have distinguishing features that are likely determined by their proximity to the oocyte and theca cells and by the paracrine substances that they produce. The mural granulosa cells in the antral follicle express the greatest steroidogenic activity, showing the highest levels of 3β-hydroxysteroid dehydrogenase and aromatase (Fig. 8-9). In addition, mural granulosa cells in the preovulatory follicle have the highest level of LH receptors. The granulosa cells closest to the antral cavity have a lower expression of steroidogenic enzymes, whereas those in the middle region have greater mitotic activity than the antral and mural granulosa cells.

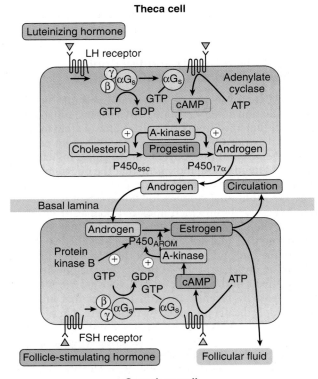

Figure 8-8. *The two-cell–two-gonadotropin system for estradiol synthesis in the follicle. Luteinizing hormone (LH) and follicle-stimulating hormone (FSH) are shown to stimulate adenylate cyclase via G-protein–coupled receptors. The cyclic AMP (cAMP) generated from ATP activates protein kinase A to stimulate expression of the respective steroidogenic enzymes in theca and granulosa cells. In addition, in granulosa cells, FSH binding to the FSH receptor leads to activation of protein kinase B, probably via a phosphatidyl inositol second message, which augments aromatase expression. GDP, guanosine diphosphate; GTP, guanosine triphosphate. (Modified from Erickson CF, Shimasaki S. The physiology of folliculogenesis: the role of novel growth factors. Fertil Steril 76:943-949, 2001, with permission.)*

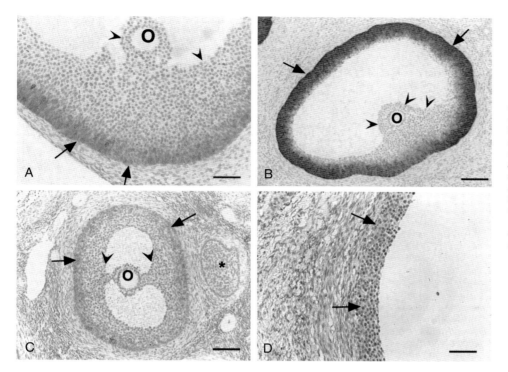

Figure 8-9. Heterogeneity of granulosa cell function in the developing follicle. Differential expression of aromatase is shown in a rat ovary (**A** and **B**) and a marmoset ovary (**C** and **D**). Arrows point to immunostained granulosa cells; arrowheads indicate absent staining in cumulus cells. *, preantral follicle; o, oocyte. Bar = 50 μm in **A**, **C**, and **D**, and 100 μm in **B**. (From Turner KJ, Macpherson S, Millar MR, et al. Development and validation of a new monoclonal antibody. J Endocrinol 172:21-30, 2002, with permission.)

The cumulus cells, which are released with the oocyte at ovulation, do not express aromatase, and their LH receptor content and level of LH responsiveness are substantially lower than those of their mural counterparts. These cells are active in producing an extracellular matrix consisting of hyaluronan, proteoglycans, and proteoglycan-binding proteins when stimulated by the prostaglandins generated in response to the ovulatory stimulus. The elaboration of this matrix leads to the preovulatory expansion of the cumulus–oocyte complex (Fig. 8-10).

THE THECA CELLS

The theca and interstitial cells are believed to arise from mesenchymal cells in the stromal compartment. Several phenotypes of theca and interstitial cells have been described.[86]

Primary interstitial cells, which resemble Leydig cells in morphology, are located in the medullary compartment of the fetal ovary. Evident at approximately 12 weeks of gestation, they disappear by 20 weeks. The primary interstitial cells are functionally limited; they are not responsive to gonadotropins and appear to be incapable of de novo steroidogenesis due to the lack of cholesterol side-chain cleavage activity. They may, however, metabolize circulating steroidogenic precursors into androgens.

Theca–interstitial cells are the main androgen-producing cells of the ovary. Production of GDF-9 by the oocyte is required for development of the theca layer. Theca cells also express kit ligand receptor, and researchers have postulated that kit ligand produced by granulosa cells is important in organizing the theca layer around the developing follicle. Theca cells engage in a bidirectional dialogue with granulosa cells through the production of keratinocyte-derived growth factor (KGF) and hepatocyte growth factor (HGF). KGF and HGF, like FSH, stimulate granulosa cells to produce kit ligand, whereas kit ligand acts on the theca cells to promote expression of KGF and HGF in a positive feedback loop (Fig. 8-11). Thus, kit ligand, KGF, and HGF achieve their highest concentrations in large antral follicles. As the oocyte expresses kit receptor, this feed-forward loop also affects oocyte function. Moreover, as described later in the section "Oocyte Maturation," theca-derived insulin-like factor-3 (INSL3) acts on the oocyte to promote maturation.

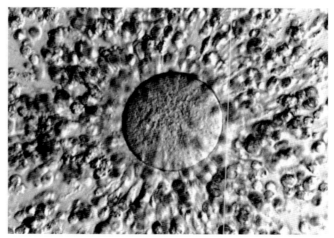

Figure 8-10. Appearance of a mature ovulated human oocyte. This metaphase II–arrested oocyte is surrounded by a highly expanded cumulus cell layer. The zona pellucida is visible only as a blurred region immediately around the oocyte (100×). (Adapted from Veeck LL. An Atlas of Human Gametes and Conceptuses. New York, Parthenon Publishing, 1999.)

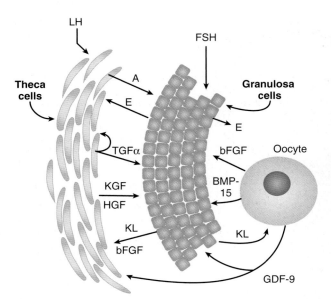

Figure 8-11. *Paracrine and autocrine interactions between theca cells, granulosa cells, and the oocyte. A, androstenedione; BMP, bone morphogenetic protein; E, estradiol; FGF, fibroblast growth factor; FSH, follicle-stimulating hormone; GDF, growth differentiation factor; HGF, hepatocyte growth factor; KGF, keratinocyte-derived growth factor; KL, kit ligand. LH, luteinizing hormone; TGF, transforming growth factor. (From Nillson E, Skinner MK. Cellular interactions that control primordial follicle development and folliculogenesis. J Soc Gynecol Investig 8[Suppl 1]:S17-S20, 2001, with permission.)*

Secondary interstitial cells are hypertrophied theca interna cell remnants of atretic follicles. These cells remain functionally and structurally unchanged in the locations of the original follicle. They are targets of noradrenergic innervation (see the section "Ovarian Innervation").

Hilar interstitial cells are large lutein-like cells with structural and functional characteristics indistinguishable from those of differentiated Leydig cells. Like Leydig cells, they contain the hexagonal Reinke crystals. Hilar cells are intimately associated with nonmyelinated sympathetic nerve fibers. The endocrine activity of these cells is assumed to be correlated with their prominence at the time of puberty, during pregnancy, and around menopause.

THE OVARIAN STROMA

The ovarian stroma contains fibroblastic cells that do not have significant steroidogenic activity (Fig. 8-12).[87] These cells express androgen receptors and may proliferate under the influence of androgens, contributing to the increased stromal density characteristic of hyperandrogenemia of ovarian origin (e.g., polycystic ovary syndrome [PCOS] and androgen-producing ovarian tumors). The stromal cells serve as insulators in the ovary, separating follicles and corpora lutea from adjacent structures physically, as well as biochemically. They produce growth factors and growth factor–binding proteins, the latter perhaps being key to the proposed insulator role. Ovarian stromal cells express substantial levels of gremlin, a protein that binds and inactivates BMPs; follistatin, which binds and inactivates activin;

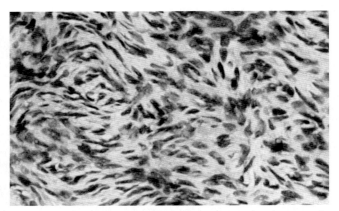

Figure 8-12. *Ovarian stroma consisting of whorls of fibroblastic cells. (Reproduced from Kurman RJ. Blaustein's Pathology of the Female Genital Tract, 3rd ed. New York, Springer-Verlag, 1989.)*

insulin-like growth factor (IGF)-binding proteins, and secreted frizzled-related proteins, which bind members of the WNT signaling family.

THE OVARIAN SURFACE EPITHELIUM

The ovarian surface epithelium, a flat to cuboidal epithelial layer of mesodermally derived cells, is also known as the *ovarian mesothelium* and by the misnomer of "germinal epithelium" because of the erroneous belief that it gave rise to germ cells.[88-89] During development, the ovarian surface epithelium may be one source of granulosa cells in addition to the rete ovarii, which has a common origin with the surface epithelium. In the adult ovary, the surface epithelium is characterized by expression of the mucus gene *MUC1* and the presence of cilia and apical microvilli. The cells sit on a basement membrane that covers a dense connective tissue layer.

The ovarian surface epithelium plays a role in the transport of material to and from the peritoneal cavity and in the repair of surface defects resulting from ovulation. During the ovulatory process, epithelial cells overlying the follicle undergo apoptotic cell death, followed by activation of a subsequent repair process. This process includes cell proliferation, which begins right after ovulation, and the resynthesis of extracellular matrix components. Proinflammatory cytokines may initiate these events.

Invaginations of surface epithelium into the ovary result in the formation of inclusion cysts. The ovarian surface epithelium in these inclusion cysts has the propensity to undergo metaplasia and neoplasia. Although some researchers have suggested that these inclusion cysts form from invaginations around the site of ovulation, they have been reported to be prominent in polycystic ovary syndrome (PCOS), a condition characterized by oligoovulation or anovulation that may also carry an increased risk of ovarian cancer. Others have proposed that inclusion cysts form as a result of inflammation, which could also explain their genesis in the periovulatory period because many features of the ovulatory process resemble an inflammatory process.

OVARIAN LEUKOCYTES AND MACROPHAGES

Macrophages, lymphocytes, and polymorphonuclear granulocytes are present in the ovary at various stages of its life cycle.[90] These cells have roles in normal ovarian function as well as in ovarian pathology, where for example, lymphocyte infiltration, particularly in the theca interna, is a characteristic feature of autoimmune ovarian failure.

Macrophages are a major cellular component of the interstitium, usually found near the perifollicular capillaries. Few other white blood cells are observed in the ovary in the early phases of follicular development, but a substantial infiltration of white blood cells occurs in the periovulatory period and in association with follicular atresia.[91] Mast cells increase progressively in number during the latter portion of the follicular phase.[92-93] In the rodent ovary, the mast cell invasion and subsequent degranulation in response to the proestrous LH surge causes a histamine-triggered hyperemia propagated by prostaglandin E_2.

After ovulation, eosinophils and T lymphocytes migrate into the corpus luteum, recruited by the expression of chemoattractants.[94-95] The infiltration and subsequent activation of these cells occurs before there is evidence of either functional or structural luteal regression. Activated T cells produce lymphokines that attract and activate macrophages. The dark stellate K cells that are scattered among the luteal cells are probably macrophages.[96] They influence luteal cell function through discrete cell–cell contacts and the production of growth factors and cytokines.[97-98] The importance of invasion of T lymphocytes and macrophages into the corpus luteum in the process of luteolysis is highlighted by the fact that pregnancy delays this invasion.

OVARIAN INNERVATION

The ovary has both extrinsic and intrinsic innervation. The extrinsic nerves, which are mainly sympathetic and sensory fibers with a small parasympathetic component, enter the ovary via the hilar perivascular plexus.[99-101] The main function of this extrinsic innervation is to regulate ovarian blood flow; however, it also affects endocrine function of ovarian cells. Electrical stimulation of the hypothalamus in hypophysectomized and adrenalectomized rats results in the alteration of ovarian steroid biosynthesis, independent of changes in ovarian blood flow. These findings suggest the existence, at least in animals, of an independent central nervous system–ovarian neural axis distinct from and parallel to the hypothalamic–pituitary–ovarian hormonal axis.

Theca–interstitial cells have direct sympathetic innervation by noradrenergic nerve terminals in the rodent. Electrical stimulation of the ovarian plexus of hypophysectomized rats causes theca–interstitial cells to take on the ultrastructural features of active steroid-secreting cells.[102] Conversely, ovarian denervation decreases the activity of 3β-hydroxysteroid dehydrogenase. Catecholamines, acting through β_2-selective adrenergic receptors, synergize with gonadotropins to promote ovarian androgen production.[103] Excessive activation of thecal adrenergic receptors possibly plays a role in the pathogenesis of ovarian hyperandrogenism. Consistent with this notion, histochemical evaluation of ovarian tissue obtained from

patients with PCOS suggested enhanced innervation of the theca–interstitial cell compartment.[104]

The human ovary also has intrinsic innervation. Most of these neurons express the low-affinity neurotrophin receptor p75 nerve growth factor (NGF) receptor. Some are catecholaminergic, as identified by the expression of tyrosine hydroxylase, the rate-limiting enzyme in catecholamine synthesis. The presence of intrinsic neurons in the human ovary parallels the findings in animals, where there is more extensive information about the function of ovarian nerves. As described later, an intraovarian neurotropic system involving germ and somatic cells operates in the ovaries. Thus, the functions of the intrinsic and extrinsic ovarian innervation and the ovarian germ and somatic cells are intertwined through a paracrine and autocrine signaling system.

The Follicular Life Cycle

Gougeon proposed that the various follicular classes, defined largely by size and the number of granulosa cells, represent sequential stages of development on the way to maturity (Fig. 8-13).[105] Based on this schema, approximately 1 year may elapse in the maturation of a primordial follicle to a dominant follicle. During much of this remarkably long period (approximately 300 days), follicles are believed to grow in a gonadotropin-independent manner. Gonadotropins influence the last 50 days of the maturation process.

INITIATION OF FOLLICULAR GROWTH

Follicular growth, which begins when primordial follicles emerge from their quiescent state, occurs continuously from the fifth to sixth month of intrauterine life until menopause. Although some researchers have suggested that the first formed follicles are the first ovulated, transition into the growth phase is more likely to be a random event independent of the sequence in which follicles formed during development.

The initiation of follicular growth is characterized by morphologic changes, including a change in granulosa cell shape from flattened to cuboidal, proliferation of granulosa cells, enlargement of the oocyte, and formation of the zona pellucida (see Fig. 8-5). The transformation of flattened granulosa cells to a cuboidal shape has functional correlates, including the expression of certain mRNAs (e.g., follistatin mRNA). Granulosa cell proliferation and the change to a cuboidal shape precede increases in oocyte diameter. In the human, the first substantial increase in oocyte diameter occurs when there are 15 granulosa cells in the largest follicle cross-section. Oocyte growth is accompanied by elaboration of the zona pellucida, first evident as islands of periodic acid-Schiff–positive material. Subsequent increases in oocyte and follicular diameters are positively correlated until well into the secondary follicle stage, when oocytes reach a mean diameter of 80 μm. This stage corresponds to a follicular diameter of 110 to 120 μm and a granulosa cell endowment of approximately 600 cells. The germinal vesicle attains a mean maximal diameter of 26 to 27 μm at this follicular size.

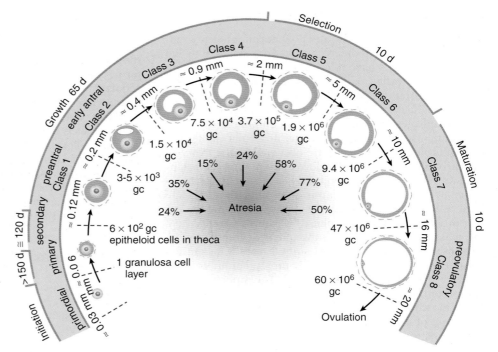

Figure 8-13. Stages of follicular development in the adult human ovary and extent of atresia in the eight classes of growing follicles. The classes are defined by the granulosa cell (gc) numbers and the corresponding estimated follicular diameter (mm). d, days. (From Gougeon A. Dynamics of follicular growth in the human: a model from preliminary results. Hum Reprod 1: 81-87, 1986.)

The early theca interna is acquired at the end of the primary follicle stage. The theca externa forms as the follicle expands and compresses the surrounding stroma (see Fig. 8-4). The migration of pretheca cells to the outer surface of the follicle is triggered by signals that remain unknown, although GDF-9 likely plays a role because the theca does not develop in the absence of this oocyte-derived factor.

As a secondary follicle is being formed, the granulosa cells develop FSH, estrogen, and androgen receptors and become coupled by gap junctions. The formation of the thecal layer is associated with the development of a follicular blood supply from arterioles that terminate in a wreath-like network of capillaries adjacent to the basement membrane. Concomitantly, the theca cells acquire LH receptors and the capacity to synthesize steroid hormones. The secondary follicles constitute the pool of preantral follicles from which FSH-dependent recruitment of follicles takes place.

OOCYTE GROWTH

A significant component of the secondary follicle growth phase is dedicated to oocyte differentiation and growth. The growing oocyte is a metabolically active cell, synthesizing mRNAs and proteins that support growth and development through the early preimplantation embryo stages. Indeed, the oocyte contributes the vast majority of the cytoplasm and nuclear components to the developing embryo. The oocyte is supported in its growth by bidirectional transport of nutrients, growth factors, and other molecules across the gap junctions that directly connect the transzonal projections of the surrounding granulosa cells to the oocyte (see Fig. 8-7).[106]

Morphologic alterations in the oocyte that occur during the growth phase include complete elaboration of the zona pellucida by the active production, assembly, and secretion of its component proteins. The quantity of several cytoplasmic organelles increases, particularly the mitochondria, which are estimated to number approximately 500,000 in a fully grown human oocyte.[107] In contrast, the centrioles that were present in oogonia are lost during the oocyte growth phase.[108] The distribution of the organelles changes, with clustering of the mitochondria, endoplasmic reticulum, and Golgi complex in the region immediately surrounding the germinal vesicle.[109]

During the growth phase, oocytes become competent to undergo meiotic maturation, or acquire "meiotic competence." The molecular basis for the acquisition of meiotic competence is not completely understood. However, it occurs only after the oocyte has reached a certain critical size. Meiotically competent oocytes do have certain attributes, including increased levels of the cell cycle proteins CDK1, cyclin B, and CDC25.[110-111] A minimum threshold amount of these proteins must likely be acquired before cell cycle resumption can occur. Importantly, proper meiotic chromosome segregation depends on successful folliculogenesis and oocyte growth, processes that have substantial energy requirements. These requirements are met by transport of ATP and energy substrates from granulosa cells via gap junctions and also by oxidative phosphorylation of pyruvate within the oocyte proper. Indeed, mouse oocytes lacking PDH1A, an enzymatic subunit of pyruvate dehydrogenase, have decreased levels of ATP and nicotinamide adenine dinucleotide phosphate (NADPH) because they cannot perform oxidative phosphorylation of pyruvate. These oocytes grow and are ovulated, but do not successfully complete meiotic maturation.[112] Similar processes may be compromised in the ovaries of older women, resulting in nondisjunction errors and aneuploidy in the embryo.[113-114]

Although it is not completed until late in preimplantation embryo development, reestablishment of genomic imprints begins to occur during oocyte growth, at least partially due to the activity of DNA methyltransferases.[115-118] Failure of the imprinting process in either oocytes or male germ cells results in aberrant expression of genes from the maternal or paternal alleles. These alterations in gene expression are associated with several inherited human diseases, including Beckwith-Wiedemann, Prader-Willi, and Angelman syndromes.[119-120] A global loss of maternal imprinting in the oocyte results in the formation of a complete hydatidiform mole.[121]

In addition to developing meiotic competence, oocytes in the growth phase begin to acquire the ability to support preimplantation embryo development and development to term, known as "developmental competence." Functional aspects of developmental competence are poorly defined, but include the ability of the oocyte cytoplasm to remodel sperm DNA and an enhanced ability to generate calcium oscillations.[122-123] Generation of a pool of maternal mRNAs that are highly stable but translationally repressed until maturation or fertilization is an important aspect of developmental competence.

At the completion of oocyte growth, transcription is actively silenced and protein translation slows substantially. Transcriptional silencing requires patent gap junctional communication with cumulus granulosa cells and is accompanied by changes in large-scale chromatin structure that are essential to confer growing oocytes with meiotic and developmental competence.[124-125] Maintenance of these chromatin changes requires the activity of histone deacetylases.[126] After transcriptional silencing, preovulatory oocytes rely on maternally derived proteins and mRNA stores to support the resumption of meiosis and the first cleavage divisions after fertilization.

FACTORS INITIATING FOLLICULAR GROWTH

Intraovarian factors are believed to play key roles in regulating the early phases of follicular growth (see Figs. 8-6 and 8-11). Among these are proteins of somatic cell origin, including activin A and the forkhead transcription factor, FOXO3, which inhibits follicular growth, and basic fibroblast growth factor (FGF) and kit ligand, which are believed to act as stimulators. Kit ligand, which is produced by granulosa cells and acts on kit, a receptor on the oocyte and theca cells, is required for initiation of follicular growth and growth of the oocyte. The oocyte-derived proteins GDF-9 and BMP-15 are important for granulosa cell proliferation in a species-specific manner, as shown by the ovarian phenotypes of the *Gdf9* knockout mouse and Inverdale sheep with homozygous mutations in the *Bmp15* gene. In both cases, granulosa cells cease proliferating after approximately two doublings. The oocytes continue to grow, however, resulting in large oocytes that ultimately degenerate and are surrounded by a single layer of granulosa cells. A requirement for estrogen in follicular development is supported by studies in laboratory animals, but whether this requirement extends to primates is a subject of debate. Müllerian inhibitory substance (MIS) produced by granulosa cells restrains follicles from entering

the growing pool; in its absence, follicular depletion is accelerated (see Fig. 8-4).[127-128]

Effector genes involved in follicular growth include transcription factors and RNA-binding proteins. Mice homozygous for mutations in the previously mentioned oocyte-specific transcription factor *Figla* and in *Dazl*, a gene encoding an RNA-binding protein, have arrested follicular development. In contrast, mice with null mutations for *Foxo3* do not restrain primordial follicle activation, this results in global follicle activation soon after birth and subsequent premature follicle depletion and ovarian failure.[129] FOXO3A activity is likely controlled by PTEN (phosphatase and tensin homologue deleted on chromosome 10), a negative regulator of phosphatidylinositol 3-kinase, which controls phosphorylation of FOXO3 and its export from the nucleus, an event that triggers follicle growth. The deletion of PTEN in the oocyte results in activation of primordial follicular growth and early depletion of follicles.

Evidence suggesting that FSH is not required for initiation of follicular growth includes the fact that the process occurs in hypophysectomized animals. In humans and mice with inactivating mutations in the FSH β subunit or FSH receptor gene, follicular development can occur to the secondary and early antral stages, but more slowly and with markedly reduced frequency than when normal levels of FSH activity are present. However, the importance of pituitary-derived factors (not necessarily FSH) in follicular growth and survival in the primate fetus was illustrated by the observation that hypophysectomy of the fetal Rhesus monkey results in oocyte depletion. Moreover, studies on rodent ovaries suggest that preantral follicles are gonadotropin-responsive. In human ovarian xenografts transplanted to immunodeficient and hypogonadal mice, FSH was shown to be required for growth of follicles beyond the two-granulosa–layer stage.[130] Thus, follicle growth before the antral stage, although possible in the absence of gonadotropins, may be facilitated by FSH.

FORMATION OF ANTRAL FOLLICLES

There is little doubt that the transition from the secondary-follicle to the antral-follicle stage is promoted by FSH. Antral follicles are rarely observed in animals or humans with FSH deficiency (unless exogenous FSH is administered) or ovaries lacking FSH receptors. The antrum and its fluid may facilitate the process of release of the cumulus–oocyte complex at ovulation and serve as a vehicle for nutrient exchange and waste removal in the avascular compartment.[131] The antrum also serves as a unique environment in which the cumulus–oocyte complex completes growth and maturation.

The development of the antrum requires the rapid influx of water, which occurs primarily through a transcellular process. This may be mediated by the water channels formed by aquaporins 7, 8, and 9, which are expressed by granulosa cells.[132] Because net transfer of water via the aquaporins requires an osmotic gradient, granulosa cells also are believed to actively transport ions to create this gradient. Alternately, the hydrolysis of glycosaminoglycans in the antrum could increase the osmolarity of follicular fluid and support the influx of water.

Between 5 and 6 days before ovulation, the follicle undergoes rapid expansion—as a result of granulosa cell proliferation and the accumulation of antral fluid—and moves to the ovarian surface. The accelerated expansion of the follicle destined to ovulate can cause midcycle pelvic pain (mittelschmerz). The expression of the cell cycle gene, cyclin D2, is important for this expansion, because cyclin D2 null mice show impaired granulosa cell proliferation and consequently have an ovulation defect. On completion of this growth phase, the follicle, now referred to as a Graafian follicle, is prepared for ovulation (see Fig. 8-4).

FOLLICULAR RECRUITMENT, SELECTION, AND DOMINANCE

The term "recruitment" has been used to describe the process by which the follicle departs from the resting pool to initiate growth. However, some authors also use this term to describe the engagement of a cohort of antral follicles into further growth. To avoid confusion, McGee and Hsueh suggested that the first situation be called *initial recruitment* and the latter, *cyclic recruitment*.[133] Cyclic recruitment, although obligatory, does not guarantee ovulation because growing follicles are vulnerable to atresia and thus may fall out from the growth trajectory. *Selection* refers to the process by which the maturing follicular cohort is reduced to a number appropriate for the species-specific ovulatory quota. This process entails negative selection against the subordinate follicles as well as positive selection of the follicles that will determine dominance. Although traditional thinking argues for a single wave of follicular development during the menstrual cycle, recent ultrasound studies suggest that multiple waves of follicular development occur.[134]

In the early follicular phase, no gross morphologic differences exist between the selected follicle and other healthy members of the cohort. However, the leading follicle can be distinguished from other members of the cohort by its size and the high mitotic index of its granulosa cells. Only the leading follicle has detectable levels of FSH in its follicular fluid. The leading follicle also contains significant levels of estradiol, a hallmark of the chosen follicle. Selection does not guarantee progression to ovulation, but given its temporal proximity to this event, ovulation usually does occur.

Dominance refers to the status of the follicle destined to ovulate and its role in regulating the size of the ovulatory quota. The follicle destined to ovulate attains dominance 5 to 7 days after the demise of the corpus luteum of the previous cycle.[135] This conclusion is supported by the observation that the levels of estradiol in the ovarian vein are remarkably different between ovaries by day 5 to 7 of the cycle, attesting to the emergence of the dominant follicle. This follicle continues to thrive under circumstances that it has made inhospitable for competing follicles in both ovaries.

The control of the temporal sequence of events leading up to follicular dominance has been elucidated by ablation studies in infrahuman primates and also in women in which the dominant follicle or corpus luteum was destroyed or removed. Destruction of the largest follicle on day 8 to 12 in the primate ovary delays the next preovulatory surge of pituitary gonadotropins. Conversely, luteectomy in the midluteal phase (days 16 to 19) advances the gonadotropin surge. In women, the interval from ablation of the dominant follicle or corpus luteum to the next ovulation is 14 days. These findings are consistent with the notion that the cyclic structures of the dominant ovary (i.e., the ovary containing the dominant follicle or corpus luteum) are the timekeepers of the menstrual cycle. The 28-day menstrual cycle is thus the result of the intrinsic life span of the dominant follicle (follicular phase) and corpus luteum (luteal phase), not timing dictated by the brain or pituitary.

Studies on primate ovaries indicate that the selection of the follicle destined to ovulate already has occurred as early as day 8 of the cycle.[136] No other member of the follicular cohort is competent to serve as a surrogate for a destroyed follicle, and a timely midcycle gonadotropin surge is not achieved. In the case of the corpus luteum, the next round of follicular growth occurs only after its interference is removed—either naturally (luteolysis) or artificially (luteectomy). Studies on hormone-replaced luteectomized primates suggest that progesterone is the principal agent responsible for the inhibition of follicular growth in the luteal phase.[137] However, inhibin A secreted by the corpus luteum may also play a role in the suppression of FSH and thus follicular maturation. Also central to the process of follicular development is its vasculature. Inhibition of the action of vascular endothelial growth factor (VEGF) blocks follicular maturation secondary to an attenuation of follicular vascular density or reduced vascular permeability, which may limit access of critical growth factors or hormones necessary for follicular growth.[138]

Endocrine Characteristics of Follicles on the Way to Dominance

Follicles with a diameter of less than 8 mm have a relatively low intrafollicular estrogen-to-androgen ratio, but from the midfollicular phase onward, this ratio is reversed (Fig. 8-14). The chosen follicle is able to synthesize estradiol in sufficient quantities to result in appreciable passage of this hormone into the general circulation and asymmetry of ovarian function as early as day 5 to 7 of the cycle.[138-139] In the late follicular phase, the intrafollicular concentrations of estradiol are directly correlated with follicular size and achieve concentrations of approximately 1 μg/mL at a time when circulating estradiol levels reach their peak.[140-141] After the ovulatory surge of LH, intrafollicular concentrations of estradiol decline and there is a parallel decrease in the concentration of androstenedione. Concurrently, progesterone and 17α-hydroxyprogesterone concentrations increase, reflecting early granulosa cell luteinization.

Inhibin A concentrations in follicular fluid increase with follicular maturation, whereas inhibin B, activin A, and free follistatin do not show variations with follicular size. Thus, as follicles mature, there is a switch from an environment dominated by activin to one dominated by inhibin A. The increase in inhibin A levels is correlated with increased expression of inhibin A α and β subunit mRNAs in granulosa cells.[142]

Higher follicular fluid concentrations of estrogens and progestogens and lower concentrations of androgens are

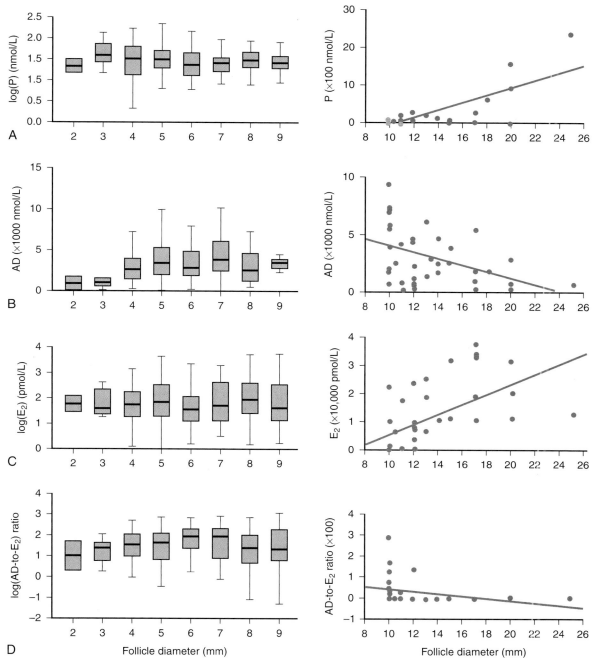

Figure 8-14. *Follicular fluid steroid levels and follicular diameter. AD, androstenedione; E_2, estradiol; P, progesterone. (From Van Dessel HJ, Schipperi, Pache TD, et al. Normal human follicle development: an evaluation of correlations with oestadiol, androstenedione, and progesterone levels in individual follicles. Clin Endocrinol 44:191-198, 1996, with permission.)*

characteristics of preovulatory follicles.[143] The hormone profiles of smaller follicles late in the follicular phase are characterized by higher concentrations of androgens and lower concentrations of estrogens and progesterone. Antral fluid FSH concentrations tend to be higher in larger follicles compared with serum levels, and estradiol levels are higher in antral fluids marked by measurable levels of FSH. These data are consistent with the concept that follicular hormone concentrations are regulated by the microenvironment of individual follicles. The expression of

functional LH receptors on granulosa cells of the preovulatory primate follicle allows LH to substitute for FSH in the promotion of the terminal stages of maturation.[144]

OVULATION

As midcycle approaches, the rise in estrogen emanating from the dominant follicle initiates an LH surge and, to a lesser extent, an FSH surge. This triggers the resumption of meiosis, ovulation, and luteinization (Fig. 8-15).[145]

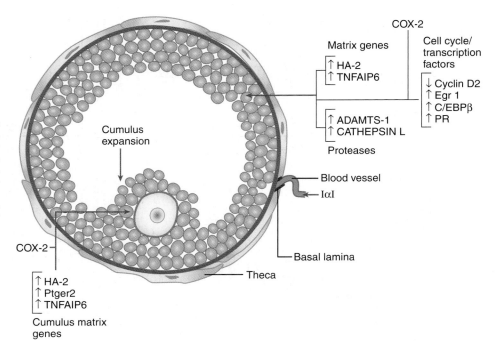

Figure 8-15. *Luteinizing hormone (LH) regulation of genes involved in ovulation. Arrows indicate up-regulation (↑) or down-regulation (↓). Iαl, inter-α-trypsin inhibitor; C/EBP, CCAT/enhancer binding protein; Egr 1, early growth response 1; HA-2, hyaluronic acid synthase-2; PR, progesterone receptor; Ptger2, prostaglandin E$_2$ receptor 2; TNFAIP6, tumor necrosis α-induced protein 6.*

The preovulatory LH surge precedes follicular rupture by as much as 36 hours. Before rupture, a number of critical changes take place in the granulosa cells and oocytes, including the suppression of transcription of genes that control granulosa cell proliferation; the loss of gap junctions, which uncouples the electrophysiologic syncytium of the granulosa cells and the oocyte; and the induction of genes essential for ovulation in granulosa cells, including the genes encoding the epidermal growth factor–like factors amphiregulin, epiregulin, and betacellulin. The latter growth factors activate endothelial growth factor (EGF) receptors, resulting in the induction of the gene encoding cyclooxygenase-2 (COX-2; *Ptgs2*) in granulosa cells and, consequently, prostaglandin E$_2$ synthesis. These act in concert with the EGF-like factors to trigger the cumulus cells to elaborate a hyaluronan-rich matrix that causes expansion of the cumulus. As described later, mice deficient in *Ptgs2* and the prostaglandin receptor EP2 (*Ptger2*) have ovulation defects that are related to an abnormality in cumulus expansion.[145-146]

Alterations in the extracellular matrix that promote expansion of the cumulus, a critical process for ovulation, are mediated by genes encoding hyaluron synthase 2 (*Has2*), required for production of the hyaluron backbone; the hyaluron-binding proteoglycan versican (*Cpg2*); tumor necrosis factor (TNF)-α–induced protein 6 (*Tnfaip6*); and pentraxin (*Ptx3*).[145-146] The matrix supporting cumulus expansion is composed of a meshlike network of hyaluronan chains that bind TNFAIP6, which transfers to hyaluronan the heavy chains of serum-derived inter-α-trypsin inhibitor, a complex macromolecule consisting of two heavy chains that are covalently bound to chondroitin sulfate and bikunin, a trypsin inhibitor. Pentraxin 3, a protein that forms pentamers, is another component that organizes the hyaluronan matrix. Mice deficient in TNFAIP6 and bikunin, one of the components of inter-α-trypsin inhibitor, have an ovulation defect associated with failed

cumulus expansion. The transcription factor liver receptor homolog 1 (*hrh1*) plays an essential role in this process as mice lacking hrh1 in granulosa cells fail to ovulate.

A conical stigma eventually rises on the surface of the protruding follicle in preparation for rupture. The rupture of the stigma is accompanied by gentle (rather than explosive) expulsion of the egg and follicular fluid, which suggests that the fluid is not under high pressure.

In primates, ovulation is believed to alternate between ovaries due to the local actions of progesterone produced by the corpus luteum on follicular dynamics; however, this belief has not been supported by definitive evidence. Although some studies suggest that ovulation occurs with equal frequency in the right and left ovaries, others suggest that right-sided ovulation is more frequent.[147-149]

Requirements for Progesterone

An early action of LH in the ovulatory process, which occurs within hours of the surge, is the induction of progesterone receptors in granulosa cells.[150] The functional importance of progesterone receptor up-regulation is documented by the fact that progesterone receptor antagonists and drugs that inhibit progesterone synthesis prevent ovulation in laboratory animals and the Rhesus monkey. Moreover, ovulation does not occur in mice with targeted deletions of the progesterone receptor gene, more specifically, the A form of the receptor.

These observations indicate that progesterone regulates the expression of ovulation genes by a classic mechanism. However, the A form of the progesterone receptor is generally a repressor of transcription, raising the possibility that an important part of progesterone's action in the preovulatory period includes suppression of gene expression. A number of candidate genes that appear to be dependent on periovulatory progesterone have been identified, including a metalloproteinase (see the section "Mechanism of Follicular Rupture"). COX-2 expression in progesterone receptor–deficient mice is normal, suggesting that prostanoids are not part of the progesterone-regulated ovulation program.

Requirements for Prostaglandins

The LH surge stimulates prostaglandin biosynthesis by ovarian follicles as a result of induction of the COX-2 enzyme in the preovulatory granulosa cells. COX-1 is not expressed by granulosa cells, and levels of this enzyme in the Graafian follicle do not change in response to an ovulatory stimulus.[151]

The requirement for prostaglandins in the process of ovulation has been revealed through pharmacologic studies and gene targeting in mice.[152] Inhibitors of prostaglandin synthesis, administered systemically or locally into the antrum, inhibit ovulation in laboratory animals and Rhesus monkeys and lead to luteinized, but unruptured follicles. Evidence for a role for prostaglandins in human ovulation derives from studies in which rofecoxib, the orally administered selective COX-2 inhibitor, delayed the time of ultrasonographic signs of follicular rupture by more than 48 hours after the LH peak. Signs of rupture were evident within 36 hours in a placebo-treated group.[153-154]

Mice with targeted mutations in the *Ptgs2* gene have defects in ovulation that can be overcome by administration of exogenous prostaglandin E_2, which is believed to be the key prostaglandin involved in ovulation. One of the abnormalities in *Ptgs2* knockout mice is a failure of the cumulus to expand. Mice deficient in the EP2 receptor for prostaglandin E_2 also have an ovulation defect and a postovulatory abnormality in cumulus expansion. These observations implicate prostaglandin E_2 in the process of ovulation and cumulus expansion. Progesterone receptors are induced in the follicles of COX-2–deficient mice, providing further evidence that the roles of progesterone and prostaglandins in ovulation are separable.

Other Nuclear Factors and Transcription Factors

The nuclear receptor interacting protein RIP40 (NRIP1), which was originally described as a transcriptional repressor, is important for ovulation in the mouse. Mice lacking this nuclear protein are anovulatory, and many LH-induced genes are reduced in the mutant ovaries. The mutant mice show defects in cumulus cell function and the expression of genes controlling expansion of the cumulus–oocyte complex. Mice lacking *PPARγ*, another gene regulated by the progesterone receptor, show ovulatory defects.

Requirement for EGF-like Factors

Luteinizing hormone stimulation induces the transient and sequential expression of the EGF-like growth factors amphiregulin, epiregulin, and betacellulin. Incubation of rodent follicles in vitro with these growth factors recapitulates the morphologic and biochemical events triggered by LH, including the necessary process of cumulus expansion and oocyte maturation. Thus, the EGF-like growth factors are essential mediators of the follicular response to LH leading to ovulation.[155-156]

Mechanisms of Follicular Rupture

Several hypotheses have been advanced to explain the process of follicular rupture. An increase in hydrostatic pressure is evidently not involved, because direct measurements have demonstrated that intrafollicular pressure is low in periovulatory follicles.[157-158] An increase in colloid osmotic pressure has been described, in part due to granulosa cell–derived proteoglycans. However, a cause-and-effect relationship between the altered composition of antral fluid and the enlargement and rupture of the follicle remains to be established.

Stigma formation and rupture undoubtedly also reflect the actions of enzymes working locally on the follicle wall. Consistent with this notion, instillation of protease inhibitors into the antral fluid inhibits ovulation. Among the candidate proteases proposed to be involved in ovulation are the plasminogen activators and members of the matrix metalloproteinase (MMP) family. Plasminogen activator has been localized in increasing concentrations in the walls of rat ovarian follicles just before ovulation.[145,159] Although there is little doubt that ovarian cells produce this protease under hormonal regulation, its functional role is questionable. Studies in knockout mice deficient in urokinase, tissue plasminogen activator, and plasminogen indicate that plasmin is not necessary for follicular rupture or, for that matter, for the activation of other proteases required for ovulation.[159]

Mice deficient in MMP-3 (stromelysin-1), MMP-7 (matrilysin), MMP-9, and MMP-11 (stromelysin-3) reproduce normally, suggesting that, individually, these enzymes do not have an obligatory role in ovulation. The involvement of other members of the MMP family (e.g., MT1-MMP, ADAM-17) cannot yet be determined from existing knockout mice, because the mutant animals die either in utero or shortly after birth.

Members of the ADAMTS (*A* disintegrin and metalloproteinase and thrombospondin motifs) family appear to play a key role in ovulation. ADAMTS1 is induced in granulosa cells of the preovulatory follicle, but not in progesterone receptor knockout mice. Consequently, this gene has been implicated as a progesterone-regulated factor involved in ovulation.[145-146,159] Targeted deletion of the *Adamts1* gene in mice results in defects in follicular growth, ovulation, and consequently, female infertility, possibly as a result of abnormal cumulus expansion or release of active growth factors. ADAMTS4 may have a related role. Cathepsin L is another progesterone-regulated gene that degrades type I and type IV collagens, elastin, and fibronectin, all components of the follicle wall, and consequently, it could play a role in ovulation.

OOCYTE MATURATION

Maintenance of Meiotic Arrest

Although the exact biochemical nature of the oocyte maturation inhibitor remains a mystery, its existence has been proposed in an effort to address the otherwise enigmatic

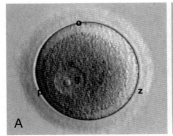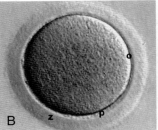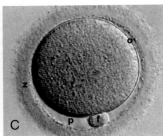

Figure 8-16. *Appearance of human oocytes during meiotic maturation. **A,** Immature, germinal vesicle–intact stage. The chromatin is arrested in prophase of meiosis I; meiotic maturation has not begun. **B,** Germinal vesicle breakdown stage. Meiosis I has resumed, with breakdown of the germinal vesicle; the chromatin is progressing through the remainder of meiosis I. **C,** Mature oocyte. The first polar body has been emitted, and the remaining chromatin is arrested in metaphase of meiosis II. f, first polar body; g, germinal vesicle; o, oolemma (oocyte plasma membrane); p, perivitelline space; z, zona pellucida (200×). (Adapted from Veeck LL. An Atlas of Human Gametes and Conceptuses. New York: Parthenon Publishing, 1999.)*

process of meiotic arrest. Indeed, relatively little is known with respect to the mechanisms responsible for holding the mammalian oocyte in abeyance in the late diplotene stage. That an inhibitor is involved is suggested by the fact that the removal of an oocyte from its intrafollicular environment results in the spontaneous resumption of meiosis once it is in culture. Thus, meiotic inhibition requires the intermediacy of the surrounding granulosa cumulus cells.

There is strong evidence that oocyte maturation is controlled by oocyte cAMP, which maintains maturation arrest.[160-161] In turn, oocyte cAMP levels are controlled by receptors on the cell surface and phosphodiesterase activity. G-protein–coupled receptor 3 (GPR3), which is coupled to the stimulatory G protein Gs, constitutively activates adenylate cyclase in the oocyte, resulting in cAMP production. Oocytes from *Gpr3* knockout mice resume meiosis independently of an increase in LH. This phenotype can be reversed by injection of *Gpr3* RNA into the oocytes. Another receptor expressed on the oocytes, GPR12, may have a similar role. LGR8, which is coupled to an inhibitory G protein, is the receptor for insulin-like factor 3 (INSL3), which is produced by theca cells. LGR8 is localized to the oocyte, and when it is activated, cAMP levels decline, initiating the resumption of meiosis. The cGMP-inhibited cAMP phosphodiesterase 3A (PDE3A) is expressed in mouse oocytes. It is indispensable for meiotic maturation because oocytes lacking the enzyme do not undergo spontaneous maturation and inhibitors of the enzyme block the resumption of meiosis.[162-163]

Nuclear Maturation

The primary oocyte is converted into a secondary oocyte, or egg, by completion of the first meiotic metaphase and formation of the first polar body (Fig. 8-16 and Table 8-2). Oocytes within fully developed antral follicles resume meiotic maturation in response to the midcycle LH surge. As described in the section "Maintenance of Meiotic Arrest," modulation of the level of cAMP within both the follicle cells and the oocyte is a critical factor. Stimulation of LH receptors on follicular cells results in the activation of Gs and the subsequent generation of cAMP by transmembrane adenylyl cyclases. The activation of this signaling pathway results in the transcription of specific genes that are important in modulating follicular cell function during oocyte maturation and ovulation. In addition, a signal is transmitted from the follicle cells to the oocyte that is responsible for inducing the resumption of meiosis. One possibility is that this signal is a molecule (e.g., cAMP), which passes into the oocyte via gap junctions between the oocyte and follicle cells. Evidence supporting this notion includes the fact that pharmacologic inhibition of PDE3, the phosphodiesterase of the oocyte that breaks down cAMP, completely blocks oocyte maturation in vivo and in vitro.[162-163] Alternatively, follicle cells secrete paracrine factors (e.g., INSL3) that activate an oocyte cell surface receptor that could be responsible for promoting maturation. In response to this signal, the level of cAMP within the oocyte decreases, and both nuclear and cytoplasmic maturation occur.

TABLE 8-2						
The Acquisition of Meiotic and Developmental Competence in the Oocyte						
	Primordial Oocytes	*Primary*	*Preantral*	*Antral*	*Fully Grown Oocytes*	*MII-Arrested Eggs*
Growth	Resting	Early growth	Mid growth	Late growth	Complete	Complete
Transcription	Limited	Active	Active	Active	Limited	Limited
GVBD	Incompetent	Incompetent	Competent	Competent	Competent	Complete
MII	Incompetent	Incompetent	Incompetent	Competent	Competent	Complete
Embryogenesis	Incompetent	Incompetent	Incompetent	Limited	Limited	Competent

GVBD, germinal vesicle breakdown; MII, metaphase of meiosis II.

There is clear evidence in lower species that steroid hormones are responsible for inducing oocyte maturation. Although steroids have been proposed to induce meiotic maturation in mammals, inhibition of follicular steroid production or action does not prevent resumption of meiosis in response to LH, so steroids cannot be obligatory for this process.

Nuclear maturation is first visible morphologically when the germinal vesicle breaks down as a result of disruption of the nuclear lamins (see Fig. 8-16). With exposure to the cytoplasm, the chromatin condenses and moves toward the cortical region, and the meiosis I spindle forms. Progression through the remainder of meiosis I, with extrusion of the first polar body, soon follows. The chromatin proceeds immediately to metaphase of meiosis II and then becomes arrested at this stage, now referred to as a *secondary oocyte* or *metaphase II–arrested egg* (see Fig. 8-16). Arrest in metaphase II occurs before physical release of the egg from the follicle during ovulation. Completion of meiosis, with extrusion of the second polar body, does not occur until fertilization.

Cytoplasmic Maturation

A process of "cytoplasmic maturation," less obvious than the morphologic changes of nuclear maturation, also occurs subsequent to the LH surge and is critical for successful egg activation and preimplantation embryo development should the egg be fertilized. At the ultrastructural level, there are changes in the distribution of the organelles, with movement of the endoplasmic reticulum, mitochondria, and cortical granules toward the oocyte cortex.[164] A loss of the Golgi complex occurs, explaining the extensive decline in the ability of the mature egg to synthesize new proteins. With movement of chromatin to the cortical region, the oocyte becomes highly asymmetric. The actin cytoskeleton is altered, with a thickening of cortical actin overlying the metaphase II spindle. This region of the plasma membrane is devoid of microvilli—unlike the rest of the oocyte plasma membrane, which is enriched with microvilli. This loss of microvilli may reduce the chance of sperm entering the region of the metaphase II spindle, potentially interfering with the normal progression of meiosis.

At the molecular level, cytoplasmic maturation is accompanied by the recruitment of specific dormant maternal mRNAs that are translated into protein. Examples of these recruited mRNAs are tissue plasminogen activator (*tPA*), *Mos*, and the inositol trisphosphate receptor type I (*IP3R-I*). Translation of *Mos* is critical for activation of the cell cycle proteins required for nuclear maturation. Recent evidence from studies in the mouse suggests that the maturation-associated increase in IP3R-I protein is important for successful egg activation by increasing the ability of the egg to exhibit calcium oscillations,[165] but the role of tPA has yet to be clarified.

The molecular mechanism by which maternal mRNAs are recruited is cytoplasmic polyadenylation. Specific nucleotide sequences in the 3′ untranslated region of the mRNAs, known as *cytoplasmic polyadenylation elements*, direct the binding of poly(A) polymerase with those mRNAs and the addition of poly(A) tracts to the mRNAs. Polyadenylation leads to the association of these mRNAs with polysomes and to subsequent translation and increases in the levels of the encoded proteins.

Post-translational modification of cytoplasmic proteins also occurs during oocyte maturation. For example, microtubules undergo alterations in acetylation during the transition from metaphase I to metaphase II.[166] In addition, phosphorylation and dephosphorylation of cytoplasmic proteins, particularly those involved in regulating the cell cycle, are required for successful cytoplasmic maturation.

Control of the Oocyte Cell Cycle

As in somatic cells, the oocyte cell cycle is controlled by alterations in the levels and activities of proteins now known as *cyclins* and *cyclin-dependent kinases*.[167-168] One of these proteins, maturation-promoting factor (MPF), was defined in bioassays as an activity that induced resumption of meiosis when microinjected into oocytes. MPF later was found to be a heterodimer of two proteins: cyclin B and p34cdc2 (now known as *cyclin-dependent kinase-1*, or cdk1).[169-170] Activation of MPF occurs in response to the LH surge, inducing resumption of meiosis I, germinal vesicle breakdown, and entry into meiosis II. The phosphatase CDC25B was recently shown to be required for the activation of MPF, because mice lacking this protein display normal folliculogenesis, but the oocytes do not undergo germinal vesicle breakdown.[171] The remainder of the signaling pathway connecting the LH surge to activation of MPF has not been delineated.

The LH surge also induces recruitment of maternal mRNA encoding MOS, resulting in an accumulation of this protein as the oocyte progresses toward meiosis II.[172-177] MOS is a component of a biologic activity known as *cytostatic factor*, defined by its ability to induce metaphase arrest when microinjected into an actively dividing cell. It is a serine–threonine kinase that indirectly activates a mitogen-activated protein (MAP) kinase that is responsible, at least in part, for the arrest of the oocyte cell cycle at metaphase of meiosis II. Mice deficient in MOS are subfertile because their oocytes do not arrest at metaphase II. Their ovaries have cysts, show parthenogenetic activation of eggs, and develop teratomas. After ovulation, the fertilizing sperm induces calcium oscillations that cause cyclin destruction and degradation of MOS, resulting in resumption of meiosis II and extrusion of the second polar body.

ATRESIA

Atresia occurs at all stages of follicular development, spontaneously or in response to environmental factors or drugs.[178] Spontaneous atresia is primarily a reflection of the absence of essential trophic factors at critical times in follicular formation or maturation.[179-180] Apoptotic death is largely responsible for elimination of oocytes as well as granulosa cells; it is most prominent in the germ cells of the fetal ovary and the granulosa cells of the adult ovary.[181] The Fas-Fas ligand system has been implicated as a key mediator of these events.[181-183]

The importance of apoptosis in the control of follicular dynamics is illustrated in the phenotypes of mutant mice. Mice lacking acid sphingomyelinase, an enzyme that produces the proapoptotic signaling molecule ceramide, have an enlarged oocyte reserve and are resistant to oocyte depletion by anticancer drugs and radiation. Fas-deficient mice (lpr/lpr mice) have increased numbers of secondary follicles, reduced numbers of large antral follicles, and defective oocyte and granulosa cell death in response to Fas ligand. The pattern of expression of Fas antigen in the human ovary, with abundant staining in oocytes of atretic primordial and primary follicles and granulosa cells of atretic antral follicles, is consistent with a role for Fas in atresia.[169] In mice lacking the proapoptotic protein Bax, oocyte reserve is augmented due to reduced postnatal apoptosis and defective granulosa cell apoptosis.[184] Conversely, mice lacking the antiapoptotic protein Bcl-2 have a diminished oocyte reserve. The same is true for mice lacking Bcl-w or mice engineered with a hypomorph Bcl-x allele. Mice lacking the death effector enzymes caspase-2, caspase-9, and caspase-11 have enlarged oocyte reserves as a result of attenuated fetal germ cell apoptosis. Caspase-12–deficient mice are resistant to anticancer drug–induced germ cell death. Caspase-3–deficient mice display aberrant atresia as a result of defective granulosa cell apoptosis.

SPONTANEOUS TWINNING

Spontaneous dizygotic twinning, a result of multiple follicular maturation, is associated with elevated FSH levels, is more prevalent in older women, and is also a genetic trait.[185] The highest rate of spontaneous dizygotic twinning has been recorded in the Yoruba people of Nigeria, with an incidence fourfold greater than in white individuals.[186] The genes governing this trait, which presumably control either FSH levels or follicle sensitivity to FSH, have not yet been determined; however, mutations and variants in several obvious candidate genes—including the FSH receptor, the inhibin α subunit, and the BMPRIB receptor—have been excluded from being major contributors to familial dizygotic twinning. Rare mutations and variants in the GDF9 gene have been reported in mothers of dizygotic twins.[185,187-189] A region on chromosome 3 near the peroxisome proliferator–activation receptor γ (PPARγ) has been linked to dizygotic twinning, and the PPARγ locus has been suggested to be the candidate gene.[190] However, this finding has yet to be confirmed.

CORPUS LUTEUM FORMATION AND DEMISE

Initial Stages of Corpus Luteum Formation

After ovulation, the ruptured follicle is reorganized into the corpus luteum. The process of luteinization and formation of a corpus luteum is associated with significant alterations in gene expression, encompassing hundreds of different genes in the granulosa cells alone.[191] A prominent feature of this reorganization is the establishment of a rich vascular network. The hemorrhage into the ovulatory cavity associated with follicular rupture is accompanied by proliferation and penetration of capillaries and fibroblasts from the surrounding stroma. The resulting neovascularization of the developing corpus luteum makes it possible for large blood-borne molecules, such as LDL, which provides cholesterol substrate for progesterone production, to reach the granulosa and theca–lutein cells, and for secretory products to be efficiently transported into the circulation. The development of the corpus luteum blood supply thus parallels progesterone production. By the time the corpus luteum is fully formed, endothelial cells make up approximately 50% of the cellular content.

The vascularization of the corpus luteum is directed by angiogenic factors, including VEGF and basic FGF triggered by LH.[192-194] There is a sixfold rise in VEGF in monkey follicular fluid within 6 hours of an ovulatory stimulus, with sustained elevations in VEGF concentrations lasting up to 36 hours. The granulosa cells appear to be a primary source of VEGF. Because there are no significant changes in VEGF mRNA during this time, the rise in VEGF protein appears to be a consequence of a post-transcriptional mechanism.

Evidence for an important role for VEGF in the development of the corpus luteum vascular network includes the finding that soluble VEGF receptor (FLT-1) administered to gonadotropin-treated rats almost completely suppresses luteal angiogenesis. Moreover, as noted previously, VEGF appears to play an important role in follicular development before the LH surge because inhibition of VEGF by neutralizing antibodies or truncated FLT-1 interrupts preovulatory follicle development. The angiopoietins and the TIE-2 receptor expressed on endothelial cells also appear to contribute to the development and maintenance of the luteal vascular network, based on their spatial and temporal patterns of expression.

The mural granulosa cells undergo significant morphologic changes in response to the LH surge, collectively referred to as luteinization. The mitotic potential of these cells is lost, as reflected in changes in the genes involved in granulosa cell proliferation: cyclin D2 expression is terminated, whereas cell cycle inhibitors p21cip and p21kip are increased.[195] The expression of genes encoding proteins involved in progestin synthesis (including StAR, P450scc, and type 2 3β-hydroxysteroid dehydrogenase) is dramatically increased.

The human steroidogenic cells of the corpus luteum are heterogeneous in size and function.[196-198] Luteinized granulosa and theca cells are both present. These two different cell types have different functional characteristics, as defined by immunohistochemistry and studies of their steroidogenic activity after purification. The granulosa–lutein cells display greater basal production of progesterone and are the presumed sites of luteal estrogen synthesis because they express aromatase. They also stain for the protein hormone relaxin. The theca–lutein cells express 17α-hydroxylase/17-20 lyase activity. These cells presumably produce the androgen precursors that are aromatized by granulosa–lutein cells, and they are probably the main site of luteal 17α-hydroxyprogesterone production. Thus, a two-cell system for estrogen synthesis exists in the corpus luteum as it does in the follicle.

With respect to progesterone production, there are differences in the characteristics of cells of different sizes

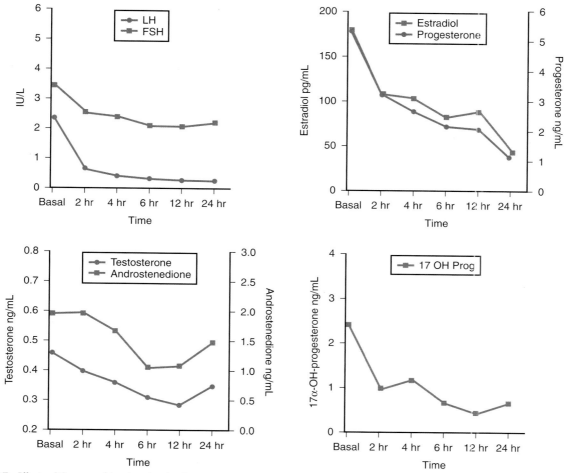

Figure 8-17. *Effects of the gonadotropin-releasing hormone receptor antagonist cetrorelix (2 mg subcutaneously) on function of the midluteal phase corpus luteum. Plasma gonadotropin and steroid concentrations in a woman receiving cetrorelix in the midluteal phase. FSH, follicle-stimulating hormone; LH, luteinizing hormone.*

within the corpus luteum and their in vitro responses to trophic stimulation. These variations have been shown by studies on dispersed cell preparations purified on density gradients.

The Role of Luteinizing Hormone

In addition to inducing ovulation and luteinization, LH has a central role in the maintenance of corpus luteum function. Long-term withdrawal of LH support in a variety of experimental circumstances almost invariably results in luteal regression. Withdrawal of LH during the monkey luteal phase, either by passive immunization or by termination of gonadotropin-releasing hormone (GnRH) infusions in animals dependent on GnRH to drive gonadotropin secretion, leads to a pronounced decline in progesterone and other steroid hormone levels.[199] Administration of a GnRH antagonist to women in the luteal phase also causes a marked fall in peripheral progesterone levels within 6 hours of treatment (Fig. 8-17). In the monkey model, luteal progesterone production is restored when LH levels recover if the LH deprivation has not been prolonged. The trophic role of LH in controlling

luteal progesterone secretion is evident during the human mid- and late luteal phases, when LH secretion is characterized by distinct pulses and a corresponding pulsatile pattern of progesterone secretion is observed.[200]

It is notable that the monkey corpus luteum can be deprived of LH support for several days but can recover its endocrine function when LH is restored, remembering its temporal history and surviving for the usual 14-day duration.[199] This intrinsic memory suggests that the process of luteinization triggers a preprogrammed life cycle that will play out in the absence of conception. The molecular and cellular mechanisms of this clock remain to be elucidated. One hypothesis is that the timekeeping is the result of sequential events that include steroid modulation of infiltration of leukocytes and immune cells that eventually suppress luteal function through the elaboration of cytokines (described later in the section "Luteolysis").

Levels of LH and human chorionic gonadotropin (hCG) receptors in the corpus luteum membranes rise progressively during the human luteal phase and then decline, but remain detectable by binding assays, even in the late luteal phase. This receptor system is evidently fully operational immediately after the endogenous LH surge, because injection of 10,000 IU hCG within the first few days after ovulation does not elicit a substantial increase in progesterone production (Fig. 8-18).[201] However, by the mid- and late luteal phases, the corpora lutea show substantial steroidogenic responses to exogenous hCG. LH and hCG receptor mRNA expression tends to follow the same pattern as LH and hCG binding, with an increase in transcript abundance from the early to midluteal phases and a decline at the time of menses.[202-203] However, LH and hCG receptor transcripts are maintained should pregnancy occur.[204] In the Rhesus monkey, LH receptor mRNA expression is maintained in the late luteal phase and only declines after menstruation.[205-206]

Progesterone as a Luteotropin

The human corpus luteum produces 25 to 50 mg of progesterone daily. The luteal cells also appear to respond to this steroid, so it has both an endocrine and an intracrine role in reproduction. As discussed in the next section, progesterone helps to support luteal function in the Rhesus monkey, and antagonism to progesterone action diminishes hCG-stimulated steroidogenesis by human luteal cells.

Luteolysis

The functional life span of the corpus luteum in a nonfertile cycle is normally 14 ± 2 days. Unless pregnancy occurs, the corpus luteum is transformed into an avascular scar referred to as the *corpus albicans*. Regression of the corpus luteum, known as *luteolysis,* encompasses functional changes (i.e., endocrine changes, most prominently a decline in progesterone production) as well as structural changes (i.e., apoptosis and tissue involution).

Withdrawal of LH and a decline in LH receptors do not account for luteolysis in primates. However, there is a postreceptor loss of LH and hCG signaling efficiency that is reflected by the reduced response of the primate corpus luteum to hCG stimulation.[205-206] This reduced signaling efficiency in the late luteal phase leads to a decline in progesterone production associated with a fall in expression of the *StAR* gene, in terms of both mRNA and protein.[201]

The decline in *StAR* expression precedes a fall in expression of other steroidogenic enzymes. Administration of a large dose of hCG in the late luteal phase restores *StAR* mRNA and protein levels to those found in the midluteal phase and causes a dramatic increase in plasma progesterone levels.[201] Infusion of exponentially increasing doses of LH or hCG also prolongs the life of the monkey corpus luteum.[207] These observations suggest that one important feature of functional luteolysis in the human is a decline in *StAR* expression. High levels of hCG can prevent this decline, maintaining progesterone-producing capacity.

Structural regression of the corpus luteum is brought about by two processes: apoptosis and autophagolysis. Early corpora lutea show no evidence of DNA fragmentation, whereas midluteal and late luteal corpora display DNA fragmentation; the frequency of apoptotic cells is increased in the regressing corpus luteum compared with the midluteal phase. In contrast, the corpora lutea of early pregnancy show no detectable apoptotic DNA fragmentation.

The factors that control cell survival and death in the human corpus luteum remain debatable.[208-215] BCL2, a cell survival factor, has been localized in granulosa–lutein cells, theca–lutein cells, endothelial cells, and blood vessels. Some researchers find no evidence of changes in BCL2 levels during the normal luteal phase or after hCG administration; however, others describe substantial changes with a decline in the late luteal phase. The proapoptotic protein Bax has been reported to remain unchanged throughout the luteal phase—and to increase from low levels in the midluteal phase to high levels in regressing corpora lutea, while being undetectable in corpora lutea of pregnancy. As described later in this section, expression of FAS and FAS ligand increases at the time of luteal regression. The existing data indicate that apoptosis is an important feature of human luteal regression, and some reports describe reciprocal changes in the expression of cell survival (*BCL2*) and proapoptotic (*BAX* and *FAS*) genes; however, morphologic studies strongly suggest that autophagy contributes to luteal regression. These two processes may, of course, coexist in the regressing corpus luteum.

What triggers the diminished sensitivity of the primate corpus luteum to LH and subsequent luteal regression in a nonfertile cycle? Although prostaglandin F2α (PGF2α) is a recognized luteolysin in animals, its role in regulating primate corpus luteum regression is less certain.[209] In vitro, PGF2α reduces gonadotropin-stimulated progesterone secretion by luteinized granulosa cells. PGF2α also suppresses *StAR* expression in cultured human luteal cells. In vivo, infusion of PGF2α transiently reduces progesterone levels during the luteal phase in humans, and intraluteal injection of PGF2α causes a fall in progesterone production and tissue involution. Human corpora lutea in the late luteal phase express higher levels of the receptor for PGF2α and have higher PGF2α contents than in the early luteal phase. Moreover, the inhibitory effects of PGF2α on hCG-stimulated progesterone production are most notable in the late luteal phase. Collectively, these observations speak for a potential role for PGF2α in the initiation of human luteolysis, perhaps in the inhibition of luteal progesterone production. However, this is probably not the only mediator of primate corpus luteum regression.

Figure 8-18. *Effect of human chorionic gonadotropin (hCG) administration on the ovarian steroidogenic response at different stages of the luteal phase. Plasma concentrations of hCG, progesterone (P4), 17α-hydroxyprogesterone (17-OHP), testosterone, and estradiol after an injection of hCG (10,000 IU) in women at varying times in the luteal phase are shown. The area under the curve (AUC) for the 24-hour time course was determined for each steroid at each stage of the luteal phase. Values are mean ± standard error of the mean. (Reprinted from Kohen P, Castro O, Palomino A, et al. The steroidogenic response and corpus luteum expression of the steroidogenic acute regulatory protein after human chorionic gonadotropin administration at different times in the human luteal phase. J Clin Endocrinol Metab 88:3421-3430, 2003, with permission.)*

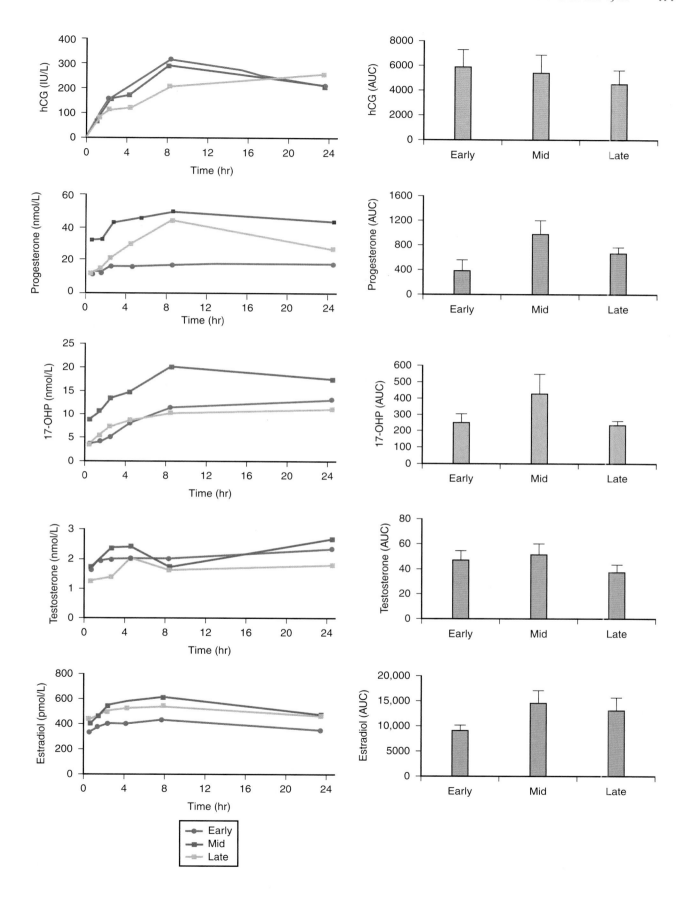

Unlike domestic species, in which PGF2α of uterine origin is involved in triggering luteal regression, hysterectomy in the human has no effect on luteal life span.[209] Thus, if prostanoids are involved in human luteal regression, they are not of uterine origin. The corpus luteum itself may be the source. In the monkey, estrogen promotes luteolysis and also raises PGF2α levels in ovarian blood. The luteolytic action of estrogens is reportedly blocked by indomethacin; however, other researchers have suggested that the luteolytic action of estradiol in the primate is mediated by effects on gonadotropin secretion.

There is good evidence that cytokines of the TNF-α superfamily and interferon γ play roles in human luteolysis.[209] The temporal and spatial expression of *FAS* and *FAS* ligand mRNA and protein is strongly correlated with luteolysis in animal and human corpora lutea. The Fas-Fas ligand system can trigger apoptotic cell death. During the late luteal phase, the expression of FAS protein increases, diminishing only as the structure transitions into a corpus albicans. Mice with a naturally occurring mutation in the Fas ligand gene (*Gld/Gld* mice) show defective luteolysis.

Tumor necrosis factor-α inhibits steroidogenesis by human luteal cells in vitro.[209-210,212] Mice lacking TNFR1, one of the receptors to which TNF-α binds, do not progress through the estrous cycle and remain in permanent diestrus, suggesting a role for TNF-α in luteal regression. TNF-α, derived from macrophages and leukocytes and also possibly endothelial cells, increases in the late luteal phase corpus luteum.[212] TNF-α–producing macrophages and leukocytes accumulate in the late luteal phase and regressing corpora lutea, probably due in part to up-regulation of monocyte chemoattractant protein-1 (MCP-1) derived from endothelial cells.[209,213] Other proinflammatory cytokines produced by leukocytes could also contribute to the inhibition of steroid production. Interferon γ inhibits gonadotropin-stimulated progesterone production by human luteal cells in vitro and also induces cell death. It is another product of macrophages and leukocytes that could contribute to functional and structural luteolysis.

The vascular component of the corpus luteum may contribute to luteal regression through production of factors directly or indirectly involved in the luteolytic mechanism, including TNF-α, endothelin-1, and MCP-1.[209] Effects of luteolytic substances on endothelial cell function, including endothelial cell survival, can affect luteal perfusion. The endothelial cells may also be a target of PGF2α, and their role in the luteolytic process, best exemplified by studies in domestic species, has yet to be comprehensively evaluated in the human corpus luteum.

Reactive oxygen species produced by leukocytes infiltrating the corpus luteum are another potentially important factor in luteolysis.[209,215] Immunosuppressive levels of dexamethasone block luteolysis in a rat model. Both human and rat luteal cells respond to H_2O_2 with a rapid reduction in progesterone secretion and gonadotropin responsiveness. The action of H_2O_2 appears to be mediated by OH^-, which inhibits protein synthesis, depletes ATP, and induces DNA damage. The LH receptor also is uncoupled from adenylate cyclase by H_2O_2, and there is impaired mitochondrial use of cholesterol for steroidogenesis.

RESCUE OF THE CORPUS LUTEUM IN THE CYCLE OF CONCEPTION

In a cycle of conception, the human corpus luteum is rescued from luteolysis by the appearance of trophoblast-derived hCG.[216] In the corpus luteum of late pregnancy, hCG suppresses apoptosis, with a lesser effect on autophagy, allowing structural maintenance of the gland and sustaining expression of the *StAR* gene.[217] The progressively rising concentrations of this luteotropin, first detectable in peripheral blood 8 days after ovulation, both stimulates steroidogenesis and prevents structural involution of the gland, which is the major source of progesterone for the first 10 weeks of gestation. The corpus luteum doubles in volume during the first 6 weeks of gestation as a result of hypertrophy of the luteinized granulosa and theca cells and accumulation of connective tissue and nonsteroidogenic cells, particularly endothelial cells.[208] Experimentally, a protocol of ever-increasing doses of hCG rescues both the human and monkey corpus luteum. Recent observations suggest that hCG stimulates luteal 11β-hydroxysteroid dehydrogenase type 1 expression, resulting in increased intraluteal generation of cortisol, which is proposed to act through the lutein cell glucocorticoid receptor to promote corpus luteum survival in the cycle of conception.[218]

The corpus luteum is essential for the first few weeks of pregnancy, and luteectomy results in miscarriage if performed before 7 weeks of gestation. Its secretory function, however, is not sustained at high levels throughout gestation, despite the presence of hCG. This characteristic has been documented by monitoring levels of 17α-hydroxyprogesterone, a steroid that is not produced by the placenta and therefore largely reflects corpus luteum function. Levels of 17α-hydroxyprogesterone rise to peak concentrations at 6 weeks of pregnancy and then decline. Part of the decline in steroidogenic activity is due to the fact that the early hypertrophy of the corpus luteum is later followed by shrinkage. The biochemical changes underlying the functional and structural changes in the corpus luteum of pregnancy have not been elucidated.

The corpus luteum of pregnancy also secretes protein hormones, including inhibin A and relaxin. Relaxin may function to promote the decidualization of the endometrium and suppress uterine smooth muscle contractile activity.

The Gonadotropins and Ovarian Function

FOLLICLE-STIMULATING HORMONE

Follicle-stimulating hormone is required for the transition of secondary preantral follicles to the antral stage. It also is a survival factor for antral follicles, and its withdrawal triggers programmed cell death in the absence of local factors that sensitize the follicle to FSH action or amplify its effects.[219-220] Follicular maturation initiated at the start of a new menstrual cycle is driven by an increase in FSH levels in the late luteal phase as progesterone, estradiol, and inhibin A levels fall. Preantral follicles apparently require a threshold FSH concentration to sustain growth, and this threshold level is reached during the late luteal phase. Remarkably, the threshold can be crossed with as little as a 10% to 30% increment in FSH, indicating that granulosa cells have a highly sensitive, but still mysterious, detection system with which they interpret circulating FSH levels. FSH can induce follicular growth to the preovulatory size of at least 17 mm in the virtual absence of LH. Although estradiol production is severely impaired under these circumstances, inhibin production is induced—reflecting the normal response of granulosa cells to FSH.

Granulosa cell division is promoted by FSH, possibly by an indirect mechanism. This action is mediated by growth factors produced by either somatic cells or the oocyte. For example, in rodents, estrogens produced in response to FSH are an important mitogen for granulosa cells. FSH also increases the number of gap junctions as well as the amount of junctional membrane between granulosa cells. An early sign that a dominant follicle has been selected is that its granulosa cells proliferate at a greater rate than the cells in the nondominant follicles. The differential mitotic rates can be detected in the late follicular phase.

One of the major actions of FSH is the induction of aromatase in granulosa cells (see Fig. 8-8). Thus, little or no estrogen can be produced by FSH-unprimed granulosa cells, even if they are supplied with aromatizable androgen precursors. FSH also induces expression of cytochrome P450 reductase, which transfers electrons to aromatase, and by type 1 17β-hydroxysteroid dehydrogenase, the "estrogenic" 17β-hydroxysteroid dehydrogenase that reduces estrone to estradiol.

In vivo studies in rodents have shown that FSH increases the number of its cognate receptors in the granulosa cells. In rodents, estrogens act synergistically with FSH in this regard, resulting in a feed-forward system that augments FSH responsiveness. However, a similar feed-forward mechanism has yet to be demonstrated in primate follicle development.

Follicle-stimulating hormone induces LH receptors in the granulosa cells of the preovulatory follicle. Consequently, in the late stages of follicular maturation, LH can subserve FSH's function in propelling follicular maturation.[144] This attribute may allow the dominant follicle to complete its maturation cycle in the face of declining FSH levels; in addition, the dominant follicle is prepared to respond to the ovulatory LH surge.

The FSH receptor is a seven-transmembrane, G-protein–coupled receptor encoded by a single gene located on chromosome 2p21.[221] The primary signal transduction cascade initiated by the FSH receptor involves cAMP. However, increases in cAMP alone evidently cannot replicate all actions of FSH on granulosa cell function, and alternate signaling pathways are likely activated by the FSH receptor (either directly or indirectly), including MAP kinases and protein kinase B.[222-225] FSH receptor variants that activate calcium and protein kinase C signal transduction systems have been identified in the ovary by some authors. The variants contain the extracellular FSH-binding domain of the receptor coupled to a single-pass growth factor–type membrane-spanning domain. However, their existence in

the human ovary has not yet been verified, and their specific roles in FSH signaling have yet to be defined.

The importance of FSH in follicular development has been documented by the discovery of mutations that inactivate the FSH β subunit and the FSH receptor in humans, and by targeted deletions of these genes in mice.[226-227] Women who are homozygous for FSH receptor mutations have the features of hypergonadotropic hypogonadism, with absent or poor development of secondary sexual characteristics and high FSH and LH levels. The ovarian phenotypes of humans with these mutations and those of FSH receptor and FSH β subunit knockout mice are remarkably consistent. In the absence of functional FSH β subunit or FSH receptor, the ovaries are small and follicular development generally goes no further than the preantral stage. The genotype–phenotype correlation in humans with FSH receptor mutations is mirrored by the mouse knockout model, in which haploinsufficiency of the FSH receptor accelerates loss of oocytes and results in premature reproductive senescence.

Mutations in the transmembrane helices of the FSH receptor and the extracellular domain cause spontaneous ovarian hyperstimulation syndrome in which the ovaries respond excessively to hCG.[228] Mutations in the transmembrane helices result in ligand promiscuity, allowing the receptor to respond to hCG and TSH, whereas mutations in the extracellular domain (S128Y) display increased specificity and sensitivity to hCG, but not to TSH.

LUTEINIZING HORMONE

In the follicular phase of the ovarian cycle, LH stimulates thecal cell steroidogenesis, which provides the androgen substrate for granulosa cell aromatization (see Fig. 8-8). As noted previously, LH is not needed for follicular expansion because exogenous purified FSH can drive follicular growth to the preovulatory stage, when LH is undetectable or markedly suppressed by pharmacologic means (i.e., GnRH agonists or antagonists).

In a normal menstrual cycle, the FSH-induced appearance of LH receptors on preovulatory granulosa cells allows LH to take over FSH's functions in the terminal stages of follicular maturation. These receptors also enable the granulosa cells to become competent to respond to the LH surge that initiates the resumption of meiosis, ovulation, and subsequent luteinization of the granulosa and theca cells. These events are triggered only when a threshold concentration of LH is achieved and not before that time. Notably, granulosa cells respond to FSH with activation of adenylate cyclase, but genes or events that constitute the program for ovulation and luteinization are not induced. The necessity for some LH to stimulate thecal androgen production and synergize with FSH for follicular maturation, together with the potential for high levels of LH to promote premature luteinization and possibly atresia of follicles that have not reached the Graafian stage, has led to the notion of an "LH window" for follicular maturation. This concept has pharmacologic and clinical relevance with respect to ovulation induction.[229] Levels of LH that are capable of stimulating maturation of the dominant follicle[144] retard the growth of smaller follicles and suppress aromatase activity. This effect has led to the theoretical possibility of minimizing multifollicular development using LH or hCG to drive terminal stages of follicular maturation.[230]

The threshold for activation of the ovulation–luteinization program may be sensed by granulosa and theca cells as a result of the intensity of the signal (i.e., the magnitude of the increase in cAMP); it may also be sensed by the activation of adjunctive signal transduction cascades that supplement the increase in cAMP (e.g., phospholipase C, MAP kinase signaling, protein kinase C, and calcium signaling). There is evidence that FSH and LH receptors differentially activate signal transduction cascades. Moreover, LH receptor activation of cAMP and IP3 signaling are dependent on LH dose, with a 10- to 100-fold higher level of LH needed to activate phospholipase C. After ovulation, LH is essential for the maintenance of corpus luteum function, as previously discussed.

The LH receptor is a seven-transmembrane domain, G-protein–coupled receptor encoded by a gene on chromosome 2p21, near the gene encoding the FSH receptor.[231] Like the FSH receptor, its primary signaling intermediary is cAMP, but as noted previously, other signal transduction pathways can be activated, either directly or indirectly. There are multiple splice variants of the LH receptor transcript, and their abundance tends to change in parallel. The physiologic significance of the different receptor isoforms encoded by the splice variants with respect to human luteal function has not been determined.

Luteinizing hormone receptor knockout mice have a relatively normal theca layer around developing follicles.[217] However, follicular maturation is arrested at the early antral stage, and there are no signs of ovulation or luteinization. This phenotype is similar to that found in women with homozygous inactivating mutations in the LH receptor gene. The clinical phenotype of affected women includes normal primary and secondary sexual characteristics, amenorrhea, and elevated circulating FSH and LH. The ovaries contain follicles in stages of development from primordial to antral, with well-developed theca layers, but no preovulatory follicles or corpora lutea. This phenotype supports the notion that LH is required for normal estrogen production by follicles, for ovulation, and for luteinization, but not for the formation of the theca layer.

Activating mutations of the human LH receptor are also informative regarding the role of LH in ovarian function.[232] Women with these mutations have no obvious reproductive phenotype, in contrast to the precocious puberty found in men. One might have anticipated a hyperandrogenemic state in females, mimicking PCOS with thecal hyperplasia. However, follicular compartments evidently develop in a coordinated fashion such that thecal responses to LH receptor activation do not occur prematurely. Moreover, levels of cAMP or other second-messenger molecules required for luteinization must be different from those generated by the constitutively active mutant receptor because premature luteinization of follicles does not occur.

PROLACTIN

Prolactin is an important luteotropin in rodents.[233] Although prolactin receptors are present in the human ovary, this hormone appears to have minimal effects on primate ovarian function when it is present in the physiologic range.[234] High concentrations of prolactin inhibit trophic hormone–stimulated progestin production by human luteinized granulosa cells in vitro. This is undoubtedly a minor action of prolactin with respect to the reproductive disturbances associated with excessive prolactin levels (see Chapter 3).

Endocrine Activity of the Ovary in Reproductive Life

STEROIDOGENESIS

Compared with the fetal testis, the human fetal ovary is generally believed to be steroidogenically quiescent, although cholesterol side-chain cleavage activity and 17α-hydroxylase/17, 20-desmolase activities are detectable. Even though follicles are present in the fetal and infant ovary, their steroidogenic capacity becomes evident only at puberty.

Estrogen Biosynthesis

The biosynthesis of estrogens requires cooperation between granulosa cells and their adjacent thecal neighbors (see Fig. 8-8). The requirement for these two cell types, and for their respective main gonadotropins (FSH and LH), has been formulated into the two-cell–two-gonadotropin model of ovarian estrogen biosynthesis. Thecal androgen production stimulated by LH yields the substrate for FSH-dependent aromatase in granulosa cells.

Studies of isolated granulosa cells have shown that FSH, but not LH, stimulates estrogen production when the cells are provided with an aromatizable substrate.[235] In contrast, isolated human theca cells do not produce substantial amounts of estrogens, but instead secrete dehydroepiandrosterone, androstenedione, and smaller amounts of testosterone when adenylate cyclase activity is stimulated. The aromatase activity of granulosa cells is estimated to be at least 700 times greater in the granulosa cells of large preovulatory follicles than in theca cells, arguing strongly for the cellular compartmentalization of estrogen synthesis outlined in the two-cell–two-gonadotropin model.

Androgen Biosynthesis

Studies of isolated human theca cells showed that the thecal layer is the major source of follicular androgens (see Fig. 8-8). The theca layer expresses STAR, P450SCC, P450C17, and type 2 3β-hydroxysteroid dehydrogenase, all under the regulation of LH. In contrast, androgen production by isolated cultured human granulosa cells is negligible, with or without added gonadotropins.

Progesterone Biosynthesis

The granulosa cell, like the theca–interstitial cell, is well prepared for progestin biosynthesis after the LH surge. This surge triggers expression of the genes encoding STAR, P450SCC, and type 2 3β-hydroxysteroid dehydrogenase, the triad of proteins required for efficient synthesis of progesterone (see Chapter 4).

PROTEIN HORMONES OF OVARIAN ORIGIN

Inhibin

Inhibin is a member of the TGF-β protein superfamily. It is a heterodimeric 32-kDa glycoprotein composed of two subunits, α (18 kDa) and β (12 kDa), linked by disulfide bonds. There is a common α subunit, but there are different β subunits, denoted β_A and β_B. The $\alpha\beta_A$ and $\alpha\beta_B$ heterodimers are named inhibin A and B, respectively. Although inhibin is produced by a number of tissues, the major site of production is the gonad. In the ovary, the primary source of inhibin is granulosa cells. The main endocrine role for inhibin, for which it was discovered and named, is to suppress pituitary FSH production.[236-237] In vitro, it augments LH- and IGF-stimulated androgen production by theca cells.

Although both isoforms of inhibin seem to have similar biologic properties, their synthesis is regulated differently during the follicular and luteal phases. Inhibin B is secreted mainly during the early follicular phase, with levels decreasing in the midfollicular phase and becoming undetectable after the LH surge. Concentrations of inhibin A are low during the first half of the follicular phase, but increase during the midfollicular phase and peak during the luteal phase.

The secretion of inhibin A is regulated by gonadotropins, but production of inhibin B evidently is not. This differential regulation of inhibin A and B production was exemplified in measurements made on follicles of different sizes that showed that inhibin A was present in follicles down to a size of 6 mm, with levels increasing with increased follicular size.[124] In contrast, inhibin B levels showed no relationship to follicle size or maturation state.

Relaxin and Relaxin-like Factors

Relaxin, a hormone that may play a role in facilitating decidualization of the endometrium and suppression of myometrial contractile activity, is produced by the large luteal cells of the corpus luteum.[238] Immunohistochemical studies show progressive accumulation from the early to late luteal phases, with corpora lutea in the late luteal phase containing the most intensely stained cells. The highest circulating levels of relaxin are achieved in the first trimester, and levels then decrease by approximately 20% and remain constant throughout pregnancy.

INSL3 (previously called *relaxin-like factor*) is produced by the theca interna and acts on the LGR8 G-protein–coupled receptor of the oocyte to suppress cAMP production. INSL3 is also expressed in the corpus luteum and ovarian stroma.[239]

Intraovarian Regulators

The growth of follicles and the function of the corpus luteum, although under the primary direction of the pituitary, are highly influenced by intraovarian factors that modulate the action of gonadotropins. These intraovarian factors most likely account for gonadotropin-independent follicular growth, observed differences in the rate and extent of development of ovarian follicles, arrest and initiation of meiosis, dominant follicle selection, and luteolysis. The intraovarian regulators include steroid hormones, growth factors, and cytokines, the latter produced by ovarian cells, endothelial cells, and resident macrophages and leukocytes. Several intraovarian regulators are believed to act in concert to modulate the growth and function of the ovarian compartments, either in their own right or as amplifiers or attenuators of gonadotropin action. These intraovarian regulators participate in paracrine communication, in which regulators produced by one cell act on other local target cells, and in autocrine communication, which involves the action of the regulator on its cell of origin.

Minimal criteria have been proposed to qualify a molecule as an intraovarian regulator. The criteria include local production, local reception, and local action. Finally, there should be evidence of physiologic importance with respect to ovarian function in vivo. Although a number of molecules meet the former criteria, much remains to be learned about the physiologic importance of specific intraovarian regulatory pathways. This task is challenging because these pathways may be redundant or modulatory, so a dramatic phenotype may not emerge from perturbation of a particular intraovarian regulatory system. Moreover, the usual gene targeting approaches may not be revealing and conditional knockouts may be needed to disclose the specific roles of these molecules.

OOCYTE-DERIVED FACTORS

Growth Differentiation Factor-9

Growth differentiation factor-9, a member of the TGF-β superfamily, is highly expressed by oocytes and, to a lesser extent, by primate granulosa cells. The follicles of GDF-9–deficient mice arrest in growth at the primary stage, yet the oocytes continue to grow at a faster rate than wild-type oocytes, progressing to advanced stages of differentiation seen in the antral follicles of normal mice. However, there are ultrastructural abnormalities in the interconnections between granulosa cells and oocytes; the oocytes ultimately die, leaving a ribbon of zona pellucida behind. The theca also does not form around the follicles, implicating GDF-9 in the organization or proliferation of this follicular component. Studies in the rat also indicate that GDF-9 stimulates the growth of primary follicles, consistent with the block to progression at the primary stage in GDF-9–deficient mice.[240]

In vitro, GDF-9 has a variety of effects on granulosa cells and theca cells that are species-specific, acting at least in part through interaction with the ALK5 (TGF-βRI) and BMP receptor type 2 (BMPRII) receptor complex.[241] In rodents, GDF-9 stimulates granulosa cell differentiation, including induction of LH receptors and steroidogenesis. In cumulus cells, GDF-9 promotes expression of hyaluronan synthase 2, pentraxin 3, and *TNFAIP6*, genes that encode proteins incorporated into the proteoglycan extracellular matrix of the cumulus oophorus complex and follicular fluid. It also suppresses urokinase expression while stimulating COX-2 and prostaglandin synthesis and progesterone formation.[242-243] LH receptor expression is suppressed, which would discourage luteinization of the cumulus cells.

These actions of GDF-9 give a unique phenotype to the granulosa cells surrounding the oocyte, which would be exposed to the highest GDF-9 concentrations. GDF-9 inhibits human granulosa–lutein and theca cell steroidogenesis in vitro, with the inhibitory effect on theca cells being more pronounced.[244] It also stimulates theca cell proliferation, a finding consonant with the apparent role of GDF-9 in the murine ovary in controlling thecal development.

Bone Morphogenetic Protein-15

Bone morphogenetic protein-15, also known as GDF-9b, encoded by a gene on the X chromosome, is another member of the TGF-β superfamily produced by oocytes.[245] It is related structurally to GDF-9 and shares a similar pattern of expression. Targeted deletion of the murine *Bmp15* gene causes a modest ovarian phenotype in nullizygous animals of subfertility with diminished ovulation and fertilization rates. However, mice nullizygous for *Bmp15* and heterozygous for a *Gdf9* mutation have severely impaired fertility, with abnormalities in folliculogenesis and cumulus cell function. Spontaneous point mutations in the ovine *Bmp15* gene (Inverdale and Hanna sheep) result in phenotypes that differ from those in *Bmp15* knockout mice.[246] In the heterozygous state, the number of follicles ovulating is increased, and thus there is an increase in fecundity. However, primary ovarian failure, with a phenotype resembling the murine *Gdf9* knockout, is observed in ewes homozygous for the mutations. In vitro, BMP-15 stimulates granulosa cell mitosis. Thus, its absence in vivo would be predicted to impair follicular growth, which is consistent with the ovarian abnormalities in homozygous mutant sheep.

In Booroola sheep, a point mutation in the BMPR1B (activin-like receptor kinase, or ALK6) receptor for BMP-15 is associated with an additive increase in ovulation rate, based on the copy number of mutant alleles. As with GDF-9, BMPRII is part of the BMP-15 receptor complex.[241] It is not known whether this point mutation activates, inactivates, or changes the specificity of the receptor. Targeted deletion of the homologous gene in mice does not affect follicular development, but it does yield an infertility phenotype as a result of defects in cumulus cell expansion that prevent in vivo fertilization. Mutations in the human homologues of the *GDF9*, *BMP15,* and *BMP1R* genes have yet to be identified and linked to alterations in ovarian function.

Both BMP-15 and kit ligand participate in a negative feedback loop: BMP-15 stimulates kit ligand expression by granulosa cells, whereas kit ligand inhibits BMP-15 expression in oocytes. In the presence of an oocyte, both BMP-15 and kit ligand stimulate granulosa cell mitosis. The observations that only the oocyte expresses kit, the kit ligand receptor, and that kit ligand suppresses expression of BMP-15, a granulosa cell mitogen, suggest that the oocyte must be involved in producing another granulosa cell mitogen.

Both GDF-9 and BMP-15 are synthesized as proproteins that form dimers and are then proteolytically processed to yield the bioactive molecules. There is evidence that GDF-9 and BMP-15 can form heterodimers and that processing of the heterodimers is impaired.[247] Notably, the Inverdale mutation that inactivates BMP-15 dramatically impairs the proteolytic processing of both the mutant BMP-15 and wild-type GDF-9 in coexpressing cells. This observation suggests that the phenotype of the Inverdale sheep may be the result, at least in part, of GDF-9 deficiency due to interference by mutant BMP-15 with wild-type GDF-9 processing. Oocyte-derived basic FGF, a factor that is not oocyte-specific, also is believed to play an important role in orchestrating follicular development, as discussed later.

STEROID HORMONES AND REGULATION OF OVARIAN FUNCTION

Role for Cholesterol Precursors

A family of C29 4,4-dimethylsterol intermediates in the cholesterol biosynthetic pathway from lanosterol has been found to induce oocytes to resume meiosis.[248] One of these sterols, 4,4-dimethyl-5α-cholest-8,14,24-triene-3β-ol, was extracted from human follicular fluid and named follicular fluid meiosis–activating substance (FF-MAS). A related compound, 4,4-dimethyl-5α-cholest-8,24-diene-3β-ol, was isolated from bull testis and called T-MAS. These compounds are synthesized from lanosterol by P450 14α-demethylase, which is encoded by the *CYP51* gene. FF-MAS and T-MAS are present in micromolar concentrations in preovulatory follicle follicular fluid: 1.6 μM for FF-MAS and about half that for T-MAS.

The accumulation of FF-MAS and T-MAS in mature follicles may be the result of increased synthesis as well as inhibition of cholesterol synthesis at steps beyond the formation of FF-MAS and T-MAS. Gonadotropins have been reported to cause a several-fold increase in *Cyp51* gene expression in rodent ovaries, which could contribute to enhanced MAS formation.[249] Additionally, progestins at concentrations found in follicular fluid in the preovulatory period block cholesterol synthesis at late steps, which would result in an accumulation of FF-MAS and T-MAS.

When perfused into rodent ovaries, FF-MAS can induce maturation of cumulus cell–deprived oocytes or oocyte maturation. However, experiments using various inhibitors of sterol synthesis—including drugs that block 14α-demethylase and those that inhibit enzymes that metabolize MAS—have yielded conflicting results. Inhibitors of 14α-demethylase block gonadotropin-stimulated, but not spontaneous, meiosis in rodents, whereas drugs that block MAS metabolism generally result in germinal vesicle breakdown of cumulus-enclosed oocytes. Consequently, the physiologic roles of FF-MAS and T-MAS in oocyte maturation, if any, remain uncertain. The pharmacologic value of FF-MAS and T-MAS also is uncertain. Some, but not all, studies on in vitro oocyte maturation suggest effects of these compounds on maturation by stimulating progression to metaphase II or increasing the survival of oocytes without affecting maturation.

Role of Estrogens

In addition to their systemic effects on the reproductive tract, hypothalamus, and pituitary, estrogens have important actions on granulosa, theca, and luteal cells in the ovaries of laboratory animals and domestic species. There are conflicting reports in the literature regarding the expression of estrogen receptor α and β in the primate ovary.[250] The most convincing of these studies indicates that both estrogen receptor α and estrogen receptor β are expressed by the surface epithelium, granulosa cells (with estrogen receptor β predominating over estrogen receptor α in medium-sized and preovulatory follicles), theca cells, and luteinized granulosa cells.

Estrogen receptor α transcripts also have been detected by polymerase chain reaction (PCR) in human oocytes by some authors, but these findings have not been confirmed by others. Although there are differences among the various reports that probably reflect the sensitivity of the method of detection of estrogen receptor expression (i.e., reverse transcriptase PCR, Northern blotting, Western blotting, immunohistochemistry), and in the case of immunochemical methods, the specific antibodies employed, the existing data support the notion that the ovary is a site of estrogen action via the classic receptor-mediated signaling pathways.

The physiologic roles of estrogen within the primate ovary are matters of current debate, as are the mechanisms by which they might influence cellular function (i.e., genomic versus nongenomic actions), given the very high concentrations achieved during follicular maturation and corpus luteum function.[250] Indeed, the extremely high levels of estradiol reached in the antrum of the preovulatory follicle (approximately 1 μg/mL) raise serious questions as to the function of the classic estrogen receptor system, which would be fully saturated by ligand during the later stages of follicular maturation.

In animal granulosa cells, estrogens have pleiotropic actions. They promote proliferation and exert antiatretic effects. Estrogens augment intercellular gap junction and antrum formation, and they also increase the estrogen receptor content of granulosa cells. Estrogens synergize with gonadotropins at several levels, including the promotion of ovarian growth, LH and FSH receptor expression, and the augmentation of aromatase activity.

Insight into the importance of estrogens in ovarian function in women comes from the study of subjects in whom estrogen synthesis is impaired. Limited studies have been performed on women with 17α-hydroxylase/17-20 desmolase deficiency who are incapable of producing thecal androgens to support granulosa cell estradiol synthesis. Promotion of follicular growth to the preovulatory stage in an estrogen-impoverished environment is possible in these individuals with exogenous gonadotropins after pituitary desensitization. The same is true in severely hypogonadotropic women given exogenous FSH. Follicles grow, but in the absence of exogenous LH, estradiol synthesis is minimal. Moreover, the development of follicular cysts with low estrogen levels is common in women with STAR, 17α-hydroxylase/17-20 desmolase, and aromatase deficiency.[251] Hence, one can conclude that the high levels of estrogen associated with normal follicular maturation are not required for the growth of follicles to the size equivalent to the preovulatory stage.

Whether the oocytes that are recovered from such follicles are endowed with the properties that will lead to successful embryonic development after fertilization is less certain. Successful in vitro fertilization of oocytes recovered from estrogen-poor follicles of a woman with 17α-hydroxylase-17/20 desmolase deficiency has been described, with the formation of cleavage-stage embryos, but a pregnancy was not achieved after embryo transfer.

There are pharmacologic data suggesting that estrogens are important for oocyte function.[252] Monkeys treated during follicular maturation with doses of an aromatase inhibitor that substantially reduces circulating estradiol levels showed no effects on follicular growth. A greater proportion of the oocytes recovered from follicles of the aromatase-treated animals were in prophase I, however, and there was retarded completion of maturation to MII. Whether this is a direct reflection of estradiol deficiency, a consequence of the aromatase inhibitor (1,4,6-androstatrien-3,17-dione), or the result of compensatory changes in endocrine status due to the decline in estradiol is not known. The implication of these observations for ovulation induction in women using aromatase inhibitors is not clear.

In vitro studies on primate granulosa cells have yielded inconsistent findings with respect to the actions of estrogens. Estradiol inhibits progesterone secretion by Rhesus monkey granulosa cells, whereas in marmoset granulosa cells, it has no effect on progesterone production, but stimulates aromatase when added in the presence of IGF-I. As discussed previously, exogenous estrogen exerts a luteolytic effect in the primate corpus luteum, probably through actions on the central nervous system.

In summary, although the primate ovary expresses the receptors that allow a variety of cells to respond to estradiol, the physiologic significance of estrogen in follicular maturation and luteal function in the primate ovary is still unknown. Evidently, follicle growth per se does not require high levels of estradiol, but the orchestration of events that result in a mature oocyte capable of developing into a viable embryo after fertilization may require estrogen action on either the granulosa cells or the oocyte.

Role of Androgens

In addition to serving as substrates for estrogen production, androgens have a number of effects on the primate ovary.[253-255] Administration of testosterone or 5α-dihydrotestosterone to Rhesus monkeys promotes accumulation of primary follicles as well as follicle survival, suggesting a folliculotropic action. In this model, androgen receptors are abundant in the granulosa cells of healthy preantral and antral follicles, with lesser expression in the theca and stroma. Moreover, androgen receptors were positively correlated with a marker of cell proliferation (Ki-67) and negatively correlated with apoptosis. These observations contrast with the view that androgens are atretogenic, a concept that emerged primarily from studies on the rodent ovary in which androgens block granulosa cell proliferation in vitro in some systems and promote follicular atresia. For example, in the absence of gonadotropins, androgens provoke follicular atresia and antagonize estrogen-associated ovarian weight increases in hypophysectomized immature rats. Similarly, treatment with

5α-dihydrotestosterone abolishes the ability of FSH to induce LH receptors in granulosa cells and inhibits granulosa cell proliferation.[256]

Studies in the marmoset indicated stage-dependent effects of androgens on granulosa cell function in vitro.[257] Androgen enhanced FSH-stimulated aromatase expression and progesterone production while inhibiting hCG-stimulated aromatase activity and progestin synthesis in cells from large preovulatory follicles. Evidence that androgens have a detrimental effect on human follicular function includes the observation that follicular fluid enriched in 5α-dihydrotestosterone and poor in estradiol is characteristic of atresia. However, this steroid profile may be a consequence rather than a cause of atresia. Favoring a causal relationship are reports that high follicular concentrations of 5α-reduced androgens, such as 5α-dihydrotestosterone, act as competitive inhibitors of granulosa cell aromatase activity.[258] In this regard, follicles from patients with PCOS have greater 5α-reductase activity than follicles from normal ovaries. Thus, androgens may exert both positive and negative effects on follicular growth and function in a stage-dependent manner through androgen receptors as well as by non–receptor-mediated mechanisms.

Role of Progesterone

Progesterone production by the preovulatory follicle is required for ovulation, as discussed previously. It also may have a role in regulating corpus luteum function. Pharmacologic blockade of ovarian progesterone production with a 3β-hydroxysteroid dehydrogenase inhibitor indicated that progesterone exerts antiapoptotic and prodifferentiation effects on luteinizing cells and maintains luteal function. The progesterone receptor antagonists mifepristone and HRP2000 inhibit hCG-stimulated progesterone and relaxin secretion by human granulosa–lutein cells.[259] Progesterone receptors, both the A and B forms, are present in the Rhesus monkey and human corpus luteum, with progesterone receptor mRNA increasing from the early to the midluteal phase. The ratio of progesterone receptor B to progesterone receptor A increases from the early to the late luteal phase. The action of progesterone receptor antagonists on lutein cell steroidogenesis is presumably a reflection of altered transcription regulated by these nuclear receptors.

THE INSULIN-LIKE GROWTH FACTORS

The IGFs are members of a family of low–molecular-weight, single-chain polypeptide growth factors named for their structural and functional similarity to insulin (Fig. 8-19).[260] Both IGF-1 and IGF-2 are present in human follicular fluid.[261-263] Follicular fluid IGF-1 is most likely derived predominantly from plasma. IGF-2, however, is produced by the theca and perifollicular vessels of all follicles and the granulosa and theca cells of small antral follicles, and is abundantly expressed by preovulatory granulosa cells.[264] In mice lacking IGF-1, follicular maturation is arrested; in addition, the animals are infertile, and granulosa cell proliferation in the basal state and in response to estrogen is impaired.[265] In women with Laron dwarfism, a disease characterized by IGF-1 deficiency, ovulation

induction with human menopausal gonadotropins after administration of a GnRH analog resulted in development of mature follicles and fertilizable oocytes. This finding indicates that, in the human, IGF-1 is not essential for normal follicular development. IGF-2, however, would be present in this situation.

In situ hybridization studies showed that IGF-1 receptors, which are activated by both IGF-1 and IGF-2, are present in the granulosa cells of dominant follicles. IGF-2 receptors, which probably are not involved in signaling, are found in theca and granulosa cells. IGF-1 and IGF-2 stimulate DNA synthesis, granulosa cell proliferation, and estradiol secretion by cultured human granulosa and granulosa–lutein cells. IGFs stimulate progesterone secretion by cultured cells, in part by increasing *StAR* gene expression. However, these in vitro experiments have been conducted in restricted culture medium, so the addition of general trophic factors might be expected to increase cellular function. Indeed, infusion of IGF-1 at levels that raise blood concentrations twofold above normal have no effect on ovarian function in Rhesus monkeys.[266] Thus, the locally produced IGFs appear to be sufficient to promote normal ovarian activity, and elevated IGF levels do not disrupt ovarian function.

The action of IGFs is modulated by the local elaboration of binding proteins. Of the six IGF-binding proteins (IGFBPs) that have been described to date, five are expressed in the human ovary. The IGFBPs bind IGFs and neutralize their activity, and they also may have direct actions on ovarian cells. IGFBP-1, -2, -3, -4, and -5 have been identified either in follicular fluid or by analysis of mRNA from granulosa cells. Of these binding proteins, IGFBP-4 is of particular interest because it is a potent antagonist of FSH-stimulated estradiol production by human granulosa cells. IGFBP-4 also is present in atretic follicles, implicating this protein in the pathway leading to follicular atresia.

Secretion of IGFBPs is inhibited by gonadotropins and IGFs, resulting in enhanced IGF bioavailability and

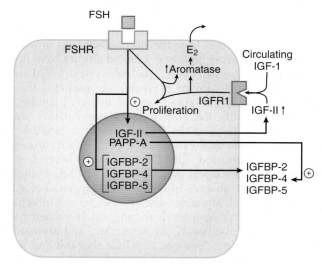

Figure 8-19. *Intraovarian role of insulin-like growth factors (IGFs) and IGF-binding proteins (IGFBPs) in regulating granulosa cell function. E₂, estradiol; FSH, follicle-stimulating hormone; FSHR, follicle-stimulating hormone receptor; IGFR1, IGF receptor type 1; PAPP-A, pregnancy-associated plasma protein-A.*

gonadotropin action. The proteolytic cleavage of IGFBPs is another mechanism controlling IGF bioavailability. IGFBP-4 protease expression is restricted to healthy follicles and corpora lutea.[267] A metalloproteinase activity contained in pregnancy-associated plasma protein A (PAPP-A), a large dimeric glycoprotein, degrades IGFBP-4 into inactive fragments. Granulosa cells from small follicles secrete low levels of PAPP-A, whereas granulosa cells from dominant follicles secrete high levels of this protein.

TGF-β SUPERFAMILY

The TGF-β superfamily includes TGF-β molecules, MIS (also known as *anti-müllerian hormone* [AMH]) activins, inhibins, BMP-2, BMP-4, BMP-5, BMP-6, and BMP-7, and the previously described oocyte-derived proteins GDF-9 and BMP-15.[241,268] These proteins are elaborated by all ovarian cell types, including the stroma and theca cells (BMP-4, BMP-7), granulosa cells (activin, inhibin, TGF-β, AMH, BMP-6) and the oocyte (TFGβ, GDF-9, BMP-15). These molecules act in autocrine and paracrine loops to integrate follicular growth and endocrine activity.

Inhibin and Activin

Although inhibin is a secretory product of the ovary, it also has intraovarian roles.[269-271] It augments LH- and IGF-stimulated androgen production by theca cells, as noted previously. Activin, composed of dimers of the β subunits of inhibin ($\beta_A\beta_B$, $\beta_A\beta_A$, or $\beta_B\beta_B$), was named because it stimulates FSH secretion by cultured pituitary cells. Almost all immunoreactive activin in human serum is bound to proteins (primarily follistatin) and is therefore inactive. Activin A levels are highest during midcycle and the late luteal phase/early follicular phase and are substantially higher in pregnancy. In follicular aspirates, activin A concentrations do not correlate with follicle size or maturity. Because inhibin A levels increase with increasing follicular size and maturation, however, follicular development is characterized by a transition from an activin-dominant to an inhibin A–dominant environment.

Activin has stage-dependent actions on follicular maturation and granulosa cell function. Immature granulosa cells proliferate in response to activin, and FSH receptors and aromatase are induced. More mature granulosa cells differentiate in response to activin. Granulosa cell–derived activin enhances the FSH-supported induction of granulosa cell LH receptors. In theca cells, activin opposes the stimulatory effects of inhibin and suppresses LH-stimulated androgen synthesis. In human granulosa cells, activin suppresses basal and gonadotropin-stimulated progesterone and estrogen production.

The oocyte expresses activin receptors, and this may be a pathway by which granulosa cells regulate oocyte development through paracrine action. There is some evidence that activin can promote oocyte maturation. Gene "knockin" studies in mice suggest that activins A and B do not have overlapping functions in the ovary and that the βA subunit is essential for normal follicular development.

Follistatin was isolated from porcine follicular fluid and named on the basis of its FSH-suppressing activity.

Follistatin exists in several forms (315 and 288 amino acids) as a result of alternate splicing, glycosylation, and proteolytic processing of the C-terminus. Follistatin binds activin nearly irreversibly and effectively neutralizes its activity. Follistatin is produced by small antral and pre-ovulatory follicles. Free follistatin levels in follicular fluid vary consistently with follicular size or maturity. Circulating concentrations of follistatin are relatively constant throughout the menstrual cycle.

Follistatin stimulates progesterone production by human granulosa cells, although it is not clear whether this is a direct effect of follistatin or a consequence of its binding of activin. Overexpression of follistatin in transgenic mice results in arrested follicular maturation at the secondary stage, confirming an important interovarian role for activin in follicular maturation.

Müllerian-Inhibiting Substance (Anti-müllerian Hormone)

Müllerian-inhibiting substance, also known as *anti-müllerian hormone*, is a dimeric glycoprotein member of the TGF-β superfamily.[272-274] MIS has newly discovered roles in the adult female ovary, in addition to its established function in inducing degeneration of the müllerian ducts during male sexual differentiation. MIS is produced by granulosa cells of small follicles, and it signals through two serine/threonine kinase receptors, of which type II is specific and type I is shared with the BMP family. Female mice lacking MIS show accelerated depletion of follicles. This effect is a reflection of MIS inhibition of recruitment of primordial follicles into the growing pool and the MIS-induced reduction in the response of the growing follicles to FSH. Thus, FSH-stimulated preantral follicular growth in vitro is suppressed in the presence of MIS.

GONADOTROPIN-RELEASING HORMONE

The expression of GnRH-1, GnRH-2, and the GnRH receptor has been demonstrated by analysis of RNA in human granulosa–lutein cells and surface epithelial cells, albeit at much lower levels than found in the hypothalamus and pituitary, respectively.[275-277] Several in vitro studies have described dose-dependent inhibitory effects of GnRH-1 and GnRH-2 on trophic hormone-stimulated steroidogenesis and inhibition of ovarian surface epithelial cell proliferation. Collectively, these findings indicate that an intraovarian GnRH system exists in the human ovary. However, this system has more profound activity in the rodent ovary. The presence of GnRH receptors also raises the possibility that the ovary is a target for GnRH agonists and antagonists. However, most clinical studies suggest that if there is an effect on ovarian function, it is minor and is confined to GnRH agonists because GnRH antagonists do not appear to have a direct effect on human ovarian cells.[278]

INTERLEUKINS

The cytokine interleukin-1 (IL-1) is predominantly produced and secreted by activated macrophages. The rodent ovary has a highly compartmentalized, hormonally dependent intraovarian IL-1 system, including ligands, receptor, and receptor antagonist.[279-280] Substantial amounts of IL-1–like activity have been detected in human follicular fluid. IL-1 suppresses the functional and morphologic luteinization of murine and porcine granulosa cells. The antigonadotropic activity of IL-1 appears to involve sites of action both proximal and distal to cAMP generation. Theca–interstitial cells also may be a site of IL-1 (but not IL-2) action. However, mice lacking IL-1α, IL-1β, and IL-1 receptors are fertile, indicating that the IL-1 system is not likely to be critical for ovarian function.

TUMOR NECROSIS FACTOR-α

As has been shown in regressing corpora lutea, TNF-α can be derived locally from activated resident ovarian macrophages. TNF-α also has been found in the antral layer of granulosa cells and in follicular fluid. TNF-α inhibits the differentiation of cultured granulosa cells from immature rats by blocking FSH action at sites proximal to cAMP generation. It also exerts dose-dependent inhibitory effects on steroidogenesis by cultured granulosa and lutein cells, and as noted previously, may be an important factor causing luteolysis.

THE NEUROTROPHINS

The neurotrophins are a family of nerve survival and differentiation factors. These molecules act on the TRK proto-oncogene family of high-affinity receptors and the low-affinity p75 nerve growth factor receptor.[281] NGF is apparently required for early follicular development because NGF-deficient mice exhibit a substantial reduction in primary and secondary follicles and an increased number of oocytes that are not incorporated into a follicular structure, despite normal gonadotropin levels.[282] The defect appears to be the result of diminished proliferation of somatic cells, implicating NGF action on non-neuronal elements in the ovary.

Part of the action of NGF is the induction of FSH receptors in developing follicles. Neurotrophins and their receptors are also expressed in the human fetal ovary, with the TRK-B receptor being localized to germ cells and p75 NGF receptor in the stroma.[283] NT-4 is expressed in germ cells as well as in granulosa cells. Brain-derived neurotrophic factor (BDNF), NT-4/5, and NT-3 are detectable in human follicular fluid aspirated from women undergoing controlled ovarian hyperstimulation. Mouse oocytes express the BDNF receptor TRK-B. BDNF, which is produced by granulosa cells in response to LH and NT-4/5, but not NT-3, stimulates mouse oocyte maturation, including extrusion of the first polar body, and promotes early embryonic development in vitro.[284] Collectively, these findings suggest that the intraovarian neurotrophin system is important for early follicular development and later oocyte maturation.

Endocrine Disruptors and Ovarian Function

An endocrine disruptor is an exogenous substance or mixture that alters the function of the endocrine system and consequently causes adverse health effects in an organism or its progeny. Almost 1000 chemicals have been proposed to be endocrine disruptors, but fewer than 100 of these have clearly established endocrine-disrupting activity.[285] The sources of these chemicals vary widely, from substances naturally occurring in the environment (e.g., phytoestrogens), to industrial chemicals and byproducts (e.g., dioxins, polychlorinated biphenyl [PCB], bisphenol A), consumer products (e.g., cosmetics, plastics), pharmaceuticals (e.g., oral contraceptives), and organochlorine pesticides (e.g., dichloro-diphenyl-trichloroethane [DDT], methoxychlor). Exposure can occur through contaminated food, contaminated groundwater, combustion sources, and direct exposure to contaminants in consumer products. Many endocrine disruptors have estrogenic properties, but some have anti-estrogenic or anti-androgenic activity.

Ovarian development, folliculogenesis, and follicle function are highly susceptible to endocrine disruption because they are precisely regulated by steroid hormones, paracrine factors, and gonadotropins. Both timing of exposure to endocrine disruptors and dose are key determinants of the specific pathologies observed in animal model systems; it is likely that this would also be the case for women. For example, prenatal exposure to an endocrine disruptor could affect ovarian development, including early stages of meiosis, whereas early postnatal exposure would affect folliculogenesis and adult exposure would be most likely to affect steroidogenesis and other aspects of follicular function. Of note, dosage effects of endocrine disruptors are frequently nonlinear in that lower doses can have significant effects not seen at higher doses and vice versa. These issues have made the effects of specific endocrine disruptors difficult to establish definitively, particularly in human studies, where robust, well-controlled data are difficult to obtain. Nevertheless, there is a substantial body of evidence to support the notion that a few specific endocrine disruptors affect women's reproductive health, mainly by effects on the reproductive tract, and based on animal studies, effects on the ovary are likely as well.

A classic example of an endocrine-disrupting chemical is diethylstilbestrol (DES). This estrogenic compound is well known for its effects on the reproductive tracts of daughters of mothers who took oral DES during pregnancy. DES also has been shown to affect ovarian function in animal model systems. In the mouse, perinatal exposure to DES causes a high frequency of multioocytic follicles: two or more oocytes surrounded by a single follicular envelope of granulosa cells.[286] In addition, prenatal DES exposure in mice results in an overall decrease in oocyte number and abnormal oocyte maturation that could be explained by abnormal oocyte–granulosa cell communication in the multioocytic follicles.[287] Of note, multioocytic follicles are also induced by genistein, the primary soy phytoestrogen, when given to mouse neonates at doses that result in blood levels similar to those in human infants fed soy-based infant formula.[288] This phenotype is explained at least in part by genistein exposure inhibiting oocyte nest breakdown and attenuating oocyte cell death during development.[289]

Bisphenol A (BPA) is another estrogenic endocrine disruptor for which there is evidence that exposure causes direct effects on the mouse ovary. Oocytes from mice exposed to BPA have a high incidence of abnormal meiosis characterized by congression failure (a defect in chromosome alignment) and aneuploidy.[290] Mouse granulosa cells undergo apoptosis in response to environmentally relevant doses of BPA; it is possible that the effects of BPA on oocytes are mediated by its effects on somatic cells.[291]

In addition to its use in polycarbonate plastic and epoxy resins, BPA is present in dental materials and plastic food and beverage containers, so there is significant human exposure to this compound. It remains to be determined whether exposure to BPA or other endocrine disruptors affects ovarian or oocyte function.

Ovarian Aging

With age, there is a decline in both the quantity and quality of the pool of follicles and oocytes. Linear extrapolation of follicular depletion in women with regular menses predicts that, by 50 years of age, each ovary would contain 2500 to 4000 primordial follicles. Because the menopausal ovary is largely devoid of follicles, follicular depletion apparently accelerates in the last decade of reproductive life (Fig. 8-20). Below a critical number of some thousand follicles, which is reached at a mean age of 45 to 46 years, menstrual irregularity occurs. In some studies, unilateral oophorectomy and nulliparity are associated with an earlier occurrence of menopause and increasing parity with later menopause.

The postmenopausal ovary, weighing less than 10 g, is a lusterless structure with a wrinkled surface.[292-293] Morphologically, the main changes in the aging ovary are a decrease in volume and increasing fibrosis of the stroma, with accumulation of connective and scar tissue. A few primordial follicles and follicles undergoing maturation and atresia may be found up to 5 years after the last menses. A reduced vascular network, with smaller vessel lumens and thickening or sclerosis of the vessel walls, is characteristic,

leading to reduced ovarian stromal blood flow, as assessed by Doppler ultrasonography.

With aging, the ovarian surface epithelium changes. Papillae and crypts are seen less frequently, and the surface epithelial cells become flatter, with fewer and shorter microvilli. Increased numbers of apoptotic and necrotic cells are observed.

MECHANISMS OF NATURAL OVARIAN AGING

Ovarian aging reflects the combined interaction of genetic factors that determine the follicular complement (described previously), the additive effects of insults secondary to normal cellular metabolism, and environmental factors that affect follicular viability.[294-297] The importance of genetic factors is highlighted by the positive correlation in age of menopause between mothers and daughters, sisters, and monozygotic twins. Studies of sister pairs suggested that approximately 85% of the variation in age of menopause could be attributed to genetics. The genes that are involved remain to be determined, although some of the candidates that have been suggested include variants of the estrogen receptor α, superoxide dismutase-1, and apolipoprotein E genes.

The increased rate of loss of follicles that evidently occurs after age 38 years suggests that some nonlinear function of aging accelerates follicular depletion (see Fig. 8-20). This "broken-stick" pattern can be accounted for by a model of an exponential rate of follicular depletion that changes gradually during aging. A rise in FSH levels at this time may be a contributing factor, although a cause-and-effect relationship cannot be confirmed.

Oocyte aging is associated with increased meiotic nondisjunction.[295] The explanation for this phenomenon is not yet known, although oocytes apparently become more error-prone with respect to meiosis with age, probably because of a decline in chromosome cohesion. A two-hit model has been offered, which holds that there is a reduced frequency and pattern of recombination in a proportion of oocytes from the beginning; a second hit associated with an increased frequency of nondisjunction results from age-related damage due to oxidative stress and impaired microcirculation around the selected follicles. Hypo-oxygenation of the preovulatory follicle, assessed by the dissolved oxygen content of follicular fluid and hypoxia-responsive genes (VEGF), is associated with a high frequency of oocyte cytoplasmic defects, impaired postfertilization cleavage, and chromosome segregation defects. Centromeres have been reported to undergo a putative premature division at meiosis I in oocytes collected from older women. Moreover, examination of oocytes from older women at meiosis II showed a diffuse spindle and lack of bipolarity, with chromosomes irregularly and loosely attached to the spindle. These observations suggest that irregularities in the meiotic apparatus, including loss of key proteins in the spindle assembly checkpoint and chromosome cohesive ties, predispose aging oocytes to nondisjunction.[295]

Spontaneous deletions in the mitochondrial genome accumulate in muscle during aging, accelerating between the ages of 30 and 40 years. These deletions have been

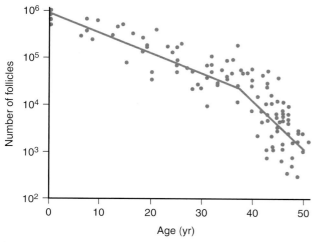

Figure 8-20. *Number of follicles in the human ovary as a function of chronologic age. The figure depicts the "broken-stick" regression. (Reprinted from Faddy MJ. Follicle dynamics during ovarian aging. Mol Cell Endocrinol 163:43-48, 2000, with permission.)*

associated with a number of diseases and pathologic processes, possibly arising as a consequence of damage resulting from the oxidative activity of mitochondria that is not adequately defended by cellular antioxidant mechanisms. Luteinized granulosa cells collected from women older than 38 years have a greater frequency of mitochondrial DNA deletions than those from women younger than 38 years of age.

Accumulation of these deletions in the oocyte mitochondria is another potential cause of ovarian aging. Indeed, the common delta mtDNA4977 deletion is found in 33% to 50.5% of oocytes, but in a smaller number of embryos (8% to 32.5%). This finding suggests that oocytes harboring these mitochondrial DNA deletions have an impaired ability to support embryonic development. Moreover, oocytes from older women have been found to be more likely to contain mitochondrial DNA deletions than those of younger women in some studies. Oxidative stress is hypothesized to be a cause of these DNA deletions, as well as induction of apoptosis. However, oxidative stress markers assessed in follicular fluid (e.g., conjugated dienes, lipid hydroperoxides, thiobarbituric acid–reactive substances) have not been correlated with the reproductive potential of oocytes in the setting of an in vitro fertilization/embryo transfer program.

Cigarette smoking represents an environmental factor that is associated with increased ovarian aging.[298] Smoking reduces the size of the ovarian follicular pool and advances the age of menopause by 2 years. It is also associated with reduced spontaneous fertility, poorer outcomes in assisted reproduction, and an increased incidence of trisomy 21. Follicular fluid cotinine levels, measures of a woman's exposure to cigarette smoke, are positively correlated with lipid peroxidation and negatively correlated with antioxidant activity. Because inhibitors of oxidative stress mimic the ability of FSH to prevent follicular apoptosis, the shift in peroxidant and antioxidant activities in the follicular fluid of smoke-exposed women suggests a mechanism underlying smoking-associated ovarian aging. Smoking also may lead to the accumulation of mitochondrial DNA deletions as a result of oxidative stress. In an animal model, polycyclic aryl hydrocarbons, a component of cigarette smoke, up-regulated expression of the proapoptotic gene *Bax* in the ovary, resulting in follicular atresia.[299]

Emerging evidence from longitudinal studies of women in the menopausal transition strongly suggests that obesity negatively affects ovarian reserve.[300] There is a significant inverse relationship between MIS levels and body mass index. This is true also for estradiol levels, particularly in African American women. The mechanisms underlying this inverse relationship between body mass index and markers of ovarian reserve have not been elucidated.

CLINICAL ASSESSMENT OF FOLLICULAR RESERVE

The number of follicles detected in the ovary by sonography is highly correlated with chronologic age and ovarian response to controlled ovarian stimulation. However, central follicle counts are operator-dependent and therefore difficult to standardize. Reductions in serum inhibin B levels and elevated day 3 FSH and estradiol levels also are predictive of reduced ovarian reserve.[301] It should be noted, however, that there are wide variations in inhibin B and FSH levels, with considerable overlap among values measured in older and younger women. Generally accepted criteria for normal ovarian reserve include a cycle day 3 FSH level of less than 10 mIU/mL and an estradiol level of less than 80 pg/mL. Women with reduced ovarian reserve reflected in a poor response to gonadotropin stimulation may have normal FSH and estradiol levels on cycle day 3, but show reduced inhibin B concentrations in serum. Moreover, elevated FSH levels reflect primarily the egg quantity that can be expected in stimulated cycles; this is not directly linked to egg quality, which is primarily affected by aging, although egg quantity and egg quality are frequently linked in older women.[302-305]

The clomiphene citrate challenge test is a provocative assessment of ovarian reserve in which a cycle day 3 FSH level is determined, followed by administration of clomiphene citrate (100 mg/day) on days 5 to 9. A second FSH determination is obtained on cycle day 10. The test indicates reduced ovarian reserve if either initial or final FSH values are elevated. This is a relatively cumbersome test, and its predictive value relative to a basal FSH and estradiol screen has not been established. Other tests of ovarian reserve, such as the GnRH agonist challenge test, are not yet recommended for routine use because their prognostic value has yet to be determined.

Anti-müllerian hormone is a valuable marker for ovarian aging.[306] This substance is produced by granulosa cells of small follicles and does not show major fluctuations during the cycle. Levels of MIS decline with aging and are highly correlated with the number of antral follicles observed by ultrasonography. MIS levels are consistently elevated in PCOS, even in adolescents. Of all of the potential biomarkers of ovarian reserve, MIS is the earliest to change with age. Moreover, because MIS production appears to be independent of gonadotropin secretion, its levels show low intercycle and intracycle variability; thus, MIS levels can be informative when sampled at random times during the cycle. Unfortunately, standardized assays for MIS with established normative values are not yet available to clinicians. Finally, there is an ongoing debate as to whether any of the current tests of ovarian reserve are useful as routine screening tools.[307-310]

ENDOCRINE ACTIVITY OF THE POSTMENOPAUSAL OVARY

Although devoid of follicles, the menopausal ovary is not a completely defunct endocrine organ in that it has a variable capacity to produce androgens.[311-313] The postmenopausal ovary is believed to be a source of testosterone, although there may be considerable variation among individuals with respect to androgen production (Fig. 8-21). This may be a reflection of variable numbers or activity of hilar cells. The circulating level of testosterone in postmenopausal women is only slightly lower than that observed in premenopausal women. Serum testosterone decreases approximately 50% after oophorectomy, and there is a significant level of testosterone in the ovarian

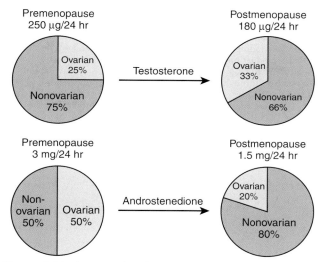

Figure 8-21. Sources of androgens in pre- and postmenopausal women.

vein compared with the peripheral blood in postmenopausal women.[314]

The postmenopausal ovary probably contributes no more than 20% of the daily production of androstenedione, with the adrenal being the predominant source. This proposal is supported by the following observations: (1) Serum androstenedione is minimally reduced after oophorectomy; (2) blood androstenedione has a diurnal rhythm (suggesting a substantial adrenal contribution); (3) serum androstenedione is markedly reduced after treatment with dexamethasone; (4) levels of androstenedione increase after the systemic administration of adrenocorticotropic hormone (ACTH), but not of hCG; and (5) the difference between androstenedione levels in the ovarian veins of menopausal women and levels in peripheral blood is of a lesser magnitude than that found in premenopausal women.

Some authors have concluded that the postmenopausal ovary is not a major site of androgen biosynthesis. Cauley and coworkers[315] examined hormone levels in postmenopausal women with and without ovaries and observed no statistically significant differences in circulating levels of testosterone and androstenedione between the two groups. Couzinet and colleagues[316] reported that plasma androgen levels were very low in all postmenopausal women with adrenal insufficiency and were similar between oophorectomized and nonoophorectomized postmenopausal women with normal adrenal function. These investigators also showed that dexamethasone dramatically suppressed plasma androgen production, whereas hCG treatment had no effect on plasma sex steroid levels, findings that are consistent with an adrenal source of androgens.

Estrogens in postmenopausal women arise almost exclusively from extraglandular aromatization of androstenedione.[317] Oophorectomy results in no substantial reduction in urinary estrogen excretion by postmenopausal women. However, adrenalectomy after oophorectomy virtually eliminates measurable estrogens from the urine. Longcope and colleagues[318] found a significant estradiol concentration gradient across the postmenopausal ovary in less than 20% of the women they studied. From in vitro

studies, researchers concluded that the postmenopausal ovarian stroma is unable to aromatize androgens.[319]

Incubation of postmenopausal ovarian stromal slices with pregnenolone yielded progesterone, dehydroepiandrosterone, and testosterone. Incubation of strips of ovarian hilar tissue from postmenopausal women showed a steroidogenic pattern similar to that of the postmenopausal ovarian stroma. However, the overall amount of steroid produced was substantially greater compared with stroma. These findings imply that the hilar cells have greater importance than the stromal cells in the overall steroidogenic potential of the postmenopausal ovary. Consistent with this view, immunohistochemical studies of most postmenopausal ovaries show that stromal cells are rarely positive for expression of P450SCC, 3β-hydroxysteroid dehydrogenase, and P450C17, three steroidogenic enzymes necessary for biosynthesis of androgens. Expression of steroidogenic enzymes involved in androgen biosynthesis is greatest in women with endometrial cancer or endometrial hyperplasia.[320]

There is some evidence that ovarian androgen production in postmenopausal women is gonadotropin-dependent. Administration of hCG to postmenopausal women results in a small increase in the circulating levels of testosterone.[321] Daily injection of hCG causes hyperplasia of the ovarian hilar cells and histochemical evidence suggesting active steroidogenesis.[322] The administration of hCG, but not ACTH, resulted in increased production of androgen, but not estrogen, by the ovaries.[323] Treatment of postmenopausal women with a long-acting GnRH agonist caused a decrease in circulating levels of testosterone, as well as a 22% decline in the levels of estradiol. The fall in serum estradiol levels was presumed to be the consequence of the reduction in serum testosterone levels. Taken together, these observations suggest that ovarian androgen biosynthesis is at least partially gonadotropin-dependent.

As suggested from the summaries of these studies, the main site of steroidogenesis may be the hilar cells. Binding sites for both LH and FSH were identified in the cortical stroma and in hilar cells.[324] Addition of hCG to hilar cells results in increased cAMP formation and steroid biosynthesis, indicating preserved responsiveness to gonadotropins.

Stromal hyperplasia can occur in the postmenopausal ovary, with the ovary enlarging with hyperplastic stromal nodules consisting of lipid-rich, luteinized cells that resemble theca interna. The ovaries with stromal hyperplasia produce large amounts of androstenedione, resulting in hirsutism and virilization.[325] Hilar cells can give rise to functional neoplasms (i.e., hilar cell tumors).[326-327] These tumors usually produce excess amounts of androgens, leading to virilization, but signs and symptoms of estrogen excess can also be evident when there is significant peripheral aromatization.

The complete reference list can be found on the companion Expert Consult Web site at www.expertconsultbook.com.

Suggested Readings

Davis JS, Rueda BR. The corpus luteum: an ovarian structure with maternal instincts and suicidal tendencies. Front Biosci 7:d1949-d1978, 2002.

Epifano O, Dean J. Genetic control of early folliculogenesis in mice. Trends Endocrinol Metab 13:169-173, 2002.

Fraser HM. Regulation of the ovarian follicular vasculature. BMC Reprod Biol Endocrinol 4:18, 2006.

Hoekstra C, Zhao ZZ, Lambalk CB, et al. Dizygotic twinning. Hum Reprod Update 14:37-47, 2008.

Jones KT. Meiosis in oocytes: predisposition to aneuploidy and its increased incidence with age. Hum Reprod Update 14:143-158, 2008.

Knight PG, Glister C. TGF-beta superfamily members and ovarian follicle development. Reproduction 132(2):191-206, 2006.

Lobo RA. Androgens in postmenopausal women: production, possible role, and replacement options. Obstet Gynecol Surv 56:361-376, 2001.

Macklon NS, Fauser BC. Ovarian reserve. Semin Reprod Med 23(3):248-256, 2005.

Mehlmann LM. Stops and starts in mammalian oocytes: recent advances in understanding the regulation of meiotic arrest and oocyte maturation. Reproduction 130(6):791-799, 2005.

Russell DL, Robker RL. Molecular mechanisms of ovulation: coordination through the cumulus complex. Hum Reprod Update 13:289-312, 2007.

Seifer DB, MacLaughlin DT. Mullerian inhibiting substance is an ovarian growth factor of emerging clinical significance. Fertil Steril 88:539-546, 2007.

Zinn AR, Ross JL. Molecular analysis of genes on Xp controlling Turner syndrome and premature ovarian failure (POF). Semin Reprod Med 19:141-146, 2001.

CHAPTER 9

The Structure, Function, and Evaluation of the Female Reproductive Tract

Jerome F. Strauss III and Bruce A. Lessey

The fallopian tubes, endometrium and myometrium, and uterine cervix function in concert to receive gametes, facilitate fertilization, support embryo growth, and ultimately orchestrate the timely expulsion of the mature fetus. The preparation of a receptive reproductive tract is programmed by ovarian steroid hormones acting directly on their cognate receptors and indirectly through the intermediacy of various steroid-regulated growth factors and cytokines. This chapter describes the structural and biochemical changes in the human reproductive tract during the normal menstrual cycle and pregnancy, the clinical evaluation of reproductive tract function, and the pathophysiology of some relevant disorders (see also Chapters 24, 25, and 33).

The components of a receptive endometrium include the luminal epithelium, which undergoes apical surface specialization expressing cell adhesion molecules that permit adherence of the blastocyst; glandular epithelial cells, which secrete substances that support blastocyst development; decidual cells and large granular lymphocytes that modulate trophoblast function and endometrial angiogenesis through the secretion of growth factors, growth factor–binding proteins, angiogenic factors, and cytokines; and a stromal extracellular matrix that facilitates trophoblast invasion. The combined actions of the locally acting molecules and extracellular matrix promote trophoblast proliferation, yet prevent uncontrolled penetration.

Innate and adaptive immune systems under the regulation of steroid hormones collectively defend the reproductive tract environment, but are also regulated to allow the fetal semiallograft to be accepted by the maternal host. The vascular system nourishes the endometrium in the initial receptive phase and is subsequently remodeled by invading trophoblasts to establish the placental blood supply. The coordinated contractile activity of the myometrium promotes sperm migration in a cycle of conception and facilitates embryo transport and placement before attachment. During pregnancy, the myometrium experiences hormone-directed hyperplasia and contractile quiescence that accommodate fetal growth. In the absence of conception, the endometrium is shed through a controlled inflammatory-like reaction involving matrix metalloproteinases (MMPs), the production of vasoactive substances, and uterine contractions that, respectively, promote remodeling, hemostasis, and the expulsion of the shed endometrial lining. Compartmentalized and specialized endometrial cells at the menstrual interface provide remarkable regenerative capacity, assuring that a new intact luminal surface is prepared for the next round of oocyte release and potential fertilization.

Structure and Morphology

MORPHOGENESIS OF THE FEMALE REPRODUCTIVE TRACT

The female reproductive tract is derived from the urogenital ridge, which during week 6 of gestation, gives rise to paired mesodermal (paramesonephric) tubes (müllerian ducts) from longitudinal invaginations of the coelomic epithelium.[1-3] These form the fallopian tubes, with the caudal ends fusing by week 10 of gestation to produce the primordial uterus and the upper portion of the vagina. A thin septum remaining after fusion eventually resorbs, yielding a single uterine cavity. The primordial uterus is initially lined by a simple cuboidal epithelium that subsequently becomes columnar and pseudostratified. Beneath this epithelium lies a condensed mesenchyme that yields the endometrial stroma and the surrounding myometrium. Glandular epithelium buds from the luminal epithelium, invaginating into the stroma. By week 22 of gestation, the uterus has taken on the structure of the adult organ. Glandular secretory activity, glycogen accumulation, and stromal edema are evident by week 32 under the influence of placentally derived steroid hormones. After delivery, with the precipitous fall in placental estrogens and progesterone, the endometrium regresses to an atrophic state, containing a few small-caliber glands and a poorly vascularized stroma.

THE ROLE OF THE WNT FAMILY AND HOMEOBOX GENES

The embryonic events described earlier are driven, in large measure, by the expression of secreted ligands of the wingless (WNT) family (WNT4, WNT5A, WNT7A) and transcriptional regulators of the homeobox (HOX) gene family (Fig. 9-1).[4-6] This morphogenetic program can only be played out in the absence of müllerian-inhibiting substance. The study of mice with targeted inactivation of Wnt genes showed the importance of these signaling molecules in the development of the reproductive tract.[4] The müllerian ducts are absent in female mice lacking Wnt4, a gene expressed in the mesenchyme.[5] Moreover, female mice lacking Wnt4 are partially sex-reversed due to the retention of the wolffian ducts. Cases of WNT4 null mutations associated with müllerian duct regression and a phenotype, including hyperandrogenemia, resembling that of the Wnt4 knockout mouse, have been reported in women.[7]

Deficiency of Wnt5a, a gene expressed in the genital tubercle and genital tract mesenchyme, results in mice with stunted genital tubercles and the absence of external genitalia.[4] Although WNT7A mutations have has not been found in women with müllerian anomalies,[8] in mice lacking Wnt7a, the oviduct is not clearly demarcated from the upper uterine horn, the uterus develops cellular characteristics that are similar to those of the vagina (including a stratified epithelium without uterine glands), and the uterine smooth muscle is disorganized.[8-9] Postnatal expression of HOXA10 and HOXA11 in the uterus is also lost. Mesenchymal β-catenin appears to be the essential downstream effector of the Wnt7a pathway and mediates its effects on the oviduct and proper development of the uterus.[9] The WNT family of genes, including receptors and downstream signaling molecules, are also expressed in a regulated fashion in the adult reproductive tract, indicating that they have additional roles beyond those involved in early morphogenetic events, including the regulation of steroid hormone action in adult tissues (discussed later).[4-6,10-13]

The HOX genes encode an evolutionarily conserved family of transcription factors that contain a signature 60–amino acid DNA-binding homeodomain.[6] They play critical roles in organizing cells along the anterior–posterior axis and directing them to select a particular pathway of development. Mammalian HOX genes are arranged in four different clusters, designated A through D, with each cluster organized in a linear arrangement that parallels the order of expression along the anterior–posterior body axis. The expression of HOXA genes in the human and mouse reproductive tract is conserved, with HOXA9 being expressed in the fallopian tubes, HOXA10 and HOXA11 in the uterus, HOXA11 in the cervix, and HOXA13 in the upper vagina.[6] Although there is a consistent regional distribution of HOX gene expression along the reproductive tract, there is evidence for some functional redundancy among the adjacent genes. Like the WNT genes, the HOX genes are also expressed in the adult uterus, and their expression is under steroid hormone (estrogen and progesterone) regulation. HOXA10 and HOXA11 have both been implicated in the process of implantation.[14]

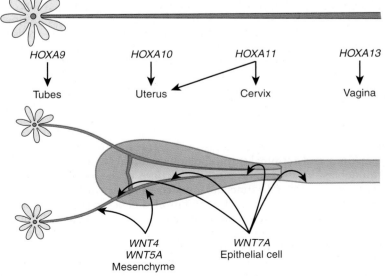

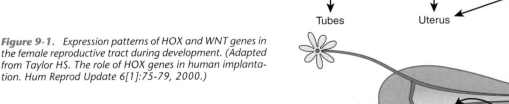

Figure 9-1. Expression patterns of HOX and WNT genes in the female reproductive tract during development. (Adapted from Taylor HS. The role of HOX genes in human implantation. Hum Reprod Update 6[1]:75-79, 2000.)

The importance of the homeobox gene family in reproductive tract function has been demonstrated through targeted deletions in specific HOXAd genes. Another significant discovery was that hand–foot–genital syndrome and Guttmacher syndrome, autosomal dominant conditions that affect bones in the hands and feet and cause reproductive tract abnormalities (including bicornuate uterus), are caused by mutations in the *HOXA13* gene.[15,16] However, to date, mutations in *HOXA7* to *HOXA13* and HOX gene cofactor PBXI have yet to be found in subjects with congenital absence of the uterus and vagina. Mice with targeted deletions in the *HOXA10* and *HOXA11* genes have subtle abnormalities in uterine morphology, including transformation of the upper uterine segment into an oviduct-like histology (*HOXA10* mutants); reduced endometrial stromal development and expression of leukemia inhibitory factor (LIF) are seen in *HOXA11* mutants.[14,17] Notably, both *HOXA10* and *HOXA11* nullizygous females are infertile due to a uterine factor, implicating these genes in the implantation process in the adult. Mice lacking *Hmx 3*, another homeobox domain gene product, are also infertile due to an implantation defect associated with perturbations in *Wnt* and *Lif* gene expression.[18]

Given their common embryonic origin, early development of the kidneys, ureters, and reproductive tract are tightly linked and involve other specific genes, including *Pax2*, *Lim1*, and *Emx2*, as well as members of the *Wnt* and abdominal-B *Hoxa* families of genes.[19] *Lim1* (Lhx1) encodes a transcription factor that, along with Pax2, is essential for urogenital tract development. *Lim1* null mice lack uteri and oviducts.[20] *Pax2* null mice lack kidneys, ureters, and genital tracts.[21] Caudal elongation of the paramesonephric duct is absent. Emx2 is another transcription factor of the homeodomain gene family that appears to be essential for urogenital tract development.[22] Emx2 is highly expressed in the adult uterus and its expression is correlated with cell proliferation and appears to be inhibited by *HOXA10*. There is decreased expression of *PAX2* and *Lim1*, and mesenchymal Wnt4 is also absent in mice lacking Emx2, suggesting the essential role for this transcription factor.

STEROID HORMONES AND FEMALE REPRODUCTIVE TRACT MORPHOGENESIS

As discussed in the next section, steroid hormones play a central role in differentiation of the reproductive tract. The morphogenesis of the female reproductive tract, however, does not require the action of estrogen mediated via the estrogen receptor α (ERα) or β (ERβ) proteins, because the oviducts, uterus, cervix, and vagina form in mice with inactivating mutations in both of these genes.[23] Even though it is independent of the ovaries and maternal or neonatal estrogen, the normal program of differentiation of the female reproductive tract can, paradoxically, be disrupted by exogenous estrogens.[24] Diethylstilbestrol (DES), a synthetic estrogen that causes uterine and cervical anomalies in exposed females (discussed later in this chapter), and polychlorinated biphenyls suppress expression of *Wnt7a* and alter the pattern of expression of *HOXA9* and *HOXA10* in the murine reproductive tract acting through ERα.[23-25] This suggests that alterations in *HOXA* and *WNT* gene expression are the likely molecular mechanisms underlying the anatomic defects observed in women exposed to DES in utero.

Mesenchymal–epithelial interactions are crucial to the formation of the reproductive tract.[26] In isolation, the epithelial and mesenchymal components of the reproductive tract will not undergo normal morphogenesis. The mesenchyme appears to be a major target for factors that govern organ formation; it also mediates many of the responses to sex steroid hormones.[27,28] Thus, estrogen receptors are detected in the embryonic mesenchyme of the female reproductive tract well before these receptors appear in epithelial cells. The mesenchyme communicates with the epithelium through paracrine effectors that encompass local growth regulators, differentiation factors, and extracellular matrix components that signal the epithelial cells through integrins and other cell adhesion molecules.[29,30] The nature of these epithelial–stromal interactions is discussed in greater detail later in this chapter.

Steroid Hormone Regulation of Female Reproductive Tract Growth and Differentiation

STEROID HORMONE ACTION IN THE REPRODUCTIVE TRACT

Many, but not all, of the reproductive tract responses to steroid hormones are mediated by nuclear receptors. These nuclear transcription factors undergo striking spatial and temporal changes in expression during the primate menstrual cycle.[31-34] The uterine response to steroid hormones is determined by the amount of bioavailable hormone, which is influenced by hormone production rates as well as local steroid metabolism; the repertoire of steroid receptors, coactivators, and corepressors expressed; and the action of growth factors and cytokines that modulate the action of steroid hormone receptors. The discovery of multiple forms of steroid hormone receptors with different transcriptional activities and cell- and tissue-specific patterns of expression revealed new levels of complexity in the control of reproductive tract function. The patterns of expression of coactivators and corepressors add another level of intricacy, which is now being explored.[35,36] The presence of membrane-bound receptors that recognize steroid hormones coordinates the paracrine, autocrine, and juxtacrine cellular mechanisms and provides an explanation for rapid effects of steroid hormones as well as the relationship between steroid hormones and growth factor responses.[37,38] Together, these layered mechanisms of steroid hormone action provide a diversity of responses that modulate the exquisite complexity required for establishment of a successful pregnancy.

Estradiol is the primary trophic hormone for the uterus. The uterine growth response is mediated by ERα, whose concentrations are highest during the proliferative phase of the cycle and decline after ovulation (Fig. 9-2).[39] These changes correlate with the proliferative activity of the endometrium. Immunohistochemical studies show estrogen receptors in the nuclei of epithelial, stromal, and myometrial cells during the proliferative phase, with the epithelial cell staining being the most prominent.[32,33] After progesterone levels rise in the luteal stage, estrogen receptor staining is restricted to the deep basal glands and vascular smooth muscle. In situ hybridization studies to distinguish patterns of expression of ERα and ERβ show that transcripts for both receptor forms are expressed in the epithelial, stromal, and smooth muscle cells at all stages of the cycle.[40] However, ERα expression is more abundant in the endometrium. In the proliferative phase, ERα messenger ribonucleic acid (mRNA) is detectable in epithelial cells and stroma, whereas ERβ mRNA is found predominantly in the glandular epithelium and is the

only estrogen receptor found in the vascular endothelium of the endometrium.[41] Expression of both transcripts falls in the secretory phase, with the decline in ERα expression being least in the basalis, consistent with the previously noted results of immunocytochemical studies. This fall in ERα at the time of implantation may be physiologically important and is a common finding across many species.[33,34,42] Failure to down-regulate estrogen receptors indicates an imbalance in regulatory mechanisms of steroid hormone interactions, and is associated with endometrial dysfunction and infertility (discussed later in the chapter).[43]

A variant of ERβ has been described (ERβcx/β2) and is formed by alternative splicing of the eighth exon of the "classic" ERβ (ERB1) transcript.[44] These isoforms have different selectivity for ligands and different affinities for coactivators. The patterns of ERβ1 and ERβ2 protein expression in the endometrium differ: ERβ1 expression appears to be more intense than ERβ2 expression; ERβ1 protein levels are unchanged throughout the menstrual cycle, whereas ERB2 levels decline in the glands of the functionalis layer, but not in the basalis layer, in the mid-secretory phase. The physiologic significance of these ERβ isoforms in the endometrium remains to be determined.

Studies on mice with targeted deletions in the genes encoding ERα and ERβ have provided clues as to the roles of the two molecules in mediating uterine responses to estrogen.[23] ERα is responsible for the main uterotrophic actions of estradiol; the uteri of mice lacking this receptor are hypoplastic and do not show the classic cell proliferation, increase in uterine wet weight, and edema in response to estradiol.[45] In mice lacking ERβ, there is an exaggerated response to estradiol, including increased accumulation of uterine secretions and uterine dilation.[46] This suggests that ERβ may function to attenuate the transcriptional activity of ERα in the uterus.[47] Severe uterine hypoplasia is observed in mice lacking both ERα and ERβ.[23] Progesterone receptors, which are up-regulated by estrogen, are reduced in the uteri of estrogen receptor knockout mice, but this reduction does not prevent the induction of progesterone-regulated genes.

Is there a threshold dose of estrogen required to elicit a uterine growth response? Key and Pike proposed that there is a threshold estrogen level of approximately 50 to 100 pg/mL at which endometrial proliferation is triggered, and above which there is no further stimulation of endometrial proliferation. This estimation was made on the basis of comparing endometrial proliferation assessed through ex vivo thymidine incorporation into endometrial explants from different stages of the menstrual cycle with corresponding estradiol levels at the different days of sampling.[48] This hypothesis finds support from studies on endometrial proliferation in postmenopausal women in response to different doses of exogenous estrogen.

Progesterone antagonizes the actions of estrogen and promotes glandular and stromal differentiation via progesterone receptors. The antagonism of the uterotrophic actions of estradiol involves several events, including alterations in estrogen receptor expression, inhibition of estrogen-induced translocation of the cell cycle regulators, and induction of enzymes that catabolize estradiol.[49-51]

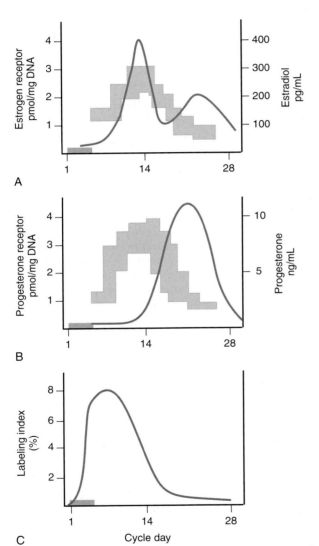

Figure 9-2. Estrogen and progesterone receptors in endometrial cells during the normal menstrual cycle. The concentrations of estrogen receptor (A) and progesterone receptor (B), mean values of plasma estradiol and progesterone, and endometrial proliferation as assessed by incorporation of [³H]thymidine in vitro (labeling index, C). The blue bar indicates menses. (Modified from Frolich M, Brand EC, van Hall EV. Serum levels of unconjugated aetiocholanolone, androstenedione, testosterone, dehydroepiandrosterone, aldosterone, progesterone, and oestrogens during the normal menstrual cycle. Acta Endocrinol [Copenh] 81:548-562, 1976.)

Three forms of the progesterone receptor, designated A (PRA), B (PRB), and C (PRC), have been identified.[49] These isoforms are derived from a single gene through use of alternative promoters and alternate translation start sites. PRA lacks a 164–amino acid N-terminal sequence present in PRB. PRC, the smallest of the progesterone receptors, also appears to be derived from an alternative translation start site. PRA and PRB have different functions, and the differential expression of these two isoforms determines tissue response. PRB is a strong transcriptional activator of several progesterone-responsive genes that do not respond to PRA. Further, PRB contains a motif that interacts with the SH3 domain of the intracytoplasmic signaling component Src; rapid activation of the Src and mitogen-activated protein (MAP) kinase signaling pathways are believed to involve this novel form of steroid receptor signaling.[52] PRA can function as a transcriptional repressor of PRB and other steroid receptors, including the estrogen receptor. PRC, of which relatively little is known, binds progesterone, but has no evident transcriptional activity. PRC may act as a repressor or modulator of PRA and PRB activity through heterodimerization, or it may serve as a progesterone-binding "sink." Differential subcellular localization of PRB outside the nucleus and PRA inside the nucleus may dictate the actions that these receptors undertake.[53,54] For example, when PRB was tagged with SV40 nuclear localization signals and forced into the nucleus, it no longer was able to interact with Src or to activate MAP kinase signaling pathways.[55]

Endometrial progesterone receptors peak at the time of ovulation and then decline, a reflection of the ability of estradiol to induce progesterone receptor expression and the down-regulatory actions of progesterone on its own receptor.[31,33,56] These receptors are localized to both epithelial and stromal cells. By day 4 after ovulation, progesterone receptor staining declines markedly in the epithelial compartment and remains weak or absent during the remainder of the secretory phase. In contrast, staining of stromal cells remains moderate to strong. PRA and PRB are coexpressed in uterine cells. PRA, however, predominates in the stroma, whereas PRB is more abundant than PRA in the midsecretory phase of the cycle.[57] Progesterone receptors have not been detected in vascular endothelial cells or vascular smooth muscle, but they are abundant in perivascular stroma. Consequently, the effects of progesterone or its withdrawal on the vasculature are likely indirect.

The significance of the different ratios of the two progesterone receptor forms with respect to regulation of gene expression in the human uterus is not yet known. However, some clues are being provided from the study of mice with targeted deletion of the receptor isoforms. The uteri of mice lacking both PRA and PRB are hyperplastic and contain inflammatory infiltrates.[50,51] Hyperplasia reflects the lack of antagonism to the uterotrophic actions of estradiol. Selective targeting of PRA showed that it is essential for progesterone-mediated actions on implantation and the decidual response. However, examination of genes associated with the window of uterine receptivity that are known to be regulated by progesterone indicated that PRA controls expression of only a subset and that the others

appear to be under the control of PRB. Ablation of PRA in mice uncovered an unexpected role for PRB in inducing epithelial proliferation. Administration of estradiol to the PRA-deficient mice resulted in uterine hyperplasia, but the combination of estradiol and progesterone resulted in even greater hyperplasia. It thus appears that PRA antagonizes the uterotrophic responses mediated by both ERα and PRB. Clinically, reductions in PRB have been associated with proliferative states, such as endometriosis,[58] supporting the paradigm of counter-regulatory mechanisms involving PR isoforms.

There is additional evidence for a dichotomous action of progesterone on uterine cell proliferation. DNA synthesis assessed by [^{3}H] thymidine incorporation into cells of the endometrium of the Rhesus monkey in vivo or into explants of human endometrium in vitro is greatest in the epithelial cells of the functionalis and least in the deep zona basalis during the proliferative phase.[59] Labeling indices fall dramatically in the luteal phase, with the exception of the basalis, where thymidine incorporation increases as progesterone levels rise, suggesting that progestins stimulate the formation of precursor cells in preparation for the next cycle. Moreover, in vitro studies using animal stromal cells have also shown progesterone-stimulated cell proliferation in the presence of a variety of growth factors.

In addition to steroid hormone receptors, coactivators probably have an important effect on the uterine response to estrogens and progestagens.[35] The uterine expression of p160 coactivators, steroid receptor coactivator-1 (SRC1), amplified in breast cancer 1 (AIB1), and transcriptional intermediary factor 2 (TIF2), has been examined by immunocytochemistry. AIB1 levels increased in the glandular epithelium in the late secretory phase, whereas SRC1 and TIF2 expression did not change. However, in endometrial biopsy specimens obtained from women with polycystic ovary syndrome (PCOS), AIB1 and TIF2, along with ERα, were elevated in the stroma and glandular epithelium, showing that an abnormal endocrine milieu can alter coactivator levels, which could, in turn, result in endometrial dysfunction.

Many of the effects of estrogen on epithelial proliferation and progesterone receptor expression are indirect, involving activation of estrogen receptors in the stroma, which produces paracrine substances that act on the epithelium to promote DNA synthesis.[27] Moreover, there is a reciprocal paracrine interaction between the epithelium and the stroma. For example, under the influence of progesterone, the epithelium produces substances that affect the response of the underlying stroma to estrogen.[60] Conversely, the stroma responds to progesterone by exerting an inhibitory effect on estrogen-induced epithelial cell DNA synthesis.[61]

The indirect actions of estradiol on epithelial proliferation have been shown in elegant reconstitution and grafting experiments employing stroma and epithelium from wild-type and estrogen receptor knockout mice. Epithelial cell proliferation does not occur when stroma from ERα knockout mouse uterus is paired with epithelium from wild-type mouse uterus.[27,60] Conversely, epithelial cell DNA synthesis in response to estrogen occurs when wild-type stroma is paired with epithelium from ERα knockout mice. Studies on human endometrial cells in culture are consistent with the mouse studies.[62] Estradiol increases epithelial cell proliferation when cocultured with stroma, but does not increase proliferation in epithelial cells cultured in the absence of stromal cells.

What is the estrogen-stimulated signal from the stroma that promotes epithelial cell proliferation? Candidates include growth factors under the transcriptional control of the estradiol receptor, including insulin-like growth factor 1 (IGF-1), transforming growth factor alpha (TGF-α), and epidermal growth factor (EGF).[63] Alternately, estradiol might suppress the production of stromal factors that restrain epithelial cell proliferation. Among the growth factors, there has been particular interest in EGF and IGF-1. Studies using mouse models, including transplantation of EGF receptor knockout mice uterus and vagina, indicate that this receptor is required for maximal fibromuscular stroma growth, but not for the epithelial cell proliferative response to estrogen.[64]

Both IGF-1 and IGF-2 stimulate the proliferation of human endometrial stromal cells via the type 1 IGF receptor. IGF-1 expression is greatest in the late proliferative and early secretory phases, whereas IGF-2 is most abundant in the midsecretory endometrium and decidua in the first trimester of pregnancy. The IGFs are bound by a family of binding proteins (IGFBPs) that modulate IGF activities in target tissues. One of the binding proteins, insulin-like growth factor–binding protein-1 (IGFBP-1), is a major secretory product of decidualized stromal cells, and it has been hypothesized to play a role in controlling trophoblast invasion.[65]

Estrogen is the primary regulator of IGF-1 expression in the uterus, which occurs predominantly in the stroma.[66,67] Estrogen also increases the expression of IGF-1 receptors, which are primarily found on epithelial cells. The mitogenic response of the mouse uterus to estrogen is absent in mice with targeted deletion of the gene encoding IGF-1. Moreover, mice overexpressing IGFBP-1, which results in reduced IGF-1 bioavailability, have a blunted DNA synthesis response to estrogen treatment.[68] Collectively, these observations suggest that IGF-1 produced in the uterine stroma in response to estrogen acts on the epithelial cells to stimulate DNA synthesis. However, tissue grafting experiments showed that IGF-1 knockout mouse uterus responds to estrogen when placed into a wild-type animal, whereas wild-type uterus placed into a IGF-1 knockout mouse showed minimal growth, indicating that systemic IGF-1 is sufficient to support estrogen-driven uterine growth.[69] These findings substantiate the importance of IGF-1 in the uterine growth response to estrogen. Although uterine growth can occur in the absence of a paracrine IGF-1 system, these studies do not preclude a role for locally generated IGF-1 as a redundant signaling mechanism or the role of other locally produced growth factors.

Some of the inhibitory effects of progesterone on epithelial cell proliferation and cell survival are mediated by stromal progesterone receptors.[61] Uterine stromal cells from progesterone receptor–deficient mice cannot suppress epithelial cell apoptosis in response to progesterone, whereas the progesterone receptor status of the epithelium did not influence the anti-apoptotic action of progesterone.

The uterus is also a target for androgens.[70] Androgen receptors are expressed in the endometrium and myometrium, most prominently in the stromal cells during the proliferative phase and in the epithelial cells of the secretory phase. Interestingly, 5α-reductase types 1 and 2, which convert testosterone to dihydrotestosterone, are expressed in epithelial cells throughout the cycle.[71] Estradiol treatment increases androgen receptor expression in the stroma of the Rhesus monkey uterus, and estradiol—in combination with either testosterone or progesterone—augments epithelial and myometrial androgen receptor levels. Consistent with these observations, androgen receptor expression is elevated in the endometrium of women with PCOS; this finding may explain, in part, the implantation defects and early pregnancy loss reported to be associated with this syndrome.[72]

There is increasing interest in functional, nontraditional estrogen and progesterone receptors and their role in reproductive tract biology.[73-75] Rapid actions of estrogen have been known since the discovery of the estrogen receptor, but a thorough understanding of these actions is only now being achieved. Estradiol can act within minutes to stimulate second messenger generation and phosphorylation of kinases. One candidate for the rapid action of estrogen is the orphan seven-transmembrane–spanning G-protein-coupled receptor 30 (GPR30). This plasma membrane protein is believed to serve as an alternative steroid receptor. Evidence suggests that this protein serves as a receptor for estrogen and mediates activation of EGF and downstream kinase activity,[76,77] likely involving release of the growth factor EGF and MAP kinase activation.[78] Progestins may also use this pathway, adding further complexity to our understanding of estrogen–progesterone interactions.[79] It is not clear whether this receptor is on the outer plasma membrane or within the endoplasmic reticulum.[37] Membrane forms of the progesterone receptor have also been identified, including mPRα, mPRβ, and mPRγ.[80] Membrane progesterone receptors have been shown to rapidly activate MAP kinase and inhibit cAMP signaling.[81] Both mPRα and mPRβ have been localized to the myometrium of humans and function to inhibit cAMP signaling, with a possible role of facilitating uterine contractions at term.[82]

STEROID HORMONE METABOLISM IN THE REPRODUCTIVE TRACT

The level of bioactive steroid hormone in the uterus is determined in part by the activities of uterine enzymes that form active molecules from prohormones and catabolize active hormones (Fig. 9-3).[83] The enzymes that carry out transformations of steroid hormones are subject to regulation during the menstrual cycle. Estradiol taken up from plasma can be converted into estrone by the action of 17β-hydroxysteroid dehydrogenases (17β-HSD) or converted to sulfated conjugates by estrogen sulfotransferase.[84] Three different forms of 17β-HSD capable of oxidizing estradiol to estrone have been detected in primate endometrium: type 2, type 4, and type 8 enzymes.[85] Type 2 and type 8 enzymes are associated with microsomes; type 4 enzyme is found in peroxisomes. Type 2 and type 4

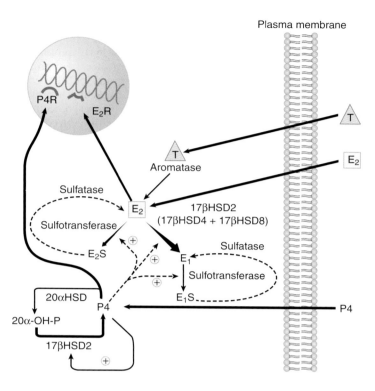

Figure 9-3. Steroid metabolism and action in the endometrium. P4 prevents the E_2-stimulated translocation of cell cycle control proteins into the nucleus, which inhibits the mitrogen effects of E_2. (+) stimulation; E_1, estrone; E_1S, estrone sulfate; E_2, estradiol; E_2R, estrogen receptor; E_2S, estradiol sulfate; HSD, hydroxysteroid dehydrogenase; P4, progesterone; P4R, progesterone receptor; T, testosterone.

enzymes use the oxidized form of nicotinamide adenine dinucleotide as a cofactor and are predominantly localized to glandular epithelium in the secretory phase. Endometrial type 2 enzyme shows the greatest change in expression during the cycle, peaking in the secretory phase. Type 8 enzyme appears to be constitutively expressed. Progesterone enhances the conversion of estradiol to estrone in endometrial cells by inducing expression of type 2 17β-HSD and, to a much lesser degree, type 4 enzyme. Progesterone also increases endometrial estradiol sulfation by increasing estrogen sulfotransferase activity. Thus, progesterone activates several enzymatic pathways that inactivate estradiol. However, there are regional differences in the balance of systems removing and restoring estradiol in the uterus. For example, estrogen sulfatase is detected only in the glandular epithelium of the basalis, where it may function to increase the level of estradiol from estradiol sulfate.[86] The normal human uterus does not appear to have the capacity to produce significant amounts of estrogen locally (either de novo or from circulating prohormones), but endometrial cancers, endometriotic lesions, and to a lesser extent, the eutopic endometrium of women with endometriosis aberrantly express components of the steroidogenic machinery that endows the tissue with the capacity to synthesize estrogens from circulating adrenal or ovarian androgens or from de novo synthesis. Endometriosis lesions have been found to express steroidogenic acute regulatory protein (StAR), the cholesterol side-chain cleavage enzyme, P450c17, aromatase, and type 1 17β-HSD in stromal cells (see Chapters 4 and 24). The estradiol produced in these lesions can enhance production of prostaglandin E_2, which in turn stimulates transcription of the aromatase gene, resulting in a feed-forward mechanism for increasing local

estrogen levels. In addition, endometriotic lesions do not express the progesterone-regulated type 2 17β-HSD that converts estradiol to estrone, which effectively increases the bioavailability of estradiol. Eutopic endometrium from patients with endometriosis and those with PCOS exhibits progesterone resistance, as measured by decreased type 2 17β-HSD[87,88]; this lack of deactivation of estradiol leads to increased estrogen action and may explain the endometrial receptivity defects noted in these conditions.

The unscheduled expression of aromatase in endometriosis is believed to be due, in part, to the presence of SF-1, a transcription factor that is not usually present in normal endometrium.[89] It has been proposed that SF-1 in stromal cells of patients with endometriosis displaces an inhibitory transcription factor, COUP-TF (which is abundant in endometrial stromal cells), from SF-1 binding sites on the aromatase promoter, propelling assembly of the general transcription machinery and aromatase expression. Other steroidogenic proteins found in endometriosis lesions, including StAR, P450scc, and P450c17, are also encoded by SF-1–regulated genes; a similar mechanism may underlie their expression in endometriosis.[90] The lack of type 2 17β-HSD in endometriosis has been attributed to abnormal expression of PRA, which generally suppresses transactivation, predominating over PRB in endometriosis.[58,91] Studies also suggest aberrant expression of ERα[43] and ERβ,[92,93] perhaps another feature of endometriosis that promotes proliferation and cell survival.[94,95]

Progesterone is catabolized in the uterus to inactive 20α-hydroxyprogesterone by 20α-HSDs. Type 2 17β-HSD, which is increased in the secretory phase, is also a 20α-hydroxysteroid oxidase that converts 20α-hydroxyprogesterone back into progesterone.[83] The induction of type 2

17β-HSD by progesterone in the secretory phase therefore contributes not only to the catabolism of estradiol, but also to the maintenance of endometrial progesterone levels.

The Adult Female Reproductive Tract and Dynamic Changes During the Menstrual Cycle

THE FALLOPIAN TUBES

The fallopian tubes facilitate gamete transport and serve as the venue for fertilization and early embryo transport. These functions are accomplished by the tubal epithelium and underlying smooth muscle. Although in vitro fertilization/embryo transfer has clearly shown that the fallopian tubes are not essential for animal and human conception, an understanding of tubal physiology was essential to the development of the modern practice of assisted reproduction. Moreover, further elucidation of the oviductal environment could improve the outcome of assisted reproduction.

The oviduct has four anatomic regions spanning from the distal to the proximal end: the *fimbria* and *infundibulum,* the *ampulla,* the *isthmus,* and the *intramural segment.* The structures of the endosalpinx and myosalpinx in these segments are distinctive and correlate with their functional roles in gamete transport and fertilization.[96] In addition, the junctions between the ampulla and isthmus and the uterus and tube are important physiologic sphincters that regulate the residence time of eggs and early embryos in the oviduct.

Gamete Transport

At the time of ovulation, the fimbriae become tumescent and congested, exhibiting pulsatile and sweeping movements.[97] The fimbriae and infundibulum have the highest density of ciliated cells in the oviduct, and these cells beat in a centripetal direction in the periovulatory period. The concerted movements of the fimbriae and ciliary strokes facilitate the pick-up of the ovulated egg and its entrance into the ampulla, which has a thin, muscular layer and a mucosa that is arranged in numerous folds, providing a large surface area for transport and exchange. Transport is arrested when the egg reaches the ampullary–isthmus junction, the site where fertilization occurs. Transport through the isthmus, which, in contrast to the ampulla, has only a few primary mucosal folds, but a thicker myosalpinx, takes several days.[98]

The intramural segment of the tube, surrounded by abundant smooth muscle, serves as a second physiologic sphincter. The activity of this sphincter is regulated by adrenergic innervation, steroid hormones, and prostanoids. Gamete and embryo transport is facilitated by contraction and relaxation of the myosalpinx.

Light microscopic studies distinguish between longitudinal and circular smooth muscle layers in the tube, but the ampulla appears to have a different organization, consisting of a continuous network of randomly anastomosed smooth muscle bundles that are repeatedly intertwined, branching into different orientations.[99] It has been proposed that this single network of muscular fibers generates random contractile waves that cause "stirring" of the tubal contents, a process that may facilitate fertilization and early embryo development by enhancing access of growth factors and nutrients and exchange of metabolites. Local production of prostaglandins $F_{2\alpha}$ and E_2 (which stimulate contraction) and prostacyclin (which causes relaxation) probably plays an important role in regulating the contraction and relaxation pattern of both the longitudinal and the circular muscle of the tubes.[100] Human chorionic gonadotropin (hCG) released by the early embryo can induce cyclooxygenase (COX)-2 mRNA expression in the tubal epithelium, which can lead to increased prostacyclin production that would favor the opening of tubal sphincters.

Studies of laboratory and domestic species have shown that sperm reaching the oviduct are stored in the caudal part of the isthmic region through surface-associated sperm lectins that bind to oviductal epithelial cell glycoconjugates.[101] These interactions appear to increase the viability of sperm and to suppress capacitation and sperm motility, evidently by modifying intracellular calcium concentrations in the spermatozoa. Near the time that the egg enters the ampulla of the tube, sperm initiate the capacitation process and are released from the oviduct epithelium in a hyperactivated state. Although there is a substantial body of literature documenting sperm binding to the oviduct in animals, there is no conclusive evidence that this occurs in humans. However, human sperm viability in vitro is promoted by coculture with oviductal epithelial cells, despite the lack of tight binding.

THE TUBAL EPITHELIUM AND TUBAL FLUID

The human tubal epithelium is composed of ciliated and secretory cells that undergo cyclic alterations in response to changes in ovarian steroid hormone levels.[102] In both the fimbriae and the ampulla, epithelial cells attain their greatest height, extent of ciliation, and beat frequency in the late follicular phase. At the end of the luteal phase, some cellular atrophy and loss of cilia are observed, particularly in the fimbriae, with hypertrophy and reciliation occurring in the subsequent follicular phase. In contrast, if pregnancy is achieved, further atrophy and loss of cilia occur. These observations indicate that estrogen dominance promotes ciliogenesis, whereas progesterone dominance leads to atrophy and deciliation. Female infertility, presumed to be of tubal origin, is a variable feature of primary ciliary dyskinesia and Kartagener syndrome, indicating that ciliary function in the female reproductive tract is important, but not absolutely essential, for in vivo fertilization.[103,104]

Gamete transport, fertilization, and early embryo development occur in a fluid environment created by the tubal epithelium. The production of oviductal fluid by selective transudation and secretion changes during the cycle in primates.[105,106] Tubal fluid accumulates at a rate of 1 to 3 mL every 24 hours, with a significant increase in accumulation around the time of ovulation. The primary cells responsible for fluid secretion in the oviduct are believed to be the nonciliated cells, which maintain a transmural electrical potential through flux of chloride ions. The mechanisms of tubal fluid secretion and its regulation by steroid hormones, neurotransmitters, and inflammatory mediators are incompletely understood.

Knowledge of tubal fluid composition has informed the development of culture media for in vitro fertilization and early embryo development.[106-109] Tubal fluid is enriched in bicarbonate compared with plasma, which facilitates sperm capacitation by activating a sperm soluble adenylyl cyclase; bicarbonate also promotes separation of the corona radiata of the egg. The high bicarbonate content of tubal fluid is maintained by carbonic anhydrase activity in tubal epithelial cells.

There are cyclic variations in the nutrient content of tubal fluid that can influence human embryo development in vitro.[109] Such variation is exemplified by a sixfold decline in glucose, from 3.1 mM to 0.5 mM, from the follicular phase to the time of ovulation, and an increase in lactate from 4.9 mM to 10.5 mM during the same time. The levels of pyruvate in tubal fluid (0.14 to 0.17 mM), an important initial embryo energy substrate, do not change during the cycle. Arginine, alanine, and glutamine are the most abundant amino acids in the tubal fluid; these and most other amino acids, except asparagine, are generally present in highest concentrations during the secretory phase. Taurine and hypotaurine are also major constituents that have been implicated in improved viability of gametes and preimplantation embryos.

Albumin is the major protein in tubal fluid that also contains secretory proteins from the epithelium. A high–molecular-weight mucin-like glycoprotein called *oviductin* (also known as *oviduct-specific glycoprotein*) is expressed exclusively by the oviduct epithelium under the regulation of estrogen.[110] Oviductin has chitinase-like domains that may facilitate its binding to oligosaccharides on the zona pellucida. This coating of oviductin may prevent ectopic pregnancy by forming a barrier between the embryo and the tubal epithelium. Oviducts also express a variety of growth factors and cytokines that could influence embryo growth and development.

The metabolic and secretory activity of animal and human tubal epithelial cells has been employed in human assisted reproduction. Several coculture protocols have resulted in increased implantation and pregnancy rates, indicating a beneficial effect of a "tube-like" microenvironment. However, it is not known whether any beneficial effects of coculture are specific to oviductal epithelium as opposed to being a general salutary effect of a somatic cell layer.

THE ENDOMETRIUM

In discussions of structure and function, the primate endometrium is commonly described as consisting of two major layers, the *functionalis* and *basalis* (Fig. 9-4). The functionalis is a transient layer, consisting of a compact zone that includes the stroma subjacent to the luminal epithelium and an intermediate spongy zone containing more densely packed tortuous glands, giving it a lacy histologic appearance. The basalis, or basal layer, lies beneath the spongy zone and adjacent to the myometrium. It contains the gland fundi and supporting vasculature and can generate the entire endometrium after menstrual shedding of the *functionalis*. These endometrial layers are histologically definable during the secretory phase. However, in terms of function, the endometrium is best considered as a polarized gradient of cells with different phenotypes. The upper layers undergo a striking progression of histologic change during the

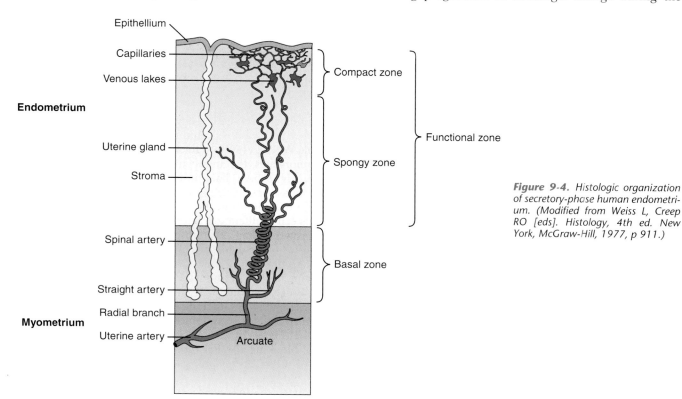

Figure 9-4. Histologic organization of secretory-phase human endometrium. (Modified from Weiss L, Creep RO [eds]. Histology, 4th ed. New York, McGraw-Hill, 1977, p 911.)

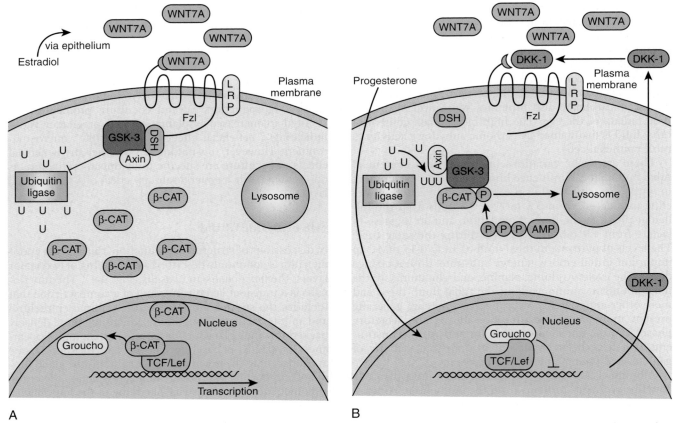

A   B

Figure 9-5. *Wnt signaling pathways in the proliferative and secretory phases of the menstrual cycle. WNT7A is a soluble factor believed to arise from the luminal epithelium.* **A,** *Under conditions of estrogen action WNT7A binds to the receptor Frizzled (Fzl), initiating signaling through the intracytoplasmic protein dishevelled (DSH). Dishevelled binds axin and glycogen synthase kinase beta (GSK), allowing beta catenin (β-CAT) to accumulate and stimulate gene transcription, leading to cell proliferation.* **B,** *When progesterone levels increase, cellular Dickkopf (DKK)-1 accumulates and inactivates Fzl through an accessory receptor, LRP. Without WNT7A, GSK facilitates the ubiquitinization of β-CAT by a ubiquitin (U) ligase, which makes it unavailable as a transcription factor.*

menstrual cycle, whereas the basal region shows only modest alterations. Patterns of cell proliferation, programmed cell death, and gene expression also show gradients across the layers, as described in the next sections. The majority of epithelial cell proliferation occurs in the upper regions of the functionalis during the proliferative phase of the cycle. Proliferative activity in glands in the basalis is modest, reaching its highest level during the midsecretory phase.

The Early Proliferative Phase

During the early proliferative phase, the endometrium is usually less than 2 mm thick. Proliferation of cells in the basal zones and epithelial cells persisting in the lower uterine and cornual segments result in the restoration of the luminal epithelium by day 5 of the menstrual cycle. At that time, mitotic activity is evident in both the glandular epithelium and the stroma. Remarkably, this recurrent "wound healing" process does not normally produce scarring. Endometrial stem cells capable of yielding progenitors of both the stromal and the epithelial components of the endometrium presumably contribute to the regenerative process.[111]

Rapid rejuvenation of the endometrium depends on many of the same factors that were involved in the ontogeny of the reproductive tract. WNT7A, a member of the Wingless family, is expressed solely by the luminal epithelium and is a diffusible factor that triggers cell proliferation through complex pathways.[12,13] Acting on the underlying stroma, soluble WNT7A binds to the receptor Frizzled (Fzl), which phosphorylates the intracytoplasmic protein Dishevelled (DSH; Fig. 9-5A). This protein inactivates glycogen synthase kinase beta (GSKβ), turning off the breakdown of beta catenin by ubiquitination. Accumulation of beta catenin signals cell proliferation activities associated with endometrial growth acting as a transcription factor in the nucleus. The diffusion gradient of WNT7A downward into the growing endometrium is an attractive model for self-regulatory mechanisms to determine the growth of the endometrium.

Counter-regulatory mechanisms to disable WNT7A/Fzl/DSH pathways include the action of progesterone, which stimulates secretion of a protein called Dickkopf-1 (DKK-1; Fig. 9-5B).[12,13] Dickkopf-1 binds to a coreceptor, LRP6, blocking the Fzl receptor and turning off the action of WNT7A by preventing beta catenin accumulation. Defects in DKK-1 production have been described in endometriosis, reflect progesterone resistance, and might

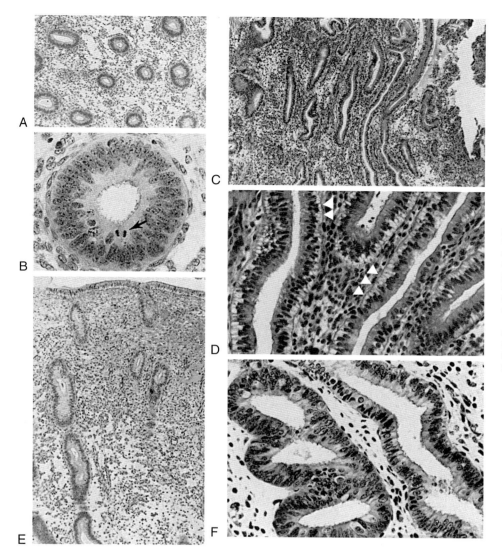

Figure 9-6. Histology of the endometrium during the menstrual cycle. **A** and **B**, Proliferative endometrium. Mitoses are present (arrow). Nuclei in the glandular epithelium are pseudostratified. **C** and **D**, Secretory endometrium, day 18. Subnuclear glycogen vacuoles are uniformly present in the glandular epithelium (arrowheads). **E** and **F**, Midsecretory endometrium. Glandular secretory activity is present, and the stroma is edematous. The stromal cells in the more superficial layers as well as around vessels have become pseudodecidualized and exhibit a flattened, polygonal configuration, with distinct cell borders.

explain the proliferative phenotype of the endometrium in this condition.[112,113]

During the early proliferative phase, the glands are narrow, straight, and tubular, and are lined with low columnar cells that have round nuclei located near the cell base (Fig. 9-6). At the ultrastructural level, the epithelial cell cytoplasm contains numerous polyribosomes, but the endoplasmic reticulum and Golgi complexes of these cells are not well developed.

The Late Proliferative Phase

The endometrium thickens in the late proliferative phase as a result of glandular hyperplasia and an increase in stromal extracellular matrix. The glands are widely separated near the endometrial surface and more crowded and tortuous deeper into the endometrium. The glandular epithelial cells increase in height and become pseudostratified as ovulation approaches (see Fig. 9-6).

The effects of steroid hormones on proliferation and secretion within the endometrium are highly dependent on the zone (basalis versus functionalis layers). Studies from the Rhesus macaque endometrium using specific labeling techniques show that proliferation during the "proliferative" phase is confined to the functional layer.[114] By the midsecretory phase, this proliferation has shifted to the basalis layer, presumably in response to progesterone.

The Early Secretory Phase

Ovulation marks the beginning of the secretory phase of the endometrial cycle, although it should be noted that the endometrial luminal and glandular epithelial cells also display secretory activity during the proliferative phase. Mitotic activity in epithelial and stromal cells is restricted to the first 3 days after ovulation and is rarely observed later in the cycle. The nuclei of glandular epithelial cells and stromal cells develop heterochromatin in the early secretory phase (see Fig. 9-6). The glandular epithelial cells begin to accumulate glycogen-rich vacuoles at their base, displacing the nuclei to the midregions of the columnar cells. Evidence of modest secretory activity is seen in

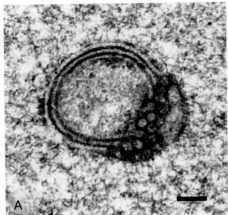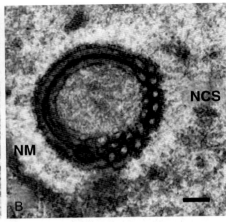

Figure 9-7. *Images of the nucleolar channel system (NCS) at the electron microscope level.* **A,** *A nucleolar channel–like structure in COS cells transfected with a Nopp140 construct.* **B,** *A nucleolar channel system induced by progesterone in endometrial cells. NM, nuclear membrane. (Reprinted with permission from Isaac C, Pollard JW, Meier UT. Intranuclear endoplasmic reticulum induced by Nopp140 mimics the nucleolar channel system of human endometrium. Cell Sci 114:4253-4264, 2001.)*

histologic preparations as a light eosinophilic collection in the gland lumina. Ultrastructural studies of endometrial epithelia show abundant endoplasmic reticulum and unusually large mitochondria, with prominent cristae. A reticular network of argyrophilic fibers containing fibrillar collagens (collagen fiber types I and III) is established in the stroma by the early secretory phase. Stromal edema contributes to the thickening of the endometrium at this time.

The Midsecretory Phase

A characteristic feature of the midsecretory phase of the cycle is the development of the spiral arteries. These vessels become increasingly coiled as they lengthen more rapidly than the endometrium thickens. The endometrial glands are tortuous in the midsecretory and late secretory phases. Their secretory activity reaches a maximum approximately 6 days after ovulation, as reflected by loss of vacuoles from the epithelial cell cytoplasm (see Fig. 9-6).

An ordered spherical stack of interdigitating tubules, the nucleolar channel system appears transiently in the nucleoli of approximately 5% to 10% of the secretory phase epithelial cells between days 16 and 24 (Fig. 9-7).[115] The nuclear channel system is believed to form from an invagination of the inner nuclear membrane, providing a direct connection to the perinuclear space for transport of mRNA to the cytoplasm. Nopp140, encoded by the *NOLC1* gene, a highly phosphorylated protein that associates with small nucleolar ribonucleoprotein particles that are required for RNA processing, appears to induce formation of this intranuclear endoplasmic reticulum.[116] The nucleolar channel system forms in response to progesterone and is an ultrastructural hallmark of the secretory phase during the expected time of implantation.

Stromal cells around blood vessels enlarge and acquire an eosinophilic cytoplasm and a pericellular extracellular matrix in the mid- to late secretory phase. These changes, referred to as *predecidualization* to distinguish them from the further transformation of the stroma that occurs in a fertile cycle, subsequently spreads, accentuating the demarcation between the subepithelial compact zone and the spongy zone. Unlike in many laboratory animal species, an embryonic signal is not required for initiation of decidualization in the human uterus.

The fact that the predecidual changes occur first near blood vessels suggests that humoral or local factors provoke them. Among the local factors may be interactions with decidual granular lymphocytes, also referred to as uterine *natural killer* (NK) cells. NK cells encircle arterioles and closely associate with stromal cells through contacts that are remarkably similar to gap junctions.[117] At the ultrastructural level, the predecidual stromal cells display well-developed Golgi complexes and parallel lamellae of endoplasmic reticulum. Their surrounding matrix consists of laminin, fibronectin, heparan sulfate, and type IV collagen.[118,119] The profile of gene expression decidualizing human stroma cells in vitro has been mapped by microarray analysis and includes induction of 121 genes, downregulation of 110 genes, and 50 genes showing a biphasic response.[120]

The stromal cells of the midsecretory and late secretory phases also express a repertoire of proteins that promote hemostasis, including tissue factor, a membrane-associated protein that initiates coagulation when it contacts blood, and plasminogen activator inhibitor type 1 (PAI-1), which restrains fibrinolysis.[121,122] This pattern of gene expression prevents focal hemorrhage that might result from trophoblast invasion during implantation.

The Premenstrual Phase

The main histologic features of the premenstrual phase are degradation of the stromal reticular network, which is catalyzed by MMPs; infiltration of the stroma by polymorphonuclear and mononuclear leukocytes; and "secretory exhaustion" of the endometrial glands, whose epithelial cells now have basal nuclei. Morphologic changes in the nuclei of granular lymphocytes, including pyknosis and karyorrhexis suggesting apoptosis, have been proposed to be some of the first events presaging menses; these changes occur before the breakdown of extracellular matrix and leukocyte infiltration.[123] In the glandular epithelium, the nucleolar channel system and giant mitochondria characteristic of the early and midsecretory phases have vanished. The endometrium shrinks preceding menstruation, partly as a result of the diminished secretory activity and the catabolism of extracellular matrix.

MENSTRUATION

Menstruation, caused by progesterone and estrogen withdrawal, marks a failure to achieve pregnancy and the need to shed the specialized uterine lining that results from spontaneous decidualization. The uniqueness of this process is highlighted by the fact that, although circulating progesterone and estrogen levels decline with corpus luteum regression in nonfertile cycles in all mammals, menstruation occurs only in humans and some Old World primates. In menstruating species, moreover, tissues that respond to estrogen and progesterone, such as the fallopian tubes, vagina, and breast, do not shed as ovarian steroid levels decline. The molecular mechanisms triggered by progesterone withdrawal include activation of the NF-Kβ transcriptional pathway (a major target of cytokines) and the resulting expression of genes such as endometrial bleeding–associated factor (EBAF), an anti–TGF-β cytokine that interferes with the action of other members of the TGF-β family that promote endometrial integrity. This orchestrated blockade of the actions of TGF-β appears to initiate many of the subsequent events of menstruation, including the elaboration of MMPs.[124]

The functional zone of the human endometrium is supplied by spiral arterioles that, in contradistinction to the radial and basal arteries that feed them, are highly sensitive to steroid hormones, which most likely influence vessel function through actions on perivascular cells. The classic studies of Markee[125] that observed the structure of autologous endometrial transplants into the anterior eye chamber suggested that an ischemic phase caused by vasoconstriction of the arterioles and spiral arteries precedes the onset of menstrual bleeding by 4 to 24 hours. It has been proposed that bleeding occurs after the arterioles and arteries relax, leading to hypoxia or reperfusion injury.

The findings of Markee form the basis of the vasoconstriction model of menstruation.[125] However, the notion that menstruation is a consequence of generalized vasoconstriction and hypoxia/anoxia in the functionalis is not supported by studies of endometrial perfusion that did not show any significant reduction in endometrial blood flow in the perimenstrual phase and during menstruation.[126] In addition, an analysis of the expression and localization of hypoxia-inducible factor (HIF), a heterodimeric transcription factor induced by hypoxia and thus a biochemical marker of reduced oxygen availability, was unrevealing. No upregulation of the two HIF component subunits, HIF-lα and HIF-lβ, was observed, and no nuclear localization of HIF subunits took place in the perimenstrual human endometrium.[127] These studies do not, however, exclude the possibility of localized regions of vasoconstriction and hypoxia.

An alternative hypothesis to the vasoconstriction model is that menstruation is an inflammatory response engendered by the withdrawal of progesterone. The inflammation hypothesis is supported by two features: the prominent accumulation of leukocytes in the endometrium in the premenstrual phase[117] and the release of matrix-degrading enzymes characteristic of an inflammatory response.[128-131]

The hypothesis of progesterone withdrawal–induced inflammation is supported by the uterine inflammation observed in mice lacking progesterone receptors. Apoptotic cell death, which can be triggered by inflammatory mediators, occurs in the late secretory phase, first in stromal cells and then gradually spreading throughout the functionalis.[132-134] Rescue from apoptosis has been shown to occur in vivo with the administration of progesterone or exogenous hCG.[135]

Changes in proteins involved in apoptosis appear to contribute to the regional programmed death in the endometrium. The anti-apoptotic protein Bcl-2 is prominently expressed in the glandular epithelium during the proliferative phase; expression declines in the secretory phase to reach low levels in the late secretory phase when apoptosis occurs.[134] Studies report an inverse pattern of expression of survivin, a recently discovered inhibitor of apoptosis. Survivin binds to and blocks the effector cell death proteases caspase-3 and -7. The activities of caspase-3, -8, and -9 are higher in the secretory phase. Low rates of survivin expression in the glandular epithelium are found in the proliferative phase, rising to peak expression in the late secretory phase. The protein was localized to the nuclei of cells in the functionalis and to the cytoplasm in cells in the basalis. This differential distribution may indicate that survivin is not capable of suppressing apoptotic death in the functionalis in the late secretory phase, but performs this role in the basalis, consistent with the observed patterns of apoptotic cell death. Elevated levels of survivin in endometriotic lesions correlate with reduced apoptotic death of cells in these lesions.[136]

Although the vasoconstriction and inflammation hypotheses of menstruation might appear to be distinct, there are several overlapping biochemical features of hypoxia and inflammation, including the release of proinflammatory cytokines and apoptotic cell death that tend to blur the distinctions between these models. The vascular changes in the endometrium in the perimenstrual phase, resulting either from ischemia/hypoxia or from inflammatory reaction, lead to extravasation of blood. Autophagy and heterophagy are evident, as is apoptotic cell death. The superficial endometrial layers become distended by the formation of hematomas; fissures subsequently develop, leading to the detachment of tissue fragments and the ultimate shedding of the functionalis. The resulting menstrual effluent contains the fragments of tissue mixed with blood, liquefied by the fibrinolytic activity of the endometrium. Clots of varying size may be present if blood flow is excessive.

The duration of menses in ovulatory cycles is variable, generally 4 to 8 days and usually similar from cycle to cycle in any individual ovulatory woman. The duration of flow is considered abnormal if it is less than 2 days or more than 7. The amount of blood lost in a normal menses ranges from 25 to 60 mL, being greater when coagulation and platelet disorders are present. Loss of more than 60 mL/month is associated with iron deficiency anemia.

Menstruation and the subsequent regeneration of the functionalis layer are notable for the lack of development of synechiae. The majority of cases of uterine synechiae causing Asherman's syndrome occur after pregnancy-related curettage, especially when curettage is performed during the first 4 weeks of the postpartum period, when the uterus is particularly vulnerable.[137]

Vascular Remodeling and Angiogenesis

Angiogenesis, the formation of new blood vessels from preexisting vessels, rarely occurs in the normal adult, except in the female reproductive tract and ovary. Here, the cyclic processes of endometrial shedding and regeneration and corpus luteum formation entail remarkable changes in vessel growth and remodeling. The angiogenic process involves multiple steps and is tightly regulated by activators and inhibitors.[138-140] There are four phases of the endometrial cycle when important events relating to angiogenesis occur: (1) at menstruation, when there is repair of ruptured blood vessels; (2) during the proliferative phase, when there is rapid growth of endometrial tissue; (3) during the secretory phase, with the development of the spiral arterioles that feed a subepithelial capillary plexus; (4) in the premenstrual phase, when there is evidence of vascular regression. If this angiogenic remodeling program is not properly executed, abnormalities in endometrial function, including menorrhagia, can result.

Angiogenesis during the proliferative phase is by vessel elongation.[141] In the secretory phase, intussusception appears to account for the increase in vessel branching; this proliferation of endothelial cells inside of vessels ultimately produces a wide lumen that can be divided by transcapillary pillars, or alternatively, may lead to capillary fusion or splitting. Although most prominent in the late menstrual and early and late proliferative phases, endothelial cell proliferation is continuous during the menstrual cycle. Thus, vessel growth continues during the secretory phase, despite the fact that the surrounding endometrial tissue has ceased to grow, resulting in the coiling of spiral arterioles.

Endometrial angiogenesis and vessel remodeling are directed by a network of signaling molecules and receptors that include members of the vascular endothelial growth factor family, fibroblast growth factors, angiopoietins, angiogenin, and the ephrins and their cognate receptors, which can also exist as secreted ligand-binding domains, as a result of alternative splicing that function as inhibitors.[138-140,142] Although the temporal and spatial patterns of expression of several other angiogenic factors and their receptors have been defined in the endometrium, the specific roles of each of these factors in the endometrial angiogenesis–vessel remodeling cycle remain to be elucidated.

Of the members of the vascular endothelial growth factor (VEGF) family that includes VEGF-A, VEGF-B, VEGF-C, and VEGF-D, VEGF-A is the most important for endometrial angiogenesis.[141-143] VEGF-A acts on two different receptors: VEGF receptor-2 (VEGFR2), which may play the dominant role in signaling endothelial cell proliferation, and another tyrosine kinase receptor, VEGFR1 (also known as FLT-1), which may play the dominant role in mediating the effects of VEGF on vascular permeability.[144-147] Both receptors are present on endothelial cells. VEGFR2, also known as *kinase domain receptor* (KDR), has been detected in stromal and epithelial cells of the premenstrual endometrium; this presence suggests actions on nonvascular compartments.

The premenstrual phase is characterized by a dramatic up-regulation of the VEGFR2 receptor in stromal cells of the superficial layers of the endometrium in response to progesterone withdrawal. The action of VEGF on VEGFR2 may participate in the increased expression of MMP-1 in the stroma in the premenstrual phase.

Expression of VEGF-A is detectable in glandular epithelial and stromal cells in the proliferative phase, presumably stimulated by estrogen. VEGF released from neutrophils in intimate contact with the endothelial cells is believed to stimulate endometrial vessel growth. It is also present in uterine NK cells. The release of VEGF from subepithelial NK cells has been suggested to play a role in directing the development of the subepithelial capillary network in the secretory phase. During the secretory phase, VEGF-A can be identified in surface epithelial cells, which presumably secrete it into the uterine cavity.

VEGF-A has four common splice variants (VEGF121, VEGF165, VEGF189, and VEGF 206). After ovulation, there is a remarkable shift in VEGF-A isoforms expressed in the uterus with the appearance of VEGF-A189 in the perivascular stromal cells; the VEGF-A189 isoform can be processed by proteolytic cleavage by plasminogen activator.[100] VEGF-A189 increases vascular permeability acting on VEGFR1, whereas its processed form binds to the VEGFR2 receptor, which mediates the mitogenic action on endothelial cells.

The highest levels of VEGF-A are found in the menstrual phase, probably in response to proinflammatory cytokines. The surge might also be attributed to focal hypoxia, which is a potent stimulus to *VEGF-A* gene transcription. Expression of *VEGFR1* and *VEGFR2* is also greatest in the menstrual phase. The elevated levels of VEGF and cognate receptor expression at this time are presumed to be important for vessel repair and preparation for angiogenesis in the proliferative phase. Notably, the functional activity of VEGFR2 (as assessed by receptor phosphorylation), a signature indicating ligand activation, is relatively low in the early menstrual phase, when levels of soluble VEGFR1 (sFLT-1), which sequesters VEGF, are highest. VEGFR2 receptor phosphorylation increases substantially in the late menstrual phase, remaining modestly elevated in the early and late proliferative phases, when sFLT-1 levels decline.[148]

The fibroblast growth factor (FGF) family of proteins may also participate in endometrial angiogenesis through interactions with the VEGF system. FGFs up-regulate VEGFR2 and VEGF-A expression, and in a feed-forward loop, VEGF-A promotes the release of FGFs from the extracellular matrix. Basic FGF is a potent stimulus for $\alpha v \beta 3$ integrin expression. This integrin is present at the site of active angiogenesis and is fundamental to endothelial invasion and vessel elongation during angiogenesis.[149]

The angiopoietins (Ang) regulate vessel stability. Ang-1, expressed in vascular smooth muscle cells, binds to a cognate receptor, Tie-2, on endothelial cells, resulting in vessel stabilization. Ang-2 is a physiologic antagonist of Ang-1. It also binds to the same Tie-2 receptor. Vessels atrophy when Ang-2 acts in the absence of VEGF-A, whereas angiogenesis is promoted in the presence of VEGF-A. In situ hybridization studies indicate that Ang-1 expression is most abundant in the glands and stroma of the early and midproliferative phases and is reduced in the late proliferative phase.[150] Ang-2 expression is detected in the glands and stroma throughout the cycle, with highest expression in the early proliferative and mid- to late secretory phases. In endometrium from women with menorrhagia, Ang-1 expression is consistently down-regulated; as a result, the ratio of Ang-1 to Ang-2 is reduced, which contributes to vessel instability.[150]

Angiogenin is a heparin-binding molecule that is expressed by endometrial epithelial and stromal cells at greatest levels in the mid- to late secretory phases and in the decidua of early pregnancy. Angiogenin is believed to contribute to the proliferation of vascular smooth muscle cells around the spiral arterioles. Like VEGF-A, expression of angiogenin is stimulated by hypoxia. It is also increased by progesterone.

Ephrins, a family of molecules and their cognate tyrosine kinase receptors, are believed to guide endothelial cells to specific targets. Ephrins have been detected in endometrial endothelial and stromal cells, but the functional roles of these molecules and their receptors in the uterus remain to be clarified.

The physiologic consequences of angiogenesis are reflected in changes in endometrial blood flow. By measuring the clearance of radioactive xenon gas, the highest endometrial perfusion was reported between days 10 and 12 and days 21 and 26 of the cycle.[86] Microvascular perfusion has been assessed by laser Doppler fluximetry with transvaginal placement of a fiber optic probe into the uterine cavity.[151] With use of this technique, endometrial perfusion was found to be highest during the proliferative phase and the early secretory phase, not too dissimilar from the finding based on xenon clearance. Uterine blood flow is greatest in the fundus, and higher flow rates are associated with better outcomes in assisted reproduction. Notably, diminished uterine blood flow has not been found in the perimenstrual period, but these methods cannot easily identify localized areas of vasoconstriction.

Extracellular Matrix Remodeling

The biochemical basis for the dramatic structural changes in the endometrium in the perimenstrual period includes the action of specific matrix-degrading proteases, the MMPs.[124,128-131] Studies on human endometrial explants in culture showed that degradation of the extracellular matrix occurs in the absence of progesterone and estrogen, which suppress the expression of MMPs. Moreover, this degradative process can be blocked by MMP inhibitors, but not by inhibitors of lysosomal cysteine proteinases, directly implicating MMPs in the catabolism of the endometrial extracellular matrix.

Enzymes of the fibrinolytic system, urokinase and tissue plasminogen activator, are increased in the endometrium as progesterone is withdrawn in the perimenstrual period. Moreover, plasminogen activator inhibitor (PAI)-1 expression is reduced, allowing the plasminogen activators to activate plasmin and proteolytically cleave and activate the latent MMP proenzymes.[152]

The MMPs represent a large family of proteinases that play a major role in remodeling of the extracellular matrix (Fig. 9-8). In situ hybridization and immunocytochemistry have been used to map the expression of MMPs and the endogenous inhibitors, tissue inhibitors of the metalloproteinases (TIMPs), in the primate endometrium. Cell-specific and menstrual cycle–specific patterns were revealed, with the most profound changes occurring during the perimenstrual period.[129,153] After ovulation, the expression of interstitial collagenase (MMP-1), stromelysin-1 (MMP-3), and stromelysin-2 (MMP-10) in the endometrial stroma is essentially restricted to the perimenstrual and menstrual phases.

Other MMPs are detected during the proliferative and secretory phases, but are significantly increased in expression perimenstrually. These include the type IV collagen-degrading enzymes MMP-2 and MMP-9. The membrane-bound MMP MMP-14 (which activates MMP-2) is detected during menstruation in stromal inflammatory cells and epithelial cells. TIMP-1, which is detectable in the endometrium throughout the cycle, is increased in the stroma, epithelium, and arterioles at menstruation.

The importance of progesterone withdrawal in regulating endometrial MMPs and the different temporal patterns of expression have been well documented in in vivo and

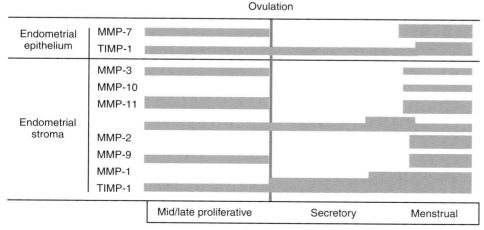

Figure 9-8. *Schematic of matrix metalloproteinase (MMP) expression in the human endometrium during the menstrual cycle. TIMP, tissue inhibitor of the matrix metalloproteinases. (Modified from Rodgers WH, Matrisian LM, Giudice LC, et al. Patterns of matrix metalloproteinase expression in cycling endometrium imply differential functions and regulation by steroid hormones. J Clin Invest 94:946-953, 1994.)*

Ovulation

| Endometrial epithelium | MMP-7 |
| | TIMP-1 |

Endometrial stroma	MMP-3
	MMP-10
	MMP-11
	MMP-2
	MMP-9
	MMP-1
	TIMP-1

Mid/late proliferative　　Secretory　　Menstrual

Phase of the endometrial cycle

in vitro systems.[91] In a primate model in which hormone levels were manipulated by steroid implants, progesterone withdrawal resulted in up-regulation of MMP-1, -2, -3, -7, -10, -11, and -14.

It is important to note that the expression of MMPs in the endometrium is heterogeneous.[124,153] At the start of menstruation, MMP-1 is found in patches of stromal cells in the superficial zone; these patches are colocalized with areas of reduced stromal and epithelial expression of estrogen and progesterone receptors and focal disruption of the extracellular argyrophilic fibrillar network, reflecting the degradative activity of MMP-1. As the process of menstruation proceeds, MMP-1 expression spreads to include the entire functionalis. Expression of MMP-2 and MMP-3 is also limited to the stromal cells in the functionalis. During menses, MMP-1, -2, -3, and -9 localize primarily in and around arteriolar walls. The heterogeneity of MMP expression suggests that MMP gene transcription is under the control of local rather than systemic (steroidal) factors. In other words, steroids are indirectly influencing MMP expression.

Progesterone, particularly in the presence of estradiol, can suppress the expression of certain MMPs (i.e., MMP-1, -2, -7, -9, and -11) in endometrial explant culture.[131] This action is most likely explained by changes in autocrine/paracrine signals, particularly proinflammatory cytokines or members of the transforming growth factor family, which respectively, are potent inducers and suppressors of MMP gene transcription. In culture systems, interleukin (IL)-1α has been implicated as the mediator of MMP-1, MMP-3, and MMP-7 expression in response to withdrawal of progesterone. Neutralizing antibodies to TGF-β prevent the action of progesterone in blocking MMP-3 and MMP-7 expression.

Endometrial bleeding factor (EBAF) is the orthologue of the murine gene named *Lefty* and another likely candidate for a progesterone-regulated cytokine controlling MMP expression.[154-156] EBAF, encoded by *LEFTY2*, was originally identified in human endometrium as a gene up-regulated in the late secretory and menstrual phases of the normal cycle, being absent in the proliferative, early, and midsecretory endometrium. EBAF expression, which is predominantly found in the endometrial stroma and, to a much lesser extent, in the glandular epithelium, is suppressed by progesterone. Interestingly, endometrium from women with a history of abnormal bleeding and endometriosis expressed EBAF at unusual times, including the proliferative, early, and midsecretory phases.[157]

Unlike other members of the TGF-β family that promote the formation and stability of the extracellular matrix, EBAF down-regulates the elaboration of collagen in association with reduced expression of connective tissue growth factor while up-regulating expression of collagenolytic and elastinolytic enzymes.[158] These actions of EBAF are the result of antagonism of the Smad signaling pathway that is activated by the other TGF-β growth factors. Thus, the decline in progesterone and estradiol in the late luteal phase initiates alterations in the endometrium that include up-regulation of proinflammatory cytokines (some of which may be contributed by immune cells that accumulate in the endometrium) and a natural TGF-β antagonist. The collective result is focal and then widespread expression of matrix-degrading enzymes that result in the remodeling of stroma and blood vessels in the functionalis.

Lysosomal involvement in the process of menstruation has been proposed because of three observations: an increase in the abundance of lysosomes in the endometrium during the late secretory phase, the cytochemical demonstration of acid phosphatase in the perimenstrual endometrium, and the high specific activity of certain lysosomal hydrolases in endometrial tissue in the menstrual phase.[159] However, inhibitors of these enzymes, leupeptin and E-64, do not prevent the progesterone withdrawal–induced breakdown of extracellular matrix in endometrial explants as do the inhibitors of MMP activity. These observations suggest that lysosomal proteinases are not major contributors to the remodeling of the perimenstrual endometrium.

Vasoactive Substances

The *endothelins* are a family of potent vasoconstrictors produced by endothelial cells that act on two types of receptors present on vascular smooth muscle. Endothelin-1, produced by endometrial epithelial or stromal cells, may act on spiral artery smooth muscle cells to promote vasoconstriction. Enkephalinase, a membrane-bound metalloendopeptidase, degrades endothelin-1 and other vasoactive peptides, and is present in highest levels in the midsecretory endometrium.[116] Expression of the gene encoding enkephalinase is up-regulated by progesterone. The decline in progesterone levels at the end of the luteal phase results in a subsequent fall in enkephalinase, which prolongs the biologic life of endothelin-1. Vasopressin may also function as a vasoconstrictor in the endometrium during the menstrual phase of the cycle.[160]

The production of prostaglandins, particularly $PGF_{2\alpha}$ and other eicosanoids in the endometrium, is enhanced by lysosomal phospholipases that liberate the arachidonic acid that accumulates in endometrium during the secretory phase; in turn, arachidonic acid is metabolized into prostanoids (see Chapter 6).[161] The premenstrual decrease in progesterone is also followed by induction of the prostaglandin synthase COX-2 and a decline in 15-hydroxyprostaglandin dehydrogenase activity, which inactivates $PGF_{2\alpha}$. This induction of the prostaglandin synthase COX-2 and the decline in 15-hydroxyprostaglandin dehydrogenase leads to increased production and bioavailability of $PGF_{2\alpha}$, which triggers myometrial contractions that compress the endometrial vasculature and promote hemostasis (Fig. 9-9).[162]

Hemostatic and Fibrinolytic Mechanisms

The relative activities of the hemostatic and fibrinolytic systems in the endometrium are shifted in the perimenstrual period such that clotting activity is reduced and fibrinolytic activity is increased. Consequently, menstrual fluid does not normally clot, even on prolonged storage. Decidualized stromal cells express tissue factor, the primary trigger of thrombin formation and hemostasis, under the influence of progesterone.[121] Tissue factor production by the

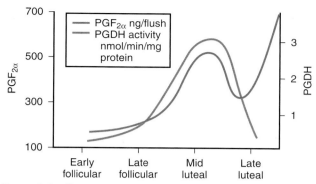

Figure 9-9. *Changes in (PCF₂ₐ) levels and endometrial 15-hydroxy-prostoglandin dehydrogenase (PGDH) activity. (From Casey ML, Hemsell DL, MacDonald PC, et al. NAD+ dependent 15-hydroxy prostaglandin dehydrogenase activity in human endometrium. Prostaglandins 19: 115-122, 1980; and Demers LM, Halbert DR, Jones DF, Fontana J. Prostaglandin F levels in endometrial jet wash specimens during the normal human menstrual cycle. Prostaglandins 10[6]:1057-1065, 1975.)*

decidualized stromal cells declines with withdrawal of progesterone.

The endometrial fibrinolytic system includes urokinase-type plasminogen activator and tissue-type plasminogen activator, which cleave plasminogen to yield the fibrinolytic enzyme plasmin.[121,163,164] Progesterone reduces expression of urokinase and increases that of PAI-1 in cultured endometrial cells. Removal of progesterone or the addition of the anti-progestin, mifepristone, reverses these responses.[164]

THE UTERUS IN THE CYCLE OF CONCEPTION AND PREGNANCY

The examination of hysterectomy specimens revealed that the first consistent structural changes in the endometrium of early pregnancy are recrudescence or accentuation of glandular secretory activity, edema, and the predecidual reaction.[165] The increased prominence of the vasculature is considered to be a manifestation of increased blood flow, which may account for the associated edema. Endometrial biopsies in a cycle of conception suggest that stromal edema and vascular congestion are the earliest persistent morphologic features of the endometrium of pregnancy.[166]

Within the first weeks of gestation, the endometrium undergoes characteristic changes in which the epithelial cells become distended with a clear cytoplasm (Fig. 9-10). Many of the epithelial cells develop enlarged and hyperchromatic nuclei. The enlarged nuclei are polyploid. These changes are commonly referred to as the *Arias-Stella reaction.*[167,168] The ultrastructural characteristics of the endometrium are consistent with a hypersecretory state. Parallel channels of endoplasmic reticulum and large mitochondria are abundant in the epithelial cells, and the Golgi complexes have numerous stacked saccules.

The Arias-Stella reaction has an irregular distribution in the uterus and is present in approximately 50% of the uteri of women with ectopic pregnancies. It could reflect changes in steroid hormone levels as well as the direct action of hCG on the endometrium, a subject discussed

later in this chapter. The endometrium exhibits significant changes in cellular composition that are reflected in the marked alterations in the synthesis and secretion of endometrial proteins. As gestation advances, endometrial glands atrophy and are scarce at term.

The decidua develops with continued exposure of the uterus to progesterone, secreted initially by the corpus luteum and later by the trophoblast of the placenta. Based on in vitro studies, other factors (including hCG and relaxin) may act synergistically with progesterone to promote decidualization. Because exogenous cyclic AMP (cAMP) in the presence of progesterone represents a sufficient in vitro stimulus to induce stromal cell differentiation into decidual cells, relaxin and hCG possibly increase levels of this second messenger. Extrapolating from studies on the mouse, including findings on knockout animals that have been found to be defective in decidualization, it is possible that amphiregulin, HOXA10, HOXA11, IL-11, LIF, and prostaglandins have a role in human decidual response.

The decidualized stroma represents a tissue plane that is both permissive and simultaneously restrictive of trophoblast invasion and placentation; its remodeling is crucial to the morphogenesis of the placenta and the establishment of the uteroplacental circulation. Moreover, the decidualized stroma represents the arena where the fetal semiallograft is exposed to maternal immunologically competent cells. While creating a hospitable environment for trophoblast invasion, the decidua also sets limits on this process to prevent excessive penetration and tissue destruction beyond its bounds.

The plump, polygonal decidual cells are arranged in a cobblestone configuration. The ultrastructural features of the decidual cells—including prominent Golgi complexes, dilated rough endoplasmic reticulum, and dense membrane-bound secretory granules—are characteristic of secretory cells. The histologically distinct cell borders around decidual cells reflect the accumulation of a pericellular matrix (Fig. 9-11).[118,119] The abundant decidual cell prolyl hydroxylase, an enzyme involved in collagen synthesis, indicates the important role of these cells in extracellular matrix production. There is also an abundance of amorphous components, including high–molecular-weight proteins with voluminous saccharide moieties (e.g., heparin sulfate proteoglycan). Fibrillar collagens are partially broken down and reorganized. Type V collagen epitopes are unmasked; collagen type 4 "stiff" short collagen fibers that bridge other fibrillar collagens, disappears from most of the stroma and persists only in association with vessels and the basement membrane of the glands.

The deposition of a basement membrane–type matrix containing laminin and type IV collagens around the decidual cells contributes to the formation of a "looser stroma" that serves as a substrate for the invading trophoblasts. For example, entactin, a component of this basement membrane–like matrix, promotes trophoblast cell adhesion and migration. The decidual matrix is also a rich source of cytokines, protease inhibitors, protease precursors, and other factors that modulate cell behavior. These are derived, at least in part, from the decidual cells whose secretory products also include IGFBP-1 and TGF-β, which may restrain the invasion of trophoblast cells.[169,170]

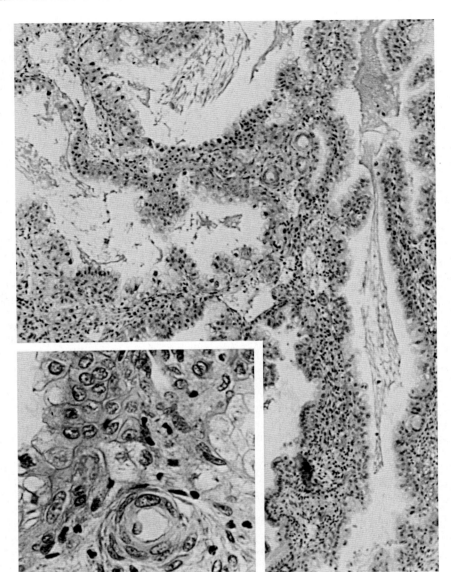

Figure 9-10. *Arias-Stella reaction. Hypersecretory glands with enlarged hyperchromatic nuclei are present. The glands have scalloped borders.* Inset, *High-power view.*

THE ENDOMETRIUM IN ADVANCING AGE

Based on donor oocyte pregnancies achieved in postmenopausal women whose reproductive tract was programmed with exogenous steroid hormones, uterine aging in the absence of acquired pathology does not preclude successful implantation and carriage of a pregnancy to term. The relentless ability of the endometrium to restore itself may hint at its longevity. A rich source of the enzyme telomerase,[171] the endometrium may have the ability to delay the normal aging process. However, there are structural changes that take place in the uterus with advancing age, pregnancy, and the cessation of ovarian function. Whether these changes affect the "reproductive potential" of the uterus or contribute to the increased incidence of pregnancy complications associated with advanced maternal age is not known.

The basal endometrium interdigitates with the myometrium with advancing age, resulting in a degree of superficial adenomyosis that is a normal finding in the uterus in the fifth decade of life. The infiltrating endometrium does not undergo normal cyclic changes. This may be a consequence of a uterus hosting a past pregnancy.[172]

After menopause, in the absence of hormone replacement, endometrial atrophy is apparent and mitotic activity ceases. Epithelial cells shrink, and the stroma becomes fibrotic. A compact eosinophilic material is found in the lumina of the endometrial glands, occasionally engorging them and giving rise to the histologic pattern referred to as *cystic atrophy* (Fig. 9-12).

THE UTERINE CERVIX

The cervix functions as a biologic valve that controls the access of sperm and microorganisms into the uterine cavity.[173] During pregnancy, it helps to retain the fetus and extraembryonic tissues and fluids in the uterus until the time of parturition. The endocervix is lined by tall columnar ciliated and nonciliated secretory cells. A rich extracellular matrix consisting of fibrillar collagens and elastin with embedded fibroblasts and a small percentage of smooth

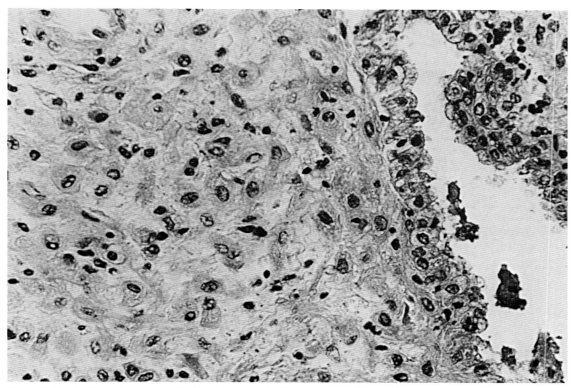

Figure 9-11. Decidua of pregnancy. Decidualized stromal cells are plump and have distinct cell borders. Glands are atrophic.

muscle cells (approximately 10%) lies beneath the endocervical epithelium. There are no true glands in the endocervix, but rather an intricate system of crypts or grooves. These endocervical cells stop at a sharply demarcated junction with the stratified squamous epithelium that covers the portio vaginalis at the external os.

The secretory cells of the endocervix elaborate mucus, with an average production of 20 to 60 mg daily in a woman of reproductive age. At midcycle, this production rate increases 10-fold to 20-fold. The mucus is a complex mixture of water, electrolytes, and mucins, which are large glycoproteins that are heavily laden with O-linked oligosaccharides. Human cervical mucus is approximately 92% to 94% water, but the water content rises to 98% at the time of ovulation. Inorganic salts make up approximately 1% of the mucus by weight.

Mucins represent 45% of the protein content of cervical mucus.[174,175] The mucin core proteins typically contain tandem repeat domains enriched in serine, threonine, and proline residues. These molecules have a role in protecting the upper reproductive tract from bacterial colonization by trapping microorganisms; they also protect the epithelial cell surface, and as a result of their hydration, form a gel that keeps the cervical canal open.

The cervix expresses a number of mucin genes, including *MUCl, M17C4, M17C5AC, M17C5B, MUC6,* and *MUC8*. The periovulatory mucins form a hydrogel, a large mesh that facilitates penetration by motile sperm. The abundance of the mRNA encoding the major cervical gel–forming mucin, MUC5B, is greatest right before ovulation; the amount of MUC5B protein per unit protein in the cervical mucus reaches a peak at ovulation. Cervical expression of MUC5B mRNA declines markedly after ovulation.

The composition of mucus determines its rheologic properties, including consistency, flow elasticity, Spinnbarkeit (the capacity of liquids to be drawn into threads), thixotropy, and tack, as well as its ability to form a ferning pattern when dried as a result of crystallization of salts (sodium chloride and potassium chloride) in the presence of protein. In the preovulatory phase, the mucus is profuse, thin, clear, and acellular, with an alkaline pH. Semiquantitative scoring schemes that assess quantity, rheologic properties such as Spinnbarkeit, ferning, and the appearance of the cervix and cervical os have been used to assess the estrogen status of women. Progestin-only contraceptives, including long-acting injectables and progestins delivered in implants, result in a viscous cervical mucus that impedes sperm penetration. These effects on cervical mucus and sperm penetration can be seen 3 days after insertion of a levonorgestrel-releasing implant.[176]

THE MYOMETRIUM

The myometrium is organized into strata: an external hood-like layer covering the fundus, a dense network of fibers beneath it, and an innermost layer surrounding the internal os and tubal ostia. Magnetic resonance imaging (MRI) of the uterus of women of reproductive age shows two distinct myometrial zones: the junctional zone underlying the endometrium (which has low signal intensity) and the outer myometrium (which has relatively high signal intensity)[177] (see Chapter 33). The junctional zone

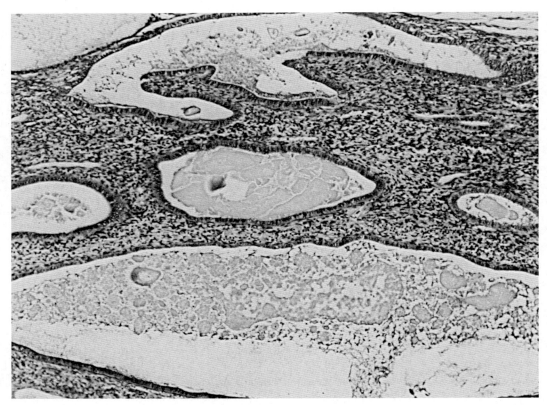

Figure 9-12. Postmenopausal endometrium. Epithelial cells are flat. The stroma is fibrotic and compact. Eosinophilic material has accumulated in the gland lumina.

corresponds to the hypoechogenic layer of the myometrium, the subendometrial halo observed in ultrasound images. The lower T2-weighted signal intensity of the junctional zone is due to the lower water content (mostly a consequence of contractile activity of this zone that decreases its blood volume), smaller quantity of extracellular matrix, and more tightly packed smooth muscle cells. This zonal anatomy is apparently dependent on sex hormones because it is not evident before menarche or in postmenopausal women who are not receiving hormone replacement therapy. MRI images show that the junctional zone is altered in early pregnancy, evidently as a consequence of embryo-derived factors.

The functions of the junctional zone of the myometrium appear to be linked to events in the menstrual cycle and the establishment of early pregnancy; those of the outer myometrium are related to pregnancy and parturition. The junctional zone has several unique features that distinguish it biochemically and functionally from the outer myometrium. Although steroid hormone receptors are expressed throughout the myometrium, the junctional zone exhibits cyclic changes in expression of estrogen and progesterone receptors that parallel those of the endometrium. This differs from the "outer" myometrium, which does not show marked cyclic changes in receptor expression.

During the menstrual cycle, subendometrial peristalsis can be observed by ultrasonography and ultrafast MRI[178-181] (see Chapter 33). The frequency, intensity, and direction of the subendometrial contractions vary during the menstrual cycle. They average two to three cycles per minute and flow from cervix to fundus at midcycle,

diminish in the luteal phase, and increase again during menstruation, but in a fundal-to-cervical direction. Changes in steroid hormone levels, expression of hormone receptors, and prostanoids govern the peristaltic activity. Some authors have suggested that the contractile activity of the junctional zone alters uterine shape from an elongated configuration in the follicular phase to a piriform configuration in the luteal phase, changes that make the uterine cavity more spherical after ovulation.[182]

In some pathologic states, including endometriosis or adenomyosis, dystonic uterine contractions have been observed.[183-185] Whether these aberrant contraction patterns contribute to infertility and other symptoms of endometriosis remains to be determined. It is tempting to speculate that disruptions in the normal fundal-to-cervical contractions during menstruation might worsen the sensation of uterine cramping associated with endometriosis and perhaps even contribute to the retrograde menstruation believed to underlie the pathogenesis of this disorder.

The myometrial compartment changes dramatically during pregnancy, primarily as a result of muscle hypertrophy, the elaboration of extracellular matrix, and an increase in lymphatics and blood vessels. The wet weight of the human uterus increases 10-fold during pregnancy, and its carrying capacity increases from 300 mL to 4.5 L, largely owing to hypertrophy and hyperplasia of the myometrium. The myometrial hyperplasia is steroid hormone–dependent and is probably mediated by growth factors, particularly the IGFs.[68] The primate myometrium expresses all components of the IGF signaling system, including IGF-1, IGF-2, and the type 1 growth factor receptor, as well as IGF-binding proteins (IGFBPs 2, 3, 4, and 5). Progesterone enhances expression of IGF-1 mRNA stimulated by estrogen. The stimulation of IGF-1 expression is accompanied by an increased number of Ki-67–positive myometrial cells, indicating myometrial cell proliferation.

Immunology of the Reproductive Tract

The uterus is an immunologically privileged organ: it can accommodate the fetus and extraembryonic tissues as a semiallograft, yet it also is endowed with mucosal immunity, defenses against ascending foreign organisms, and a system to efficiently clear the endometrial detritus that results from menstruation (see Chapter 6). The human reproductive tract has both an innate and an adaptive immune system. Uterine epithelial cells express members of the Toll-like receptor family (TLR 2-6, 9, and 10), which detect pathogen products and trigger a cellular response to these "foreign" molecules, including peptidoglycans from Gram-positive bacteria (TLR2), lipopolysaccharide from Gram-negative bacteria (TLR4), and unmethylated CpG islands found in bacterial DNA (TLR9). The endometrium also produces host defense molecules, defensins, as well as cytokines and chemokines. Uterine lymphoid and myeloid cells play roles in tissue defense, immune modulation, angiogenesis, and tissue remodeling.[117,186-189] These cells are present in the fallopian tubes, uterus, and cervix, with the fallopian tubes and uterus containing a higher proportion of leukocytes than the normal vagina.[190] The endometrial innate and adaptive immune systems are regulated by steroid hormones. For example, progesterone induces a local Th2-type cytokine response in the uterus, which includes an increase in IL-4, IL-5, and IL-15, and down-regulation of the IL-13 receptor α_2, which is a negative regulator of the anti-inflammatory cytokine, IL-13. This Th2 response is believed to counter proinflammatory processes in the endometrium that could lead to rejection of the embryo. Steroid hormone–directed alterations in endometrial chemokine production also influence the trafficking of blood leukocytes in the reproductive tract.

LEUKOCYTES AND LYMPHOCYTES

There are striking menstrual cycle–dependent changes in the immune cell population of the endometrium. Neutrophils, the most abundant leukocytes of the immune system, are rare in the normal endometrium until the perimenstrual phase, when they accumulate and account for 6% to 15% of the total cell number. Eosinophils are also rarely found in the normal endometrium until the perimenstrual phase, when they also accumulate—usually in aggregates—and show evidence of activation, as revealed by the extracellular location of eosinophil cationic proteins. Macrophages are present in the endometrium throughout the cycle, increasing in number from the proliferative phase to the menstrual phase. Immediately before menstruation, the number of macrophages in the functional layer of the endometrium is equivalent to that of neutrophils.

Mast cells expressing tryptase (a characteristic of mucosal mast cells) and chymase (a characteristic of connective tissue mast cells) are found in the human endometrium. In the functionalis, mast cells are positive only for tryptase, whereas those in the basalis express both enzymes. Degranulation of these cells may initiate activation of MMPs as a result of tryptase and chymase action on proMMP-1 and proMMP-3.

The endometrial lymphoid system has a distinctive composition and activity. There is good reason to believe that endometrial T cells are activated in situ, as judged by their expression of antigens that are characteristic of the activated state; these antigens include the major histocompatibility complex (MHC) class II molecules HLA-DR, HLA-DP, and HLA-DQ, and very late antigen 1. CD3+ T cells represent only 1% to 2% of the lymphomyeloid cells detectable in the human endometrium. They are present throughout the cycle in aggregates in the basalis, as well as singly throughout the stroma and in intraepithelial sites. The number of these cells increases before menstruation. The ratio of CD4+ T helper lymphocytes to CD8+ cytotoxic T cells in the endometrium is inverted compared with peripheral blood. The latter are cytolytically active during the proliferative phase, but this activity diminishes in the secretory phase. This decline might reflect the influence of the tissue environment programmed by steroid hormones, or possibly an alteration in the cell population through deletion or recruitment of CD8+ cells with a different phenotype. Few B cells and plasma cells are present in the human endometrium.

UTERINE NATURAL KILLER CELLS

The uterine NK cell, also known as the *granular lymphocyte*, is a unique member of the lymphoid lineage found in the endometrium.[186] These are round cells that characteristically have bilobed or indented nuclei and a pale cytoplasm containing acidophilic granules. They are a specialized subset of NK cells, based on their expression of cell surface antigens (CD3−, CD16+, and NCAM/CD-56bright). This pattern is different from that of blood NK cells, which have a phenotype of CD56dim CD16+.

Uterine NK cells are among the most abundant lymphomyeloid cells in the perimenstrual endometrium. Very few are present in the proliferative phase endometrium; they accumulate during the secretory phase, at which time they comprise 15% to 25% of the cells in the endometrial stroma. It has been postulated that the dynamic changes in uterine NK cell number during the cycle are determined by changes in endometrial prolactin production, which is controlled by ovarian steroid hormones. This notion is based on the known roles of prolactin as an immunomodulator and the correlation between endometrial prolactin levels and NK cells.[191,192]

The NK cells persist in the decidua during the first trimester of pregnancy, when they represent 70% of the decidual leukocyte population. Their close association with stromal cells has led to the suggestion that they have an important role in initiating and maintaining decidualization. In a nonfertile cycle, the NK cells that amass during the secretory phase undergo programmed cell death.

When activated by IL-2 in vitro, NK cells become competent to kill malignant cells (and some normal ones) through the release of cytotoxic proteins such as perforin. Beginning in the late proliferative phase, the NK cells express cytotoxic activity and are believed to play a role in protecting the endometrium against infection. The cells have also been proposed to modulate trophoblast invasion during implantation and placentation because of their abundance in the decidua during the first trimester.

Although in vitro studies document the killing activity of cytokine-activated NK cells, there is little evidence of destruction of trophoblast cells in vivo. Thus, any restraining activity that NK cells exert on invading trophoblast cells appears to be through a noncytotoxic mechanism that may involve secreted cytokines, including colony-stimulating factor-1 (CSF-1), IL-1, LIF, and interferon-γ. The apparent in vitro and in vivo resistance of trophoblast cells to killing by NK cells may be explained by the fact that trophoblast cells express a nonclassic and nonpolymorphic MHC class I antigen, HLA-G. NK killing activity is also suppressed by endometrial stromal cells, which may help spare trophoblast.

In the transgenic mouse line, TgE26, which lacks NK cells, abnormal implantation sites are found. Fetal demise follows, in association with changes in uterine arterioles suggestive of arteriosclerosis and hypertension.[192] These histopathologic changes are reminiscent of preeclampsia in humans. In contrast, mice lacking IL-15, and consequently, circulating and decidual NK cells, are fertile, but show a thickening in uterine vessels. These findings collectively implicate NK cells in vessel remodeling, a role consistent with their expression of angiogenic factors.

FACTORS REGULATING UTERINE IMMUNE CELL DYNAMICS

The changes in lymphomyeloid cell populations in the endometrium, particularly their accumulation in the premenstrual phase, appear to be the result of recruitment from the peripheral circulation and intraendometrial proliferation. The accumulation of migratory cells is directed by chemoattractant cytokines, chemokines, and the expression of intercellular adhesion molecules that attach leukocytes to the endothelium in preparation for extravasation and trafficking through the endometrium.[193] Expression of these molecules changes during the menstrual cycle, at least partly under the influence of steroid hormones.

The expression of several chemokines has been documented in the human endometrium, including fractalkine (CX3CL1), RANTES (CCL5), IL-8, MCP-1 (CCL2), MCP-2 (CCL8), and eotaxin (CCL11). These chemokines bind to receptors on leukocytes, promoting the appearance of molecules that mediate adhesion to the endothelium, extravasation, and chemotaxis along the concentration gradient of the chemokine, thus targeting specific leukocyte types to specific endometrial compartments. A repertoire of cell adhesion molecules expressed in the endometrium, including ICAM-1, ICAM-2, VCAM-1, E-selectin, and PECAM, specifies the recruitment and location of leukocyte and platelet accumulation. ICAM-1 is present in the functionalis in the menstrual phase; ICAM-2 is restricted to the vascular endothelium and does not appear to change during the cycle,

VCAM-1 and E-selectin appear in the upper layer of the functionalis in the secretory phase, and the platelet endothelial cell adhesion molecule PECAM is abundant in the stroma during the menstrual phase.

Evidence of leukocyte proliferation in the endometrium includes the expression of Ki-67 and the incorporation of BrdU (both proliferation markers) by NK cells, with a marked increase in the secretory phase. Uterine NK cell proliferation may be driven by progesterone-regulated stromal factors because CD56+ cells proliferate in vitro in the presence of progesterone-treated endometrial tissue.

THE COMPLEMENT SYSTEM

The human fallopian tube, endometrium, and cervical mucosa express components of the complement system.[194-198] Activation of the third (C3) and fourth (C4) components of complement induces chemotaxis of inflammatory cells, enhances phagocytosis, and mediates cell lysis. This system of natural immunity must be tightly regulated so that it can target foreign organisms and cells while avoiding untoward tissue damage. This is especially important during early pregnancy, when the process of implantation might be disrupted. Complement activation is regulated by decay-accelerating factor (DAF, also known as CD55), which inactivates the C3 convertase enzymes that activate C3, and by membrane cofactor protein (MCP, also known as CD46), which serves as a cofactor for factor I–mediated degradation of activated C3 and C4.

A third protein, present only in rodents, complement regulator decay–accelerating factor (Crry), has DAF- and MCP-like activities. Crry controls the deposition of activated C3 and C4 on the surface of autologous cells. Fetal demise due to complement deposition and placental inflammation was observed in mice lacking Crry, reflecting unchecked activation of the complement system.[199] Complement activation appears to be an essential event in pregnancy loss associated with antiphospholipid syndrome and can be prevented by administration of heparin.[200-202] These observations suggest that control of the complement system is essential for fetomaternal tolerance against attack by the innate immune system.

In the endometrium, complement component C3, factor B, and DAF are present in the glandular epithelium, and their expression is up-regulated in the secretory phase. MCP is expressed in the glandular epithelium throughout the menstrual cycle. Complement receptor 1 is present in the stroma during the secretory phase; complement receptor 2 is not detectable, and complement receptor 3 is associated with infiltrating leukocytes in the luteal phase. The cyclic changes in C3, factor B, and DAF expression suggest progesterone regulation. In model human endometrial epithelial cell culture systems, however, steroid hormones did not alter decay-accelerating factor expression, but heparin-binding epidermal-like growth factor (HB-EGF) did increase it.[151] Thus, the steroid hormone effects on expression of some of the complement system proteins may be indirect, perhaps acting through the stromal compartment.

Members of the integrin family are now believed to be involved in the regulation of C3, as some of the protective proteins that prevent the cascade of complement activation. DAF or factor H may interact with these cell surface receptors (including αvβ3 integrin and perhaps CD44) through binding to osteopontin (OPN) to limit C3 activation by digesting bound C3b. The αvβ3 integrin, OPN, and DAF all appear synchronously at the time of implantation in human endometrium and may serve as a primary safeguard against complement activation at the time of embryonic attachment, thus avoiding destruction of the early pregnancy by the host's defenses.

ANTIMICROBIAL PEPTIDES

Epithelial cells of the female reproductive tract elaborate antimicrobial peptides that presumably guard against ascending infection.[203,204] These peptides coat the epithelial surface and enter the cervical mucus. Among the antimicrobial peptides expressed other than complement are lactoferrin, lysozyme, secretory leukocyte protease inhibitor (SLP1), and defensins. The α-defensins are elaborated by leukocytes and epithelial cells and the β-defensins by epithelial cells. Defensin-5 and α-defensin are expressed in the upper half of the stratified squamous epithelium of the vagina and ectocervix and in columnar epithelial cells of the fallopian tube and endometrium. β-Defensin-1 and -2 and secretory leukocyte protease inhibitors are produced by endometrial glandular epithelial cells. β-Defensin-2 expression is increased by proinflammatory cytokines, and defensin-5 is also evidently up-regulated by inflammation. Defensin-5 and secretory leukocyte protease inhibitor levels in the endometrium also fluctuate during the endometrial cycle, being highest in the secretory phase.

Uterine Receptivity and Embryo Implantation

The timing of conception is exquisitely synchronized to ovarian events. With ovulation, progesterone from the nascent corpus luteum transforms the proliferative phase endometrium into a secretory structure and readies it for the newly fertilized ovum (Fig. 9-13A and 9-13B).[113,205] With the appropriate endocrine milieu, the growing embryo will interact with the surface epithelium and invade the underlying stroma, initiating gestation (Fig. 9-13C). Implantation can be divided into distinct and separate stages, timed precisely to the steroid-mediated changes ongoing in the endometrium (Fig. 9-14).[206] After ovulation, the ovum enters the fallopian tube, where fertilization occurs. The early cell divisions ensue and the embryo enters the uterine cavity at the morula stage, approximately 2 to 3 days after being fertilized.

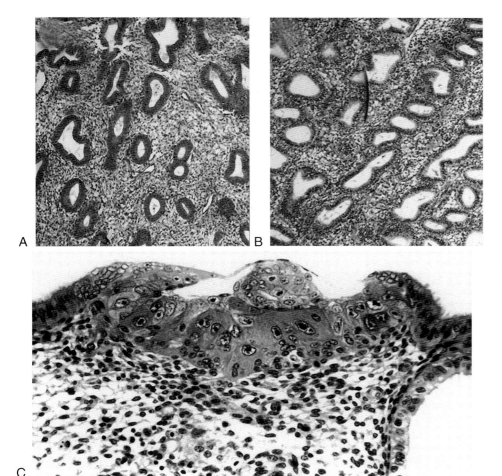

Figure 9-13. *Proliferative (**A**, prereceptive) and midsecretory (**B**, receptive) endometrium is regulated by ovarian steroids, resulting in successful implantation of the human embryo (**C**). (Generously provided by Dr. Allen Enders, from the Carnegie Collection of early human implantation sites. Used with permission from Human Reproduction.)*

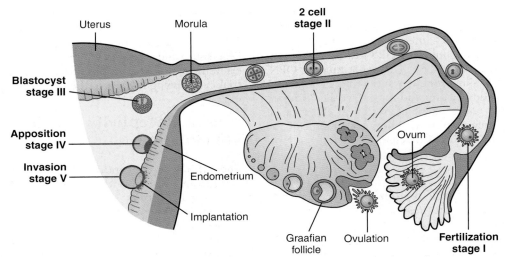

Figure 9-14. *Stages of implantation, beginning with ovulation and followed by fertilization and transport to the waiting endometrium. Implantation depends on synchronous development between the endometrium and the embryo.*

Implantation begins several days later, around the sixth to seventh day after fertilization. The initial attachment reaction (apposition) may be the rate-limiting step, and failure to adhere may preclude the subsequent stages of implantation.

Studies in experimental and domestic animals have shown that there must be synchronous development of the embryo and endometrium for normal implantation and development to occur.[207-211] In laboratory animals, there is a discrete "window" of time for implantation, which in some species lasts only a matter of hours.[211] The concept of a "window" for implantation has also been proposed in the human,[209,212-214] but the molecular basis for the alterations in human endometrium leading to uterine receptivity remains to be firmly elucidated.

Uterine receptivity is defined as the period of endometrial maturation during which the trophectoderm of the blastocyst can attach to the endometrial epithelial cells and subsequently proceed to invade the endometrial stroma. The transition from the nonreceptive to the receptive endometrial state is presumably determined by the regulated expression of membrane-bound, soluble, or secretory factors that are permissive to trophoblast attachment and subsequent migration. Factors expressed during this temporal window can be considered as either biomarkers or functional mediators of the receptive state.

Because the human blastocyst can implant at ectopic sites, it may not have such rigorous requirements for nidation. Although human embryos are capable of attachment and spreading on various extracellular matrix components or other cells, it is evident that there is a defined period during which such a process can occur in vivo and within the uterus. In the rodent model, the luminal surface may define the barrier to implantation, as its removal allows for implantation outside this restricted period of receptivity.[215]

The timing of implantation has been examined with increasing scrutiny over the last 50 years. In the 1950s, luteal phase hysterectomy samples in pregnant subjects suggested that embryos did not attach until day 20 of a 28-day cycle.[165] Using fertilized donor oocytes transferred into hormonally prepared recipients, Navot and Bergh later suggested that implantation occurred between cycle days 20 and 24.[216] More recently, by examining the time of pregnancy in 221 normal cycling women who were attempting pregnancy, Wilcox and coworkers showed that implantation normally occurred between 7 and 10 days after ovulation (days 21 to 24).[214] In these studies, delayed implantation was associated with a higher miscarriage rate, possibly due to a shift in the time of implantation and the concomitant loss of synchrony between endometrium and embryo (Fig. 9-15). This explanation may provide insights into some cases of otherwise unexplained infertility and recurrent pregnancy loss.

Implantation can be viewed as a highly complex and orchestrated interaction between the maternal endometrium and the newly formed embryo.[206,217] As seen in Figure 9-16, multiple soluble and membrane-bound factors have been elucidated that facilitate embryo growth, differentiation, attachment, invasion, and defense against immunologic rejection. Maternal factors appear to simultaneously permit intrusion while limiting the degree of embryonic invasion into maternal tissue. Many of the embryonic signals or receptors have complementary ligands or coreceptors on the maternal surface. Mimicking of maternal antigens by the invading embryo is a strategy that is also used by the embryo to penetrate the endometrium, without triggering host defenses.[218]

Major Uterine Secretory Products

The endometrium produces a large number of secreted proteins that serve autocrine, paracrine, and juxtacrine roles for the developing endometrium and embryo.[211,217] In addition to secretory proteins and glycoproteins, the uterus is highly endowed with members of the adenosine triphosphate–binding cassette transporter family; these proteins are involved in the secretion or exclusion of a

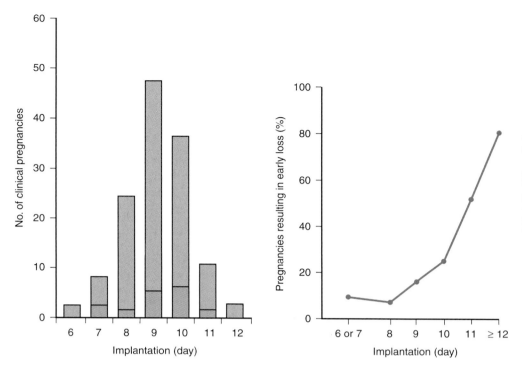

Figure 9-15. The timing of implantation in a population of fertile women. Fifteen of these clinical pregnancies ended in miscarriage (blue bars). (Reproduced with permission from Wilcox AJ, Baird DD, Weinberg CR. Time of implantation of the conceptus and loss of pregnancy. N Engl J Med 340:1796-1799, 1999.)

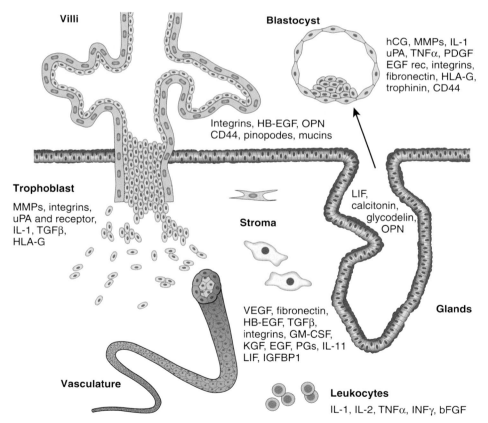

Figure 9-16. Schematic showing some of the factors and their cells of origin during normal implantation in women. EGF, epidermal growth factor; EGF rec, EGF receptor; FGF, fibroblast growth factor; GM-CSF, granulocyte–macrophage colony-stimulating factor; HB-EGF, heparin-binding epidermal-like growth factor; hCG, human chorionic gonadotropin; HLA-G, IGFB, insulin-like growth factor; IL, interleukin; INF, KGF, MMPs, matrix metalloproteinases; OPN, osteopontin; PDGF, platelet-derived growth factor; PGs, TGF, transforming growth factor; TNF, tumor necrosis factor; UF, uPA, VEGF, vascular endothelial growth factor.

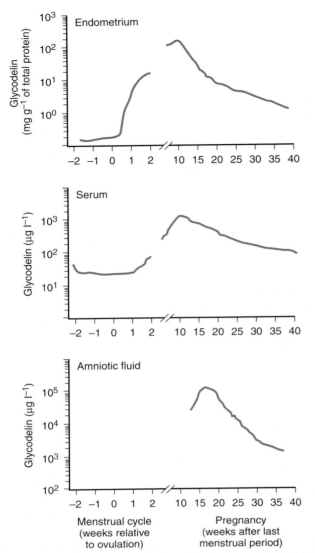

Figure 9-17. *Glycodelin levels in endometrium, serum, and amniotic fluid. (Reprinted with permission from Seppala M, Koistinen H, Koistinen R. Glycodelins. Trends Endocrinol Metab 72:111-117, 2001.)*

variety of small molecules from cells, including drugs, lipids, and conjugated molecules.[219]

The secretory proteins of the uterus have been most thoroughly studied. Some of these proteins enter the general circulation and can be detected in the serum, whereas others are localized within the lumen of the uterine cavity; these probably function to nurture or direct growth and differentiation of the early embryo (see Fig. 9-16). A remarkable increase in secretory activity is associated with the luteal phase and early pregnancy, primarily in the glandular epithelial cells and later in the decidua. Many of these secreted proteins are expressed either directly or indirectly in response to progesterone.[205,220,221] Several secretory proteins produced by the endometrium deserve special attention because of their potential physiologic relevance to endometrial and trophoblast function or their utility as markers of endometrial function.

GLYCODELIN

Glycodelin, one of the most abundant products of the secretory phase endometrial glands and decidua, is known by several names: *progesterone-associated endometrial protein, α-uterine protein, pregnancy-associated endometrial α₂ globulin, endometrial protein 15, chorionic α₂ macroglobulin,* and *placental protein 14* (an erroneous designation because glycodelin is an endometrial/decidual protein).[221,222] The mature form of glycodelin contains 162 amino acid residues and is 17.5% carbohydrate by weight. It has extensive structural homology with the β-lactoglobulins and, to a lesser extent, with retinol-binding proteins.

Glycodelin exists as isoforms, depending on its glycosylation pattern. Glycodelin A is the major progesterone-regulated protein secreted into the uterine lumen. However, its functions with respect to the endometrium, implantation, and pregnancy are still largely unknown. Glycodelin A is a potent inhibitor of sperm–egg binding, and researchers have postulated that it may play a role as an immunomodulator because of its ability to suppress NK cells.[223,224] The absence of glycodelin A during the time of fertilization and its appearance during the time of implantation and placentation are consistent with these proposed functions.[225]

Glycodelin levels in uterine flushings are tightly correlated with the histologic date of the endometrium (Fig. 9-17). It is not detectable in significant amounts in uterine flushings during the follicular and early luteal phases. Six days after ovulation, however, the levels rise rapidly to reach a concentration 100 times higher than plasma levels. In peripheral serum, glycodelin appears 5 days after ovulation, reaching peak concentrations in nonfertile cycles at approximately the time of menstruation; levels reach a nadir during the midfollicular phase of the subsequent cycle. In a cycle of conception, glycodelin levels increase rapidly after implantation, reaching a maximum at 8 to 10 weeks of gestation and subsequently declining in a pattern that mimics the changes in hCG.

The discordant pattern of glycodelin and progesterone in serum may reflect the slower turnover of the protein. Levels of glycodelin in serum do not rise in women using combination-type oral contraceptives and in some patients with luteal phase defects.[226] There is good—but not perfect—correlation between the progestational activity of steroids and their ability to stimulate endometrial glycodelin synthesis.

Relaxin has also been implicated as a stimulus for glycodelin expression.[225,227] Some histone deacetylase inhibitors have been shown to potentiate the action of progesterone on both endometrial epithelium and stroma and modulate glycodelin production.[228] The histone deacetylase inhibitor trichostatin (TSA) induces glycodelin in Ishikawa cells. Using an in vitro model of implantation, Uchida et al showed that induction of glycodelin by another histone deacetylase inhibitor enhanced placental cell (JAR) spheroid attachment to Ishikawa cells.[229] This and other studies suggest a role for glycodelin in both the differentiation and function of the receptive endometrium.

Glycodelin has been shown to be decreased in the endometrium of women with infertility, including those with luteal phase defects[226] and PCOS.[230] In women exposed to the levonorgestrel-containing intrauterine device or the Yuzpe emergency contraception regimen, glycodelin expression was unaffected or increased.[231,232]

INSULIN-LIKE GROWTH FACTOR–BINDING PROTEIN-1

Insulin-like growth factor–binding protein-1, also known as pregnancy-associated α_1-protein and placental protein 12, is a major secretory product of decidual cells.[233] It is one of several proteins that bind IGF-1 and IGF-2, affecting the ability of these growth factors to interact with the IGF receptors. Consequently, the binding proteins can have significant roles in modulating IGF effects. The protein undergoes post-translational modification by phosphorylation, which increases its affinity for IGF-1 and therefore its ability to neutralize IGF-1 action.

Insulin-like growth factor–binding protein-1 derived from the decidua has been proposed to control the invasion and proliferation of trophoblast cells during implantation and placentation by sequestering IGFs. In a transgenic mouse model, overexpression of IGFBP-1 in the decidua resulted in abnormal placental morphology due to defects in trophoblast invasion and differentiation.[234] Because IGFBP-1 contains the Arg-Gly-Asp (RGD) motif recognized by cell surface integrins that bind fibronectin, its actions may be more complex than simple IGF sequestration when it is presented to cells that express the RGD-binding integrins.[235]

Stromal cell IGFBP-1 mRNA levels are regulated by progesterone as well as by IGFs, insulin, relaxin, and other growth factors as well as by hypoxia.[236-238] Both IGF and insulin decrease decidual IGFBP-1 release, whereas relaxin increases its release in a dose-dependent manner. HOXA10 may have a modest effect on IGFBP-1 expression, but in the presence of the forkhead/winged-helix transcription factor, FOXO1, IGFBP-1 is markedly stimulated.[239] FOXO1, prolactin, and IGFBP1 all promote decidualization and likely are involved in the progesterone-mediated stromal differentiation and prevention of apoptosis in preparation for nidation.

Intrauterine microdialysis studies showed that IGFBP-1 is released into the uterine lumen in the late secretory phase (10 days after ovulation or later)[240] and its secretion increases in response to hCG.[240] IGFBP-1 expression is increased between the midsecretory phase and 6 weeks of pregnancy, as demonstrated by DNA microarray analysis on endometrium from ectopic pregnancy.[241] IGFBP-1 levels then decline in the second trimester, only to rise again in late pregnancy, also accumulating in amniotic fluid. Pregnancy termination with the anti-progestin mifepristone causes a marked decline in IGFBP-1 levels before a decrease in hCG levels, confirming the progesterone dependence of IGFBP-1 production by decidual cells.

Alterations in IGFBP-1 expression have been noted in certain conditions associated with infertility and pregnancy loss, including PCOS and endometriosis.[230,242] Such observations may reflect an altered endocrine milieu, higher insulin levels, or a relative progesterone resistance in these conditions. In vitro, insulin inhibits the normal process of endometrial stromal differentiation (decidualization). In addition, hyperinsulinemia down-regulates hepatic IGFBP-1, resulting in elevated free IGF-1 in the circulation. Thus, the elevated androgens and estrogen seen in PCOS, along with decreased progesterone in the absence of ovulation, could contribute to the endometrial dysfunction, infertility, increased miscarriage rate, endometrial hyperplasia, and endometrial cancer common in women with PCOS.

OSTEOPONTIN

Osteopontin is a member of the SIBLING family of proteins.[243,244] Each protein in this large family contains the three–amino acid sequence Arg-Gly-Asp, and each has binding sites specific for two major cell surface receptors, $\alpha v \beta 3$ and CD44.[243] OPN is a 70-kDa glycosylated phosphoprotein secreted by the glandular epithelium and is expressed during the midsecretory phase, localized to the luminal endometrial epithelium.[245] OPN is regulated by progesterone.[245,246] The secretion of OPN and subsequent binding to the luminal surface suggests that direct interaction is occurring between integrins and this molecule. A role as a "sandwich" ligand that serves as a bridge between surface receptors on the endometrial and embryonal surfaces has been proposed. Alternative roles for OPN and these receptors include the prevention of complement fixation as part of a protective mechanism involving the innate immune system.[247]

PROLACTIN

Prolactin is produced by both the endometrium and the myometrium.[248,249] Serum levels of prolactin do not change across the menstrual cycle, but rise markedly during the first trimester of pregnancy in parallel with the decidual response, reaching peak concentrations at 15 to 20 weeks of gestation. Prolactin, like IGFBP-1, is a downstream biomarker of decidualization of human endometrial stromal cells. Regulators of decidualization include ovarian steroids, cAMP, forskolin, and IL-11. Recent studies suggest that upstream mediators of decidualization may regulate prolactin expression, including various proteins expressed during the secretory phase, such as ghrelin, IGFBP-related protein-1, leptin, and oncostatin-M.[250-254] The proliferation of endometrial cells is inhibited during decidualization, perhaps through stromal factors, such as IL-6 and oncostatin-M.[250,255] The role of prolactin in the decidualization process remains unclear. The prolactin receptor (PRL-R) is expressed on the endometrial stroma. Whereas PRL-R knockout mice had defects in decidualization, the phenotype, including reduced expression of LIF, amphiregulin, HB-EGF, COX-1, COX-2, PPARδ, HOXA10, cyclin-D3, VEGF, and its receptors, Flk-1 and neuropilin-1, could be rescued by exogenous progesterone. This suggests that ovarian PRL-R stimulation by prolactin, inducing progesterone secretion, is the critical event rather than any direct effect of prolactin acting directly on the decidualizing stroma.[256] A role for uterine prolactin in controlling NK cells has recently been suggested, as noted above.[257] Prolactin produced by the decidua during pregnancy accumulates in the amniotic fluid, where it has been postulated to affect osmoregulation and fetal lung development.

The Role of Growth Factors, Cytokines, and Gonadotropins in Establishing a Receptive State

Various growth factors have been implicated in the dramatic morphologic changes that occur in the endometrium during the menstrual cycle and pregnancy. Among the growth factors whose expression has been demonstrated in the human endometrium and decidua are EGF and EGF-like molecules, including TGF-α and HB-EGF; acidic and basic fibroblast growth factor (FGF); IGF-1 and IGF-2; IL-1, IL-11, and IL-6; LIF; macrophage colony-stimulating factor (M-CSF, also known as CSF-1); granulocyte–macrophage colony-stimulating factor (GM-CSF); members of the TGF-β superfamily; platelet-derived growth factor (PDGF); tumor necrosis factor-α (TNF-α); and endothelins 1, 2, and 3. Many of these factors have been proposed to play crucial roles in endometrial function and during pregnancy.[206,233,258] The endometrium, decidua, and embryo/trophoblast have also been shown to express receptors for many of these factors, including the EGF/TGF-α, IGF-1 and IGF-2, IL-1, CSF-1, GM-CSF, PDGF, and VEGE. With such a wide array of growth factors, it has become difficult to determine with clarity the role of each factor in endometrial growth and differentiation or their importance in processes involving maternal embryonic interaction and placental development.[259]

Several growth factors have been shown to exert regulatory effects on the expression of extracellular matrix proteins, their cellular receptors (integrins, selectins, cadherins), and enzymes (MMPs) that also influence cell growth, differentiation, and remodeling.[260-262]

THE TGF-β FAMILY

The TGF-β family, which includes multifunctional proteins that regulate cell growth and differentiation, includes five dimeric polypeptides encoded by related genes.[258,263-266] They bind to three cell surface proteins designated *type I, II, and III receptors.* The type I and type II receptors are believed to mediate the actions of TGF-β through the SMAD signaling pathway. All three isoforms of TGF-β can be found in human endometrium, including TGF-β1, TGF-β2, and TGF-β3. Null mutant mice bearing mutations for each of the three genes have a distinct phenotype, suggesting a separate role for each member of this growth factor family.[267] All three isoforms and the type II receptor were identified in all cell types of the endometrium.[268] TGF-β1 and TGF-β3 are found in both epithelial and stromal cells, whereas TGF-β2 is found primarily in the stroma and increases during the secretory phase.[266,269] TGF-β3 increases at menstruation and remains high throughout the proliferative phase, whereas TGF-β1 is maximal at menstruation. Ovarian steroids strongly repress TGF-β2 and TGF-β3 in the stroma, but only TGF-β2 is repressed in glandular epithelium. Although cAMP prevents this inhibition of TGF-β2 by progesterone, MAP kinase inhibitors differentially stimulate TGF-β2 and TGF-β3. These opposite effects provide insight into the discrete and highly temporal and spatial expression of the TGF cytokines during the menstrual cycle.

In addition, TGF-β has profound effects on the extracellular matrix, increasing the synthesis of collagen while decreasing its degradation.[124,270] In the secretory phase, TGF-β is a potent inhibitor of MMP activity in both stroma (MMP-3) and epithelium (MMP-7) while simultaneously promoting TIMP expression. This cytokine is induced by progesterone, acting in concert with retinoic acid to maintain these profibrogenic activities. In the event of pregnancy, progesterone acting through TGF-β maintains the integrity of the endometrium throughout gestation. In the absence of pregnancy, the fall in progesterone releases the MMP inhibitory factors, resulting in programmed breakdown of the extracellular matrix and subsequent menstruation.

Other members of the TGF-β family are expressed in the endometrium.[258] EBAF may participate in the menstruation process, acting as a potent inhibitor to TGF-β.[154] Antagonism of TGF-β1 by overexpression of EBAF reduces the number of implantation sites in rodent models,[271] consistent with human data showing high levels of EBAF in infertile women.[157]

Activins are highly abundant in the endometrium. Activin β (βA and βB) is found in the glandular epithelium, with peak expression during the secretory phase. Activin A promotes decidualization in vivo, whereas follistatin opposes the actions of activin.[272] Activin A enhances production of LIF and enhances MMP-22 during decidualization. Activity of both MMP and LIF is crucial for decidualization in the rat and primate.

Both TGF-β1 and TGF-β2 have been reported at the interface between embryo and endometrium, and they likely play multiple roles during embryo attachment and invasion.[265,273] In pregnancy, TGF-β is most abundant in the decidua in the first trimester, where it is believed to restrain trophoblast invasion by promoting trophoblast differentiation away from the invasive phenotype. TGF-β is sequestered in the extracellular matrix, where it can be activated by embryo-derived proteases. TGF-β up-regulates the expression of cellular fibronectin by trophoblast cells and induces integrins on the trophoblast that interact with the extracellular matrix during invasion, promoting MMP activity.[274,275] TGF-β also induces TIMPs and PAI-1 activity to counterbalance the invasiveness of the trophoblast.

TGF-β is a potent immunosuppressant that may prevent maternal immune rejection of the fetal allograft. Its actions include suppression of chemotaxis and macrophage and T-cell activity. ADAMTS (A disintegrin and metalloproteinase with thrombospondin repeats) is believed to play a critical role in extracellular matrix remodeling during implantation. IL-1 increases ADAMTS expression, whereas the anti-inflammatory effects of TGF-β1 decrease its expression.[276] These opposing actions illustrate the balance between factors favoring embryonic invasion and maternal efforts to control this invasion and reflect the essential role of TGF-β in this process.

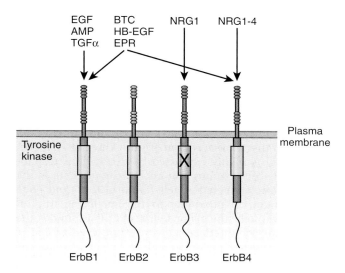

Figure 9-18. *The EGF family of growth factors and receptors. EGF and its family members associate with specific receptors that signal through intracellular tyrosine kinase action. The four receptors can dimerize is predictable ways. BTC, betacellulin; EPR, epiregulin; HB-EGF, heparin-binding epidermal-like growth factor; NRG, neuregulin; TGF, transforming growth factor.*

THE EGF FAMILY OF GROWTH FACTORS

The EGF family of growth factors appears to play a major role in uterine development and physiology.[206,233] The EGF ligands are produced by a family of genes, epidermal growth factor (EGF), heparin-binding EGF-like growth factor (HB-EGF), amphiregulin (AMP), betacellulin (BTC), epiregulin (EPR), tumor growth factor α (TGF-α), and neuregulin (NRG). This EGF family of ligands has the ability to bind and activate one or more of four homologous ErbB receptors via a conserved 60–amino acid "EGF-like" binding domain. These four receptors differ in their activities and dimerize with each other to further expand the diversity of this growth factor family. Interacting with their receptors, members of the EGF family act as autocrine and juxtacrine factors, and some exist as membrane-bound forms that are released by proteolytic cleavage to function in a paracrine or endocrine manner. The proteolytic cleavage is accomplished by cell surface metalloproteases, similar to those involved in L-selectin ligand and MUC-1 cleavage, suggesting an important role for metalloprotease action at the maternal–fetal interface.[277-279]

The receptors for the EGF ligand family, ErbB1, ErbB2, ErbB3, and ErbB4, are structurally homologous, and the specificity of ligand binding is determined by differences in extracellular domain sequences (Fig. 9-18). The ErbB proteins function as hetero- or homodimers and possibly also as higher-order multimers.[280] ErbB2 lacks ligand-binding activity and ErbB3 lacks functional tyrosine kinase activity. Thus, ErbB2 and ErbB3 likely function only as heterodimers, with another ErbB protein supplying the missing function in a dimer.

Both EGF and TGF-α stimulate the proliferation of endometrial stromal cells.[233] The synthesis of fibronectin and vitronectin by epithelial cells is enhanced by EGF.

EGF also stimulates stromal cell differentiation and enhances the synthesis of laminin and fibronectin. These growth factors also enhance the morphologic and functional differentiation of decidual cells in vitro. EGF has not been identified in the circulation of cycling or menopausal women, but it has been detected in the serum of pregnant women, with peak concentrations occurring in early pregnancy. Binding studies indicate that EGF receptor peaks at the time of ovulation (or shortly thereafter) and declines during the secretory phase, reaching a nadir immediately before menses. The binding sites are present on both stromal and epithelial cells, as well as in the decidua of pregnancy. Studies using immunohistochemistry suggest that decidualization is associated with an increase in EGF-R. Abnormal EGF and EGF-R activity has been reported in cases of intrauterine growth retardation. It has been hypothesized that EGF and related molecules play a role in the induction of trophoblast differentiation.

Multiple EGF family members appear to participate directly in the process of implantation.[281] HB-EGF exists as a transmembrane-anchored precursor (HB-EGF™) that gives rise to a soluble processed form. These proteins can bind to two different EGF receptors, HER1/ErbB1 and HER4/ErbB4. HB-EGF mRNA is found in the stroma during the proliferative phase, but in the midsecretory phase, it is also detected in the luminal and glandular epithelium.[282,283] This expression pattern appears to be driven by a combination of progesterone and estrogen.

HB-EGF is postulated to play roles both in adhesion via its membrane-anchored precursor (which binds to HER4/ErbB4 on the apical surface of the trophectoderm) and in stimulating embryo growth. In the rodent, HB-EGF is one of the first cytokines found around the implanting embryo.[284,285] In the human endometrium, HB-EGF mRNA levels increase during the secretory phase, reaching a peak at the time of implantation.[282] HB-EGF™ can mediate attachment of human embryos in an in vitro assay of implantation.[286] HB-EGF also may promote embryonic development. When added to serum-free medium, it increases the number of embryos reaching the blastocyst stage and stimulates hatching. HB-EGF may also participate in paracrine actions within the endometrium. Stromal derived HB-EGF promotes expression of LIF, HOXA10, αvβ3 integrin, and DAF by endometrial cells in vitro. Other members of the EGF family presumably play important roles during early pregnancy as well.[287]

OTHER CYTOKINES PARTICIPATE IN ENDOMETRIAL GROWTH AND DIFFERENTIATION

Platelet-derived growth factor (PDGF) is produced by endometrial stromal cells and also released in the endometrium by activated platelets.[288] PDGF is a potent mitogen that acts on endometrial receptors that are most abundant in the proliferative phase of the cycle.

The FGFs encompass a family of growth factors that can stimulate growth of endometrial cells and smooth muscle cells.[289,290] Acidic and basic FGFs bind to proteoglycans. Because these proteins do not contain secretory signal sequences, they may be most important in the endometrium during menstruation, when they could be released from dying cells. Basic FGF is angiogenic, but also stimulates stromal cell proliferation in the presence of progesterone. FGF-7, also known as *keratinocyte growth factor,* stimulates epithelial cell proliferation. FGF-7 mRNA is expressed at highest level in the late secretory phase endometrium in the stroma; its receptor is most abundant in the glandular epithelium in the late proliferative phase. These findings suggest that FGF-7 is progesterone-dependent, whereas its receptor is estrogen-sensitive. FGF-8 is a uterine growth factor isolated from bovine uterus, and FGF-9 was recently described in the late proliferative phase of human endometrium.[290]

The IGF system of growth factors encompasses not only IGF-1 and IGF-2 hormones, but also two distinct receptors and multiple binding proteins that modulate IGF activity.[234,235,291-295] IGF-1 and IGF-2 are mitogenic growth factors that share structural similarities to insulin and are present in the mouse uterus and throughout the menstrual cycle in women.[296] Both hormones are present in the stroma, although the receptors are present in both epithelial and stromal cells. IGF-1 is more abundant in the proliferative phase and may function in epithelial proliferation, whereas IGF-2 is expressed in a more robust fashion in the secretory phase and is believed to be a mitogen for the stroma of pregnancy.

The hormone IGF-1 binds to both the type 1 IGF receptor (IGF-1 receptor), which is structurally similar to the insulin receptor, and the type 2 receptor (IGF-2 receptor) with high affinity. IGF-2 binds the latter with higher affinity.[297]

IGF-1 mRNA is localized by in situ hybridization primarily in the syncytial trophoblast. IGF-2 mRNA has been found in mesenchymal fibroblasts of the villous core and is also expressed in first-trimester and term cytotrophoblasts. The expression of IGFs in the placenta seems to be under the regulatory control of hormones (insulin, human placental lactogen, and estrogens) as well as growth factors, including PDGF. IGF-1 receptors have been detected in the placenta during the earliest periods of gestation, and it has been hypothesized that IGFs promote trophoblast proliferation.

The pleiotropic factor TNF-α exerts inflammatory, mitogenic, mitostatic, angiogenic, and immunomodulatory effects in a variety of tissues.[298] It is a membrane-bound 14-kDa polypeptide that is derived by proteolytic cleavage from the 26-kDa precursor. Expression of TNF-α mRNA and protein has been shown in human endometrium, decidua, and trophoblasts; its receptors have also been found in all of these tissues. TNF-α in the human endometrium is subject to regulation by steroid hormones—namely, estrogens and progesterone.

Both TNF-α and its receptors (TNF-R) are expressed by trophoblasts during early and late gestation.[299] There is differential expression of the two genes encoding TNF-R, allowing some regulation of TNF-α activity. In cultured human chorionic cells, TNF-α affects cellular fibronectin secretion. Scientists have hypothesized that, along with other endometrial and trophoblast factors, TNF-α controls trophoblast adhesion and invasion and alters the integrin expression pattern in endometrial stroma.[300,301]

Colony-stimulating factors are a family of cytokines that were initially identified by their ability to stimulate hematopoietic stem cells to form colonies in semisolid culture media. CSF-1 is a glycosylated disulfide-linked homodimer. CSF-1 and its receptor are expressed in the endometrium, decidua, and placenta.[233,302] CSF-1 levels in the endometrial glands are higher in the secretory phase compared with the proliferative phase, and the decidua expresses higher levels of CSF-1 mRNA and protein than the proliferative phase endometrium. The CSF-1 receptor (CSF1R) is highly expressed by extravillous trophoblasts in the cell columns that anchor the placenta to the uterus.[303] The endometrial cells, both of local and bone marrow origin, in proximity to the anchoring trophoblasts, appear to be the major source of CSF-1 found at the placental–uterine interface. Lower serum levels of CSF-1 have been reported in women with recurrent spontaneous abortions. Although CSF-1 has been proposed to regulate trophoblast proliferation and differentiation, this role is not confirmed by the phenotype of the *op/op* (osteopetrotic) mouse that lacks CSF-1. This mouse has reduced fertility and smaller litter sizes, evidently due to a defect in ovulation, not implantation or placentation.

LEUKEMIA INHIBITORY FACTOR AND IL-11

The glycoproteins IL-6, LIF, and IL-11 belong to the same family of cytokines whose receptors use gp130 as a common signaling molecule.[304,305] LIF acquired its name by its capacity to inhibit the proliferation of a mouse leukemic cell line. LIF is expressed constitutively in the ampullary region of the fallopian tube and in a cyclic fashion in both the epithelial and stromal cells of the endometrium, with epithelial expression being greater.[287,306-312] The functional LIF receptor, a complex consisting of LIF receptor β (which binds LIF) and gp130 (which mediates signal transduction) is present throughout the menstrual cycle in the luminal epithelium. LIF receptors are expressed by all trophoblast types, particularly the villous syncytiotrophoblast and cytotrophoblasts and, to a lesser extent, the extravillous trophoblast cells.

Sentinel observations in the mouse have clearly shown that LIF of endometrial origin is crucial for the process of implantation, particularly the decidualization response.[307] LIF-deficient female mice did not become pregnant or respond to a uterine decidualizing stimulus. However, transfer of their embryos to pseudopregnant, wild-type females resulted in viable pregnancies, as did infusion of LIF into the uteri of LIF-deficient females. The primary action of LIF appears to be on the uterus. However, in mice, subsequent placentation is disrupted, perhaps because the role of LIF in modulating trophoblast differentiation and expression of MMPs cannot be executed. Implantation of LIF receptor–deficient human embryos occurs, but these offspring suffer from Stüve-Wiedemann/Schwartz-Jampel type 2 syndrome.[310]

The LIF mRNA and protein are present in human endometrium, being most abundant in the glandular and luminal epithelium and peaking in the secretory phase of the cycle.[313-315] The cycle-dependent expression of LIF in human endometrium may be a function of other growth factors rather than a direct effect of steroid hormones. If implantation occurs, LIF expression by the endometrial glands is down-regulated and there is a concomitant increase in LIF expression by endometrial NK and T cells. LIF has been found to enhance human blastocyst formation and to modulate trophoblast differentiation in vitro.[306] LIF levels in uterine flushings rise 7 days after ovulation, reaching a maximum 5 days later. LIF levels in uterine flushings and secretion of LIF from cultured endometrium obtained from patients with repeated implantation failures or unexplained infertility are decreased,[287,316] and defects in LIF have been implicated in some cases of recurrent pregnancy loss.[306]

The mechanisms underlying implementation failure in LIF-deficient states include a cascade of key regulatory proteins. LIF has been implicated in the activation of STAT-3; mice homozygous for a mutation in the STAT activation site on gp130 have a defect nearly identical to that in LIF-deficient mice.[317] Suppressor of cytokine signaling protein-3 (SOCS-3) is stimulated by LIF and blocks phosphorylation of gp130 and STATs. In LIF null mice, stromal COX-2 and epithelial HB-EGF are absent at the site of implantation.[318,319] Two other EGF family members, amphiregulin and epiregulin, are also reduced in LIF knockout mice. IL-1 has been shown to induce COX-2.[320-322] Prostacyclin, acting through the peroxisome proliferator–activated receptor γ, is essential for decidualizaton.[323-324] COX-2 null mice have multiple defects in ovulation, fertilization, and implantation.[325] Together, the observations suggest that LIF stimulation of the luminal epithelium and blastocysts may trigger IL-1 that triggers decidual changes.

Mutations in the coding sequence of one copy of the *LIF* gene were identified in a small number of infertile women (3 of 74 infertile nulligravid subjects), and a presumed polymorphism was found in 1 of 75 fertile control subjects and none of 131 nonobstetric patients.[326] One of the mutations in the infertile group was in the 5′-regulatory region of the *LIF* gene; the two others were in the coding sequence in a domain believed to be important for LIF binding to its receptor. Unfortunately, the authors did not determine whether LIF levels or bioactivity in uterine flushings or endometrial biopsy material were correlated with genotype. Although these observations are consistent with an important role for LIF in human implantation, trophoblast differentiation, or placentation, a definitive link between the genetic variants/ mutations and infertility remains to be established.

IL-11 is another member of the IL-6 family that is implicated in the decidual response.[305,327,328] As with the LIF knockout mice, female mice lacking the IL-11 receptor alpha chain are infertile because of defective decidualization.[327] Further, IL-11 is present in the human endometrium and it advances progesterone-induced decidualization of cultured endometrial stromal cells. Both relaxin and prostaglandin E_2 increase IL-11 expression. An inhibitor of IL-11 (W147AIL-11) reduces prolactin secretion by endometrial stromal cells in response to relaxin and PGE_2, suggesting that IL-11 is the critical factor in this signaling cascade.[329] Like LIF, IL-11 is an activator of the JAK/ STAT signaling pathway through STAT3, which stimulates SOCS3, a negative feedback mechanism for receptor activity. Ovarian steroids and cAMP differentially stimulate STAT3 and SOCS3, respectively, in vitro, whereas IL-11 activates both by phosphorylation.[330] The anti-progestin onapristone increases SOCS3, attenuating IL-11–induced STAT3. Recent investigations in women suggest that IL-11 and phosphorylated STAT3 are significantly lower in the infertile endometrium compared with control subjects, whereas IL-11 receptor and LIF were not different.[331]

HUMAN CHORIONIC GONADOTROPIN

In in vitro studies, the addition of follicle-stimulating hormone, luteinizing hormone (LH), hCG, thyroid-stimulating hormone, and free β subunit have been shown to affect human reproductive tract tissues—including the stimulation of prolactin production, enhancement of decidualization, and myometrial relaxation.[332,333] The presence of LH/hCG receptors in the fallopian tube, myometrium, and endometrium has also been reported. However, the transcripts detected are smaller than those encoding the gonadal LH/hCG receptors; the proteins are also smaller, detected as 50- to 60-kDa molecules compared with the observed receptor molecular weights in gonadal tissue (83-95 kDa). Thus, extragonadal LH/hCG receptors appear to be truncated, evidently lacking extracellular domains, but still retaining the capacity to signal after binding LH and hCG. The primary signal transduction cascade initiated by the truncated endometrial LH/ hCG receptors may not involve the classic cAMP/protein kinase A system as the primary pathway, but rather the mitogen-activated protein kinase pathway or the activation of prostaglandin synthesis.

Although extragonadal LH/hCG receptors have been proposed to play various roles in the reproductive tract, they are probably most important in the context of pregnancy, where high levels of hCG are present. Thus, hCG could be an important embryonic signal in the bidirectional dialogue between conceptus and uterus. The best evidence that extragonadal LH/hCG receptors have an important role in primate reproduction is derived from the study of the baboon, where administration of recombinant hCG causes alterations in both epithelial and stromal cells. Preliminary studies in women indicate that hCG can also affect the human endometrium in vivo.[334]

In the baboon, the response to intrauterine administration of hCG by osmotic minipump over a 4-day period, starting on day 6 after ovulation, includes the formation of an epithelial plaque, hypertrophy of the surface epithelium, and rounding off of the glands characteristic of pregnancy in this species.[333] Glycodelin expression in the endometrial glandular epithelium is enhanced, and α-smooth muscle cell actin is expressed in the stroma. In vitro, hCG inhibits stromal cell apoptosis and stimulates decidual changes—reflected by increased IGFBP-1 expression as well as increased expression of COX-2. As previously noted, in vitro studies have shown that the glycoprotein α subunit stimulates production of prolactin, another uterine secretory product. Activation of myometrial LH/hCG receptors in vitro causes myometrial relaxation, which could facilitate nidation in vivo.[334] With the use of intrauterine microdialysis in the human, it was recently shown that administration of hCG significantly reduces

IGFBP1 and M-CSF expression after postovulatory day 10, whereas LIF, VEGF, and MMP-9 were all dramatically increased.[240,335] This finding suggests that hCG is an important modulating factor during early pregnancy. In vitro studies, using hCG-coated beads, have shown an induction of trophinin on the endometrial epithelium when IL-1 is present, suggesting a mechanism for enhanced embryonic–endometrial interactions at the maternal–fetal interface.[336] As an endocrine factor, hCG likely has independent effects on a wide variety of endometrial genes, independent of direct trophoblast interactions.[241]

PROSTANOIDS AND OTHER LIPIDS

The role of prostaglandins in the implantation process has long been suspected because of their effects on the vascular system and association with inflammatory processes. The fact that mice deficient in COX-2 display abnormalities in the implantation process—particularly the early decidual response—is consistent with this notion.[334] Evidence suggestive of a role of prostanoids in human implantation includes the presence of COX-1 and COX-2 in the human endometrium (mainly the glandular epithelium) during the presumptive implantation period.[337] A study of prenatal use of nonsteroidal anti-inflammatory drugs (NSAIDs), drugs that inhibit COX enzymes, indicated an increased risk of miscarriage in users of aspirin and other NSAIDs.[338] One of the key prostanoids involved in implantation is believed to be prostacyclin, a ligand for the peroxisome proliferator–activated receptor delta (PPARδ), a nuclear receptor family member expressed in subluminal stromal cells in the rodent uterus.[323,339-341] This transcription factor is implicated in the implantation process as well.

Another lipid implicated in implantation is the arachidonate derivative known as *arachidonylethanolamide* or *anandamide*, a ligand for the cannabinoid receptors.[342-345] Anandamide, referred to as an *endocannabinoid*, binds to cannabinoid receptors CB1-R and CB2-R, which are expressed in the preimplantation embryo and in the reproductive tract. The embryo is enriched in CB1-R, and in the blastocyst, the expression of this receptor is most abundant in the trophectoderm. Uterine anandamide levels in the mouse are reduced at the time of implantation and are highest at interimplantation sites. Endocannabinoids at low levels accelerate trophoblast differentiation, but at high levels, they inhibit trophoblast differentiation and arrest embryonic development. Tetrahydrocannabinol and synthetic agonists of the cannabinoid receptors have similar effects. Thus, it has been postulated that endocannabinoids play an important role in controlling the synchrony of embryonic development for implantation in rodents. Anandamide is present in human reproductive tract fluids,[344] and high anandamide levels are associated with in vitro fertilization failures.[345]

Early Implantation Events in the Human

Before it interacts with the surface epithelium, the blastocyst must hatch from the confines of the zona pellucida. Gradual zona thinning, as well as complete hatching of embryos, can be observed in vitro. The existence of ectopic implantation suggests that the endometrium is not obligatory for this process to be successfully completed. Nevertheless, there may be more subtle regulation of hatching within the endometrial cavity. Although degradation of the zona pellucida is a process controlled by the embryo, inhibitors or agents that induce "zona hardening" may affect the timing of the process.

Work on subhuman primates shows that mononuclear cytotrophoblasts of the trophectoderm of the blastocyst have fused into syncytia before these cells attach to the endometrial epithelium.[346] Careful histologic descriptions of very early human implantation sites (such as those studied by Hertig and colleagues[165]) indicate that the syncytial trophoblast layer of the human embryo comprises the invading front during the first few days of implantation. Thus, the consensus appears to be that it is a syncytial trophoblast cell that initially interacts with and adheres to the endometrial epithelium; only after the human embryo is completely embedded in the endometrium do the cytotrophoblast cell columns start to stream out of the trophoblastic shell and further invade the uterus.[347,348] This process starts approximately 1 week after the initiation of implantation and continues well into the second trimester of pregnancy.

The early human implantation sites that have been examined histologically show that by day 12 after ovulation, the embryo is almost completely covered by endometrium. The endometrial stroma around the implantation site displays the predecidual reaction and is edematous. By the classic histologic criteria of Noyes and associates,[349] the endometrium of the implantation site is not that different from the nonpregnant midsecretory phase endometrium. The glands adjacent to the embryo are themselves deflected by invading trophoblasts, but maintain the tortuosity and secretion-filled appearance typical for this stage of the menstrual cycle.

In vitro observations using human embryos or human trophoblasts have attempted to characterize some morphologic features of the early events of trophoblastic–endometrial interactions.[350-354] There is growing consensus that initial apposition and attachment is an evanescent and rate-limiting step in the initiation of implantation. A receptor-mediated paradigm for embryo attachment and invasion has long been postulated.[355] Numerous endometrial and trophoblastic cell adhesion molecules and associated moieties have been suggested as candidates to serve as attachment receptors.[286,356-359] Historically, surface modification of the glycocalyx was a subject of much interest,[360-362] but more recently, the molecules that populate the luminal surface have come under scrutiny. As shown in Figure 9-19, a limited number of adhesion/attachment components have been suggested to play key roles. MUC1 is a large glycoprotein that is down-regulated on the endometrial surface in most species at the time of implantation,[363] but expressed throughout the menstrual cycle in humans.[359] Nevertheless, debate continues regarding this large glycoprotein as a possible attachment receptor for the human embryo. Other smaller molecules are present and may serve the purpose of initial attachment—including trophinin, integrins, CD44, L-selectins, and HB-EGF™.[364,365]

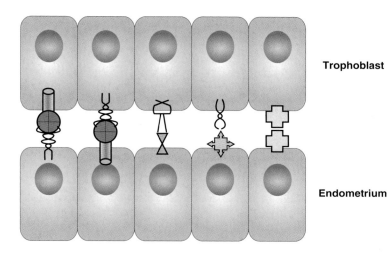

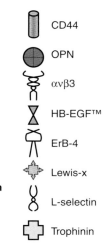

Figure 9-19. *Luminal surface proteins that may interact with complementary proteins on the embryonic surface. Experimental evidence exists for each of these possible attachment reactions. It is likely that there is redundancy in these systems and that each may serve specific functions, such as signaling or attachment during the initial stages of implantation. HB-EGF™, heparin-binding epidermal-like growth factor; OPN, osteopontin.*

The cascade of events leading to successful implantation probably requires many critical proteins with different functional contributions. A novel cell surface protein called *trophinin* has been suggested as a homologous pairing partner between trophoblast and endometrium during implantation.[357] The αvβ3 integrin and its ligand OPN are expressed at the time of implantation on the luminal surface of receptive endometrium. Secreted OPN binds to this integrin through an RGD sequence.[245,366] Because OPN can also bind to the CD44 hyaluronate receptor through non-RGD binding sites, it was suggested that these serve in a "sandwich"-pairing mechanism at the point of interface.[367,368] In the human, surface epithelial cells on both the embryo and the endometrium express both the αvβ3 integrin and CD44.[369] There is also ample evidence that RGD binding is vital to the process of implantation.[370,371] Peptides containing this sequence reduce implantation efficiency in animal models, including the rabbit and mouse.[372,373] Thus, integrin-mediated adhesion may somehow play a role in successful implantation. More recently, it has been suggested that OPN, αvβ3 integrin, and CD44 binding serves to suppress the innate immune system through decay-accelerating factor (DAF)–mediated interference with complement subunit C3,[243,247] a role that could be critical for the protection of the embryo at the time of initial attachment and invasion.

The transmembrane form of HB-EGF™ and its receptor ErbB-4 are expressed on the surface of endometrium and on the outer cells of the embryo, respectively. Evidence in both rodents and human suggests that these molecules could serve as an attachment receptor–ligand pair during implantation.[284,286] Soluble HB-EGF interferes with this process, perhaps through competitive inhibition. HB-EGF™ could also play a paracrine role, especially if cleaved from its transmembrane location when the embryo enters the uterine cavity.

Perhaps the most promising mechanism involves that previously elucidated for leukocyte–endothelial interaction. L-selectin and an oligosaccharide ligand are expressed on the blastocyst and endometrial surface in the human, respectively.[358] This type of adhesion reaction between embryo and endometrium at the time of implantation is quite appealing and likely involves integrin mechanisms for embryo invasion, similar to leukocyte intercalation at sites of inflammation.

Evidence from humans shows a temporal and spatial regulation of L-selectin ligand expression on the luminal and glandular epithelium.[374] Likewise, each mechanism could be disrupted in infertile women, leading to a failure of implantation.[375]

Structural alterations accompany the biochemical changes noted on the surface epithelium. Scanning electron microscopic examination shows that the human endometrial epithelium consists of secretory and ciliated cells (Fig. 9-20). The ratio of nonciliated to ciliated cells changes during the menstrual cycle, decreasing in the late proliferative phase and increasing in the secretory phase. In general, estradiol levels correlate directly with the presence of ciliated cells, and withdrawal of estrogen is associated with loss of cilia. The ciliated cells do not undergo surface morphologic changes during the menstrual cycle, whereas the secretory cells show significant cycle-dependent surface modifications.

Transient surface specializations of the secretory cells called *pinopodes*, also known as *pinopods* or *uterodomes*, have been a focus of research because the temporal patterns of expression seemed to coincide with the time of maximal uterine receptivity.[376] These surface structures were first identified on the luminal epithelium of rodent endometrium during the limited period (approximately 12 hours) when the uterus is receptive to implantation; they were shown to be involved in pinocytosis—hence, the appellation of *pinopode* (from the Greek word meaning "drinking foot").[377] Similar structures, although with different morphologic features, were subsequently discovered in numerous species, including humans; their appearance again generally correlated with the time of implantation.

Although it is certain that pinopodes are involved in pinocytosis in the rodent uterus, in vitro studies did not show that they serve this function in women—hence, the suggestion that the structures should be designated "uterodomes" as opposed to "pinopodes."[378,379]

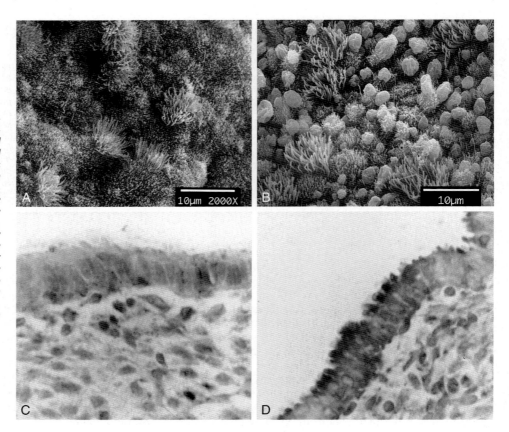

Figure 9-20. A, The surface epithelium of human endometrium is composed of ciliated and secretory cell types. B, During the time of maximal receptivity, the surface of these cells transforms into a sac-like protrusion seen in many species, now called pinopodes. During the prereceptive phase, surface receptors, such as the $\alpha v \beta 3$ integrin, are not present (C), but are expressed during the window of implantation on these pinopode structures (D). (Diedrich K, Fauser BCJM, Devroey P, Griesinger G. The role of the endometrium and embryo in human implantation. Human Reproduction 15(suppl 16):39-50, 2000, used with permission of Human Reproduction.)

Mechanisms underlying the formation of pinopodes in the human endometrium have not been elucidated. They may form from the accumulation of membrane components, as a consequence of secretory activity, or from reorganization of the cell cytoskeleton. Some researchers have suggested that they serve to elevate the endometrium above the ciliated cells, providing a platform with the necessary complement of surface adhesion receptors.

The role of pinopodes in human embryo implantation (beyond the temporal correlation between their appearance and the estimated time of nidation) is supported by in vitro studies showing that human blastocysts implant on human endometrial epithelial cells only in areas bearing pinopodes (Fig. 9-21). Other studies have shown that surface biomarkers are present on the pinopodes. HB-EGF™, a molecule implicated as a membrane-bound ligand and a juxtacrine/paracrine factor important in signaling to the embryo, is on the surface of pinopodes at the expected time of implantation.[380] The $\alpha v \beta 3$ integrin and its ligand are also both present on these apical protrusions during the window of implantation (Figs. 9-20 and 9-22).[381] MUC-1 and OPN appear to be on different cell types of the luminal surface, based on findings with electron immunohistochemistry; MUC-1 is present solely on the ciliated cells, whereas OPN is present on the secretory or pinopode-bearing cells.

The formation of pinopodes appears to be dependent on progesterone, whereas estrogen causes them to regress. The earlier appearance of pinopodes in controlled ovarian stimulation cycles is correlated with the preovulatory rise in plasma progesterone. Administration of a low dose of the progesterone receptor antagonist mifepristone on cycle days 14 and 15 delays pinopode formation. Studies in the mouse suggest that *HOXA10,* a progesterone-regulated gene, is required for pinopode formation,[382] although pinopodes have been described in both *LIF* and *HOXA10* null mice.[383]

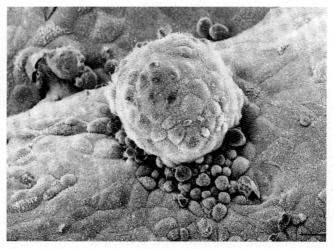

Figure 9-21. In vitro culture of human embryos on cultured endometrial epithelium appears to show that embryos prefer to attach to areas with pinopode expression. (Reproduced with permission from Bentin-Ley U. Relevance of endometrial pinopodes for human blastocyst implantation. Hum Reprod 15[Suppl 6]:67-73, 2000.)

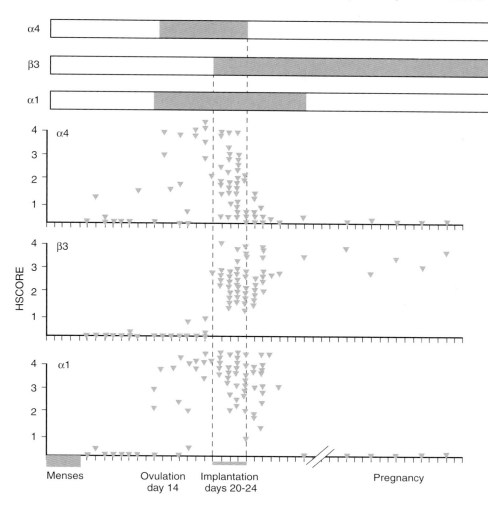

Figure 9-22. Scattergram showing distribution of three cycle-dependent epithelial integrin subunits in cycling endometrium. Although each of the integrin subunits has a unique pattern of expression, all three are coexpressed during the time of maximal receptivity between cycle days 20 and 24. HSCORE is a semiquantitative measure of immunostaining from 0 (negative) to 4 (maximal staining). (Used with permission of the American Society for Reproductive Medicine.)

The actual temporal distribution of pinopodes has been brought into question in the last several years, with several studies showing little correlation with the actual window of implantation.[384-386] Although pinopodes could be involved in embryonic–endometrial interactions, the utility of these structures as markers of uterine receptivity appears limited.

Biochemical Evaluation of the Endometrium

BIOMARKERS OF ENDOMETRIAL RECEPTIVITY

Attempts have been made to find suitable biomarkers of endometrial receptivity[387,388]; an illustration of the best characterized candidate biomarkers is provided in Figure 9-23. Each of these endometrial factors has been selected on the basis of temporal patterns of expression that correlate with the putative window of implantation on cycle days 20 to 24. Although certain biomarkers, such as calcitonin or LIF, are aligned closely within this window, others have a pattern of expression that is inversely related to the time of maximal endometrial receptivity (epithelial estrogen receptor alpha [ERα], progesterone receptors, EBAF, and telomerase).

Among the best-characterized biomarkers for assessment of uterine receptivity are the integrins. As shown in Figure 9-22, three epithelial integrins undergo changes in expression during the luteal phase. This pattern has now been consistently observed in multiple studies.[365,389-394] Of these, αvβ3 is the most extensively studied. Dyssynchronous or delayed maturation of the endometrium is associated with delayed expression of the αvβ3 integrin. Although patterns of integrin expression suggest roles in cell adhesion and maintenance of tissue architecture, the αvβ3 integrin is present on the uppermost portion of the luminal epithelium, corresponding to the localization of OPN and pinopodes (see Fig. 9-20). This integrin has been used for the assessment of the endometrium in women with endometriosis and other benign conditions—including hydrosalpinges, unexplained infertility, and PCOS—although not all studies agree on its usefulness.[365]

Based on the use of biomarkers such as the integrins, two distinct types of deficiencies have been identified in women with infertility. This model fits well with data presented by Wilcox and coworkers that suggest that delayed implantation may reduce cycle fecundability.[214] The normal uterine receptivity provides the opportunity for the embryo to attach and invade the maternal lining. In some cases, as in luteal phase defect, this window may

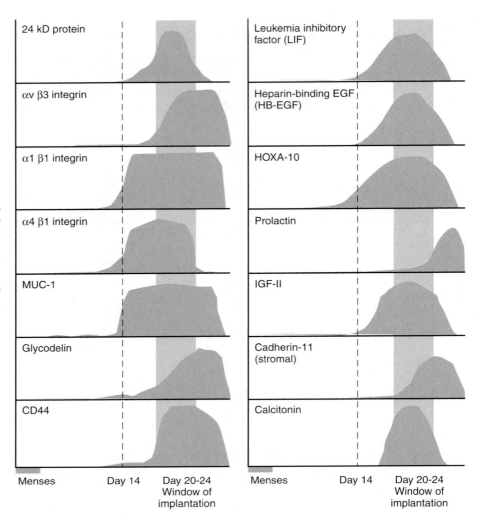

Figure 9-23. Candidate biomarkers of uterine receptivity showing their period of maximal expression relative to the presumptive window of implantation (gray bar). (Used with permission from Lessey BA. The use of biomarkers for the assessment of uterine receptivity. In Gardner DK, Weissman A, Howles CM, Shoham Z (eds). Textbook of Assisted Reproductive Technologies. London: Dunitz, 2001, p. 357.)

be shifted or delayed, resulting in pregnancy loss or failure to conceive. This can occur when progesterone levels are suboptimal or when the response to progesterone is decreased. In other cases, histologic development is normal, but the biochemical changes associated with a receptive endometrium do not develop in a timely fashion. Such a mechanism of occult defects has been suggested to be the underlying implantation defect in women with endometriosis and hydrosalpinges.[365] The cause of this type of receptivity defect remains a topic of debate and an active area of research.

GLOBAL GENE EXPRESSION PATTERNS DURING THE WINDOW OF IMPLANTATION

The dramatic changes in growth, secretion, and then cell death have been studied at the molecular level using DNA microarrays. The key patterns of gene expression between the prereceptive (early secretory) phase and the receptive (midsecretory) phase were first defined in 2002; 370 genes (3.1%) displayed decreases ranging from 2- to more than 100-fold, whereas 323 genes (2.7%) showed increases ranging from 2- to more than 45-fold.[395] A survey of the gene expression patterns has recently been completed in

normal fertile women.[396] The patterns of up- and down-regulated genes define four stages of endometrial development, and suggest that the functional characteristics of each phase are determined largely by the proteins that are expressed during each phase. Cell cycle proteins are the predominant feature of the proliferating endometrium, whereas a secretory profile of gene expression characterizes the early secretory phase. Preparation for implantation involves changes in the extracellular matrix, cell communication and adhesion, negative effectors of cell proliferation, synthesis of amino acids, cell ion homeostasis, and appearance of genes involved in innate immunity; all of these are up-regulated during this time. Finally, with menstruation, there are dramatic changes in gene expression toward cell death, enzymatic digestive processes and endocytosis/phagocytosis, hemostasis, and antimicrobial actions.

The molecular phenotype of the human endometrium in the midsecretory phase has been characterized using DNA microarray analysis of RNA extracted from endometrial biopsy specimens obtained from fertile women.[395-398] The published data have been generated from chips that now contain sequences from up to 54,600 known human genes or expressed sequence tags. A relatively small percentage of genes (<6%) represented on the chips had significant increases or decreases in expression (at least twofold) in the presumed receptive phase. The microarray analysis confirmed the up-regulation of transcripts previously known to be increased during the window of implantation (including OPN, DAF, glycodelin, and IGFBP-1) and the down-regulation of others (including MMP-7 and cyclin B). However, several previously unappreciated genes changed in expression during the presumed window of implantation, most notably, members of the WNT signaling pathway (see Figs. 9-5A and 9-5B). Such changes included the increased expression of the WNT pathway inhibitor DKK-1 and a striking decline in the soluble form of FrpHE (SFRP4), another WNT pathway inhibitor. Carson and colleagues also reported a large increase in WNT-10B expression and a large decrease in soluble FrpHE, an interesting observation given existing evidence implicating this signaling molecule in glandular development and hyperplasia in the mammary glands.

The microarray analysis also showed significant alterations in genes encoding water and ion transporters, including up-regulation of claudin-4/*Clostridium perfringens* enterotoxin receptor; prostaglandin synthesis and action were also found to be altered, including up-regulation of phospholipase A_2 and prostaglandin E_2 receptor (EP_1). The functional significance of these genes and the alterations in others remains to be determined. Moreover, the interpretation of the findings is complicated by the fact that alterations in specific endometrial cellular compartments could not be ascertained for the majority of the genes of interest. The data sets do, however, provide a first approximation of the molecular signature of the human endometrium during the putative time of implantation in a small group of fertile women. This information could be used to develop a diagnostic "chip" profile for establishing normal uterine function.

Of note, with these efforts to identify the endometrial transcriptome across the entire menstrual cycle, investigators can now view each segment of the menstrual cycle as a unique fingerprint detailing the role of steroid hormones and their receptors in the endometrium.[396] The genes that are expressed during the proliferative phase in response to estrogen play roles in cell adhesion, cell–cell signaling, cell cycle regulation, and cell division. After ovulation, in the early secretory phase, in response to ovarian estrogen and progesterone, gene expression shifts globally to include metabolic enzymes, transporter proteins, and inhibitors of WNT signaling with marked up-regulation of lipid metabolism, phospholipase activity, and prostaglandin metabolism. There is increased EGF signaling noted during this time. The midsecretory phase is distinct from the other phases due to the down-regulation of ER and PR in the epithelial compartment, and this difference is reflected in the gene expression profiling. With this loss of estrogen action and a dominance of progesterone action in the stroma comes a shift to cell adhesion, communication, and motility. There is an increase in intracellular signaling, antiapoptosis, and immune response, including DAF, defensin, complement component 4, and glycodelin.

During the late secretory phase, progesterone withdrawal leads increased expression of MMPs, EBAF, and bone morphogenetic protein-2, and increased signaling through the IL-2 receptor. Evidence of leukocyte infiltration appears with gene expression patterns reflecting leukocyte integrins. Genes encoding proteins for the humoral immune response are further up-regulated at this time, whereas the most down-regulated genes reflect a passing window of receptivity, with loss of LIF, DKK-1, IGF-1, and complement proteins. It is remarkable how well defined the four segments of the menstrual cycle are with DNA microarray, again reflecting the shifts in ovarian steroids and their receptors throughout the phases of the menstrual cycle.

DIFFERENCES IN GENE EXPRESSION IN WOMEN WITH ENDOMETRIOSIS

Global comparisons of the endometrium from women with and without endometriosis have also been performed.[112,113] When midluteal endometrium from each group was compared, the overall impression was that of progesterone insensitivity in endometrium from women with endometriosis. Changes in gene expression were small, with an increase in expression of 91 genes (0.7%) and a decrease in expression of 115 genes (0.9%). Collagen α2 type I and bile salt export pumps are examples of genes that were overexpressed. Interestingly, down-regulation of an enzyme necessary for L-selectin ligands (*N*-acetylglucosamine-6-*O*-sulfotransferase) may be significant because L-selectins have been postulated to be receptors on the embryo necessary for adhesion to the surface epithelium. Glycodelin, a major progesterone-induced secretory product, was also reduced. These differences may provide a profile for endometrial dysfunction in this and other diagnoses that have been associated with implantation defects. Multiple studies have also examined the difference between eutopic and ectopic endometrium in women with endometriosis.[399-403] Interestingly, when mild endometriosis was compared with moderate to severe endometriosis, there was a shift in progesterone resistance toward the early luteal phase, suggesting that stage of endometriosis matters when considering the effects on the eutopic endometrium.[113]

Clinical Evaluation of the Endometrium

ENDOMETRIAL BIOPSY

Endometrial biopsy is used to assess endometrial histology. Although this technique is employed extensively in the setting of abnormal bleeding as a diagnostic tool for endometrial cancer or hyperplasia, its primary role in the evaluation of the infertile couple has been the assessment of the luteal phase. However, as described later, the clinical utility of endometrial biopsy as a routine test is questionable. The literature reflects a wide range of opinions regarding the use of this test,[404-407] including when to perform the biopsy, the number of days' lag time that should be required to consider a sample abnormal, and the utility of other modalities to evaluate the luteal phase.[408] Rigorous standardization of endometrial biopsy to evaluate histologic criteria has never been established, despite more than 50 years of use.[404,409] The chronologic reference point, crucial to the interpretation of results, has shifted from retrospective to prospective determination during that time.[410] These variations in the use of the endometrial "dating" may explain, in part, the wide diversity of opinion in the literature regarding the incidence and clinical importance of luteal phase deficiency (LPD).[405]

Luteal phase deficiency is uncommon and probably accounts for no more than 3% to 5% of infertility in the population. The high prevalence of LPD in some reports is understandable, given the variability of endometrial histology between women and even in the same woman in subsequent cycles. Add to that the variation in timing of the biopsy and inter- and intraobserver variation in evaluating the histologic findings, and the real significance of luteal phase biopsy may become of historic interest only.

The histologic changes that serve as the basis for this technique were described in 1950 in the now classic paper by Noyes and associates.[349] Unfortunately, these criteria are only an approximation of the cumulative effect of progesterone on the endometrium. Cycle-to-cycle variability and high inter- and intra-observer variation also reduce the overall reliability of these dating criteria. The original indices, as defined, were only obtained in an *infertile* population, making it somewhat difficult to know whether the same histologic changes occur in normal fertile women. Indeed, recent studies in normal fertile control subjects do not support this technique of dating endometrium as a precise or reproducible method of endometrial assessment.[404] Currently, the best method for diagnosing luteal phase defects may be the presence of a shortened luteal phase, as shown by methods such as basal body temperature charting (Fig. 9-24). Although the normal luteal phase should be approximately 12 to 14 days long, premature luteolysis could potentially compromise the establishment of pregnancy. Such charting can also demonstrate anovulatory cycles.

Some of the observations regarding luteal function may have a basis that is worthy of further consideration. With the completion of the human genome project and the availability of high-throughput DNA microarray analyses, it appears that progesterone resistance does occur, based on patterns of gene expression in women with endometriosis compared with fertile control subject.[113] Whether this precedes or is a result of endometrial pathology has not been settled. Although endometriosis appears to be the primary example of this phenomenon, it also appears to be common in ovulatory women with PCOS.[35,411] Such changes may account for the infertility or pregnancy loss associated with these conditions. Defects in progesterone receptors or in progesterone-mediated regulators of cell growth or differentiation have all been implicated in progesterone resistance, including changes in HOXA genes, integrins, Mig-6, FKBP52, PRB, or DKK-1.[12,43,58,112,412,413] These findings provide new information to aid in the understanding of subtle defects in progesterone responsiveness and help to keep attention focused on LPD, even 60 years after its original description.

ULTRASONOGRAPHY

Abnormalities of the structure of the uterus as a result of congenital defects, neoplasia, or synechiae can impair fertility. Diagnostic imaging methods play an important role in the assessment of these uterine defects[414] (see Chapter 33).

Transvaginal sonography (TVS) has become widely accepted as a tool for high-resolution imaging of the female internal reproductive organs.[415] This noninvasive, convenient, and safe technology provides rapid diagnoses with high correlation with pathology. TVS is used primarily to monitor follicular development and endometrial thickness during exogenous hormone treatment of infertile patients. The method might offer significant advantages for use as a diagnostic aid in various other endometrial conditions, such as endometrial polyps, submucous and intramural leiomyomata, endometrial hyperplasia, and carcinoma. TVS has certainly found its use in the assessment of early pregnancy.

Growth of the endometrium can easily be measured using ultrasound. Endometrial thickness and texture are commonly assessed, especially when women are sequentially monitored as part of treatment with human menopausal gonadotropins. Endometrium in the early proliferative phase immediately after menses is typically thin; in response to estrogen, the endometrium thickens and becomes trilaminar in appearance, growing between 0.1 and 0.5 mm daily. After ovulation, the endometrium becomes hyperechoic as secretory changes ensue. Various attempts have been made to classify these patterns on the basis of thickness and texture. Most authors suggest that a thickness of 8 mm or greater with a trilaminar appearance is adequate for implantation in an in vitro fertilization cycle.[416-420] Beyond a certain threshold, however, there is no correlation between implantation rates and endometrial thickness.

The cyclic endometrial changes induced by varying estrogen and progesterone levels result in predictable sonographic changes, especially in blood flow and vessel density. Both endometrial thickness and echogenic pattern have been studied as potential markers of uterine receptivity and predictors of successful embryo implantation. Transvaginal pulsed Doppler ultrasound measures uterine artery blood flow (or the impedance to flow) and is expressed as the *pulsatility index* (PI). The PI varies across the menstrual cycle and may be an additional index to predict implantation after assisted reproductive techniques. Aside from endometrial thickness, morphology, blood flow, and uterine artery pulsatility have all been examined as possible markers of a receptive endometrium. Increased PI has been associated with elevated markers of pregnancy loss, including anticardiolipin antibodies.[421,422] Studies in pregnancy using Doppler flow ultrasound and pregnancy rates have been inconclusive.[423]

SONOHYSTEROGRAPHY AND THREE-DIMENSIONAL ULTRASOUND

Identification of uterine fibroids, endometriomas, and uterine septa are now fairly routine (see Chapter 33). Lesions such as polyps within the uterine cavity may be misinterpreted as thickened endometrium and therefore go undiagnosed. Instillation of sterile saline into the uterine cavity as part of sonohysterography provides an enhanced view of the uterine cavity and may detect even small lesions. This approach is valuable in assessing the effects of selective estrogen receptor modulators, such as tamoxifen, on the endometrium.[424] A sonohysterogram in a normal uterus shows a smooth contour (Fig. 9-25A). In some cases, abnormalities can be more clearly seen with installation of sterile saline solution (Fig.

9-25B). Three-dimensional sonohysterograms can provide dramatic three-dimensional rendering of the uterine cavity, giving a better overall appreciation of such lesions, and can better determine the location and point of attachment (Fig. 9-25C).[425] This evolving technology may further improve the sensitivity and specificity of the technique used to detect small polyps or fibroids. With the advent of three-dimensional ultrasound, differential diagnoses between a septate versus a bicornuate uterus can also be more readily

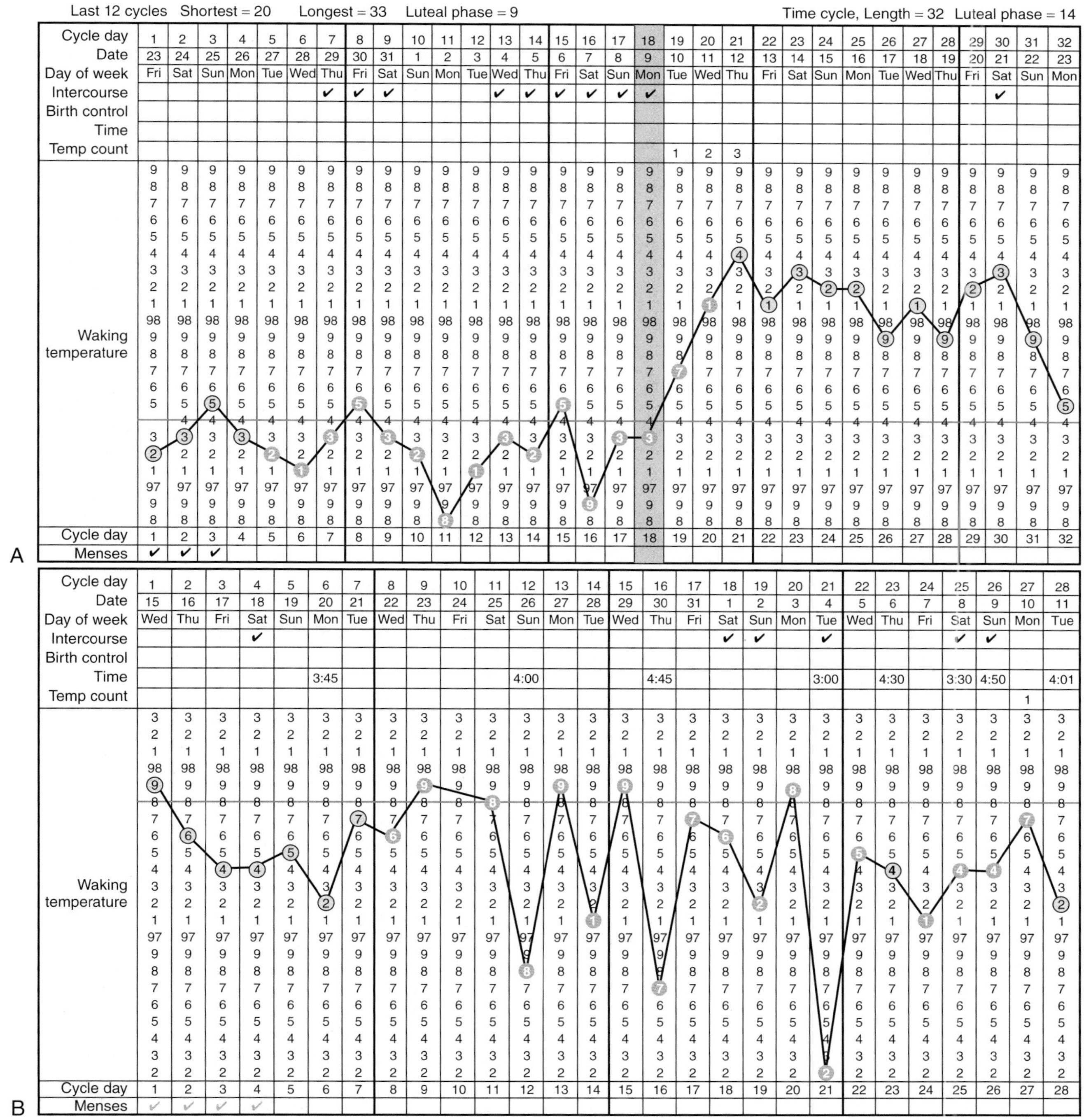

Figure 9-24. Basal body temperature charts can be helpful for the diagnosis of ovulatory dysfunction. Compared with the normal 14-day luteal phase (**A**), anovulatory cycles do not show a normal thermogenic shift (**B**).   *Continued*

Last 12 cycles   Shortest = 20   Longest = 33   Luteal phase = 9   Time cycle, Length = 32   Luteal phase = 14

Cycle day	1	2	3	4	5	6	7	8	9	10	11	12	13	14	15	16	17	18	19	20	21	22	23	24	25	26	27
Date	23	24	25	26	27	28	29	30	31	1	2	3	4	5	6	7	8	9	10	11	12	13	14	15	16	17	18
Day of week	Fri	Sat	Sun	Mon	Tue	Wed	Thu	Fri	Sat	Sun	Mon	Tue	Wed	Thu	Fri	Sat	Sun	Mon	Tue	Wed	Thu	Fri	Sat	Sun	Mon	Tue	Wed
Intercourse							4	4	4				4	4	4	4	4	4									
Birth control																											
Time								7:30					7:30														
Temp count																			1	2	3						

Waking temperature (°F scale 97–99)

Cycle day: 1–27, Menses: 4, 4, 4

Figure 9-24, cont'd *In some cases, a short luteal phase is evident (C).*

determined, avoiding the need for more expensive modalities, such as MRI. The use of three-dimensional ultrasound for the assessment of uterine receptivity is also evolving.[426]

HYSTEROSCOPY

Hysteroscopy is a highly useful tool to identify and correct lesions identified by hysterosalpingography or sonohysterography (Fig. 9-25D).[427,428] Visualization of the endometrial cavity has proven useful for the inspection of the uterine cavity in women with abnormal bleeding, infertility, and recurrent pregnancy loss. Direct visualization allows the operator to resect lesions or obtain a biopsy specimen, once a lesion is identified. Resection of uterine septa in müllerian fusion defects is commonly performed. More recently, hysteroscopic sterilization techniques have been refined to a point that challenges other techniques, and this method is readily available in many centers around the world.[429]

MAGNETIC RESONANCE IMAGING

Occasionally, MRI may be useful for the diagnosis of myometrial lesions, including fibroids and adenomyosis (see Chapter 33). T2-weighted images may provide evidence of endometriotic lesions outside the uterine fundus and aid in the diagnosis of congenital uterine anomalies before surgical correction.

Endometrial Neoplasia

Clinicopathologic correlation strongly suggests that there are two major types of endometrial cancers, type 1 (most endometrioid and mucinous adenocarcinomas) and type 2 (mostly serous and clear cell adenocarcinomas), which have different molecular and biologic characteristics and are believed to arise by different pathogenetic mechanisms.[430,431] Type 1 tumors are associated with estrogen, whereas type 2 cancers are unrelated to estrogen. Endometrioid cancers, the most common malignancy, accounting for more than 80% of endometrial cancers, are almost always type 1 tumors, whereas the rarer and more aggressive serous carcinomas are primarily type 2 cancers. Tumor grade, assessed by the morphology of the glandular components of the tumor, is generally high in type 2 cancers.

Risk factors for type 1 cancers are largely related to quantity or duration of exposure to estrogen.[432] They include estrogen and tamoxifen therapy, estrogen-producing tumors, and PCOS. Nulliparity, early menarche, and late menopause, all related to greater duration of estrogen exposure and, in the case of nulliparity, shorter duration of progesterone dominance, are also risk factors.

Obesity has long been identified as a risk factor. It potentially contributes to excess estrogen as a result of extraglandular aromatization of androgen precursors and the storage of fatty acid esters of estrogen in adipose tissue. Sex hormone–binding globulin levels are also diminished, resulting in more bioavailable estrogen and androgen for aromatization. Obese women have also been found to have alterations in estrogen catabolism that favor the formation of estriol and epiestriol, as opposed to less estrogenic catechol estrogens.

Diabetes is an acknowledged risk factor, probably because of reduced sex hormone–binding globulin levels associated with insulin resistance. The compensatory hyperinsulinemia may also be a factor, as well as the diminished IGF-binding protein expression that results in more bioavailable IGF-1. The relative risk associated with type 1

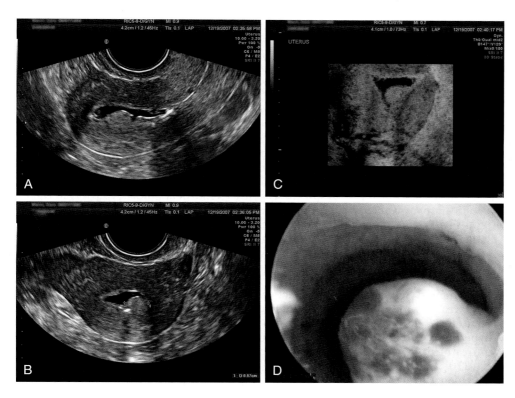

Figure 9-25. Sonohysterography can be used to visualize intracavitary lesions. Injection of sterile saline shows the uterine cavity to be free of polyps or fibroids (*A*). In the case of intrauterine pathology, lesions such as a polyp can be easily delineativated in either two-dimensional (*B*) or three-dimensional rendering (*C*). Hysteroscopy confirms a polyp (*D*) that can then be easily resected.

versus type 2 diabetes is not yet known because only one study has addressed this issue (finding a greater odds ratio for type 1 diabetes). Pregnancy, the use of combination-type oral contraceptives and intrauterine devices, and diets rich in isoflavones seem to protect against type 1 endometrial cancers. The only known risk factor for type 2 cancers, which usually occur in women older than 60 years, is age. Unlike type 1 tumors, progestins do not retard the growth of type 2 cancers.

Endometrial hyperplasia is believed to represent a histologic and biologic continuum extending from exaggerated proliferation of normal endometrium to endometrioid carcinoma. In contrast, type 2 tumors, such as the serous carcinomas, typically develop in atrophic endometrium. Endometrial hyperplasia is directly related to dose and duration of estrogen exposure; 20% of women receiving unopposed estrogen hormone replacement therapy have endometrial hyperplasia after 1 year.[329] Substantial literature indicates that endometrial hyperplasia associated with nuclear atypia, characterized by large round nuclei with prominent nucleoli and complex glandular crowding, is a precursor of endometrioid cancers.[432] The progression of endometrial hyperplasia with cytologic atypia to endometrioid carcinoma is impressive; endometrioid cancer developed in 24% to 57% of patients sequentially monitored over time after atypical endometrial hyperplasia was identified and left untreated.

In contrast, there is a relatively low likelihood of progression of simple or complex hyperplasia without atypia to cancer. In one large study, fewer than 2% of women with endometrial hyperplasia without atypia subsequently had cancer more than 1 year after the diagnosis of hyperplasia was made. In contrast, cancer developed in 23% of subjects with hyperplasia and cellular atypia.[432] There is, however,

an apparent age-related biologic difference in atypical hyperplasias; this lesion in premenopausal women is effectively reversed with progesterone treatment, whereas it is less responsive in postmenopausal subjects.

The concept that atypical endometrial hyperplasia is a precursor to endometrioid cancer is also consonant with several other observations: the frequent coexistence of adenocarcinoma and hyperplasia, the similar appearance of atypical endometrial hyperplasia and low-grade endometrioid carcinoma, and the sharing of molecular phenotypes. Further, unlike benign hyperplasia, atypical hyperplasia is usually a clonal lesion and coexisting endometrioid carcinoma is derived from the same clone. Indeed, the histopathologic diagnosis of endometrial hyperplasia and well-differentiated endometrioid carcinoma is problematic in the absence of frank invasion.

Endometrial hyperplasia with atypia and endometrioid cancers usually contain estrogen and progesterone receptors, whereas serous endometrial cancers do not. Although normal endometrium does not express aromatase, the stroma of endometrioid cancers does express the enzyme, providing a local source of estrogen to fuel tumor proliferation. Endometrial hyperplasias and endometrioid cancers also express progesterone receptors. Progestins inhibit endometrial epithelial cell proliferation in part by blocking cell cycle protein activation and nuclear translocation, thereby reducing endometrial estrogen receptor content by increasing receptor turnover and decreasing receptor synthesis. Progestins also induce the expression of type 2 17β-hydroxysteroid dehydrogenase (which converts estradiol to estrone) and sulfotransferase (which converts estrogens to inactive sulfonates). Progesterone exerts some of these effects via stromal progesterone receptors.

Elevated risk of endometrial hyperplasia and cancer has been associated with PCOS.[433,434] Although infrequent ovulation and prolonged exposure to unopposed estrogen undoubtedly play a role, there appear to be intrinsic differences in the endometrium of women with this disorder. Increased steroid receptors and receptor coactivators have been described in PCOS endometrium.[35,72] Elevated expression of the estrogen-responsive protein, Cyr61, cFos, and markers of cell proliferation provides further evidence of increased estrogen activity throughout the luteal phase.[435] Loss of Mig-6, a negative modulator of the EGF receptor, has also been identified in PCOS endometrium, suggesting a fundamental mechanism for the heightened risk of hyperplasia and cancer in women with this condition.[411] The absence of this EGF receptor inhibitor is associated with hyperplasia in Mig-6 knockout mice.[436]

The effect of progestogens on the human endometrial response to exogenous estrogens has been well documented.[431,432,437] The incidence of endometrial hyperplasia ranges from 16% to 32% in women treated with cyclic estrogens, but progestogen treatment for 7 days each month reduces the incidence of hyperplasia to between 3% and 4%. Extending progestogen treatment to 10 days reduces the incidence even further (2%), and treatment for 13 days each month reduces the incidence to zero. The risk of endometrial cancer mirrors these findings, with odds ratios of more than 6.0 for women using estrogens without progestins for 5 years or more being reduced to 1.6 when progestins are administered cyclically or continuously. However, in the cohort of women using cyclical progestin therapy for approximately 10 days per cycle, the odds ratio is slightly higher, at 2.5.

It is important to note that the dose of progestin needed to prevent endometrial hyperplasia depends on the dose of estrogen, with higher progestin doses needed to protect the endometrium when high doses of estrogen are administered. Tissue response to progesterone may also influence progression to neoplasia; a functional polymorphism in the progesterone receptor promoter that favors transcription of PRB has been associated with increased risk of endometrial cancer.[438] This finding is consistent with the observation that highly malignant endometrial cancers overexpress PRB.

Endometrial hyperplasias and endometrioid cancers display microsatellite instability in approximately 20% of lesions.[438] These alterations in lengths of repetitive sequences reflect defects in DNA mismatch repair mechanisms that result in genome instability. Epigenetic inactivation, rather than mutations, appears to account for altered activity of the principal mismatch repair genes (hMLH1 and hMSH2) in endometrial cancers. Genomic instability is also reflected in loss of heterozygosity at specific chromosomal locations (indicating the presence of tumor suppressor genes), with the greatest frequency reported for endometrial cancers on chromosome 10q.

The PTEN tumor suppressor gene, located on 10q23-q26, acts as a phosphatase implicated in control of cell survival, partly through antagonism of Akt/protein kinase B, which provides a signal that protects cells from apoptosis. Mutations in this gene are found in atypical hyperplasias and endometrioid cancers, particularly when there is microsatellite instability.[439,440] All female mice lacking one copy of the Pten gene have a complex atypical endometrial hyperplasia, and in nearly one fourth of these animals, this lesion progresses to endometrial carcinoma.[441] DNA repair mismatch deficiency accelerates the formation of endometrial tumors in the Pten heterozygous mice.

The presence of PTEN mutations in endometrial hyperplasia, even without atypia, suggests that mutation of this gene is an early event in the pathway of type 1 endometrial carcinogenesis. Elevated Akt/protein kinase B activity is a characteristic feature of PTEN inactivation and results in a decreased rate of apoptosis. PTEN is normally expressed in a cyclic fashion in the endometrium, with its highest expression in the secretory phase, suggesting progesterone regulation and the presence of another mechanism whereby progestins can reverse hyperplasia.[336] In addition to PTEN, other putative tumor suppressor genes on 10q have been implicated in endometrial cancer, as have inactivating mutations in the ras oncogene.[431] Microsatellite instability and mutations in PTEN and ras are rarely found in serous cancers, which usually show histochemical staining for p53, which correlates with the presence of p53 mutations leading to overexpression of the protein.

Early investigators suggested that estrone was more likely than estradiol or estriol to promote endometrial carcinoma. This conclusion was reached on the basis of retrospective epidemiologic studies suggesting an association between exogenous estrogens and endometrial malignant neoplasia, in which most women had received conjugated estrogens consisting of approximately 65% estrone sulfate. However, equivalent doses of conjugated estrogens and estradiol evidently produce the same degree of endometrial stimulation and the same incidence of hyperplasia.[432] Even when the regimen takes into account estriol's rapid absorption and metabolic clearance, endometrial hyperplasia still has been found to develop. Moreover, no significant differences in the effects of estradiol on the endometrium are found when it is administered with or without estriol, dispelling the notion that estriol protects against estradiol-induced endometrial stimulation.

A model pathway for the development of type 1 endometrial cancers has been suggested by Sherman.[431] It is proposed that estrogen, presumably acting on the endometrial stroma, promotes the production of growth factors that stimulate epithelial proliferation. In the absence of an adequate progestogenic "brake," epithelial proliferation progresses to hyperplasia without atypia. Mutations acquired in the ras and PTEN genes lead to expansion of a clone of cells with atypia, and subsequent DNA mismatch repair defects result in a further progression from atypical hyperplasia to endometrioid carcinoma.

The serous carcinomas are proposed to develop from endometrial intraepithelial carcinoma, a distinctive histopathologic lesion characterized by replacement of benign surface endometrium and underlying glands containing cells with anaplastic nuclei. Endometrial intraepithelial carcinoma is believed to arise as a result of genotoxic stress, with genomic instability leading to the progression of invasive serous carcinoma.

The complete reference list can be found on the companion Expert Consult Web site at www.expertconsultbook.com.

Suggested Readings

Achache H, Revel A. Endometrial receptivity markers, the journey to successful embryo implantation. Hum Reprod Update 12:731-746, 2006.

Conneely OM, Mulac-Jericevic B, DeMayo F, et al. Reproductive functions of progesterone receptors. Recent Prog Horm Res 57:339-355, 2002.

Croxatto HB. Physiology of gamete and embryo transport through the fallopian tube. Reprod Biomed Online 4:160-169, 2002.

Donaghay M, Lessey BA. Uterine receptivity: alterations associated with benign gynecological disease. Semin Reprod Med 25:461-475, 2007.

King A. Uterine leukocytes and decidualization. Hum Reprod Update 6:28-36, 2000.

Leese HJ, Tay JI, Reischl J, et al. Formation of fallopian tubal fluid: role of a neglected epithelium. Reproduction 121:339-346, 2001.

Morcel K, Camborieux L, Guerrier D. Mayer-Rokitansky-Kuster-Hauser (MRKH) syndrome. Orphanet J Rare Dis 2:13, 2007.

Norwitz ER, Schust DJ, Fisher SJ. Implantation and survival of early pregnancy. N Engl J Med 345:1400-1408, 2001.

Paria BC, Reese J, Das SK, et al. Deciphering the cross-talk of implantation: advances and challenges. Science 296:2185-2188, 2002.

Seppala M, Taylor RN, Koistinen H, et al. Glycodelin: a major lipocalin protein of the reproductive axis with diverse actions in cell recognition and differentiation. Endocr Rev 23:401-430, 2002.

Silverberg SG. The endometrium. Arch Pathol Lab Med 131:372-382, 2007.

Slayden OD, Keator CS. Role of progesterone in nonhuman primate implantation. Semin Reprod Med 25:418-430, 2007.

Wang H, Dey SK. Roadmap to embryo implantation: clues from mouse models. Nature Rev Genetics 7:185-199, 2006.

CHAPTER 10

The Breast

Robert L. Barbieri

The breast overlies the second to the sixth ribs. The medial border of the breast is the sternum, and the lateral border is the latissimus dorsi. The superior and inferior borders are the clavicle and the costal margin and upper rectus sheath. The breast consists of glandular, adipose, and connective tissues.

The glandular tissue of the breast is arranged in approximately 15 to 20 lobes (Fig. 10-1). Each lobe consists of a branching structure made up of lobules and acini (also referred to as *alveoli*). The acini are lined by a single layer of milk-secreting epithelial cells. Each acinus is encased in an interwoven pattern of contractile myoepithelial cells. The lumens of the acini connect to collecting intralobular ducts, which empty into the main 15 to 20 lobar collecting ducts. In turn, each lobe drains into the nipple. The nipple is surrounded by a pigmented areola. The sebaceous glands located on the perimeter of the areola are referred to as the *glands of Montgomery*. The glandular tissue is embedded in fat, which accounts for most of the mass of the breast. The lobules are separated by connective tissue septa (Cooper's ligaments) that run from the subcutaneous tissue to the chest wall.

The breast is sensitive to the sex steroids estradiol, progesterone, and testosterone, and to numerous protein hormones, including prolactin and oxytocin.[1] During puberty and pregnancy, the breast is stimulated to grow. In many mammals, estradiol is especially important in stimulating the growth of the ductal system, and progesterone is important in stimulating the growth of the acini and stromal elements. During pregnancy, estradiol, progesterone, and prolactin are important factors stimulating breast growth. Androgens tend to inhibit breast growth, an effect that can be characterized as anti-estrogenic.

A genetic experiment of nature, *androgen insensitivity syndrome*, provides a clinical example of the important interplay between estrogens and androgens in the regulation of breast growth.[2] In androgen insensitivity, due to mutations in the androgen receptor, genetic males (46,XY) do not have a functional androgen receptor. Testosterone is produced by the testis, but target tissues are not capable of responding to the high levels of circulating androgens. In this syndrome, estradiol levels are in the range of 50 pg/mL, comparable to levels in the early follicular phase.[3]

Breast volume in individuals with androgen insensitivity is typically above average. This suggests that, in the complete absence of androgen inhibition, modest levels of estradiol are capable of stimulating significant breast growth. Progesterone levels are low in individuals with loss of the androgen receptor. This suggests that breast volume is not absolutely dependent on progesterone stimulation. The anti-estrogenic effect of androgen on breast growth is the basis for therapies used to treat fibrocystic disease.

Development of the Breast

The development of the breast occurs in three major phases: in utero, at puberty, and during pregnancy. This process has been best studied in the rodent. During in utero development of the breast, the growth of epithelial elements into the underlying mesenchyme results in the development of a rudimentary ductal system. In the mouse, the majority of mammary morphogenesis occurs in the postnatal period. Immediately after birth, the mammary ducts are quiescent. At sexual maturity, the distal ends of the ducts proliferate and develop into the end buds, a structure similar to the human acinus. With the onset of pregnancy, a second round of proliferation occurs. Numerous hormones play roles in this process, including estradiol, progesterone, androgens, prolactin and other lactogenic factors, thyroxine, glucocorticoid, insulin, growth hormone, transforming growth factor-β, and epidermal growth factor (EGF).[4-6]

During the normal menstrual cycle, the breast undergoes cycles of growth and quiescence. In the early follicular

Anatomic Structures

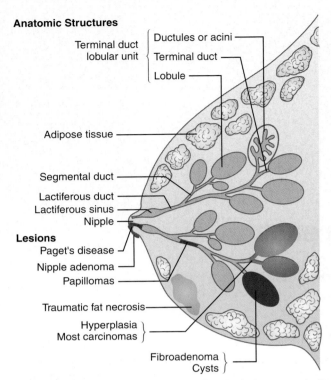

Figure 10-1. Anatomy of the breast and major lesions at each site within the breast. (From Cotran RS, Kumar V, Robbins SL. Pathologic Basis of Disease, 5th ed. Philadelphia, WB Saunders, 1994, p 1090.)

phase, the ductal cells proliferate and continue to develop throughout the remainder of the cycle. In the luteal phase of the cycle, progesterone stimulates the proliferation of the terminal duct structure, basal epithelial cells, and stromal cells. Accompanying these proliferative changes are an increase in stromal edema and vacuolization of epithelial cells. These effects may account, in part, for the sense of breast fullness women experience during the late luteal phase. At menses, the decrease in estradiol and progesterone is associated with a decrease in cell proliferation, stromal edema, and the size of the ducts and acini.

The two most common congenital anomalies of the breast are supernumerary nipples and accessory axillary breast tissue. Supernumerary nipples result from the persistence of epidermal thickenings along the embryologic milk line. Supernumerary nipples can extend from the axilla to the suprapubic area. On occasion, breast tissue extends into the axillary fossa. Ectopic breast tissue in this region can be mistaken for an axillary mass or may cause pain after pregnancy because of engorgement of the tissue with milk.[4,5,7]

Lactation, Prolactin, and Oxytocin

In reproduction, the main role of the breast is secretion of milk. Breast milk consists of milk proteins, including casein and lactalbumin, free fatty acids, and the milk sugar lactose. *Lactose* is a disaccharide consisting of glucose and galactose. During pregnancy, the breast is prepared for lactation by the actions of estradiol, progesterone, prolactin, and other factors—including placental lactogen.

In pregnancy, the breast is exposed to high levels of lactogenic hormones, including prolactin, human placental lactogen, and placental growth hormone. In the nonpregnant woman, prolactin levels are typically less than 25 ng/mL. During the third trimester of pregnancy, prolactin levels are typically 15-fold higher, in the range of 200 to 450 ng/mL.[7] Human placental lactogen reaches concentrations in the range of 6000 ng/mL during the third trimester.

These lactogenic stimuli cause the breast to grow and prepare the alveoli for lactation. During pregnancy, the high concentration of progesterone blocks lactogenesis. After delivery, the decrease in circulating estradiol and progesterone concentrations and the continued elevated prolactin concentration result in an increase in the production of all of the components of milk.[8] The molecular mechanisms subserving these effects are discussed later.

After the decrease in estradiol and progesterone, milk production requires 2 to 5 days to become established. In the postpartum interval, milk production can be suppressed by replacing estradiol and progesterone, or by suppressing prolactin secretion.[9] Milk production also requires the synergistic action of growth hormone, insulin, thyroxine, and cortisol.

During suckling, sensory signals originating in the nipple travel through thoracic nerves 4, 5, and 6 to the central nervous system. When the suckling-induced signals reach the paraventricular and supraoptic nuclei, they stimulate the release of oxytocin from the posterior pituitary. Suckling-induced signals also cause the hypothalamus to induce an acute release of prolactin, in part by suppressing dopamine secretion.[10]

Prolactin maintains lactogenesis by stimulating the transcription of the casein and lactalbumin genes and other genes needed for the synthesis of free fatty acids and lactose. Oxytocin release during suckling causes contraction of the myoepithelial cells of the mammary acini and ducts, which induces the flow of milk. In addition to suckling, visual and auditory stimuli can cause oxytocin to be released from the posterior pituitary.

THE EFFECT OF PROLACTIN ON *β-CASEIN* GENE FUNCTION

The cellular mechanisms that control milk protein production have been best elucidated for the β-casein and whey acidic protein genes. For the *β-casein* gene, gene function is regulated by prolactin, progesterone, estradiol, insulin, glucocorticoids, thyroxine, cell substratum proteins, and growth factors, such as EGF. In the murine mammary epithelial cell line HC11, expression of the β-casein milk protein gene is largely regulated at the transcriptional level.

Prolactin is the key endocrine regulator of *β-casein* gene transcription. The prolactin receptor is a member of the cytokine receptor family.[11] These receptors are characterized by extracellular cysteine motifs, a single transmembrane-spanning domain, and the absence of an intrinsic receptor-associated tyrosine kinase in the intracellular domain. Prolactin binding to its cognate receptor results in dimerization of the receptor and activation of the tyrosine Janus

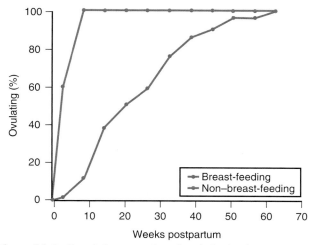

Figure 10-2. Cumulative proportion of ovulation by time postpartum for non–breast-feeding and breast-feeding women. (From Campbell OMR, Gray RH. Characteristics and determinants of postpartum ovarian function in women in the United States. Am J Obstet Gynecol 169:55-60, 1993.)

kinase 2 (JAK2) associated with the membrane-proximal, intracellular domain of the receptor.

In turn, JAK2 phosphorylates and activates STAT5, one of the signal transducers and activators of the transcription (STAT) family. STAT5, previously known as *mammary growth factor,* increases transcription of the β-casein gene.[12] Various phosphatases, which are themselves regulated, dephosphorylate STAT5 and reduce the transcription of β-casein gene transcription.[13]

The addition of prolactin to cultures of mammary epithelial cells results in *casein* gene transcription within 30 minutes. This effect requires the presence of both insulin and glucocorticoid. Deletion and point mutagenesis studies in HC11 cells transfected with the rat *β-casein* promoter have shown that a region of approximately 340 bases immediately upstream of the transcription start site is a major site for gene regulation.[14,15] The 340 bases 5′ of the transcription start site contain the bases that confer gene inducibility by insulin, glucocorticoids, and prolactin.

LACTATION AND AMENORRHEA

Suckling activates multiple systems that inhibit gonadotropin-releasing hormone (GnRH) secretion (see Chapters 1 and 3). The inhibitory systems activated during suckling include dopamine, serotonin, γ-aminobutyric acid, and corticotropin-releasing factor. In turn, inhibition of GnRH secretion results in oligo- or anovulation. The degree to which breast-feeding suppresses GnRH secretion is modulated by the intensity of the breast-feeding, the nutritional status of the mother, and the body mass of the mother.[16-18] Lactation represents a metabolic energy burden. When nutrition is adequate and the basal body mass and composition are normal, intensive lactation is less likely to result in prolonged suppression of GnRH. When nutrition is inadequate to meet the energy demands of both daily living and lactation, oligo- or anovulation is more likely to persist for an extended period.[19,20] During exclusive breast-feeding, approximately

40% of women remain amenorrheic at 6 months postpartum (Fig. 10-2).[21] Women who remain amenorrheic during breast-feeding may have higher prolactin levels than do women who become ovulatory while breast-feeding.[22]

Women who are breast-feeding and are amenorrheic have circulating estradiol levels in the range of 20 to 40 pg/mL. In contrast, normally cycling women have a preovulatory estradiol concentration in the range of 250 to 300 pg/mL. The hypoestrogenic state that is associated with breast-feeding and amenorrhea can produce symptoms such as vaginal dryness. Transdermal estradiol treatment results in a dose-dependent increase in circulating estradiol concentration, but does not appear to significantly increase the estradiol concentration in breast milk.[23] Many gynecologic diseases, such as endometriosis and uterine leiomyomas, are stimulated by high estradiol levels. The hypoestrogenic effect associated with amenorrhea and breast-feeding may have a beneficial effect on these estrogen-dependent disease processes and may account for the laboratory and epidemiologic observation that the risk of estrogen-dependent disease is reduced in women who have breast-fed.[24,25] In one study of the relationship between lactation and the risk of laparoscopically proven endometriosis, a lifetime duration of lactation of greater than 23 months resulted in an 80% decrease in the risk of being diagnosed with endometriosis.[26] The protective effect of lactation disappeared 5 years after the woman's last delivery.

Lactation may also have long-term effects on the metabolic and immune systems. In the Nurses Health Study, 1 year of lactation was associated with a 15% reduction in the risk of being diagnosed with diabetes[27] and a 20% reduction in the risk of being diagnosed with rheumatoid arthritis.[28]

LACTATION AND STEROID CONTRACEPTIVES

In the puerperium, the episodic release of prolactin that is induced by suckling is important in maintaining the production of breast milk. High doses of estrogen, progestins, and androgens suppress lactation.[29] Steroid contraceptives, especially those containing both estrogen and progestin, significantly alter the daily volume and composition of breast milk.

In one study of more than 170 lactating women, the combination of 30 μg ethinyl estradiol and 150 μg levonorgestrel reduced daily milk volume by 42%. In contrast, a progestin-only minipill containing 75 μg norgestrel reduced daily milk volume by only 12%.[30] Combination estrogen–progestin contraceptives also decrease the concentration of nitrogen, lactalbumin, lactoferrin, and lactose in breast milk. These changes in the composition of breast milk are modest and within the normal range of physiologic variation observed in lactating women who are not taking contraceptive steroids.[31]

The development of the newborn does not appear to be significantly affected by the changes in milk composition and volume associated with the use of combination estrogen–progestin oral contraceptives. In one study, the weight and neurologic development of newborns of lactating mothers who took oral contraceptives were similar to those whose mothers did not take oral contraceptives.[30,32] A comparative study of the effects on lactation of a progestin-only contraceptive implant versus a copper intrauterine device (IUD) showed that infant growth was similar for both treatments.[33] Medicated and nonmedicated IUDs do not appear to affect the growth of breast-fed children.[34] If a steroid contraceptive is to be recommended for a lactating woman, it is probably best to use a progestin-only regimen, such as a minipill or depot medroxyprogesterone acetate.

The combination of lactation plus a progestin-only contraceptive is likely to be associated with a prolonged interval of amenorrhea compared with the use of an IUD for contraception.[35]

LACTATION SUPPRESSION

Prolactin secretion is crucial to the maintenance of lactation. Suppression of prolactin secretion with dopamine agonists such as bromocriptine also suppresses lactation.[36] The frequency of adverse effects associated with bromocriptine use in the puerperium is low.[36] However, there are a few case reports of severe hypertension and seizures that occurred in postpartum women who used bromocriptine.[37,38] Owing to these adverse outcomes, many authorities do not recommend bromocriptine as a first-line agent to suppress lactation. There may be a few clinical situations, such as placement of a newborn for adoption, in which bromocriptine or cabergoline could be considered for the suppression of lactation. In most mothers, lactation suppression can be achieved with minimization of the mechanical stimulation of the breast and nipple, ice packs, and anti-prostaglandin treatment. Milk stasis appears to decrease the production of STAT5, the main intracellular activator of milk protein production.[39,40]

INDUCTION OF LACTATION

Induced lactation is defined as breast-feeding in the absence of a recent pregnancy. On occasion, adoptive mothers desire to breast-feed.[41] In countries where access to formula is limited, induced lactation in a surrogate may be important if the biologic mother cannot continue to breast-feed.[42] The key hormone involved in lactation is prolactin. Medications that raise prolactin levels can be used to help induce lactation. For example, metoclopramide, 10 mg three times daily, causes an increase in prolactin secretion.[43] When metoclopramide is coupled with nipple stimulation every few hours using an electronic breast pump, lactation can be established in the majority of women. In many cases, the amount of milk produced may be insufficient to breast-feed the infant exclusively. Agents such as sulpiride and chlorpromazine can also be used to induce lactation, but these agents may be associated with drowsiness and extrapyramidal symptoms.[44]

LACTION AND BONE METABOLISM

During pregnancy, calcium is mobilized from bone, in part, to provide a stable source of calcium for fetal development. Pregnancy is associated with a 1% to 2% decrease in bone mineral density, as determined by dual x-ray absorptiometry. After birth, women who breast-feed lose additional bone mineral from the lumbar spine. Women who bottle-feed their infants typically regain the bone they lost during pregnancy. After breast-feeding is discontinued, bone density returns to prepregnancy values.[45]

LACTATION AND TRANSMISSION OF HUMAN IMMUNODEFICIENCY VIRUS

Human immunodeficiency virus (HIV) can be transmitted from mother to child through breast milk.[46,47] In developed countries where women have access to clean water and the rate of infant death from diarrheal-related illnesses is low, the consensus recommendation is for HIV-infected women to avoid breast-feeding their children. However, in countries with a high rate of infant death from diarrheal-related illnesses due to lack of access to clean water, breast-feeding may be preferred to formula-feeding.

If access to clean water is possible, formula-feeding is probably better than breast-feeding. For example, in one study in Kenya, HIV-positive, postpartum women were randomized to use formula or to breast-feed their infants. The women assigned to the formula-feeding group were educated about diarrheal illnesses and given access to clean water. In this study, the rate of HIV infection in the infants at follow-up 2 years later was 17% in the formula-fed group and 33% in the breast-fed group. In this study, where the women had access to clean water, there was no increase in diarrheal-related illnesses in the formula-fed group.[48] Lactating HIV-positive women who are administered highly active antiretroviral drugs have a low rate of vertical transmission of HIV to their breast-feeding child.[49] The metabolic energy burden of HIV disease plus lactation is often associated with weight loss among these women.[50]

GALACTORRHEA

Galactorrhea is the secretion of breast milk at a time remote from nursing. In contrast to other breast secretions, the unique feature of galactorrhea is that the secretion contains milk. This can be demonstrated by drying the secretion on a glass slide and staining for the presence of fat. Galactorrhea is usually due to hyperprolactinemia or excessive sensitivity of the breast to normal circulating levels of prolactin. When galactorrhea is associated with normal ovulatory menses, the most likely cause of the galactorrhea is excessive sensitivity of the breast to normal circulating levels of prolactin. When galactorrhea is associated with amenorrhea, it is likely that the circulating prolactin level is elevated. Approximately 75% of women with both galactorrhea and amenorrhea have hyperprolactinemia. The causes of hyperprolactinemia are reviewed in detail in Chapter 3. Briefly, the most common causes of hyperprolactinemia are a prolactin-secreting pituitary tumor, the use of dopamine antagonist medications (such as phenothiazines), pregnancy, renal disease, and primary hypothyroidism.

Galactorrhea of any cause can be suppressed by the use of dopamine agonist medications, such as bromocriptine. In women with galactorrhea, normal ovulatory menses, and normal prolactin concentration, low doses of bromocriptine (1.25 to 2.5 mg) are often effective in the suppression of galactorrhea. Patients with unilateral nipple discharge or nipple discharge containing blood should be referred to a breast surgeon.

Benign Breast Disease

Fibrocystic change is the most common benign breast abnormality. It is characterized histologically by hyperplastic changes of the lobular epithelium, ductal epithelium, or connective tissue.[51] The disorder is characterized clinically by breast tenderness that is particularly severe in the premenstrual phase of the menstrual cycle. Fibrocystic changes in the breast occur in a high percentage of women. Some authorities contend that fibrocystic change is a variant of normal breast physiology, not a disease state.

The medical management of fibrocystic disease continues to evolve. Danazol is an attenuated androgen that is effective in reducing symptoms associated with fibrocystic disease in 80% of patients.[52] Danazol is effective in the treatment of fibrocystic disease, probably because of its anti-estrogenic effects. Danazol is a teratogen, and doses of less than 400 mg daily do not reliably suppress ovulation; the recommended dosage is between 100 and 400 mg daily. Women taking danazol should use a barrier contraceptive. Tibolone, gestrinone, tamoxifen, and GnRH-agonist analogs are also effective in the treatment of breast pain.

Benign breast disease is associated with an increased risk of breast cancer. The histologic appearance of the benign lesion influences cancer risk. For example, in a study of more than 9000 women with benign breast disease who were followed for 15 years, nonproliferative histologic findings were associated with a 1.27 (95% confidence interval [CI], 1.15 to 1.41) risk of breast cancer and proliferative histologic findings in the absence of cellular atypia were associated with a 1.88 (95% CI, 1.66 to 2.12) risk of breast cancer. The histologic presence of atypia increases the risk to 4.24 (95% CI, 3.26 to 5.41).[53] Women with fibrocystic breast disease typically have nonproliferative changes on breast biopsy.

Breast Cancer: An Endocrine Disease

GENETIC CONTRIBUTIONS

In developed countries, breast cancer is the most common cancer of women. Worldwide, breast cancer is the cause of more than 500,000 deaths annually.[54] In developed countries, the lifetime risk of breast cancer is approximately 10%. Approximately 20% of cases are diagnosed before the age of 50 years, and 80% are diagnosed after the age of 50 years. Numerous factors, including genetics, hormones, diet, lifestyle, and reproductive and other environmental exposures, contribute to the risk of breast cancer.

Cancer is caused by the sequential accumulation of mutations in genes that regulate cell proliferation. Genetic factors are major contributors to breast cancer risk. In

1866, French physician Paul Broca reported 10 cases of breast cancer in four generations of his wife's family. It has taken more than 130 years to begin to characterize some of the genes involved in familial breast cancer.[55] In women with one affected first-degree relative, the risk of breast cancer is increased twofold to threefold.[56] If two first-degree relatives are affected, or if the disease was diagnosed in a family member before age 45 years, the risk is further increased.[56,57] Overall, approximately 15% of cases of breast cancer are related to family history, and approximately half of this risk is attributed to cancer susceptibility genes.[57] Germline mutations in *BRCA1*, *BRCA2*, the gene encoding ataxia-telangiectasia, and *TP53* are associated with breast cancer risk.

BRCA1 is a tumor suppressor gene on chromosome 17 that is mutated in the germline in approximately 5% of women with breast cancer.[58] Because the mutation is inherited in an autosomal dominant manner, many generations of women in an affected family may have breast and ovarian cancer. The *BRCA1* gene is composed of 22 coding exons distributed over 100 kilobases of genomic DNA. The gene encodes a protein of 1863 amino acids.[59] The BRCA1 protein contains a zinc finger motif and is a nucleic acid–binding protein that acts as a tumor suppressor by repairing breaks in double-stranded DNA (the main genetic insult is caused by radiation and some mutagens).[60] Approximately 0.1% to 0.2% of all women have a germline allele of a *BRCA1* gene that contains an inactivating mutation.[61] If the second allele of *BRCA1* undergoes an inactivating somatic mutation, the affected woman has a high risk of breast cancer. Women who have a germline mutation of one *BRCA1* allele have a 65% to 85% chance of having breast cancer by the age of 70 years.[62] Some population-based studies have reported lower risks in the range of 40% to 50%.[63] More than half of *BRCA1*-associated breast cancers occur before age 50 years.

In families at high risk for breast cancer, many mutations in *BRCA1* have been reported.[58] In a study of more than 1400 sequence variants in the *BRCA1* and *BRCA2* genes, more than 40 variants were strongly associated with breast cancer risk.[64] Most of the mutations are inactivating, which is consistent with *BRCA1* being a tumor suppressor gene. Most of the mutations are frameshift or nonsense mutations that prematurely truncate the protein and result in loss of protein function.

Women with a critical *BRCA1* mutation are at high risk for ovarian cancer. It is estimated that approximately 40% to 50% of women with a critical *BRCA1* mutation will have ovarian cancer by age 60 years.[65] Among women of Ashkenazi Jewish origin, a frameshift mutation of the *BRCA1* gene, 185delAG, occurs with a carrier frequency of 1%. In a study of 31 Jewish women with ovarian cancer, 6 women had the 185delAG mutation (19%). In contrast, none of the control Jewish women without ovarian cancer had the mutation. For the Jewish women with ovarian cancer diagnosed before age 50 years, 38% had the 185delAG mutation.[66]

BRCA2 is a breast cancer susceptibility gene on 13q12-13.[67] *BRCA2* mutations are associated with a higher risk of male breast cancer and a lower risk of ovarian cancer than are *BRCA1* mutations.[68] *Ataxia-telangiectasia* is an autosomal recessive disorder with a phenotype of cerebellar ataxia and oculocutaneous telangiectasias.[69] Approximately 1% of the population carries one copy of a mutated gene for ataxia-telangiectasia. Female relatives of patients with ataxia-telangiectasia are at two to three times greater risk for breast cancer than are women who do not have the disorder.[70] Li-Fraumeni syndrome is associated with premenopausal breast cancers, brain tumors, adrenocortical cancers, and other tumors.[71] Germline mutations in *TP53* have been identified in more than 50% of Li-Fraumeni families.[72] The risk of breast cancer in mutation carriers is approximately 50%.

Other genes that have been associated with an increased risk of breast cancer include the *Cowden, HRAS1 VNTR, HCHK2,* and transforming growth factor-β1 genes.[73] Recent genome-wide scans have identified *FGFR2, TNRC9, MAP3K1,* and *LSP1* as genes associated with breast cancer risk.[74] A major public health issue is whether genetic testing for *BRCA* mutations should be widely deployed among low- to medium-risk women.

REPRODUCTIVE RISK FACTORS

Reproductive exposures play a major role in breast cancer risk. Early age at menarche (before age 12 years) and late age at menopause are associated with an increased risk of breast cancer.[75,76] For every 2-year delay in menarche, there is a 10% reduction in the risk of breast cancer.[77] For each year that menopause is delayed, there is a 3% increase in the risk of breast cancer.[78] Parity decreases the risk of breast cancer.[79] However, delaying first birth until after age 35 years increases the risk of breast cancer. Breast-feeding, a natural hypoestrogenic state, is associated with a reduced risk of breast cancer.[80] Bilateral oophorectomy before age 40 years reduces the risk of breast cancer by 50%.[81]

In an analysis of 47 studies including 50,302 women with breast cancer and 96,973 women without breast cancer, the role of parity and breast-feeding was highlighted. The relative risk of breast cancer decreased by 4.3% for every 12 months of breast-feeding and by 7% for each birth. In this study, the beneficial effect of breast-feeding did not differ by country (developed versus undeveloped), maternal age, menopausal status, or ethnic origin. The investigators estimated that the cumulative incidence of breast cancer in developed countries would be reduced by 50% if women had the average number of births and lifetime duration of breast-feeding that was prevalent in developing countries (Figs. 10-3 and 10-4).[82]

Obesity has differing effects on the risk of breast cancer in premenopausal and postmenopausal women. In premenopausal women, obesity is associated with an increased risk of anovulation, which is associated with an increase in circulating androgen and a decrease in total integrated exposure to estrogen. Not surprisingly, obesity in premenopausal women is associated with a decreased risk of breast cancer.[82] However, in postmenopausal women, obesity is associated with an increase in the peripheral aromatization of androstenedione to estrone and an increase in the total integrated exposure to estrogen. Postmenopausal women have little or no ovarian production of estrogen, so most of the estrogen in the circulation of postmenopausal women is derived from peripheral aromatization. Obesity in postmenopausal women is associated with an increased risk of breast cancer.

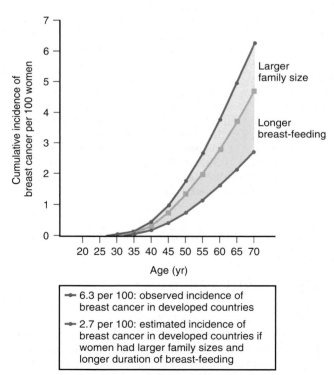

Figure 10-4. *Estimated cumulative incidence of breast cancer in developed countries if women had family sizes and breast-feeding patterns typical for developing countries. Gold line represents estimated incidence of breast cancer in developed countries if women had, on average, 6.5 births instead of 2.5 births, and if women breast-fed each child, on average, for 24 months instead of a lifetime mean of 8.7 months. (From Collaborative Group on Hormonal Risk Factors in Breast Cancer. Breast cancer and breastfeeding. Lancet 360:187-195, 2002.)*

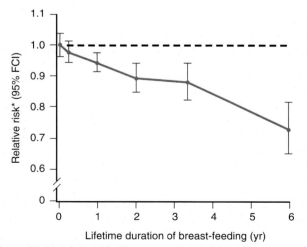

Figure 10-3. *Relative risk of breast cancer (green line) in parous women in relation to lifetime duration of breast-feeding. The relative risk was calculated as floating absolute risk and stratified by study, age, parity, age at first birth, and menopausal status. Hashed line represents the control nulliparous group. FCI, formal confidence interval. (From Collaborative Group on Hormonal Risk Factors in Breast Cancer. Breast cancer and breastfeeding. Lancet 360:187-195, 2002.)*

THE ROLE OF ESTROGEN, ANDROGEN, AND PROGESTERONE

Reproductive hormones clearly play an important role in the development of breast cancer. In men, the lifetime risk of breast cancer is 100 times less than the risk in women. In women who have had a bilateral oophorectomy early in life, the risk of breast cancer is very low. Data from prospective cohort studies indicate that postmenopausal women with serum estradiol, estrone, estrone sulfate, or dehydroepiandrosterone sulfate (DHEAS) levels in the upper quartile of the population have an approximately two-fold increase in the risk of breast cancer.[83]

In this study, serum was obtained from 11,169 postmenopausal women without diagnosed breast cancer. Over the next 4 years, 156 new cases of breast cancer were diagnosed. Serum collected at the beginning of the study was then assayed for estradiol, estrone, estrone sulfate, androstenedione, testosterone, DHEAS, and DHEA from both cases (patients newly diagnosed with breast cancer) and controls (disease-free subjects). The absolute differences in the steroid hormone concentrations between cases and controls were small, in the range of 10% to 15%. The risk of breast cancer was greatest in the women with the highest levels of estrone sulfate and DHEAS. Both of these steroids can be converted to estradiol in breast tissue.[84] Similar results have been reported by other investigators.[85,86] The association between endogenous steroid hormones and breast cancer risk is probably limited to estrogen receptor–positive cancers.[87] The majority of data linking endogenous steroid hormones and breast cancer risk have been generated in studies focused on menopausal women. Recent studies in premenopausal women have reported a positive association between follicular phase estradiol concentration and the risk of breast cancer.[88] The relationship between endogenous steroid hormones and breast cancer appears to be greatest for estrogen receptor–positive breast cancers. Endogenous steroid hormones do not appear to increase the risk for estrogen receptor–negative breast cancers.[89]

Multiple randomized trials have shown that when the anti-estrogens tamoxifen and raloxifene are given to women at above average risk for breast cancer, their risk of primary breast cancer is significantly reduced. For example, in the Breast Cancer Prevention Trial, 4 years of treatment with tamoxifen was associated with a 45% reduction in breast cancer incidence.[90] In the Multiple Outcomes of Raloxifene Evaluation (MORE) trial, 3 years of raloxifene treatment was associated with a 70% reduction in breast cancer incidence in menopausal women.[91]

In the MORE study, raloxifene treatment was the most effective in preventing breast cancer in the women with the highest levels of endogenous serum estrogen and least effective in the women with the lowest levels of serum estrogen at the beginning of the study. In this study, serum estradiol levels were measured in a baseline fasting blood specimen obtained before entry into the study. The baseline estradiol level was a strong predictor of subsequent breast cancer risk. Women with serum estradiol concentrations greater than 2.7 pg/mL had a risk of breast cancer that was five times greater than that in women with undetectable serum estradiol (3% had breast cancer in 4 years versus 0.6%, respectively).

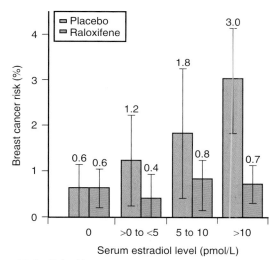

Figure 10-5. *Risk of breast cancer over 4 years is shown among patients in the placebo* (purple) *and raloxifene* (blue) *groups with various baseline serum concentrations of estradiol. (From Cummings SR, Duong R, Kenyon E, et al. Serum estradiol level and risk of breast cancer during treatment with raloxifene. JAMA 287:216-220, 2002.)*

Women with an estradiol level greater than 2.7 pg/mL had a 76% reduction in breast cancer incidence when treated with raloxifene for 4 years. In contrast, women with undetectable serum estradiol had no decrease in breast cancer incidence when treated with raloxifene (Fig. 10-5).[92]

The administration of aromatase inhibitors to women with breast cancer appears to reduce the rate of development of a new cancer in the contralateral breast.[93] Aromatase inhibitors are being studied in clinical trials for their efficacy in reducing the risk of breast cancer in women at high risk.

THE ROLE OF PROLACTIN, INSULIN-LIKE GROWTH FACTORS, AND INSULIN-LIKE GROWTH FACTOR–BINDING PROTEINS

In animal studies, prolactin has been shown to induce mammary tumors. In a large-scale prospective trial, prolactin levels, measured at study entry in postmenopausal women, were found to be positively associated with the risk of breast cancer. Women with baseline prolactin levels in the highest quartile were 2.03 times more likely to have breast cancer (95% CI, 1.24 to 3.31; $P < 0.01$) than women with prolactin levels in the lowest quartile. The relationship was independent of plasma levels of estradiol, estrone, estrone sulfate, testosterone, and DHEAS. This study suggests that higher plasma prolactin levels are associated with an increased risk of breast cancer in postmenopausal women.[94]

Insulin-like growth factor 1 (IGF-1) is a mitogenic and anti-apoptotic protein that can increase proliferation in breast epithelial cells. In a large prospective epidemiologic study, plasma IGF-1 levels were not associated with the risk of breast cancer in postmenopausal women. However, in premenopausal women younger than 50 years of age, the relative risk of breast cancer was significantly increased for women with IGF-1 levels in the top quartile versus those in the bottom quartile (relative risk [RR], 4.58; 95% CI, 1.75 to 12; $P < 0.02$). When adjustments were made for bioavailable

IGF-1 by including IGF-binding protein 3 (IGFBP-3) levels in the analysis, the relative risk increased to 7.28.

This study showed a positive relationship between circulating IGF-1 concentration and the IGF-l/IGFBP-3 ratio and the risk of breast cancer in premenopausal women, but *not* in postmenopausal women.[95] Taken as a whole, these studies suggest that measurement of IGF-1, IGFBP-3, prolactin, estrone sulfate, DHEAS, and possibly estradiol could be used to identify women at the highest risk of breast cancer for chemoprevention interventions.

Recent genome-wide studies have reported that variants in the FGFR2 gene, whose protein product may have an important role in mesenchymal–epithelial growth regulations, are associated with significant increased risk of breast cancer.[96]

ORAL CONTRACEPTIVES AND BREAST CANCER RISK

The use of modern, low-dose monophasic oral contraceptives is not associated with an increased risk of breast cancer (see also Chapter 34).[97] For example, in one case–control study, 4575 women with breast cancer and 4682 control subjects who ranged from 35 to 64 years of age were interviewed regarding their use of oral contraceptives and other relevant exposures. Neither current (RR, 1; 95% CI, 0.8 to 1.3) nor past use of oral contraceptives (RR, 0.9; 95% CI, 0.8 to 1) was associated with the development of breast cancer. Long periods of oral contraceptive use (>15 years) and initiation of use at a young age (<15 years of age) did not correlate with an increased risk. Use of oral contraceptives by women with a family history of breast cancer was not associated with the development of breast cancer. The results were similar among white and black women. This study shows that the use of modern, low-dose oral contraceptives is not associated with breast cancer.

Many previous epidemiologic studies combined women using low-dose and those using high-dose oral contraceptives. Use of oral contraceptives containing higher doses of estrogen and progestin may have been associated with a very slight increase in the risk of breast cancer.[98] How can high levels of endogenous estrogens be associated with an increased risk of breast cancer, if oral contraceptives are not associated with an increased risk of breast cancer? One possible explanation is that the increased risk of breast cancer conferred by estrogen is dependent on the dose, the duration of treatment, and the endogenous hormonal milieu. In a premenopausal woman, the use of oral contraceptives (exogenous estrogen) causes suppression of ovarian production of estrogen (endogenous estrogen), resulting in a neutral effect on integrated circulating estrogen from all sources. Consequently, there is no increase in breast cancer with oral contraceptive use.[98,99]

HORMONE REPLACEMENT THERAPY AND BREAST CANCER RISK

One of the greatest health concerns of women is their fear of breast cancer. This worry is probably exaggerated relative to the actual quantitative risk.[100] For many years, women have been concerned that hormone replacement

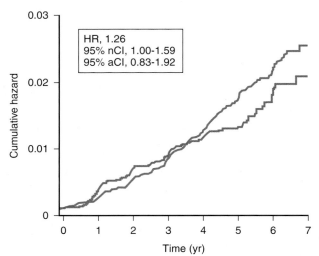

Figure 10-6. *The incidence of breast cancer in women treated with conjugated equine estrogen (0.625 mg daily) plus medroxyprogesterone acetate (2.5 mg daily) (green line) versus women treated with placebo (purple line) in the Women's Health Initiative. The incidence of breast cancer is similar in the two groups until year 4 of the study, when the women treated with hormone therapy start to show a higher rate of breast cancer than women treated with placebo. aCI, adjusted confidence interval; HR, hazard ratio; nCI, nominal confidence interval. (From Writing Group for the Women's Health Initiative Investigators. Risks and benefits of estrogen plus progestin in healthy postmenopausal women. JAMA 288:321-333, 2002.)*

therapy may be associated with an increased risk of breast cancer. Evidence from the Women's Health Initiative clinical trial indicates that long-term use of combination conjugated equine estrogen plus medroxyprogesterone acetate is associated with an increased risk of breast cancer, but use of conjugated equine estrogen only, for less than 5 years, is not associated with an increased risk. In the Women's Health Initiative, women randomized to receive combination conjugated equine estrogen plus medroxyprogesterone acetate had a 24% increased risk of breast cancer after taking hormone therapy for an average of 5.2 years (Fig. 10-6).[101,102] In contrast, women who had a hysterectomy and were randomized to receive equine estrogen–only hormone therapy had a 23% reduction in risk of breast cancer.[103]

Many observational epidemiologic studies also report that long-term use of estrogen plus progestin is associated with an increased risk of breast cancer.[104] In addition, some epidemiologic studies report that long-term use of estrogen therapy alone, especially estradiol, in postmenopausal women is associated with a small increase in the risk of breast cancer.[105] In contrast, the use of low doses of conjugated equine estrogen alone, especially for intervals less than 5 years, may not be associated with an increased risk of breast cancer.[106] The paradox of the finding of an increased risk of breast cancer with estradiol therapy and a decreased risk of breast cancer with conjugated equine estrogen therapy has not yet been adequately explained. One possibility is that conjugated equine estrogens act as both an estrogen agonist and a selective estrogen receptor modulator (SERM).

The functional biology of the estrogen receptor system has not been fully characterized. The selective tissue effects of various estrogenic compounds are believed to be mediated by at least three factors: (1) the relative activity of the alpha and beta estrogen receptors in target tissues[107]; (2) the differential changes in estrogen receptor conformation and functional activity induced by various estrogen-like ligands[108]; and (3) the relative activity of intracellular coactivators and corepressors that bind to the estrogen receptor and modulate the activity of the ligand-bound estrogen receptor complex on gene transcription.[109] Conjugated equine estrogen is a complex mixture of estrogen compounds that includes estrone sulphate, equiline sulphate, delta 8,9-dehydroestrone sulphate, 17-alpha estradiol sulphate, and 17-alpha dihydroequilin sulphate. Each compound may have different estrogen agonist–antagonist prosperities in various tissues. For example, some studies report that delta 8,9-dehydroestrone sulphate is a potent estrogen agonist in the brain, but a weak estrogen agonist in the liver.[110] In contrast, estrone sulphate is a potent estrogen agonist in both the brain and liver. In addition, 17-alpha estradiol and 17-alpha estrone, components of conjugated equine estrogen, may be estrogen antagonists because they can bind to the estrogen receptor, but do not promote transcriptional activity. One interpretation of the available data is that there is a spectrum of estrogen activity from the pure estrogen agonist estradiol to the pure estrogen antagonist fulvestrant. Agents such as conjugated equine estrogen, tamoxifen, and raloxifene are arrayed on the spectrum as SERMs, with varying estrogen agonist and antagonist effects in various tissues, depending on the hormonal milieu.[111]

The type of progestin used in hormone therapy may also influence the risk of breast cancer. The use of native progesterone appeared to be associated with a lower risk of breast cancer than the use of C-19 nortestosterone derivatives.[112]

ALCOHOL USE AND BREAST CANCER RISK

Alcohol use by women appears to be associated with a decreased risk of heart disease and an increased risk of breast cancer. Fuchs and colleagues[113] reported on the association between alcohol use and mortality from heart disease and breast cancer in the Nurses' Health Study. During 12 years of follow-up of 85,709 nurses (for a total of 1,010,209 person-years of follow-up), 2658 women died. A total of 503 women died of cardiovascular disease; 1495 died of cancer, including 350 of breast cancer. Accidents and suicides resulted in 203 deaths, and 52 deaths occurred because of cirrhosis of the liver.

Alcohol at doses of 1.5 to 29.9 g/day reduced the risk of death (a 4-ounce glass of wine contains approximately 10.8 g alcohol; a standard drink of spirits contains 15.1 g alcohol; 12 ounce of beer contains 13.2 g alcohol). At all doses, alcohol consumption reduced the risk of death as a result of cardiovascular disease. At high doses (>30 g daily), alcohol consumption increased the risk of death from breast cancer (RR, 1.67) and liver cirrhosis (RR, 2.55).

These data suggest that alcohol consumption is an independent risk factor for breast cancer. Alcohol may increase the risk of breast cancer by increasing the bioavailability of estrogen[114] and increasing the circulating concentration of estrone sulfate and DHEAS.[115] Alcohol may also enhance mammary gland susceptibility to carcinogenic DNA damage and increase the metastatic potential of breast cancer cells.[116]

Interestingly, consumption of folate appears to reduce the association between alcohol and breast cancer. In one large prospective epidemiologic study, the relationship between alcohol intake (>15 g daily) and breast cancer risk was strongest for those women with daily folate consumption of less than 300 μg daily. For those women with folate consumption of greater than 300 μg daily, the relationship between alcohol intake and breast cancer was markedly attenuated.[117]

Recent data suggest that alcohol consumption may alter estrogen metabolism in women using estrogen replacement therapy. Ginsburg and colleagues[118] studied the effects of alcohol consumption on the half-life of estradiol in menopausal women using transdermal estradiol. In women using transdermal estradiol who consumed a carbohydrate beverage, the apparent half-life of estradiol was 245 minutes. After consumption of a large dose of ethanol (approximately 0.7 g/kg), the apparent half-life of estradiol was 378 minutes. This suggests that alcohol decreases the clearance rate of estradiol.

In a follow-up study, Ginsburg and colleagues[119] showed that in women taking oral micronized estradiol, the acute consumption of alcohol resulted in an approximately 300% increase in circulating estradiol levels (Fig. 10-7). This suggests that alcohol may also increase the efficiency of absorption of estrogen from the gastrointestinal tract.

These studies were performed with high doses of alcohol. Additional studies are needed to determine whether alcohol consumed alone or with meals can also produce a rise in circulating estradiol. If these studies show an effect of dietary alcohol intake on estradiol in women taking oral estradiol hormone replacement, it may be reasonable to adjust the estrogen replacement dose downward. The "Napa Valley" rule is to reduce by half the estrogen dose prescribed to women if they consume significant quantities of alcohol.

Breast Cancer Treatment

Treatment of breast cancer has three main goals (see also Chapter 27):

1. Control of the primary tumor site
2. Minimization of the risk of metastatic disease or new disease in the contralateral breast
3. Maintenance of the woman's quality of life

Surgical treatment, including lumpectomy or mastectomy combined with radiation therapy, is the main method for controlling tumor recurrence at the site of the primary tumor. Lumpectomy combined with radiation therapy is as effective as mastectomy or radical mastectomy in controlling local disease.[120] Hormonal treatment and chemotherapy are the main approaches to reduce the risk of metastatic tumors and to treat existing metastatic disease.

The Early Breast Cancer Trialists' Collaborative Group[121] reviewed the efficacy of various treatment regimens for breast cancer. Data were available from 133 trials

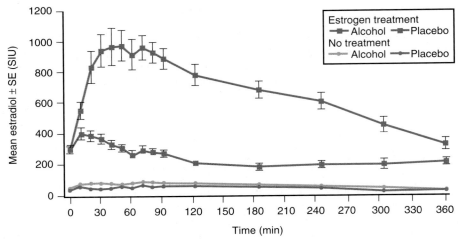

Figure 10-7. *Serum estradiol levels after alcohol or carbohydrate drink in postmenopausal women. Alcohol administration (0.7 g/kg) is represented by the* blue *and* yellow. *Carbohydrate drink (Polycose) administration is represented by the* blue *and* purple. *After administration of alcohol or carbohydrate drink, blood samples were obtained for 6 hours. Estradiol levels for women who were receiving micronized estradiol, 1 mg daily, are shown as* squares. *Estradiol levels for women not receiving hormone replacement therapy are shown as* circles. *Mean ± standard error of the mean; N = 12. In menopausal women receiving micronized estradiol, serum estradiol significantly increased after administration of alcohol (P < 0.001). (From Ginsburg ES, Mello NK, Mendelson JH, et al. Effects of alcohol ingestion on estrogens in postmenopausal women. JAMA 276:1747-1751, 1996. Copyright 1997, American Medical Association.)*

that involved 75,000 women with early breast cancer, of whom 32% died during treatment and follow-up and 10% had new recurrences. The women participated in clinical trials that evaluated the efficacy of tamoxifen (30,000 women), oophorectomy (3000 women), polychemotherapy (11,000 women), single-agent chemotherapy (15,000 women), and immunotherapy (6000 women).

Tamoxifen, oophorectomy in women younger than 50 years, and polychemotherapy all reduced the recurrence of disease and mortality. Recurrence rates were reduced by 25%, 26%, and 25% by tamoxifen, oophorectomy in women younger than 50 years, and polychemotherapy, respectively. The mortality rate was reduced by 17%, 25%, and 16% by tamoxifen, oophorectomy in women younger than 50 years, and polychemotherapy. Oophorectomy after age 50 years and immunotherapy were not effective. Long courses of tamoxifen (2 to 5 years) were more effective than short courses. Courses of polychemotherapy of 4 to 6 months were more effective than courses of 3 months and equally as effective as longer courses or very high-dose regimens. In general, adjuvant treatment is offered to women with greater than a 20% risk of recurrent disease. Clinical characteristics of this population of patients include positive lymph nodes, large primary tumor (>2 cm), and invasion of lymphatic or vascular channels in the breast.

The probability of breast cancer recurrence is higher for women with histologically positive axillary lymph nodes. In the past, axillary lymph node dissection was used to define the risk of recurrence. Such dissections, although useful for predicting future risk of metastatic disease, do not reduce the risk of recurrence and can be associated with significant complications, such as lymphedema of the arm. A new approach to determining the risk of breast cancer recurrence is to perform biopsy on a sentinel node. Sentinel lymph node mapping is performed by injecting a radioactive substance or a blue dye in the area around the tumor. At surgery, the lower ipsilateral axilla is explored

and the lymph node that has taken up the dye is excised. If the lymph node is negative, it is likely that all of the remaining axillary lymph nodes are also negative.[122,123]

THE ROLE OF TAMOXIFEN AND OTHER ANTI-ESTROGENS

Tamoxifen is a triphenylethylene derivative that is structurally related to clomiphene (Fig. 10-8). At the standard dose of 20 mg daily, steady-state plasma concentrations are reached after approximately 4 weeks of therapy.[124,125] Tamoxifen undergoes extensive hepatic metabolism, mainly by hydroxylation and conjugation pathways. One of tamoxifen's main bioactive metabolites, N-desmethyltamoxifen, reaches steady-state concentration after 8 weeks of therapy.[124] N-desmethyltamoxifen has affinity for the estrogen receptor that is comparable to that of tamoxifen.[126] A metabolite that is present at low concentrations, 4-hydroxytamoxifen has affinity for the estradiol receptor similar to that of estradiol.[127,128] Some authorities believe that 4-hydroxytamoxifen may account for a substantial portion of the anti-estrogenic properties of tamoxifen.

Tamoxifen is both an estrogen agonist and an estrogen antagonist. The observed effects of tamoxifen are dependent on endogenous estradiol concentration and the specific organ or cell type being studied. For example, in hypoestrogenic states, tamoxifen can be shown to have estrogen agonist properties in the liver as demonstrated by increases in circulating high-density lipoprotein cholesterol and sex hormone–binding globulin.[129,130] In hypoestrogenic states, tamoxifen can be shown to increase progesterone receptors in the endometrium[131] and increase vaginal cornification,[132] both estrogen agonist effects. Finally, tamoxifen has been found to increase bone density in menopausal women.[133]

In contrast to these estrogen agonistic effects on the liver, bone, endometrium, and vaginal epithelium, tamoxifen

Estradiol

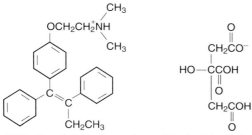

Clomiphene citrate

Tamoxifen citrate

Figure 10-8. Chemical structures of estradiol, clomiphene citrate, and tamoxifen citrate. Note the similarity in the structure of clomiphene, an agent used to induce ovulation, and tamoxifen, an anti-estrogen used in the treatment of breast cancer.

has estrogen antagonist effects in breast tumor cells. Tamoxifen blocks human breast tumor growth in immunodeficient mice.[133,134] Tamoxifen also blocks estradiol-stimulated DNA synthesis and transforming growth factor-β and EGF synthesis in breast cancer cells in vitro.[135,136]

As noted earlier, tamoxifen delays the time to first relapse and significantly increases overall survival in both premenopausal and postmenopausal women with breast cancer. In patients with node-negative, estrogen receptor–positive breast cancer, tamoxifen is as effective as chemotherapy in increasing survival and time to first relapse.[137] The current recommendation is for tamoxifen therapy for approximately 5 years. This recommendation is the result of more than 20 years of investigation.

Initially, investigators showed that 2 years of tamoxifen therapy was clearly better than placebo at extending disease-free and overall survival.[121] Comparative trials of tamoxifen therapy for 2 years versus 5 years demonstrated that 5 years of treatment resulted in longer disease-free intervals and better overall survival than did treatment for 2 years. In addition, second primary breast tumors were reduced by 50% in women treated for 5 years.[138]

Studies have also compared the effects of 5 years versus 10 years of tamoxifen treatment. Two studies suggested that 10 years of tamoxifen treatment is not associated with

shorter disease-free intervals than 5 years of treatment.[139] Consequently, the National Cancer Institute has recommended no more than 5 years of tamoxifen treatment.[139] Some experts have interpreted these findings to indicate that the estrogen antagonist tamoxifen may have agonistic properties in breast tumors with long-term use.[140]

A major advantage of tamoxifen therapy is that it has no major life-threatening effects and has a beneficial effect on the quality of life. It is important to contrast this record of safety and acceptability with that of polychemotherapy. Many authorities recommend that in patients with metastatic breast cancer, tamoxifen or another hormone treatment should be the first line of therapy if the tumor is hormone-responsive (estrogen receptor–positive). If the tumor is estrogen receptor–negative, then polychemotherapy should be used. The most common side effects of tamoxifen are nausea and vomiting, which occur in up to 20% of women. Vaginal bleeding, irregular menses, and rash are reported in fewer than 10% of women.

Tamoxifen clearly increases the risk of endometrial polyps and endometrial cancer. In one study of 4914 women participating in tamoxifen clinical trials, there was a sixfold increase in endometrial cancer and a threefold increase in gastrointestinal tract cancer in the women receiving tamoxifen.[141] In another study, there was an eightfold increase in the risk of endometrial cancer occurrence.[142] In this study, the rate of new endometrial cancer was 1.6 per 1000 woman-years in patients treated with tamoxifen versus 0.2 per 1000 woman-years in the placebo group.[142]

In addition, tamoxifen therapy is associated with a 1.9-fold increase in the risk of colon cancer and a threefold increase in the risk of stomach cancer. These studies suggest that the endometrium and gastrointestinal tract may be targets for tamoxifen-induced carcinogenesis. An international consensus conference concluded that tamoxifen should be labeled a potential carcinogenic agent.

Types of endometrial disease reported in women receiving tamoxifen include endometrial hyperplasia, polyps, endometrial cancer, clear cell cancer, and leiomyosarcoma.[143] These findings suggest that women receiving tamoxifen must be carefully monitored by a gynecologist. An aggressive clinical strategy is to perform office hysteroscopy and directed endometrial biopsy on a yearly basis for women receiving tamoxifen. This strategy is expensive, but provides high sensitivity and specificity in detecting endometrial abnormalities. Two less aggressive strategies are yearly sonography and hysterosonography, with biopsy as indicated. The least aggressive strategy is to perform only biopsy and hysteroscopy in women with genital bleeding.

Clinicians should exercise caution when prescribing tamoxifen to premenopausal women. Tamoxifen is an anti-estrogen in the central nervous and pituitary systems, which control GnRH and gonadotropin secretion. In normal ovulatory premenopausal women treated with tamoxifen, elevations in gonadotropin levels result in multifollicular development, multiple follicular ovulation, and elevated concentrations of estradiol and progesterone (Fig. 10-9).[144-146] In premenopausal women, long-term tamoxifen therapy can be associated with enlargement of the ovary due to multifollicular development and ovarian torsion. For premenopausal women, the combination of

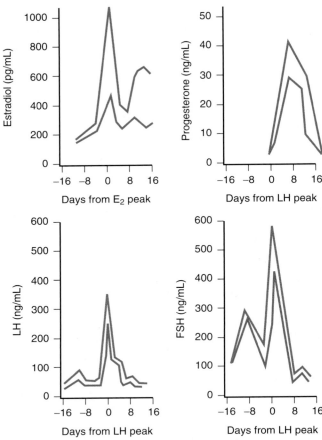

Figure 10-9. *The effects of tamoxifen treatment on luteinizing hormone (LH), follicle-stimulating hormone (FSH), estradiol (E₂), and progesterone levels in five normal premenopausal women during one baseline cycle (upper limit of response, green lines) and two tamoxifen treatment cycles (average response, purple lines). Treatment of premenopausal women with tamoxifen resulted in an increase in circulating estradiol and progesterone. No significant changes in circulating LH or FSH were detected in this small study. In premenopausal women, tamoxifen treatment probably results in multifollicular development. (Adapted from Sherman BM, Chapler FK, Crickard K. Endocrine consequences of continuous antiestrogen therapy with tamoxifen in premenopausal women. J Clin Invest 64:398-404, 1979. Reproduced by copyright permission from The American Society for Clinical Investigation.)*

tamoxifen plus a GnRH agonist analog may be superior to either agent alone in terms of tumor suppression and survival.[147,148]

Raloxifene is an estrogen receptor ligand that appears to act as an estrogen agonist in bone and liver and as an antagonist in breast and uterus.[149] In studies of women with osteoporosis, raloxifene clearly decreases the incidence of breast cancer. Unlike tamoxifen, raloxifene does not appear to be associated with the development of endometrial cancer.

Toremifene and fulvestrant are anti-estrogens that have been approved for the treatment of breast cancer. For the treatment of metastatic breast cancer, toremifene has efficacy and toxicity similar to those of tamoxifen.[150] Toremifene displays cross-resistance with tamoxifen. It should not be used in women with documented tamoxifen-resistance disease. Fulvestrant is an anti-estrogen that blocks estrogen receptor

function before coactivator binding. Theoretically, this agent should be especially effective in tamoxifen-resistant breast cancers.[151] In two studies of hormone treatment of women with tamoxifen-resistant breast cancer, both fulvestrant and anastrozole were similarly effective.[152]

Anti-progestins also appear to be effective in the treatment of breast cancer. The anti-progestin onapristone appears to be effective in the treatment of breast cancer and appears to have increased efficacy when it is combined with an anti-estrogen.[153]

AROMATASE INHIBITORS

The aromatase inhibitors, such as anastrozole, letrozole, and exemestane, appear to be as effective as or more effective than tamoxifen for the treatment of estrogen receptor–positive breast cancer in postmenopausal women. One study found that anastrozole was associated with a significantly longer time to disease progression than tamoxifen (11.1 months versus 5.6 months) in the treatment of postmenopausal women with newly diagnosed metastatic breast cancer.[154] Similarly, letrozole was found to be superior to tamoxifen for first-line hormonal treatment of postmenopausal women with advanced breast cancer with respect to overall response rate (30% versus 20%) and time to tumor progression (41 versus 26 weeks).[155,156]

In a recent trial (ATAC), 9366 postmenopausal women with breast cancer were randomized to receive tamoxifen (20 mg daily), anastrozole (1 mg daily), or a combination of the two. Anastrozole was associated with a 17% reduction in the risk of recurrence and a 58% decrease in the risk of contralateral breast cancer compared with tamoxifen. In addition, compared with anastrozole, tamoxifen was associated with a higher risk of deep venous thrombosis (8.1% versus 4.5%), endometrial cancer (0.5% versus 0.1%), and vaginal bleeding (8.1% versus 4.5%). Compared with tamoxifen, anastrozole was associated with an increased risk of osteoporotic fractures (5.8% versus 3.7%) and increased vasomotor symptoms and bone pain. Compared with tamoxifen, anastrozole was also associated with fewer endometrial abnormalities, such as endometrial polyps.[157]

Interestingly, the combination of anastrozole plus tamoxifen was inferior to anastrozole alone in reducing the risk of recurrence. This suggests that profound suppression of estrogen is required to treat breast cancer effectively and that the weak estrogen agonist activity of tamoxifen may contribute to the recurrence of breast cancer.[158] Aromatase inhibitors have become the first-line agent for adjuvant endocrine therapy in women with breast cancer. Most trials show that both anastrozole and letrozole are more effective than tamoxifen, with fewer side effects. A major disadvantage of the aromatase inhibitors is that they cause more osteoporotic fractures than tamoxifen. In the ATAC trial, osteoporotic fracture occurred in 7% of the women taking anastrozole and in 4% of those taking tamoxifen. Most women with breast cancer who are taking aromatase inhibitors are screened for osteoporosis and treated with calcium, vitamin D, and a bisphosphonate if the results of bone density testing show osteoporosis. A recent hypothesis suggesting that sequential use of tamoxifen followed by an aromatase inhibitor is especially effective in some women with breast cancer has not been supported by further analyses.[159]

PROPHYLACTIC MASTECTOMY AND PROPHYLACTIC SALPINGO-OOPHORECTOMY FOR WOMEN AT HIGH RISK OF BREAST AND OVARIAN CANCER

Women with *BRCA1* or *BRCA2* mutations are at high risk for breast and ovarian cancer. Recent studies have shown that in women at high risk, prophylactic mastectomy or oophorectomy reduces the risk of breast cancer and salpingo-oophorectomy reduces the risk of ovarian cancer.[160] In one study, 139 women with *BRCA1* or *BRCA2* mutations were offered prophylactic bilateral mastectomy or intensive diagnostic follow-up. Mastectomy was chosen by 76 women, whereas 63 chose diagnostic follow-up. During approximately 3 years of follow-up, none of the women in the mastectomy group and eight women in the surveillance group had breast cancer.[161] In a second study involving 639 women, prophylactic mastectomy was associated with an approximate 90% reduction in the incidence of breast cancer.[162] Currently, total (simple) mastectomy is recommended. The vast majority of women who underwent bilateral mastectomy were very pleased with their treatment choice.

Women with *BRCA1* mutations are at high risk for both breast and ovarian cancer. An alternative to mastectomy is the use of bilateral salpingo-oophorectomy, to attempt to reduce the risk of breast and ovarian cancer simultaneously.[163,164] In one study, bilateral salpingo-oophorectomy reduced the risk of ovarian cancer by 95% and the risk of breast cancer by 50%.[165] For women who choose this option, the bilateral salpingo-oophorectomy is typically performed after age 35 years or when childbearing is completed. In *BRCA1* carriers, histologic studies indicate that ovarian cancer actually begins in the fallopian tube as small microscopic areas of cancer.[166] These studies indicate that the distal portion of the fallopian tube must be removed to obtain maximal protection against ovarian cancer.

PREMENOPAUSAL OOPHORECTOMY: AN EFFECTIVE TREATMENT OF BREAST CANCER

In 1896, Beatson reported that oophorectomy was effective for the treatment of breast cancer.[167] Polychemotherapy for breast cancer is associated with many adverse effects, including nausea, vomiting, alopecia, myelosuppression, thrombophlebitis, and mucositis. For premenopausal women with estrogen receptor–positive breast cancer, oophorectomy has efficacy similar to that of polychemotherapy in the reduction of recurrence and mortality rates.

In one trial, 332 premenopausal women with node-positive breast cancer were randomized to receive either bilateral oophorectomy or polychemotherapy with cyclophosphamide, methotrexate, and 5-fluorouracil. After a maximum of 12 years of follow-up, there was no significant difference in disease-free survival or recurrence rates in the two groups. Actuarial survival at 8 years was 60%. Oophorectomy was associated with better survival than polychemotherapy in women with tumor estrogen–receptor concentrations greater than 20 fmol/mg protein (estrogen receptor–positive). Polychemotherapy was more effective than oophorectomy for women with tumors that were estrogen receptor–negative.[168] In another study, tamoxifen plus ovarian suppression (oophorectomy or GnRH agonist analogs) was as effective as six cycles of cyclophosphamide, methotrexate, and 5-fluorouracil in the treatment of early-stage estrogen receptor–positive breast cancer.[169]

A large clinical trial randomized 2144 women with breast cancer who were receiving tamoxifen (with or without chemotherapy) to receive either ovarian ablation (oophorectomy, ovarian radiation, or GnRH analog treatment) or no ovarian ablation. Ovarian ablation did not improve long-term outcomes, including relapse-free survival or overall survival rates. The study design was complicated by the fact that some of the women were given chemotherapy, which caused them to enter menopause. Ablating the ovaries in these women is unlikely to provide any endocrine benefit. However, the overall findings of the study suggest that adjuvant hormone therapy is a better first-line endocrine intervention than oophorectomy, except in patients with breast cancer who are at high risk for ovarian cancer.[170]

CHEMOTHERAPY-RELATED AMENORRHEA

The definition of chemotherapy-related amenorrhea varies by investigator, ranging from 3 to 12 months of amenorrhea in women undergoing chemotherapy who had menses within the 12 months preceding the initiation of chemotherapy.[171] A review of approximately 3000 premenopausal women receiving adjuvant chemotherapy for breast cancer showed a 70% rate of chemotherapy-related amenorrhea.[125] The rate of chemotherapy-induced amenorrhea was 40% for women younger than 40 years of age and 70% for women older than 40 years for cyclophosphamide, methotrexate, and 5-fluorouracil–based regimens.[171]

The interval between the initiation of chemotherapy and the cessation of menses was dependent on the age of the women treated. For women younger than 40 years, the onset of cessation of menses ranged from 6 to 16 months after the initiation of chemotherapy. For women older than 40 years, the cessation of menses occurred 2 to 4 months after the initiation of chemotherapy. Alkylating agents, such as cyclophosphamide, melphalan, and thiotepa, are the agents most likely to cause ovarian dysfunction and depletion of the oocyte pool. The antimetabolites, such as methotrexate and 5-fluorouracil, are less likely to cause ovarian dysfunction.

There is a relationship between the dose of cyclophosphamide and the rate of chemotherapy-related amenorrhea. For women who received a cumulative dose of cyclophosphamide in the range of 400 mg/m^2, the rate of chemotherapy-related amenorrhea was 10% to 30%, depending on the age of the woman. At cumulative cyclophosphamide doses in the range of 8000 mg/m^2, the rate of amenorrhea was 60% and 95% in younger and older age groups, respectively.[172]

Many women with chemotherapy-related amenorrhea have elevated follicle-stimulating hormone levels.

Curiously, a significant number of women with breast cancer and chemotherapy-related amenorrhea resume menses 6 to 24 months after completing chemotherapy.[173] Approximately 50% of women younger than 40 years resume menses, whereas only approximately 10% of women older than 40 years resume menses. Interestingly, recurrence of breast cancer appears to be somewhat more common in women who resume menses after adjuvant chemotherapy.[173] Premenopausal women who become amenorrheic after chemotherapy appear to have a better long-term prognosis.[174]

Hormone Replacement Therapy in Survivors of Breast Cancer

Many breast cancers are estrogen receptor–positive. Some authorities believe that a goal of breast cancer treatment is to minimize the exposure of these tumors to estrogen. However, the hypoestrogenic state is associated with significant and often disabling symptoms, such as hot flashes, sleep disturbance, and urogenital discomfort. The decision to treat a survivor of breast cancer with estrogen is an exceedingly complex one. It involves weighing the risk of tumor recurrence and progression against the benefits of symptom treatment. Observational studies reported that the risk of hormone therapy in postmenopausal women with breast cancer was minimal or modest. Recent clinical trials reported adverse effects of hormone therapy in women with breast cancer.

In a review of four observational studies, 214 women with breast cancer and a mean disease-free interval of 52 months were given hormone therapy. Among these women, 4.2% had a recurrence compared with 5.4% in a group of matched controls.[175] Similar results were reported in another observational study.[176]

In one clinical trial, 434 women with breast cancer were randomly assigned to receive 2 years of hormone therapy (estrogen alone in women with a hysterectomy and estrogen–progestin in women with an intact uterus) versus nonhormonal treatment.[177] After a median follow-up of 2 years, 26 women in the hormone therapy group and 7 in the nonhormone group had a breast cancer recurrence, yielding a relative risk of 3.5 (95% CI, 1.5 to 8.1) in the hormone-treated women. The study was stopped because of the statistically significant increased risk. Most oncologists prefer that women with breast cancer not receive hormone therapy.[178]

Pregnancy in Survivors of Breast Cancer

No randomized clinical trials are available concerning the effects of pregnancy on breast cancer. A limited number of case series have been published.[179-183] These studies reported that pregnancy does not have an adverse effect on women who have survived breast cancer. For example, Von Schoultz and coworkers[184] observed 50 women who became pregnant after treatment for breast cancer. Eight percent of the women who became pregnant after breast cancer treatment had metastatic disease. In a cohort of comparable women who did not become pregnant, 24% had metastatic disease. In most reports, women with breast cancer were advised to wait 2 to 3 years before becoming pregnant. Adherence to this advice will prevent pregnancy in women who are destined to have a recurrence shortly after primary treatment. Women with the most rapid recurrences after primary treatment are at the highest risk for death as a result of breast cancer.

For women, one of the most feared diseases is breast cancer. A popular perception is that women would rather die 10 times of heart disease than once of breast cancer. Genetic predisposition and endocrine exposure are dominant factors in the etiology of breast cancer. Both the geneticist and the reproductive endocrinologist will play major roles in developing strategies to cure this devastating disease.

The complete reference list can be found on the companion Expert Consult Web site at www.expertconsultbook.com.

Suggested Readings

Abe O, Abe R, Enomoto K, et al. Effects of chemotherapy and hormonal therapy for early breast cancer on recurrence and 15-year survival. Lancet 365:1687-1717, 2005.

Cuzick J. Aromatase inhibitors for breast cancer prevention. J Clin Oncol 23:1636-1643, 2005.

Dorgan JF, Longcope C, Franz C, et al. Endogenous sex hormones and breast cancer in postmenopausal women: reanalysis of nine prospective studies. J Natl Cancer Inst 94:606-616, 2002.

Guray M, Sahin AA. Benign breast diseases: classification, diagnosis and management. Oncologist 11:435-449, 2006.

Hankinson SE, Eliassen AH. Endogenous estrogen, testosterone and progesterone levels in relation to breast cancer risk. J Steroid Biochem Mol Biol 106:24-30, 2007.

Stuebe AM, Rich-Edwards JW, Willett WC, et al. Duration of lactation and incidence of type 2 diabetes. JAMA 294:2601-2610, 2005.

Winer EP, Hudis C, Burstein HJ, et al. American Society of Clinical Oncology Technology Assessment on the use of aromatase inhibitors. J Clin Oncol 23:619-629, 2005.

CHAPTER 11

The Endocrinology of Human Pregnancy and Fetoplacental Neuroendocrine Development

Sam Mesiano

The birth of a healthy baby is dependent on an ordered sequence of biologic events during pregnancy. Important among these events are

1. Successful implantation of the developing embryo
2. Adaptation of maternal physiology to accept the fetal allograft and satisfy its nutritional, metabolic, and physical demands
3. Appropriate growth and functional development of fetal neuroendocrine systems
4. Proper timing of birth so that it occurs when the fetus is mature enough to survive outside the uterus

The hormonal interactions between the fetus/placenta and mother that control the establishment and progression of pregnancy, fetal development, and the process of parturition are discussed in this chapter.

The chapter begins with a brief review of the hormonal events that control endometrial growth and function during the menstrual cycle so that it becomes receptive to blactocyst implantation and the establishment of pregnancy. This discussion includes the processes of implantation, placental development, and the mechanism by which the fetal allograft subverts the maternal immune system.

Once pregnancy is established, the fetus, placenta, and mother initiate and maintain communication by means of the endocrine system. The endocrine milieu of human pregnancy is dominated by placental hormones, the major function of which is to modify maternal physiology to satisfy the nutritional and physical demands of the growing fetus. In this context, the physiologic role of the principal placental hormones is discussed.

The fetal neuroendocrine system must become functionally competent by term so that the neonate can maintain homeostasis after birth. The developmental program of the fetal neuroendocrine system is therefore discussed separately.

Finally, the endocrine interactions between the fetus, placenta and mother that culminate in the induction of parturition are discussed. The appropriate timing of birth, so that it occurs when the fetus is sufficiently mature to survive as a newborn, is a major determinant of postnatal survival. This section addresses current understanding of the hormonal interactions that control the process and timing of human parturition.

Establishment of Pregnancy

ENDOMETRIAL RECEPTIVITY

During the menstrual cycle, the ovarian steroid hormones, estrogen and progesterone, induce structural and functional changes in the endometrium essential for implantation and the establishment of pregnancy (see Chapter 9). During the luteal phase and under the influence primarily of progesterone, the proliferative endometrium is converted to a secretory phenotype; it becomes thick (5 to 6 mm), spongy, and well vascularized with the development of specialized spiral arterioles. In addition, the glandular epithelium produce a variety of chemokines, growth factors, and cell adhesion molecules (CAMs) that provide a favorable intrauterine environment for embryo survival. The expression of chemokines and CAMs attract the blastocyst to specific docking sites for implantation and increased vascularization and development of spiral arterioles within the endometrial stroma provide an optimal substrate for invasion and placentation.

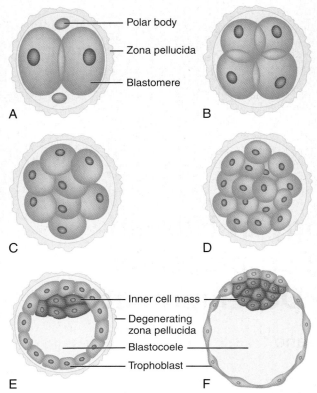

Figure 11-1. *Cleavage of the zygote and formation of the blastocyst. A to D, Various stages of cell division. E, Formation of the blastocoele. F, Fully formed blastocyst. (From Jones RE. Human Reproductive Biology. San Diego, Academic Press, 1997, p 186.)*

The receptivity of the endometrium to embryonic implantation has temporal and spatial characteristics. In humans, implantation between days 20 and 24 of the menstrual cycle is associated with a high (85%) success rate for continuing pregnancy, whereas implantation after day 25 has a low success rate (11%).[1]

During days 20 to 24, the endometrial epithelium develops dome-like structures known as pinopodes, which correlate with implantation sites.[2] The tips of the pinopodes appear to be the preferred site for embryo adherence and express chemokines and CAMs that attract the embryo. Interestingly, areas between the pinopodes express a repellent molecule, MUC-1, that prevents embryo adhesion.[3] Analysis of the transcriptosome of the human endometrium during the implantation window using microarray technology has revealed numerous genes that are up- and down-regulated in comparison with late proliferative phase endometrium,[4] demonstrating the remarkable complexity of molecular interactions underlying endometrial differentiation.

A complex array of growth factors, cytokines, and transcription factors produced within the endometrium mediate the qualitative and quantitative responses to ovarian steroid.[5] For example, the homeobox gene, *HOXA10*, is an important regulator of endometrial differentiation[6,7] and its expression is essential for steroid hormone-induced differentiation and the establishment of a receptive phenotype.[8] Endometrial expression of *HOXA10* increases

during the midsecretory phase of the menstrual cycle, corresponding to the time of implantation and increase in circulating progesterone.[9]

IMPLANTATION

After fertilization, the embryo undergoes an intrinsic developmental program. The sequence of cell divisions and differentiation is not dependent on the hormonal milieu of the fallopian tube or the uterus, as fertilization and early embryonic development occur successfully in vitro. By the third to fourth day after fertilization, the embryo comprises a solid ball of cells encapsulated by the translucent remnant of the zona pellucida. At about the fourth or fifth day after fertilization, a fluid-filled cavity, the blastocele, forms within the embryo. At this stage the embryo is referred to as a blastocyst. The outer layer of blastocyst cells adjacent to the zona pellucida is known as the trophectoderm. These cells eventually give rise to the placenta and chorion. The fetus, amnion, and mesenchymal and vascular components of the placenta are derived from the inner cell mass, a group of cells lying under the trophectoderm at one end of the blastocele (Fig. 11-1).

Although there is considerable variation in the process of implantation between eutherian mammals, the end result is the same: the blastocyst becomes fixed in position and forms a physical and functional contact with the uterus (Fig. 11-2).

In humans, the blastocyst enters the uterus at around the fifth day after fertilization and floats freely for 2 to 3 days. By this stage, the embryo has "hatched" from the zona pellucida and is in an optimal condition to implant. The developing blastocyst interacts in a paracrine manner with the endometrial epithelium by producing multiple cytokines, chemokines, and CAMs that facilitate adherence. Almost immediately after fertilization hormonal signals from the conceptus are transmitted to the mother. A platelet activating factor–like substance produced by the ovum soon after fertilization is one of the earliest factors produced by the conceptus in high enough amounts to be detected in the maternal circulation.[10] During its journey through the fallopian tube the cumulus cells surrounding the conceptus produces progesterone and estrogen. These steroids are thought to act locally to modulate tubal motility to facilitate transport of the conceptus toward the uterine cavity.[11]

Any delay in embryo development or in its transit through the oviduct will disrupt the synchrony between the blastocyst development and endometrial receptivity and increase the likelihood of reproductive failure. Thus, development of the "seed" and conditioning of the "soil" are synchronized. Given this delicate balance, it is not surprising that the highest rate of embryo loss occurs during the peri-implantation period.

The embryo implants in a polarized fashion such that trophoblast cells overlying the embryonic pole are the first to interact with the uterine epithelium (see Fig. 11-2). After hatching from the zona pellucida the trophectoderm cells overlying the embryonic pole become adhesive and dock with specific sites in the epithelial lining of the endometrium, most likely at the pinopodes. The trophoblast

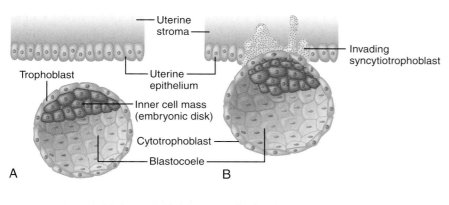

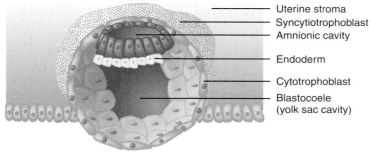

Figure 11-2. *Implantation of the human embryo.* **A,** *Floating blastocyst.* **B,** *Attachment to the uterine epithelium and initial invasion of the syncytiotrophoblast cells.* **C,** *The blastocyst penetrates deeper into the uterine stroma and develops an amniotic cavity.* **D,** *The fully implanted embryo invades the maternal vasculature and the uterine epithelium grows over the implantation site and undergoes the decidualization. (From Jones RE. Human Reproductive Biology. San Diego, Academic Press, 1997, p 189.)*

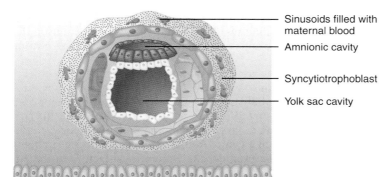

cells aggregate and fuse their plasma membranes to become a single multinucleated cell know as the syncytiotrophoblast, which becomes the leading edge of implantation. The syncytiotrophoblast secretes proteases that degrade the endometrial extracellular matrix forming a path for the blastocyst to infiltrate the uterine stroma. The blastocyst then penetrates into the endometrium and becomes completely surrounded by the endometrial stroma. The embryo then embarks on a remarkable invasion into the uterine wall.

Implantation involves a complex paracrine dialogue between the embryo and the endometrium/decidua. Many of the molecules (produced by the endometrial cells and/or the blastocyst) involved in the implantation process have been identified.[12-14] These substances include the following:

- Leukemia inhibiting factor (LIF)
- Interleukin 11 (IL-11)
- Heparin-binding epidermal growth factor (HB-EGF)
- Prostacyclin (PGI_2)
- Prostaglandin E_2 (PGE_2)
- Peroxisome-proliferator-activator receptor (PPARδ)
- Products of the *HOXA10* and *HOXA11* genes
- Metalloproteinase-2 and -9 (MMP-2 and MMP-9)
- Basic and acidic fibroblast growth factor
- Bone morphogenetic proteins (BMPs) and the BMP antagonist Noggin
- Wnt and Indian Hedgehog signaling molecules (see Chapter 9)

DECIDUALIZATION OF THE ENDOMETRIUM

Late in the luteal phase the endometrial stroma undergoes a series of morphologic and functional changes collectively referred to as decidualization. The process of decidualization is dependent on progesterone and occurs independently of conception and implantation. It initiates around blood vessels during the midsecretory phase and progressively encompasses the entire endometrial stroma during the latter part of the secretory phase. The fully decidualized endometrial stroma is composed of large polyhedral cells, containing high levels of glycogen and lipids that secrete a tough pericellular capsule composed of collagen, laminin, fibronectin, and heparan sulfate proteoglycan. There also is an accumulation of bone marrow–derived immune cells, primarily large granular lymphocytes (LGLs), and formation of extensive cell-cell contacts between the lymphocytes and the stromal cells, especially in the vicinity of blood vessels.[15]

The decidualized endometrium is hostile to implantation. Therefore, the blastocyst has a limited window of opportunity to establish a successful implantation before the decidual barrier is established. Attachment of the blastocyst to the uterine epithelium accelerates the decidualization process further limiting the window of opportunity for implantation. In an infertile cycle menstruation occurs to eliminate the nonreceptive decidualized endometrium. The endometrium is renewed to a receptive state in the subsequent cycle. Thus, the term decidua is highly appropriate because this tissue is cast off at menstruation, miscarriage, and delivery.

The decidua is thought to form a critical barrier between the mother and the conceptus and represent an attempt by the mother to restrict blastocyst invasion. The large component of immune cells (mainly LGLs) within the decidual tissue may also restrict the passage of fetal antigens to the maternal compartment.[16] Interestingly, decidualization of the endometrium appears limited to species with interstitial implantation in which the blastocyst is completely imbedded in the endometrial stroma, further supporting the argument that it limits the invasiveness of the blastocyst during implantation.

Once pregnancy is established the decidua can be divided into three types, depending upon anatomic location: (1) the decidua basalis, which underlies the site of implantation and forms the maternal component of the placenta; (2) the decidua capsularis, which overlies the gestational sac (this portion disappears in the later stages of pregnancy); and (3) the decidua vera, which lines the remainder of the uterine cavity and becomes intimately approximated to the chorion.

The decidua of pregnancy is associated with the fetal membranes and is considered to be an endocrine organ.[17] Hormones produced by the decidua can act on the adjacent tissue (chorion and myometrium) or communicate with the fetus by means of the amniotic fluid. The decidua produces prolactin,[18-20] relaxin,[21] and prostaglandins[22,23] that are thought to be involved in the process of parturition. Its close proximity to the myometrium is ideal in this regard.

PLACENTATION

Early in the implantation process some trophoblast cells aggregate and form migrating columns, which penetrate into the inner third of the myometrium. The invading trophoblasts target maternal blood vessels and, via interstitial and endovascular routes, completely surround and plug spiral arterioles. They then displace maternal endothelial cells and musculoelastic tissue and effectively create a low-resistance arteriolar system by increasing vessel diameter.

According to Poiseuille's law of fluid dynamics, flow through a cylinder is proportional to the radius multiplied to the fourth power. On average, the radii of arterioles in the pregnant human uterus are around 10-fold greater than in the nonpregnant state. Such a change would increase flow 10,000-fold, ample to serve the future requirements of the growing fetus. Moreover, the trophoblasts that occupy the vasculature sites prevent maternal vasomotor control of uterine blood flow and therefore eliminate maternal control of the placental blood supply.[24]

Placentation across all eutherian mammals is characterized by high angiogenic activity and blood vessel growth. This is particularly the case for the site of placental attachment. To this end, the human placenta produces several known angiogenic factors, including platelet-derived endothelial cell growth factor, vascular endothelial growth factor (VEGF), angiopoietin-1, and angiopoietin-2.[25,26] In addition, two potent inhibitors of angiogenesis have been isolated from mouse placenta.[27] The specific interplay between angiogenic factors and their inhibitors in the placenta is not well understood. However, it is possible that the presence of anti-angiogenic factors within the placenta may serve to control vessel growth. This may be important for preventing maternal endothelial cells from resealing the ends of spiral arterioles that have been occupied by trophoblasts. In addition, anti-angiogenic factors may prevent the overgrowth of maternal and fetal vessels, thereby precluding maternal blood vessels from entering the fetal compartment and fetal vessels from growing out into the uterus.[28]

The extent and depth of the placental incursion appears to be the sum of the intrinsic pro-invasive characteristics of trophoblasts and the physical and biochemical barriers mounted by the decidua. Imbalances in this equation can lead to failed implantation and pathologic conditions. The angiogenic events occurring during implantation and placentation likely are critical factors in the etiology of hemodynamic disorders in pregnancy. For example, in preeclampsia, cytotrophoblast invasion is restricted to the superficial decidual segments, leaving the myometrial spiral arterioles undisturbed and still responsive to maternal vasomotor influences.[29] These pathologic changes result in shallow implantation and impaired blood supply to the placental unit, which then attempts to compensate by increasing maternal systemic blood pressure, leading to preeclampsia.

Because trophoblasts are genetically distinct from maternal tissue, implantation represents an extraordinary breach of maternal immune defenses. The mother must distinguish between the fetal allograft as being immunogenically foreign or self and the placental trophoblasts must protect themselves from immune destruction by activated T cells. The decidua is composed mainly of a uterus-specific subset of LGLs with a natural killer (NK) cell phenotype.[15,16] NK cells preferentially attack targets that lack polymorphic class I or class II HLA antigens. Trophoblasts do not express polymorphic class I or class II HLA antigens and therefore are highly susceptible to attack by decidual NK cells.[30] However, differentiated cytotrophoblasts that lie at the maternal/fetal interface produce HLA-G, a unique MHC (major histocompatibility complex) class I molecule.[31] Because of its reduced polymorphism, HLA-G is less immunogenic and could prevent immunologic recognition by activated T cells and NK cells. In addition, trophoblasts express the Fas ligand, which induces apoptosis in immune cells that carry the Fas receptor.[32] Thus, the fetal allograft may escape immune attack by presenting the unique HLA-G camouflage or by actively subverting immune recognition by means of the Fas ligand.

The functional unit of the human placenta is the chorionic villus, which is formed by a sprouting of syncytiotrophoblasts that project into the intervillous space, a pool of maternal blood surrounding the blastocyst. The finger-like chorionic villi have a central core of loose connective tissue with an extensive capillary network linking it with the fetal circulation. Surrounding the core are the inner syncytiotrophoblast and outer cytotrophoblast cells that form the functional barrier between the maternal and fetal circulations. This arrangement is referred to as a hemochorial placentation because the syncytiotrophoblast layer separates the maternal and fetal circulations.

The Endocrine Placenta

Placental hormones dominate the endocrine milieu of human pregnancy. This remarkable organ not only provides the conduit for alimentation, gas exchange, and excretion for the fetus, it also is a major endocrine organ, producing a plethora of protein (including cytokines and growth factors) and steroid hormones, which it secretes in large quantities primarily into the maternal circulation (Table 11-1).

Most hormones produced by the placenta are counterparts to those produced in the nonpregnant adult. In particular, the human placenta simulates a hypothalamic-pituitary axis; it produces and responds to functional cohorts of hypothalamic and pituitary hormones.[33,34]

As placental hormones can bind to maternal hormone receptors, they can be regarded as allocrine factors, that is, hormones produced by one organism (the fetus) to act on the receptors of another (the mother). In general, placental hormones modify maternal homeostatic mechanisms to meet the nutritional, metabolic, and physical demands of the rapidly growing fetus. Maternal targets cannot discriminate between hormones of placental or maternal origin and as such, placental hormones can readily influence maternal physiology. Thus, the placenta represents a secondary neuroendocrine control center that tends to override the maternal system in favor of maintaining the pregnant state and adjusting maternal homeostasis to support the developing fetus.

Most placental hormones are secreted in large amounts into the maternal circulation. The hemochorial anatomic arrangement of the human placenta is ideal for this purpose. Cyto- and syncytiotrophoblast cells of the placenta have direct access to the maternal circulation. In contrast, the trophoblast layer prevents most maternal hormones from entering the fetal compartment, and consequently the fetal/placental endocrine system generally develops and functions independently of that of the mother. The roles of some of the principal placental hormones in the endocrine control of human pregnancy are discussed in the following section.

TABLE 11-1

Peptides, Steroid Hormones, and Monoamines Produced by the Human Placenta

Neuropeptides	Pituitary-like Hormones	Steroid Hormones	Monoamines and Adrenal-like Peptides
CRH	ACTH	Progesterone	Epinephrine
TRH	TSH	Estradiol	Norepinephrine
GnRH	GH	Estrone	Dopamine
Melatonin	PL	Estriol	Serotonin
Cholecystokinin	CG	Estetrol	Adrenomedullin
Met-enkephalin	LH	2-Methoxyestradiol	
Dynorphin	FSH	Allopregnanolone	
Neurotensin	β-Endorphin	Pregnenolone	
VIP	Prolactin	5α-Dihydroprogesterone	
Galanin	Oxytocin		
Somatostatin	Leptin		
CGRP	Activin		
Neuropeptide Y	Follistatin		
Substance P	Inhibin		
Endothelin			
ANP			
Renin			
Angiotensin			
Urocortin			

ACTH, adrenocorticotropic hormone (corticotropin); ANP, atrial natriuretic peptide; CG, chorionic gonadotropin; CGRP, calcitonin gene-related peptide; CRH, corticotropin-releasing hormone; FSH, follicle-stimulating hormone; GH, growth hormone; LH, luteinizing hormone; PL, placental lactogen, TRH, thyrotropin-releasing hormone; TSH, thyroid-stimulating hormone; VIP, vasoactive intestinal peptide.
From Reis FM, Petraglia F. The placenta as a neuroendocrine organ. Front Horm Res 27:216, 2001.

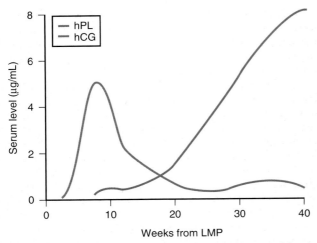

Figure 11-3. Schematic representation of concentrations of human chorionic gonadotropin (hCG) and placental lactogen (hPL) throughout gestation. Note differences in the magnitude of the concentrations of the two hormones in early and late gestation. LMP, last menstrual period.

PLACENTAL GONADOTROPIN

Progesterone is essential for endometrial differentiation and the establishment of pregnancy and is produced exclusively by the corpus luteum (CL) during initial weeks of pregnancy. In nonconceptive cycles, the CL usually regresses at about the second week after ovulation and the subsequent decline in progesterone leads to menstruation. For pregnancy to establish, the demise of the CL and the associated withdrawal of progesterone must be prevented. Thus, one of the first endocrine interactions between the conceptus and the mother involves signaling by the early embryo that pregnancy is occurring and that the functional life span of the CL must be extended. This event is referred to as the maternal recognition of pregnancy and is mediated by chorionic gonadotropin (CG) produced by the trophoblast cells.

During the first 5 to 7 weeks of pregnancy progesterone is produced exclusively by the CL in response to CG. Consequently, the ovaries are obligate organs for pregnancy maintenance during this time, and abortion rapidly ensues if they are removed. However, after weeks 6 to 7 of pregnancy the placenta begins producing large amounts of progesterone and at around the same time progesterone production by the CL decreases. This transition in the source of progesterone is referred to as the luteal-placental shift. Consequently, removal of the ovaries after the ninth week has no impact on pregnancy.[35] The placenta supplies progesterone for the remainder of pregnancy.

Chorionic Gonadotropin

Human chorionic gonadotropin (hCG) is a 36- to 40-kDa glycoprotein hormone that is biologically and immunologically similar to pituitary luteinizing hormone (LH). It is produced by trophoblasts almost immediately after implantation.[36] As with LH and follicle-stimulating hormone (FSH), hCG is a heterodimer composed of an α and β subunit. The α subunits of hCG, LH, and FSH are identical, whereas the β subunits differ, conferring specificity to each hormone.

Like LH, hCG is a potent luteotropin, and as such, it stimulates progesterone secretion by the CL. Importantly, hCG prolongs the functional life of the CL and converts the CL of the menstrual cycle into the CL of pregnancy, ensuring the production of progesterone necessary for the establishment of pregnancy. In an evolutionary context, this role may provide a basis for selection, as pregnancy will not ensue if the embryo is defective and cannot gain control of the CL. The capacity of the embryo to produce large amounts of hCG may represent a selective test of the embryo's endocrine competence. Furthermore, the maternal level of resistance to the embryo's efforts to control the CL would select embryos with more robust endocrine function.[37]

In normal pregnancies, hCG is detectable 9 to 11 days after the midcycle LH peak, which is around 8 days after ovulation and only 1 day after implantation.[36] Therefore, pregnancy can be detected before the first missed menstrual period. This has clinical utility when it is important to determine the presence of pregnancy at an early stage. In early pregnancy, there is an approximate doubling of levels every 2 to 3 days and concentrations of hCG rise to peak values by 60 to 90 days of gestation. Thereafter, hCG levels decrease to a plateau that persists during the remainder of the pregnancy (Fig. 11-3). Maternal immunoassayable LH and FSH levels are virtually undetectable throughout pregnancy.

Other Actions of Chorionic Gonadotropin

The actions of hCG may not be limited to maintaining progesterone production. Much of the increased thyroid activity that occurs in pregnancy has been attributed to hCG,[38,39] which binds specifically to thyroid gland membranes and displaces thyroid-stimulating hormone (TSH).[39-41] hCG also influences the development and function of the fetal adrenals and testes[42-44] (discussed subsequently). In addition, hCG may have actions on the maternal reproductive tract, including the decidual response, relaxin production by the CL, and relaxation of uterine smooth muscle.[45,46] hCG receptors have been detected on myometrial cells,[47] and in vitro hCG directly relaxes human myometrial strips.[48] These effects are mediated by a decrease in gap junction formation, a reduction in intracellular calcium levels, and increased phosphodiesterase activity.[49]

Production of hCG by the invading blastocyst may contribute in a paracrine manner to the implantation process. In vitro and in vivo studies in nonhuman primates demonstrate that CG can promote decidualization of the endometrial stroma.[50,51] The hormone appears to have marked effects on the endometrial physiology at the implantation site before its levels are detectable in the circulation. Studies suggest that CG produced by the blastocyst prolongs the window of implantation by inhibiting endometrial insulin-like growth factor binding protein (IGFBP-1) production, augmenting angiogenesis at the implantation site by increasing VEGF expression, modulating local cytokine and chemokine expression, augmenting local protease activity, and by means of an autocrine effects on the trophoblasts themselves, promoting differentiation and augmenting invasive potential.[46]

The placenta may not be the only source of hCG. The fetal kidney and fetal pituitary gland synthesize and secrete biologically active hCG.[44,52-55] It is possible that the finding of hCG in some adult nontrophoblastic tumors represents an atavistic reversion to a fetal form of hormone synthesis.

Placental trophoblasts may have an autoregulatory mechanism for hCG synthesis that involves intrinsic hormonal axes analogous to those operating in the hypothalamic-pituitary-gonadal (HPG) axis. Regulators of pituitary gonadotropin can also influence placental hCG production (at least in vitro). These regulators include progesterone, inhibin, activin, and gonadotropin-releasing hormone (GnRH).

Gonadotropin-Releasing Hormone

The human placenta produces gonadotropin-releasing hormone (GnRH), which is identical to that produced by the hypothalamus.[56,57] Levels of GnRH in the circulation of pregnant women are highest in the first trimester and correlate closely with hCG levels.[58] The close relation between GnRH and hCG suggests a role for GnRH in regulating hCG production. GnRH stimulates the production of both the α and β subunits of hCG in placental explants and specific GnRH-binding sites are present in the human placenta.[59] Thus, there appears to be autoregulation of hCG production within the placenta.

hCG also may influence placental steroidogenesis, suggesting a complete internal regulatory system within the placenta. This concept is further strengthened by the presence of other regulators of GnRH expression, including inhibins and activins, in the human placenta.

Inhibins and Activins

Inhibin is a heterodimer composed of an α subunit and one of two β subunits, βA or βB. Inhibins (αβA and αβB) derive their name from their ability to preferentially inhibit pituitary FSH secretion. In contrast to inhibins, the homodimers βA βA and βB βB stimulate FSH production. These compounds have been termed activins.

Inhibins are produced by the human placenta; all three subunits are expressed in the syncytiotrophoblast and the levels of expression do not change with advancing gestation.[60-62] Activin-A is also produced by the corpus luteum, decidua, and fetal membranes during human pregnancy.[63] The placenta also produces follistatin, the binding protein for activin. These factors are secreted into the maternal and fetal circulations and amniotic fluid and their production varies with stage of gestation.[64]

Although the exact function of the inhibin/activin system in human pregnancy is not known, several studies indicate their involvement in the pathogenesis of gestational diseases. Levels of inhibin-A and activin-A in the maternal circulation can be indicative, albeit with relatively weak predictive value, of disorders such as placental tumors, hypertensive disorders of pregnancy, intrauterine growth restriction, fetal hypoxia, Down syndrome, fetal demise, preterm delivery, and intrauterine growth restriction.[65]

In cultured human placental cells, production of inhibin is stimulated by hCG, vasoactive intestinal peptide and neuropeptide Y (NPY), analogs of cAMP, and adenylate cyclase activators.[61,66] Because inhibin and activin are synthesized in the cytotrophoblast,[66] they may be involved in autoregulating placental hCG production by modulating local GnRH activity. In vitro studies have shown that inhibin decreases GnRH-stimulated hCG production by placental cell cultures,[67] whereas inhibin antiserum increases GnRH release and causes a parallel rise in hCG secretion. Further, this effect of blocking endogenous inhibin action is reduced by the addition of a GnRH antagonist, pointing to an interaction of endogenous inhibin and GnRH on hCG secretion.[68] Therefore, it is possible that inhibin exerts an autocrine or paracrine effect on hCG secretion by suppressing GnRH action. In contrast, activin augments the GnRH-induced release of hCG in cultured trophoblast cells, an effect that can be reduced by the addition of inhibin.[67] Thus, at least in vitro, activin and inhibin, by means of their paracrine effect on placental GnRH production, contribute to the regulation of hCG secretion.

PLACENTAL SOMATOTROPINS

In most eutherian mammals, the placenta expresses and secretes members of the growth hormone (GH)/placental lactogen (PL) gene family.[69] These genes are encoded by a 66 kb segment of chromosome 17q22-q24. This locus includes five closely related genes: *GH1*, *GH2*, *CSH1*, *CSH2*, and *CSHL1*, each derived from the duplication of a common ancestral gene. The *GH1* gene encodes pituitary GH and is expressed only in the pituitary. The other four are expressed exclusively in the placenta. The *GH2* gene encodes a placental GH variant, which differs from human pituitary GH at 13 amino acids. The *CSH1* and *CSH2* genes are identical and encode human placental lactogen (hPL). The *CSHL1* gene has a high degree of homology with *CSH1* and *CSH2*; however, it is considered a pseudogene due to a G to A transversion at the second intron splice site.

Historical Perspective on Nomenclature

In 1961, Ito and Higashi[70] described a substance in the placenta with mammotropic activity. The following year, Josimovich and MacLaren[71] demonstrated that this material had immunologic similarity with hGH. Because of its lactogenic actions in the pigeon crop sac assay and its ability to promote milk production in rabbits, they named the substance placental lactogen.

Thereafter, many investigators explored the physiology and pathophysiology of PL and it was soon realized that it also has somatotropic actions. The existence of a placental GH variant was unknown when many of the early studies of PL action were performed. In fact, there was much debate as to whether the material identified as PL was more like GH than prolactin. The term placental lactogen was therefore considered inadequate by many investigators, and other designations were proposed. These terms included chorionic growth hormone-prolactin, purified placental protein, and human chorionic somatomammotropin (hCS). Presently, the term PL has attained common usage, and will be used herein to refer to the product of the *CSH1* and *CSH2* genes, even though these genes are assigned the chorionic somatomammotropin acronym. The product of the *GH2* gene will be referred to as human placental growth hormone (hPGH).

Human Placental Lactogen

hPL is a single-chain polypeptide of 191 amino acids with two disulfide bridges and has a 96% homology with hGH. It can be detected in the placenta from around day 18 of pregnancy and in the maternal circulation by the third week of pregnancy. Low levels of hPL (7 to 10 ng/mL) are present in the maternal circulation by 20 to 40 days of gestation. Thereafter, hPL levels in the maternal circulation increase exponentially, reaching levels of 5 to 10 µg/mL at term.[72]

In contrast to the elevated levels of hPL in the maternal circulation, concentrations of hPL in the fetal circulation range from 4 to 500 ng/mL at midgestation and only 20 to 30 ng/mL at term.[73] This indicates that hPL is preferentially secreted into the maternal compartment. The concentration of hPL in maternal peripheral blood is about 300 times that in umbilical vein blood, and the concentration of hPL in the blood leaving the gravid uterus is markedly greater than that in the peripheral circulation.

hPL is detectable in the serum and urine in both normal and molar pregnancies, and it disappears rapidly from the serum and urine after delivery of the placenta; it cannot be detected after the first postpartum day. After removal of the placenta, the half-life of the disappearance of circulating hPL is 9 to 15 minutes. To maintain circulating concentrations, this would imply placental production of between 1 and 4 g of the hormone per day at term.[74] This remarkable rate of gene expression is reflected by the observation at term 5% of the total mRNA in the placenta encodes hPL.[75] Therefore, production of hPL represents one of the major metabolic and biosynthetic activities of the syncytiotrophoblast.

In normal pregnancy, hPL is first synthesized by the cytotrophoblasts of the developing placenta up to 6 weeks. Thereafter, expression switches to the syncytiotrophoblasts, which eventually become the exclusive source of hPL. The extent of hPL expression by syncytiotrophoblasts does not change during the course of pregnancy, although total placental production increases substantially.[76] Therefore, the rise in hPL production is thought to be due to the increase in placental mass, as circulating maternal hPL levels rises concordantly with the amount of syncytiotrophoblast tissue as gestation progresses[77] (Fig. 11-4). Like hCG, hPL appears to be expressed by all types of trophoblastic tissue; it has been found in the urine of patients harboring trophoblastic tumors and in men with choriocarcinoma of the testis.

Factors that regulate hPL production have been assessed in cultured syncytiotrophoblast cells. Insulin and growth hormone-releasing factor (GHRF) stimulate hPL secretion, whereas somatostatin (SS) appears to inhibit its secretion. The presence of hPL, hPGH, SS, and GRF in the same cell suggests that an autoregulatory loop, analogous to the hypothalamic-pituitary axis, may operate within the placenta. In the third trimester, maternal hPL and GRF levels are closely correlated.[78] Interestingly, SS expression is maximal in early pregnancy and decreases during the second and third trimesters, a pattern opposite to that of hPL secretory activity.[79,80] Thus, locally produced GRF and SS may regulate placental hPL expression.

Several studies have demonstrated changes in maternal hPL levels in response to metabolic stress. Specifically, prolonged fasting at midgestation[81,82] and insulin-induced hypoglycemia raise maternal hPL concentrations.[83] However, hPL levels do not change in association with normal metabolic fluctuations during a typical 24-hour period.[84,85] Although extreme metabolic stress influences hPL production, hPL expression does not appear to be modulated by metabolic status within the normal range.

Human Placental Growth Hormone

Two forms of hPGH have been identified, both of which are expressed in syncytiotrophoblast cells.[86,87] The smaller, 22-kDa form is almost identical to pituitary GH, differing by only 13 amino acids. The larger 26-kDa hPGH is a splice variant that retains intron 4. The extent of hPGH production is significantly less than that of hPL, and hPGH is not secreted into the fetal compartment.[88] Consequently, circulating levels of hPGH are approximately 1000-fold less than hPL and can be detected in the maternal circulation later in gestation (between 21 and 26 weeks). During the third trimester, maternal hPGH levels increase exponentially, in concert with hPL, and reach a maximum of approximately 20 ng/mL by term.

During the course of human pregnancy, hPGH becomes the dominant GH, and maternal pituitary GH production gradually declines. In the first trimester, pituitary GH is measurable and secreted in a highly pulsatile manner.[89] However, pituitary GH production decreases progressively from about week 15 and by 30 weeks cannot be detected. In addition, the responsiveness of maternal somatotropes

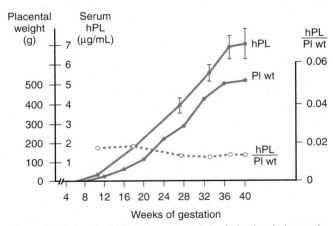

Figure 11-4. *Levels of hPL in the maternal circulation in relation to placental weight (Pl wt). (From Selenkow HA, Saxena BM, Dana CL, Emerson K Jr. Measurement and pathologic significance of human placental lactogen. In Pecile A, Fenzi C [ed]. The Foeto-placental Unit. Amsterdam, Excerpta Medica, 1969, pp 340-362.)*

to secretogogues decreases dramatically.[90,91] During the same period, nonpulsatile secretion of hPGH by the placenta increases markedly. Thus, maternal pituitary GH production declines during the second trimester and is not detectable during the third. By this stage, the hPGH serves as the GH of pregnancy.

Biologic Actions of hPL and hPGH

Several cases of hPL and hPGH deficiency have revealed their potential roles in human pregnancy.[92,93] In all cases of complete hPL deficiency (lack of detectable hPL in the mother's blood or in the placenta) pregnancy and fetal development were normal. Thus, despite the remarkably high levels of hPL, it is not essential for normal pregnancy. However, deficiency of both hPL and hPGH due to a mutation in the GH/PL gene cluster, results in severe fetal growth retardation, but an otherwise normal pregnancy. Pregnancies in which only hPGH is deficient have not been identified. These experiments of nature indicate that hPL is not necessary for normal pregnancy, whereas fetal growth is dependent on hPGH.[69,94,95] Alternatively, such findings may indicate that fetal growth is dependent on either hPGH or hPL and that these hormones constitute a redundant system.

As mentioned above, the initial identification of hPL was based in its lactogenic activity in bioassays; therefore, it would be reasonable to surmise that hPL acts as a lactogen in human pregnancy. However, it is important to distinguish "activity" in heterologous assays from "function" physiologically. Notably, administration of hPL to nonpregnant women in sufficient quantities to mimic pregnancy levels did not induce lactation.[96] However, this does rule out hPL as a lactogen, as its actions on the mammary gland may be dependent on other factors in the endocrine milieu of pregnancy (e.g., estrogen and progesterone). Nevertheless, the in vivo lactogenic properties, if any, of hPL in human pregnancy remain to be established.

In addition, maternal prolactin levels increase significantly in the later stages of pregnancy and, together with estrogen and progesterone, are likely sufficient to induce mammary growth and lactation. Thus, although hPL is produced in very large quantities, it appears to be a redundant hormone.

As hPL and hPGH share a high degree of homology, it would be reasonable to surmise that they act through a common membrane-bound receptor. Indeed, both hPGH and hPL bind the growth hormone receptor, although the affinity of hPL is around 2000-fold less than that of hGH.[97] However, the high levels of hPL in the maternal circulation compared with those of hPGH would, in part, compensate for the reduced receptor affinity. Both hormones have equal affinity for the prolactin receptor. To date, no specific hPL receptor has been identified. Thus, it is likely that the absence of hPL can be compensated for by hPGH and vice versa, whereas the absence of both is detrimental to fetal growth.

As hPGH does not enter the fetal compartment, its principal action may be on the mother. In contrast, hPL is present in the mother and the fetus. However, deficiency in hPL alone has no effect on fetal growth, whereas deficiency in both hPL and hPGH is associated with severe fetal growth retardation. Taken together, these observations indicate that hPL and hPGH influence fetal growth through effects on the mother. This is consistent with the thesis that hPL and hPGH modulate maternal metabolism to meet fetal energy requirements.

A stronger case, as proposed by Kaplan and colleagues, can be made for hPL and hPGH as modulators of maternal metabolism.[98] Pregnancy simulates a diabetogenic state, with impaired maternal glucose tolerance, relative insulin insensitivity, and elevated levels of circulating free fatty acids. Such a state is advantageous to the fetus, as it increases maternal energy supplies available for fetal use. This is particularly important for the fetal brain, which uses glucose exclusively as an energy source. In nonpregnant subjects, hPL impairs carbohydrate tolerance and increases insulin and free fatty acid levels,[99-101] actions consistent with the diabetogenic state of pregnancy. These properties of hPL, together with its high level of secretion into the maternal compartment, suggest that it is an important regulator of metabolic homeostasis during pregnancy.

Soon after birth insulin resistance reverts to the normal nonpregnant state, suggesting that maternal glucose homeostasis is influenced by hormonal factors produced by the fetus/placenta. To maintain glucose homeostasis during pregnancy maternal insulin secretion increases to compensate for the decrease in insulin sensitivity. In women with gestational diabetes insulin secretion is insufficient to balance the decrease in insulin sensitivity, and consequently blood glucose levels increase, leading to pathophysiologic disorders, including fetal macrosomia (see Chapter 26).

As pregnancy progresses, the fetus increases its substrate requirements, which leads to an increased functional role for hPL and hPGH in the second and third trimesters. The GH-like and contra-insulin effects of these hormones would lead to impaired glucose uptake and stimulation of free fatty acid release. Free fatty acids can cross the placenta, and the increased ketones induced by their metabolism are an important energy source for the fetus. As a consequence of insulin resistance, muscle proteolysis and the formation of ketones may be enhanced. In addition, the decreased maternal glucose consumption induced by hPL and hPGH would ensure a steady supply of glucose for the fetus. These effects of hPL and hPGH on fat and carbohydrate metabolism are similar to those after treatment with hGH. In this manner maternal metabolism would be directed toward mobilization of resources to furnish the needs of the developing fetus.

This hormonal interaction represents an example of fetal/maternal conflict as proposed by David Haig.[37] That model suggests that through natural selection the fetus has acquired traits (e.g., somatotropin production) that extract resources from the maternal organism. Conversely, mothers have evolved a mechanism to counteract fetal demand. Through natural selection a compromise is attained between fetal requirements and maternal health. Disorders on either side of this equation lead to pathophysiologic events of pregnancy including preterm birth.

PLACENTAL CORTICOTROPINS

POMC and POMC-Derived Hormones

The human placenta expresses pro-opiomelanocortin (POMC).[101] In pituitary corticotropes, this 31-kDa glycoprotein is the precursor for the adrenocorticotropic hormone (ACTH)–endorphin family of peptides. POMC is enzymatically cleaved into several peptide hormones, including ACTH, β-lipotrophic hormone (β-LPH), α-melanocyte-stimulating hormone (α-MSH), and β-endorphin (β-EP). These neuroendocrine hormones play major roles in the physiologic response to stress and the control of behavior. Each of these peptides, including full-length POMC, has been detected in the human placenta.[103-105]

Placental syncytiotrophoblasts express POMC in a transcriptional pattern similar to that of extrapituitary tumors.[104] However, the processing of POMC in placental cells is different than that in pituitary corticotropes. Although some placental POMC is cleaved, a significant amount of intact POMC is secreted by the placenta into the maternal circulation. This is unusual, as POMC, at least in pituitary corticotropes, is processed completely; in nonpregnant adults, plasma POMC is undetectable in the circulation.[105] During pregnancy, however, maternal circulating POMC levels are readily detectable by the third month and then increase steadily until midgestation, reaching a plateau of around 300 U/mL between 28 weeks and term. Soon after birth, POMC returns to undetectable levels. Placental POMC production is constant with no diurnal variability, unlike in the pituitary, and it is not inhibited by glucocorticoids. Interestingly, maternal POMC levels do not correlate with plasma or cortisol levels. However, plasma POMC levels are closely correlated with plasma corticotropin-releasing hormone (CRH) levels during the third trimester.[105]

The physiologic role, if any, of placental ACTH and other POMC-derived proteins in the control of human pregnancy remains to be elucidated. With regard to fetal adrenal growth, placental ACTH plays a negligible role, because it is not sufficient to prevent adrenal hypoplasia in fetal hypopituitarism due to anencephaly. However, placental ACTH may influence maternal physiology and could be responsible for the relative resistance to negative feedback suppression of pituitary ACTH by glucocorticoids during pregnancy.[106]

Similarly, the role of placenta-derived β-EP is unclear. Immunoreactive β-EP in the maternal circulation remains relatively low throughout pregnancy, with mean levels of approximately 15 pg/mL.[107] Levels rise to approximately 70 pg/mL during late labor and rise further (mean, 113 pg/mL) at delivery.[107] Similar concentrations of β-EP (mean, 105 pg/mL) also are detectable in cord plasma at term, suggesting secretion by the placenta into the fetal compartment or secretion by the fetal pituitary. Many factors that cause an increase in pituitary ACTH (e.g., hypoxia and acidosis) also increase β-EP production.[108]

In addition to β-EP and β-LPH, there are two other families of endogenous opioids: enkephalins and dynorphins. Immunoreactive methionine-enkephalin has been found in the human placenta and is chemically identical to the native molecule. Circulating levels of methionine-enkephalin do not change appreciably throughout pregnancy.[109] Three forms of dynorphin have been found in the human placenta.[110] The placental content of dynorphin at term is of similar magnitude to that found in the pituitary gland and brain.[110] Relatively high concentrations of dynorphin are found in amniotic fluid and umbilical venous plasma, and maternal plasma levels in the third trimester and at delivery are higher than in nonpregnant women.[110] Dynorphin binds to kappa opiate receptors, which are abundant in the human placenta and increase at term. Because kappa receptor agonists stimulate the release of hPL,[111] it is possible that dynorphin exerts local regulatory effects on hPL production.

Corticotropin-Releasing Hormone

First identified in the hypothalamus, CRH is a 41–amino acid peptide that stimulates the expression and processing of POMC by pituitary corticotropes and, as its name implies, the secretion of ACTH. The human placenta, fetal membranes, and decidua also express CRH that is identical to that produced by the hypothalamus.[112] Expression of placental CRH can be detected from the seventh week of pregnancy and increases progressively until term. In the last 5 to 7 weeks of pregnancy, placental expression of CRH increases more than 20-fold[113] (Fig. 11-5).

Placental CRH is released mainly into the maternal compartment. Levels of CRH in the maternal circulation can be detected as early as 15 weeks of gestation and then increase throughout gestation (see Fig. 11-5). Remarkably, this top level is about 1000-fold higher than peripheral CRH levels in nonpregnant women. Placental CRH also is secreted into the fetal circulation, albeit to a lesser extent, resulting in elevated CRH levels in the fetus throughout gestation.[114,115]

A binding protein (BP) for CRH also exists, and for most of pregnancy it is present in excess of CRH in the maternal circulation. As the CRH-BP binds CRH with greater affinity than the CRH receptor, it effectively suppresses CRH activity. Thus, for most of pregnancy the bulk of the placental CRH is sequestered by CRH-BP. However, during the last 4 weeks of pregnancy CRH-BP levels decrease markedly.[116] This coincides with the exponential increase in placental CRH production, which could result in a dramatic increase in CRH biologic activity (Fig. 11-6).

Despite the elevated concentrations of CRH during pregnancy, maternal ACTH secretion does not increase concordantly. In fact, pituitary ACTH levels remain low throughout pregnancy. The lack of CRH stimulation could be due to inhibition by the CRH-BP. However, maternal ACTH production remains low late in gestation when CRH increases and CRH-BP decreases. In vivo studies have shown that CRH responsiveness of the maternal pituitary is markedly attenuated during pregnancy, and in vitro studies have shown that CRH down-regulates expression of its receptor in pituitary corticotropes.[117]

Actions of CRH are mediated by specific cell membrane receptors. Two major CRH receptor (CRH-R) subtypes have been identified, CRH-R1 and CRH-R2.[118-120] CRH binds to CRH-R1 with greater affinity than CRH-R2. These receptors and various subtypes within each group exhibit tissue-specific expression and possibly contribute to differential actions of CRH on different cell types.

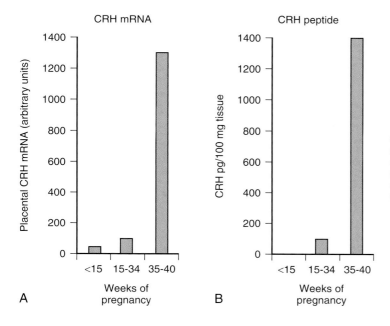

Figure 11-5. *Changes in placental corticotropin-releasing hormone (CRH) mRNA (**A**) and CRH peptide (**B**) during gestation. (From Frim DM, Emanuel RL, Robinson BG, et al. Characterization and gestational regulation of corticotropin-releasing hormone messenger RNA in human placenta. J Clin Invest 82:287, 1988, copyright American Society of Clinical Investigation.)*

In vitro studies indicate that agents that increase CRH production by the hypothalamus also increase CRH production by cultured placental cells.[121] These agents include prostaglandins E_2 and $F_{2\alpha}$ (PGE$_2$ and PGF$_{2\alpha}$), norepinephrine, acetylcholine, vasopressin, angiotensin II, oxytocin (OT), interleukin I, and NPY. In contrast, progesterone[121] and nitric oxide donors[122] inhibit placental CRH expression in vitro.

Interestingly, expression and secretion of placental CRH are increased by glucocorticoids. This response is in contrast to hypothalamic CRH expression, which is decreased by glucocorticoids. This stimulatory action has been observed in vivo in women who receive glucocorticoid treatment during the third trimester[123,124] and in vitro in cultured placental cells.[125] As placental and hypothalamic CRH are products of the same gene, the molecular basis for this difference in glucocorticoid regulation is thought to involve placental-specific transcription factors acting through distinct response elements in the CRH promoter region.[126]

The stimulation of placental CRH production by glucocorticoids may result in a positive feedback endocrine loop. Placental CRH may stimulate ACTH production by the fetal pituitary, which would increase cortisol secretion by the fetal adrenals. Fetal adrenal cortisol could then further stimulate placental CRH production. The marked rise in placental CRH during the last 10 weeks of pregnancy could be due to such a positive feedback interaction. This endocrine loop may be involved in the process of parturition.

CRH also may influence fetal adrenal steroidogenesis by directly increasing dehydroepiandrosterone sulfate (DHEA-S) production.[127,128] Interestingly, CRH is as effective as ACTH in stimulating dehydroepiandrosterone sulfate (DHEA-S) production but 70% less potent than ACTH in stimulating cortisol production (Fig. 11-7). The capacity for CRH to act as an adrenal androgen secretagogue also has been demonstrated in vivo in adult men.[129] The preferential induction of adrenal androgen synthesis indicates that placental CRH indirectly augments placental estrogen synthesis, because fetal adrenal DHEA-S is the principal substrate for placental estrogen production. Placental CRH and fetal adrenal DHEA-S increase concordantly during the third trimester, suggesting that production of these two hormones is related. The implication of this endocrine axis in the regulation of parturition is discussed later in this chapter.

Several actions have been ascribed to placental CRH in the control of human pregnancy. CRH may serve an autocrine-paracrine function within the placenta by regulating expression and processing of POMC. The formation of ACTH, β-LPH, β-EP, and α-MSH by cultured placental cells can be stimulated by CRH, an effect that is inhibited by CRH antagonists.[130]

Placental CRH may be part of the fetal-placental stress response mechanism. The placenta is comparable to the hypothalamus in its production of CRH in response to stress. Neurotransmitters and neuropeptides activated in response to stress stimulate placental CRH release in vitro.[131,132] The physiologic implications of this are that the fetus may be able to mount a stress response by means of

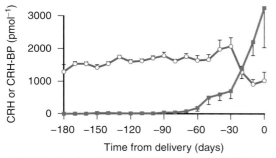

Figure 11-6. *Levels of corticotropin-releasing hormone (CRH) and CRH binding protein (CRH-BP) in the maternal circulation during human pregnancy (From McLean M, Bisits A, Davies J, et al. A placental clock controlling the length of human pregnancy. Nat Med 1:460, 1995.)*

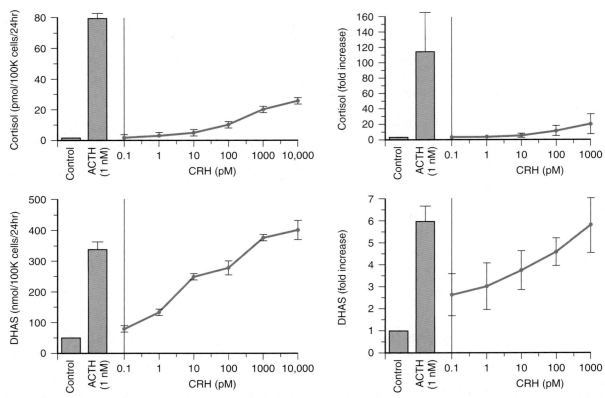

Figure 11-7. *Effect of corticotropin-releasing hormone (CRH) on cortisol and dehydroepiandrosterone sulfate (DHEA-S) production in cultured human fetal (midgestation) adrenal cortical cells. ACTH, adrenocorticotropic hormone. (From Smith R, Mesiano S, Chan EC, et al. Corticotropin-releasing hormone directly and preferentially stimulates dehydroepiandrosterone sulfate secretion by human fetal adrenal cortical cells. J Clin Endocrinol Metab 83:2916, 1998.)*

placental CRH. This may be critical in conditions of fetal stress such as preeclampsia, placental vascular insufficiency, and intrauterine infection.

The human placenta also produces urocortin, a 40–amino acid peptide that is a member of the CRH family, has the same biologic actions as CRH, and binds to CRHR1.[133-135] The role of placental urocortin in human pregnancy is uncertain.[136]

THYROTROPIN-RELEASING HORMONE

A substance similar to the hypothalamic thyrotropin-releasing hormone (TRH) has been found in the human placenta.[57,137] It stimulates pituitary thyrotropin (TSH) release in the rat both in vitro and in vivo, but is not identical to hypothalamic TRH.[138] To date, a placental TSH has not been identified. Whether placental TRH plays a role in stimulating fetal or maternal pituitary TSH remains to be ascertained. As discussed earlier, the thyroid-stimulating activity of the placenta has been ascribed to hCG.

LEPTIN

Leptin, a 146–amino acid protein produced primarily by adipocytes, is a key regulator of satiety and body mass index, and its levels are thought to reflect the amount of energy stores and nutritional state.[139] Leptin decreases food intake and body weight by means of its hypothalamic

receptor.[140] In the reproductive system, leptin is thought to coordinate body mass status with reproductive function.[141] In general, leptin acts as a permissive factor in reproduction; pulsatile hypothalamic GnRH secretion does not occur unless leptin levels reach a threshold value. Such a mechanism may ensure that energy stores are sufficient to support a pregnancy.

The actions of leptin may not be limited to regulation of satiety and energy stores, as its expression and that of its receptor have been identified in a variety of tissue types. This multifocal distribution of expression and targets suggests that leptin plays a paracrine role in a variety of physiologic processes.[142]

The placenta is the principal source of leptin during pregnancy.[143] Most of the leptin produced by the placenta is secreted into the maternal circulation, and as a consequence leptin levels are elevated during pregnancy. In the first trimester, maternal plasma leptin levels are double nonpregnant values and continue to increase during the second and third trimesters.[144-148] In the second and third trimesters, leptin is also expressed by the chorion and amnion.[149] The proportion of placental leptin directed to the fetus is uncertain, and its role in fetal development is unknown. Leptin levels decline to normal nonpregnant values within 24 hours of delivery.[144]

The influence of placental leptin on maternal biology also is unclear. Interestingly, leptin levels during pregnancy do not correlate with body mass index as they do in the nonpregnant state.[150] Pregnancy appears to be a state of hyperleptinemia and leptin resistance, with uncoupling of eating behavior, satiety, and metabolic activity.[151] Leptin is lipolytic and favors fatty acid mobilization from adipose tissue. Based on its actions in the hypothalamus, leptin may regulate satiety and maternal energy expenditure during pregnancy. It also may act in the liver, pancreas, and muscle to decrease insulin sensitivity and mobilize glucose. Thus, leptin appears to be another hormone utilized by the placenta to modulate maternal metabolism and partition energy supplies to the fetus.[152]

The human placenta expresses leptin receptors and therefore leptin can act in a paracrine manner to modulate placental function. Leptin induces hCG production in trophoblast cells. Leptin is also thought to increase placental growth by augmenting mitogenesis, animo acid uptake, and extracellular matrix synthesis.[153,154]

NEUROPEPTIDE Y

Found in the central and peripheral nervous systems, NPY is a 36–amino acid protein that influences neuroendocrine function and behavioral events such as eating and satiety.[155,156] Immunoreactive NPY and binding sites for NPY have been found in the term human placenta.[157] In women with preeclampsia, placental NPY expression is decreased compared with normal pregnancies.[158] Interestingly, this decrease is associated with increased expression of leptin.[158] The inverse relationship between placental NPY and leptin resembles hypothalamic regulation of NPY, whereby leptin suppresses hypothalamic NPY release.[159]

Maternal NPY levels are increased above those of nonpregnant women beginning early in gestation. They remain elevated until term and rise still further during labor, reaching their acme with cervical dilation and parturition.[160] There is no significant change in NPY concentrations in the circulation of women undergoing cesarean section who are not in labor.[160] NPY levels decline rapidly after delivery, again suggesting a placental source of this neuropeptide. Elevated concentrations of NPY are also found in amniotic fluid.[160]

Because NPY can stimulate CRH release from cultured placental cells,[161] but not the release of GnRH, hCG, or hPL, it may play a role in the regulation of placental CRH release.

GROWTH FACTORS AND CYTOKINES

Many growth factors, cytokines, and their cognate receptors have been found in the human placenta.[162-164] These factors likely play a role in controlling the growth, development, and differentiated function of the placenta and fetus. In this regard the insulin-like growth factors (IGFs) are notable. Studies in mice, using homologous recombination, have shown that IGF-I and IGF-II are critical for placental and fetal growth. Disruption of placenta-expressed IGF-II[165] or overexpression of decidual IGFBP-1 (an IGF binding protein that inhibits IGF action)[166] leads to restriction of placental and fetal growth.

Interestingly, IGF-II is imprinted; only the paternal allele is expressed in the fetus and placenta.[167] The finding that a paternal gene promotes placental growth supports the concept of genetic conflict between the maternal and

fetal genomes.[37] The size and ultimate health of the fetus depends greatly on the size of the placenta. Growth factors that increase placenta size are an advantage to the fetus because they allow it to more efficiently extract resources from the mother. Passage of paternal genes to the next generation is favored if nutrient supply to the fetus is maximized. Maternal genes, on the other hand, not only must survive to the next generation, but also must ensure that the current pregnancy does not compromise the mother's future reproductive capacity. Maternal genes would therefore be selected to counter and control the effects of paternally imprinted genes such as IGF-II. Interestingly, IGFBP-1 is produced by the decidua, a maternal tissue, and essentially all of the IGFBP-1 in amniotic fluid is maternally derived.[166] Thus, placental, and ultimately fetal, growth appears to be the net result of a balance between factors that stimulate (e.g., IGF-II) and those that restrict (e,g., IGFBP-1) growth.

STEROID HORMONES AND THE FETOPLACENTAL UNIT

In regard to steroid hormone formation in pregnancy, two aspects must be considered: the integrated role of the fetus, placenta, and mother in the formation of the large quantities of estrogens and progesterone; and steroid hormone formation and regulation within the fetus itself.

The placenta is an incomplete steroid-producing organ—unlike the adult adrenal, testis, and ovary—and must rely on precursors reaching it from the fetal and maternal circulations. The interdependence of fetus, placenta, and mother for steroid hormone production in pregnancy led to the concept of an integrated fetoplacental-maternal unit. To understand this concept, the reader will find it useful to review the general biosynthetic pathways in steroid hormone formation and the unique features that distinguish placental steroidogenesis from the process in the adrenal cortex and gonads (Fig. 11-8; see also Chapter 4).

Progesterone and Estrogens

The human placenta expresses cholesterol side-chain cleavage (P450scc) and 3β-hydroxysteriod dehydrogenase (3βHSD) but lacks the 17α-hydroxylase/17,20-lyase (P450c17) enzyme (Fig. 11-9), and therefore steroidogenesis derived from cholesterol terminates at progesterone. Maternal low-density lipoprotein cholesterol is converted first to pregnenolone and then rapidly and efficiently to progesterone.[168] Production of progesterone approximates 250 mg/day by the end of pregnancy, at which time circulating levels are on the order of 130 ng/mL.[169]

To form estrogens, the placenta, which has a highly active aromatizing capacity, uses circulating C19 androgens, primarily from the fetus but also from the mother. The major precursor used for placental estrogen formation is DHEA-S, mainly from the fetal adrenal gland. Because the placenta has an abundance of the sulfatase (sulfate-cleaving) enzyme, DHEA-S is converted to free (unconjugated) DHEA and then to androstenedione, thereafter to testosterone, and, by means of these androgens, to estrone and 17β-estradiol (see Fig. 11-9).

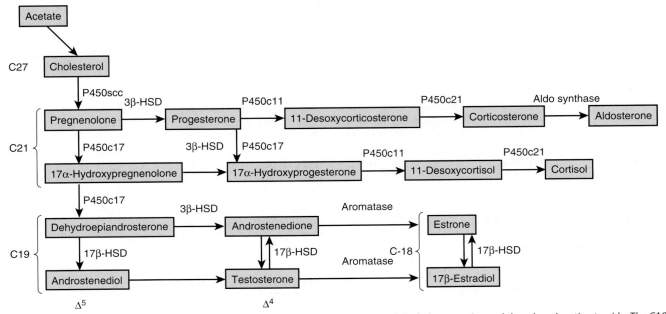

Figure 11-8. *Biosynthetic pathways in steroid hormone formation. The C21 compounds include progestins and the adrenal corticosteroids. The C19 compounds include androgens, and the C18 compounds include estrogens. Steroids with a double bond between the 5 and 6 positions in the steroid nucleus (Δ5-steroids) are shown on the left, and those with a double bond between the 4 and 5 positions (Δ4-steroids) are depicted on the right. Aldo, aldosterone; HSD, hydroxysteroid dehydrogenase; P450c11, 11β-hydroxylase; P450c17, 17α-hydroxylase; P450c21, 21α-hydroxylase; P450scc, cholesterol side-chain cleavage.*

An interesting facet of steroid hormone metabolism in the human fetus is the formation of sulfate conjugates of the steroid hormones. The process of sulfoconjugation of hydroxylated steroids is ubiquitous in the fetus, occurring in a variety of sites, including lung, gut, liver, and adrenal gland. In the adrenal, sulfurylation leads to the formation of a variety of steroid sulfates, including pregnenolone sulfate, 17α-hydroxypregnenolone sulfate, and DHEA-S.[170]

By far the major estrogen formed during human pregnancy is estriol, which has an additional hydroxyl group at position 16. Estriol constitutes more than 90% of the estrogen in pregnancy urine, into which it is excreted as sulfate and glucuronide conjugates. Concentrations increase with advancing gestation, and range from approximately 2 mg/24 hours at 26 weeks to 35 to 45 mg/24 hours at term.[171] The concentration of estriol in the maternal circulation at term is 8 to 13 ng/dL.[172] In contrast, the ovary of nonpregnant women does not secrete estriol.[172]

Estriol is formed by a biosynthetic process unique to human (and higher primate) pregnancy (Fig. 11-10). When DHEA-S of either fetal or maternal origin reaches the placenta, estrone and estradiol are formed. However, little of either is converted to estriol by the placenta. Instead, some of the DHEA-S undergoes 16α-hydroxylation, primarily in the fetal liver and, to a limited extent, in the fetal adrenal gland itself. When the newly formed 16α-hydroxy-DHEA-S (16α-OH-DHEA-S) reaches the placenta, the placental sulfatase enzyme cleaves the sulfate side chain. The unconjugated 16α-OH-DHEA, after further metabolism, is aromatized to form estriol, which is then secreted into the maternal circulation. Estriol is conjugated to form estriol sulfate and estriol glucosiduronate in the maternal liver and excreted via the maternal urine.[173] Another placental estrogen derived from a fetal precursor is estetrol, formed after 15-hydroxylation of 16α-OH-DHEA-S. Its function is not known. Levels of progesterone and estrogens in the maternal circulation during human pregnancy are shown in Figure 11-11.

Estrogen and progesterone cause dramatic changes in maternal physiology, which provide advantages for the developing conceptus and are central to the adaptation of the mother to the pregnant state.[174]

Progesterone. As its name implies, progesterone is a "pro-gestational" hormone; it promotes and sustains the pregnant state. Progesterone has been aptly called the "hormone of pregnancy" because it is essential for pregnancy maintenance in all mammals examined. Any interference of progesterone synthesis or action during pregnancy rapidly induces abortion. Progesterone suppresses T-lymphocyte cell-mediated responses involved in tissue rejection and may contribute to preventing the rejection of the conceptus by the maternal immune system.[175] The high local (intrauterine) concentrations of progesterone may effectively block maternal cellular immune responses to foreign antigens.

Actions of progesterone are mediated through genomic and nongenomic pathways. Genomic effects of progesterone are mediated by the classic nuclear progesterone receptors (nPRs) that function as ligand-activated transcription factors. The human nPR gene encodes two major products, the full-length PR-B and the N-terminally truncated (by 164 amino acids) PR-A, that are independently regulated by separate promoters. Each nPR is a member of the nuclear receptor superfamily (see Chapter 5).

Nongenomic actions of progesterone are mediated by its interaction with membrane-bound PRs (mPRs) that are functionally linked to intracellular signal transduction

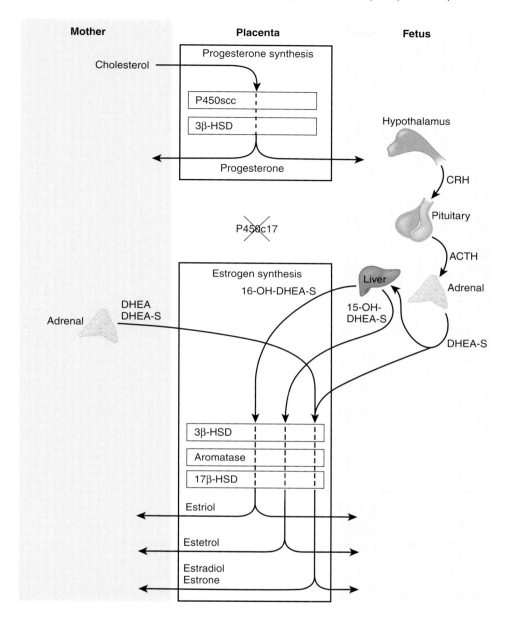

Figure 11-9. *Biosynthesis of progesterone and estrogens by the human placenta. Progesterone is produced mainly from maternal cholesterol. P450c17 is not expressed in the human placenta, and therefore, progesterone cannot be converted to C19 androgens. Instead, estrogens are biosynthesized from C19-androgen precursors (mainly dehydroepiandrosterone sulfate [DHEA-S]) provided by the maternal and fetal adrenals. ACTH, adrenocorticotropic hormone; CRH, corticotropin-releasing hormone; HSD, hydroxysteroid dehydrogenase (From Mesiano S. Roles of estrogen and progesterone in human parturition. Front Horm Res 27:86, 2001.)*

pathways.[176] Several specific mPRs have recently been identified, but their roles mediating progesterone actions during pregnancy are uncertain.

A major function of progesterone during pregnancy is to promote myometrial relaxation and quiescence. Progesterone relaxes the pregnancy myometrium genomically by repressing the expression of genes encoding contraction-associated proteins (CAPs) and by inhibiting estrogenic actions on the pregnancy myometrium. The induction of labor and delivery by nPR-specific antagonists such as RU486 reflects the importance of nPR-mediated progesterone actions for the maintenance pregnancy and, in particular, myometrial relaxation.

Studies examining the rapid effects of progesterone on isolated myometrial strips from various species generally showed that it inhibits OT-induced contractions and that it uncouples the excitation-contraction process (for review see Perusquia[176]). However, in vitro studies using human pregnancy myometrium yielded mixed results with some investigators reporting a rapid relaxatory effect of progesterone and progesterone metabolites[177-181] and others reporting that progesterone augments contraction frequency but decreases duration and amplitude.[182-184] The reason for this variability could be due to difference in the progestins used and how they were prepared, and the contractile state of the tissue before it was mounted on the myograph. Nonetheless, the studies clearly demonstrated that progesterone has a rapid nongenomic effect on myometrial contractility.

Studies of progesterone action in dispersed myometrial cells and on myometrial strips suggest that it inhibits basal and uterotonin-induced contractility by suppressing intracellular free Ca^{2+} ($[Ca^{2+}]_i$) levels[179,185] and increasing intracellular cAMP ($[cAMP]_i$).[186,187] This may be vital for the maintenance of relaxation since an increase in $[Ca^{2+}]_i$ induces contraction, whereas an increase in $[cAMP]_i$ relaxes the myometrium.

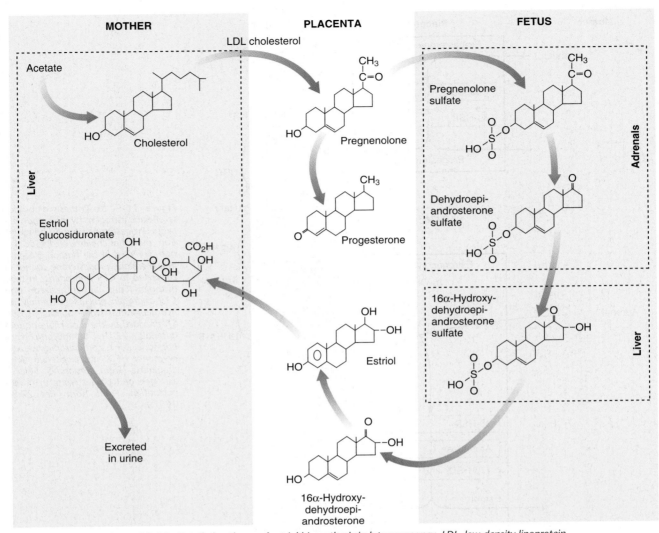

Figure 11-10. *Detailed pathway of estriol biosynthesis in late pregnancy. LDL, low-density lipoprotein.*

The molecular mechanisms that mediate nongenomic effects of progesterone on myometrial contractility are not clearly understood and are therefore somewhat controversial. Progesterone may exert these effects by interacting with specific mPRs[188] or other receptors such as the oxytocin receptor[189-191] and the GABA$_A$ receptor.[192]

It is especially intriguing in this regard that the nongenomic and genomic actions of progesterone cooperate to promote myometrial relaxation. It is possible that genomic progesterone actions establish the long-term quiescent phenotype (e.g., by suppressing CAP genes expression), and nongenomic progesterone actions may prevent any acute challenge to this relaxed state by directly inhibiting $[Ca^{2+}]_i$ or augmenting $[cAMP]_i$.

Use of Progesterone Treatment to Prevent Preterm Birth. Studies in the 1950s and 1960s showed that administration of high doses of progesterone (as an IV bolus or into the amniotic fluid) decreased the frequency of spontaneous contractions and attenuated OT responsiveness.[193,194] These findings suggested that progesterone could be used therapeutically to prevent preterm birth.

Clinical trials of chronic progestin therapy to prevent preterm birth have produced mixed outcomes. Long-term prophylactic treatment with natural progesterone administered vaginally[195] or a synthetic caproate ester of 17α-hydroxyprogesterone (17HPC) given as a long-acting intramuscular injection[196] decreased the incidence of preterm birth in women with an increased risk for preterm birth (based on a prior preterm birth) and improved neonatal outcome. However, those findings were not confirmed in some subsequent studies. In a large multinational study, vaginal administration of progesterone failed to alter preterm birth rates[197] and administration of 17HPC to women with twin pregnancies failed to decrease the incidence of preterm birth in this subgroup.[198] The only positive data to emerge from recent clinical trials was that vaginal progesterone therapy decreases the incidence of preterm birth in women with a short cervix.[199] The mechanism of this effect is unclear and the value of progestin therapy to prevent preterm birth is a subject of debate.[200]

Estrogen. Estrogenic actions during pregnancy are mediated by the nuclear estrogen receptors (ERs: ERα and

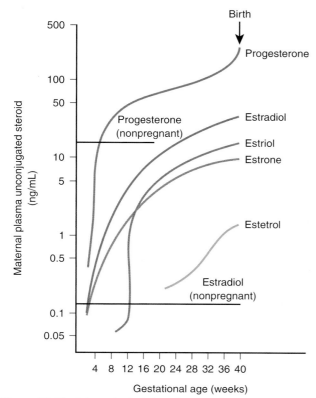

Figure 11-11. *Schematic depiction of maternal progesterone and estrogen (estradiol, estrone, and estriol) concentrations throughout human pregnancy compared with average levels in normal cycling women.*

estriol is a weak estrogen with approximately 1% the potency of estradiol and 10% that of estrone, on a weight basis. However, there is one function for which estriol appears to be as effective as the other estrogens: its ability to increase uteroplacental blood flow. Therefore, this may be a primary function of the large amounts of placental estriol.[202] Its relatively weak estrogenic effects on other organ systems may make it an ideal candidate for this purpose.

In the parturitional process, estrogens are thought to oppose the actions of progesterone by stimulating biochemical and physical changes in the uterus and fetal membranes needed for labor and delivery.[203] Estrogens increase uterine contractions by increasing myometrial excitability through changes in the resting membrane potential and formation of gap junctions between myometrial cells. These changes increase myometrial responsiveness to stimulatory uterotonins and the capacity for synchronous contractions. In addition, estrogens increase the production and release of prostaglandins (PGs) by the fetal membranes. In the cervix, estrogens stimulate expression of proteolytic enzymes (e.g., collagenase), which degrade the extracellular matrix to allow cervical dilation.

PLACENTAL GLUCOCORTICOID METABOLISM

For most of gestation the placenta expresses the 11β-hydroxysteroid dehydrogenase type 2 (11β-HSD-2) enzyme, which inactivates cortisol by catalyzing its conversion to cortisone.[204-206] Thus, the placenta forms a biochemical barrier to maternal cortisol, inactivating it before it enters the fetal compartment. As maternal cortisol levels are three times those of the fetus, this barrier serves to prevent excess cortisol from entering the fetal compartment. This is important because exposure of the fetus to high levels of cortisol not only could interfere with the fetal hypothalamic-pituitary axis, but also is associated with decreased birth weight and hypertension.[207-209]

Studies in the baboon placenta suggest that estrogen upregulates 11β-HSD-2 expression in the placenta. Because estrogen synthesis by the placenta requires fetal adrenal androgen precursors (produced in part by fetal pituitary ACTH stimulation) the estrogen regulation of placental 11β-HSD-2 represents a regulatory loop that ensures that maternal cortisol does not affect the fetal hypothalamic-pituitary-adrenal (HPA) axis.[203]

Development of the Fetal Neuroendocrine System

ONTOGENY OF FETAL HYPOTHALAMIC AND PITUITARY HORMONES

Hypothalamus

By the end of the fifth week of gestation, the primitive hypothalamus can be identified as a swelling on the inner surface of the diencephalic neural canal. It then differentiates to form a complex of interconnecting nuclei. By 9 to 10 weeks, the median eminence of the hypothalamus is evident. The interconnecting fiber tracts of hypothalamic nuclei can be identified by 15 to 18 weeks.

ERβ). The role of the placental estrogens in human pregnancy has been revealed by conditions in which placental estrogen synthesis is markedly decreased (e.g., anencephaly, congenital adrenal lipoid hyperplasia, placental aromatase deficiency, and placenta sulfatase deficiency). Although pregnancy was prolonged in some cases of placental sulfatase deficiency and anencephaly, in most cases a marked decrease in placental estrogen synthesis had little effect on fetal and placental development and the timing of parturition. In the studies of placental aromatase deficiency, it was concluded that estrogens of placental origin are not essential for normal pregnancy and parturition, but rather a critical role of placental aromatase is to act as a sink for circulating androgens to protect the female fetus and mother from virilization.[201]

These observations do not exclude a role for estrogen in the control of human pregnancy. In all cases of decreased placental estrogen synthesis, the levels of maternal estrogens, although low compared with normal pregnancies, were still in a physiologically significant range (1 to 1.6 nmol/L) and comparable to levels reached in the midcycle and luteal phase of the menstrual cycle (0.6 to 2 nmol/L). Thus, despite the inability of the placenta to produce estrogens in certain abnormalities of pregnancy such as aromatase deficiency, the estrogen target tissues are still exposed to moderately high levels of estradiol. The reason that the fetoplacental unit produces such high levels of estrogens through most of pregnancy remains unclear.

The functional role of estriol in pregnancy has attracted a great deal of speculation. In many biologic systems,

Pituitary Gland

The pituitary primordium appears as the epithelial evagination of Rathke's pouch arising from a diverticulum of the stomadeum. The evaginated pituitary primordium appears at 4 weeks and separates from the stomadeum by 5 weeks. The floor of the sella turcica is in place by the seventh week and separates the pituitary from its epithelial origins. The progenitors of pituitary hormone-secreting cells originate in the ventral neural ridges of the primitive neural tube. This region also gives rise to the diencephalon, suggesting that the hypothalamus and anterior pituitary share a common embryonic origin.

The pituitary increases in size and cell number through proliferation of cell cords into mesenchyme beginning during the sixth week. Capillaries interdigitate among the mesenchymal tissue of Rathke's pouch and the diencephalon at 8 weeks and the median eminence is distinguishable by 9 weeks. The hypothalamic-hypophyseal vascular system in fetuses is intact by 11 to 16 weeks.

HYPOTHALAMIC HORMONES

The hypothalamic nuclei and fiber tracts can be distinguished at 14 to 16 weeks, and the hypophysiotropic hormones GnRH, TRH, CRH, growth hormone-releasing hormone (GHRH), and SS appear in the fetal hypothalamus during this period (Table 11-2).

Gonadotropin-Releasing Hormone

The human fetal hypothalamus produces immunoreactive and bioactive GnRH by 10 weeks of gestation.[210] Between 10 and 22 weeks, the concentration of GnRH in the fetal hypothalamus remains constant (0.27 to 13.1 pg/mg) and is not different between sexes. GnRH release from human fetal hypothalamic explants is pulsatile.[211]

In male Rhesus monkey fetuses, GnRH increases LH and testosterone levels.[210] Thus, by at least the last third of gestation, the pituitary-gonadal axis of the male monkey fetus responds to GnRH stimulation. It is likely that a similar situation exists in the human male fetus. Whether this also is the case for the female fetus is unresolved.

Thyrotropin-Releasing Hormone

Significant levels of immunoreactive TRH are found in the human fetal hypothalamus early in gestation.[212] As with GnRH, fetal hypothalamic TRH levels do not correlate with sex or gestational age. The presence of TRH in the fetal hypothalamus in early and midgestation suggests its possible role in the regulation of TSH, and possibly PRL, secretion.

Growth Hormone–Releasing Hormone and Somatostatin

GHRH can be detected in fetal hypothalamic neurons and fiber tracts at 18 weeks, with increasing levels found up to 30 weeks.[213] The simultaneous detection of GHRH in neuron cell bodies and fiber tracts indicates its release into portal vessels by midgestation.

TABLE 11-2

Ontogeny of Human Fetal Hypothalamic and Pituitary Hormones

Hormone	Age Detected (wk)
Hypothalamic	
Gonadotropin-releasing hormone	14
Thyrotropin-releasing hormone	10
Somatostatin	14
Dopamine	11
Growth hormone–releasing hormone	18
Corticotropin-releasing hormone	16
Pituitary	
Prolactin	16.5
Growth hormone	10.5
Corticotropin (ACTH)	7
Thyroid-stimulating hormone (thyrotropin)	13
Luteinizing hormone	10.5
Follicle-stimulating hormone	10.5

Immunoreactive SS can be identified in the hypothalamus of human fetuses from 10 to 22 weeks.[212] In contrast to GnRH and TRH, fetal hypothalamic SS increases with advancing gestational age.

Corticotropin-Releasing Hormone and Arginine Vasopressin

CRH is a potent secretagogue for ACTH and β-endorphin release by the human fetal pituitary gland.[214] Arginine vasopressin (AVP) also directly stimulates ACTH secretion by the fetal pituitary and can synergize with CRH.[211] CRH-immunoreactive fibers can be detected in the median eminence between 14 and 16 weeks.[215,216] CRH immunoactivity and bioactivity and AVP immunoactivity have been detected in human hypothalamic extracts from 12 to 13 weeks.[217]

Hypothalamic CRH and AVP increase with gestational age, and the CRH bioactivity of fetal hypothalamic extracts, measured in isolated rat anterior pituitary cells, is augmented by AVP. Thus, the human fetal hypothalamus has the capacity to regulate pituitary ACTH production from early in the second trimester. The extent to which fetal hypothalamic CRH and AVP and placental CRH interact in regulating fetal ACTH release remains uncertain.

Catecholamine/Dopamine

Catecholamine fluorescence in cells projecting from the arcuate nuclei to the internal and external layers of the median eminence appears during the interval from 12 to 16 weeks.[218] Dopamine is present in the fetal hypothalamus at weeks 11 to 15 at a concentration twice that of the adult. Consistent with the effects of dopamine functioning as the PRL release-inhibiting factor, fetal hypothalami taken within this interval display a PRL release-inhibiting activity.[219]

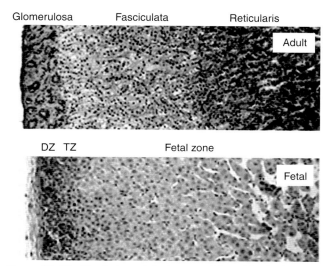

Glomerulosa   Fasciculata   Reticularis

Adult

DZ   TZ   Fetal zone

Fetal

Figure 11-12. Morphology of the human adult and fetal adrenal cortex. DZ, definitive zone; TZ, transitional zone.

PITUITARY HORMONES

The anterior pituitary gland comprises five types of specialized epithelium-derived secretory cells:

1. Lactotropes producing PRL
2. Somatotropes producing GH
3. Corticotropes producing ACTH
4. Thyrotropes producing TSH
5. Gonadotropes producing LH and FSH

Within the pituitary, ACTH-containing cells have been detected at 7 weeks, β-lipotropin and β-endorphin at 8 weeks, GH-containing and LH-containing cells both at 10.5 weeks, and TSH-containing cells at 13 weeks. MSH-containing cells, which probably contain β-lipotropin, have also been reported to appear at 14 weeks, and PRL-containing cells appear at 16.5 weeks (see Table 11-2).[220] Many of the components required for the normal regulated function of the secretory cells of the anterior pituitary, the hypophysiotropic factors elaborated by the hypothalamus, and the neurohemal link connecting the hypothalamus and pituitary, are present in the fetus well before the end of the first half of pregnancy.

The functional relationship between these components is not clearly established. The primate fetal pituitary is competent to respond in vitro to virtually all of the known hypophysiotropic factors by midgestation. Whether it responds to these compounds in vivo remains to be demonstrated directly, although studies in the catheterized Rhesus monkey fetus in utero suggest that responses to at least one of the hypophysiotropic factors, GnRH, can occur.[210]

THE FETAL PITUITARY-ADRENAL AXIS

The anlage of the human adrenal cortex is first identified at about the fourth week of gestation as a thickening of the coelomic epithelium in the notch between the primitive urogenital ridge and the dorsal mesentery. By the fifth week, these primitive cells begin to migrate toward the cranial end of the mesonephros where they condense to

form the earliest recognizable manifestation of the adrenal gland. Cells destined to become the steroidogenic cells of the adrenals and gonads are derived from neighboring areas of the coelomic epithelium and are morphologically identical. In general, the portion medial to the mesonephros produces cells destined for the adrenal cortex, whereas the portion ventral to the mesonephros produces cells destined for the gonad.

During the last two thirds of gestation in humans and higher primates, the fetal adrenal glands are disproportionately enlarged and exhibit extraordinary growth and steroidogenic activity. The growth is attributable to adrenal cortical hypertrophy.

For much of gestation, the human fetal adrenal cortex is composed of two morphologically distinct zones, the fetal zone and the definitive zone (Fig. 11-12). The fetal zone accounts for 80% to 90% of the cortex and is the primary site of growth and steroidogenesis. During midgestation, the fetal zone produces 100 to 200 mg/day of DHEA-S, which is quantitatively the principal steroid product of the human fetal adrenal gland throughout gestation. As its name implies, the fetal zone exists only during fetal life; it involutes or undergoes remodeling soon after birth. Clusters of immature neuroblasts are present between the innermost fetal zone cells. These cells aggregate at birth to form a functional adrenal medulla.

The definitive zone (also referred to as the adult cortex, neocortex, or permanent zone) comprises a narrow band of small, tightly packed basophilic cells that exhibit structural characteristics typical of cells in a proliferative state. Its inner layers form arched cords that send finger-like columns of cells into the outer rim of the fetal zone. Definitive zone cells begin to resemble steroidogenically active cells later in pregnancy, and appear to secrete mineralocorticoids late in the third trimester.

Ultrastructural and functional studies have revealed a third zone between the fetal and definitive zones, referred to as the transitional zone, the cells of which have intermediate characteristics between the fetal and adult zones (see Fig. 11-12). After midgestation, transitional zone cells have the capacity to synthesize cortisol and thus may be analogous to cells of the zona fasciculata of the adult adrenal. By week 30 of gestation, the definitive zone and transitional zone begin to take on the appearance of the zona glomerulosa and the zona fasciculata, respectively. Thus, by late gestation, the fetal adrenal cortex resembles a rudimentary form of the adult adrenal cortex.

The postnatal remodeling of the primate adrenal cortex involves a complex wave of differentiation such that the inner portion of the fetal zone atrophies and the zonae glomerulosa and fasciculata develop.[221] Fetal zone remodeling in the human is an apoptotic process.[222] It has generally been thought that the adult cortical zones develop from the persistent definitive zone. However, there is no evidence of adrenal cortical insufficiency during the perinatal period and the postnatal remodeling process. Thus, it is likely that the nascent adult cortical zones are present and functional before birth. Indeed, morphologic and functional studies have identified rudimentary zonae glomerulosa and fasciculata during late gestation.[223] This lends support to the notion that the postnatal remodeling of the primate adrenal cortex involves apoptosis of a portion of the fetal zone and the simultaneous expansion of preexisting zonae glomerulosa and fasciculata.

ACTH secreted from the fetal pituitary is the principal trophic regulator of the fetal adrenal cortex. However, ACTH may not be acting directly. During the last two thirds of gestation, the fetal zone grows rapidly and produces large amounts of steroids, even though circulating ACTH concentrations do not rise significantly. Soon after birth the fetal zone rapidly involutes but exposure to ACTH continues, albeit at lower concentrations.

Other factors, possibly specific to the intrauterine environment, appear to play a role in the regulation of fetal adrenal cortical growth and function. Substances produced by the placenta (e.g., hCG) have been implicated,[43,224] and peptide growth factors produced locally within the fetal adrenal[225] appear to influence fetal adrenal cortical growth and function by mediating or modulating the trophic actions of ACTH. Specific orphan nuclear receptor transcription factors, including SF-1 (NR5A1) and DAX1 (NR0B1), also appear to be important regulators of adrenal cortical development by influencing early embryonic differentiation of adrenal cortical progenitors and the maintenance of steroidogenic function.[226,227]

Evidence of fetal adrenal steroidogenesis is first seen at 6 to 8 weeks, when the cells in the developing adrenal differentiate and acquire steroidogenic characteristics. At around week 12 of gestation, estriol concentrations in the maternal circulation rapidly increase (approximately 100-fold). This increase coincides with the initiation of fetal zone enlargement and ACTH secretion by the fetal pituitary gland.[220]

These observations indicate that the human fetal adrenal cortex produces DHEA-S beginning at around 8 to 10 weeks in sufficient quantities to cause increases in maternal estrogen levels. Production of DHEA-S by the fetal adrenal cortex continues for the remainder of pregnancy and increases considerably during the second and third trimesters; by term, the human fetal adrenal produces around 200 mg DHEA-S per day. Thus, placental production of estriol directly reflects the steroidogenic activity of the fetal HPA axis. For this reason, maternal estriol previously was used as an endocrine marker to evaluate fetal well-being.

The point at which the fetal adrenal cortex begins producing physiologically relevant amounts of cortisol has yet to be definitively identified. This question has been partially answered, however, by observations of infants with congenital adrenal hyperplasia (CAH). In CAH due to a deficiency of the 21-hydroxylase (P450c21) enzyme, the fetal adrenals cannot synthesize cortisol. As a result, excess ACTH is produced because of loss of glucocorticoid-negative feedback. Female infants with CAH often are born with urogenital sinus defects and virilization primarily caused by exposure of the urogenital sinus to excessive amounts of adrenal androgen. Because this condition derives from adrenal glucocorticoid deficiency, these observations imply that the adrenal produces enough cortisol in female fetuses to regulate ACTH levels and to prevent overproduction of adrenal androgens that may masculinize the female urogenital sinus. These observations also suggest that the human fetal pituitary produces ACTH before 10 weeks of gestation, permitting regulation of fetal adrenal

steroidogenesis. Expression of key steroid metabolizing enzymes suggests that the human fetal adrenal cortex does not produce cortisol de novo from cholesterol until around week 30 of gestation. However, this does not preclude the possibility that cortisol is produced by using progesterone as a precursor early in gestation.[228]

Because the fate of pregnenolone metabolism is initially determined by the branch point steroidogenic enzymes cytochrome P450 17α-hydroxylase/17,20-lyase (P450c17) and 3β-hydroxysteroid dehydrogenase/Δ$^{4-5}$ isomerase (3β-HSD), the steroidogenic potential of cells may be inferred by the pattern of expression of these two enzymes (see Fig. 11-8). Expression of 3β-HSD by the human fetal adrenal cortex is a critical step in the metabolism of pregnenolone because it confers on cells the ability to convert Δ^5-3β-hydroxysteroids to Δ^4-3-ketosteroids essential for mineralocorticoid and glucocorticoid production.

Between 12 and 22 weeks of gestation, the human fetal adrenal cortex does not express 3β-HSD. After 22 weeks, 3β-HSD expression can be detected first in the definitive zone cells and later in gestation in the definitive and transitional zone cells. At no time in gestation is 3β-HSD expression detected in the fetal zone. In contrast, expression of P450c17 is highly abundant in the transitional and fetal zones and is lacking in the definitive zone at all gestational ages.[223,229]

The persistent lack of 3β-HSD and expression of large amounts of P450c17 in the fetal zone is consistent with this cortical compartment producing only C19/Δ^5 steroids, particularly DHEA. The lack of P450c17 in the definitive zone, and the eventual expression of 3β-HSD in this compartment, is consistent with this zone producing mineralocorticoids late in gestation. The co-expression of 3β-HSD and P450c17 in the transitional zone indicates that this zone has the capacity for glucocorticoid production.

Thus, the human fetal adrenal cortex appears to be composed of three functionally distinct zones:

1. The definitive zone, which is the likely site of mineralocorticoid synthesis late in gestation
2. The transitional zone, which appears to be the site of glucocorticoid synthesis late in gestation when it expresses both P450c17 and 3β-HSD
3. The fetal zone, which is the site of Δ^5-steroid production, particularly DHEA (Fig. 11-13)

Steroidogenic enzymes downstream of P450c17 and 3β-HSD also have been examined.[230] Their localization and ontogeny are consistent with the concept that the definitive zone develops to form the zona glomerulosa, the transitional zone is analogous to the zona fasciculata, and the fetal zone is analogous to the zona reticularis.

Mineralocorticoid production by the primate fetal adrenal cortex is low early in gestation but increases during the third trimester. At term, 80% of the aldosterone in human and Rhesus monkey fetal blood appears to originate from the fetal adrenal.[231] In 18- to 21-week human fetal adrenals, the mineralocorticoid metabolic pathway is localized to the definitive zone, but its activity is low and unresponsive to secretagogues.[232,233]

The angiotensin II receptors, AT1 and AT2, are present on human fetal adrenal cortical cells after 16 weeks.[234] The

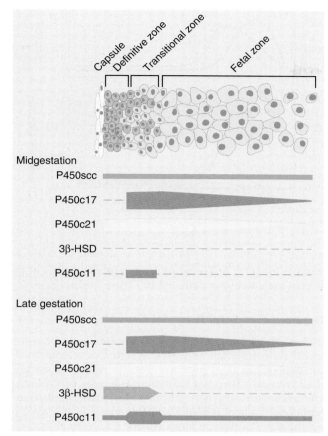

Figure 11-13. *Schematic representation of the localization of expression of P450scc, 3β-hydroxysteroid dehydrogenase (HSD), P450c17, P450c21, and P450c11 in the primate fetal adrenal cortex during midgestation and late gestation. Thickness of the line indicates relative abundance of expression. Dashed line indicates lack of expression. Note the lack of P450c17 expression in the definitive zone at all stages of gestation and the ontogenetic expression of 3β-HSD only in the definitive and transitional zones late in gestation (From Mesiano S, Jaffe RB. Developmental and functional biology of the primate fetal adrenal cortex. Endocr Rev 18:378, 1997.)*

AT2 receptor is localized mainly on definitive zone cells, whereas the AT1 receptor is detectable to a lesser extent in cells from both fetal and definitive zones. Thus, during the first and second trimesters, the ability of the human fetal adrenal cortex to synthesize mineralocorticoids is minimal even though the cells express AT receptors.

THE FETAL PITUITARY-GONADAL AXIS

The foundation for normal puberty and adult reproductive function is established during fetal life. Intrauterine gonadal development is essential for normal sexual development. The consequence of impairment of this system can be irreparable loss of germ cells and reproductive potential. The development of the fetal testis is described in Chapter 16 and that of the fetal ovary in Chapters 8 and 16. Therefore, their development is only encapsulated here from a slightly different perspective.

Sexual development in humans, as in most mammals, can be divided into four stages:

1. Pregonadal
2. Indifferent
3. Primary sex differentiation
4. Secondary sex differentiation

The first three stages and part of the fourth occur in the embryo in the human (first 8 weeks after conception). These facets of embryonic development are pivotal to understanding the subsequent events occurring during human fetal life.

Pregonadal Stage

The pregonadal stage begins with the differentiation of primordial germ cells in 4.5-day-old blastocysts. At this point, there are no specific gonadal structures.

Indifferent Stage

The indifferent stage is the period during embryonic development during which the gonads, sex accessory ducts, and external genitalia of both sexes are morphologically identical. By 5 to 6 weeks the indifferent gonad is composed of primordial germ cells, supporting cells of the coelomic epithelium, and gonadal ridge mesenchyme.

Primary (Gonadal) Sex Differentiation

If the primordial germ cells possess a Y chromosome, testes develop from the indifferent gonads. As described in Chapter 16 and illustrated in Figure 16-4, the development of a male gonad is directed by the sex-determining region of the Y chromosome (SRY). This region encodes a testis-determining factor that, as its name implies, induces the differentiation of the indifferent gonadal cells to form testicular structures.

Development of the Testes. Initially, the primordial germ cells concentrate in the medulla of the indifferent gonad and the cortex regresses. Structures known as medullary cords then develop, which contain germ cells and Sertoli cells; these cords eventually become the seminiferous tubules and rete testes. This is followed by production of müllerian-inhibiting substance (MIS) by the Sertoli cells and the differentiation of mesenchymal somatic cells into Leydig cells. Throughout embryonic and fetal development the Sertoli cells perform important paracrine (MIS) and endocrine (inhibin/activin) functions.[235] Androgen-secreting Leydig cells develop in the testis at 8 weeks. Concentrations of androgens in testicular tissue, blood, and amniotic fluid reach a maximum at 15 to 18 weeks,[236,237] paralleled by an increase in Leydig cell number. Their numbers subsequently decrease, and only a few Leydig cells are seen at term.[238]

Development of the Ovaries. Differentiation of the ovaries occurs several weeks later than that of the testes. If the primordial germ cells lack a Y chromosome, ovaries develop from the indifferent gonads. In this case, the medulla of the indifferent gonad partially regresses and the cortex forms focal structures known as cortical cords in which the primordial germ cells concentrate.

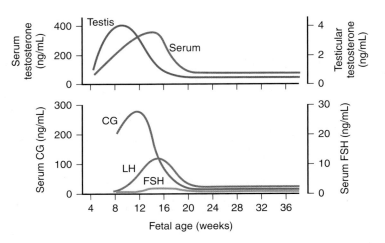

Figure 11-14. *Schematic depiction of serum human chorionic gonadotropin (CG) and pituitary gonadotropin levels in the human fetus and their temporal relationship to testicular and circulating testosterone levels. FSH, follicular-stimulating hormone; LH, luteinizing hormone. (From Wartenberg H Differentiation and development of the testes. In Burger H, DeKretzer D [eds]. The Testis. New York, Raven Press, 1989, p 41.)*

Between 7 and 9 weeks, large ameboid-appearing cells, the majority of which are oogonia, are scattered throughout the ovarian parenchyma. The oogonia then enter the meiotic prophase at around 11 to 12 weeks. With increasing gestational age, more germ cells enter meiosis and go through leptotene, zygotene, and pachytene stages.[239] The diplotene stage of prophase is completed shortly after birth, and oocytes enter a resting stage until puberty. The peak number of germ cells is reached at 16 to 20 weeks, at which time their number increases to about 6 million, with subsequent progressive reduction to about 2 million at term[196] (for a more detailed discussion of this process, see Chapter 8).

At 13.5 to 14 weeks, diplotene oocytes begin to be surrounded by an incomplete layer of flattened follicular cells. After 16 weeks, follicular development intensifies, and shortly thereafter all diplotene oocytes are in primordial follicles (oocytes surrounded by a single layer of flat granulosa cells and a basement membrane without a defined theca cell layer).[240]

Interstitial cells possessing ultrastructural characteristics of steroid-producing cells can be seen after 12 weeks, perhaps accounting for the steroidogenic capacity of the early fetal ovary. During the last trimester, theca cells with steroidogenic capacity surround the developing follicles. Despite this steroidogenic capacity, significant secretion of fetal ovarian steroids is unlikely to occur during most of pregnancy. Few steroids, if any, are produced de novo in the ovary during its development. In fact, there is no apparent need for ovarian steroidogenic function during female fetal and neonatal development.

Secondary (Phenotypic) Sex Differentiation

During secondary sex differentiation, androgen and MIS (see Chapter 16) production by the male testis causes müllerian duct regression and stabilization of the wolffian duct and its derivatives. Androgen produced by the testes then induces the differentiation of the urogenital sinus into the male phenotype. In the absence of these testicular products, the wolffian ducts regress, the müllerian ducts persist, and the female genitalia form in the absence of androgenic exposure. Levels of testicular testosterone and the temporal

relationship with hCG and pituitary gonadotropins in the human male fetus are depicted in Figure 11-14.

Regulation of Fetal Gonadal Growth

Studies of anencephalic fetuses indicate that embryonic sexual differentiation and early gonadal development do not depend on fetal pituitary gonadotropes. In anencephalic fetuses, there is a reduction in Leydig cell number, whereas a reduction in the number of spermatogonia is uncommon.[241] There is also a similar time of appearance of seminiferous tubules in anencephalic and normal fetuses.

In female anencephalic fetuses, the ovary appears to develop normally until 32 weeks; testicular development is impaired earlier. At term, ovaries of anencephalic fetuses are smaller than normal, and central follicles are absent, and proliferation of oogonia with progression through meiosis until development of primordial follicles is not initiated.[241] Thus, pituitary gonadotropins are necessary for granulosa cell/follicular proliferation near term; they are also needed to a lesser extent, through granulosa cell regulation, for oocyte survival.

In at least some mammalian species, Kit ligand (stem cell factor), produced locally by the granulosa cell, influences oocyte development. The receptor for Kit ligand, c-kit, is located on the oocyte.[242-244] On the basis of studies in fetal Rhesus monkeys, fetal pituitary gonadotropins appear necessary for granulosa cell proliferation and follicular fluid formation during the latter part of pregnancy.[245]

Gonadotropic regulation differs for males and females in human and monkey (a model for late gestation) fetal gonads. FSH receptors are present in the second-trimester human and late gestational Rhesus monkey fetal testes.[246] Specific FSH binding is not found in human second-trimester ovaries, but it is present in near-term monkey fetal ovaries.[246] Thus, the ovary develops gonadotropin receptors only at a later stage of pregnancy.

Regulation of Fetal Gonadal Steroidogenesis

In contrast to the ovary, fetal testes exhibit steroidogenic activity and synthesize testosterone de novo.[247,248] Testosterone secretion by Leydig cells is necessary at different stages of pregnancy for adequate growth of internal and external genitalia. In the fetal Rhesus monkey in utero, testosterone production can be elicited by hCG injection and by stimulating the fetal pituitary-testicular axis with GnRH.[210,249] Low-density lipoprotein cholesterol can serve as a precursor for steroid synthesis in the fetal testis and may function as an inducer of testicular steroidogenesis as well.[250] The gradual decline of Leydig cells in the fetus is accompanied by the decline of the mRNA levels of the steroidogenic enzymes P450scc and P450c17.[251] Levels of aromatase activity, necessary for estrogen formation, are low in the fetal testis.[252]

In contrast to the male, ovarian steroid production is not essential for female phenotypic development. Furthermore, meiosis in the ovary begins relatively early, but significant estrogen production does not occur until late in fetal life—although the capacity for aromatization exists by the eighth week.[253] The preponderance of data indicates that although certain enzymatic activity can be demonstrated in the fetal ovary, it cannot form estrogen de novo and is probably steroidogenically quiescent through most of pregnancy.

As with the fetal adrenal cortex, locally produced growth factors, acting in an autocrine/paracrine manner, may play critical roles in controlling the growth and development of the fetal gonads. However, this function has not been studied extensively to date in the human.

THE FETAL PITUITARY-THYROID AXIS

In the human fetus, the thyroid gland acquires its characteristic morphologic appearance and the capacity to concentrate radioiodine and to synthesize iodothyronines by 10 to 12 weeks of gestation.[254] Coincidentally, hypothalamic TRH is detectable at 10 to 12 weeks; by this stage, thyrotropes can be detected in the fetal pituitary and TSH can be found by radioimmunoassay in the fetal pituitary and serum. Thyroxine (T_4) has also been found in the fetal circulation.[254]

Thyroid function remains in a basal state until midgestation. At this time, secretory activity of the thyroid gland and serum T_4 concentrations begin to increase. This rise is likely to be related to the establishment of continuity between the hypothalamic and pituitary portions of the portal vascular system. Pituitary and serum TSH concentrations begin to rise shortly before the rise in T_4 levels. Maximal TSH concentrations are reached early in the third trimester and do not increase further until term.

In the Rhesus monkey, a TSH response to TRH administration is present early in the equivalent of the third trimester.[255] In contrast to the adult, triiodothyronine (T_3) administration to the fetus does not suppress the pituitary TSH response to TRH in primates.[255] The human infant born after 26 to 28 weeks of gestation responds to exogenous administration of TRH with an increase of circulating TSH levels similar to those seen in adults.[254,256]

At term, TSH secretion by the human fetus can be inhibited by the administration of T_4.[256,257] In addition, the elevated cord T_4 is associated with marked suppression of the neonatal TSH surge.[257] This inhibitory effect of T_4 is presumably mediated through pituitary conversion of T_4

to T_3. Human fetal serum T_4 and free T_4 levels increase progressively during the last trimester, although serum TSH levels do not.[257]

Serum T_3 concentrations are usually not measurable in the human fetus until approximately the 30th week of gestation.[257] Thereafter, concentrations rise to a mean level of approximately 50 ng/dL at term. The prenatal increase in serum T_3 concentration occurs during several weeks and may be related to increased cortisol concentration.[258] Immediately after birth (during the first 4 to 6 hours), circulating T_3 levels increase still further to concentrations three to six times those occurring in utero.[258,259]

Reverse T_3 (3,3',5'-triiodothyronine) reaches concentrations in the human fetus greater than 250 ng/dL early in the last trimester and then decreases progressively until term.[257,259,260] In contrast with T_3 levels, serum reverse T_3 concentrations remain virtually unchanged during early neonatal life in term infants.

An acute increase in pituitary TSH levels occurs when the term fetus is exposed to the extrauterine environment. This, in turn, stimulates thyroidal iodine uptake and evokes release of thyroid hormones. The maximal TSH concentrations are attained 30 minutes after birth. Thereafter, there is a rapid decrease in serum TSH during the first day of extrauterine life and a slower decrease during the succeeding 2 days. Serum T_4 and free T_4 levels reach a peak at 24 hours and then decrease slowly during the first weeks of life.[261]

Binding of iodothyronine and maturation of thyroid hormone receptors have not been reported in the human fetus. In the rat, hepatic nuclear T_3 receptors mature during the first few weeks after birth.[262] T_3 receptor capacity, and possibly affinity, increases during the first 3 to 4 weeks. In the brain (in contrast with the liver) T_3 nuclear receptor binding develops early, is comparable with that in the adult brain, and increases still further in the first 3 days of neonatal life.[263]

However, there appears to be a discrepancy between T_3 nuclear receptor binding and brain tissue responsiveness in both the neonate and the adult. Neither appears to respond to exogenous T_3 administration with an increase in oxygen, α-glycerophosphate dehydrogenase, or malic enzyme consumption.[263] Of interest is the observation that thyroid hormones increase nerve growth factor concentrations in adult and newborn mouse brain[264]; it has been postulated that this nerve growth factor may mediate the effects of thyroid hormones on brain development.[263]

FETAL PITUITARY GROWTH HORMONE

GH is produced and secreted by the human fetal pituitary from around 8 to 10 weeks of gestation.[265,266] Levels of GH in the fetal circulation peak at around 6 nmol/L at midgestation, then gradually decrease for the remainder of gestation to around 1.5 nmol/L at term. The peak in GH at midgestation is thought to be due to unrestrained secretion because cultured pituitary cells from 9- to 16-week fetuses respond to GHRH with increased GH secretion; they are far less responsive to inhibition by SS.[267] Alternatively, negative feedback pathways for the regulation of GH secretion may develop later than GHRH stimulation. The physiologic control of pituitary GH production and secretion is mature by term, and circulating GH responds appropriately to GHRH, SS, insulin, and arginine.[265,266]

The role of fetal pituitary GH is unclear. Anencephalic fetuses on average are of normal size and weight, suggesting that fetal growth is controlled by factors other than fetal pituitary GH. Placental GH and PL are likely candidates. Clearly, pituitary GH is required for postnatal growth and development, and therefore this system must be mature at birth. However, it likely plays a minimal role in the control of fetal somatic growth.

FETAL PITUITARY PROLACTIN

Levels of PRL in the fetal circulation are very low during the first half of human pregnancy. The pituitary begins secreting PRL at 25 to 30 weeks, gradually secreting more for the remainder of gestation and reaches a peak at term.[266] The level of *PRL* gene expression by the fetal pituitary increases progressively from around 15 weeks. In anencephalic fetuses, pituitary PRL content is within the normal range, indicating that its production by the pituitary is independent of hypothalamic control during most of gestation.[266]

Control of PRL secretion by TRH and dopamine matures late in pregnancy and during the first few months after birth.[265,266] In cultured pituitary cells obtained from midgestation human fetuses, estrogen stimulates and dopamine inhibits PRL secretion.[265] Interestingly, the increase in fetal PRL levels with ongoing gestation coincides with increases in estrogen levels, indicating that its production by the fetal pituitary is primarily regulated by estrogen during most of pregnancy. The role of PRL in fetal development remains uncertain.

LONG-TERM EFFECTS OF FETAL NEUROENDOCRINE MATURATION

The appropriate functional maturation of neuroendocrine systems during fetal life has profound effects on long-term health into adulthood. This phenomenon, referred to as developmental origins of adult disease, arose through epidemiologic observations that show an association between perturbations of intrauterine nutritional status and the development of hypertension, insulin resistance, and obesity that predispose to cardiovascular disease, diabetes, and the metabolic syndrome in adulthood.[268-276]

The developmental origins model predicts functional plasticity in the development of fetal neuroendocrine and organ systems such that a single genotype gives rise to multiple "normal" phenotypes in response to environmental cues (e.g., extent of maternal nutrition and stress) mediated through the maternal organism. Thus, the fetus prepares itself for the extrauterine environment by modulating its physiologic set points to match the anticipated environmental based in maternal cues. Interestingly, the period of neuroendocrine plasticity is limited and the physiologic changes appear to be permanent; plasticity does not continue later in life. For example, studies in animals show that changes in basal and stress-induced fetal HPA activity induced in utero by maternal starvation

persist after birth. The altered stress-response pathway may underpin pathophysiologic conditions that develop during adulthood.[273] Detrimental effects occur when there is a mismatch between the neuroendocrine program determined in utero and the environmental conditions encountered after birth.

The physiologic, biochemical, and genetic mechanisms that mediate the reactive plasticity of fetal neuroendocrine development are not clearly defined. The placenta is thought to play an active role, although it remains uncertain how information regarding the environment is transmitted from the mother through the placenta to the fetus. As described earlier in the chapter, the placenta produced a plethora of hormones that could influence the developmental trajectories of fetal neuroendocrine axes. For example, CRH production by the placenta may modulate the responsiveness of the fetal adrenal cortex to ACTH and therefore contribute to the establishment of the HPA setpoint.[277] Clearly, further studies are needed to unravel the endocrine interactions that underlie this critical developmental process.

Nevertheless, accumulating evidence from animal studies and human epidemiologic studies demonstrate that the fetus can adjust its physiology in response to variations in maternal nutrition status and that these changes persist into adulthood and can sometimes underlie pathologic conditions. Remarkably, studies in sheep indicate that maternal nutrition status before conception influences fetal growth and length of gestation, suggesting that pre-implantation blastocyst or the endometrium might be programmed by nutritional status.[278] Whether the findings from animal studies can be extrapolated to the human condition is not certain; however, the consensus is that the central tenet of the developmental origins of adult disease model likely applies to human pregnancy.

Fetal Maturation and Timing of Parturition

FETAL ORGAN MATURATION AND PREPARATION FOR EXTRAUTERINE LIFE

At birth the fetus is abruptly required to establish and maintain physiologic homeostasis independently of the placenta and in a markedly altered environment. Therefore, survival of the neonate is dependent upon the functional maturation of organ systems essential for the transition from intrauterine to extrauterine life. Critical among these are organs that interface with the environment and extract resources (e.g., lungs, gut, and immune system) and those that maintain homeostasis (e.g., the HPA axis, kidneys, liver, and pancreas). The coordination of fetal maturation and the timing of parturition such that birth occurs when the fetus is sufficiently mature to survive as a newborn is therefore critical for neonatal survival.

Many studies in multiple species have demonstrated that glucocorticoids promote the functional maturation of fetal organ systems.[279,280] Critical processes induced by glucocorticoids include surfactant production by the fetal lungs; activity of enzyme systems in the fetal gut, retina, pancreas, thyroid gland and brain; and deposition of glycogen in the fetal liver. In sheep, fetal organ maturation is induced by a prepartum surge in cortisol secretion by the fetal adrenals.[281] The cortisol surge also triggers the onset of labor. Thus, in sheep, the fetal HPA axis, by means of cortisol, mediates a physiologic link between the timing of parturition and fetal organ maturation.

The effect of glucocorticoids on the maturation of the fetal lungs is especially important. The inability to exchange gases due to pulmonary immaturity (respiratory distress syndrome) is the leading cause of neonatal morbidity and death among preterm infants. Synthetic glucocorticoids that readily cross the placenta are a standard form of therapy administered to women in preterm labor. This treatment significantly increases survival rates among preterm infants mainly by promoting lung maturation and decreasing the severity of respiratory distress syndrome.

In the human, maturation of fetal organ systems is accelerated by treatment with synthetic glucocorticoids. However, the extent to which cortisol from the fetal adrenals regulate fetal organ maturation is uncertain. Experiments of nature suggest that maturation of the human fetus during late gestation is independent of fetal adrenal cortisol production. Fetuses with CAH due to P450c21 deficiency produce markedly reduced levels of cortisol, yet these infants are usually born at term without any apparent signs of organ immaturity.[282] This observation suggests that cortisol produced by the fetal adrenal gland is not essential for fetal organ maturation; another source of glucocorticoid, possibly from the maternal adrenals, could contribute to the stimulation of fetal organ maturation at the end of human gestation; or maturation of the human fetus is not dependent upon glucocorticoids alone and other factors may be involved.

Although cortisol stimulates maturation of fetal organ systems, it also can have adverse effects on fetal development. As described previously, to protect the fetus from these negative effects the human placenta prevents maternal cortisol from entering the fetal compartment throughout most of human pregnancy by expressing the 11β-HSD-2 enzyme that converts cortisol to the inactive cortisone.[204] Thus, for most of pregnancy the placenta forms a biochemical barrier to maternal cortisol.

Late in human pregnancy (around 34 to 35 weeks), however, the placental barrier to maternal cortisol weakens, at least partially. The evidence for this is that estriol levels in the maternal circulation during late pregnancy are inversely related to the circadian changes in circulating maternal cortisol levels.[283] Thus, when maternal cortisol goes up, estriol goes down. This implies that, late in gestation, some maternal cortisol crosses the placenta to the fetal compartment and suppresses ACTH production by the fetal pituitary gland that leads to decreased DHEA-S production by the fetal adrenals and in turn decreased estriol production by the placenta. Increased transfer of maternal cortisol to the fetus may represent a backup mechanism to ensure fetal lung maturation. This may explain why fetuses with glucocorticoid deficiency are born without overt signs of organ system immaturity.

THE PROCESS OF HUMAN PARTURITION

The process of parturition involves (1) transformation of the myometrium from a quiescent to a highly contractile phenotype; (2) remodeling of the uterine cervix such that it softens and dilates to allow passage of the fetus; and (3) rupture of the fetal membranes. These temporally coordinated events can be divided into distinct phases based on the contractile activity of the myometrium[284] (Fig. 11-15).

Phase 0 (Quiescence)

For most of pregnancy the myometrium is in a state of relaxation and relatively insensitive to stimulatory uterotonins, such as prostaglandins (PGs) and oxytocin (OT). In addition the uterine cervix remains closed and rigid. This period, referred to as Phase 0 or quiescence, is controlled by pro-pregnancy relaxatory uterotropins (factors that modulate uterine function and growth) and uterotonins

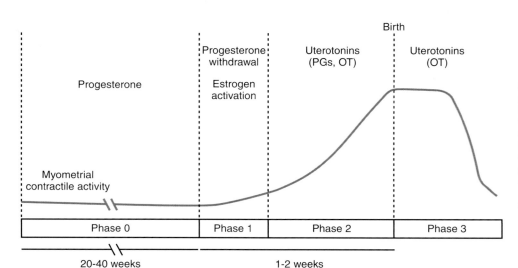

Figure 11-15. Phases of human parturition based on myometrial contractile activity and the principal regulatory uterotropins and uterotonins involved. OT, oxytocin; PGs, prostaglandins (Adapted from Casey ML, Macdonald PC. Endocrine changes of pregnancy. In Wilson JD, Foster DW, Kronenberg HM, Larsen PR [eds]. Williams Textbook of Endocrinology. Philadelphia, WB Saunders, 1998, p 1259.)

(factors that modulate uterine contraction) such as progesterone, β-adrenergic agents, prostacyclin (PGI$_2$), relaxin, CRH, parathyroid hormone-related peptide, and nitric oxide. In general, factors that activate adenylate cyclase and increase intracellular cAMP (e.g., by means of G$_{\alpha s}$-protein–coupled receptors) promote myometrial relaxation.

Phase 1 (Transformation)

Parturition begins with the transition from Phase 0 to Phase 1. As an essential prelude to active labor, the myometrium undergoes a phenotypic transformation whereby it gains the capacity to contract forcibly and rhythmically and becomes more responsive to uterotonins. The awakening of the quiescent uterus is initiated by progesterone withdrawal and increased estrogenic drive and is characterized by distinct biophysical changes in the myometrium.

Transformation of the myometrium involves the increased expression of a specific cohort of genes, collectively referred to as *contraction-associated proteins* (CAPs).[279] Some important CAPs include connexins (e.g., connexin-43), which form gap junctions between myometrial cells, allowing rapid electrical and chemical signaling between adjacent cells to permit coordinated contractions; ion channels (e.g., calcium channels), which determine the resting membrane potential and excitability; uterotonin receptors (e.g., OT and PG receptors); and enzymes that determine the rate of local uterotonin synthesis (e.g., PG synthase type 2 [PGHS-2]). Concurrently, the uterine cervix gradually softens and becomes more elastic due to increased expression of collagenase enzymes. In addition, intrauterine production of PGE$_2$ and PGF$_{2\alpha}$ increases.

Phase 2 (Activation)

The increased myometrial exposure to PGs and its augmented responsiveness to PGs and OT eventually initiate Phase 2, which is defined by the onset of active labor. During Phase 2, uterotonic drive induces coordinated rhythmic contractions that eventually become more forceful as labor progresses. At the peak of active labor the myometrium is one of the strongest muscles (on a per weight basis) in the human body. As the cervix effaces and becomes more compliant, the contractions progressively move the fetus toward the birth canal. As contractions become more pronounced the force of the fetus against the lower uterine segment dilates the softened cervix enough for it and the placenta to pass through the birth canal.

Phase 3 (Hemostasis and Involution)

Phase 3 begins after the placenta is expelled. Importantly, myometrial contraction is sustained (mainly in response to OT) during this time, which helps constrict the spiral arterioles to facilitate postpartum uterine hemostasis. During the following weeks the uterus gradually reverts back to the menstrual state through a combination of myometrial cell apoptosis and atrophy. In addition, the cervix remodels and reverts to the closed and rigid state.

THE HORMONAL CONTROL OF PARTURITION

Efforts to unravel the hormonal control of parturition were pioneered in the 1930s and 1940s by George Corner and Willard Allen, who identified the progestational substance produced by the CL that sustains pregnancy in rabbits.[285] The so-called "progestin" was found to be a steroid and was therefore named progesterone. Subsequent studies by Arpad Csapo, in a variety of species, led to the progesterone block hypothesis,[286] which posits that for most of pregnancy progesterone actively blocks parturition by promoting myometrial quiescence, and that labor is initiated by progesterone withdrawal.

Early studies also found that estrogens (mainly estradiol) oppose the actions of progesterone by stimulating biochemical and physical changes in the uterus and fetal membranes needed for labor and delivery. In general, estrogens increase myometrial contractile capacity and excitability by increasing CAP gene expression. Estrogens also increase collagenase expression by in the cervix and PG production by the fetal membranes.

Thus, the contractile activity of the pregnancy myometrium is determined by the balance between the relaxatory actions of progesterone and the stimulatory actions of estrogens. During most of pregnancy the relaxatory actions of progesterone (i.e., the progesterone block) prevail. Parturition is initiated by progesterone withdrawal, which permits the stimulatory estrogenic actions to increase myometrial contractility and excitability and promote cervical softening.

The hormonal control of parturition involves fetal and maternal signals that induce progesterone withdrawal. For example, parturition in sheep is triggered by an exponential rise in cortisol production 1 to 2 weeks before term due to increased activity of the fetal hypothalamic-pituitary-adrenal (HPA) axis.[287-290] The prepartum cortisol surge induces expression of the P450c17 enzyme in the ovine placenta.[291] This enzyme converts progesterone to androstenedione, which can then be used as substrate for estrogen synthesis (see Fig. 11-8). The net effect of P450c17 induction is that placental progesterone production declines (systemic progesterone withdrawal) and estrogen production increases (systemic estrogen activation)—changes that transform the uterus and cervix and initiate the onset of labor. Thus, in sheep the fetus controls the timing of its birth through the activity of its HPA axis. This system ensures that parturition is coordinated with fetal maturation, because cortisol is the principal regulator of both events.[292,293]

A role for the fetal hypothalamic-pituitary axis in the control of human parturition was first proposed by Malpas in 1933[294] based on observations that gestation was prolonged in some pregnancies in which the fetus was anencephalic. However, the specificity and severity of the hypothalamic-pituitary lesions varied markedly, and information regarding the functional status of the fetal HPA axis was scant. Subsequent studies showed that human parturition is not exclusively controlled by the activity of the fetal HPA axis.[282,295,296] These inconsistencies highlight the fact that hormonal interactions that control the timing of parturition differ markedly between species. In contrast to the sheep, the human placenta lacks P450c17

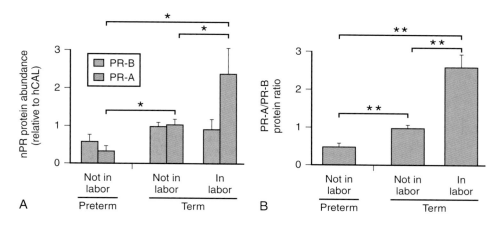

Figure 11-16. *Relative abundance of progesterone receptor (PR)-A and PR-B proteins (A) and the PR-A/PR-B protein ratio (B) in lower uterine segment myometrium obtained from term and preterm cesarean section deliveries. Each bar is mean ± SEM. * P < 0.05; ** P < 0.001. (From Merlino AA, Welsh TN, Tan H, et al. Nuclear progesterone receptors in the human pregnancy myometrium: evidence that parturition involves functional progesterone withdrawal mediated by increased expression of progesterone receptor-A. J Clin Endocrinol Metab 92:1927, 2007.)*

and therefore placental progesterone and estrogen production is sustained during parturition.

Factors that trigger parturition were likely selected through evolution to match the overall reproductive strategy employed by a particular species. For example, sheep give birth to relatively mature neonates on a seasonal basis, whereas humans give birth to remarkably immature babies throughout the year. The evolutionary forces that led to such differences are likely to have influenced the hormonal mechanisms controlling the timing of parturition. Multiple redundant physiologic triggers for parturition may have evolved in the human. In this context, it is likely that the uniquely human traits of bipedalism, which decreased the size of the pelvic outlet, and encephalization, which increased the size of the fetal head, exerted strong selective pressure on the birth timing mechanism so that the big-headed fetus is born before it outgrows the narrowed pelvic opening. This could explain why the human neonate is so immature.

Despite the multiple strategies for parturition control, several hormonal interactions have been preserved in all viviparous species:

1. The initiation of parturition by progesterone withdrawal and estrogen activation
2. A contribution by the fetoplacental unit to the hormonal control of pregnancy to establish a link between fetal organ maturation and the timing of parturition
3. The involvement of uterotonins, particularly prostaglandins and oxytocin, in the induction and progression of labor

PROGESTERONE WITHDRAWAL AND ESTROGEN ACTIVATION IN HUMAN PARTURITION

The onset of labor in most species is preceded by a dramatic decrease in maternal progesterone levels and a concomitant increase in maternal estradiol. In humans, however, progesterone withdrawal and estrogen activation are not mediated by changes in circulating progesterone and estrogen levels (see Fig. 11-11), which are high during most of pregnancy and remain elevated during labor

and delivery. To explain this conundrum it is proposed that progesterone withdrawal and estrogen activation in human parturition are mediated by functional changes in myometrial progesterone and estrogen responsiveness.

Functional Progesterone Withdrawal

Myometrial progesterone responsiveness is primarily determined by the extent and activity of nPRs and associated co-regulators. In most human cell types and in the majority of promoter systems examined to date, PR-B is the principal ligand-dependent transcriptional modulator of progesterone-responsive genes. The relaxatory actions of progesterone on the pregnancy myometrium are thought to be mediated by PR-B. In contrast, PR-A binds progesterone with equal affinity, but in most cells and promoter constructs it represses the transcriptional activity mediated by PR-B.[297-300] Thus, PR-A and PR-B form a dual system of target cell-mediated control of progesterone action whereby PR-B mediates, and PR-A suppresses, progesterone responsiveness. In most cells, the extent to which PR-A suppresses progesterone responsiveness depends upon its abundance relative to PR-B (i.e., the PR-A/PR-B expression ratio). Thus, genomic progesterone responsiveness is determined by the PR-A/PR-B ratio.

This general observation led to the PR-A/PR-B hypothesis, which posits that progesterone withdrawal in human parturition is mediated by an increase in the myometrial PR-A/PR-B ratio and that PR-A represses the relaxatory and progestational actions of progesterone mediated through PR-B. Consistent with this hypothesis several studies have found that the PR-A represses the transcriptional activity of PR-B in myometrial cells and that the onset of labor is associated with a significant increase in myometrial PR-A expression and a rise in the PR-A/PR-B expression ratio (Fig. 11-16).[301-303]

Functional progesterone withdrawal could also be mediated by the inhibition of PR-B interaction with target DNA. Studies in term human decidua indicate that the onset of labor involves changes in the nPR transcriptional complex leading to a decrease in DNA association.[304] In the myometrium, labor is associated with a decline in specific nPR coactivators, particularly cAMP-response element-binding protein-binding protein and steroid receptor coactivators-2 and -3.[305] The reduction in coactivators may decrease histone acetylation that effectively closes chromatin around the progesterone response element, making it inaccessible to the nPR transcriptional complex. Such a scenario would explain the decrease in nPR binding to nuclear response elements in decidual cells.[304]

As a variation on this theme, Dong and colleagues[306] identified a protein known as polypirimidine tract-binding protein-associated splicing factor (PTB) that specifically inhibits nPR transactivation and whose expression in rat myometrium increases at term. They proposed that this factor contributes to functional progesterone withdrawal by acting as an additional nPR co-repressor.

Functional Estrogen Activation

In most species, maternal estrogen levels rise prior to delivery, indicating the involvement of circulating estrogens in the initiation of parturition. In humans, this rise occurs gradually over the final weeks of pregnancy and is dependent on fetal adrenal steroidogenic activity. However, congenital abnormalities affecting function of the fetoplacental unit (such as anencephaly, congenital adrenal lipoid hyperplasia, placental aromatase deficiency, and placenta sulfatase deficiency) do not affect the timing of birth. Thus, relatively little estrogen is required for normal human pregnancy and parturition.

The effect of augmented placental estrogen synthesis on the timing of parturition can be observed in pregnancies in which the fetus has CAH due to P450c21 deficiency. In these pregnancies, cortisol production by the fetal adrenals is markedly reduced, leading to abnormally high ACTH production by the fetal pituitary. This in turn increases DHEA-S production because C19 androgen production is not affected by P450c21 deficiency. The increased DHEA-S permits increased estrogen production by the placenta. Despite markedly elevated placental estrogen production throughout most of pregnancy, individuals with CAH generally do not deliver before term.[282] This outcome is inconsistent with studies in the Rhesus monkey in which preterm birth was induced by increased placental estrogen production.[307,308] Thus, increased estrogen synthetic activity by the human fetoplacental unit beyond the already high level does not appear to be involved in the initiation of human parturition. These observations suggest that, as with functional progesterone withdrawal, estrogenic actions in human parturition are mediated by changes in myometrial responsiveness (i.e., functional estrogen activation) rather than by circulating estrogen levels.

The human estrogen receptor exists as two major subtypes, ERα and ERβ[309] (see Chapter 5). Expression of ERα by the human pregnancy myometrium increases significantly at term in association with the onset of labor, whereas ERβ expression in the human myometrium is very low and not affected by the onset of labor.[302] The rise in ERα expression is directly associated with Cx43 expression, a key estrogen-responsive CAP gene. This suggests that the increase in ERα expression at parturition increased myometrial responsiveness to circulating estrogen (i.e., functional estrogen activation).[302]

Coordination of Functional Progesterone Withdrawal and Functional Estrogen Activation

Numerous studies in a variety of species have demonstrated functional interaction between the ER and PR systems such that progesterone decreases uterine estrogen responsiveness by decreasing ER expression, and estrogen increases uterine progesterone responsiveness by increasing PR expression. This interaction may have evolved to ensure an appropriate physiologic outcome despite wide variability in the circulating hormone levels. For example, during the menstrual cycle autoregulation of responsiveness to estrogen and progesterone may ensure an intrauterine environment conducive to embryo survival and implantation, even though estrogen and progesterone levels vary markedly between cycles.

Similarly, during human pregnancy, the myometrium is exposed to elevated and highly variable levels of progesterone and estrogens, yet outcome is usually consistent (i.e., delivery at term). In this context, interaction between the myometrial ER and PR systems may be of major importance. Levels of ERα expression in quiescent term human myometrium correlate positively with the PR-A/PR-B expression ratio.[302] These findings suggest that as myometrial progesterone responsiveness decreases due to increases expression of PR-A, expression of ERα increases.

It is possible that during most of human pregnancy progesterone decreases estrogen responsiveness by inhibiting myometrial ERα expression. This would explain why the myometrium is refractory to the estrogenic drive for most of pregnancy. Early in the parturition cascade myometrial PR-A expression increases leading to a decrease in genomic progesterone responsiveness due to the repression of PR-B transcriptional activity. The gradual inhibition of PR-B–mediated progesterone actions removes the inhibition of ERα expression leading to a concomitant increase in ERα expression levels, which would allow circulating estrogens to increase expression of CAP genes and transform the uterus to a contractile phenotype. Thus, during human pregnancy, progesterone may not only suppress expression of CAP genes directly involved with myometrial contractility but also diminish responsiveness of the myometrium to estrogenic drive (Fig. 11-17).

Such a system, in which hormone action is principally controlled by target cell responsiveness, requires circulating hormone to be present; however, the level is not critical, provided that it is above a minimal value. This paradigm would explain why inhibition of progesterone action alone (e.g., with RU486) is sufficient to initiate the full parturition cascade. In addition, suppression of estrogen responsiveness by progesterone may explain why parturition is not initiated prematurely by naturally occurring conditions in which estrogen levels are increased above normal.

CONTROL OF PROGESTERONE WITHDRAWAL

The general paradigm regarding the physiologic control of human birth timing is that multiple and possibly redundant hormonal signals initiate parturition by converging to

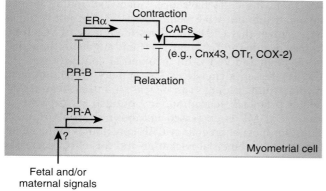

Figure 11-17. *Theoretical model for the role of the myometrial estrogen receptor (ER) and progesterone receptor (PR) systems in the regulation of human pregnancy and parturition. For most of pregnancy, progesterone acting through PR-B inhibits contraction-associated protein (CAP) gene expression and expression of ERα. At term, expression of PR-A increases leading to functional progesterone withdrawal through its inhibition of PR-B action. As a consequence, expression of ERα increases, leading to increased myometrial responsiveness to circulating estrogens, i.e., estrogen activation. Estrogens increase CAP expression leading to increased myometrial contractility and excitability (From Mesiano S. Myometrial progesterone responsiveness and the control of human parturition. J Soc Gynecol Invest 11:193, 2004.)*

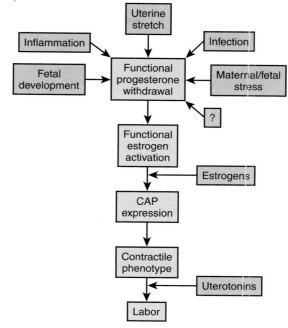

Figure 11-18. *Theoretical model for how various physiologic inputs initiate the human parturition cascade by inducing functional progesterone withdrawal in the myometrium. CAP, contraction-associated protein.*

induce functional progesterone withdrawal. In this context the hormonal control of myometrial progesterone responsiveness, and especially PR-A expression, is a central issue.

Studies in human myometrial cell lines showed that $PGF_{2\alpha}$ stimulates PR-A expression and increases the PR-A/PR-B expression ratio.[310] This finding suggests that functional progesterone withdrawal in human parturition is induced by $PGF_{2\alpha}$.

In women, administration of $PGF_{2\alpha}$ induces labor and delivery at all stages of pregnancy. However, in contrast to its potent and almost instantaneous uterotonic actions when administered to women in active labor (Phase 2), the induction of labor by $PGF_{2\alpha}$ in a quiescent (Phase 0) uterus occurs after a latency of 15 to 20 hours.[311,312] This likely represents the time needed for the myometrium to transform to a contractile state and indicates that $PGF_{2\alpha}$ has uterotrophic as well as a uterotonic actions.

The induction of Phase 1 by a hormone involved in Phase 2 suggests the existence of a positive feedback hormonal loop in the process of human parturition. The following hormonal cascade has been suggested: (1) progesterone maintains myometrial relaxation via genomic pathways mediated by specific PRs; (2) functional genomic progesterone withdrawal is mediated by increased myometrial expression of PR-A; (3) functional progesterone withdrawal induces functional estrogen activation by means of increased myometrial ERα expression, (4) circulating estrogens increase myometrial CAP expression and uterotonin (including $PGF_{2\alpha}$) production and responsiveness, and (5) a variety of factors (including $PGF_{2\alpha}$) induce functional progesterone withdrawal by increasing myometrial PR-A expression (Fig. 11-18).

Normal term labor is associated with, and possibly preceded by, increased PG production by the fetal membranes

and decidua.[313] Importantly, abnormal parturition could also involve the same process and this interaction may underlie infection/inflammation-associated preterm labor. For example, the laboring myometrium contains a large number of infiltrating lymphocytes[314] that could produce enough $PGF_{2\alpha}$ and possibly other inflammatory cytokines to cause functional progesterone withdrawal and initiate the parturition cascade.

This model predicts that pro-inflammatory cytokines produced locally as part of an inflammatory response within the gestational tissues initiate parturition by inducing functional progesterone withdrawal in the myometrium. A significant proportion of preterm births are associated with clinically silent upper genital tract infection and bacterial vaginosis.[315-317] The inflammatory drive to the myometrium need not be local; maternal periodontal disease has also been identified as a risk factor for preterm birth.[318-321] In the Rhesus monkey activation of the inflammatory system precedes the onset of labor,[322] and studies in mice have shown that administration of the key inflammatory cytokine interleukin 1 (IL-1) initiates preterm labor.[323] Thus, a considerable body of data supports the concept that the maternal immune system represents a key trigger for the initiation of human parturition. It is possible that fetal stress initiates parturition via a similar mechanism.

Uterine stretch has also been proposed as a signal for the induction of parturition. Such a mechanism would ensure that the fetus does not grow larger than the pelvic opening. In general, gestation is shorter in twin pregnancies,[324,325] presumably in part due to the increased stretch imposed on the uterine wall. Studies in rats have shown that distention of a nonpregnant uterine horn induces changes

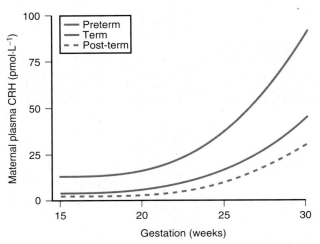

Figure 11-19. *Schematic representation of the association between changes in maternal plasma corticotropin-releasing hormone (CRH) levels between 15 and 30 weeks of gestation and the timing of birth. (From McLean M, Bisits A, Davies J, et al. A placental clock controlling the length of human pregnancy. Nat Med 1:460, 1995.)*

in CAP gene expression similar to those in the pregnant horn and that progesterone inhibits stretch-induced CAP gene expression.[326-328] The stimulatory effect of stretch on CAP gene expression was also observed in cultured human myometrial cells.[329-333] These data show that myometrial stretch contributes to the parturition process.

Thus, multiple physiologic signals (normal and pathologic) may converge on the pregnancy myometrium to induce functional progesterone withdrawal either directly (e.g., by increasing PR-A expression or altering the cohort of nPR co-regulators) or indirectly (e.g., by increasing local $PGF_{2\alpha}$ production or sensitivity to PGs). The induction of functional progesterone withdrawal may be a pivotal integrative step in the hormonal control of human parturition.

ROLE OF PLACENTAL CRH IN THE CONTROL OF HUMAN PARTURITION

A unique feature of primate pregnancy is that the placenta produces CRH in increasing amounts during gestation.[334] Studies of maternal CRH levels during human pregnancy suggest that placental CRH plays a role in the physiology of parturition. Concentrations of CRH in the maternal circulation and the rate of change as gestation progresses are predictive of the gestation length.[116] The trajectory of maternal CRH levels at midgestation are indicative of whether parturition will occur at term, preterm, or post-term (Fig. 11-19).

Interestingly, the exponential rise in maternal plasma CRH concentrations with advancing pregnancy is associated with a concomitant fall in the concentrations of the CRH-binding protein in late pregnancy.[116] The implication of these reciprocal concentration curves is that there is a rapid increase in circulating levels of bioavailable CRH concurrent with the onset of parturition.

CRH may be involved directly in the regulation of human parturition by modulating myometrial contractility.

Receptors for CRH have been identified in the human myometrium and fetal membranes.[335-338] In vitro studies have shown that CRH stimulates the release of PGs from human decidua and amnion,[339,340] and augments the action of oxytocin and $PGF_{2\alpha}$ on myometrial contractility.[341-343] CRH increases adenylate cyclase activity in the quiescent myometrium, leading to an increase in intracellular cAMP, which promotes relaxation. In contrast, its capacity to increase cAMP is decreased in laboring myometrium.[344] Thus, for most of pregnancy CRH contributes to the maintenance of myometrial relaxation and this effect decreases as part of the parturition process. Whether changes in CRH receptor signaling contribute to the onset of labor remains unknown.

As previously mentioned, the existence of an extrahypothalamic source of CRH may have profound effects on the activity of the fetoplacental unit. In particular, a positive feedback endocrine loop may develop between placental CRH and the fetal adrenal cortex as a consequence of the direct action of CRH on the fetal adrenal cortex and the stimulation of placental CRH expression by cortisol. In addition, CRH may increase ACTH responsiveness in fetal adrenal cortical cells (especially cells in the transitional zone) by increasing ACTH receptor expression in fetal adrenal cortical cells.[277] As a result, fetal adrenal cortisol and placental estrogen synthesis increase through a positive feedback loop involving placental CRH (Fig. 11-20). The role of this hormonal loop in the physiology of human parturition is not clearly understood.

ROLE OF UTEROTONINS IN HUMAN PARTURITION

Uterotonins are substances that modulate myometrial tone and contractility (see also Chapter 26). These factors play pivotal roles in human pregnancy and parturition by controlling myometrial contractility. The main uterotonins involved in human labor are OT and PGs (mainly PGE_2 and $PGF_{2\alpha}$). In addition, the PGs (especially PGE_2) also promote cervical ripening. The physiologic actions of PGs and oxytocin are thought to be terminal events in the human parturitional cascade and occur distal to progesterone withdrawal and estrogen activation. Therefore, disruption of PG and OT action has attracted considerable attention as tocolytic strategies for the treatment of preterm labor.

Prostaglandins

A considerable body of data has accumulated in the last 30 to 40 years demonstrating that PGs produced by intrauterine tissues are critical regulators of myometrial contractility (see Chapter 6). Key among these are the following observations:

- Administration of $PGF_{2\alpha}$ at any stage of human pregnancy will induce uterine contractions and cervical ripening and cause labor and delivery.[345,346]
- Inhibition of PG biosynthesis with aspirin, indomethacin, or specific PGHS-2 inhibitors suppresses labor and prolongs gestation.[347,348]

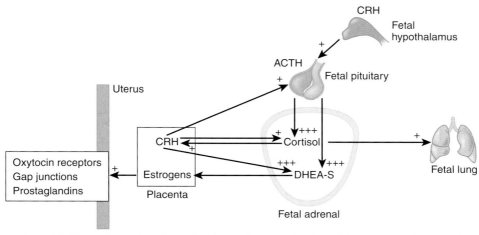

Figure 11-20. *Schematic model of how placental corticotropin-releasing hormone (CRH) modulates activity of the fetoplacental unit. An increase in bioactive placental CRH at term has effects on both the fetus and the mother. In the fetus, CRH stimulates the fetal adrenal directly, to stimulate production of dehydroepiandrosterone sulfate (DHEA-S), which is converted by the placenta to estrogen, which in turn, drives expression of contraction-associated proteins (CAPs) necessary for uterine contractions and parturition. The placental CRH may also act on the fetal adrenal cortex by up-regulating adrenocorticotropic hormone (ACTH) receptor expression and increasing responsiveness to ACTH, which evokes fetal adrenal cortisol production from the definitive transitional zones and DHEA-S production from the fetal zone. A positive-feedback loop is thus started as fetal adrenal cortisol production, in turn, stimulates CRH production by the placenta. (From Smith R, Mesiano S, Chan EC, et al. Corticotropin-releasing hormone directly and preferentially stimulates dehydroepiandrosterone sulfate secretion by human fetal adrenal cortical cells. J Clin Endocrinol Metab 83:2916, 1998.)*

- Production of PGE_2 and $PGF_{2\alpha}$ by intrauterine tissues (particularly the amnion, chorion, decidua, and myometrium) increases late in gestation and in association with the onset of labor.[313]

The regulation of intrauterine PG production is considered to be a pivotal event in human parturition. The rate-limiting step in PGE and PGF biosynthesis is catalyzed by PGHS-1 and PGHS-2 enzymes also known as cyclooxygenase-1 (COX-1) and cyclooxygenase-2 (COX-2), respectively (see Chapter 6). PGHS-1 appears to be constitutively expressed in most tissue types, whereas PGHS-2 expression is inducible, increasing in response to various physiologic conditions such as inflammation.

PGs are metabolized by the prostaglandin dehydrogenase (PGDH) enzyme, which irreversibly converts PGE_2 and $PGF_{2\alpha}$ to inactive forms. Intrauterine biosynthesis of PGs occurs mainly in the amnion and, to a lesser extent, in the chorion. Both tissues express PGHS-2, which increases in association with the onset of term and preterm labor (Fig. 11-21).

PGs also are produced in the decidua and in the myometrium, and in both sites, production increases with labor. In the fetal membranes, PGHS-2 expression increases during the third trimester and several weeks before the onset of labor.[349] This finding supports the notion that intrauterine PG production rises as part of the parturitional process rather than as a consequence of labor.

PGs produced by the amnion, and their accumulation in amniotic fluid, do not necessarily gain access to myometrial targets. The specific localization of PG synthesizing and metabolizing enzymes within the fetal membranes may control exposure of the myometrium to fetal-derived PGs. The chorion, which lies between the amnion and the maternal tissues of the uterus, expresses high levels of PDGH.[350] Thus, through most of pregnancy the chorion acts as a barrier, preventing amnion-derived PGs from activating the myometrium (Fig. 11-22).

Exposure of the myometrium to fetal membrane-derived PGs is dependent on the balance between PGHS-2 and PGHD activities in the chorion. Several studies have indicated that pro-pregnancy factors such as progesterone prevent myometrial exposure to PGs by stimulating PGHD and inhibiting PGHS-2. In contrast, cortisol, CRH, and several immune cytokines may inhibit PGDH and stimulate PGHS-2, leading to a net increase in active PGs accessing the myometrium (Fig. 11-23).[351,352] Thus, the balance of PG synthesis and metabolizing activities in the fetal membranes may be pivotal in the control of uterine contractility.[313,351-361]

Actions of PGs are mediated by a cohort of specific prostanoid receptors.[362] During pregnancy, the human myometrium expresses receptors for PGE_2, $PGF_{2\alpha}$, PGI_2, and thromboxane.[363-365] The pleiotropic actions of PGs in diverse tissue types can be explained by the existence of multiple receptor species linked to different intracellular signaling pathways.[366,367] For example, PGE_2 interacts with four subtypes of the EP receptor: EP1, EP2, EP3, and EP4. In addition, eight splice variants of the EP3 receptor have been identified.[368]

With regard to myometrial contraction, the diversity of PGE_2 receptor types may have important physiologic ramifications. Interaction of PGE_2 with the EP1 and EP3 receptors increases intracellular calcium and decreases cAMP, leading to contraction. In contrast, interaction of PGE_2 with the EP2 and EP4 receptors activates adenylate cyclase, leading to increased cAMP and relaxation. Thus, PGE_2 can cause uterine contraction or relaxation depending on the types of EP receptors expressed. $PGF_{2\alpha}$ interacts with a single receptor, known as the FP receptor, that increases intracellular calcium leading to contraction. PGI_2 binds the IP receptor that is linked to adenylate cyclase,

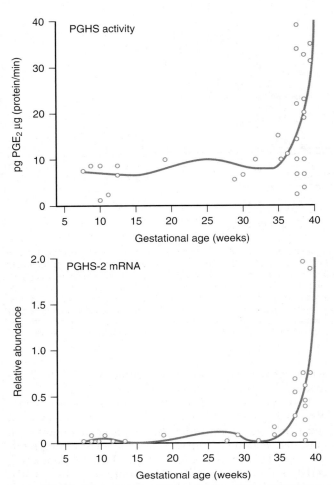

Figure 11-21. *Prostaglandin endoperoxide H synthase (PGHS)-2 activity and expression increase in the amnion at term before the onset of labor. (From Mijovic JE, Zakar T, Nairn TK, et al. Prostaglandin endoperoxide H synthase (PGHS) activity and PGHS-1 and -2 messenger ribonucleic acid abundance in human chorion throughout gestation and with preterm labor. J Clin Endocrinol Metab 83:1358, 1998.)*

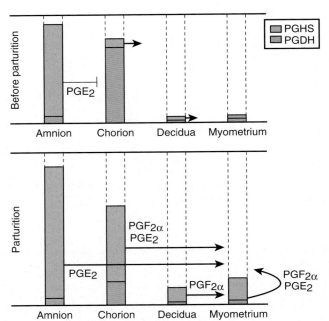

Figure 11-22. *Changes in prostaglandin endoperoxide H synthase (PGHS) and prostaglandin dehydrogenase (PGDH) activities in the fetal membranes decidua and myometrium associated with the onset of human labor. Parturition is associated with a marked increased in PGHS activity in all tissues. PGDH is predominantly expressed by the chorion and effectively blocks amnion prostaglandins (PGs) from accessing the myometrium. Parturition is associated with decreased PGDH activity in the chorion which could allow more active PG to reach the myometrium.*

leading to increased intracellular cAMP and relaxation. Thromboxane binds to the TP receptors and increases calcium. A more detailed description of PG receptors can be found in Chapter 6.

The regulation and localization of specific PG receptors in the myometrium and cervix is thought to be an important component in the endocrine control of pregnancy and parturition. Recent studies of EP and FP receptor expression in the term human uterus have shown that EP2 expression is greater than FP before the onset of labor and decreases with increasing gestation; expression of the FP receptor is low before labor and increases significantly in association with the onset of labor.[369] These findings indicate that myometrial relaxation through most of pregnancy is maintained at least in part by the EP2 receptor, whereas the onset of labor involves an increase in myometrial FP receptor, allowing $PGF_{2\alpha}$ to stimulate contraction. Thus, the balance between PG receptors mediating relaxation and contraction and their distribution in the uterus (fundal or cervical) may determine the net effect of PGs on uterine contractility.

Oxytocin

Oxytocin (OT) is one of the most potent and specific stimulants of uterine contraction. It is routinely administered by means of intravenous infusion to induce labor and treat postpartum hemorrhage. OT is a 9–amino acid peptide secreted by the posterior pituitary and is also produced in a number of peripheral tissues, including the ovary. During pregnancy, OT is produced by the amnion, chorion, and decidua.[370] OT is not generally considered to be involved in the initiation of labor because its circulating levels do not increase until the expulsive phase of labor.[371-373] This is not unexpected, because vaginal distention is a principal stimulus for the release of pituitary OT in human labor. This is known as the Ferguson reflex.

However, as with PGs, OT produced by intrauterine sites may play a significant paracrine role in regulating uterine contractions at parturition. The mechanisms underlying the control of intrauterine OT production and its potential to stimulate uterine contractions remain uncertain. Despite this, it is clear that OT contributes to the uterotonic milieu of human parturition because inhibition of OT action by specific synthetic antagonists disrupts the normal pattern of labor, decreases uterine contractility in women with threatened preterm labor, and significantly prolongs gestation.[374,375]

OT action appears to be regulated at the level of target tissue responsiveness by changes in OT receptor expression. In the human, myometrial and decidual OT receptor content and expression increase gradually toward the

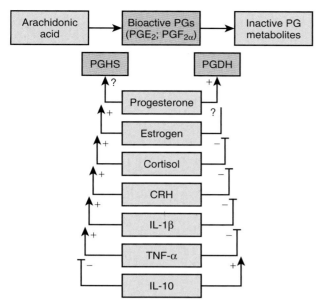

Figure 11-23. *Potential hormonal regulators of prostaglandin (PG) synthesis. Inhibition of prostaglandin dehydrogenase (PGDH) and/or stimulation of prostaglandin endoperoxide H synthase (PGHS) would increase net synthesis of bioactive prostaglandins (PGs) (PGE$_2$ and PGF$_{2\alpha}$).*

end of pregnancy and then rise significantly in association with the onset of labor.[376] Expression of the OT receptor by myometrial cells is up-regulated by estrogen and is part of the cassette of contraction-associated genes required to transform the myometrium to a contractile phenotype. Thus, induction of OT responsiveness by increased OT

receptor expression may be the principal mechanism underlying the uterotonic actions of locally produced and pituitary OT in human pregnancy. After birth, pituitary oxytocin contributes to uterine involution and the preparation of the breast for lactation (see Chapters 3 and 10).

The complete reference list can be found on the companion Expert Consult Web site at www.expertconsultbook.com.

Suggested Reading

Achache H, Revel A. Endometrial receptivity markers, the journey to successful embryo implantation. Hum Reprod Update 12:731, 2006.

Catalano PM, Hollenbeck C. Energy requirements in pregnancy: a review. Obstet Gynecol Surv 47:368, 1992.

Challis JRG, Matthews SG, Gibb W, et al. Endocrine and paracrine regulation of birth at term and preterm. Endocr Rev 21:514, 2000.

Diedrich K, Fauser BC, Devroey P, et al. The role of the endometrium and embryo in human implantation. Hum Reprod Update 13:365, 2007.

Giudice LC. Growth factors and growth modulators in human uterine endometrium: their potential relevance to reproductive medicine. Fertil Steril 61:1, 1994.

Gluckman PD, Hanson MA, Pinal C. The developmental origins of adult disease. Matern Child Nutr 1:130, 2005.

Haig D. Genetic conflicts in human pregnancy. Q Rev Biol 68:495, 1993.

Hertelendy F, Zakar T. Regulation of myometrial smooth muscle functions. Curr Pharm Des 10:2499, 2004.

Keelan JA, Blumenstein M, Helliwell RJ, et al. Cytokines, prostaglandins and parturition: a review. Placenta 24(Suppl A). S33, 2003.

Kliman HJ. Uteroplacental blood flow. The story of decidualization, menstruation, and trophoblast invasion. Am J Pathol 157:1759, 2000.

Mesiano S, Jaffe RB. Developmental and functional biology of the primate fetal adrenal cortex. Endocr Rev 18:378, 1997.

Rabinovici J, Jaffe RB. Development and regulation of growth and differentiated function in human and subhuman primate fetal gonads. Endocr Rev 11:532, 1990.

CHAPTER 12

The Hypothalamo-Pituitary Unit, Testes, and Male Accessory Organs

Peter Y. Liu and Johannes D. Veldhuis

The function of the hypothalamo-pituitary-testicular-accessory organ axis is to ensure normal androgenization (including embryonic, infantile, pubertal, and adult sexual maturation), male sexual behavior, and reproductively competent sperm output. Thus, the system is important for both the health of individuals and preservation of humankind. All elements in the system acting together as an integrative regulatory network are critical for male reproductive health. Dysfunction may result in ambiguous genitalia, sex reversal, pubertal delay, eunuchism, impaired spermatogenesis, and reduced systemic androgen exposure. Furthermore, partial deficiency of reproductive hormones may contribute to some of the features of male aging, impair recovery from protracted critical illness, and heighten visceral adiposity with insulin resistance. This chapter reviews the hypothalamo-pituitary-testicular axis, its components, and their joint regulation. Where practicable, emphasis is on newer discoveries in humans. Hormonal methods to regulate male fertility and to limit age-associated frailty constitute examples of how knowledge of male reproductive physiology is being translated into clinical practice.

Physiology of the Male Gonadal Axis

OVERVIEW: ENSEMBLE NATURE OF REPRODUCTIVE SYSTEM

Male reproductive hormones consist of the hypothalamic decapeptide gonadotropin-releasing hormone (GnRH), pituitary gonadotropins, luteinizing and follicle-stimulating hormones (LH and FSH), testicular steroids, testosterone and estradiol (Te and E_2), and putatively systemically active gonadal peptides, such as inhibin B. Integration requires repeated incremental and decremental feedforward (stimulatory) and feedback (inhibitory) signaling among neural and hormonal components of the axis (Fig. 12-1). The negative-feedback system can be exploited to regulate male fertility by suppressing spermatogenesis with exogenous sex hormones. Gonadotropin and Te deficiency can result in infertility or subfertility, impaired sexual maturation, reduced muscle and bone mass, insulin resistance, visceral fat accumulation, and diminished erythropoiesis, libido, potency, and general well-being.[1]

ESSENTIAL ROLES OF GNRH AND UPSTREAM KISS1 NEURONS

In the adult, specialized neurons (approximately 1200 neurons in the human) located in the arcuate nucleus of the mediobasal hypothalamus secrete GnRH in a pulsatile fashion into a portal microvasculature system. GnRH pulses stimulate gonadotropes located in the anterior pituitary to secrete LH and FSH.[2] In the embryo, migration of GnRH neurons from the olfactory placode into the upper diencephalon is essential to establish the anatomic proximity required for effectual hypothalmo-pituitary signaling. Several genes (*KAL1*, *KAL2*, and *PROK2*) are critical for both olfactory bulb morphogenesis and proper GnRH neuronal migration. *KAL1*, *KAL2*, and *PROK2* are located on chromosomes X, 8, and 3, and respectively encode anosmin-1, fibroblast growth factor (FGF) receptor 1, and prokineticin 2.[3] Inactivating mutations of any of these genes and less commonly neuroembryonic LHRH factor (NELF) cause Kallmann syndrome.[4] The syndrome is characterized clinically by hyposmia or anosmia and isolated gonadotropin deficiency.[5] Inheritance patterns are respectively X-linked, autosomal dominant, and recessive for defects in anosmin, FGF-receptor 1, and prokineticin or its receptor.

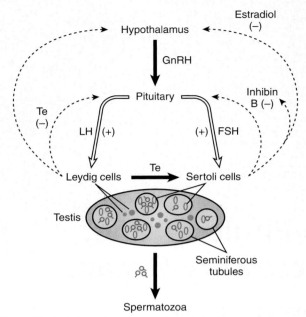

Figure 12-1. *Schematic representation of the human male gonadal axis. The left side highlights feedforward (stimulation) by gonadotropin-releasing hormone (GnRH) on luteinizing hormone (LH) secretion and LH on testosterone (Te) secretion as well as feedback (inhibition) by Te onto hypothalamic GnRH and pituitary LH outflow. The right side presents GnRH → follicle-stimulating hormone (FSH) drive and FSH → inhibin B/estradiol (E$_2$) feedforward, and conversely feedback by inhibin B and E$_2$. The inhibin B feedback loop has not been demonstrated directly in men. (Adapted from Liu PY, Takahashi PY, Nehra AX, et al. Neuroendocrine aging: Pituitary-testis: LH/FSH/prolactin. In Squire LR, Albright TD, Bloom FE, et al [eds]. New Encyclopedia of Neuroscience. Oxford, Elsevier, 2008, Fig. 6.)*

Pulsatile GnRH release is both intrinsic to clusters of GnRH neurons and essential to stimulate LH secretion over the long term. Continuous GnRH delivery down-regulates gonadotrope GnRH receptors and signaling pathways; this action forms the basis for treating prostatic cancer and precocious puberty with long-acting GnRH agonists.[6] Episodic GnRH secretion begins during fetal development when GnRH neurons first populate the mediobasal hypothalamus. A second surge of high-amplitude LH pulsatility emerges in infant boys during the first several months of age.[7] GnRH secretion declines during childhood only to be reinstated at markedly higher amplitude and slightly higher frequency in puberty.[8,9]

The kisspeptin-GPR54 system controls the timing of puberty, and may also regulate GnRH secretion in other epochs of life.[10,11] GPR54 is a G-protein coupled receptor expressed on GnRH neurons.[12] *KiSS1* is the gene that encodes kisspeptin-121, which is proteolytically cleaved to a 54–amino acid peptide named kisspeptin-54 (also known as metastin) and kisspeptin-14 and -13. Kisspeptin-54 is the natural ligand for the receptor GPR54. Inactivating mutations of either *KiSS1* or GPR54 in mice and of *KiSS1* in men result in normosmic hypogonadotropic hypogonadism, thus establishing that kisspeptin and cognate receptor are necessary upstream activators of GnRH neurons.[13] Proximate control of kisspeptin neurons and GPR54 receptors by sex steroids and neurotransmitters

is under intensive study. Table 12-1 highlights some of a myriad of GnRH regulators, whose sites of action require more precise definition. Regulators include seasonal, appetitive, anorexigenic, stress-associated, and anabolic (trophic) factors.

KiSS1 gene expression is regulated by sex steroids in a brain region–specific manner, consistent with its postulated role in mediating gonadal-feedback inhibition.[47] Estrogen and androgen repress KiSS1 in the arcuate nucleus, thereby inferably transducing sex-steroidal inhibition of GnRH outflow. This is not true in the anteroventral periventricular nucleus, which directs positive feedback by estrogen in females (Fig. 12-2). The latter site contains few KiSS1 neurons in the male. Other neurotransmitters may be important, because the administration of antihypertensive agents (particularly alpha-adrenergic blockers, selective serotonin

TABLE 12-1

Selected Putative Nonsteroidal Regulators of GnRH Neurons

Ligand	Role	Reference
GnRH	Autoinhibit (or stimulate)	14-16
Kisspeptin	Activate GPR54 receptor on GnRH neurons	17, 50
Galanin, neuromedin B	Stimulatory of GnRH release‡	15, 18, 19
Glutamate	Activate N-methyl-D-aspartate receptor	20, 21
Nonrepinephrine	Excitatory (beta-1 receptor) or inhibitory (alpha-1 receptor)	22-24
GABA*	Inhibit or stimulate	25-29
Nitric oxide	Stimulatory	30, 31
Dopamine	Repressor or activator	32, 33
Neuropeptide Y	Activate or inhibit via distinct receptor subtypes	34-36
CART†	Stimulate	37, 38
Opiatergic peptides	Repress	39
Prolactin	Inhibit via cognate receptor	40
Calcitonin gene-related peptide	Inhibit	41
Ciliary neuro-trophic factor	Stimulate	42
Leptin, orexin A/B	Stimulate GnRH outflow fasting	43
Somatostatin	Inhibit GnRH neurons	15
Serotonin	Inhibit or stimulate (via 5HT-1A or 2C and 4)	44

*γ-Aminobutyric acid (GABA) acts via a type A or type B receptor.
†Cocaine- and amphetamine-regulated transcript.
‡Carticotropin-releasing hormone (CRH), arginine vasopressin (AVP), and γ-melanocyte-simulating hormone (MSH), inhibit, whereas melanin-concentrating hormone stimulates, GnRH release. GnRH, gonadotropin-releasing hormone.
Data from Murray JF, Hahn JD, Kennedy AR, et al. Evidence for a stimulatory action of melanin-concentrating hormone on luteinizing hormone release involving MCH1 and melanocortin-5 receptors. J Neuroendocrinol 18:157, 2006; and Chen MD, Ordog T, O'Byrne KT, et al. The insulin hypoglycemia-induced inhibition of gonadotropin-releasing hormone pulse generator activity in the rhesus monkey: role of vasopressin and corticotropin-releasing factor. Endocrinology 137:2012, 1996.

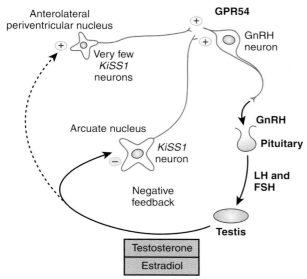

Figure 12-2. *Model of kisspeptin-GPR54 signaling in the brain of male rodent. KiSS1 neurons in the arcuate nucleus (ARC) secrete kisspeptin, which acts as a stimulatory input to gonadotropin-releasing hormone (GnRH) neurons. Kisspeptin signals via GPR54 expresses on GnRH neurons. The KiSS1 gene is negatively regulated by gonadal sex steroids, thereby providing a plausible mechanistic basis for inhibitory effects of testosterone and estradiol on hypothalamic GnRH, and secondarily on pituitary luteinizing hormone (LH) and follicle-stimulating hormone (FSH) secretion. Males possess very few, whereas females possess numerous, KiSS1 neurons in the anteroventral periventricular nucleus (AVPV). (Adapted from Kauffman AS, Clifton DK, Steiner RA. Emerging ideas about kisspeptin-GPR54 signaling in the neuroendocrine regulation of reproduction. Trends Neurosci 30:504, 2007, Fig. 12-1.)*

reuptake inhibitors, γ-aminobutyric acid agonists, and dopamine) can influence LH secretion. However, whether such effects are direct or indirect with respect to KiSS1 and GnRH neurons remains largely unexplored.[48]

DIFFERENTIAL CONTROL OF LH AND FSH SECRETION

GnRH preferentially stimulates FSH secretion in childhood and LH secretion in infancy, puberty, and adulthood.[49] Like GnRH, kisspeptin stimulates LH release twofold more than FSH release in healthy men.[50] The putative bases for these distinctions include feedforward and feedback factors. With respect to feedforward, slower GnRH pulse frequencies prior to puberty favor gonadotrope biosynthesis of specific FSHβ over LHβ subunits.[51-53] In addition, the dimeric glycoprotein, activin A, may stimulate FSH secretion in the prepubertal rat and nonhuman primate.[54-56] At a second level of feedforward, blood-borne FSH acts on Sertoli cells in spermatogenic tubules to drive inhibin B and E_2 secretion, and LH acts on Leydig cells in the testis interstitium to cause Te production.[57] There is some indirect evidence that FSH can also increase Te production, possibly via Sertoli cell–secreted nonsteroidal factors,[58,59] but the effect is quantitatively small.[60] In relation to resultant feedback,[61-63] pubertal elevations in inhibin B and E_2 concentrations would tend to restrict FSH responses to GnRH.[64-66] Elevated Te concentrations would likewise

tend to repress the rise in LH concentrations. The fact that the latter does not occur suggests muting of Te's feedback or strong central GnRH drive. Both mechanisms are inferable from mathematical feedback analyses performed in transpubertal cohorts of boys.[9]

Te's negative feedback on LH is mediated primarily[67] but not exclusively[68] via aromatization to E_2.[69] Significant feedback occurs at the pituitary level. Sex steroids repress GnRH secretion, but inhibition is not likely to be direct because GnRH neurons do not express the androgen receptor (AR) or estrogen receptor-α (ERα). Although ERβ is detectable and might enhance Ca^{2+}-dependent synchrony of GnRH neurons,[70] transgenic silencing of AR or ERα rather than ERβ is needed to elevate LH and Te concentrations in the adult animal.[71,72] These data favor a feedback role of KiSS1 neurons, which express both AR and ERα.[73] In addition, nongenomic actions of Te and E_2 transduced via membrane-dependent signaling may contribute to feedback in some species.[74]

GNRH AND GNRH RECEPTORS

More than 23 different GnRH peptides exist among species.[75] Human GnRH decapeptide exists in at least two forms, designated GnRH I and GnRH II, cloned initially in mammals and chickens, respectively.[76] The genes encoding these peptides are located on chromosomes 8p11-21 and 20p13, respectively.[77] Rapid and slow GnRH half-lives in men are about 2.6 and 5.2 minutes.[78] GnRH I is the predominant agonistic peptide regulating gonadotropin secretion in humans.[79] In animals GnRH II seems to stimulate sexual arousal and courting behavior,[80] whereas GnRH III (lamprey) induces significant FSH release.[81] Truncational mutation of the GnRH-I gene occurs in the *hpg/hpg* mouse, but has not been described in humans.[82]

At least 23 GnRH-receptor types have been cloned to date.[76] GnRH receptors are calcium-dependent G-protein coupled receptors (GPRs),[83,84] which control the activity of intracellular heterotrimeric G proteins by promoting guanine-nucleotide exchange and activation of adenylate cyclase, transmembrane Ca^{2+} influx, or intracellular Ca^{2+} mobilization.[83] GPRs contain seven transmembrane segments that form α helices connected by three extracellular and three intracellular loops. Receptor activation causes a conformational change in the associated G protein α subunit, promoting the release of GDP and binding of the activator nucleotide, GTP. The GTP-bound α subunit dissociates from the receptor leaving a stable $\beta\gamma$ dimer. Dissociated subunits modulate cellular signaling as proximate messengers in the cyclic AMP--protein kinase A (α subunit) and phospholipase C–protein kinase C ($\beta\gamma$ dimer) pathways. High intrahypothalamic concentrations of GnRH may mediate autoinhibition via a G_i subunit.[85]

Two distinct GnRH receptors have been identified in humans. GnRH I receptor is the hypophyseal receptor coupled to LH and FSH synthesis, which is encoded by a gene located on chromosome 4. Two splice variants of the GnRH I receptor exist.[86] Both GnRH I (secreted) and GnRH II (brain) peptides can activate the GnRH I receptor. The GnRH II receptor gene is located on chromosome 1,[77] but is silenced in the human, chimpanzee, cow, and sheep.[80] GnRH regulates neurotransmission and sexual behavior in the rodent via the GnRH II receptor.[76] Truncational, nonsense, and missense mutations in the GnRH receptor I gene or homeobox genes (*LHX3*) can lead to nonexpression, inactivation, misfolding, and misrouting of nascent receptors, and thereby autosomal recessive hypogonadotropic hypogonadism without anosmia.[87,88] Activating mutations of the GnRH receptor could result in isosexual precocious puberty, but have not yet been identified.[89] Other non-GnRH signals (e.g., IGF-I, galanin, activin A, inhibin B, follistatin, cytokines, gonadotropin-inhibitory hormone) may potentiate or inhibit GnRH action in the pituitary in animal models.[76,90-95]

GONADOTROPINS AND COGNATE RECEPTORS

Gonadotropins include lutropins (LH and human chorionic gonadotropin, hCG) and follitropin (FSH). Gonadotropins and thyroid-stimulating hormone (TSH) are oligosaccharide-modified dimeric proteins with a molecular mass of 30 to 40 kDa. All four corresponding genes are expressed in the human pituitary gland, albeit minimally in the case of hCG.[96] Each contains a common α subunit and a hormone-specific β subunit. Subunits are associated by noncovalent interactions, but cysteine residues (10 in the α subunit and 12 in the β subunit) permit disulfide linkages within subunits. The α subunit is encoded by a single gene localized at 6q12.21.[97] Mutations of this gene have not been identified, possibly because simultaneous loss of all glycoprotein hormones may be lethal in utero. The α subunit gene is larger than the β subunit gene because of a noncoding exon 1 and a long first intron, but the translated proteins are comparable in size. The β subunit genes are located on chromosomes 19q13.32 (LH/hCG cluster) and 11p13 (FSH). The human LH/hCG cluster consists of one LHβ and 6 hCGβ genes and pseudogenes. Glycosylation and terminal sialylation or sulfation via critical N- and O-linked sites within α (two sites) and β (one site in LH, two in FSH and TSH) subunits influence in vivo bioactivity, receptor binding, and metabolic clearance.[98] In particular, four O-linked glycosylation linkages present in an extended C-terminal portion of hCGβ (but not LHβ) increase intact hCG half-life to 24 to 30 hours compared with 1 hour for LH, and augment biopotency by limiting hCG-receptor dissociation.[99]

Exonic polymorphisms and mutations have been described for each gonadotropin β subunit (hCG, LH, and FSH) gene.[100] In mice, knockout of LHβ results in decreased production of Te and fewer elongated spermatids.[100] One polymorphism of LHβ, termed variant LHβ, occurs in as many as 30% of some Northern European and Australian aboriginal populations, and contains two amino acid transversions (Ile15Thr and Trp8Arg) and a supernumerary consensus glycosylation site (Asn13AlaThr) reminiscent of hCGβ. Variant LH is more biopotent, but has a shorter in vivo half-life than wild-type LH putatively due to resistance to peptidases or impaired sialylation and sulfation of terminal oligosaccharides.[101] In contrast, mutations of the FSHβ gene are rare in men. There are only three reported cases, each being associated with azoospermia[59,102,103] and one with hypoandrogenism.[103]

The LH/hCG receptor is a G-protein coupled receptor that is encoded by an 11-exon gene located on chromosome 2p21.[104] Unlike the FSH receptor, the lutropin receptor expressed is widely outside the gonad, including in the brain, leading to speculative extragonadal actions of LH or hCG.[105,106] Men with inactivating LH-receptor mutations present with male pseudohermaphroditism and a phenotype ranging from micropenis and hypospadias to complete feminization, in each case without an extragonadal phenotype. Activating mutations of the LH/hCG receptor become manifest as gonadotropin-independent (familial) male sexual precocity or testotoxicosis.[107] LH-receptor polymorphisms have also been described (such as Asn291Ser and Asn312Ser) in association with undermasculinization[108] and Leydig cell hypoplasia.[109] A rare splice variant (deleted exon 9) is marked by inhibitory properties.[110] Thus, structural analyses of interactions among LH receptor, ligand, and relevant G proteins should lead to targeted ligand discovery.[111]

The FSH receptor is also a G-protein coupled receptor, but is encoded by a 10-exon gene located on chromosome 2p21.[112] The crystal structure has been determined, revealing a hand-clasp interaction between the receptor and FSH (follitropin) that orients the glycoprotein hormone perpendicular to the long axis of the ligand-binding domain.[113] The follitropin receptors appears to be expressed exclusively on Sertoli cells located within the blood-testis barrier formed by tight junctions.[114] For this reason FSH is believed to regulate spermatogenesis primarily. A few controversial reports exist of FSH-receptor expression elsewhere, such as on spermatogonia[114] or skeletal osteoclasts.[115] Replication of these preliminary findings is required.[116]

Polymorphisms of the FSH receptor occur, but their influence on signal transduction and spermatogenesis remains unclear.[97] Inactivating mutations of the FSH receptor in five men were associated with subfertility (three cases) and fertility (two cases) with phenotypic variations ranging from oligozoospermia to euspermia.[117] Such data suggest that very low receptor activity is sufficient for spermatogenesis or that other endocrine or intratesticular factors may compensate to varying degrees.[118] An activating mutation of the FSH receptor was reported,[119] but functional significance has not been corroborated.

In young men, FSH seems necessary for the formation of spermatogonia type B and pachytene spermatocytes, and LH/hCG for round spermatids.[120] In contrast, LH is the dominant agonist of steroidogenesis.[121]

TESTICULAR STEROIDOGENESIS

Testosterone (Te) is the most important local and systemic androgen produced by the testes. Te concentrations are similar by race and ethnicity[122] but decline with increased abdominal visceral fat and with age.[123,124] In contrast, African-American men have higher E_2 and SHBG (sex hormone–binding globulin) concentrations than their white counterparts.[122] Androgens are crucial for male reproduction and general health. Testosterone triggers the development of male secondary sexual characteristics at puberty, maintains adult sexual behavior and function, and drives late stages of spermatogenesis independently of its metabolite 5α-dihydrotestosterone (DHT).[125] During fetal development Te is essential for differentiation of the internal and DHT the external male urogenital system. Inactivation of 5α-reductase type I in mice is lethal to the embryo (putatively due to unopposed brain estrogen toxicity), whereas inactivation of 5α-reductase type II in mice and men leads to male pseudohermaphroditism (perineoscrotal pseudovaginal hypospadias, hypoplastic prostate tissue, and decreased male-pattern balding and beard growth).[126] Despite low or absent DHT in such XY individuals, Te is sufficient to ensure wolffian duct differentiation (epididymides, vasa deferentia, seminal vesicles). Other androgens, such as the reduced metabolite 5α-androstane-3α,17β-diol, are important for fetal sexual maturation in marsupials, but their roles in primates are unknown.[127,128]

Leydig cells are located in the interstitial compartment of the testis, which allows secretion of Te and E_2 into seminiferous tubules, gonadal lymphatics, and venules. Fetal Leydig cells and maternal hCG are responsible for an intrauterine peak in Te secretion at 12 to 14 weeks of gestation. This peak is critical for male urogenital tract organogenesis. Testosterone production declines during the remainder of in utero life as fetal Leydig cells begin to degenerate. Augmented pulsatile LH secretion and neonatal proliferation of Leydig cells result in a second peak of androgen production at 2 to 3 months of postnatal age.[7] The neonatal peak is putatively important for imprinting masculine behavior at least in animals. Fetal Leydig cells undergo apoptosis, but are slowly replaced as mesenchymal stem cells populate the interstitium, and differentiate into initially immature Leydig cells that secrete 3α- and 5α-reduced androgens rather than Te. Further division and differentiation occur in puberty, when mature (adult) Leydig cells secrete large amounts of Te (Fig. 12-3). Beginning in young adulthood and progressively thereafter, total Te concentrations fall gradually by 0.6% to 1.1% annually,[129,130] resulting in a net decrement of 35% to 50% from the young adult maximum by the eighth decade in life.[123,131]

Testosterone is synthesized from cholesterol through sequential reactions that are catalyzed by cytochrome P450-containing complexes. A defect in any step results in variably severe male pseudohermaphroditism (46,XY

infant with undermasculinization of the external genitalia). Five major steps are involved, namely, (1) cholesterol C20,22-desmolase (CYP11A cholesterol side-chain cleavage), (2) 3β-hydroxysteroid dehydrogenase/Δ⁴,⁵-isomerase (3β-OHSDH), (3 and 4) C17,20-desmolase/17α-hydroxylase (CYP17A), and (5) 17β-hydroxysteroid dehydrogenase type III (Fig. 12-4). Cytochrome P450 refers to a 450-nm light-absorbing heme-binding peptide sequence that is critical for stoichiometry. The enzymatically rate-limiting step in steroidogenesis is encoded by *CYP11A*, which converts cholesterol to pregnenolone in the inner mitochondrial membrane. However, the kinetically rate-limiting step is delivery of LDL-, membrane-, and cholesteryl ester-derived free cholesterol to the inner mitochondrial leaflet by steroidogenic acute regulatory (StAR) protein.[132,133] LH activates StAR rapidly via posttranslational modification and slowly via increased gene transcription. Combined responses ensure both immediate and sustained access of cholesterol to mitochondrial side-chain cleavage system.

Pregnenolone leaves mitochondria and enters endoplasmic reticulum, where subsequent enzymatic modifications occur. Pregnenolone (or its 3β-reduced metabolite, progesterone) undergoes sequential cleavage and hydroxylation via *CYP17A*-encoded C17,20 lyase/17α-hydroxylase (a single enzyme with dual functions), which constitutes the androgen-committing step. The product is a weak ketosteroid, androstenedione, which must be converted to the potent hydroxysteroid, Te, via 17β-hydroxysteroid dehydrogenase type 3.[134,135]

In men, gonadal steroidogenesis accounts for over 95% of Te production, with the remainder produced by the adrenal gland and extraglandular conversion of the weak androgenic precursors, dehydroepiandrosterone and androstenedione, to Te.[136,137] Te production in young men averages 15 to 30 μmol (4 to 9 mg) per day. Estimates are consistent when determined by infusion of stable or radioactive isotopes and recent noninvasive analytical methods.[138-144] Testosterone secretion is determined genetically and environmentally. For example, men convert more Te to E_2 by peripheral aromatization and more androstenedione to Te via 17β-hydroxysteroid dehydrogenation than women.[145] In addition, Te concentrations differ between ethnic Chinese men living in an Asian environment compared with those in a Western environment.[140,146] Combined factors also may explain some populational differences in 5α reduced metabolites and prostate volume.[147]

Intratesticular regulation of Leydig cells is complex, and not yet fully understood.[148] All three of spermatogonial, peritubular myoid, and Sertoli cells exert effects on Leydig cell steroidogenesis.[121,149] Central nervous system and spinal cord pathways that innervate the testes further modulate testicular steroid production, particularly in the settings of inflammatory stress, alcohol intoxication, and central adrenergic modulation.[150]

AROMATIZATION, 5A-REDUCTION, AND INACTIVATION OF Te

Untransformed Te exerts potent anabolic effects. Te also functions as a prohormone, which undergoes conversion to other steroids, such as E_2 and DHT.[1] Converted steroids

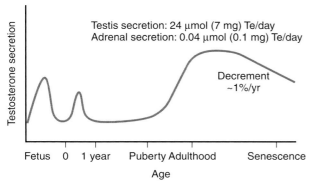

Figure 12-3. *Schematic profile of testosterone (Te) secretion over the human male lifetime. There are three prominent intervals of amplified Te production.*

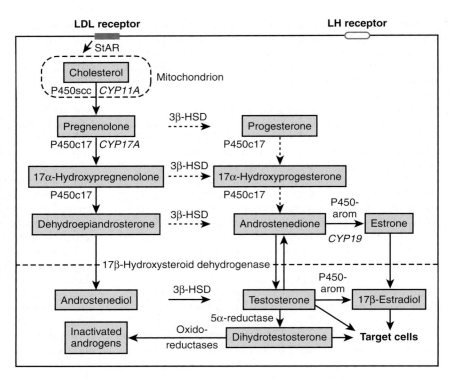

Figure 12-4. *Testosterone (Te) biosynthesis in Leydig cells. The principal (Δ⁵) pathway in humans is indicated by continuous arrows. The Δ⁴ route (dashed arrows) is more important in other species. Some Te is taken up by Sertoli cells, which convert the androgen to estradiol and dihydrotestosterone (DHT). LDL, low-density lipoprotein; P450scc, cytochrome P450 cholesterol side-chain-cleavage enzyme (CYP11A); 3β-HSDH, 3-hydroxysteroid dehydrogenase; P450c17, C17,20-lyase/17α-hydroxylase (CYP17A); P450arom, aromatase (CYP19); StAR, steroidogenic acute regulatory protein. DHT is inactivated to 3α- and 3β-diol metabolites. (From McLachlan RI, O'Donnell L, Meachem SJ, et al. Identification of specific sites of hormonal regulation in spermatogenesis in rats, monkeys, and man. Recent Prog Horm Res 57:149, 2002.)*

can mute or amplify, and thus diversify, Te's actions through ligand-receptor and coactivator specificities (Fig. 12-5). In particular, DHT binds ERα negligibly,[151] whereas E$_2$ binds AR with an affinity one order of magnitude less than that of Te.[151] Testosterone directly stimulates AR, but with a potency 2- to 30-fold less than that of DHT, depending upon target tissue. Thus, by being reduced or aromatized, Te may oppose or potentiate the actions of E$_2$ on certain genes.

Estradiol acts via two primary (and multiple variant) ERs, whereas Te and DHT act via a single AR. Heterogeneity of tissue responses is presumably conferred via cellular differences in the expression of AR and important corepressors and coactivators. The existence of tissue-selective modulators of nuclear AR action confers a basis for designing pharmacologically selective AR modulators (SARMs) to target anabolism in osteoblasts, erythropoietic

precursors, and stellate cells in skeletal muscle and brain while exerting little or no effect on adipocytes or the prostate gland.[152-155] A subset of SARMs may be suitable for use in male contraception.[156,157] Compared with Te, DHT is more potent due to both higher affinity for and slower dissociation from AR.[158-160] DHT is considered a pure androgen in that it is nonaromatizable. Only 4% of blood Te is converted to DHT,[146,161,162] less than 1% is transformed to E$_2$,[141,163] and approximately 2% to androstenedione[146] (see Fig. 12-5). Although systemic transformation is minimal, tissue-specific conversion of androstenedione to Te and of Te to DHT or E$_2$ may be critical in organs expressing AR or ER.[160] For example, systemic Te administration elevates intraprostatic DHT concentrations by providing substrate for local 5α-reductase type II, whereas exogenous DHT lowers prostatic DHT concentrations by suppressing LH and thereby

Figure 12-5. *Amplification, diversification, and inactivation of testosterone by means of its conversion to dihydrotestosterone (DHT) or estradiol, and subsequent receptor-specific drive. *, Potentially activated by DHT metbolites. AR, androgen receptor; ER, estrogen receptor. (Adapted from Liu PY, Death AK, Handelsman DJ. Androgens and cardiovascular disease. Endocr Rev 24:313, 2003.)*

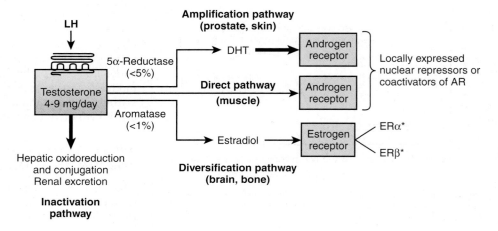

Te secretion.[164] Other hormones such as vitamin D, glucocorticoids, and progesterone also modify 5α-reductase under pharmacologic conditions.

The *CYP19* gene, located on chromosome 15q21.1, encodes the enzyme aromatase, which converts Te to E_2 and androstenedione to estrone.[165,166] Aromatase is widely distributed in the testes (Leydig cells, Sertoli cells, spermatid lineage), bone, brain, pituitary, liver, intestine, skin fibroblasts, adipocytes, and breast stromal cells.[167] Systemic aromatization predominantly (>60%) proceeds in extra-abdominal adipose tissue.[141,168] The coexistence of *CYP19* and ER in the brain, pituitary, and testes suggests that locally produced E_2 is physiologically important in these key sites. Evidence favors a role for E_2 and ERα in stimulating libido and mating frequency, especially in animals, inhibiting testis descent into the scrotum by repressing the *INSL3* gene, opposing germ cell apoptosis in older animals, decreasing LH secretion, inhibiting Leydig cell growth and differentiation, maintaining efferent spermatogenic ductule water reabsorption and endocytosis, and stimulating male breast anlagen[169-171] (Table 12-2). Moreover, transgenic silencing and rare human mutations of *CYP19* or ERα have unmasked important roles for E_2 in bone mineral density, fat deposition patterns, appetitive behavior, and feedback on LH and FSH. Splice variants and polymorphisms of *CYP19* exist,[180,181] and might modify the risks of prostatic cancer or osteoporosis.[181,182]

Two isoforms (type I and type II) of 5α-reductase are present in the human, encoded by separate genes located on chromosomes 5p15 and 2p23.[159,183] Type I is found mainly in skin, liver, and brain, and type II primarily in male accessory sex glands, liver, and brain.[184] The isoenzymes share approximately 50% structural peptide homology. Polymorphisms of both isoenzymes have been reported, some of which (e.g., V89L) alter enzymatic activity[185] or correlate with sperm output (A49TT and V89LV).[186] Genetic variations in DHT synthesis or catabolism may thus contribute to interindividual variability in spermatogenic suppression by Te in male contraceptive regimens.[187] Prospective assessment of this postulate is needed.[188,189]

Testosterone and DHT are inactivated in the liver, kidney, and prostate by mixed-function oxidoreductases (e.g., 3α- and 3β-hydroxysteroid dehydrogenases) or glucuronidases (conjugation reactions).[190] 3α-Reduction of DHT decreases its affinity for AR by a factor of 100,000-fold. The oxidoreduced and conjugated metabolites are lost into urine and bile, respectively. Certain metabolites of DHT, such as 5α-androstane-3β,17β-diol may mimic E_2 action via ERβ or modulate neurotransmission[128] (see Fig. 12-5).

Progesterone

Although gonadotropes and KiSS1 neurons express nuclear progesterone receptors, there is no established role of progesterone in adult human male reproductive physiology. Exogenous progesterone and synthetic progestins can suppress gonadotropin output in vivo through the hypothalamic progesterone receptor,[191] and inhibit Te biosynthesis in vitro by down-regulating Leydig cell LH

TABLE 12-2
Estrogen Effects on Male Gonadal Axis

Action	Mechanism*
↓ GnRH gene transcription	GnRH neuronal ERβ and kisspeptin ERα[172]
↓ gonadotropin concentrations	↓ LH and FSH pulse size
↓ GnRH-stimulated LH secretion	↓ GnRH efficacy at pituitary level
↓ Testosterone biosynthesis	↓ CYP17A, StAR, and LH receptor[173]
↓ Testis descent	↓ Insulin-like factor 3 in Leydig cells via ERα[174,175]
↓ Spermatogenesis	↓ FSH by feedback in adult
↓ Epididymal and seminiferoustubule fluid aborption	Putatively via ERα, which maintains aquaporin-1 expression[176]
↓ Germ-cell apoptosis	Older male animal[177]
↓ Leydig cell proliferation	Fetal and puberal testis[178]
↑ Male sexual arousal and aggressive behavior	Neonatal brain ERα pathways[179]

*Male ERβ-knockout and mice are fertile.

ER, estrogen receptor; FSH, follicle-stimulating hormone; GnRH, gonadotropin-releasing hormone; LH, luteinizing hormone; StAR, steroidogenic acute regulatory.

Data from O'Donnell L, Robertson KM, Jones ME, et al. Estrogen and spermatogenesis. Endocr Rev 22:289, 2001.

receptors.[192] Reduced metabolites of pregnenolone and progesterone exert inhibitory effects on neurotransmission in experimental models, but the relevance of these actions in men is unknown.

Sex-Steroid Receptors

Sex-steroid hormones are lipophilic, thus allowing passive transmembrane diffusion into the cell before interaction with specific high-affinity nuclear receptors. Whether active transmembrane transport also occurs is possible but unproved. Ligand-receptor binding prompts dissociation of chaperone proteins (heat shock protein [Hsp] 90 and immunophilin Hsp 56), receptor dimerization, and interaction with distinct palindromic DNA sequences known as steroid-responsive elements.[193] Typical motifs consist of hexanucleotide sequences arranged as inverted repeats that are separated by three nonconserved base pairs (GGTACAnnnTGTTCT). The classical genomic mode of action is represented by this pathway, in which steroid hormone receptors function as ligand-activated transcription factors.

Circumstantial evidence in many cell systems suggests that steroids may also act through nongenomic membrane-associated signaling mechanisms.[194,195] In general, nongenomic pathways are inferred when responses are (1) too rapid to arise by nuclear effects; (2) evident in cells lacking sex-steroid receptors; (3) persistent in the presence of inhibitors of transcription and protein synthesis; or (4) elicited by steroids bound to substances that preclude entry into the cell.[194,195] When defined in this manner, membrane-associated pathways trigger calcium flux, cyclic AMP generation, and extracellular-regulated or mitogen-activated protein kinases.[196-198] However, the precise molecular relationship between putative membrane and known nuclear receptors is not clear.

ANDROGEN RECEPTOR IN TESTES

The androgen receptor (AR) is encoded by a gene located on the X chromosome.[199] Splice variants of the AR exist,[199] but the full-length isoform is the predominant or only form expressed in many tissues, including male reproductive organs.[200] In the testis, AR expression is prominent in early-stage Sertoli cells associated with stage III of the spermatogenic cycle,[201] and to a lesser extent Leydig and myoid but not germ cells.[201] Murine knockout models indicate that AR activity is essential in Sertoli and Leydig cells for fertility due to AR's role in spermatogenesis and steroidogenesis, respectively. In contrast, functional AR in peritubular myoid cells is not critical for reproduction.[202-205] Other tissues expressing AR include prostate, seminal vesicles, skin, fat, liver, all three of smooth, skeletal, and cardiac muscle, brain, pineal gland, bone, and cartilage.[147,206-211] Leydig cell Te stimulates AR in spinal motor neurons, thereby activating gonadal descent into the scrotum via muscles in the outer layer of the gubernaculums ("rudder") of the testis.[212] A Leydig cell–derived peptide, insulin-like factor (INSL3), albeit insufficient without Te, is necessary for development of gubernacular ligaments and prevention of cryptorchidism.[213] INSL3 is a relaxin-like ligand, which signals by the LGR8/GREAT receptor.[214,215]

Inactivating mutations of AR result in the androgen-insensitivity (testicular-feminization) syndrome in the genetic male, and are the most common cause of male intersex.[199,216] Genotype and phenotype are strongly correlated, and mutations that increasingly impair receptor function result in more marked androgen insensitivity. A regularly updated electronic database of AR mutations is available at the Androgen Receptor Gene Mutations Database (http://androgendb.mcgill.ca).

Polymorphisms that modify AR function have been described, such as polymorphic polyglycine (GGC) and polyglutamine (CAG) repeats. Increasing polyglutamine-repeat length is associated with decreasing AR transcriptional activity,[217] impaired spermatogenesis or subfertility,[218] and genital abnormalities[219] in some but not all studies.[220,221] Polyglutamine-repeat length may contribute to nonuniform suppression of sperm output during male hormonal contraception.[221,222] Selected nuclear coregulators of AR could be targets of tissue-specific androgen-receptor modulators.[223-228]

ESTROGEN RECEPTORS

The genes encoding ERα and ERβ have been mapped to chromosomes 6 and 14, respectively.[229,230] There are striking similarities in both the DNA-recognition and ligand-binding domains of the expressed receptor proteins. ERα is expressed in pituitary, brain, kisspeptin (but not GnRH) neurons, fat, skin, bone, seminal vesicles, Leydig cells, round spermatocytes, and spermatids,[167,231] whereas ERβ is detectable in gonadotropes, kisspeptin and GnRH neurons, prostatic epithelium, and Sertoli, Leydig, and spermatogonial cells in several mammals.[231-233] Male ERα-knockout mice exhibit elevated LH concentrations due to impaired negative feedback, enhanced Leydig cell steroidogenesis and oligo/azoospermia associated with efferent ductule occlusion.[234,235] In contrast, ERβ-disabled mice maintain normal LH and Te concentrations, have decreased germ cell apoptosis in later adulthood, Leydig cell hyperplasia, and normal fertility.[230,236-238] ERα and ERβ can act individually or as heterodimers, and can exert opposing or synergistic effects upon target genes, thus creating signaling diversity (Fig. 12-5). Splice variants and polymorphisms are described for both ER subtypes, some of which may be linked to reduced sperm output and infertility.[239,240] Environmental xenoestrogens and phytoestrogens could in principle influence spermatogenesis further in genotypically susceptible individuals.[241] Estradiol may also activate membrane-bound receptors, such as GRP30 linked to camp,[242] and others coupled to extracellularly regulated kinases or Ca^{2+}.[243-246] Some but not all E_2 actions depend upon estrogen-response elements (ERE). For example, ERα and ERE are together necessary to maintain male sexual behavior, whereas either ERα or non-ERE-mediated pathways can suppress LH and Te secretion in mice.[247]

PROGESTERONE RECEPTOR

A single gene located on chromosome 11q22-3 encodes two progesterone receptor isoforms (termed A and B) through alternative transcriptional initiation sites.[248-250] The isoforms exert reciprocal effects via interactions with selected DNA motifs, defined as progesterone-responsive elements. Progesterone receptors are expressed widely including in KiSS1 neurons, gonadotropes, breast, brain, and adipose tissue.[249,251] Whether progesterone receptors are expressed in the testis is debated. Although physiologic actions of progesterone remain to be elucidated in men, pharmacologic amounts of progesterone and progestins suppress gonadotropin output, which has utility in the design of male hormonal contraception.[191]

SEX HORMONE–BINDING GLOBULIN: STEROID TRANSPORTER AND PUTATIVE LIGAND

SHBG in the male primate is expressed in the liver, adrenal cortex, prostatic alveoli, epididymides, and seminiferous tubules.[252] Infusion of SHBG acutely reduces the metabolic clearance of Te and E_2 in male monkeys.[253] Crystallographic studies show that SHBG is a homodimer structurally similar to the pentraxin family of proteins. Each monomeric subunit contains one hydrophobic steroid-binding pocket as well as tandem laminin G–like domains near the N-terminus that are critical for dimerization.[254-256] Homodimerization is induced by the presence of steroid ligand, and stabilized by calcium ions. Both potential steroid-binding regions in the dimer are occupied by Te.[257] SHBG contains several glycosylation sites, which give rise to multiple posttranslational isoelectric isoforms,[258] and by common variants (polymorphisms) or mutations that alter glycosylation sites resulting in inefficient secretion or metabolic clearance of secreted SHBG.[259-261] Mutagenesis studies suggest that glycosylation sites in the C-terminus of SHBG may be important for cell-surface recognition.[262]

Te, E_2, and progesterone bind SHBG[254,263] and to a lesser degree corticosteroid-binding globulin.[263] About 45% of blood Te is bound to high-affinity SHBG, 4% to corticosteroid-binding globulin, and the remaining 50% to lower-affinity high-capacity binding proteins, such as albumin. Approximately 1% to 2% remains free/unbound.[264] DHT and anabolic steroids have greater affinity for SHBG than Te.[264] Although of higher affinity, the 1000-fold lower molarity of plasma E_2 than Te in men limits any substantial depression by E_2 of Te's binding to SHBG at physiologic pH and temperature.[265,266] Low-affinity binding of Te (or E_2) to albumin may create a reservoir from which free Te (or E_2) arises rapidly due to an equilibrium dissociation half-time of about 0.2 second compared with 3.8 seconds for SHBG.[243,267] Significant one-pass dissociation is inferable in the liver, brain, and splanchnic circulation,[145] but whether capillary-bed dissociation kinetics are organ selective is unknown. In one study, experimentally controlled free, bioavailable, and total Te concentrations equally predicted feedback onto GnRH/LH outflow in healthy men.[268]

The traditional perspective is that protein binding mediates steroid hormone retention and transportation in plasma, and restricts metabolism and inactivation.[269] This view has been challenged by recent experimental data,[270-272] since SHBG and albumin-bound steroids may also be biologically available for tissue-specific uptake.[262,267,273] Although only free (unbound) hormone is believed to enter the cell by diffusion, SHBG may associate with presumptive high-affinity membrane-binding receptors, such as megalin, which may facilitate SHBG-bound Te's entry into cells.[274] Mutagenetic studies suggest that certain glycosylation sites in the C-terminus of SHBG are important for cell-surface (albeit not necessarily megalin) receptor recognition.[254] Megalin-knockout mice exhibit apparent androgen resistance, inferable from impaired testicular descent into the scrotum.[271] In addition, occupancy of membrane-bound SHBG by Te, DHT, or E_2 may activate intracellular Ca^{2+} or cAMP signaling purportedly via G-protein coupled and mitogen-kinase pathways.[275]

SHBG and testicular androgen-binding protein (ABP) are both encoded by a single gene located on the short arm of chromosome 17.[276] The proteins differ in their sites of production (SHBG by hepatocytes, brain, and placenta and ABP by Sertoli cells and possibly brain), as well as oligosaccharide composition.[277,278] SHBG secretion by hepatocytes is induced prominently by estrogens, thyroxine, and some anticonvulsant drugs and repressed by insulin, growth hormone/IGF-I, and nonaromatizable androgens. The presumptive intratesticular role of testicular ABP is to maintain high intratubular total Te concentrations required for spermatogenesis.[279-282] This notion is endorsed by the findings of increased germ cell apoptosis and decreased fertility after transgenic overexpression of ABP in mouse testes.[279]

PHYSIOLOGY OF HYPOTHALAMO-PITUITARY-TESTICULAR NETWORK

None of kisspeptin, GnRH, LH, or Te acts alone. Rather, all four signals are interlinked in a network or ensemble (Fig. 12-6A). Pulsatile GnRH secretion drives pulsatile LH secretion, which stimulates pulsatile Te production.[282-284] Direct sampling of human spermatic-vein blood suggests that (1) Te feeds back onto both LH and FSH secretion within 30 to 45 minutes (LH) or longer (FSH); (2) LH, but not FSH, feeds forward onto Te secretion after a delay of 40 to 90 minutes; and (3) secreted Te distributes rapidly among free (aqueous), albumin-bound, and SHBG-bound compartments[138,284-286] (Fig. 12-6B). These concepts form the basis for constructing biomathematical models of time-delayed, nonlinear interactions among GnRH, LH, and Te with ultradian (pulsatile) and circadian (24-hour rhythmic) features.[138,268,287] Further model advances require inclusion of locally modulated Te actions via ER subtypes, AR, and membrane receptors.

Both GnRH outflow and LH secretion are subject to feedback inhibition by Te and E_2. Te feedback is substantially,[67,288] but not completely,[68,289] mediated by aromatization to E_2 systemically and/or within the hypothalamo-pituitary unit. Exogenous E_2 by acting on the pituitary reduces LH pulse amplitude without altering pulse frequency,[290] whereas exogenous Te by acting on the hypothalamus and the pituitary gland decreases GnRH/LH pulse frequency and amplitude.[68] Conversely, depletion of endogenous E_2 concentrations with an aromatase inhibitor or blockade of E_2 action with an ERα antagonist augments LH pulse size and number,[67,291,292] therein mimicking the effects of nonsteroidal anti-androgens.[289,293] Inasmuch as E_2 depletion but not E_2 excess modulates GnRH/LH pulse frequency, endogenous estrogenic inhibition of the GnRH pulsing process (but not GnRH-driven LH pulse size) may be already maximal in normal men.

The characteristics of Te delivery may modulate inhibition of LH, because greater suppression is enforced by continuous than pulsatile Te infusions.[294] This outcome supports the male hormonal contraceptive approach of sustained Te administration to suppress LH and thereby intragonadal Te concentrations. Endogenous DHT plays a lesser role in feedback onto GnRH and LH, given that patients with 5α-reductase type II deficiency exhibit minimally elevated LH concentrations.[295] Administration of a potent combined type I and II 5α-reductase inhibitor, dutasteride, in healthy young men, reduced systemic DHT concentrations by 95% and stimulated basal (constitutive) LH (and Te) secretion.[296] This mechanism could explain the rise in all three of mean, nadir, and peak LH concentrations in patients with 5α-reductase deficiency.

FSH concentrations are also regulated by negative feedback. Aromatization of Te to E_2 appears to be critical because (1) combined deprivation of Te and E_2 and isolated depletion of E_2 elevate FSH concentrations to comparable degrees[63]; (2) physiologic replacement of either Te or E_2 in hypogonadal men normalizes FSH concentrations; and (3) an aromatase inhibitor fully reverses suppression of FSH by Te.[67] Although nonaromatizable

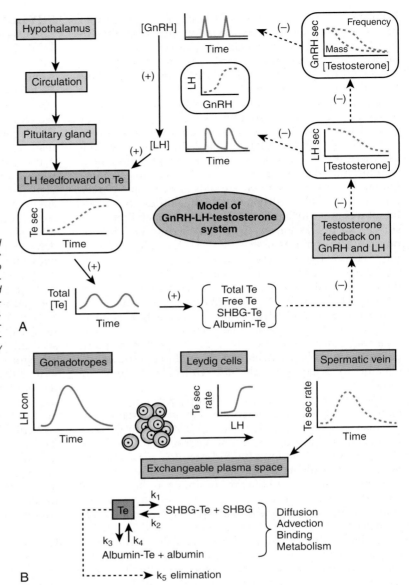

Figure 12-6. A, *Ensemble construct of GnRH → LH and LH → Te feedforward and time-delayed Te → LH and Te → GnRH feedback. No single pathway or signal acts alone to maintain male reproductive function.* **B,** *Schema of regulated secretion, plasma distribution, protein binding, and elimination of secreted Te by LH pulses. GnRH, gonadotropin-releasing hormone; LH, luteinizing hormone; sec, secretion; SHBG, sex hormone–binding globulin; Te, testosterone. (From Keenan DM, Veldhuis JD. Divergent gonadotropin-gonadal dose-responsive coupling in healthy young and aging men. Am J Physiol 286:R381, 2004.)*

androgens can also suppress FSH and LH secretion, the study paradigms have been pharmacologic rather than physiologic.[68,297-299]

Nonsteroidal testicular products, such as inhibin B secreted by Sertoli cells, may be involved in feedback regulation in animals.[64] In humans, inhibin B concentrations exhibit a multimodal lifetime pattern. Values in umbilical cord blood are comparable to peripheral venous levels in men, increase further in infancy, decline during subsequent childhood, rise in puberty, and fall by 25% by the eighth decade of life.[300] The changes are paradoxically concordant (birth through puberty) and reciprocal (adulthood) with FSH, LH, and Te secretion, indicating that other factors modulate both FSH and inhibin B. Albeit supported by corollary data, the role of inhibin B in restraining FSH production in vivo has been inferable only in the adult male rodent and monkey. To date, no clinical studies have infused or neutralized inhibin B in men, and no human

mutations of inhibin B or its receptor have been described. The same qualifications apply to the roles of activin A, a homodimer that stimulates FSHβ gene expression, and follistatin, a linear peptide that binds to and antagonizes feedforward by activin.[301,302] Inhibins and activins signal via transforming growth factor (TGF) β receptors and β-glycan co-receptors.[301] TGF receptors also strongly regulate cell proliferation, apoptosis, tumorigenesis, and hematopoiesis.[303] Contraceptive applications of safe and effective mimetics of inhibin B and antagonists of activin A remain to be exploited.

The Testes

The adult testes are paired ovoid structures suspended in the scrotum by the spermatic cord. Prepubertal testis volume is less than 7 mL, and postpubertal volume exceeds

12 mL. Each is encapsulated by the fibrous tunica albuginea ("white cloak"), which is invaginated posteriorly to form the mediastinum testis perforated by neurovascular and lymphatic vessels and efferent ductules. Efferent ductules form from the rete (net-like) testis, which represents the convergence of all seminiferous tubules. Fibrous septa project from the tunica albuginea into the testis dividing it into 250 to 300 lobules. Each lobule contains 1 to 4 segments of seminiferous tubules. The latter develop at the time of puberty through canalization of the seminiferous cords. Peritubular myoid and Sertoli cell interactions mediate formation of seminiferous cords. Spermatogenic tubules are lined internally by Sertoli cells, which support the proliferation and differentiation of spermatogonial cells by secreting trophic and prosurvival factors, like stem cell factor (c-kit ligand), which nourish and inhibit apoptosis of germ cells.[304] Sertoli cells protect spermatogonia by maintaining an unique tubular microenvironment through tight junctional complexes that constitute the blood-testis barrier. Conversely, spermatogonia and peritubular myoid cells both signal to Sertoli cells.[305,306] Sertoli cells abut a basement membrane, which is lined externally by peritubular myoid cells. Myoid cells are surrounded by an interstitium containing Leydig cells, lymphatics, venules, and nerve fibers. Peritubular myoid, Leydig, and Sertoli cells together regulate spermatogenesis.

Testes develop intra-abdominally, and descend into the scrotum perinatally. Insulin-like growth factor 3 induction of gubernacular development is essential for transinguinal migration.[307] Male sex determination and testicular morphogenesis are orchestrated by the SRY (sex-determining region of the Y chromosome), which is both necessary and sufficient for testis formation (Fig. 12-7). SRY in turn activates a family of homeobox-related genes, in particular *Lim1* and *SOX9*, as well as steroidogenic factor 1 (SF1; also designated NR5A1). SF1 is a member of the NR5A subfamily of nuclear receptors required for testis, adrenal, and gonadotrope development. Mutations in SRY, *SOX9*, and SF1 or its repressor, the dosage-sensitive X-linked sex-reversal (*DAX1*; also designated NR0B1) gene, are responsible for the majority of known causes of aberrant sexual development.

ACCESSORY ORGANS

Under the influence of Te, embryonic wolffian (mesonephric) ducts develop into the internal male reproductive tract, namely the epididymis (upper segment), vas deferens (middle), and ejaculatory duct and seminal vesicles (lower). By the fourth week of embryonic life, the ejaculatory ducts arch anteriorly to join the ventral portion of the cloaca. The cloaca subsequently differentiates into the urogenital sinus. DHT is required for development of the prostate gland, urethra, scrotum, and penis from the urogenital sinus.

VAS DEFERENS

Vasa deferentia transport sperm by means of muscular layers that propel spermatozoa during ejaculation. In the absence of ejaculation, spermatozoa stored in each vas deferens dribble through the terminal dilated ampulla into

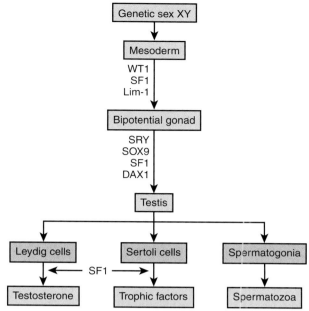

Figure 12-7. *Critical embryogenetic determinants of testis formation given the genetic sex 46XY. The bipotential gonad of mesonephric origin must be directed definitively by SRY (sex-determining region of Y chromosome). DAX1, dosage-sensitive sex-reversal; SF1, steroidogenic factor 1; SOX9, SRY-related HMG-box 9; WT1, Wilms' tumor. Further differentiation of the primitive male gonad entails development of Leydig, Sertoli, and germ cells. (From Rajender S, Thangaraj K, Gupta NJ, et al. A novel human sex-determining gene linked to Xp11.21-11.23. J Clin Endocrinol Metab 91:4028, 2006.)*

the ejaculatory duct where they are washed away during micturition. The distal urethral meatus discharges urine or semen from the body.

EPIDIDYMIS

The epididymis is formed from a single duct through which all spermatozoa pass, mature, gain fertilizing capability, and become motile before entering the vas deferens and ejaculatory duct. The human epididymis is 4 to 5 cm long and consists of the caput, corpus, and cauda. The cauda in man appears to differ from that in other species by way of more rapid transit of spermatozoa (2 to 4 days) and a less differentiated initial segment. Peptides and nonproteinaceous molecules are secreted into the epididymal lumen by principal cells. Although little is known in any species about precise regulation of luminal fluids that modulate sperm maturation and motility, microarray profiling of human epididymal tissue has demonstrated highly regionalized gene expression with maximal complexity in the caput and least in the corpus.[308] The maturation process is complete by the time spermatozoa enter the proximal (caudal) epididymis and are able to hyperactivate, bind the zona pellucida of the oocyte, and undergo the acrosome reaction.

The micromilieu of spermatozoa stored in the cauda epididymidis remains poorly understood. Ductal mucosa must play a critical role in controlling solute concentrations and degree of sperm hydration. Muscular cells exist only in the cauda epididymides and ductus deferens, and hence repeated ejaculation increases the rate of sperm transport from these regions only.

Epididymal growth, development, and function are dependent on androgens, estrogens, and other nonsteroidal luminal factors. Luminal androgen concentrations exceed those in peripheral blood, and for this reason systemic androgen exposure may not be critical for epididymal development and function. Amplification of luminal Te effects occurs by local synthesis of DHT via gonadal 5α-reductase type II.

SEMINAL VESICLES

The seminal vesicles secrete the majority of fluid found in the ejaculate. Secretion includes fructose, prostaglandin, semenogelin I (responsible for coagulation of the seminal fluid), reactive-oxygen scavengers (superoxide dismutase, catalase), and immunoglobulin G receptor III. During embryogenesis, androgens transform simple saccular anlagen into active secretory epithelium by branching morphogenesis, yielding a highly folded internal structure

with an expanded surface area. The precise molecular mechanisms are not yet defined.

PROSTATE GLAND

The prostate is the largest accessory gland, but unlike the epididymis and seminal vesicles arises from the urogenital sinus rather than mesonephric ducts and requires DHT action (Fig. 12-8). Prostatic fluids, which compose about one third of the volume of the ejaculate, contain high concentrations of zinc, citric acid, choline, and proteins such as acid phosphatase, seminin, plasminogen activator, and prostate-specific antigen (PSA). PSA is an important blood marker of prostate size and proliferation. PSA concentrations are elevated in benign prostate hypertrophy, inflammation, and prostatic cancer. The prostate gland develops from distinct sets of tubules that initially form discrete lobes, which become confluent by adulthood. Thus, the adult prostate gland is generally divided into peripheral, central, and transitional zones according to morphologic and functional properties rather than lobular structure. The peripheral zone is subcapsular and

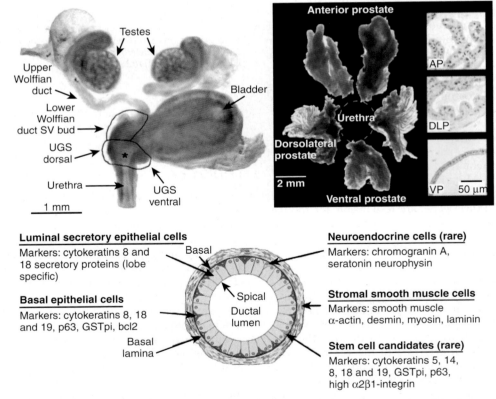

Figure 12-8. *Micromorphometric features of the prostate gland. Portion of the urogenital tract from a male embryonic mouse day 16.5 (top left). The prostate develops from the urogenital sinus (UGS), which is located at the base of the developing bladder. UGS epithelium is visible as a dilation of the urethra (lighter area containing asterisk) surrounded on the dorsal and ventral sides by condensed UGS mesenchyme (darker areas). AP, anterior prostate; DLP, dorsolateral prostate; SV, superoventral; VP, ventral prostate. Lobes of the adult mouse prostate (top right) are seen together with hematoxylin and eosin stained sections of prostatic ducts from each lobe (inset micrographs). Each lobe has a distinct shape and histologic appearance. Diagram of a ductal cross section (bottom) with labels indicates cell types present in prostatic ducts: luminal secretory epithelial cells, basal epithelial cells, neuroendocrine cells, stromal smooth muscle cells, and stem cell candidates. Below the label for each cell type is a list of differentiation markers commonly used to distinguish these cell types. Prostatic epithelial stem cell candidate markers include cytokeratins 5, 14, 8, 18, and 19, GSTpi, p63, and α2β1-integrin. (Adapted from Marker PC, Donjacour AA, Dahiya R, Cunha GR. Hormonal, cellular, and molecular control of prostatic development. Dev Biol. 253[2]:165, 2003, Fig. 1.)*

surrounds the distal urethra, the central zone encircles the ejaculatory ducts, and the transition zone envelops the proximal urethra. The peripheral and central zones make up 70% and 25%, respectively, of total prostate gland volume in young men, accounting for equivalent proportions of prostate cancer in later life. In contrast, prostate cancer rarely arises from the transition zone (5% of volume), where benign prostate hypertrophy usually develops.

Spermatogenesis

Spermatogenesis is a dynamic complex process contingent on systemic hormone support and local cellular, autocrine, and paracrine interactions directed ab initio via SRY and *SOX9*.[309,310] Sperm production proceeds in an orderly stage-specific fashion in all species (Fig. 12-9). Seminiferous tubules exhibit a stratified and layered arrangement of germ cells wherein spermatogonia rest on the basement membrane and more mature germ cells fill the apical luminal regions. In humans and some other primates, stages follow an intertwined helical pattern so that a single tubular cross section may contain up to six distinguishable stages.

Embryonic spermatogonia develop from primordial germ cells, which first appear in the yolk sac and then migrate to the hindgut and genital ridge during the fourth week of fetal life to form sex cords. The resultant seminiferous tubule permits spermatogenesis to proceed via four basic stages: (1) development and repopulation of spermatogonia from stem cells accomplished via mitotic divisions that renew the stem cell population and yield type A and B spermatogonia; (2) meiosis requiring DNA synthesis and two meiotic divisions to produce haploid spermatids, specified as primary and secondary spermatocytes; (3) spermiogenesis, defined by development and differentiation of the spermatid head and tail; and (4) spermiation, denoting release of mature spermatozoa into the seminiferous tubule lumen.[311-315]

Type A spermatogonia are divided into A dark and A pale according to morphologic criteria of chromatin staining. The A-dark spermatogonia exhibit uniform dark nuclei and are presumptive adult stem cells, but other theories claim that both A-pale and A-dark spermatogonia are capable of self-renewal.[311] Spermatogonial niches in the seminiferous tubules are thought to provide the necessary microenvironment to maintain self-renewal in the presence of relevant systemic and locally secreted Sertoli

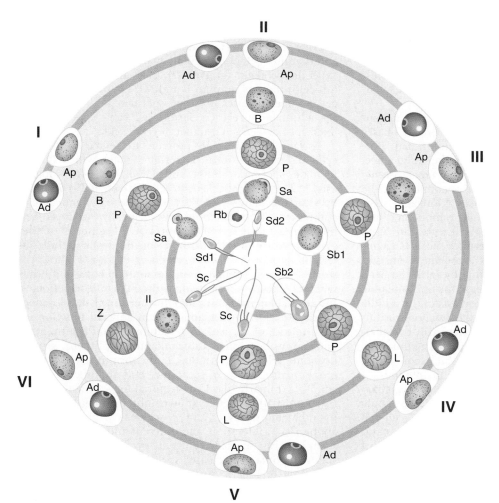

Figure 12-9. Spermatogenic cycle. Schematic representation of the six stages of the human spermatogenic cycle and with associated germ cells positioned to show sequence of development as a spiral pathway of ever-increasing radius. In actual tubules, some cell associations would be more superficial or deeper levels. Ad, Ap, and B denote, respectively, dark and pale type A and B spermatogonia; PL, L, Z, P, and II, preleptotene, leptotene, zygotene, pachytene, and meiotic division I and II spermatocytes; Sa, Sb1, Sb2, Sc, Sd1, and Sd2, steps in spermiogenesis; Rb, excess residual body cytoplasm. (From Kerr JB. Functional cytology of the human testis. Baillieres Clin Endocrinol Metab 6[2]:235, 1992, Fig. 4.)

cell factors. Endocrine, paracrine, and autocrine signals to spermatogonial mitosis include FSH, retinoic acid, stem cell factor (*kit* ligand), and glial cell line–derived neurotropic factor. The last two peptides are produced by Sertoli cells. Inactivating mutations of the *c-kit* gene (stem cell factor receptor) cause azoospermia, bone marrow failure, and absence of mast cells.[316,317]

Type B spermatogonia are characterized by granulated nuclear chromatin and a nucleolus, consistent with greater differentiation and commitment to meiosis. Meiosis requires 3.5 weeks in humans, comprising a prophase (leptotene, zygotene, pachytene, and diplotene), metaphase, and anaphase. Cells undergoing meiosis are primary spermatocytes, in which the preleptotene stage is characterized by DNA synthesis (occurring for the last time during spermatogenesis). Chromosome number remains diploid but DNA content doubles in association with finely granulated and uniformly distributed nuclear chromatin. Spermatocytes then lose contact with the basement membrane of the tubule (see Fig. 12-9). Leptotene (thin and thread-like) spermatocytes begin in prophase, and then gradually enter the zygotene phase when homologous chromosomes pair and synapse. Cells continue to increase in volume until the pachytene (large size) stage of premeiotic chromosomal recombination that introduces genetic diversity. The subsequent first meiotic division produces secondary spermatocytes, in which chromosome number is halved, thereby defining haploidy, and DNA content per cell is reduced from 4N to 2N. Secondary spermatocytes are rarely identified histologically, because the second meiotic division follows rapidly without an intervening S phase of DNA synthesis to form 1N spermatids.

Round and elongated spermatids undergo spermiogenesis, which can be divided into three interlinked phases referred to as Golgi, acrosomal, and maturational. Protein synthesis increases markedly during the Golgi stage, and the acrosome forms by coalescence of proacrosomic vesicles from the Golgi apparatus. Concomitantly, the nucleus of round spermatids condenses. Elongated spermatids emerge by further structural remodeling and differentiation. Although morphologic features are used to stage spermatid development, spermiogenesis is a continuous, not a discrete, process. As acrosome formation proceeds at one nuclear pole to eventually form the head of the spermatozoon, centrioles gather at the opposite pole to form the flagellum (tail). The tail consists of the middle piece, principal piece. and end piece. Mitochondria migrate along the developing axoneme, the main cytoskeletal component of the sperm tail. Collapse of cytoplasmic volume results in a residual cytoplasmic body containing obsolete organelles and redundant nuclear membranes.

As the spermatid elongates, an ectoplasmic specialization orients the flagellum toward the seminiferous tubule lumen. The ectoplasmic specialization is a unique cell-cell junction joining the plasma membranes of the spermatid acrosome and the Sertoli cell. Spermiation, or release of spermatids into the lumen of the seminiferous tubules, involves disassembly of these ectoplasmic specializations. During spermiation, the residual cytoplasmic body is retained by Sertoli cells, and eventually phagocytosed.

Meiosis and spermiogenesis are hormonally regulated in rodents, whereas spermatogonial division and spermiation are so regulated in primates. Adequate FSH and LH secretion and action are required to initiate spermatogenesis in primates. The relative importance of FSH, unlike Te, in maintaining spermatogenesis remains controversial.[318,319] LH elevates intratesticular Te concentrations by 65-fold more than systemic Te concentrations, as is necessary to maintain spermatogenesis. Sertoli cells express an FSH-inducible aromatase system, thus permitting intratubular synthesis of E_2 as well. Te stimulates Sertoli cells expressing AR rather than germ cells, which probably do not express AR.[320]

Sertoli Cells

Adult Sertoli cells are nondividing asymmetrical columnar cells with an elongated typically tripartite nucleus, a prominent nucleolus, abundant smooth endoplasmic reticulum, Golgi complexes, mitochondria, lysosomes, and cytoskeletal components. Immature Sertoli cells proliferate during fetal and neonatal life until the age of 12 to 18 months, and then again during the peripubertal period.[321] Secretion of müllerian-inhibiting substance by fetal Sertoli cells is critical for the regression of embryonic müllerian ducts, leaving the prostatic utricle as a remnant. Proliferation and maturation are subject to endocrine control. FSH stimulates proliferation, whereas Te and thyroid hormones regulate maturation of Sertoli cells. With the neonatal surge of LH, FSH, and Te, the two Sertoli cell products, inhibin B and MIS, both rise.[322] Sertoli cell number dictates maximal spermatogenic capacity in the adult, because each Sertoli cell can support only a fixed species-defined number of germ cells.

Estradiol and multiple proteins are secreted by Sertoli cells and serve as local paracrine signals, which further regulate spermatogenesis and Leydig-cell steroidogenesis.[118] For example, Sertoli cell–derived IGF-I induced by systemic delivery of FSH to the testis enhances LH-stimulated Te production synergistically, whereas Sertoli cell–secreted IGFBP-3 mutes IGF-I action.[148] Other systemic hormones that can act on the testis include interleukins, leptin, growth hormone, L-thyroxine, and cortisol.[323-325] In the human, a large amount of cortisol inhibits whereas growth hormone does not affect Te secretion.[326] Intratesticular mediators may further direct developmental and stress-related adaptations in gonadal function via local release of E_2, activin A, inhibin A, follistatin, atrial natriuretic hormone, catecholamines, ghrelin, growth hormone releasing hormone, corticotropin-releasing hormone, neuropeptide Y, serotonin, and arginine vasopressin.[327-331] In particular E_2 is required for spermatogenesis, in contrast to its better known inhibitory effects on the hypothalamo-pituitary unit,[238] whereas activins influence apoptosis, proliferation, and differentiation.[303]

In humans, the spermatogenic cycle (transit time from spermatogonia to ejaculated spermatozoa) is 60 to 70 days according to kinetic studies using stable isotopes.[312,332] This cycle length is shorter than earlier estimates of 90 days.[333] Cross-species germ cell transplantation experiments suggest that cycle length is dictated by the germ cell, rather than Sertoli cell.[334] Physiologic principles of spermatogenesis confer a basis for understanding male-directed (hormonal and nonhormonal) contraceptive methods, because repression of spermatogonial proliferation only becomes evident 2 months later in ejaculated sperm.

Regulation of Male Fertility

Child rearing imposes major life demands, and consequently fertile couples practice family planning to obviate unintended pregnancies and to conform childbearing with personal desires and financial abilities. Accordingly, broadening contraceptive choices to allow men and women the option to share family-planning responsibilities satisfies important individual and societal needs. Surveys reveal that effective and safe male-directed contraceptive methods, if available and reversible, would be acceptable to many men and women.[335,336]

Hormonal methods that exploit exogenous feedback-based suppression of gonadotropin secretion, analogous to ovulation inhibition by combined estrogen-progestin contraceptives, are effective, reversible, and safe in the short term.[337-342] Androgen or androgen-progestin treatment combinations promote germ cell apoptosis and inhibit spermatogenesis, resulting in azoospermia (no sperm in ejaculate) or near-azoospermia (≤1 million sperm/mL semen) with acceptable safety parameters.[343] Dual-hormone regimens are more effective and white populations more responsive than Asian cohorts.[344] Marked suppression of sperm output confers contraception with efficacy rates of 97% to 100%.[337-340] Subsequent restoration of spermatogenes to levels consistent with normal male fertility has been observed in all men.[341]

Additional approaches to male contraception are under active investigation. Long-acting GnRH-receptor antagonists with Te addback are candidate agents. Epididymal targets are plausible, because spermatozoal maturation is critical for fully motile sperm.[345,346] Other studies have explored contraceptive vaccines using GnRH or zona pellucida (oocyte) proteins as antigenic targets.

Decremental Changes in GnRH-LH-Te Axis in Aging

The fundamental mechanisms that cause hypoandrogenemia in the aging male remain unknown. However, recent animal experiments and clinical investigations have disclosed multiple alterations in the aging gonadal axis, such as (1) lower amplitude LH pulses, suggesting reduced drive by GnRH or excessive sex-steroid inhibition; (2) more frequent LH pulses and less orderly patterns of LH release, pointing to diminished negative feedback; (3) preserved LH and heightened FSH responses to exogenous GnRH pulses, indicating intact gonadotrope function; (4) reduced pulsatile and thereby total daily Te secretion; and (5) impaired Te secretion in response to both elevated endogenous LH concentrations (stimulated by flutamide, tamoxifen, GnRH, or anastrozole) and infused pulses of recombinant human LH.[131,347] These alterations are summarized in Figure 12-10.

Collective clinical findings allow the hypothesis that relative androgen deficiency in older men reflects multisite failure of the GnRH-LH-Te axis. This postulate has not yet been tested in individual men. One noninvasive strategy is to exploit an integrative biomathematical model of reciprocal interactions among GnRH, LH, and Te via estimable feedback and feedforward interactions.[287] The analytical rationale is to reconstruct aging-related adaptations among all three interlinked signals, rather than any one signal in isolation.[268] According to such ensemble analyses, the most parsimonious explication of available clinical data is that aging (1) attenuates hypothalamic GnRH outflow, (2) impairs testicular responsiveness to LH pulses, and (3) decreases androgenic negative feedback.[138,268]

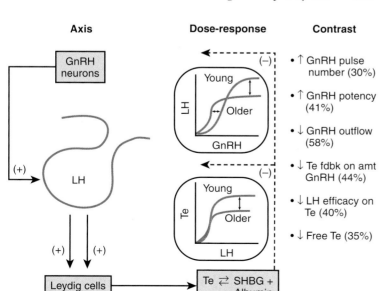

Axis   **Dose-response**   **Contrast**

- ↑ GnRH pulse number (30%)
- ↑ GnRH potency (41%)
- ↓ GnRH outflow (58%)
- ↓ Te fdbk on amt GnRH (44%)
- ↓ LH efficacy on Te (40%)
- ↓ Free Te (35%)

Figure 12-10. Schema of inferred anatomic sites (left) and adaptive mechanisms (right) that subserve relative testosterone deficiency in healthy older (age > 60 years) compared with young (age < 35 years) men. Arrows define stimulation (+) and inhibition (–). The two circled insets depict age-related contrasts in GnRH → LH drive [top center] and LH → Te feedforward [bottom center]. GnRH, gonadotropin-releasing hormone; LH, luteinizing hormone; SHBG, sex hormone–binding globulin; Te, testosterone. (Adapted from Liu PY, Takahashi PY, Nehra AX, et al. Neuroendocrine aging: Pituitary-testis: LH/FSH/Prolactin. In Squire LR, Albright TD, Bloom FE, et al [eds]. New Encyclopedia of Neuroscience. Oxford, Elsevier, 2008, Fig. 8.)

Longitudinal studies will be required to establish the relative importance of inferred regulatory deficits in healthy aging men. In addition, the degree to which mechanisms associated with aging emerge in other clinical syndromes of hypogonadotropic hypogonadism, such as those associated with visceral adiposity, type II diabetes mellitus, uremia, hepatic failure, or chronic stress-anxiety states, has not been investigated.

ACKNOWLEDGMENTS: We thank Kay Nevinger for support of manuscript preparation and Ashley Bryant for graphical presentations. Supported in part via the Center for Translational Science Activities (CTSA) Grant Number 1 UL 1 RR024150 from the National Center for Research Resources (Rockville, MD); AG029362, DK072095, and DK063609 from the National Institutes of Health (Bethesda, MD); and Career Development Award 511929 from the National Health and Medical Research Council of Australia.

The complete reference list can be found on the companion Expert Consult Web site at www.expertconsultbook.com.

Suggested Reading

Adham IM, Agoulnik AI. Insulin-like 3 signalling in testicular descent. Int J Androl 27:257, 2004.

Cunha GR, Ricke W, Thomson A, et al. Hormonal, cellular, and molecular regulation of normal and neoplastic prostatic development. J Steroid Biochem Mol Biol 92:221, 2004.

Heinlein CA, Chang C. Androgen receptor (AR) coregulators: an overview. Endocr Rev 23:175, 2002.

Keenan DM, Takahashi PY, Liu PY, et al. An ensemble model of the male gonadal axis: illustrative application in aging men. Endocrinology 147:2817, 2006.

Liu PY, Iranmanesh A, Nehra AX, et al. Mechanisms of hypoandrogenemia in healthy aging men. Endocrinol Clin North Am 34:935, 2005.

Liu PY, Swerdloff RS, Christenson PD, et al. Rate, extent, and modifiers of spermatogenic recovery after hormonal male contraception: an integrated analysis. Lancet 367:1412, 2006.

Matzuk MM, Lamb DJ. Genetic dissection of mammalian fertility pathways. Nat Cell Biol 4(Suppl):S41, 2002.

McLachlan RI, Rajpert-De ME, Hoei-Hansen CE, et al. Histological evaluation of the human testis: approaches to optimizing the clinical value of the assessment: mini review. Hum Reprod 22:2, 2007.

O'Donnell L, Robertson KM, Jones ME, et al. Estrogen and spermatogenesis. Endocr Rev 22:289, 2001.

Phillips DJ. Activins, inhibins and follistatins in the large domestic species. Domest Anim Endocrinol 28:1, 2005.

Plant TM. The role of KiSS-1 in the regulation of puberty in higher primates. Eur J Endocrinol 155(Suppl 1):S11, 2006.

Revelli A, Massobrio M, Tesarik J. Nongenomic actions of steroid hormones in reproductive tissues. Endocr Rev 19:3, 1998.

Schnorr JA, Bray MJ, Veldhuis JD. Aromatization mediates testosterone's short-term feedback restraint of 24-hour endogenously driven and acute exogenous GnRH-stimulated LH and FSH secretion in young men. J Clin Endocrinol Metab 86:2600, 2001.

Sharpe RM, McKinnell C, Kivlin C et al. Proliferation and functional maturation of Sertoli cells, and their relevance to disorders of testis function in adulthood. Reproduction 125:769, 2003.

Stocco DM, Clark BJ. Regulation of the acute production of steroids in steroidogenic cells. Endocr Rev 17:221, 1996.

Trarbach EB, Silveira LG, Latronico AC. Genetic insights into human isolated gonadotropin deficiency. Pituitary 10:381, 2007.

Tsai MY, Yeh SD, Wang RS, et al. Differential effects on spermatogenesis and fertility in mice lacking androgen receptor in individual testis cells. Proc Natl Acad Sci U S A 103:18975, 2006.

Winters SJ, Moore JP. Paracrine control of gonadotrophs. Semin Reprod Med 25:379, 2007.

Wu FCW, Butler GE, Kelnar CJH, et al. Patterns of pulsatile luteinizing hormone secretion from childhood to adulthood in the human male: a study using deconvolution analysis and an ultrasensitive immunofluorometric assay. J Clin Endocrinol Metab 81:1798, 1996.

Yu B, Handelsman DJ. Pharmacogenetic polymorphisms of the AR and metabolism and susceptibility to hormone-induced azoospermia. J Clin Endocrinol Metab 86:4406, 2001.

CHAPTER 13

Reproductive Immunology and Its Disorders

Breton F. Barrier, Antonio R. Gargiulo, and Danny J. Schust

The immune system plays a central role in maternal-placental-fetal cross-talk, and its involvement in the pathophysiology of a growing number of reproductive disorders is well described. The involvement of the immune system in normal and abnormal pregnancy processes underscores the importance of a detailed understanding of basic principles of immunology to the field of reproductive medicine. The contribution of experimental immunology to clinical reproductive medicine has evolved and expanded rapidly. This evolution of knowledge, in concert with the frequently confusing terminology characteristic of the field, often hinders its ready access to the practicing physician. This chapter will review key immunologic concepts, the role of the immune system in the pathophysiology of human reproductive disorders, and current diagnostic and therapeutic options for immune-mediated infertility and recurrent pregnancy loss.

Basic Immune Principles

Historically, immune responses have been characterized by their location, timing, target, or specificity (Table 13-1). Antigen-specific immune responses can be divided into cellular and humoral arms. *Cellular immunity* is defined as a response to a particular antigen that can be transferred to a naive (nonimmunized) individual via the lymphocytes (but not the plasma or serum) from another immunized subject. Conversely, *humoral immune responsiveness* to a particular antigen can be transferred to a naive subject using only the plasma or serum from an immunized individual. The response is known to be dependent on the presence of antibodies in the immunizing sera. Put simply,

cellular responses require cell-to-cell interactions, whereas humoral responses are antibody-mediated.

Immune responses have also classically been divided into acquired (also called adaptive) and innate subtypes. *Acquired immune responses* are antigen-specific and are largely mediated by T cells and B cells. Acquired responses involve the development of immunologic memory and can be classified as either primary (a response associated with initial antigen contact) or secondary (a rapid and powerful amnestic response associated with repeated contact to the same antigen). In contrast, *innate immune responses* are rapid but not antigen-specific. As recently as 10 years ago, innate responses were understood only as the body's first line of defense against pathogenic invasion. We now know that innate responders not only destroy invaders, but also detect the type of pathologic threat they pose and then appropriately polarize the acquired immune response to respond accordingly. Therefore, innate immunity is particularly important at sites of common pathogen contact, such as the skin, the intestine, and the reproductive tract.

In the first section covering basic immune principles, we will (1) introduce innate immunity and inflammation; (2) give a brief overview of acquired immunity; and (3) review the current understanding of immune regulation. Each is important for the proper understanding of the immunology of reproduction.

INNATE IMMUNITY AND INFLAMMATION

Vital to innate immunity are secretion of certain cytokines; activation of the complement cascade; phagocytosis of pathogens by macrophages and polymorphonuclear

(PMN) leukocytes such as neutrophils, basophils, and eosinophils; and the killing of infected or abnormal cells by natural killer (NK) cells.

The initial entry of foreign organisms or cells into a host is met by an inflammatory response. This is true for pathogens such as bacteria and also for necessary invaders such as sperm or the blastocyst. The difference in the response is determined by the invader—some, such as bacteria and viruses, cause inflammation that promotes an offensive environment, a call to arms.[1] Others, such as sperm or some cancer cells, appear to cause inflammation that is accommodating to the invader.[2,3] Elements of inflammation common to all responses include an increase in the local blood supply, influx of leukocytes, and an increase in local tissue edema. Local edema leads to an increase in intracellular hydrostatic pressure promoting lymphatic flow toward draining lymph nodes.

Cellular Mediators of the Innate Immune Response

The leukocytes initially recruited to inflamed tissues include polymorphonuclear leukocytes (PMNs—neutrophils, basophils, and eosinophils), NK cells, and monocytes. The PMNs target pathogens that have been *opsonized*—tagged or coated—by complement components, antibodies, or the two in combination. PMNs kill by releasing toxic granules containing effector molecules and enzymes in close proximity to the target.[4] The local killing is thus nonspecific and bystander damage can occur, including the sacrifice of the PMN. PMNs have a lifespan in the resting state measured in hours, not days.

NK cells, on the other hand, are very selective innate killers, employing the same method of killing as their close relatives, the cytotoxic T cells. This method includes identification of an abnormal cell, formation of an *immunologic*

TABLE 13-1
Dichotomous Concepts in Immunology

Concept	Dichotomous Variables	
General Mediators of Antibody Response	**Innate** Antigen nonspecific; rapid Sentinel function: antigen-presenting cells; acquired immune polarization Effector cell function: mediated by NK cells, macrophages; antibody dependent and independent cytotoxicity; no "memory"	**Acquired/Adaptive** Antigen-specific; primary and secondary responses Effector cell function: mediated by T and B lymphocytes; capable of developing "memory" Regulatory function: mediated by CD4+ CD25+ regulatory T cells
	Cellular Acquired immunity transferred to naive recipient via the cellular fraction; lymphocyte-mediated	**Humoral** Immunity transferred to naive recipient via the soluble fraction; antibody-mediated
	Primary Peaks at 5-10 days IgM > IgG Lower magnitude	**Secondary** Peaks at 2-5 days IgG > IgM Robust response; immunologic memory; antibody isotype switching
Immune Subsystems	**Peripheral** Immune interactions in the spleen, lymph nodes, lymphatic system, and peripheral blood; promote the recognition and destruction of pathogenic organisms	**Mucosal** Immune interactions in the respiratory tract, gastrointestinal tract, genitourinary tract and lacrimal ducts; IgA secretion; promote the induction of active immune tolerance toward innocuous factors
Antigen Presentation	**MHC Class I** Expressed on nearly all cells; includes HLA-A, -B, and -C tissue antigens; involved in viral infections and transplant recognition; interact with T-cell receptor on CD8+ T lymphocytes; interact with specific NK cell receptors	**MHC Class II** Expressed on antigen presenting cells—dendritic cells, macrophages, B lymphocytes, and epithelia; upregulated by interferon-γ; includes HLA-DR tissue antigen interact with T-cell receptor on CD4+ T-lymphocytes Extracellular pathogens Bacterial infections
Education	**B cells** Bone marrow Single step Negative selection against self-antigen	**T cells** Thymus Two steps Positive selection for self MHC Recognition/negative selection against self-antigen

HLA, human leukocyte antigen; MHC, major histocompatibility complex; NK, natural killer.

synapse, release of *perforin* to form channels in the cell membrane, and the release of *granzyme* into the cell to activate the *caspase cascade* within the target. This cascade results in *apoptosis* or programmed cell death of the targeted cell. Abnormal cells are recognized by NK cells through several known mechanisms. It has been classically understood that NK cells recognize and kill cells that do not express major histocompatibility complex (MHC) class I antigens, such as some transformed cells. This process is referred to as the *null cell hypothesis*. However that is only part of the story. Some MHC class I negative cells are ignored by NK cells. This can be explained because, although NK cells recognize distress proteins expressed on somatic cells, it is the balance in signaling between activating and inhibitory receptors that determines NK cell behavior.[5]

NK cells are important to the establishment of early pregnancy. At least two NK cell subsets have been described. The majority (~90%) of human NK cells have low-density expression of CD56 (CD56dim) and express high levels of CD16, the immunoglobin receptor responsible for NK-mediated, antibody-dependent cellular cytotoxicity. Conversely, approximately 10% of NK cells are CD56bright, CD16dim, or CD56bright, CD16−.[6] Human CD56bright NK cells are considered to be poorly cytotoxic but are potent cytokine producers, whereas CD56dim NK cells display higher levels of cytotoxicity but are poor cytokine producers. Low levels of CD56bright, CD16− NK cells are found in the nonpregnant endometrium throughout the follicular phase of the menstrual cycle. Their numbers increase during the luteal phase. In pregnancy, these NK cells aggregate in the decidua basalis at the implantation site, remain at high numbers during early gestation, decrease after 20 weeks of gestation, and are absent in term decidua.[7-9]

Antigen-presenting cells (APCs) bridge the gap between innate and acquired immunity. APCs, including dendritic cells and macrophages, initiate adaptive processes by phagocytizing pathogens. They then process these pathogens and present the resulting antigens to T lymphocytes in draining lymph nodes. For completeness, it is mentioned here that B lymphocytes—members of the acquired immune system—are also capable of presenting antigen to helper T (T$_H$) cells that, in turn, release programming cytokines that facilitate proper antibody production.

Monocytes are the precursors of macrophages and of dendritic cells (DCs) of myeloid lineage. Another class of DCs appear to be derived from a lymphocyte lineage. Different types of DCs appear to promote different types of immune responses, including the development of peripheral self-tolerance. Our understanding of the biology of DCs is still in its infancy, but evolves rapidly. For more information on the subject the reader is directed to current reviews, such as that by Iwasaki.[10]

Most tissues already contain differentiated cells important for antigen presentation. Proteins called *pattern recognition receptors* (PRRs), such as the *toll-like receptors*, are utilized by the APCs to detect conserved pathogen-specific molecules such as lipopolysaccharide or double-stranded RNA. The detected *pathogen-associated molecular patterns* (PAMPs) then activate and mature the APC and dictate which cytokines are secreted by this cell to polarize the acquired immune response.[1]

Complement

The *complement cascade* is a vital part of innate immunity. It may be useful to compare the complement cascade to a more familiar clinical entity, the coagulation cascade. Both have components that circulate in inactive forms. Activation of each pathway can occur via two mechanisms. Reminiscent of the intrinsic and extrinsic coagulation pathways, the complement cascade can be activated via classical and alternative pathways (Fig. 13-1).[11] The classical pathway is activated when a complement component C1 binds to antigen-antibody complexes (IgG or IgM). The alternative pathway is activated when complement component C3b binds to activating surfaces such as the cell wall of a bacterial pathogen. Each pathway sets off a series of activating enzymatic digestions of subsequent complement cascade components.

Like the coagulation cascade, both of the activation pathways in the complement cascade intersect, joining in a final common effector pathway. Late components of the

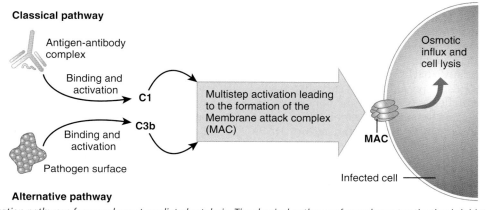

Figure 13-1. *Activation pathways for complement-mediated cytolysis. The classical pathway of complement activation is initiated by the binding of antigen-antibody complexes to complement factor C1. The binding of C3b to activating surfaces such as a bacterial cell wall activates the alternative pathway. Activation of either pathway results in a cascade of subsequent enzymatic activations. These pathways converge, forming the membrane attack complex (MAC). The MAC allows osmotic shifts that lyse the affected target cell. Complement-mediated activities can also include promotion of inflammatory responses, direct opsinization of pathogenic substances, and clearance of unwanted immune complexes.*

TABLE 13-2

Representative Cytokines, Source, and Function

Cytokine	Source	Function
IFN-γ	T_H1 cells, CTLs, NK cells	Recruits NK cells Up-regulates MHC Promotes T_H1 cells Suppresses T_H17 and T_H2 cells
IL-2	T_H1 cells, CTLs	Lymphocyte proliferation Receptor is CD25
IL-17	T_H17 cells	Induces stromal cells to produce IL-8 and IL-6 Suppresses T_H1 cells
IL-4	T_H2 cells, dendritic cells	Promotes B-cell antibody production Promotes T_H2 cells Suppresses T_H1 cells
IL-13	T_H2 cells	Promotes B-cell antibody isotype switching Up-regulates MHC II
TNF-α	Primarily macrophages	Recruits PMN leukocytes Causes cardinal signs of inflammation Causes apoptosis in some cells
IL-6	Stromal cells and macrophages	Promotes acute-phase protein production
IL-8	Stromal cells and macrophages	Recruits neutrophils
IL-10	T_{reg} cells, dendritic cells	Anti-inflammatory Inhibits production of IFN-γ, IL-2, and TNF-α
TGF-β	T_{reg} cells, dendritic cells	Promotes the differentiation of T_{reg} cells Suppresses T_H1 and T_H2 cells

CTLs, cytolytic T cells; IFN, interferon; IL, interleukin; MHC, major histocompatibility complex; NK, natural killer; PMN, polymorphonuclear; TGF, transforming growth factor; T_H, T helper cell; TNF, tumor necrosis factors; T_{reg}, regulatory T cell.

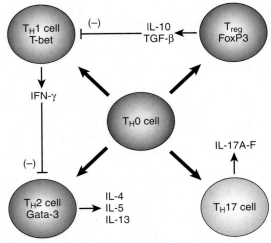

Figure 13-2. *The T_H1/T_H2 polarization paradigm. The cytokine microenvironment in which antigen is presented by antigen-presenting cells to immature (T_H0) T helper cells promotes development into T_H1, T_H2, T_H17, and T_{reg} phenotypes. It appears that each T helper phenotype supports further development of itself while opposing development of its counterparts.*

complement cascade can interact with specific complement receptors, resulting in pathogen phagocytosis or activation of the humoral immune system. Alternatively, activation of the complement cascade can result in the formation of a membrane attack complex (MAC) that results in indirect osmotic lysis of a target cell through the formation of an ion permeable transmembrane pore in that target cell.

Because complement provides a potent tool for opsonizing targets, recruiting immune effectors and directly damaging tissues, it is imperative that it be controlled. Complement regulatory proteins exist to protect against excessive or unwanted complement effects. CD59 is a membrane-bound inhibitor of C5b-9 formation and aggregation of the membrane attack complex. Decay accelerating factor (DAF; CD55) is a membrane-bound complement regulator that inhibits the C3/C5 convertase step. Yet another enzyme called factor I is capable of cleaving and inactivating C3b and C4b in combination with an array of other cofactors, including membrane cofactor protein (MCP; CD46). Many of these factors are present on the early developing syncytiotrophoblast and extravillous cytotrophoblast cell, underscoring the importance of protecting the early placenta from nonspecific complement activation.[12,13]

Cytokines

The rapidly enlarging and pleomorphic family of cytokines are important soluble mediators of immune responses. *Cytokines* are a family of secreted proteins generated by immune cells and even by some tissues. They include the interleukins (ILs), the interferons (IFNs), tumor necrosis factors (TNFs), transforming growth factors (TGFs), and the chemokines. Cytokines may act through autocrine, paracrine, or endocrine mechanisms, and effects are mediated by specific cytokine receptors. Most cytokines have short half-lives, so direct actions are typically of short duration. Cytokines, however, often stimulate additional immune cell activity with cascading cytokine secretion and effects. Members of this large family of soluble immune mediators often have complementary or redundant activities. A list of representative cytokines and their source and function is found in Table 13-2.

A helpful way to understand cytokine function is to think of different combinations of cytokines as analogous to a chord on a piano that elicits not a musical sound, but rather a specific immune response (Fig. 13-2). For example, when the "chord" of IL-10 and TGF-β is "played" by regulatory T cells, a local tolerogenic response is aroused. When the "chord" of IL-4, IL-5, and IL-13 is "played" by a T_H2 cell, a B cell is told to develop an antibody-mediated response, especially an IgE response. And when IFN-γ and IL-12 are "played" in combination by a DC, a responding T_H0 cell becomes a T1 cell. Many variations of these signals likely exist, contributing to the beauty and complexity of the immune response.

ADAPTIVE IMMUNITY

The cellular effectors of adaptive immunity include the lymphocytes, which can be divided into subclasses based on function and upon cell surface markers called *cluster*

TABLE 13-3

CD4+ T Helper Cell (T$_H$) Penotypes

T$_H$1	T$_H$17	T$_H$2	T$_{reg}$
Promotes inflammation	Promotes inflammation	Promotes antibody responses	Suppresses inflammation
Characterized by IFN-γ and IL-2 secretion	Characterized by IL-17 secretion	Characterized by IL-4, IL-5, and IL-13 secretion	Characterized by IL-10 and TGF-β secretion
Promoted by IL-12, and IFN-γ	Promoted by IL-23	Promoted by IL-4	Promoted by TGF-β
Associated with T-bet	Associated with RORγt	Associated with Gata-3	Associated with FoxP3

IFN, interferon; IL, interleukin; TGF, transforming growth factor; T$_{reg}$, regulatory T cell.

of differentiation (or CD) markers. Lymphocyte subclasses include T cells and B cells. The close relatives of these lymphocytes include the natural killer (NK) cells and a subset of dendritic cells. Both B and T lymphocytes originate in the bone marrow and participate in antigen-specific immune responses.

In humans, *T cells* circulate through the thymus, where they gain specific CD markers, antigen specificity, and tolerance to self. T lymphocytes maturing in the thymus express both CD8 and CD4 cell surface receptors during early development, but those exiting the thymus express only one of these cell surface markers.

The majority of CD8+ T cells leaving the thymus are destined to mature into cytolytic T cells (CTLs), which are intended to kill infected or otherwise altered target cells. The CD8+ CTLs are important for clearing intracytoplasmic infections. These CTLs bind to the infected cell and induce *apoptosis*, or programmed cell death. The apoptotic cells are then cleared by antigen-presenting cells, such as macrophages, further reinforcing the acquired immune response.

The majority of circulating CD4+ lymphocytes are naïve, functionally immature T helper cells (T$_H$0).[14] The T$_H$0 cell is matured at the time of exposure to antigen presented by an APC. The type of APC presenting antigen and the conditions of exposure, including the presence of the local cytokine microenvironment, directs the differentiation pathway of a CD4 T helper cell. CD4+ T$_H$ cell subsets are defined by the secretion of specific cytokines that affect the local immunologic microenvironment (Table 13-3; see also Fig. 13-2).

T helper subsets with reciprocal patterns of immunity were first proposed by Mosmann and Coffman in their T$_H$1/T$_H$2 hypothesis,[15] although the array of CD4+ T helper cell subsets continues to be defined. If antigen is recognized by T$_H$0 cells in a microenvironment dominated by the cytokine interleukin 12 (IL-12), the resulting T helper effector phenotype is characterized by the secretion of cytokines that potentiate cell-mediated cytotoxicity, including IFN-γ and IL-2. This type of response is called a *T helper 1 (T$_H$1) response*.[16] Alternatively, if T$_H$0 cells recognize antigen in a microenvironment dominated by IL-4, the predominant T helper response is of the T$_H$2 type and is characterized by secretion of IL-4, IL-5, IL-9, and IL-13.[17,18] These T$_H$2 cytokines, in turn, stimulate allergic-type responses, including mast cell and eosinophil activation and B-cell antibody production. In general, T$_H$1 responses enhance T$_H$1 responses while inhibiting T$_H$2 responses. T$_H$2 responses initiate a positive feedback loop that promotes further T$_H$2 activity while inhibiting T$_H$1 effects.

Pioneering literature suggests that T$_H$1 and T$_H$2 responses represent a cytotoxic/humoral balance within the immune system, with pregnancy supported by a T$_H$2 but threatened by a T$_H$1 balance.[19] Some cases of spontaneous, isolated, or recurrent pregnancy loss have been hypothesized to be the result of an abnormal polarization of maternal lymphocytes upon exposure to placental antigens.[20-23] The universal applicability of this view has been modified as challenging new data have emerged.[24] Recently, additional fundamental helper cell subtypes have been described, including the so-called T$_H$17 and regulatory T-cell (T$_{reg}$) subsets. Both of these important T helper subtypes may be found to play and important role in normal and pathologic immune processes during implantation and pregnancy.

The T$_H$17 cell is a CD4+ cell subset that preferentially produces IL-17 family cytokines (including IL-17A and IL-17F) that cause local neutrophilic inflammation by upregulating stromal IL-8 and IL-6. These cells play a critical role in sustaining the inflammatory response, and their presence is closely associated with autoimmune diseases (reviewed by Harrington and colleagues).[25]

The T$_{reg}$ cell is a recently described CD4+ T-cell subtype that appears to play an important role in protection against autoimmunity and in successful allotransplantation through its secretion of regulatory cytokines such as IL-10 and/or TGF-β.[26,27] T$_{reg}$ cells are identified as CD4+ cells that are also constitutively positive for CD25 even in their resting state.[28] CD25 is the IL-2 receptor α chain that is upregulated on all activated lymphocytes. For this reason, T$_{reg}$ cells can be confused with other activated lymphocytes. It is therefore prudent to use other factors in their identification, such as the intracellular presence of the forkhead box P3 (FoxP3) transcription factor which seems to be relatively specific for this T helper subtype.[29,30] Emerging evidence also suggests that T$_{reg}$ cells may play a role in the prevention of immunologically mediated abortion. In the abortion-prone mouse model, Zenclussen and colleagues performed experiments in which the adoptive transfer of T$_{reg}$ cells from normal pregnant mice into abortion-prone mice was sufficient to prevent immunologically mediated abortion.[31]

B Cells

B cells appear to be educated in the bone marrow prior to exit into the peripheral immune system.[32] Like T lymphocytes, B lymphocytes are antigen specific. Unlike T lymphocytes, B cells function to secrete antibodies, which characterize humoral immune responses.

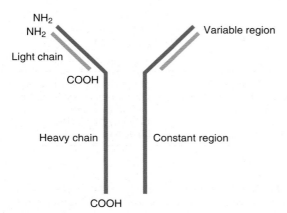

Figure 13-3. *A typical immunoglobulin molecule. The constant region (carboxy [COOH] terminal) isotype of the heavy chain determines function. The combined variable regions (amino [NH₂] terminal) of the heavy and light chains determine antigen specificity. IgC, IgE, and IgD isotypes are typically monomers of this basic structure.*

Immunoglobulins and Humoral Immunity

Immunoglobulin (Ig) molecules are composed of dimerized subunits of heavy and light chains (Fig. 13-3). The N-terminal portions of each of the heavy and light chains are highly polymorphic and are termed their *variable* regions. The variable region of one heavy chain combines with the variable region of one light chain to give the immunoglobulin its antigen specificity. The C-terminal segments of the immunoglobulin heavy and light chains are called their *constant segments* and have minimal polymorphism.

The constant portion of the immunoglobulin heavy chain interacts with other immune response components. Because these interactions are governed by heavy chain–constant region isotype, so too is immunoglobulin effector function. Ig molecule isotypes include IgA, IgD, IgE, IgG, and IgM. IgG, IgE, and IgD molecules are typically present as single Ig molecules (monomers). IgA molecules usually

circulate as dimers, and IgM molecules as pentamers (Figs. 13-3 and 13-4).

Each Ig isotype has distinctive functions. IgA dimers are often found at mucosal surfaces. These dimers, connected by *a joining* or J *chain*, have been best described in the mucosa of the intestine. They are actively transported into the gut lumen by interaction of the J chain with mucosally derived secretory component, thus exposing IgA to antigens within the intestinal lumen. IgE molecules interact with eosinophils in parasitic infections, allowing eosinophil-mediated target lysis. IgE molecules are also implicated in delayed-type hypersensitivity through mast cell interactions. Membrane-bound IgD and IgM monomers are components of the antigen-recognizing B cell receptor on naive B cells. Pentavalent IgM molecules activate the complement cascade. Secreted IgM multimers are also characteristic of the early antigen-specific responses of naive B cells.

Primary and Secondary Immune Responses

If the antigen recognized by the naive B lymphocyte is not a peptide, T-cell help will be absent. In turn, the initial response, albeit antigen specific, will be of lower affinity, will involve more IgM secretion than IgG, and will not generate immunologic memory. In contrast, if the naive B cell recognizes peptide antigen, the associated help from CD4+ T cells will promote the generation of both primary and secondary humoral immune responses.

The initial or primary immune response requires fairly significant antigenic stimulus and typically peaks approximately 5 to 10 days after antigen exposure. Primary responses usually involve more IgM secretion than IgG, and the magnitude of the response is often lower than that after a second exposure to peptide antigen. Primary exposure to peptide antigen promotes the generation of memory B cells, which drive the characteristics of the secondary humoral immune response.

Antigen exposure, in combination with T-cell help, simultaneously activates B cells, leading to the antibody isotype switching that characterizes secondary responses.

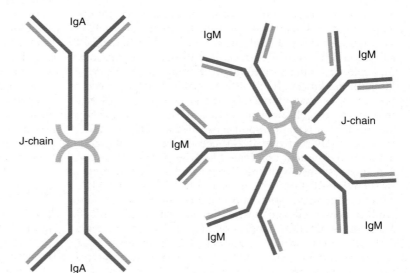

Figure 13-4. *IgA dimers and IgM pentamers. Each structure is connected by a joining chain (J-chain).*

Upon reexposure to the same peptide antigen, this secondary response ensues. Secondary responses require less antigenic exposure than primary responses, they peak more rapidly (2 to 5 days after exposure), and they are typically more robust than primary responses. As a result of isotype switching, IgG rather than IgM molecules represent the predominant immunoglobulin subtype in secondary immune responses.

These IgG molecules have multiple immune effector functions. They can cross the placenta, allowing immune transfer from mother to fetus. IgG can directly bind antigen via its variable region, allowing the free-constant portion of the IgG heavy chain (Fc portion) to be recognized and internalized by phagocytic cells in a process termed *opsonization* (discussed earlier in this chapter). Similarly, IgG bound to cell-associated antigen can signal lytic attack by cytotoxic T cells or NK cells, promoting a process called *antibody-dependent cellular cytotoxicity*. Finally, IgG molecules can activate the complement cascade.

IMMUNE SPECIFICITY AND IMMUNE CELL EDUCATION

While many of the salient attributes of the immune system can be addressed in a description of the cellular and soluble components of immune responses, there are two additional defining features of immune responses that require specific discussion: the specificity of immunologic antigen recognition, and T-lymphocyte education.

Antigen Presentation

Most of the antigens recognized by the effector cells involved in acquired immune responses cannot be detected in isolation. Rather, antigens must be specifically presented to effector cells. This presentation process places antigens into a context in which the cell presenting the antigen can be recognized by the effector cell as "self-derived" and the antigen can be seen as foreign. This process, called *antigen presentation*, is essential to antigen-specific development of both cellular and humoral immune responses.[33,34]

Two sets of genes within the major histocompatibility complex (MHC) region of the human leukocyte antigen (HLA) locus on human chromosome 6 play major roles in antigen presentation. These genetic loci encode the MHC class Ia and MHC class II products (Fig. 13-5), as well as many other molecules involved in antigen presentation. MHC class Ia molecules (e.g., HLA-A, HLA-B, and HLA-C) are present on the surface of nearly every cell in the human body. They aid in defending against intracellular pathogens, such as viruses, by presenting virus-derived antigens at the surface of infected cells. MHC class I molecules also aid in the detection of oncogenically transformed cells by presenting abnormal cellular proteins that occur as a result of oncogenic transformation.

Class I products also play a central role in transplant recognition and rejection. In each case, MHC class I molecules act as important ligands for the T-cell receptor (TCR) on CD8+ cytotoxic T cells. They may also act as important ligands for a variety of receptors on NK cells. MHC class I–mediated intercellular interactions generally activate the

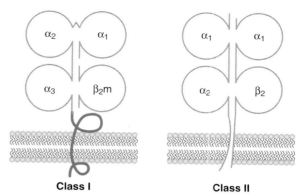

Figure 13-5. Molecular structure of the class I and class II molecules of the HLA system.

cellular portion of the immune response and result in killing of the antigen-presenting (i.e., virally infected, cancerous, or transplanted) cell expressing the class I molecule.

Unlike the globally expressed MHC class I molecules, MHC class II molecules (HLA-DR, HLA-DP, and HLA-DQ) are present on the surface of a limited number of "professional" antigen-presenting cells. These cells include dendritic cells, macrophages, monocytes, B cells, and tissue-specific antigen presenters (e.g., Langerhans' cells in the skin). MHC class II molecules are important in defense against extracellular pathogens, typically bacterial in origin. The T-cell receptor on CD4+ T helper cells acts as the major ligand for MHC class II products. Accordingly, MHC class II–mediated interactions with these T helper cells typically modulate humoral immune responses.

The remarkable polymorphism of the classical MHC class I and class II genes allows for the recognition and presentation of an enormous diversity of peptides. In fact, the MHC genes are typically the most polymorphic of all loci in each species. Between the MHC class I (intracellular pathogens/proteins) and class II (extracellular pathogens/proteins) antigen presentation pathways, nearly every protein in the human body can be sampled. Those derived from foreign (nonself) antigens or altered self are recognized as such and trigger an immune response. In the absence of an autoimmune disorder, peptides derived from unaltered self do not trigger a strong response.

A large number of immune related genes are located within the HLA locus. These genes include many of the complement component and cytokine genes, as well as the classical MHC class Ia and MHC class II products. Other MHC molecules are also encoded within the HLA region of human chromosome 6 and include nonclassical MHC class Ib products and MHC class I–like products. These molecules tend to be less polymorphic than their classical counterparts and are thus predicted to have a less important role in antigen presentation. Nonclassical and MHC class I–related products are thought to play a central role in immune responses at mucosal surfaces, including those within the reproductive tract (these types of responses will be described in more detail later in the section "Antigen Presentation in the Placenta").

Lymphocyte Education

The ability of cells in the immune system to differentiate self from nonself is essential. The education of B lymphocytes in this regard may involve only a single step process—one of negative selection. Those immature B cells that express receptors that recognize self-antigen with high affinity do not survive to exit the bone marrow. This process of negative selection against self-antigen promotes B-cell tolerance to recognition of self-antigens. Self-tolerance by B cells is independent of MHC molecules.[35,36]

T lymphocytes, in contrast, are educated in the thymus via a two-step process.[37,38] Immature T cells entering the thymus express neither the T-cell receptor (TCR) nor the CD4 or CD8 co-receptors. Upon entering the thymus, all three cell surface molecules come to be expressed. During a process called *thymic education*, CD4/CD8 double-positive cells undergo both positive and negative selection events in which T cells mature from CD4/CD8 double-positive cells to single-positive (CD4+ or CD8+) cells.

This two-step maturation positively selects those T cells with T-cell receptors that recognize self-MHC products. Those recognizing self-MHC class I molecules are destined to become CD8 single-positive cytotoxic T cells. Those recognizing self-MHC class II molecules are destined to mature into CD4+ T helper cells. The immature CD4/CD8 double-positive thymocytes that do not recognize self-MHC will die by apoptotic mechanisms.

The second portion of the two-step intrathymic T-cell maturation process is one of negative selection. Negative selection of T cells within the thymus appears to depend on the strength of the recognition of MHC/peptide antigen complexes by the TCR of the developing T lymphocyte. If recognition is particularly strong, the cells undergo apoptosis. This functions to eliminate cells reactive against self-peptide antigens, which are likely to be fairly abundant within the antigen-binding clefts of the thymic antigen-presenting cells. T lymphocytes exiting the thymus should therefore recognize self-MHC but ignore self-antigen.

PERIPHERAL AND MUCOSAL IMMUNE SYSTEMS

The peripheral immune system is composed of those immune cells populating the spleen, lymph nodes, lymphatic system, and peripheral blood. Its basic function is to eliminate blood-borne pathogens and to recognize foreign or oncogenically transformed tissues. Classical immunology and much of modern-day immune investigation have been limited to the study of the peripheral immune system and its responses.

More recently described, and more directly relevant to the reproductive biologist, is the mucosal immune system. The *mucosal immune system* monitors the entry of pathogens across the extensive surface area of mucosal tissues, including the lacrimal ducts, the respiratory and gastrointestinal tracts, the mammary ducts, and the genitourinary tract. Mucosal surfaces typically serve as the initial point of entry for most pathogens. The other major point of pathogen entry is via the surface of the skin which, although sharing many similarities with the mucosal immune system, has its own characteristic effector mechanisms.[39] The cutaneous and mucosal immune systems are largely responsible for providing initial immunologic protection against the majority of exogenous pathogens. Both rely heavily upon innate immune responses.

Many of the properties described here for the peripheral immune system deserve additional description as they apply to mucosal surfaces. Effector cells within the mucosal immune system include all those components found within the peripheral system. However, when compared to peripheral sites, the proportions of leukocyte subpopulations at mucosal sites differ dramatically. Some cell types that are fairly rare within the peripheral circulation are comparatively abundant at mucosal surfaces.

For instance, in the peripheral immune compartment, the vast majority of T cells express a T-cell receptor that has an αβ heterodimer (TCRαβ+) subunit. A very small proportion of T cells in the periphery express a TCR that has a γδ heterodimer (TCRγδ+). In contrast, TCRγδ+ T cells are much more abundant at mucosal surfaces, accounting for as much as 5% of immune cells at some sites. Although the function of TCRγδ+ T cells is incompletely understood, they appear to fulfill functions quite distinct from their TCRαβ+ counterparts. These functions may include direct, non-MHC restricted recognition of antigens within tissues.[40] TCRγδ+ T cells may play an important role in innate immune reactions, consistent with their increased prevalence at mucosal immune sites. They may fill a protective niche missed or poorly addressed by B cells and TCRαβ+ T cells.

Much of what is known about mucosal immunity was initially described within the gastrointestinal tract. Three concepts are important to note. First, the education and trafficking of the immune effector cells populating mucosal sites is often quite distinct from that of the periphery.[41] For instance, some of the effector cells present at sites within the epithelia of the gastrointestinal and reproductive tracts appear to be educated at sites other than within the thymus, a process referred to as *extrathymic education*.[42] Some investigators believe this education may occur within the mucosal epithelia itself.

A second important concept in mucosal immunology is that of cellular recruitment or homing. How is it that the specialized effector cells of particular mucosal immune sites find their way from the peripheral immune system? That question has been best studied within the intestine. Here, cellular recruitment (homing) has been shown to rely on the presence of receptors (integrins) on the surface of immune cell subpopulations. These integrins specifically interact with ligands on the surface of the endothelial cells of blood vessels within the intestine (e.g., selectins, vascular cell adhesion molecule).[43,44] Similar homing characteristics also appear to define immune cell types and vascular structures within the reproductive tract.[45,46]

The third concept to be stressed concerning mucosal site immune reactions is that, although similar in many regards, not all mucosal sites function identically. For instance, both animal and human data suggest that the immune cells at the maternal-fetal interface are selected and maintained in ways that differ both from peripheral immune cells and from cells populating other mucosal sites, such as the intestine.[47]

Reproduction and Immunology: The Fetal Allograft

Application of the basic immune concepts described herein to the process of reproduction generates multiple questions, many of which continue to be actively investigated. In the five decades since Sir Peter Medawar[48] first remarked upon the ability of the implanting fetus to avoid rejection by a maternal host who is typically immunocompetent and semi-allogeneic, studies of reproductive mucosal immunity have often been predicated on the concept of the fetus as an allograft.

Why doesn't the pregnant mother recognize paternal antigens and reject the partially foreign and remarkably invasive tissues implanting in her uterus? Are there special immune cell types or soluble immune mediators at the site of implantation? Is antigen presentation at the maternal-fetal interface distinct from that at other mucosal immune sites? Do unique immunologic control systems exist within the reproductive tract that allow survival of the fetal allograft?[49,50] The answers to such mechanistic questions may be revealed through description of some of the unique aspects of immune responses at the maternal-fetal interface.

CELLULAR AND SOLUBLE MEDIATORS OF IMMUNE RESPONSES AT THE MATERNAL-FETAL INTERFACE

Immune Cell Subtypes

Unlike the peripheral immune system, the human endometrium is populated by very few B lymphocytes. To illustrate this fact, the gynecologist knows well from clinical practice that the presence of plasma cells within the endometrium is abnormal and suggestive of chronic endometritis. The endometrium is, however, normally populated by T cells,[51] macrophages, NK-like cells, and a number of more specialized immune effector cell subtypes.[52-54] The relative proportions of these resident cells demonstrate remarkable menstrual cyclicity. A few of these cellular populations deserve specific description, because their presence in both the female reproductive tract and in the peri-implantation decidua implicate a particularly important role for innate immune interactions during implantation and early pregnancy.[53,55,56]

Peripheral immune cells have been described that have characteristics of both NK cells and T cells.[57] Known as NKT cells, these cells and their ligands (e.g., GDI) have been documented within the decidua of animals[58-60] and have been implicated in some forms of pregnancy loss.[60] Initial investigations in humans have also demonstrated the presence of NKT cells within the endometrium and decidua.[61] The NK-like phenotype of these cells suggests innate immune function.

A more prevalent NK-like cell population is found in the endometrium during the late luteal phase and early pregnancy in the decidua of women. These unusual cells have been variably called *large granular lymphocytes* (LGLs), *decidual granular lymphocytes* (DGLs), and *decidual natural killer cells*.[62] LGLs differ phenotypically from typical NK cells found in the periphery in their content of large numbers of cytoplasmic granules and in their cell surface CD expression. Still, most investigators consider them to be NK cell variants. The signature CD expression of this cell type is CD56bright, CD16⁻ (discussed in detail earlier in the section "Cellular Mediators of the Innate Immune Response").

The proportion of LGLs in the decidua of early pregnancy rises to nearly 70% to 90% of the total decidual lymphocyte population.[52,54,63] The luteal timing of the initial increase suggests regulation by progesterone, but LGLs do not express a classical progesterone receptor, and their function is not directly altered by progesterone.[64,65] These cells are closely associated with endometrial stromal cell decidualization that first occurs in the spiral artery perivascular areas during the late luteal phase of the menstrual cycle. Decidualized endometrial stromal cells produce IL-15 under some degree of influence by progesterone.[66,67] IL-15 is important for normal NK cell development in vivo.[68] Interestingly, the finding of normal numbers of LGLs in the uterine decidua of patients with ectopic pregnancy and in endometriotic lesions suggests that their presence is not dependent on contact with or local influence by trophoblast.[69,70]

LGLs are potent producers of many different cytokines and growth factors including TNF-α, IL-10, GM-CSF, IL-1β, TGF-β1, CSF-1, LIF, IFN-γ, VEGF-C, PlGF, and Ang-2.[71-74] The cytokine profile of LGLs appears to change depending on the local microenvironment, such as when these cells come into direct contact with cells expressing HLA-G. LGLs express receptors for the nonclassical HLA antigens expressed by extravillous trophoblast.[75] The nonclassical HLA antigen, HLA-G, has been shown in vitro to selectively increase the proliferation and production of IFN-γ by LGLs when compared to all other endometrial mononuclear cells. To this point, the production of IFN-γ appears to be different in decidua basalis compared with decidua parietalis.[76] Although the origin, functional capabilities, and physiologic purpose of these cells remains enigmatic, their abundance at sites of implantation suggests importance in pregnancy maintenance and compels further study.[56-63,75]

Animal and human data have also suggested roles for suppressor macrophages and TCRγδ⁺ T lymphocytes in the immunology of early pregnancy. *Suppressor macrophages* are present within the murine placenta.[77] Suppressor macrophages characteristically secrete cytokines that inhibit inflammation, a quality that differentiates them from their more typical and abundant macrophage counterparts. As mentioned previously, TCRγδ⁺ T cells have proposed importance in innate immunity. Their presence within the human endometrium increases dramatically in early pregnancy,[78-80] again indicating an important role for innate immune interactions at the maternal-fetal interface.

Soluble Immune Effectors

The human endometrium and decidua are replete with immune and inflammatory cells capable of cytokine secretion.[7,81-87] Many cytokine genes have been deleted in animal models, and few of these factors appear to be absolutely required in pregnancy maintenance. However, one cytokine, *leukemia inhibitory factor* (LIF), has been demonstrated to be required for blastocyst implantation[88,89] but not for subsequent embryogenesis.[90,91] The fact that an essential role for many of the individual cytokines in pregnancy maintenance has not been demonstrated may reflect the redundancy of this system. These results suggest that future studies should address the integrated effects of multiple cytokines.

Application of the T_H1/T_H2 paradigm to pregnancy maintenance has led to the hypothesis that the intrauterine environment surrounding normal human pregnancies is T_H2-dominant. This hypothesis is based almost solely on in vitro data. For instance, when peripheral blood cells from women with normal pregnancy histories are exposed to placental antigens in vitro, the measured cytokine responses are typically of the T_H2 type. In contrast, some women with histories of recurrent pregnancy losses have T_H1 responses in the same in vitro assay systems.[20,92-95] Inflammatory cytokines characteristic of T_H1 responses (e.g., IFN-γ) have also been shown to be harmful to the implanting embryo.[92,96]

As mentioned previously in this chapter, two additional distinct T helper subsets, T_H17 and T_{reg}, have emerged and may contribute to a better understanding of pregnancy maintenance. Many of the autoimmune effects previously attributed to T_H1 cells in the past are now being attributed to T_H17 cells.[97] To date, no studies of the role of T_H17 cells in normal or abnormal pregnancy have been published. T_{reg} cells are emerging as a potentially important contributor to the development of specific immune tolerance necessary for the establishment of normal murine pregnancy.[31] In humans, Mjösberg and colleagues recently demonstrated that T_{reg} cells purified from pregnant women suppressed autologous peripheral blood mononuclear cell (PMBC) secretion of IFN-γ when challenged by paternal or unrelated PMBCs in mixed culture. Interestingly, T_{reg} cells also suppressed IL-4 secretion against paternal but not unrelated alloantigens during pregnancy, suggesting that T_H2 cells were are able to escape suppression by T_{reg} cells and aid them in inhibiting potentially detrimental local IFN-γ secretion.[98]

Despite these promising studies, the antigen recognized at the site of implantation that might cause dysregulation of the local T helper response phenotype has never been definitively identified in vivo. In vitro studies have been based on the supposition that the antigen is placental in origin, a reasonable but unverified hypothesis. Cytokine profiles in the microenvironment of the implantation site are also difficult to document, and dysregulation in the presence of a failing pregnancy will always be obfuscated by the question of cause versus effect. The possibility of a T helper response dysregulation as a cause of pregnancy loss, therefore, remains intriguing but undocumented.

ANTIGEN PRESENTATION IN THE PLACENTA

It is generally accepted that the characteristics of antigen presentation in the placenta are unique. For many years, Medawar's paradox of the fetal allograft[48] appeared consistent with the assumption that the placenta lacked MHC class I and class II transplantation antigens. This assumption, however, was only partially correct. True, the MHC class II molecules are not expressed on the surface of placental trophoblast cells,[99,100] nor are the classical MHC class I transplantation antigens HLA-A and HLA-B. However, the classical MHC class I product HLA-C and two nonclassical products, HLA-G and HLA-E, *are* found on particular subpopulations of trophoblast cells.[101-106]

The placental cotyledon is composed of a core of fetal vessels surrounded by maternally derived cytotrophoblast cells.[107] Villous cytotrophoblast cells, in turn, are covered by the multinucleated cells of the syncytiotrophoblast layer. Placenta villi that contact the maternal decidua are termed *anchoring villi*; these structures contain a third trophoblast cellular subpopulation—the extravillous trophoblast. Extravillous trophoblast cells are derived from the villous cytotrophoblast, but during the course of early placental maturation, these cells leave the tip of the anchoring villi to invade the maternal decidua.

Continued invasion allows these cells to reach their ultimate destination: the maternal decidual vasculature. Here the extravillous trophoblast cells will ultimately replace cells within the walls of arterial decidual vessels and be termed *endovascular trophoblast cells*.[108,109] At this site, these fetally derived extravillous trophoblast cells intimately contact maternal immune effector cells, thereby exposing the fetus to potential MHC-restricted recognition as nonself. Invasion of extravillous trophoblast cells is regulated by a number of factors such as MHC expression patterns, integrin expression patterns and integrin switching,[110] matrix metalloproteinase (MMP) production,[111-113] and in situ oxygen tension.[114]

The unique MHC class I expression pattern of the extravillous trophoblast cell and its contact with the maternal immune system have led to numerous hypotheses to explain why all placental cells down-regulate expression of the classical transplantation antigens (HLA-A and HLA-B), but invasive extravillous trophoblast express HLA-C, HLA-E, and HLA-G.[52,53,63,102,115-117] No conclusive or unifying hypothesis has gained full acceptance, although many have merit.

Some authors have recently promoted a reconsideration of these questions in the context of innate, rather than acquired T cell–mediated immunity.[56] This novel approach, although radically shifting attention away from the Medawar allotransplantation paradigm, does have attractive evolutionary support. For instance, because NK cells will recognize and kill cells that lack MHC class I products, the expression of class I products with limited polymorphism (HLA-G and HLA-E) or limited expression half-life (HLA-C) may protect extravillous trophoblast cells from NK-like LGL-mediated attack.[102]

With deference to Medawar,[48] down-regulation of more classical transplantation antigens (HLA-A and HLA-B) may protect from allogenic T-cell attack.

Alternatively, interactions of trophoblast-expressed HLA-C, HLA-E, or HLA-G with surface receptors on maternal immune effector cells may modulate immune cell cytokine expression profiles.[63,75,118] Evidence that decidual and peripheral immune cells shift toward the T_H2 phenotype when exposed to HLA-G[116] supports this hypothesis and evokes a link between T helper dysregulation at the maternal-fetal interface and the unique MHC class I expression pattern in trophoblast. Moreover, at least one group of investigators has suggested that HLA-G expression may play a role in the development of regulatory T cells (T_{reg} cells).[119,120]

Trophoblast MHC class I expression might also promote essential decidual and vascular invasion by cells of placental origin.[116] To this point, altered trophoblast expression of HLA-G has been linked to disorders of placental invasion, such as preeclampsia.[121,122] Finally, the effects of trophoblast MHC class I products on maternal adaptation to implantation of the allogeneic pregnancy need not be direct. For instance, circulating soluble forms of MHC class I products such as HLA-B have been shown to promote tolerance.[123,124] If secreted into the maternal circulation, similar soluble forms of trophoblast HLA-C, HLA-E, or HLA-G might be hypothesized to promote maternal tolerance to pregnancy-associated tissues.[125,126]

IMMUNOMODULATION AND PREGNANCY MAINTENANCE

Many investigators believe that during a normal pregnancy, the fetus is usually recognized by the maternal immune system. Immune responses to fetal antigens have been demonstrated in both animal models and in humans.[127,128] These responses, however, occur in an environment characterized by dramatic systemic and local hormonal and metabolic alterations. Many of these alterations have potential immunomodulatory effects, and any or all may be critical for pregnancy maintenance. In fact, the pregnant state has long been considered a state of relative immunosuppression.

Although consistent with the hypothesis that local immunosuppression could protect the allogenic fetus, this philosophy appears to overly simplify the immunology of pregnancy. Pregnancy is *not* a state of systemic immunosuppression. Rather, pregnancy should be considered a state of dramatic immune *modulation*.

Some evidence supports the concept that a decrease in systemic maternal immune responses occurs in normal pregnancy and may be essential to pregnancy maintenance. For instance, failure to down-regulate maternal responses to recall antigens, such as tetanus toxoid and influenza, has been linked to poor pregnancy outcome among patients with recurrent pregnancy loss.[129] Autoimmune disorders such as rheumatoid arthritis are less symptomatic during pregnancy, but symptoms often flare post partum.[130] Progression of multiple sclerosis is typically retarded during pregnancy.[131] Furthermore, some viral diseases, including varicella, are particularly aggressive when first encountered during pregnancy.[132] However, pregnant women are not more susceptible to most infectious diseases, nor are they safeguarded from the effects of the majority of autoimmune disorders.

Whether pregnant or not, women are, in general, more susceptible to autoimmune diseases than men. This striking gender difference in immune responsiveness[133-136] is thought to reflect effects of reproductive hormones on peripheral cell-mediated immunity. Reproductive steroid hormones (e.g., estrogen, progesterone, and testosterone) and protein hormones (e.g., prolactin) are all potent immune modulators.[135,138-140] The effects of reproductive hormones within the microenvironment of the maternal-fetal interface may be further enhanced because their concentrations are significantly higher than those in the maternal circulation.[141]

Circulating levels of maternal estrogens and progesterone are elevated early in pregnancy and this elevation continues through most of gestation. Many of the described immunomodulatory effects of these hormones can be considered to support pregnancy. Progesterone's immunosuppressive characteristics include an inhibition of mitogen-induced proliferation of $CD8^+$ T cells and of cytokine secretion by these cells.[142] Progesterone's effects on T helper cell function promote T_H2-type responses and increase expression of LIF.[22,143,144] Both responses would be predicted to promote an immune environment favoring pregnancy maintenance.

Interestingly, the effects of progesterone in immune cell function are not necessarily receptor-mediated,[64,145] but rather can occur via direct cell membrane alterations.[146] Estrogen-related immune alterations that would be pre-dicted to promote pregnancy maintenance include the down-regulation of delayed-type hypersensitivity reactions, the promotion of T_H2-type immune responses, and demonstrated protection against chronic allograft rejection.[138,147-151] Prolactin has stimulatory effects on both cell-mediated and humoral immune responsiveness.[137,139,140] The magnitude of these effects depends on post-translational modifications of the prolactin molecule and may extend to innate immune effector cells such as $\gamma\delta$ T cells.[152]

Application of the principles of general immune function, of mucosal immune reactivity, and of the immunology of the reproductive tract described herein should allow a more informed approach to the rapidly evolving field of reproductive immunology. The concepts presented should likewise serve as a reference for the following sections describing evidence-based approaches to the diagnosis and treatment of immune-associated pregnancy loss and of immune-related subfertility.

Evidence-Based Diagnosis and Treatment of Immune-Associated Reproductive Disorders

Clinical reproductive immunology remains vexed by heated controversies. Disagreement among experts in the field has reached unprecedented levels in the medical literature and continues to generate confusion among physicians and patients alike.[153] It is currently impossible to define the extent of immune cause and the absolute standard of care for most of the reproductive disorders associated with immune dysregulation.

The following sections discuss the main clinical endocrinologic aspects of reproductive immunology. They present evidence supporting an autoimmune cause for some cases of idiopathic premature ovarian failure (POF) and evaluate the roles of autoimmunity in the pathogenesis of polycystic ovary syndrome, endometriosis, and unexplained infertility. Finally, they review the immunologic factors associated with sporadic and recurrent pregnancy losses.

PREMATURE OVARIAN FAILURE

The classic definition of POF as hypergonadotropic hypogonadism with persistent secondary amenorrhea between puberty and age 40[154] is a conservative one. The incidence of POF as defined by such classic criteria is estimated to be about 1%.[155] In fact, even at age 43, the onset of menopause lies two standard deviations below the mean,[156] which, according to conventional medical statistics, could be considered abnormal. A more modern description of this condition also acknowledges that the onset of ovarian failure can precede or coincide with puberty, thereby presenting as primary rather than secondary amenorrhea.[157]

The pathophysiology of POF usually involves untimely follicular exhaustion caused by genetic, enzymatic, iatrogenic, infectious, or immunologic factors.[158] Substantial evidence indicates that POF can result from autoimmune processes directed against the steroidogenic cells of the ovarian follicle. This is reminiscent of other destructive autoimmune endocrinopathies such as adrenal insufficiency (Addison's disease). Two distinct clinical scenarios can be identified: (1) idiopathic POF with associated manifestations of adrenal autoimmunity and (2) idiopathic POF without manifestations of adrenal autoimmunity (Table 13-4).

Idiopathic Premature Ovarian Failure Associated with Adrenal Autoimmunity

Adrenal insufficiency, which results from a destruction of over 90% of the adrenal cortex by infectious, neoplastic, or autoimmune causes, is commonly known as Addison's disease. The condition has an autoimmune cause in over 80% of cases in developed countries but is quite rare, with a reported prevalence of 3 to 6 per 100,000.[159]

Addison's disease is often a component of multiorgan disorders known as autoimmune polyglandular syndromes (APGS) (Table 13-5). APGS type 1 is an extremely rare autosomal recessive disorder also known as Blizzard's syndrome, or autoimmune polyendocrinopathy-candidiasis-ectodermal dystrophy (APECED). Patients with APGS type 1 mainly present with Addison's disease (72% to 100%), chronic mucocutaneous candidiasis (73% to 100%), and hypoparathyroidism (79% to 76%). Less frequently associated endocrinopathies include POF (17% to 60%).[160,161] APGS type 2 is an autosomal dominant disorder also known as Schmidt's syndrome. Addison's disease is invariably present, in association with autoimmune thyroid disease (69%), type 1 diabetes mellitus (52%), POF (4%), and other more rare autoimmune features. The condition has incomplete penetrance; therefore, affected siblings may display different components of the syndrome.[161,162]

Longitudinal observations of women with Addison's disease have shown that up to 10% will develop frank POF during the course of the disease, and up to 25% will experience amenorrhea not associated with ovarian failure.[163,164] Conversely, when women with POF are studied, 2% to 10% of cases are associated with idiopathic Addison's or with serologic evidence of adrenal autoimmunity.[165]

Pathogenic Antibodies. Indirect immunofluorescence assays (IIF) have demonstrated that peripheral serum from most patients with Addison's disease contains immunoglobulins that specifically bind antigens on human adrenal cortex. Adrenal autoantibodies (AA) have exclusive specificity for the adrenal cortex, whereas steroid cell autoantibodies (SCA) cross-react with other steroidogenic tissues such as placental syncytiotrophoblast, Leydig cells of the testis, and the theca interna/granulosa layers of ovarian follicles[163,166,167] (Table 13-6). Immunoblotting techniques have recently characterized some

TABLE 13-4

Characteristics of Autoimmune Premature Ovarian Failure (POF)

Characteristic	Idiopathic POF with Adrenal Autoimmunity	Idiopathic POF without Adrenal Autoimmunity
Occurrence among idiopathic POF patients	Rare	Common
Autoantibodies present	Antibodies against steroid-secreting cells Adrenal antibodies	Thyroid antibodies Antibodies against the zona pellucida (e.g., ZP3) Antibodies against 3β-hydroxysteroid dehydrogenase
Ovarian histopathologic findings	Lymphocytic oophoritis	Little immune cell infiltration

TABLE 13-5

Characteristics of Autoimmune Polyglandular Syndromes

Characteristic	Type 1	Type 2
Name	Blizzard's syndrome	Schmidt's syndrome
Inheritance	Autosomal recessive	Autosomal dominant, incomplete penetrance
Associated immune disorders	Addison's disease (72-100%) Chronic mucocutaneous candidiasis (73-100%) Hypoparathyroidism (79-86%) Premature ovarian failure (17-60%)	Addison's disease (100%) Autoimmune thyroid disease (69%) Type I diabetes mellitus (52%) Premature ovarian failure (4%)

TABLE 13-6

Antibodies in Premature Ovarian Failure Associated with Adrenal Autoimmunity

	Adrenal Autoantibodies	Antibodies Against Steroid-Secreting Cells
Specificity	Adrenal cortex	Cross-react with multiple steroidogenic tissues
Enzymes targeted	Cytochrome P450 21-hydroxylase	Cytochrome P450 17β-hydroxylase
		Cytochrome P450 side-chain cleavage enzyme

of the specific tissue antigens representing the targets of the AA and SCA detected by IIF assay: these are microsomal enzymes catalyzing key steps of steroid hormone synthesis. Cytochrome P450 21-hydroxylase, an adrenal-specific antigen, appears as the natural target responsible for the AA binding.[168,169] Other microsomal components which are present in the adrenal cortex, the gonads, and the placenta, such as cytochrome P450 17-β-hydroxylase and cytochrome P450 side-chain cleavage enzyme, seem to represent the main SCA targets.[168-170]

Data on SCA support the hypothesis of an autoimmune cause for a number of cases of idiopathic POF and provide important prognostic information.[171] SCA are not good markers of POF per se; however, when POF is associated with Addison's disease the frequency of SCA is very high (60% to 80% of subjects).[167,171,172] The presence of SCA is therefore a marker for the association of Addison's disease and POF. In the few SCA-positive POF patients without adrenal insufficiency, longitudinal observation reveals a high risk of progression to adrenal insufficiency.[173,174] Thus, prolonged observation of adrenal function in these individuals may allow early diagnosis of autoimmune adrenocortical failure. This rationale may justify obtaining AA and SCA studies in women with idiopathic POF: however, the cost-effectiveness of such an approach has not been studied. Clinical follow-up of all women with idiopathic POF is warranted in any case. Overall the prevalence of associated endocrinopathies in women with idiopathic POF is low. For example, a study of 119 women with idiopathic POF undergoing a one-time screening for adrenal, thyroid, and pancreatic islet function did not identify any cases of adrenal failure.[175]

SCA-positive Addison's patients without POF are at significant risk of developing POF.[173,176,177] As is typical of autoimmune conditions, there is a long latency from the appearance of circulating autoantibodies (SCA) to the clinically apparent condition (POF). This observation supports the autoimmune cause of some cases of idiopathic POF. For a woman with Addison's disease and SCA who has not completed childbearing, the risk of developing POF justifies IIF testing.

Ovarian histopathologic studies in SCA-positive POF patients consistently show lymphocytic oophoritis. CD4+ and CD8+ T lymphocytes and plasma cells make up most of the infiltrate, but B lymphocytes and antigen-presenting cells are less common.[178] T lymphocytes and plasma cells spare primordial follicles and increase in number around more mature and active steroid-secreting follicles.[179-181]

Animal Models. Animal models of experimental autoimmune oophoritis also support the hypothesis of an autoimmune cause of POF in SCA-positive patients. In mice, oophoritis is observed, along with other organ-specific autoimmune derangements, if thymectomy is performed between neonatal days 2 and 5.[182-184] In this model, the pattern of lymphocyte infiltration at the level of the ovary is strikingly similar to that described in SCA-positive women with POF. There is no histologic or serologic evidence of adrenal autoimmunity in these mice. Autoimmune oophoritis induced by transfer of CD4+/CD8− thymocytes from normal mice to athymic nude mice is histologically identical to that induced by neonatal thymectomy.[185] Ovarian follicle depletion in athymic girls and in newborn Rhesus monkeys thymectomized in utero suggest that findings in the murine model may be indicative of primate pathophysiology.[186,187]

Based on these findings, active production of CD4+ thymic lymphocytes with suppressor activity in euthymic animals is thought to counteract the effect of naturally occurring effector autoimmune CD4+ T cells, thereby avoiding a default autoimmune response. Because thymic production of suppressor T cells occurs later in fetal life compared to effector T-cell production, early thymectomy may promote a low suppressor/effector T-cell ratio. The induction of autoimmune oophoritis in mice recipient of circulating CD4+ T cells from thymectomized donors lends further credit to this hypothesis.[188,189] Ovarian autoantibodies, including steroid-secreting cell antibodies, are continually detectable in this animal model but may become undetectable following ovarian atrophy.[182-184] Taken together, these findings support the hypothesis that, in women with autoimmune POF, SCA may or may not be detectable, depending upon the stage of the disease. Data generated in these animal models are also consistent with an autoimmune cause of POF not associated to Addison's disease.

In conclusion, several lines of evidence support the hypothesis that POF, when associated with serologic or clinical evidence of adrenal autoimmunity, is an autoimmune endocrinopathy. The epidemiologic and histologic data and the observations of the time course of autoimmune oophoritis in animal models suggest that the presence of autoantibodies against steroidogenic enzymes of the adrenal gland and ovary may be involved in the pathogenesis of POF.

Idiopathic Premature Ovarian Failure in the Absence of Adrenal Autoimmunity

Most women with idiopathic POF (90% to 98%) have neither Addison's disease nor SCA.[165] Still, complete follicular atrophy is noted in 60% of cases, and some residual follicular presence is observed in the remainder. Ten percent of women with idiopathic POF have numerous ovarian follicles. Ovarian lymphocytic infiltration is consistently absent in these patients. However, a lack of lymphocytic infiltration and atrophy do not exclude the possibility of prior autoimmune damage which has led to functional loss.

Pathogenic Antibodies. Antibodies to other endocrine and systemic antigens are found in some women with idiopathic POF.[165] In particular, thyroid autoantibodies and autoimmune thyroid disease have been described in 14% of patients with idiopathic POF but without adrenal autoimmunity. The most readily tested autoantibodies against ovarian steroid-secreting cells (SCA) are typically absent in these women when assessed with IIF.[167,172,176]

Immunoblotting studies have demonstrated that autoantibodies to microsomal ovarian enzymes may be present in the absence of detectable AA and SCA activity. A recent study screened an adrenal complementary DNA expression library using SCA-positive serum from a patient with idiopathic POF and no evidence of Addison's disease.[190] The authors identified recombinant 3β-hydroxysteroid dehydrogenase (3β-OHSD) as the target of SCA in this patient. They then tested SCA-negative sera from another 47 patients with idiopathic POF and no evidence of Addison's disease and found that autoantibodies to 3β-OHSD were detected by immunoblotting in 21% of these women compared to 5% of healthy controls ($P = 0.002$). The autoantibody identified in this study was associated with idiopathic POF but not with SCA. Because molecular biology techniques appear to be more accurate and sensitive compared to IIF to define autoantibody targets in steroid-secreting cells, eventually tests like SCA and AA may be abandoned in favor of more specific panels of antibodies to individual steroidogenic cell antigens. A more recent study on 48 patients with POF identified autoantibodies to 3β-OHSD in only one of the subjects: moreover, this was one of two patients with detectable titers of SCA.[191] Although further studies are needed to correlate the presence of autoantibodies detected by immunoblotting with autoimmune conditions, their low prevalence makes them an unlikely candidate for clinical testing.

Some women with idiopathic POF but no manifestations of adrenal autoimmunity may form ovarian autoantibodies against antigens of the zona pellucida such as ZP3, the primary sperm receptor on human oocytes.[192,193] During the repeated process of follicular atresia, ZP3 can act as a potentially sensitizing immune epitope throughout a woman's life. In experimental murine autoimmune oophoritis, purified ZP3 antigens induce follicular depletion and ovarian failure.[194,195]

Autoantibodies that block gonadotropin receptors have been proposed as autoimmune etiologic factors in isolated POF and in resistant ovary syndrome. Data supporting this hypothesis are inconclusive because most of the studies have employed binding assays with nonhuman tissue as the substrate. The only study employing human recombinant LH and FSH receptors as the substrate demonstrated no binding of autoantibodies in POF patients or in control subjects.[196] Generally speaking, however, inactivation of gonadotropin receptors is not a mechanism associated with POF. For example: recent genetic studies have demonstrated that an FSH receptor gene mis-sense mutation originally described in Finnish women with POF has not been confirmed in several studies in other countries.[197-201] Taken cumulatively, these studies suggest that neither immunologic nor genetic inactivation of gonadotropin receptors is a significant factor in the etiology of POF.

Cellular Alterations. In an effort to test whether a cellular immune abnormality may be associated with the POF, several studies have compared peripheral leukocyte counts between patients with idiopathic POF and healthy volunteers.[178] In these studies, patients with POF did display an increase in activated peripheral T cells when compared to control subjects. This finding, however, has been subsequently attributed to a immunostimulatory effect of the characteristic hypoestrogenemia documented in women with POF.[202]

In conclusion, there is sufficient evidence to suggest an autoimmune cause in some cases of idiopathic POF that are not associated with adrenal autoimmunity. The roles of peripheral leukocyte abnormalities and of autoantibodies against gonadotropin receptors in the etiology of this condition remain unclear.

Special Considerations in the Management of Idiopathic Premature Ovarian Failure

Although there is convincing evidence that idiopathic POF can be caused by an autoimmune process, proposed nonimmunologic causes of idiopathic POF abound. Particularly well studied are genetic defects of the gonadotropin hormones or their receptors, X chromosome deletions, and fragile X mutations. Fortunately, most of these genetic conditions do not carry the medical risks of autoimmune endocrinopathies.

Despite the importance of correctly diagnosing autoimmune POF, there is currently no serum antibody marker that will predictably confirm this clinical diagnosis. Therefore, serologic testing should only be offered within investigational trials.[203] A histologic diagnosis is also unnecessary in the management of women with idiopathic POF and is only justified within the limits of experimental medicine. For clinical management purposes, the presence or absence of antral and preantral follicles can be assessed by transvaginal sonography[204] and may be useful in predicting the possibility of a spontaneous remission. In fact, recent reports indicate that the number of antral and preantral follicles assessed ultrasonographically has a direct correlation with the number of histologically identifiable primordial follicles.[205] Currently, techniques are being developed for the in vitro maturation of oocytes. In the future, when primordial follicles can be readily extracted by laparoscopic ovarian biopsy and matured in vitro, this approach may become important in the treatment of patients with immunogenic POF.

For clinical management, it currently seems safest to assume a possible autoimmune cause in all women with idiopathic POF so that a baseline screening for associated endocrinopathies can be offered. Adrenal insufficiency is 300 times more common in women with POF than in the general population[206] and is the most important potential concomitant medical condition to be identified. The adrenocorticotropic hormone (ACTH) stimulation test with measurement of cortisol levels remains the gold standard for the diagnosis of adrenal insufficiency. It should be offered to all patients with idiopathic POF. A recent study comparing the ACTH stimulation test to a widely available adrenal-antibody test suggested that the latter represents a more efficient tool in the clinical setting. The antibody test had a higher negative predictive value and comparable positive predictive value compared to the ACTH stimulation test.[206]

The association of POF with other endocrine disorders in APGS types 1 and 2 may warrant initial screening for diabetes mellitus, thyroid disorders, and hypoparathyroidism. This can be accomplished using a fasting glucose level, a thyroid-stimulating hormone (TSH) level, and serum levels of calcium, phosphate, and total protein, respectively. The cost effectiveness of such broad screening has never been established, and with the exception of an annual TSH and fasting glucose evaluation, periodic screening is not currently considered standard of care.[175] Nevertheless, the threshold for suspicion of associated endocrinopathies should remain low in physicians caring for women with idiopathic POF.

Idiopathic POF is often a waxing and waning condition, susceptible to spontaneous remissions in over half of the women diagnosed. As such, it cannot be equated with premature menopause, which defines a final and irreversible loss of ovarian function. Remissions in idiopathic POF may occur at any time from the onset of ovarian failure to the physiologic age of menopause.[207] Remission can be limited to spontaneous estrogen production or may allow normal ovulation. Pregnancies occur in 5% to 10% of young women with POF.[157,208]

No therapeutic intervention has been proved safe and effective in restoring fertility in patients with POF. Because some cases of POF can be caused by an active immunologic factor, autoimmune ovarian failure is theoretically amenable to treatment with immunomodulating agents.[209-211] Some studies have employed corticosteroids to induce immunosuppression. This may carry serious medical risks. Moreover, most of these studies lack controls and, because of their small size, may have been confounded by spontaneous temporary remissions. Theoretically, these unproved therapies could even have adverse reproductive effects, including prevention of spontaneous ovulation and pregnancy. Currently, ovum donation remains the only reliable method to establish a pregnancy in women with POF. Gonadal steroid supplementation in women with POF is described elsewhere in this volume.

The specialist considering a diagnosis of POF, particularly of idiopathic POF, should plan a conclusive diagnostic workup, provide thorough patient education, and arrange follow-up with a licensed counselor. A recent random survey of women with POF suggests that diagnosis is often delayed for several years and that patient counseling is typically suboptimal.[212]

POLYCYSTIC OVARY SYNDROME

The simplest definition of this common ovarian dysfunction is that of oligoamenorrhea associated with hyperandrogenism. Such broad diagnostic criteria

improve clinical sensitivity in the identification of patients with a metabolic rather than a classic neuroendocrine etiology of the condition.[213] The lack of a clear etiologic mechanism in the great majority of cases has led to a multitude of symptom-oriented treatments. An exception to this is the use of insulin-lowering agents in those patients with clinical signs of hyperinsulinemia.[214]

Two aspects of a potential immune system involvement in the pathogenesis of PCOS have been studied: the presence of serum autoantibodies and ovarian follicular fluid cytokine profiles. Autoantibodies against the insulin receptor are an uncommon but well-characterized cause of insulin resistance and hyperinsulinemia and have been described in association with cases of severe PCOS.[215] Antibodies directed to the ovary itself have also been described. Early reports of autoimmune oophoritis in association with polycystic ovaries and antiovarian antibodies did not necessarily apply to true PCOS, but rather to a multifollicular stage that possibly preceded ovarian failure.[216] Later studies in which PCOS was better characterized clinically have produced conflicting results. At the time of this publication the best evidence comes from a recent study assessing the incidence of antiovarian antibodies in women with PCOS compared to eumenorrheic and postmenopausal women. Because the frequency of ovarian autoantibodies in this study was similar in the three groups, it seems unlikely that these antibodies have a causal role in the condition.[217] Limited studies comparing the follicular fluid of women with PCOS to that of control subjects have highlighted some differences in the concentrations of certain cytokines. In particular, leukemia inhibiting factor and insulin-like growth factors I and II are reduced in women with PCOS.[218,219] It should be noted that cytokines can function within reproductive tissues independently of immunologic mechanisms. Therefore, differences in cytokine concentrations cannot be equated with immune dysregulation. In fact, these same studies could not demonstrate a difference in concentrations of immunomodulatory cytokines such as TNF, IFN-γ, IL-11, and TGF-β2. In conclusion, current evidence does not support a central role for autoimmunity in the pathogenesis of PCOS.

ENDOMETRIOSIS

This enigmatic condition with protean clinical and pathologic manifestations is defined by the presence of ectopic endometrial glands and stroma and is extremely prevalent in women of reproductive age.[220,221] One of a number of pathogenetic theories is the menstrual dissemination theory. According to this theory, eutopic endometrium shed in retrograde fashion through the fallopian tubes is transplanted onto the pelvic peritoneum.[222] However, retrograde menstruation is a physiologic event occurring with the same frequency in women with and without endometriosis.[223-225] In most women peritoneal monocytes suppress implantation of endometrial cells, and NK cells, activated macrophages, and cytotoxic T lymphocytes perform immunologic clearance of ectopic endometrium. Possibly, endometrial transplantation occurs only in women who have impaired peritoneal clearance of endometrial cells.[226-229]

Altered Cellular Immune Responses and the Initiation of Endometriosis

Altered cell-mediated immunity has been described in women with endometriosis. The number and ratio of circulating immune cell subsets do not differ between normal women and women with endometriosis.[230] However, in women diagnosed with endometriosis, a decreased recognition of autologous endometrial antigens by peripheral blood lymphocytes has been observed in in vitro proliferation assays.[226,231] Cytotoxicity studies employing autologous endometrial cells from subfertile women have shown decreased peripheral cytotoxic T-lymphocyte activity in patients with endometriosis.[228,229,232] Interpretation of data from circulating leukocytes in normal adults is limited by variables such as smoking, medications, and exercise. Moreover, functional studies on peripheral lymphocytes may not reflect local immune cell behavior in the peritoneum. In fact, data from in vivo studies in the baboon endometriosis model from D'Hooghe and coworkers have provided persuasive evidence that NK and cytotoxic T-lymphocyte activity are unlikely to be causally related to the disease.[233,234] In a recent study, the same investigators have demonstrated that recombinant TNF-α can effectively inhibit the development of endometriosis in the baboon model without the hypoestrogenic effects observed with GnRH-analogs.[235]

Altered Humoral Immune Responses and the Initiation of Endometriosis

In women with endometriosis, ectopic endometrial implantation may be allowed or even stimulated by abnormal monocyte function. After successful endometrial transplantation, activated macrophages may recognize endometrial tissue as displaying modified self-antigens and begin a cytokine response involving chemoattraction, activation of T cells, and eventual activation of B cells. These B cells then differentiate into plasma cells with specific antibody secretion against endometrial antigens.

Some data appear to support this attractive hypothesis, but the interpretation remains a matter of controversy. For example, the hypothesis assumes that endometrial cells, either eutopic or ectopic, are antigenic; this has never been proved. Studies have, however, demonstrated a high incidence of autoantibodies, including anti-endometrial antibodies, in women with endometriosis.[236-243] Nevertheless, most of these studies are flawed by the inclusion of heterogeneous study groups, by inappropriate selection of control subjects, and by unspecified timing of laparoscopic biopsies. The lack of standardization of the antibody assays employed makes comparison between studies almost impossible.

Finally, epidemiologic considerations such as the familial occurrence of endometriosis do not offer strong support to the theory of an autoimmune cause. Unlike other autoimmune disorders, endometriosis is not linked to a specific HLA haplotype, although it can run in families.[244,245]

Immunologic Alterations and the Maintenance of Endometriotic Lesions

Data do not support a prominent role of immunologic derangement in the etiology of endometriosis. However, once endometriosis is established, a dysfunctional peritoneal monocyte/macrophage system may contribute to the maintenance of the inflammatory state and to progression of the disease. Monocytes migrate from the peripheral blood to the peritoneal cavity to become macrophages in response to the local irritation caused by retrograde menstrual flow. In peritoneal fluid obtained from women with endometriosis, macrophages are increased in concentration and activation status compared to control subjects.[246-249] Macrophages secrete chemokines such as complement component 3, RANTES, and IL-8, which attract other immune cells into the peritoneal fluid.[250-252] These cells in turn secrete a wide range of inflammatory cytokines among which the best studied is TNF-α.

When ascertained by immunoassay or bioassay, peritoneal fluid concentrations of TNF-α are significantly increased in fertile and infertile patients with endometriosis when compared to matched control subjects.[253,254] TNF-α concentrations are significantly suppressed in the peritoneal fluid of women with endometriosis after treatment with danazol or a gonadotropin-releasing hormone (GnRH) analog.[255] Physiologic levels of TNF-α significantly enhance adhesion of endometrial stromal cells onto a mesothelial cell layer in vitro.[256] Therefore, abnormal local production of TNF-α by macrophages and activated lymphocytes may facilitate peritoneal implantation of endometrial debris.

TNF-α is currently considered as a major mediator of endometrial cell dyscohesion and apoptotic processes during the late secretory and menstrual phase.[257-260] A generalized TNF-α up-regulation might therefore be responsible for an untimely shedding of basalis endometrium, a pluripotent tissue with higher implantation potential than the functionalis layer. Although definitive data are still lacking, the hypothesis that local peritoneal inflammatory cells may contribute to the histogenesis and maintenance of endometriotic lesions appears promising.

UNEXPLAINED INFERTILITY

Infertility is conventionally defined as the failure to conceive after 12 months of unprotected intercourse. Unexplained infertility is a diagnosis of exclusion. It has been variably defined based on the changing perceptions of clinicians regarding the validity of available diagnostic tests. The role of antibodies in unexplained infertility remains controversial. Several studies have demonstrated that autoantibodies to nuclear and thyroid antigens and antiphospholipid antibodies (APAb) are present more often in infertile patients than in fertile women.[208,261-263] However, when one compares the findings for specific antibody types among these studies, conflicting results appear. Moreover, no study has shown a causal relationship between such antibodies and infertility. Both APAb and antisperm antibodies (ASAb) have been studied extensively and are discussed in detail in the following sections.

Antiphospholipid Antibodies

Antiphospholipid antibodies bind negatively charged cell membrane phospholipids and have been conclusively associated with recurrent pregnancy loss. Many investigators have proposed that APAb affect the initial stages of implantation by causing microthrombotic events within decidual spiral arteries. Deposition of specific antibodies has been demonstrated in decidual vessels of patients with APAb.[264] Damage within the placenta is, in theory, possible only after the fetoplacental circulation is established. Although the timing of this transition is a matter of dispute, it is certainly completed by the tenth week of gestation.[265-267] Still, it is conceivable that APAb may disrupt a pregnancy much before this transition by altering the early endometrial-trophoblast paracrine milieu. The ensuing recurrent preclinical pregnancy loss might be perceived as unexplained infertility.[261]

Two factors should be considered when interpreting antiphospholipid antibody testing in the infertile couple. First, many laboratories employ assays that are not standardized. Instead, a certain number of standard deviations above the mean is arbitrarily set to define abnormally high values. Therefore, a percentage of the general population must be above the cut-off value. In a case where 2 standard deviations from the mean define abnormality, 97.5% of the distribution values lay below the +2 standard deviation threshold: in such a case, the probability that a test result is positive by chance is 0.025. The formula $1 - (0.975)n$, where n is the number of independent tests, may be used to calculate the probability of a false positive result when multiple independent tests are performed. In a hypothetical case in which 11 antibodies are tested, the probability that a test will be positive by chance alone is as high as 0.24. In clinical practice, it is common to encounter much larger antibody panels. Only the assays for the anticardiolipin antibodies (ACA) and the lupus anticoagulant (LAC) are currently well standardized. A second consideration is that antiphospholipid antibodies occur in up to 4% of healthy individuals with no reproductive dysfunction. For these two reasons, testing for multiple antibodies and isotypes will yield a high incidence of false positive results.[268]

Currently available assisted reproduction technologies (ART) are not expected to overcome the proposed immunopathophysiologic mechanisms of implantation failure. Therefore, studies on patients undergoing in vitro fertilization (IVF) and intrauterine embryo transfer (ET) provide a unique opportunity to study the effect of APAb at this early stage of pregnancy. Studies assessing a putative correlation between autoantibody status and pregnancy rates from ART cycles abound. Because of the shortcomings of antibody testing, the results are conflicting and difficult to interpret.[269-280] A recent meta-analysis[281] included all available cohort studies (three prospective and four retrospective) on patients with and without elevated APAb who underwent IVF without immunomodulating therapy, and

for whom outcome data included the clinical pregnancy rate. Cumulatively, the studies involved 2053 patients, of whom 703 (34%) had at least one abnormal APAb test result. Abnormal levels of APAb were not associated with a reduction in IVF success rates. In addition, other studies have shown that previous IVF procedures do not appear to be causally linked to the induction of autoantibodies.[269,282] Taken together, these findings do not support a role for the routine testing of APAb in all patients undergoing IVF. Larger prospective studies are needed to identify a potential prognostic role of APAb testing in specific subsets of patients, such as those with pelvic disease or those with multiple failed IVF cycles. To be definitive, these studies may need to include high-specificity APAb tests, such as the anti-β_2-glycoprotein 1 ELISA (enzyme-linked immunosorbent assay) or the newer ELISA for antibodies against a mixture of negatively charged phospholipids.[283]

Despite the lack of evidence for APAb as a causative factor in the pathophysiology of infertility, clinical trials have been conducted to evaluate the efficacy of immunomodulating therapy in improving IVF outcome in women with APAb.[270,278,280] These trials were relatively small, were nonrandomized, and were not appropriately controlled (no comparisons were made between antibody-positive treated and antibody-positive untreated, or between antibody-negative treated and antibody-negative untreated). Currently there is no treatment of proven efficacy to improve clinical pregnancy rates in patients with APAb undergoing IVF.

Antisperm Antibodies

Sperm are rich with complex antigens serving as modulators of spermatogenesis, inducers of capacitation, and regulators of sperm and oocyte interactions. Most of these are foreign to women and men. It is evident how sperm antigens could induce an immune response in women. In fact, it is unclear how most sexually active women avoid producing ASAb. The risk of developing ASAb does not seem to increase with exposure to sperm from multiple sources. This is suggested by the finding of a similar prevalence of ASAb in the serum of women who completed donor sperm inseminations from an average of 14.5 different donors sources and women undergoing various ART procedures with husband sperm.[284]

The explanation for the presence of ASAb in men is less obvious. The clonal selection theory suggests that antigens that are not present during the development of the immune system in early fetal life will subsequently be recognized as nonself. Indeed, sperm are nonexistent in men until puberty and spermatogenesis is a requisite for ASAb development in men. Even after the pubertal initiation of spermatogenesis, sperm remain physically separate from immune-competent cells. Effective compartmentalization is provided by the tight junctions of Sertoli cells that compose the blood-testis barrier. Sperm antigens can escape their immunologic sanctuary in cases of mechanical obstruction due to vasectomy, trauma, surgery, or congenital anomalies. For example, up to 70% of vasectomized men and over 50% of men with vas deferens obstruction following childhood inguinal herniorrhaphy have sera positive for ASAb.[285,286] Similarly, 71% of men with cystic fibrosis and associated congenital bilateral absence of the vas deferens have ASAb bound to motile sperm.[287] In addition, inflammation from past or current infections of the genital tract may lead to ASAb formation. Orchitis, epididymitis, vasitis deferentitis, and prostatitis can cause tissue disruption with extravasation of sperm. In this case, particles derived from microbiologic agents may adhere to sperm and further enhance the immune response by acting as haptens. For instance, *Chlamydia trachomatis* infections have been closely associated with the development of ASAb. A recent study comparing the seroprevalence of antibodies to *Chlamydia* with the prevalence of ASAb in semen noted antichlamydial antibodies in 51.4% of men with ASAb compared with 16.8% of men without ASAb.[288]

ASAb may disrupt reproductive processes prior to and after fertilization. They may interfere with sperm transport by causing sperm agglutination or frank asthenozoospermia. Alternatively, ASAb may disrupt oocyte-sperm interactions by inhibiting capacitation, the acrosome reaction, sperm penetration of the zona pellucida, and sperm fusion with the oolemma. Finally, these antibodies may hinder zygote development by inhibiting pronuclear formation or embryo cleavage.

For several reasons it is impossible to estimate the prevalence of ASAb in the general populace based on currently available data. First, a vast array of different ASAb tests is currently employed. Second, ASAb exist as IgM, IgA, or IgG antibody isotypes. IgG and secreted IgA are clinically relevant, but IgM are confined to serum and cannot interact with sperm. Third, ASAb have been measured in seminal plasma, serum, cervical mucus, and follicular fluid, and on live or fixed sperm. Only antibodies within the semen or cervical mucus interfere with reproduction.[289] Fourth, various diagnostic inclusion criteria have been employed by different authors studying ASAb. Lastly, sperm antigens are protean in nature, may change during sperm maturation, and can be intracellular or extracellular. Intracellular antigens and those which are lost during sperm maturation are not relevant to fertility.

Testing for ASAb

The clinical usefulness of ASAb testing of cervical mucus was assessed in a large cohort of women with a median of 5 years of infertility. The prevalence of ASAb in cervical mucus of these women was only 1.6%. All women with ASAb had unfavorable postcoital tests and none of them conceived in the year following testing.[290] The finding of cervical mucus antibodies prompts the same recommendation of intrauterine insemination (IUI) as does a diagnosis of unexplained infertility. For this reason, and because the postcoital test is not a valid screening test in infertility patients,[291] ASAb measurements in cervical mucus are not clinically useful.

Identification of IgG or IgA ASAb on sperm is the sole test that carries potential clinical value. This test should be performed only on untreated live sperm because the use of fixed or otherwise prepared sperm can expose internal antigens, which are unlikely to have a role in infertility. Among the 10 or so techniques described to detect sperm-bound ASAb, the most widely used by reproductive endocrinologists in the United States is the immunobead (IBD) test.[292,293] The mixed antiglobulin reaction (MAR) test standardized by the World Health Organization is the preferred method internationally[294] (Fig. 13-6). The IBD test employs polyacrylamide beads coated with antibodies specific for either human IgG or IgA. The beads are exposed to viable sperm (usually washed) and bind to sperm-bound ASAb if these are present. Light microscopy is used to assess the percentage of sperm bound to beads and the location of binding (head, midpiece, or tail). The MAR test is similar to the IBD test in principle. It uses Rh-positive erythrocytes

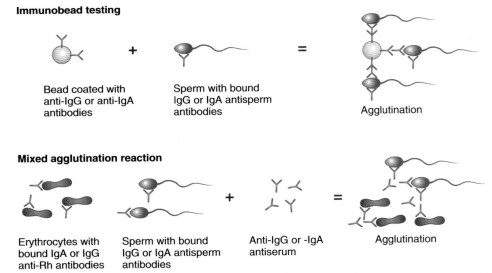

Immunobead testing

Bead coated with anti-IgG or anti-IgA antibodies   +   Sperm with bound IgG or IgA antisperm antibodies   =   Agglutination

Mixed agglutination reaction

Erythrocytes with bound IgA or IgG anti-Rh antibodies   Sperm with bound IgG or IgA antisperm antibodies   +   Anti-IgG or -IgA antiserum   =   Agglutination

Figure 13-6. *Antisperm antibody testing. Both the immunobead test (IBD) and the mixed agglutination reaction (MAR) are used to assay semen specimens for the presence of antisperm antibodies (ASAb). In the IBD, polyacrylamide beads are coated with anti-IgG or anti-IgA antibodies. Beads are then mixed with sample sperm. Sperm with bound ASAb (IgC or IgA) will agglutinate with the immunobeads and can be visualized microscopically. In the MAR, erythrocytes are coated with IgC or IgA anti-Rh antibodies. These coated erythrocytes are mixed with sample sperm and with anti-IgG or anti-IgA antiserum. Agglutination of erythrocytes acts as an internal positive control. ASAb-coated sperm will also agglutinate with erythrocytes and with other antibody-bound sperm and can be visualized microscopically.*

bound to anti-Rh antibodies of either IgA or IgG isotype. These are mixed with viable sperm (usually washed) and with either anti-IgA or anti-IgG antiserum. The erythrocytes serve as a positive control and clump in the presence of the appropriate anti-Ig antibody. If ASAb of IgG or IgM isotypes exist, these will be bound to the sperm and cause sperm agglutination in the presence of the corresponding anti-Ig. The percentage of sperm agglutination is estimated by light microscopy. The physical location of binding is impossible to assess with accuracy. An IBD or MAR is usually defined as positive if at least 20% of the sperm show signs of binding to ASAb. This threshold however is arbitrary. Most laboratories adopt a value between 10% and 50%. Despite good evidence for a role of ASAb in unexplained infertility, the lack of standard methodology for the detection, interpretation and reporting of ASAb levels limits the clinical value of these tests. These considerations aside, the majority of reproductive endocrinologists in the United States currently employ the IBD test in their clinical practice.[293]

Therapies for ASAb

Some strategies have been devised to counteract the potential deleterious effects of ASAb on fertility. Immunosuppression aims at decreasing ASAb production and is largely limited to corticosteroid administration. This therapy is of uncertain efficacy and carries significant risks. Two placebo-controlled, double blind studies (both including exactly 43 infertile men with ASAb) stand out as the best designed to date. The shorter study employed 32 mg of methylprednisolone or placebo administered three times a day for a week, with a 2-day taper. This regimen was repeated a total of three times at monthly intervals on the basis of the female partner's menstrual cycle. In spite of a decrease in sperm-bound IgG in the treatment group, there was no difference in sperm-bound secretory IgA, sperm parameters, or pregnancy rate compared to the placebo group.[295] The longer study employed 20 mg of prednisolone or placebo, administered twice daily on days 1 to 10 of the female partner's menstrual cycle, with a 2-day taper. This was repeated for nine consecutive months, after which a cross-over was performed. A significant difference in pregnancy rate occurred in women whose partners were in the steroid arm (31%) versus those whose partners were taking placebo (9%).[296] The different results in these two very similar studies may be reconciled if immunosuppression takes longer than 3 months to affect ASAb effects on fertility. Another possible explanation for the disparate results is that, even when ASAb activity is removed, baseline human fecundity may not be high enough to result in an observable difference in pregnancy rates given the size and brevity of these studies (i.e., the shorter study is particularly prone to a beta error).

Sperm washing prior to ART might theoretically circumvent the deleterious effects of ASAb. Although sperm washing does remove free antibodies from the seminal plasma, sperm-bound antibodies persist after as many as 18 consecutive sperm washing cycles.[297] Therefore, pregnancies that result from use of washed sperm in ART cycles do so in the presence of sperm-bound ASAb.

Intrauterine insemination successfully overcomes the inhibitory effect of ASAb on sperm penetration of the cervical mucus. However, this procedure may not prevent the disruption of sperm-oocyte interactions due to sperm-bound antibodies. The efficacy of IUI in overcoming unexplained infertility associated with ASAb remains controversial due to the lack of prospective and appropriately controlled studies. One recent study compared pregnancy rates among couples with unexplained infertility and sperm-bound ASAb who underwent IUI or IVF. All 29 couples enrolled in the study had primary infertility and each of the male partners had IgG or IgA ASAb demonstrated by a positive MAR test (>50% binding). Couples were given a choice between IVF (up to three cycles) and superovulation with IUI (up to three cycles) before proceeding to IVF.[298] The cumulative live birth rate was 64.3% after three IUI cycles versus 93.3% after three IVF cycles. However, the live birth rate after one IVF cycle was only 46.6%. Based on a previously published cost-benefit analysis,[299] the authors advocate superovulation with IUI as an effective first-line therapy in male immunologic infertility. This study was prospective but small and nonrandomized. If larger randomized studies confirm these findings, the algorithms for treatment of unexplained infertility and male immunologic infertility will become quite similar. This would further limit the clinical relevance of measuring ASAb.

Studies reporting conventional IVF outcome in couples with ASAb are generally small and not controlled. Early studies included patients with abnormal semen parameters,[300] and couples with ASAb measured in the female partner's serum.[301] Overall, these early studies do not suggest an important effect of ASAb on IVF outcome. A more recent, small, case control study reported significantly decreased fertilization rates (44.2% versus 84.4%) and decreased early embryonic cleavage in couples with positive MAR test (>20% binding) compared to control subjects. The effect on clinical pregnancy rate was not statistically significant (11% versus 44%),[302] although this may represent a beta error due to study size. Finally, a cost effectiveness study employed the IBD test to screen patients undergoing IVF. The IBD test demonstrated poor sensitivity (11.4%) in predicting low or absent fertilization and there was a low incidence of positive tests. The positive predictive value for a positive IBD test was only 25%. The IBD test was not deemed cost effective. IBD testing of all patients would have been more expensive than performing intracytoplasmic sperm injection (ICSI) on patients experiencing one IVF cycle with failed fertilization.[303]

ICSI will allow some couples to avoid fertilization failure secondary to ASAb. Retrospective studies of ICSI report high fertilization rates in couples with ASAb who had poor fertilization rates with conventional IVF.[304,305] Unfortunately, decreased embryo quality is frequently observed in such studies. This suggests that the effect of ASAb on postfertilization events is not amenable to treatment with ICSI.

IMMUNE-ASSOCIATED PREGNANCY LOSS

Spontaneous abortion occurs in approximately 15% of all clinically recognized pregnancies and recurrent pregnancy loss occurs in approximately 1% to 2% of the population experiencing spontaneous pregnancy loss.[306] An identifiable cause of recurrent pregnancy loss (RPL) will be detected in an estimated 50% to 60% of couples.[307,308]

The only undisputed causes of recurrent pregnancy loss are parental chromosomal structural abnormalities[310] and the antiphospholipid antibody syndrome (APAS),[311,312] although other frequently cited causes include advanced maternal age,[313] luteal phase deficiency with abnormal expression of $\alpha v \beta 3$ integrin,[314] untreated hypothyroidism,[315] hyperprolactinemia,[316] polycystic ovary syndrome,[317] uncontrolled diabetes mellitus,[318] and uterine anatomic abnormalities.[319,320] This leaves a significant proportion of patients with RPL due to miscellaneous or unknown causes. Presumably, a proportion of these patients have immunologic causation. The estimated proportion of patients with immunogenic recurrent pregnancy loss varies dramatically, often reflecting research or referral biases of the reporting sites.

The appropriate diagnosis and treatment of recurrent pregnancy loss remain hotly debated. In fact, there are few truly evidence-based interventions for immunologic recurrent pregnancy. There are several reasons why this field remains so controversial:

- Pregnancy loss is very common, and is most likely the final outcome of a number of heterogeneous, and potentially unrelated, disorders.
- Early pregnancy is commonly referred to as a "black box." In reality, it may be more accurately described as a "gray box." The intricate molecular pathways that operate during implantation and early pregnancy are now being described. Still, reproductive scientists face the challenge of piecing together current knowledge into a more global understanding of the interactions during early pregnancy.
- The published literature concerning recurrent pregnancy loss is remarkably inconsistent. There has been no consensus as to the clinical definition of recurrent pregnancy loss so variable criteria have been used in directing study subject inclusion. In addition, the diagnostic tests performed prior to investigational treatments have not been uniform or have been poorly described. Collectively, these factors conspire to make evaluation of the existing literature difficult.
- The prognosis for most patients with a history of recurrent pregnancy loss is good. Although there is variability in the published literature, a reasonable estimation of prognosis for patients with recurrent pregnancy loss reveals that approximately 76% of couples who have had a single spontaneous loss will have a term gestation in their next pregnancy. After two spontaneous losses, chances for a term gestation decrease to 70% in the subsequent pregnancy; the prognosis of a term pregnancy decreases to 65% after three losses. The patient who has experienced four spontaneous losses has a 60% chance of carrying to term in the next pregnancy.[307,321]
- Recruitment of patients with recurrent pregnancy loss into placebo-controlled double-blinded studies is often difficult. Thus, the existing literature is plagued by small and typically uncontrolled studies. Use of meta-analyses has begun to address this difficulty.

- Distinguishing between immune alterations that cause pregnancy loss and those that occur in response to pregnancy loss is problematic.
- Peripheral measurements of immune parameters may not appropriately reflect the immunology of the maternal-fetal interface.

Some of the confusion surrounding the immunologic causes and treatments for recurrent pregnancy loss is inherent to the disease process. However, acceptance of a standardized definition for RPL and improved documentation of the timing of spontaneous pregnancy failure might facilitate comparison and interpretation of future studies.

The clinician needs to consider several factors when deciding whether an evaluation for recurrent pregnancy loss should be initiated:

1. The probability that a subsequent miscarriage will occur
2. The probability that the practitioner will succeed in finding a cause for the couple's previous losses
3. The potential that medical therapy based on this evaluation will improve a couple's chance for a successful pregnancy

Defining Recurrent Pregnancy Loss

In the past, recurrent pregnancy loss was defined as three or more spontaneous, consecutive losses. This criterion was used to select couples who warranted an evaluation. However, the best available data suggest that, in a patient with no prior live births, the risk of subsequent pregnancy loss after two prior miscarriages is a clinically significant 35%.[321] In a patient with one prior live-born child, the risk of a subsequent loss does not reach 32% until after the third miscarriage.

Based upon these probabilities of an unwanted outcome, evaluation for recurrent pregnancy loss may be reasonably begun after two prior miscarriages in a patient with primary RPL. In a patient with secondary RPL, waiting until three miscarriages to begin an evaluation is appropriate. In support of this, in a study of over 1000 patients with a history of pregnancy losses, the probability of finding a cause for RPL in a population with two versus three miscarriages was nearly identical.[322]

The Timing of Pregnancy Demise

Pregnancy can be divided into pre-embryonic, embryonic, and fetal stages. The *pre-embryonic stage* begins at conception and extends to the end of the fourth week from the last menstrual period. During this stage, implantation occurs and the pre-embryo develops into a trilaminar disk of cells with a defined central neural axis.

The *embryonic stage* begins at the fifth week of gestation and ends at the ninth week of gestation. During this stage, the trilaminar disk folds to become cylindrical and the head and tail regions of the embryo are defined. Organogenesis also occurs during this stage. Of particular importance during the embryonic stage are the development of the heart, and the provision of oxygen and nutrients through the umbilical cord and placenta.

The *fetal stage* begins at 10 weeks of gestation and extends through delivery. Its beginning coincides with the initiation of maternal blood contact with villous trophoblast cells.[265,266,323-325]

Although pregnancy loss may occur during any of these gestational stages, the temporal distribution of loss is apparently somewhat biphasic. One study of over 200 women with suspected normal pregnancies revealed an overall loss rate of 13.4%.[326] Of these losses, 87% occurred in the pre-embryonic and embryonic stages, no losses occurred between 8.5 weeks' and 14 weeks' gestation, 2% were lost between 14 and 20 weeks' gestation, and the remainder of the pregnancy losses (11%) occurred after 20 weeks' gestation.

The timing of a loss may suggest its etiology. Pre-embryonic and early embryonic losses are overwhelmingly attributed to genetic factors, but autoimmune, thrombotic, and anatomic causes are more commonly associated with late fetal losses.[308] However, in a clinical setting, defining the stage at which pregnancy loss occurs can be difficult. The symptoms of miscarriage may begin several days to weeks after the demise of the conceptus. For example, the onset of bleeding or uterine cramps at 10 to 12 weeks from the last menses may represent a pre-embryonic or embryonic pregnancy loss, not a fetal loss. Close monitoring of RPL patients during early pregnancy may provide a more accurate assessment of the timing of pregnancy loss.

An Evidence-Based Evaluation for Recurrent Pregnancy Loss

An accepted evaluation of a couple experiencing recurrent pregnancy losses begins with taking a complete medical history, performing a directed physical examination, and documenting prior pregnancies with their associated testing and procedures. Initial diagnostic testing will often include parental peripheral blood karyotyping, assessment of the intrauterine cavity, thyroid function testing, a platelet count, and testing for the APAS (if indicated).

Other testing may be appropriate in a limited number of couples, including luteal phase endometrial biopsy, testing for insulin resistance, and evaluation of ovarian reserve. Screening for selected inherited disorders that predispose to arterial or venous thrombosis may also be useful among patients with otherwise unexplained first and second trimester pregnancy losses or with suggestive personal or family history of thrombophilia.[308,309,327,328]

Diagnostic Testing for Immune-Associated Pregnancy Loss

Immune responses can be divided into *autoimmune responses* (reactions against self-antigens) and *alloimmune responses* (reactions against nonself antigens). Both autoimmunity and alloimmunity have been evaluated in association with RPL. Still, whether or not these immune responses are beneficial or detrimental to placental growth and pregnancy maintenance remains unclear.

Alloimmunity. Because the fetus is antigenically different from the mother, the mother's immune system might be predicted to identify the fetus as foreign and to execute an immune response. The abundance of immune cells within the decidua and the production of numerous immunologic cytokines at the maternal-fetal interface make the potential for an immune-associated pregnancy rejection plausible. Unless the appropriate mechanisms are in place to modify adverse maternal immune processes, the semi-allogeneic fetus should be rejected.

Several different analyses have been performed to address the potential role of alloimmune factors in RPL, including anti-paternal cytotoxic antibody testing, mixed lymphocyte culture reactivity testing, embryotoxicity evaluations, immune cell phenotyping, peripheral cytokine phenotyping, and HLA profiling (Table 13-7). Although none of these tests has been proved clinically useful, many continue to be employed in clinical practice.

Embryotoxicity assays have been proposed as a means to detect abnormal peripheral cellular immune responses to human trophoblast-derived antigens.[20,96,329] The embryo-toxic factor (ETF) assay reflects the development of an inflammatory reaction to the presence of placental antigens and may predict similar in vivo responses during a subsequent pregnancy. Still, although the theoretical basis for the use of the ETF assay may have some merit, the commercially available test has proved to be neither consistent in predicting pregnancy outcome nor useful in clinical management.

Immune phenotyping using flow cytometric analysis of peripheral blood cells, especially NK cells (CD56[+]), has been evaluated in RPL.[330,331] Although the basic scientific literature regarding NK cells in pregnancy is intriguing, the current clinical literature is conflicting and supports

TABLE 13-7

Immunologic Evaluation and Interventions for Patients with Recurrent Pregnancy Loss

Description	Testing	Treatment
Proven	Lupus anticoagulant Anticardiolipin antibody levels (IgG or IgM) Anti-β_2-glycoprotein-1 levels	Anticoagulation for the antiphospholipid antibody syndrome Progesterone supplementation
Potentially promising but incompletely studied	Antiphosphatidyl-serine levels NK cell testing	Intravenous immunoglobulins in very limited patient subgroups
Misleading, ineffective, or potentially harmful	Use of extensive antibody panels Anti-paternal cytotoxic antibodies Mixed lymphocyte culture reactivity Leukocyte antibody testing Parental HLA typing Peripheral T_H1/T_H2 cytokine profiling Antinuclear antibody assays	Prednisone Leukocyte infusion therapy

HLA, human leukocyte antigen; NK, natural killer; T_H, T helper Cells.

neither testing for peripheral NK cell activity nor immunomodulatory intervention based on assay results.

Assays aimed at detecting anti-paternal cytotoxic antibodies and anti-leukocyte antibodies are likewise of little value in the assessment of couples with recurrent pregnancy wastage. These antibodies are usually not detected before 28 weeks' gestation and are often not detectable in nonpregnant women. Because of these characteristics, tests for these antibodies cannot prospectively and predictably direct interventions, making them poor screening tools.

Testing for peripheral evidence of T_H1/T_H2 cytokine dysregulation (peripheral cytokine profiling) has never been demonstrated to be consistently useful in the evaluation of RPL couples.[21,332,333] Peripheral cytokine profiling studies are plagued by questions about the correlation between peripheral findings and events at the maternal-fetal interface. There also remain concerns that T_H1/T_H2 dysregulation may represent a response to pregnancy demise rather than its primary cause.

Many investigators have proposed that maternal recognition of pregnancy is essential to its maintenance. A lack of this essential recognition was then linked to immune-mediated pregnancy loss. These authors proposed that immune recognition resulted in the production of soluble factors (presumably antibodies) that blocked maternal cell-mediated responses toward her implanting fetus. The production of "blocking antibodies" was considered essential to pregnancy maintenance and testing for these factors was pursued.[334-336] One proposed test of the development of blocking antibodies is the mixed lymphocyte culture reactivity test. This test does not aid in the prediction of pregnancy outcome but, rather, reflects the number and duration of prior pregnancies. Its use has no clinical role in the evaluation or management of recurrent pregnancy loss.

The role of HLA typing in the diagnostic workup of recurrent pregnancy loss patients has also been investigated. Like supporters of the "blocking antibody" hypothesis, those posing the importance of HLA-mediated pregnancy loss believe that maternal immune recognition of the conceptus is *beneficial* to pregnancy. Theoretically, if the maternal and paternal HLA molecules are too similar, pregnancy loss will ensue. Investigations of this hypothesis involved the Hutterite religious sect in South Dakota. From this circumscribed, stable, and in-bred population came initial data refuting a role for HLA matching in adverse pregnancy outcome.[337] However, a more recent and expanded investigation of the same population reported that exact HLA matching can be associated with adverse pregnancy outcome.[338] As noted in the conclusions and discussions of this paper, HLA matching is virtually never seen in out-bred populations. Therefore, HLA typing is not recommended in the evaluation of patients with RPL.

Autoimmunity. A variety of autoimmune causes of RPL have been suggested. Antibodies to phospholipids, nuclear antigens, thyroid proteins, histones, and single-stranded and double-stranded DNA have all been evaluated in relation to RPL (see Table 13-7). At present, there is no consistent evidence supporting testing for antithyroid antibodies.[339-342] In the absence of coexistent rheumatic or autoimmune disease, testing for antinuclear antibodies is nonspecific and seldom, if ever, indicated. Extensive immune testing that involves large panels of autoantibodies or alloantibodies is expensive, unproven, and potentially misleading. The poor standardization of many of these tests, in combination with their false positive rates, may lead to unwarranted and invasive interventions.

Antiphospholipid Antibody Syndrome. APAS is the only widely accepted, readily diagnosed, and effectively treated autoimmune cause of RPL. Clinicians have recognized for over 2 decades that pregnancy loss is associated with the presence of antiphospholipid antibodies. While early definitions that included pregnancy loss in the criteria for APAS limited these losses to the second trimester,[311] the most recent definitions include both early and late pregnancy complications.[312,343]

Currently accepted clinical criteria for pregnancy complications attributable to antiphospholipid antibodies include the following:

1. Three or more consecutive spontaneous abortions before 10 weeks' gestation with exclusion of maternal anatomic and hormonal abnormalities and exclusion of paternal and maternal chromosomal abnormalities
2. One or more unexplained deaths of a morphologically normal fetus at or beyond 10 weeks' gestation (normal fetal morphology documented by ultrasound or direct examination of the fetus)
3. One or more premature births of a morphologically normal neonate at or before 34 weeks' gestation due to severe preeclampsia or placental insufficiency[312,343]

The pregnancy-related clinical criteria for APAS imply that, although early and late losses may be caused by phospholipid antibodies, this association is stronger for fetal losses. In fact, as many as 50% of the pregnancy losses among women with high titers of ACA antibodies and LAC were found to be fetal deaths, compared with less than 15% of those in women without antiphospholipid antibodies.[344,345]

Laboratory criteria for the diagnosis of APAS have recently been expanded.[343] They now include (1) positive plasma levels of the lupus anticoagulant, (2) ACA of the IgG or IgM isotype at medium to high levels, or (3) anti-β_2-glycoprotein-I antibody of the IgG or IgM isotype in titers greater than the 99th percentile.[343,346] Testing must be positive on two or more occasions with evaluations 12 or more weeks apart.

Clinical testing for the presence of ACA typically uses solid phase immunoassays, such as an ELISA, conducted on plates coated with cardiolipin. To differentiate infectious etiologies of positive results from APAS-associated etiologies, bovine beta-2 glycoprotein-1 (β_2GPl) is often added to these ELISAs. Infectious ACA are typically β_2GPl-independent, while those from patients with APAS are dependent.[345]

Although antiphospholipid antibodies are not associated with sporadic pregnancy losses that occur at less than 20 weeks' gestation, many studies have demonstrated positive tests for LAC and IgG or IgM ACA in up to 20%

of women with RPL.[347-350] In most studies of pregnancy loss, women who are positive for ACA are positive for both the IgG and IgM antibody subtypes. Although an isolated (but repeated) medium- to high-positive IgM level meets standard laboratory criteria, its clinical significance in recurrent pregnancy loss patients remains unclear. In one study, women with low-positive IgG ACA or isolated IgM ACA titers had no greater risk of antiphospholipid-related events than women whose test results were negative.[351]

β_2-Glycoprotein-l is found in large amounts in human plasma and may be the antigen directly recognized by antiphospholipid antibodies.[352] Its presence enhances the binding of antiphospholipid antibodies to phospholipids.[353] These characteristics, in conjunction with the known association of APAS with pregnancy losses, made testing for these anti-β_2-glycoprotein-l antibodies attractive. This testing was recently added to the diagnostic laboratory criteria for APAS and should be included in the evaluation of patients with RPL.[343] Anti-β_2-glycoprotein-l antibodies are an independent risk factor for thrombotic events and for pregnancy loss in APAS patients.[346,354-356] In addition, they are more specific than anticardiolipin antibodies in the diagnosis of APAS and are the sole antibody found in 3% to 10% of APAS patients.[357,358]

Testing for the presence of the lupus anticoagulant (LAC) is indirect. In fact, the term *lupus anticoagulant* refers to in vitro testing results only. In screening tests, LAC is associated with prolonged coagulation; clinically, patients with LAC have increased thrombotic risk. Testing for LAC typically begins with a variety of screening tests for prolongation of coagulation using platelet-poor plasma. Screening tests vary by institution, but may include any of the following:

1. The dilute prothrombin time (a test of the extrinsic clotting pathway)
2. An activated partial thromboplastin time or kaolin clotting time (tests of the intrinsic clotting pathway)
3. The dilute Russell viper venom time, the Taipan venom time, or alternate snake venom-induced coagulation tests (all assess the final common clotting pathway)

Abnormalities detected on one or more of these screening assays should be investigated further. To determine if the abnormality is due to a deficiency of a coagulation factor rather than the presence of a coagulation inhibitor, the patient's sera is mixed with normal patient sera. If the prolongation in coagulation is not corrected, the presence of a coagulation inhibitor is assumed. The phospholipid dependence of this inhibitor is next assessed by adding excess phospholipid to the coagulation assay. Partial or complete correction of prolonged coagulation upon addition of phospholipid is consistent with the presence of a lupus anticoagulant.[345]

Other antibodies have been demonstrated to have potential mechanistic associations with RPL, although testing for their presence has yet to be shown of proven diagnostic or prognostic utility. For instance, antiphosphatidylserine antibodies have been demonstrated to inhibit trophoblast invasion in vitro,[359] but the clinical utility of tests for these antibodies in the evaluation of women with RPL has never been proved.[360-363]

In conclusion, existing data support the assessment of the LAC, the IgG and IgM titers of ACA, and anti-β_2-glycoprotein-l antibodies in the evaluation of immune-associated recurrent pregnancy loss. No other test related to autoimmune-associated miscarriage is presently recommended for clinical use (see Table 13-7).

Management of Immune-Associated Recurrent Pregnancy Loss

Both immune stimulation and immune suppression have been proposed as appropriate interventions in the treatment of presumed immune-mediated RPL. Leukocyte transfusion, intravenous immunoglobulin administration, progesterone supplementation, and prednisone administration have all been evaluated or employed in the treatment of autoimmune and alloimmune-associated or unexplained RPL (see Table 13-7).

Leukocyte immunization has involved maternal transfusion with either paternal lymphocytes (paternal white blood cell immunization) or with pooled donor white blood cells. Immunization was thought to be immunostimulating and aimed to promote the maternal production of protective blocking factors. Leukocyte immunization therapy has no demonstrable role in the treatment of couples with recurrent pregnancy loss.[364-368] In fact, a large, multicenter, randomized, placebo-controlled, and double-blinded trial demonstrated that leukocyte infusion therapy resulted in an increase in pregnancy loss in women with unexplained RPL.[369]

Intravenous immunoglobulin (IVIG) administration has a variety of immunomodulatory effects. Although many of these effects are incompletely understood, they may include decreased production and increased clearance of autoantibodies, T cell and Fc receptor regulation,[370] complement inactivation,[371] enhanced T suppressor cell function, decreased T-cell adhesion to the extracellular matrix,[372] and suppression of T_H1 cytokine production.[373] Individual studies on the efficacy of IVIG in the treatment of patients with RPL have provided conflicting results; a meta-analysis of many of these investigations revealed that IVIG therapy lacked efficacy in the treatment of RPL patients.[374] This conclusion was substantiated by the results of a more recent multicenter clinical trial,[375] although the results of a continuing large, randomized, muticentered trial based at the University of Chicago remain unreleased at the time of this publication.

Based on its safely profile during early pregnancy, progesterone supplementation has been widely used in the empiric treatment of presumed immune-associated or unexplained RPL. As previously mentioned, progesterone has demonstrable immunomodulatory effects. Its efficacy in the treatment of patients with RPL has not yet been appropriately studied in a single randomized trial. Still, a meta-analysis of the published data has supported its use in patients with a history of recurrent, but not isolated, pregnancy losses.[376]

One large study has focused on the utility of immunosuppression with prednisone to address adverse pregnancy outcome in women with a history of RPL and concomitant autoantibodies (anticardiolipin, antinuclear, antilympho-cyte, or anti-DNA) or LAC. Treatment of these women with low-dose aspirin and prednisone did not produce any noteworthy improvements in pregnancy outcome. Rather, there was a substantial increase in maternal complications (gestational diabetes, hypertension) and fetal complica-tions (premature delivery) among those women receiving prednisone and aspirin.[377]

Only tests for LAC, ACA, and anti-β_2-glycoprotein-l antibodies are currently recommended in evaluating im-mune-associated recurrent pregnancy loss. Accordingly, only therapies for antiphospholipid antibody-associated RPL will be considered in detail. Notably, the current in-tervention for APAS (the only proven immune cause of recurrent pregnancy loss) is not immune-based. Treatment is aimed at mitigating the effects of circulating antibodies rather than at preventing antibody production.

Studies have revealed decidual vasculopathy and exten-sive placental infarction among patients with recurrent fetal loss and either lupus or LAC.[378-380] Numerous thrombogenic mechanisms have been reported.[381-383] Because thrombosis within the uleroplacental circulation appeared to link ad-verse pregnancy outcomes and APAS, the therapeutic use of antithrombotic agents appeared reasonable. Thrombogenic mechanisms, however, are only part of the pathophysiology of APAS as it relates to pregnancy. Antiphospholipid anti-bodies have direct adverse effects on implantation. They alter signal transduction during decidual cell differentia-tion,[384,385] they inhibit hCG production by the syncytiotro-phoblast,[386,387] they inhibit trophoblast invasion[388,389] and trophoblast fusion,[390] and they activate the complement cascade.[391] In addition to its antithrombotic effects, hepa-rin promotes trophoblast invasion,[392] inhibits trophoblast apoptosis,[393] restores placental hCG production,[387,392] and directly alters cellular immune responses.[394]

Heparin and Aspirin. Heparin and aspirin have been suc-cessfully used in the treatment of women with RPL who have positive serum LAC or ACA (reviewed by Stephen-son[309] and Ware Branch[395]). Although the mechanism of heparins effect is likely a combination of antithrombotic, immunomodulatory, and direct actions, that of low-dose as-pirin therapy relies on reduced platelet aggregation and ben-eficial alterations in the thromboxane:prostacyclin ratio.

Because of its low cost and relatively innocuous side effect profile, aspirin has commonly been used in com-bination with heparin in the successful treatment of ACA-associated RPL. The safety of low-dose aspirin in pregnancy has been confirmed in a study of more than 20,000 women.[396] Heparin does not cross the placenta. Empson and colleagues[397] demonstrated in a meta-analysis that the combination of low-dose aspirin and unfrac-tionated heparin was superior to steroids and aspirin or aspirin alone in the treatment of patients with recurrent pregnancy loss.

At the present time, all women with APAS are advised to be treated with a combination of low-dose aspirin and subcutaneous heparin, in either thromboprophylactic or anticoagulant doses.[398] Women with APAS and previ-ous venous or arterial thrombosis should be treated with

subcutaneously administered heparin every 12 hours to prolong the activated partial thromboplastin time (aPTT) in the therapeutic range. Thromboprophylactic doses of heparin should be used in women with ACA, RPL, and no previous vascular thrombotic event.

With reference to the published literature, the favored thromboprophylactic regimen includes subcutaneous ad-ministration of 15,000 to 20,000 units per day of unfrac-tionated sodium heparin and 60 to 100 mg of aspirin per day. Low-molecular-weight heparin may also be used in pregnancy and appears to have an improved safety profile in comparison to its unfractionated counterpart.[399] Some investigators suggest that doses of low-molecular-weight heparins should produce trough anti-factor Xa activity levels of 0.1 to 0.15 U/mL. Others use empiric thrombo-prophylactic dosages.[400]

Treatment with aspirin can logically begin when one is attempting pregnancy. Heparin therapy entails more risks and typically should not be initiated until the pa-tient has conceived. The adverse effects of heparin include osteoporosis, thrombocytopenia, and local ecchymosis. Heparin-induced osteoporotic fracture occurs in 1% to 2% of pregnant women treated with unfractionated hepa-rin.[401] Therefore, women undergoing unfractionated hep-arin therapy should receive 1000 to 1500 mg of calcium and 600 IU of vitamin D daily; these doses can be found in most prenatal vitamins. Weight-bearing exercise should also be encouraged.

Heparin-induced thrombocytopenia[402] is immune-mediated and begins 3 to 15 days after initiation of therapy. Thrombocytopenia occurs in up to 5% of women treated with unfractionated heparin and is usually mild. A more severe form of thrombocytopenia occurs in 0.5% of patients treated with unfractionated heparin. Both osteoporotic changes and thrombocytopenia occur less frequently with low-molecular-weight heparin than with unfractionated sodium heparin. Some argue, however, that the immuno-modulatory and direct placental effects of unfractionated heparin may not be recapitulated by low-molecular-weight heparins, making the latter less beneficial in patients with APAb-related disease. Trials comparing unfractionated and low-molecular-weight heparins in the treatment of APAS-related pregnancy loss remain small.[399]

Conclusion

Attempts to define interactions between the complex hu-man reproductive and immune systems will be predictably complex. Although a great many details are known about each system, in most cases the link between dysregulation of the immune system and disease of the reproductive sys-tem is incompletely understood. For many disorders, in-cluding immune-associated recurrent pregnancy loss, this uncertainty has delayed the formulation of standard test-ing and treatment procedures. Regrettably, some clinicians have forged ahead with diagnostic tests and treatments that have not been adequately supported by scientific data.

It is an exciting time for reproductive immunologists. The study of the effects of immune processes on reproduc-tion is well established and is certain to be increasingly fruitful. There is the hope of developing a wider array of more effective treatments for patients suffering with immune-related reproductive difficulties. Studies of the effects of reproductive hormones on immune responses are gaining momentum and highlighting the importance of gender-specific approaches to health and disease. In a world characterized by an increasingly subfertile and aging population, realizing the potential benefits of testing and treatments involving reproductive immunology is more challenging and rewarding than ever before.

ACKNOWLEDGMENTS: The authors would like to extend their gratitude to Dr. Linda Graziadei Schust for her expert editorial comments and Alisha Johnson for her administrative assistance.

The complete reference list can be found on the companion Expert Consult Web site at www.expertconsultbook.com.

Suggested Readings

Clarke GN, Elliott PJ, Smaila C. Detection of sperm antibodies in semen using the immunobead test: a survey of 813 consecutive patients. Am J Reprod Immunol 3:118-123, 1985.

Culligan PJ, Crane MM, Boone WR, et al. Validity and cost-effectiveness of antisperm antibody testing before in vitro fertilization. Fertil Steril 5:894-898, 1998.

Empson M, Lassere M, Craig JC, et al. Recurrent pregnancy loss with antiphospholipid antibody: a systematic review of therapeutic trials. Obstet Gynecol 1:135-144, 2002.

Gleicher N, Vidali A, Karande V, et al. The immunological "Wars of the Roses": disagreements amongst reproductive immunologists. Idiotype and anti-idiotype specific T cell responses on transplantation with hybridomas reactive to viral hemagglutinin and human tumor antigen. Hum Reprod 3:539-542, 2002.

Hornstein MD, Davis OK, Massey JB, et al. Antiphospholipid antibodies and in vitro fertilization success: a meta-analysis. Fertil Steril 73(2):330-333, 2000.

Jager S, Kremer J, van Slochteren-Draaisma T. A simple method of screening for antisperm antibodies in the human male. Detection of spermatozoal surface IgG with the direct mixed antiglobulin reaction carried out on untreated fresh human semen. Int J Fertil 1:12-21, 1978.

Mellor AL, Munn DH. Immunology at the maternal-fetal interface: lessons for T cell tolerance and suppression. Annu Rev Immunol 18:367-391, 2000.

Miyakis S, Lockshin MD, Atsumi T, et al. International consensus statement on an update of the classification criteria for definite antiphospholipid syndrome (APS). J Thromb Haemost 2:295-306, 2006.

Moffett-King A. Natural killer cells and pregnancy. Nat Rev Immunol 9:656-663, 2002.

Neurath M, Finotto S, Glimcher L. The role of Th1/Th2 polarization in mucosal immunity. Nat Med 6:567-573, 2002.

Oates-Whitehead RM, Haas DM, Carrier JA. Progestogen for preventing miscarriage. Cochrane Database Syst Rev 4:CD003511, 2003.

Ober C, Hyslop T, Elias S, et al. Human leukocyte antigen matching and fetal loss: results of a 10 year prospective study. Hum Reprod 1:33-38, 1998.

Ober C, Karrison T, Odem R, et al. Mononuclear-cell immunization in prevention of recurrent miscarriage: a randomized trial. Lancet:365-369, 1999.

Stephenson M, Kutteh W. Evaluation and management of recurrent early pregnancy loss. Clin Obstet Gynecol 1:132-145, 2007.

Thellin O, Coumans B, Zorzi W, et al. Tolerance to the foeto-placental 'graft': ten ways to support a child for nine months. Curr Opin Immunol 6:731-737, 2000.

CHAPTER 14

Menopause and Aging

Rogerio A. Lobo

Epidemiology

Menopause is defined by the last menstrual period. Because cessation of menses is variable and many of the symptoms thought to be related to menopause may occur prior to cessation of menses, there is seldom a precise timing of this event. Other terms used are *perimenopause*, which refers to a variable time beginning a few years before and continuing after the event of menopause, and *climacteric*, which merely refers to the time after the cessation of reproductive function. While the terms *menopausal* and *postmenopausal* are used interchangeably, the former term is less correct because "menopausal" should only relate to the time around the cessation of menses.

As life expectancy increases beyond the eighth decade worldwide, particularly in developed countries, an increasing proportion of the female population is postmenopausal. With the average age of menopause being 51 years, more than a third of a woman's life is now spent after menopause. Here symptoms and signs of estrogen deficiency merge with issues encountered with natural aging. As the world population increases and a larger proportion of this population is made up of individuals over 50, medical care specifically directed at postmenopausal women becomes an important aspect of modern medicine. Between the years 2000 and 2005, the world population older than 60 years doubled, from 590 million to 1 billion. In the United States, the number of women entering menopause will almost double in the 30 years between 1990 and 2020 (Table 14-1).[1]

Age of menopause, which is a genetically programmed event, is subject to some variability. The age of menopause in Western countries (between 51 and 52 years)[2,3] is thought to correlate with general health status.[4-6] Lower socioeconomic status is associated with an earlier age of menopause.[3] Higher parity, on the other hand, has been found to be associated with a later menopause.[7] Smoking has consistently been found to be associated with menopause onset taking place 1 to 2 years earlier.[3,8] Although body mass has been thought to be related to age of menopause (greater mass with later menopause),[9] the data have not been consistent. Malnourishment and vegetarianism have both been found to be associated with earlier onset of menopause.[10,11] However, physical and athletic activity has not been found consistently to influence the age of menopause.

There also appear to be ethnic differences in the onset of menopause. In the United States, African-American and Hispanic women have been found to have menopause approximately 2 years earlier than white women.[12,13] Although parity is generally greater around the world than in the United States, the age of menopause appears to be somewhat earlier. Malay women have menopause at approximately age 45, Thai women at age 49.5 years, and Filipina women between ages 47 and 48.[14-16] Countries at higher altitude (Himalayas or Andes) have been shown to have menopause 1 to 1.5 years earlier.[17,18] Because the average age of menopause in the United States is 51 to 53 years with an age distribution weighted toward white women, menopause prior to age 40 is considered premature. Conversely, by age 58, 97% of women will have gone through menopause.

The primary determinate of age of menopause is genetic. Based on family studies, heritability for age of menopause averaged 0.87—suggesting that genetics explain up to 87% of the variance in menopausal age.[19] Other than gene mutations that cause premature ovarian failure (explained later in this chapter), no specific genes have been discovered to date that account for this genetic influence. However, several genes are likely involved, including genes coding telomerase, which is involved in aging.

TABLE 14-1

U.S. Population Entering the Postmenopausal Years, Ages 55 to 64

Year	Population
1990	10.8 million
2000	12.1 million
2010	17.1 million
2020	19.3 million

Adapted from U.S. Bureau of the Census. Current population reports: projections of the population of the United States 1977 to 2050. Washington, D.C., U.S. Government Printing Office, 1993.

Premature Ovarian Failure

Premature ovarian failure (POF) is defined as hypergonadotropic ovarian failure occurring prior to age 40. POF has occurred in 5% to 10% of women who are evaluated for amenorrhea,[20,21] thus the incidence varies according to the prevalence of amenorrhea in various populations. Estimates of the overall prevalence of POF in the general population range between 0.3% and 0.9% of women.[22,23]

Throughout life, there is an ongoing rate of atresia of oocytes. Because this process is accelerated with various forms of gonadal dysgenesis due to defective X chromosomes, one possible etiologic factor in POF is an increased rate of atresia that has yet to be explained. A decreased germ cell endowment or an increased rate of germ cell destruction can also explain POF.[20] Nevertheless, some 1000 (of the original 2 million) primarily follicles may remain.[24,25] Even though most of these oocytes are likely to be functionally deficient, occasionally spontaneous pregnancies occur in young women in the first few years after the diagnosis of POF.

There are several possible causes of POF:

* Genetic
* Enzymatic
* Immune
* Gonadotropin defects
* Ovarian insults
* Idiopathic

Defects in the X chromosome may result in various types of gonadal dysgenesis with varied times of expression of ovarian failure. Even patients with classical gonadal dysgenesis (e.g., 45,XO) may undergo a normal puberty, and occasionally a pregnancy may ensue[26-29] as a result of genetic mosaicism. Very small defects in the X chromosome may be sufficient to cause POF.[30] Familial forms of POF may be related to either autosomal-dominant or sex-linked modes of inheritance.[31-33]

Mutations in the gene encoding the follicle-stimulating hormone (FSH)-receptor (e.g., mutation in exon 7 in the gene on chromosome 2p) have been described,[34] but these are extremely rare outside the Finnish population in which these mutations were originally described. An expansion of a trinucleotide repeat sequence in the first exon on the *FMR1* gene (Xq27.3) leads to fragile X syndrome, a major cause of developmental disabilities in males.[35] The permutation in fragile X syndrome has been shown to be

associated with POF.[36,37] Type 1 blepharophimosis/ptosis/epicanthus inversus syndrome (BPES), an autosomal dominant disorder due to mutations in the forkhead transcription factor FOXL2, includes POF.[38] Triple X syndrome has also been associated with POF. Dystrophic myotonia has also been linked to POF, although the mechanism underlying this relationship is unclear.[39] Other POF candidate genes are reviewed in Chapter 8.

Under the category of enzymatic defects, galactosemia is a major cause of POF that is related to the toxic buildup of galactose in women who are unable to metabolize the sugar. Even in women with fairly well controlled galactose-free diets, POF tends to occur.[40,41] Another enzymatic defect linked to POF is 17α-hydroxylase deficiency. This rare condition manifests differently from the other causes discussed here because the defect in the production of sex steroids leads to sexual infantilism and hypertension.[42-44]

Because of the prevalence of autoimmune disorders in women, the degree to which autoimmunity may be responsible for POF is unclear (see Chapter 13). One study has suggested an association in 17.5% of cases.[45] Virtually all autoimmune disorders have been found to be associated with POF, including autoimmune polyendocrinopathies such as autoimmune polyendocrinopathy–candidiasis-ectodermal dystrophy (APECED), which is caused by mutations in the autoimmune (*AIRE*) gene on band 21q22.3.[46] The presence of the thymus gland appears to be required for normal ovarian function as POF has been associated with hypoplasia of the thymus.[47] In patients who have undergone ovarian biopsy as part of their evaluation, lymphocytic infiltration surrounding follicles has been described, as well as resumption of menses after immunosuppression.[48-51]

Immunoassays utilizing antibodies directed at ovarian antigens have been developed and have demonstrated positive findings in some patients with POF,[52] although the relevance of these findings remains unsettled. Ovarian autoantibodies could also conceivably be a secondary phenomenon to a primary cell-mediated form of immunity. Specific enzymes such as 3β-hydroxysteroid dehydrogenase (3β-HSD) may also be the target of ovarian autoimmunity.[53] From a practical standpoint, screening for the common autoimmune disorders is appropriate in women found to have POF. Although relatively rare, as many as 2% to 4% of women with POF have anti-adrenal antibodies[54] and may be at risk for adrenal failure. Commercial antibodies to 21-hydroxylase are available and agree with other assays for adrenal cortex antibodies.[55] It has been suggested that screening women using dehydroepiandrosterone sulfate (DHEAS) may also be useful to detect signs of adrenal insufficiency.

More from a theoretical standpoint, abnormalities in the structure of gonadotropins, in their receptors, or in receptor binding could be associated with POF. Although abnormal urinary forms of gonadotropins have been reported in women with POF,[56] these data have not been replicated. Abnormalities of FSH-receptor binding, as mediated by a serum inhibitor, have been described.[57] A genetic defect that may lead to alterations in FSH-receptor structure was mentioned previously.[34]

Under the category of ovarian insults, POF may be induced by ionizing radiation, chemotherapy, or overly aggressive ovarian surgery. Although not well documented, viral infections have been suggested to play a role, particularly mumps.[58] A dose of 400 to 500 rads is known to cause ovarian failure 50% of the time,[59,60] and older women are more vulnerable to experiencing permanent failure. A dose of approximately 800 rads is associated with failure in all women.[60,61] Ovarian failure (transient or permanent) may be induced by chemotherapeutic agents, although younger women receiving this insult have a better prognosis.[61,63] Alkalyzing agents, particularly cyclophosphamide, appear to be most toxic.[64]

By exclusion, the majority of women are considered to have idiopathic POF because no demonstrable cause can be pinpointed. Among these women, small mutations in genes lying on the X chromosome or yet to be identified autosomal genes may be the cause.

MANAGEMENT OF PRIMARY OVARIAN FAILURE

Evaluation of women under age 30 who have POF should include screening for autoimmune disorders and a karyotype; detailed recommendations for screening of such women are available.[65] In addition, vaginal ultrasound may be useful for assessing the size of the ovaries and the degree of follicular development, which, if present, may signify an immunologic defect.

Treatment usually consists of estrogen replacement. If fertility is a concern, the most efficacious treatment is oocyte donation. Various attempts at ovarian stimulation are usually unsuccessful, and the sporadic pregnancies that may occur are just as likely to occur spontaneously (~5%) as with any intervention.[66,67] These spontaneous pregnancies are frequently encountered while receiving estrogen replacement. Noting irregular or unscheduled bleeding (while receiving hormonal treatment) is important as a sign of endogenous sex steroid production.

It has been well established that POF as well as bilateral oophorectomy prior to the usual age of menopause is associated with an increased risk[68] of cardiovascular disease (CVD) as well as increased mortality rate (Fig. 14-1). CVD mortality rate specifically is increased two- to fourfold, and observational studies have suggested that using hormone therapy (HT) reduces this risk. Accordingly, unless there are contraindications, estrogen should be considered in all young women with POF, at least until the age of natural menopause.

The Menopausal Transition (Perimenopause)

A workshop was convened in 2001 to build consensus on describing various stages of the menopausal transition.[69] As depicted in Figure 14-2, the menopausal transition (perimenopause) is divided into early and late phases according to menstrual acyclicity. These changes signify a varying period of time (years) during which rapid oocyte depletion occurs, followed by hypoestrogenism.

The ovary changes markedly from birth to the onset of menopause (Fig. 14-3).[70] The greatest number of primordial follicles is present in utero at 20 weeks' gestation and undergoes a regular rate of atresia until around the age of 37. After this time, the decline in primordial follicles appears to become more rapid between age 37 and menopause (Fig. 14-4), when no more than a thousand follicles remain.[71] These remaining follicles are primarily atresic in nature.

TYPES OF OVARIAN CHANGES

Although perimenopausal changes are generally thought to be endocrine in nature and result in menstrual changes, a marked diminution of reproductive capacity precedes this period by several years. This decline may be referred to

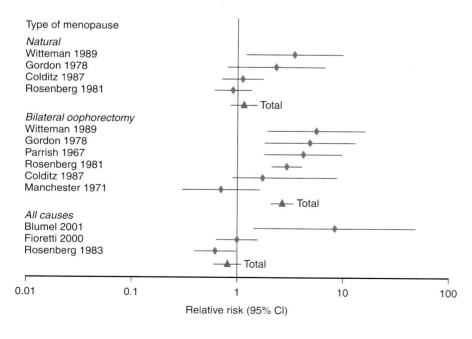

Figure 14-1. Effect of type of "early" menopause on cardiovascular disease. Data taken from a meta-analysis. (From Atsma F, Bartelink ML, Grobbee DE, et al. Postmenopausal status and early menopause as independent risk factors for cardiovascular disease: a meta-analysis. Menopause 13[2]:265-279, 2006 [review]. See reference 329 for data sources.)

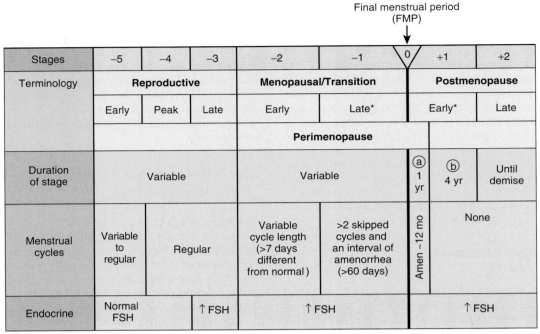

Stages	−5	−4	−3	−2	−1	0	+1	+2
Terminology	**Reproductive**			**Menopausal/Transition**			**Postmenopause**	
	Early	Peak	Late	Early	Late*		Early*	Late
				Perimenopause				
Duration of stage	Variable			Variable		ⓐ 1 yr	ⓑ 4 yr	Until demise
Menstrual cycles	Variable to regular	Regular		Variable cycle length (>7 days different from normal)	>2 skipped cycles and an interval of amenorrhea (>60 days)	Amen ~12 mo	None	
Endocrine	Normal FSH	↑FSH		↑FSH			↑FSH	

Final menstrual period (FMP)

Figure 14-2. *The Stages of Reproductive Aging Workshop (STRAW) staging system. ↑ FSH, elevated follicle-stimulating hormone. *, Stages most likely to be characterized by vasomotor symptoms. (From Soules MR, Sherman S, Parrott E, et al. Executive summary: Stages of Reproductive Aging Workshop [STRAW]. Fertil Steril 76:874-878, 2001.)*

as *gametogenic ovarian failure.* The concept of dissociation in ovarian function is appropriate. Gametogenic failure is signified by reduced early follicular phase inhibin secretion, rising serum FSH levels, and a marked reduction in fecundity. These changes may occur with normal menstrual function and no obvious endocrine deficiency, however, and they may occur in some women as early as age 35 (10 or more years before endocrine deficiency ensues).

Although subtle changes in endocrine and menstrual function can occur for up to 3 years before menopause,

it has been shown that the major reduction in ovarian estrogen production does not occur until approximately 6 months before menopause (Fig. 14-5).[72] There is also a very slow decline in androgen status (i.e., androstenedione and testosterone), which cannot be adequately detected at the time of the perimenopause.

Products of the granulosa cell are most important for the feedback control of FSH. As the functional capacity of the follicular units decreases, secretion of substances that suppress FSH also decreases. Most notably, inhibin

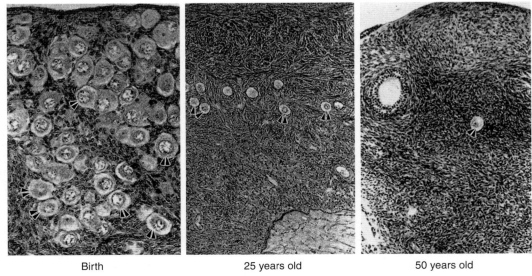

Birth   25 years old   50 years old

Figure 14-3. *Photomicrographs of the cortex of human ovaries from birth to 50 years of age. Small nongrowing primordial follicles (arrows) have a single layer of squamous granulosa cells. (Adapted from Erickson CF. An analysis of follicle development and ovum maturation. Semin Reprod Endocrinol 4:233-254, 1986.)*

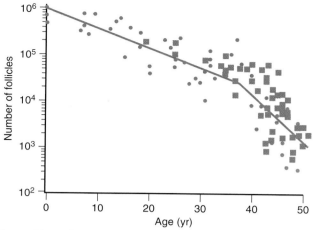

Figure 14-4. *The age-related decrease in the total number of primordial follicles (PFs) within both human ovaries from birth to menopause. As a result of recruitment (initiation of PF growth), the number of PFs decreases progressively from about 1 million at birth to 25,000 at 37 years. At 37 years, the rate of recruitment increases sharply, and the number of PFs declines to 1000 at menopause (about 51 years of age). Note: The different colors and shapes in the graph represent different studies. (Adapted from Faddy MJ, Gosden RJ, Gougeon A, et al. Accelerated disappearance of ovarian follicles in mid-life: implications for forecasting menopause. Hum Reprod 7:1342-1346, 1992.)*

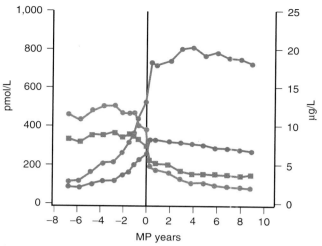

Figure 14-5. *Mean serum levels of follicle-stimulating hormone (FSH, blue), luteinizing hormone (LH, green), estradiol (E_2, brown), and estrone (E_1, purple), showing the perimenopausal transition. MP, menopause. (Adapted from Rannevik G, Jeppsson S, Johnell O, et al. A longitudinal study of the perimenopausal transition: altered profiles of steroid and pituitary hormones, SHBG, and bone mineral density. Maturitas 21:103-113, 1995.)*

B levels are lower in the early follicular phase in women in their late 30s (Fig. 14-6).[73,74] Indeed, FSH levels are higher throughout the cycle in older ovulatory women than in younger women (Fig. 14-7).[75]

The functional capacity of the ovary is also diminished as women enter into the perimenopause. With gonadotropin stimulation, although estradiol (E_2) levels are not very different between younger and older women, total inhibin production by granulosa cells is decreased in women over age 35.[76] From a clinical perspective, subtle increases in FSH on day 3 of the cycle, or increases in the clomiphene challenge test, correlate with decreased ovarian responses to stimulation and decreased fecundity.[77,78]

Although there is a general decline in oocyte number with age, an accelerated atresia occurs around age 37 or 38 (see Fig. 14-4).[71] The reason for this acceleration is not clear, but one possible explanation relates to activin secretion. Because granulosa cell–derived activin is important for stimulating FSH-receptor expression,[79] the rise in FSH levels could result in more activin production, which in turn enhances FSH action. A profile of elevated activin with lower inhibin B has been found in older women (Fig. 14-8).[80] This autocrine action of activin, involving enhanced FSH action, might be expected to lead to accelerated growth and differentiation of granulosa cells. Further, activin has been shown to increase the size of the pool of preantral follicles in the rat. At the same time, these follicles become more atretic.[81]

Clinical management of women in the perimenopause should address three general areas of concern:

1. Irregular bleeding
2. Symptoms of early menopause, such as hot flushes
3. The inability to conceive

Treatment of irregular bleeding is complicated by the fluctuating hormonal status. Estrogen levels may be higher than normal in the early follicular phase[72] and progesterone secretion may be normal, although not all cycles are ovulatory. For these reasons, short-term use of an oral contraceptive (usually 20 μg ethinyl estradiol) may be an option for otherwise healthy women who do not smoke to help them cope with irregular bleeding.

Early symptoms of menopause, particularly vasomotor changes, may occur as the result of fluctuating hormonal levels. In this setting, an oral contraceptive again may be an option if symptoms warrant therapy. Alternatively, lower doses of estrogen used alone may be another option.

Reproductive concerns often require more aggressive treatment because of decreased cycle fecundity. Once day 3 FSH levels increase, the prognosis for pregnancy is markedly reduced.

Hormonal Changes with Established Menopause

Depicted in Figure 14-9 are the typical hormonal levels of postmenopausal women compared with those of ovulatory women in the early follicular phase.[82] The most significant findings are the marked reductions in E_2 and estrone (E_1). Serum E_2 is reduced to a greater extent than E_1. Serum E_1, on the other hand, is produced primarily by peripheral aromatization from androgens, which decline principally as a function of age. Levels of E_2 average 15 pg/mL and range from 10 to 25 pg/mL, but are closer to 10 pg/mL in women who have undergone oophorectomy. Serum E_1 values average 30 pg/mL but may be higher in obese women because aromatization increases as a function of the mass of adipose tissue.

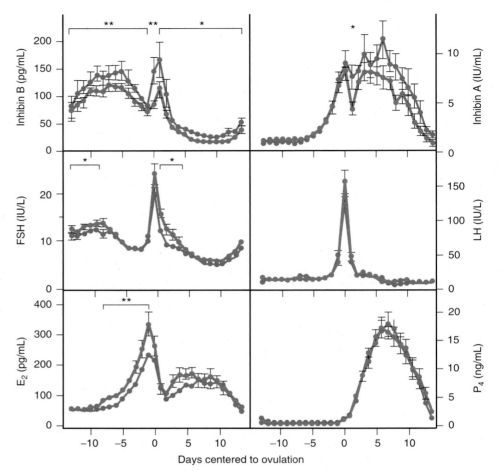

Figure 14-6. Mean inhibin B, follicle-stimulating hormone (FSH), estradiol (E_2), inhibin A, and progesterone (P_4) levels in cycling women 20 to 34 years old (purple) and 35 to 46 years old (green). Hormone levels are depicted as centered to the day of ovulation (*, P < 0.04;**, P < 0.02) when comparing the two age groups. (Adapted from Welt CK, McNicholl DJ, Taylor AE, Hall JE. Female reproductive aging is marked by decreased secretion of dimeric inhibin. J Clin Endocrinol Metab 84:105-111, 1999.)

Estrone sulfate (E_1S) is an estrogen conjugate that serves as a stable circulating reservoir of estrogen, and levels of E_1S are the highest among estrogens in postmenopausal women. In premenopausal women, values are usually above 1000 pg/mL; in postmenopausal women, levels average 350 pg/mL.

Apart from elevations in FSH and luteinizing hormone (LH), other pituitary hormones are not affected. The rise in FSH, beginning in stage –3 as early as age 38 (see Fig. 14-2), fluctuates considerably until approximately 4 years after menopause (stage +1) when values are consistently greater than 20 mIU/mL. Specifically, growth hormone (GH), TSH, and adrenocorticotropic hormone (ACTH) levels are normal. Serum prolactin levels may be very slightly decreased because prolactin levels are influenced by estrogen status.

Both the postmenopausal ovary and the adrenal gland continue to produce androgen. The ovary continues to produce androstenedione and testosterone but not E_2, and this production has been shown to be at least partially dependent on LH.[83,84] Androstenedione and testosterone levels are lower in women who have experienced bilateral oophorectomy, with values averaging 0.8 ng/mL and 0.1 ng/mL, respectively. The adrenal gland also continues to produce androstenedione, dehydroepiandrosterone (DHEA), and dehydroepiandrosterone sulfate (DHEAS); primarily as a function of aging, these values decrease somewhat (adrenopause), although cortisol (ACTH) secretion remains unaffected. Some data suggest that much "ovarian" testosterone production may actually arise from the adrenal.[85] Most likely, this production is by indirect mechanisms due to the adrenal supplying precursor substrate (DHEA and androstenedione).

Although DHEAS levels decrease with age (approximately 2% per year),[86] recent data have suggested that levels transiently rise in the perimenopause before the continuous decline thereafter (Fig. 14-10).[87] This interesting finding from the Study of Women Across the Nation (SWAN) also suggested that DHEAS levels are highest in Chinese women and lowest in African-American women.[87]

Testosterone levels also decline as a function of age, which is best demonstrated by the reduction in 24-hour mean levels (Fig. 14-11).[88] Because of the role of the adrenal in determining levels of testosterone after menopause,[83] adrenalectomy or dexamethasone treatment results in undetectable levels of serum testosterone. Compared with total testosterone, the measurement of bioavailable or "free" testosterone is more useful in postmenopausal women. After menopause, sex hormone–binding globulin (SHBG) levels decrease, resulting in relatively higher levels of bioavailable testosterone or a higher free androgen index (Fig. 14-12).[89] In women receiving oral estrogen, bioavailable testosterone levels are extremely low because

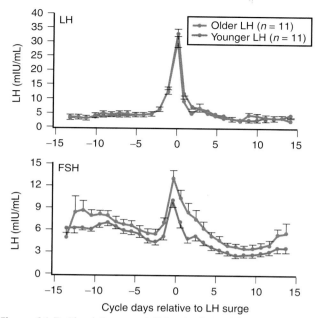

Figure 14-7. The daily serum follicle-stimulating hormone (FSH) and luteinizing hormone (LH) levels throughout the menstrual cycle of two groups (older and younger) of 11 women each (mean ± SE). The gonadotropin secretion pattern in normal women of advanced reproductive age is shown in relation to the monotropic FSH rise. (Adapted from Klein NA, Battaglia DE, Clifton DK, et al. The gonadotropin secretion pattern in normal women of advanced reproductive age in relation to the monotropic FSH rise. J Soc Gynecol Investig 3:27-32, 1996.)

SHBG levels are increased. How this relates to the decision to begin androgen therapy in postmenopausal women will be discussed later in this chapter.

Elevated gonadotropin (FSH/LH) levels arise from reduced secretion of E_2 and inhibin as described earlier. Estrogen is important in controlling the production of GnRH mRNA in type 1 neurons.[90,91] In addition, the increase in gonadotropins observed at menopause appears to be enhanced by substance P[92] as well as by tachykinins produced in hypertrophied neurons,[93,94] which result from the decrease in E_2.

Unlike the rodent, where there is evidence for a hypothalamic factor involved in ovarian senescence,[95-97] no such clear evidence exists for women. The hypothesis proposed by Wise and colleagues suggested that the effects of aging in the brain affect neurotransmitter systems that regulate GnRH, disrupting ovarian folliculogenesis, and ultimately promote senescence. Thus, the accelerated follicular loss that is apparent in the late 30s is postulated to be due to age-related desynchronization in the rhythmicity of GnRH secretion.[97]

Although some aging effects of the brain are likely to exist, there is abundant human evidence for an ovarian-induced menopause. In rodents there is slowing of LH pulsatility with aging, but LH pulse frequency and amplitude increase with age as menopause approaches in women (Fig. 14-13).[98] Most recently, a sleep-entrained alteration in GnRH pulse dynamics has been observed in postmenopausal women, namely the inability to increase

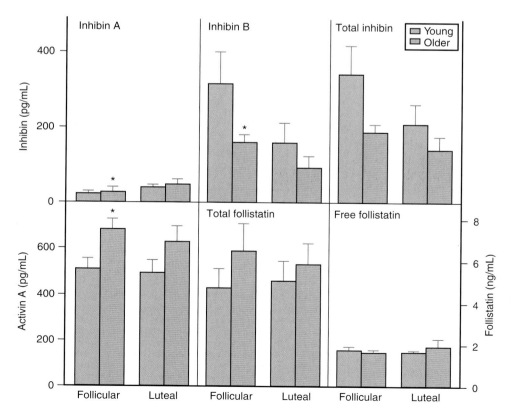

Figure 14-8. Mean concentrations of gonadal proteins from the same subjects. Total inhibin is a derived number from the sum of inhibin A and inhibin B. *, Group differences; P < 0.05. Net increase in stimulatory input resulting from a decrease in inhibin B and an increase in activin A may contribute in part to the rise in follicular phase follicle-stimulating hormone of aging cyclic women. (Adapted from Reame NE, Wyman TL, Phillips DJ, et al. Net increase in stimulatory input resulting from a decrease in inhibin B and an increase in activin A may contribute in part to the rise in follicular phase follicle-stimulating of hormone of aging cyclic women. J Clin Endocrinol Metab 83:3302-3307, 1998.)

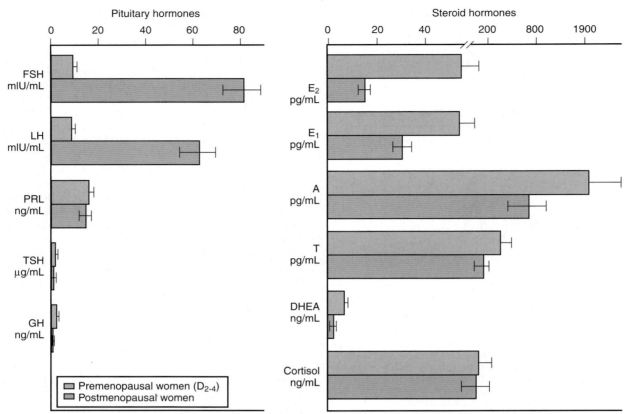

Figure 14-9. *Circulating levels of pituitary and steroid hormones in postmenopausal women compared with levels in premenopausal women studied during the first week (days 2 to 4 [D$_{2-4}$]) of the menstrual cycle. A, androstenedione; DHEA, dehydroepiandrosterone; E$_1$, estrogen; E$_2$, estradiol; FSH, follicle-stimulating hormone; GH, growth hormone; LH, luteinizing hormone; PRL, prolactin; T, testosterone; TSH, thyroid-stimulating hormone. (Adapted from Yen SSC. The biology of menopause. J Reprod Med 18:287, 1977.)*

GnRH pulse amplitude at night.[99] There is some evidence that the high-frequency and high-amplitude pulses of LH observed in the first few years in postmenopausal women slows down in late menopause[100]; this latter effect is clearly related to aging per se.

Ovarian aging is a programmed event; the return of atresia, accelerating at around age 37.5 years until the natural age of menopause, has now been shown to occur in almost the exact way in the chimpanzee.[101] Ovarian aging from a hormonal standpoint is best characterized by small elevations in serum FSH occurring at the beginning of the menstrual cycle (days 2 to 3), reductions in inhibin B, as well as steep declines in serum müllerian inhibiting substance (MIS) or anti-müllerian hormone (AMH)[102] (Fig. 14-14). The latter is a very useful and practical determinant in that it tends to undergo less cycle to cycle variation compared to FSH, and can be measured at any phase of the cycle.[103]

EFFECTS ON VARIOUS ORGAN SYSTEMS

Central Nervous System

The brain is an active site for estrogen action as well as estrogen formation.[104] Estrogen activity in the brain is mediated via ERα and ERβ receptors. Whether or not a novel membrane receptor (non-ERα/ERβ) exists is still being debated.[105] However, both genomic and nongenomic

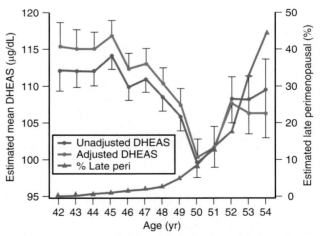

Figure 14-10. *Mean (± SE) circulating dehydroepiandrosterone sulfate (DHEAS) at each year of age of the entire study population before and after adjustment for age, current smoking, menopausal status, log body mass index (BMI), ethnicity, site, and the interaction between ethnicity and log BMI. Also shown is the percentage of women at each year of age who have transitioned to late perimenopausal status. (Adapted from Lasley BL, Santoro N, Randolf JF, et al. The relationship of circulating dehydroepiandrosterone, testosterone, and estradiol to stages of the menopausal transition and ethnicity. J Clin Endocrinol Metab 87:3760-3767, 2002.)*

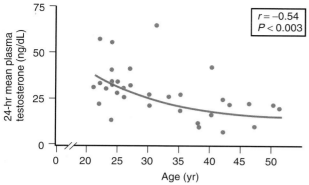

Figure 14-11. *The 24-hour mean plasma total testosterone (T) level compared with age in normal women. The regression equation was T (nmol/L) = 37.8 × age (years)$^{-1.12}$ (r = −0.54; P < 0.003). (Adapted from Zumoff B, Strain GW, Miller LK, et al. Twenty-four hour mean plasma testosterone concentration declines with age in normal premenopausal women. J Clin Endocrinol Metab 80:1429-1430, 1995.)*

mechanisms of estrogen action clearly exist in the brain. Figure 14-15 illustrates the predominance of ERβ in the cortex (frontal and parietal) and the cerebellum, based on work in the rat.[106,107] While 17β-E$_2$ is a specific ligand for both receptors, certain synthetic estrogens have a greater affinity for ERβ.

There are multiple actions of estrogen on the brain, as reviewed by Henderson (Box 14-1),[108] and thus, there are important functions linked to estrogen that contribute to well-being in general and, more specifically, to cognition and mood. The hallmark feature of declining estrogen status in the brain is the hot flush, which is more generically referred to as a vasomotor episode.

The *hot flush* usually refers to the acute sensation of heat, and the flush or vasomotor episode includes changes in the early perception of this event and other skin changes (including diaphoresis). Hot flushes usually occur for 2 years after the onset of estrogen deficiency, but can persist for 10 or more years.[109,110] In 10% to 15% of women these symptoms are severe and disabling.[109-111] In the United States the incidence of these episodes varies in different ethnic groups. Symptoms are greatest in Hispanic and African-American women, intermediate in white women, and lowest among Asian women (Fig. 14-16).[112]

The fall in estrogen levels precipitates the vasomotor symptoms. Although the proximate cause of the flush remains elusive, the episodes result from a hypothalamic response (probably mediated by catecholamines) to the change in estrogen status. The flush has been well characterized physiologically. It results in heat dissipation as witnessed by an increase in peripheral temperature (fingers, toes); a decrease in skin resistance, associated with diaphoresis; and a reduction in core body temperature (Fig. 14-17).[113] There are hormonal correlates of flush activity, such as an increase in serum LH and in plasma levels of pro-opiomelanocortin peptides (ACTH, β-endorphin) at the time of the flush,[114] but these occurrences are thought to be epiphenomena that result as a consequence of the flush and are not related to its etiology. Data from Friedman has suggested that the major physiologic finding in women with and without hot flushes is a narrowing of

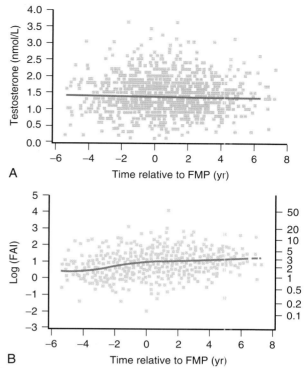

Figure 14-12. *A, Linear regression model: observed testosterone and fitted levels of mean T across the menopausal transition. B, Double logistic model: observed free androgen index (FAI) and fitted levels of mean FAI across the menopausal transition. The left and right axes show FAI levels on the log and antilog scales, respectively. The horizontal axis represents time (years) with respect to first menstrual period (FMP); negative (positive) numbers indicate time before (after) FMP. (From Burger HG, Dudley EC, Cui J, et al. A prospective longitudinal study of serum testosterone, dehydroepiandrosterone sulfate, and sex hormone-binding globulin levels through the menopause transition. J Clin Endocrinol Metab 85:2832-2838, 2000.)*

the threshold for sweating and shivering in symptomatic women (Fig. 14-18).[115]

One of the primary complaints of women with hot flushes is sleep disruption. They may awaken several times during the night, and require a change of bedding and clothes because of diaphoresis. Nocturnal sleep disruption in postmenopausal women with hot flushes has been well documented by electroencephalographic (EEG) recordings.[116] Sleep efficiency is lower, and the latency to rapid eye movement (REM) sleep is longer in women with hot flushes compared with asymptomatic women.[117,118] This disturbed sleep often leads to fatigue and irritability during the day. The frequency of awakenings and of hot flushes are reduced appreciably with estrogen treatment (Fig. 14-19).[116,119,120] Sleep may be disrupted even if the woman is not conscious of being awakened from sleep. In this setting, EEG monitoring has indicated sleep disruption in concert with physiologic measures of vasomotor episodes.

In postmenopausal women, estrogen has been found to improve depressed mood regardless of whether or not this is a specific complaint[121-127] (critics of some of this work point out that mood is affected by the symptomatology and by sleep deprivation). Blinded studies carried out in asymptomatic women have also shown benefit.[126] In an

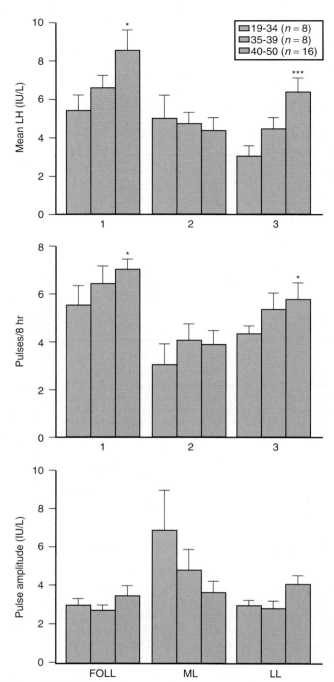

Figure 14-13. *Effects of age on pulsatile luteinizing hormone (LH) secretory characteristics (age groups are in years). All subjects were studied across the same menstrual cycle. FOLL, early follicular phase; ML, mid-luteal phase; LL, late luteal phase. *, P < 0.05; ***, P < 0.001. (From Reame NE, Kelche RP, Beitins IZ, et al. Age effects on follicle-stimulating hormone and pulsatile LH secretion across the menstrual cycle of premenopausal women. J Clin Endocrinol Metab 81:1512-1518, 1996.)*

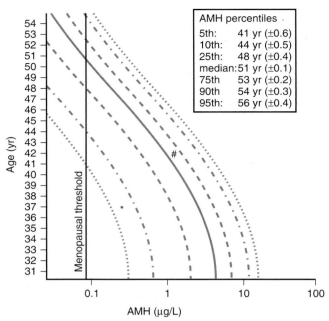

Figure 14-14. *Rapid decline in levels of anti-müllerian hormone (AMH) with aging. Levels are undetectable prior to menopause. (From van Disseldorp J, Faddy MJ, Themmen AP, et al. Relationship of serum anti-mullerian hormone concentration to age of menopause. J Clin Endocrinol Metab 93[6]:2129-2134, 2008.)*

estrogen-deficient state such as occurs after the menopause, a higher incidence of depression (clinical or subclinical) is often manifest. However, menopause per se does *not* cause depression, and while estrogen does generally improve depressive mood, it should *not* be used for psychiatric disorders. Nevertheless, very high pharmacologic doses of estrogen have been used to treat certain types of psychiatric depression in the past.[128-130] Progestogens as a class generally attenuate the beneficial effects of estrogen on mood, although this effect is highly variable.[131,132]

Cognitive decline in postmenopausal women is related to aging as well as to estrogen deficiency. The literature is somewhat mixed in showing whether there are benefits of estrogen in terms of cognition. In more recent studies, verbal memory appears to be enhanced with estrogen[133-136] and has been found to correlate with acute changes in brain imaging signifying brain activation.[135-137]

Dementia increases as women age, and the most common form of dementia is Alzheimer's disease (AD). Listed in Box 14-1 are several neurotrophic and neuroprotective factors that relate to how estrogen deficiency may be expected to result in the loss of protection against the development of AD. In addition, estrogen has a positive role in enhancing neurotransmitter function, which is deficient in women with AD. This function of estrogen has particular importance and relevance for the cholinergic system that is affected in AD.[138,139]

Estrogen use after menopause appears to decrease the likelihood of developing or delays the onset of AD (Fig. 14-20).[140-157] However, once a woman is affected by AD, estrogen is unlikely to provide any benefit.[158]

Collagen

Estrogen has a positive effect on *collagen*, which is an important component of bone and skin and serves as a major support tissue for the structures of the pelvis and urinary system. Both estrogen and androgen receptors have been identified in skin fibroblasts. Nearly 30% of skin collagen is lost within the first 5 years after menopause, and

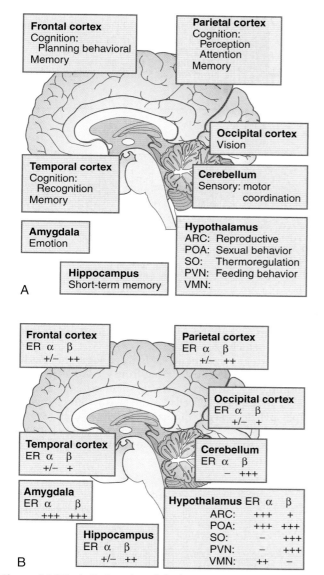

Figure 14-15. *A, Each region of the brain has an important role in specific brain functions. Optimal brain activity is maintained by means of the integration of different areas by neural tracts. B, Distribution of estrogen receptors ERα and ERβ mRNA in the rat brain. ARC, arcuate nucleus; POA, preoptic area; PVN, paraventricular nucleus; SO, supraoptic nucleus; VMN, ventromedial nucleus. (B, Adapted from Cela V, Naftolin F. Clinical effects of sex steroids on the brain. In Lobo RA [ed]. The Treatment of Postmenopausal Woman: Basic and Clinical Aspects, 2nd ed. Philadelphia, Lippincott Williams & Wilkins, 1999, pp 247-262.)*

BOX 14-1

Effects of Estrogen on Brain Function

Organizational actions
   Effects on neuronal number, morphology, and connections occurring during critical stage of development
Neurotrophic actions
   Neuronal differentiation
   Neurite extension
   Synapse formation
   Interactions with neurotrophins
Neuroprotective actions
   Protection against apoptosis
   Antioxidant properties
   Anti-inflammatory properties
   Augmentation of cerebral blood flow
   Enhancement of glucose transport into the brain
   Blunting of corticosteroid response to behavioral stress
   Interactions with neurotrophins
Effects on neurotransmitters
   Acetylcholine
   Noradrenaline
   Serotonin
   Dopamine
   Glutamate
   γ-Aminobutyric acid
   Neuropeptides
Effects on glial cells
Effects on proteins involved in Alzheimer's disease
   Amyloid precursor protein
   Tau protein
   Apolipoprotein E

Adapted from Henderson VW: Estrogen, cognition, and a woman's risk of Alzheimer's disease. Am J Med 103 (suppl 3A): 11-18, 1997.

---

collagen decreases approximately 2% per year for the first 10 years after menopause.[159] This statistic, which is similar to that of bone loss after menopause, strongly suggests a link between skin thickness, bone loss, and the risk of osteoporosis.[160]

Although the literature is not entirely consistent, estrogen therapy generally improves collagen content after menopause and improves skin thickness substantially after about 2 years of treatment.[159,161-165] There is a possible biomodal effect with high doses of estrogen causing a reduction in skin thickness.[159-166] The supportive effect of estrogen on collagen has important implications for

bone homeostasis and for the pelvis after menopause. Here, reductions in collagen support and atrophy of the vaginal and urethral mucosa have been implicated in a variety of symptoms, including prolapse and urinary incontinence.[167,168]

Symptoms of urinary incontinence and irritative bladder symptoms occur in 20% to 40% of perimenopausal and postmenopausal women.[169-171] Uterine prolapse and other gynecologic symptoms related to poor collagen support, as well as urinary complaints, may improve with estrogen therapy.[112,172-174] Although estrogen generally improves symptoms, urodynamic changes have not been shown to be altered.[175,176] Estrogen has also been shown to decrease the incidence of recurrence of urinary tract infections.[177] Restoration of bladder control in older women with estrogen has been shown to decrease the need for admission to nursing homes in Sweden.[178] Estrogen may also have an important role in normal wound healing. In this setting, estrogen enhances the effects of growth factors such as transforming growth factor-β (TGF-β).[179,180]

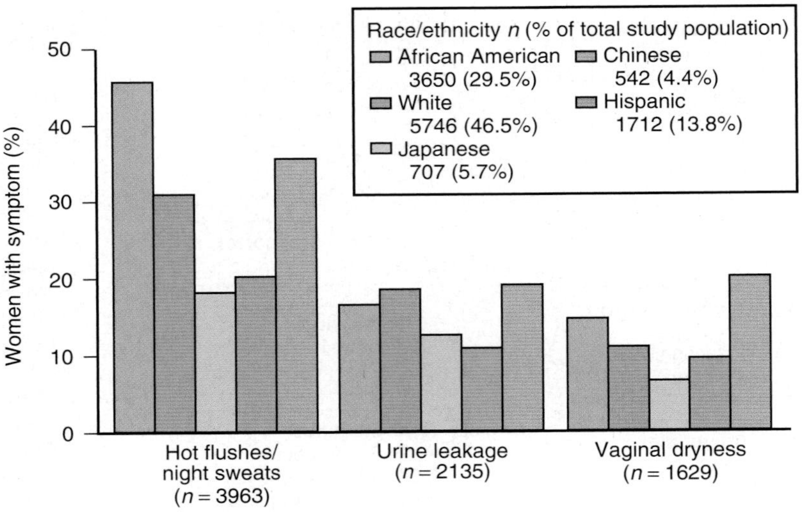

Figure 14-16. *Study of Women's Health Across the Nation (SWAN): Symptom severity. (Adapted from Gold EB, Sternfeld B, Kelsey JL, et al. Relation of demographic and lifestyle factors to symptoms in a multi-racial/ethnic population of women 40-55 years of age. Am J Epidemiol 152:463, 2000.)*

Genital Atrophy

Vulvovaginal complaints are often associated with estrogen deficiency. In the perimenopause, symptoms of dryness and atrophic changes occur in 21% and 15% of women, respectively. However, these findings increase with time, and by 4 years these incidences are 47% and 55%, respectively.[181,182] With this change, an increase in sexual complaints also occurs, with an incidence of dyspareunia of 41% in sexually active 60-year-old women.[183] Estrogen deficiency results in a thin and more pale vaginal mucosa.

The moisture content is low, the pH increases (usually greater than 5), and the mucosa may exhibit inflammation and small petechiae.

With estrogen treatment, vaginal cytologic changes have been documented, transforming from a cellular pattern of predominantly parabasal cells to one with an increased number of superficial cells. Along with this change, the vaginal pH decreases, vaginal blood flow increases, and the electropotential difference across the vaginal mucosa increases to that found in premenopausal women.[184]

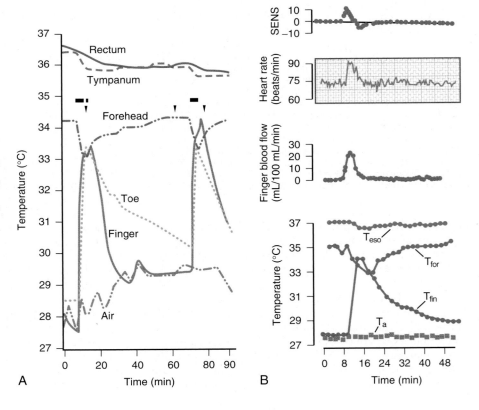

Figure 14-17. *Temperature responses to two spontaneous flashes and evoked flash. Down arrow indicates finger stab for blood sample. Black bars indicate time of hot flush. SENS (Data adapted from Molnar GW. Body temperature during menopausal hot flashes. J Appl Physiol 38:499-503, 1975.)*

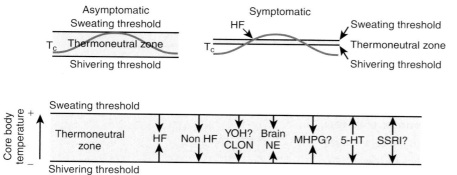

Figure 14-18. Narrowing of the thermoregulatory zone in symptomatic women. HF, hot flush. (Data from Freedman RR. Menopausal hot flashes. In Lobo RA (ed). Treatment of the Postmenopausal Woman, 3rd ed. New York, Academic Press, 2007, pp 187-198.)

Bone Loss

Estrogen deficiency has been well established as a cause of bone loss. This loss can be noted for the first time when menstrual cycles become irregular in the perimenopause. From 1.5 years before the menopause to 1.5 years after menopause, spine bone mineral density has been shown to decrease by 2.5% per year, compared with a premenopausal loss rate of 0.13% per year.[185,186] Loss of trabecular bone (spine) is greater with estrogen deficiency than is loss of cortical bone.

Postmenopausal bone loss leading to osteoporosis is a substantial health care problem. In white women, 35% of all postmenopausal women have been estimated to have osteoporosis based on bone mineral density.[187] Further, the lifetime fracture risk for these women is 40%.[188] The morbidity rate and economic burden of osteoporosis is well documented.[189] Interestingly, there are data to suggest that up to 19% of white men also have osteoporosis.

Bone mass is substantially affected by sex steroids through classic mechanisms to be described later in this chapter. Attainment of peak bone mass in the late second decade (Fig. 14-21)[190] is key to ensuring that the subsequent loss of bone mass with aging and estrogen deficiency does not lead to early osteoporosis. Estradiol, together with GH and insulin-like growth factor-1, act to double bone mass at the time of puberty,[191] beginning the process of attaining peak bone mass. Postpubertal estrogen deficiency (amenorrhea from various causes) substantially jeopardizes peak bone mass. Adequate nutrition and calcium intake are also key determinants. Although estrogen is of predominant importance for bone mass in both women and men, testosterone is important in stimulating periosteal apposition; as a result, cortical bone in men is larger and thicker.[192,193]

Estrogen receptors are present in osteoblasts,[194,195] osteoclasts,[196,197] and osteocystes.[198,199] Both ERα and ERβ are present in cortical bone, but ERβ predominates in cancellous or trabecular bone.[200] However, the more important actions of estradiol are believed to be mediated by means of ERα.

Estrogens suppress bone turnover and maintain a certain rate of bone formation.[201] Bone is remodeled in functional units, called *bone multicenter units* (BMUs), where resorption and formation should be in balance.[202] Multiple sites of bone go through this turnover process over time. Estrogen decreases osteoclasts by increasing apoptosis and thus reduces their lifespan.[203] The effect on the osteoblast is less consistent, but E_2 antagonizes glucocorticoid-induced osteoblast apoptosis.[201,204] Estrogen deficiency increases the activities of remodeling units, prolongs resorption, and shortens the phase of bone formation[201]; it also increases osteoclast recruitment in BMUs—thus, resorption outstrips formation.

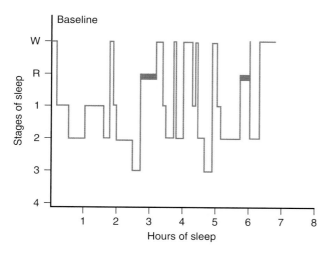

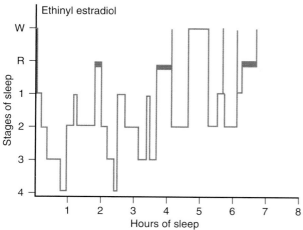

Figure 14-19. Sleepgrams measured in symptomatic patient before and after 30 days' administration of ethinyl estradiol, 50 μg four times daily. (Adapted from Erlik Y, Tataryn IV, Meldrum DR, et al. Association of waking episodes with menopausal hot flushes. JAMA 245:1741-1744, 1981.)

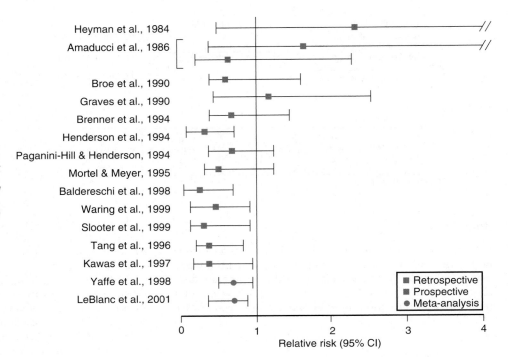

Figure 14-20. Estrogen/hormone replacement therapy use and Alzheimer's disease risk. *(Adapted from LeBlanc ES, Janoowsky J, Chan BK, Nelson HD. Hormone replacement therapy and cognition: systematic review and meta-analysis. JAMA 285:1489-1499, 2001.)*

The molecular mechanisms of estrogen action on bone involve the inhibition of production of proinflammatory cytokines including interleukin 1, interleukin 6, tumor necrosis factor-α, colony-stimulating factor-1, macrophage colony-stimulating factor, and prostaglandin E_2, which lead to increased resorption.[201-203] Estradiol also up-regulates TGF-β in bone,[204] which inhibits bone resorption. Receptor-activation of NF-kB ligand (RANKL) is responsible for osteoclast differentiation and action.[205,206] A scheme for how all these factors interact has been proposed by Riggs (Fig. 14-22).[207]

In women, Riggs has suggested that bone loss occurs in two phases. With estrogen levels declining at the onset of menopause—leading to an accelerated phase of bone loss—predominantly cancellous bone loss occurs. Here 20% to 30% of cancellous bone and 5% to 10% of cortical bone can be lost in a span of 4 to 8 years.[208] Thereafter a slower phase of loss (1% to 2% per year) ensues when more cortical bone is lost. This phase is thought to be induced primarily by secondary hyperparathyroidism.[209]

The first phase is also accentuated by the decreased influence of stretching or mechanical factors, which generally promote bone homeostasis, as a result of estrogen deficiency.[210-212]

Genetic influences on bone mass are more important for attainment of peak bone mass (heritable component, 50% to 70%) than for bone loss. Polymorphisms of the vitamin D receptor gene, TGF-β gene, and the Spl-binding site in the collagen type 1 AI gene have all been implicated[213] as being important for bone mass. Although testosterone is important for bone formation and stimulation of bone mass, even in men estrogen action is of paramount importance.[214-216] Bone mass was shown to increase in aromatase-deficient men upon estrogen administration.[217]

Bone mass can be detected by a variety of radiographic methods (Table 14-2).[218] *Dual energy x-ray absorptiometry (DEXA) scans* have become the standard of care for detection of osteopenia and osteoporosis. By convention, the *T score* is used to reflect the number of standard deviations of bone loss from the peak bone mass of a young adult. Osteopenia is defined by a T score of −1 to −2.5 standard deviations; osteoporosis is defined as greater than 2.5 standard deviations. Because bone mass does not completely reflect bone strength, which is really what matters in terms of fracture risk, several approaches have been made to assess bone strength. An assessment of biochemical bone turnover (discussed later) as well as bone mass is deemed important. One newer approach is to assess bone microarchitecture, a so-called virtual bone biopsy, by using high-resolution peripheral quantitative computed tomography (pQCT) (Fig. 14-23).[219] This technique is only available as a research tool at present.

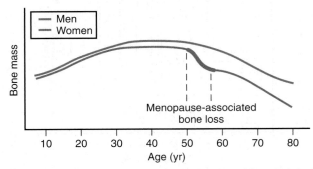

Figure 14-21. Bone mass by age and sex. *(Adapted from Finkelstein JS. In Cecil RL, Goldman L, Bennett JC [eds]. Cecil Textbook of Medicine, 21st ed. Philadelphia, Saunders, 1999, pp 1366-1373; and Riggs BL, Melton LJ III. Involutional osteoporosis. N Engl J Med 314:1676-1686, 1986.)*

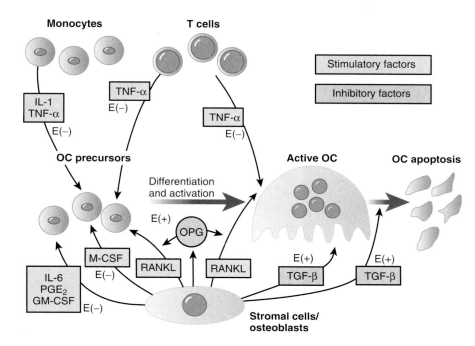

Figure 14-22. *Model for mediation of effects of estrogen (E) on osteoclast formation and function by cytokines in bone marrow microenvironment. Stimulatory factors are shown in orange and inhibitory factors are shown in blue. Positive (+) and negative (–) effects of E on these regulatory factors are shown in red. The model assumes that regulation is accomplished by multiple cytokines working together in concert. (Adapted from Riggs BL. The mechanisms of estrogen regulation of bone resorption. J Clin Invest 106:1203-1204, 2000.)*

Various biochemical assays are also available to assess bone resorption and formation in both blood and urine (Table 14-3).[220] At present, serum markers appear to be most useful for assessing changes with antiresorptive therapy.

There are now many agents that can prevent osteoporosis. The use of estrogen will depend on whether or not there are other indications for estrogen treatment and whether there are contraindications. Estrogen has been shown to reduce the risk of osteoporosis as well as to reduce osteoporotic fractures. In the Women's Health Initiative, hip fractures as well as all fractures were reduced with conjugated equine estrogens (CEE)/medroxyprogesterone acetate (MPA) and CEE alone, and this occurred in a nonosteoporotic population. A dose equivalent to 0.625 mg of CEE was once thought to prevent osteoporosis, but we now know that lower doses (0.3 mg of CEE or its equivalent) in combination with progestogens are able to prevent bone loss[221,222] although there are no data on fractures.

Whether or not the addition of progestogens, by stimulating bone formation, increases bone mass over that of estrogen alone is unclear. The androgenic activity of certain progestogens, such as northindrone acetate, also has been suggested to play a role.[223]

Selective estrogen receptor modulators (SERMs) such as raloxifene, droloxifene, and tamoxifen have all been shown to decrease bone resorption. Raloxifene has been shown to decrease vertebral fractures in a large prospective trial.[224] Tibolone has also been shown to be an effective treatment for osteoporosis. Tibolone (not yet marketed in the United States) has SERM-like properties, but it is not specifically a SERM because it has mixed estrogenic, antiestrogenic, androgenic, and progestogenic properties. The drug does not cause uterine or breast cell proliferation but is beneficial for vasomotor symptoms. It prevents osteoporosis and has been shown to be beneficial in treatment of osteoporosis as well.[225,226]

TABLE 14-2				
Techniques for the Detection of Osteopenia				
Technique	*Anatomic Site of Interest*	*Precision in Vivo (%)*	*Examination and Analysis Time (min)*	*Estimated Effective Dose Equivalent (μSv)*
Conventional radiography	Spine, hip	NA	<5	2000
Radiogrammetry	Hand	1-3	5-10	<1
Radiographic absorptiometry	Hand	1-2	5-10	<1
Single x-ray absorptiometry	Forearm, heel	1-2	5-10	<1
Dual x-ray absorptiometry	Spine, hip, forearm, total body	1-3	5-20	1-10
Quantitative computed tomography	Spine, forearm, hip	2-4	10-15	50-100
Quantitative ultrasound	Heel, hand, lower leg	1-3	5-10	None

NA, not applicable.
Adapted from van Kuijk C, Genant HK: Detection of osteopenia. *In* Lobo RA (ed). Treatment of the Postmenopausal Woman: Basic and Clinical Aspects, 2nd ed. Philadelphia, Lippincott Williams & Wilkins, 1999, pp 287-292.

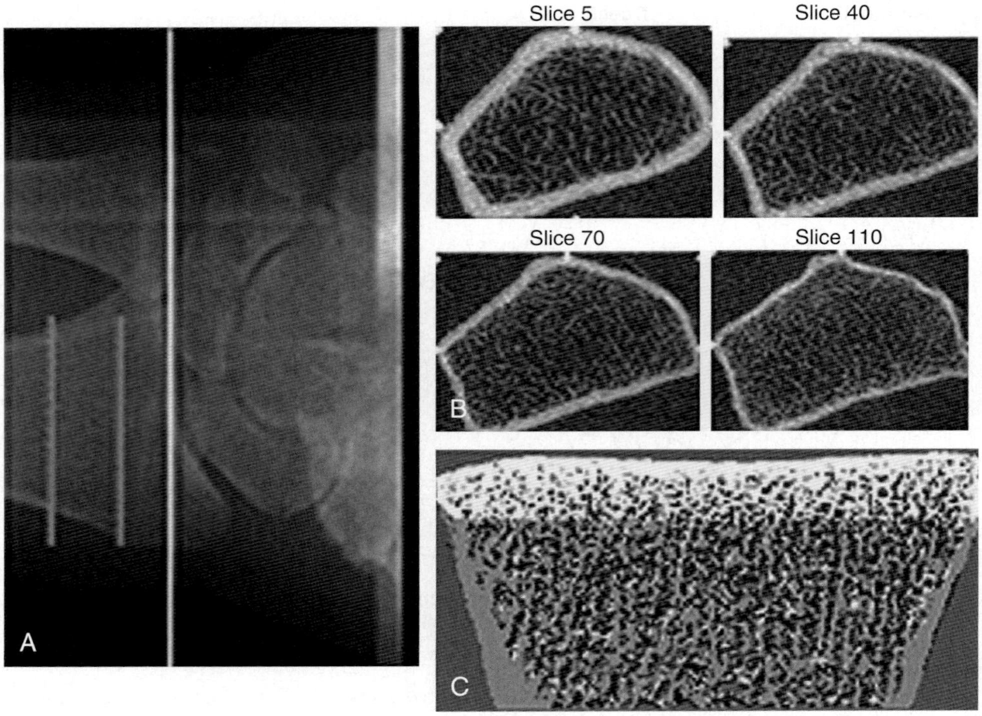

Figure 14-23. High-resolution peripheral quantitative computed tomography (pQCT). *A,* Radiograph of distal radius; lines indicate the section analyzed. *B,* Representative cross-sectional images from computed tomography slices. *C,* Representative three-dimensional image. (Adapted from Khosla S, Riggs BL, Atkinson EJ, et al. Effects of sex and age on bone microstructure at the ultradistal radius: a population-based noninvasive in vivo assessment. J Bone Miner Res; 21:124-131, 2006.)

TABLE 14-3	
Bone Turnover Markers	
Marker	*Specimen*
Bone Resorption Markers	
Cross-linked N-telopeptide of type 1 collagen (NTX)	Urine, serum
Cross-linked C-telopeptide of type 1 collagen (CTX)	Urine ($\alpha\alpha$ and $\beta\beta$ forms) Serum ($\beta\beta$ form)
MMP-generated telopeptide of type 1 collagen (ICTP or CTX-MMP)	Serum
Deoxypyridinoline, free and peptide bound (fDPD, DPD)	Urine, serum
Pyridinoline, free and peptide bound (fPYD, PYD)	Urine, serum
Hydroxyproline (OHP)	Urine
Glycosyl hydroxylysine (GylHyl)	Urine, serum
Helical peptide (HelP)	Urine
Tartrate-resistant acid phospharase 5b Isoform specific for osteoclasts (TRACP 5b)	Serum, plasma
Cathepsin K (Cath K)	Urine, serum
Osteocalcin fragments (uOC)	Urine
Bone Formation Markers	
Osteocalcin (OC)	Serum
Procollagen type 1 C-terminal propeptide (PICP)	Serum
Procollagen type 1 N-terminal propeptide (PINP)	Serum
Bone-specific alkaline phosphatase (bone ALP)	Serum

Bisphosphonates have been shown to have a significant effect on the prevention and treatment of osteoporosis. With this class of agents (etidronate, alendronate, residronate, and ibandronate), incorporation of the bisphosphonate with hydroxyapatite in bone increases bone mass. The skeletal half-life of bisphosphonates in bone can be as long as 10 years.[227] Most data have been derived with alendronate, which, at a dosage of 5 mg daily (35 mg weekly), prevents bone loss; at 10 mg daily (70 mg weekly), alendronate is an effective treatment for osteoporosis, with evidence available that this treatment reduces vertebral and hip fractures.[228] Ibandronate is available as a monthly pill and by injection. It has primary efficiency for vertebral fracture protection. Zoledronic acid, 5 mg, is expected to be available as an annual parenteral therapy.

Calcitonin, 50 IU subcutaneous injections daily, or 200 IU intranasally has been shown to inhibit bone resorption. Vertebral fractures have been shown to decrease[229,230] with calcitonin therapy. Long-term effects, however have not been established.

Fluoride has been used for women with osteoporosis because it increases bone density.[231] Currently, a lower dose (50 µg daily) of slow-release sodium fluoride does not seem to cause adverse effects (gastritis) and has efficacy in preventing vertebral fractures.[232,233]

Intermittent parathyroid hormone (PTH) offers promise as an agent to increase bone mass in women with osteoporosis. In a randomized trial lasting 3 years, average bone density increased in the hip and spine with fewer fractures observed.[234] This therapy is now available in the United States.

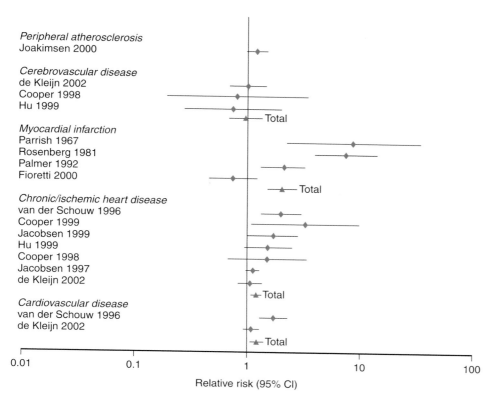

Peripheral atherosclerosis
Joakimsen 2000

Cerebrovascular disease
de Kleijn 2002
Cooper 1998
Hu 1999
— Total

Myocardial infarction
Parrish 1967
Rosenberg 1981
Palmer 1992
Fioretti 2000
— Total

Chronic/ischemic heart disease
van der Schouw 1996
Cooper 1999
Jacobsen 1999
Hu 1999
Cooper 1998
Jacobsen 1997
de Kleijn 2002
Total

Cardiovascular disease
van der Schouw 1996
de Kleijn 2002
Total

0.01   0.1   1   10   100

Relative risk (95% CI)

Figure 14-24. Effect of "early" menopause on types of cardiovascular disease. (From Atsma F, Bartelink ML, Grobbee DE, et al. Postmenopausal status and early menopause as independent risk factors for cardiovascular disease: a meta-analysis. Menopause 13[2]: 265-279, 2006 [review]. See reference 330 for data sources.)

Adjunctive measures for prevention of osteoporosis are calcium, vitamin D, and exercise. Calcium with vitamin D treatment has been shown to increase bone only in older individuals.[235] These modalities alone are not thought to be effective for the treatment of osteoporosis. A woman's total intake of elemental calcium should be 1500 mg daily if no agents are being used to inhibit resorption, and 400 to 800 IU of vitamin D should also be ingested. Exercise has been shown to be beneficial for building muscle and bone mass and for reducing risk of falls.[236,237] The reader should know that the most up to date guidelines regarding management of osteoporosis were published by the National Osteoporosis Foundation in February 2008 (www.nof.org). Also, WHO has produced guidelines for assessing an individual's risk of osteoporosis based on history, anthropometry, and bone mineral density. This new paradigm, called Fracture Risk Assessment Tool, may be obtained at www.shef.ac.uk/FRAX.

Cardiovascular Effects

Clearly, after menopause, the risk of cardiovascular disease in women is increased. Data from the Framingham study[238] have shown that the incidence is three times lower in women before menopause than in men (3.1 per 1000 per year in women aged 45 to 49). The incidence is approximately equal in men and women aged 75 to 79 (53 and 50.4 per 1000 per year, respectively). This trend also pertains to gender differences in mortality rate due to cardiovascular disease. Coronary artery disease is the leading cause of death in women, and the lifetime risk of death is 31% in postmenopausal women versus a 3% risk of dying of breast cancer.[239]

Although cardiovascular disease becomes more prevalent only in the later years following a natural menopause, premature cessation of ovarian function (before the average age of menopause) constitutes a significant risk. Premature menopause, occurring before age 35, has been shown to increase the risk of myocardial infarction two- to threefold, and oophorectomy before age 35 increases the risk severalfold.[240]

An analysis of several studies on this issue has been conducted and reviewed[241] with the data depicted in Figures 14-1 and 14-24. It has been suggested that total mortality rate is increased if bilateral oophorectomy occurs even after the natural menopause, until around age 60. This change in total mortality rate is due to an excess in coronary disease, suggesting a protective effect of the ovary even beyond the normal age of menopause.[242]

When the possible reasons for the increase in cardiovascular disease are examined, the most prevalent finding is that of the accelerated rise in total cholesterol in postmenopausal women. The changes of weight, blood pressure, and blood glucose with aging, while important, are not thought to be as important as the rate of rise in total cholesterol, which is substantially different in women versus men. This increase in total cholesterol is explained by increases in levels of low-density lipoprotein cholesterol (LDL-C). The oxidation of LDL-C is also enhanced, as are levels of very low density lipoproteins and lipoprotein a. HDL-C levels trend downward with time, but these changes are small and inconsistent relative to the increases in LDL-C.[243]

Coagulation balance is not substantially altered as counterbalancing changes occurs. Some procoagulation factors increase (factor VII, fibrinogen, and plasminogen activator inhibitor, PA1-1), but so do counterbalancing

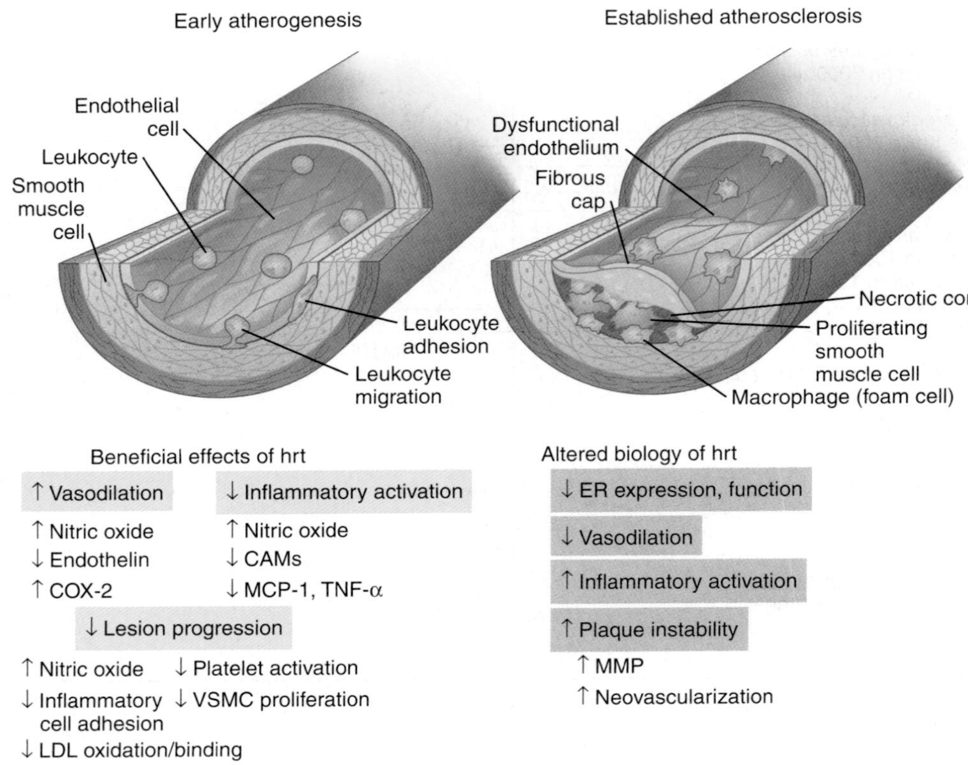

Early atherogenesis

Established atherosclerosis

Figure 14-25. Early and esterified atherosclerosis with aging and the beneficial and negative effects of estrogen during these stages. ER, estrogen receptor; MMP, matrix metalloproteinase; TNF, tumor necrosis factor. (From Mendelsohn ME, Karas RH. Molecular and cellular basis of cardiovascular gender differences. Science 308[5728]:1583-1587, 2005 [review].)

Beneficial effects of hrt

↑ Vasodilation   ↓ Inflammatory activation

↑ Nitric oxide   ↑ Nitric oxide
↓ Endothelin   ↓ CAMs
↑ COX-2   ↓ MCP-1, TNF-α

↓ Lesion progression

↑ Nitric oxide   ↓ Platelet activation
↓ Inflammatory   ↓ VSMC proliferation
  cell adhesion
↓ LDL oxidation/binding

Altered biology of hrt

↓ ER expression, function

↓ Vasodilation

↑ Inflammatory activation

↑ Plaque instability

↑ MMP
↑ Neovascularization

factors such as antithrombin III, plasminogen, protein C, and protein S.[244] Blood flow in all vascular beds decreases after menopause; prostacyclin production decreases, endothelin levels increase, and vasomotor responses to acetylcholine are constrictive, reflecting reduced nitric oxide synthetase activity. With estrogen, all these parameters (generally) improve and coronary arterial responses to acetylcholine are dilatory with a commensurate increase in blood flow.[245-252]

Circulating plasma nitrites and nitrates have also been shown to increase with estrogen, and angiotensin-converting enzyme levels tend to decrease. Estrogen and progesterone receptors have been found in vascular tissues, including coronary arteries (predominantly ERβ). In addition, there are membrane effects mediated by estrogen—which may or may not relate to either ERα or ERβ.[253,254]

Overall, the direct vascular effects of estrogen are viewed to be as important as, or more important than, the changes in lipid and lipoproteins after menopause. Although replacing estrogen has been thought to be beneficial for the mechanisms previously cited, these beneficial arterial effects may only be seen in younger (stage +1) postmenopausal women. Women with significant atherosclerosis or risk factors such as those studied in a secondary prevention trial do not respond in a beneficial manner[255-260] (Fig. 14-25). Some of this lack of effect may be accounted for by increased methylation of the promoter region of ERα, which occurs with atherosclerosis and aging.[261]

Another recent theory proposed to explain differences in the effects of estrogen when given early rather than later is the interfering effect of endogenous 27-hydroxycholesterol. This endogenous metabolite of cholesterol increases with advancing levels of cholesterol and competes for binding with E_2 at the ER in the endothelium. Thus, when cholesterol is elevated, high levels of 27-HC may prevent estrogen action[262] (Fig. 14-26).

In normal, nonobese postmenopausal women, carbohydrate tolerance also decreases as a result of an increase in insulin resistance. This, too, may be partially reversed by estrogen.[263] Biophysical and neurohormonal responses to stress (stress reactivity) are exaggerated in postmenopausal women compared with premenopausal women, and this heightened reactivity is blunted by estrogen.[264] Whether or not these changes influence cardiovascular risk with estrogen deficiency is not known, but clearly estrogen treatment returns many parameters into the range of premenopausal women in early postmenopausal women.

These consistently strong basic science and clinical data for the protective effects of estrogen on the cardiovascular system, together with strong epidemiologic evidence for a protective effect of estrogen (Fig. 14-27),[265] led to the belief that estrogen should be prescribed to prevent cardiovascular disease in women. However, randomized controlled trials (RCTs) have refuted this notion in women with established disease as noted previously. Results from several randomized trials in women,[255-257] have found there to be more coronary events in older women given estrogen for the first time.[266]

This trend toward increased cardiovascular events in women with diseased coronary arteries ("early harm") occurs within the first 1 to 2 years.[267,268] The Women's Health Initiative (WHI) trial, which compared CEE/MPA with placebo, came to similar conclusions[269] (Table 14-4). This trial was considered to be a primary prevention trial

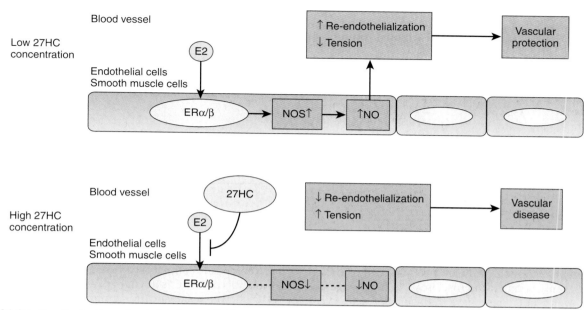

Figure 14-26. *Hypothesis of how elevated cholesterol (27-hydroxycholesterol, 27HC) can influence the effect of estradiol (E₂). ER, estrogen receptor; NO, nitric oxide; NOS, nitric oxide synthase. (From Umetani M, Domoto H, Gormley AK, et al. 27-Hydroxycholesterol as an endogenous SERM that inhibits the cardiovascular effects of estrogen. Nat Med 13[10]:1185-1192, 2007.)*

that evaluated younger women without cardiovascular risk factors; the higher frequency of cardiovascular events was reported in an older cohort of women (mean age 63). These women did not have vasomotor symptoms and had more risk factors than the healthy women studied in observational cohorts.

The protective effect of estrogen demonstrated in the Nurses' Health Study (see Fig. 14-27)[265] occurred predominantly in young healthy symptomatic women. Table 14-5 compares the demographics of the participants of WHI and the Nurses' Health Study. Trials carried out in the monkey model have shown that there is a 50% to 70% protective effect against coronary atherosclerosis when estrogen is begun at the time of oophorectomy, with or without an atherogenic diet; delaying the initiation of hormonal therapy for even 2 years (in the monkey) prevents this protective effect (Fig. 14-28).[270-274]

No clear explanation exists for what the observed "early harm" may be due to, but these effects were not observed in those women receiving statins concurrently.[275] This finding suggests that hormone replacement therapy (HRT) (in the doses used) may lead to plaque destabilization and thrombosis in some women with coronary disease. The molecular mechanisms for this may be due to estrogen up-regulating matrix metalloproteinase-9 (MMP-9) within the mural area of the plaque; the resultant disruption of the gelatinous covering then leads to thrombosis. This process is inhibited by statins. In women who had been receiving estrogen for a prolonged time, mortality rate was decreased in those who sustained a myocardial infarction.[276] No increase in cardiovascular events has been found in young healthy symptomatic women during the first 2 years of various ERT/HRT regimens in clinical trials.[277]

It is now well established that the late treatment of postmenopausal women with standard doses of estrogen may be harmful and affords no coronary protection. This finding pertains to various trials with end-points of coronary events, or angiographically determined disease,

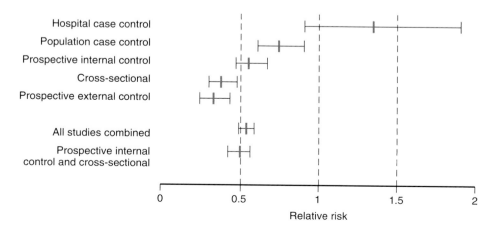

Figure 14-27. *Estrogen replacement therapy and coronary heart disease. Relationship between relative risk and study type. (Adapted from Stampfer MJ, Colditz GA. Estrogen replacement therapy and coronary heart disease: a quantitative assessment of the epidemiologic evidence. Prev Med 20:47-63, 1991.)*

TABLE 14-4

Women's Health Initiative (WHI) Results: Summary of Main Outcomes

Outcome	Relative Risk versus Placebo n (95% CI)	Increased Absolute Risk per 10,000 Women-Years	Increased Absolute Benefit per 10,000 Women-Years
Coronary heart disease	1.29 (1.02-1.63)	+7	—
Invasive breast cancer	1.26 (1.00-1.63)	+8	—
Stroke	1.41 (1.07-1.85)	+8	—
Pulmonary embolism	1.41 (1.39-3.25)	+8	—
Colorectal cancer	0.63 (0.43-0.92)	—	–8
Hip fracture	0.66 (0.45-0.98)	—	–5
Global index	1.15 (1.03-1.28)	—	—

as noted above, and does not appear to be modified by the hormonal regimen or route of administration. This is also true whether or not the woman has sustained a known coronary event. Because atherosclerosis is highly age-dependent, even women who have not had a coronary event may have diseased arteries (Fig. 14-29). Also, as shown in Figure 14-28, well over 70% of the women studied in WHI would have been expected to have atherosclerotic vessels.

In concert with the view that estrogen given to early (and younger) postmenopausal women may have different effects, data have been analyzed in the 50- to 59-year-old age group in WHI, and in those less than 10 years from menopause. The definitions of menopause in WHI were not precise, and more women in the 50- to 59-year-old age group were over 55 years. The data are in strong contrast to the results of the entire group (two thirds over 60 years). In the estrogen-only arm of WHI (hysterectomized women)

TABLE 14-5

Baseline Characteristics: Nurses' Health Study (NHS) Compared with Women's Health Initiative (WHI)

Characteristic	NHS	WHI
Mean age or age range at enrollment (years)	30-55	63
Smokers (past and current)	55%	49.9%
BMI (mean)	25.1 kg/m²	28.5 kg/m²*
Aspirin users	43.9%	19.1%
HT regimen	Unopposed or sequential	Continuous-combined
Menopausal symptoms (flushing)	Predominant	Uncommon

*34.1% had BMI ≥30 kg/m2.
BMI, body mass index; HT, hormone therapy.
Data from Colditz GA, Stampher MJ, Willet WC, et al. A prospective study of parental history of myocardial infarction and coronary heart disease in women. Am J Epidemiol 123:48-58, 1986; Grodstein F, Manson JE, Colditz GA, et al. A prospective, observational study of postmenopausal hormone therapy and primary prevention of cardiovascular disease. Ann Intern Med 133:933-941, 2001; Grodstein F, Stampfer MJ, Manson JE, et al. Postmenopausal estrogen and progestin use and the risk of cardiovascular disease. N Engl J Med 335:453-461, 1996; and Writing Group for the WHI Investigators. Risks and benefits of estrogen plus progestin in healthy postmenopausal women. JAMA 288:321-333, 2002.

receiving CEE 0.625 mg, the 50- to 59-year age group had reduced coronary event scores of borderline significance and a composite coronary score of statistical significance.[278] An analysis of 20 RCTs in younger women (which included WHI) showed a statistically significant benefit in a reduction of coronary events[279] and mortality rate.[280] Younger women in WHI using estrogen only also had significantly reduced coronary calcium.[281] Although the data are not as strong for the use of combined HT (CEE/MPA) in WHI, it is difficult to conclude that MPA attenuates the benefit or may add harm in that the two trials in WHI were different and studied different populations of women. The WHI conducted an observational trial in parallel with the RCTs. The results of the observational trials are more in keeping with the older observational data suggesting coronary protection and with no adverse effects on stroke.[282,283] These data could not be reconciled with the RCT data but reinforce the notion that early initiation of therapy and length of treatment influence these findings.[283]

The overall results of WHI for the 50- 59-year-old age group in the two trials (CEE and CEE/MPA) were recently reanalyzed[284] (Table 14-6). These data are more useful to assess in that this is the relevant population of symptomatic postmenopausal women who may be candidates for HT. For CHD, in the 50- to 59-year age group, the hazards ratio (HR) was 0.93 (0.65 to 1.33) for women receiving CEE and MPA; and was 0.63 (0.36 to 1.09) for those receiving CEE alone. For the entire group total mortality rate was significantly decreased in this age group, to 0.7 (0.51 to 0.96). These findings and point estimates are very much in line with the older observational data.

In the original papers of WHI overall stroke was significantly increased in women receiving CEE/MPA or CEE. However, this was not the case in younger women.[284] Age, obviously, and particularly hypertension, influences the risk of stroke in postmenopausal women; and this is significantly influenced by the dose of estrogen.[285] It is ischemic stroke, and not hemorrhagic stroke, which is influenced by the use of HT. Overall, it has to be acknowledged that there is a small "rare" increase in ischemic stroke, in women of the ages studied in WHI receiving oral estrogen in standard doses (8 more strokes/10,000 woman-years). This risk is lower or nonsignificant in younger normotensive women, and the overall risk is reduced with the use of lower doses.[285]

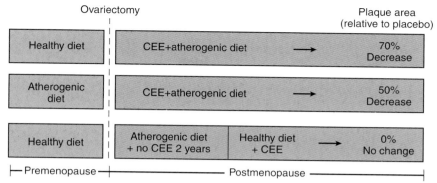

Figure 14-28. Importance of timing of intervention on the effect of estrogens on atherogenesis in nonhuman primates. CEE, conjugated equine estrogens. (Adapted from Clarkson TB, Anthony MS, Jerome CP. Lack of effect of raloxifene on coronary artery atherosclerosis of postmenopausal monkeys. J Clin Endocrinol Metab 83:721-726, 1998; Adams MR, Register TC, Golden DL, et al. Medroxyprogesterone acetate antagonizes inhibitory effects of conjugated equine estrogens on coronary artery atherosclerosis. Arterioscler Thromb Vasc Biol 17:217-221, 1997; Clarkson TB, Anthony MS, Morgan TM. Inhibition of postmenopausal atherosclerosis progression: a comparison of the effects of conjugated equine estrogens and soy phytoestrogens. J Clin Endocrinol Metab 86:41-47, 2001; and Williams JK, Anthony MS, Honore EK, et al. Regression of atherosclerosis in female monkeys. Arterioscler Thromb Vasc Biol 15:827-836, 1995.)

It has been acknowledged for some time that oral estrogen increases the risk of venous thrombosis/thromboembolism (VTE) in postmenopausal women. This risk tends to occur early (within the first 1 to 2 years of therapy) and is markedly increased if there is an underlying thrombophilia (about a 15-fold increased risk).[286] However, in the absence of a family history or a prior thrombotic event, it is not standard practice to screen for factor V Leiden mutation or other abnormalities. Although the relative risk of thrombosis with oral estrogen is two- to threefold, the prevalence of this is low, particularly in a younger population. For example, the risk of pulmonary embolism may increase from 20 to 40 cases per 100,000 women-years with HT, but this is less than the general risk of 60 per 100,000 women-years observed in pregnancy. The overall relative risk of VTE reported in WHI was in the range of two- to threefold (as noted earlier), but did not achieve statistical significance in the hysterectomized group using estrogen alone. Although this was a more obese group who could have been considered at very high risk, two other possibilities exist. The first is that approximately 50% of women had used estrogen in the past, and it is possible that this population of exposed women had received therapy beyond the first year or two when VTE usually occurs in susceptible women, and were not susceptible. Second, there is a possibility that the progestogen addition with CEE with MPA

increases the risk further. In a larger French observational study, the type of progestogen was considered to confer an additional risk of VTE.[287] Further data from this cohort of women in the ESTHER study showed no increase in VTE risk with transdermal estrogen.[287,288]

As noted earlier, blood pressure increases after menopause increase CVD risk. Apart from an idiosyncratic hypertensive response to oral estrogen in some women, the overall effect of estrogen on blood pressure is neutral, including women who are already hypertensive. There are studies showing some small increase, others showing no changes, and others showing a decrease even in hypertensive women.[289] Uncontrolled hypertension in postmenopausal women constitutes a major concern for stroke, and this may be aggravated in some women with the use of HT.

Breast Cancer

Because of the enormous importance of this topic, breast cancer and its relationship to HT use will be reviewed separately as well as in the context of the risk-benefit assessment discussed later. Listed in Table 14-7 are the approximate rates of breast cancer by decade of life; clearly, age is a major determinant of risk. More baseline risk information may be found in Chapter 27. However, postmenopausal breast cancer, fortunately, is not as lethal as

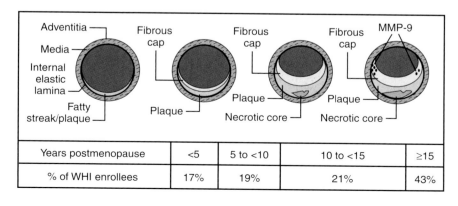

Figure 14-29. Relationship between number of years since menopause to progression of atherosclerosis in Women's Health Initiative (WHI) enrollees. MMP-9, matrix metalloproteinase-9. (Adapted from Clarkson TB. The new conundrum: Do estrogens have any cardiovascular benefits? Int J Fertil 47:61-68, 2002.)

Years postmenopause	<5	5 to <10	10 to <15	≥15
% of WHI enrollees	17%	19%	21%	43%

TABLE 14-6

Cardiovascular and Global Index Events by Age at Baseline

	Age Group at Randomization									
	50-59 yr			60-69 yr			70-79 yr			
	No. of Cases			No. of Cases			No. of Cases			
Event	Hormone Therapy (n = 4476)	Placebo (n = 4356)	HR (95% CI)*	Hormone Therapy (n = 6240)	Placebo (n = 6122)	HR (95% CI)*	Hormone Therapy (n = 3100)	Placebo (n = 3053)	HR (95% CI)*	P Value for Trend†
CHD‡	59	61	0.93 (0.65-1.33)	174	178	0.98 (0.79-1.21)	163	131	1.26 (1.00-1.59)	0.16
Stroke	44	37	1.13 (0.73-1.76)	156	102	1.50 (1.17-1.92)	127	100	1.21 (0.93-1.58)	0.97
Total mortality	69	95	0.70 (0.51-0.96)	240	225	1.05 (0.87-1.26)	237	208	1.14 (0.94-1.37)	0.06
Global index§	278	278	0.96 (0.81-1.14)	717	661	1.08 (0.97-1.20)	606	528	1.14 (1.02-1.29)	0.09
	CEE Trial									
Event	CEE (n = 1637)	Placebo (n = 1673)	HR (95% CI)*	CEE (n = 2387)	Placebo (n = 2465)	HR (95% CI)*	CEE (n = 1286)	Placebo (n = 1291)	HR (95% CI)*	P Value for Trend†
CHD‡	21	34	0.63 (0.36-1.09)	96	106	0.94 (071-1.24)	84	77	1.13 (0.82-1.54)	0.12
Stroke	18	21	0.89 (0.47-1.69)	84	54	1.62 (1.15-2.27)	66	52	1.21 (0.84-1.75)	0.62
Total mortality	34	48	0.71 (0.46-1.11)	129	131	1.02 (0.80-1.30)	134	113	1.20 (0.93-1.55)	0.18
Global index§	114	140	0.82 (0.64-1.05)	333	342	1.01 (0.86-1.17)	300	262	1.16 (0.98-1.37)	0.01

Event	CEE+MPA (n = 2839)	Placebo (n = 2683)	HR (95% CI)*	CEE+MPA (n = 3853)	Placebo (n = 3657)	HR (95% CI)*	CEE+MPA (n = 1814)	Placebo (n = 1762)	HR (95% CI)*	P Value for Trend†
					CEE + MPA Trial					
CHD‡	38	27	1.29 (0.79-2.12)	78	72	1.03 (0.74-1.43)	79	54	1.48 (1.04-2.11)	0.70
Stroke	26	16	1.41 (0.75-2.65)	72	48	1.37 (0.95-1.97)	61	48	1.21 (0.82-1.78)	0.56
Total mortality	35	47	0.69 (0.44-1.07)	111	94	1.09 (0.83-1.44)	103	95	1.06 (0.80-1.41)	0.19
Global index§	164	138	1.10 (0.87-1.38)	384	319	1.15 (0.99-1.34)	306	266	1.13 (0.95-1.33)	0.96

*Cox regression models stratified according to prior cardiovascular disease and randomization status in the Dietary Modification Trial.
†Test for trend (interation) using age as continuous (linear) form of categorical coded values. Cox regression models stratified according to active versus placebo trial, including terms for age and the interaction between trials and age.
‡Defined as CHD death, nonfatal myocardial infarction, or definite silent myocardial infarction (Novacode 5.1 or 5.2).
§Defined as CHD, stroke, pulmonary embolism, breast cancer, colorectal cancer, endometrial cancer for CEE plus MPA trial only, hip fracture, or death from other causes.
CEE, conjugated equine strogens; CHD, coronary heart disease, CI, confidence interval; HR, hazard ratio; MPA, medroxyprogesterone acetate.
From Rossouw JE, Prentice RL, Manson JE, et al. Postmenopausal hormone therapy and cardiovascular disease by age and years since menopause. JAMA 297(13):1465-1477, 2007.

TABLE 14-7

Women Who Will Develop Breast Cancer: Risk According to Age

Decade of Life	Incidence
Third	1 of 250
Fourth	1 of 77
Fifth	1 of 42
Sixth	1 of 36
Seventh	1 of 34
Eighth	1 of 45

From Adapted from Lobo RA: Treatment of the postmenopausal woman: where we are today . *In* Lobo RA (ed). Treatment of the Postmenopausal Woman: Basic and Clinical Aspects, 2nd ed. Philadelphia, Lippincott Williams & Wilkins, 1999, pp 655-659.

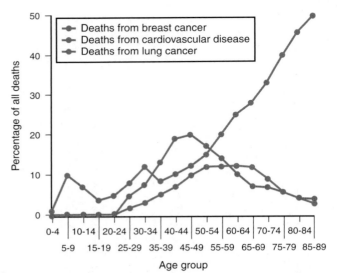

Figure 14-30. *Risks of breast cancer and lung cancer versus cardiovascular disease in various age categories. (Adapted from Phillips KA, Glendon G, Knight JA. Putting the risk of breast cancer in perspective. N Engl J Med 340:141-144, 1999.)*

lung cancer or CVD. In Figure 14-30 the age-specific mortality rate is depicted and shows that breast cancer mortality rate decreases after the initial age of menopause, while deaths from lung cancer are higher after menopause, and the rates of CVD mortality increase dramatically from this time onward. The effect of HT on breast cancer risk has been studied for at least 30 years, and only recently has there been a little more clarity on the issue.[290-293] Most of the data on breast cancer risk have been derived from case control and cohort observational studies. Because now we also have a few prospective RCTs, such as data from WHI (at least for the use of two specific regimens)[291,292] these will be presented separately as well.

In summary, RCTs show lower point estimates than observational data and little increased risk of estrogen alone.[292,293] With estrogen alone, the WHI showed reduced risk,[292] and others, including the Million Women's Study, showed some increased risk.[294] This latter study, although large, has been widely criticized on methodologic grounds. An update of the Nurses' Health Study (NHS) showed no increasing risk for up to 20 years in hysterectomied women using CEE 0.625 mg.[293] As shown in Table 14-8, the overall risk going out 15 to 20 years is principally

TABLE 14-8

Risk of Invasive Breast Cancer by Duration of ET Use Among All Postmenopausal Women Who Had Undergone Hysterectomy and Those With ER+/PR+ Cancers Only*

ET Use and Duration (yr)	All Postmenopausal Women Who Had Undergone Hysterectomy				ER+/PR+ Cancers Only			
	All		Screened Cohort[†]		All		Screened Cohort[†]	
	Cases	Risk	Cases	Risk	Cases	Risk	Cases	Risk
Never current	226	1.00	104	—	87	—	48	—
<5	99	0.96 (0.75-1.22)	59	1.06 (0.76-1.47)	38	1.00 (0.67-1.49)	26	1.04 (0.64-1.70)
5-9.9	145	0.90 (0.73-1.12)	95	0.91 (0.68-1.21)	70	1.19 (0.86-1.66)	50	1.08 (0.72-1.62)
10-14.9	190	1.06 (0.87-1.30)	141	1.11 (0.85-1.44)	85	1.27 (0.93-1.73)	77	1.29 (0.89-1.86)
15-19.9	129	1.18 (0.95-1.48)	95	1.19 (0.89-1.58)	61	1.48 (1.05-2.07)	58	1.50 (1.02-2.21)
≥20	145	1.42 (1.13-1.77)	127	1.58 (1.20-2.07)	69	1.73 (1.24-2.43)	74	1.83 (1.25-2.68)
P for trend for current use	—	<0.001	—	<0.001	—	<0.001	—	<0.001

*All cases are reported as number of cases; risks are reported as multivariate relative risk (95% CI), controlled for age (continuous), age at menopause (continuous), age at menarche (continuous), BMI (quintiles), history of benign breast disease (yes or no), family history of breast cancer in first-degree relative (yes or no), average daily alcohol consumption (0, 0.5-5, 5-10, 10-20, or ≥20 g/day), parity/age at first birth (nulliparous; 1-2 children and age at first birth ≤22 years; ≥3 children and age at first birth 23-25 years; ≥3 children and age at first birth >25 years).
†Screened cohort defined as those women starting in 1988 who reported either a screening mammogram or clinical breast examination in the previous 2 years.
All cases before 1988 are excluded.
BMI, body mass index; CI, confidence interval; ER+/PR+, positive for both estrogen and progesterone receptors; ET, unopposed estrogen therapy.
From Chen WY, Manson JE, Hankinson SE, et al. Unapposed estrogen therapy and the risk of invasive breast cancer. Arch Intern Med 166: 1027-1032, 2006.

in lean women. Because obesity itself is associated with an increased risk of breast cancer, an additional risk with HT has not been demonstrated.

In the CEE-alone trial of WHI, there was a borderline significant reduction in breast cancer risk, which was statistically significant for adherent women (Fig. 14-31) and for ductal cancers.[292] These data are reassuring for a negligible effect of estrogen alone on breast cancer risk, but should not be interpreted as estrogen being protective for breast cancer.

There seem to be consistent findings of increased risk with estrogen and progestogen regimens after 5 years of use. This risk estimate ranges from 1.2 to 1.7 and is related to dose, possibly the type of progestogen,[295] and duration of use. However, there are no clear data showing a difference between continuous combined and sequential regimens of progestogen therapy. In a less well-known publication from WHI, when adjustments were made for breast cancer risk factors, the overall risk for the 5 to 6 years of CEE/MPA use was not significant 1.20 (0.94 to 1.53).[291] Of great importance was the finding that in women who had never received HT (70% of the WHI population), the relative risk (RR) was 1.02 (0.77 to 1.36);[291] that is, the trend for an increased risk was accounted for by prior use and a longer cumulative exposure to estrogen and progestogen.[295] There also has been a suggestion that estrogen and progestogen therapy increases the relative frequency of lobular cancers which are normally more rare, but generally more well differentiated and less aggressive. This, however, has not been proved.

If estrogen and progestogen therapy over 5 years, with standard doses, increases the risk of breast cancer by 24% (RR 1.24), what does this translate into in absolute terms? If the background risk between the ages of 50 and 60 is 2.8% (2.8 women out of 100 will be expected to get breast cancer over this 10-year span), then the rate would increase to 3.4% (less than 1% increase). Clearly there is probably no increased risk in those who were never users for up to 5 years and particularly if lower than the standard dose is used. Also, recent observational data from France have suggested that progesterone and dydrogesterone are not associated with an increased risk, as opposed to synthetic progestogens. These data, however, remain to be confirmed.

This RR of 1.2 to 1.6 for 5 years of estrogen and progestogen use as discussed previously should also be compared to other experiences such as having a waist/hip ratio of greater than 0.8:3.3 (range, 1.1 to 10.4) or being an airline flight attendant with a ratio of 1.87 (1.15 to 2.23).

A recent report showing a downward trend in breast cancer rates in the United States suggested that this might be related to a reduction in hormone use after the WHI and other reports.[296] However, there are several other possible explanations as well, including a reduction in mammography use and other variables reviewed elsewhere. Of interest is that the reduction in breast cancer in the United States also occurred in older women (70s) as well (not users of hormones) and has not been reported in other countries, such as the United Kingdom, where HT use has dropped as well. A recent 3-year follow-up of WHI showed that the breast cancer risk also persisted (nonsignificantly) over this follow-up period.[297]

The Decision to Use Estrogen

Whether or not hormonal therapy should be considered is a very individual decision. The woman must take into account symptoms, risk factors, and individual preferences and needs. The predominant indication for estrogen is for symptoms (vasomotor and vulvovaginal). Alternatives should also be considered. If hormonal therapy is chosen, there should be flexibility in prescribing because there is no ideal regimen for every woman, and each woman has individual risks and needs.

RISK-BENEFIT ASSESSMENT

Several recent guidelines have endorsed the use of HT for control of symptoms (International Menopause Society,[298] North American Menopause Society,[299] Medscape,[300] and American Association of Clinical Endocrinologists[301]). These guidelines stress the relative safety in symptomatic women, and that lower doses should be used with individualization regarding the length of treatment. Whether osteoporosis prevention alone is a sufficient indication for HT is controversial, but this should be considered as well.

At present there is no indication for using HT for the prevention of CVD or Alzheimer's risk. Nevertheless, for both of these diseases there is the suggestion that early initiation of therapy (as was carried out in observational trials) may show protective effects.

Individualization of therapy is what is key in that there is no way to tally the risks and benefits of therapy in a global way. The "global index" used by WHI is an unvalidated instrument which gives equal weight to a number of parameters that are not expected to be equal in terms of risks for

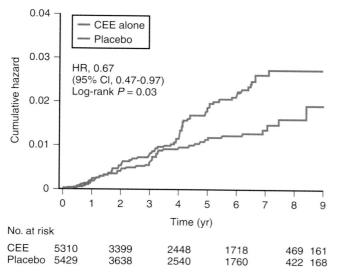

Figure 14-31. *Sensitivity analysis of invasive breast cancer in women receiving conjugated equine estrogens (CEE) alone compared to placebo. CI, confidence interval; HR, hazard ratio. (From Stefanick ML, Anderson GL, Margolis KL, et al. Effects of conjugated equine estrogens on breast cancer and mammography screening in postmenopausal women with hysterectomy. JAMA 295[14]:1647-1657, 2006.)*

an individual woman. Further, data obtained to generate the global index for the trials (+ or – a certain number of events) included findings which were not statistically significant, making numbers of absolute risk inapplicable, although they were applied as such to create the composite score.

CHANGES IN MORTALITY RATE WITH ESTROGEN USE

In several cohort studies,[302-304] an overall 40% reduction in all-cause mortality rate has been observed with long-term estrogen use. Two studies have shown that the benefit in mortality rate is related to the duration of use; one study has suggested that the effect is decreased beyond 10 years of use because of an increase in breast cancer mortality rate (only reported in this cohort and not in the others).[304] Most studies have shown either no change in breast cancer mortality rate with estrogen use, or a decrease in mortality rate. In the reanalysis of data from WHI, in the 50- to 59-year-old age group, total mortality rate in the two trials was reduced significantly by 30% (hazard ratio [HR] 0.7) (0.51 to 0.96), corroborating the findings of the earlier observational data.[284]

In these observational cohorts looking at all-cause mortality rate, the overall reduction was found to be attributable to a reduction in cardiovascular mortality rate, although there was a small effect in cancer mortality rate as well. It is important to note that the women in these observational (epidemiologic) trials received ET/estrogen-progestogen therapy (EPT) at the onset of menopause, and the women observed were healthier. In older women (10 or more years after menopause) who may have silent or established cardiovascular disease, there may not be a protective effect on mortality rate.

RISKS ASSOCIATED WITH ESTROGEN THERAPY

Among the risks that have been associated with estrogen are endometrial disease; breast cancer; side effects such as vaginal bleeding; somatic complaints; and idiosyncratic reactions, including hypertension. Cardiovascular events and thrombosis risk have been discussed earlier. All of the risks are, in part, dose-related, lending credence to the practice of using lower doses. Endometrial disease occurs with unopposed estrogen therapy in women who have a uterus. Although a woman's risk for endometrial cancer with unopposed estrogen use is twofold to eightfold higher than that for the general population, precursor lesions (primarily endometrial hyperplasia) signal the presence of an abnormality in most patients. Thus, the risk is far less for endometrial cancer than it is for varying degrees of hyperplasia.

One study showed that the risk of endometrial hyperplasia was 20% after 1 year of use of 0.625 mg of oral CEE.[305] In another study, the 3-year postmenopausal Estrogen/Progestin Interventions Trial,[306] this risk was approximately 40% at the end of 3 years. No cancers were reported in either of these two studies, and the addition of a progestin essentially eliminated the hyperplasia. Using a dose of 0.3 mg of CEE results in a risk in the range of 5%

to 10% after 2 to 3 years. With the same dose of esterified estrogens (which is less potent), no hyperplasia was found after 2 years.[221]

The risk for endometrial cancer is the same for a woman taking estrogen and progestin EPT as for the general population. The addition of a progestin merely eliminates the excess risk attributed to estrogen. However, there are a few studies published suggesting a reduced risk with continuous combined HT. Other endometrial cancers occurring in postmenopausal women are not thought to be hormonally related (see Chapter 9). Although the risk for endometrial cancer is increased substantially in estrogen users, the risk of death from this type of endometrial cancer does not increase proportionately.[307,308] Endometrial cancers associated with estrogen use are thought to be less aggressive than spontaneously occurring cancers, in part because tumors in women taking estrogen are more likely to be discovered and treated at an earlier stage, thus improving survival rates.

Several studies have also suggested an increased risk of ovarian cancer with long duration of use of ET/HT. However, the data are inconsistent and the purported risk is in the range of less than a twofold relative risk.[309,310] An analysis found no association, and there was no increase reported in the WHI studies.[311]

One of the concerns of women receiving estrogen is the return of menstrual bleeding. Somatic complaints such as breast tenderness and bloating may also occur with ET, but these can be alleviated by alterations in the dose and type of preparation. Such concerns should be discussed with the patient, and the choice of the regimen should remain flexible.

Idiosyncratic reactions like hypertension and allergic manifestations have been observed in users of estrogen, particularly oral estrogen. Hypertension with estrogen use, the cause of which is not entirely clear, occurs in about 5% of women using the oral route. Otherwise, estrogen usually causes no change in blood pressure; it may actually reduce blood pressure, a finding that has relevance for normotensive as well as hypertensive individuals. However, an increase in both diastolic and systolic blood pressure has been noted in susceptible individuals and is rapidly reversible with discontinuation of the regimen. A different form of estrogen may eliminate the problem, and alterations in the route of estrogen administration have also resulted in normal blood pressure responses in such individuals.

In unsusceptible individuals, ET does not increase procoagulant factors outside the normal range; for many years, ET was not considered to increase the risk of venous thrombosis—unlike oral contraceptive use. However, several recent observational studies and the results of HERS[255] and WHI[269] have suggested a twofold increase in venous thromboembolic phenomena with oral estrogen. This risk has not been definitively related to an unknown thrombophilia, but some women, based on an individual sensitivity, are clearly at increased risk for thrombosis. The observed events all tend to occur in the first 1 or 2 years of estrogen exposure. The increased risk does not increase mortality rate. As discussed earlier, it has been suggested that there is no increased risk with transdermal estrogen.

A meta-analysis estimated that the absolute increased risk for venous thromboembolic events is 15 per 100,000 women per year which is categorized as an uncommon finding.[312] Nevertheless, all patients must be informed of these findings. Women who have a family history of thrombosis or have had thrombotic events linked to oral contraceptives or any prior estrogen use should be counseled very carefully and monitored closely. A low-dose, nonoral form of estrogen would be a consideration for these patients; again, the need for choosing estrogen as a treatment should be clearly documented.

As noted previously, the risk of unstable angina and potentially myocardial infarction is increased within the first 2 years of initiating ET in older women with silent or established coronary disease. As stated earlier, there is evidence that concurrent statin use may decrease or eliminate this early risk.[275] Nevertheless, standard ET should not be initiated within 2 years of a coronary event, particularly not for the indication of preventing heart disease. It is generally not recommended to use HT in this setting.

APPROACH TO THERAPY

In developed countries, much of what women know about health care is gleaned from the mass media.[313] In general, the more sensational an item is, the more noteworthy. For example, breast cancer risk is a real and serious concern for all women, but the fear of breast cancer seems to drive *all* decision making, particularly regarding hormonal options.

American women believe that the leading cause of death in women is breast cancer and attribute only a small percentage of deaths to cardiovascular disease. In reality, the opposite is true. Statistics indicate that one in three women older than age 65 has some evidence of cardiovascular disease. Despite public perception, the overall incidence of breast cancer has remained constant in recent years. Nevertheless, what is not commonly appreciated by those health care professionals counseling patients is the age-associated relationship in the incidence of breast cancer.

The rationale for choosing estrogen at the onset of menopause for symptom control is expected to have a minimal effect on breast cancer incidence, particularly if the dose of estrogen is lowered and with a reduction in progestogen exposure in women with a uterus. Whether or not there is also some cardiovascular benefit in this setting cannot be determined at this time.

HORMONE REGIMENS

The various hormonal preparations available for treatment are listed in Box 14-2. Also included are the SERM raloxifene and other compounds like bisphosphonates, tibolone, and human parathyroid hormone (1-34). For the clinician and patient, the decision to start estrogen therapy need not involve a long-term commitment. For short-term treatment of symptoms, estrogen should be used at the lowest dose that can control hot flushes or can be administered via the vaginal route for symptoms of dryness or dyspareunia.

BOX 14-2

Hormonal Treatment Available for Postmenopausal Women

Estrogens
Oral
  Oral CEE, 0.3, 0.625, 0.9, 1.25, and 2.5 mg
  Piperazine estrone sulfate, equivalent of 0.625, 1.25, and 2.5 mg
  Esterified, 0.3, 0.625, 0.9, 1.25, and 2.5 mg
  Micronized estradiol, 0.5, 1, and 2 mg
Transdermal
  Estradiol patches, 0.025, 0.0375, 0.05, 0.75, and 0.10 mg/day
  Estradiol gel, 1.5 and 3 mg (not yet available)
Vaginal
  Cream, CEE (0.0625%), estradiol (0.01%)
  Estradiol ring, 2 mg; vaginal tablets, 25 μg
Parenteral
  Intramuscular injections should be avoided

Progestins
Oral
  Medroxyprogesterone acetate, 2.5, 5, and 10 mg
  Norethindrone acetate, 5 mg
  Micronized progesterone, 100 and 200 mg
Vaginal
  Micronized progesterone, 100 mg
  Progesterone gel, 4% and 8%

Combinations
Oral
  CEE + MPA (0.625 mg) + MPA (2.5 or 5 mg)
  CEE + MPA (0.45 mg) + MPA (1.5 mg) (not yet available)
  Micronized estradiol (1 mg) + norethindrone acetate (0.5 mg)
  Ethinyl estradiol 5 μg; norethindrone, 1 mg
Transdermal
  Patch, 0.05 mg estradiol with 140 μg or 250 μg norethindrone acetate

Androgens
Oral
  Esterified estrogen and methyltestosterone (0.625/1/25 mg and 1.25/2.5 mg)
Transdermal
  Patch, 150 μg/300 μg in development

Bisphosphonates
  Alendronate, 5 and 10 mg daily; 35 and 70 mg weekly
  Risedronate, 5 mg
  Etidronate, 200 mg (intermittent)

Selective Estrogen Receptor Modulators
  Raloxifene, 60 mg

Others for Osteoporosis
  Tibolone, 2.5 mg
  Human parathyroid hormone I-34

CEE, conjugated equine estrogens; MPA, medroxyprogesterone acetate.

TABLE 14-9

Mean Serum Estradiol (E$_2$) and Estrone (E$_1$)

Estrogen Dose (mg)	Level (pg/mL)	
	E$_2$	E$_1$
CEE (0.3)*	18	76
CEE (0.625)	39	153
CEE (1.25)	60	220
Micronized E$_2$ (1)	35	190
Micronized E$_2$ (2)	63	300
E$_1$ sulfate (0.625)	34	125
E$_1$ sulfate (1.25)	42	220

*Conjugated equine estrogen (CEE) contains biologically active estrogens other than E$_2$ and E$_1$.

Oral ET results in higher levels of E$_1$ than E$_2$; this is true for oral estradiol as well as estrone products. CEE is a mixture of at least 10 conjugated estrogens derived from equine pregnant urine. Estrone sulfate is the major component, but the biologic activities of equilin, 17β-dihydroequilin, and several other B-ring unsaturated estrogens, including -dihydroestrone, have been documented. Table 14-9 compares the standard doses of the most frequently prescribed oral estrogens and the levels of E$_1$ and E$_2$ achieved.[314,315] Much of the clinical information contained below may be found in systematic reviews.[316]

Synthetic estrogens, given orally, are more potent than natural estradiol. Ethinyl estradiol is used in oral contraceptives, with a dose of 5 μg being equivalent to the standard ERT doses used (0.625 mg CEE or 1 mg micronized estradiol). Standard ERT doses are five or six times less than the amount of estrogen used in oral contraceptives.[317] For hepatic markers, CEE 0.625 mg. is generally more potent than E$_2$ and is closer to 1.5 mg E$_2$.

Oral estrogens have a potent hepatic "first pass" effect that results in the loss of approximately 30% of their activity with a single passage after oral administration. However, this results in stimulation of hepatic proteins and enzymes. Some of these changes are not particularly beneficial (an increase in procoagulation factors), whereas other changes are beneficial (an increase in HDL-C and a decrease in fibrinogen and plasminogen activator inhibitor-1).

E$_2$ can be administered in patches, gels, and subcutaneously. These routes of administration are not subject to major hepatic effects as with oral therapy. Standard doses in the United States of alcohol-based or matrix patches are 0.05 mg or 0.1 mg. Lower-dose patches of 0.025 mg are also available for administration once or twice weekly. Matrix patches are preferable because there is less skin reaction and estrogen delivery is more reliable. Whereas levels of E$_2$ vary widely among women, levels with transdermal therapy are more constant in individual women than with oral ET. With the 0.05-mg patch, E$_2$ levels are in the 40- to 50-pg/mL range; with the 0.1-mg patch, levels are typically 70 to 100 pg/mL. Levels in excess of 200 pg/mL are not unusual for some women.[318] An ultralow dose patch, 0.014 mg, has been approved for osteoporosis protection in older women.

In women with vulvovaginal or urinary complaints, vaginal therapy is most appropriate. Creams of estradiol or CEE are available, as well as tablets and an estrogen ring. With creams, systemic absorption occurs but with levels that are one fourth of that achieved after similar doses administered orally. Absorption decreases as the mucosa becomes more estrogenized. For CEE, only 0.5 g (0.3 mg) or less is necessary; for micronized E$_2$, doses as low as 0.25 mg are sufficient. Other products (tablets and rings) are available that have been designed to limit systemic absorption.[319,320] A Silastic ring of E$_2$ is now available that delivers E$_2$ to the vagina for 3 months with only minimal systemic absorption.[321]

Estrogen may be administered continuously (daily) or for 21 to 26 days each month. If the woman has a uterus, a progestin should be added to the regimen.[322] For women who are totally intolerant of progestins (regardless of the dose and route of administration) and take unopposed estrogen, annual endometrial sampling is necessary. Alternatively, a different progestin may be tried, micronized progesterone can be used vaginally, or an intrauterine system (IUS) can be used. The current IUS, releasing 20 μg levonorgestrel, is too large a dose for routine HRT and the 10 μg IUS, although well studied, will not be marketed as such.[323]

Colon Cancer and Other Changes

Observational studies have reported a reduced risk of colorectal cancer in menopausal women who are current and past users of EPT. This was confirmed in the WHI trial using EPT (HR 0.65). This protective effect is believed to increase with duration of use. With aging, there is a decline in macular function.[324] In observational studies, estrogen therapy has been reported to reduce macular degeneration and maintain visual acuity in menopausal women. There are also several studies showing that estrogen is associated with a reduction in tooth loss.[325,326]

Androgen Therapy

In a very subtle way, some women are relatively androgen deficient.[327] Clinicians have proposed adding androgen to ET or EPT for complaints or problems relating to libido and energy which are not relieved by adequate estrogen,[328] though well-controlled trials using parenteral testosterone have shown benefit in younger oophorectomized women; there have been few data showing benefit using more physiologic therapy until recently. Recent data using a testosterone patch (with near physiologic levels) have shown improvement in several scales of well-being and sexual function.[329-333] An oral preparation (esterified estrogens 0.625 mg with 1.25 mg of methyl testosterone) was shown to improve sexual motivation and enjoyment in women with hypoactive sexual desire who were unresponsive to estrogen alone.[334] The latter findings correlated with an increase in circulating unbound testosterone levels. As newer forms and doses of androgen become available, perhaps more women may benefit from this approach. At present, androgen therapy should be individualized and considered for those women who have symptoms that are not adequately relieved with traditional ET or EPT.[328]At lower doses, androgenizing side effects are very infrequent but should be discussed before prescribing testosterone. At present, small doses of methyltestosterone (1.25 and 2.5 mg) added to esterified estrogens are available in tablets, as are testosterone patches that are available for men (and therefore require dose reductions) and testosterone subcutaneous pellets. The testosterone patch (300 μg) has not been approved for use in women in the United States but is available in Europe. Administration of dehydroepiandrosterone at 25 to 50 mg/day may also be an option.[335]

Another SERM-like compound that is used worldwide but is not yet approved in the United States is tibolone. This progestin-like compound exhibits estrogenic, antiestrogenic, and androgenic effects by virtue of its structure and metabolites. At 2.5 mg, tibolone suppresses hot flushes, prevents osteoporosis, and has a positive effect on mood and sexual function.[336] There is also very limited (or no) uterine stimulation. However, there is a suppression of HDL-C, but at the same time a decrease in triglycerides. In the monkey, there is no deleterious effect of tibolone on coronary arteries.[337] In older women it may increase the risk of stroke.

Alternative Therapies for Menopause

PHYTOESTROGENS

Phytoestrogens are a class of plant-derived estrogen-like compounds conjugated to glycoside moieties. Phytoestrogens are not biologically active in their native forms unless taken orally. After oral ingestion, colonic bacteria cleave the glycosides, producing active compounds that are subject to the enterohepatic circulation. These compounds can produce estrogen-agonistic effects in some tissues, whereas in other tissues they can produce antagonistic effects.

Few randomized trials have examined the efficacy of phytoestrogens. For large daily doses (60 mg isoflavone) there appears to be some limited efficacy in relieving hot flushes.[338] With doses of 30 to 40 mg, cholesterol levels are reduced, but it is no longer recommended as a strategy for lowering cholesterol as it was previously.[339] It should be noted that there is an important reduction in hot flushes with *any* placebo treatment. Phytoestrogens do not appear to have much of an effect on bone loss or on vaginal atrophy.

Estimates are that between 30% and 60% of women use so-called alternative interventions for the symptoms of menopause, including "natural" estrogens, plant estrogens, herbal medicines, and acupuncture. Botanicals, herbals, and many steroid products are sold over the counter, and some do in fact exert significant hormonal activity. The use of botanicals to alleviate the symptoms of menopause is extremely popular. This popularity is fostered by the notion that plant sterols might provide all the benefits of estrogen replacement therapy without the risks. However, most plant products recommended for menopause have performed poorly in clinical trials. The Dietary Supplement Health and Education Act of 1994 classifies most

botanical medicines as food supplements and removes them from regulatory oversight and scrutiny by the U.S. Food and Drug Administration (FDA). Adulteration, contamination, and poor quality control in their harvesting, manufacture, and formulation yield products of questionable efficacy and safety.

The FDA has determined that more than 25% of Chinese patent medicines are adulterated with hidden pharmaceutical drugs. These kinds of deficiencies make it difficult for consumers and practitioners to employ botanicals with confidence and security. Furthermore, clinical trial data obtained using one brand of herbal product cannot necessarily be extrapolated to other brands using the same plant. DHEA is marketed as a dietary supplement for a variety of purported benefits. There are no data in women to support its role in well-being or immune function. As an androgen, DHEA is converted to androstenedione and testosterone. Doses of 25 to 50 mg raised testosterone and have been mentioned as an option for androgen therapy.[335] However, these doses can reduce HDL-C levels.

USE OF A PROGESTOGEN

There are many ways to administer progestogens. The most commonly used oral progestins are MPA in doses of 5 to 10 mg, norethindrone (NET) in doses of 0.3 to 1 mg, and micronized progesterone in doses of 100 to 300 mg. Equivalent doses to prevent hyperplasia when administered for at least 10 days in a woman receiving ET (equivalent to 0.625 mg CEE) are as follows: MPA, 5 mg; NET, 0.35 mg; and micronized progesterone, 200 mg.[340] Larger doses of estrogen may require larger doses and more prolonged regimens of progestins. In sequential administration of progestins, the number of days (length of exposure) is more important than the dose. Thus, if a woman is receiving oral ERT continuously, a regimen of at least 10 to 12 days of exposure is preferable to a 7-day regimen.

When progestins are administered sequentially (10 to 14 days each month), withdrawal bleeding occurs in about 80% of women. Continuous administration of both estrogen and progestin (continuous combined therapy) was developed to achieve amenorrhea. In the first 3 to 6 months, breakthrough bleeding and spotting is common. In some women on this regimen, amenorrhea is never completely achieved. The most common combinations in the United States are single tablets containing 0.625 mg CEE and 2.5 mg (or 5 mg) MPA, and the lower dose combination with 0.45 mg and 0.3 mg (CEE); 5 μg of EE with 1 mg NET; 1 mg micronized E$_2$ with 0.5 mg NET; and 1 mg of E$_2$ with 0.5 mg of drosperinone. Patches with E$_2$ NET of levonorgesterone are also available. Currently, the only marketed sequential regimen is one that contains 0.625 mg CEE and 5 mg MPA, which is added for 14 days each cycle.

Equal efficacy to standard doses has been demonstrated for several low-dose combinations in terms of reduction of hot flushes, maintenance of bone mass, metabolic profiles, and a reduction in the incidence of bleeding in the first year of treatment has been observed.

Progesterone administered vaginally (in low doses) avoids systemic effects and results in high concentrations of progesterone in the uterus. Intrauterine delivery of progestins is ideal for targeting the uterus but is not approved in the United States.

Progestins, particularly when taken orally, may lead to problems of continuance or compliance because of adverse effects, including mood alterations and bleeding. These have to be dealt with effectively, and they usually require more flexibility in prescribing habits. Most short-term clinical trials have demonstrated an attenuating effect of progestins on cardiovascular end-points that are improved with estrogen; these effects include lipoprotein changes (an attenuation of the rise in HDL-C) and arterial and metabolic effects. A reduction in blood flow and some brain effects may also be found.

How progestins influence cardiovascular risk is not clear at present. The observational studies, which showed a benefit for ET, did not find any diminution of this effect with EPT. Although there were differences in the effects of CEE/MPA and CEE along in WHI, there were separate trials which are difficult to compare. The addition of progestin probably is responsible for the observed increase in the risk of breast cancer in susceptible women. Progestogens should not be prescribed in women who have undergone hysterectomy.

Aging

It is extremely difficult to separate the effects of menopause from that of natural aging. Some of these problems have been reviewed in detail elsewhere, and the much needed research in this area has been outlined.[341] The key areas where it is important to dissect out aging effects from the effects of estrogen deficiency are in bone loss and

osteoporosis, cardiovascular disease, cognitive decline, decline in sexual function, and depression. Although premenopausal estrogen therapy may play a role in protecting against these entities, aging also has significant effects.

From a reproductive endocrine perspective, the hormonal systems that are most notably affected by aging are declines in the somatotropic axis, declines in adrenal steroids, and changes in cortisol secretion. Table 14-10 outlines the endocrine metabolic changes with aging.

THE SOMATOTROPHIC AXIS

In men and women GH decreases with aging,[341] beginning around age 40[342,343]; this decrease may be responsible for some of the changes in body composition. A redifferentiated proportion of body fat increases by 100%. Concomitantly there is a 20% to 50% decrease in muscle mass and a 20% decrease in body fat. In women, declines in GH-releasing hormone secretion and a loss of the priming effect of estrogen explain the decline in GH.[344-347]

The anabolic effects of replacing GH can result in stimulated muscle development and strength, a loss of fat, and an increase in bone mass.[348] Accordingly GH releasing peptides have been studied for this purpose.[349,350]

METABOLIC CHANGES

With aging, weight gain and fat accumulation occurs, as stated previously. These changes begin a few years before menopause and parallel increases in FSH[355] (Fig. 14-32). These changes are associated with increases in leptin. In early menopause, associated with normal BMI, adiponectin increases.[356] However, in late menopause, as with

TABLE 14-10

Endocrine-Metabolic Changes With Aging

Substance	Change
Luteinizing hormone	↑
Follicle-stimulating hormone	↑
Growth hormone	↓
Adrenocorticotropic hormone	→*
Prolactin	↓
Thyroid-stimulating hormone	→*
Estradiol	↓
Estrone	↓
Progesterone	↓
Triiodothyronine	→
Thyroxine	→*
Cortisol	↑
Dehydroepiandrosterone	↓
Dehydroepiandrosterone sulfate	↓
Testosterone	↓
Androstenedione	↓
Inhibin	↓
Melatonin	↓
Insulin-like growth factor-1	↓
Dopamine	↓
Norepinephrine	↑

*May be slightly increased or decreased in response to specific secretagogue (e.g., corticotropin-releasing hormone, thyrotropin-releasing hormone, somatostatin, growth hormone-releasing hormone, adrenocorticotropin) with age.

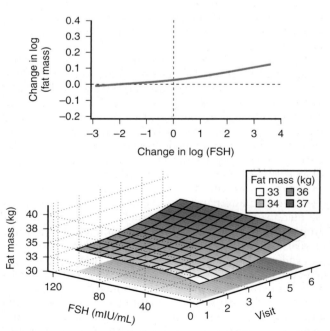

Figure 14-32 *Changes in fat mass during the perimenopause and relationship to follicle-stimulating hormone (FSH). FMP, final menstrual period.*

obesity, adiponectin is reduced increasing CVD risk.[357] With aging, there is a reduction in pancreatic β cell secretion increasing the risk of diabetes mellitus. Adding to this risk, insulin resistance increases with age but is accelerated with weight gain and obesity.

ADRENAL STEROIDS

The age-related decline in adrenal androgens has been noted previously, as well as the possibility of administering DHEA for androgen support in postmenopausal women.[335] While higher DHEAS levels in men are associated with a better cardiovascular survival, this correlation has not been found in women. Similarly, the data on enhancing insulin sensitivity and immune function, as well as quality of life assessments in postmenopausal women, are inconsistent,[354,355] requiring more study.

Because DHEA/DHEAS may be produced locally in the brain[356,357] and bind to the γ-aminobutyric (GABA) receptors,[358] there may be an important role for DHEA in remedying the mood and cognition declines that come with aging. Positive effects of DHEA on mood and cognition in the elderly have been reported.[359,360]

Cortisol levels are higher in older postmenopausal women.[361] This relates to a higher nocturnal rhythmicity which has been related to loss of resiliency and could explain sleep disturbances in the elderly.

The complete reference list can be found on the companion Expert Consult Web site at www.expertconsultbook.com.

Suggested Readings

Hsia J, Langer RD, Manson JE, et al. Conjugated equine estrogens and coronary heart disease: the Women's Health Initiative. Arch Intern Med 166:357-365, 2006.

Lobo RA. Evidence-based medicine and the management of menopause. Clin Obstet Gynecol 51(3):534-538, 2008.

Lobo RA (ed): Treatment of the Postmenopausal Woman, 3rd ed. New York, Academic Press, 2007.

Manson JE, Allison MA, Rossouw JE, et al. Estrogen therapy and coronary-artery calcification. N Engl J Med 356:2591-2602, 2007.

Mendelsohn ME, Karas RH. Molecular and cellular basis of cardiovascular gender differences. Science 308(5728):1583-1587, 2005 (review).

Rossouw JE, Prentice RL, Manson JE, et al. Postmenopausal hormone therapy and cardiovascular disease by age and years since menopause. JAMA 297(13):1465-1477, 2007.

Stefanick ML, Anderson GL, Margolis KL, et al. Effects of conjugated equine estrogens on breast cancer and mammography screening in postmenopausal women with hysterectomy. JAMA 295(14):1647-1657, 2006.

Sowers MF, Zheng H, Tomey K, et al. Changes in body composition in women over six years at midlife: ovarian and chronological aging. J Clin Endocrinol Metab 92(3):895-901, 2007.

Writing Group for the Women's Health Initiative Investigators. Risks and benefits of estrogen plus progestin in healthy postmenopausal women: principal results from the Women's Health Initiative randomized controlled trial. JAMA 288:321-333, 2002.

CHAPTER 15

Male Reproductive Aging

Peter J. Snyder

As men age, reproductive function declines in several ways. Although the change is gradual, unlike the relatively abrupt decline that occurs in women at the time of menopause, it is progressive and probably has some adverse consequences. The decline is sometimes called "andropause" or "male menopause." This chapter reviews the changes in male reproductive function with aging and what is known about the consequences of attempting to prevent the changes by treatment with testosterone.

Changes in Male Reproductive Function with Age

SPERMATOGENESIS AND SEMEN PARAMETERS

The little information available suggests that spermatogenesis does not decline severely with increasing age. Testicular volume, which reflects largely seminiferous tubular volume, averaged 20.6 mL, as determined by ultrasound, in 114 elderly men compared to 29.7 mL in 42 young men.[1] Sperm production was studied in an autopsy study of 89 men aged 21 to 50 years and 43 men aged 51 to 80 years who died suddenly. The older men had a daily sperm production rate per testis that was approximately 30% less than that in the younger men.[2] Ejaculated sperm were studied in 20 fathers aged 24 to 37 years old and 22 grandfathers aged 60 to 88 years old. Sperm density was somewhat higher in the older men, and percentage of sperm motility was somewhat lower in the older men, so that total number of motile sperm was similar in the two groups.[3] The serum inhibin concentration is an indicator of Sertoli cell function, which in turn, reflects seminiferous tubular function. In 189 ambulatory men, the serum concentration of inhibin B in men over 70 years old was about 75% of that in men younger than 35 years old ($P = 0.002$).[4] In

the same study, the serum follicle-stimulating hormone (FSH) concentration was more than three times as high in the men over 70 years old than in the men under 35 years old ($P < 0.001$). From these data it appears that if sperm production declines with age, it does so marginally.

SEX STEROID HORMONE AND GONADOTROPIN CONCENTRATIONS

Serum Testosterone Concentration

The serum testosterone concentration has been found to decrease with age in both cross-sectional and longitudinal studies. The decrease appears to occur gradually beginning in the third decade of life. The magnitude of the decrease appears to be greater in longitudinal than cross-sectional studies, and greater in the free testosterone concentration than in the total. This decrease reflects a decrease in testicular secretion of testosterone, since in men testosterone is principally of testicular origin.

Several cross-sectional studies show a decrease in serum testosterone concentration with age. One study was performed in 83 healthy, community-dwelling men, 20 to 88 years old, who volunteered for the New Mexico Aging Process Study.[5] Their serum concentrations of total testosterone decreased gradually with increasing age, but the fall was quite modest and did not reach statistical significance. The serum concentration of sex hormone–binding globulin (SHBG), however, increased about 75% from the youngest to the oldest men, which explains why the serum free testosterone concentration fell to a much greater degree than did the total. The free testosterone concentration at age 80 was approximately one third of that at age 20. Another cross-sectional study was performed in 302 healthy men in Belgium, in whom the serum testosterone concentrations decreased with increasing age.[6] The mean (± SD) total testosterone

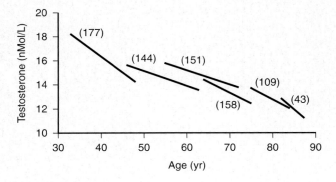

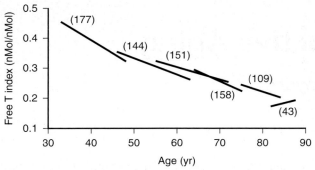

Figure 15-1. Serum testosterone concentration and free testosterone index as functions of aging in men. Linear segment slopes by decade are shown for 890 men who participated in the Baltimore Longitudinal Study on Aging and had testosterone measurements on two or more occasions during an interval of 1 to 30 years. Each line represents a cohort, and the numbers in parentheses represent the number of men in each cohort. (From Harman SM, Metter EJ, Tobin JD, et al. Longitudinal effects of aging on serum total and free testosterone levels in healthy men. Baltimore Longitudinal Study of Aging. J Clin Endocrinol Metab 86[2]:724, 2001.)

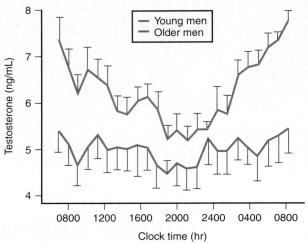

Figure 15-2. This graph shows pronounced diurnal variation in the serum testosterone concentration in young men but much less pronounced variation in elderly men. (From Bremner WJ, Vitiello V, Prinz PN. Loss of circadian rhythmicity in blood testosterone levels with aging in normal men. J Clin Endocrinol Metab 56:1278, 1983.)

concentration in that study in the 70 men 20 to 39 years old was 683 ± 289 ng/dL and that in 51 men 70 to 79 years old was 428 ± 128 ng/dL. The calculated free testosterone concentration fell by a relatively greater amount; in 70- to 79-year-old men it was approximately half of that in 20- to 39-year-old men. In a study of 4263 men 70 to over 85 years old, total serum testosterone remained stable with age, but SHBG increased and free testosterone decreased.[7]

Longitudinal studies all show a decrease in testosterone with increasing age. In the New Mexico Aging Process Study, 77 of the subjects, age 60 to 75 at entry, were followed for up to 15 years.[8] The average rate of fall of serum total testosterone concentration was 110 ng/dL per decade during this 15-year period of observation. In the Baltimore Longitudinal Study of Aging, the serum total testosterone concentration and a calculated free testosterone index fell from the third to the ninth decades in 890 men who were followed longitudinally (Fig. 15-1).[9] By the eighth decade, approximately 30% of men were hypogonadal using the total testosterone concentration and 70% were hypogonadal by the free testosterone index. In the Massachusetts Male Aging Study, a population-based, random sample cohort of men aged 40 to 70 at baseline, 1156 men were followed for 7 to 10 years.[10] The serum concentration of total testosterone fell at a rate of 0.8% per year cross-sectionally, but 1.6% per year longitudinally.

The decrease in serum testosterone concentration with increasing age appears to be primarily the result of a decrease in the morning peak that younger men experience (Fig. 15-2).[11] When the serum testosterone concentration was measured once an hour for 24 hours in 17 men aged 23 to 28 years and 12 men aged 58 to 82 years, the young men exhibited a clear diurnal variation, the peak at 8 AM and the nadir at 8 PM. The older men exhibited much less of a diurnal variation, so that the young men had a significantly higher serum testosterone concentration than the older men from 2 AM to 1 PM but not from 2 PM to 1 AM. The decrease in serum testosterone concentration with increasing age also appears to be affected by other health factors. In the Massachusetts Male Aging Study, a decrease in body mass index of 4 to 5 kg/m² or a loss of a spouse resulted in a similar decrease in testosterone as 10 years of aging.[12]

Serum Estradiol Concentration

The serum total estradiol concentration does not appear to change with increasing age, but the serum bioavailable estradiol concentration, that not bound to SHBG, appears to decrease slightly. In a study of 810 men aged 24 to 90 years old in Rancho Bernardo, California, the serum concentration of total estradiol decreased by only 0.3 pg/mL per year of age, but the concentration of bioavailable estradiol decreased by 0.12 pg/mL per year of age.[13] In Rochester, Minnesota, 130 men, aged 66 to 90 years old, did not have a significantly different concentration of total estradiol than did 88 men 22 to 39 years old, but the older men had a significantly lower serum bioavailable estradiol concentration than did the younger men, 40 pmol/L compared to 59 pmol/L.[14] In a study of 206 men 18 to 95 years old in Parma, Italy, both the total and free serum concentrations of free estradiol fell with age.[15]

Serum Gonadotropin Concentration

Both cross-sectional and longitudinal studies show an increase in the serum concentrations of luteinizing hormone (LH) and FSH with increasing age. In 15 years of observation in the New Mexico Aging Process Study, the mean serum LH concentration increased from 9.4 mIU/mL to 13.7 mIU/mL and the FSH from 14.1 mIU/mL to 27.4 mIU/mL.[8] In the Massachusetts Male Aging Study, LH increased by 0.9% per year and FSH by 3.1% per year.[10] This increase in serum gonadotropins suggests that a degree of primary hypogonadism is responsible for the decline in testosterone, which is supported by the smaller testosterone response to hCG[16] or recombinant human LH[17] stimulation of elderly men than young men. The increase in basal serum LH, however, is not as great as one would expect for the magnitude of testosterone decline, suggesting secondary hypogonadism as well. In several aspects of LH secretion, the magnitude appears to be less in elderly men than in younger men. The LH response to a bolus dose of gonadotropin-releasing hormone (GnRH) is slightly less in older men than in younger men, and the peak response is somewhat delayed.[18] Spontaneous LH pulses are also different in elderly men compared to young men. LH secretory burst amplitude is less in elderly men than in young men.[19] The fall in testosterone with increasing age, therefore, appears to be the result of a combination of Leydig cell and hypothalamic-pituitary deficiencies.

CONSEQUENCES OF DECREASED SERUM TESTOSTERONE CONCENTRATIONS

The parallels between the consequences of frank hypogonadism due to known hypothalamic-pituitary or testicular disease and the consequences of normal aging in men suggest that the fall in testosterone with increasing age might contribute, at least in part, to the consequences of aging in men. These consequences include decreases in bone density, muscle mass and strength, physical function, energy, and sexual function, and an increase in heart disease. Treatment of these deficiencies in frankly hypogonadal men often reverses those consequences.

Bone

The bone mineral density of men who are evaluated because of hypogonadism is lower than that of eugonadal men.[20,21] When men are made hypogonadal by orchiectomy[22] or GnRH agonist treatment, their bone mineral density decreases.[23,24] As men age, bone mineral density also decreases. In a study of normal men who had no history of hip fracture, bone mineral density of the spine and hip deceased linearly from age 20 to more than 80 years (Fig. 15-3); the decline was less than that in women,[25] similar to the findings of other cross-sectional studies.[26,27] However, a cross-sectional study in which bone density was measured by quantitated computed tomography (QCT) showed a greater rate of bone loss[28] than did the studies cited earlier, perhaps

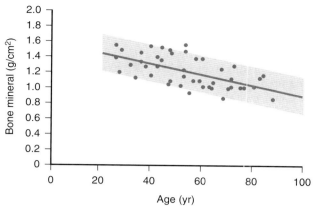

Figure 15-3. Decrease in bone mineral density of the intertrochanteric region of the proximal femur in 52 men with increasing age. (From Riggs BL, Wahner HW, Seeman E, et al. Changes in bone mineral density of the proximal femur and spine with aging. J Clin Invest 70:716, 1982.)

reflecting the greater sensitivity of QCT in detecting changes in trabecular bone than bone densitometry. A longitudinal study showed as rapid a loss of bone density in men as in women.[29] Within the 2908 men of average age 75.4 years in the Swedish Osteoporotic Fractures in Men (MrOS) study, serum free testosterone was a modest predictor of bone density and prevalent osteoporotic fractures.[30]

Replacement of testosterone in frankly hypogonadal men greatly increases bone mineral density. Administration of 100 mg of testosterone enanthate for 18 months to 29 men with previously untreated hypogonadism resulted in a 5% increase in bone mineral density in the lumbar spine as determined by dual energy x-ray absorptiometry (DEXA).[21] Trabecular bone mineral density, as measured by quantitative computed tomography, increased by 14%. Administration of testosterone transdermally for 3 years to 18 hypogonadal men who had previously untreated hypogonadism resulted in increases in bone mineral density by DEXA of 7.7% at the lumbar spine and 4.0% at the trochanter.[31]

Body Composition

When men become hypogonadal as the result of hypothalamic-pituitary or testicular disease, they experience a decrease in lean body mass and an increase in fat mass, and testosterone treatment of hypogonadal men usually reverses those changes. The same changes occur as men age. Whole-body lean mass in one study was about 15% less at age 70 than at age 20, and whole body fat mass was about 100% more.[32] In another study, appendicular skeletal muscle mass was 16% less in men over 75 years old than in men 18 to 34 years old.[33] Percentage of body fat was 26% in 36 hypogonadal men compared to 19% in 44 eugonadal men.[21] When six normal young men were made hypogonadal for 10 weeks by the administration of the GnRH agonist leuprolide, their fat-free mass decreased from 56.5 to 54.4 kg and their fat mass increased from 15.8 to 16.9 kg.[34]

Administration of testosterone reverses these changes in body composition. Administration of 100 mg of testosterone enanthate to previously untreated hypogonadal men resulted in a 14% decrease in total body fat and a 12% decrease in subcutaneous fat, as assessed by quantitated computed tomography.[21] Lean muscle mass, assessed by the same technique, increased 6.8%. When testosterone was administered transdermally to 18 previously untreated hypogonadal men, lean body mass increased 5.8%.[31]

Muscle Strength

Muscle strength has long been known to decrease with increasing age, but demonstration that hypogonadism leads to decreased muscle strength and that testosterone treatment improves strength have been much more difficult to demonstrate. In a study of 72 normal men in three age groups ages 20 to 86, strength of knee extension, both isometric and isokinetic, decreased with increasing age.[35] In another study in 114 men ages 11 to 70 years old, quadriceps strength increased up to the third decade, was stable until age 50, then declined with increasing age.[36] The only clear demonstration that hypogonadal men have lower muscle strength than eugonadal men was provided by the study, described earlier, in which six healthy young men were made severely hypogonadal for 10 weeks by administration of leuprolide. At the end of the 10 weeks, their strength of knee extension was 6% less than prior to treatment when measured isokinetically at 60 degrees angular velocity, but was not significantly different during treatment than before when measured isokinetically at 180 degrees angular velocity or isometrically at either angular velocity.[34]

Administration of testosterone transdermally to 18 previously untreated hypogonadal men did not increase their strength of knee extension or flexion or handgrip strength.[31] Administration of 100 mg testosterone enanthate once a week to men with wasting secondary to HIV infection resulted in a 16% increase in leg press strength compared to no significant change in those treated with placebo, whereas men who were treated with testosterone and resistance exercise did not exhibit a greater increase than those treated with placebo and exercise.[37] In short, it is clear that muscle strength decreases with increasing age, but it is not clear how much, if any, the decline in testosterone contributes to the decrease in muscle strength.

Cardiovascular and Metabolic Risk

Because the prevalence of heart disease is greater in men than in women, the possible role of testosterone in the development of arteriosclerotic cardiovascular disease has long been discussed. An alternative explanation for the difference is higher estradiol concentrations in women before menopause. This possibility is suggested by the gradual decrease in the gap between the genders the greater the length of time after menopause. A recent study, however, suggests that it may be low testosterone that is harmful. When 794 men of median age 73.6 years had a serum testosterone measurement and were followed for an average of 11.8 years, men whose serum testosterone concentrations were in the lowest quartile (<241 ng/dL)

were 40% more likely to die of all causes and 38% more likely to die of cardiovascular causes[38] than men with higher values. This association was independent of age, adiposity, and lifestyle.

If low testosterone does cause increased mortality rate, one possible mechanism is via metabolic risk factors, because in epidemiologic studies low testosterone precedes the development of central obesity, the metabolic syndrome, and diabetes.[39-41] However, in the study cited earlier, the association between low testosterone and higher mortality rate persisted even after adjusting for metabolic syndrome and diabetes mellitus. Further, associations between testosterone and metabolic syndrome and diabetes are equivocal. In the Baltimore Longitudinal Study of Aging, the prevalence of the metabolic syndrome was associated with a lower total testosterone but a higher index of free testosterone.[42] Conversely, in an analysis of data from the Third National Health and Nutrition Survey (NHANES III), men in the lowest tertile of an index of free testosterone were four times as likely to have a diagnosis of diabetes mellitus than men in the highest tertile, but that relationship was not observed with total testosterone.[43] Perhaps the best evidence that testosterone influences glucose metabolism is a randomized, placebo-controlled crossover trial in which testosterone treatment for 3 months of men who had type II diabetes and low-normal to low serum testosterone concentrations improved their fasting glucose, hemoglobin A_{1c}, and HOMA index, compared to placebo treatment.[44]

Other possible mechanisms by which testosterone could affect cardiovascular disease are via serum lipids, clotting factors, and markers of inflammation, but treatment of hypogonadal men with testosterone does not consistently change these parameters.[31,45-50]

Energy

Men's sense of energy decreases with increasing age, and when men who are hypogonadal due to known disease are treated with testosterone, their self-reported energy increases markedly. Administration of testosterone transdermally to 18 men with severe, untreated hypogonadism resulted in an increase in self-reported energy, reaching an apparent peak in about 3 months.[31]

Cognition

The association of low testosterone with declining cognitive function was evaluated in the Baltimore Longitudinal Study of Aging, in which 407 men ages 50 to 91 years at baseline assessment were followed for an average of 10 years. Men who were classified as hypogonadal, defined for this study as a free testosterone index (total testosterone/SHBG) below the 2.5 percentile, had significantly lower scores on measures of memory and visuospatial performance and a faster decline in verbal memory.[51]

Sexual Function

Libido, as self-reported on a questionnaire, decreases with increasing age.[52] (Erectile dysfunction increases with increasing age, but this is the result of influences other than a decrease in testosterone, such as neurologic and vascular disease and certain medications.) Hypogonadism also causes a decrease in libido. When men who were frankly hypogonadal were treated with a single dose of testosterone enanthate, sexual function increased much more within a few weeks after a dose of 100 mg than a dose of placebo, and even more after a dose of 400 mg than 100 mg.[53] When 18 severely hypogonadal men were treated with testosterone transdermally, sexual function had increased markedly when first reassessed at 3 months but did not increase further when the observation was continued for a total of 3 years.[31]

Attempts to Reverse the Consequences of Aging by Testosterone Treatment

A few attempts have been made to administer testosterone to relatively small numbers of elderly men to raise their serum testosterone concentration to that of young men to determine if the changes of aging can be reversed. Improvements in some parameters occurred.

PARAMETERS OF IMPROVEMENT

Bone

In one study, 108 healthy elderly men over 65 years old with a serum testosterone concentration below 475 ng/dL were randomized to receive testosterone or placebo transdermally for 3 years. Bone mineral density of the lumbar spine increased somewhat more in the testosterone-treated group than in the placebo-treated group, but overall the difference was not statistically significant. When the data were analyzed by a linear regression model, there was an inverse correlation between the pretreatment serum testosterone concentration and the effect of testosterone on bone mineral density above that of placebo, called the testosterone treatment effect (Fig. 15-4). For example, for a pretreatment serum testosterone of 400 ng/dL, the testosterone treatment effect on the percentage of increase in bone mineral density above baseline was only 0.9%, but when the pretreatment serum testosterone concentration was 300 ng/dL, the testosterone treatment effect was 3.4%, and when the pretreatment serum testosterone was 200 ng/dL, the testosterone treatment effect was 5.9%.[54] No significant difference was observed in hip bone mineral density. In another study, 67 men over 65 years old who had subnormal bioavailable testosterone concentrations were randomized to receive testosterone transdermally for 1 year. In the 44 men who completed the trial, femoral neck bone mineral density increased 0.3% in the testosterone-treated group and decreased 1.6% in the placebo-treated group, a difference that was statistically significant, but there were no significant differences in bone mineral density at other sites in the hip or in the spine.[55] In a third study, in which elderly men were randomized to receive testosterone enanthate alone (24 men), testosterone enanthate plus finasteride (22 men), or placebo (24 men) for 3 years, the men treated with testosterone alone or with finasteride exhibited 10.2% and

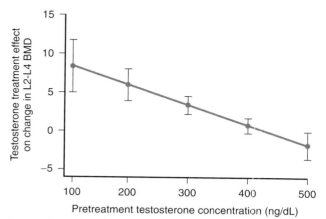

Figure 15-4. *Effect of testosterone treatment for 3 years on spine bone mineral density (BMD) of elderly men. Shown is a linear regression model of the testosterone treatment effect (the effect of testosterone over placebo) as a function of the pretreatment serum testosterone concentration, showing that only men who have a lower than normal serum testosterone concentration would be expected to experience an increase in spine bone mineral density if treated with testosterone. (From Snyder PJ, Peachey H, Hannoush P, et al. Effect of testosterone treatment on bone mineral density in men over 65 years of age. J Clin Endocrinol Metab 84[6]:1966, 1999.)*

9.3% increases in spine bone density, whereas the men treated with placebo increased only 1.3%.[56] Increases in the total hip were less, 2.7% and 2.2% versus –0.2%, but still statistically significant.

Body Composition

Several studies show that testosterone treatment of elderly men increases lean body mass and decreases fat mass. In the 108 elderly men described earlier,[57] lean mass increased by 1.9 kg and fat mass decreased by 3.0 kg in the testosterone-treated men during the 3 years of treatment (Fig. 15-5). In the study of 67 men described earlier,[55] lean mass increased by 1.0 kg and fat mass decreased by 1.7% in the 1 year of treatment. In a study of elderly men treated with placebo or testosterone enanthate for 6 months,[58] 21 testosterone-treated men experienced a 1.4 kg increase in lean mass and a 1.2 kg decrease in fat mass, whereas 17 placebo-treated men experienced no change. In the study of 70 men treated with testosterone enanthate with or without finasteride or with placebo for 3 years, lean body mass increased by about 4 kg and fat mass decreased by about 5 kg in the two testosterone-treated groups.[59,60]

Muscle Strength

Although an increase in muscle mass should result in an increase in muscle strength, controlled studies in which a physiologic dose of testosterone has been administered to elderly men have generally not demonstrated an increase in muscle strength compared to placebo-treated men. In the study of 108 men described earlier[57] who were randomized to receive either testosterone or placebo for 3 years, the testosterone-treated men did not differ from the placebo-treated men in change from baseline

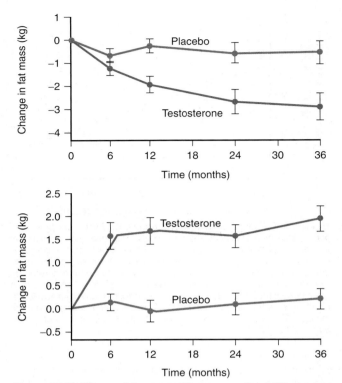

Figure 15-5. *Effect on fat mass and lean mass when 108 men were treated with testosterone or placebo for 3 years. (From Snyder PJ, Peachey H, Hannoush P, et al. Effect of testosterone treatment on body composition and muscle strength in men over 65 years of age. J Clin Endocrinol Metab 84[8]:2647, 1999.)*

in strength of knee extension or flexion at 60 degrees or 180 degrees angular velocity at 3 years or earlier, nor in handgrip strength. In the study of 67 men described earlier[55] who were randomized to receive testosterone or placebo for 1 year, strength of knee extension by leg press was no different at the end of the year in the testosterone-treated group than in the placebo-treated group. In 40 men randomized to receive human chorionic gonadotropin (hCG) or placebo for 3 months,[60] shoulder and knee strength as measured by dynamometry did not differ in the two groups at the end of treatment. In the 70 men treated with testosterone enanthate with or without finasteride or treated with placebo, the testosterone-treated men exhibited a greater improvement than placebo-treated in right handgrip strength but not in left handgrip strength or in ankle or knee strength.[59]

Physical Function

Parameters of physical function also have not changed significantly following administration of testosterone to elderly men. In 108 men randomized to receive testosterone or placebo, walking time and stair climbing did not differ between the two groups at the end of 3 years of treatment.[57] The testosterone-treated men, however, had a more favorable perception of their physical function than the placebo-treated men had of theirs. In 67 men randomized to receive testosterone or placebo, physical function, as estimated activity by Physical Activity for the Elderly

questionnaire, did not differ between the two groups.[55] In 40 men who were randomized to receive hCG or placebo, maximum reach, static and dynamic balance, gait, and chair rise did not differ between the two groups at the end of 3 months of treatment.[60] In the men treated with testosterone enanthate with or without finasteride or treated with placebo, the testosterone-treated men exhibited greater improvement than placebo-treated men after 3 years.[59]

Energy

Testosterone treatment of elderly hypogonadal men has generally not affected their energy. In 108 elderly men randomized to receive either testosterone or placebo, self-reported energy and sense of well-being was no different in the two groups at the end of 3 years of treatment.[57] In 67 men randomized to receive testosterone or placebo, sense of well-being was no different between the two groups at the end of 1 year of treatment.[61]

Cognition

The effects of testosterone treatment on cognition have been studied in elderly men who have low-normal serum testosterone concentrations, but the results have been variable. Some studies have shown in improvement in various aspects of cognitive function,[62] but others have not.[61]

Libido

Testosterone treatment of elderly men has not been shown to increase libido. In 108 men randomized to receive testosterone or placebo for 3 years, the two groups did not differ in libido, as determined by questionnaire, either at the end of treatment or at any earlier time.[57] In 40 men randomized to receive either hCG or placebo for 1 year, libido also did not differ at the end of treatment.[60]

POTENTIAL DELETERIOUS CONSEQUENCES OF TESTOSTERONE TREATMENT OF ELDERLY MEN

Several diseases to which elderly men are prone are testosterone-dependent. These diseases include prostate cancer and benign prostatic hyperplasia, and possibly erythrocytosis and sleep apnea. Prostate cancer, for example, was the first cancer shown to be hormonally dependent,[63] and treatment of metastatic prostate cancer even now is based on blocking the secretion and action of testosterone.[64,65] An additional reason for concern that testosterone treatment of elderly men might increase the risk of prostate cancer is that approximately 50% of men who are 50 to 60 years old harbor clinically silent prostate cancer.[66] If these men were treated with testosterone, would these clinically silent tumors become clinically significant? Benign prostatic hyperplasia has been known to be testosterone-dependent for over a century, and a current treatment for this condition is also based on blocking the action of testosterone in the prostate.[67,68] Testosterone stimulates erythropoiesis, which is why men have higher hemoglobin concentrations than do women, but it probably does not cause erythrocytosis unless the dose is excessive or there is a concomitant illness that treatment of hypogonadism unmasks. The evidence that testosterone exacerbates sleep apnea is based on studies of small numbers of patients.[69]

Prostate Events

Testosterone treatment of elderly men has generally not been associated with a significant increase in prostate disease, but the studies performed so far have been far too small to draw any conclusions from these results. In a study of 108 men randomized to receive testosterone or placebo, the serum prostate specific antigen (PSA) concentration increased from 1.4 ng/mL to 2.1 ng/mL, which was statistically significant but still well within the normal range.[54] The testosterone-treated men experienced somewhat more prostate events,[18] such as persistently elevated PSA, urinary retention, and urosepsis, than did the placebo-treated men.[11] In subjects treated for a shorter period, PSA did not differ between the two groups at the end of treatment.[55,60]

Erythrocytosis

In 108 men randomized to receive either testosterone or placebo transdermally, hemoglobin and hematocrit increased significantly in the men treated with testosterone, although within the normal range, but not in men treated with placebo.[54] In men treated with 200 mg of testosterone enanthate every 2 weeks, 30% experienced an increase in hematocrit above the upper limit of normal (52%).[56]

Cardiovascular Risk Factors

Administration of testosterone to elderly hypogonadal men has little effect on serum lipid or apolipoprotein concentrations, but other cardiovascular risk factors have not been well studied. In 108 elderly men randomized to receive either testosterone or placebo, there was no difference between the two groups in serum concentrations of total cholesterol, low-density lipoprotein (LDL) cholesterol, high-density lipoprotein (HDL) cholesterol, apolipoprotein A_2, apolipoprotein B, triglycerides, or lipoprotein a at the end of 3 years of treatment.[70] In 67 men randomized to receive testosterone or placebo, total and LDL cholesterol did not differ between the two groups after a year, but HDL cholesterol decreased in the men who received testosterone.[71] Endothelial brachial artery reactivity did not change in either group.

Sleep Apnea

Although there are a few reports that men with frank hypogonadism who were treated with testosterone experienced an increase in apneic episodes during sleep, sleep apnea has not been shown to increase in elderly men treated with testosterone.[54,60]

Conclusions

Although the serum testosterone concentration falls as men age, the potential beneficial effects and potential risks of reversing that fall are still being discovered. Small, placebo-controlled trials of raising the serum testosterone of elderly men to that of normal young men suggest that this treatment increases lean muscle mass and decreases fat mass. They also suggest that testosterone treatment increases bone mineral density of the spine. Whether or not this treatment increases the risks of prostate cancer, benign prostatic hyperplasia, erythrocytosis, or sleep apnea, however, remains to be determined.

The complete reference list can be found on the companion Expert Consult Web site at www.expertconsultbook.com.

Suggested Readings

Bremner WJ, Vitiello V, Prinz PN. Loss of circadian rhythmicity in blood testosterone levels with aging in normal men. J Clin Endocrinol Metab 56:1278, 1983.

Harman SM, Metter EJ, Tobin JD, et al. Longitudinal effects of aging on serum total and free testosterone levels in healthy men. Baltimore Longitudinal Study of Aging. J Clin Endocrinol Metab 86(2):724, 2001.

Huggins C, Hodges CV. Studies on prostatic cancer. I. The effect of castration, of estrogen and androgen injection on serum phosphatases in metastatic carcinoma of the prostate. Cancer Res 1:293, 1941.

Laughlin GA, Barrett-Connor E, Bergstrom J. Low serum testosterone and mortality in older men. J Clin Endocrinol Metab 93(1):68, 2008.

McConnell JD, Bruskewitz R, Walsh P, et al. The effect of finasteride on the risk of acute urinary retention and the need for surgical treatment among men with benign prostatic hyperplasia. Finasteride Long-Term Efficacy and Safety Study Group. N Engl J Med 338(9):557, 1998.

Moffat SD, Zonderman AB, Metter EJ, et al. Longitudinal assessment of serum free testosterone concentration predicts memory performance and cognitive status in elderly men. J Clin Endocrinol Metab 87(11):5001, 2002.

Snyder PJ, Peachey H, Berlin JA, et al. Effects of testosterone replacement in hypogonadal men. J Clin Endocrinol Metab 85(8):2670, 2000.

Snyder PJ, Peachey H, Hannoush P, et al. Effect of testosterone treatment on body composition and muscle strength in men over 65 years of age. J Clin Endocrinol Metab 84(8):2647, 1999.

Snyder PJ, Peachey H, Hannoush P, et al. Effect of testosterone treatment on bone mineral density in men over 65 years of age. J Clin Endocrinol Metab 84(6):1966, 1999.

Travison TG, Araujo AB, Kupelian V, et al. The relative contributions of aging, health, and lifestyle factors to serum testosterone decline in men. J Clin Endocrinol Metab 92(2):549, 2007.

PART II

Pathophysiology and Therapy

CHAPTER 16

Disorders of Sex Development

Valerie A. Arboleda and Eric Vilain

Introduction to Human Sex Development

From the moment of conception, each of us has a sex. Our individual sex has a major role in determining the physical attributes of our bodies, the structure of our brains, our behavioral tendencies, and our self-concept. Understanding the development of sex differences has informed and been informed by advances in the molecular dissection of genes responsible for disorders of sex development (DSDs). New genes have been identified, allowing for rapid diagnosis, understanding of pathophysiology, and prediction of future fertility.

In parallel to the progress in the biology of sex development, the management of individuals with DSDs has started a gentle revolution. From a practice based on the opinions of a few leaders in the field, the clinical approach to DSDs is slowly entering the era of evidence-based medicine, under the pressure of patient advocacy groups, who have been highly instrumental in establishing a dialogue between practitioners and patients. As a result, physicians are beginning to understand the difficulties involved in defining normalcy as well as the ethical importance of acting medically on children before they reach the age of consent.

For the first time in 2005, a consensus on the management of "intersex" disorders emerged, bringing together experts from a variety of fields (endocrinology, genetics, surgery, psychology, and advocacy groups). The consensus statement provides guidelines for all aspects of management of "intersex," including genital surgery, the need for a multidisciplinary team of mental health professionals, and the diagnostic approach. This chapter reflects the advances made in the field as well as the recommendations of the consensus statement.[1] One area that changed considerably was the nomenclature of intersexuality. The term *disorders of sex development* was proposed, as defined by "congenital conditions in which development of chromosomal, gonadal or anatomical sex is atypical." This broad definition replaces the word "intersex," which has social connotations and reflects a concept of sexual identity. It includes patients who do not necessarily have ambiguous external genitalia (e.g., complete androgen insensitivity, or Turner syndrome) and yet belong to the broad family of DSDs.

The new nomenclature was guided by the following principles. First, although a modern categorization should integrate the important progress in the molecular genetic aspects of sex determination and differentiation, it should not overemphasize one particular aspect of the biology of sex (e.g., gonadal sex) and should accommodate the spectrum of phenotypic variations. Second, terms should be as precise as possible and should reflect the genetic etiology when available. Finally, the new nomenclature should be understandable by patients and families and should be psychologically sensitive. In particular, gender labeling in the diagnosis should be avoided, and use of the words "hermaphrodite," "pseudohermaphrodite," and "intersex" should be abandoned, because they either are confusing or have a negative social connotation that may be perceived as harmful by some patients and parents.

The new nomenclature is summarized in Tables 16-1 and 16-2. This chapter refers to the new rather than the old nomenclature.

NORMAL HUMAN SEX DEVELOPMENT

Sex determination refers to the developmental decision that directs the orientation of the biopotential, undifferentiated embryo into a sexually dimorphic individual. In mammals, this decision occurs during the development of the gonads. In 1947, physiologist Alfred Jost performed a series of elegant experiments showing that all mammalian

TABLE 16-1
Proposed Revised Nomenclature

Previous	Proposed
Intersex	DSD
Male pseudohermaphrodite, undervirilization of an XY male, and undermasculinization of an XY male	46,XY DSD
Female pseudohermaphrodite, overvirilization of an XX female, and masculinization of an XX female	46,XX DSD
True hermaphrodite	Ovotesticular DSD
XX male or XX sex reversal	46,XX testicular DSD
XY sex reversal	46,XY complete gonadal dysgenesis

DSD, disorder of sex development.

From Lee PA, et al. Consensus statement on management of intersex disorders. International Consensus Conference on Intersex. Pediatrics 118(2):e488-e500, 2006.

embryos that are castrated early in development and reimplanted into the uterus develop into females, regardless of genetic sex (Fig. 16-1).[2,3] This study established the current paradigm of sex determination and differentiation in placental mammals: genetic sex determines gonad development, and gonadal sex in turn governs anatomic sex.

At conception, genetic sex is determined based on whether the X or Y chromosome was paternally inherited.[4-7] *Sex determination* is defined by the developmental choice of the biopotential and undifferentiated gonad to become either testis or ovary. After this sex determination decision, the process of *sex differentiation* begins and the testes start producing the male hormones testosterone and anti-müllerian hormone (AMH) which are responsible for male internal and external genitalia, whereas the lack of these hormones results in female internal and external genitalia (Fig. 16-2).

The molecular mechanisms of mammalian sex determination are still poorly understood. The vast majority (approximately 75%) of sex-reversed patients cannot be explained at the molecular level, suggesting the existence of a number of unknown sex-determining genes.[8] The next section outlines the known molecular mechanisms affecting sex determination and sex differentiation.

Sex Determination: Testes or Ovary?

This paradigm for sex development established by Jost led to the search for a sex-determining gene that was a testis-determining factor. When the karyotypes of male patients with Klinefelter syndrome (47,XXY)[9] and female patients with Turner syndrome (45,X)[10] were determined, it became clear that the Y chromosome was sex-determining and that the testis-determining factor had to be located on the Y chromosome.

In the early 1990s, a series of elegant experiments found *SRY* to be the elusive mammalian testis-determining gene. Positional cloning located a 35-kb fragment of the Y chromosome translocated to the X chromosome of the XX male and true hermaphrodite patients.[11,12] Further sequence analysis defined a conserved sequence within this region. *Sry* gene expression analysis showed a male-specific

TABLE 16-2
Example of a DSD Classification

Sex Chromosome DSD	46,XY DSD	46,XX DSD
45,X (Turner syndrome and variants)	Disorders of gonadal (testicular) development: (1) complete gonadal dysgenesis (Swyer syndrome); (2) partial gonadal dysgenesis; (3) gonadal regression; (4) ovotesticular DSD	Disorders of gonadal (ovarian development: (1) ovotesticular DSD (e.g., SRY translocation, RSPO1 mutation); (2) testicular DSD (e.g., SRY+; dupSOX9); (3) gonadal dysgenesis
47,XXY (Klinefelter syndrome and variants)	Disorders of androgen synthesis of actions; (1) androgen biosynthesis defect (e.g., CYP17 deficiency, SRD5A2 deficiency, StAR mutations); (2) defect of androgen action (CAIS, PAIS); (3) luteinizing hormone receptor defects (Leydig cell hypoplasia); (4) disorders of anti-müllerian hormone and anti-müllerian hormone receptor	Androgen excess: (1) fetal (e.g., 21-hydroxylase deficiency, 11-hydroxylast deficiency); (2) fetoplacental (aromatase deficiency, POR deficiency); (3) maternal (luteoma)
45,X/46,XY (mixed gonadal dysgenesis, ovotesticular DSD)		
46,XX/46,XY (chimeric, ovotesticular DSD)		

CAIS, complete androgen insensitivity syndrome; DSD, disorder of sex development; PAIS, partial androgen insensitivity syndrome; POR, cytochrome P450 oxidoreductase; StAR, steroidogenic acute regulatory.

Adapted from Lee PA, et al. Consensus statement on management of intersex disorders. International Consensus Conference on Intersex. Pediatrics 118(2): e488-e500 2006.

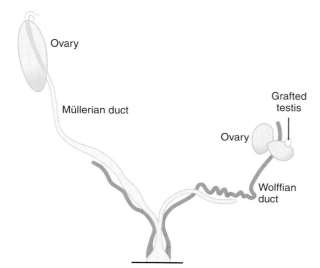

Figure 16-1. *Alfred Jost's classic experiment defined the current paradigm of sex development by grafting testicular tissue to the right ovary of a rabbit fetus. The testis was able to stimulate the wolffian duct and inhibit müllerian development, but the effect was only ipsliateral to the grafted testes. (From Embryonic and fetal development. In Austin C, Short RV [eds]. Reproduction in Mammals, Book 2. New York, Cambridge University Press, 1972, p 58.)*

increase in transcript, consistent with the earliest known divergence of male and female gonadal development. Furthermore, XX mice transgenic for the 14-kb fragment containing *Sry* developed testes and the full male phenotype. This work was followed with experiments showing that deletions and mutations in *SRY/Sry* result in XY sex reversal in both humans and mice.[13-15]

In humans, 8 weeks after conception, the biopotential gonad progresses toward testis organogenesis in the presence of *SRY* and can be recognized on ultrasound by week 10.[16-19] *SRY* expression in the Sertoli cell precursors initiates testes determination by activating downstream effectors, such as *SOX9* (SRY-related HMG-box 9). Sertoli cell proliferation and organization into tubular cords is directed by *SOX9* (SRY-related HMG-box 9) and *SF1* (steroidogenic factor-1; NR5A1). At 9 weeks of gestation, after the organization of discrete tubules, Sertoli cells begin the secretion of AMH.[20,21] Other genes involved in sex determination are *DAX-1*, in which a single copy is required for testes development; however, the presence of two copies in XY fetuses results in XY gonadal dysgenesis by repressing testis organogenesis.[22] Another gene involved in sex determination is *desert hedgehog* (*DHH*), which up-regulates SF1,which in turn regulates Leydig cell proliferation.[23,24]

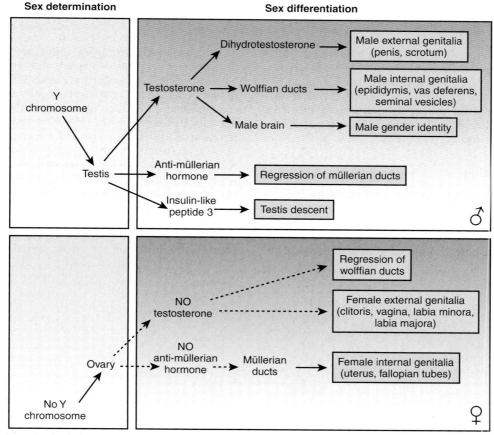

Figure 16-2. *Sex determination is the process by which genetic sex (presence or absence of the Y chromosome) results in gonadal sex. Sex determination refers to the development of internal and external genitalia directed by the presence or absence of testicular tissue. In XY males, sex differentiation is an active process requiring testis-derived hormones, testosterone, anti-müllerian hormone, and insulin-3. In XX females, sex differentiation is a default pathway that occurs in the absence of testis-derived hormones.*

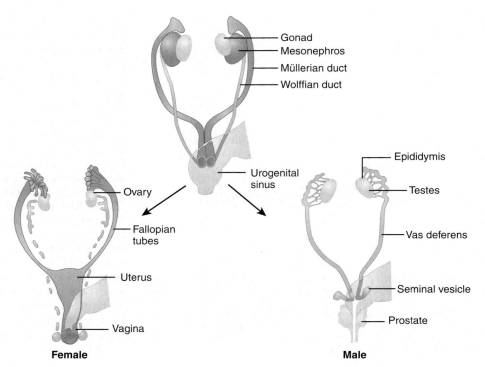

Figure 16-3. *Internal genital development of the male and female ductal systems. (Courtesy of Dr. J. Wilson, University of Texas, Southwestern Medical School, Dallas, TX.)*

Relative to testis organogenesis, there is much less information on the genes involved in ovary organogenesis. Studies suggesting that ovary development does not require a large number of genes are incomplete in that they look at time points that are important in testis determination, but may not be critical in ovarian determination.[25,26] Despite this, researchers have uncovered several autosomal genes required for proper ovarian development, including *WNT-4* (wingless-related MMTV integration site 4), *RSPONDIN-1,* and *FOLLISTATIN.*[27]

Sex Differentiation

The type of internal and external genitalia is decided by the presence of a viable testis. Therefore, the testis actively governs *sexual differentiation.* Conversely, the growth of female genitalia is the default process in sexual differentiation. The biopotential ductal system consists of the paramesonephric (müllerian) and wolffian ducts that give rise to female and male internal genitalia, respectively (Fig. 16-3).

Hormones secreted from testes are essential to the development of male internal and external genitalia. Normally developed testes have both Sertoli cells and testicular cords. Sertoli cells secrete AMH, causing müllerian (paramesonephric) duct regression. At the same time, Leydig cells, the steroidogenic cells of the testes, secrete testosterone and insulin-like peptide 3, to promote development of wolffian structures (epididymis, vas deferens, and seminal vesicles) and mediate transabdominal descent of the testes to the internal inguinal ring, respectively.[28] To mediate the development of the male external genitalia, testosterone is converted into 5α-dihydrotestosterone (DHT), a more potent androgen, by the enzyme 5α-reductase (Fig. 16-4). Except for phallic growth and inguinoscrotal descent in the third trimester, male sexual differentiation is

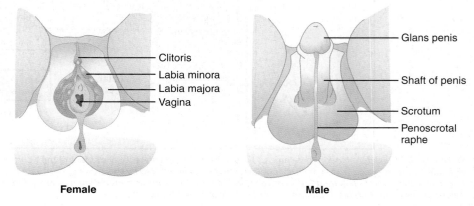

Figure 16-4. *External genital development, demonstrating homologies and common anlagen in males and females. (Courtesy of Dr. J. Wilson, University of Texas, Southwestern Medical School, Dallas, TX.)*

essentially complete. Defects in labioscrotal fusion and urogenital sinus growth cannot be modified by high doses of androgens after week 14 of gestation.

In females, the absence of testicular tissue and its associated hormones, such as AMH or testosterone, results in müllerian structure development (fallopian tubes, uterus, and upper vagina) and wolffian duct regression, at approximately 12 weeks of gestation. Additionally, the lack of DHT results in no further virilization of external genitalia.

Disorders that can cause ambiguous genitalia but are not associated with dysgenic gonads (e.g., complete androgen insensitivity syndrome, partial androgen insensitivity syndrome, congenital adrenal hyperplasia) are considered disorders of sexual differentiation, not disorders of sex determination. Overview of the diagnostic differences in DSDs, including disorders of sex determination and disorders of sex differentiation, are presented in Table 16-3.

SEX CHROMOSOME DISORDERS OF SEX DEVELOPMENT

Sex chromosome DSDs are defined by aneuploidy of the sex chromosomes X and Y. In disorders of autosomal aneuploidy (i.e., trisomy 21), maternal errors in meiotic nondisjunction account for the majority of cases. However, paternal errors in meiosis are the etiology of sex chromosome aneuploidy of sex chromosomes.

Turner Syndrome

In 1938, Turner described a group of females with short stature, primary amenorrhea, and a lack of secondary sex characteristics. Turner syndrome is classified as a sex chromosome DSD, with the majority having a 45,X karyotype and the remaining patients having a 46,XX karyotype, with a deletion in part of one X chromosome, or having various mosaics involving 45,X and 46,XX, and 46,XY cells or more complex combinations. In 100% of patients with 45,X and 80% of patients with a mosaic variant, the universal feature is short stature (Fig. 16-5). Patients are usually less than 58 inches tall. The genetic locus for short stature in both Turner syndrome and idiopathic short stature lies in the pseudoautosomal region (PAR1) of the X chromosome. This region is deleted in individuals with short stature caused by the lack of one copy of the homeobox gene *SHOX*.

The classic Turner 45,X karyotype is believed to be one of the most common human chromosomal abnormalities and is estimated to occur in 0.8% of all zygotes. However, fewer than 3% of these zygotes survive to term, and this karyotype is commonly found in spontaneous abortions.[29] The incidence of 45,X karyotypes is approximately 1:2000 live newborn phenotypic females.[30]

The gonads of females with Turner syndrome do not develop normally and have reduced follicle formation and growth in utero.[31] A normal number of eggs develop in girls with Turner syndrome, but for unknown reasons, they disappear prematurely.[32] Interestingly, the gonads appear as streaks of white tissue next to the fallopian tubes—called "streak gonads." Histologic examination shows primitive connective tissue stroma without primary follicles. Patients with Turner syndrome have fewer follicles and therefore less estrogen secretion from granulosa cells than normal females, resulting in delayed puberty.

Presentation and Diagnosis. In the prenatal period, fetuses with 45,X DSD and its variants frequently have intrauterine growth restriction. Turner syndrome should be suspected if large septate cystic hygromas, nuchal thickening, short femur, total body lymphangiectasia, or cardiac defects are detected by ultrasound. At birth, infants with Turner syndrome often have low birth weight; 30% of infants present with lymphedema of the upper and lower extremities (Fig. 16-6), an extension of the lymphangiectasias in utero, which disappears in the first few months of life. Additionally, 45,XX DSD should be suspected in patients with a webbed neck (pterygium colli; see Fig. 16-5) and dysmorphic features, including high arched palate, low-set prominent ears, low posterior hairline, epicanthal folds, micrognatia, hypoplastic nail beds, or hypoplastic fourth and fifth metacarpals at birth.[33] Patients with Turner syndrome may have increased carrying angle of the arms (cubitus valgus), a shield-like chest with wide-set nipples, hearing loss, and a higher frequency of cardiovascular disease, such as coarctation of the aorta. Furthermore, the incidence of renal anomalies is between 30% and 50%, with the most common being a horseshoe kidney, followed by abnormal vasculature.

During adolescence, the most common presentation is short stature, amenorrhea, and lack of secondary sex characteristics. Patients may also have any of the other characteristics mentioned earlier. Patients with 45,X DSD have normal intelligence. Depending on the degree of gonadal dysgenesis, up to 30% of patients with Turner syndrome undergo some degree of spontaneous puberty.[34]

Diagnosis is made by karyotype, which shows a 45,X or mosaic variant of cells. If the karyotype appears normal, but the presentation is suggestive of Turner syndrome, fluorescence in situ hybridization (FISH) or comparative genomic hybridization (CGH) study should be done because there may be a cryptic deletion in the pseudoautosomal region in one of the X chromosomes. Typically, patients with 45,X or 46,XX with a chromosomal abnormality in one X chromosome have more prominent phenotypic features than those with a mosaic variant.

Management. For most patients with 45,X DSD, the greatest concern is for short stature and secondary sex development. The treatment of both of these should be carefully titrated. For cases diagnosed in childhood, the use of low-dose anabolic steroid, coupled with growth hormone, has been shown to increase final adult height, with increased beneficial effects compared with those who started therapy late.[35-37] At the onset of the age of puberty, high-dose estrogen and progesterone should be given to promote the development of secondary sex characteristics. Estrogens and progesterone should be taken throughout life to prevent complications, such as osteoporosis.[38]

In young patients diagnosed with Turner syndrome, spontaneous puberty is a good indicator of the presence of ovarian tissue. Overall, it is estimated that 2% to 5% of

TABLE 16-3

Syndromes Associated with Disorders of Sex Development (DSD)

Syndromes Associated with Ambiguous Genitalia	Phenotype	Gene	Locus	OMIM #
Syndromes Associated with Gonadal Dysgenesis (GD)				
Denys-Drash	Diffuse mesangial sclerosis of kidneys in infancy, Wilms' tumor, XY gonadal dysgenesis	WT-1	11p13	194080
Frasier	Focal segmental glomerulosclerosis in adolescence, gonadoblastoma, XY gonadal dysgenesis	WT-1	11p13	136680
Camptomelic dysplasia	Congenital bowing of long bones, hypoplastic scapulae, hypoplastic pedicles of thoracic vertebrae, variable genitalia	SOX9	17q24.3-q25.1	114290
GD with neuropathy	XY gonadal dysgenesis with associated minifascicular neuropathy (1 of 4 cases)	DHH	12q12-13.1	607080
X-linked alpha-thalassemia/mental retardation	Hemoglobin H disease, mental retardation, dysmorphic facies, genital abnormalities	XH2	Xq13.3	301040
Palmoplantar hyperkeratosis with squamous cell carcinoma and XX sex reversal	Variable degrees of XX sex reversal, with palmoplantar keratosis and squamous cell carcinoma	RSPO1	1p34.3	610644
Blepharophimosis-ptosis-epicanthus inversus syndrome type I	Blepharophimosis, ptosis, epicanthus inversus syndrome, either with or without premature ovarian failure	FOXL2	3q23	110100
Syndromes Associated with Small Penis or Cryptorchidism				
VACTERL/VATER	Vertebral defects, anal atresia, tracheo-esophageal fistula with esophageal atresia, radial dysplasia, limb anomalies	Unknown	10q23	192350
Goldenhar syndrome (hemifacial microsomia)	Unilateral deformity of the external ear and small ipsilateral half of the face, with epibulbar dermoid, vertebral anomalies, and congenital cardiac anomalies	Unknown	14q32	164210
Smith Lemli Opitz syndrome	Multiple congenital malformations, mental retardation syndrome	DHCR7	11q12-q13	270400
Pallister Hall syndrome	Hypothalamic hamartoblastoma, postaxial polydactyly, imperforate anus	GLI3	7p13	146510
Robinow syndrome	Mesomelic limb shortening associated with facial and genital abnormalities	ROR2	9q22	180700
Prader Willi syndrome	Obesity, muscular hypotonia, mental retardation, short stature, hypogonadotropic hypogonadism	SNRPN	15q12, 15q11-q13	17620
Kallmann syndrome	Hypogonadotropic hypogonadism, anosmia	FGFR-1	8p11.2-p11.1	147950
Holoprosencephaly	Craniofacial dysmorphology	Many	21q22.3, 2q37.1-q37.3	236100
Malpeuch facial clefting syndrome	Short stature, hypertelorism, eye anomalies, facial clefting, hearing loss, urogenital abnormalities, mental retardation	Unknown	Unknown	248340
Najjar syndrome	Genital anomaly, mental retardation, cardiomyopathy	Unknown	Unknown	212120
Varadi-Papp syndrome	Big toes, hexadactyly, cleft lip/palate or lingual nodule, somatic and psychomotor retardation; some show absent olfactory bulbs and tracts, cryptorchidism	Unknown	Unknown	277170
Juberg-Marsidi syndrome	Cleft lip/palate, with abnormal thumbs and microcephaly	Unknown	Unknown	216100
Johanson-Blizzard syndrome	Aplasia or hypoplasia of the nasal alae, congenital deafness, hypothyroidism, postnatal growth retardation, malabsorption, mental retardation, midline ectodermal scalp defects, absent permanent teeth	Unknown	15q15-q21.1	243800

Continued

TABLE 16-3

Syndromes Associated with Disorders of Sex Development (DSD)—continued

Syndromes Associated with Ambiguous Genitalia	Phenotype	Gene	Locus	OMIM #
Borjeson-Forssman-Lehmann syndrome	Severe mental defect, epilepsy, hypogonadism, hypometabolism, marked obesity	Unknown	Xq26.3	301900
Torticollis, keloids, cryptorchidism, renal dysplasia	Torticollis, keloids, cryptorchidism, renal dysplasia	Unknown	Xq28	314300
Hypertelorism with esophageal abnormality and hypospadias	Laryngotracheoesophageal cleft; clefts of lip, palate, and uvula; difficulty swallowing, hoarse cry; genitourinary defects, mental retardation; congenital heart defects	Unknown	22q11.2	145410
Faciogenitopopliteal syndrome	Cleft palate, webbing of the intercrural pterygium	Unknown	1q32-q41	119500
Dubowitz syndrome	Short stature, microcephaly, mild mental retardation with behavior problems, eczema, distinctive facies	Unknown	Unknown	223370
Noonan syndrome	Hypertelorism, downward eye slant, low-set, posteriorly rotated ears; short stature; webbed neck; cardiac anomalies	PTPN11	12q24.1	163950
Aarskog syndrome (faciogenital dysplasia)	Embryonic ocular hypertelorism, anteverted nostrils, broad upper lip, peculiar penoscrotal relation	FGD1	Xp11.21	305400
Cornelia de Lange syndrome	Low anterior hairline, anteverted nares, maxillary prognathism, long philtrum, "carp" mouth) in association with prenatal and postnatal growth retardation, mental retardation	NIPBL	5p13.1	122470
Rubinstein-Taybi syndrome	Mental retardation, broad thumbs and toes, facial abnormalities	CREBBP	16p13.3, 22q13	180849
Seckel syndrome	Growth retardation, microcephaly with mental retardation, a characteristic "bird-headed" facial appearance.	SCKL1	3q22-q24	210600
Miller Dieker syndrome	Microcephaly, a thickened cortex with 4-6 layers	LIS1	17p13.3	247200
Lenz-Majewski hyperostosis syndrome	High palate; short, yellow, carious teeth; progeroid appearance; short stature; increased venous pattern of the forehead and thorax	Unknown	Unknown	151050
Lowe syndrome	Ophthalmia, cataract, mental retardation, vitamin D–resistant rickets, amino aciduria	OCRL1	Xq26.1	309000
Syndromes Associated with Müllerian Malformations				
MURCS association	Müllerian duct aplasia, renal aplasia, cervicothoracic somite dysplasia	Unknown	Unknown	601076
Mayer-Rokitansky-Kuster-Hauser syndrome	Müllerian duct aplasia	WNT4 (in subset with hyperandrogenism)	Unknown, 1p35	277000
McKusick Kaufman syndrome	Hydrometrocolpos, congenital heart malformations, postaxial polydactyly	Unknown	20p12	236700

OMIM, Online Mendelian Inheritance in Man.

patients with Turner syndrome have the potential for spontaneous pregnancy.[39]

Klinefelter Syndrome

In utero, the XXY fetal testis has the normal complement of primordial germ cells in the XXY testes. However, these germ cells degenerate during childhood, most likely due to a defect in Sertoli cell and germ cell communication during testes maturation.[40] In theory, the etiology of the nondisjunction in Klinefelter syndrome can be maternal meiosis I or II or paternal meiosis II; therefore, each situation should contribute 33% of cases. However, nearly 50% of cases of Klinefelter syndrome show a paternal origin,[41] with some studies showing increased frequency of XY sperm with advanced paternal age.[42]

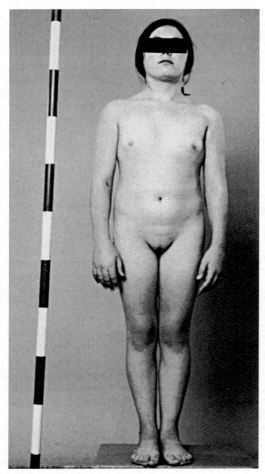

Figure 16-5. Patient with Turner syndrome. Note the short stature, webbed neck, and lack of secondary sex development.

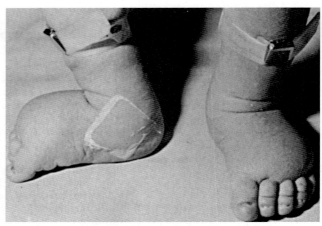

Figure 16-6. Lymphedema in the lower extremities of an infant with Turner syndrome.

Presentation and Diagnosis. Klinefelter syndrome is largely undiagnosed in the general population.[43] In early life, Klinefelter syndrome may be diagnosed in boys with behavioral disorders, abnormally small testes, and long legs (Fig. 16-7). The presence of long lower extremities with normal upper extremities distinguishes Klinefelter syndrome from the other forms of eunuchoidism that result in equally long upper and lower extremities. In patients with Klinefelter syndrome, IQ typically falls within the normal range; however, it tends to be below that of other siblings. Most patients present in adolescence with small, firm testes and hypogonadism, with varying degrees of androgen deficiency.[44] In later life, many men present at infertility centers with azoospermia.

Diagnosis of Klinefelter syndrome is performed by karyotype of lymphocytes. Some mosaic cases are detected only by karyotype of skin fibroblasts and occasionally of testicular biopsy specimens.

Management. Early detection of Klinefelter syndrome allows for early intervention for cognitive and behavioral disorders. Current studies are exploring the role of androgen replacement therapy in childhood, to help with cognitive and behavioral disabilities. Replacement of androgens

allows for development of masculine secondary sex characteristics, improved self-esteem, and increased libido, strength, and bone mineral density.[45] With regard to fertility, testicular mosaicism is an important factor in determining spermatogenesis and the potential for fertility. The vast majority of 47,XXY patients are azoospermic, but since the advent of intracytoplasmic sperm injection technology, they have the potential to be fertile. It should be noted that there is a higher rate of sex chromosomal hyperploidy and autosomal aneupoloidy[46] in the sperm of patients with Klinefelter syndrome. However the risk of passing sex chromosome aneuploidy to the offspring remains unclear. Regardless, preimplantation genetic diagnosis or fetal karyotype should be implemented to prevent chromosomal abnormalities in the progeny. Using testicular sperm extraction technology, sperm can be successfully extracted from the testes[47] and injected into a donor oocyte.

46,XY Disorders of Sex Development

46,XY DISORDERS OF GONADAL DETERMINATION

46,XY Gonadal Dysgenesis

Etiology and Pathophysiology of Pure/Complete Gonadal Dysgenesis. XY gonadal dysgenesis (GD) is a result of abnormal testis development in utero. There are three types of GD, pure (or complete), partial, and mixed, all of which can be differentiated by the extent of normal testicular tissue within the gonad and the karyotype of the individual. In pure/complete GD, individuals have intra-abdominal bilateral fibrous streaks that do not secrete AMH or testosterone. Phenotypically, pure XY GD individuals are unambiguously phenotypic females (previously known as *Swyer syndrome*), but usually possess internally hypoplastic müllerian structures.

Given the primary importance of *SRY* in human testes determination, it is surprising that mutations in *SRY* account for only approximately 15% of cases of pure XY

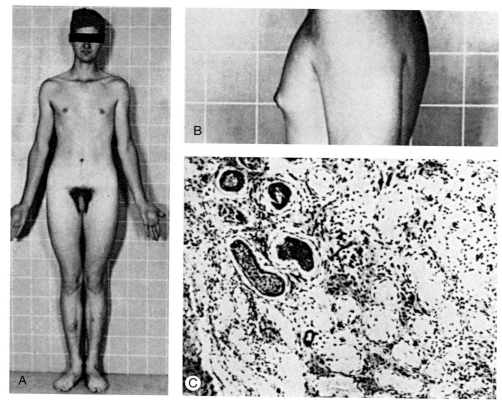

Figure 16-7. *Klinefelter syndrome.* **A,** *Phenotypic male with XXY. Note the long lower extremities compared with the upper extremities.* **B,** *XXY patient with gynecomastia.* **C,** *Testicular biopsy of the patient shown in* **B.** *Note the marked hyalinization of the seminiferous tubules and Leydig cell hyperplasia. (From Gumbach MM, Conte FA. Disorders of sex differentiation. In Wilson JS, Foster DW, Kronenberg HM, Larsen PR [eds]. Williams Textbook of Endocrinology. Philadelphia, WB Saunders, 1998, p 1368.)*

GD.[15,48-50] This suggests the existence of many other genes involved in primary human sex determination. SRY is a transcription factor, but its mechanism of action remains poorly understood. For instance, it is still unclear whether it acts as an activator or a repressor[51] and which genes are downstream targets. The most direct target for Sry is Sox9, another transcription factor from the Sox (Sry-box) family of genes. To date, there are 50 verified mutations within the *SRY* gene. Mutations that result in streak gonads primarily occur within the high-mobility group (HMG) box. These mutations cause reduced DNA binding,[50] alter DNA binding,[52] or prevent nuclear import of the *SRY* protein.[53] There are more than 50 known mutations of the *SRY* open reading frame (ORF). Larger cytogenetic deletions of Yp, which include *SRY*, have also been implicated in XY GD.[48,49,54]

Steroidogenic factor 1 (SF1) is an orphan nuclear receptor (NR5A1) that is necessary for adrenal and testicular development. Interactions between SF1 and the transcription factors GATA-4 and FOG2 appear to be necessary for SRY expression in developing testes.[55,56] Recent studies have underlined the importance of SF1 in testicular development because nearly 15% of isolated cases of XY GD can be attributed to SF1 haploinsufficiency.[57] However, in three cases, SF1 mutations have been reported with XY GD and adrenal hypoplasia congenita, which reflects the role of SF1 in adrenal development. Together, mutations or deletions of *SRY* and SF1 account for 30% of cases of XY

GD, indicating that other genes critical to testes determination cascade remain to be discovered.

Mutations in genes involved in testis sex determination (*XH2, SOX9, WT-1, DHH*) and duplications of putative "anti-testis" genes (*WNT-4, DAX1*) are responsible for a small minority of cases of XY GD,[58-60] but are usually associated with other syndromic features, which are outlined in Table 16-3.

Etiology and Pathophysiology of Partial or Mixed Gonadal Dysgenesis. As with many developmental disorders, with GD, there is a wide range in phenotypic variability. When testis dysgenesis does not involve the entirety of both gonads and the phenotype is unambiguous rather than female, the condition is called "partial" GD. The internal genitalia show varying degrees of wolffian and müllerian development and genital ambiguity, corresponding to the percentage of the gonads that is dysgenic, or "streak." The medical literature is often confusing in regard to the difference between "partial" and "mixed" GD, and the terms are often used interchangeably. *Partial XY GD* refers to intermediate stages of dysgenic testes, between streak gonads and normal testes, and patients usually have a 46,XY nonmosaic karyotype. However, *mixed 46,XY GD* typically refers to a situation in which one gonad is a streak gonad, whereas the opposite gonad is partially dysgenic or is even a normal testis. Mosaicism for 45,X/46,XY is the most frequent cause of mixed GD, although a minority of patients have a 46,Xi(Yq) karyotype.[7] The evidence of the variable phenotypic spectrum of individuals with 45,X/46,XY mosaicism was reported in a series of 10 45,X/46,XY patients, of whom 4 individuals were undervirilized males with bilateral testes, 3 were diagnosed with mixed GD and genital ambiguity, and 3 were diagnosed with Turner syndrome.[61] Although not proven, there is preliminary evidence that the percentage of normal testicular tissue and phenotypic maleness is correlated with an increase in the proportion of gonadal Y chromosome.[62,63]

Familial cases of pure and partial 46,XY, GD have been reported.[50,64-66] In some of these cases, *SRY* mutations present with phenotypic variability, in which the father and male relatives are phenotypically normal and fertile and their XY offspring have GD.[50,64] Additionally, there are cases of fathers with mosaic mutant and normal *SRY* transmitting the mutation to their XY daughters.[67,68] Presumably, the normal father's mosaicism reflects a postzygotic mutation event. From these cases, it is clear that autosomal genetic modifiers influence the sex determination cascade. These unique cases provide more hints about the molecular basis of sex determination. This is particularly relevant because the genetic cause of 70% of cases of 46,XY GD is unknown.

Presentation and Diagnosis of Gonadal Dysgenesis.
Pure XY GD presents as a phenotypic female with normal or tall stature, bilateral streak gonads, delayed puberty, amenorrhea, and small or normal müllerian structures, with no signs of Turner syndrome. If they are not diagnosed at birth (e.g., when the in utero karyotype does not match the phenotypic sex at birth), most patients are diagnosed during adolescence due to pubertal delay and primary amenorrhea. Patients rarely present with an abdominal or pelvic mass, which often is a gonadoblastoma. Occasionally, XY GD can be part of a constellation of other symptoms that are outlined in Table 16-3.

Individuals with partial or mixed 46,XY GD typically present at birth with varying degrees of masculinization of the external and internal genitalia. Depending on the percentage of testicular tissue, dysgenetic testes can be found anywhere along the line of testis descent, from the abdomen, and in cases of normal testes, in the scrotum. However, the streak gonad in mixed 46,XY GD is always abdominally located. Patients with partial 46,XY GD usually have female external genitalia, with some degree of virilization, such as clitoromegaly or a bifid scrotum (see Fig. 16-8). The uterus and fallopian tubes are usually well formed, but occasionally may be hypoplastic. In mixed GD, the development of wolffian and müllerian structures, as well as the virilization of external genitalia, correlates with the degree of development of the ipsilateral testis, resulting in asymmetric virilization of the external or internal genitalia and unilateral cryptorchidism. Pelvic ultrasound often can detect the presence of absence of male or female internal genitalia, and in the case of mixed XY GD, asymmetry in the development of the müllerian and wolffian structures. There are rare reported cases of patients presenting with premature adrenarche in an otherwise unambiguous female, due to a testosterone-producing gonadal tumor.[69]

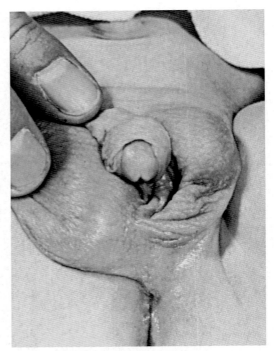

Figure 16-8. *External genitalia of an infant with XO/XY mosaicism. Note the enlarged phallus, labioscrotal fusion, and gonadal bulges (histologically, testes) in the labioscrotum.*

Isolated 46,XY pure GD is considered in an adolescent with primary amenorrhea and sexual immaturity with a full female external phenotype, whereas partial or mixed GD should be considered more likely in the differential diagnosis of a 46,XY patient with ambiguous genitalia. The biochemical changes in complete, partial, and mixed GD are outlined in Table 16-4.

The major criteria for the diagnosis of pure, partial, or mixed GD are the appearance and histologic features of both gonads. Therefore, the ultimate diagnosis of any type of GD, particularly the distinction between mixed and partial GD, requires biopsy of both gonads. Because the risk of gonadoblastoma in these patients is so high, precise diagnosis of the type of GD is usually determined after prophylactic or therapeutic gonadectomy. In pure 46,XY GD, both gonads are streak gonads. Partial GD is defined by bilateral dysgenetic gonads, whereas mixed GD typically has one streak gonad. Karyotype of peripheral leukocytes shows 46,XY in pure and partial GD and mosaic 45,X/46,XY is frequent in mixed GD. However, if there is a streak gonad on one side and a normal testis contralaterally, but the peripheral karyotype is 46,XY, cryptic mosaicism is often found within the gonad.

Once a presumptive diagnosis is made in 46,XY patients, FISH for *SRY* or for Yp can be performed. Only a minority of cases of XY GD can be explained by complete or partial *SRY* deletion or mutation, or *SF1* mutation. The majority of patients are 46,XY and positive for *SRY* and *SF1*. Sequencing of *SRY* or *SF1* ORF for mutations is positive in up to 30% of cases of 46,XY pure GD.[49,50,57,70] Certain isolated and syndromic forms of XY GD can be diagnosed molecularly with cytogenetics, comparative

TABLE 16-4

Diagnostic Criteria for Disorders of Sex Development

DSD	Biochemical Changes	Differentiating Features	Major Diagnostic Criteria
46,XY Disorders of Gonadal Development			
46,XY pure/partial/ mixed GD	Pure/partial/mixed ↑ FSH, LH Nml to ↓ AMH No ↑ with hCG Nml adrenal hormones and precursors Pure ↓↓; T, DHT, E$_2$ ↓↓ AMH Partial/mixed ↓ T, DHT, E$_2$	Presence of partial testicular function (T, AMH) points toward partial or mixed GD. However, histologic examination of the testes after prophylactic gonadectomy can differentiate among pure, partial, and mixed GD. There is little genotype-phenotype correlation; however, the presence of mosaicism 45,X/46,XY is often associated with mixed GD.	Sequencing for *SF1* and *SRY* mutations, if no mutation is found If partial/mixed GD is suspected, patient should be tested for mosaicism. CGH should be performed to look for copy number variants as a source for XY GD.
Testicular regression	↑ FSH, LH ↓↓ T, DHT, E$_2$ ↓↓ AMH No hCG response	Complete absence of gonad or fibrosis of gonad (as opposed to streak of dysgenic testes in patients with GD). Completely virilized male phenotype	Fibrous nodules on laporoscopic examination (not streak of dysgenic testes)
Disorders of Sex Differentiation: Disorders of Androgen Synthesis and Action			
StAR deficiency; P450scc deficiency	↑ Renin ↓ Aldo ↑ K ↓ Na ↓ All adrenal hormones ↓ 17-OHProg	Histologic presence of lipid vacuoles in adrenals. P450scc deficiency presents with enlarged adrenals. No HTN and hyperkalemia differentiates from CYP17 deficiency	Histologic presence of lipid-filled vacuoles; sequencing of a mutation of the StAR or *CYP11A1* gene gives definitive diagnosis.
3βHSD type II	↑ Renin ↓ Aldo, F ↑ K ↓ Na ↑ Ratio 17-OHProg: cortisol ↓ A4, T	Baseline and ACTH-stimulated ratios of 17-hydroxypregnenolone: cortisol consistently distinguished between affected and non-affected patients	Sequencing of the *HSD3B2* gene
17α-hydroxylase/ 17,20-lyase	↓ Renin ↓ Aldo, F ↓ 17-OHP ↑ LH, FSH ↑ Progesterone, DOC, B ↑ Na ↓ K ↓ DHEA-S, A4, T; no response to hCG stimulation	HTN and hypokalemic alkalosis in the presence of low 17-hydroxyprogesterone	Sequencing for mutations of the *CYP17* gene
P450 oxido-reductase	↑ 17-OHProg ↑ Progesterone ↓ F, DHEA-S ↓ A4, T	HTN in the presence of elevated 17-hydroxyprogesterone (differentiates from CYP17 deficiency) sometimes Antley-Bixler skeletal malformations are present.	Sequencing for *CYP450 oxidoreductase*
17βHSD type 3	Nml to +A4 ↑ Ratio A4/T (>15) ↓ T, DHT	Differentiated from 5α-reductase type 2 by levels and ratios of serum hormones	Sequencing of the *HSD17B1* gene for deletions, insertions, and point mutations
Leydig cell hypoplasia	↑ LH Nml FSH ↑ AMH ↓ T, DHT, E$_2$ ↓ hCG response Nml A4/T ratio	To differentiate LCH from GD, AMH is used as a marker of testicular function.	Sequencing of the *LHCGR* gene for deletions, insertions, and point mutations
5α-reductase type 2	Nml FSH, LH Nml T, E$_2$ ↓ DHT ↑ Ratio T/DHT (>30)	Development of male secondary sex characteristics in puberty, with fine and sparse facial hair. These can be differentiated clinically from 17βHSD and AIS by the lack of gynecomastia during puberty.	Sequencing of *SRD5A2*
Androgen receptor	Nml FSH, LH (PAIS) ↓ FSH, LH (CAIS) Nml to ↑ AMH Nml A4, T, DHT ↑↑ hCG response	Female phenotype with breast development at puberty, with sparse pubic and axillary hair	Sequencing of the *AR* gene looking for single–amino acid substitutions, which account for 90% of reported cases

Continued

TABLE 16-4

Diagnostic Criteria for Disorders of Sex Development—continued

DSD	Biochemical Changes	Differentiating Features	Major Diagnostic Criteria
AMH/AMHR	Nml hormonal profile	Presence of both müllerian and wolffian derivatives, usually discovered incidentally	
46,XX Disorders of Sex Determination			
XX Testicular/ovo-testicular DSD	↑ FSH, LH ↓ T, DHT Nml AMH No ↑ with hCG	The only way to differentiate between 46,XX testicular and ovotesticular DSD is by complete gonadal histologic examination looking for ovarian tissue.	Testicular DSD: FISH for *SRY* or *SOX9* or if the clinical phenotype is appropriate, sequence the *RSPO1* gene. If no molecular diagnostic test is successful, CGH should be performed. Ovotesticular DSD: Search for XX/XY mosaicism (30% to 33% ovotesticular DSD) and sequencing for *SRY* (7% to 10% of ovotesticular DSD).
XX GD	↑ FSH, LH No ↑ with hCG No AMH	Full female phenotype with amenorrhea and lack of secondary sex development	Isolated 46,XX GD: Sequencing for *FSH* mutations can be performed. If the clinical presentation matches, sequence the *FOXL2* mutation. CGH can also be done to identify delirious duplications or mutations.
Disorders of Androgen Excess			
21α-hydroxylase (CYP21)	↑ Renin ↓ Aldo, DOC, cortisol ↑ K ↓ Na ↑ 17-OHProg ↑ DHEA-S, A4, T	17-OHProg elevated in the absence of HTN, which is typical in 11βHSD1 deficiency	Sequencing of *CYP21* gene gives a definitive diagnosis. Knowledge of the mutation can inform parents about genetic counseling and fetal diagnosis to prevent adverse effects of hyperandrogenism in utero.
11β-Dehydrogenase (CYP11B1)	↓ Aldo, cortisol, Renin ↑ DOC ↑ K ↓ Na ↑ 17-OHProg ↑ DHEA-S, A4, T	Differentiate from CYP21 deficiency by hypertension and hypokalemic alkalosis.	Sequencing of *CYP11B1*.
P450 aromatase (CYP19A1)	↑ 16-OHAn (maternal) ↑ FSH, LH, A4, T ↓ Estrone, E_2	Presence of maternal virilization during pregnancy and XX virilization, which stops after delivery	Presence of maternal virilization during pregnancy and XX virilization, which stops after delivery. Sequencing of CYP19A1 gives a definitive diagnosis.

16-OHAn, 16-hydroxyandrostenedione; 17-OHPreg, 17-hydroxypregnenolone; 17-OHProg, 17-hydroxyprogesterone; A4, androstenedione; ACTH, adrenocorticotropic hormone; AIS, androgen insensitivity syndrome; Aldo, aldosterone; AMH, anti-müllerian hormone; AMHR, anti-müllerian hormone receptor; AR, androgen receptor; CAIS, complete androgen insensitivity syndrome; CGH, comparative genomic hybridization; DHEA, dehydroepiandrosterone; DHT, 5α-dehydrotestosterone; DOC, 11-deoxycorticosterone; DSD, disorder of sex development; E_2, estradiol; FISH, fluorescence in situ hybridization; FSH, follicle-stimulating hormone; GD, gonadal dysgenesis; hCG, human chorionic gonadotropin; HSD, hydroxysteroid dehydrogenase; HTN, hypertension; LCH, Leydig cell hypoplasia; LH, luteinizing hormone; LHCGR, luteinizing hormone chorionic gonadotropin receptor; Nml, normal; PAIS, partial androgen insensitivity syndrome; SF1, steroidogenic factor-1; StAR, steroidogenic acute regulatory; T, testosterone.

genomic hybridization, or sequencing of known genes (see Table 16-4).

If a mutation or translocation involving *SRY* is found, the father should be tested for a possible familial mutation because *SRY* mutations can result in a full spectrum of phenotypes, from 46,XY fertile males to ambiguous individuals to females with partial and pure GD. Due to potential autosomal modifiers, it is very difficult to predict the risk of recurrence of a GD phenotype in XY offspring.

Management of XY Gonadal Dysgenesis. The major concern in the treatment of patients with XY GD is the risk of gonadoblastoma, a mixed germ cell–sex cord tumor. The risk of gonadoblastoma formation in patients with XY GD increases with age and has been estimated to be as high as 30% by 30 years of age.[49,54,71,72] Due to the high risk of gonadoblastoma formation, patients should undergo prophylactic or therapeutic gonadectomy, preferably in the first decade of life. Patients are followed with regular ultrasound every 6 months, starting at age 2, until gonadectomy can be performed. With the advent of laparoscopic techniques, the invasiveness of these surgeries is decreasing and the results are improving.[72]

In patients with XY pure GD, genitals and gender identity are unambiguously female. There are no reported cases of gender dysphoria. In patients with partial or mixed GD, the degree of genital masculinization can be used for initial gender assignment. However, issues of gender identity arise in partial and mixed GD and are outlined later in the chapter.[73]

To complete secondary sex development, sex steroid replacement should be initiated at puberty. Sex steroid replacement is essential not only for the development of secondary sex characteristics, but also for the growth spurt and normal accrual of bone mineral density. Height, weight, and bone density should be monitored regularly. Furthermore, a DEXA scan for bone density should be performed before induction of puberty with exogenous hormone replacement, and yearly thereafter for the first 2 years. As long as the first three DEXA scans are reported as normal, they can be done every 2 to 3 years.

Because a normal uterus is often present, hysterectomies are not common to preserve childbearing potential with in vitro fertilization methods. Despite this, most patients do not carry successful pregnancies for unknown reasons.[7] Individuals with mixed XY GD with more masculinization of the external genitalia are often raised as males and consequently require lifetime testosterone administration, through intramuscular injections or transdermal patches or gel.

Testicular Regression Syndrome

In some cases, initial testicular development occurs normally, but there is an insult to the developing testes during sex differentiation, resulting in variable degrees of masculinization of the internal and external genitalia. Testicular regression syndrome (TRS) is distinct in that the insult occurs after initial testes determination.[74-76] Internal and external genitalia are variably developed, which presumably depends on when the loss of fetal testes occurred in

utero.[74,75,77,79] Rarely, patients can present in adulthood as females with primary amenorrhea.[77,78] Typically, however, TRS is characterized by primitive epididymis and spermatic cord in the presence of a fibrous nodule rather than streak, or dysgenetic, gonads.[75,76,79] The presence of spermatic cord structures, the absence of müllerian derivatives, and a normal male external phenotype suggest that viable testes existed early in development, and imply a late fetal or early neonatal regression. Diagnostic criteria are outlined in Table 16-4. In the literature, this variant is often called "vanishing testes."[76]

The incidence of TRS has been estimated at 5% of males presenting with cryptorchidism,[77] and as high as 12% of cryptorchid patients older than 1 year.[76,80] Correct diagnosis of TRS versus XY GD is essential because of the significant malignant potential of abdominal or dysgenic testes.

DISORDERS IN SEX DIFFERENTIATION: 46,XY DISORDERS OF ANDROGEN BIOSYNTHESIS AND ACTION

The occurrence of 46,XY DSD, with phenotypes ranging from full sex reversal to undervirilized XY males, can be a result of defects in steroidogenic enzymes (Fig. 16-9) or their receptor action. The biosynthesis of testosterone is essential for the development of secondary sex characteristics in XY individuals, including differentiation of wolffian structures, inguinoscrotal testes descent, and masculinization of external genitalia after conversion to DHT. Additionally, mutations in Sertoli cell products, such as anti-müllerian hormone or its respective receptor, can result in incomplete regression of female internal genitalia. Mutations in the synthesis and action of testosterone or upstream regulators of testosterone production can all cause incomplete virilization or müllerian regression in the XY male. However, in these individuals, the testes are of normal size.

Congenital Lipoid Adrenal Hyperplasia

Mutations in enzymes involved in the initial enzymatic regions of steroidogenesis, such as steroidogenic acute regulatory (StAR) protein and cytochrome P450 side chain cleavage P450scc (*CYP11A*),[81,82] result in global silencing of adrenal and gonadal steroidogenesis. The accumulation of cholesterol in the adrenals and gonads ultimately results in primary adrenal and gonadal failure.[83] StAR protein transports cholesterol across the inner and outer mitochondrial membranes of steroidogenic cells. P450scc catalyzes the initial reaction in all steroidogenic tissues, the conversion of cholesterol to pregnenolone (see Fig. 16-9).[84,85] On histologic examination, patients with mutations in StAR protein or P450scc have lipid vacuoles in the adrenals. However, patients with StAR protein mutations have adrenal hyperplasia, whereas the six patients with P450scc mutations did not exhibit adrenal enlargement.

Presentation and Diagnosis. Newborns with congenital lipoid adrenal hyperplasia typically present with a salt-wasting adrenal crisis at birth that is usually fatal if not

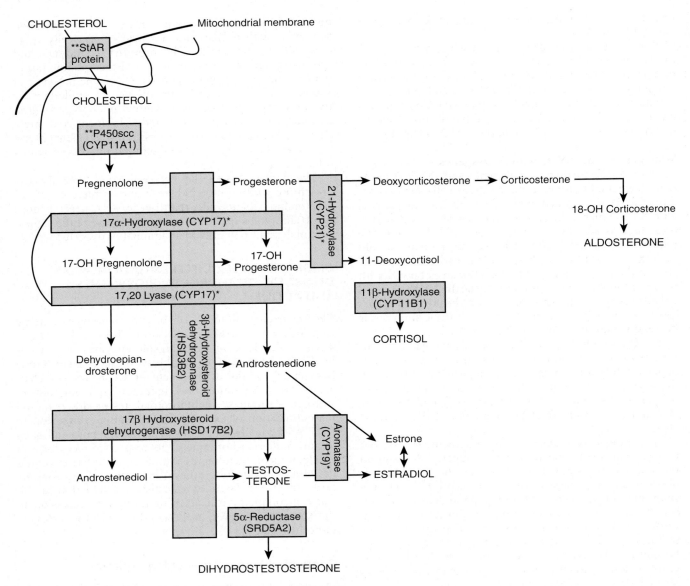

*P450 oxidoreductase deficiency results in partial activity of this enzyme.
**Both of these proteins result in congenital lipoid adrenal hyperplasia.

Figure 16-9. *Adrenal steroidogenesis pathways. Many disorders of sex differentiation are due to defects in steroidogenesis, with the majority of them occurring in the adrenal gland. StAR, steroidogenic acute regulatory.*

immediately diagnosed and treated; however, there are reports of delayed presentation. All XY patients present with a female phenotype, or in cases of partial defect, some degree of genital ambiguity. XX patients only exhibit the features of adrenal insufficiency at birth.

Usually, 46,XY patients have testes, no müllerian structures due to the presence of AMH, partial or absent wolffian derivates as a lack of testosterone biosynthesis, and a blind vaginal pouch. The spectrum of external genital phenotype ranges from female external genitalia to ambiguous genitals. Testes can be found in the abdomen, inguinal canal, or labia. Additionally, intrauterine glucocorticoid deficiency often results in elevated adrenocorticotropic hormone (ACTH) levels that manifest as generalized

hyperpigmentation at birth. Partial deficiency of StAR protein may result in 46,XX. Unlike 46,XY patients, 46,XX patients can experience spontaneous puberty, menarche, and anovulatory menses because their ovaries are able to produce estrogen through StAR-independent pathways.[83,86,87] Because the ovaries do not produce steroids until puberty, they are spared from the cholesterol-induced damage that occurs from birth in the adrenals.[86] However, at puberty, XX females have multiple cysts in their ovaries, possibly from anovulation.

Definitive diagnosis of congenital lipoid adrenal hyperplasia is done by sequencing of StAR or CYP11A1. Characteristic biochemical abnormalities are outlined in Table 16-4. Furthermore, adrenal enlargement has only been found in patients with StAR protein mutations and not in six patients with proven p450scc mutations.

Management. Patients should be given physiologic replacement doses of glucocorticoid and mineralocorticoids. Patients should be given sex hormones at the onset of puberty in concordance with phenotypic sex.

3β-Hydroxysteroid Dehydrogenase Deficiency

3β-Hydroxysteroid dehydrogenase deficiency is a rare variant of congenital adrenal hyperplasia that can have a wide range of phenotypes, ranging from the classic presentation (salt wasting, with a range of female external genitalia to ambiguous genitalia in genetic XY individuals) to nonclassic (no salt wasting and later presentation). Rare defects in adrenal and gonadal 3β-hydroxysteroid dehydrogenase (*HSD3B2* gene) affect the three major adrenal steroid hormones: cortisol, aldosterone, and testosterone synthesis. The resulting phenotype is adrenal insufficiency in XX and XY patients and genital ambiguity only in XY patients. 3βHSD2 is the enzyme responsible for the conversion of Δ^5 steroids (pregnenolone, 17-OH pregnenolone, DHEA) → Δ^4 steroids (progesterone, 17-OH progesterone, androstenedione) in all steroidogenic tissues, including the testes, ovaries, and adrenal glands (see Fig. 16-9).

17α-Hydroxylase/17,20-Lyase Deficiency

Biosynthesis of adrenal and sex hormones requires cytochrome P450 17α-hydroxylase/17,20-lyase (*CYP17* gene). Here, a single gene, *CYP17*, catalyzes two steps in the steroidogenic pathway that are essential for sex steroid and glucocorticoid synthesis. Mutations in this gene ultimately result in decreased cortisol synthesis, with shunting of steroidogenesis toward a mineralocorticoid precursor, Doc, that has mineralocorticoid activity (see Fig. 16-9).

Presentation and Diagnosis. Most patients present at puberty with primary amenorrhea, low-renin hypertension, and hypokalemia (due to elevated mineralocorticoids). This autosomal recessive disorder results in ambiguous genitalia only in 46,XY patients. 46,XY individuals have phenotypes ranging from female external genitalia, with no wolffian duct development, to ambiguous genitalia with partial development of the male ductal system, depending on the severity of the enzymatic defect. All patients show müllerian structure regression, due to the presence of functional Sertoli cells. In contrast to individuals with 3βHSD deficiency or lipoid congenital adrenal hyperplasia (CLAH), patients do not have adrenal crisis due to the presence of glucocorticoid precursors that maintain some activity.[88] Serum diagnostic criteria are outlined in Table 16-4. Some rare *CYP17* mutations cause isolated 17,20-lyase deficiency[89] that only affects sex steroid biosynthesis and results in variably feminized 46,XY individuals with normal levels of cortisol.

Management. Patients should be treated with physiologic levels of glucocorticoids and appropriate sex steroid replacement to develop secondary sex characteristics.

P450 Oxidoreductase Deficiency

Cytochrome P450 oxidoreductase (POR) deficiency is a recently characterized cause of congenital adrenal hyperplasia, which affects the enzymatic activity of all microsomal P450 enzymes, including the steroidogenic enzymes CYP17, CYP21, CYP19.[90-93] POR is a flavoprotein that is required for the action of all microsomal p450 enzymes. Unlike other genetic defects, which only affect one enzyme in the steroidogenesis pathway (see Fig. 16-9), POR causes partial enzymatic activity in multiple enzymes. Therefore, POR deficiency presents with a wide range of phenotypes and is particularly difficult to diagnose using serum hormone levels. Partial enzymatic deficiencies in 21α-hydroxylase account for the CAH phenotype and virilization in XX females, whereas partial 17α-hydroxylase deficiency accounts for undervirilization of XY individuals. Aromatase deficiency as a result of POR deficiency is believed to be the cause of virilization of mothers carrying fetuses with POR deficiency.

Presentation and Diagnosis. The unique pathophysiology of POR deficiency results in a wide phenotypic spectrum, in which patients present during the prenatal period as newborns with ambiguous genitalia, or as XX adolescents with amenorrhea and/or polycystic ovary syndrome. During prenatal screening, this diagnosis should be considered in the differential diagnosis of a virilized pregnant woman with low estriol levels, but normal ultrasound findings. Endocrine changes are shown in Table 16-4.

17β-Hydroxysteroid Dehydrogenase Deficiency

The 17β-HSD3 enzyme is a member of the 17β-HSD family, which catalyzes the conversion of androstendione (Δ^4A) to testosterone in the testes (see Fig. 16-9). The gene *HSD17B3* maps to chromosome 9q22 and is primarily expressed in the gonads, unlike other isoenzymes, which are expressed postnatally in peripheral tissues. This is a rare cause of 46,XY DSD, with only 10 reported cases in the United States.[94]

Presentation and Diagnosis. In XY individuals with female external genitalia, HSD17B3 deficiency may be difficult to recognize in infancy because patients manifest no other significant clinical problems and have near-normal laboratory values. However, depending on the degree of residual enzyme activity, HSD17B3 deficiency can cause a range of undervirilization of XY individuals at birth, from an empty bifid scrotum with perineoscrotal hypospadias to clitoromegaly and posterior labioscrotal fusion. Testes can be undescended or labial. Müllerian ducts are absent, but interestingly, wolffian ducts derivatives are present, despite the decreased testosterone production. During puberty, 46,XY patients may experience progressive adrenarche. Patients may experience increasing virilization, clitoral or phallic enlargement, muscle development, breast development, testicular descent, and plasma testosterone levels within the normal range of pubertal males.[94-96] To date, no affected 46,XX females have been reported. Biochemical changes in patients with mutations in *HSD17B3* are outlined in Table 16-4.

Management. XY patients are usually raised as females.[95,97] In one study, up to 40% of affected XY individuals who were raised as females successfully switched gender roles at puberty.[97] General management is discussed later.

Defects in 5α-ReductaseType 2

Steroid 5α-reductase deficiency (SRD5A2) results from a defect in the enzyme converting testosterone to DHT. DHT is responsible for the differentiation of male external genitalia (see Fig. 16-2). The peripheral conversion of testosterone to DHT is an irreversible reaction catalyzed by the two isoenzymes of 5α-reductase, SRD5A1 and SRD5A2. During puberty, the SRD5A1 isozyme is active in skin fibroblasts. During fetal development, the SRD5A2 isozyme is expressed in the genital skin tissue and male accessory sex organs. Consequently, inactivating mutations in SRD5A2 result in undermasculinized external genitalia (e.g., micropenis, perineal hypospadias). The internal genitalia show normally differentiated wolffian ducts, no müllerian structures, and a blind vaginal pouch.[98,99] Adrenal and gonadal biosynthesis remains normal.

Presentation and Diagnosis. In 46,XY infants with mutations in SRD5A2, the degree of ambiguity ranges from isolated hypospadias to severe undermasculinization, complete with perineal hypospadias, micropenis, bifid scrotum, and hypoplastic prostate.[100] At puberty, 46,XY patients experience a surge of testosterone, which can cause development of male secondary sex characteristics, such as male body habitus, deepening of the voice, and penile enlargement. However, these individuals have unusually fine upper lip hair. Due to the underdevelopment of the prostate and seminal vesicles, their semen is highly viscous and their ejaculate volume is extremely low (<0.5-1 mL). Despite the low ejaculate volume, sperm counts are normal. Patients who are unambiguously female at birth often present in puberty with amenorrhea, a deepening voice, clitoromegaly, and increased musculature. In contrast to patients with 17β-HSD3 deficiency and androgen insensitivity syndrome, those with mutations in 5RDA2 do not have gynecomastia during puberty. Females with 46,XX and SRD5A2 deficiency have normal sexual differentiation and fertility, but delayed puberty and sparse pubic hair.

Diagnosis of *SRD5A2* deficiency during early infancy and puberty can be made based on an elevated ratio of testosterone to DHT (normal < 30:1), with or without human chorionic gonadotropin (hCG) stimulation.[98,101] DHT is low in infants, but can reach near-normal levels during adolescence without treatment, presumably by peripheral SRD5A1 activity. If the diagnosis is suspected during prepubertal childhood or during adolescence, hCG stimulation is necessary to elicit the diagnostic hormone levels because the hypothalamo–pituitary–gonadal axis is inactive. Affected females, although phenotypically normal, have the same biochemical abnormalities (outlined in Table 16-4) as affected males.

Mutational analysis of the *SR5A2* gene can be performed, and mutations have been reported in all five exons. To date, more than 50 mutations in *SR5A2* have been found, ranging from point mutations to deletions, but genotype–phenotype correlations are poor.

Management. The autosomal recessive disorder SRD5A2 has been described in a number of consanguineous families in Turkey, New Guinea, Saudi Arabia, and the Dominican Republic. Many XY patients with this disorder are raised as female during childhood, but at the onset of puberty, identify with the male gender.[102-104] It is unclear why individuals with this disorder have a high prevalence of gender identity change. However, given the geographic clustering of this disorder, the gender switch may be attributed in part to cultural and societal beliefs. Topical application of DHT cream in the pubic area promotes phallic growth before puberty, and local application results in increases in both facial and body hair. Fertility is possible with surgical correction of the male ductal system or through assisted reproductive technology.

DEFECT IN ANDROGEN ACTIVITY

Complete and Partial Androgen Insensitivity Syndrome

In the presence of normal gonads and steroid biosynthesis, mutations in the steroid hormone receptors can mute the effects of circulating steroids on specific tissues. Mutations in the androgen receptor (AR), which is located on the X chromosome, result in androgen insensitivity syndrome (AIS). Both testosterone and DHT can activate the AR, and when the AR is bound to either steroid hormone, it has organizational within an organ and an activational role for specific genes. The AR plays important roles in the differentiation of male internal and external genitalia and in the maintenance of spermatogenesis. Currently, there is an estimated incidence of 1:20,400 liveborn XY individuals, in which more than 300 mutations have been identified.

In 46,XY individuals, AIS is characterized by a range of phenotypes, from unambiguous XY females, termed *complete AIS (CAIS)*, to phenotypic XY males. In CAIS, the only manifestation is infertility and amenorrhea, typically presenting in puberty.[105,106] At the other extreme is minimal AIS (MAIS), in which phenotypically male patients often present with infertility, gynecomastia, or hypospadias. Patients who exhibit various degrees of XY ambiguity are referred to as having *partial AIS (PAIS)*. All known forms of AIS are caused by disruption of AR activity. CAIS is generally associated with a complete absence of androgen binding and AR activation. Beyond this, there is almost no genotype–phenotype correlation between the percentage of residual AR activity and phenotype.[107] This suggests that there are other genetic modifiers that modulate the phenotype. Even within families, the phenotype resulting from the same mutation can vary between PAIS and CAIS.[108,109]

The majority of mutations resulting in AIS are caused by single–amino acid substitutions, which account for approximately 90% of cases. Mutations are spread throughout the gene, and there is no single mutation that appears to be prevalent over others.[110] Interestingly, exon 1 rarely possesses a causative mutation.[110] The majority of cases are inherited, but 30% of all cases are de novo mutations. Because de novo mutations originate in a single germ cell as a result of germ cell mosaicism, the risk of recurrence in future offspring is low.

In familial PAIS, and in both familial and sporadic types of CAIS, mutations in *AR* exonic sequences are found in 85% to 90% of cases.[109,110] In contrast, detectable mutations in *AR* account for only 10% to 15% of sporadic cases, with the hormonal profile and clinical presentation suggestive of de novo PAIS.[109] The molecular defect in these cases remains unknown. Although the genotypes causing CAIS are consistent in phenotypic presentation, in PAIS, there is phenotypic variability among affected individuals carrying the same mutation.

Presentation and Diagnosis.   The phenotype of patients with PAIS is extremely heterogeneous. Patients present in infancy or childhood with variable degrees of virilization, such as micropenis, cryptorchidism, and perineoscrotal hypospadias. Infants and children may present with unilateral or bilateral inguinal hernias. Testes are present and functional, producing high levels of testosterone and AMH, resulting in variable wolffian derivative development and regression of müllerian structures in most patients.[111] In patients presenting at puberty, breast development and sparse pubic hair are suggestive of PAIS, and these manifestations help to differentiate it from 5α-R2 deficiency.

Usually, CAIS presents at puberty with primary amenorrhea. Physical examination shows a short, blind vagina, absent uterus, and sometimes palpable inguinal or labial testes. Testosterone-dependent wolffian derivatives and prostate are absent or vestigial. Additionally, height, bone maturation, and breast development are normal, but pubic and axillary hair, an androgen-mediated feature, is absent or sparse. Patients' identity and behavior are feminine without gender dysphoria.[112] Less commonly, CAIS may present in infancy with phenotypic female genitalia and inguinal or labial masses representing testes.

Diagnostic criteria for serum hormone levels are outlined in Table 16-4. Examination and pelvic ultrasound show abdominal testes and the absence of müllerian structures.

Molecular genetic testing of the *AR* gene detects mutations in more than 95% of probands with CAIS. Molecular testing has been shown to be more consistent than biochemical functional assays of AR function, which have been discredited based on the high degree of variation due to biopsy site and testing laboratory.[113] Sequencing of *AR* exons 2 to 10 can be routinely performed,[114] as well as sequencing of the much longer exon 1, and some intronic and promoter regions. Prenatal testing by mutation analysis is available for families in which the AIS-causing allele has been identified in an affected family member.[109]

LUTEINIZING HORMONE RECEPTOR DEFECTS

Leydig Cell Hypoplasia/Agenesis

Leydig cell hypoplasia (LCH) is a disorder caused by inactivating mutations of the luteinizing hormone/chorionic gonadotropin receptor (LHCGR) and characterized by impaired Leydig cell differentiation and testosterone production. LH and hCG activate a shared G-protein–coupled receptor, LHCGR. In utero, placental hCG stimulates Leydig cells to produce testosterone, resulting in male internal and external genitalia. LH takes over during the third trimester of gestation through neonatal life to complete Leydig development and continue testosterone production.

More than 20 inactivating mutations of LHCGR have been identified scattered throughout the gene.[115,116] These cause variable degrees of loss of receptor activity. More severe mutations, resulting in truncation, decreased surface expression, or decreased coupling efficiency, are usually associated with unambiguous female phenotype. Partial inactivating mutations often result in an undervirilized phenotype, such as micropenis or hypospadias.[117] One specific mutation highlights the differential binding sites of hCG and LH to the same receptor. A splicing variant resulting in the absence of exon 10 was described in an 18-year-old man who presented with normal male phenotype, pubertal delay, small testicles, and delayed bone age.[118] The receptors responding to hCG were normal, inferred from normal sex differentiation. However, LHCGR was not activated by LH, resulting in delayed puberty and bone age.

Presentation and Diagnosis.   Patients with severe inactivating mutations in LHCGR are often missed at birth and present at puberty with amenorrhea. Partially inactivating mutations present at birth, with undervirilization of the external genitals (e.g., micropenis, hypospadias, cryptorchidism). In XX females, LHCGR mutations result in hypergonadotropic hypogonadism, with primary amenorrhea or oligoamenorrhea, cystic ovaries, and infertility.[119-122] However, XX females undergo spontaneous breast and pubic hair development during puberty.

Pelvic ultrasound shows absence of the uterus and fallopian tubes. To distinguish LHCGR from XY GD, AMH is used as a marker of testicular Sertoli cell function and is normal to high in patients with LCH and low to undetectable in patients with XY GD.[123] Histologic analysis of the testis shows normal Sertoli cells and hyalinized seminiferous tubules, without mature Leydig cells or spermatogenesis. Patients with partially inactivating mutations may show some early spermatogenesis, but do not produce viable sperm. Therefore, patients have the potential for fertility with assisted reproductive technology.

Biochemical changes are outlined in Table 16-4. Definitive diagnosis requires sequencing of the LHCGR gene for deletions, insertions, and point mutations.

DISORDERS OF ANTI-MÜLLERIAN HORMONE OR THE ANTI-MÜLLERIAN HORMONE RECEPTOR

Persistent Müllerian Duct Syndrome

Unlike many of the conditions mentioned previously, there is no underdevelopment of the male internal genitalia, but rather the incomplete destruction of female precursors. Mutant AMH or AMH receptor type II in XY individuals does not cause müllerian duct regression, causing mixed (male and female) internal genitalia called *persistent müllerian duct syndrome* (PMDS). During the critical time in sex differentiation, between weeks 10 and 12 of gestation, testicular AMH causes regression of the müllerian derivatives. However, inactivating mutations can prevent this regression, resulting in both male and female internal genitalia, but normal male external genitalia.

Presentation and Diagnosis. The diagnosis of PMDS is commonly made incidentally during abdominal imaging studies or surgical exploration of the abdomen.[124] XY patients with PMDS are phenotypically male. Other than having a uterus and fallopian tubes in addition to the male external genitalia, they often have no clinical abnormalities. Therefore, the true prevalence of PMDS is difficult to ascertain. The vast majority of cases of PMDS have mutations in *AMH* and *AMHR2* in approximately equal proportions.[125,126] Inheritance is autosomal recessive for both loci.

Boys can also present with cryptorchidism (20%) or with an inguinal hernia[127] containing müllerian structures, but normal virilization.[125,128] The increased likelihood of abdominal testes in PMDS results in increased incidence of gonadoblastoma.[129]

46,XX Disorders of Sex Development

46,XX DISORDERS OF GONADAL DEVELOPMENT

46,XX Testicular Disorder of Sex Development

Individuals who are XX and have a disorder of sex determination have a range of phenotypes, from phenotypic males to all degrees of genital ambiguity. Histologic features of the gonads range from immature testes to combinations of testicular and ovarian tissue within an individual. Compared with XY DSDs, XX testicular DSDs and XX ovotesticular DSDs are estimated to be much less common, at 1:20,000. Eighty-five percent of all patients with XX testicular DSDs are unambiguously male[130] and possess an Xp:Yp translocation, including *SRY*. One third of all recombination occurs at the *PRKX* locus hot spot on Xp22.3 and the Y homologue *PRKY*.[131] In these cases, there is often skewed X inactivation in favor of the X chromosome without Y chromosome translocation,[130,132,133] cryptic mosaicism,[130,134] or duplication of the region of chromosome 17 with SOX9.[135] The rare families in which XX DSDs are inherited are typically *SRY*-negative, and family members can present with 46,XX partial or complete testicular DSD, or ovotesticular DSD.[136]

Presentation and Diagnosis. In the classic medical literature, individuals with 46,XX DSD who have fully masculinized genitals have been referred to as having *de la Chapelle syndrome*. Although some characteristics of XX testicular DSD, such as small testes, azoospermia, gynecomastia, and lack of secondary sex development, are similar between 47,XXY (Klinefelter syndrome) and XX testicular DSD,[133] these patients are not short and do not exhibit the same learning and behavioral issues. In XX testicular DSD, the phallus is small to normal, and these patients exhibit normal sexual function.

The majority of cases are discovered during adolescence because most patients are unambiguously male. Occasionally, patients present earlier with undervirilized genitalia. Typically, the presence of *SRY* is correlated with completely masculinized genitalia. The diagnosis of most patients with XX testicular DSD is outlined in the next section.

46,XX Ovotesticular Disorder of Sex Development

Patients with ovotesticular DSD (previously known as *true hermaphrodites*) are identified by the presence of both testicular and ovarian gonadal tissue within a single individual. Testicular tissue is characterized by the presence of seminiferous tubules and ovarian tissue by the presence of follicles. Both tissue types can occur within the same gonad, which is known as an *ovotestis*. Among patients with 46,XX ovotesticular DSD, bilateral ovotestis occurs 20% of the time, an ovotestis with a contralateral ovary or testis occurs 50% of the time, and an ovary and testis opposite each other occurs 30% of the time.[137]

The predominant tissue within the individual gonad typically determines where in the abdominal or pelvic region the gonad can be found. Gonads with a high percentage of testis material are typically found in the scrotal sac, whereas gonads with more ovarian tissue can be found in the abdomen.[137] Both the side and the amount of testicular tissue determine the virilization of the internal and external genitalia. The degree of internal genitalia development correlates with the ipsilateral gonad, and as in cases of XY DSDs, can be asymmetrical. The development of a uterus and fallopian tubes can occur in the presence of an ovary or ovotestis. However, the male wolffian structures require a well-formed testis to develop fully. Development of external genitalia is governed by testis hormone production.

Patients with XX ovotesticular DSD lie on the spectrum with XX testicular DSD. Both of these conditions can be caused by skewed X inactivation of the SRY-carrying X chromosome,[132,138] or by cryptic mosaicism.[130,134,139] However, 90% of all patients with XX ovotesticular DSD are not SRY-positive.

A fraction of cases of ovotesticular DSD are found in patients with a 46,XY karyotype, and in these, there have been two reports of mutations found in *SRY*.[49,137,139] Approximately one third of cases of ovotesticular DSD are mosaics, with one of the cell lines containing Yp material.[137,139] Some of these mosaics are 46,XX/46,XY and may actually represent chimeras.[140-145] Recently, a form of syndromic true hermaphroditism has been shown to be due to a single gene mutation in *Rspondin1*[146] and is associated with hyperkeratosis and squamous cell carcinoma.

Presentation. The majority of patients with ovotesticular DSD present in infancy because of underdeveloped genitalia. The phenotype of the internal and external genitalia is controlled by the gonad's hormonal status and often reflects the asymmetrical mixture of ovarian and testicular tissue within the gonads. In all patients, müllerian duct regression is incomplete, yet the uterus remains immature, and a unicornate uterus is a common finding. However, in more phenotypically female patients, the adnexa and vagina are generally better developed, and approximately half of phenotypic females menstruate.[147,148]

Patients with a high degree of masculinization and a male phenotype may have some uterine remnants, such as a prostatic utricle (prostatic vagina). Phenotypic males also tend to have bilateral palpable gonads, or at least one descended gonad. The undescended gonad may be an intra-abdominal ovary or an ovotestis and may be located at any point of the pathway of testicular descent.

In some rare cases, patients with unambiguous genitalia present with atypical secondary sex characteristics, opposite their assigned gender. For example, at puberty, phenotypically female patients may experience clitoromegaly and deepening voice, whereas phenotypic males may experience gynecomastia. In these cases, ultrasound may not fully demonstrate the testicular or gonadal nature of either gonad, but gonadal biopsy can definitively show the presence of both ovarian and testicular tissue.

Diagnosis of 46,XX Testicular and 46,XX Ovotesticular DSD.

In males without genital ambiguity, a diagnosis is often made during evaluation of infertility or delayed puberty. Patients with XX testicular DSD have hypergonadotropic hypogonadism with elevated FSH and LH, decreased testosterone, DHT, and a less than twofold increase in response to the hCG stimulation test. Unlike individuals with GD or XX testicular DSD, the gonads of patients with ovotesticular DSD have some degree of function and therefore show normal levels of FSH, LH, estradiol, testosterone, and DHT. In children with 46,XX karyotype and genital ambiguity, the biochemical diagnostic criteria are the same as those for 46,XX testicular DSD. However, SRY is positive in only 10% of patients with 46,XX ovotesticular DSD.

Serum AMH levels are a good biochemical indicator of functioning testicular tissue, suggestive of XX testicular DSD or ovotesticular DSD.[123] Pelvic ultrasound shows absence of a uterus, and semen analysis shows normal semen volume with azoospermia. A combination of male and female internal and external genitalia is suggestive of 46,XX ovotesticular DSD.

Genetic tests that should be performed are FISH for SRY, which is positive in 90% of phenotypically male patients with XX testicular DSD. The 10% of patients with XX testicular DSD who are negative for SRY should undergo further cytogenetic testing for SOX9 microduplication or cryptic mosaicism for Yp.

It is important to note that the only way to obtain definitive diagnosis of either ovotesticular or testicular DSD is by gonadal tissue confirmation in which both gonads are extensively examined for the presence of ovarian tissue. Complete absence of ovarian tissue allows for definitive diagnosis of 46,XX testicular DSD, whereas the slightest presence of ovarian tissue gives rise to 46,XX ovotesticular DSD. If gonadal biopsy material is available, it should be

tested for karyotype, cryptic mosaicism, and SRY mutations because SRY expression in the gonads has been seen despite the lack of Yp in the karyotype.[130,134,149] Patients who are mosaic for 46,XX and 46,XY should be tested for potential chimerism, particularly those conceived with in vitro fertilization.

Management of 46,XX Testicular and Ovotesticular DSD.

Of primary concern in patients with testicular and ovotesticular DSDs is the surgical repair of medically concerning issues, such as inguinal hernias, fistulas, and malignancies. Continuing management is determined by the gender assignment of these patients, which is discussed later.

There is a 5% incidence of gonadal tumors in ovotesticular DSD,[150,151] which likely represents an increased risk associated with abdominal gonads possessing testicular tissue, as well as the increased risk of gonadoblastomas in dysgenic gonads with Yp material. Phenotypically male patients with XX testicular DSD who are SRY-positive are not at increased risk for gonadoblastomas because they lack a complete Y chromosome. Some reports also indicate that the risk of breast cancer may be increased in patients with XX testicular and ovotesticular DSD.[152,153]

Patients with 46,XX ovotesticular DSD with partially developed müllerian structures can also have ovarian follicles, with the potential to carry a biologic pregnancy to term.[138] There are eight reported pregnancies in patients with ovotesticular DSD. In all of these patients, the karyotype was 46,XX, which contributes to the belief that patients with the Y chromosome cannot become pregnant. However, one case report describes a 20% 46,XX/80% 46,XY patient with ovotesticular DSD who carried a successful pregnancy to term.[151] Males with ovotesticular DSD are generally azoospermic, but there have been infrequent cases of males with mature sperm,[137,154] and even more rare cases of men with ovotesticular DSD who have fathered children.[137]

Because the majority of individuals with XX testicular DSD carry the Xp:Yp translocation, paternal karyotype and FISH for SRY should also be performed to determine whether the father carries a balanced translocation, or if the translocation occurred in the germline or de novo. Fathers who carry the balanced translocation can only produce offspring with 46,XX SRY-positive testicular DSD or 46,XY SRY-negative complete GD.

46,XX Gonadal Dysgenesis

Most cases of ovarian dysgenesis involve abnormal complements of X chromosomes in phenotypic females.[156] The most common of these is Turner syndrome, discussed earlier as a sex chromosome DSD. Impaired ovary development can occur with a normal female sex chromosome complement, referred to as *46,XX GD*, which can occur either as an isolated entity or as part of a syndrome. Patients possess normal female genitalia at birth, but remain sexually infantile and do not experience normal puberty. Ovarian failure with hypergonadotropic hypogonadism at puberty is highly suggestive of ovarian dysgenesis. Müllerian structures are normal, and histologic study of the

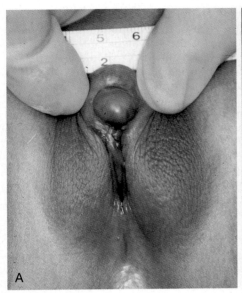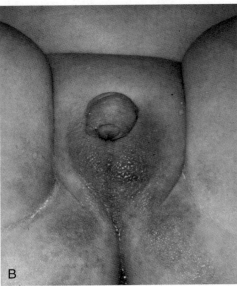

Figure 16-10. External genitalia of two patients with congenital adrenal hyperplasia, with CYP21 mutations with varying degrees of virilization. **A,** The labia appear partially fused posteriorly, and show some rugae. The clitoris is moderately hypertrophic. **B,** The labia are completely fused and have a scrotal appearance. No gonads are palpated. The clitoris is very hypertrophic, and has a penis-like appearance.

gonads shows bilateral streaks. Absent associated somatic abnormalities, patients present with amenorrhea and infertility.

Several studies of familial ovarian dysgenesis have noted the frequent reports of consanguinity, suggesting that isolated 46,XX GD is inherited as an autosomal recessive condition.[156-159] Mutations in the gene for the FSH receptor (gene *FSHR*, 2p16) have been implicated in some cases,[158,160,161] but do not explain the phenotype in all populations studied.[162,163] Translocations involving the critical region Xq13.3-q26 have also been described.[164] However, the molecular basis for 46,XX GD remains unknown for the majority of patients.

46,XX DISORDERS OF SEX DIFFERENTIATION: ANDROGEN EXCESS

High levels of intrauterine androgens or androgenic precursors result in masculinization of the internal and external genitalia of 46,XX fetuses. In these patients, development of the wolffian ducts and virilization of the external genitalia occur to varying degrees. Patients often present with clitoromegaly, "scrotalization" of the labia, urogenital sinus, and phallic urethra, along with fully developed müllerian derivatives.

In XX infants with normally developed gonads and müllerian structures, the most common cause of genital ambiguity in newborns is virilizing CAH.[165] Inactivating mutations of any enzyme steroidogenic pathway, shown in Figure 16-9, are the most common cause of virilization in XX infants and are discussed later. Rare causes of CAH that can result in both 46,XY DSD and 46,XX DSD, such as P450scc deficiency, StAR protein mutations, 3βHSD2 deficiency, and 17-βHSD3 were described earlier.

There are three major sources of excess androgens in utero: fetal steroidogenesis, fetoplacental steroidogenesis, and maternal causes of excess androgens (i.e., iatrogenic, androgenic tumors).

FETAL SOURCES OF ANDROGEN EXCESS

Congenital Adrenal Hyperplasia

Depending on the enzyme implicated, CAH can cause either 46,XY DSD or 46,XX DSD. Deficiency of 21-hydroxylase (*CYP21*) accounts for more than 90% of cases of CAH and is the most common etiology of ambiguous genitalia in the newborn.[165-167] CYP21 deficiency results in blockage of both aldosterone and cortisol biosynthetic pathways. The build-up of 17-OH progesterone is shunted toward androgen biosynthesis, resulting in virilization of XX fetuses. The disease frequency in the general population is 1:15,000, but is much higher in certain ethnic groups, including Hispanics and Ashkenazi Jews.[168]

Mutations in 11β-hydroxylase (*CYP11B1* gene) account for another 5% of cases of virilizing CAH.[165,169] As in 21-hydroxylase deficiency, XX neonates are virilized, but XY neonates have normal genitalia. Blockage of *CYP11B1* results in elevated levels of aldosterone and androgens, by shunting of cortisol precursors to biosynthesis of other hormones. Other adrenal causes of excess androgen, such as 3βHSD2 and P450 oxidoreductase defects,[91,92] were discussed earlier.

Presentation and Diagnosis. Fetuses with XX typically present at birth with ambiguous genitalia. XY fetuses do not exhibit any degree of undervirilization. However, there is a wide range of phenotypes, from the classic salt-wasting or simple virilizing phenotype to nonclassic forms that present with hyperandrogenism and precocious puberty. There is a strong correlation between the degree of enzymatic activity and the severity of clinical phenotype.[170] Figure 16-10 shows the wide range of genital phenotypes in CAH.

Individuals with XY and 21-hydroxylase deficiency often are not detected in the newborn period, unless accompanied by a salt-wasting crisis. XY patients often present with premature masculinization and accelerated physical development. If left untreated, there is premature fusion of epiphyses, resulting in short stature.

Diagnosis of 21-hydroxylase deficiency can be initially identified by elevated 17-OH progesterone. Biochemical changes are outlined in Table 16-4. Clinically, 11-beta hydroxylase deficiency can be differentiated from 21-hydroxylase deficiency by the presence of hypertension with hypokalemic alkalosis. Molecular diagnosis can be ascertained by sequencing of the disease gene.

Management. Treatment of 21-hydroxylase deficiency can begin in utero to prevent overvirilization of XX fetuses. Due to the timing of genital development, oral treatment with dexamethasone begins at 4 weeks' gestation, even before determination of sex and the presence of disease genes in the fetus. Maternal dexamethasone can be continued until chorionic villous sampling or amniocentesis shows a XY karyotype or lack of homozygosity of the 21-hydroxylase mutation. If the fetus is XX and is affected, treatment with oral dexamethasone continues until delivery.[171] This treatment remains controversial because of a high likelihood of unnecessary treatment of unaffected fetuses, with little knowledge of the long-term effects.

Newborns diagnosed with 21-hydroxylase deficiency should be monitored carefully for salt-wasting crises in early life. For newborns with either CYP21 or CYP11B1 deficiency, glucocorticoid replacement is essential to preventing adrenal crisis and normalizing serum levels of steroidogenic precursors.

FETOPLACENTAL CAUSES OF ANDROGEN EXCESS

P450 Aromatase Deficiency

Aromatase (*CYP19A1*) catalyzes the conversion of androgens to estrogen. Mutations that affect aromatase activity have effects on both males and females. Estrogen is required for spermatogenesis in males and for the development of secondary sex characteristics in females.

Presentation and Diagnosis. The initial manifestation of aromatase deficiency is placental, with maternal virilization.[172-174] These mothers have elevated levels of androgenic precursors in the liver, causing their own virilization and that of their XX fetuses. Biochemical findings are outlined in Table 16-4. CAH is the major differential diagnosis considered and can be excluded with an ACTH stimulation test showing an increase in adrenal hormones but not in androgens.

Patients with XX do not undergo spontaneous puberty and often have polycystic ovaries, increased virilization, and amenorrhea, without breast development.[172,175,176] XY males experience normal puberty, but are infertile because of the lack of estrogen, which is essential to spermatogenesis.[174,177,178]

With regard to growth, both XX and XY patients do not experience a growth spurt during puberty, instead experiencing linear growth, but are considered tall. Skeletal maturity is delayed and osteoporosis develops early.[174,179] Patients often have bone pain.[174] The use of sex hormone replacement therapy at puberty is discussed later.

P450 Oxidoreductase Deficiency

A rare cause of ambiguous genitalia in 46,XX and 46,XY infants is POR. The pathophysiology and presentation were described earlier.

MATERNAL ETIOLOGIES OF ANDROGEN EXCESS

Maternal ingestion of androgens is a potential cause of virilization of XX newborns. However, current progestin-containing oral contraceptives are not highly androgenic, and this cause of XX virilization is rare.[182-184] Hormonally active tumors, such as luteomas, are another uncommon cause of maternal virilization and ambiguous genitalia in an XX infant.[180] Hyperreactio luteinalis, a cystic ovarian condition associated with virilization of the mother and fetus, is associated with XX virilization in 15% of cases.[180] Although CAH causes most cases of XX virilization, oncologic and iatrogenic causes of maternal and fetal virilization should always be considered.

General Management of Patients with Disorders of Sex Development

Patients with DSDs have grown up. What was once viewed as a rare phenomenon, seen only in a few, highly specialized academic centers, has become global. First, the issues generated by the management of DSDs have had wide exposure in the media, feeding societal debates on gender assignment and patients' rights to be involved in medical decision-making. Then, the clinical issues that were limited to genital surgery have expanded to the management of low fertility, cancer, and psychosexual dysfunction of adulthood, informing knowledge of many other, more frequent conditions.

MULTIDISCIPLINARY APPROACH

An essential aspect of care for children with DSDs is an experienced multidisciplinary team that typically includes an endocrinologist, a pediatric surgeon or urologist, a psychologist or psychiatrist, a gynecologist, a geneticist, a pediatrician or neonatologist, and if available, a social worker, a nurse, and a medical ethicist.[181] Open communication between the team and the family, as well as participation in decision-making, is essential. Support groups may have an important role in the delivery of care. Transition to adult care is also a key element of care. Fundamental concepts to establish with the family include the following: children with DSDs have the potential to become fully functional members of society; DSDs are not shameful; and the situation is often complex, so that the best plan may not be obvious initially.

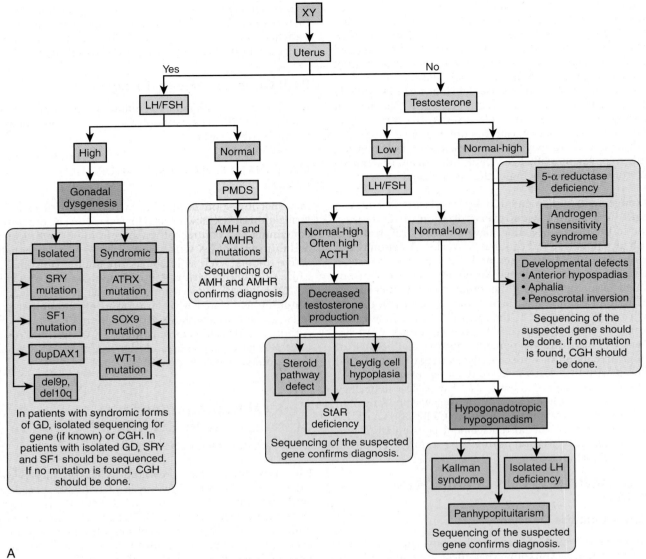

A

Figure 16-11. **A,** *Diagnostic flowchart of the major disorders of sexual development in undervirilized XY individuals.*

Continued

DIAGNOSIS

Extraordinary progress has been made in the molecular and endocrine evaluation of patients with DSDs. After a thorough interview for family and prenatal history, the initial testing includes sex genotyping, which can be performed rapidly by FISH with X and Y probes, or by regular karyotype. This testing is followed by pelvic imaging (with ultrasound increasingly being replaced by pelvic magnetic resonance imaging) and measurement of levels of 17-hydroxyprogesterone, testosterone, LH, FSH, AMH, and electrolytes. Subsequent and more specialized testing is guided by algorithms, such as the ones proposed in Figure 16-11. One recent advance in molecular testing is CGH, a microarray-based technology used to screen for small deletions or duplications that typically are not seen on regular karyotype. CGH should be offered if the most frequent and easily testable causes of DSD have been excluded.

GENDER ASSIGNMENT

Until the mid-1950s, the medical management of individuals with DSDs was based on the assumption that the "true sex" was equivalent to the sex of the gonads. Human sexual anatomy was indeed classified in five categories in the 19th century: (1) male and (2) female (with typical feminine or masculine external genitalia, respectively); (3) male and (4) female pseudohermaphrodites (with ambiguous genitalia and the presence of testes or ovaries, respectively); and (5) true hermaphrodites (with both testicular and ovarian tissue).[182] It was assumed that a person's identification as male or female would naturally conform to the individual's "true sex."

In the late 1950s, however, under the influence of psychologist John Money and pediatric endocrinologist Lawson Wilkins, gender assignment began to be influenced by the "optimal gender" principle. It became standard practice in the 1970s, and was only challenged recently, starting in the mid-1990s.

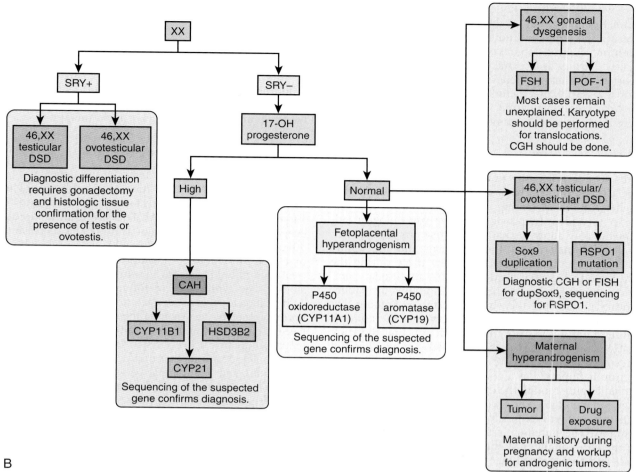

B

Figure 16-11, cont'd B, Diagnostic flowchart of the major disorders of sexual development in XX individuals. ACTH, adrenocorticotropic hormone; AMH, anti-müllerian hormone; AMHR, anti-müllerian hormone receptor; CAH, congenital adrenal hyperplasia; CGH, comparative genomic hybridization; DSD, disorder of sex development; FISH, fluorescence in situ hybridization; FSH, follicle-stimulating hormone; GD, gonadal dysgenesis; HSD, hydroxysteroid dehydrogenase; LH, luteinizing hormone; PMDS, persistent müllerian duct syndrome; POF-1, SF1, steroidogenic factor-1; StAR, steroidogenic acute regulatory. (Adapted from Fleming A, Vilain E. The endless quest for sex determination genes. Clin Genet 67:15-25, 2004.)

The "optimal gender" approach considered multiple aspects of outcome, giving greatest consideration to the potential for complete sexual functioning. It is based on two assumptions: (1) gender identity is not firmly established at birth, but rather is influenced by socialization and sex of rearing; and (2) stabilization of gender identity and favorable psychological outcome depend on the congruence between genital appearance and assigned gender. The clinical consequences of the "optimal gender" policy are that gender should be assigned as early as possible, during a window of gender flexibility that ends at 18 to 24 months of age; reconstructive genital surgery should be performed equally early to match the chosen gender; the assignment should be made to the gender that carries the best prognosis for reproductive and sexual function; and uncertainty on the part of parents and health care providers about the gender of rearing should be minimized. Recent challenges to this paradigm view the determination of gender identity and gender role as biologic (with prenatal androgens as the best candidate),[183] and the appearance of genitals as

a reflection of brain masculinization, and not the reverse. What was seen as an absolute requirement for gender assignment (a typical penis and scrotum for males, a typical clitoris and labia for females) was questioned by outcome studies of XY patients born with cloacal exstrophy, a complex abdominal malformation resulting in de facto absence of a functional penis, but normal testicular function. Only 5 of 14 patients assigned as female at birth had a clear female gender identity at follow-up in the teen years.[184] On balance, cases of ablatio penis in early childhood, caused by botched circumcision, have had diverse outcomes. Although the most famous example in the literature (the "John/Joan" case), which prompted the recent challenges to the "optimal gender" policy, ended in a disastrous outcome (gender dysphoria, and ultimately suicide),[185] another case resulted in a clear, stable female gender identity in an otherwise bisexual woman with a history of "tomboyism" during childhood. On two occasions (at ages 16 and 26 years), this patient requested a vaginoplasty. This case shows that female gender identity can develop in a genetic male.

So, what is the best way to assign gender in this post– "optimal gender" era? As before, based on the medical literature and outcome studies for specific diagnoses, consideration of chromosomal constitution, hormone levels, potential fertility, and sexual function are, as always, quite important. The main difference is that early genital surgery is not necessarily directly linked to the gender assignment. One clear recommendation is that all individuals should receive early gender assignment.

GENITAL SURGERY

As discussed earlier, the traditional perspective, at least since the 1950s, has been to provide an anatomy that matches the sex of rearing. The goal has been to influence gender identity, provide positive psychological adjustment, and allow sexual intercourse. In this model, the decision-makers are the physician and the family because the genital surgery must take place during the early period of gender flexibility. This traditional paradigm was challenged in the 1990s, initially by patient advocacy groups and then by physicians,[186] arguing that the rationale for early genital surgery was the comfort of others, not necessarily the patient, and that there are negative consequences if the assigned gender does not correspond to the ultimate gender identity or if sexual function is impaired as a consequence of the surgery. In the challenging model, the decision-maker is the patient, when old enough. The 2005 consensus statement on DSDs provides guidelines for a more cautious approach to surgery. The statement requires that the surgeons outline the consequences of surgery, from infancy to adulthood, and that only surgeons with specific training in the treatment of DSDs perform genital surgery. It is also argued that clitoral surgery should only be considered in severe cases (Prader III to V), that no vaginoplasty in patients with short or absent vaginas be performed in infancy, and that no vaginal dilation be performed before puberty.

HORMONAL THERAPY

Hormonal therapy may be used for several purposes. In the case of classic CAH, glucocorticoids and mineralocorticoids are used as life-saving replacement therapy. In the case of patients with DSDs who are raised as males, testosterone may be used to increase penile tissue growth, as well as to induce puberty. In the case of patients with DSDs who are raised as females, estrogens are used for induction of puberty and bone protection.

Glucocorticoid Replacement Therapy

In CAH, hydrocortisone (10-20 mg/m^2/24 hour) is given orally in two or three daily doses. The treatment must provide enough hormones to replace the adrenal steroids and suppress the adrenal androgens while avoiding iatrogenic Cushing's syndrome and its effect on growth rate and bone maturation. Daily doses are increased by two to three times during periods of stress (e.g., fever, surgery).

More potent glucocorticoids (e.g., prednisone) can be used in adulthood, after growth is complete.

Mineralocorticoid Replacement Therapy

In the salt-wasting form of CAH, treatment with 9-fluorohydrocortisone (Florinef; 0.05-0.3 mg/day orally) and sodium chloride (1-3 g/day as a supplement) is often required, in addition to glucocorticoid therapy.

Testosterone Replacement Therapy

Treatment of patients with testosterone deficiency (e.g., 46,XX testicular DSD or Klinefelter syndrome) includes the initiation of low-dose testosterone therapy after age 14 years. Testosterone enanthate is given intramuscularly every 3 to 4 weeks, starting at 100 mg and increasing by 50 mg every 6 months to 200 to 400 mg. Initial high doses of testosterone should be avoided to prevent priapism. The treatment should plateau, in adulthood, at the best possible dosage, typically 50 to 400 mg every 2 to 4 weeks.

If an individual has short stature and is eligible for growth hormone therapy, testosterone therapy should be either delayed or given at lower doses initially to maximize growth potential. Alternative delivery systems to injections that result in a more stable dosing include transdermal patches (scrotal and nonscrotal) and transdermal gels. Testosterone-containing gels have an increased risk of interpersonal transfer, which can be reduced by the use of the new hydroalcoholic gels.[187]

Estrogen Therapy

To develop and maintain secondary sexual characteristics in women who are hypogonadic (or in postgonadectomy patients with CAIS) and to prevent osteoporosis, estrogen treatment is initiated at the lowest available dose and progressively increased (e.g., starting at 0.3 mg/day of conjugated estrogens orally and increasing to 0.625 mg/day). Other delivery systems include transdermal patches.

DISCLOSURE

The traditional paradigm of the "optimal gender" policy calls on practitioners to limit disclosure, based on the rationale that it prevents gender identity confusion, within the reasoning that nurture influences gender identity. The challenging view favors full disclosure, in the interest of patient autonomy, and with the rationale of preventing secrecy and shame. Studies of chronic medical disorders and of adoptees shows that disclosure is associated with enhanced psychosocial adaptation.[188] Although there is no rule about the appropriate age to fully disclose a condition, it is recommended to proceed gradually and recurrently with children, and to adapt disclosure to the child's cognitive and psychological development.[1]

MENTAL HEALTH

Psychological care should be integral to the medical management of patients with DSDs. Multidisciplinary teams caring for children with DSDs should include a mental health professional, who should inform decisions about gender assignment and reassignment as well as the timing of surgery. Although atypical gender role behavior is more common in children with DSDs, it should not be taken as an indicator for gender reassignment. The mental health professional should help parents cope with their child's condition, should help in the process of full disclosure, and most importantly, should provide long-term behavioral support to the patient. This includes support for quality-of-life items, such as falling in love, dating, intimacy, sexual functioning, and ability to build relationships and raise children.

FERTILITY

Not long ago, infertility was seen as an immutable feature of DSDs. Advances in assisted reproductive technologies have changed this view. Some patients with DSDs, who were previously infertile or subfertile, have the opportunity to have biologic children. If germ cells are present, sperm or oocytes can be obtained from the gonads and used in intracytoplasmic sperm injection and in vitro fertilization. Table 16-5 outlines the fertility levels and assisted reproductive technology options for patients with various DSDs.

The ability to produce biologic offspring in females is solely dependent on the presence of oocytes. Adolescent patients who undergo premature ovarian failure (i.e., Turner syndrome) can cryopreserve their oocytes for future use. Furthermore, phenotypic female patients with a uterus can undergo donor embryo transfer, with a 30% rate of pregnancy. For phenotypic female patients, carrying a pregnancy to term is associated with an increased risk of maternal complications. Therefore, these patients should be followed closely by an obstetrician specializing in high-risk patients.

CANCER

The various DSDs are accompanied by variable risks of germ cell tumor, which should be taken into consideration in the long-term management of these patients. Higher risks of gonadal tumors have been shown in GD positive for the presence of testis-specific protein Y encoded on the Y chromosome, and for PAIS with intra-abdominal gonads. Lower risks are observed in ovotesticular DSD and

TABLE 16-5

Fertility in Patients with Disorders of Sex Development

Disorder	Level of Fertility	Potential Use of Assisted Reproductive Technology
Sex Chromosome Disorders of Sex Development		
Turner syndrome	• Only 2-5% of Turner patients are spontaneously fertile.[189] • There have been ~170 reported spontaneous pregnancies in patients with mosaic variants of Turner.[190] Recently, 2 cases of spontaneous pregnancy in nonmosaic variants were reported.[191,192] • Pregnancy rates of 30-60% after oocyte donation; high risk of pregnancy complications (i.e., hypertension, preeclampsia)[39]	Cryopreservation of follicles in youth Single embryo transfer from donor oocytes
Klinefelter syndrome	• 3 case reports of spontaneous pregnancy in 47,XXY patients.[193–195] • 43 reports of pregnancy after ICSI, leading to liveborn children.[44]	Cryopreservation of sperm Testicular sperm extraction ICSI
46,XY DSD: Testes Development		
46,XY gonadal dysgenesis (pure, partial, mixed)	• 7 case reports of successful pregnancy after oocyte donation in patient with complete 46,XY GD[196–202] • No reports in 46,XY partial or mixed GD. Patients with mixed GD are usually infertile.	Single embryo transfer from donor oocytes
Testicular regression syndrome	• Infertile	None
46,XY DSD: Adrenal Synthesis and Action		
Disorders of androgen biosynthesis	• In XY patients with forms of CAH, infertility is often caused by testicular adrenal rest tumors.[203] • 3β-HSD: XY: Lower levels of spermatogenesis; 2 case reports of severely affected male fathering 2 children. Fertility in XX females unknown[204-205]	Glucocorticoid therapy to optimize fertility; ICSI and in vitro fertilization
Leydig cell hypoplasia 5α-Reductase deficiency	• Untreated patients are azoospermic and infertile.[206] • Fertility is possible with surgical reconstruction of the male ductal system.[207]	Unknown ICSI
Complete/partial androgen insensitivity syndrome	• Male infertility: no uterus; therefore, cannot carry pregnancy	

Continued

TABLE 16-5

Fertility in Patients with Disorders of Sex Development—continued

Disorder	Level of Fertility	Potential Use of Assisted Reproductive Technology
Persistent müllerian duct syndrome	• In patients with cryptorchidism, fertility is better preserved in adulthood if orchiopexy is done before age 2.[208]	ICSI
46,XX DSD: Ovarian Determination		
XX Testicular DSD XX Ovotesticular DSD	• Case report of patients with 46, ovotesticular DSD with 1 ovary and 1 ovotestis who became spontaneously pregnant after removal of ovotestis.[209,210] • Fertility and pregnancy has been reported after removal of the testicular portion of the ovotestis.[148]	Potential for biologic children using in vitro fertilization techniques or selective removal of only testicular tissue to stimulate spontaneous ovulation
46,XX DSD: Adrenal Excess		
Congenital adrenal hyperplasia 21-Hydroxylase 11β-Hydroxylase	• In XX patients, excess adrenal steroids, ovarian hyperandrogenism, PCOS, ovarian adrenal rest tumors, neuroendocrine factors, genital surgery, and psychological factors contribute to decrease in fertility. Normalization of hormonal factors can increase chance for spontaneous pregnancy in these women.[204,211]	Long-acting glucocorticoids can be used to regulate menstrual cycles and maximize fertility. ICSI and in vitro for patients who cannot conceive spontaneously Single embryo transfer in patients with stenotic vaginas due to genital surgery
P450 aromatase P450 oxidoreductase Maternal sources of DSD	• XX patients have polycystic ovaries and do not undergo spontaneous puberty.[212] • XY individuals undergo normal puberty, but are sterile due to the lack of estrogen. • No reports of spontaneous pregnancy to date; however, long-term studies of these patients have not been completed. • No known effect on adult fertility • Fertility in XX individuals is affected by management of ambiguous genitalia, such as genital surgery and psychological factors.	In theory, single embryo transfers (from biologic or donor oocytes) for XX,DSD patients

CAH, congenital adrenal hyperplasia; DSD, disorder of sex development; GD, gonadal dysgenesis; HSD, hydroxysteroid dehydrogenase; ICSI, intracytoplasmic sperm injection; PCOS, polycystic ovarian syndrome.
Adapted from Lee PA, et al. Consensus statement on management of intersex disorders. International consensus conference on intersex. Pediatrics 118(2): e488-e500, 2006.

TABLE 16-6

Gonadoblastoma Risk

Risk Group	Disorder	Malignancy Risk (%)	Recommended Action	Patients (n)	Studies (n)
High	GD* (+Y)† intra-abdominal	15-35	Gonadectomy	12	>350
	PAIS nonscrotal	50	Gonadectomy	2	24
	Frasier	60	Gonadectomy	1	15
	Denys-Drash (+Y)	40	Gonadectomy	1	5
Intermediate	Turner (+Y)	12	Gonadectomy	11	43
	17β-hydroxysteroid dehydrogenase	28	Watchful waiting	2	7
Low	CAIS	2	Biopsy and possible gonadectomy	2	55
	Ovotesticular DSD	3	Testicular tissue removal	3	426
	Turner (-Y)	11	None	11	557
No (?)	SRD5A2	1	Unresolved	1	3
	Leydig cell hypoplasia	1	Unresolved	1	2

CAIS, complete androgen insensitivity syndrome; DSD, disorder of sex development; GD, gonadal dysgenesis; PAIS, partial androgen insensitivity syndrome.
*Gonadal dysgenesis (including not further specified 46,XY, 45,X/46,XY, mixed, partial, complete).
†GBY region–positive, including the testis-specific protein Y–encoded (TSPY) gene.
Adapted from Lee PA, et al. Consensus statement on management of intersex disorders. International Consensus Conference on Intersex. Pediatrics 118(2): e488-e500, 2006.

CAIS. A review of the risk of germ cell tumor, according to diagnosis, is shown in Table 16-6.

PATIENT-CENTERED CARE

A patient-centered model of care should be used in the treatment of patients with DSDs. In this model, open communication with patients and family should be promoted, especially at times of decision-making. Gender change should be supported by the multidisciplinary team, as needed, in accord with the patient's wishes. The consensus statement also calls for a limit on genital examinations and medical photography.

The complete reference list can be found on the companion Expert Consult Web site at www.expertconsultbook.com.

Suggested Readings

Hughes IA, Deeb A. Androgen resistance. Best Pract Res Clin Endocrinol Metab 20(4):577-598, 2006.

Lanfranco F, et al. Klinefelter's syndrome. Lancet:273-283, 2004.

Lee PA, Houk CP, Ahmed SF, Hughes IA. International Consensus Conference on Intersex organized by the Lawson Wilkins Pediatric Endocrine Society and the European Society for Paediatric Endocrinology. Consensus statement on management of intersex disorders. International Consensus Conference on Intersex. Pediatrics 18(2):e488-e500, 2006.

Nikolova G, Vilain E. Mechanisms of disease: transcription factors in sex determination: relevance to human disorders of sex development. Nat Clin Pract Endocrinol Metab 2(4):231-238, 2006.

Ogilvie CM, Crouch NS, Rumsby G, et al. Congenital adrenal hyperplasia in adults: a review of medical, surgical and psychological issues. Clin Endocrinol (Oxf) 64(1):2-11, 2006.

Speiser PW. Prenatal and neonatal diagnosis and treatment of congenital adrenal hyperplasia. Horm Res 68(Suppl 5):90-92, 2007.

Turner Syndrome Study Group. Care of girls and women with Turner syndrome: a guideline of the Turner Syndrome Study Group. J Clin Endocrinol Metab 92(1):10-25, 2007.

Wilhelm D, Palmer S, Koopman P. Sex determination and gonadal development in mammals. Physiol Rev 87(1):1-28, 2007.

CHAPTER 17

Puberty: Gonadarche and Adrenarche

Selma Feldman Witchel and Tony M. Plant

Introduction

Puberty in humans is defined as the period of first becoming capable of reproducing, and is marked by maturation of the genital organs, development of secondary sex characteristics, acceleration in growth, changes in affect and, in the female, the occurrence of menarche.[1] In humans, the transition into puberty is driven by two physiologic processes: gonadarche and adrenarche. *Gonadarche* comprises growth and maturation of the gonads and is associated with increased secretion of sex steroids and with the initiation of folliculogenesis and ovulation in the female and spermatogenesis in the male. Gonadarche leads to thelarche and menarche in girls and testicular enlargement in boys.

Adrenarche, which typically precedes gonadarche,[2] comprises maturation of the adrenal cortex associated with increased secretion of adrenal androgens—namely, dehydroepiandrosterone (DHEA), dehydroepiandrosterone sulfate (DHEAS), and androstenedione—and leads to the appearance of sexual hair (pubarche). Adrenarche late in prepubertal development appears to be peculiar to our own species and to the great apes[3] and, in humans, the absence of adrenarche does not prevent gonadarche or the attainment of fertility.[4,5]

The age at onset of puberty and the tempo at which puberty unfolds is dependent on many factors. In girls, increased ovarian and adrenal sex steroid secretion leads to the physical manifestations of puberty, thelarche and pubarche. In general, these changes occur between 8 and 13 years of age. The mean age at menarche among multiple ethnic groups is between 12 and 13 years.[6] In boys, the earliest physical manifestation of puberty is an increase in testicular volume, and this usually occurs between 9 and 14 years of age.

Traditionally, diagnosis of precocious puberty is considered when signs of puberty develop before 8 years of age in girls and 9.5 years in boys, but these criteria should be used as guidelines to complement the evaluation of individual patients.[7] For girls, the absence of thelarche or menarche by age 13 and 16 years, respectively, is considered delayed puberty.[8] For boys, delayed puberty is defined as absence of testicular enlargement by age 14 years.

Although the mechanism underlying the onset of adrenarche remains to be elucidated, it is now established that gonadarche results from the resurgence of activity in the hypothalamic–pituitary axis, which has been relatively quiescent since early childhood. The neuroendocrine regulation of gonadarche in humans is similar to that observed in other higher primates,[5] and nonhuman primates (in particular, the Rhesus monkey) have been extensively employed as paradigms for the study of human puberty. Subsequently, our discussion of the control of the onset of gonadarche will be based on both the human and nonhuman primate literature.

Stages of Pubertal Development, Secular Trends, and Racial and Ethnic Differences

PUBERTAL STAGING

For both sexes, the genital and pubic hair changes that unfold at puberty are classified into five stages: stage 1 is prepubertal and stage 5 is adult (Fig. 17-1 and Table 17-1). These physical changes may be the result of either gonadarche (as in the case of breast or testicular enlargement) or adrenarche (as in the case of pubic hair development).

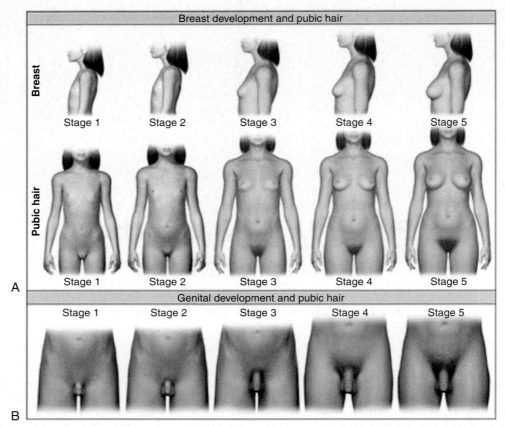

Figure 17-1. *Pubertal rating according to Tanner stages. **A,** Breast development in girls is rated from 1 (prepubertal) to 5 (adult). Stage 2 breast development (appearance of the breast bud) marks the onset of gonadarche. For girls, pubic hair stages are rated from 1 (prepubertal) to 5 (adult). Stage 2 marks the onset of adrenarche. **B,** Genital development in boys is rated from 1 (prepubertal) to 5 (adult). Stage 2 genital development, characterized by enlargement of the testes and scrotum accompanied by a change in the texture of the scrotal skin, marks the onset of gonadarche. Pubic hair development in boys is rated from stage 1 (prepubertal) to 5 (adult). Stage 2 represents the onset of pubarche, which can reflect adrenarche or gonadarche. Although pubic hair and genital or breast development are represented as synchronous in the figure, they do not necessarily take place simultaneously and should be scored separately. In normal boys, stage 2 pubic hair generally develops 1 to 1.5 years after stage 2 genital development. (From Carel JC, Léger J. Clinical practice. Precocious puberty. N Engl J Med 358:2366, 2008. Reproduced with permission of the* New England Journal of Medicine.*)*

Although the physical sequelae of gonadarche and adrenarche generally occur concomitantly, a discordance of the two processes may also occur in normal development.

Increased estrogen secretion promotes breast development in girls. The development of breast buds with increased areolar diameter is considered to be stage 2; greater enlargement of the breasts occurs in stage 3, accompanied by increased pigmentation of the areolae and nipples. During stage 4, the areolae are mounded above the breast tissue. Recession of the areola to the general breast contour represents breast stage 5. Additional effects of estrogen at this stage of development include cornification of the vaginal mucosa, uterine growth, and morphogenesis of an adult female body habitus.

Menarche follows an anovulatory cycle and generally occurs 2 to 3 years after the onset of breast development. Menstrual cycles during the first year after menarche are typically irregular and anovulatory, with most ranging in duration from 21 to 45 days. Within 5 years of menarche, most cycles are regular and range from 21 to 35 days. Although primordial and preantral follicles predominate during the prepubertal years, small antral follicles develop during this phase of maturation. With further development, the adolescent ovary may appear on ultrasound to be multicystic or polycystic.[9]

In girls, increased adrenal androgen secretion is considered to be responsible for the development of darker hairs along the labia, which is classified as pubic hair stage 2. The hair becomes darker and coarser during pubic hair stage 3, spreading over the pubic symphysis, with gradual progression to a full female escutcheon. Apocrine odor may precede or accompany the development of pubic hair. Associated findings include acne and oiliness of skin and hair.

For boys, genital stage 2 comprises an increase in testicular volume and enlargement of the scrotum. At stage 2, the testes are approximately 4 to 8 mL in volume, with the longest axis being approximately 2.5 cm. The volume of the mature human testis is approximately 20 to 30 mL and represents increased growth of the seminiferous tubule due to Sertoli cell proliferation and differentiation, and initiation of spermatogenesis. At genital stage 3, further growth of the testes has occurred, and the length and diameter of the penis has increased. At genital stage 4, penile size has increased and the scrotal skin has become darkened.

TABLE 17-1

Stages of Pubertal Development (Tanner)

		Girls	
Stage	*Breast*	*Pubic Hair*	
1	Prepubertal	No pigmented hair	
2	Budding, with larger areolae	Small amount of coarse, pigmented hair, mostly along the labia majora	
3	Enlargement of breast and areolae	Spread of coarse, pigmented hair over the mons pubis	
4	Secondary mound of areolae	Almost adult pattern	
5	Mature contour	Adult pattern	
		Boys	
Stage	*Genitalia*	*Pubic Hair*	*Testicular Volume (mL)*
1	Prepubertal	No pigmented hair	<3
2	Thinning and darkening of the scrotum, increased size of the penis	Small amount of coarse, pigmented hair at the base of the penis	3-8
3	Increased diameter of the penis	Coarse, pigmented hair extends above the penis	10-15
4	Increased diameter and length of the penis	Almost adult pattern	15-20
5	Adult size and shape	Adult pattern	>25

In stage 2, male pubic hair consists of downy hair at the base of the penis. For pubic hair stage 3, the hair is longer and darker, and extends over the junction of the pubic bones. In pubic hair stage 4, the extent of hair has increased, but has not yet achieved the adult male escutcheon. Other secondary sexual characteristics in boys include increased size of the larynx, deepening of the voice, increased bone mass, and increased muscle strength. Approximately 3 years after the appearance of pubic hair, terminal hair appears in androgen-dependent regions on the face and trunk, where it may develop for years thereafter. There is considerable variation in the distribution and density of beard, chest, abdominal, and back hair, presumably reflecting genetic differences. The appearance of spermatozoa in early morning urine specimens (spermaturia) occurs during genital stage 3. Gynecomastia is observed in 50% of boys.[10] Typically, this is most prominent in midpuberty, when the ratio of circulating concentrations of estradiol to testosterone is relatively high. In most instances, gynecomastia resolves spontaneously by 16 years of age.

The pubertal growth spurt in girls occurs concurrently with the onset of breast development. Usually, only 4 to 6 cm of growth occurs after menarche. The pubertal growth spurt in boys, with an average height velocity of 9.5 cm/year, occurs around genital stages 3 and 4. In general, the age at peak height velocity shows an inverse relationship with the magnitude of the growth spurt.[11,12] Schemata for the temporal development of the secondary sexual characteristic and their relationship to growth velocity are shown for girls and boys in Figures 17-2 and 17-3, respectively.

SECULAR TRENDS AND RACIAL AND ETHNIC DIFFERENCES IN THE ONSET AND TEMPO OF PUBERTY

Reports of secular changes in the onset of puberty have focused on girls, and it is generally viewed as axiomatic that there was a decline in the age of menarche in Europe and North America from the early 19th century (16-17 years of age) to the later half of the 20th century (13 years of age). This trend has been attributed to the improving socioeconomic conditions during this epoch.[4] Although the most recent data from North America, several European countries, and other regions of the industrialized world indicate that the trend toward earlier menarche has been reduced or halted,[6,13-17] breast and pubic hair development are apparently occurring earlier than they were 50 years ago.[6] The biology underlying this continued positive secular trend in sexual development in girls, which in some populations is loosely associated with a similar trend in growth, is unclear, and may or may not involve an earlier onset of gonadarche or adrenarche. Analogous studies of boys are limited, but no striking sex differences in secular trends in puberty and growth are apparent. In a recent study of American boys who were taller and heavier than those in previous cohorts, pubic hair and testicular development was reported to occur earlier than previously recognized.[18]

It is important to recognize that the age at onset of puberty varies between ethnic groups. In a recent study of American girls, mean ages for breast development, pubic hair development, and menarche were, respectively, 9.5, 9.5, and 12.1 years for African-American girls; 9.8, 10.3, and 12.2 years for Mexican-American girls; and 10.3, 10.5, and 12.7 years for white girls.[19] Data obtained through the Third National Health and Nutrition Examination Survey (NHANES III) between 1988 and 1994 showed that African-American girls enter puberty first, followed by Mexican-American and white girls.[19,20] For boys in NHANES III, median estimated ages for genital and pubic hair stage 2 were, respectively, 9.3 and 11.1 years for African-American boys, 10.4 and 12.3 years for Mexican-American boys, and 10.1 and 12 years for white youths. For genital and pubic hair stage 5, median ages were, respectively, 14.9 and 15.2 years for African-American boys, 15.8 and 15.7 years for Mexican Americans, and 16 and 15.6 years for white boys.[21]

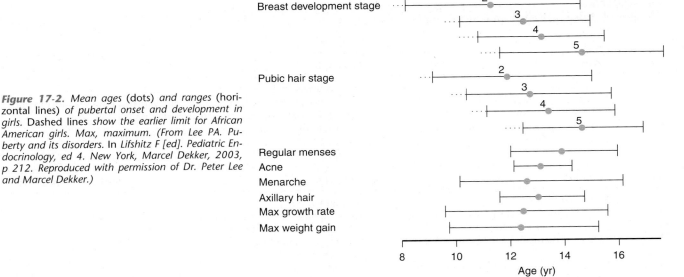

Figure 17-2. *Mean ages* (dots) *and ranges* (horizontal lines) *of pubertal onset and development in girls. Dashed lines show the earlier limit for African American girls. Max, maximum. (From Lee PA. Puberty and its disorders.* In *Lifshitz F [ed]. Pediatric Endocrinology, ed 4. New York, Marcel Dekker, 2003, p 212. Reproduced with permission of Dr. Peter Lee and Marcel Dekker.)*

Physiology of Puberty

STEROIDOGENESIS

The biosynthetic pathways for gonadal and adrenal steroids are considered together because of their similarities and importance in understanding the physiology and pathophysiology of puberty (Fig. 17-4; see also Chapter 4). Synthesis of sex steroids from cholesterol requires

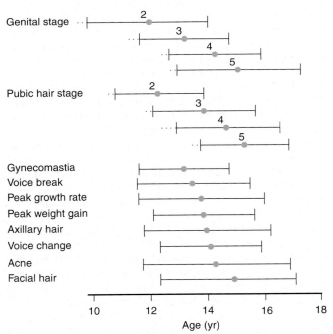

Figure 17-3. *Mean ages* (dots) *and ranges* (horizontal lines) *of pubertal onset and development in boys.* Dashed lines *show the earlier limit for African American boys. (From Lee PA. Puberty and its disorders.* In *Lifshitz F [ed]. Pediatric Endocrinology, ed 4. New York, Marcel Dekker, 2003, p 213. Reproduced with permission of Dr. Peter Lee and Marcel Dekker.)*

expression of specific enzymes and other proteins in the gonads and adrenal glands. The rate-limiting step of steroidogenesis is transport of cholesterol into mitochondria mediated by steroidogenic acute regulatory protein (StAR). Within the mitochondria, cholesterol desmolase (also known as *side-chain cleavage*) converts cholesterol into pregnenolone. One enzyme, 17 α-hydroxylase/17,20-lyase (P450c17), is the qualitative regulator of adrenal and gonadal steroidogenesis. This enzyme mediates 17α-hydroxylation to convert pregnenolone into 17α-hydroxypregnenolone. In the adrenal zona reticularis, ovarian theca, and Leydig cells, this same enzyme catalyzes scission of the C17-20 bond to produce DHEA. Although one protein is capable of two distinct enzymatic reactions, these enzyme activities are differentially regulated. Cytochrome b_5 modulates adrenal androgen secretion by increasing the 17,20-lyase activity of P450c17.[22-24] P450 oxidoreductase (POR) is a protein that transfers electrons from nicotinamide adenine dinucleotide phosphate to microsomal cytochrome P450 enzymes, such as P450c17, P450c21, and aromatase.

The Δ^5-steroids are converted to the Δ^4-steroids by 3β-hydroxysteroid dehydrogenase type 2, the adrenal and gonadal isoform, resulting in conversion of DHEA to androstenedione. In the zona fasciculata, 17-hydroxypregnenolone is converted to 17-hydroxyprogesterone (17-OHP) by 3β-hydroxysteroid dehydrogenase. Subsequently, 17-OHP is converted to 11-deoxycortisol by 21-hydroxylase (P450c21) and to cortisol by 11β-hydroxylase (CYP11B1).

In the zona reticularis of the adrenal cortex, DHEA sulfotransferase converts DHEA to DHEAS; this enzyme is also expressed in the liver. In the ovary, androstenedione is synthesized in the theca cell and diffuses into the granulosa cell, where it is aromatized by aromatase (CYParo) to estrone and converted to estradiol by 17β-hydroxysteroid dehydrogenase type 1. In Leydig cells, androstenedione is converted to testosterone by 17β-hydroxysteroid dehydrogenase type 3. In many androgen target cells, such as those in the external genitalia and prostate, testosterone is

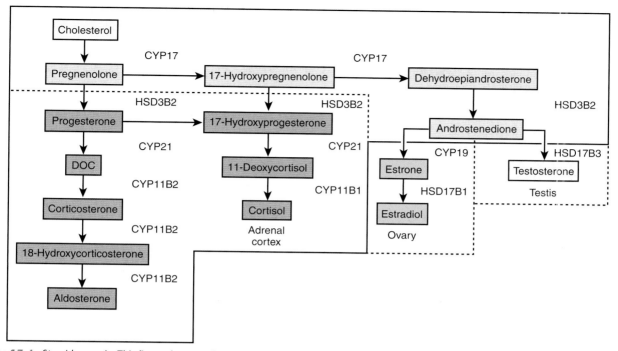

Figure 17-4. *Steroidogenesis. This figure shows pathways of adrenal, ovarian, and testicular steroidogenesis.* Dark solid lines *indicate the predominant pathways for adrenal steroidogenesis.* Dashed lines *indicate the predominant pathways for gonadal steroidogenesis. DOC, deoxycorticosterone. (From Witchel SF, Lee PA. Ambiguous genitalia.* In *Sperling MA [ed]. Pediatric Endocrinology, ed 2. Philadelphia, WB Saunders, 2002, p 119.)*

converted to dihydrotestosterone (DHT) by 5α-reductase type 2. In other androgen-sensitive tissue, such as bone, testosterone is converted to estradiol.

The 17β-hydroxysteroid dehydrogenase enzymes comprise a large family of enzymes involved in steroid biosynthesis and metabolism. Seventeen different enzymes have been described.[25] Differences in tissue distribution, substrate preferences, subcellular localization, and mechanisms of regulation lead to microenvironment adjustment of sex steroids.[26] The type 1 isozyme is expressed in ovaries, placenta, endometrium, and liver, where it favors conversion of estrone to estradiol. The type 3 isozyme is expressed in the testis, where it preferentially converts androstenedione to testosterone.[27]

Once secreted, sex steroids circulate bound to sex hormone-binding globulin (SHBG) and to albumin.[28] The unbound or free hormone is considered to be the bioavailable form that diffuses passively into target cells and interacts with nuclear steroid receptors. These are ligand-dependent transcription factors, comprising three functional domains: the N-terminal domain serves to modulate function; the DNA-binding domain mediates binding of the receptor to DNA; and the ligand-binding domain binds to steroids.[29] Steroid receptor activation also requires expression of coactivators, which may be tissue-specific.

It should also be noted that nongenomic actions of steroids have been reported.[30] Sex steroids can be metabolized to inactive forms by a variety of enzymes. Glucuronidation decreases the biologic activity of steroid hormones and increases solubility to facilitate renal excretion. This process, catalyzed by uridine diphosphate-glucuronosyl-glucuronyltransferase (UGT) enzymes, involves the transfer of glucuronic acid from uridine diphosphoglucuronic acid to steroid hormones. In humans, the UGT2B isoforms show greater specificity for C19 androgens.[31] A second mechanism is sulfoconjugation, in which DHEA sulfotransferase catalyzes conversion of DHEA to DHEAS and estrogen sulfotransferase converts estrogens to estrone sulfate. The inactive sulfated steroids can be hydrolyzed to active forms by steroid sulfatase.

ACTIVATION OF GONADARCHE

Increased gonadal steroidogenesis and the completion of gametogenesis during gonadarche are stimulated by enhanced secretion of the gonadotropins luteinizing hormone (LH) and follicle-stimulating hormone (FSH). LH and FSH are heterodimeric proteins composed of a common α-subunit and a unique β-subunit; all are glycosylated peptides.[32] The temporal increments in circulating LH and FSH concentrations at the time of puberty, and their relationships to those of the gonadal steroids at this stage of development, have been well documented in both boys and girls.[4,5]

The actions of LH and FSH are mediated by their cognate seven-transmembrane domain G-protein–coupled receptors: the LH receptor (LH-R) and FSH receptor (FSH-R), respectively (see also Chapter 2). In girls, LH stimulates androgen production by the thecal cells of the ovarian follicles and progesterone secretion from luteinized granulosa cells of the corpus luteum. FSH is critical for the process of follicular recruitment and selection.[33] In granulosa cells of the developing follicle, FSH induces expression of aromatase, which is responsible for aromatization of androgens secreted by the theca cells. FSH also induces LH-R in granulosa cells of the dominant follicle, which selectively amplifies the effect of declining FSH concentrations on the dominant follicle.[33] In the male, LH regulates the secretion of testosterone from Leydig cells in the interstitium of the testis. FSH, together with testosterone, is responsible for initiating and maintaining spermatogenesis.[34] The actions of FSH and testosterone to stimulate spermatogenesis are indirectly exerted on the somatic Sertoli cell of the seminiferous tubule.

Activation of the ovary and testis during gonadarche also results in the increased secretion of the gonadal proteins, known as *inhibins*. Mature inhibins are dimers composed of a common α-subunit covalently linked with one of two β-subunits (β_A and β_B). The α/β_A and α/β_B dimers are known as inhibin A and inhibin B, respectively.[35] The gonadal inhibins, similar to the gonadal steroids, play both an endocrine role in the regulation of gonadotropin secretion and a paracrine role within the gonads. Inhibin B, which is synthesized in part by the Sertoli cell, is the principal inhibin secreted by the testis.[36] In prepubertal boys, mean concentrations of circulating inhibin B are approximately 60 pg/mL, which compare with adult values that vary considerably around an average of 200 pg/mL.[37,38] The pubertal increase in inhibin B may be attributed to Sertoli cell proliferation and to the initiation of spermatogenesis, both of which result from the increased gonadotropin drive to the testis at the time of gonadarche.[34]

In girls, circulating levels of inhibin A and B are low or undetectable before puberty.[39] Inhibin B begins to rise with the onset of puberty, as does inhibin A in breast stages 3 and 4. Adult levels are attained at approximately 14 to 15 years of age.[40] During the menstrual cycle, inhibin A levels are elevated in the luteal phase, whereas inhibin B predominates in the circulation of the follicular phase.[41,42]

Müllerian-inhibiting hormone (MIH), also known as anti-müllerian hormone (AMH), plays a critical role in the regression of the müllerian ducts during fetal development. MIH is secreted postnatally by the testis and, to a lesser extent, by the ovary.[43] At puberty, circulating concentrations of MIH in boys decline in association with increasing testosterone secretion to reach low values characteristic of those observed in girls.

The pubertal drive to the pituitary–gonadal axis is generated by a diffusely distributed network of hypothalamic neurons expressing the *GnRH-I* gene (see also Chapters 1 and 7).[44] By mechanisms that are not entirely understood, this neuronal network, known as the "hypothalamic gonadotropin-releasing hormone (GnRH) pulse generator," produces an intermittent discharge of GnRH into the hypophysial portal circulation that is obligatory for gonadotropin secretion by the pituitary gonadotrophs.[33] LH and FSH secretion is stimulated by pulsatile secretion of GnRH acting through its receptor, GnRH-R (a seven-transmembrane–domain G-protein–coupled receptor), located on gonadotropin-secreting cells (gonadotrophs) in the pituitary gland.[45] A second GnRH gene (*GnRH-II*) is also expressed by neurons in the primate brain and, recently, a GnRH-II receptor has been cloned from the pituitary.[46,47] However, the significance, if any, of this second GnRH system in the control of the human

pituitary–gonadal axis has not been delineated. Similarly, a hypothalamic gonadotropin-inhibiting hormone (GnIH) has been identified in avian and mammalian species,[48] but its neuroendocrine role in humans is unclear. In conditions under which pulsatile GnRH release is compromised, such as occurs in anorexia nervosa and during periods of strenuous physical training in young women, gonadotropin secretion is attenuated and pubertal development is arrested. Thus, the pituitary–gonadal axis in both males and females may be viewed as being a slave to the hypothalamic GnRH pulse generator, and this analogy should be kept in mind when considering the mechanisms triggering the onset of gonadarche.

In pubertal and postpubertal individuals, the ovaries and testes are governed by feedback control systems.[49] GnRH and the gonadotropins comprise the feedforward components from hypothalamus to pituitary and from pituitary to gonad, respectively. Steroid and protein hormones from the gonads, in turn, provide the feedback signals that regulate the secretion of LH and FSH. The feedback actions of these gonadal hormones, which involve both negative and stimulatory (positive) actions, may be exerted directly at the level of the pituitary gonadotrophs to modulate expression of the genes encoding LHβ and FSHβ.[45] Feedback may also be exerted indirectly at the level of the hypothalamus to regulate the release of GnRH (see Chapters 7 and 12).

In the male, negative feedback actions of testosterone and inhibin B are the major regulators of LH and FSH secretion, respectively.[34,49,50] The action of testosterone is predominantly exerted at the hypothalamic level, whereas that of inhibin appears to occur directly at the pituitary. The role of aromatization of testosterone to estradiol in mediating the negative feedback action of this androgen on LH secretion continues to be an area of active investigation.[51,52] The feedback control of LH and FSH throughout the menstrual cycle is complicated and involves both negative and positive feedback actions of ovarian steroids at both the hypothalamic and pituitary levels[33] (see also Chapter 7). The maintenance of normal ratios of circulating LH and FSH concentrations is important for gonadal function, particularly for folliculogenesis and ovulation. The role of ovarian inhibins in regulating gonadotropin secretion in pubertal and premenopausal women remains to be fully elucidated.

NEUROBIOLOGY OF GONADARCHE

The 1000 or so GnRH neurons that comprise the GnRH pulse generator are born in the olfactory placode and migrate during early fetal development from the nose through the forebrain to the hypothalamus.[53] Several guidance molecules have been implicated in this process, including anosmin-1, fibroblast growth factor 1, and prokineticin 2.[53-56] LH and FSH reach detectable levels by the 10th week of gestation in the human pituitary, peak in midgestation, and are higher in female fetuses than in male fetuses.[4,5] Although the hypothalamic control of the fetal gonad has not been extensively studied in higher primates, by midgestation, the GnRH pulse generator is clearly driving the gonadotrophs of the fetal pituitary.[5] As gestation progresses, the secretion of estradiol and other steroids by the fetoplacental unit increases dramatically. This increase suppresses gonadotropin secretion from the fetal pituitary by exerting an inhibitory action either directly at the pituitary or indirectly on the hypothalamus to restrain GnRH release.

After parturition, GnRH pulse generator activity is robustly expressed as a result of a loss in fetoplacental steroid inhibition, and the pituitary gonadotrophs of the infant respond with LH and FSH secretion.[5] Moreover, in a male infant, the Leydig cells of the testis are stimulated and circulating testosterone levels are similar to those observed in adult men. The GnRH pulse generator is brought into check within the first year or two of life, leading to the hypogonadotropic state that guarantees gonadal quiescence until the prepubertal phase of development is terminated by a resurgence of GnRH pulse generator activity.[57,58] It should be noted that the onset of gonadarche is not limited by the GnRH neurons, the pituitary gonadotrophs, or the cells of the gonads.[5] During childhood and juvenile development, when the hypothalamus or pituitary is provided with pulsatile neurochemical (N-methyl-D-aspartate [NMDA], a glutamate receptor agonist)[59,60] or GnRH stimulation, respectively, or when the ovary and testis are stimulated directly with LH and FSH, gonadarche may be readily elicited. This phenomenon is graphically illustrated in children with GnRH-dependent precocious puberty, which is discussed later in this chapter. The observation that the GnRH neuronal network in the juvenile hypothalamus is able, on NMDA stimulation, to immediately elicit an adult hypophysiotropic GnRH drive is consistent with the finding that, in the monkey, hypothalamic GnRH gene expression and peptide content are maintained throughout this phase of prepubertal development.[59] Thus, transcriptional regulation of the gene encoding GnRH from birth to puberty appears to be minimal, and the locus of developmental control of GnRH release must lie upstream of the GnRH neuronal network.

Because GnRH is secreted in only picogram quantities into the hypophysial portal circulation, changes in the concentration of this neuropeptide in the peripheral circulation do not reflect hypothalamic activity. Therefore, studies of the dynamics of the pubertal resurgence of GnRH pulse generator activity in humans and other higher primates have generally used the high-fidelity relationship that exists between the frequencies of pulsatile GnRH release and episodic LH secretion.[61] The latter may be tracked with relative ease by measuring moment-to-moment changes in LH concentrations in the peripheral circulation.[49] Although the pubertal increase in hypothalamic GnRH drive to the gonadotroph probably involves both frequency and amplitude modulation of the GnRH pulse generator, the relationship between GnRH and LH pulse amplitudes is more complex than the relationship between frequencies; amplitude modulation of LH release may not reflect changes in GnRH pulse amplitude. During initiation of gonadarche in boys and girls, an acceleration in LH pulse frequency and an increase in LH pulse amplitude is observed in association with an amplification of a preexisting sleep-related diurnal pattern in release.[5,62-66] This change in neuroendocrine activity may occur before the physical changes of gonadarche are manifest. In boys in particular, LH pulse frequency appears to decline later in pubertal development, probably due to a negative feedback action of rising testosterone concentrations.[67] A longitudinal study of the agonadal monkey[68] suggests that, as in humans, the pubertal acceleration of pulsatile GnRH release is an early neurobiologic event in the initiation of gonadarche, and that it is a rapidly completed process. Thus, the slow tempo of the overall progression of puberty probably results from mechanisms downstream from the hypothalamus. A model illustrating the ontogeny of GnRH pulse generator activity from fetal to pubertal development in the male and female is shown in Figure 17-5.

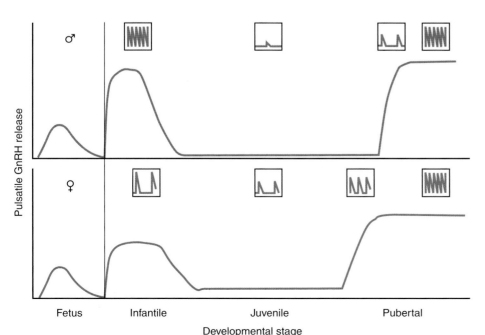

Figure 17-5. A model of the effect of the neurobiologic brake on pulsatile gonadotropin-releasing hormone (GnRH) release during juvenile development (childhood) in boys (top) and girls (bottom). Insets indicate the frequency of pulsatile GnRH release at respective stages of development. (From Plant TM. Control of onset of puberty in primates. Topic Endocrinol 20:1, 2002.)

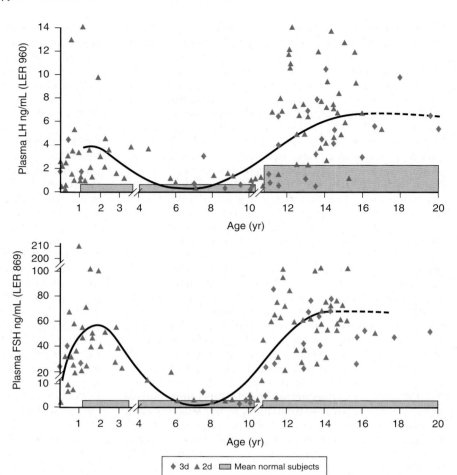

Figure 17-6. *The neurobiologic restraint that holds the gonadotropin-releasing hormone (GnRH) pulse generator in check during childhood is imposed in the absence of the gonads, as reflected by the time courses of circulating concentrations of luteinizing hormone (LH; top) and follicle-stimulating hormone (FSH; bottom) in 58 patients with gonadal dysgenesis. Closed triangles, 45, X karyotype; circles, X chromosome mosaicism or structural abnormalities; cross-hatching, mean plasma gonadotropin concentrations in normal girls. Bold curves, polynomial regressions of gonadotropin concentration with age. (From Conte FA, Crumbach MM, Kaplan SL. A diphasic pattern of gonadotropin secretion in patients with the syndrome of gonadal dysgenesis. J Clin Endocrinol Metab 40:670, 1975.)*

The control system that dictates the up-down-up pattern of GnRH pulse generator activity from birth until puberty may be viewed as a neurobiologic "brake" (or "central restraint," as it has been previously described in the pediatric literature[4]) that holds GnRH neuronal activity in check during the greater part of prepubertal development.[59] Here it is important to recognize that the notion of a brake is conceptual (i.e., the pubertal resurgence in robust GnRH pulsatility could be occasioned either from the removal of an inhibitory input or by the application of a stimulatory signal to the GnRH neuronal network, or a combination of the two). A similar argument may be applied to the earlier transition between infancy and childhood, when GnRH pulsatility is markedly diminished. The neurobiologic brake on pulsatile GnRH release throughout childhood and juvenile development is imposed in the absence of the ovary or testis. Consequently, the characteristic pattern of gonadotropin secretion observed during postnatal development in humans—with robust gonadotropin secretion during infancy and puberty, separated by a prolonged hiatus in LH and FSH secretion—is maintained in the agonadal situation (Fig. 17-6).[69] In such children, however, the degree of prepubertal suppression of gonadotropin release is less than that observed in eugonadal individuals.[4]

Interestingly, in agonadal children, circulating gonadotropin levels are higher in girls than in boys, indicating that the intensity of the neurobiologic brake imposed on the GnRH pulse generator during prepubertal development is less in the female than in the male. As a result, the gonadotropin drive to the prepubertal ovary stimulates a low level of estradiol secretion, which through negative feedback action on LH and FSH release, amplifies the relatively weaker neurobiologic brake restraining gonadotropin secretion in the prepubertal girl. This sex difference in the strength of the neurobiologic brake on prepubertal GnRH release is associated with a shorter duration of the brake in girls, which probably accounts for the relatively earlier age of gonadarche in the female. These and other sex differences in the developmental control of the GnRH pulse generator are presumed to result from greater exposure of the fetal male hypothalamus to testosterone.[5]

A major component of the neurobiologic brake imposed on pulsatile GnRH release during the greater part of prepubertal development is composed of a hiatus in stimulatory kisspeptin and glutamate input to the GnRH neuronal network. Such a role for glutamate is based on findings in the monkey that hypothalamic glutamate release is increased at the time of puberty in the female,[70]

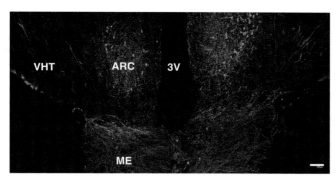

Figure 17-7. *A coronal section through the medial basal hypothalamus of an adult Rhesus monkey showing the relationship between kisspeptin (green) and GnRH-1 (red) neurons shown by double-label fluorescence immunohistochemistry. Note the medial location of kisspeptin cell bodies in the arcuate nucleus (ARC, termed the infundibular nucleus in humans) and the more lateral location of GnRH perikarya in the ventral hypothalamic tract (VHT). Both populations of these peptidergic neurons send axonal projections to the median eminence (ME). 3V, third ventricle. Scale bar, 100 um. (From Ramaswamy S, Guerriero KA, Gibbs RB, Plant TM. Structural interactions between kisspeptin and GnRH neurons in the mediobasal hypothalamus of the male monkey [Macaca mulatta] as revealed by double immunoflourescence and confocal microscopy. Endocrinology 149[9]:4387, 2008.)*

and that repetitive activation of glutamate receptors in the juvenile monkey leads rapidly to the onset of precocious gonadarche (discussed earlier). The kisspeptins, which are encoded by *KiSS1* and signal at the kisspeptin receptor (KiSS1R), also known as G-protein–coupled receptor 54 (GPR54), have recently been identified as major regulators of the hypothalamic–pituitary–gonadal axis.[71-74] Kisspeptins are highly potent GnRH secretagogs.[75,76] Loss-of-function mutations of *KiSS1R* are associated with hypogonadotropic hypogonadism during infancy and at later stages of development in conjunction with absent or delayed puberty.[77-79] In such patients, pituitary response to exogenous GnRH does not appear to be compromised,[78] indicating a hypothalamic locus for the genetic deficit. On the other hand, a gain-of-function mutation of *KiSS1R* (nonconstitutive) has been reported in a 7-year-old girl with GnRH-dependent precocious breast development.[80]

In the monkey, hypothalamic *KiSS1* expression and kisspeptin release increase at the time of the pubertal resurgence in GnRH pulsatility.[81,82] Intermittent administration of kisspeptin at hourly intervals during juvenile development elicits a precocious and sustained adult-like pulsatile pattern of GnRH activity.[83] As shown in Figure 17-7, kisspeptin neurons in the primate hypothalamus are located primarily in the infundibular nucleus,[84,85] and they communicate directly with GnRH neurons via inputs to both GnRH perikarya and dendrites, and to axonal terminals in the median eminence.[85] The regulation of GnRH release at the level of the median eminence[86] is consistent with the absence of major developmental changes in hypothalamic GnRH gene expression and peptide content (discussed earlier). In GnRH neurons, ligand binding to KiSS1R results in phosphatidylinositol 4,5-biphosphate (PIP2) hydrolysis, calcium mobilization, and mitogen-activated

protein (MAP) kinase phosphorylation that is associated with activation of a canonical transient receptor potential (TRPC)-like cationic channel.[87,88] Continuous exposure of KiSS1R to kisspeptin leads to down-regulation of the receptor.[89]

Although neuroglia have classically been regarded as subserving only a "supporting role" in the central nervous system (CNS), contemporary views hold that these non-neuronal cells play important functional roles within the brain.[90] Moreover, in the context of the hypothalamus, secretion of transforming growth factor-α (TGFα) by astroglia has been postulated to provide the GnRH neuronal network with a stimulatory input at the time of puberty.[91]

In addition to the removal of stimulatory inputs to the GnRH neuronal network during childhood and juvenile development, studies of the female Rhesus monkey provide evidence that γ-aminobutyric acid (GABA), the major inhibitory neurotransmitter in the brain, is upregulated during juvenile development.[69] Inhibition of GABA tone in the median eminence of the prepubertal monkey leads to precocious menarche and ovulation. In the male Rhesus monkey, neuropeptide Y (NPY) appears to be an important component of the neurobiologic brake. NPY neurons are found in close proximity to GnRH neurons in the hypothalamus, and NPY gene expression in the hypothalamus is inversely related to the up-down-up pattern of GnRH pulse generator activity from birth to puberty.[92,93] NPY receptors are inhibitory G-protein receptors, and their activation leads to hyperpolarization and inhibition of neural activity.[94,95] Systematic studies of GABA in the male and of NPY in the female have not been conducted.

The developmental changes in inhibitory and stimulatory inputs that dictate the up-down-up pattern of pulsatile GnRH release from birth until puberty are likely to be associated with a corresponding structural remodeling in those hypothalamic neuronal and glial circuits underlying the inhibitory and excitatory signals regulating the postnatal ontogeny of GnRH release.[96,97] In this regard, the hypothalamus of the postnatal brain retains its capacity for plasticity, as reflected by the expression of polysialic acid-NCAM.[98]

Although attempts have been made to develop an integrative model of the neurobiologic brake that holds pulsatile GnRH release in check during prepubertal development, these have not been entirely successful.[59,70,99] A recent proposal argues that developmental changes in a network of genes coding for transcriptional factors that, in a molecular sense, lie upstream of the genes coding for the neuropeptides (or enzymes regulating GABA and glutamate synthesis and release) serve as a governing hierarchy to orchestrate the timing of when excitatory and inhibitory inputs are brought into play.[100] Because such networks of genes are further proposed to function in the absence of signals derived from the periphery, conceptually, they may be viewed at a systems level as comprising a pubertal clock (discussed later). Three transcriptional regulators, Oct2, thyroid transcription factor 1 (TTF1), and enhanced at puberty 1 (EAP1), have been implicated.[100]

PUTATIVE SIGNALS TRIGGERING GONADARCHE

The mechanisms that regulate the timing of the pubertal resurgence of pulsatile GnRH release have intrigued investigators for decades, but this fundamental developmental event in humans remains largely a mystery. Two basic schemata, however, may be proposed.[101] In the first, a cue to reawaken the GnRH pulse generator is provided by the attainment of a particular state of somatic maturation. According to this hypothesis, the brain receives this information by way of a signal in the circulation that is tracked by a somatometer resident within the CNS. In the second schema, a pubertal clock (presumably resident in the CNS) generates the signal. The latter idea has not been explored in either humans or higher primates.

In the case of the somatometer hypothesis, the attainment of a particular proportion of body fat has long been argued to be necessary for the onset of gonadarche,[102] and girls who are overweight tend to mature earlier.[103] Interest in the latter hypothesis was rekindled with the discovery of leptin, a protein that is secreted by adipocytes and regulates feeding behavior and body weight by providing the hypothalamus with information on fat mass.[104,105] In girls, it is generally recognized that plasma leptin levels increase progressively through breast stages 1 to 5.[106-108] In boys, plasma leptin levels increase during early puberty also, to reach peak levels at 10 to 12 years of age, but they subsequently decline as blood levels of testosterone rise into the adult range.[106,109,110] The recent finding that circulating concentrations of the soluble form of the leptin receptor progressively decrease during childhood until approximately 11 years of age suggests that the increase in bioavailable leptin during early puberty may be greater than that reflected in total leptin concentrations.[110,111]

Several individuals with mutations of the leptin gene (*LEP*) associated with low leptin concentrations and obesity have not progressed through puberty.[112,113] Over the last 10 years, Farooqi and colleagues have reported that leptin replacement to seven patients with leptin deficiency due to mutations of *LEP* was closely associated with the onset of puberty when individuals were of pubertal age at the time of initiating treatment (three children). However, significantly, in younger children, there has been no evidence of premature puberty after replacement treatment[113,114] (I. S. Farooqi, unpublished observations). Moreover, among children with GnRH-dependent precocious puberty, leptin concentrations correlated with body mass index and not with pubertal status.[115] These findings provide compelling evidence for the view that the action of leptin, albeit obligatory for the onset of puberty, is nevertheless permissive.[116-118] The permissive action of leptin that allows gonadarche to unfold once the cue for increased GnRH release has been received by the hypothalamus may require only low circulating levels of the adipocyte hormone because pubertal development in three female subjects with various lipodystrophies despite low leptin concentrations was reported to be normal.[119,120] With the recent finding that KiSS1 neurons in the murine hypothalamus express the major signaling isoform of the leptin receptor,[121] it is tempting to speculate that kisspeptin neurons mediate, at least in part, the action of leptin to permit puberty to unfold.

Other somatic factors have been proposed to serve as signals to the somatometer. The hypothesis that such a factor is skeletal in origin[101] is based on the finding that, in children with an accelerated or retarded maturational tempo, menarche and testicular enlargement correlate better with skeletal age than with chronologic age.[122,123] Skeletal age, also known as "bone age," is determined by comparing a radiograph of the left hand with gender-specific standards obtained at various chronologic ages. Several caveats are relevant when assessing skeletal maturity. The degree of skeletal maturation at various sites, such as the hands, elbows, and knees, may differ. Skeletal maturation of the carpal bones, distal radius, and distal ulna often lags behind that of the metacarpals and phalanges.[124] Nevertheless, the association between bone age and the onset of gonadarche is maintained in disorders of growth. In children with constitutional delay of growth and true isolated growth hormone (GH) deficiency, gonadarche occurs at a late chronologic age but at a normal skeletal age.[125-127] On the other hand, when skeletal maturation is advanced, as may occur in association with congenital adrenal hyperplasia (CAH) or familial testotoxicosis, secondary GnRH-dependent precocious puberty may develop.[127] Although proteins synthesized in bone enter the vascular compartment,[128] the question of whether such factors are able to modulate the activity of the GnRH pulse generator has not been addressed.

During childhood, GH secretion is relatively stable, but GH release is amplified up to threefold in boys and girls with the initiation of gonadarche and the rise in circulating levels of sex steroids.[129] The pubertal increase in GH, in combination with the increased circulating concentrations of insulin-like growth factor-1 (IGF-1),[130] estrogens, and androgens, contributes to the adolescent growth spurt. The increased secretion of GH at the time of gonadarche is not sustained; by late puberty, GH levels begin to decline,[129] a phenomenon known as the *somatopause*. Because the increases in GH and IGF-1 appear to be in response to the initiation of gonadarche and particularly to increased gonadal steroid secretion at this time,[129] neither GH nor IGF-1 represents a compelling candidate for the signal responsible for the resurgence of GnRH release.[5]

At the time of gonadarche, insulin sensitivity decreases. This insulin resistance is greatest among children in Tanner stages 2 and 3 compared with prepubertal children and adults.[131] The manifestations of insulin resistance appear to be limited to effects on carbohydrate metabolism and are associated with compensatory hyperinsulinemia. Using euglycemic-hyperinsulinemic clamp studies in conjunction with investigation of substrate use, one longitudinal study found that puberty was associated with decreased insulin sensitivity, increased insulin secretion, increased total body lipolysis, decreased glucose oxidation, and increased IGF-1 concentrations.[132] The changes in IGF-1 concentrations during puberty have been reported to mirror those in insulin sensitivity.[133] The ability of insulin to suppress hepatic glucose production was noted to be preserved during puberty,[134] indicating that decreased insulin sensitivity is limited to peripheral glucose uptake. Although cross-sectional studies suggest that the magnitude of insulin resistance is influenced by body mass index (BMI; body weight/height^2 [kg/m^2]), sex, and ethnic background, these associations have not been consistently noted in longitudinal studies. Mean 24-hour serum GH and IGF-1 concentrations positively correlate with the degree of insulin resistance during puberty, and the pubertal changes in insulin sensitivity may be partially mediated by increased GH and IGF-1 concentrations.[132] On the other hand, although it is generally recognized that increased gonadal steroid levels are responsible for activation of the GH/IGF-1 axis at puberty (discussed earlier), a causal relationship between testosterone or estradiol and insulin resistance has not been shown.[135]

Treatment of nonobese Catalunyan girls with premature adrenarche and advanced skeletal maturation with the insulin sensitizer metformin was associated with later onset of breast development and menarche.[136] Moreover, in this relatively homogenous ethnic population, metformin treatment for 3 years slowed pubertal tempo among low–birth weight girls, who are at risk for early puberty and shorter adult stature.[137,138] Taken together, the foregoing considerations raise the possibility that decreased insulin sensitivity may represent a component of the cue that times the onset of gonadarche.

Ghrelin is a small acylated peptide that is secreted predominantly by the stomach and promotes GH secretion.[139] Circulating ghrelin concentrations are higher during fasting and decrease after food intake, suggesting that ghrelin signals energy-deficient states and modulates appetite and carbohydrate metabolism. Fasting morning ghrelin concentrations appear to be independent of age and pubertal status, but show negative correlation with weight.[140] Ghrelin and leptin appear to act as reciprocal regulators of energy homeostasis exerting opposing influences on the hypothalamic–pituitary–gonadal axis.[141] Resistin and adiponectin are two recently described hormones secreted by adipocytes that appear to provide metabolic and nutritional status information.[142,143] The respective roles, if any, of these hormones on gonadarche or adrenarche remain to be determined.

ACTIVATION AND TIMING OF ADRENARCHE

Whereas increased DHEAS secretion is the earliest hormonal manifestation of adrenarche, changes in pituitary adrenocorticotrophin (ACTH) secretion have not been detected nor have specific adrenal androgen-stimulating factors been isolated from the pituitary. ACTH is a peptide derived after proteolytic cleavages of proopiomelanocortin (POMC). In the adrenal cortex, ACTH binds to its cognate receptor, a G-protein–coupled seven-transmembrane–domain receptor that signals via cyclic adenosine monophosphate (cAMP) and protein kinase A. ACTH has both acute and chronic effects on the adrenal cortex. Acutely, it promotes uptake of low-density lipoprotein, stimulates cholesterol esterase activity, enhances synthesis and phosphorylation of StAR, and promotes cortisol secretion. The chronic effects of ACTH involve stimulation of transcription and translation of steroidogenic enzyme genes.

The onset of adrenarche is associated with increased 17,20-lyase activity and decreased 3β-hydroxysteroid dehydrogenase activity.[144] Available data suggest that, at the time of adrenarche, changes in expression of cytochrome b$_5$, DHEA sulfotransferase, and 3β-hydroxysteroid dehydrogenase play essential roles in DHEA/DHEAS production.[145] Histologically, increased thickness of the zona reticularis occurs concurrently with the increase in DHEAS concentration. DHEAS concentrations peak between 20 and 25 years of age, followed by continuous decline. Although the findings have been inconsistent, clinical studies suggest that insulin, IGF-1, and GH concentrations influence the timing, onset, and progression of adrenarche.[146] Comparisons of IGF-1 concentrations among prepubertal children have shown higher concentrations in African-American children.[147] Whether these ethnic differences contribute to the earlier onset of adrenarche or increased incidence of premature pubarche in African-American girls is unknown. Clinical observations regarding associations between adrenarche and body size and fatness have been inconsistent; one longitudinal study showed that DHEAS concentrations increased commensurate with the largest increase in BMI, whereas another longitudinal study found no association between DHEAS and weight, BMI, or body surface area.[148,149] Available data suggest that undefined gradual developmental changes within the adrenal cortex underlie the onset of adrenarche.

Hypothalamic releasing factors, such as corticotropin-releasing hormone (CRH) and vasopressin (ADH), play important roles in governing hypothalamic–pituitary–adrenal axis function. In contrast to the role of hypothalamic GnRH in gonadarche, however, CRH and ADH do not appear to trigger the onset of adrenarche. Moreover, adrenarche occurs independently of developmental changes in the hypothalamic–pituitary–gonadal axis. For example, children with gonadal dysgenesis experience normal adrenarche and pubarche, whereas children with primary adrenal insufficiency may have normal gonadarche.[150]

GENETICS AND PUBERTY GENES

As pointed out by others,[151] the observations that the temporal correlation in somatic maturation and attainment of pubertal stages in monozygotic twins is more robust than that in dizygotic twins, that the age of menarche in mothers and daughters is correlated, that parents of children with constitutional delay recall a later age of menarche and of the adolescent growth spurt than those of a control group of children,[152,153] that precocious gonadarche in girls may be familial and transmitted in an autosomal dominant mode,[154] and that the age of menarche varies with racial group imply the existence of a major genetic component to puberty. When a genetic influence is established, however, it remains unclear whether the genotype is directly dictating the timing of the pubertal resurgence of GnRH release (perhaps a clock gene in analogy to circadian timekeeping)[155] or simply controlling permissive factors that are required for expression of pubertal mechanisms. We suggest that the term "puberty" gene should therefore be restricted to those genes that are specifically involved in the timing of either adrenarche or gonadarche.[5] For gonadarche, such genes would determine the age of the pubertal resurgence of pulsatile GnRH release by regulating the timing of the application or withdrawal of the neurobiologic brake to the GnRH neuronal network of the juvenile hypothalamus. Puberty genes could time the resurgence of pulsatile GnRH release, not only by triggering a hypothalamic signal at puberty but also potentially by determining the duration of the prepubertal brake on pulsatile GnRH release or by timing the "turn off" of the GnRH pulse generator during infancy. In the case of adrenarche, the developmental increase in adrenal androgen secretion would presumably be timed by genes that are expressed in the adrenal and unrelated to any brain genes controlling the onset of gonadarche. Despite the accelerating pace of elucidation into the genetic causes of disorders of pubertal development,[156] the identity of specific puberty genes, that is, those that dictate the timing of the resumption of pulsatile GnRH release (and therefore determine the age of gonadarche) and those that regulate the developmental increase in adrenal androgen secretion that determines the age of pubarche, have not been identified. A gene that has recently attracted much attention in this regard is *KiSS1R* (discussed earlier). Although a gain-of-function mutation of *KiSS1R* has been recently reported in a 7-year-old girl with GnRH-dependent precocious breast development,[80] the report of hypogonadotropism in an infantile boy with a loss-of-function mutation of *KiSS1R*[79] suggests that the receptor encoded by this gene is probably critical for pulsatile GnRH release at all stages of development. Therefore, it does not meet the criteria for a puberty gene. Similarly, mutations of several other genes have profound effects on both gonadarche and adrenarche,[157] but their effect on the reproductive axis involves more than just timing the onset of puberty. For example, mutations of the *KAL-1* gene, which encodes anosmin (an extracellular glycoprotein that appears to be involved in the migration of GnRH neurons from the olfactory bulb to the hypothalamus during fetal development), may lead to profound hypogonadotropic hypogonadism[158] and, therefore, to the absence of gonadarche.

In addition to nucleotide sequence variation, genetic information can be transmitted by other mechanisms such as DNA (CpG) methylation, chromatin packaging, and small RNA/micro-RNA effects on transcription. Whereas most autosomal genes are expressed from the alleles of both parents, a number of growth regulatory genes show parent-of-origin effects due to genomic imprinting.[159] Environmental factors such as nutrition, hormone and chemical exposures, and physical factors can alter gene expression through these epigenetic modifications.[160,161] Maternal nutritional status can influence fetal gene expression through epigenetic mechanisms; animal studies suggest that this effect may be transmitted to subsequent generations.[162] Developmental disorders, such as

Prader-Willi syndrome, in which the timing and tempo of puberty are altered (discussed later), are associated with abnormal expression of imprinted genes.[159] These disorders may represent the "tip of the iceberg" for epigenetic influences on the genes that dictate or modulate the timing puberty.

FACTORS MODULATING THE TIMING OF PUBERTY

In general, the majority of studies that have examined the influence of various parameters on the onset and tempo of puberty have focused on the process of gonadarche. Considerably less attention has been paid to the timing and progression of adrenarche. Additionally, many factors that influence the onset and tempo of puberty (e.g., nutritional status) also modulate hypothalamic GnRH pulse generator activity in the majority of adults. Therefore, a modulator of puberty is not necessarily a component of the mechanism that initiates this developmental event. Rather, it is more likely that such factors play permissive, albeit in some cases, obligatory, roles to allow the process of puberty to unfold once the signal responsible for the resurgence in pulsatile GnRH secretion has been activated.

Nutrition and Diet

Nutritional state will modulate the onset of gonadarche in girls,[163] as reflected by the findings that menarche is delayed in malnourished girls,[164] obesity is associated with early breast development and menarche,[165] and menarche tends to occur at a particular or "critical" body weight rather than at a set age.[166] The delay in gonadarche in malnourished girls is probably mediated at the hypothalamic level by reduced availability of metabolic fuels or altered hormonal signals that interrupt or attenuate the pubertal resurgence of GnRH pulse generator activity.[167] Although the effect of undernutrition on gonadarche in boys has received less attention, there is no reason to suspect that the male axis is unaffected. The timing of adrenarche may also be influenced by nutritional status.

Differences unrelated to racial or ethnic background in the timing and tempo of gonadarche have been reported in well-nourished girls. Researchers have suggested that dietary habits may account for such variations.[168-170] Specifically, attention is drawn to subtle relationships between diets high in animal protein and early menarche, and between diets high in vegetable grains and delayed onset or tempo of gonadarche. Phytoestrogens, which have the potential to function as selective estrogen receptor modulators (SERMs), are found in soybeans, flaxseed, peanuts, and some vegetables. Most are diphenolic compounds with structural features common to estrogenic steroid agonists and antagonists. They, therefore, have mixed activities.[171] The issue of whether (or under what circumstances) these naturally occurring SERMs should be viewed as endocrine disruptors[172] rather than as "physiologic" modulators of the pubertal process merits discussion.

Moderate to vigorous exercise in the absence of weight restriction appears to have a negligible effect on the timing and tempo of puberty in either sex. However, breast development, menarche, and skeletal maturation are frequently reported to be delayed in girls involved in strenuous physical training.[173] The association between extreme energy expenditure and delayed gonadarche in the female is particularly marked in ballerinas, long-distance runners, and figure skaters, who must maintain their body weight within strict limits. Such girls have amenorrhea secondary to hypothalamic hypogonadism. The factors responsible for compromising pulsatile GnRH release in pubertal children who exercise vigorously are probably similar to those resulting from undernutrition. The life of the young female dancer or athlete is stressful; therefore, stress may also represent a contributing factor underlying exercise-induced delayed gonadarche. Because certain physical and psychological characteristics are necessary for outstanding athletic performances, there may be a significant contribution of self-selection involved in the decision of girls to participate at such an exceptional level. In a study of young female gymnasts and their parents, menarche in the mothers was found to be delayed relative to that of mothers of sedentary girls.[174] Therefore, the possibility of a genetic contribution to this phenomenon cannot be excluded. The effect of physical training on the timing of pubarche in girls has been less studied, and the available data are contradictory.[175,176]

Although the relationship between strenuous physical training and male puberty has received less attention, this developmental process is apparently less susceptible in boys than it is in girls.[177] This may be related, in part, to sex differences in the age at which training is initiated, and to the intensity of the exercise. Nevertheless, in sports, such as wrestling, that require weight control achieved with a combination of strenuous exercise and dietary restriction, impaired testosterone secretion may occur.[177]

Prenatal Influences

Some children with intrauterine growth retardation or who are born small for gestational age (SGA) have decreased insulin sensitivity.[138,178,179] These children appear to have an increased risk of hypertension, diabetes, and coronary artery disease in adulthood.[180] Increased adrenal androgen levels and, in some cases, precocious or exaggerated adrenarche have been reported in both boys and girls born SGA.[181-183] Some, but not all, girls with precocious adrenarche are at increased risk for ovarian hyperinsulinemic hyperandrogenism (early polycystic ovarian syndrome) at the time of gonadarche.[181,182,184] Despite inconsistent reports, the majority of studies indicate that the timing of menarche in girls born SGA does not appear to be markedly different from that of girls born at an appropriate size for gestational age.[185-188] The timing of puberty in boys born SGA appears to be normal,[187] although subfertility has been reported after they reached adulthood.[189]

Adoption or Migration from Developing to Developed Countries

Several European countries have reported precocious gonadarche in a relatively dramatic proportion of children—particularly girls—adopted from developing regions, such as Asia and South America.[190,191] This precocity is preceded by increased endocrine activity in the pituitary–ovarian axis before the onset of physical manifestations of puberty, indicating a central origin to the condition.[192] Although it was initially argued that improved nutritional and social conditions were in some way responsible for this phenomenon, the cause of the precocity appears to be complex. Precocious gonadarche is also seen in immigrant girls arriving with their parents and without evidence of earlier compromised growth and nutrition.[193] Moreover, ethnic background does not appear to be involved. A study of immigrant girls in Belgium with premature gonadarche found an association with previous exposure to organochlorine pesticides.[193] Although most reports of this form of precocity have not raised the possibility that the precise age of the adopted children may be in doubt, birth records are not always well documented.

Disorders of Early Puberty

The terminology used to describe disorders of puberty has evolved as the pathophysiology and molecular etiologies of these disorders have been clarified (Box 17-1 and Table 17-2). The term "central precocious puberty" or "GnRH-dependent precocious puberty" refers to premature resurgence of GnRH pulse generator activity, which we have labeled as *GnRH-dependent precocious gonadarche*. The terms "partial," "incomplete," "peripheral," "pseudo-," and "GnRH-independent" precocious puberty have been used to describe other etiologies of premature sexual development. We refer to these disorders as *GnRH-independent precocious puberty*. *Isosexual* refers to the development of sexual characteristics typical for the patient's gender. *Heterosexual* refers to the development of sexual characteristics typical of the other gender (e.g., feminizing tumors in males). Delayed puberty has been categorized as being either *hypogonadotropic* (low gonadotropin concentrations) or *hypergonadotropic* (elevated gonadotropin concentrations). With expanding knowledge of the functional genomics of the pubertal process and the molecular genetics underlying its pathophysiology, the classification of the etiologies of disorders of puberty will continue to evolve.

GnRH-DEPENDENT PRECOCIOUS PUBERTAL DEVELOPMENT

Progressive Precocious Gonadarche

Despite its name, GnRH-dependent precocious puberty represents precocious gonadarche due to either premature resurgence or incomplete suppression of the hypothalamic GnRH pulse generator. It occurs more often in girls than in boys. This sex difference is probably related to the lesser prepubertal suppression of the GnRH pulse generator in girls than in boys. The sequence of pubertal development is typical of normal puberty, including adrenarche in some cases, but it begins at an earlier-than-normal age.

Useful laboratory studies include x-ray assessment of skeletal maturation (bone age) and serum sex steroid concentrations. A GnRH (gonadorelin [Factrel] or a GnRH-R agonist [GnRH-Ra], such as leuprolide) stimulation test

BOX 17-1

Etiologies of Precocious Puberty

Gonadotropin-Releasing Hormone (GnRH)-Dependent Gonadarche
Idiopathic: Progressive, nonprogressive
Congenital central nervous system (CNS) lesions: Hypothalamic hamartoma, septo-optic dysplasia, arachnoid cysts, suprasellar cysts
Acquired CNS disorders: Postinflammatory, postradiation therapy, abscess, hydrocephalus, trauma, tumors
Chronic exposure to androgens: Congenital adrenal hyperplasia, familial male-limited precocious puberty
Other conditions: Williams-Beuren syndrome, maternal uniparental disomy of chromosome 14, histiocytosis X

GnRH-Independent Gonadarche
McCune-Albright syndrome
Feminizing disorders, estrogen-secreting tumors: Ovarian (granulosa cell, Peutz-Jeghers syndrome, gonadoblastoma/dysgerminoma, carcinoma, cystadenoma, theca cell, lipoid) and adrenal
Feminizing disorders, estrogen secretion unrelated to tumors: Aromatase mutation
Isolated premature menarche: Estrogen-secreting cyst, tumor, McCune-Albright syndrome, primary hypothyroidism
Premature thelarche: Variant of normal development, Rubinstein-Taybi syndrome, Kabuki syndrome
Primary hypothyroidism
Exposure to exogenous sex steroids or endocrine disruptors
Virilizing disorders: Premature adrenarche, congenital adrenal hyperplasias (21-hydroxylase deficiency, 3β-hydroxysteroid dehydrogenase deficiency, 11β-hydroxylase deficiency), inherited glucocorticoid resistance, familial male-limited precocious puberty (testotoxicosis), androgen-secreting tumors (adrenal sex steroid–secreting tumors, such as adenoma and carcinoma; ovarian tumors, such as arrhenoblastoma; testicular Leydig cell), human chorionic gonadotropin–secreting tumors (hepatoblastoma/hepatoma, dysgerminoma, teratoma, choriocarcinoma), Cushing syndrome (Cushing disease associated with increased adrenocorticotrophin [ACTH] secretion, adrenal disease, ectopic secretion of corticotropin-releasing hormone or ACTH)

TABLE 17-2

Monogenic Disorders Associated with Precocious Puberty

Gene	Locus	Phenotype
GNAS1	20q13.2	McCune-Albright syndrome
STK11/LKB1	19p13.3	Peutz-Jeghers syndrome
CYP21	6p21	CAH due to 21-hydroxylase deficiency
HSD3B2	1p13.1	CAH due to 3β-hydroxysteroid dehydrogenase deficiency
CYP11B1	8q21	CAH due to 11β-hydroxylase deficiency
LHR	2p21	Familial male-limited precocious puberty
CYP19	15q21.1	Precocious puberty/gynecomastia
GRL	5q31	Inherited glucocorticoid resistance
GPR54	19p13.3	Precocious puberty associated with activating mutations

CAH, congenital adrenal hyperplasia.

expectations regarding psychosocial development and abilities. Cognitive and emotional development, however, are normal for chronologic age. Thus, the guilelessness and naïveté of such children exposes them to an increased risk of sexual abuse, with affected girls at risk for becoming pregnant.

Hypothalamic hamartomas, congenital malformations composed of a heterotropic mass of nerve tissue, usually located on the floor of the third ventricle or attached to the tuber cinereum, are a common etiology of precocious gonadarche. The tumors can be classified as *parahypothalamic*, attached to or suspended from the floor of the third ventricle, or as *intrahypothalamic*, in which the mass is enveloped by the hypothalamus and distorts the third ventricle. The lesions do not grow over time and do not metastasize. Extreme precocity or the absence of circulating tumor markers, such as β-human chorionic gonadotropin (hCG) and α-fetoprotein,[195,196] suggests a hamartoma. Although gelastic or laughing seizures can be associated with precocious puberty due to hypothalamic hamartomas, the majority of patients do not exhibit neurologic symptoms.

On computerized tomography (CT) or magnetic resonance imaging (MRI) scans, hamartomas appear as an isodense, abnormal fullness. Imaging with MRI is superior to CT, but the lesions do not enhance with contrast material. Histologic examination of hypothalamic hamartoma tissue has shown immunoreactivity for GnRH and for astroglial-derived factors, such as TGFα.[197] Two potential mechanisms have been hypothesized, with one being

is important to demonstrate a pubertal pattern of gonadotropin responses with LH secretion predominating and thus to verify increased GnRH pulse generator activity. In girls, when gonadotropins are measured using third-generation monoclonal fluorometric assays, basal and GnRH-stimulated LH concentrations greater than 0.6 and 6.9 U/L, respectively, are 70% and 92% sensitive for the diagnosis of GnRH-dependent precocious gonadarche.[194] Although it is often considered idiopathic in girls, an organic etiology can usually be identified in boys.

Because affected children appear older than their chronologic age, parents and teachers may have inappropriate increased GnRH secretion from tissue emancipated from suppression by the prepubertal brake. The other possibility is that factors such as TGFα provide an ectopic drive to GnRH neurons, with a normal distribution in the hypothalamus. Gene expression profiling of hypothalamic hamartomas associated with precocity may provide clues about genes, proteins, and regulatory pathways associated with the timing of puberty.[198]

Optic gliomas, suprasellar cysts, arachnoid cysts, previous head trauma, static cerebral encephalopathy, CNS infections, CNS radiation, hydrocephalus, meningomyelocele, and neurodevelopmental disabilities may also be associated with progressive precocious gonadarche.[199-201] If the precocity is due to CNS tumors, neurologic symptoms usually precede the premature pubertal development. Optic gliomas are associated with neurofibromatosis type 1 (NF-1), an autosomal dominant disorder that is diagnosed based on clinical features that include size and number of café-au-lait spots, macrocephaly, and family history of the disorder. The type of CNS lesion influences the presentation of GnRH-dependent precocious puberty, presumably due to differences in the mechanisms inducing puberty and the hypothalamic–pituitary deficiencies associated with the initial lesion or its treatment.[202] CNS radiation used to treat intracranial tumors or used prophylactically for malignancies can induce precocious gonadarche, perhaps as a result of an astroglial response, with increased TGFα production.[203] In this situation, it is important to note that simultaneous GH deficiency may be masked by accelerated growth velocity due to precocious gonadarche.

Precocious gonadarche, which appears to be GnRH-dependent, has been reported in Williams-Beuren syndrome, histiocytosis X,[204,205] and maternal uniparental disomy for chromosome 14.[206] An imprinted domain located at chromosome 14q32 appears to be the critical region for the phenotype associated with maternal uniparental disomy. In addition to precocious puberty, clinical features include pre- and postnatal growth retardation, developmental delay, hypotonia, and joint laxity. Deletion of the paternal allele and imprinting defects involving this region can result in a similar phenotype.[207] Other situations associated with progressive precocious gonadarche include virilizing disorders (such as CAH) and familial male-limited precocious puberty (testotoxicosis), in which skeletal maturation is usually markedly advanced. In these situations, the precocious gonadarche is considered secondary to the virilizing disorder, but the mechanism through which the GnRH pulse generator is prematurely activated is unclear. The increase in sex steroids in children with either primary or secondary precocious gonadarche is associated with elevated IGF-1 and IGF-binding protein-3 (IGFBP3) concentrations, which do not decrease to prepubertal values with treatment of the underlying disorder.[208]

The treatment of choice for children with progressive precocious gonadarche is a GnRH-Ra. In situations of coexisting GH deficiency, combined treatment with recombinant human GH may be helpful to preserve height potential. GnRH-Ras are modifications of the native GnRH decapeptide, have greater resistance to degradation, and possess increased affinity for the GnRH-R. They are, therefore, perceived by the pituitary as a continuous GnRH stimulation, which induces down-regulation of GnRH-R function and leads to decreased gonadotropin secretion. GnRH-Ras are available as daily injections or depot forms that are currently administered every 28 days. The depot formulation of leuprolide acetate is commonly used in the United States; the recommended dose is 0.3 mg/kg administered every 28 days. Another GnRH-Ra, histrelin, has been formulated as a hydrogel subdermal implant that is surgically inserted into the inner aspect of the upper arm.[209] Over the course of 1 year, histrelin diffuses from the 50-mg implant. Early studies indicate excellent gonadotropin suppression; prospective longitudinal studies are needed to confirm safety and efficacy.[209]

When the progressive nature of the disorder is equivocal, serial evaluations are necessary to detect a sustained acceleration in the tempo of pubertal development, including skeletal maturation (and therefore loss of height potential), before initiation of therapy. This strategy is necessary because children with nonprogressive precocious puberty do not benefit from treatment. The major goals of treatment are to prevent further pubertal progression until appropriate for chronologic age and to attain normal adult height.

Clinically, the cessation of gonadarcheal progression is apparent within 3 months of initiation of treatment. Signs related to adrenarche neither regress nor are prevented, and may progress. In girls, breast size typically decreases, but may not completely regress. Vaginal bleeding secondary to estrogen withdrawal as well as acne may occur during the first month of treatment. Subsequently, there should be no further vaginal bleeding, even if menarche occurred before the initiation of therapy. The ovaries and uterus decrease in size. In boys, testicular volume decreases. Linear growth velocity and the rate of bone mineral accretion decrease. Longitudinal evaluation of a cohort of children with precocious gonadarche showed increased lumbar bone mineral density and BMI standard deviation scores at initiation of therapy. Two years after cessation of therapy in these children, bone mass, bone turnover, and percent body fat were normal, suggesting that peak bone mass will be appropriate.[210]

Adequacy of treatment is judged by prepubertal estradiol/testosterone concentrations and prepubertal gonadotropin response to GnRH stimulation. Monitoring to confirm the efficacy of therapy includes interim history; physical examination to ascertain height, weight, and stage of pubertal development; and bone age x-rays. In addition, GnRH stimulation tests should be repeated at regular intervals (3-6 months) to document gonadotropin suppression. This monitoring is necessary because bone maturation may progress despite regression of the clinical features associated with gonadarche. Urinary gonadotropin determinations do not provide adequate sensitivity to judge the efficacy of therapy.[211]

The duration of GnRH-Ra therapy should be individualized, with the decision to discontinue therapy based on chronologic age, skeletal maturation, projected adult height, and psychosocial readiness for resumption of puberty. For girls, menstruation usually occurs 9 to 15 months after discontinuation of GnRH-Ra therapy, with earlier onset in those who had experienced menarche before treatment. Studies indicate that final height is improved over initial predicted height at diagnosis, but is still less than that based on midparental height. Rapidly progressive pubertal development, advanced skeletal maturation, predicted compromise of adult height, and psychosocial considerations justify treatment.[212,213]

Among the adverse effects of treatment, parents may note increased emotional lability and moodiness just before the GnRH-Ra injection. Local or systemic allergic reactions or sterile abscesses may occur, but are uncommon. Some children show increased weight gain disproportionate to their linear growth. Intermittent therapy, often due to poor compliance, may have the deleterious effect of increasing gonadotropin and gonadal steroid secretion, leading to progressive skeletal maturation and further compromise of adult height.

Long-term experience (>20 years) has now accrued for GnRH-Ras. No major adverse effects on reproductive function have been noted.[214,215] Pregnancies with normal offspring have been observed.[216]

Nonprogressive Precocious Gonadarche

Some children experience a nonprogressive (or slowly progressing) form of precocious gonadarche attributed to a premature but intermittent or transient activation of the hypothalamic GnRH pulse generator.[217] Among this latter group of children, basal gonadotropin concentrations and gonadotropin responses to GnRH stimulation may be normal for chronologic age, but can overlap values observed among children with progressive precocious gonadarche. Because the physical signs of pubertal development do not always correlate with GnRH-stimulated gonadotropin responses, physical findings alone cannot differentiate between the two forms of precocious gonadarche.[218] In general, children with this nonprogressive form of precocious gonadarche show no evidence of pubertal responsiveness to GnRH stimulation and no loss of height potential, and do not usually benefit from GnRH-Ra therapy.[219]

GnRH-INDEPENDENT PRECOCIOUS PUBERTAL DEVELOPMENT

Precocious pubertal development may occur in the absence of an elevation of pulsatile GnRH secretion. In these situations, inappropriate gonadal or adrenal steroid secretion or exposure to exogenous steroids induces the physical signs of puberty. In most instances, the pubertal development is incomplete and fertility is not attained.

McCune-Albright Syndrome

The classic clinical triad of McCune-Albright syndrome is precocious pubertal development, café-au-lait spots, and bony fibrous dysplasia. Premature pubertal development is not observed in all cases and appears to be more common among girls than among boys. This disorder is due to constitutive activation of the $G_s\alpha$ protein that is coupled to membrane-bound glycoprotein hormone receptors and is associated with autonomous function of endocrine glands. The syndrome is due to somatic cell mutations in the *GNAS1* gene, with missense mutations R201H and R201C being among the most common.[220] These gain-of-function mutations in the $G_{s\alpha}$ gene lead to constitutive activation of gonadotropin receptors and subsequent increased ovarian estrogen and testicular testosterone secretion in affected girls and boys, respectively.[221] Partial or atypical forms are increasingly recognized; among 113 children with one to three features typical of McCune-Albright syndrome, a polymerase chain reaction–based mutation analysis protocol identified a missense mutation at codon 201 in 90% when an affected tissue (e.g., ovarian, bone, adrenal tissue) was analyzed.[222]

Because the precocious pubertal development is GnRH-independent, GnRH-Ra treatment is ineffective. However, treatment with testolactone (aromatase inhibitor), tamoxifen (anti-estrogen), or medroxyprogesterone acetate can be helpful.[223,224] Although safe, treatment with anastrozole for 1 year did not halt vaginal bleeding or attenuate rates of skeletal maturation and linear growth in girls with McCune-Albright syndrome, suggesting that aromatase inhibitors may not be useful in the treatment of this form of precosity.[225] One outcome study showed variable gonadal function in affected adult women, with some having regular menses and fertility, whereas others had persistent autonomous gonadal function associated with irregular menses and infertility.[226]

The café-au-lait lesions are usually large, do not cross the midline, and have irregular "coast of Maine" margins. The typical bone lesion is polyostotic fibrous dysplasia and tends to be asymmetrical, affecting any bone, including the skull. The cystic bone lesions can lead to pathologic fractures and deformities. Pseudoarthrosis can occur. With involvement of the skull, hyperproliferation of the preosteoblastic cells results in impingement into cranial foramina, leading to compression of cranial nerves. Blindness, deafness, facial asymmetry, or ptosis can result. Rather than being associated with a single abnormality of bone, the specific histopathology varies, depending on the anatomic location: axial/appendicular skeleton, cranial bones, or gnathic bones.[227] Bone lesions may be apparent on bone scans before they are visible on x-rays. Hypermetabolic bone disease is indicated by increased serum osteocalcin and alkaline phosphatase concentrations, as well as by increased urinary hydroxyproline concentrations.

Short-term studies suggest that bisphosphonate therapy may benefit the bone disease. In one small series, bone pain decreased without apparent change in the bone lesions by radiography or scintigraphy.[228] However, other patients showed increased bone mineral density and radiographic evidence of bone healing with pamidronate treatment.[229]

Other endocrine manifestations include nodular thyroid hyperplasia with hyperthyroidism; multiple pituitary adenomas associated with gigantism, acromegaly, or hyperprolactinemia; parathyroid adenoma or hyperplasia with hyperparathyroidism; and adrenal nodules associated with Cushing syndrome.

Feminizing Disorders

Estrogen-Secreting Tumors. Estrogen-secreting tumors are a rare cause of premature or abnormal pubertal development. Types of tumors include granulosa cell, gonadal stromal cell, ovarian sex cord stromal, and theca cell.[230,231] The majority of juvenile granulosa cell tumors can be palpated on bimanual examination. Estrogen concentrations may be very elevated, and circulating tumor markers, such as α-fetoprotein or hCG, may be detected. Rarely, gonadoblastomas in streak gonads, lipoid tumors, cystadenomas, and ovarian carcinomas can secrete estrogens, androgens, or both. Elevated serum inhibin and MIH concentrations, and the finding of MIH immunoreactivity in the tumor, indicate that the tumor cells are of granulosa or Sertoli cell origin.[232-234] If originally positive, these markers may be useful to recognize recurrence. Assessment of specific gene expression can help to identify the histologic origin of gonadal tumors, providing greater precision in tumor classification.[235]

Sex cord tumors with annular tubules are common in patients with Peutz-Jeghers syndrome, an autosomal dominant disorder characterized by mucocutaneous pigmentation and gastrointestinal polyposis. These tumors, which are multifocal and bilateral, may differentiate into granulosa or Sertoli cell tumors with the potential to secrete estrogen. Thus, affected males may present with gynecomastia.[236] Although usually benign, granulosa and Sertoli cell tumors can undergo malignant changes.[237] Affected individuals have an increased risk of cancers of the colon, stomach, small intestine, breast, and pancreas. Inactivating mutations involving the *STK11/LKB1* gene have been identified in approximately 50% of patients with Peutz-Jeghers syndrome.[238]

Among boys, adrenal, testicular, or hepatocellular tumors can express aromatase, leading to secretion of estradiol and estrone.[239-241] When gynecomastia is excessive, prolonged, and apparent at a time other than midpuberty (approximately stage 3), further evaluation may be warranted.[242] The evaluation should include testosterone, estradiol, hCG, LH, FSH, thyroid-stimulating hormone (TSH), and DHEAS measurements. In addition to tumors, the differential diagnosis of gynecomastia includes Klinefelter syndrome, impaired testosterone biosynthesis, androgen insensitivity, and hyperprolactinemia.

Estrogen Secretion Unrelated to Tumors. In one family, autosomal dominant familial gynecomastia was due to aberrant transcription of the aromatase gene; the affected girl had GnRH-independent precocious pubertal development.[243] Autosomal dominant aromatase excess syndrome is characterized by high systemic estrogen levels, short stature, prepubertal gynecomastia, and testicular failure in males, and premature breast development, macromastia, and uterine pathology in females. Small chromosomal arrangements in the promoter region of the aromatase gene appear to be associated with increased promoter activity, resulting in increased aromatase activity.[244] Pathologic gynecomastia in males may be observed in association with hypogonadism, especially Klinefelter syndrome (see Chapter 16).

Isolated Premature Menarche. *Isolated premature menarche* is vaginal bleeding at an inappropriately early age in the absence of other signs of puberty. The duration of bleeding is usually limited to a few days. The most common endocrine etiology is spontaneous resolution of an estrogen-secreting ovarian cyst. Often, ultrasound shows no abnormality because the cyst has resolved by the time the study is obtained. Most cases are self-limited, remit spontaneously, and are associated with normal pubertal development. Typically, isolated menarche due to an estrogen-secreting cyst is a sporadic event that usually occurs once. However, such cysts and episodes of vaginal bleeding may recur. The bloody vaginal discharge noted in female infants during the first week of life is a physiologic event secondary to estrogen withdrawal.

Tumors and trauma usually do not cause cyclic bleeding. The other major differential diagnoses of isolated vaginal bleeding include sexual abuse, vaginal foreign bodies, neoplasms such as rhabdomyosarcoma, vaginal infection, McCune-Albright syndrome, and primary hypothyroidism.

Premature Thelarche. *Premature thelarche* is isolated breast development without other signs of pubertal maturation. Typically, the parents or pediatrician note breast development, either unilateral or bilateral, between 9 and 18 months of age. No significant nipple development or pigmentation occurs, and the vaginal mucosa remains pink and shiny.

Breast ultrasound can help distinguish breast tissue from cysts, fibroadenomas, neurofibromas, or other less common lesions, but is usually not needed.[245] Pelvic ultrasound may show a bilateral increase in the number of ovarian follicular cysts. Using a recombinant cell bioassay with increased sensitivity, estradiol concentrations are higher among girls with premature thelarche than among healthy control subjects. However, estradiol concentrations in such patients are still low and remain below assay detection limit for most radioimmunoassays.[246] FSH concentrations may be increased for chronologic age, but LH concentrations and LH responses to GnRH stimulation are prepubertal. No acceleration in linear growth velocity or skeletal maturation occurs, and the breast development usually regresses spontaneously over time.[247] In most instances, onset of puberty, adult height, and adult reproductive function are normal.[248] Premature thelarche can be considered a normal variant, and longitudinal evaluation is helpful to ensure the nonprogressive nature of this disorder. Rarely, some girls with premature thelarche subsequently show progressive gonadarche.[249]

Premature thelarche has been described in Rubinstein-Taybi syndrome, an autosomal dominant disorder characterized by short stature, psychosocial retardation, a characteristic facies, broad thumbs and halluces, and increased risk of neoplasia. Premature breast development is also observed in approximately 23% of female infants with the Kabuki syndrome, which is characterized by a peculiar facies with eyes reminiscent of Kabuki actors, mental retardation, and decreased growth velocity.[250]

Hypothyroidism. Girls with primary hypothyroidism can, on rare occasions, present with breast development or isolated vaginal bleeding.[251] This constellation of clinical features was first described by Van Wyk and Grumbach in 1960.[252] On ultrasound, enlarged multicystic ovaries may be noted.[253,254] Additional features may include delayed bone age, ascites, and pleural and pericardial effusions.[255] This is the only etiology of precocious puberty associated with delayed bone age. Thyroid hormone replacement therapy is associated with regression and resolution of the cysts; surgical treatment is not indicated. The mechanism underlying the ovarian stimulation is unclear. One possibility is that the excessively elevated TSH concentrations cross-react with the FSH receptor to promote estrogen secretion.[256] Another explanation is that increased FSH secretion observed in the hypothyroid state is responsible.

Hypothyroid boys may show increased testicular volume (macroorchidism) for age. Interestingly, after thyroxine replacement to a cohort of such boys and the subsequent attainment of stage 5, testicular volume was found to be considerably greater than that in control subjects.[257] The macroorchidism associated with prepubertal hypothyroidism is probably the result of an expanded population of undifferentiated Sertoli cells resulting from increased FSH signaling in response to elevated concentrations of either FSH or TSH.[257-260]

At the hypothalamic–pituitary level, hypothyroidism leads to a delay in the pubertal resurgence of LH secretion,[261] which presumably accounts for the delayed puberty that is generally associated with chronic hypothyroidism (discussed later).

Exogenous Estrogens and Other Endocrine Disruptors with Estrogen Activity. Exposure to exogenous estrogenic steroids or estrogen receptor agonists can induce pubertal development.[17,262] Potential sources of estrogenic steroids include oral contraceptives, creams, shampoos, and various lotions. In addition, phytoestrogens found in a variety of foods and phthalate esters present in plastics are environmental endocrine disruptors with estrogen agonist activity.

Epidemics of premature breast development reported in Puerto Rico and Italy have been attributed to increased exposure to estrogenic steroids, phthalates, phytoestrogens, or estrogenic mycotoxins.[263] Mycotoxins are naturally occurring substances that can be found as environmental contaminants in cereals, corn, and nuts.[264] In the Puerto Rico epidemic, 69% of samples from girls with premature thelarche contained phthalates compared with 3% of samples from control children.[262] It has been suggested that prenatal exposure to endocrine disruptors may influence fetal programming of the endocrine system and, therefore, may influence the timing and tempo of puberty. Certain drugs, such as marijuana, isoniazid, spironolactone, ketoconazole, and cimetidine, can induce gynecomastia by a variety of mechanisms.

Virilizing Disorders

Premature Adrenarche. Although the age of adrenarche varies considerably among ethnic groups, it is generally considered premature when it occurs before age 8 years in girls and age 9.5 years in boys. As in normal adrenarche, pubarche, axillary hair, adult-type apocrine odor, and acne may develop, whereas skeletal maturation may be appropriate for chronologic age or slightly advanced. Clitoromegaly and marked phallic enlargement are unusual findings in patients with premature adrenarche. Usually, gonadarche occurs at an appropriate chronologic age and subsequent pubertal development proceeds normally. Girls tend to be referred for evaluation more often than boys. Despite BMI comparable to that of control subjects, one recent study reported that girls with premature pubarche appear to have increased total and central fat mass.[265] In one study of Spanish and Italian girls, mean age at menarche for girls with documented premature pubarche was 6 months earlier than that of healthy control subjects.[266]

Typically, androgen concentrations are elevated for chronologic age, but within normal limits for the stage of pubic hair development. However, some girls with premature adrenarche show persistent hyperandrogenism on gonadarche.[267,268] Insulin resistance, hyperinsulinemia, and dyslipidemia have been described in these girls. Such girls have chronic anovulation, hirsutism, insulin resistance, hyperinsulinemia, severe acne, and aberrant patterns of gonadotropin secretion characterized by a high LH/FSH ratio. These features are suggestive of incipient polycystic ovary syndrome. Subsequently, some of these adolescent girls with PCOS have impaired glucose tolerance and type 2 diabetes mellitus.[269] In some populations, the frequency of heterozygosity in mutations in the 21-hydroxylase (*CYP21*) gene is higher among children with premature pubarche and adolescent girls with incipient PCOS.[270] Genetic markers, which appear to be associated with an increased risk of progression from premature pubarche to incipient PCOS, are the P12A variant of the peroxisome proliferator–activated receptor γ2 (*PPAR γ2*) and the G972R variant of the insulin receptor substrate-1 (*IRS-I*) genes.[271,272]

Premature pubarche due to premature adrenarche is a diagnosis of exclusion. The majority of children with premature adrenarche require no pharmacologic intervention. However, the ability to predict outcome and risk of PCOS is imperfect. Because lifestyle interventions involving food choices and exercise programs decrease the progression from impaired glucose tolerance to diabetes mellitus among adults,[273,274] it seems prudent to counsel children with premature pubarche to adopt healthy lifestyles.

Virilizing Congenital Adrenal Hyperplasias. The virilizing CAHs are a group of autosomal recessive disorders in which cortisol synthesis is impaired due to decreased 21-hydroxylase, 3β-hydroxysteroid dehydrogenase, or 11β-hydroxylase activity (see also Chapters 4 and 16). The specific pattern of circulating steroid hormone concentrations reflects which steroid enzyme is involved. Approximately 90% to 95% of cases are due to 21-hydroxylase deficiency, which is due to mutations in the *CYP21* gene.[275,276] Mutations in 3β-hydroxysteroid dehydrogenase type 2 (*HSD3B2*) and 11β-hydroxylase (*CYP11B1*) genes account for the remaining 5% to 10% of patients with virilizing CAH.[277]

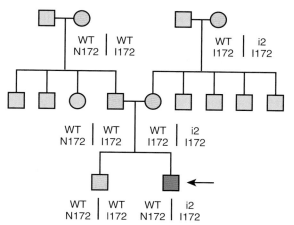

Figure 17-8. Molecular genetics of congenital adrenal hyperplasia. The proband presented with premature pubarche at age 5 years, 9 months. His height and weight were greater than the 95th percentile. He had Tanner stage 3 pubic hair, phallic enlargement, prepubertal testes, and a small amount of axillary hair. His bone age was 73 years. Laboratory findings showed elevated 17α-hydroxyprogesterone (10,735 ng/dL), androstenedione (1372 ng/dL), and testosterone (220 ng/dL). Molecular genotype analysis showed that he was a compound heterozygote with I172N on his paternal allele and the intron 2 splicing mutation on his maternal allele.

In all cases, decreased cortisol concentrations lead to loss of negative feedback inhibition, increased ACTH secretion, and increased adrenal androgen biosynthesis. The clinical spectrum of these disorders ranges from complete loss of function mutations, which typically present during infancy with genital ambiguity, to partial loss of function mutation, which may present in childhood, adolescence, or adulthood. Here, discussion is limited to the milder, "nonclassic" or "late-onset" forms of CAH, in which the major symptoms are secondary to hyperandrogenism, rather than to adrenal cortical insufficiency, as in the classic forms of this disease.

During childhood, boys or girls with milder forms of CAH may have premature pubarche, adult-type apocrine odor, increased growth velocity, and tall stature. In contrast to premature adrenarche, clitoromegaly or phallic enlargement and advanced skeletal maturation are more common. In female patients, the symptoms of late-onset CAH are similar to those of PCOS. Chronic hyperandrogenism associated with mutations involving any of the three steroidogenic enzymes can be associated with increased LH/FSH ratios and polycystic ovaries on ultrasound, but such patients typically lack the magnitude of insulin resistance associated with PCOS. The late onset of hyperandrogenic signs and symptoms of the milder forms of CAH (i.e., hirsutism and amenorrhea) result in an ascertainment bias such that affected males with normal testicular size for age are usually not detected by clinical features.

21-Hydroxylase Deficiency. The milder form (nonclassic, or late-onset form) of this disorder is reported to affect 1 in 1000 patients, whereas the reported incidence of the more severe forms is approximately 1 in 14,000. In 21-hydroxylase deficiency, decreased 21-hydroxylase activity leads to increased concentrations of 17-OH-hydroxyprogesterone, 17-OH-hydroxypregnenolone,

DHEA, androstenedione, and testosterone. The gene coding for 21-hydroxylase, *CYP21*, maps to chromosome 6p21. A highly homologous nonfunctional pseudogene, CYP21P, is located in close proximity to the functional gene. The *CYP21* and *CYP21P* genes show greater than 95% homology within coding regions.[278] The majority of mutations associated with 21-hydroxylase deficiency represent gene conversion events in which the functional gene has acquired deleterious nucleotide sequences from the pseudogene. To date, more than 100 mutations have been reported, but approximately 10 mutations account for the majority of affected alleles.[279] Most affected individuals are compound heterozygotes and carry different *CYP21* mutations on each allele (Fig. 17-8). Phenotype–genotype correlations are fairly consistent, with the phenotype usually representing the least severe mutation.[280-283] However, phenotypic heterogeneity does occur and is most commonly identified with either the intron 2 splicing mutation or I172N.[284-286] A single *CYP21* allele can carry multiple mutations; two mutations on the same allele can act synergistically to impair enzyme activity to a greater extent than would be anticipated for each mutation individually.[287]

Although random 17α-hydroxyprogesterone concentrations can be diagnostic (especially in the more severe forms), ACTH stimulation tests may be necessary to confirm the diagnosis of milder forms. Despite the availability of *CYP21* genotype analyses, the complexity of this locus precludes routine use of molecular diagnostics; therefore, ACTH stimulation tests may be necessary to confirm CAH. Techniques that genotype each allele and inclusion of parental DNA samples to segregate the alleles are helpful.

3β-Hydroxysteroid Dehydrogenase Deficiency. In this form of virilizing CAH, decreased activity of the specific adrenal and gonadal form of 3β-hydroxysteroid dehydrogenase leads to increased concentrations of 17α-hydroxypregnenolone and DHEA.[288] This disorder is due to mutations in the gene coding for 3β-hydroxysteroid dehydrogenase type 2, *HSD3B2*. Patients with classic 3β-hydroxysteroid dehydrogenase deficiency have been found to have mutations in the *HSD3B2* gene.[289-291] However, nonclassic CAH due to *HSD3B2* mutations is extremely rare.[292-294] Thus, molecular genetics have shown that nonclassic 3β-hydroxysteroid dehydrogenase deficiency is not a common allelic variant. Consequently, correlation of molecular genotype data with hormonal responses has led to the adoption of more stringent criteria for the diagnosis of 3β-HSD deficiency. In general, ACTH-stimulated 17-OH-hydroxypregnenolone and DHEA responses are elevated.

11β-Hydroxylase Deficiency. The clinical features of 11β-hydroxylase deficiency are similar to those of 21-hydroxylase deficiency. Patients with this type of virilizing adrenal hyperplasia may have hypertension attributed to increased deoxycorticosterone secretion. This disorder is due to mutations in the *CYP11B1* gene located on chromosome 8. Nonclassic CAH due to *CYP11B1* mutations is extremely rare. The incidence of 11β-hydroxylase deficiency has been estimated to be 1:100,000 among white populations, but the incidence among Israeli Jews of Moroccan origin is reported to be as high as 1:7000.[295,296] Elevated basal and ACTH-stimulated 11-deoxycortisol concentrations are typically found in this form of CAH. Serum 17-OHP, androstenedione, and testosterone concentrations may be mildly elevated. Plasma renin activity concentrations are low or suppressed.

Oxidoreductase Deficiency. Oxidoreductase deficiency is a newly described autosomal recessive type of CAH that is characterized by a steroid profile suggesting combined 17α-hydroxylase and 21-hydroxylase deficiencies.[297,298] The more severe phenotype is characterized by ambiguous genitalia, adrenal insufficiency, and skeletal anomalies, and is known as Antley-Bixler syndrome. The skeletal abnormalities can include craniosynostosis, midface hypoplasia, choanal atresia, low-set ears, pear-shaped nose, arachnodactyly, clinodactyly, and radiohumeral synostosis. This disorder is due to mutations in the P450 oxidoreductase (POR) gene located at chromosome 7q11.2.[299] The protein encoded by the POR gene functions as an electron donor to cytochrome P450 enzymes. Loss-of-function mutations influence the activities of 21-hydroxylase, 17α-hydroxylase, and aromatase enzymes.

Maternal virilization during pregnancy may occur and has been attributed to the aromatase deficiency. One woman was found to be a compound heterozygote with loss-of-function mutations on both alleles; she had breast development, primary amenorrhea, and cystic ovaries.[300] Prenatal virilization of female fetuses occurs, but there is minimal postnatal virilization. Basal and ACTH-stimulated steroid profiles are variable because POR deficiency affects multiple steroidogenic enzymes; serum 17-OH-hydroxyprogesterone concentrations tend to be elevated. Urinary analysis of steroid excretion using gas chromatography and mass spectroscopy can provide hormonal confirmation of the diagnosis. Cortisol deficiency may occur; affected individuals may benefit from glucocorticoid replacement therapy.[298] Mutations in the FGFR2 gene are associated with similar skeletal anomalies, but those affected have normal steroidogenesis and normal external genitalia.[301]

Diagnosis and Treatment of CAH. Steroid hormone responses to ACTH stimulation help to differentiate between premature adrenarche and CAH. To perform an ACTH stimulation test, a pharmacologic dose of synthetic ACTH (0.25 mg cosyntropin) is administered after a basal blood sample has been obtained. A second sample is collected 30 to 60 minutes later. Basal and stimulated steroid hormone concentrations and hormone ratios provide important information. Stimulated 17-OH-hydroxyprogesterone responses of less than 500 ng/dL at 30 minutes are within normal limits. Responses greater than 1500 ng/dL are consistent with 21-hydroxylase deficiency.[302] Intermediate responses, 500 to 1500 ng/dL, are consistent with heterozygosity for 21-hydroxylase deficiency. Children with premature pubarche due to HSD3B2 mutations have had ACTH-stimulated 17-OH-hydroxypregnenolone values greater than 9000 ng/dL.[303]

Treatment of the virilizing CAHs involves hormone replacement therapy with glucocorticoids. The goal of treatment is suppression of excessive ACTH and adrenal androgen secretion without hypercortisolism. Hydrocortisone or a synthetic glucocorticoid, such as prednisone or dexamethasone, can be used. During childhood, hydrocortisone is often considered to be the preferred glucocorticoid because linear growth in the growing child is extremely sensitive to glucocortcoid levels. Longer-acting glucocorticoids, such as prednisone and dexamethasone, may interfere with linear growth velocity. Typically, hydrocortisone dosages range from 7 to 15 mg/m^2/day and must be administered three times daily because of the hormone's short duration of action. This relatively short duration of action is the major disadvantage of hydrocortisone because patients may have significant variation in serum hormone concentrations between doses.

Some suggest the use of a reverse diurnal dosing such that the highest dose is administered at night, whereas others suggest that the highest dose should be administered in the morning.[304] Older adolescents and young adults may like the convenience of fewer daily doses and use prednisone (5-7.5 mg divided into two daily doses) or dexamethasone (0.25-0.5 mg daily). The growth-suppressive potencies of prednisone and dexamethasone are greater than their anti-inflammatory potencies.[305] It is also important to remember that the mineralocorticoid activity of these glucocorticoids varies, with prednisolone having less mineralocorticoid activity than hydrocortisone and dexamethasone having no mineralocorticoid activity.

Long-term management involves an interim medical history, physical examination with assessment of growth velocity, and hormone measurements to assess for adequate adrenal suppression.[306] Glucocorticoid therapy alone is generally sufficient for children with milder forms of CAH. Stress doses are indicated for fever, persistent vomiting, serious injuries, and surgery. Families should have injectable hydrocortisone readily available for situations in which oral medications are not tolerated. All affected individuals should wear a MedicAlert (MedicAlert Foundation, Turlock, CA) identification badge to alert emergency health care providers to their disorder.

Children with CAH who have a secondary GnRH-dependent precocious gonadarche may benefit from GnRH-Ra treatment. Children with overt salt loss, as well as those with simple virilizing forms, benefit from receiving mineralocorticoid replacement therapy.

Now that increased numbers of children with CAH or other disorders of sexual differentiation survive into adulthood, the medical and psychosocial aspects of their health care are undergoing reevaluation. Thus, interest in the determinants of gender identity, approach to genital reconstructive surgery, and outcome has increased.[307] Hence, issues related to gender identity, surgery, sexuality, and outcome may be discussed when evaluating patients with these disorders.

Because CAH is one of the most common disorders associated with aberrant external genital differentiation, most of the literature in this area relates to outcome in women with classic CAH. One study reported that adult women with CAH tended to be unmarried, have fewer children than healthy control subjects, and have negative self-images. The frequency of homosexuality, however, was not increased.[308] Girls with CAH tend to have female gender identity with preferences for male-type play and male career choices.[309] Gender identity in adolescent girls with CAH was not associated with the extent of prenatal androgen exposure, magnitude of virilization of the external genitalia, or age at reconstructive surgery.[310] Preliminary data from a limited number of outcome studies indicate that honesty, extensive education, and counseling benefit these patients with disorders of sexual differentiation and their families.[311-313]

Gonadal adrenal rest tumors may develop in the testes of boys with CAH. These testicular tumors are more common in boys who are undertreated or poorly compliant. The tumors tend to be benign and bilateral, and are believed to arise from aberrant ACTH-responsive adrenal cells. Due to their location in the mediastinum testis, obstruction of the seminiferous tubules, leading to gonadal dysfunction and infertility, can occur.

Inherited Glucocorticoid Resistance. Familial glucocorticoid resistance is an autosomal dominant disorder caused by loss-of-function mutations in the glucocorticoid receptor (GRL) gene. Consequently, in the face of normal or elevated cortisol concentrations, there is loss of negative feedback inhibition, leading to increased ACTH secretion and adrenal androgen biosynthesis, similar to that seen in CAH. The predominant symptoms of this disorder are due to excessive androgen and mineralocorticoid secretion rather than glucocorticoid deficiency. Affected children may present with premature pubarche, hypertension, fatigue, or hypokalemia.[314] Laboratory investigation shows elevated plasma concentrations of cortisol, adrenal androgens, aldosterone, and ACTH; these levels recede after administration of a high dose of dexamethasone. Treatment involves high-dose therapy with a potent glucocorticoid (i.e., dexamethasone), leading to suppression of ACTH release and decreased adrenal androgen secretion.

Familial Male-Limited Precocious Puberty. This autosomal dominant disorder is caused by constitutive activating mutations of the LHR gene[315,316] that alter the tertiary confirmation of the receptor protein, leading to increased cAMP signaling in the absence of ligand.[317] Clinical manifestations are limited to male patients and include phallic enlargement, increased testicular volume, pubic hair, body odor, accelerated growth velocity, and advanced skeletal maturation. These characteristics may present within the first few years of life. Testosterone concentrations are high, whereas gonadotropin concentrations are low. Short-term treatment with steroid synthesis inhibitors, such as testolactone, spironolactone, or ketoconazole, can be used. If a secondary GnRH-dependent gonadarche develops, GnRH-Ra treatment can improve height prediction.[318] Long-term treatment with cyproterone acetate or ketoconazole showed similar outcomes without major side effects in 10 boys with testotoxicosis; effects on final height outcome were variable.[319,320] The

lack of a female phenotype[321] is a mystery; perhaps the most attractive possibility is that expression of LHR by the prepubertal ovary is low.

Androgen-Secreting Tumors. Leydig cell tumors secrete testosterone, leading to precocious pubertal development in boys. Testicular volume may be asymmetrical because the tumors are often unilateral. Because some tumors are too small to be palpated, ultrasonography may be helpful to localize the tumor. The majority of Leydig cell tumors are benign. Malignant tumors tend to be larger, show greater cell atypia, and infiltrate beyond the testis. In rare instances, the tumor can secrete large quantities of other steroids, such as 17-OH-hydroxyprogesterone, which may confound the diagnosis.[322] A novel somatic cell–activating mutation of the LHR gene has been found in some adenomas.[323] Alterations in other factors, such as MIH, inhibin, and other growth factors, may also contribute to the development of such tumors. Hence, the etiologies of tumors at the molecular level are heterogeneous.[324] If possible, the tumor can be excised without removing the testis. Ovarian androgen-secreting tumors are a rare cause of virilization in girls. Such tumors can occur at an anatomic location distinct from the ovary, such as the round ligament.[325]

hCG-Secreting Tumors. In boys, hCG-secreting tumors induce testicular testosterone secretion, leading to precocious pubertal development. These tumors are frequently hepatic in origin. In girls, hCG-secreting tumors in the absence of pubertal levels of FSH are not usually associated with precocious pubertal development. Although exceptions have been described,[326] this finding is consistent with the idea that LHR expression in the prepubertal ovary is low.

Cushing Syndrome. Cushing syndrome is characterized by excessive glucocorticoid concentrations, whether endogenous or exogenous in origin. Although the predominant features of glucocorticoid excess in children and adolescents are arrested pubertal development and growth failure, precocious virilization may occur when the hypercortisolism is accompanied by hyperandrogenism. This occurs in Cushing disease, in cases of ectopic secretion of ACTH or CRH, and in rare cases of adrenal tumors. The combination of pubertal development and hypercortisolism suggests an adrenal tumor. Such tumors, which are rare, secrete a mixed array of steroid hormones. However, virilization is a common presentation for childhood adrenocortical tumors. There is a female predominance. Complete surgical excision is the treatment of choice; complete resection is required for cure. Residual or metastatic disease is associated with a poorer prognosis.[327] Histologic examination may not be able to accurately differentiate benign adenomas from carcinomas. The majority of benign lesions of the adrenal cortex appear to be associated with abnormalities of the cAMP signaling pathway, whereas adrenocortical carcinomas are linked to aberrant expression of insulin-like growth factor II, tumor protein p53, and related molecules.[328,329]

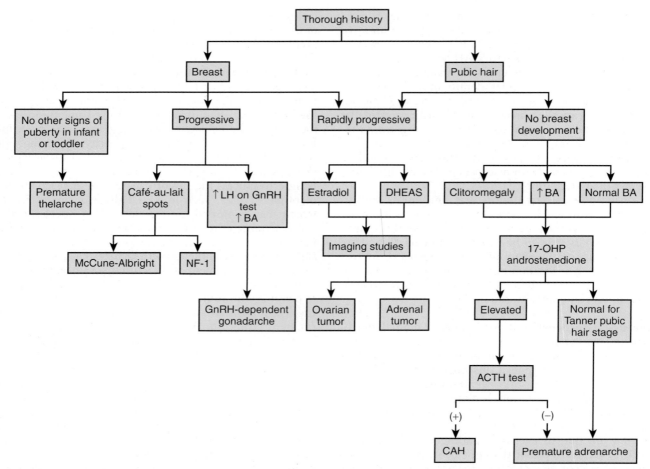

Figure 17-9. *Algorithm for precocious puberty in girls. Beginning with a thorough medical history, this flowchart provides guidelines for the differential diagnosis of the most common causes of precocious puberty in girls. As seen in Figure 17-10, assessment for hypercortisolism should be considered in patients with premature pubic hair, advanced bone age, and increased adrenal hormone concentrations. ACTH, adrenocorticotrophin; BA, bone age; CAH, congenital adrenal hyperplasia; DHEAS, dehydroepiandrosterone sulfate; GnRH, gonadotropin-releasing hormone; LH, luteinizing hormone; NF-1, neurofibromatosis type 1.*

Approach to the Child with Precocious Pubertal Development

Identification of the etiology of sexual precocity begins with a thorough medical history, with questions focusing on the physical manifestations of puberty and the age and sequence of their appearance (Figs. 17-9 and 17-10). Does the patient have neurologic symptoms or gelastic seizures? Has the patient received radiation therapy? Was the patient exposed to exogenous hormones? Obtaining a complete family history is important because some disorders, such as familial male-limited precocious puberty, glucocorticoid resistance, and neurofibromatosis type 1, show autosomal dominant inheritance.

Next, a complete physical examination, including auxologic measures, should be performed; particular attention should be paid to development of secondary sexual characteristics. For girls, is breast or pubic hair development present? For boys, is testicular volume increased? Because increased growth velocity occurs concomitantly with

breast development among girls, observation of accelerated growth velocity helps to differentiate GnRH-dependent precocious gonadarche from nonprogressive gonadarche or premature thelarche. The physical examination should be directed to detect physical signs indicating onset of gonadarche or adrenarche, as well as features suggestive of specific disorders—such as café-au-lait spots in McCune-Albright syndrome. Does the patient have manifestations of hypothyroidism?

Laboratory studies are used to confirm or exclude specific disorders based on the possible differential diagnoses. Bone age is usually, but not always, advanced among patients with GnRH-dependent precocious gonadarche and the CAHs. Typically, bone maturation is not significantly advanced among those with premature thelarche or premature adrenarche.

Because gonadotropin secretion is pulsatile, random concentrations usually provide only limited information. GnRH stimulation tests help to differentiate GnRH-dependent precocious gonadarche from premature thelarche, because an LH-predominant response is typical

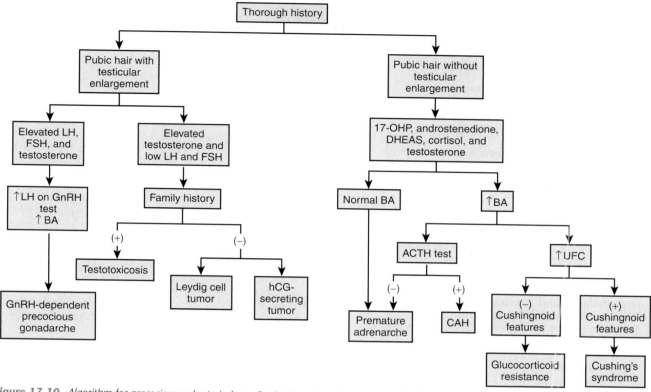

Figure 17-10. *Algorithm for precocious puberty in boys. Beginning with a thorough medical history, this flowchart provides guidelines for the differential diagnosis of the most common causes of precocious puberty in boys. ACTH, adrenocorticotrophin; BA, bone age; CAH, congenital adrenal hyperplasia; DHEAS, dehydroepiandrosterone sulfate; FSH, follicle-stimulating hormone; GnRH, gonadotropin-releasing hormone; hCG, human chorionic gonadotropin; LH, luteinizing hormone; UFC, urinary free cortisol.*

of GnRH-dependent precocious gonadarche, whereas an FSH-predominant response is typical of premature thelarche.[330] The limited availability of GnRH (gonadorelin) has led to development of stimulation tests using leuprolide (Lupron) as the provocative agent.[331] Comparison of immunochemiluminometric assay (ICMA) and immunofluorometric assay (IFMA) indicated that for prepubertal children, the upper limit of normal for LH after a GnRH stimulation test by ICMA was 4.1 IU/L for boys and 3.3I IU/L for girls, and that for IFMA was 3.3 IU/L for boys and 4.2 IU/L for girls.[332] It is important to be aware of the normal values for the specific method used. Most current assays for gonadotropins are sandwich assays specific to the β-subunit.

For patients with GnRH-dependent precocious gonadarche, MRI of the head is helpful. Boys with elevated hCG concentrations may require imaging of the head, chest, and abdomen to detect an extratesticular hCG-secreting tumor. Among girls, pelvic ultrasound can ascertain pubertal development of the ovaries and uterus; it can also detect tumors and ovarian cysts.[333]

Adrenal ultrasound to assess for adrenal tumors is appropriate for children with premature pubarche and extremely elevated DHEAS concentrations.

Individuals with chronic conditions, such as rheumatoid arthritis, steroid-dependent nephropathies, and asthma requiring high-dose steroid treatment, may have signs and symptoms of glucocorticoid excess. Intranasal steroids can cause iatrogenic Cushing syndrome and adrenal suppression.[334]

Disorders of Delayed Puberty

In most cases, delayed puberty is the result of delayed gonadarche and is defined as secondary sexual characteristic development at an age greater than two standard deviations more than for the normal population. Thus, for girls, lack of breast development by age 13 years or menarche by 16 years may be viewed as delayed. For boys, prepubertal testicular volume at age 14 years is considered delayed. Pubertal delay can be broadly subclassified into six groups:

1. Constitutional
2. GnRH-dependent (hypothalamic hypogonadotropism)
3. Pituitary-dependent
4. Hypothalamic and pituitary-dependent
5. Gonad-dependent
6. Steroid receptor–dependent

Patients with gonad-dependent delayed puberty may be further subdivided into those with primary gonadal failure and those with impaired steroidogenesis. Inappropriate pubertal development during the adolescent years may also reveal disorders of sexual differentiation that escape diagnosis during infancy. Failure to complete puberty within 5 years

---

BOX 17-2

Etiologies of Delayed Puberty

Constitutional Delay

Gonadotropin-Releasing Hormone (GnRH)-Dependent (Hypothalamic Hypogonadotropic Hypogonadism)
Kallmann syndrome and related disorders
Anorexia nervosa
Undernutrition/chronic disease/intensive exercise
Leptin-dependent

Pituitary-Dependent (Pituitary Hypogonadotropic Hypogonadism)
GnRH-R gene mutation
FSHβ gene mutation
LHβ gene mutation
Developmental anomalies: *Hesxl* gene mutation (septo-optic dysplasia), *Pitx2* gene mutation (Rieger syndrome), *PROP-1* gene mutation, maternal cocaine abuse, valproate toxicity, intrauterine vascular events

Hypothalamic and Pituitary-Dependent Hypogonadotropic Hypogonadism
Adrenal hypoplasia congenital (*DAX1* mutation)
Intracranial tumors
Histiocytosis X
Hyperprolactinemia
Steroidogenic factor-1 (*NR5A1* mutation)
Prader-Willi syndrome

Bardet-Biedl syndrome
Bloom syndrome
Hereditary hemochromatosis

Gonad-Dependent
Primary gonadal failure: Gonadal dysgenesis (Turner syndrome, mixed 45,X/46,XY, pure 46,XY gonadal dysgenesis such as SR/gene mutations, pure 46,XX gonadal dysgenesis, Denys-Drash syndrome, Frasier syndrome, 46,XX male, *SOX9* gene mutation), Klinefelter syndrome, testicular regression syndrome (vanishing testis), autoimmune ovarian failure, galactosemia, Noonan syndrome, Down syndrome, trauma, torsion, postinfectious (e.g., mumps)
Defects in steroidogenesis: *LH-R* gene mutation, *FSH-R* gene mutation, congenital lipoid adrenal hyperplasia *StAR* gene mutation, 17α-hydroxylase/17-20-lyase deficiency (*CYP17* gene mutation), aromatase deficiency (*CYP19* gene mutation), 17β-hydroxysteroid dehydrogenase deficiency (*HSD17B3* gene mutation), 5α-reductase deficiency (*SRD5A2* gene mutation)
Steroid hormone receptor–dependent: Androgen insensitivity (*AR* gene mutation), estrogen receptor mutation

Anatomic Abnormalities
Mayer-Rokitansky-Kuster-Hauser syndrome

Chemotherapy

Radiation Therapy

---

also warrants evaluation.[335] In general, treatment of delayed puberty involves steroid hormone replacement, which is discussed in detail later (Box 17-2 and Table 17-3).

CONSTITUTIONAL

Rather than being a truly pathologic condition, constitutional delay of puberty is currently considered an extreme of the normal variation of pubertal timing. Typically, both gonadarche and adrenarche are delayed. There is no definitive diagnostic test and, therefore, constitutional delay of puberty is a diagnosis of exclusion. Often, linear growth velocity during the first few years of life is decreased. Subsequently, growth velocity normalizes and tracks close to the fifth percentile during childhood. Growth velocity again decreases during the early adolescent years, associated with an apparent transient decrease in GH secretion. Typically, the family history is positive for delayed puberty. Skeletal maturation is retarded,[336] and the predicted height is often greater than the final adult height, which is usually in the lower range of genetic height potential, based on midparental height calculations.[336]

GnRH-DEPENDENT (HYPOTHALAMIC HYPOGONADOTROPISM)

Delayed puberty as a consequence of impaired GnRH secretion may result from either primary developmental anomalies of the hypothalamus or secondary pathophysiologic conditions.

Kallmann Syndrome and Related Disorders

Kallmann syndrome and related disorders are reported to affect 1 in 7500 male patients and 1 in 70,000 female patients.[337] They can be subclassified into three major categories:

1. Kallmann syndrome with anosmia
2. Hypogonadotropic hypogonadism without anosmia
3. Acquired hypogonadotropic hypogonadism with onset after the initiation of puberty

Kallmann syndrome is characterized by isolated gonadotropin deficiency, due to the failure of GnRH neurons to migrate from the olfactory bulb into the hypothalamus during embryonic development.[158] Typically, the syndrome is associated with anosmia, which is usually due to defective olfactory bulb development and can be confirmed by MRI. In addition to sporadic forms, inheritance has been reported as being X-linked recessive, autosomal dominant, and autosomal recessive. Sporadic cases are more common than inherited forms.

Approximately half of families with the X-linked form have mutations in the gene that encodes anosmin-1 (*KAL-1*), which is located in the pseudoautosomal region of the X chromosome.[338-340] Ansomin-1 is a protein that contains motifs found in other molecules involved in neuronal guidance activity, including fibronectin III repeats and a whey-acidic protein domain. Patients with *KAL-1* mutations show complete loss of LH pulsatility, suggesting greater deficits in the GnRH system than patients with autosomal forms, in whom low-amplitude LH pulses can often be

TABLE 17-3

Monogenic Disorders Associated with Delayed Puberty

Gene	Locus	Phenotype
KAL-1	Xp22.3	Hypogonadotropic hypogonadism (Kallmann syndrome)
FGFR1	8p11.2-p11.1	Hypogonadotropic hypogonadism (Kallmann syndrome)
PROK2	3p21.1	Hypogonadotropic hypogonadism (Kallmann syndrome)
PROKR2	20p13	Hypogonadotropic hypogonadism (Kallmann syndrome)
GPR54	19p13.3	Hypogonadotropic hypogonadism
GnRHR	4q21.2	Hypogonadism
FSHβ	11p13	Hypogonadism
LHβ	19q13.32	Hypogonadism
HESX1	3p21.2-p21.1	Hypopituitarism (septo-optic dysplasia)
P1TX2	4q25-q26	Hypopituitarism (Rieger syndrome)
PROP-1	5q	Hypopituitarism
LHX3	9q34.4	Hypopituitarism
LEP	7q31.3	Obesity
LEPR	1p31	Obesity
DAX-1	Xp21.3-p21.2	Adrenal hypoplasia congenita
SF-1	9q33	Adrenal insufficiency, hypogonadism
PTPN11	12q24.1	Noonan syndrome

detected.[341] Men with X-linked Kallmann syndrome have been found to have a higher incidence of cryptorchidism and microphallus, lower inhibin B concentrations, higher MIH concentrations, and increased frequency of immature testicular morphology.[252] Other features associated with the X-linked form include unilateral renal agenesis, synkinesia, and sensorineural hearing loss. Phenotypic heterogeneity, even with the same mutation, suggests that modifier loci or epigenetic factors modulate the clinical manifestations.[342,343]

The majority of cases of Kallmann syndrome, however, are not associated with KAL-1 mutations. Some autosomal dominant cases of Kallmann syndrome result from inactivating mutations of the gene encoding the fibroblast growth factor receptor-1 (FGFR1, or KAL-2). As observed with KAL-1 mutations, development of the olfactory bulbs is impaired and bimanual synkinesis may occur.[344] In general, clinical manifestations are more severe among men with KAL-1 mutations compared with those carrying FGFR1 mutations.[345,346] Female carriers of either KAL-1 or FGFR1 mutations generally do not manifest a reproductive phenotype. Cerebellar ataxia (Gordon-Holmes syndrome) is an associated clinical feature in some families in which autosomal recessive inheritance occurs.[347]

As noted earlier, investigation of familial autosomal recessive hypogonadotropic hypogonadism led to the identification of mutations in the GPR54 gene and to the subsequent elucidation of the kisspeptin-GPR54 system. To date, several loss-of-function mutations have been reported in the GPR54 gene. Mutations in the prokinetin 2 (PROK2) gene have been identified in siblings with autosomal recessive hypogonadotropic hypogonadism; two siblings had anosmia and an affected female sibling was normosmic.[348] PROK2 is a secreted protein that signals through two G-protein–coupled receptors, prokineticin receptors 1 and 2. Mutations have been identified in the PROKR2 gene in patients with hypogonadotropic hypogonadism.[349] In addition to single gene defects, two families have been reported to carry digenic mutations. In other words, mutations in two different genes associated with hypogonadism were identified in these families.[350]

Curiously, a few individuals with hypogonadotropic hypogonadism associated with loss-of-function mutations have reversible hypogonadotropic hypogonadism.[351,352] The question arises as to whether constitutional delay and idiopathic hypogonadotropic hypogonadism may represent a spectrum of disorders characterized by delayed reactivation of the GnRH pulse generator.[353]

Anorexia Nervosa

Anorexia nervosa is a chronic psychiatric disorder characterized by decreased caloric intake, weight loss, distorted body image, and excessive physical activity (see also Chapter 18). Approximately 90% of individuals with this disorder are females. Delayed puberty and associated oligomenorrhea or amenorrhea are secondary to deficient GnRH secretion. Primary or secondary amenorrhea can precede weight loss and can persist despite weight gain. This condition would suggest that factors other than metabolic and nutritional determinants are involved in the suppression of the GnRH pulse generator. Other hormone findings include elevated cortisol and GH concentrations and decreased IGF-1 concentrations. The "low T_3 syndrome" is also common, in which T_3 is decreased, T_4 is normal or subnormal, and TSH is normal.[354] Osteopenia and osteoporosis are serious and persistent consequences of anorexia nervosa in both sexes. Bulimia nervosa, characterized by hinging and purging induced by vomiting or laxative abuse, is a variant of anorexia nervosa.

Undernutrition, Chronic Disease, and Intensive Exercise

Undernutrition and chronic disease, such as inflammatory bowel disease, cystic fibrosis, hypothyroidism, and poorly controlled type 1 diabetes mellitus, are associated with delayed or arrested puberty (see also Chapters 18, 19, and 23). Primary or secondary amenorrhea can occur. In many chronic illnesses, inadequate nutrition leads to impaired GnRH secretion, resulting in hypothalamic hypogonadism. Effective treatment of the underlying disorder is associated with pubertal progression. For example, after successful renal transplantation, children with chronic renal disease manifest resumption of gonadotropin secretion and progressive pubertal development. Anemias, such as sickle cell anemia and thalassemia, are also associated with compromised GnRH release. Treatment of these anemias with frequent transfusions may lead to iron overload, iron deposition in the pituitary, and exacerbation of the hypogonadotropism.

Intensive exercise and other athletic training schedules—including caloric restriction to maintain a weight class—may delay or interrupt pubertal development due to decreased GnRH secretion. Long-distance runners, gymnasts, ballerinas, and wrestlers are among the most commonly affected athletes. During the competitive season, male wrestlers lose body weight, fat mass, and lean body mass, and disruption of the neuroendocrine axes governing testicular function and growth may be observed. These changes, however, reverse within months after conclusion of the wrestling season.[355] Administration of leptin to eight women with hypothalamic amenorrhea was associated with improvement in reproductive, growth hormone, and thyroid function, providing additional evidence for leptin's important role as a signal indicating energy status.[356]

Leptin-Dependent Obesity

Retarded pubertal development has been associated with early-onset morbid obesity due to autosomal homozygous mutations of LEP gene or the gene encoding for the leptin receptor (LEPR).[112,357,358] A 9-year-old girl with a homozygous mutation of the LEPR gene was treated with recombinant human leptin for a 12-month period.[113] At the time of initiation of treatment, the patient showed no signs of pubertal development. Although bone age was advanced by 3.5 years, gonadotropin and estradiol levels were in the prepubertal range. At the end of leptin treatment, a pulsatile pattern of nocturnal gonadotropin secretion characteristic of early puberty was observed. As discussed earlier, this finding should not necessarily be taken as evidence that leptin triggers the pubertal resurgence of GnRH release.

PITUITARY-DEPENDENT (PITUITARY HYPOGONADOTROPISM)

Pituitary hypogonadotropism in subjects with delayed puberty may be due to either mutation in specific genes encoding the GnRH-R or one of the gonadotropin subunits, or to more generalized developmental anomalies of the pituitary.

GnRH-R Gene Mutations

The inheritance pattern of hypogonadotropic hypogonadism secondary to mutations in the GnRH-R gene is autosomal recessive, but sporadic cases are observed. Reported phenotypes range from complete to partial hypogonadism.[359] In general, the clinical phenotype correlates with biochemical LH pulsatility profiles and responses to exogenous GnRH. Complete hypogonadotropic hypogonadism is usually associated with low levels of apulsatile LH, whereas some spontaneous LH pulses, albeit reduced in amplitude, may be seen in patients with partial forms. The clinical phenotype correlates with the magnitude of the functional consequence of the mutation on receptor function. Nevertheless, phenotypic heterogeneity for the same mutation has been observed.[360,361] The mutations in GnRH-R reported to date appear to impair receptor folding and ligand binding and to decrease activation of the inositol phosphate/phospholipase C signaling pathways.[362,363]

FSHβ Gene Mutations

Women found to have mutations in the FSHβ gene have presented with absent breast development and primary amenorrhea. Circulating FSH and estrogen concentrations were low, whereas LH secretion was elevated.[364,365] Three affected males have been reported, with phenotypes ranging from absent to normal secondary sexual development. All three had azoospermia[366-368] and, as in females, FSH concentrations were low, whereas LH levels tended to be elevated.[369]

LHβ Gene Mutations

One male homozygous for a missense mutation, Q54R, in the LHβ gene had delayed puberty, elevated immunoreactive LH concentrations, few Leydig cells, and arrested spermatogenesis; treatment with hCG stimulated testosterone synthesis and spermatogenesis (see Chapter 2).[370] Another variant, G102S, has been associated with male and female infertility.[371] Functional characterization of the G102S variant at high LH concentrations showed impaired receptor binding and decreased ability to stimulate progesterone biosynthesis compared with wild-type LH.[372] Homozygosity for a splicing mutation in the LHβ gene was associated with hypogonadism in the affected male siblings and spontaneous pubertal development with secondary amenorrhea and infertility in the female sibling.[373]

One LHβ variant appears to be relatively common; the frequency varies widely between ethnic groups, ranging from near 0% in the Kotas of Southern India to 50% in Australian aborigines.[374] This variant has two single-nucleotide polymorphisms (SNPs) in the coding region, which are predicted to generate the missense mutations, Y8R and I15T, and eight SNPs in the promoter region. Differences in transcriptional activity between the variant and wild-type forms have been attributed to the SNPs in the promoter of the variant.[375] Comparisons of the recombinant variant peptide subunit with the native subunit showed differences in carbohydrate side chains and in intracellular trafficking.[376] Among healthy boys, heterozygosity for the Y8R/I15T variant was associated with smaller testicular volumes, slower growth rates, and lower IGFBP3 concentrations, suggesting that this variant affects the tempo of puberty.[377] Existing data suggest that, in girls, this variant may be associated with subfertility, lower frequency of PCOS, and delayed appearance of breast cancer.

Developmental Anomalies of the Pituitary

Developmental anomalies of the CNS, such as midline defects or septo-optic dysplasia, may be associated with gonadotropin and other pituitary hormone deficiencies and, therefore, with delays in pubertal development. Septo-optic dysplasia, also known as *de Morsier syndrome,* is characterized by abnormalities of the septum pellucidum, thinning of the corpus callosum, and hypoplasia of the optic nerve. With optic nerve hypoplasia, physical examination shows pendular nystagmus and pale hypoplastic optic discs. Mutations in the *HESX1* gene have been reported in familial cases of septo-optic dysplasia.[378] HESX1 is an early marker of pituitary differentiation, with limited spatiotemporal expression early in gestation.

Mutations in other genes involved in pituitary differentiation have been identified among patients with multiple anterior pituitary hormone deficiencies. Rieger syndrome is an autosomal dominant disorder characterized by eye anomalies, dental hypoplasia, and anterior pituitary hormone deficiencies associated with mutations in the *PITX2* gene, which encodes a transcription factor involved in pituitary cell differentiation and maintenance.

Delayed puberty associated with impaired gonadotropin secretion has been reported in patients with mutations in the *LHX3* gene, which codes for a homeodomain-containing transcription factor expressed early in the differentiation of the anterior pituitary.[379] Mutations in the *PROP-1* (paired-like homeodomain factor 1, prophet of Pit1) gene are associated with combined pituitary hormone deficiencies. The *PROP-1* gene codes for a transcription factor involved in the development of somatotrophs, thyrotrophs, and lactotrophs.[380] Most patients with *PROP-1* gene mutations have presented in childhood with TSH and GH deficiencies. LH and FSH deficiencies develop later, with a variable age of onset, such that the clinical presentation ranges from delayed puberty to secondary amenorrhea. Corticotroph dysfunction associated with ACTH deficiency and acquired adrenal insufficiency can also develop over time.[381,382] Thus, phenotypic heterogeneity occurs with regard to age at presentation and the spectrum of anterior pituitary hormone deficiencies.[383]

Nongenetic factors may also lead to CNS developmental abnormalities with hypogonadotropism and should therefore be considered in the etiology of pituitary-dependent delayed puberty. Three such entities—maternal cocaine abuse, valproate toxicity, and intrauterine vascular disruptive events—have been implicated as possible etiologies of septo-optic dysplasia.[384-386]

HYPOTHALAMIC AND PITUITARY-DEPENDENT HYPOGONADISM

This section discusses disorders that involve both the hypothalamus and pituitary. Some disorders, such as adrenal hypoplasia congenita (AHC), also affect the development of the adrenal cortex. For some disorders, inconsistency of investigative reports precludes precise definition of the anatomic localization.

Adrenal Hypoplasia Congenita

Characterized by primary adrenal insufficiency and hypogonadotropic hypogonadism, AHC is an X-linked recessive disorder caused by mutations in the *DAX-1* (dosage-sensitive sex reversal, AHC-critical region of the X chromosome, gene 1, which is also known as *NROB1*) gene located on the short arm of the X chromosome.[387,388] In AHC, the development of the fetal zone of the adrenal cortex during fetal development and its regression during the first year of postnatal life occur normally. The adult zone of the adrenal cortex, on the other hand, does not develop. Thus, symptoms of adrenal insufficiency in AHC generally do not manifest until after 6 to 8 weeks of age, and affected males can present in infancy or childhood with primary adrenal insufficiency. Delayed adrenarche may occur. In addition, the complete or partial hypogonadotropic hypogonadism associated with the adrenal insufficiency can lead to delayed gonadarche. Isolated hypogonadotropic hypogonadism due to *DAX-1* mutations may occur rarely in the absence of adrenal insufficiency or a family history of hypogonadism.[389] Heterozygotic females may have delayed puberty, but show normal fertility.[390]

The *DAX-1* gene codes for a receptor protein expressed in the hypothalamus, pituitary, adrenal, and gonads. Because no ligand has been identified for the receptor, it is classified as an orphan nuclear receptor. Through its C-terminus transcriptional repression domain, the protein silences transcription of many genes involved in steroid hormone metabolism. The majority of mutations detected in patients with AHC cluster in the region encoding the C terminal of the protein.[391] Structure–function analysis suggests that the mechanism through which *DAX-1* mutations cause AHC involves abnormal folding of the receptor, leading to impaired nuclear translocation and transcriptional silencing.[392] Mutations in this region of the X chromosome may be part of a contiguous gene deletion syndrome, which includes glycerol kinase deficiency and Duchenne muscular dystrophy. Phenotypic heterogeneity can occur, even within a family.[393]

Intracranial Tumors

Depending on their precise location and size, intracranial tumors can suppress gonadotropin secretion either directly or indirectly, via interruption of GnRH release. Those that present before or during puberty, therefore, lead to delayed or arrested gonadarche. Deficiencies of other pituitary hormones may be present or develop later. Thus, concurrent GH, TSH, ACTH, and ADH deficiencies may be present. Acquired pituitary hormone deficiencies, especially if accompanied by diabetes insipidus, suggest the presence of a CNS tumor.

The most common neoplasm is a craniopharyngioma, which is believed to arise from remnants of Rathke's pouch, the embryonic anlagen of the anterior pituitary. These tumors account for approximately 10% of childhood CNS tumors, with the peak chronologic age at presentation between 5 and 20 years.[394] In addition to delayed pubertal development, signs and symptoms suggestive of a craniopharyngioma are decreasing growth velocity, headache, polyuria, and visual disturbance (bilateral temporal field deficits, optic atrophy, or papilledema). Suprasellar or intrasellar calcifications may be seen on skull radiographs. MRI and CT scans confirm the presence of the tumor and show whether it is cystic or solid. Treatment usually involves surgical resection, with outcome dependent on the size and precise location of the tumor. Radiation therapy may be used as adjunctive therapy. Recurrences are common.

Other types of tumors include germ cell tumors, epidermoid and dermoid cysts, chromophobe adenomas, prolactinomas, and optic gliomas. Germ cell tumors include germinomas, dysgerminomas, embryonal cell carcinomas, and teratomas. Such tumors account for approximately 6.5% of intracranial neoplasms in children. Diabetes insipidus is a common manifestation; however, other anterior pituitary hormone deficiencies may occur. Germ cell tumors often originate in the suprasellar hypothalamus or pineal gland, and they may show subependymal spread along the lining of the third ventricle such that seeding of the cerebrospinal fluid leads to involvement of the lower spinal cord and cauda equina. Elevated β-hCG or α-fetoprotein concentrations may be detected secondary to secretion by the tumor cells. Usually, the response to radiation therapy is good and surgery is not needed unless a tissue diagnosis is necessary.

Epidermoid and dermoid cysts are epithelial-lined intracranial cysts that are often located in the suprasellar region or at the cerebellopontine angle. Chromophobe adenomas are rare in children, but may occur in older adolescents, leading to delayed puberty, secondary amenorrhea, or acquired testosterone deficiency. Optic nerve and chiasmatic gliomas (astrocytomas) account for approximately 5% of pediatric brain tumors and tend to present during the first two decades of life.[395] Although optic nerve gliomas are often associated with NF-1 and precocious puberty, delayed puberty due to hypogonadotropism (with other anterior pituitary hormone deficiencies) may also occur.

Histiocytosis X

Histiocytosis X, also known as *Langerhans' cell histiocytosis or Hand-Schüller-Christian disease,* is characterized by infiltration of lipid-laden histiocytes into skin, bone, or visceral organs. These specific dendritic cells can infiltrate almost any organ. The clinical course can be unpredictable such that spontaneous resolution or progression to a disseminated form may occur. Infiltration of the orbit can cause exophthalmos. The typical radiographic findings include cyst-like areas involving flat bones of the skull, ribs, pelvis, scapula, and lower spine, and long bones of the limbs. Pituitary MRI imaging shows loss of the posterior pituitary bright spot and thickening of the infundibulum. Although not cancerous, the histiocytes can invade adjacent tissues.

Diabetes insipidus is the most common endocrine manifestation, occurring in approximately 25% of affected children, but other pituitary hormone deficiencies can occur. Once established, anterior pituitary hormone deficiencies are generally permanent. Gonadotropin deficiency may develop several years after the initial diagnosis. Thus, delayed puberty may be seen. Hypothalamic infiltration can manifest as neuropsychiatric and behavioral disorders as well as autonomic dysregulation.[396]

Hyperprolactinemia

Hyperprolactinemia can lead to hypogonadotropism as a result of the action of prolactin to directly suppress pulsatile GnRH secretion (see Chapter 3).[397] Thus, if hyperprolactinemia occurs before puberty, delayed or interrupted gonadarche with galactorrhea may be observed. Even if galactorrhea is not readily apparent, nipple manipulation may induce fluid release. Because prolactin release may be stimulated by nipple manipulation, evaluation of serum prolactin levels should be conducted on blood samples collected in the morning from fasting subjects before breast examination. Hyperprolactinemia can be due to microadenomas (adenomas larger than 10 mm) and macroadenomas (>10 mm).[398] Although CT scans can be used to identify pituitary adenomas, MRI provides more anatomic detail. Individuals taking antipsychotic medications and patients with primary hypothyroidism may also have hyperprolactinemia.[399] Prolactin secretion is tonically inhibited by hypothalamic dopamine release, and dopamine receptor agonists (bromocriptine or cabergoline) are effective to decrease tumor size and prolactin concentrations.[400]

Steroidogenic Factor-1/*NR5A1* Mutations

The gene that encodes steroidogenic factor-1 (*NR5A1/ SF1*) plays a major role in male sexual differentiation, steroidogenesis, and development of the hypothalamus, pituitary, adrenal glands, and testes. Because inactivating mutations impair testicular differentiation and testosterone secretion, affected 46,XY individuals would be predicted to have undervirilization of the external genitalia. The phenotype reported for one 46,XY patient who was heterozygous for an inactivating mutation included undervirilization of the external genitalia (46,XY male to female sex reversal), adrenal insufficiency in the neonatal period, and delayed puberty.[401] A 46,XX patient presented with adrenal insufficiency and apparently normal ovarian differentiation, but whether she will undergo spontaneous pubertal development remains to be seen.[402] Heterozygous mutations in *SF1* have been reported among patients with 46,XY partial gonadal dysgenesis and underandrogenization but normal adrenal function.[403,404] Thus, the specific role, if any, of this protein in human puberty remains to be established.

Other Syndromes Associated with Delayed Puberty

Delayed puberty due to hypogonadotropic hypogonadism is observed in several unrelated syndromes, such as Prader-Willi, Bardet-Biedel, Rud, Alstrom, and Bloom syndromes. Although both premature pubarche and GnRH-dependent premature gonadarche have been reported to occur in Prader-Willi syndrome, the majority of affected boys have cryptorchidism. When spontaneous pubertal development occurs, it generally progresses slowly and is often incomplete.[405] Hormone replacement therapy may not be necessary for all patients with Prader-Willi syndrome. Prader-Willi syndrome is also characterized by short stature, hypotonia, hyperphagia, obesity, mental retardation, and decreased fetal movements. It is a contiguous gene deletion syndrome involving loss of the paternal allele or uniparental disomy of the maternal allele for several genes, including the necdin and small nuclear ribonucleoprotein polypeptide N (*SNRPN*) genes located in the region of chromosome 15q11-13.[406,407]

Typical features of Bardet-Biedl syndrome include retinal dystrophy, dystrophic extremities (polydactyly, syndactyly, brachydactyly), mental retardation, and obesity. Affected females may have structural abnormalities involving the internal genitalia, and they may experience hydrometrocolpos.[408] Inheritance is autosomal recessive, with linkage to at least six distinct loci.[409]

Rud syndrome is characterized by hypogonadotropic hypogonadism, congenital ichthyosis, epilepsy, and mental retardation. Given the close proximity of genetic loci for the *KAL-1* gene and X-linked ichthyosis on the short arm of the X chromosome, this disorder may represent a contiguous gene deletion syndrome.

Alstrom syndrome is an autosomal recessive disorder characterized by cone–rod retinal dystrophy, cardiomyopathy, and type 2 diabetes mellitus. Hypogonadism is an inconsistent feature. The syndrome has been mapped to chromosome 2p13, and it has been recently attributed to mutations in the *ALMS* gene.[410,411] Evaluation of 15 young adults with Alstrom syndrome showed short stature, increased obesity, fasting hyperinsulinemia, and decreased testosterone concentrations in males. Gonadotropin levels were normal among affected females.[412]

Bloom syndrome is an autosomal recessive disorder characterized by impaired prenatal and postnatal growth, predisposition to neoplasia, chromosomal instability, and hypogonadism due to inactivating mutations in the gene coding for DNA helicase RecQ protein-like-3.

In addition, hereditary hemochromatosis is associated with iron overload and iron deposition in endocrine organs. The typical endocrine manifestations include hypogonadotropic hypogonadism, impaired glucose tolerance, and diabetes mellitus. At least five subtypes have been identified on the basis of different genetic loci. Hypogonadism is a common presentation for type 2 or juvenile hemochromatosis.[413]

GONADAL CAUSES OF DELAYED PUBERTY (PRIMARY GONADAL FAILURE)

Primary gonadal failure is associated with hypergonadotropic hypogonadism (see also Chapter 16). Etiologies include sex chromosome abnormalities leading to aberrant differentiation of the gonads (gonadal dysgenesis), absence of the gonads, and injury to the gonads. The hypergonadotropism associated with primary gonadal failure and with disorders of steroidogenesis or steroid hormone action is a result of loss of negative feedback inhibition by gonadal steroids at both the hypothalamic and the pituitary level.

Gonadal Dysgenesis

Gonadal dysgenesis is used to describe disorders in which gonadal differentiation is aberrant (see also Chapter 16). Gonadal dysgenesis can be due to haploinsufficiency for the X chromosome (i.e., Turner syndrome). Other forms may result from mutations in genes involved in the process of sexual differentiation.

Turner Syndrome

Turner syndrome is due to deletions or structural rearrangements of the X chromosome. The reported incidence of liveborn females with this form of gonadal dysgenesis is 1:2000 to 1:5000.[414] Although follicles develop during fetal ovarian differentiation, accelerated postnatal follicular atresia frequently leads to ovarian failure, and the majority of girls with Turner syndrome do not enter puberty. Nevertheless, 25% to 30% of girls with Turner syndrome spontaneously show partial pubertal development at the appropriate time, and 2% to 5% may have spontaneous menses. As described earlier, LH and FSH secretion is amplified at all stages of postnatal development (see Fig. 17-6) due to the primary ovarian failure with loss of negative feedback inhibition of gonadotropin release by estradiol.

Short stature is also a characteristic feature of Turner syndrome.[415] Common skeletal features include cubitus valgus, shortened fourth metacarpals, short neck, high-arched palate, and Madelung's deformity. Scoliosis may develop during the adolescent years.[416] Haploinsufficiency for the short stature homeobox-containing (*SHOX*) gene, located in the pseudoautosomal region of the X chromosome, contributes to the short stature and skeletal abnormalities associated with Turner syndrome.[417] Because the majority of patients with Turner syndrome present with short stature, exclusion of this form of gonadal dysgenesis is essential in the evaluation of all girls with short stature.[418] Bone mineral density is decreased, with bone markers indicating both increased resorption and normal to decreased bone formation.[419]

Aberrant development of the lymphatic system, especially in the nuchal region, is associated with a short, webbed neck; peripheral lymphedema; and a low posterior hairline. Additional features include bilateral otitis media, sensorineural hearing loss, cardiac malformations (especially of the left side of the heart), renal abnormalities, hypoplastic and hyperconvex nails, and multiple pigmented nevi. Phenotypic heterogeneity is common among girls with Turner syndrome. Only approximately 25% of affected girls are diagnosed with Turner syndrome as infants or toddlers.

Mosaicism with coexistence of multiple cell lines is not uncommon, although detection may require evaluation of multiple tissues. It has been speculated that mosaicism in critical cell lines is essential for fetal viability.[420,421] If clinical suspicion of Turner syndrome is high despite a normal peripheral blood karyotype, it may be worthwhile to examine a second tissue, such as skin. When a cell line containing a Y chromosome is present, the external genital phenotype may vary from female to ambiguous to male and the gonadal structure can range from a streak to a functional testis. In some cases, Y chromosome–specific sequences can be detected using sensitive molecular techniques.[422] Currently, assessment for the *SRY* gene or other Y chromosomal material can be limited to girls with evidence of virilization or presence of a marker chromosome. If Y chromosomal sequences are present, the risk of gonadoblastoma is estimated to be 7% to 10%.[423] Such gonadoblastomas may secrete testosterone or estrogens and become calcified, but rarely become malignant.

Girls with Turner syndrome tend to have normal verbal abilities. As a group, however, they show specific deficits in visuospatial processing, visuoperceptual skills, motor function, and nonverbal memory compared with normal girls. These deficits may be associated with one or more deletions of a critical region in the pseudoautosomal region of the X chromosome.[424] For example, some girls with Turner syndrome may experience difficulty with interpretation of body language and facial expressions and trouble maintaining relationships with peers, reading maps, and understanding geometry. Although most deficits persist into adulthood, some cognitive deficiencies improve due to a maturational or developmental lag, or due to the effects of estrogen therapy. Nevertheless, the neurocognitive deficits, psychosocial issues, and school difficulties can lead to frustration and poor self-esteem.[425] Mental retardation is typical for girls with ring X chromosomes lacking the *XIST* gene (the gene responsible for X inactivation) because of failure to inactivate one copy of certain genes.[426]

Estrogen replacement therapy is necessary to induce pubertal development.[427] Yet, despite adequate estrogen replacement therapy, uterine maturation may be incomplete and may contribute to a high rate of miscarriage in both spontaneous and assisted pregnancies among women with Turner syndrome.[428] The growth deficit in girls with Turner syndrome can be partially ameliorated by GH treatment. Earlier treatment and use of GH doses of 0.36 mg/kg/week are associated with improved final height outcome.[429] Management of girls with Turner syndrome includes regular monitoring of thyroid function (free T$_4$, TSH, and anti-thyroid antibodies) because of an increased risk of chronic lymphocytic thyroiditis. Screening for renal structural abnormalities, skeletal malformations (congenital dislocated hips, Madelung's deformity, scoliosis), hypertension, and celiac disease is also necessary.[430] Evaluation by a cardiologist is necessary to ascertain whether certain cardiovascular abnormalities are present, such as coarctation of the aorta, bicuspid aortic valve, or mitral valve prolapse. Prophylactic antibiotic therapy is generally indicated if bicuspid aortic valve or mitral valve prolapse is detected. Repeat echocardiograms for adolescent and young adult women are important to assess for dilation of the aortic root because of the increased risk of aortic dissection.[431] With the vast diversity of clinical features, a multidisciplinary approach is essential for long-term clinical management.[416]

46,XY Gonadal Dysgenesis

Aberrant testicular differentiation in 46,XY fetuses is one cause of gonadal dysgenesis (see also Chapter 16). Because the degrees of gonadal dysgenesis and testosterone deficiency vary, the external genital development can range from normal-appearing female external genitalia to undervirilization of male external genitalia. In "complete" or "pure" 46,XY gonadal dysgenesis, affected individuals appear to be normal females at birth. This disorder of gonadal differentiation is also known as *Swyer syndrome* or *46,XY sex reversal disorder of sexual differentiation*. Affected individuals usually present with delayed puberty and primary amenorrhea; they are usually found to have streak gonads. The internal genital structures are usually female due to prenatal testosterone and MIH deficiencies. "Partial" or "incomplete" 46,XY gonadal dysgenesis is characterized by defective testicular differentiation, ambiguous external genitalia, and a combination of wolffian and müllerian duct structures. Patients with 46,XY sex reversal have an increased risk of gonadoblastoma. In one series of 22 patients, 32% were found to have dysgerminoma and 14% had gonadoblastoma.[432] Compared with healthy control subjects, women with complete gonadal dysgenesis were taller and had smaller uterine sizes.[432] Spontaneous breast development in patients with gonadal dysgenesis may be secondary to estrogen secretion by these gonadal tumors.[433,434] Early diagnosis is beneficial to detect gonadal neoplasia and initiate hormone replacement therapy.

Laboratory evaluation shows elevated gonadotropin concentrations, low testosterone concentrations, and 46,XY karyotype. Approximately 15% of patients with 46,XY gonadal dysgenesis have mutations in the testis-determining *SRY* gene. Most *SRY* mutations are de novo events. Curiously, some mutations are familial and present in unaffected fathers.[435,436] Because the majority of patients with 46,XY sex reversal do not have mutations in the *SRY* gene, it is presumed that they carry mutations involving other genes either upstream or downstream of SRY in the process of sexual differentiation.

Other Forms of Gonadal Dysgenesis

Denys-Drash and Frasier syndromes are associated with gonadal dysgenesis. Both disorders are due to heterozygous mutations in the Wilms' tumor-1 (*WT1*) gene.[437,438] Denys-Drash syndrome is characterized by 46,XY male-to-female sex reversal, Wilms' tumor, and chronic renal failure due to diffuse mesangial sclerosis. In addition to 46,XY male-to-female sex reversal and renal disease, patients with Frasier syndrome have a higher incidence of gonadoblastomas than patients with Denys-Drash syndrome. Patients with either of these syndromes and 46,XX karyotypes tend to have normal female external genitalia.

Ovotesticular disorder of sexual differentiation (previously known as *true hermaphroditism*) is characterized by the concurrent presence of testicular tissue with seminiferous tubules and ovarian tissue with follicles. Although an ovotestis is the most commonly identified gonad, an ovary may be present on one side, with a testis on the other side. The development of müllerian and wolffian duct derivatives is variable and depends on the amount of functional testicular tissue. Patients with true hermaphroditism are usually recognized in infancy due to genital ambiguity. The most frequent karyotypes are 46,XX (60%), 46,XX/46,XY (33%), and 46,XY (7%).[439]

Heterozygous inactivating mutations in the *SOX9* gene are associated with camptomelic dwarfism and 46,XY male-to-female sex reversal.[440] Because some of the related skeletal abnormalities (such as small thoracic cage, undermineralized ribs, and tracheobronchomalacia) can cause respiratory distress, affected individuals often die early. However, milder forms could present with delayed puberty due to primary gonadal failure.[441] Another form of gonadal dysgenesis is 46,XX gonadal dysgenesis, which is characterized by female internal and external genital structures, delayed puberty, and streak gonads.

46,XX Males

Testicular differentiation can occur in the absence of the Y chromosome. Because 46,XX males often have normal male external genital development, they typically seek medical attention for delayed puberty, infertility, or gynecomastia. On physical examination, the testes are usually small. Some present in the newborn period with genital ambiguity or hypospadias. In approximately 80% of 46,XX males, the *SRY* gene is detected by molecular genotype analysis.[442] Neither Leydig cell function nor response to hCG stimulation correlates with the amount of Y chromosome–specific DNA.[443]

Klinefelter Syndrome

Klinefelter syndrome is a chromosomal abnormality characterized by a 47,XXY karyotype and primary testicular failure that may manifest before or after puberty (see also Chapter 16). Gonadarche may be variable, ranging from normal to absent. In one study, the incidence of Klinefelter syndrome was 1 in 667 males when diagnosed by prenatal cytogenetic analysis, whereas the incidence was much lower when patients were detected by clinical features alone. This finding suggests incomplete clinical ascertainment of patients with Klinefelter syndrome.[444] Clinical features include gynecomastia; small, firm testes; and tall stature, with a disproportionate increase in limb lengths. As would be anticipated, gonadotropin concentrations are elevated and testosterone concentrations tend to be low. Among men with Klinefelter syndrome undergoing fertility treatment, testicular volume, testosterone concentrations, and hCG-stimulated testosterone responses correlated with sperm production after testicular sperm extraction.[445] In one longitudinal study, prepubertal boys had inhibin B concentrations within the normal range, which decreased during late puberty, consistent with progressive testicular failure at the time

of gonadarche.[446] Because the magnitude of primary testicular failure varies between patients, dosage and age at initiation of hormone replacement therapy must be individualized. Affected boys may experience academic difficulties and fulfill criteria to be considered mentally retarded.[447] They tend to have generalized learning disabilities, with underachievement in arithmetic, reading, and spelling, which become more apparent and limiting over time.[448]

One study involving 55 boys with Klinefelter syndrome reported that affected boys often had reduced penile length and small testes in childhood. In addition, the phenotype in boys with Klinefelter syndrome did not differ according to presenting clinical features or parental origin of the extra X chromosome. Before puberty, affected boys can be detected by tall stature, relatively decreased penile length, clinodactyly, hypotonia, and the need for speech therapy.[449]

Testicular Regression Syndrome

This disorder, also known as "vanishing testis syndrome," affects at least 5% of boys who present with cryptorchidism. Typically, the external genitalia are male, but one or both testes cannot be identified. Rather, a nubbin of discrete vascularized fibrosis, usually located in close proximity to a blind-ending spermatic cord structure, is found at the time of orchidopexy. Histologic examination often shows calcification or hemosiderin deposits.[450] Often attributed to testicular torsion, the precise etiology of this condition that is responsible for primary testicular failure remains to be established. A novel heterozygous missense mutation (V355M) in the steroidogenic factor-1 gene (*NR5A1*) was identified in a single boy with a micropenis and testicular regression syndrome.[451]

Autoimmune Ovarian Failure

Autosomal recessive type I autoimmune polyglandular syndrome (APS-1) is characterized by mucocutaneous candidiasis, hyperparathyroidism, and adrenal insufficiency. APS-1 is due to mutations in the *AIRE* gene located at chromosome 21p22.3.[452] Ovarian failure is common in APS-1 and may be associated with autoantibodies to the P450 steroidogenic enzymes expressed in the gonads and adrenal glands, such as 3β-hydroxysteroid dehydrogenase.[453] Autoimmune testicular failure may also occur. The incidence of autoimmune primary gonadal failure is low in APS-2, which is characterized by immune-mediated type 1 diabetes mellitus, chronic lymphocytic thyroiditis, vitiligo, and pernicious anemia.[453] Some researchers have suggested that, in unexplained infertility, ovarian antibodies are an independent marker of ovarian failure that may precede changes in FSH and inhibin B concentrations.[454]

Noonan Syndrome

Clinical features of Noonan syndrome include short stature; hypertelorism; a short, webbed neck; mental retardation; bleeding disorders; and right-sided cardiac anomalies.

The estimated incidence ranges from 1:1000 to 1:2500 live births. Although it is inherited in an autosomal dominant manner, 60% of cases are sporadic.[455] Cryptorchidism is common in affected males. At least 50% of cases have missense mutations in the *PTPN11* gene, which encodes the nonreceptor protein tyrosine phosphatase SHP2.[456] Other genes in the Ras-MAP kinase pathway have been found to be associated with Noonan syndrome; these include *KRAS*, *SOS1*, and *NF1*.[457] Reproductive function tends to be normal in women. Elevated FSH concentrations and an exaggerated gonadotropin response after GnRH stimulation in males with Noonan syndrome suggest primary gonadal dysfunction.[458]

Galactosemia

Galactosemia is an autosomal recessive metabolic disorder characterized by abnormal galactose metabolism. Three different genes encode proteins involved in galactose metabolism: galactokinase (*GALK*), galactose-1-phosphate uridyl transferase (*GALT*), and UDP-galactose 4-epimerase (*GALE*). Mutations in any of these genes can result in human disease. Affected women have elevated FSH concentrations and ovarian failure.[459] In three women with galactosemia, the glycosylation of FSH was abnormal, suggesting the hypothesis that FSH signal transduction was impaired.[460] Affected males appear to have normal testicular function.

Down Syndrome

The occasional child with Down syndrome presents with abnormal pubertal development. Normal uterine size and the presence of follicles in ovaries have been documented.[461] However, for both sexes, gonadal failure with elevated gonadotropins may develop in adulthood.[462] For counseling purposes, women with Down syndrome can conceive, but affected men tend to be infertile. Children with Down syndrome are at increased risk for other chronic disorders that may affect onset and progression of puberty. These disorders include hypothyroidism, celiac disease, and diabetes mellitus.[463]

DEFECTS IN STEROIDOGENESIS OR STEROID HORMONE ACTION

LH-R Gene Mutations

In males, inactivating *LH-R* mutations impair testosterone biosynthesis; such patients may present with delayed puberty (see Chapter 2). Inherited as an autosomal recessive disorder, the most severe form is characterized by Leydig cell hypoplasia, testosterone deficiency, and 46,XY male-to-female sex reversal. Müllerian duct derivatives are absent. Milder forms may present with hypogonadism in 46,XY individuals. The typical presentation for 46,XX individuals who carry severe inactivating mutations of this gene is the absence of puberty, with primary amenorrhea, which may be associated with LH hypersecretion, cystic ovaries, and infertility.[464,465] A 46,XY patient who presented with delayed puberty was found to have a homozygous deletion of exon 10. Functional analysis to determine the consequences of the mutation showed that, despite being able to bind LH, the mutant receptor was less effective at stimulating increased cAMP production than the normal receptor.[466]

FSH-R Gene Mutations

Although inactivating mutations of the *FSH-R* gene are associated with primary ovarian failure and infertility, the development of secondary sex characteristics is variable in this autosomal recessive disorder (see Chapter 2).[467-469] Although pubarche appears to occur normally, breast development varies from absent to normal. Menarche is typically absent, although early secondary amenorrhea is occasionally observed. The variation in phenotype would suggest that the *FSH-R* gene is not completely inactivated and that low levels of estradiol may be secreted. The phenotype is less severe in males, and pubertal development has occurred in the cases reported to date.[470] Testicular volume and sperm count, however, were decreased.

Congenital Lipoid Adrenal Hyperplasia

Mutations in the *StAR* gene are the molecular basis of congenital lipoid adrenal hyperplasia (see also Chapter 4). Consequently, sustained trophic hormone stimulation of the adrenal gland and the testis or ovary leads to the accumulation of cholesterol esters and cholesterol auto-oxidation in the cytoplasm of steroidogenically active cells. Cell destruction ensues because the accumulated lipid droplets lead to both physical engorgement and chemical damage from the cholesterol auto-oxidation products. Thus, the phenotype of congenital lipoid adrenal hyperplasia reflects the consequences of two separate events—the inactivating mutation and subsequent cellular damage.[471] These two hits interfere with fetal testicular testosterone biosynthesis, leading to androgen deficiency and undervirilization of affected 46,XY fetuses. Yet, despite the genetic mutation in the *StAR* gene, StAR-independent steroidogenesis allows for normal placental steroidogenesis and low, but measurable, adrenal steroid concentrations in the immediate newborn period. Subsequent cellular damage, however, leads to complete loss of adrenal steroidogenesis. Because the fetal, neonatal, and prepubertal ovary are relatively quiescent, ovarian lipid accumulation is minimal at these stages of development, and gonadarche may be initiated in affected 46,XX individuals.[472] Milder nonclassic forms of congenital lipoid adrenal hyperplasia have been reported.[473]

17α-Hydroxylase/17,20-Lyase Deficiency

The clinical features of decreased 17α-hydroxylase/17,20-lyase activity, resulting from mutations in the *CYP17* gene, can include glucocorticoid and sex steroid hormone deficiencies (see also Chapters 4 and 16). Because mineralocorticoid biosynthesis is unaffected, patients may have hypertension due to increased aldosterone production. Affected males may present with complete or partial male-to-female sex reversal due to impaired testosterone secretion. Affected females have normal female internal and external genitalia; they typically present with delayed puberty secondary to inadequate estrogen production.

In some patients, the lyase activity of the enzyme is more impaired than its hydroxylase activity. The molecular basis for this differential effect appears to be related to the consequences of mutations in specific domains of the mature protein such that mutations in the steroid-binding domain are associated with deleterious effects on both activities. Mutations in the redox partner–interaction domain impair lyase activity to a greater extent than the hydroxylase activity.[474,475]

Aromatase Deficiency

Aromatase deficiency is an autosomal recessive disorder due to inactivating mutations in the aromatase gene, *CYP19* (see Chapter 4). The consequence of decreased aromatase activity is impaired conversion of androgens to estrogens. Affected female infants may present with genital ambiguity due to excessive androgen exposure in utero. Subsequently, affected females show absence of breast development, estrogen deficiency, progressive virilization, and hypergonadotropic hypogonadism.[476] From the small number of male patients who have been reported with this mutation, gonadarche appears to be initiated and male secondary sexual characteristics are normal.[477] When semen analysis has been performed, oligozoospermia or azoospermia has been noted. The cardinal feature of the mutation in the male is delayed bone maturation and decreased bone mineralization. Interestingly, women pregnant with affected fetuses can virilize due to impaired placental aromatase activity, leading to hyperandrogenism.

17β-Hydroxysteroid Dehydrogenase Deficiency

In 17β-hydroxysteroid dehydrogenase deficiency, an autosomal recessive disorder, testicular conversion of androstenedione to testosterone is impaired secondary to mutations in the *HSD17B3* gene (see Chapters 4 and 16). Affected 46,XY individuals show varying degrees of external genital ambiguity at birth, ranging from microphallus to perineoscrotal hypospadias with bilateral labial gonads. Affected 46,XY individuals have hypoplastic wolffian duct development. Progressive virilization occurs at puberty and is presumed to be due to increased peripheral conversion of sex steroids to testosterone. Affected individuals, raised as females, may convert to male gender roles as puberty progresses. Appropriate gender assignment can be made when the diagnosis is made in the neonatal period. Phenotypic heterogeneity, even within a single family, has been reported.[478] Although increased basal androstenedione-to-testosterone ratios are anticipated, hCG stimulation and molecular genetic analysis may be necessary to confirm the diagnosis.

5α-Reductase Deficiency

In specific androgen target cells, such as the developing external genitalia and prostate, testosterone is converted to DHT by 5α-reductase type 2 (see Chapters 4 and 16).

In this autosomal recessive disorder, the conversion of testosterone to DHT is impaired due to mutations in the 5α-reductase type 2 (*SRD5A2*) gene. Affected 46,XY individuals show phenotypic heterogeneity, with varying degrees of male-to-female sex reversal at birth.[479] Typically, they have perineoscrotal hypospadias and bilateral labial gonads at birth. At puberty, affected individuals virilize, with phallic enlargement and development of pubic hair. When initially raised as girls, some affected individuals change to a male gender when virilization occurs. Spermatogenesis is usually impaired. Although random testosterone-to-DHT ratios may be elevated, hCG stimulation testing may be necessary to confirm the diagnosis.

Androgen Receptor Gene Mutations

The phenotype of 46,XY individuals with mutations in the *AR* gene varies from male-to-female sex reversal to male infertility (see Chapter 16). Inheritance is X-linked recessive; the *AR* gene is located in the region of chromosome Xq. More than 300 mutations have been reported in the *AR* gene. Mutations in the ligand-binding domain interfere with androgen binding. Although ligand binding is normal, if the mutation is located in the DNA-binding domain, AR activity is impaired.

Individuals with complete androgen insensitivity have female external genitalia with labial masses or undescended testes. Müllerian-derived structures are absent because testicular MIH secretion in utero is normal. Patients are often considered female at birth and can present with either inguinal hernias in childhood or delayed menarche, with sparse sexual hair development in adolescence. In partial androgen insensitivity, the phenotype is often that of an undervirilized male. Those with partial androgen insensitivity may have gynecomastia, decreased sexual hair, hypospadias, cryptorchidism, small penis, and infertility. Typically, LH and testosterone concentrations are elevated. FSH concentrations may be normal or elevated.

Even within a family, phenotypic heterogeneity can occur.[480] In some instances, phenotypic heterogeneity appears to be secondary to somatic cell mosaicism.[481] Based on one case report, some researchers have speculated that some cases of apparent androgen insensitivity may also result from abnormalities of receptor cofactors, in addition to being due to mutations in the *AR* gene itself.[482]

MAYER-ROKITANSKY-KUSTER-HAUSER SYNDROME

Mayer-Rokitansky-Kuster-Hauser syndrome is a congenital disorder characterized by anatomic abnormalities of müllerian duct derivatives, with a prevalence of between 1:4000 and 1:10,000 female patients. Affected patients usually have normal ovarian function, but present with primary amenorrhea or cyclic abdominal pain. Müllerian duct remnants may be palpable on bimanual rectoabdominal examination as a midline band of tissue. Although ultrasound and MRI are helpful, laparoscopy may be needed to confirm the diagnosis.[483-485] Renal abnormalities—especially ectopic kidneys or unilateral renal agenesis—and skeletal abnormalities may be present. Vaginal development is

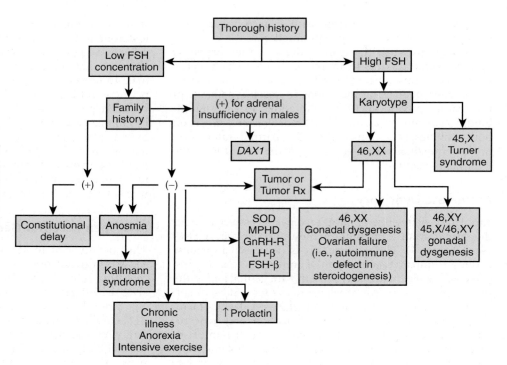

Figure 17-11. *Algorithm for delayed puberty in girls. Beginning with a thorough medical history, this flowchart provides guidelines for the differential diagnosis of the most common causes of delayed puberty in girls. FSH, follicle-stimulating hormone; MPHD, multiple pituitary hormone deficiencies; SOD, septo-optic dysplasia.*

variable, and often vaginal dilation is helpful to enlarge the vagina for intercourse. Successful outcome of vaginal dilation depends on the patient's motivation and compliance.

CHEMOTHERAPY AND RADIATION THERAPY

Chemotherapy and radiation therapy for tumors before puberty can affect multiple components of the hypothalamic–pituitary–gonadal axis, depending on the specific drugs and radiation fields. The germ cells of the gonads are particularly vulnerable to radiation. For example, spermatogenesis is more sensitive to the effects of low-dose irradiation (>1-2 Gy) than Leydig cell steroidogenesis (approximately 12 Gy).[486,487] Alkylating agents such as cyclophosphamide can injure germ cells in both sexes, causing delayed or absent pubertal development, especially among girls.[488] CNS irradiation may lead to gonadotropin deficiency and other pituitary hormone deficiencies. Boys with brain tumors who received cranial irradiation and adjuvant chemotherapy are at increased risk for hypogonadotropic hypogonadism. In such patients, low inhibin B concentrations suggest damage to the seminiferous tubules and impaired spermatogenesis.[489]

Because the indications for bone marrow transplant are expanding to include malignant and nonmalignant hematologic disorders, solid tumors, and inherited metabolic disorders, more children are undergoing this procedure. After total body irradiation and bone marrow transplant, boys tend to have normal pubertal development, whereas girls tend to have delayed puberty. However, low serum testosterone and elevated FSH concentrations among boys suggest that the prognosis for fertility is poor.[490] Other anterior pituitary hormones can be affected by cancer treatment in childhood.[491]

Approach to the Child with Delayed Puberty

As with sexual precocity, a thorough medical history is crucial to the identification of the etiology of delayed puberty (Figs. 17-11 and 17-12). Is the patient undergoing treatment for any other disorder? What, if any, pubertal development has occurred? Is there a family history of delayed puberty? What were the age of onset and the sequence of any pubertal development? Is the delay associated with anosmia and neurologic abnormalities?

Growth records to assess for stature, changes in growth velocity, weight loss, and decreased weight for height should be examined. A thorough physical examination, focusing on consequences of estrogen and androgen actions, should be performed. In boys, testicular length greater than 2.5 cm along the longitudinal axis suggests the onset of gonadarche. Features suggestive of specific disorders should be sought on physical examination (e.g., Turner syndrome, midline defects, and Prader-Willi syndrome). Short stature in a girl is suggestive of Turner syndrome and warrants measurement of gonadotropin concentrations and a karyotype, even in the absence of other stigmata of the condition. Small, firm testes, especially when gynecomastia is present, suggest Klinefelter syndrome. Height, upper-to-lower segment ratios, and arm span help to define eunuchoid habitus. Tall stature, especially with long limbs, suggests hypogonadism, such as Kallmann syndrome or 46,XY gonadal dysgenesis.

Useful laboratory studies include LH, FSH, DHEAS, sex steroid, and prolactin measurements. Hypothyroidism should be excluded by measurement of free T_4 and TSH concentrations. Bone age determinations are used to assess

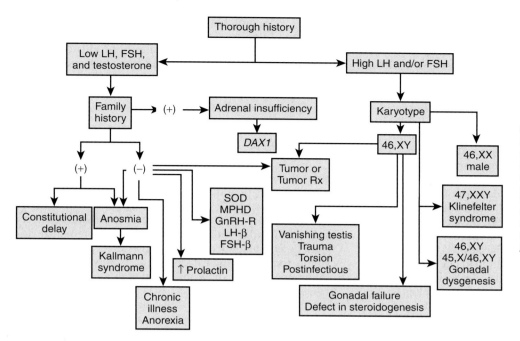

Figure 17-12. Algorithm for delayed puberty in boys. Beginning with a thorough medical history, this flowchart provides guidelines for the differential diagnosis of the most common causes of delayed puberty in girls. FSH, follicle-stimulating hormone; LH, luteinizing hormone; MPHD, multiple pituitary hormones deficiencies; SOD, septo-optic dysplasia.

the degree of delay, monitor subsequent development, and estimate final adult height. Urinalysis, erythrocyte sedimentation rate, and renal function studies help to exclude chronic disorders. Assessment for celiac disease or chronic inflammatory bowel disease may be indicated.

Elevated basal gonadotropin concentrations confirm primary gonadal failure, but this assessment is less reliable when skeletal maturation is less than 11 years in girls and 12.5 years in boys. In most cases, when gonadotropin concentrations are elevated, a karyotype determination is indicated to assess for Turner syndrome in girls, Klinefelter syndrome in boys, gonadal dysgenesis, or defects in sex steroid synthesis or action. After ensuring that pregnancy is not the cause of primary amenorrhea, progesterone withdrawal can be performed to assess estrogenization of the uterus and patency of the vaginal outflow tract. Withdrawal bleeding generally occurs within 24 to 72 hours of completing a course of progesterone (5-10 mg daily for 10 days). Imaging studies may be warranted, depending on the differential diagnosis formulated from the history and physical examination.

If random gonadotropin concentrations are not elevated, testing with hCG may be indicated when the testes are not palpable or if defects in testosterone biosynthesis are suspected. Multiple regimens have been described for hCG stimulation tests, ranging from daily injections for 5 days to biweekly injections over several weeks. At least 5000 units should be administered over the treatment period, with total dosage not exceeding 3000 units per injection or 15,000 units over the treatment period. A blood sample to measure testosterone, dihydrotestosterone, DHEA, and androstenedione should be obtained within 24 hours of the last injection. When *CYP17* mutations are being considered, serum pregnenolone and 17-OH-hydroxyprogesterone levels should also be determined.

Differentiation of hypothalamic and pituitary gonadotropin disorders from constitutional delay may be difficult.

In both situations, basal gonadotropin concentrations and GnRH-stimulated (100 μg GnRH) gonadotropin responses are low and show considerable overlap. In this regard, the presence of coincidental disorders, such as other anterior pituitary hormone deficiencies, decreases the chances of the delay being constitutional. In addition, constitutional delay of puberty is usually associated with delayed adrenarche; however, adrenarche may also be delayed among subjects with ACTH deficiency. No single blood test, stimulation study, or imaging study accurately distinguishes between these entities. Thus, serial observation remains the best way to distinguish constitutional delay from hypogonadotropic hypogonadism.

ESTROGEN REPLACEMENT

The goal of estrogen replacement therapy is to mimic the normal pattern of ovarian estradiol secretion to induce development of secondary sexual characteristics. Considerations such as chronologic age, actual height, and predicted height are factored into the decision as to when to initiate therapy. It is important for girls to experience menarche at the same time as their peers; for this reason, estrogen therapy is generally initiated at approximately age 12 years. Estrogen treatment alone can be administered initially by transcutaneous absorption or by oral administration. Transdermal patches (0.025 mg estradiol, applied either once or twice weekly), ethinyl estradiol in doses of 3 to 5 μg/day (100 ng/kg daily), or conjugated estrogens (0.3 mg daily) can be used to induce breast development. Two types of transdermal patches are available: reservoir and matrix. One advantage of matrix patches is the ability to cut the patches into pieces to administer lower doses. Nocturnal application of pieces of transdermal matrix patches can mimic the spontaneous estrogen concentrations and diurnal variation observed in early gonadarche.[492]

Once breakthrough bleeding occurs, or after 1 year of unopposed estrogen, a progestogen should be added. The patient can then be switched to an oral contraceptive, or a combination of patches and pills can be used for cyclic estrogen-progesterone therapy. Alternatively, estrogen alone can be administered for the first 11 days of each month and estrogen and progesterone can be administered on days 12 through 21 of each month, with no medication administered from day 22 until the end of the month. The estrogen dosage can be titrated according to the tempo and adequacy of pubertal development. Initial daily estrogen doses can range from 6-12 µg/day administered as transdermal estradiol, 0.25 mg/day administered as oral micronized estradiol, or 0.2-0.4 mg/month as intramuscular depot estradiol. The estradiol dose can be gradually increased over 2 years to achieve adult replacement doses, which approximate 100-200 µg/day administered as transdermal estradiol, 2-4 mg/day administered as micronized estradiol, 20 µg/day administered as oral ethinyl estradiol, or 1.25-2.5 mg/day administered as concentrated equine estrogens. In this regimen, micronized oral progesterone (200 mg/day) or medroxyprogesterone (5-10 mg/day) can be used.[427] On completion of pubertal development, the estrogen dose should be the minimum necessary to prevent breakthrough bleeding, support regular menstrual cycles, and promote calcium deposition. For females with complete androgen insensitivity, congenital adrenal hyperplasia, or Mayer-Rokitansky-Kuster-Hauser syndrome, nonsurgical self-vaginal dilation supervised by a multidisciplinary team is an effective alternative to vaginal surgery and often improves vaginal length.[493]

ANDROGEN REPLACEMENT

Testosterone replacement therapy will induce and maintain secondary sexual characteristics in boys. Testosterone can be administered by intramuscular injection or transcutaneous absorption. To induce pubertal genital changes, intramuscular depot testosterone esters (such as testosterone enanthate or testosterone cypionate) are administered monthly, initially at low doses, such as 50 mg/month, with subsequent increases in dose. Medication-impregnated patches or testosterone gel can be used. Some individuals complain of itchiness or inadequate adherence of the patches. Studies in adult men showed achievement of steady-state testosterone concentration within 72 hours of therapy with the gel.[494] However, optimal dosing regimens have not been established for induction of puberty with these newer forms of testosterone. Adult testosterone replacement therapy consists of weekly depot injections of 100 mg given at 1-, 2-, or 3-week intervals. When the interval between injections is increased beyond 3 weeks, testosterone concentrations may be supraphysiologic immediately after the injection and decline to subtherapeutic concentrations before the next injection. Transdermal testosterone-impregnated patches and testosterone gel provide less variable serum concentrations. Testosterone gels must be allowed to dry completely to avoid transfer of the gel to clothing or bedding, with the potential for accidental exposure to female family members and younger siblings.

Boys with anorchia can be offered the option of having saline-filled testicular prostheses surgically placed into the scrotum. The scrotum should be able to accommodate adult-sized prostheses so that only a single operation is necessary to minimize the risk of infection and scarring.

Psychosocial Considerations for Precocious and Delayed Puberty

Early puberty, especially among girls, negatively influences self-esteem and is associated with increased risks of psychosocial stress.[495,496] Thus, older girls with residual behavioral issues as a consequence of precocious puberty may benefit from counseling.[497] Although premature adrenarche is usually benign, some girls meet the diagnostic criteria for psychological disorders.[498] Boys with precocious puberty may show increased activity and increased aggressive behavior, and may masturbate. Parents report decreased self-esteem and self-confidence in some late-maturing boys. Because early or late puberty can create stress for the child and the child's family, discussion to ascertain how the deviation from the normal timing of puberty affects the patient is crucial. Importantly, maturation of cognitive function appears to correlate better with chronologic age than biologic maturation.[499]

Among children with delayed puberty, in the absence of major psychosocial issues, longitudinal reevaluations to ensure pubertal development and progression may be sufficient. For those children with significant consequences, short courses of sex-appropriate steroids in small doses may be beneficial. For prepubertal boys, intramuscular depot testosterone (50-75 mg) can be administered monthly for three injections. After a medication-free period of at least 2 months, testosterone concentrations should be measured to assess for gonadarche. If the testosterone concentration remains low, a second course of therapy may be indicated. When used in small doses, testosterone increases growth velocity (by direct steroid action on bone and indirectly by stimulating GH secretion) and does not compromise adult height.[335] If testosterone, LH, and FSH concentrations remain low after a second course of testosterone therapy, the boy may have hypogonadotropic hypogonadism and require long-term testosterone replacement therapy.

The ability to reproduce is presumed, and is closely linked to self-esteem, gender identity, and body image. Thus, when infertility is likely to occur based on the underlying disorder, it is important to be honest and discuss the possibility of infertility. Patients and their families may need to mourn this loss of fertility, and thus involuntary childlessness, without the availability of established religious and social rituals that are extant in the case of death.[500] Subsequent discussion should include alternative ways to achieve a family, such as adoption or marriage to someone with children from an earlier relationship. Advancements in assisted reproductive technologies offer the opportunity for parenthood. For example, girls with Turner syndrome can carry pregnancies. Short-term hCG treatment successfully stimulated spermatogenesis in a man homozygous for a *GnRH* mutation.[501]

Conclusion

Puberty, which normally unfolds toward the end of the first, or the beginning of the second, decade of life, results from initiation of two independent developmental processes: gonadarche and adrenarche. *Gonadarche* describes the pubertal activation of the gonad that results in gametogenesis and the production of adult patterns in gonadal steroid synthesis. Gonadarche results from increased gonadotropin secretion, which in turn, is triggered by a resurgence in the pulsatile mode of hypothalamic GnRH-1 release that has been held in check by a neurobiologic brake from the time of late infancy.

According to current knowledge, this brake (considered conceptual in nature) is composed of a hiatus in stimulatory kisspeptin and glutamate inputs coordinated with an increased GABA and NPY tone to the GnRH neuronal network, and primarily regulates the release of GnRH-1 rather than transcription of the *GnRH-1* gene. The lifting of the brake, and therefore the timing of the pubertal resurgence of pulsatile GnRH-1, probably involves somatic cues—although the identity of these signals remains unclear. *Adrenarche* describes the pubertal increase in adrenal androgen production that is responsible for pubarche. The timing of adrenarche, in contrast to that of gonadarche, does not appear to require a signal from the brain. The timing and tempo of puberty may be modulated by genetic and environmental factors. Understanding the genomics of puberty and the interaction of environmental determinants to time the onset of human fertility is critical to improved therapeutic approaches for disorders of pubertal development.

With an appreciation and understanding of the physiology underlying gonadarche and adrenarche, a differential diagnosis can be derived for patients presenting with disorders of pubertal development. With the tools of molecular genetics, the molecular bases and risk for recurrence can often be determined. Evaluation and treatment include consideration of the psychosocial complications of "off-time" pubertal development or possible infertility.

Note Added to Proofs: In December 2008, Topaloglu et al. (Nature Genetics doi 10.1038/ng.306) reported that inactivating mutations of the gene coding for neurokinin B (*TAC3*) and its receptor (*TAC3R*) were associated with normosmic hypogonadotropic hypogonadism, that is, the identical phenotype observed in patients with inactivating GPR54 mutations.[77,78] This is intriguing because it suggests that concomitant kisspeptin and neurokinin B release may be essential for initiation of puberty.

The complete reference list can be found on the companion Expert Consult Web site at www.expertconsultbook.com.

Suggested Readings

Bondy CA, Turner Syndrome Study Group. Care of girls and women with Turner syndrome: A guideline of the Turner Syndrome Study Group. J Clin Endocrinol Metab 92:10, 2007.

Buck Louis GM, Gray LE Jr, Marcus M, et al. Environmental factors and puberty timing: expert panel research needs. Pediatrics 121(Suppl 3): S192, 2008.

Cole LW, Sidis Y, Zhang C, et al. Mutations in prokineticin 2 and prokineticin receptor 2 genes in human gonadotrophin-releasing hormone deficiency: Molecular genetics and clinical spectrum. J Clin Endocrinol Metab 93:3551, 2008.

Dodé C, Hardelin JP. Kallmann syndrome. Eur J Hum Genet 17:139, 2009.

Gajdos ZK, Hirschhorn JN, Palmert MR. What controls the timing of puberty? An update on progress from genetic investigation. Curr Opin Endocrinol Diabetes Obes 16:16, 2009.

Partsch CJ, Heger S, Sippell WG. Management and outcome of central precocious puberty. Clin Endocrinol (Oxf) 56:129, 2002.

Plant TM. The role of *KiSS-1* in the regulation of puberty in higher primates. European J Endocrinology 155:S11, 2006.

Raivio T, Falardeau J, Dwyer A, et al. Reversal of idiopathic hypogonadotropic hypogonadism. N Engl J Med 357:863, 2007.

CHAPTER 18

Nutrition and the Pubertal Transition

Nanette Santoro, Alex Polotsky, Jessica Rieder,
and Staci Pollack

The process of puberty is believed to represent the culmination of a series of developmental events. The end result of these events is the full maturation of the hypothalamic–pituitary–gonadal (HPG) axis to its adult state. In males, this means that pulsatile gonadotropin-releasing hormone (GnRH) and gonadotropin secretion occurs at a mean interval of every 2 hours,[1] and testosterone secretion, normal virilization, and spermatogenesis are maintained. In females, a more complex series of gonadal tasks must be accomplished, including maturation of a single follicle, follicular rupture and ovulation, and corpus luteum formation. The mature female hypothalamic–pituitary–ovarian (HPO) axis must respond dynamically with negative, then positive (bimodal) feedback to rising estradiol, which is secreted by the developing follicle.[2] The positive feedback response, in the form of a luteinizing hormone (LH) surge, must be sufficient to initiate the molecular events of follicle rupture and subsequent luteinization. Optimal functioning of the female reproductive system requires more versatility of the HPO axis and this system is therefore more vulnerable to disruption.[3]

Pulsatile secretion of hypothalamic GnRH and pituitary LH occurs before birth, and continues throughout the prepubertal period.[4] The system is both amplitude- and frequency-modulated. Pulsatile LH secretion has been detected in children and occurs at a normal, adult frequency in boys and girls[5]; however, the amplitude of the signal is minuscule and requires highly sensitive measurement methods to detect. The suppression of pulsatile GnRH–LH secretory amplitude in prepuberty has been attributed to a combination of enhanced sensitivity of the childhood reproductive axis to estradiol, as well as a predominance of inhibitory neural and neuroendocrine signals that ultimately dampen the amplitude of the central GnRH pulse generator.[6] This working model hypothesizes that, prepubertally, the hypothalamic–pituitary axis is inhibited, and during puberty, the axis is released from this inhibition.

The mechanisms by which the gonadostat is set have been remarkably resistant to detection, but there are promising clues that have been obtained by elegant human and animal experiments. There are three general themes to the areas of exploration: (1) neuroendocrine regulation of GnRH secretion; (2) integration and organization of neuronal networks; and (3) permissive inputs to the GnRH–LH secretory apparatus. These signals will be addressed briefly in this introduction, but the chapter will focus largely on the data that have been most recently acquired about factors that modify the human pubertal transition.

The GnRH neurons are inherently pulsatile and are subject to short- and long-loop feedback. They provide pulsatile release throughout the prepubertal years, albeit at a very low level that is clinically undetectable. GnRH neurons are responsible for reproductive failure only when they are absent or when other, permissive signals are lacking, such as occurs in starvation or with excessive exercise. The amplitude modulation of GnRH–LH secretion that occurs during puberty has been linked to the action of the kisspeptin and its cognate receptor, GPR54.[7] Kisspeptin appears to act directly on GnRH neurons and amplifies GnRH and consequently LH and follicle-stimulating hormone (FSH) secretion. Both kisspeptin and its receptor, GPR54, increase coincident with the onset of puberty. In addition to kisspeptin, there are many other upstream regulators of GnRH that appear to provide redundancy to prevent reproductive failure. These are discussed in detail in Chapter 17.

In addition to enhancement of the amplitude of GnRH by direct stimulatory molecules, the acquisition of functional networks of neurons and glial cells provides the necessary communication pathways through which signaling can occur. The acquisition of these networks may involve anatomic changes in cell populations or recruitment as well as increases in neuronal connectivity. For example, glial cells, long believed to be inert but helpful in providing scaffolding, may play a more critical role in GnRH secretion. Microglia, macrophages that differentiate into glial cells, are necessary for optimal GnRH secretion. Colony stimulating factor-1 (CSF-1) knockout mice, who lack adequate macrophage function, do not have adequate microglial development and are deficient in hypothalamic GnRH secretion.[8]

Finally, peripheral signals to the hypothalamic–pituitary axis provide a series of permissive signals that may assist in the peripubertal activation of the reproductive axis. It has long been known that body weight influences the onset of reproductive maturation, inasmuch as very underweight girls and boys would not undergo the normal pubertal process and had apparent deficiency of central GnRH secretion.[9] The peripheral signal that has been most investigated as communicating nutritional status to the hypothalamus is leptin. It has been shown in both animal models[10] and humans that inadequate leptin is associated with lack of GnRH secretion, and leptin replacement can restore normal cycles in women who have hypothalamic amenorrhea and hypoleptinemia.[11] However, leptin alone is insufficient to initiate pubertal maturation of the HPG axis, and a specific leptin concentration or threshold, above which maturation occurs, has not been defined.[12] Additional adipose signals have been proposed, but rarely tested.

A role for peripheral adrenal gland signaling to the HPG axis has also been proposed. Prepubertal girls with higher dehydroepiandrosterone (DHEA) and DHEA sulfate (DHEAS) levels and earlier adrenarche attain menarche at younger ages, suggesting that androgens can accelerate the process.[13] Interestingly, body size and androgen exposure may be linked. With increasing body mass index (BMI), there is increasing insulin resistance and progressive reduction in sex hormone–binding globulin (SHBG), the principal high-affinity plasma carrier protein for testosterone and estradiol. Decreased SHBG leads to increases in bioavailable androgen and estradiol. In this way, adiposity and BMI may interact to stimulate the pubertal process further. Low–birth-weight children, who have more body fat, appear to be at higher risk for adrenal androgen elevations in the peripubertal period.[14]

Under physiologic conditions, the interplay of these three sets of signals is concurrent and integrated. The process of HPG axis maturation in the human typically takes years. The chronology of events in humans has been partially characterized and follows a general pattern, which has been separated into stages. Attainment of pubertal stages varies by race and ethnicity in girls, although boys appear to have a stable rate of pubertal progression over recent recording of trends. African-American girls begin puberty earlier than white girls, at approximately ages 8 to 9 years compared with 10 years, respectively.[15,16] Although there is some debate about whether pubertal progression is occurring at earlier ages, most data show that, in girls, the overall process was initiated earlier in 2007 than it was in the early part of the 20th century, when the first published reports of normative data appeared.

These modifications in the pubertal process appear to be attributable to environmental or peripheral factors that modulate the process, rather than to a fundamental change in neuronal networks or GnRH neuronal function. This chapter will discuss the role of the various environmental influences that have been proposed to modulate the pubertal process, most notably in girls, and will seek to explain how these factors have interacted in recent decades.

The Normal Pubertal Process

The known and conjectured mechanisms initiating puberty are reviewed in Chapter 17. Herein, we will focus on the epidemiology of normal puberty in girls. Puberty appears to be imminent when hypothalamic–pituitary sensitivity to negative feedback inhibition by estradiol is reduced,[17] and attendant inhibitory neural networks diminish in activity. These processes lead to increased GnRH secretion[18] as well as increased gonadotropin pulsatility, initially at night, and then extending throughout 24 hours.[19] The result is folliculogenesis in girls, spermatogenesis and testosterone production in boys, and the attainment of fertility milestones. In females, the ultimate maturation of the HPO axis is the manifestation of positive hypothalamic–pituitary feedback to increasing estradiol, which initiates an LH surge and ovulation of the preovulatory dominant follicle.[2]

There is evidence that maturation is not a linear process, however. Girls who have their first menstrual period do not always continue to ovulate monthly thereafter. It is also not certain whether menarche routinely reflects an antecedent ovulatory cycle, or if it is merely indicative of a rise and fall in estradiol. Epidemiologic studies have observed that the attainment of regular menstruation takes from as few as 2 to as many as 7 years after menarche.[20-23] However, many such studies were conducted in populations of girls who differ from the current U.S. population. These studies included few young women of color, yet African-American girls are known to attain menarche and to undergo pubertal maturation earlier than white girls. This has been related in part to increased BMI, but may also be due to other factors.[24] It is possible that earlier populations studied included many girls who were nutritionally marginal, certainly by today's standards. However, weight and BMI data are not available from these earlier studies.[22,25,26] Given the high rates of obesity among adolescents in the current U.S. population and the increase in body fat in U.S. adolescents over the last century,[27] it is likely that any restraint that low body weight might place on the HPO axis is minimally operative in our current society.[28] The virtual elimination of undernutrition might be expected to reduce the overall age at menarche in population studies. However, this has not been uniformly the case. In one 50-year cohort and family study of a population sample in Ohio, BMI was not shown to be independently related to an earlier age at menarche.[29] However, this population reflects minimal minority representation and had a mean age at menarche of 12.7 years before 1954 and 12.6 years after 1954, a minimal decrease. Body composition or BMI in this sample may have been optimal before 1954.

One study of 112 white girls, followed every 6 months perimenarcheally, found elevated urinary progesterone levels, consistent with regular ovulation, within 1 year of menarche.[30] However, in this study, sampling was performed only every 6 months, a frequency inadequate for the detection of monthly ovulatory events. Our group has recently completed a study of perimenarcheal girls using daily sampling, and the findings reinforce the notion that regular ovulation occurs relatively rapidly, within months instead of years after menarche.[31] Both Metcalf et al.[21] and Borsos et al.,[32] who also conducted weekly hormonal assessments in perimenarcheal girls, concluded that a mature pattern of ovulatory cycles was established in 23% and 13% women within 1 year of menarche, respectively. However, weekly urine sampling may be inadequate for the detection of brief excursions of progesterone, or its urinary metabolite, pregnanediol glucuronide (Pdg). Luteal phases may also be shorter than the adult norm of 14 days when adolescents are observed. Recent data from our group indicate that the capacity to produce an ovulatory LH surge in response to estrogen is present, even before the onset of the first menses.[31] These findings indicate that, at least in some girls, a biphasic feedback response to estradiol is not the rate-limiting step in attaining regular, ovulatory menses. Irregular menstruation has been associated with low gynecologic age, low BMI, chronic nonspecific lung disease or allergic disease, weight loss, and stress.[33]

Rosenfield[34] hypothesized that low-amplitude hormonal cycles occur in early puberty, with nighttime levels greater than daytime levels. Indeed, it may be that all of the hormonal components of the HPO axis are functioning at an adult frequency, but the hormonal signals are dampened and slowly increase to detectable levels. It is also possible that the ovary is less capable of responding to appropriate hypothalamic–pituitary signals, and that ovarian maturation is also required for the initiation of puberty. This latter hypothesis is relatively untested.

The notion that body weight or body fat is a permissive maturational signal to the hypothalamic–pituitary axis in girls is also supported by clinical data showing an increase in leptin associated with puberty.

The onset of puberty around the world shows a 4- to 5-year variation that involves genetic factors, ethnicity, nutritional conditions, secular trends, physical activity, and endocrine-disrupting chemicals.[35] Between the mid-19th century and the mid-20th century, a rapid decline in mean menarcheal age has been noted, from 17 years to younger than 14 years, in the United States and some Western European countries. A North–South European gradient exists, with earlier menarche occurring in France and Mediterranean countries compared with Scandinavia. After the 1960s, these downward trends seemed to stabilize, with mean menarcheal ages reported to be approximately 12.7 years according to data in the United States and most European countries.[35] However, in 1997, data from the

American Academy of Pediatrics Pediatric Research in Office Settings network, a cross-sectional study of more than 17,000 girls, reported a continuation of a downward trend in the age of onset of puberty, noting breast development occurring at a mean age of 10 years in white girls and 8.9 years in African-American girls, trends confirmed by the National Health and Nutrition Examination Survey.[15,16] Although the methods of assessing breast development (inspection versus palpation) have called some of these data into question, the recommended guidelines for evaluating girls with sexual precocity have been changed, with the lower age limit for nonphysiologic breast development 7 years in white girls and 6 years in African-American girls.[36] The reasons for this new downward trend are unclear. As noted earlier, the roles of increasing weight, body fat, and BMI in the Western world provide compelling hypothetical sources for these findings. However, other scenarios that could lead to earlier puberty imply that additional factors are also at play.

It has been shown that, within developing countries, pubertal timing variations exist between girls in well-off versus underprivileged conditions, with earlier ages at menarche in well-off girls.[35] Whether these differences relate to nutritional status or physical activity or energy expenditure or to perceived environmental stressors is not known.

Internationally adopted girls from developing countries into Western households display an increased prevalence of precocious puberty, compared with girls from their native countries and girls within their adoptive countries.[4,37] The risk of precocious puberty appears greater the older the age at adoption (especially so for girls adopted when they were older than 2 years old as opposed to girls adopted when they were younger than 2 years old), and is lower in girls who immigrate with their families, arguing against a direct role for immigration per se.[37] A recent study has suggested that the mechanism is centrally driven because higher levels of FSH, an age-dependent rise in measurable LH, and higher serum estradiol levels have all been observed in adopted girls without clinical signs of puberty, compared with control subjects.[38]

There is an evolutionary "reproductive strategy" theory of prepubertal childhood experiences and stressors influencing early pubertal progression and precocious sexuality. Girls reared in the absence of fathers in the first 7 years of life show an earlier onset of puberty and precocious sexuality.[39,40] This theory hypothesizes that father absence leads to depression and weight gain in the abandoned daughters, hastening the timing of the permissive signaling provided by leptin (or other adipose-signaling molecules), which in turn inhibit neuropeptide Y (NPY) and help to trigger the pubertal process. Another theory posits that the X-linked androgen receptor GGC repeat polymorphisms predispose fathers to behaviors such as conflict and family abandonment and also predispose daughters to early menarche and precocious sexuality.[40,41]

Environmental exposures are also hypothesized to contribute to the trend of earlier puberty in Western societies. Endocrine disruptors, or xenoestrogens, contained in plastics or agricultural pesticides, are ubiquitous in industrialized societies, and most individuals demonstrate appreciable levels of exposure. In general, these compounds bind weakly to sex steroid receptors and their signaling is likely to be overridden by endogenous sex steroids in gonadally intact, reproductive-age males and females. However, at the extremes of reproductive life in women and prepubertally in men, these mixed sex steroid agonists may play a role in providing nonphysiologic input to the reproductive axis. In the past, tainted milk, veal, or poultry has led to transient increases in premature thelarche, with the geographic distribution of central precocious puberty suggesting that these environmental exposures activate the hypothalamic–pituitary axis.[42]

How Does Fat Signal the HPO Axis?

Leptin is the putative "missing link" between the metabolic and reproductive axes. Leptin is a 16-kD protein secreted primarily by adipocytes. Initially described as a satiety factor,[43] it conveys an afferent signal to the central nervous system on body fat status. Mice deficient in leptin (ob/ob) or leptin receptor (db/db) exhibit hyperphagia, profound obesity, and sexual infantilism. In humans, leptin levels are markedly elevated in obesity[44] and pregnancy,[45] and are higher in women than in men.[46] A theory of dual regulation of energy balance by leptin was proposed. In a state of energy equilibrium (input = output), leptin concentrations reflect total body fat mass. Alternatively, in conditions of energy disequilibrium, leptin functions as a sensor of energy imbalance, whereby its concentrations decrease in states of net weight loss and increase in conditions of positive weight balance (reviewed in Meier and Gressner[47]).

The actions of leptin on the HPO axis are believed to have differential effects on the central and peripheral components of the reproductive system. In the central nervous system, leptin has been shown to modulate GnRH pulse frequency in vitro.[48] It does not act directly on GnRH neurons, but rather acts via indirect mechanisms through interneurons secreting hypothalamic neuropeptides, such as NPY, galanin-like protein, melanocyte-stimulating hormone, and endogenous opioids (reviewed in Moschos et al.[49]). On the gonadal level, leptin has been found in ovarian follicular fluid and leptin receptor has been localized to human granulosa, theca, and Leydig cells. In the bovine model, leptin decreases sex steroid production from granulosa and theca cells.[50] In humans, leptin may interrupt normal oocyte maturation[51] and has been correlated with poor implantation potential.[52] The dual low-leptin/high-leptin mechanism has been proposed to take into account the complex nature of leptin–HPG axis interactions.[53] According to this theory, the predominant effect of leptin action on the HPG axis is determined by its concentration, whereby low levels of leptin exert a negative influence centrally and elevated levels of leptin yield a negative effect peripherally at the gonadal or embryonal level.

The exciting discovery of leptin as an indicator of fat mass gave rise to speculation that it may represent the missing link in the Frisch hypothesis[54] and, thus, serve as a trigger of pubertal development. Leptin administration results in reversal of pubertal arrest in leptin-deficient mice.[55] When given to normal prepubertal animals, leptin hastens sexual development, as manifested by the advancement of vaginal opening.[56] Cheung et al. assessed the temporal sequence of pubertal events in rodents[57,58] and showed that serum leptin elevation did not precede pubertal development in rats. Similarly, expression of leptin messenger RNA receptor in the hypothalamus of female mice did not increase with pubertal development. Finally, administration of leptin to starved animals advanced estrus compared with food-restricted untreated control subjects, but occurred at the same time as in the mice fed ad libitum. Taken together, these results imply that leptin appears to provide a necessary input of adequacy of energy stores to the brain, thus authorizing, but not initiating, progression to puberty.

In humans, congenital deficiencies of leptin or leptin receptor are rare conditions that are characterized with early-onset obesity and, variably, hypogonadism.[59,60] Dramatic reversal of pubertal delay with leptin administration in a leptin-deficient girl has been described.[61] Interestingly, unexplained spontaneous correction of sexual infantilism and menarche were reported in two women with congenital leptin deficiency.[62] In leptin-replete individuals, serum leptin increases during childhood, with the highest concentrations in children who gain the most weight; higher serum leptin concentrations are associated with earlier menarche in girls.[63] In boys with constitutional delay of puberty, leptin elevation was not a prerequisite for progression to puberty.[64] Furthermore, a case report of two women with lipoatrophic diabetes and chronic hypoleptinemia showed normal menarche and childbearing, suggesting that normal pubertal maturation is possible even with very low serum levels.[65] Thus, both animal and human data support the notion that leptin is necessary, but not sufficient, for pubertal development. Although leptin does not act as a "trigger," it conveys an essential metabolic permission for the body to develop its reproductive function and prepare for procreation.

Other Potential Molecules That Communicate Metabolic Signals to the HPO Axis

Adiponectin, another major adipokine, is the most abundant gene transcript of adipose tissue.[66] It plays a role in the development of insulin resistance and, most notably, is profoundly decreased in obesity and type II diabetes.[67] Adiponectin plasma concentrations show a sexual dimorphism, with women having significantly higher levels,[67] whereas prepubertal children show no sex difference. Adiponectin levels significantly decrease after puberty[68]; however, it remains to be seen whether this represents a consequence of the increasing body mass or a distinct phenomenon.

Ghrelin, a 28–amino acid, stomach-secreted peptide, is a ligand for the growth hormone secretagogue receptor.[69] Ghrelin is a central appetite stimulator that regulates hunger and stimulates meal initiation[70] and has recently attracted attention as another putative link between the metabolic and reproductive axes. In cross-sectional studies, ghrelin concentrations decreased from childhood to adolescence.[71] In contrast, children with central precocious puberty do not exhibit an increase in serum ghrelin after treatment with a GnRH analog.[72] In children evaluated for short stature, administration of exogenous sex steroids decreased serum ghrelin in boys, but not in girls.[73] Although one group reported that the fall in ghrelin levels during childhood is a putative mechanism of pubertal growth acceleration,[74] larger longitudinal studies are needed to evaluate ghrelin's role in pubertal development.

Inflammatory cytokines, most notably tumor necrosis factor-α and interleukin-6, exhibit alteration in concentration in obesity and are regulated by leptin. In monkeys, leptin has been shown to modulate the inflammatory response, suggesting that low-grade inflammation may play a role in the pathogenesis of obesity.[75] Weight loss results in decreased infiltration of adipose tissue by macrophages and improvement of the cytokine profile (reviewed in Bastard et al.[76]). In obese adolescents, C-reactive protein concentrations were significantly elevated, providing the first indication of the low-grade inflammation hypothesis starting at a young age.[77] Further study of this rapidly evolving field may provide new molecules that could take part in the cross-talk between nutrition and reproduction.

Neuropeptide Y, a member of the pancreatic polypeptide family, is a 36–amino acid neurotransmitter that is predominantly found in sympathetic neurons.[78] NPY is one of the most potent orexigenic peptides and was recently shown to stimulate fat angiogenesis and proliferation and differentiation of adipocytes in the periphery.[79] Leptin decreases NPY gene transcription in the arcuate nucleus,[80] thereby sending a signal to decrease food intake. In the male Rhesus monkey, antagonism of an NPY receptor led to precocious GnRH release, suggesting a role for NPY in maintenance of the prepubertal brake of the GnRH pulse generator.[81]

The arcuate nucleus of the medial basal hypothalamus is a central relay station for body fat signaling and is a site of GnRH release. It functions to converge the influences of orexigenic stimuli, such as NPY and agouti-related protein (Agrp), and anorexic stimuli, such as alpha-melanocyte–stimulating protein, corticotropin-releasing hormone, and opioids. In rats, exogenous leptin administration results in down-regulation of NPY and Agrp.[82] Expression of leptin receptors in the arcuate and ventromedial hypothalamic nuclei suggests that this is a site of modulation of leptin effects on the reproductive axis.[51,83]

The Role of Body Weight as a Modifier of Puberty

INTRAUTERINE NUTRITION AND EARLY POSTNATAL EFFECTS ON PUBERTY

The principle of prenatal programming relates to the nutritional, hormonal, and metabolic effect of the prenatal in utero environment on offspring. As it relates to puberty, changes to the nutritional, hormonal, or metabolic environment during a "critical" developmental period may have

an effect on reproductive functional capacity. Although the mechanism for this programming remains uncertain, birth weight and prematurity have been linked to the timing and progression of puberty, although associations are variable. Low–birth-weight and small-for-gestational-age (SGA) status have been associated with precocious pubarche (appearance of pubic hair earlier than 8 years of age) and early and exaggerated adrenarche in girls.[84-87] Prematurity alone or in the presence of SGA status has also been associated with premature pubarche.[87] The role of prenatal stress associated with prematurity may have an independent or additive effect on the prenatal programming effect resulting from growth restriction. Low–birth-weight children have been found to have higher dehydroepiandrosterone levels compared with children of normal weight, indicating amplified adrenarche.[86,88] Low birth weight has also been associated with an increased likelihood of polycystic ovary syndrome (PCOS) and hyperinsulinemia and future development of diabetes mellitus and coronary artery disease. Although the majority of studies indicate that SGA status is associated with premature pubarche and earlier onset of menarche,[89] Van Weissenbruch et al., in one longitudinal study, found no differences in the timing and progression of puberty, including age at menarche, between girls born SGA and girls born appropriate for gestational age.[88] Another study found SGA status to be associated with pubertal delay.[90] Studies evaluating birth weight associations with age at menarche in the general population have also been variable, with some studies finding no significant association between birth weight and age at menarche and others finding lower birth weight associated with earlier pubertal onset.[91-93] Although the prenatal environment clearly influences the timing and onset of puberty, the variable evidence relating gestational size and pubarche requires further longitudinal study to elucidate the nature of the relationship and identify the mechanisms underlying this influence.

CHILDHOOD NUTRITION AND MODIFICATION OF PUBERTY

Nutritional status may play a role in pubertal onset and reproduction through its influence on pituitary–gonadal function. The hypothalamic mechanisms controlling food intake and energy balance and the onset of puberty involve common local and peripheral regulators, which are numerous and act through redundant pathways. Thus, although nutritional status may not be a direct determinant of physiologic variations in the timing of puberty, it may play a permissive role in its timing, or may simply be evidence of concurrent developmental hypothalamic processes (i.e., adult food intake and nutritional balance and reproductive maturation). The effect of malnutrition in children and adolescents on pubertal timing has been studied primarily in youth with anorexia nervosa, elite athletes, and underfed children adopted from developing countries. The focus has largely been on the progress of reproductive maturation in a nutritionally deprived environment. The effect of obesity on pubertal timing has more recently been addressed in obese youth with premature pubarche and in children with low birth weight and rapid postnatal catch-up in weight.

Suboptimal caloric intake associated with disordered eating habits can influence pubertal onset. Pugliese et al. evaluated 14 boys (9) and girls (5), ages 9 to 17 years, with growth failure and delay in puberty (7 of the 14) due to malnutrition resulting from self-imposed caloric restriction.[94] Although caloric intake was restricted for fear of becoming obese, psychiatric screening showed no psychiatric disease or anorexia nervosa, and increased linear growth and pubertal progression resumed with the resumption of age-appropriate caloric intake. Matejek et al. studied the relationship among leptin levels, fat stores, and reproductive hormone levels in 13 female juvenile elite gymnasts and 9 adolescent girls with anorexia nervosa.[95] Leptin levels were subnormal and were related to body fat mass in girls with anorexia nervosa. Leptin levels were lowest in the elite gymnasts, who had even lower body fat mass than the girls with anorexia nervosa. In both groups, estradiol levels were low and menarche was delayed. The findings suggest that low leptin levels are associated with low caloric intake, and the finding of parallel leptin and reproductive hormone patterns suggests a similar mechanism for the dysregulation of the HPO axis in girls with anorexia nervosa and elite athletes, primarily in relation to low body fat.

Underfed children have also been shown to have delays in pubertal onset. Catch-up height and weight in immigrant and adopted children who move from developing countries to developed countries are associated with precocious menarche.[96] "Hypothalamic priming," which results when catch-up growth stimulates hypothalamic maturation and leads to puberty, is believed to occur at a critical period. Girls who are malnourished for longer periods and who undergo catch-up growth at a later age are more likely to experience precocious menarche than those who undergo catch-up growth at a younger age.[97] Further, Johnson et al. found that Romanian adoptees brought to the United States had less weight compromise than height compromise.[98] These findings suggest that, although nutritional deprivation may play a significant role in altering the timing of puberty, other factors, such as genetics, prematurity, intrauterine growth restriction, medical illness, stress, and even endocrine-disrupting chemicals, may play an even more determinant role than nutritional status in puberty initiation. Studies that compare the timing and progression of puberty in developed and developing countries will better elucidate the effects of migration and nutritional status on puberty initiation.

Longitudinal and cross-sectional data from studies conducted since the 1970s have shown an overall close association between obesity and early pubarche in girls, although there is a paucity of such evidence for boys. Precocious puberty has been linked to childhood obesity,[85] and girls with precocious pubarche tend to be hyperinsulinemic, especially if their birth weight was low and if they showed a rapid postnatal catch-up in weight.[86] Decreased insulin sensitivity has been documented in children with a history of low birth weight[99] and in girls of normal body weight with precocious puberty.[100-102] The hyperinsulinemia has been associated with low levels of sex hormone–binding globulin and excess total and central adiposity.[84,100] Girls of normal weight with a history of low birth weight and

premature pubarche who are treated with an insulin sensitizer show improvement in body composition, decrease in lipid abnormalities, and delay or prevention of the progression to PCOS.[101] Further longitudinal data are needed to test causality in the association between obesity and early-onset pubarche.

Young Adult and Adult Associations

There are a number of different theories as to how nutritional status may influence the timing of menarche. Frisch and Revelle noted a direct relationship between body weight and age at onset of puberty[103,104] and concluded that a critical amount of body fat was needed for the onset of puberty.[105] Although Frisch and Revelle proposed that a critical amount of body fatness is needed for menarche, it is not clear whether the degree of fatness causes menarche or whether an increase in body fat is the consequence of the onset of puberty and the two findings may be coincidentally and independently related to endocrine or genetic factors. Others have argued that physiologic variations in body fat mass are more relevant than a critical fat mass, a notion supported by the fact that girls with early menarche are more likely to be obese than those with late menarche.[91] In comparison with nonobese girls, obese girls have been found to have earlier menarche in Japan (9 months earlier)[106] and Thailand (10.8 months earlier).[107] Early menarche has also been associated with an increased risk of obesity in adulthood, indicating that early menarche may precede the development of obesity.[108,109] However, other studies have shown that obesity precedes early menarche. Cooper et al. found that age at menarche was inversely associated with weight at 7 years,[110] and He and Karlberg noted that incremental increases in BMI between the ages of 2 and 8 years were associated with early onset of the pubertal growth spurt in both boys and girls.[111]

Several authors have argued that the association between menarcheal age and body fatness may be due to correlated genetic effects and are influenced by separate environmental correlates independent of each other.[112] Karlberg noted that peak height velocity and menarche can occur simultaneously or up to 2 years apart, supporting the notion that the parameters of pubarche and body fat are associated coincidentally, but are not necessarily associated causally.[113] The Fels longitudinal study examined the relationship between the mean age of menarche and the simultaneous change in BMI from age 3 to 35 years in successive birth cohorts (born from 1929-1990).[114] Although the age at menarche in the 1980s cohort was significantly lower than that in girls born previously, and these findings match the findings of several recent reports that suggest a decline in the mean age at menarche of U.S. girls over the last 20 years, the decline in age at menarche was not associated with a significant concurrent increase in BMI in childhood or adolescence. Girls born in the 1960s and 1970s, however, showed significant increases in BMI in adulthood, relative to girls born in earlier cohorts, without a concurrent significant change in the age at menarche. The authors concluded that the secular trends in increasing

BMI and decreasing age at menarche cannot be casually related, and are in fact independent, yet coincident processes. The major argument against this conclusion relates to the fact that the authors did not document a significant secular trend toward increasing BMI during childhood and adolescence in this predominantly white cohort. The BMIs reported were in the normal range, and thus the authors could not address the question as to whether large increases in BMI in childhood might be associated with changes in age at menarche. The most significant decline in age at menarche occurred in the 1980 cohort relative to the 1930 cohort, which more closely approximates the commencement of the rising obesity epidemic. Further, the study lacks information on body composition, and thus it cannot be determined whether the findings relate to changes in body composition versus changes in BMI.

Beyond pubarche, reproductive functioning in adolescents and young adult women appears to have an association with body fatness. The secular trend in the decline in menarcheal age has been found to occur together with an opposite trend in the time interval to regular cycling after the onset of menarche. Over a 25-year period, Clavel-Chapelon showed that the interval between menarche and regular cycling increased from 1.9 to 3 years and the proportion of women with an interval of 5 years increased from 9% to 21%.[115] Furthermore, the prevalence of ovulatory disorders in adolescents also appears to be on the rise.[116] Concurrent with these menstrual and reproductive changes, rates of overweight and obesity have been steadily climbing in the United States as well as in other developed and developing countries. Data from the 2003-2004 National Health and Nutrition Examination Survey indicated that 17.1% of U.S. children and adolescents were overweight.[117] The prevalence of overweight in female youth increased from 13.8% in 1999-2000 to 16% in 2003-2004 and in male youth from 14% to 18.2% in the same period. Overweight youth are at risk for becoming obese adults, and this risk increases with age: the probability for overweight adolescents to become overweight or obese adults may exceed 80%.[118]

Because of the association between obesity and ovulatory abnormalities and the increased degree of obesity in patients with PCOS, obesity may only minimally increase the risk of PCOS.[119] Obesity in adults[120] as well as in peripubertal children[121] has been associated with hyperandrogenemia. Obesity and elevated serum androgens are known to have independent, deleterious effects on glucose tolerance and androgen production, and these effects may also be synergistic.[122-124] Obesity begets insulin resistance, the associated hyperinsulinemia suppresses hepatic production of SHBG, and in turn free or unbound plasma testosterone becomes elevated.[123,125,126] Women with PCOS have insulin resistance that is more severe than can be accounted for by obesity alone,[127-129] and this leads to even greater reductions in SHBG and higher levels of free androgens. In turn, insulin may drive androgen secretion in PCOS, causing a feedforward mechanism promoting hyperandrogenemia. According to the 2003 Rotterdam Consensus Group, the free androgen index, which increases as SHBG levels decrease, is the preferred method for assessing hyperandrogenemia in adults.[130] Although there is little consensus regarding the diagnostic utility of depressed SHBG levels, in the Study of Women's Health Across the Nation (SWAN), Santoro et al. recently showed that SHBG is strongly inversely associated with a metabolic syndrome phenotype and increased bioavailable androgens.[131] More research is needed to better elucidate the relationship between obesity and SHBG in reproductive function in adolescent girls.

Conclusions

Maturation of the reproductive axis remains a somewhat enigmatic process. A series of neuroendocrine signals and networks appear to act cooperatively to initiate the final events of HPO axis maturation in females. Amplification of the pulsatile GnRH signal appears to be an obligatory final pathway; however, the existence of many inputs into the hypothalamus implies that there are a number of concurrent factors that act as permissive signals. Moreover, it is likely that these signaling pathways are redundant because it is in the best interests of the survival of the human species to assure that reproductive maturation will take place. It now seems clearer that environmental modifiers of the pubertal transition also contribute to the process. Psychological stressors, xenoestrogens, and body fat are but three such factors. It appears that none of these factors bears a simple relationship to the pubertal process, in that both accelerations and delays are associated with various stressors and increasing body fat. Further research is needed to understand the nature of these associations and the pathways through which they operate.

The complete reference list can be found on the companion Expert Consult Web site at www.expertconsultbook.com.

Suggested Readings

Demerath D, Li J, Sun S, et al. Fifty year trends in serial body mass index in adolescent girls: the Fels Longitudinal Study. Am J Clin Nutr 80:441-446, 2004.

El Majdoubi M, Sahu A, Ramaswamy S, Plant TM. Neuropeptide Y: a hypothalamic brake restraining the onset of puberty in primates. Proc Natl Acad Sci U S A 97(11):6179-6184, 2000.

Frisch RE, McArthur JW. Menstrual cycles: fatness as a determinant of minimum weight for height necessary for their maintenance or onset. Science 185(4155):949-951, 1974.

Kaplowitz P, Oberfeld S. Reexamination of the age limit for defining when puberty is precocious in girls in the United States: implications for evaluation and treatment. Drug and Therapeutics Executive Committees of the Lawson Wilkins Pediatric Endocrine Society. Pediatrics 104:936-941, 1999.

Legro R, Lin H, Demers L, Lloyd T. Rapid maturation of the reproductive axis during perimenarche independent of body composition. J Clin Endocrinol Metab 85:1021-1025, 2000.

McCartney CR, Prendergast KA, Chhabra S, et al. The association of obesity and hyperandrogenemia during the pubertal transition in girls: obesity as a potential factor in the genesis of postpubertal hyperandrogenism. J Clin Endocrinol Metab 91(5):1714-1722, 2006.

Messinis IE. From menarche to regular menstruation: endocrinological background. Ann NY Acad Sci 1092:49-56, 2006.

Parent A-S, Teilmann G, Juul A, et al. The timing of normal puberty and the age limits of sexual precocity: variations around the world, secular trends, and changes after migration. Endocr Rev 24:668-693, 2003.

van Weissenbruch MM. Delemarre-van de Waal HA. Early influences on the tempo of puberty. Horm Res 65(Suppl 3):105-111, 2006.

Zhang K, Pollack S, Ghods A, et al. Onset of ovulation after menarche in girls: a longitudinal study. J Clin Endocrinol Metab 93(4):1186-1194, 2008.

Physiologic and Pathophysiologic Alterations of the Neuroendocrine Components of the Reproductive Axis

Kristin D. Helm, Ralf M. Nass, and William S. Evans

Reproductive dysfunction of central etiology can result from any process that disturbs the tightly regulated hypothalamic–pituitary system. The reproductive axis itself relies on pulsatile release of gonadotropin-releasing hormone (GnRH) from a collection of neurons that are distributed diffusely throughout the hypothalamus rather than within a discrete nucleus.[1] Control of GnRH secretion is complex. Neuropeptide Y (NPY) facilitates GnRH release and gonadotropin responsiveness to GnRH. Substance P, beta-endorphin, leuenkephalin, and other endogenous opiates inhibit hypothalamic GnRH release, both acutely and tonically (in the case of beta-endorphin).[2,3] Stress-related surges in corticotrophin-releasing hormone (CRH) suppress GnRH gene transcription as well as GnRH release, as do inflammatory cytokines, such as tumor necrosis factor-α (TNF-α).[4] This CRH-induced suppression may be mediated by endogenous opiates.[5,6] The effects of catecholamines (norepinephrine, epinephrine, dopamine) are more controversial and likely depend on the prevailing endocrine milieu and the stage of sexual maturation.[2] Neurotransmitters, such as gamma-aminobutyric acid (GABA), have been shown to have both excitatory[7,8] and inhibitory[9,10] effects in animal studies, and use of the GABA-ergic drug valproic acid (VPA) in women did not affect hypothalamic–pituitary hormones.[9] Such conflicting data on the role of GABA in modulating GnRH release illustrate the challenges inherent in using rodent models to understand GnRH regulation in humans.[2]

Integration of these multiple signals ultimately results in neuronal release of GnRH, which then travels via the hypothalamic–hypophyseal portal circulation to the anterior pituitary gland, where it binds to the GnRH receptor 1 and up-regulates synthesis and secretion of two pituitary hormones—luteinizing hormone (LH) and follicle-stimulating hormone (FSH). GnRH secretion is pulsatile, with discrete bursts of GnRH affecting the release of pulses of LH and FSH by the pituitary. Moreover, the frequency of GnRH secretion has been shown in animal models to differentially affect the synthesis of LH and FSH, with rapid-frequency GnRH pulses (1 pulse/hour) favoring LH synthesis and slow-frequency GnRH pulses favoring the synthesis of FSH.[10] The secretion of LH and FSH is also regulated by direct negative feedback from gonadal products (estradiol [E_2], inhibin A and B). Once released from the pituitary, LH and FSH travel through the systemic circulation to stimulate sex steroid production and gametogenesis by the gonads. The patterns of hypothalamic, pituitary, and gonadal activity are responsible for the transition from childhood to adulthood, as well as for normal ovulatory cycles in postmenarchal women and normal sexual function in males.

The presence of appropriate quantities of these hormones is not enough to maintain a normal reproductive axis. Frequent sampling of plasma hormone concentrations has led to the belief that most hypothalamic hormones are secreted episodically, and often in a circadian rhythm. Hormonal release may be linked primarily to the sleep–wake cycle, synchronized with food ingestion, or related to the dark–light cycle. Thus, integrity of the hypothalamic suprachiasmatic nucleus, which maintains both the circadian rhythm and the sleep–wake cycle, is an important factor for regulating gonadal function in men and women.

Patients with abnormalities of this complex hypothalamic–pituitary axis often show undetectable or inappropriately low levels of pituitary gonadotropins (FSH and LH) in combination with low sex steroid levels (testosterone < 100 ng/dL in males and E_2 < 20 pg/mL in females). This combination of laboratory findings defines the condition *hypogonadotropic hypogonadism*. In contrast, patients with primary gonadal pathology have elevated FSH and LH levels in combination with low testosterone or E_2 levels, a disorder referred to as *hypergonadotropic hypogonadism*. The clinical presentation of hypogonadotropic hypogonadism varies with age of onset and degree of hormonal deficiency. Males may present with micropenis and cryptorchidism. Testicular function can be completely impaired, with Leydig cell atrophy, or testicular size can approach normal, with only mild Leydig cell impairment. The phenotype of hypogonadotropic hypogonadism in women is also quite variable, ranging from a classic eunuchoid appearance in some women (lower body segment [floor to pubis] > 2 cm longer than the upper body segment [pubis to crown] and arm span > 2 cm longer than height) to moderate breast development in others.[11] Amenorrhea, whether primary or secondary, frequently is the reason why women seek medical attention. The degree of ovarian follicular development depends on the duration of gonadotropin deficiency; in cases of congenital hypogonadotropic hypogonadism, few follicles beyond the primordial stage may be present.[12] The administration of exogenous gonadotropins (or exogenous pulsatile GnRH, when it was available) can affect ovulation and pregnancy.[13]

Although some patients with hypogonadotropic hypogonadism have no evidence of pulsatile LH secretion, others have detectable LH secretory pulses that are of insufficient frequency and amplitude to trigger gonadal steroid synthesis. A small number of patients show nearly normal patterns of LH secretion, but the LH molecules are inactive and consist only of the uncoupled α subunit.[10] This heterogeneity of basal LH secretion in patients with hypogonadotropic hypogonadism is mirrored in their responses to exogenous GnRH stimulation. Complete unresponsiveness to GnRH is rare,[14] but many patients show subnormal increases of FSH and LH. In other cases, FSH or LH levels may rise in isolation, or both may increase normally.[13,15]

Hypogonadotropic hypogonadism may be physiologic, as occurs during puberty and lactation, or it may be a manifestation of congenital or acquired pathology. Congenital hypogonadotropic hypogonadism usually occurs in the absence of other pituitary hormonal deficits, whereas acquired GnRH deficiency may be caused by tumors, infiltrative diseases, infection, trauma, or radiation, all of which can also cause other hormonal deficiencies. Epilepsy is frequently associated with reproductive dysfunction, often polycystic ovary syndrome (PCOS). Abnormalities of other hormones (i.e., thyroid hormone, cortisol, prolactin [PRL]), over- and undernutrition, exercise, stress, and medications can also cause functional hypogonadotropic hypogonadism. Hypogonadotropic hypogonadism commonly occurs with pituitary disease due to tumors and apoplexy, as well as other autoimmune and inflammatory disorders.

Hypothalamic Dysfunction

Reproductive integrity requires an intact hypothalamus, which secretes GnRH from neurons that are distributed diffusely throughout the hypothalamus rather than in a discrete nucleus.[1] As discussed earlier, GnRH is secreted in a pulsatile fashion, the frequency of which differentially affects the pulsatile secretion of the gonadotropins. Moreover, the frequency of GnRH secretion is known to affect gene expression, with rapid-frequency GnRH pulses (1 pulse/hour) favoring LH synthesis, and slow-frequency GnRH pulses favoring FSH synthesis. Pituitary LH and FSH secretion are also regulated by direct negative feedback from gonadal products (E_2, inhibin A and B). The patterns of hypothalamic, pituitary, and gonadal activity are responsible for the transition from childhood to adulthood, as well as for normal ovulatory cycles in postmenarchal females and sexual function and spermatogenesis in males. Disruption of hypothalamic GnRH secretion at any point during development can have transient or permanent effects on fertility. Such disturbances can result from congenital, structural, or functional abnormalities of the central nervous system (CNS)/hypothalamic component of the reproductive axis.

CONGENITAL DISEASE OF THE HYPOTHALAMUS

Hypogonadotropic hypogonadism resulting from abnormal development of GnRH neurons is relatively rare, affecting 1:10,000 males and 1:50,000 females.[16] GnRH neurons originate during embryonic life outside of the CNS in the nasal placode. Olfactory neurons have a similar embryonic origin in humans and many other vertebrate species. Migration of olfactory axons toward the olfactory bulb anlage is required for normal olfactory bulb (OB) development.[17] GnRH neurons then migrate across the cribriform plate toward the OB in two phases—one before OB formation and one in association with OB formation.[18] The latter wave of migration occurs in association with olfactory, vomeronasal, and terminal nerves as well as neural cell adhesion molecules, ultimately resulting in GnRH neuronal cell dispersion in the arcuate nucleus of the medial basal hypothalamus by 14 weeks of gestation.[19,20] The mature GnRH axonal neuron network eventually coordinates pulsatile secretion of GnRH into the hypothalamic–hypophyseal portal circulation.[21] Disruption of this complex series of events can result in varying degrees of hypothalamic dysfunction, which manifests clinically as hypogonadotropic hypogonadism.

Congenital hypogonadotropic hypogonadism is usually divided into two categories: that which is accompanied by olfactory deficits (anosmic idiopathic hypogonadotropic hypogonadism [IHH] or Kallmann syndrome [KS]) and that which is associated with an intact sense of smell (normosmic IHH). As discussed later, exciting progress has been made in identifying genetic causes for both anosmic

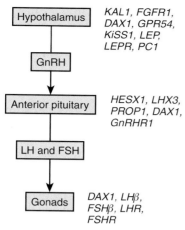

Hypothalamus	*KAL1, FGFR1,*
	DAX1, GPR54,
	KiSS1, LEP,
	LEPR, PC1

| GnRH |

Anterior pituitary	*HESX1, LHX3,*
	PROP1, DAX1,
	GnRHR1

| LH and FSH |

Gonads	*DAX1, LHβ,*
	FSHβ, LHR,
	FSHR

Figure 19-1. *Schematic diagram of the hypothalamic–pituitary–gonadal axis showing genetic mutations that are responsible for some cases of hypogonadotropic hypogonadism. FSH, follicle-stimulating hormone; GnRH, gonadotropin-releasing hormone; LH, luteinizing hormone. (Modified from Cadman SM, Kim SH, Hu Y, Gonzalez-Martinez D, Bouloux P. Molecular pathogenesis of Kallmann's syndrome. Horm Res 67:231, 2007. With permission from S. Karger AG, Basel.)*

and normosmic IHH, as summarized in Figure 19-1 and Table 19-1. However, most cases of GnRH deficiency in humans are sporadic. In the cohort of 106 patients with GnRH deficiency with and without anosmia reported by Waldstreicher et al., only 30% of cases were familial.[22] Because

IHH predominantly impairs fertility, families with multiple affected members are few, but the availability of gonadotropin therapy to induce fertility in both affected males and females may increase vertical transmission of the condition.

Anosmic Idiopathic Hypogonadotropic Hypogonadism *KAL1* Mutations

The pathologic association between IHH and olfactory dysfunction was originally recognized in the 19th century, but Kallmann and Schoenfeld first suggested a genetic basis for this group of patients in 1944.[23] In 1989, Schwanzel-Fukuda et al. discovered a tangle of GnRH neurons on the surface of the cribriform plate in a human fetus with X-linked KS.[24] The finding of the neurons in this location rather than in the typical location in the hypothalamus established defective GnRH neuronal migration as the cause of hypogonadotropic hypogonadism in KS.[24,25] Because the initial differentiation and migration were normal, research then focused on factors affecting axonal growth, path-finding, and maturation. The *KAL1* (also known as *FGFR1*) gene on the X chromosome (Xp22.3) was subsequently identified in 1991 by two groups, and both deletions and point mutations have since been found in patients with KS.[26,27] The product of *KAL1*, anosmin-1, is transiently expressed in numerous tissues of the developing human fetus, including the OB and along the migratory pathway for GnRH neurons. In the absence of anosmin-1

TABLE 19-1

Genes and Idiopathic Hypogonadotropic Hypogonadism

Clinical Features	Condition	Gene	Localization	Inheritance	Site of GnRH Impairment
HH + anosmia	Kallmann syndrome	*KAL1*	Xp22.3	X-linked	Hypothalamus (incomplete GnRH neuronal migration)
HH ± anosmia ± midline facial defects	Kallmann syndrome	*KAL2*	8p11.2	Autosomal dominant	
HH + anosmia	Kallmann syndrome			Autosomal recessive	
HH		*GnRH-R*	4q21.2	Autosomal recessive	Pituitary (↓ GnRH-R activity)
HH		*GPR54*	19p13	Autosomal recessive	Hypothalamus
HH + adrenal insufficiency	Adrenal hypoplasia congenital	*AHC*	Xp21	X-linked	Hypothalamus Pituitary
HH		*LHβ*	19q13.3	Autosomal recessive	Pituitary
HH		*FSHβ*	11p13	Autosomal recessive	
Optic atrophy + midline CNS abnormalities + HH	Septo-optic dysplasia	*HESX1*	3q21.1-21.2	Autosomal recessive	Pituitary
Obesity + HH	Obesity syndrome	*Leptin*	7q31.3	Autosomal recessive	Hypothalamus
Obesity + HH	Obesity syndrome	Leptin receptor	1q31	Autosomal recessive	
Combined hormone deficiencies (short stature, hypo-thyroidism, HH)		*PROP1*	5q	Autosomal recessive	Pituitary

AHC, adrenal hypoplasia congenital; CNS, central nervous system; FSH, follicle-stimulating hormone; GnRH, gonadotropin-releasing hormone; GnRH-R, gonadotropin-releasing hormone receptor; HH, hypogonadotropic hypogonadism; LH, luteinizing hormone.
Modified with permission from Hay C, Wu F. Genetics and hypogonadotropic hypogondism. Curr Opin Obstet Gynecol 14:303, 2002.

(with the *KAL1* mutation), OB differentiation and early olfactory axon navigation are impaired. Without olfactory nerve synaptogenesis in the OB, GnRH neurons have no migratory pathway to follow to the forebrain, resulting in the anosmia and hypogonadotropic hypogonadism typical of KS.[28] *KAL1* expression also occurs in the mesonephric tubules, ureteric bud, and corticospinal tract by 7 weeks of age, and in the retina and kidney by 11 weeks of age.[29] This tissue-specific expression accounts for the high prevalence of renal, neurologic, and midline facial abnormalities in patients with KS. Unilateral renal agenesis is believed to occur because of developmental failure of the collecting duct system in the absence of mesonephric tubule anosmin-1. Synkinesia ("mirror movements," or the involuntary movements of one extremity when an individual is asked to perform rapid, repetitive motions with the other extremity) results from abnormal fast-conducting ipsilateral corticospinal tract projections.[30] Absence of anosmin-1 expression in the facial mesenchyme leads to a high incidence of cleft palate in patients with *KAL1* mutations. Renal agenesis and synkinesia were present in 31% and 85% of patients, respectively, of a British cohort of patients with KS.[30] These abnormalities were not present in any patients with KS without the *KAL1* mutation or in patients with normosmic IHH.

As is the case with all forms of hypogonadotropic hypogonadism, KS is much more common in males, with prevalence estimated at 1:7500 males versus 1:70000 females.[31] The *KAL1* mutation accounts for only 3% to 15% of cases of anosmic IHH[16,32] and no more than one third of familial cases of IHH,[22] but it is highly penetrant. No cases of *KAL1* mutations have been described in female patients or in normosmic males.[32] Patients with KS usually do not undergo puberty, but a minority may have some degree of testicular growth or breast development, suggesting that GnRH deficiency is not always complete. Additional reproductive features may include cryptorchidism and microphallus. As is the case with other genetic defects discussed later, there is no clear genotype-to-phenotype relationship in those with a *KAL1* mutation,[31] illustrating the importance of modifier genes and environmental factors.

***FGFR1* Mutations.** Autosomal mutations cause the majority of familial anosmic hypogonadotropic hypogonadism (KS). Mutations in the gene encoding fibroblast growth factor receptor 1, *KAL2*, appear to be inherited in an autosomal dominant pattern and are seen in 7% to 10% of individuals with KS.[32] Fibroblast growth factor signaling is involved with the formation, growth, and shaping of a variety of tissues and organs, including the OB.[33] Fibroblast growth factor (FGF) receptor-1 (FGFR1) has been detected in both the nasal placode and the developing OBs of mice as well as along the migratory pathway for GnRH neurons and in the mature hypothalamus. Studies in rodents with targeted abolition of FGFR1 signaling resulted in aplasia of the OB. Both FGFR1 and anosmin-1 are coexpressed in the olfactory placode of human embryos by 4.5 weeks' gestation, and again at 8 weeks in the terminal nerve portion that guides GnRH neuronal migration to the hypothalamus.[25] Studies suggest that FGFR1 is a ligand for anosmin-1.[33] Loss-of-function mutations in the *FGFR1*

gene located on chromosome 8p11.2 can cause IHH, with or without anosmia.[34,35] At least 12 missense mutations have been identified in this gene thus far, and loss of function of the isoform FGFR1c is present in approximately 10% of male and female patients with KS.[21] Isoform FGFR1c is also important for palate morphogenesis as well as olfactory development.[36]

Unlike *KAL1* mutations, *FGFR1* mutations are not always associated with a severe reproductive phenotype. A minority of patients may have delayed puberty or normal reproductive function, suggesting that the *FGFR1* mutation may not prevent GnRH migration entirely, but may affect neuronal maturation in the hypothalamus. This variable expressivity of *FGFR1* suggests a role for other genes or the environment in modifying the phenotypic expression of this mutation. It also raises the possibility that *FGFR1* mutations account for other reproductive phenotypes associated with hypothalamic dysfunction, such as hypothalamic amenorrhea and delayed puberty.[34]

Identification of *FGFR1* mutations and the relationship between FGF signaling and anosmin-1 may explain the male predominance of hypogonadotropic hypogonadism despite the low prevalence of the X-linked form of the disease. Females have two copies of the *KAL1* gene and, therefore, higher levels of anosmin-1, which may compensate for inadequate *FGFR1* function in the presence of an *FGFR1* mutation. Thus, women with *FGFR1* mutations often have a milder, if not a normal, reproductive phenotype. On the other hand, males have a lower level of *KAL1*/anosmin-1 expression and are unable to compensate for impaired FGF signaling in the presence of an *FGFR1* mutation. Thus, their reproductive phenotypes tend to be more severe.[21,33]

As is the case for IHH as a whole, most cases of KS are sporadic and cannot be traced to familial transmission. Autosomal recessive transmission of KS does exist, but the responsible gene has yet to be cloned. Other candidate genes that may be involved in cases of anosmic IHH without *KAL1* mutations include: (1) *CHD7*, mutations of which can cause CHARGE syndrome (coloboma, congential heart disease, choanal atresia, mental and growth retardation, genital hypoplasia, and ear malformations or deafness); (2) *NELF*, the murine form of which is involved in olfactory and GnRH neuronal migration; and (3) *Pkr2*, which encodes a G-protein–coupled receptor critical for OB and reproductive organ development in mice.[25] FGF receptor mutations have also been identified in normosmic individuals with IHH, suggesting that anosmic IHH and normosmic IHH are part of a spectrum of disease rather than distinct clinical entities.[21,35]

Normosmic Idiopathic Hypogonadotropic Hypogonadism

Not all patients with hypogonadotropic hypogonadism have an impaired sense of smell. Those with a normal sense of smell are given the diagnosis of IHH. In the American cohort reported by Waldstreicher et al., approximately half of patients with hypogonadotropic hypogonadism were normosmic.[22] Nasal mucosal biopsy specimens from patients with normosmic IHH showed immunologically recognizable GnRH, providing evidence that the GnRH gene itself is intact and that defective GnRH synthesis is not the cause of IHH in these patients.[20] Other etiologies for IHH have since been identified in this group of patients, in whom the frequency of cryptorchidism[30] and nonreproductive phenotypes (synkinesia, palate abnormalities, hearing loss) is much less common than in anosmic IHH.[34]

GnRH Receptor Mutations. Attempts to identify congenital defects that would explain normosmic IHH have led to the discovery of loss-of-function missense mutations in the gene encoding the GnRH *receptor* (GnRH-R) on chromosome 4q21.2. These mutations are transmitted in an autosomal recessive pattern. The GnRH receptor is a G-protein–coupled transmembrane receptor involved with signal transduction. Mutations in this protein were initially considered unlikely because patients with normosmic IHH showed increased FSH and LH secretion in response to exogenous GnRH stimulation. However, in the study by de Roux et al., the index cases both had partial IHH and likely responded normally to GnRH stimulation because the exogenous dose was high enough to overcome their partial receptor defects.[37] *GnRH-R* mutations are estimated to occur in 40% of autosomal recessive cases of normosmic IHH and in 10% to 15% of sporadic cases.[38,39] Heterozygotes are unaffected.[25]

Identical mutations can produce different clinical phenotypes, suggesting that gonadotroph function depends on other genes as well. The clinical presentation of patients with *GnRH-R* mutations can include microphallus, cryptorchidism, gynecomastia, and delayed puberty in males, and primary amenorrhea, incomplete thelarche, and delayed puberty in females.[38] Phenotypes can also be milder, as in men with normal adult-sized testes as well as intact spermatogenesis, but impaired LH-dependent Leydig cell testosterone secretion ("fertile eunuch syndrome").[40] It is now believed that GnRH secretion in these cases is sufficient to trigger enough Leydig cell testosterone production locally to maintain spermatogenesis and testicular growth, but insufficient to generate systemic testosterone levels capable of achieving full virilization.[41]

Screening for *GnRH-R* mutations at the time of diagnosis of IHH is not clinically useful unless fertility is an immediate treatment goal. In these cases, knowledge of a *GnRH-R* mutation would guide one toward gonadotropin therapy and away from pulsatile GnRH therapy (when it was available for clinical use), as the latter was less effective in restoring reproductive function. As with other confirmed genetic abnormalities, identification of a *GnRH-R* mutation would also allow screening and treatment of family members.[38]

GPR54 Mutations. Homozygous deletions in the gene *GPR54* on chromosome 19 (19p13) were first reported in 2003 in a large consanguineous family with multiple members affected by IHH but with normal GnRH receptors. *GPR54* encodes an orphan G-protein–coupled receptor that is expressed widely across the reproductive axis, including the hypothalamus, pituitary, gonads, and placenta.[42] The ligand for GPR54 is metastin, which is derived from kisspeptin-1. Metastin was originally discovered because of its ability to inhibit metastatic melanoma and breast cancer cell lines. Continued study of this protein suggests that it may play an important role in regulating central puberty through its ability to signal through *GPR54* and stimulate GnRH release. Both male and female *GPR54*-deficient mice had a hypogonadotropic hypogonadal phenotype (males with small testes, females with delayed vaginal opening and delayed follicular maturation), but had normal levels of hypothalamic GnRH and responded to exogenous GnRH.[43,44] Similarly, spermatogenesis and successful ovulation have been achieved in *GPR54*-deficient patients treated with exogenous GnRH. *GPR54* does appear to have tissue-specific effects, because the in vitro administration of metastin did not have the same stimulatory effects on pituitary gonadotrophs as it did on the hypothalamus, and homozygous mutations in *GPR54* did not affect spermatogenesis or ovarian steroidogenesis.[42] The exact mechanism by which *GPR54* regulates puberty remains the subject of ongoing investigation.

Gonadotropin Mutations. Both FSH and LH are composed of a common α subunit and a beta subunit that is unique to FSH, LH, thyroid-stimulating hormone (TSH), and human chorionic gonadotropin (hCG). Alpha subunit mutations have not been reported and likely are not compatible with life.[25] However, beta subunit mutations in both the LH[45] and FSH molecules[46] have been identified and are associated with delayed puberty.

Pituitary Transcription Factors. Mutations in various homeobox transcription factors involved with normal adenohypophyseal development have been reported. Homozygous mutations in *LHX3* have been described in two consanguineous families who presented with combined pituitary hormone deficiencies, including deficits in LH and FSH.[47] Mutations in *PROP1* are also associated with variable degrees of FSH and LH insufficiency and other pituitary hormone deficiencies.[48,49] Homozygous and heterozygous mutations of *HESX1* have been implicated in some cases of septo-optic dysplasia, a disease that includes optic nerve hypoplasia, pituitary gland hypoplasia, and midline CNS anomalies. Children with septo-optic dysplasia can have either precocious puberty or pubertal failure.[50,51]

Hypogonadotropic Hypogonadism and Adrenal Failure. Normosmic hypogonadotropic hypogonadism can occur in association with adrenal failure due to loss-of-function mutations in *DAX1* (adrenal hypoplasia congenital). *DAX1* encodes an orphan nuclear receptor on chromosome Xp21 and is critical for the development and function of both the adrenal gland and the hypothalamic–pituitary–gonadal axis. In the presence of *DAX1* mutations, adrenal failure usually presents in male infants or boys, and is followed by impaired pubertal development due to failure of hypothalamic and pituitary gonadotropin production. Males with this mutation are often resistant to gonadotropin stimulation because of impaired spermatogenesis. Steroidogenic factor 1 (SF1), another nuclear receptor that regulates gene transcription in both the adrenal gland and the gonads, caused both adrenal and gonadal agenesis when knocked out in a murine model.[52] Human SF1 mutations were associated with XY sex reversal and adrenal failure.[53] It is now thought that *DAX1* represses transcription of nuclear receptors, including SF1, and that loss of *DAX1* function causes a variety of adrenal, pituitary, and hypothalamic abnormalities.[41]

Hypogonadotropic Hypogonadism and Obesity Syndromes. Mutations in leptin[54] and the leptin receptor[55] have been identified in morbidly obese patients with normosmic IHH. It is leptin's effects on the release of NPY that are likely responsible for its effects on GnRH secretion.[56] Mutations in prohormone convertase 1 (PC1) also cause morbid obesity and hypogonadotropic hypogonadism, as well as hypocortisolemia (with elevated proopiomelanocortin) and hypoinsulinemia (with elevated proinsulin).[57]

Adult-Onset Idiopathic Hypogonadotropic Hypogonadism. An acquired form of GnRH deficiency was described in 1997 in 10 men who presented with decreased libido, impotence, and infertility at a mean age of 35 years, after undergoing normal puberty. None had features of congenital GnRH deficiency (anosmia, synkinesia, cleft palate, or a family history of GnRH deficiency), and none had a tumor, a history of radiation, infection, or infiltrative disease that might have explained their abnormal gonadotropin and sex steroid levels. Treatment with pulsatile GnRH reversed the hypogonadism and restored fertility in the subset of men who received long-term therapy. The cause of this acquired GnRH deficiency remains unknown.[58]

Diagnosis of Idiopathic Hypogonadotropic Hypogonadism

Hypogonadotropic hypogonadism should be included in the differential diagnosis for any patient with absent or incomplete pubertal development. In males, this can include microphallus, cryptorchidism, absence of facial hair, and small testes, and in women, incomplete or absent breast development, amenorrhea, or a eunuchoid body habitus. Obtaining a family history can also be helpful when considering a diagnosis of IHH. Whereas the incidence of delayed puberty in the general population is less than 1%, the incidence of delayed puberty among relatives of a series of 106 patients with IHH was 12%.[41] Because the GnRH pulse generator is quiescent until the onset of puberty (after an initial period of activation during infancy), the diagnosis of hypogonadotropic hypogonadism is usually not made until the age of 18 years, when such physical findings might prompt laboratory evaluation. Characteristic findings include low sex steroid levels (testosterone < 100 ng/dL; E_2 < 20 pg/mL) in association with low or inappropriately "normal" gonadotropin levels. Assessment of other pituitary hormones should also be performed when hypogonadotropic hypogonadism is initially discovered. To exclude structural causes of GnRH deficiency, magnetic resonance imaging (MRI) is indicated in the evaluation of such patients. When laboratory studies and negative findings on imaging studies offer no other explanation for hypogonadotropic hypogonadism, a diagnosis of IHH or isolated GnRH deficiency is appropriate.

Management of Idiopathic Hypogonadotropic Hypogonadism

Therapy for patients with IHH depends on the degree of sexual maturity and the desire for fertility. For men with severe gonadotropin deficiency who have yet to complete puberty, hCG is used as a surrogate for LH to stimulate Leydig cell testosterone secretion, typically using an intramuscular dose of 2000 IU three times weekly. Plasma testosterone and sperm counts are followed every 4 to 8 weeks, and hCG doses are adjusted to maintain normal testosterone levels. Recombinant FSH (75-150 IU three times weekly) is often required to improve the quality of the sperm produced, although it may not be required for initiation of spermatogenesis in men with partial IHH and those with postpubertal onset of hypogonadism. Inability to achieve a normal sperm count after 6 months of hCG treatment alone and declining sperm count despite hCG are indications to add FSH.[59-61] Success with this combination is possible, regardless of previous exposure to testosterone, although individuals differ in the timing of their response to induction of spermatogenesis.[62,63] Restoration of fertility occurs as early as 4 months in some men, but can take more than 1 year in others. Even if spontaneous pregnancy does not occur, adequate sperm are usually present after combined hCG/FSH therapy such that assisted reproductive techniques, including in vitro fertilization with intracytoplasmic sperm insertion, are good options. Subcutaneous or intravenous administration of GnRH via pump has been shown to achieve spermatogenesis more rapidly than treatment with gonadotropins, but it is no longer available.[64] Once pregnancy is achieved, hCG but not FSH should be continued to maintain normal serum testosterone and some spermatogenesis to facilitate future pregnancies. Men who only desire virilization can be given intramuscular or topical testosterone, depending on their preferred mode of administration.[32]

Cyclic estrogen and progesterone should be given to female patients to induce normal sexual development and preserve normal bone mineral density (BMD), although progesterone should not be added until breast development is complete.[38] Women who desire fertility should receive exogenous gonadotropins to stimulate ovulation. Recombinant FSH alone can induce follicular growth, as shown in Figure 19-2A, and has been shown to be as effective as highly purified FSH in achieving pregnancy, with a lower risk of ovarian hyperstimulation.[65] However, women with severe hypogonadotropic hypogonadism require some source of LH to generate adequate androgen precursors for aromatization to E_2, as illustrated in Figure 19-2B.[66] E_2 is required for endometrial proliferation and creation of a uterine environment optimal for implantation.[67,68]

Treatment with hCG (75 IU daily) may be used in such cases to maintain adequate E_2 concentrations. In women with baseline LH levels of greater than 1.2 IU/L, FSH alone may be sufficient to stimulate follicular growth as well as ovarian steroidogenesis. Once adequate follicular development and E_2-induced endometrial proliferation have occurred, exogenous recombinant hCG (250 μg) can be

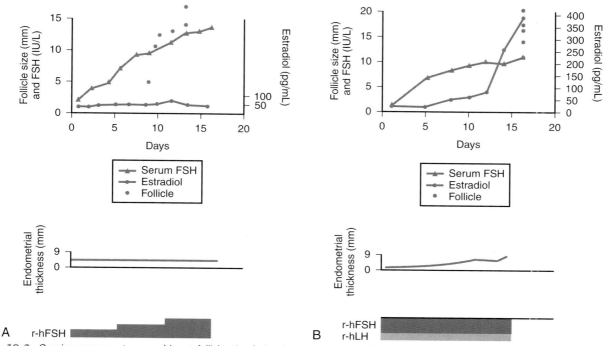

Figure 19-2. *Ovarian response to recombinant follicle-stimulating hormone (r-hFSH) [A] or a combination of recombinant FSH and luteinizing hormone (r-hLH) [B] in women with severe hypogonadotropic hypogonadism. Follicle size and endometrial thickness were monitored by transvaginal ultrasonography. (Modified from Shoham Z, Mannaerts B, Insler V, Coelingh-Bennink H. Induction of follicular growth using recombinant human follicle-stimulating hormone in two volunteer women with hypogonadotropic hypogonadism. Fertil Steril 59:738, 1993.)*

used to induce ovulation and is as effective as urinary hCG.[69] Recombinant formulations of LH are available, but their shorter half-life and higher cost preclude their widespread clinical use. Provision of luteal-phase progesterone is also recommended. When using FSH and hCG in combination, a woman's chance of conception is approximately 70% after six cycles. Such treatment does carry a risk of ovarian hyperstimulation and multiple gestations, and these risks are higher than those associated with pulsatile GnRH therapy when it was available.[70] For this reason, close monitoring with transvaginal ultrasound is required in women receiving gonadotropin therapy. In addition, pregnancies in women with hypopituitarism should be considered high risk because they are associated with higher rates of spontaneous abortion, possibly reflecting a uterine environment devoid of important endocrine growth factors.[71]

In addition to issues surrounding hormone replacement therapy and fertility treatment, there are other considerations when treating patients with IHH. Those with anosmic IHH and a family history suggestive of an X-linked mode of inheritance should have an abdominal/pelvic ultrasound at the time of diagnosis to assess for possible renal agenesis, given the relatively high frequency of this nonreproductive abnormality in patients with a *KAL1* mutation. Genetic testing is not routinely employed in patients with IHH because the majority of cases are sporadic. However, limited genetic testing is available for patients suspected of carrying a *KAL1* mutation. Research laboratories can also investigate for point mutations in *KAL1* or *FGFR1* and *GnRHR* gene mutations.[32]

Prognosis for Recovery

Until recently, it was believed that lifelong hormone therapy was required to maintain secondary sex characteristics and sexual function in men with IHH, but recent reports of testicular growth in men receiving maintenance androgen replacement therapy led to the identification of a minority of patients (10%) in whom reversal of IHH occurs. Such reversal can occur in men who underwent partial puberty or who were prepubertal at the time of diagnosis, and in men with either anosmic or normosmic IHH. It is believed that exposure to sex steroids promotes plasticity of the GnRH neuronal network, such that gradual reversal of IHH is possible, even in the face of genetic defects in men who are treated with androgen replacement therapy. Thus, men being treated for IHH should have their hypothalamic–pituitary axis reassessed periodically so that such reversal can be identified.[72,73]

STRUCTURAL DISEASE OF THE HYPOTHALAMUS

Mass lesions in the hypothalamus can also disrupt the secretion of GnRH into the hypothalamic–hypophyseal portal circulation and cause hypogonadotropic hypogonadism. Such cases usually cause other pituitary hormone abnormalities as well. Distinguishing hypothalamic mass lesions from pituitary mass lesions requires MRI. Dynamic testing with hypothalamic-releasing hormones is not used clinically, with the exception of CRH, which is used in combination with inferior petrosal sinus sampling (IPSS) to determine whether hypercortisolemia is of pituitary or ectopic origin.

Tumor

Craniopharyngioma. Craniopharyngiomas are rare epithelial tumors arising from remnants of the craniopharyngeal duct that occur with an annual incidence of 0.13 cases per 100,000 person-years.[74,75] They are the most common lesions involving the hypothalamic–pituitary region in children, and account for 5.6% to 15% of the intracranial neoplasms in this population (2% to 5% in adults).[76,77] Craniopharyngiomas affect men and women at equal rates, and no genetic susceptibility has been identified.[74] They are histologically benign lesions, usually cystic or mixed (84% to 99%) rather than solid (1% to 16%).[78] Two subtypes have been identified—adamantinomatous and papillary. The adamantinomatous type is more common in children and often contains calcification. Although tumor margins are usually sharp, adamantinomatous craniopharyngiomas tend to generate significant reactive gliosis in the adjacent normal brain tissue, making complete surgical resection difficult. Cysts may be multiloculated and contain viscous fluid rich in desquamated squamous epithelial cells and cholesterol.[75] The papillary subtype is seen almost exclusively in adults and is rarely associated with calcification. Papillary craniopharyngiomas tend to be solid or mixed rather than purely cystic, and they are less likely to infiltrate surrounding normal brain tissue, making surgical resection easier.[79]

Craniopharyngiomas almost always have a suprasellar component and are rarely purely intrasellar,[80] as the images in Figure 19-3 show. Because of their proximity to vital neural structures and their significant size at the time of diagnosis (58% to 76% are between 2 and

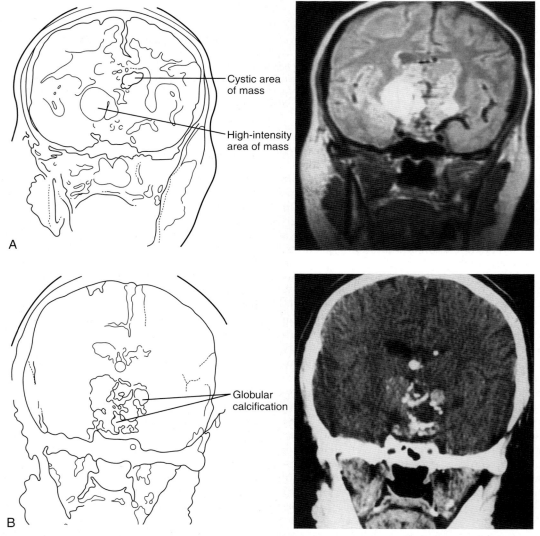

Figure 19-3. **A,** Schematic and proton-density–weighted coronal magnetic resonance imaging showing a cystic area and a high-intensity signal area in a large sellar/suprasellar mass, typical of craniopharyngiomas. **B,** Characteristic globular calcification is apparent on a coronal computerized tomography image of the same patient. (Modified from Peebles T, Haughton VM. Neuroradiology and endocrine disease. In *Besser GM, Thorner MO* [eds]. *Comprehensive Clinical Endocrinology,* 3rd ed. London, Elsevier, 2002.)

4 cm), they frequently present with headache, nausea, vomiting, visual disturbances, growth failure (in children), and hypogonadism (in adults), although the rate of tumor growth also determines the severity of symptoms.[75,79] Bitemporal hemianopsia is the most common visual complaint, occurring in almost 50% of cases. Hydrocephalus can be present, occurring more frequently in children than in adults for unclear reasons (41% to 54% versus 12% to 30%).[75] With the exception of hydrocephalus and its associated symptoms, there was no difference in symptom duration or extent of hormone deficiency between children and adults with craniopharyngiomas.[80]

Both computed tomography (CT) and MRI can be helpful in diagnosing craniopharyngiomas. CT can show calcification that is characteristic of the adamantinomatous subtype, whereas MRI with gadolinium enhancement provides better structural analysis. When the findings of imaging studies are consistent with craniopharyngioma, surgical resection is usually the initial therapy, although radiation therapy (RT) has been used for small lesions not causing pressure-related visual, neurologic, or endocrinologic damage. The surgical approach depends on tumor size, location, and degree of calcification, and the experience of the surgeon, but often involves craniotomy and sometimes a two-stage process. Preoperative drainage of large cystic components in the days before surgery can relieve pressure-related symptoms and make surgical resection easier, although cyst cavities refill if surgery is delayed by weeks. Gross total resection is the goal in all cases, but it often cannot be achieved because of tumor size and adherence to vital neurovascular structures.[75]

Unfortunately, craniopharyngiomas often recur even after gross total resection has been achieved and confirmed radiographically. Recurrence rates at 10 years vary from 0% to 62%, but improve with use of adjuvant RT. Recurrence-free survival correlates best with extent of surgical removal; age, sex, location (intrasellar versus suprasellar), and size of the tumor at the time of surgical resection do not predict recurrence. Management of recurrent disease usually involves RT rather than repeated surgery because of the perioperative morbidity and mortality associated with the latter. In fact, surgery for recurrent disease is only recommended in the event of acute pressure-related symptoms.[75] The 10-year progression-free survival rate from the time of the first recurrence was 72% in a series of 25 patients who received RT.[81] Other options for the management of recurrences include brachytherapy (for predominantly cystic lesions), bleomycin installation via an Ommaya reservoir, and stereotactic radiosurgery.[75,82]

The endocrine, visual, and neuropsychological morbidities associated with craniopharyngiomas are significant. At the time of presentation, 35% of the patients in Van Effenterre's cohort had one to three hormone deficits.[83] After treatment, the frequency of individual hormone deficits varies significantly across studies (88% to 100% for growth hormone [GH], 80% to 95% for FSH and LH, 55% to 88% for adrenocorticotropic hormone [ACTH], 39% to 95% for TSH, and 25% to 86%

for antidiuretic hormone [ADH]) and is not affected by the type of therapy. Unlike pituitary adenomas, it is very unusual for patients with pretreatment hormone deficits to experience restoration of those axes after treatment, but pituitary hormones can be replaced relatively easily. Visual defects (i.e., quadrantanopia or worse) are present in the majority of patients after surgery with or without adjuvant RT.[84] Potentially more disabling are the consequences of hypothalamic damage that occur so commonly in patients with craniopharyngiomas. Obesity secondary to hyperphagia affects 26% to 61% of patients who undergo surgery with and without adjuvant RT.[75] Diabetes insipidus (DI), with an impaired sense of thirst and resulting water and electrolyte imbalances, was present in 14% of a pediatric cohort.[85] Neuropsychological and cognitive functions often decline in patients with craniopharyngiomas. At follow-up 7 years after initial treatment, 16% of the adults and 26% of the children in Van Effenterre's cohort were not living independently and had not returned to their previous jobs or schools.[83] Mortality rates three to six times higher than those of the general population have been reported in patients with craniopharyngiomas.[75]

Germ Cell Tumors. Germ cell tumors (GCTs) are believed to result from malignant transformation and abnormal migration of primordial germ cells. They are characterized by their secretion of hCG and alpha-fetoprotein (αFP). Intracranial GCTs occur most commonly in the pineal region (50%) and in the anterior hypothalamus (30%).[86] They account for 2.9% of all intracranial tumors in children and have a peak incidence between ages 10 and 14 years.[87] Presenting symptoms depend on tumor location: nausea, vomiting, diplopia, and paralysis of upward gaze (Parinaud syndrome) occur with pineal gland tumors, whereas suprasellar lesions can cause hypopituitarism, DI, and visual deficits.[86] Histologically, GCTs are often cystic and are classified as germinomatous GCT (GGCT) or nongerminomatous GCT (NGGCT). NGGCTs account for the minority of intracranial GCTs and include choriocarcinomas, teratomas, embryonal carcinomas, and yolk sac tumors. Serum hCG and AFP levels tend to be elevated in NGGCTs, whereas only a minority of patients with GGCTs have an abnormal serum hCG.[88] Stereotactic biopsy is indicated when the diagnosis is unclear from imaging studies and serum hCG and AFP levels. If a diagnosis of GGCT is made, therapy usually consists of radiation rather than resection, given the radiosensitivity of GGCTs and the neurologic morbidity associated with surgery. Chemotherapy is an alternative therapy, but is associated with a higher recurrence rate when used in the absence of RT.[89] NGGCTs are less radiosensitive and, therefore, carry a poorer prognosis. However, platinum-based chemotherapy, in combination with craniospinal RT, is often used, followed by surgical resection if a residual mass persists.[90,91]

Other lesions occurring in the pineal region include pineal parenchymal tumors, astrocytomas, meningiomas, metastases, cysts, and vascular malformations. Hypothalamic–pituitary function can be disturbed by any of these.

Infiltrating Diseases

Sarcoidosis. Sarcoidosis is a multisystem disease of activated T lymphocytes and noncaseating granulomas that commonly affects the lungs, lymph nodes, eyes, and skin, but can involve the CNS and peripheral nervous system in 10% to 20% of cases. Neurologic symptoms can be the presenting sign of disease in 50% of the latter group of patients and can increase morbidity and mortality. CNS lesions can appear as subdural plaques or infundibular plaques, infiltrating intraparenchymal pseudotumoral masses, or as multiple nodules on MRI studies. Although hypothalamic–pituitary lesions may not be evident on MRI, 25% to 33% of patients with neurosarcoidosis have DI and autopsy studies in such patients show extensive granulomatous inflammation of the hypothalamus, with little pituitary involvement. DI results from vasopressin deficiency and destruction of neurons in the neurohypophysis, but damage to the osmoreceptor controlling thirst also contributes to polyuria and polydipsia. Other symptoms of hypothalamic disease include somnolence, body temperature dysregulation, hyperphagia, and obesity.[92,93] Impaired secretion of anterior pituitary hormones also occurs; GH and gonadotropin deficiencies occur more commonly than TSH or ACTH deficiency.[93] In Murialdo and Tamagno's Italian series of 91 patients, 39% had hypogonadotropic hypogonadism, and 59% of the women in the study (*n* = 46) reported amenorrhea.[92]

As with other forms of sarcoidosis, confirmation of neurosarcoidosis requires histologic evidence of noncaseating granulomas and lymphocyte infiltration of affected tissue, but obtaining nervous system tissue can be difficult. However, a probable diagnosis can be made with the proper clinical picture and imaging studies (i.e., MRI; Fig. 19-4). PRL elevation can be a useful screen for hypothalamic involvement. Results of cerebrospinal fluid (CSF) analysis are abnormal in 80% of patients with CNS sarcoid, and can include elevations in protein, lymphocytes, or angiotensin-converting enzyme levels.[92]

Prednisone (40-80 mg daily) is the mainstay of treatment for neurosarcoidosis, as it is for other forms of the disease, although therapy is often intensified in CNS disease. Cyclosporine A (4-6 mg/kg) is often added to minimize glucocorticoid requirements. RT is employed in patients who do not respond to oral medications. Unfortunately, anterior pituitary deficiencies usually are not restored, despite treatment. Dopaminergic agents can be used to decrease PRL levels, but they will not restore fertility if hypogonadotropic hypogonadism is also present.[92]

Sarcoidosis can also infiltrate the epididymis and testes, resulting in painless epididymitis or a scrotal mass, both of which respond to glucocorticoids. Granulomatous involvement of the uterus and fallopian tubes has also been reported in women with sarcoidosis who present with amenorrhea or menorrhagia.[93] Thus, reproductive dysfunction in patients with sarcoidosis can be both primary and secondary to CNS disease.

Langerhans Cell Histiocytosis. Langerhans cell histiocytosis (LCH) is another multisystem disease of unknown etiology that has a predilection for the hypothalamus and pituitary. It is characterized by the clonal accumulation and proliferation of abnormal dendritic histiocytes, with accompanying lymphocytes, eosinophils, and neutrophils. These cellular infiltrative lesions can destroy a variety of tissues, including skin, bone, lymph nodes, liver, spleen, lungs, and bone marrow. Known previously as *Letterer-Siwe disease, Hand-Schüller-Christian disease, eosinophilic granuloma,* and *histiocytosis X,* LCH primarily affects children between the ages of 1 and 3 years. It can remit spontaneously or disseminate, even resulting in death in rare cases.[94] Adults make up fewer than 30% of all reported cases of LCH, with an incidence of 1.8 cases per million people. LCH in adults more commonly affects the skin, lung, and bones.[95]

The hypothalamic–pituitary axis is involved in 5% to 50% of children with LCH,[94] with 15% to 50% of these children presenting with DI.[96,97] The incidence of DI

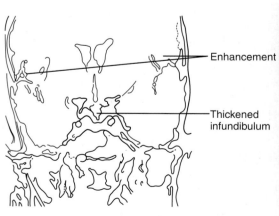
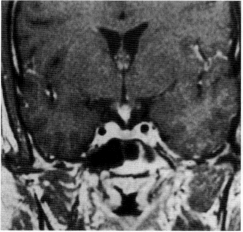

Figure 19-4. *Schematic and T1-weighted magnetic resonance imaging after contrast administration showing a thickened, enhancing infindibulum typical of granulomatous disease, such as sarcoidosis. Enhancement in the sylvian fissure on the* left *and near the inner table on the* right *identifies leptomeningeal involvement. (Modified from Peebles T, Haughton VM. Neuroradiology and endocrine disease. In Besser GM, Thorner MO [eds]. Comprehensive Clinical Endocrinology, 3rd ed. London, Elsevier, 2002.)*

Enhancement

Thickened infindibulum

increases over time. It is usually seen within 5 years of diagnosis, and occurs more often in the setting of multi-system disease.[98] DI was also the earliest hormonal abnormality in the adult cohort reported by Kaltsas et al., 33% of whom presented with DI.[95] Anterior pituitary hormone deficiency occurs in approximately 20% to 35% of patients and is usually associated with DI. In a large pediatric cohort, the estimated 5- and 10-year risks of pituitary involvement with LCH were 22% and 24%, respectively. GH deficiency is the most common pituitary endocrinopathy, occurring in 10% of patients with LCH and increasing in frequency over time. Ear, nose, and throat involvement increases the risk of GH deficiency.[97] GH deficiency in the absence of DI is unusual,[96] but 54% of patients with DI who were followed for 10 years ultimately had GH deficiency.[97] GH replacement effectively improves the final height in children with GH deficiency, although midparental height is usually not achieved because children have fairly severe growth restriction at the time therapy is initiated.[96,97] Importantly, GH therapy did not increase the risk of LCH disease activity.[97] GH replacement in adults with LCH has not been well studied.

Gonadotropin deficiency also occurs in LCH, almost always in association with other anterior pituitary hormone deficiencies. Because most patients are prepubertal at the onset of disease activity, those with gonadotropin deficiency require exogenous sex steroids to induce and maintain puberty.[96] Fifty percent of the cohort of 12 patients reported by Kaltsas et al. had gonadotropin deficiency at a median of 7 years after diagnosis of LCH, and exogenous gonadotropins successfully restored fertility in one male patient.[95]

Findings on MRI are abnormal in the majority of patients with LCH and endocrinopathy. Loss of the posterior pituitary bright spot on T1-weighted images and infundibular enlargement are the most common abnormalities, with the former observed in 100% of patients with DI.[96] As shown in Figure 19-5, other less common radiologic abnormalities include a thickened infundibular stalk,

a partially or completely empty sella, and lesions in the hypothalamus.[94]

Both children and adults with LCH and DI are at high risk for anterior pituitary deficits and should be followed closely. Unfortunately, dynamic evaluation of pituitary function was not a useful predictor of later endocrinopathies.[99] DI and other hormonal deficiencies tend to be permanent once established, despite treatment of LCH lesions with radiation therapy, chemotherapy, or both. RT may be helpful for controlling localized disease and mass effects, however. Chemotherapy was not helpful in long-term disease management in adults.[95]

Other infiltrating diseases that can cause hypothalamic infiltration with resulting reproductive dysfunction include hemochromatosis (which more commonly affects the pituitary; discussed later),[100] leukemia,[101,102] lymphoma,[103-105] and Wegener granulomatosis.[106-108] Central DI is often the presenting feature, and treatment of the underlying condition sometimes results in resolution of this and other associated hormonal abnormalities.[107,108] When associated with malignancies (leukemia, lymphoma), hypothalamic involvement is a poor prognostic feature and usually does not respond to treatment.[109]

Infections

Infections are a rare cause of hypothalamic–pituitary disease affecting the reproductive axis. They usually present acutely with fever, headache, meningismus, and change in mental status or seizure, and can be identified using culture, polymerase chain reaction, or detection of antibodies to viral antigens. Tuberculosis and atypical mycobacterial infections, viral encephalitis, mycotic infections, and bacterial meningitis can all cause infiltration of the hypothalamus or pituitary and result in hormonal deficiencies. Box 19-1 summarizes the classification of infiltrative, infectious, and other nontumoral diseases involving the hypothalamus that can cause hypogonadotropic hypogonadism.

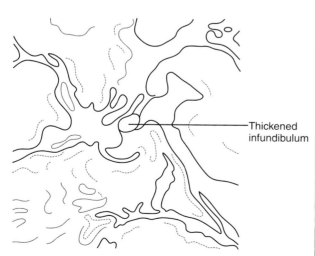
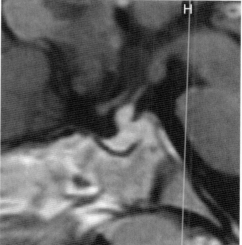

Thickened infundibulum

Figure 19-5. *Schematic and sagittal T1-weighted contrast-enhanced magnetic resonance imaging showing a thickened enhancing infundibulum from known Langerhans cell histiocytosis (H). (Modified from Peebles T, Haughton VM. Neuroradiology and endocrine disease.* In *Besser GM, Thorner MO, [eds].* Comprehensive Clinical Endocrinology, *3rd ed. London, Elsevier, 2002.)*

BOX 19-1

Classification of the Infiltrative, Infectious and Other Nontumoral Diseases Involving the Hypothalamus Causing Hypogonadotropic Hypogonadism

Infiltrative or Autoimmune Diseases
Sarcoidosis
Langerhans' cell histiocytosis
Lymphomatous diseases
Castelman disease
Wegener granulomatosis
Vasculitis

Infectious Diseases
Tuberculosis
Atypical mycobacterial infections
Bacterial meningitis
Encephalitis (viral)
Mycotic infections

Others
Trauma
Pituitary stalk section
Radiation therapy
Hydrocephalus and pseudotumor cerebri

Modified from Murialdo G, Tamagno G. Endocrine aspects of neurosarcoidosis. J Endocrinol Invest 25:650, 2002.

Head Trauma

Head trauma has been recognized as a cause of neuroendocrine dysfunction for many years, but assessment of hypothalamic–pituitary function during acute and long-term management of patients with traumatic brain injury (TBI) occurs infrequently. TBI is most common in males between the ages of 11 and 29 (5:1 male-to-female ratio), and is the leading cause of death and disability among young adults.[110] Road accidents account for 75% of cases of TBI.[111] Most patients who have post-head trauma hypopituitarism (PHTH) were comatose for a period after their injuries, and all had Glasgow Coma Scale scores of less than 13. PHTH can result from structural injury to the hypothalamus or pituitary, but a vascular insult leading to cerebral swelling is the most likely mechanism in most cases.[112] Such localized edema increases intracranial pressure in the sellar or suprasellar regions and can temporarily impair hypothalamic–pituitary function. PHTH may also be an adaptive mechanism to the acute illness often associated with TBI.[110,113]

One third of patients studied 3 months to 23 years after head injury had at least one pituitary hormonal deficiency: 18% had an inadequate GH response to insulin tolerance testing, and 20% to 25% had insufficient responses to GnRH stimulation.[112] The frequency of gonadotropin deficiency was even higher (80% to 90%) when defined by low early morning testosterone or E_2 levels and inappropriately low FSH and LH levels.[110] TBI-associated neuroendocrine dysfunction only presents with DI in the minority of cases (25% to 30%). PRL elevation occurs in approximately 50% of patients and correlates negatively with Glasgow Coma Scale score, likely because it is a marker of pituitary stalk or hypothalamic damage.[110,111]

Unfortunately, PHTH is usually not diagnosed during hospitalization unless a patient has acute ACTH deficiency or DI. Because pituitary hormone deficiency eventually recovers in approximately 60% of patients with moderate to severe head injury, some deficiencies (i.e., GH, gonadotropin) may never be recognized.[112,113] Gonadotropin-secreting cells appear to be the most sensitive to TBI, and patients with PHTH often present after hospital discharge with amenorrhea, erectile dysfunction, and infertility.[111] FSH and LH in such patients may be inappropriately low. Most hormonal deficits (75%) appear within 1 year after injury, but diagnosis can be delayed by 5 or more years in 15% of patients.[111] In patients with a known history of TBI whose anterior pituitary function is initially normal, repeat evaluation during follow-up care may be indicated, given the delayed appearance of hypopituitarism in some cases.

Radiation Therapy

Hypothalamic–pituitary dysfunction after cranial irradiation has long been recognized to occur in survivors of childhood cancer and in patients who receive high-dose RT for nasopharyngeal carcinoma[114,115] or pituitary disease.[116] However, not until recently has the high frequency of endocrine dysfunction in adult survivors of nonpituitary brain tumors who receive RT been recognized.[117] This frequency is only likely to increase with the improvements in prognosis for both children and adults with primary brain malignancies. Of a cohort of 56 patients with primary brain tumors who had received their last dose of RT at least 1 year before the time of study, 23 (41%) showed evidence of hypopituitarism with multiple (25%) or single (16%) hormone deficiencies. GH deficiency was most common, followed by gonadotropin, ACTH, and TSH deficiency.[118] DI is rarely associated with radiation-induced hypopituitarism. The risk of hormonal deficiency depends on the total dose, fraction size, number of fractions received, and total duration of RT. Panhypopituitarism can occur when the total dose exceeds 60 gray (Gy), but this risk can be reduced by administering more fractions of smaller dose, thereby extending treatment time.[119]

The rates of gonadotropin and GH deficiency in adults are significantly lower than those observed in pediatric studies, in which 20% to 50% of patients eventually have partial or severe gonadotropin deficiency[117,120] and GH deficiency occurs in 80% to 100%.[118] It is thought that the hypothalamic–pituitary axis is more radiosensitive in children than in adults.[118,121,122] Doses exceeding 50 Gy in childhood can cause gonadotropin deficiency, but smaller doses can result in precocious puberty. In low-dose cranial irradiation used prophylactically in children being treated for acute lymphocytic leukemia, girls are more susceptible to early puberty than boys, but this sexual dichotomy disappears when higher doses (25-50 Gy) are used to treat primary brain tumors.[119] In a pediatric cohort with preexisting GH deficiency, the relationship between age at time of irradiation and age at onset of puberty was linear.[123] The severity of gonadotropin deficiency varies in postpubertal subjects, from low normal to frankly low sex hormone levels.[119]

The site of radiation-induced injury is the hypothalamus, and postradiation studies show normal responses to hypothalamic-releasing hormones, including GnRH.[124] The mechanism of this radiation-induced damage is unclear, but may involve direct damage to hormonally active cells or to their surrounding microvasculature. Alternatively, radiation may damage the vascular connections between the hypothalamus and the pituitary.[117,118] Hormone deficiencies may not become evident for many years,[125] because the radiation-induced damage takes its toll on the slowly dividing cells of the hypothalamus and secondary pituitary atrophy occurs after previous hypothalamic damage.[117-119] The delayed appearance of these deficits mandates that such patients be followed annually for these late effects of radiation.

Gonadal damage is also a concern in patients treated for primary brain tumors, but usually occurs as a result of adjuvant chemotherapy or spinal RT. Alkylating agents, procarbazine, cisplatin, and vinblastine are chemotherapeutic agents often associated with gonadal toxicity, whereas gonadal damage secondary to spinal RT occurs from radiation scatter.[119] Sixty-four percent of girls who received craniospinal irradiation but no chemotherapy had evidence of primary ovarian failure over 8 years of follow-up.[126] Sex steroids and germ cells are both lost in female patients treated with RT or chemotherapy, whereas males may present with infertility with normal levels of testosterone as a result of a differential effect of cancer therapy on Leydig cell function and spermatogenesis.[119]

Treatment for radiation-associated infertility secondary to disruption of the hypothalamus or pituitary requires replacement of gonadotropins. Physiologic exogenous pulsatile GnRH therapy restored ovulation in the majority of women when it was clinically available.[127] Theoretically, cryopreservation of embryo, sperm, oocyte, or ovarian tissue can be used to preserve fertility when cancer treatment is expected to cause gonadal damage. However, each has significant drawbacks and none is routinely employed.[128,129]

SEIZURE DISORDERS

Epilepsy is a relatively common condition, with a prevalence of 5:1000 to 9:1000 and has been associated with subfertility in numerous epidemiologic studies. The background rate of menstrual dysfunction (50% to 60%) far exceeds that of the general adult female population.[130] PCOS is the most common form of reproductive dysfunction in this population and affects up to 25% of epileptic women, although hypothalamic amenorrhea and luteal phase deficiency (LPD) can also occur.[131] The diagnosis of PCOS was unrelated to the type of epilepsy.[131]

Both seizures themselves and the antiepileptic drugs (AEDs) used to treat them have been implicated as the cause for reproductive dysfunction in patients with epilepsy. Epileptiform discharges transiently increase PRL and may disrupt GnRH pulsatility, a hypothesis suggested by observations of altered LH pulse frequency in regularly menstruating women with epilepsy who were not taking AEDs.[131,132] The similar rates of PCOS among medicated and unmedicated women with epilepsy also provide evidence that seizure activity itself interferes with normal reproductive function.[130,131] In addition, the use of AEDs (specifically, VPA) in normal women and those with other conditions (bipolar affective disorder) does not increase the risk of PCOS or affect baseline LH pulse dynamics, gonadal hormones, or rates of oligomenorrhea,[133-135] arguing for the position that epilepsy itself is responsible for interfering with reproductive function in some women.

Antiepileptic drug therapy, especially VPA, appears to worsen the central reproductive dysfunction caused by epilepsy itself. VPA has been shown to augment LH secretion in response to GnRH in healthy women, presumably via its stimulatory effects on glutamic acid decarboxylase and its inhibitory effects on GABA transaminase, ultimately leading to an increase in brain GABA activity.[133,136] No association between PCOS and the use of any specific AED was apparent in a relatively lean cohort of epileptic women reported by Bilo et al., but polycystic ovaries and hyperandrogenism were observed in 70% of a Finnish cohort receiving VPA monotherapy.[137] The frequency of menstrual disorders, polycystic ovaries, and hyperandrogenism was increased in both lean and obese women, but was higher in the latter.[138] Anovulatory cycles occurred in 43% of women who were currently using VPA or had done so within the previous 3 years, whereas only 10% of cycles were anovulatory in women with generalized epilepsy who had never taken VPA.[139] Although VPA is associated with weight gain, the changes observed in serum androgens (testosterone, androstenedione) occurred as early as 1 to 3 months after initiation of VPA and before any significant changes in body weight.[140] These observations suggest that VPA-associated PCOS in women with epilepsy is likely multifactorial in origin, with genetic and environmental factors playing some role.[131,141,142] In addition, the initiation of VPA before the age of 20 years was a risk factor for future development of PCOS.[137] Although VPA has never been shown to increase LH secretion, it may have direct ovarian effects, which in combination with the GnRH pulse generator dysfunction described earlier, ultimately lead to the hyperandrogenemia characteristic of many epileptic women receiving VPA.[142]

Ovulatory dysfunction related to AEDs may also arise as a result of alterations in cytochrome P450 activity. Phenytoin, phenobarbital, and carbamazepine induce cytochrome P450 activity, thus increasing sex hormone–binding globulin (SHBG) synthesis and reducing bioavailable testosterone and E_2 levels.[142] VPA inhibits cytochrome P450 enzyme activity and increases androgen concentrations.[139] However, these changes in bioavailable hormone levels are not always significant enough to alter reproductive function, and women taking carbamazepine have never been shown to have a higher risk of menstrual dysfunction, hyperandrogenemia, or PCOS.

Unfortunately, anovulatory cycles can be the only sign of epilepsy-associated reproductive dysfunction. Thus, an awareness of the effect of the disease and its treatment on patients' reproductive health should be part of routine care for women with epilepsy.[139] Menstrual cycle duration and body weight should be monitored regularly in women taking AEDs, especially VPA, so that reproductive abnormalities are not overlooked.[142] When such changes develop, switching women to other AEDs, such as lamotrigine, in consultation with their neurologist, can reverse the adverse reproductive and metabolic phenotype associated with AED treatment.[143]

Men with epilepsy also have reproductive endocrine abnormalities and are 36% less likely than unaffected male siblings to be biologic fathers.[144] Approximately one third of men with temporolimbic epilepsy have hypogonadism,[145] and reductions in sperm count or motility as well as abnormal sperm morphology are observed in 8% to 90% of men, regardless of AED use.[146,147]

FUNCTIONAL ALTERATIONS AND DISORDERS OF THE HYPOTHALAMUS

Physiologic Hypogonadotropic Hypogonadism

Pubertal Transition. Hypogonadotropic hypogonadism can be physiologic during certain phases of life. GnRH neurons are temporarily activated during infancy, producing midpubertal levels of either testosterone or E_2. After 6 months of age, however, GnRH neurons become quiescent, and gonadotropin levels and sex steroid levels fall. This *physiologic hypogonadotropic hypogonadism of prepuberty* persists until approximately 8 to 9 years of age, when serum LH, FSH, and E_2 levels begin to rise, primarily overnight.[41,148] Over the course of puberty, mean LH increases 116-fold, FSH increases 7-fold, and E_2 increases 12-fold.[149] These changes are shown in Figure 19-6.

These gonadotropin changes directly reflect hypothalamic GnRH release because they can be simulated by exogenous GnRH administration,[150] can be blocked by GnRH antagonist administration,[148] and can occur in the absence of functioning gonadal tissue.[151] The factors mediating this reactivation of the GnRH pulse generator in early puberty are still unclear,[151] as are the factors permitting the progressive increase in daytime LH that occurs during puberty. Because hypogonadotropic hypogonadism is normal during puberty, distinguishing it from pathologic causes of hypogonadotropic hypogonadism becomes difficult during adolescence. Both are characterized by absent or incomplete sexual maturation, low gonadotropin concentrations, low sex steroid levels (testosterone < 100 ng/dL; E_2 < 20 pg/mL), and no evidence of other hypothalamic–pituitary axis abnormalities. The α subunit response to GnRH injection was used in the past to separate these two conditions; adolescents who ultimately had the former condition had little α subunit production after GnRH, indicating pituitary disease.[152] However, the current unavailability of GnRH forces clinicians to rely on clinical features and family history rather than laboratory data to distinguish constitutional delay of growth and puberty (a normal variant characterized by hypogonadotropic hypogonadism) from more sinister causes of delayed puberty.

Postpartum Period. The postpartum period is another time in life in which hypogonadotropic hypogonadism is physiologic. Amenorrhea occurs in all women after childbirth. High levels of E_2 progesterone during pregnancy are initially responsible for this hypothalamic–pituitary suppression. However, amenorrhea persists for varying durations into the puerperium and is prolonged further

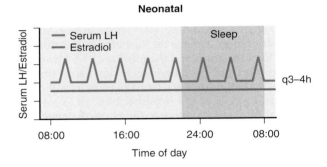

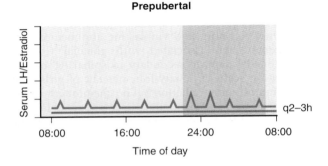

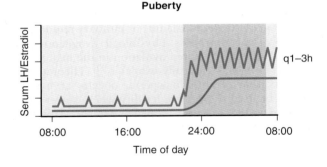

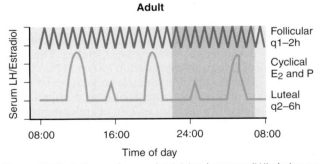

Figure 19-6. Patterns of serum luteinizing hormone (LH) during pubertal maturation in females. The duration of sleep is shown by the bar. E_2, estradiol; P, progesterone. (Modified from Marshall JC. Control of pituitary hormone secretion: role of pulsatility. In Besser GM, Thorner MO [eds]. *Comprehensive Clinical Endocrinology*, 3rd ed. London, Elsevier, 2002.)

in women who breast-feed.[153] FSH levels remain low (similar to those seen in the early follicular phase), mean LH and LH pulse frequency are reduced, and serum E_2 and progesterone are low.[154] The mechanisms responsible for this continued suppression of the hypothalamic–pituitary–gonadal axis are unknown.[155,156] PRL has been implicated because it is universally elevated in the immediate postpartum period and suppresses GnRH release. However, PRL declines long before menstrual cyclicity returns in lactating women, arguing that mechanisms other than hyperprolactinemia must be responsible for lactational amenorrhea.[157] The suckling stimulus itself increases PRL, as shown in Figure 19-7, but also increases the sensitivity of the GnRH pulse generator to the negative feedback effects of E_2, such that GnRH and LH pulse activity are nearly absent in the immediate postpartum period.[158] Both of these effects of suckling diminish with time, however.

Once they reappear, LH pulse patterns are initially erratic and are augmented by sleep, similar to the pattern observed in early puberty.[155,158] Follicle growth and associated E_2 production often return to normal before ovulation resumes because suckling impairs the normal positive feedback of E_2 that is required for the preovulatory LH surge. Thus, menses may return, but cycles may be anovulatory until the suckling stimulus decreases further and normal ovulatory cycles resume.[153,158] Additional evidence suggesting a hypothalamic etiology for lactational amenorrhea comes from studies in lactating women exposed to pulsatile exogenous GnRH. Midcycle LH surges occurred in these women, luteal phases were normal, and FSH declined appropriately in response to increasing levels of ovarian steroids.[159] The hypothalamic hypogonadism of lactation can persist for more than 12 months, depending on the frequency and intensity of suckling.[158] This endogenous contraception allows women to cope with the physiologic demands of the postpartum period before considering additional pregnancies. Both puberty and the postpartum period illustrate the neuroendocrine control mechanisms that govern GnRH, and abnormalities can be seen in a number of pathophysiologic states.

Pathophysiologic Hypogonadotropic Hypogonadism

Hypogonadotropic Hypogonadism Associated with Altered Secretion of Thyroid Hormone, Cortisol, and Prolactin.

The neuroendocrine components of the reproductive axis are highly sensitive to disturbances in other hormones, including thyroid hormone, cortisol, and PRL. Within this context, menstrual irregularity occurs in approximately 25% of women with any degree of *thyroid hormone deficiency*, although the prevalence increases with the severity of hypothyroidism. Oligomenorrhea and menorrhagia are the most common menstrual disturbances, and sexual dysfunction (hypoactive sexual desire, erectile dysfunction, and delayed ejaculation) is observed in the majority of men with hypothyroidism.[160,161] Men with hypothyroidism often have low free testosterone levels that improve with initiation of thyroid hormone replacement.[162] Hypogonadotropic hypogonadism (low FSH and LH) may be present, but the clearance rate of the gonadotropins and sex steroids is reduced in the presence of hypothyroidism.[162-165] Pituitary sensitivity to GnRH may be reduced in hypothyroid children, but appears normal in hypothyroid women.[163,165] Fewer than 10% of patients with newly diagnosed hypothyroidism (TSH > 4 mU/L) have associated hyperprolactinemia that resolves with initiation of thyroid hormone replacement. However, correction of hyperprolactinemia in these patients does not correct the menstrual dysfunction. Only with restoration of a euthyroid state does menstrual function normalize, assuming it was secondary to thyroid dysfunction originally.[166]

Thyroid hormone excess, as occurs in Graves disease, is also associated with menstrual irregularities, anovulation, and infertility in women and sexual dysfunction in men.[161,167] Amenorrhea may be present in severe hyperthyroidism. Excess thyroid hormone increases gonadotropin sensitivity to GnRH[168-170] and may impair aromatase activity.[171] Hepatic SHBG production is also increased in hyperthyroidism, resulting in higher total testosterone and E_2, but normal free testosterone.[168-170] This increase in E_2 can cause gynecomastia in men with severe hyperthyroidism. Spermatogenesis may be impaired in men with

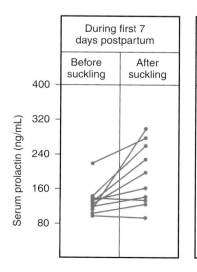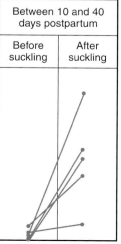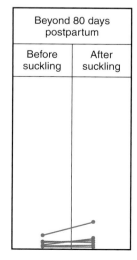

Figure 19-7. Serum prolactin concentrations basally and in response to suckling as a function of time after delivery. Within the first week after delivery, the basal value is high relative to the nonpregnant state, and there may be a further increase in response to suckling. Several weeks after delivery, the basal value is close to that of the nonpregnant state, but there is still a pronounced increase in response to suckling. Three months after delivery, the basal value is similar to that of the nonpregnant state, and there is a minimal response to suckling, if any. (From Tyson JE. Studies of prolactin secretion in human pregnancy. Am J Obstet Gynecol 113:14, 1972.)

thyroid hormone excess, but normalizes after restoration of a euthyroid state.[169,170]

Reproductive dysfunction frequently accompanies *abnormalities of cortisol secretion.* Amenorrhea develops in 25% of patients with *adrenocortical insufficiency,* although the etiology of such a severe reproductive disturbance is likely multifactorial, with chronic illness, weight loss, or autoimmune ovarian failure contributing.[172] Appropriately treated patients with autoimmune adrenal insufficiency (Addison disease) have basal LH levels and LH pulse patterns similar to those of normal healthy adults. During experimental periods with low cortisol replacement, patients with Addison disease showed elevated CRH and ACTH levels, but normal sex steroid levels (testosterone and E_2). Gonadotropin alterations were gender-specific; mean LH concentrations and LH pulse amplitudes were suppressed in men in the setting of insufficient cortisol replacement for 47 hours, whereas similar conditions had no effect on LH dynamics in pre- and postmenopausal women. These differences may reflect higher opioid receptor activation in men than in women because opioids mediate the inhibitory effects of glucocorticoids on LH release.[173] Responses to low-dose GnRH stimulation did not vary in either sex under low cortisol conditions,[173] although higher doses of GnRH did alter stimulated FSH and LH concentrations.[174] These experimental conditions do not replicate the effects of long-term hypocortisolism, however, and clinical observations would suggest that maintaining physiologic cortisol levels is crucial for preserving a normal hypothalamic–pituitary–gonadal axis.

Menstrual irregularities (amenorrhea, oligomenorrhea, polymenorrhea) are present in the majority of women with *cortisol excess* (Cushing syndrome), with only 20% reported to have normal menses in one large cohort.[175] GnRH neurons possess cortisol receptors,[176] and hypercortisolemia blocks both GnRH release and the action of gonadotropins on the gonad.[175] Gonadotropin levels are low or inappropriately normal in the presence of glucocorticoid excess, although GnRH testing showed normal or slightly increased gonadotropin reserve in hypercortisolism.[175,177,178] Thus, impaired GnRH release from the hypothalamus rather than pituitary dysfunction likely explains the reproductive pathology seen in Cushing syndrome. This reduction in gonadotropin secretion explains the radiographic appearance of the ovaries in women with Cushing syndrome, which tend to be smaller, with few primordial follicles and stromal hyperplasia.[179] Plasma E_2 and free and total testosterone are low in hypercortisolism, consistent with hypogonadotropic hypogonadism.[175,180,181] E_2 correlates inversely with the degree of cortisol elevation.[175] This hypogonadism can be reversed by restoration of normal serum cortisol levels.[178,180]

Although excess cortisol itself could explain these abnormalities of the hypothalamic–pituitary–gonadal axis, other hormones have been implicated, including *corticotrophin-releasing hormone, PRL,* and *androgens.* CRH is an important inhibitor of gonadotropin release in settings of acute stress, but it is suppressed by negative feedback in states of cortisol excess and is therefore unlikely to play a role in menstrual dysfunction in patients with Cushing disease. Similarly, hyperprolactinemia is present in the minority of patients with Cushing disease, but does not correlate with the severity of the reproductive disturbance and is unlikely to be causative. Androgens were long believed to mediate Cushing-associated menstrual abnormalities. However, in a cohort of 45 premenopausal women with newly diagnosed Cushing disease, serum testosterone and androstenedione concentrations were elevated in only 29% and 39%, respectively, and there was no correlation between androgen levels and cortisol.[175] Metyrapone treatment of women with Cushing syndrome restores regular menses despite the increase in androgen levels associated with this drug.[182,183] These data suggest that hypothalamic GnRH release is suppressed by excess cortisol itself rather than by its adverse effects on other hormonal parameters.

Hyperprolactinemia is a common cause of reproductive dysfunction in premenopausal women, and is usually caused by pituitary lactotroph adenomas that are less than 1 cm in diameter (microadenomas). Hyperprolactinemia accounts for 10% to 20% of cases of amenorrhea (after pregnancy is excluded). Menstrual disturbances of varying degrees were present in 87% of a cohort of premenopausal women, whereas galactorrhea, another manifestation of hyperprolactinemia, was only present in 47%.[184] The severity of menstrual disturbance is related directly to the degree of hyperprolactinemia. Mild hyperprolactinemia (20-50 ng/mL) may impair progesterone secretion by the corpus luteum, resulting in a shortened luteal phase, but no menstrual irregularities. Moderate increases in PRL (50-100 ng/mL) can result in oligomenorrhea, whereas amenorrhea and overt hypogonadism occur when PRL is significantly elevated (>100 ng/mL). Any degree of hyperprolactinemia can contribute to infertility, however.[185,186] The severity of reproductive dysfunction in men also relates to the degree of hyperprolactinemia and can include decreased libido, infertility, gynecomastia, and galactorrhea.[187,188] The diagnosis of hyperprolactinemia is often delayed in postmenopausal women because they are already hypoestrogenic; such patients often present with compressive symptoms related to PRL-secreting adenomas, including headache, visual symptoms, or abnormalities of other pituitary hormones.

The mechanism of PRL-associated amenorrhea is suppression of hypothalamic GnRH release, resulting in low or inappropriately normal gonadotropin levels and low sex steroid levels. This reduction in hypothalamic GnRH release results in decreased LH pulse frequency, but LH pulse amplitude is higher.[189,190] The sleep-associated slowing in LH pulse frequency that occurs in normal adults is also lost in those with hyperprolactinemia. These effects of PRL on the hypothalamus are not mediated by increased hypothalamic opioid activity, and can be overcome with provision of exogenous pulsatile GnRH, which has resulted in pregnancy.[191] These observations and others show that hyperprolactinemia, whether due to normal physiologic states (lactational amenorrhea) or pathophysiologic causes, does not interfere with pituitary–gonadal feedback mechanisms or with the actions of LH and FSH on the ovary.[191,192] Restoration of normal PRL levels, either medically or surgically, allows LH pulse frequency and amplitude to recover, thereby normalizing menses, correcting hypogonadism, and restoring fertility.[184,193]

Evaluation of any woman with menstrual dysfunction or any man with symptoms consistent with hypogonadism should include measurement of a serum PRL level. Mild increases in PRL can occur with intense breast or chest wall stimulation, strenuous exercise, and emotional or physical stress. Thus, mild elevations should be confirmed before further evaluation for a cause of hyperprolactinemia. PRL secretion is normally inhibited by tonic hypothalamic dopamine secretion; thus, use of any drug that inhibits hypothalamic release or transport of dopamine to the pituitary or that blocks pituitary dopamine receptors can cause hyperprolactinemia. Such agents include metoclopramide, phenothiazines, butyrophenones, risperidone, verapamil, and rarely, the selective serotonin reuptake inhibitors. Discontinuation of potentially offending agents should be attempted, if possible, for at least 72 hours to determine whether hyperprolactinemia is drug-induced. In the absence of drug-induced hyperprolactinemia, hypothalamic lesions (craniopharyngiomas, granulomatous infiltration) must also be considered in the differential diagnosis. Such processes can cause hyperprolactinemia by compressing the pituitary stalk and thus interfering with dopamine transport. PRL levels greater than 200 ng/mL should also be repeated after dilution to avoid the "hook" effect, which can artificially lower actual PRL values by interfering with both immunoradiometric and chemiluminescent assays.[194] Once the presence of non–drug-induced hyperprolactinemia is confirmed, pituitary imaging with MRI is preferred for identification of adenomas.

Effects of Nutrition on the Neuroendocrine Components of the Reproductive Axis

States of Undernutrition: Effects of Fasting. Nutritional status is an important regulator of reproductive health. Individual and species survival are at stake when food is scarce; thus, reproductive potential is appropriately reduced in the setting of undernutrition. The effects of undernutrition on the reproductive axis have been studied experimentally by fasting normal subjects. These studies have suggested that the hypothalamic–pituitary axis in men may be more sensitive to the effects of starvation than that in women. Mean LH and FSH decrease within 48 hours of fasting in men.[195,196] Although the mechanisms involved remain unclear, similar reductions observed in animal studies did not appear to be opioid-mediated.[197] The data on LH pulse frequency and amplitude are less consistent, however. Within this context, Veldhuis et al. did not detect any change in LH pulse frequency in healthy men during a 5-day fast, although LH pulse amplitude was attenuated.[196] In contrast, the results of Cameron et al. in healthy men who fasted for 48 hours showed a significant reduction in LH pulse frequency, but no change in pulse amplitude.[195] Serum testosterone decreased in both studies.[195,196] The GnRH pulse generator in men may be more sensitive to the effects of fasting because of the sensitizing effects of gonadal steroids.[198] Older men, whose sex steroid levels have declined with age, do not show the same fasting-induced changes in LH pulsatility that are seen in younger men.[199] Animal studies have also shown that these effects of sex steroids on neuroendocrine function may vary with the type of stressor.[200-202]

The GnRH pulse generator in women appears less susceptible to the effects of acute fasting. Despite minor perturbations in LH pulse frequency and mean LH, at the end of a 72-hour follicular-phase fast, follicle development in fasting women was similar to that in women who were fed, as illustrated in Figures 19-8 and 19-9.[203-205]

This resistance of the GnRH pulse generator to the acute effects of fasting occurs despite documented changes in cortisol and melatonin, both of which have been proposed to be critical regulators of the GnRH axis.[203] Body weight may mediate the effect of fasting on GnRH drive, and LH pulse frequency declined by 20% in lean women compared with normal weight women.[206] Attempts to determine the effects of acute undernutrition on GnRH activity during the luteal phase in women have proven more difficult, and exogenous administration of E_2 and progesterone to simulate the luteal phase also suppresses LH. As in their male counterparts, however, women showed alterations in both cortisol and melatonin when fasted during a simulated luteal phase, with dramatic increases in cortisol and duration of nocturnal melatonin secretion with fasting, evidence that this nutritional stress was not without some hormonal perturbation.[203]

Fasting can only be maintained in healthy subjects for short periods. The effects of more sustained caloric deprivation have been assessed in healthy women maintained on 800 to 1100 kcal/day diets for one menstrual cycle. Such caloric restriction was sufficient to cause weight loss[207,208] and resulted in anovulation in some women.[207,209] Dieting reduced follicular-phase LH secretion as well as follicular-phase LH pulse frequency, but luteal-phase LH patterns and FSH were unaffected.[207] Sex steroids (testosterone, androstenedione) were decreased, SHBG increased, and dehydroepiandrosterone sulfate did not change with dietary restriction.[208] These data in healthy, regularly ovulating women suggest that cortisol and melatonin may be the first hormones affected by short-term fasting,[203] but that continued caloric deprivation reduces GnRH activity within weeks. Amenorrhea can develop with loss of approximately 10% of body weight, regardless of initial body weight.[210]

States of Undernutrition: Anorexia Nervosa. Anorexia nervosa (AN) is an extreme example of the effects of undernutrition on the reproductive axis. It is difficult to separate the neuroendocrine effects of this nutritional deprivation itself from the hormonal alterations caused by the comorbid psychiatric illnesses that are frequently associated with AN. However, the effects of long-term caloric deprivation alone are also difficult to discern in other states of chronic undernutrition, such as protein–calorie malnutrition in hospitalized patients. Thus, AN has been best studied as a model of the reproductive consequences of severe caloric restriction. AN is defined by weight loss of greater than 15% for height, an intense fear of gaining weight, a disturbance in one's body image, and amenorrhea for at least 3 months. It is estimated to affect 0.5% of young women, with an even lower prevalence in males. Both primary and secondary amenorrhea can occur in AN, depending on the time of onset of the condition. A loss of 10% to 15% of normal weight for height is enough to delay the onset of menarche (primary amenorrhea), and a

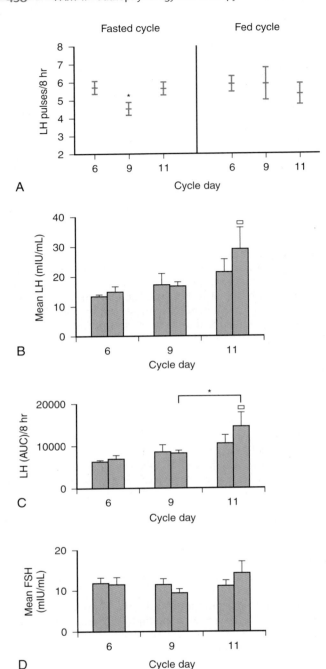

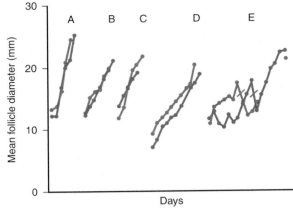

Figure 19-9. *Patterns of daily follicle growth in five women during fed (green) and fasted (purple) cycles beginning on cycle day 6 and lasting until the day before the collapse of the dominant follicle. The interrupted line in subject E in both fed and fasted curves represents the loss of the largest measured follicle not associated with a luteinizing hormone surge. A 5-day hiatus in measurements occurred before the last point in the fed cycle. (From Olson BR, Cartledge T, Sebring N, Defensor R, Nieman L. Short-term fasting affects luteinizing hormone secretory dynamics but not reproductive function in normal-weight sedentary women. J Clin Endocrinol Metab 80:1187, 1995. With permission from The Endocrine Society.)*

Figure 19-8. *Cumulative 8-hour luteinizing hormone (LH) and follicle-stimulating hormone (FSH) secretion on cycle days 6, 9, and 11 in women fasted on cycle days 7 to 9 (purple bars, n = 10) or fed (blue bars, n = 7). **A,** Mean number of LH pulses for each woman during the study for fasted (left) and fed (right) cycles. **B,** Mean LH vtalue for the groups. **C,** LH area under the curve (AUC. **D,** Mean FSH values. The rectangle indicates the effect of time within a group of P < 0.05 by repeated-measures analysis of variance. Asterisks indicate P < 0.05 significance from day 6 in part A and differences detected between days within a group in part C. (From Olson BR, Cartledge T, Sebring N, Defensor R, Nieman L. Short-term fasting affects luteinizing hormone secretory dynamics but not reproductive function in normal-weight sedentary women. J Clin Endocrinol Metab 80:1187, 1995. With permission from The Endocrine Society.)*

similar amount of weight loss disrupts normal menstrual cycles in postmenarchal girls (secondary amenorrhea). However, amenorrhea precedes weight loss in a significant percentage of patients with anorexia,[211,212] evidence that psychological stress and excessive exercise can also play a role. Other organ systems affected by AN include the cardiovascular and peripheral vascular (hypotension, arrhythmias), hematologic (anemia), dermatologic (lanugo hair), and renal systems (hypokalemia).[211]

Menstrual disturbances in anorexia result from hypothalamic rather than pituitary or ovarian dysfunction. Mean serum LH concentrations are lower than those of regularly menstruating women studied in the follicular phase,[213] and the LH secretory pattern is prepubertal, even in previously menstruating adolescents.[214] Responses to exogenous GnRH are blunted; the degree of response is greater in women who are closer to ideal body weight and in those who will ultimately resume normal menses after restoration of body weight.[215-217] Positive feedback from E_2 on the hypothalamus is also impaired in anorexic patients, as shown by studies with clomiphene citrate and exogenous estrogen that did not augment gonadotropin secretion.[218,219] The reduction in gonadotropin stimulation of the ovaries results in low estrone (E_1), E_2, progesterone, testosterone, and androstenedione levels.[215] Reduction in aromatase activity as a result of low body fat also contributes to the hypoestrogenism seen in anorexia, as does the preferential synthesis of catecholestrogen over E_2. Catecholestrogen is an endogenous antiestrogen that is capable of binding to estrogen receptors without having any biologic action. Catecholestrogen also competes with dopamine for the enzyme catechol-O-methyltransferase, thus increasing dopamine levels, further inhibiting GnRH pulsatility, and potentiating hypoestrogenism.[211] These alterations in E_2 metabolism result from changes in body weight and are not specific to anorexia.[220] Additional evidence that anorexia-associated amenorrhea is the result of hypothalamic dysfunction is the induction of menses in anorexic women with the use of pulsatile GnRH.[221]

The biochemical factors responsible for the hypothalamic amenorrhea in anorexia are unclear. Increased opioid tone is unlikely to be the only operative mechanism because administration of naloxone increased LH secretion in some,[222] but not all, studies.[216,223] Women who had reached ideal body weight and those with the highest basal LH levels had the most significant responses to opiate antagonists (naloxone).[216,222] Dopamine can also inhibit LH release, but the use of the dopamine agonist metoclopramide did not result in a significant increase in LH in a cohort with anorexia.[224] Metabolites of serotonin, such as 5-hydroxyindolacetic acid, which stimulate hypothalamic GnRH release and increase pituitary sensitivity to GnRH,[225] are low in patients with anorexia and increase during recovery, as shown in Figure 19-10.[226]

Selective serotonin reuptake inhibitors, which restore CNS serotonin levels, have been shown to be effective in reversing abnormal eating behaviors in some patients with anorexia. Thus, disturbance of the serotonin system may also play some role in anorexia-associated hypogonadotropic hypogonadism.[211,226] Another potential factor is leptin, which is secreted by adipocytes and is critical for energy homeostasis. Leptin receptors have been identified in the hypothalamus, pituitary, endometrium, ovary (granulosa, theca, and interstitial cells), and testes (Leydig cells). Leptin indirectly stimulates GnRH release, acting in concert with other molecules involved in appetite control (NPY, melanocortin). It also directly stimulates LH and FSH release from anterior pituitary cells. Leptin gene expression is promoted by estrogen and insulin. Anorexia and other states of hypoinsulinemia are characterized by reduced leptin concentrations, which correlate with body fat. Weight restoration in anorexia is associated with increases in leptin, changes that correlate with increases in serum LH and FSH. Thus, leptin may serve as a peripheral signal of adequate adipose stores that is capable of

reactivating the hypothalamic–pituitary–gonadal axis and restoring menses during recovery from AN.[227] The changes in leptin in AN are also accompanied by changes in ghrelin, another peptide intimately involved in control of feeding behavior. Ghrelin is increased in anorexic females compared with age-matched control subjects and constitutionally thin women without AN. Ghrelin correlates negatively with body mass index (BMI) and leptin,[228,229] and partial weight recovery results in a 25% decrease in ghrelin levels in patients with anorexia.[228]

Dehydroepiandrosterone sulfate and androstenedione are reduced in women with anorexia, but serum and urine cortisol levels are higher than normal. This preferential synthesis of cortisol over adrenal androgens is similar to that seen normally in prepubertal children and reflects relative 17,20-desmolase deficiency.[230] The resulting hypercortisolemia is augmented by the prolonged plasma half-life of cortisol in AN.[231] In spite of elevated cortisol, ACTH levels are not elevated at baseline or in response to CRH, as illustrated in Figure 19-11.

These findings show that the negative feedback effects of this hypercortisolemia remain intact at the level of the pituitary, and that excess secretion of CRH and decreased clearance of CRH contribute to this hypercortisolemia.[232] The lack of clinical signs of hypercortisolemia may result from diminished tissue expression of glucocorticoid receptors in patients with anorexia.[233] Importantly, these alterations of the hypothalamic–pituitary–adrenal (HPA) axis resolve with long-term weight recovery.[213,232] The hypothalamic–pituitary–gonadal axis also recovers with restoration of ideal body weight, as shown in Figure 19-12.[214]

Although no absolute BMI or percentage of body fat has been found to correlate with the resumption of menses, more than 85% of patients who achieve a weight that is 90% of their ideal body weight note return of menses within 6 months.[234] However, amenorrhea persists in a minority of women (10% to 30%), despite weight gain. Of the latter, many admit to restricting their fat intake and score higher on questionnaires designed to detect anorexic behaviors.[212] Hypoestrogenemia in such women correlates with the degree of ovarian dysfunction, and ovarian ultrasound shows small, amorphous ovaries. However, small multifollicular ovarian cysts appear once weight gain starts, with the return of a dominant ovarian follicle once premorbid weight is achieved.[235] Those who recover from anorexia, resume regular menses, and have normal eating behaviors can successfully conceive and bear healthy children.[212]

Recovery from AN and restoration of ideal body weight requires both emotional and nutritional rehabilitation, and remains quite challenging, despite improvements that have been made in understanding the pathophysiology of AN during the last century. Standardized mortality rates in patients with AN are increased 10- to 13-fold when patients are followed for 10 years.[236] The crude death rate in large meta-analyses, including more than 3000 patients with AN, was 5.9%.[237] The percentage of patients who recover entirely is less than 50%, whereas a significant proportion of patients have binge-eating behaviors at some point during their illness.[236] At least 10% still meet the criteria for AN after long-term follow-up. Factors

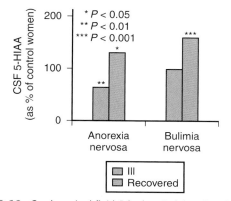

Figure 19-10. Cerebrospinal fluid 5-hydroxyindolacetic acid (5-HIAA) concentrations when ill and after recovery in people with anorexia and bulimia nervosa. Values are compared with those of healthy control women, which are set at 100%. (Modified from Kaye W, Gendall K, Strober M. Serotonin neuronal function and selective serotonin reuptake inhibitor treatment in anorexia and bulimia nervosa. Biol Psychiatry 44:825, 1998.)

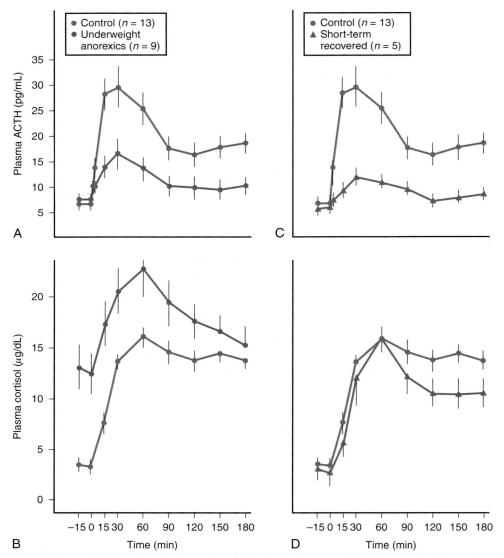

Figure 19-11. *Response of plasma (ACTH) and cortisol to corticotrophin-releasing hormone (CRH) in control subjects and patients with anorexia nervosa while chronically underweight (**A** and **B**) and while in short-term recovery (**C** and **D**). (Modified from Gold PW, Gwirtsman H, Avgerinos PC, Nieman LK, Gallucci WT, Kaye W, Jimerson D, Ebert M, Rittmaster R, Loriaux DL. Abnormal hypothalamic-pituitary-adrenal function in anorexia nervosa. Pathophysiologic mechanisms in underweight and weight-corrected patients. N Engl J Med 314:1335, 1986. Copyright © 1986 Massachusetts Medical Society. All rights reserved.)*

associated with poorer outcomes included longer duration of illness before the first inpatient treatment and a lower BMI, illustrating the importance of early diagnosis and intervention.[238]

Unfortunately, the effects of severe undernutrition on other body systems can persist, even when anorexic patients restore their body weight. Osteopenia and osteoporosis are the most serious long-term consequences of AN, and they result from both decreased bone formation (related to energy deprivation) and increased bone resorption (related to hypoestrogenism). The majority of patients presenting with amenorrhea and anorexia have some degree of low bone density, and bone mass can decline by as much as 2% to 6% per year during periods of undernutrition.[212] Unfortunately, BMD does not always normalize after restoration of a healthy body weight and

menstrual cyclicity, often because peak bone mass was not achieved during the adolescent and young adult years. The declines in bone density have been shown to correlate with the duration of anorexia and the age of onset of the disease.[211,212] Treatment of anorexia-associated osteopenia appears to require more than hormone replacement, likely because the osteopenia results from various nutritional and hormonal factors, not just estrogen deficiency.[239] For example, patients who received recombinant human insulin-like growth factor-1 (IGF-1) in combination with oral contraceptives had higher BMD than those who received oral contraceptives alone.[240]

Males account for only 5% of the anorexic population, but the diagnosis of AN in males is often delayed because the signs of reproductive dysfunction are harder to identify. Anorexia in men is strongly associated with depression

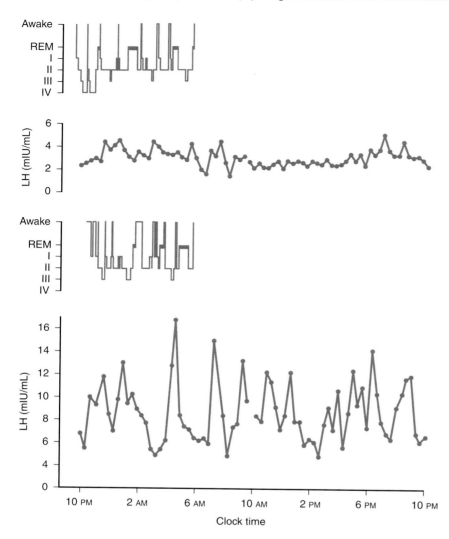

Figure 19-12. Plasma luteinizing hormone (LH) concentrations every 20 minutes for 24 hours during acute exacerbation of anorexia nervosa (top) and after clinical remission with return of body weight to normal (bottom). REM, rapid eye movement. (From Boyar RM, Katz J, Finkelstein JW, Kapen S, Weiner H, Weitzman ED, Hellman L. Anorexia nervosa. Immaturity of the 24-hour luteinizing hormone secretory pattern. N Engl J Med 291:861, 1974. Copyright © 1974 Massachusetts Medical Society. All rights reserved.)

and other underlying psychiatric disturbances, although the rate of comorbid substance abuse is higher than it is in women. Other features more prevalent in males with anorexia include a history of obesity, sexual identity concerns, and excessive exercising.[211] Boys are at higher risk for malnutrition-induced delays in growth and pubertal development, because they enter puberty later than girls. Studies in males with anorexia have shown abnormalities in the hypothalamic–pituitary–gonadal axis similar to those in women. Serum testosterone concentrations are often below normal, as are mean 24-hour LH concentrations.[196,217] GnRH-stimulated gonadotropin levels are also lower than those of normal control male subjects. Unlike gonadotropin levels in anorexic females, basal LH and FSH do not correlate with BMI (and degree of weight loss) in males with anorexia.[217] This hypogonadotropic hypogonadism is likely the result of severe caloric restriction itself because caloric restriction in obese men had similar effects on sex steroid and gonadotropin levels.[241]

States of Undernutrition: Bulimia Nervosa. *Bulimia nervosa* (BN) is another eating disorder characterized by irregular feeding patterns, specifically binge eating, in individuals of normal body weight, many of whom aspire to body weight far below normal. These episodes of binge eating are followed by periods of self-induced vomiting, laxative abuse, or extreme exercise, all driven by an abnormal body image. BN affects approximately 2% of the general female population, and approximately one third of patients with BN who present for treatment have a history of anorexia. Both anorexia and bulimia are more common in patients with coexisting low self-esteem, depression, and anxiety.[226] Disturbances in the reproductive axis can be seen in patients with bulimia, but they do not define the condition, as in anorexia. Amenorrhea occurs in 30%.[242] Approximately half of women with bulimia show hypogonadotropic hypogonadism and no evidence of follicular development associated with decreased LH pulse frequency,[243,244] whereas others have normal gonadotropin secretion and normal follicular development, but impaired luteal-phase progesterone levels.[243] Patients with purging behaviors showed more severe reductions in LH responses to GnRH infusion than nonpurging patients with bulimia and control subjects.[245] As in women with anorexia, serum cortisol is higher in bulimic women than in control subjects,[244,246] possibly related to increased CRH stimulation.

States of Overnutrition. *Overnutrition* and *obesity* pose a much greater threat to human health in most parts of the world than does food scarcity. Associated morbidities, including diabetes, obstructive sleep apnea, cardiovascular disease, and osteoarthritis, often remain undiagnosed until later in adulthood, although their foundations are established in young adulthood. However, men and women of reproductive age can have obesity-associated reproductive dysfunction that brings them to medical attention much sooner than these other conditions. For example, the most common endocrinopathy in reproductive-age women is PCOS, which affects 5% to 10% of women in this age group and is associated with reproductive as well as cardiovascular and cosmetic complications.[247,248] Many patients with PCOS are obese, and adiposity correlates linearly with testosterone levels in these women.[249] Weight reduction can restore menstrual regularity and, therefore, fertility in many patients with PCOS.[248] Both lean and obese women with PCOS show rapid LH pulse frequencies, but increasing body weight is associated with decreases in LH pulse amplitude in women with PCOS.[250] This neuroendocrine dysfunction is a product of and contributes to hyperandrogenemia, thus creating a vicious cycle in women with PCOS.

Obesity itself in the absence of PCOS-associated hyperandrogenemia also affects the hypothalamic–pituitary axis. Historical analysis of menstrual cycle data shows a higher percentage of menstrual abnormalities or hirsutism in women who were heavier.[251] The number of menstrual cycles with evidence of luteal activity was lower in overweight or obese women than in normal-weight participants in the Study of Women's Health Across the Nation (SWAN) study. Women with BMI of 25 kg/m² or greater also had statistically longer follicular phases and shorter luteal phases.[252] Consistent with these population studies, detailed hormonal sampling studies have shown that excess body weight suppresses gonadotropins. LH amplitude was reduced by 50% in morbidly obese women (mean BMI, 48.6 kg/m²) with regular cycles studied before gastric bypass surgery, although pulse frequencies did not differ. Nevertheless, the marked attenuation of pulse amplitude resulted in a lower mean LH compared with normal-weight control subjects.[253] This reduction in LH drive also results in deficient luteal stimulation and corpus luteum progesterone production, as reflected by lower urinary excretion of the progesterone metabolite pregnanediol glucuronide, illustrated in Figure 19-13.[252,253] Plasma E_2 and androstenedione concentrations are lower in obese women with regular cycles,[254] although E_1 does not change with body weight in most studies.[252,253]

Multiple factors are likely responsible for these obesity-associated neuroendocrine changes. The response to exogenous physiologic-dosed GnRH was inversely related to body weight in women with PCOS, but not in normally cycling women, suggesting that obesity may blunt the pituitary response to GnRH.[255] Insulin may also interfere with pituitary gonadotropin secretion, although no clear relationship between LH and insulin has been identified. Hyperinsulinemia clearly suppresses hepatic secretion, however, thereby increasing free E_2 levels. Free E_2 may exert more negative feedback on the pituitary because it is more biologically active, thus decreasing gonadotropin production.[252] Leptin, an adipose-derived hormone, increases hypothalamic GnRH pulsatility and pituitary

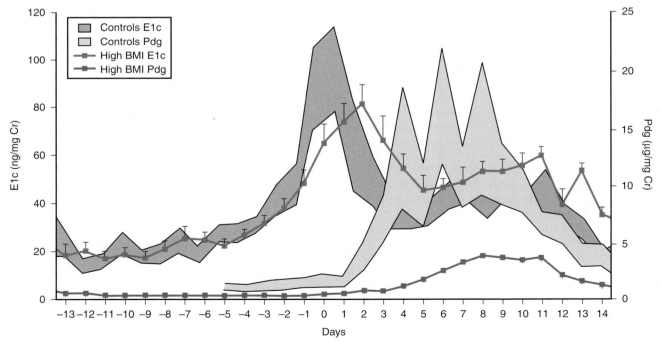

Figure 19-13. *Daily urinary estrone conjugate (E1c) and pregnanediol glucuronide (Pdg) in women with a high body mass (BMI) versus mean values of control women ± 1 standard deviation. Data are standardized to day 0, 13 days before ovulation. (Modified from Jain A, Polotsky AJ, Rochester D, Berga SL, Loucks T, Zeitlian G, Gibbs K, Polotsky HN, Feng S, Isaac B, Santoro N. Pulsatile luteinizing hormone amplitude and progesterone metabolite excretion are reduced in obese women. J Clin Endocrinol Metab 92:2468, 2007. With permission from The Endocrine Society.)*

gonadotropin release,[227] although obesity is often associated with leptin resistance. Leptin also inhibits granulosa cell responses to hCG and may interfere with oocyte maturation. Thus, the exact relationship of leptin to the neuroendocrine changes described earlier is not fully understood. Similarly, the role of other adipose-derived substances, including TNF-α and interleukin-1β, is an area of active investigation because both have the ability to reduce pituitary response to GnRH as well as to impair corpus luteum function.[253]

Obesity in men is also associated with reductions in circulating gonadotropin and sex steroid concentrations. The hyperinsulinemia-associated decrease in hepatic SHBG decreases binding affinity for testosterone and results in greater aromatization of testosterone to E_2. The subsequent increase in free E_2 and the reduction in the testosterone-to-E_2 ratio have important implications for male sexual function.[256-258] Total testosterone is lower in obese men compared with normal-weight men, but free testosterone does not change.[257,259,260] Mean LH, LH pulse frequency, and LH pulse amplitude are suppressed in severely obese men (BMI > 35), again reflecting the negative feedback effects of elevated free E_2. More moderate degrees of adiposity (BMI 30-35) do not affect gonadotropin secretion.[260,261] These alterations in the hypothalamic–pituitary–gonadal axis can decrease sperm concentrations.[256] Importantly, reducing hyperinsulinemia through weight loss allows for restoration of normal testosterone and LH levels.[261]

Effects of Exercise on the Neuroendocrine Components of the Reproductive Axis. Excessive exercise in the absence of eating disorders can result in hypogonadotropic hypogonadism due to hypothalamic dysfunction ("athletic amenorrhea"). The clinical manifestations of the reduced GnRH activity are varied and may include amenorrhea, oligomenorrhea, LPD, or anovulation. Menstrual cycle length is not a good marker of ovarian function in athletic women because it may be normal during cycles characterized by anovulation or LPD. In addition, one woman's cycle will differ over time, depending on the volume of her exercise and other environmental factors.[262] Exercise-associated menstrual dysfunction has been reported in women engaged in a variety of athletic activities, including long-distance running, rowing, skiing, tennis, gymnastics, ballet, fencing, and volleyball.[263] Dancers and long-distance runners have especially high rates of menstrual dysfunction (60% to 70%), but divers, cheerleaders, and gymnasts also have rates of amenorrhea (22%) that far exceed those in the general population.[264] Even recreational athletes are susceptible to exercise-associated menstrual dysfunction; 78% of such women had LPD or anovulation in at least one of three menstrual cycles.[262]

Risk factors for exercise-associated menstrual irregularities include the volume of training, eating behaviors, and gynecologic age. Studies of distance runners have illustrated the effect of exercise volume on menstrual function, with the prevalence of amenorrhea increasing from 3% to 60% as weekly training mileage increased.[265] Surveys of eating behaviors among female collegiate athletes show relatively low rates of diagnosed eating disorders among this population (3.3% with AN; 2.3% with bulimia

nervosa). Importantly, however, almost one third may be "at risk" for eating disorders, based on assessments of their attitudes toward eating, and these athletes are the ones most likely to report menstrual irregularities or bone injuries.[266] Although all menstruating females are susceptible to the disruptive effects of exercise on the reproductive axis, those who are younger and closer to the time of menarche (i.e., lower gynecologic age) are more sensitive, regardless of body size, body composition, training mileage, or years of training.[263,267,268] This sensitivity of the hypothalamic–pituitary–gonadal axis appears to be maximal in the first 15 years after the onset of menses and wanes thereafter.[268]

Exercise-induced menstrual dysfunction is characterized by low gonadotropin and E_2 concentrations.[269] Whereas athletic women with normal cycles had 20% to 30% reductions in LH pulse frequency compared with regularly cycling sedentary women, amenorrheic athletes experienced an additional 20% reduction in LH pulse frequency,[270-272] as shown in Figure 19-14.[270]

Reductions in LH pulse amplitude and loss of sleep-associated changes in LH pulsatility also occur in the amenorrheic group.[270,273] FSH secretion is impaired during the follicular–luteal phase transition. These gonadotropin changes may be subtle enough that menses remain regular, but they likely contribute to the high rates of anovulation (12%) seen in recreational athletes. Ultimately, ovarian steroid production is reduced in the absence of appropriate gonadotropin stimulation and corpus luteum function is impaired. The former is reflected in Figure 19-15 (*top*)[270] by a reduction in urinary E_1 (E_1G) excretion in amenorrheic athletes, whereas Figure 19-15 (*bottom*) shows urinary excretion of the progesterone metabolite prenanediol glucuronide (PdG) in these women. Reductions in PdG define luteal phase deficiency (LPD) and characterize 43% of the menstrual cycles in regularly cycling athletic women and can contribute to infertility.[270]

Provision of exogenous GnRH to women with exercise-induced amenorrhea illustrated that the etiology of this disorder is reduced hypothalamic GnRH secretion, rather than impaired pituitary or ovarian responsiveness. Submaximal graded doses of GnRH (2.5 μg, 5 μg, 10 μg, 25 μg) elicited exaggerated LH responses in athletic women compared with sedentary control women, whereas supraphysiologic doses of GnRH (100 μg) in amenorrheic athletes resulted in greater LH secretion compared with regularly menstruating athletic women.[274]

Exercise also causes hypogonadotropic hypogonadism in men, with reductions in both gonadotropins and total and free testosterone levels that correlate with the intensity of endurance exercise.[275,276] High-mileage endurance exercise can also affect sperm count, density, motility, and morphology on semen analysis.[276-278] Unlike endurance exercise, resistance exercise is associated with transient increases in androgens and dehydroepiandrosterone sulfate in men.[279] Because hypogonadism in males is less often recognized by both medical providers and patients themselves, literature on the effects of exercise on the male reproductive axis is more limited.

Physical activity is associated with hypogonadotropic hypogonadism in some, but not all, female athletes.

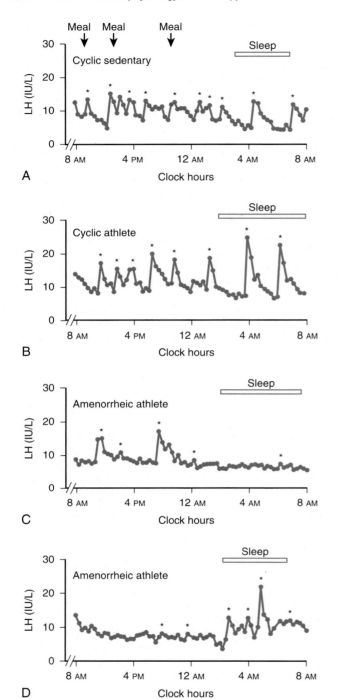

Figure 19-14. Serum luteinizing hormone (LH) levels at 20-minute intervals for 24 hours in a cycling sedentary women (**A**), a cycling athletic woman (**B**), and two amenorrheic athletic women (**C** and **D**). Asterisks indicate pulses, as identified by the Cluster pulse analysis program using a 2 × 1 cluster size and balanced T criteria of 2.1. (Modified from Loucks AB, Mortola JF, Girton L, Yen SSC. Alterations in the hypothalamic-pituitary-ovarian and the hypothalamic-pituitary-adrenal axes in athletic women. J Clin Endocrinol Metab 68:402, 1989. With permission from The Endocrine Society.)

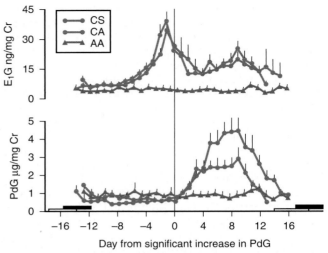

Figure 19-15. Mean (± standard error) daily urinary excretion of estrone glucuronide (E_1G) (top) and pregnanediol glucuronide (PdG) [bottom] in cycling sedentary (CS), cycling athletic (CA), and amenorrheic athletic (AA) women. Days are oriented from a significant increase in urinary PdG excretion, with day 1 being the day of the first significant increase. For urinary E_1G, 1 ng/mg creatinine (Cr) = 2.134 pmol/mg Cr; for PdG, 1 μg/mg Cr = 2.014 nmol/mg Cr. (Modified from Loucks AB, Mortola JF, Girton L, Yen SSC. Alterations in the hypothalamic-pituitary-ovarian and the hypothalamic-pituitary-adrenal axes in athletic women. J Clin Endocrinol Metab 68:402, 1989. With permission from The Endocrine Society.)

A prospective study of previously eumenorrheic women who engaged in distance running (65 miles/week) at or above the lactate threshold for 12 months or longer detected no significant changes in menstrual cycle length, follicular and luteal phase length, or integrated serum progesterone and E_2 concentrations compared with control women who were not exercise-trained. Body weight, percentage of body fat, lean body mass, and caloric intake did not change during the 12-month training period, and none of the women had oligo- or amenorrhea. Only luteal phase length was shorter in the group exercising above the lactate threshold. This stability of the reproductive axis occurred despite significant increases in oxygen consumption in the training groups.[263] Importantly, the women in this study had few risk factors for exercise-induced reproductive dysfunction because their mean gynecologic age was 17 years and they were carefully screened for coexisting psychiatric disease or eating disorders. Nevertheless, critics of this study note that the trained women may have been exercising enough at baseline to alter reproductive hormone secretion,[280] although there was little evidence that intensifying their exercise adversely affected their reproductive function.

The mechanisms whereby some women lose menstrual cyclicity when they initiate an exercise regimen are complex. Loss of body fat with intense exercise, with or without an underlying eating disorder, has long been thought to explain exercise-induced amenorrhea. Maintenance of a minimal percentage of body fat and a minimal weight for height was believed to be necessary to prevent menstrual dysfunction or restore menses in athletic women experiencing amenorrhea.[281] However, this theory has been disproved in multiple studies, none of which has been able to differentiate normally cycling athletes from oligo- or amenorrheic athletes by anthropometric features alone.[267,272,282,283] In addition, the changes in LH pulsatility are evident within 5 days,[284] much sooner than changes in adiposity appear.[285]

An imbalance between caloric intake and the amount of energy expended with exercise more likely explains the reduced hypothalamic GnRH drive observed in women with exercise-associated menstrual dysfunction.[271,286] Energy availability can be defined by the difference between energy intake and energy expenditure, with exercise being one component of energy expenditure. When energy availability is low, reproductive function suffers, as do thermoregulation, growth, and cellular maintenance.[264] Detailed nutritional assessments of athletic women who were expending 900 to 1000 kcal/day exercising showed that their daily caloric intake was similar to that of sedentary women. Thus, energy availability was significantly lower in the former, although none of these athletes had been formally diagnosed with an eating disorder. Fat and protein accounted for a smaller percentage of calories in the athletic women, and the athletic women with amenorrhea consumed 50% less fat than their regularly menstruating counterparts. This negative energy balance was reflected in insulin–glucose dynamics, with amenorrheic athletes showing marked hypoinsulinemia throughout the 24-hour observation period and glucose levels that were 10% lower. Women with more significant hypoinsulinemia had the lowest dietary fat intake and experienced greater reductions in LH pulse frequency.[271]

These effects of energy availability on hypothalamic GnRH secretion occur relatively quickly. When a negative energy balance is created experimentally, by restricting calories,[287] increasing expenditure,[288] or combining the two,[286] declines in LH pulse frequency occur within 1 week. Detailed studies in women whose energy availabilities were gradually decreased while they maintained a constant energy expenditure of 15 kcal/kg lean body mass (LBM)/day (kcal/kg LBM × day) illustrated that 30 kcal/kg LBM × day is the threshold of energy availability required to maintain normal reproductive function.[284] When energy availability falls below this threshold, LH pulse frequency declines and amplitude increases, as illustrated in Figure 19-16.[284]

The sensitivity of GnRH neurons to energy availability appears to decline with increasing gynecologic age, suggesting that hypothalamic centers become desensitized to these metabolic signals over time. Caloric restriction combined with vigorous daily aerobic exercise altered LH pulse frequency in adolescents, but not adults, changes that appeared within 5 days of energy deprivation, as shown in Figure 19-17.[268] Correction of this negative energy balance in amenorrheic exercising monkeys who continued vigorous training was achieved with overnutrition, and the rapidity of recovery was directly related to energy consumption.[289,290]

These experimental data suggest a role for a peripheral marker of adequate energy stores that can also act centrally to regulate the reproductive axis. Derived principally from adipose tissue, leptin is one such hormone whose receptors have been identified in the hypothalamus,

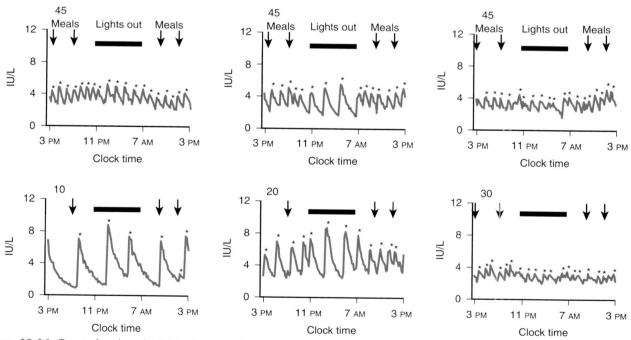

Figure 19-16. Twenty-four–hour luteinizing hormone (LH) pulse profiles for representative women after balanced energy availability treatments of 45 kcal/kg lean body mass (LBM) × day (top) and the paired restricted energy availability treatments of 10, 20, and 30 kcal/kg LBM × day, left to right, respectively (bottom). Asterisks indicate LH pulses. The black bar indicates when lights were turned off. Arrows indicate meals. (Modified from Loucks AB, Thuma JR. Luteinizing hormone pulsatility is disrupted at a threshold of energy availability in regularly menstruating women. J Clin Endocrinol Metab 88:297, 2003. With permission from The Endocrine Society.)

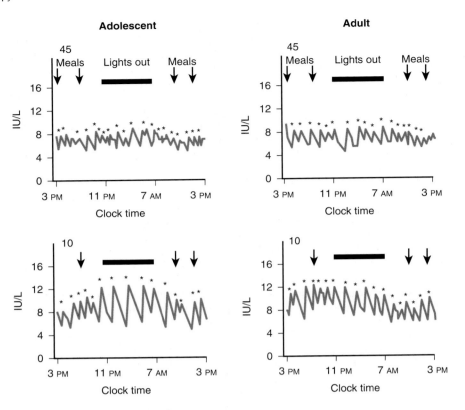

Figure 19-17. Twenty-four–hour luteinizing (LH) pulse profiles of a representative adolescent and adult after energy availability treatments of 45 and 10 kcal/kg fat-free mass/day. Asterisks indicate LH pulses. The black bar indicates when lights were turned off. Arrows indicate meals. (Modified from Loucks AB. The response of luteinizing hormone pulsatility to 5 days of low energy availability disappears by 14 years of gynecologic age. J Clin Endocrinol Metab 91:3158, 2006. With permission from The Endocrine Society.)

pituitary, ovary, and testes. Its effects are stimulatory in the CNS and inhibitory at the gonads.[227] Leptin concentrations in amenorrheic athletic women are significantly reduced compared with those in eumenorrheic athletic women,[291] and the normal diurnal pattern of leptin secretion is lost in the former.[292] Opposing the actions of leptin, ghrelin is an orexigenic hormone that stimulates the release of NPY and agouti-related protein from the arcuate nucleus of the hypothalamus. Exercise does not appear to alter ghrelin levels in the short term. Chronic exercise over 1 year in overweight sedentary women was associated with increases in ghrelin when the exercise was accompanied by weight loss. Not surprisingly, amenorrheic athletes had 85% higher levels of ghrelin than did women who were ovulatory and sedentary, ovulating and exercising, or exercising with a LPD.[293] Thus, both leptin and ghrelin are likely involved in the metabolic signaling cascade that mediates the reproductive effects of exercise.

Exercise may also impair the hypothalamic–pituitary–gonadal axis in some women by acting as a chronic stressor and activating the HPA axis. This activation mobilizes fuel stores in an attempt to maintain metabolic homeostasis. Ultimately, however, this HPA activation impairs other hypothalamic–pituitary axes, including the hypothalamic–pituitary–gonadal axis, through changes in CRH, pro-opiomelanocortin, ACTH, endogenous opiates, adrenal corticosteroids, or neurotransmitters. Both regularly menstruating and amenorrheic female athletes demonstrated higher plasma cortisol levels compared with regularly menstruating nonathletes with preservation of a diurnal pattern.[270,271] The degree of hypercortisolism correlated negatively with the magnitude of reduction in LH pulse frequency.[271] Administration of carbohydrates during prolonged exercise was shown to attenuate these increases in cortisol in both rodents[294] and humans,[295] suggesting that this HPA axis activation may occur in response to inadequate energy availability and that dietary energy restriction is more disruptive to the reproductive axis than energy expenditure through exercise.[273]

Alterations in the somatotroph axis also occur as a result of exercise-associated metabolic changes. Both GH pulse frequency and mean 24-hour mean GH are augmented in amenorrheic athletes,[271,296] changes also observed in states of nutritional deficiency, such as AN.[297] These increases in GH levels do not effect a rise in circulating serum IGF-1, which directly stimulates LH release in rodent studies.[298] This lack of increase in IGF-1 likely reflects the increases in its binding protein (IGF binding protein-1 [IGFBP-1]), which is the most metabolically response IGF-binding protein. In the prevailing hormonal milieu associated with exercise (low endogenous insulin, elevated cortisol), IGFBP-1 increases and serves as another peripheral signal of fuel shortage, slowing hypothalamic GnRH release. Unlike IGFBP-1, the concentrations of other GH-binding proteins (GHBPs) fall 35% in amenorrheic athletes and are unchanged in regularly cycling athletes, demonstrating the role that nutrient availability plays in the regulation of hepatic GHBP synthesis. Exercise-associated variations in circulating catecholamine and free fatty acid levels may also contribute to this complex regulation of hypothalamic–pituitary GH secretion.[271]

Given its role in metabolism, it is not surprising that thyroid hormone is affected by the hypothalamic dysfunction that occurs with exercise of moderate intensity. Energy imbalance as a result of carbohydrate restriction causes triiodothyronine (T_3) to decline, the result of reduced 5'-diodinase activity. In men, increased energy expenditure through moderate exercise results in a rise in reverse T_3 and a fall in serum free T_3, changes similar to those seen in the "low T_3 syndrome."[299] Exercise in women is associated with significant reductions in T_4 and T_3, although only amenorrheic athletic women have alterations in free T_3 and reverse T_3 levels, both of which are significantly decreased compared with regularly menstruating athletes or sedentary women. Mean 24-hour TSH levels are not affected by this reduction in thyroid hormone negative feedback. Thyrotropin-releasing hormone (TRH) deficiency with exercise could explain these differences in women.[300] Alternatively, the nocturnal hypermelatoninemia observed in amenorrheic athletes[301] could modulate thyroid hormone levels because melatonin secretion from the pineal gland reduces serum thyroid hormone levels in animals and humans.[300,302,303]

In summary, multiple metabolic signals are clearly involved with signaling to the GnRH pulse generator. Exercise can temporarily alter these metabolic signals if it creates an imbalance in energy availability. Such an imbalance can be prevented by supplementing dietary intake. Although most female athletes do not intentionally restrict their intake, few consume the additional calories needed to maintain a healthy energy balance. The exact nature of these interactions is complex and continues to be the subject of multiple investigations, but appears to be independent of body weight.

Long-term complications of the hypoestrogenism associated with exercise include infertility, lipid abnormalities, and premature bone loss.[264] Infertility results from poor or absent ovarian follicular development, impaired ovulation, or insufficient luteal-phase progesterone concentrations to support implantation. Amenorrheic athletes frequently have elevated low-density lipoprotein cholesterol levels[304] and endothelial dysfunction, despite their lack of body fat and low dietary fat intake.[305] Although the long-term effects of these cardiovascular risk factors in this population are not known, the adverse effects of amenorrhea on the skeletal system in young female athletes are well established. Estimates of the prevalence of osteopenia among female athletes range from 22% to 50%, whereas the prevalence of osteoporosis is much lower (0% to 13%).[306] Reductions in BMD are the result of increased bone resorption secondary to estrogen deficiency and decreased bone formation resulting from reduced energy availability.[264] Exercise itself may have differential effects on BMD, depending on the site examined. BMD at weight-bearing sites containing predominantly cortical bone, such as the femoral neck, was normal or increased in adolescent ballet dancers, whereas BMD was reduced at sites with predominantly trabecular bone, such as the spine and ribs. Sedentary amenorrheic girls with anorexia whose percentage of body fat was similar to the ballet dancers had lower BMD at all sites compared with regularly menstruating girls. Thus, weight-bearing exercise may offset the adverse effects of exercise-associated hypogonadism on cortical bone.[307] The skeletal effects of milder degrees of reproductive dysfunction, such as LPD, are unknown, and increasing

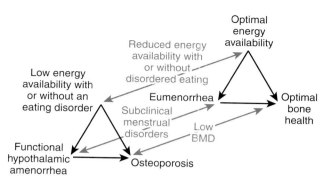

Figure 19-18. *Female athletic triad. The spectrums of energy availability, menstrual function, and bone mineral density (BMD) along which female athletes are distributed (purple arrows). An athlete's condition moves along each spectrum at a different rate according to diet and exercise habits. Energy availability, defined as dietary energy intake minus exercise energy expenditure, affects bone mineral density both directly via metabolic hormones and indirectly via effects on menstrual function and thereby estrogen (black arrows). (From Nattiv A, Loucks AB, Manore MM, Sanborn CF, Sundgot-Borgen J, Warren MP. The female athlete triad. Med Sci Sports Exer 38:1867, 2007.)*

evidence suggests that the declines in BMD associated with exercise-induced hypogonadotropic hypogonadism may not be reversible.[308]

The American College of Sports Medicine uses the term "the female athlete triad" to refer to the association of menstrual dysfunction, disordered eating, and osteoporosis in female athletes. Figure 19-18 illustrates the importance of optimal energy availability for both reproductive and skeletal health.[264]

Caloric intake that is adjusted for the energy expended during exercise maintains normal hypothalamic–pituitary–gonadal function (eumenorrhea), while also providing nutrients for normal bone formation. Athletes who maintain such homeostasis often have BMD 5% to 15% above those of age-matched individuals. However, even mild but sustained reductions in energy availability can induce subtle degrees of menstrual dysfunction. Eventually, such dysfunction impairs estrogen-mediated bone resorption and BMD begins to fall below that expected. Not surprisingly, eumenorrheic athletes have higher BMD than amenorrheic athletes, and eumenorrheic athletes with disordered eating but no formal eating disorder have lower BMD.

Identifying adolescents and women with the female athlete triad can be difficult, especially when overt amenorrhea has not developed. Even in the absence of a clinical eating disorder, restrictive eating behaviors should raise concern and should be investigated further, potentially with the help of a mental health professional. A history of multiple stress fractures or fractures with minimal trauma might also be the first clinical manifestations of nutritional deficits.[307] Health care providers should be especially mindful of menstrual dysfunction in adolescent females engaged in sports where leanness is emphasized (i.e., gymnastics, cheerleading, diving). Such athletes should be encouraged to optimize their nutrition and vitamin D status to prevent exercise-induced menstrual dysfunction.[264] Exercise-associated menstrual dysfunction is a diagnosis of exclusion, however, and women should still be evaluated for pregnancy, hyperprolactinemia, thyroid dysfunction, premature ovarian failure, and anatomic abnormalities of the uterus, even if the history is consistent with exercise as the cause of oligo- or amenorrhea.

Treatment of adolescents and adults with exercise-associated reproductive dysfunction requires a modification in diet or exercise behavior to increase energy availability, an intervention that is often difficult to implement.[309,310] Such nonpharmacologic approaches are also more effective at increasing bone density than is hormone replacement therapy (HRT).[308,311] In the absence of weight gain, HRT has not been consistently effective at increasing BMD in patients with exercise-induced hypogonadotropic hypogonadism,[312] likely because it does not correct the abnormal metabolic milieu that may be contributing to premature bone loss. In addition, many athletes refuse to take estrogen because of the associated weight gain. HRT may be indicated in a woman with continued loss of BMD on serial bone densitometry scans, despite adequate nutritional intake and body weight. Bisphosphonates are not used for the bone loss associated with exercise-induced amenorrhea because of their long residence time in bone and the harm they may cause to future developing fetuses. Recombinant IGF-1 used in combination with HRT in the form of oral contraceptive pills may be better than oral contraceptives alone at increasing BMD, but is not currently used clinically.[240]

Infertility related to exercise-induced alterations of the hypothalamus can be treated with exogenous gonadotropins, but more conservative interventions, such as restoration of body weight, are much preferred. Women with low body weight and borderline nutritional status before conception may not augment their intake enough during pregnancy to sustain normal fetal growth, thus placing them at higher risk for spontaneous fetal loss. Progesterone can be prescribed for those women with LPD that does not correct, despite increases in energy intake or decreases in exercise.[264]

Stress and Functional Hypothalamic Amenorrhea. Undernutrition, overnutrition, and exercise are well-recognized causes of functional hypothalamic amenorrhea (FHA), which is defined by hypothalamic hypogonadism in the absence of any structural hypothalamic or pituitary abnormality. The mediators of this hypothalamic dysfunction are multiple and likely include insulin, leptin, ghrelin, CRH, and cortisol. FHA accounts for 34% of cases of secondary amenorrhea in adults, making it the most common cause of this disorder.[313] FHA also exists in women who do not meet the criteria for an eating disorder and do not exercise; such cases are often attributed to stress or are termed *idiopathic*. Life-threatening stress (i.e., experiencing refugee or concentration camps, wars, air raids) has long been known to cause amenorrhea in the majority of women; it resolves once environmental conditions improve.[314] Less severe stressors also contribute to menstrual dysfunction in some women. Characterization of women with such stress-associated menstrual dysfunction is complicated by the heterogeneity of the condition.

Stress is difficult to define objectively,[315] but Selye noted in 1939 that it was accompanied by activation of the HPA axis and that it reduced reproductive capacity.[316] This physiologic response makes sense teleologically because it allows for preservation of adrenocortical function in the case of emergency at the expense of gonadal activity. Acute stress results in a brief increase in LH and testosterone, possibly as a result of a decrease in the metabolic clearance rate rather than a change in the secretory rate. However, this initial stimulatory phase is short-lived and is not nearly as clinically relevant as the response to prolonged stress, which has consistently been shown to inhibit hypothalamic GnRH secretion, to interfere with GnRH-induced LH production, and to impair gonadal response to LH and FSH. Stress-related increases in CRH, pro-opiomelanocortin, ACTH, endogenous opiates, adrenal corticosteroids, or neurotransmitters may modulate these central and peripheral effects on the reproductive axis. The interactions of each of these factors with each other and with the hypothalamus, pituitary, and gonads are extremely complex, as shown in Figure 19-19 and, therefore, difficult to distinguish experimentally.[317]

The decreased GnRH activity characteristic of FHA reflects CNS and hypothalamic responses to perceived or actual stressors. Different stressors elicit different neuromodulatory responses in different people, and the magnitude of these responses may be determined early in life by events that permanently influence the sensitivity of the HPA axis.[318] The severity of patients' self-reported psychomatic disturbance has been shown to correlate with the degree of gonadotropin suppression.[319] Most women are able to maintain normal menstrual cycles throughout stressful life events, periods of weight loss, and periods of intense exercise. In those who have amenorrhea, some degree of menstrual irregularity often precedes the complete cessation of menses, whereas women with amenorrhea related to Cushing syndrome, hypothyroidism, Sheehan syndrome, or pituitary tumors usually have no history of menstrual dysfunction.[313] Similarly, athletes who have amenorrhea during periods of intense exercise often have a history of menstrual irregularity.[320] Clearly, in some individuals, the hypothalamic–pituitary–gonadal axis is more sensitive to disturbances in homeostasis than it is in others. Men are also susceptible to stress-associated reproductive compromise, but identifying functional declines in GnRH pulsatility is quite difficult in males. Asthenospermia (decline in sperm motility) may be the mildest manifestation of altered GnRH drive, but is usually only diagnosed in the workup of infertility.[321]

Gonadotropin secretion in women with FHA is inappropriately low, but the pattern of secretion varies during the course of illness. Studies in women with FHA who were of normal weight for height, who were not being treated for an eating disorder, and who were not exercising excessively at the time of sampling showed low-frequency LH secretion in 43%, low-frequency/low-amplitude secretion in 27%, low-amplitude secretion in 8%, apulsatile secretion in 8%, and an unclassified pattern in 14%, as shown in Figure 19-20.[322]

Twelve patients participated in two to eight overnight sampling studies each, and LH secretory patterns changed in 75% of these women on repeated study. The majority of these women responded to naloxone infusion with

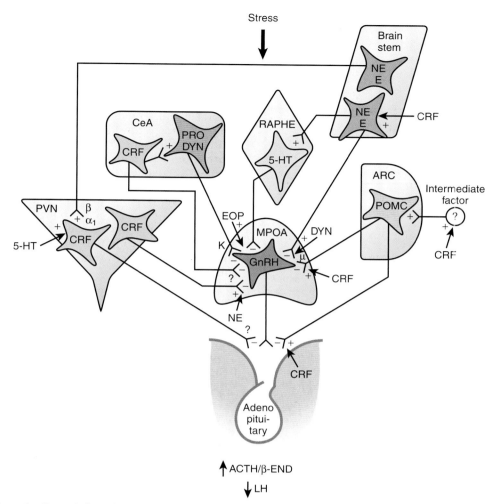

Figure 19-19. *The main effects of physical stress on different brain areas, and peptidergic or aminergic pathways directly or indirectly involved in alteration of the activity of gonadotropin-releasing hormone (GnRH) neurons. ACTH, adrenocorticotropic hormone; ARC, arcuate nucleus; β-END, β endorphin; CeA, central amygdaloid nucleus; CRF, corticotropin-releasing factor; DYN, dynorphin; E, epinephrine; EOP, endogenous opioid peptides; NE, norepinpehrine; 5-HT, 5-hydroxytryptophan; LH, luteinizing hormone; MPOA, medial preoptic area; POMC, proopiomelanocortin; PRODYN, prodynorphin; +, stimulation; PVN, paraventricular nucleus; RAPHE, –, inhibition; ?, mechanisms unclear and remain to be fully investigated. (Modified from Rivier C, Rivest S. Effect of stress on the activity of the hypothalamic-pituitary-gonadal axis: peripheral and central mechanisms. Biol Reprod 45:523, 1991.)*

increases in LH pulse frequency, implicating enhanced opioid tone as a cause of hypothalamic amenorrhea in a subset of patients. This naloxone response occurred in women regardless of their baseline neuroendocrine patterns, and has been supported by previous studies.[323] Thus, women with FHA do not appear to have a static defect of GnRH secretion. Rather, their hypothalamic sensitivity to endogenous opioids and other stress-associated factors is heightened, resulting in GnRH concentrations that rise and fall with changes in endogenous opioid levels. Such disordered GnRH pulsatility is unable to support follicular development and ovulation.[322]

Metabolic signals may also be responsible for inhibiting GnRH activity in idiopathic and stress-induced FHA. Specifically, both leptin and ghrelin have been implicated as markers of inadequate nutrition stores that are capable of signaling to the hypothalamus and suppressing the reproductive axis. In nonathletic women of normal weight with FHA, adipose-derived leptin levels are reduced compared with age-, weight-, and body fat–matched eumonorrheic control subjects, suggesting that energy deprivation may underlie menstrual dysfunction in these patients, as it does in patients with eating disorders and excessive exercise.[324,325] Administration of exogenous leptin to a small group of women with FHA increased maximal follicular diameter, ovarian volume, and endometrial thickness, as well as the number of dominant follicles, as shown in Figure 19-21.[326] LH pulse patterns normalized, and E_2, thyroid hormone, and IGF-1 levels increased in the majority of these women, despite the fact that they lost weight and experienced a decline in their percentage of body fat.[326]

Unlike the anorexigenic leptin, ghrelin is an orexigenic molecule that stimulates food intake. Ghrelin acts on the same neurohormonal pathways as leptin and is secreted by gastric oxyntic cells. Ghrelin levels correlate well with feelings of hunger and are higher in women with eating disorders and in exercising women who lose weight.[229] In

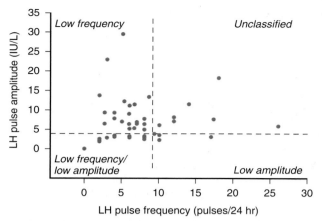

Figure 19-20. *Classification of subjects with hypothalamic amenorrhea by luteinizing (LH) pulse frequency and amplitude, defined by mean −1 standard deviation in normally cycling women (hatched lines). Low pulse amplitude was defined as less than 4 IU/L. Low pulse frequency was defined as fewer than 9 pulses/24 hr. (From Perkins RB, Hall JE, Martin KA. Neuroendocrine abnormalities in hypothalamic amenorrhea: spectrum, stability, and response to neurotransmitter modulation. J Clin Endocrinol Metab 84:1905, 1999. With permission from The Endocrine Society.)*

addition, in animal studies, ghrelin has been shown to suppress LH pulse frequency.[327] It may not be surprising that ghrelin levels are significantly higher in women with FHA, whose scores on tests of eating disordered behaviors were

significantly higher than those of control women. Ghrelin elevation may be another mechanism that the body uses to stimulate appetite and suppress reproduction in the face of a negative energy balance.[328] Studies of male Army Rangers engaged in an elite combat leadership course also support the hypothesis that low energy availability is an important mediator of FHA. In these men, alterations in metabolic and reproductive hormones during periods of semistarvation resolved after *ad libitum* refeeding, despite continued exposure to other stressors (heat, cold, sleep deprivation, extreme exercise, illness, injuries).[329] Thus, whether a reduction in energy availability occurs as the primary homeostatic insult, as it does in AN, or whether it is a secondary response to stress, it may be the proximate causes of the majority of reproductive disorders.[315] The hypogonadotropic hypogonadism associated with FHA may be the final common pathway by which the body serves to protect itself from additional stressors, such as childbearing.

Detailed overnight hormonal sampling studies in women with FHA showed the expected changes in gonadotropins. Mean serum LH concentrations, LH pulse frequency, and FSH were reduced by 30%, 53%, and 19%, respectively. Importantly, however, abnormalities in other hypothalamic–pituitary axes were also apparent. In addition, 24-hour cortisol secretion was 17% higher in women with FHA compared with eumenorrheic women,[330] but

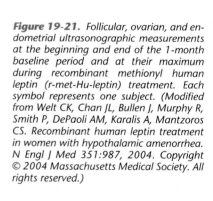

Figure 19-21. *Follicular, ovarian, and endometrial ultrasonographic measurements at the beginning and end of the 1-month baseline period and at their maximum during recombinant methionyl human leptin (r-met-Hu-leptin) treatment. Each symbol represents one subject. (Modified from Welt CK, Chan JL, Bullen J, Murphy R, Smith P, DePaoli AM, Karalis A, Mantzoros CS. Recombinant human leptin treatment in women with hypothalamic amenorrhea. N Engl J Med 351:987, 2004. Copyright © 2004 Massachusetts Medical Society. All rights reserved.)*

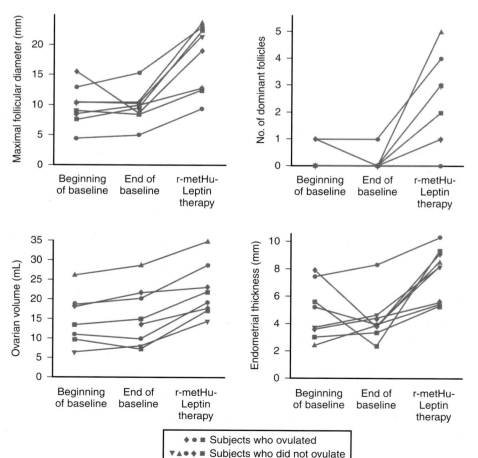

this hypercortisolemia did not suppress CSF CRH levels, suggesting hypothalamic resistance to cortisol negative feedback.[331] In addition, 24-hour PRL was lower, and nocturnal GH secretion was higher and more disordered. TSH was unchanged, but serum T_3 and T_4 were lower in the women with FHA. Administration of hypothalamic-releasing factors (GnRH, CRH, GH-releasing hormone [GHRH], TRH) showed normal pituitary responses in both groups, evidence that global hypothalamic dysfunction occurs in women with FHA.[330]

Restoring reproductive function in cases of stress-associated FHA is not as straightforward as the treatment of exercise-induced amenorrhea or anorexia-associated amenorrhea, in which case the pathologic behaviors are obvious and potentially reversible. Women with all three types of amenorrhea tend to be perfectionists who desire social approval and who possess abnormal attitudes toward eating.[332,333] Detailed questioning is often required to uncover these unhealthy eating behaviors, which tend to be of the bulimic type in adult women and of the restrictive type in adolescents.[319,325] Women and adolescents with FHA tend to have lower self-esteem and a higher prevalence of psychological disturbances compared with eumenorrheic control subjects and women with amenorrhea due to other causes.[319,334] Cognitive behavioral therapy (CBT) can help to identify stressors and maladaptive attitudes toward eating and provide patients with problem-solving techniques to better cope with stress-inducing circumstances. CBT has also been shown to restore ovulation in up to 75% of women who were previously anovulatory, whereas observation alone was effective in only one of eight women during the 20-week study period. Responses to CBT occurred relatively quickly after CBT initiation (mean, 11.2 ± 3.3 weeks)[335] and were preceded by normalization of the hypercortisolemia characteristic of FHA.[336] Such psychological intervention is also more likely to allow for recovery of all endocrine and metabolic disturbances than is targeted treatment of the hypothalamic–pituitary–gonadal axis alone with sex steroid replacement.[337] Sex steroids can be considered after amenorrhea has persisted for 6 months or more despite lifestyle changes; lumbar spine BMD may improve in such patients.[338] Recombinant leptin may also have a potential role in preventing FHA-associated bone loss in the future, either alone or in combination with E_2, although leptin's suppressive effects on appetite are concerning in this population, which is already predisposed to altered eating behaviors.[339] Exogenous gonadotropins can be used to induce ovulation and achieve pregnancy in FHA, but they will not reverse the hypothalamic hypothyroidism and hypercortisolism that often accompany the hypogonadism. If pregnancy is achieved, obstetric and fetal outcomes may be adversely affected by failure to correct these other hormonal disturbances.[337,340]

Establishing recovery rates in cases of FHA unrelated to weight loss or exercise is complicated by the difficulty in defining this subset of patients. FHA of idiopathic etiology confers a poorer prognosis, with recovery rates in small longitudinal studies of 6 to 10 years' duration ranging from 29% to 61%. FHA related to stress almost always resolves once the causal factor is reversed, especially if there is associated weight loss that improves

concurrently.[341,342] No neuroendocrine pattern was predictive of recovery.[341] The fact that few women with FHA of defined etiology do not experience recovery of menses, even after correction of the inciting factor, shows that both physiologic and environmental insults are important.[341]

Medication-Associated Hypogonadotropic Hypogonadism. A variety of medications can interfere with the hypothalamic–pituitary axis as a result of their tendency to increase PRL. Given that PRL release is under tonic inhibition by hypothalamic dopamine secretion, medications that interfere with hypothalamic release or transport of dopamine or that block pituitary dopamine receptors can raise serum PRL. The degree of PRL elevation in such cases is usually less than 100 ng/mL, a range that overlaps that seen with PRL-secreting microadenomas and with stalk deviation caused by other pituitary lesions.[343] Nevertheless, even such modest hyperprolactinemia can be enough to suppress hypothalamic GnRH release and reduce FSH, LH, E_2, and testosterone levels. Hyperprolactinemia can also interfere with gonadal response to the gonadotropins, and with conversion of testosterone to dihydrotestosterone via 5α-reductase, both of which further reduce sex steroid concentrations.[344] Thus, it is not surprising that patients with medication-induced hyperprolactinemia report high levels of sexual dysfunction, including decreased libido, decreased arousal, orgasmic dysfunction, galactorrhea, oligomenorrhea, anovulation, and subfertility.[345] These side effects frequently interfere with medication compliance. Fortunately, they resolve with discontinuation of the medication believed to be responsible for raising serum PRL. Cessation of therapy must be approached cautiously, however, especially when psychiatric illness is the underlying disease.

Metoclopramide (Reglan), which is commonly used to treat diabetic gastroparesis, blocks dopamine receptors and causes hyperprolactinemia in the majority of patients. This PRL increase appears acutely after each dose of medication and is unrelated to the cholinergic properties of the drug.[346,347] Women taking metoclopramide commonly present with galactorrhea or amenorrhea, whereas men present with impotence. These signs of PRL excess can develop within weeks of drug initiation, and similarly resolve over weeks once the medication is discontinued.[348] Because it is such a potent stimulator of PRL release, metoclopramide has been used in research settings to study the effects of PRL on other aspects of the hypothalamic–pituitary axis.[347]

Antipsychotic medications are frequently associated with hyperprolactinemia, a side effect that occurs within the first 1 to 8 weeks of treatment.[349,350] Such agents block D2 dopamine receptors in the hypothalamic tubuloinfundibular system and on pituitary lactotrophs. Medications in this class include both the older, typical antipsychotics (phenothiazines, such as perphenazine, prochlorperazine, promethazine, fluphenazine, thioridazine, chlorpromazine; and butyrophenones, such as haloperidol) and newer atypical antipsychotics. The ability of the older neuroleptic agents to elevate PRL correlates with their antipsychotic potency,[343] whereas the effect of the newer atypical antipsychotic drugs is not uniform among all drugs in the class. Clozapine (Clozaril), olanzapine (Zyprexa), quetiapine (Seroquel), ziprasidone (Geodon), and aripiprazole (Abilify) are considered PRL-sparing antipsychotics and may cause transient increases in PRL within the range of normal. On the other hand, the extent of hyperprolactinemia with risperidone (Risperdal) therapy is similar to, if not greater than, that observed with older conventional antipsychotics.[351] The differences among atypical antipsychotics may result from the differential binding of these agents to hypothalamic and pituitary dopamine receptors.[352] Table 19-2 summarizes the effects of various psychotropic medications on serum PRL.[343]

Fortunately, both PRL-sparing and non–PRL-sparing atypical antipsychotic drugs have similar efficacy in controlling psychiatric symptoms. Thus, clinically stable patients with medication-associated hyperprolactinemia can be switched to a PRL-sparing agent, such as olanzapine, and achieve PRL normalization without adversely affecting their psychiatric disease control. When such patients continue a non–PRL-sparing antipsychotic regimen, they rarely achieve euprolactinemia, as illustrated in Figure 19-22.[352]

Restoration of normal PRL levels also increases free testosterone levels in male patients, restores regular menses in female patients, and improves sexual function in both sexes.[352] However, self-reported measures of sexual dysfunction do not always correlate with improvements in serum PRL. A study of clinically stable patients with schizophrenia who were followed for 3 years showed greater sexual dysfunction scores in patients taking olanzapine and quetiapine than in those taking risperidone or haloperidol.[353] Other studies have shown no greater improvements in sexual function with the use of atypical antipsychotics compared with haloperidol.[354] Although medication compliance may improve with correction of sexual dysfunction, the adverse metabolic effects of olanzapine and other PRL-sparing antipsychotics cannot be overlooked.[352] Restoration of normal PRL levels with drug discontinuation occurs within 48 to 96 hours, but correction of the metabolic disturbances (weight gain, dyslipidemia) obviously requires weeks to months.[343]

There is increasing evidence that hyperprolactinemia occurs with *selective serotonin reuptake inhibitors* as well. One in eight outpatients with normal PRL levels at baseline had hyperprolactinemia after 12 weeks of fluoxetine treatment, regardless of medication dose. The incidence of hyperprolactinemia was much higher among women (22.2%) than among men (4.2%), illustrating the fact that the PRL response tends to be more robust in women, regardless of the clinical condition (surgical stress, primary hypothyroidism, antipsychotic drug therapy).[349,350,355] There was no decline in testosterone levels in men during this study, and the effect of selective serotonin reuptake inhibitors therapy on menstrual function was not assessed. Thus, the clinical importance of these elevations in PRL remains unclear and needs to be addressed with longer and larger studies.[355] Hyperprolactinemia also occurs with other types of *antidepressant medications,* including tricyclic agents (TCAs) and monoamine oxidase inhibitors (MAOIs), but it is most severe with agents that are no longer in widespread clinical use, such as clomipramine

TABLE 19-2

Effects of Psychotropic Medications on Prolactin Levels

Medication	Increase in Prolactin
Antipsychotics	
Typical	
Phenothiazines	+++
Butyrophenones	+++
Thioxanthenes	+++
Atypical	
Risperidone	+++
Molindone	++
Clozapine	0
Quetiapine	+
Ziprasidone	0
Aripiprazole	0
Olanzapine	+
Antidepressants	
Tricyclics	
Amitriptyline	+
Desipramine	+
Clomipramine	+++
Nortriptyline	-
Imipramine	CR
Maprotiline	CR
Amoxapine	CR
Monoamine Oxidase Inhibitors	
Pargyline	+++
Clorgyline	+++
Tranylcypromine	±
Selective Serotonin Reuptake Inhibitors	
Fluoxetine	CR
Paroxetine	±
Citalopram	±
Fluvoxamine	±
Other	
Nefazadone	0
Bupropion	0
Venlafaxine	0
Trazodone	0

CR, isolated case reports of hyperprolactinemia, but generally no increase in prolactin levels.
0, no effect; ±, minimal increase but not to abnormal levels; +, increase to abnormal levels in a small percentage of patients;
++, increase to abnormal levels in 25% to 50% of patients;
+++, increase to abnormal levels in more than 50% of patients.
From Molitch ME. Medication-induced hyperprolactinemia. Mayo Clin Proc 80:1050, 2005.

(TCA) and pargyline and clorgyline (MAOIs). Hyperprolactinemia has not been reported with long-term use of nefazodone (Serzone), bupropion (Wellbutrin), venlafaxine (Effexor), trazodone, or lithium.[343]

Other medications associated with hyperprolactinemia include *opiates, cocaine, danazol,* and *verapamil.* Long-term use of morphine and morphine analogs has been shown to increase PRL by inhibiting hypothalamic dopamine secretion, actions which are mediated by the μ receptor. Mild but sustained hyperprolactinemia has also been observed in patients abusing cocaine.[343] Danazol is an

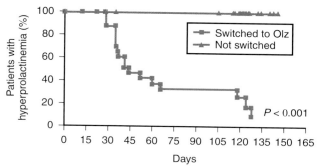

Figure 19-22. *Sustained reversal of hyperprolactinemia was achieved in 90% of patients who were switched to olanzapine (Olz) 5 to 20 mg/ day, whereas all of the patients who remained on prestudy medication continued to have elevated prolactin levels throughout the study. Normal serum prolactin levels were less than 18.8 ng/mL (0.8 nmol/L) for males and less than 24.4 ng/mL (1.05 nmol/L) for females. (Modified from Kinon BJ, Ahl J, Liu-Seifert H, Maguire GA. Improvement in hyperprolactinemia and reproductive comorbidities in patients with schizophrenia switched from conventional antipsychotics or risperidone to olanzapine. Psychoneuroendocrinology 31:577, 2006.)*

androgen whose inhibitory effects on LH and FSH are used clinically to treat endometriosis and fibrocystic breast disease, as well as hereditary angioedema. Amenorrhea and breakthrough bleeding are common side effects of danazol therapy.[356-358] Verapamil (Calan, Covera, Isoptin, Verelan), unlike other antihypertensive agents, has been shown to suppress GnRH-mediated release of LH and FSH while simultaneously increasing PRL release. These effects occur regardless of the route of drug administration and can be associated with galactorrhea.[359-361] A large population study in male outpatients showed an 8.5% prevalence of hyperprolactinemia in patients taking verapamil; the rate declined to zero after drug discontinuation.[362] Verapamil reduces central dopamine production by blocking calcium influx through slow calcium channels in the hypothalamus.[363] This effect appears to be drug-specific and has not been seen with diltiazem, another nondihydropyridine calcium channel blocker,[360] or with nifedipine and other dihydropyridine calcium channel blockers.[364,365]

Uncertainty exists regarding the ability of *exogenous estrogen* to cause hyperprolactinemia. Physiologic amounts of estrogen minimally increase PRL, but likely explain the more robust PRL responses to physiologic stimuli observed in women compared with men.[366] Studies of women taking estrogen-containing oral contraceptives have generated mixed results regarding the ability of these physiologic exogenous doses of estrogen to raise serum PRL.[343] Higher levels of estrogen, such as those that occur during pregnancy, can cause hyperprolactinemia,[367] but a thorough evaluation for other causes of PRL elevation should be completed in any patient using oral contraceptives or hormone replacement therapy who presents with hyperprolactinemia.

Case reports of hyperprolactinemia developing in response to various other drugs can be found in the literature. These drugs include *histamine receptor blockers* (cimetidine, ranitidine), *protease inhibitors*, and *1,25-dihydroxyvitamin D*. However, larger case series did not validate the association of any of these drugs with serum PRL elevations.[343]

BOX 19-2

Medications That May Cause Hyperprolactinemia

Antipsychotics (neuroleptics)
    Phenothiazines
    Thioxanthenes
    Butyrophenones
    Atypical antipsychotics
Antidepressants
    Tricyclic and tetracyclic antidepressants
    Monoamine oxidase inhibitors
    Selective serotonin reuptake inhibitors
    Other
Opiates and cocaine
Antihypertensive medications
    Verapamil
    Methyldopa
    Reserpine
Gastrointestinal medications
    Metoclopramide
    Domperidone
    Histamine receptor blockers (?)
Protease inhibitors (?)
Estrogens

?, Case reports only.
Modified from Molitch ME. Medication-induced hyperprolactinemia. Mayo Clin Proc 80:1050, 2005.

Box 19-2 summarizes the variety of medications that can cause hyperprolactinemia.[343]

Medication history is critical when evaluating a patient with reproductive dysfunction. If initial evaluation shows hyperprolactinemia and the patient is taking a drug frequently associated with hyperprolactinemia, cessation of the offending agent should result in normalization of PRL within days. However, drug discontinuation should be approached cautiously in psychiatric patients, whose underlying condition may acutely worsen with changes in medication regimen. If drug discontinuation is not believed to be a viable option, substitution of a PRL-sparing agent from the same medication class is sometimes an option. Alternatively, hypothalamic–pituitary imaging can be ordered to evaluate for mass lesions. If is the findings are normal, the hyperprolactinemia can be assumed to be medication-related.[343]

Treatment of medication-associated hyperprolactinemia depends on whether the individual is symptomatic. Patients with galactorrhea alone can often be reassured and do not need additional treatment, whereas those with sexual dysfunction associated with amenorrhea or impotence may need additional intervention. If the patient's underlying condition (i.e., schizophrenia, depression) needs treatment, the best option is to switch to a PRL-sparing agent within the same medication class. If there are no alternative agents available within the same class and hypogonadism is the concern, E_2 or testosterone can be prescribed. Bisphosphonates can be used to prevent loss of BMD if that is the concern. Dopamine agonists (bromocriptine, cabergoline) have been tried in numerous patients in whom the agent causing symptomatic hyperprolactinemia was considered necessary and there were no alternative agents. Unfortunately, these medications can exacerbate the underlying psychiatric condition and do not always normalize PRL.[343]

Pituitary Dysfunction

PITUITARY TUMORS

Development of Pituitary Tumors: Etiologic Considerations

Currently available information suggests that the majority of pituitary tumors develop from monoclonal tumor cell expansion of a mutated somatic cell.[368] Such mutations can occur in a familial setting within the germ cell line or may be sporadic. The development of a pituitary adenoma within a familial setting is known to occur in multiple endocrine neoplasia type 1 (MEN 1) and Carney complex (CNC)[369,370] as well as in familial acromegaly.[371] As discussed later, the MEN 1 syndrome is caused by mutations in the tumor suppressor gene *MEN1*, which is located on chromosome 11q13 and encodes a 610–amino acid nuclear protein. In patients with the *MEN1* gene, pituitary adenomas occur in approximately 40% of cases. Other mutations, such as that in the *CDKN1B* gene (which encodes for the cyclin-dependent kinase inhibitor p27^{Kip1}), are also considered to be possibly involved in the MEN 1 syndrome. CNC is associated with mutations in the protein kinase A1 alpha regulatory subunit gene on chromosome 2p16 in 60% of cases.[372,373]

Isolated familial somatotropinoma (IFS) is defined as more than two cases of acromegaly in a family in the absence of MEN 1 or CNC. The genetic pathophysiology is still unclear, even though a mutation in the gene encoding the aryl-hydrocarbon receptor–interacting protein has been found in some cases.[374] Somatic mutations in the $G_s\alpha$ gene (*GNAS1*) are found in a subset of GH-secreting tumors, with a prevalence ranging from 40% in white populations to 10% in Japanese populations. The oncogenic gsp mutation correlates with constitutively increased cyclic AMP response element–binding protein phosphorylation and activity, which then leads to increased Pit-1 transcription and GH synthesis.[373] An example of a sporadic mutation associated with pituitary cell tumors is the activating mutation in *GNAS1*, which is seen in McCune-Albright syndrome, a condition with multiple endocrine manifestations, including hyperplastic pituitary lesions.[375] Several in vivo and in vitro lines of evidence suggest that the clonal expansion of the mutated pituitary cell requires a secondary event for tumor progression.

This secondary event may be an additional somatic mutation or overexpression of genes in pituitary adenomas. Somatic mutations of the Ras oncogene have been associated with increased aggressiveness of prolactinomas and have been detected in metastasis of pituitary carcinomas.[376] Increased expression of cyclin E is associated with ACTH-producing pituitary adenomas. Overexpression of the pituitary tumor–transforming gene (*PTTG*) has been

thought to be involved in pituitary tumorigenesis as all pituitary adenoma subtypes, and particularly invasive adenomas express *PTTG*. *PTTG* is a member of the securin family that regulates the separation of chromatids during mitosis.[377] Overexpression of *PTTG* is thought to be at least partly responsible for the aneuploidism often observed in pituitary tumors. Promotor methylation of the retinoblastoma gene and p16INK4a and low expression of the p27Kip1 protein all cause loss of tumor suppressor gene function and have been associated with the development and the aggressiveness of pituitary adenomas.[378,379]

Several growth factors have been shown to induce pituitary hyperplasia, with or without adenoma development. FGF-β, which is expressed in the pituitary and is a potent mitogen for neuroectoderm cells and their synthesis, is induced in NIH3T3 cells overexpressing *PTTG*.[380] The heparin-binding secretory transforming gene *hst* seems to be associated with the aggressiveness of the tumor,[381] and pituitary TGF-α has been associated with estrogen-induced lactotrophic hyperplasia.

Few data concerning the effect of environmental factors on the development of pituitary tumors are available. However, the presence of the aryl hydrocarbon receptor on pituitary tumors, which is believed to mediate cell responses to toxins, such as dioxin,[382] suggests that such mechanisms may play a role in tumor development.

From both a morphologic and a mechanistic perspective, pituitary hyperplasia must be distinguished from pituitary adenomas. Mechanisms subserving hyperplasia certainly include overstimulation of particular pituitary cell types by hypothalamic factors, such as GHRH and CRH, which may be secreted ectopically and lead to somatotrophic and corticotrophic hyperplasia. Moreover, situations in which negative feedback on the hypothalamic–pituitary system is absent as well may result in hyperplasia. For example, and as discussed later, untreated hypothyroidism may result in thyrotrophic hyperplasia, and inadequate glucocorticoid replacement after adrenalectomy is thought to be involved in the development of corticotrophic hyperplasia (Nelson syndrome).[373]

Pituitary Adenomas

Nonfunctioning Adenomas and Gonadotroph Adenomas. *Nonfunctioning tumors of the pituitary* either do not secrete hormone or do so at such a low level that clinical syndromes of hormone excess do not develop. The majority of these tumors are microadenomas (<1 cm) and clinically lead to no significant symptoms. Most of the nonfunctioning adenomas that do come to medical attention are macroadenomas that compress both pituitary and nonpituitary tissues and result in hypopituitarism.

In 70% of patients with a nonfunctioning macroadenoma, visual field defects are present.[383] More than 90% of patients have at least one pituitary hormone deficiency before surgery, most commonly, GH deficiency followed by hypogonadism. In 80% of these patients, secondary hypothyroidism occurs, and in 60%, secondary adrenal insufficiency is present before surgery.[384] In the rare case in which an adenoma secretes biologically active FSH, amenorrhea, high E_2 concentrations, and multiple ovarian follicles can occur.[385] In pubertal girls, these events may result in premature breast development and vaginal bleeding.[386]

Typically, the clinical diagnosis of a *gonadotroph adenoma* is made by an absence of symptoms that would suggest a different type of pituitary adenoma (e.g., of somatotrophic, corticotrophic, lactotrophic, or thyrotrophic origin) and by basal and stimulated secretion of gonadotrophins and their subunits. Approximately 80% of clinically nonfunctioning pituitary tumors are gonadotroph adenomas, and hypersecretion of more than one monomeric subunit, with or without LH/FSH secretion, is common. β-FSH is elevated in approximately 30% of patients, whereas the α subunit is elevated in approximately 20% of patients. Intact FSH hypersecretion occurs less frequently. In rare cases, LH hypersecretion is present, but seldom is sufficient to result in abnormally elevated testosterone levels.

In the setting of primary gonadal failure in general and in postmenopausal women in particular, serum concentrations of the gonadotropins and free subunits are also increased in the absence of an adenoma. Under those conditions, intravenous administration of TRH has been reported to help to distinguish a normal hypothalamic–pituitary response to gonadal failure from a pituitary tumor. In approximately 40% of male patients and 69% of postmenopausal women with nonfunctioning pituitary adenomas, intravenous TRH results in an increase in serum concentrations of the gonadotropins or the free α/β subunit. In a study by Daneshdoost et al., none of the healthy postmenopausal women had LH-β, LH, or FSH[387] responses to TRH. Unfortunately, TRH is not currently available for clinical use in the United States. Few data exist about the utility of measuring pituitary glycoprotein hormones or their free subunits, although some literature suggests that a postsurgical decrease in circulating FSH concentration correlates with tumor size reduction. The final determination of the cellular basis of nonfunctioning pituitary tumors is based on immunohistochemistry. In most nonfunctioning tumors, immunostaining detects either intact pituitary glycoprotein hormones (FSH, LH, TSH) or the free subunits of these glycoproteins (α subunit, β-FSH, β-LH, β-TSH). In rare cases, PRL, ACTH, or GH is found. In fewer than 30% of nonfunctioning adenomas, no immunoreactive hormone or hormone subunit is seen (*null cell* pituitary tumors).[388]

With regard to therapeutic strategies, nonfunctioning pituitary adenomas may express receptors for TRH, GnRH, and dopamine, but treatment with somatostatin analogs, GnRH agonists, GnRH antagonists, and dopamine agonists have shown inconsistent results.[389] In a small number of patients, 6-month combination therapy with cabergoline and octreotide resulted in a 30% tumor size reduction, but only in those patients who had detectable baseline or stimulated LH, FSH, and α subunit levels.[390] To date, the treatment of choice remains surgical removal, with or without postsurgical radiation.

Prolactin-Secreting Adenomas. Under physiologic conditions, the regulation of PRL is inhibitory, mediated by dopamine through the type 2 isoform (D2) of the dopamine receptor. Dopaminergic neurons are primarily located in the arcuate nucleus (tuberoinfundibular system), but also in the rostral caudate and paraventricular nuclei (tuberohypophysial system).[391] Pituitary stalk injury or stalk compression interrupts these inhibitory circuits and results in increased PRL levels, which usually do not exceed 250 ng/mL. Although a primary PRL-releasing factor has yet to be identified, hypothalamic hormones known to stimulate PRL secretion include TRH, vasoactive intestinal peptide (VIP), oxytocin, PACAP, and galanin.[392-395]

Prolactin-secreting pituitary tumors include both prolactinomas and GH-producing pituitary tumors, which in 25% of cases cosecrete PRL. The latter observation reflects the fact that lactotroph and somatotroph cells derive from a common progenitor GH-expressing stem cell. Possible candidate genes involved in the pathogenesis of prolactinomas of monoclonal origin include *PTTG* as well as the heparin-binding secretory transforming (*hst*) gene. Other potential candidates include the overexpression of bone morphogenetic protein 4 and high-mobility group A2 gene (*HMGA2*).[381,396-398]

Prolactinomas are classified as microadenomas (<10 mm) or macroadenomas (≥10 mm), with the risk of progression from micro- to macroadenoma estimated at 4% to 7% over a period of 8 years.[399] Such a tumor progression has been found by Schlechte et al.[399] during an observation period of 8 years. High PRL levels, larger tumor size, cavernous sinus invasion, and resistance to dopamine agonists are associated with increased aggressiveness. A serum PRL cutoff level of 3300 ng/mL predicts an invasive tumor with a specificity of 91%.[400] Loss of tumor suppressor genes at loci 11q13, 13q12-14, 10q, and 1p is also thought to be associated with more invasive tumors. Other specific histochemical and biochemical markers associated with more aggressive prolactinomas include increased Ki-67/MIB-1 labeling indices and reduced E-cadherin/catenin expression as well as overexpression of the *hst* gene.[401]

Specific clinical symptoms of prolactinomas in premenopausal women include hypogonadism, which may present as infertility, oligomenorrhea, or amenorrhea,[402,403] and galactorrhea. However, it cannot be overemphasized that galactorrhea may also occur in normoprolactinemic women. Kleinberg et al. reported that 86% of women with idiopathic galactorrhea without amenorrhea had normal PRL levels.[404] Regardless of its cause, the degree of PRL elevation correlates with the severity of hypogonadism. Serum PRL levels greater than 100 ng/mL are associated with hypogonadism and low E_2, which result in amenorrhea, hot flashes, and vaginal dryness. PRL levels of 50 to 100 ng/mL can be associated with both oligomenorrhea and amenorrhea, and levels of 20 to 50 ng/mL can result in a shortening of the luteal phase and resultant infertility.[186] Women with hyperprolactinemia and amenorrhea exhibit lower spine and forearm BMD compared with women with hyperprolactinemia and normal menses.[405] In men, sexual dysfunction is the main clinical manifestation of prolactinomas. Galactorrhea occurs in approximately 15% to 25% of men with micro- or macroprolactinomas and is less frequent compared with women. Osteoporosis can also occur in men with increased PRL levels.[406-408]

Besides PRL-producing pituitary adenomas, other causes of hyperprolactinemia include medications such as antiemetics, antipsychotics, antidepressants, selective serotonin reuptake inhibitors, and narcotics, which antagonize dopamine action or elevate serotonin or endorphin activity.[347,409,410] Verapamil has also been shown to increase serum PRL levels.[411] Other causes of hyperprolactinemia include hypothyroidism, chest wall trauma,[412] estrogens, chest wall tumors, herpes zoster of the chest, chronic renal failure, alcoholic cirrhosis, pregnancy, nipple stimulation, and the postictal state.[413] Idiopathic hyperprolactinemia is the diagnosis when no cause can be found. In a study by Sluijmer et al.,[414] only 1 of 59 patients with idiopathic hyperprolactinemia who were followed for an average of 6.5 years had a pituitary adenoma.

In approximately 10% of patients with hyperprolactinemia, *macroprolactinemia* may be diagnosed. This condition is characterized by a predominance of high–molecular-mass circulating prolactin, which represents PRL complexed with anti-PRL immunoglobulins.[415] The cause of immunoglobulin production (mainly immunoglobulin G) is unclear. In a study that included more than 100 cases, dopaminergic treatment did not always result in normalization of serum PRL concentrations. Clinical symptoms associated with macroprolactinoma are sometimes absent because of the weak in vivo biologic activity of macroprolactin. In patients with high serum PRL levels and few or no symptoms related to PRL excess, this condition should be considered.[415]

Falsely low PRL measurements can be encountered in the presence of very high PRL levels, reflecting the hook effect. In this case, the antigen (PRL) is present in the serum in excess and there is not enough antibody to bind both sides of the antigen. The assay value is significantly lower than the real value. Dilution of the samples will resolve the problem. The hook effect should be considered in the presence of a large pituitary tumor and low levels of circulating PRL.[416]

The primary treatment objectives in patients with PRL-secreting pituitary adenomas include normalization of PRL levels, restoration of gonadal function, reduction of tumor size, and recovery of pituitary function. Both surgical and medical approaches to achieve these goals are available. Transsphenoidal surgery is effective in normalizing serum PRL levels in 70% to 91% of patients with microadenomas. Recurrence rates average 13% to 17%, and overall cure rates of 59% to 74% have been reported. In patients with macroadenomas, 32% to 38% show an initial normalization of PRL levels after surgery. However, the recurrence rate is 19% to 40% postoperatively, and the long-term cure rate is only 23% to 26%. These outcome data can vary significantly, depending on the experience of the neurosurgeon.[406]

Given that surgery does not reliably result in cure and possibly leads to pituitary deficiency, treatment with dopamine agonists has emerged as the primary therapy to both reduce tumor size and decrease PRL levels. Currently available medications to treat prolactinomas are dopamine agonists and include bromocriptine, quinagolide, and cabergoline.[417] A fourth drug, pergolide, is no longer used because of the finding that patients with Parkinson disease who were treated with this dopamine agonist had an increased risk of valvular heart disease.[418] Women who intend to become pregnant should be advised to use a mechanical form of contraception until two regular menstrual cycles

have occurred after therapy initiation and should stop taking bromocriptine in the setting of a positive pregnancy test. When fertility is not of concern, it may be reasonable to consider administering an oral contraceptive to women with microprolactinomas to prevent bone loss.[419] Even though it appears that the use of oral contraceptives is not associated with the growth of microprolactinomas, yearly PRL levels must be measured in women with microprolactinomas who are given oral contraceptives. Figure 19-23 shows an algorithm for the treatment of hyperprolactinemia.[419]

With regard to macroprolactinomas, treatment with the dopamine agonist bromocriptine restores gonadal function in 75% of cases. In the setting of chiasmal compression, studies show that medical treatment shrinks tumor size by at least 25% in most patients.[406] Visual improvement often precedes the tumor shrinkage and can occur within 12 hours. Tumor shrinkage is observed between 1 week and 1 year, with the major effect noted during the first 6 months after initiation of the treatment. In the case of chiasm herniation, visual acuity can worsen, despite a decrease in tumor size, and may require surgical intervention.[420] In most patients, lifelong treatment with dopamine agonists is necessary, although in 6% to 37% of patients, the drug may be discontinued without recurrence of hyperprolactinemia.[406,419]

A major issue related to medical treatment is intolerance to dopamine agonist therapy, which may include nausea, vomiting, postural hypotension, nasal stuffiness, and constipation. These side effects can almost always be avoided by gradually increasing the dose. Another therapeutic option in the case of intolerability to oral dopamine agonist therapy is the use of vaginal bromocriptine, which has been shown to be safe and effective and better tolerated.[421,422] Resistance to dopamine agonists is encountered on occasion and is usually an indication for surgical intervention. However, there is no clear definition of dopamine resistance, and it is difficult to assess in some cases because some tumors show a decrease in size, but no change in PRL levels and vice versa.[423]

In pregnant patients with a prolactinoma, measurement of serum PRL is not useful because PRL-secreting lactotrophs increase their contribution to the total pituitary cell population by 20% to 50% during pregnancy. Women with microprolactinomas who intend to become pregnant are at very low risk for tumor expansion during pregnancy. Patients who had a macroprolactinoma before the start of treatment, with or without chiasmal compression, may experience symptom recurrence when the medication is discontinued during pregnancy[424,425] and thus need careful monitoring. In the case of compressive symptoms, medical therapy can be reinitiated and surgical therapy may be considered. Bromocriptine is not approved for treatment during pregnancy in the United States, but its use during pregnancy has been described in isolated cases with no increase in fetal abnormalities, even though the medication does cross the placenta and suppresses fetal PRL production.[406,419] Prophylactic surgical tumor removal before pregnancy is another possibility if complications are expected.

Growth Hormone–Secreting Adenomas. Growth hormone is secreted in a pulsatile fashion by somatotrophic cells within the anterior pituitary gland. GH pulses can

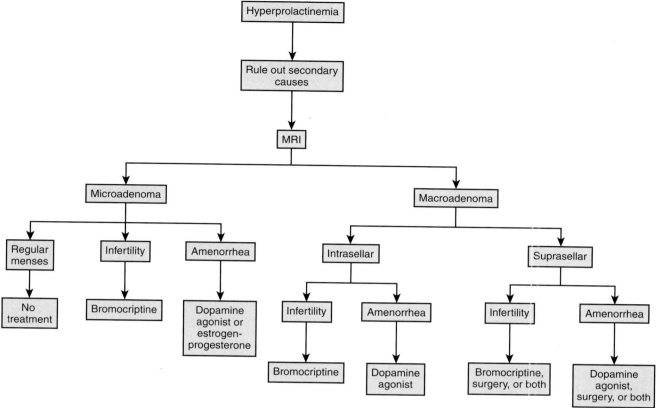

Figure 19-23. *Algorithm for the management of prolactinoma in women. (Reproduced from Schlechte JA: Clinical practice. Prolactinoma. N Engl J Med 349:2035, 2003, with permission.)*

be detected every 3 to 4 hours and are primarily regulated by the interaction between the hypothalamic peptides somatostatin and GHRH. Most GH pulses occur at night. Somatostatin determines the trough levels of GH, whereas GHRH stimulates the release of GH from the pituitary as well as the increase in GH gene transcription.[426] Approximately 75% of pituitary GH circulates in the 22-kDA form, with 5% to 10% in the 20-kDA form.[427]

Growth hormone–secreting pituitary tumors represent approximately 2.8% of all pituitary tumors,[428] and are monoclonal in origin, suggesting intrinsic genetic alterations as the cause for their development. In a subset of GH-secreting tumors, a mutation of the *gsp* gene has been found, with the prevalence ranging from 40% in whites to 10% in Japanese. Other candidate genes associated with GH adenomas include *PTTG, H-ras, MEN1*, and *P16INK4a*. *PTTG* overexpression in pituitary tumors has been shown to correlate with tumor size. In 25% of GH-secreting pituitary adenomas, PRL is co-secreted.[429,430] Adenomas with plurihormonal secretion often have no apparent clinical symptoms and are called *silent somatotroph adenomas*, with increased IGF-1 and PRL levels.

In very rare cases, *ectopic GHRH secretion* is the cause of increased GH secretion. In such cases, MRI shows a normal or mildly enlarged pituitary because GHRH leads to hyperplasia of the somatotrophs.[431] Sources of increased GHRH secretion include hypothalamic tumors, bronchial carcinoids, and tumors of the pancreas, gastrointestinal

tract, thyroid, and adrenals. Ectopic GH secretion by nonendocrine tumors has also been reported.[432]

Growth hormone–producing adenomas are phenotypically diverse, with two predominant histologic forms, *densely granulated* and *sparsely granulated*. The two forms differ in their morphologic features and respective growth patterns. *Densely granulated* GH cell adenomas show slow, expansive growth without invasion, resulting in the gradual development of acromegalic features. Such adenomas exert pressure on the surrounding nontumorous gland, resulting in the formation of a pseudocapsule, which helps with surgical removal. The *sparsely granulated* GH cell adenoma grows more rapidly and diffusely and is often invasive. Mixed adenomas expressing both GH and PRL are also more likely to invade surrounding tissues.[433]

Table 19-3 compares the most frequent symptoms found in acromegalic patients with symptoms found in patients with nonfunctioning pituitary tumors and prolactinomas. Many of the signs and symptoms of acromegaly develop slowly and insidiously, and patients are often treated for seemingly nonendocrine conditions long before the diagnosis of acromegaly is made. The average time between the onset of recognized symptoms and diagnosis is approximately 10 years.[428] Consequently, more than 70% of GH-secreting adenomas are macroadenomas at the time of diagnosis.[434] Besides the compressive symptoms of pituitary tumors, such as headache, visual field defects, and cranial nerve palsies, clinical symptoms of GH

TABLE 19-3

Comparison of Symptoms Between Acromegalic Patients and Patients with Nonfunctioning Pituitary Tumors and Prolactinomas

	Total Percentage		
Feature	Nonfunctioning (n = 99)	Acromegaly (n = 176)	Prolactinoma (n = 96)
Hypogonadal symptoms*	35	38	**70**
Headache	**48**	40	46
Galactorrhea	19	9	**49**
Visual deficit	**48**	26	19
Acral enlargement	—	**86**	—
Maxillofacial changes	—	**74**	—
Excessive perspiration	—	**48**	—
Arthralgia	—	**46**	—
Weight gain	13	18	13
Fatigue	20	26	17

*Hypogonadal symptoms include decreased libido, oligo- or amenorrhea, infertility, and erectile dysfunction.

The most frequent features observed for each tumor type are shown in **bold** print.

From Drange MR, Fram NR, Herman-Bonert V, Melmed S. Pituitary tumor registry: a novel clinical resource. J Clin Endocrinol Metab 85:168, 2000.

hypersecretion include hyperhidrosis, acral enlargement, thickness of the soft tissues of the hands and feet, prognathism, jaw malocclusion, macroglossia, arthralgias and arthritis, bilateral carpal tunnel syndrome, proximal myopathy, frontal bossing, skin tags, colon polyps, cardiomyopathy, hypertension, diabetes mellitus, sleep apnea, and visceromegaly. Cardiac disease is the primary cause of death in untreated acromegaly, with 50% of patients dying before the age of 50 years. Hypertension occurs in approximately 40% of patients, and left ventricular hypertrophy is present in more than 50% of normotensive acromegalic patients.

The serum IGF-I level is the best biochemical marker of clinical disease activity in acromegaly. Before the availability of IGF-I assays, dynamic tests were used and the oral glucose tolerance test ([OGTT] 75-g oral glucose load with serum GH sampling every 30 minutes over 2 hours) was the recommended test for the diagnosis and assessment of therapeutic outcome postoperatively. The OGTT may help diagnostically when there is a discrepancy between GH and IGF-I data, but it does not add additional diagnostic value when IGF-I levels are clearly elevated. A GH nadir during OGTT of less than 1 µg/L theoretically excludes acromegaly and indicates postoperative remission. However, the results of the OGTT must be interpreted with caution in conditions such as puberty, pregnancy, hepatic and renal disease, AN, and diabetes mellitus, all of which may cause inadequate GH suppression. A random GH level of 0.4 µg/L or less and an IGF-I level in the age- and sex-matched reference range excludes the diagnosis of acromegaly.[435] Clinicians who use the DPC Immulite GH assay (Siemens, Deerfield, IL) with an analytical sensitivity of 0.01 µg/L

should apply an OGTT nadir value of 0.04 µg/L for women and 0.01 µg/L for men.

Treatment options for GH-secreting adenomas include surgery (with or without presurgical medical treatment), medical treatment, and RT. Data on postsurgical cure rates and recurrence rates must be interpreted by carefully reviewing the specific cutoff levels used for defining cure or recurrence. Surgical cure rates also depend on the experience and workload of the surgeon.[436] Frank et al.[437] defined remission by a basal GH level of less than 2.5 ng/mL, a normal sex- and age-adjusted IGF-I level, and a GH nadir of less than 1 ng/mL after OGTT, and reported a cure rate of 83% in microadenomas and 64.5% in macroadenomas. Intraoperative invasiveness of the tumor decreased the cure rate to 44%, which was similar to the findings of other studies that reported that GH is controlled in approximately 80% of microadenomas. In macroadenomas, on the other hand, IGF-I and GH are controlled in fewer than 50% of cases. Using these criteria, long-term surgical remission rates range from 42% to 62% and multimodality (surgery followed by RT or medical treatment) remission rates vary from 52% to 97%.[434,438] Independent of which cutoff levels are used, both GH and IGF-I should be measured 3 months after surgery, although stabilization of IGF-1 levels can take up to 12 months. In addition, preoperative treatment with long-acting somatostatin analogs can have a prolonged suppressive effect on GH of up to 3 months postoperatively.[435] The postoperative GH level is the most important determinant of mortality outcome, with published data suggesting that a random GH level of less than 2 µg/L measured by radioimmunoassay is associated with the reversal of increased mortality and continued suppression of GH. Persistence of disease (using the less stringent criteria of 5 µg/L) is associated with a 2.4 to 4.8-fold enhanced mortality.[439] If GH and IGF-I are normal 3 months postsurgery, annual follow-up measurements are recommended. The postsurgical serum GH level during the OGTT should be as low as 0.3 µg/L measured by a current two-site assay. The IGF-I level should be within the age-adjusted reference interval according to the latest consensus statement of the Joint Consensus Conference of the Growth Hormone Research Society and the Pituitary Society, published in 2004.[435] Residual pituitary function should be assessed no later than 3 months postsurgery.[435]

Medical therapy includes *dopamine agonists* (e.g., cabergoline, bromocriptine), *somatostatin analogs* (e.g., octreotide, lanreotide), and the *GH receptor antagonist* pegvisomant. Dopamine agonists can provide adequate control in a minority of patients with acromegaly, and it may take 3 months to achieve maximal suppression of GH and IGF-I. Measurements should be performed annually after normalization. Vilar et al.[440] reported normalization of PRL and IGF-1 and 70% to 90% tumor shrinkage with cabergoline in two cases of somatotroph macroadenomas co-secreting PRL and GH. Cabergoline in combination with somatostatin receptor ligands may improve the responsiveness of patients with acromegaly that is otherwise resistant to maximal doses of somatostatin receptor ligands.[441] High-dose dopamine agonists used alone lead to a GH level of less than 5 ng/mL in only 15% of patients and normalize IGF-I levels in fewer than 10%. The advantage is the relatively low cost of the drugs, but disadvantages include the incidence of side effects in approximately 30% of patients.

Satisfactory GH and IGF-I levels are achieved in approximately 65% of patients, and IGF-I levels are normalized in 70% with somatostatin analogs. The effects are inversely related to pretreatment GH levels. Approximately 50% of patients show 30% average tumor volume shrinkage. Transient gastrointestinal symptoms, such as nausea, vomiting, and diarrhea, can occur during the first 2 weeks of therapy, and 25% of patients have gallbladder sludge and gallstones, which are usually diagnosed within the first 2 years after the start of treatment. Somatostatin analogs inhibit insulin secretion and may cause deterioration of glucose metabolism. Therefore, fasting blood glucose and hemoglobin A_{1C} should be measured annually. Although octreotide is given subcutaneously three times daily, there are also long-term depot somatostatin preparations (octreotide long-acting release) available that are given every 3 months.[442]

The GH receptor antagonist pegvisomant directly inhibits GH action in the periphery without inhibiting GH secretion. It normalizes circulating IGF-I levels in more than 95% of the patients treated for up to 36 months, whereas circulating GH values may rise during the first weeks, but then plateau. Pegvisomant is indicated after failure of other therapy options. Of 160 patients, 2 exhibited progression of tumor growth under pegvisomant therapy; therefore, patients should have an MRI every 6 months during the first year of pegvisamont therapy and annually thereafter. Therapy is monitored with IGF-I measurements every 6 months. In addition, liver enzymes should be monitored over the initial 6 months of therapy, given the potential transaminitis that can occur with GH antagonist therapy.[443]

Indications for the use of RT in acromegaly include conditions in which surgery or medical therapy does not lead to GH and IGF-I normalization. RT techniques include external radiation with a cyclotron or cobalt 60 source, proton-beam therapy, and stereotactic ablation by gamma knife radiosurgery. Whereas RT decreases GH levels to less than 5 ng/mL in 90% of patients within 18 years, fewer than 5% show a normalization of IGF-I.[444] An overall reduction in GH levels of 30% to 50% can be expected in the first 1 to 2 years, with a slower rate of decline after that. Pituitary deficiency develops in 50% of patients within 10 years of RT. GH and IGF-I should be measured 2 years after conventional multiple-dose RT, and pituitary function should be assessed annually. After gamma knife therapy, GH and IGF-I should be measured after 1 year and residual pituitary function measured at 6-month intervals.[435]

ACTH-Secreting Adenomas. In 70% of cases, hypercortisolism (Cushing syndrome) is caused by excessive ACTH secretion from the pituitary (Cushing disease).[445] Cushing disease is almost always caused by a solitary corticotroph adenoma[446] and presents more often in women than in men. The reported incidence is between 0.7 and 2.4 cases per million inhabitants per year, and patients have a fourfold higher mortality rate compared with age- and sex-matched peers as a result of cardiovascular complications.[447] Approximately 90% of the adenomas are microadenomas (<1 cm in diameter). The etiology of Cushing disease is unclear. Monoclonal tumor cell expansion is one possibility. Based on the findings in a patient with generalized glucocorticoid resistance due to a missense mutation of the glucocorticoid receptor preceding the development of Cushing disease,[448] others speculate that decreased negative feedback might also play a role in corticotroph adenoma formation. The cyclin-dependent kinase inhibitor p27 (Kip1) is believed to be involved in corticotroph tumorigenesis, and cytogenetic studies show loss of chromosomes 2, 15q, and 22. Brg 1 and histone deacetylase 2 (HDAC2) are considered candidates for glucocorticoid resistance and are also believed to be involved in the tumorigenic process of the adenoma.[449]

Symptoms of Cushing disease result from excessive cortisol production, with its widespread systemic effects. One of the earliest signs of Cushing disease is weight gain, often associated with increased abdominal, supraclavicular, facial, and dorsocervical fat.[450,451] However, proximal muscle weakness, with preservation of distal strength, plethora, and ecchymoses are considered the most discriminant indicators of hypercortisolism.[452,453] Such muscle weakness affects the upper arms and legs and results from cortisol-induced mobilization of amino acids from the muscle. If hypokalemia is present, muscle weakness is significantly more prominent. Cutaneous atrophy leads to wrinkling of the skin, which is especially obvious at the dorsum of the hands and elbows. The skin also can show striae around the hips, abdomen, shoulders, and breasts. These striae are purple, in contrast to the white or pink striae found in generalized obesity, and the width of hypercortisolism-associated striae often is greater than 1 cm. The skin frequently shows increased bruisability as a result of increased fragility of the capillaries. Vellus hair, especially on the upper cheeks and forehead, can also be found. Other skin manifestations include those associated with fungal infections. Many patients have emotional and cognitive changes that correlate well with the degree of hypercortisolism and include depressed mood, irritability, tearfulness, insomnia, and anxiety.[454] Osteoporosis is present in 40% to 80% of patients, and a history of fractures of the feet, ribs, and vertebrae is not unusual. Hypertension occurs in approximately 80% of patients, and type 2 diabetes is present in 20% to 30%.[455,456] Menstrual and sexual dysfunction occurs in up to 75% of patients. A summary of the clinical manifestations of Cushing disease is shown in Table 19-4.

The diagnosis of Cushing disease does not rely on a single test, but often requires the combination of several biochemical tests. The procedures used to confirm the diagnosis are based on the fact that, in hypercortisolism (Cushing syndrome), the normal circadian rhythm of cortisol is no longer present and the normal feedback characteristics of glucocorticoids on the HPA axis are disturbed. To confirm hypercortisolism, the consensus statement by Arnaldi et al. stated that the 24-hour urinary free cortisol (UFC) measurement should be the initial screening test.[452] The 24-hour UFC is reported to have specificity of 100%, but sensitivity ranges from 45% to 71%. The authors suggest that up to three 24-hour UFC measurements should be obtained. When measuring urinary cortisol high-performance liquid chromatography, interfering

TABLE 19-4

Frequency of Clinical Signs and Symptoms of Cushing Syndrome in Five Series of Adults (1952-1982) and Two Series of Children (1994, 1995)

Sign/Symptom(%)	Plotz et al. 1952 (n = 33)	Sprague et al. 1956 (n = 100)	Soffer et al. 1961 (n = 50)	Urbanic and George 1981 (n = 31)	Ross and Linch 1982 (n = 70)	Magiakou et al. 1994 (n = 59)	Weber et al. 1995 (n = 12)
Obesity or weight gain	97	84	86	79	97	90	93
Decreased linear growth	—	—	—	—	—	83	80
Hypertension	84	90	88	77	74	47	—
Plethora	89	81	78	—	94	—	—
Round face	89	92	92	—	88	—	—
Hirsutism	73	74	84	64	81	78	58
Thin skin	—	—	—	84	—	—	—
Abnormal glucose tolerance	94	—	84	39	50	—	—
Easy bruising	60	62	68	77	62	25	17
Weakness	83	—	58	90	56	45	50
Osteopenia or fracture	83	—	56	48	50	—	—
Electrocardiogram changes or atherosclerosis	66/89	—	34	—	55	—	—
Menstrual changes	86	35	72	69	84	78	20
Decreased libido (men/women)	86	—	100/33	55	100	—	—
Depression or emotional lability	67	—	40	48	62	—	25
Headache	58	—	—	—	47	—	50
Striae	60	64	50	51	56	61	—
Edema	60	—	66	48	50	—	—
Acne	82	64	—	35	21	47	58
Buffalo hump	—	67	34	—	54	—	—
Female balding	—	—	51	—	13	—	20
Lipid abnormalities	39	—	—	—	—	—	—
Decreased wound healing	42	—	—	—	—	—	—
Delayed bone age	—	—	—	—	—	11	—
Accelerated bone age	—	—	—	—	—	8	—
Pigmentation	—	—	—	—	—	14	8

From Newell-Price J. Clinical manifestations of CD. Endocr Rev 19:647, 1998.

substances, such as carbamazepine and digoxin, can produce false-positive results. Therefore, the preferred method for measurement of 24-hour UFC is tandem mass spectrometry, which is less likely to produce false-positive results. Of note, if the glomerular filtration rate is less than 30 mL/min, urinary cortisol excretion is decreased, resulting in a false-negative result.[457]

Another first-line diagnostic procedure is the low-dose (1 mg) overnight dexamethasone suppression test (DST). The recommended level for a normal plasma cortisol level after a low-dose overnight DST is less than 1.8 µg/dL (50 nmol/L), with a required cortisol assay sensitivity of 1 µg/dL.[452] Some centers suggest the 2-day low-dose DST as a first-line screening test[458] in which the patient takes 0.5 mg dexamethasone orally every 6 hours. Urine is collected for UFC on 2 baseline days and is measured on the second day of dexamethasone administration, or cortisol is measured at 9 AM and 48 hours after the first dose. A normal response consists of a decrease in UFC to less than 10 µg/24 hours on the second day after dexamethasone administration or a plasma cortisol level of less than 1.8 µg/dL on the morning of the last dose of dexamethasone.[452]

Findling and Raff[459] suggested that measurement of a late-night or bedtime salivary cortisol level is an excellent surrogate for documenting an increased midnight serum cortisol level and is the test of choice. The assay has sensitivity and specificity of greater than 90% to 95%. Although this approach may be the most useful for the practicing endocrinologist, false-positive findings may be encountered in certain conditions, such as hypertension and advanced age, and in the setting of psychiatric disease.

Exogenous hypercortisolism always must be considered in the evaluation of patients for Cushing syndrome. The use of all prescription and over-the-counter medications and herbal remedies must be assessed, including injections into joints. This diagnosis is suggested by findings of suppressed ACTH and cortisol with no response to CRH or ACTH. Screening for synthetic glucocorticoids in serum or urine may be useful. Factitious hypercortisolism due to exogenous ACTH injections shows similar laboratory data as Cushing disease, but attention to the patient's history and a search for injection sites may show the cause.[460]

Other factors to consider include the effects of exogenous compounds, such as estrogens, antiepileptic drugs, and glycyrrhetinic acid, on cortisol measurements. Estrogen administration increases corticosteroid-binding globulin levels, with a concomitant increase in total plasma cortisol levels.[461] However, free cortisol levels and 24-hour UFC levels are normal. Pharmacologic agents, such as phenytoin, barbiturates, and rifampicin, have an effect on the metabolism of dexamethasone by increasing its hepatic conjugation and biliary excretion. Thus, measurement of urinary free cortisol rather than a DST is suggested in these patients.[462,463] Glycyrrhetinic acid, an extract from licorice, has been shown to increase UFC by inhibiting 11β-hydroxysteroid dehydrogenase, which converts cortisol to cortisone. As a result, there is a cortisol excess, especially in the kidney, with increased concentrations in the urine, but not in the plasma. Therefore, urinary cortisol measurements can be misleading in patients taking licorice.[464]

Once the diagnosis of Cushing syndrome is made, the next challenge is to determine whether the hypercortisolism is ACTH-dependent or ACTH-independent. The interpretation of circulating ACTH levels depends on proper preanalytical sampling and on the use of an assay that can reliably detect plasma ACTH values of less than 10 pg/mL. ACTH values of greater than 10 pg/mL suggest ACTH-dependent Cushing syndrome (Cushing disease), whereas values of less than 10 pg/mL are most often consistent with ACTH-independent Cushing syndrome. However, caution is warranted in the interpretation of ACTH levels, given that Cushing disease can occur with ACTH values of less than 10 pg/mL in rare cases,[465] and adrenal hypercortisolism can be present with values of greater than 20 pg/mL. Values of 10 to 20 pg/mL are considered indeterminate, and it is prudent to repeat measurements of ACTH or perform a CRH test. If the ACTH response to CRH is greater than 20 pg/mL, Cushing disease is very likely.

If the diagnosis of an ACTH-dependent pituitary adenoma seems probable, MRI may help to locate the adenoma. In 65% of cases, MRI shows a pituitary tumor. However, the diagnosis of Cushing disease cannot be based on MRI imaging alone, given that some ACTH-secreting adenomas may not be visible, even after gadolinium enhancement, and nonsecreting incidentalomas may be present and misinterpreted as the source of ACTH.

Cushing disease accounts for 70% to 90% of cases of ACTH-dependent hypercortisolism. However, ectopic ACTH production must be excluded. Currently, the procedure of choice to exclude ectopic ACTH production is IPSS. In experienced centers, bilateral IPSS has very high sensitivity (95% to 99%) for diagnosing Cushing disease. The test is recommended in patients with ACTH-dependent Cushing syndrome who have clinical, biochemical, or radiologic findings that are discordant or equivocal. An IPPS-to-peripheral cortisol ratio (IPSS/P) greater than 2 in the basal state and 3 after CRH administration suggests the diagnosis of Cushing disease. False-negative results with IPSS can occur as a result of unsuccessful catheterization or anomalous venous drainage; the additional measurement of PRL can be helpful in such cases.[466] IPSS has limited utility in lateralization of ACTH-producing pituitary adenomas within the gland. In a literature review of 313 cases, the diagnostic accuracy ranged from 50% to 100%, and a gradient of 1.4 or greater across both sides of the pituitary predicted the tumor location in 78% of cases. In the case of asymmetrical drainage, IPSS predicted the lateralization of the adenoma in only 44% of patients. Cavernous sinus sampling has been proposed as an alternative to IPSS for lateralization because the cavernous sinuses are closer to the pituitary. Accurate localization was reported

in 73.3% of cases without CRH and in 93.3% of cases with CRH stimulation.[467]

A less invasive test for distinguishing ectopic ACTH production from pituitary-dependent Cushing syndrome is the single-dose, 8-mg overnight DST, which has 92% sensitivity and 100% specificity for Cushing disease when morning plasma cortisol is suppressed by 50%, according to Tyrrell et al.[468] Aron et al. reported sensitivity of 81% and specificity of 66.7%, with both the 2-day, high-dose DST (2 mg dexamethasone every 6 hours for 48 hours) and the 8-mg, single-dose overnight test using the 50% threshold.[469] Patients with ectopic ACTH secretion were significantly older (mean, 51 years versus 40.2 years), were more likely to be male (58.8% versus 27.4%), had a shorter duration of clinical findings (11.6 months versus 39.9 months), and were more likely to have hypokalemia (50% versus 8.6%). Such patients also had higher baseline 24-hour UFC levels (mean, 3015 μg/day versus 422 μg/day) and higher plasma ACTH levels (210 pg/mL versus 78 pg/mL)[469] compared with patients with Cushing disease. Figure 19-24 describes a possible diagnostic approach to determine the source of hypercortisolis.[452]

Special mention should be made of differentiating patients with Cushing syndrome from those with the much more common PCOS. Women of reproductive age who have hypercortisolism have symptoms similar to those of women with PCOS, including oligomenorrhea or amenorrhea, adrenal hyperandrogenism with acne or hirsutism, and metabolic syndrome.[452] Kaltsas et al. speculated that PCOS may be one manifestation of Cushing syndrome. In their small group of women, they found that 46% had ovaries with morphologic features of PCOS.[470] Because the prevalence of PCOS is significantly higher than that of Cushing syndrome, the latter should always be considered in the differential diagnosis of PCOS. Especially in the case of mildly elevated cortisol levels, an endocrine profile suggestive of PCOS can be present (estrogen sufficiency, normal or increased androgen levels, enlarged ovaries). The authors also found that patients with proven Cushing syndrome had significantly higher blood pressure (both systolic and diastolic) than women with PCOS.[470]

The treatment of choice of Cushing disease is selective transsphenoidal adenoma resection. The procedure has a mortality rate of less than 1%, and the most common postsurgical complication is transient DI, which may be present in up to 28% of patients.[471] The goal of surgery is selective adenomectomy and preservation of as much normal pituitary tissue as possible. If it is not possible to identify the tumor, hemihypophysectomy on the side of the gland with the ACTH gradient on IPSS is often performed. Recovery of the HPA axis after successful surgery rarely occurs before 3 to 6 months and commonly is not confirmed until 1 year after the procedure. Until recovery is confirmed, patients are treated with glucocorticoid replacement.

The definition of cure of Cushing disease is still under debate. Several reports suggest that serum morning cortisol levels of less than 5 μg/dL measured at day 1 or day 2 after surgery (first surgery) are associated with sustained remission in 93% of patients after 32 months.[472] Others suggest that postsurgical remission is likely if serum cortisol levels

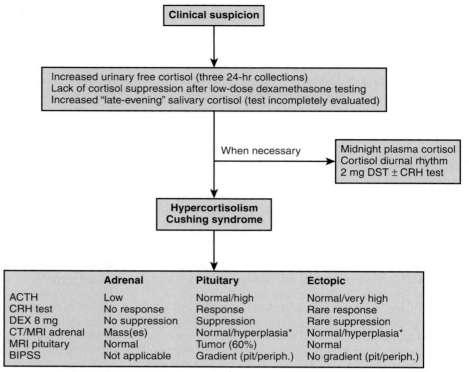

Figure 19-24. *Cascade of tests to diagnose Cushing syndrome. ACTH, adrenocorticotropic hormone; BIPSS, bilateral inferior petrosal sinus sampling; CRH, corticotrophin-releasing hormone; CT, computed tomography; MRI, magnetic resonance imaging; pit/periph, pituitary/peripheral. (Reproduced from Arnaldi G, Angeli A, Atkinson AB, et al. Diagnosis and complications of Cushing's syndrome: a consensus statement. J Clin Endocrinol Metab 88:5593, 2003, with permission.)*

Clinical suspicion

Increased urinary free cortisol (three 24-hr collections)
Lack of cortisol suppression after low-dose dexamethasone testing
Increased "late-evening" salivary cortisol (test incompletely evaluated)

When necessary → Midnight plasma cortisol
Cortisol diurnal rhythm
2 mg DST ± CRH test

Hypercortisolism
Cushing syndrome

	Adrenal	Pituitary	Ectopic
ACTH	Low	Normal/high	Normal/very high
CRH test	No response	Response	Rare response
DEX 8 mg	No suppression	Suppression	Rare suppression
CT/MRI adrenal	Mass(es)	Normal/hyperplasia*	Normal/hyperplasia*
MRI pituitary	Normal	Tumor (60%)	Normal
BIPSS	Not applicable	Gradient (pit/periph.)	No gradient (pit/periph.)

*Nodules

are 2 µg/dL or less within 72 hours of surgery.[473,474] When applying a serum cortisol threshold of 1.8 µg/dL or less measured 5 to 14 days after surgery and at least 24 hours after the last dose of hydrocortisone, the reported surgical remission rate was between 40% and 65%, and the 10-year incidence of recurrence was 25%.[472] Other studies reported postoperative remission rates of 60% to 90%.[475] Of note, postoperative detectable serum cortisol levels above those suggested earlier may still be compatible with cure and can decrease within 2 weeks. However, the absence of secondary adrenal insufficiency 4 to 6 weeks postoperatively suggests that the patient has persistent hypercortisolism or will have a recurrence.[459] When no histologic confirmation of tumor removal can be made, remission is achieved in only 50% of patients.[476] Reasons for surgical failure include residual tumor within the pituitary gland, tumor located ectopically in the intrasellar or perisellar region, and residual invasive tumor within the dura mater of the sella turcica or the cavernous sinus.[477] When surgery is unsuccessful, additional therapeutic options include repeated transsphenoidal surgery, medical treatment, RT, and bilateral adrenalectomy. A report by Locatelli et al.[475] suggests a favorable effect on remission in patients with initial surgical failure when the repeat surgery is done within 15 days. Figure 19-25 summarizes their suggested management of Cushing disease.[475]

When surgical intervention fails or is likely to be unsuccessful (e.g., in patients with cavernous sinus or dural invasion), pituitary radiation—either conventional or gamma knife—is recommended. Remission rates of 76% have been reported for gamma knife RT.[478,479] The expected normalization of cortisol levels occurs 12 to 36 months after RT; thus, adrenostatic therapy is required in the interim.[478,479]

Medical treatment targets adrenal steroid secretion and includes ketoconazole, metyrapone, aminoglutethimide, mitotane, and etomidate. *Ketoconazole* is an imidazole antifungal agent and an inhibitor of cytochrome P450 enzymes that blocks adrenal steroid synthesis at several points. The principal side effects of ketoconazole include hepatic toxicity, skin rash, gastrointestinal upset, and gynecomastia.[480,481] *Metyrapone* blocks the cortisol synthetic pathway by inhibiting the enzyme 11β-hydroxylase. The drug achieves cortisol trough levels 2 hours postdose and is given in three to four doses per day. However, the drug is not approved by the U.S. Food and Drug Administration for this use and has been withdrawn from the U.S. market. The main side effects include hirsutism, acne, edema, hypertension, and gastrointestinal upset.[183] *Aminoglutethimide* blocks the conversion of cholesterol to pregnenolone and causes a reduction in the synthesis of all hormonally active steroids, including corticosteroid production. Its side effects include a morbilliform rash, fever, and dizziness. *Mitotane* blocks adrenal cortisol synthesis and has direct cytotoxic effects on the adrenals. In high doses, it can achieve remission in up to 83% of patients. In lower doses and in combination with RT, remission can be achieved in up to 80% of patients.[482] The onset of effect can take up to 6 to 8 weeks, and effects can last for weeks and even months after discontinuation due to its lipophilic activity. Major side effects are related to gastrointestinal and neurologic toxicity. Elevated liver enzyme levels, abnormal platelet function, and hypercholesterolemia are other side effects. High doses are used for adrenocortical carcinoma and

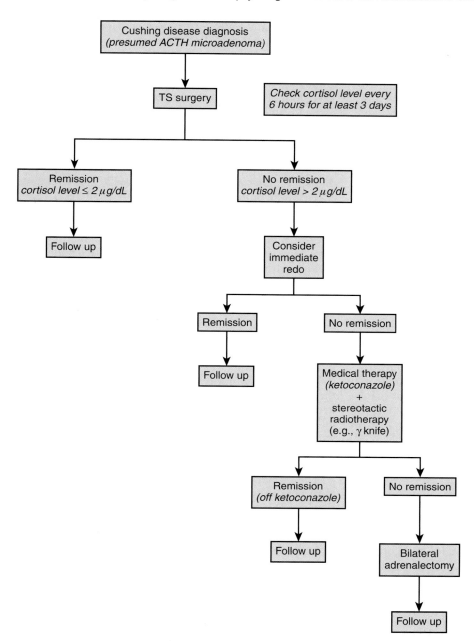

Figure 19-25. Therapeutic algorithm for the management of Cushing disease. ACTH, adrenocorticotropic hormone TS, trans-sphenoidal. (Reproduced from Locatelli M, Vance ML, Laws ER: Clinical review: the strategy of immediate reoperation for transsphenoidal surgery for Cushing's disease. J Clin Endocrinol Metab 90:5478, 2005, with permission.)

can cause anorexia and ataxia. *Etomidate* is an imidazole-derived anesthetic agent that inhibits adrenocortical 11β-hydroxylase. Given as a nonhypnotic low-dose infusion (0.1 mg/kg/hour or lower), it has been shown to control cortisol levels in severe hypercortisolemia.[483] It acts rapidly, but its use is limited because it must be given parenterally.

In cases of persistent hypercortisolism or intolerable side effects related to the adrenostatic therapy, bilateral adrenalectomy is an option. It has no risk of hypopituitarism and may be chosen over RT in younger patients who worry about postradiation hypopituitarism and loss of reproductive function. Disadvantages of bilateral adrenalectomy include the lifelong requirement to take glucocorticoid and mineralocorticoid replacement therapy as well as a 50% risk of Nelson syndrome (discussed later). Prophylactic

pituitary radiation before adrenalectomy can reduce this risk to 25%.[484]

Nelson Syndrome. The first case of Nelson syndrome (NS) was reported in 1958.[485] Since that time, various criteria have been used to define this syndrome, including: (1) the presence of a pituitary macroadenoma, and (2) the presence of high ACTH levels after bilateral adrenalectomy. Nelson et al. suggested that the definition need not include the presence of a pituitary adenoma.[486] More recently, others have used the term *corticotroph tumor progression* for NS.[487]

The pathogenetic mechanisms underlying the development of a Nelson tumor are not fully understood. NS is believed to be in part the result of lack of cortisol feedback after adrenalectomy. Other findings support a role for mutations in regulatory genes.[448] Some studies suggest that ACTH stimulation after CRH infusion is greater and more prolonged in NS compared with Cushing disease.[488] Studies of the ACTH secretion profile in NS show an altered secretion profile compared with patients with Cushing disease.[489] Immunohistochemically, tumors stain strongly positive for ACTH.

Published data suggest that the prevalence of NS after adrenalectomy ranges from 8% to 50%.[484,490] The interval between adrenalectomy and the diagnosis of NS ranges from 0.5 year to 24 years. According to Assie et al.,[491] a shorter duration of Cushing disease and a relatively high plasma ACTH concentration in the year after adrenalectomy are predictive of corticotrophic tumor progression. In their study, tumor progression was first diagnosed as early as 3 years after adrenalectomy. Others found a relationship between pretreatment urinary cortisol levels and the occurrence of NS.[492] Kelly et al.[493] reported that a shorter duration of the disease before adrenalectomy is also predictive of tumor progression.

The clinical features of NS are caused by the mass effects of the tumor on surrounding structures, secondary loss of other pituitary hormones, and the effects of the high serum alpha-melanocyte–stimulating hormone (α-MSH) concentration (a derivative of proopiomelanocortin) on the skin. Cutaneous hyperpigmentation of hand lines, scars, gingivae, and areolae is present.[494] The degree of pigmentation reflects the level of serum α-MSH.

Treatment strategies for Nelson syndrome include surgical intervention and RT, which rarely cure the disease. There have also been therapeutic approaches with drug treatment. Because the peroxisome proliferative-activated receptor (PPARγ) is expressed in corticotroph adenomas, the effect of PPARγ agonists on tumor growth has been documented. Using a rodent model, some studies have suggested that PPARγ agonists have a favorable effect on retarding tumor growth and lowering ACTH and cortisol levels.[495,496] However, studies in humans that have focused on the effects of rosiglitazone (given over 8 weeks) have not shown a reduction in ACTH. Longer-duration studies and the evaluation of PPARγ agonists with stronger agonist activity warrant consideration.[497] Other neuropharmacologic approaches, such as treatment with valproate or dopamine agonists, are rarely effective. Studies investigating neurosurgical interventions show success rates of 10% to 70%.[498] RT of the pituitary after adrenalectomy has been shown to reduce the risk of NS by 50% in some studies.[484]

Thyrotropin-Secreting Tumors and Thyrotroph Hyperplasia. The term *thyrotropin-producing pituitary tumors* describes two distinct clinical conditions: true thyrotroph neoplasia, which results in secondary hyperthyroidism, and pituitary hyperplasia, resulting from long-standing hypothyroidism.[499] It is important to distinguish one from the other because the therapeutic approaches are different.

Thyrotrophic adenomas (TSHomas) account for 0.5% to 1% of all pituitary adenomas, with a prevalence of one to two cases per million. They have no sex preference. TSHomas are almost always benign but are,

in approximately 90% of cases, macroadenomas, which are highly invasive.[500] Such tumors have been shown to be monoclonal in origin.[501] Previous thyroid ablation appears to have deleterious effects on the size of the pituitary adenoma. Approximately 72% of tumors secrete TSH alone. In 28% of cases, hypersecretion of TSH is associated with hypersecretion of the α subunit and can also be associated with hypersecretion of GH and PRL and, in rare cases, with gonadotropins. No association with ACTH is known.

Clinically, patients present with symptoms of hyperthyroidism (goiter and clinical thyrotoxicosis) and with mass effects of the pituitary adenoma (visual field defects, headache). However, the size of the tumor in the imaging study does not correlate with serum TSH levels.[499] Clinical characteristics of patients with TSHomas are shown in Table 19-5. More than 90% of patients present with a goiter. Approximately one third had an inappropriate thyroidectomy or radioiodine thyroid ablation before the TSH-secreting pituitary adenoma was discovered. Typically, the concentration of thyroid hormone is elevated in the presence of detectable TSH. Some reports suggest that TSH molecules in patients with TSHomas have increased bioactivity.[502] It has been suggested that an α subunit/TSH ratio above 1 indicates a TSHoma.[503] The TSH inhibition test using T_3 (80-100 μg) given for 8 to 10 days can be used to confirm the presence of a TSHoma. The lack of suppression confirms the autonomy of the TSH secretion by the adenoma, but the test is contraindicated in the elderly and patients with coronary heart disease.[499] In the rare cases when no pituitary adenoma is present, resistance to thyroid hormone must be considered.

The primary approach to treatment of TSHomas is surgical removal of the pituitary tumor. Approximately two thirds of TSHomas respond to surgery or irradiation.[499] An undetectable TSH level 1 week after surgery typically indicates successful surgery. A measurable TSH level after the T_3 suppression test suggests the need for additional treatment after surgery. If surgery is not an option, RT followed by somatostatin analog administration can be considered.

Pituitary hyperplasia as a consequence of untreated hypothyroidism is rarely symptomatic, but may present with hypothyroidism, headache, visual defects, hyperprolactinemia, amenorrhea, or galactorrhea. A goiter is present in 16% of cases. In children, presenting signs and symptoms include abnormal puberty, delayed bone age, and short stature. Treatment is medical, with adequate thyroid hormone replacement resulting in total tumor regression in 62% and partial regression in 29% of cases,[499] occurring sometimes within 1 or 2 months. In children, initial therapy can lead to pseudotumor cerebri; such a complication should be considered when symptoms worsen after initiation of thyroid hormone replacement.

Adenomas of Multiple Endocrine Neoplasia Type 1

The combined occurrence of tumors of the parathyroid gland, pancreatic islet cells, and the anterior pituitary is characteristic of *multiple endocrine neoplasia type 1* (MEN 1; also called *Wermer syndrome*). The *MEN1* gene is located

TABLE 19-5

Clinical Characteristics of Patients with Thyroid-Stimulating Hormone–Secreting Pituitary Adenoma Reported in the Literature (updated to January 1996)

	No thyroid ablation % (n)[*]	Previous thyroid ablation % (n)	All patients % (n)
Age (yr)[†]	41 ± 15 (156)	42 ± 13 (80)	41 ± 14 (236)
Sex (female %)	52 (168)	62 (87)	55 (255)
Goiter	92 (114)	97 (63)	94 (177)
Thyroglobulin autoantibodies or Thyroid peroxidase autoantibodies	11 (63)	2 (43)	8 (106)
Anti-thyrotropin receptor autoantibodies	5 (40)	3 (33)	4 (73)
Exophthalmos	8 (79)	4 (49)	6 (128)
Menstrual disorders[‡]	40 (30)	23 (40)	30 (70)
Galactorrhea[‡]	50 (12)	17 (18)	30 (30)
Visual field defects	40 (73)	45 (53)	42 (126)
Headache	23 (44)	13 (61)	17 (105)
Tumor size			
Microadenomas and intraseller macroadenomas	34 (155)[§,‖]	19 (88)[§,‖]	29 (243)
Macroadenoma with extrasellar extension	39 (155)[¶]	32 (88)[¶]	36 (243)
Invasive macroadenoma	27 (155)	49 (88)	35 (243)

[*]n = number of patients for whom the information was available.
[†]Mean ± standard deviation.
[‡]Data include women with or without associated prolactin hypersecretion.
[§]P = not significant versus macroadenoma with extraseller extension (by Fisher's exact test).
[‖]$P < 0.0006$ versus invasive macroadenoma (by Fisher's exact test).
[¶]$P < 0.006$ versus invasive macroadenoma (by Fisher's exact test).
From Beck-Peccoz P, Brucker-Davis F, Persani L, et al. Thyrotropin-secreting pituitary tumors. Endocr Rev 17:610, 1996.

on chromosome 11q13 and encodes the protein MENIN. More than 90% of tumors from patients with MEN 1 have loss of heterozygosity, suggesting that the MEN1 gene is a tumor-suppressor gene. The overall incidence of MEN 1 is 0.25%. It is 1% to 18% in patients with primary hyperparathyroidism and less than 3% in patients with pituitary tumors.[504,505] All forms of MEN 1 are either inherited as autosomal dominant syndromes or occur sporadically. A patient may be considered to have MEN 1 if two of the three principal related tumors (parathyroid, pancreatic islet [e.g., gastrinoma, insulinoma, glucagonoma, VIPoma], and anterior pituitary [prolactinoma, GH-producing, ACTH-producing, nonfunctioning]) are diagnosed.[506] Associated tumors include carcinoid tumors, adrenocortical tumors, lipomas, facial angiofibromas, and collagenomas, as well as thyroid tumors.[507] The incidence of pituitary tumors in patients with MEN 1 ranges from 15% to 90%. The majority of the pituitary tumors are microadenomas, and approximately 60% secrete PRL. Fewer than 25% secrete GH, and 5% secrete ACTH. The rest are nonfunctioning and secrete glycoprotein subunits. The treatment of these pituitary tumors is identical to that of other isolated pituitary tumors. Because of its autosomal dominant inheritance,[508] distinction between sporadic and familial forms is important for first-degree relatives who have a 50% risk of having the disease.

Carcinoma of the Pituitary

Pituitary carcinomas are rare neoplasms that can be distinguished from invasive adenomas by the presence of craniospinal or systemic metastasis. An unresolved question is whether pituitary carcinomas develop from pituitary adenomas or occur de novo. Studies addressing this question have been limited by the small number of patients and the lack of sufficient follow-up.[509] Pituitary carcinomas are defined by metastases. Whether extensive invasion of the brain by a pituitary tumor is a further criterion is a matter of controversy.[510] Adenomas that meet these criteria should be followed carefully.

Immunohistochemically, MIB-1 (Ki-67) and p53 staining correlate with the aggressiveness of pituitary tumors.[511] Studies of molecular markers suggest that the Ras oncogene may play a role in the anaplastic progression of GH-producing tumors. Expression of the *p53* gene has been shown to be increased during the transformation of a pituitary adenoma to a pituitary carcinoma.[512] Loss of heterozygosity on autosomes 1p, 3p, 10q26, 11q13, and 22q12 has also been shown to be present in ACTH-producing pituitary carcinomas.[513] Other factors, such as telomerase and its subunits, have been shown to be increased in PRL-producing pituitary carcinoma.[514] Animal studies have suggested a connection between the loss of the retinoblastoma gene (*Rb*) and the development of pituitary carcinomas, observations that could not be confirmed in benign ACTH-positive adenomas in humans.[515]

The prevalence of pituitary carcinoma is 0.2% of all adenohypophysial neoplasms,[516] with the majority of such tumors being endocrinologically active (88%). Available data suggest that 12% are null cell pituitary tumors, 33% are PRL-producing tumors, 42% are ACTH-producing tumors, 22% are associated with Nelson syndrome, 6% are GH-producing pituitary tumors, 5% are gonadotroph-producing tumors, and approximately 1% are TSH-producing tumors.[516,517] PRL-producing pituitary tumors (71%) and ACTH-producing tumors (57%) have the highest propensity to metastasize.[518] An average 15.3-year interval between adenoma diagnosis and the development of carcinoma has been reported in cases of Nelson syndrome.[516]

The prognosis of pituitary carcinoma is poor. In a study of 15 patients with pituitary carcinoma, 80% died of metastatic disease within 7 days to 8 years after diagnosis. Sixty-six percent of the patients died within 1 year.[516] Sironi et al. reported a mean survival time for patients with PRL-secreting carcinomas of 2.4 years.[519]

The majority of pituitary carcinomas are hormone-secreting, are invasive, and result in symptoms from local mass effect. Sites of pituitary tumor metastasis include the brain, spinal cord, bone, liver, lymph nodes, ovary, heart, and lung. In ACTH-secreting pituitary carcinomas, ACTH levels range from 145 to 280,000 pg/mL.[520] Serum PRL levels associated with PRL-secreting pituitary carcinomas range from 6 to 22,000 ng/mL, and increased levels are associated with tumor recurrence and metastasis.[516,521]

Treatment options for pituitary carcinomas include medications specific for the pituitary tumor as well as RT and chemotherapy. Dopamine agonists have a role in the treatment of PRL-producing pituitary tumors, but control serum PRL levels for a limited time. Neither adjuvant RT to the sella and distant metastases nor stereotactic radiation has been shown to have an effect on long-term outcome. Similarly, different chemotherapy protocols with agents such as carmustine, hydroxyurea, and 5-fluorouracil have not improved outcomes.[517]

Metastatic Disease Involving the Pituitary

Metastatic disease to the pituitary has been found in 1% to 3.6% patients at the time of pituitary resection.[522] If both the pituitary and the surrounding sella turcica are evaluated, metastases are found in 27% of patients with malignant tumors.[523] Of tumors known to metastasize to the pituitary, cancer of the breast is the most common (accounting for up to 33% to 40%), followed by cancer of the lung (33% to 36%). Others include prostate, colon, and other gastrointestinal tumors; lymphoma; leukemia; and thyroid tumors.[524] Most metastatic disease is found in the posterior pituitary gland (57%), followed by the anterior gland (13%) and both lobes (12%). This preference for the posterior pituitary is probably explained by its direct arterial blood supply.[525] Of interest, metastases from breast cancer seem to occur most often in the anterior as opposed to the posterior pituitary. Perhaps surprisingly, most metastases to the pituitary are clinically silent and only 7% have been found to have produced symptoms in an autopsy series. Clinical features include DI, followed by ophthalmoplegia, visual impairment, headache, and anterior hypopituitarism. Kimmel and O'Neill.[526] suggested that 14% to 20% of patients presenting with DI may have pituitary metastases.

Although there are no imaging characteristics that are specific for pituitary metastases, Fassett and Couldwell[524] have suggested that thickening of the pituitary stalk, loss of the high-intensity signal of the posterior pituitary, isointensity of T1- and T2-weighted MRI scans, invasion of the cavernous sinus, and sclerotic changes around the sella

turcica may make metastatic disease more likely. Treatment includes surgery, RT, and chemotherapy, which do not change the mean survival rate in most cases, which ranges from 6 to 22 months.[527]

PITUITARY APOPLEXY AND SHEEHAN SYNDROME

Pituitary apoplexy is a potentially life-threatening condition that results from acute expansion of an infarcted or hemorrhagic pituitary adenoma. Symptoms typically associated with pituitary apoplexy include sudden severe headache, visual field defects, decreased visual acuity, and ophthalmoplegia.[528] Other symptoms are nausea, vertigo, meningismus, facial pain, and in some cases, hemiparesis and Horner syndrome. Headache occurs in nearly 100% of cases and is believed to be a consequence of meningeal irritation from blood or dural stretching. In cases of extension to the lateral wall of the sinus, cranial nerve damage can occur in association with ophthalmoplegia. The accompanying hypopituitarism and possible pressure on the brain stem can result in decreased consciousness. The symptoms are often similar to those of other disease entities, such as ruptured intracranial aneurysms and bacterial or viral meningitis.

All types of pituitary tumors have a similar risk of apoplexy, and the incidence of apoplexy within pituitary tumors has been estimated at 2% to 7%.[529,530] Approximately 50% to 80% of cases of apoplexy occur in patients who were unaware of the presence of pituitary tumors before the apoplectic event. The ratio of men to women presenting with apoplexy is 2:1, and most patients present in the fifth or sixth decade.[528] Precipitating factors described in the literature include hypertension, hypotension, bromocriptine therapy, anticoagulation, surgery, diabetic ketoacidosis, RT, and pregnancy.[531-536]

The most reliable method to diagnose pituitary apoplexy is MRI. Early MRI images show predominant hyperintensity on T1 images and predominant hypointensity on T2-weighted images.[537] Whereas pituitary apoplexy can be confirmed by MRI in essentially all cases, CT scans may not show this disorder in 54% to 79% of patients.[528] Because vascular emergencies are more common than pituitary apoplexy, head CT is often the first procedure performed to evaluate the symptoms that are common to both conditions. Thus, the low sensitivity of CT scanning for the diagnosis of pituitary apoplexy must not be overlooked when no aneurysm is identified.

Timely surgical intervention to provide decompression is essential. Although the outcome of pituitary apoplexy is unpredictable, cranial nerves III, IV, and VI seem to recover more easily than do the chiasmal and optic nerves, especially if decompression is achieved within 7 days. DI occurs in only 2% to 3% of patients, whereas reports show that 88% of patients are GH-deficient, 76% do not secrete LH, and 66% have secondary adrenal insufficiency.[528] Verrees et al. reported that decompression within 3 days after the onset of symptoms resulted in full return of pituitary function in 73% of patients.[528]

Sheehan syndrome is a form of pituitary apoplexy that results from hypotension secondary to severe postpartum uterine hemorrhage. In rare cases, it is seen without massive bleeding or after normal bleeding. It has been suggested that the enlarged pituitary during pregnancy is more prone to have ischemic necrosis after postpartum bleeding. The presence of a small sella has also been proposed as a potential risk factor for Sheehan syndrome.[538] It may be difficult to distinguish Sheehan syndrome from postpartum autoimmune hypophysitis (AH), given that pituitary antibodies have been described in both disorders.[539] In the early stage of Sheehan syndrome, MRI shows an enlarged pituitary, and in later stages, an empty sella can be present.[540] Clinical manifestations include failure of postpartum lactation and failure to resume regular menstrual cycles postpartum, together with the loss of pubic and axillary hair. Other symptoms of anterior hypopituitarism can be present. In the case of hypopituitarism, replacement therapy (especially glucocorticoids) must be initiated as soon as possible. Partial or complete spontaneous recovery has been reported.[541]

EMPTY SELLA SYNDROME

Primary empty sella syndrome is a radiologic finding. It refers to the anatomic state that occurs as a result of intrasellar herniation of the subarachnoid space through an opening in the diaphragma sellae, allowing spinal fluid to enter the sella. The result is a compressed and often posteriorly displaced pituitary gland. The term *primary empty sella syndrome* is used when no identifiable cause can be found. The majority of patients are asymptomatic. Of those who have symptoms, 80% are middle-aged women who are overweight and hypertensive.[542] Chronic headache is the most common symptom and often the only one. Elevated intracranial pressure is believed to be an important contributing factor, and 10% of patients with benign intracranial hypertension also have empty sella syndrome.[543] In 5% of patients, moderate hyperprolactinemia resulting from stalk compression is evident. In 10% of patients, CSF rhinorrhea is present and is the result of CSF pulsation-associated thinning of the sella floor.[544]

Secondary empty sella syndrome can be the consequence of previous surgery, radionecrosis, or pituitary apoplexy. In contrast to primary empty sella syndrome, there is no association with body habitus or sex. Visual symptoms are not uncommon and are usually the result of chiasmal prolapse. Panhypopituitarism or selective pituitary hormone deficiencies can occur. Having established the diagnosis, the treatment is primarily based on the complications (endocrinologic, ophthalmologic, CSF rhinorrhea).

LYMPHOCYTIC HYPOPHYSITIS

Autoimmune hypophysitis, also referred to as *lymphocytic hypophysitis,* is the most common form of chronic inflammation that primarily affects the pituitary gland. AH is a rare disease that should be part of any differential diagnosis of a nonsecreting pituitary mass during pregnancy or postpartum. Outcomes of this disease range from spontaneous recovery to death. Women are affected much more commonly than are men (9:1 occurrence rate, and symptoms include those of sellar compression, such as headache and

visual disturbance, pituitary deficiency, and DI.[545] DI can be masked by coexisting glucocorticoid deficiency, given that glucocorticoids inhibit the secretion of ADH from the paraventricular nucleus and suppress the synthesis of aquaporin 2, which is an ADH-dependent water channel in the renal collecting tubules.[546-548] In AH, the anterior pituitary corticotrophin-secreting cells are most frequently impaired, whereas the least common finding is hyperprolactinemia. The clinical diagnosis of AH may be difficult. Indeed, 40% of cases are misdiagnosed preoperatively as pituitary adenomas. AH should always be considered when there is a temporal relationship with the identification of pituitary pathology and pregnancy or the postpartum state. The strong association between pregnancy and AH might be explained by the presence of low-titer serum antibodies, which are directed against alpha-enolase, a 49-kDa cytosolic pituitary protein that is expressed in the placenta.[549,550] However, others have found a similar association between these antibodies and nonfunctioning pituitary adenomas, thus calling into question the specificity of these antibodies. Other autoantibodies have been associated with the disease as well. AH has been associated with other autoimmune diseases, such as Hashimoto thyroiditis, polyglandular syndrome type 2, Graves disease, and systemic lupus erythromatosis.[545] Imaging studies often show an enlarged pituitary, sometimes with suprasellar extension and occasionally with thickening of the infundibulum. In rare cases, an empty sella is present.[551] The histopathology of lymphocytic hypophysitis shows lymphoplasmacytic infiltrates.

Visual loss related to AH can necessitate surgical intervention. If surgery is not urgently needed, medical treatment with corticosteroids and sequential MRI are recommended. There are also reports of successful treatment with azathioprine[552] and methotrexate[553] after unsuccessful glucocorticoid therapy. RT has been used successfully in few cases.[554]

PITUITARY HEMOCHROMATOSIS

Primary hemochromatosis is the most common form of hemochromatosis. It is an autosomal recessive disorder caused by a single site mutation of the *HEFE* gene.[555] This gene is located near the human leukocyte antigen complex and produces the HEFE glycoprotein, which binds to the transferrin receptor and decreases the affinity of this receptor for iron-bound transferrin. *Secondary hemochromatosis* may result from disorders including thalassemia, aplastic anemia, blood transfusion, long-term kidney dialysis, and chronic liver disease. Patients with hemochromatosis of both types have increased iron deposition in different organs, including the liver, skin, heart, joints, pancreas, hypothalamus, and pituitary. The most common feature of hemochromatosis is fatigue; other symptoms include arthritis, heart failure, diabetes mellitus, hepatic cirrhosis, hyperpigmentation, hypothyroidism, and hypogonadism.[556]

Iron has been found as aggregates of ferritin and hemosiderin in the cytoplasm of all five anterior pituitary cell types, but with a propensity for the gonadotrophs. The cytotoxic effect seems to correlate with the quantity of iron stored. The most common consequences of deposition of iron in the pituitary gland and hypothalamus are hypogonadotropic hypogonadism and GH deficiency.[557] Thirty percent of men with hemochromatosis have low gonadotrophin and testosterone levels resulting from impaired LH and FSH response to GnRH by the damaged gonadotrophs.[558] Siminoski et al.[100] described a patient with idiopathic hemochromatosis with no LH or FSH response after clomiphene administration, suggesting that a defect in the hypothalamic GnRH response can also occur. In patients with iron overload, MRI shows low signal intensity,[559] and some authors suggested that the MRI T2 relaxation rate of the pituitary correlates with the extent of pituitary siderosis.[560] Treatment options include phlebotomy and desferrioxamine, which is a chelating agent.[561]

IATROGENIC PITUITARY DYSFUNCTION

Hypopituitarism has been described in patients after *radiation therapy* for nonpituitary disorders, such as primary brain tumors and nasopharyngeal carcinoma, as well as in children who undergo prophylactic cranial irradiation for leukemia. GH is usually the first pituitary hormone affected by cranial RT, followed by the gonadotropins ACTH and TSH.[116] The total dose of radiation administered determines the severity of the pituitary deficiencies.[116] Children and adults differ with regard to the threshold dose for the risk of hypopituitarism.[562] Agha et al. reported that 41% of adult patients who had irradiation of a nonpituitary brain tumor had hypopituitarism.[118] After RT, regular evaluation is mandatory to check for recurrence and pituitary function, even though the site of radiation may have been distant from the hypothalamic–pituitary region.[117]

Radiation of the pituitary, most often used to treat residual disease after pituitary surgery or recurrent pituitary tumors, typically uses either gamma knife or linear accelerator–based radiosurgical techniques. Gamma knife treatment delivers a high dose (25 Gy to the periphery of secretory tumors and 12 to 20 Gy to the periphery of nonsecretory tumors) in a single fraction. Hypopituitarism occurs in approximately 30% of patients postradiation, with thyroid and GH deficiencies being the most common.[563] Data on the outcome of treatment with linear accelerator–based treatments are comparable to those for gamma knife treatment, with 20% to 40% of patients requiring hormone replacement 10 to 20 years after linear accelerator radiation.[564] Additional longer-term studies are needed to evaluate the hormonal effects of both treatment options.

Chemotherapy, alone or in combination with RT, can affect the hypothalamic–pituitary axis. Patients treated with chemotherapy (e.g., vincristine, vinblastine) may have syndrome of inappropriate antidiuretic hormone secretion as a result of cytotoxic effects on the paraventricular and supraoptic neurons, leading to increased vasopressin release.[565] Autopsy findings have related cyclophosphamide therapy to vasopressin depletion of the posterior pituitary as well as to infundibular necrosis.[566] A rare case of pituitary apoplexy after treatment with vinblastine, cisplatin, and methotrexate for squamous cell carcinoma was reported by Davies et al.[567] Prolonged high-dose exogenous glucocorticoid therapy in children with leukemia or lymphoma can lead to secondary adrenal insufficiency via suppression of the HPA axis. Children treated with chemotherapy often exhibit growth retardation after which "catch-up growth" occurs. When catch-up growth does not occur after 1.5 to 2 years, such children should be tested for GH deficiency.

The complete reference list can be found on the companion Expert Consult Web site at www.expertconsultbook.com.

Suggested Readings

Apter D, Butzow TL, Laughlin GA, et al. Gonadotropin-releasing hormone pulse generator activity during pubertal transition in girls: pulsatile and diurnal patterns of circulating gonadotropins. J Clin Endocrinol Metab 76:940, 1993.

Assie G, Bahurel H, Bertherat J, et al. The Nelson's syndrome...revisited. Pituitary 7:209, 2004.

Barker FG II, Klibanski A, Swearingen B. Transsphenoidal surgery for pituitary tumors in the United States, 1996-2000: mortality, morbidity, and the effects of hospital and surgeon volume. J Clin Endocrinol Metab 88:4709, 2003.

Bhagavath B, Podolsky RH, Ozata M, et al. Clinical and molecular characterization of a large sample of patients with hypogonadotropic hypogonadism. Fertil Steril 85:706, 2006.

Bills DC, Meyer FB, Laws ER Jr., et al. A retrospective analysis of pituitary apoplexy. Neurosurgery 33:602, 1993.

Crowley WF Jr., Filicori M, Spratt DI, et al. The physiology of gonadotropin-releasing hormone (GnRH) secretion in men and women. Recent Prog Horm Res 41:473, 1985.

Ehrmann DA. Polycystic ovary syndrome. N Engl J Med 352:1223, 2005.

Karavitaki N, Cudlip S, Adams CB, et al. Craniopharyngiomas. Endocr Rev 27:371, 2006.

Miyagawa Y, Tsujimura A, Matsumiya K, et al. Outcome of gonadotropin therapy for male hypogonadotropic hypogonadism at university affiliated male infertility centers: a 30-year retrospective study. J Urol 173:2072, 2005.

Nattiv A, Loucks AB, Manore MM, et al. American College of Sports Medicine position stand. The female athlete triad. Med Sci Sports Exerc 39:1867, 2007.

Nieman LK, Ilias I. Evaluation and treatment of Cushing's syndrome. Am J Med 118:1340, 2005.

Schlechte JA. Clinical practice. Prolactinoma. N Engl J Med 349:2035, 2003.

Thakker RV. Multiple endocrine neoplasia—syndromes of the twentieth century. J Clin Endocrinol Metab 83:2617, 1998.

CHAPTER 20

Polycystic Ovary Syndrome and Hyperandrogenic States

R. Jeffrey Chang

Understanding the clinical significance and pathophysiology of polycystic ovaries and polycystic ovary syndrome has evolved over more than 150 years. The first description of enlarged, polycystic ovaries surrounded by a smooth capsule was reported in 1844.[1] This was followed by similar observations, including a description of hyperthecosis in 1897.[2] In the early 1900s, there was a growing awareness that dysfunctional uterine bleeding was associated with multiple cystic follicles of the ovary, which in part, led to the therapeutic recommendation of bilateral ovarian wedge resection. In 1926, it was demonstrated in rodents that gonadotropic extract derived from the urine of pregnant women was capable of inducing multiple ovarian cyst formation.[3] This finding suggested that abnormal secretion of anterior pituitary hormones may be responsible for the morphologic changes in the ovary. Subsequently, in 1935, the classic description of polycystic ovaries that was reported by Stein and Leventhal codified the association with hyperandrogenism, amenorrhea, and infertility as well as established the syndrome named for the authors.[4] As investigators began to study the pathogenesis of this disorder and the number of relevant publications increased, there followed a gradual and distinct terminologic conversion to what has become known as *polycystic ovary syndrome* (PCOS).

Currently, *PCOS* refers to a multisystem reproductive–metabolic disorder that has evolved over decades and stands to be further defined. The principal clinical manifestations are hyperandrogenism and irregular menstruation, the latter of which leads to infertility. The ovaries of women with these symptoms are polycystic and conform to a specific anatomic appearance that may be detected on ultrasound imaging, although the ovarian morphology can exist in women without the overt clinical manifestations. The associated metabolic dysfunction includes insulin resistance, dyslipidemia, and in the United States, an apparent increased prevalence of obesity. The intriguing nature of PCOS rests with the underlying mechanisms responsible for the juxtaposed abnormalities of hypothalamic–pituitary–ovarian–adrenal function with those of altered metabolic physiology. All of these factors may contribute to the clinical phenotype, pose increased long-term health risks, and serve as targets for therapeutic intervention in women with PCOS.

Epidemiology

PREVALENCE

It is estimated that the prevalence of PCOS is 4% to 12% of women in their reproductive years,[5-7] which designates this disorder as the most common reproductive endocrinopathy of women. Estimates may vary among reports, based on the study population and whether ultrasound imaging of the ovary was included in the diagnostic criteria. In a study of 277 unselected black and white women in the southeastern United States, 4.6% were found to have PCOS.[5] In this study, the rate of PCOS was similar between groups. The diagnosis was based on the presence of hirsutism and irregular cycles and confirmed by hormone evaluation. These results confirmed earlier reports from the United Kingdom in which the diagnosis of PCOS was highly likely in women with hirsutism and oligomenorrhea.[8-10] In Greece, the rate has been estimated at 9%, whereas in Spain, the prevalence was 6.5%.[7,11] Among Caribbean Hispanic women, the prevalence of PCOS was found to be twice that of African-American women. Recently, it has been suggested that PCOS is more prevalent in women of South Asian descent, based on clinical findings in South Asian immigrants and white women in Britain.[12,13]

Some women with hirsutism unaccompanied by menstrual abnormalities have been shown to exhibit polycystic ovaries by pelvic ultrasonography.[9,14] In these hirsute women, observed increases in circulating androgen levels may have facilitated the development of abnormal ovarian morphology. This notion is supported by studies in which female-to-male transsexuals treated with high-dose androgen acquire the typical appearance of polycystic ovaries.[15] In the absence of hirsutism, women with anovulation appear to have a high incidence of PCOS. In 206 nonhirsute women, biochemical assessment showed elevated androgens consistent with the diagnosis in 87% of those with oligomenorrhea and 32% of those with amenorrhea.[10]

Although the sonographic demonstration of polycystic ovaries in the presence of typical clinical features is regarded as confirmatory for the syndrome, it has been clearly shown that polycystic ovaries can be found in normal ovulatory women without a history of hyperandrogenism.[16] In 257 volunteer women who considered themselves to have normal menstruation without hyperandrogenic symptoms, 22% had the characteristic image of polycystic ovaries.[8,9] However, careful reexamination of those with polycystic ovaries showed that 75% experienced some degree of menstrual disturbance and 45% had objective evidence of hirsutism. Despite the likelihood of PCOS in these unsuspecting normal individuals, many of the women with polycystic ovaries did not show evidence of the disorder. In stark contradistinction, some ovulatory women with PCOS have entirely normal follicle development, as determined by serial ultrasound.[17] Thus, although the requisite identification of polycystic ovaries to establish the diagnosis appears to be clinically appropriate, the morphogenesis of the polycystic ovary may not necessarily be unique to the disorder.

FAMILIAL OCCURRENCE

It has been well documented that PCOS tends to aggregate within families.[18] Moreover, several studies have addressed the prevalence of PCOS among first-degree relatives. Based on clinical evidence and laboratory confirmation of hyperandrogenism, anovulation, and polycystic ovaries, the likelihood of the disorder in sisters and mothers of affected women has been reported to be considerably higher than in normal control subjects. In a study of 115 sisters of 80 probands, PCOS was found in 22% of reproductive-aged siblings, whereas hyperandrogenemia was found in an additional 24%.[18] An analysis of 29 families with PCOS, as judged by polycystic ovaries and elevated androgen levels, showed that 66% of sisters and 52% of mothers had the syndrome, which was significantly greater than the prevalence in 10 control families.[19] Similar results were observed in 93 first-degree relatives of affected patients in which 16 of 50 sisters (32%) and 19 of 78 mothers (24%) had PCOS. Consideration of those individuals who were not under treatment, which could have masked symptoms of PCOS, increased the prevalence to 40% in sisters and 35% in mothers.[20] In contrast, a study of 102 sisters and mothers of 50 Turkish women with PCOS showed rates of 16% and 8%, respectively.[21] Notably, mean serum levels of testosterone, androstenedione, and dehydroepiandrosterone sulfate (DHEAS) were significantly higher in the sisters compared with values found in age- and body mass index (BMI)-matched control subjects. In most of these studies, the prevalence of insulin resistance and impaired glucose tolerance was considerably greater in the relatives compared with normal control subjects.

A PCOS phenotype for men and male siblings of women with PCOS has not been established. However, circulating DHEAS levels in first-degree male relatives have been shown to be significantly higher than those of unrelated BMI-matched controls.[22] Serum testosterone, sex hormone–binding globulin (SHBG), luteinizing hormone (LH), and follicle-stimulating hormone (FSH) were similar between groups.

Collectively, these results indicate that first-degree relatives of women with PCOS are at significant risk for PCOS. The findings support a genetic basis for hyperandrogenemia, which may account, at least in part, for the familial clustering of this disorder.

Clinical Description

HIRSUTISM

The most distinctive and visible clinical feature of PCOS is mild to severe hirsutism. The rate of hair growth is important clinically because gradual and progressive growth indicates a functional etiology, whereas the rapid appearance of thick, pigmented hair often suggests a neoplastic source of androgen production. In PCOS, increased hair growth is commonly found on the side of the face, upper lip, and chin, extending down to the neck region, lower back, and inner thighs (Fig. 20-1). This pattern of hirsutism invariably is accompanied by extension of pubic hair growth toward the umbilicus and may resemble a male escutcheon. More severe cases include the appearance of hair on the chest. Progressive hyperandrogenism may be associated with temporal balding and male pattern baldness. Excessive hair also may be found on the extremities and abdominal flank, although these areas are not considered specific sites of sexual hair growth. The degree of hair growth is commonly determined subjectively, although standardized measurement may be achieved using the Ferriman-Gallwey method, which quantifies terminal hair over nine body areas.[23] A Ferriman-Gallwey score of greater than 7 is usually regarded as hirsutism. In PCOS, the amount of hirsutism has been correlated to serum androgen concentrations. However, the rate and distribution of hair growth may vary among individuals due to altered responses to androgens based on ethnic differences, which may account for subtle changes in the prevalence of PCOS in different parts of the world.

Coexisting conditions that alter the bioactivity of androgens, such as hypothyroidism and obesity, may also give rise to excessive hair growth. These conditions are associated with lowered SHBG, which provides increased availability of free testosterone. Sequence variations within the coding region of separate SHBG alleles have been reported in a heterozygous woman who presented with severe hyperandrogenism during pregnancy.[24] Her serum SHBG

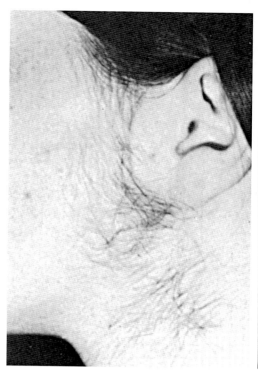
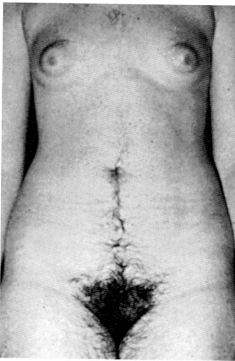

Figure 20-1. Moderately severe hirsutism in a young woman. Note the male pattern of hair distribution.

levels were barely detectable, and non–protein-bound testosterone concentrations were markedly higher than the normal reference range. A single-nucleotide polymorphism within an allele encoded a missense mutation that permitted normal steroid hormone binding, but caused abnormal glycosylation and decreased secretion of SHBG.

MENSTRUAL IRREGULARITY

In PCOS, menstrual dysfunction is primarily characterized by irregular, infrequent, or absent menstrual bleeding. Commonly, bleeding is not preceded by premenstrual symptoms, which is typical for anovulatory bleeding and therefore is unpredictable. Typically, this pattern of bleeding is an extension of postmenarchal irregularity, and monthly menstrual cyclicity is never established. In some women, the onset of chronic anovulation emerges beyond adolescence, but this is unusual. The volume of blood loss associated with menstrual irregularity is generally mild, but in women with significant endometrial proliferation, the bleeding can be substantial and may result in anemia with transient orthostatic hypotension. Prolonged heavy bleeding should raise consideration of abnormal endometrial hyperplasia and even endometrial adenocarcinoma. The thickened endometrium is prone to superficial sloughing or tissue breakdown in response to persistent secretion or spontaneous decreases in circulating estrogen, respectively. The physiologic link between anovulation and irregular menses is related to persistent estrogen production. Within the polycystic ovary, granulosa cells generate very little estrogen, based on a lack of mature follicle development. Rather, chronic unopposed estrogen secretion most likely results from extraglandular

conversion of androgen to estrogen. By comparison, a mechanism to account for arrested follicle growth has not been established.

In approximately 20% of women, there is complete absence of menses, whereas 5% to 10% of patients show regular ovulatory function. Recognition of normal ovulation in PCOS is significant in that a history of regular menstrual cycles does not exclude the diagnosis. In late reproductive life, women with PCOS have been observed to experience regular ovulation for unknown reasons.[25] Aging women with PCOS with regular menstrual cycles appear to have a smaller follicle cohort, higher serum FSH levels, and lower FSH-induced inhibin release compared with age-matched women with PCOS who have persistent anovulation.[26] Notably, in the older ovulatory women with PCOS, serum androgen levels were also significantly lower than those observed in the anovulatory women. Whether changes in the follicle population or alterations in the ovarian endocrine milieu may be responsible for resumption of ovulation in older women with PCOS women remains to be determined.

OVARIAN MORPHOLOGY

In the original description of women with PCOS, the ovaries were enlarged, with numerous peripheral small antral follicles and increased central stroma (Fig. 20-2). From this classic appearance, the definition of polycystic ovaries has been modified to include the presence of at least 12 antral follicles per ovary, with no consideration of distribution or stromal area.[27] Although the process that leads to excessive antral follicle development in PCOS is not completely understood, it has been proposed that

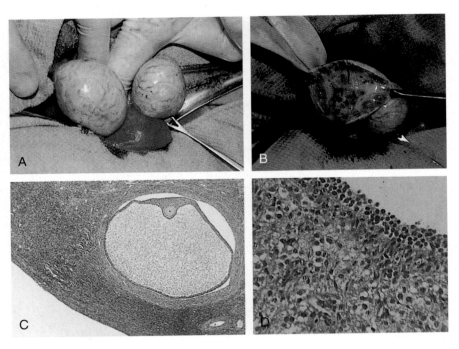

Figure 20-2. Gross and microscopic characteristics of polycystic ovaries. **A,** Bilateral enlarged ovaries with a smooth and thickened capsule. **B,** On cut section, multiple follicular cysts surrounded by abundant ovarian stroma are found throughout the cortex of the ovary. **C,** The subcapsular cysts are lined with granulosa cells, with early stages of antrum formation. **D,** Hyperplasia of the theca interna with luteinization.

normal follicular growth appears to occur up to the mid-antral stage, after which maturation ceases.[28] However, the finding that follicle development becomes arrested at the midantral stage does not necessarily signal the immediate onset of atresia. In a careful study of granulosa cells obtained by aspiration of antral follicles from unstimulated ovaries of women with PCOS, viability measures indicated robust cell survival with substantial steroidogenic potential compared with cells obtained from ovaries of normal women in the early follicular phase of their menstrual cycles.[29] It was concluded that despite the presence of apoptosis among granulosa cells, the majority of antral follicles in PCOS retain ample functional capacity. This would account, at least in part, for the progressive accumulation of follicular fluid that expands the antrum and gives rise to the classic appearance of cystic follicles. Eventually, the loss of granulosa cells is overwhelming and the follicle ceases to be steroidogenically active. Whether the rate and extent of programmed granulosa cell death exceeds that observed in follicles from normal ovaries has not been examined.

The ovarian follicle population in PCOS also is distinctive in that histomorphometric studies have revealed a two- to threefold increase in the numbers of primary, secondary, and tertiary follicles compared with those of the normal ovary.[30] Whether the ovaries are endowed with a greater number of follicles or whether the rate of programmed cell death is decelerated compared with the normal ovary has not been systematically studied. Relevant to this issue, anti-müllerian hormone (AMH) may contribute, at least in part, to the increased growing follicle population in polycystic ovaries. As a member of the transforming growth factor β superfamily, AMH is an exclusive product of granulosa cells, primarily in growing preantral and small antral follicles. Within the ovary, AMH appears to negatively regulate the advancement of follicle growth.[31,32] Its expression

in growing preantral follicles of polycystic ovaries is decreased compared with normal ovaries.[33] Thus, a lack of AMH may permit accelerated entrance and advancement of growing ovarian follicles, consistent with the altered follicular dynamics of polycystic ovaries. Paradoxically, in women with PCOS, circulating levels are elevated two- to threefold compared with those of normal women, which probably reflects the greater number of growing preantral and small antral follicles in their ovaries compared with those of normal women.[34]

Recently, it has been shown that follicles from polycystic ovaries show a decreased rate of atresia in culture, suggesting a mechanism for maintaining a larger follicle pool throughout reproductive life in women with PCOS.[35] These observations are in agreement with the finding of increased granulosa cell proliferation in primary follicles from women with PCOS compared with those of normal women.[36] Thus, it appears that several factors may be involved in the generation of increased ovarian follicle number in women with PCOS.

A mechanism for the morphogenesis of the polycystic ovary has not been established. However, a role for androgen excess in follicle growth and development has been suggested from ovarian morphology in hyperandrogenic women with congenital adrenal hyperplasia and androgen-producing ovarian tumors.[37-40] In particular, polycystic ovaries have been demonstrated in male-to-female transsexuals receiving long-term androgen treatment.[15,41,42] These ovaries contained many follicle cysts and granulosa cells exhibited intense nuclear staining for androgen receptor, which was considerably greater than that found for normal premenopausal women.[43] The underlying basis for androgen-induced follicle formation in nonhuman primates has been explored in studies that showed increased ovarian size and follicle number after subcutaneous placement of silicone (Silastic, Dow Corning, Midland, MI)

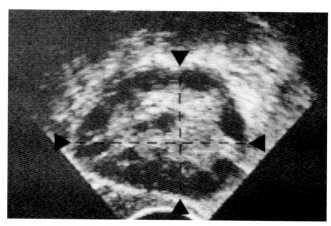

Figure 20-3. *Polycystic ovary on ultrasound.* Arrowheads *demarcate the largest vertical and horizontal diameters of the ovary.*

capsules containing testosterone.[44] In situ hybridization studies showed that androgen receptor messenger RNA was expressed primarily in healthy small and medium antral follicles compared with large preovulatory follicles.[45] Moreover, androgen receptor messenger RNA was found to colocalize with that of the FSH receptor and testosterone treatment increased the expression of FSH receptor mRNA.[46]

The polycystic ovary has been characterized by ultrasound examination (Fig. 20-3). In 1986, a description was provided to include ovarian enlargement, 10 or more antral follicles ranging from 2 to 10 mm in diameter arranged in a peripheral distribution, and increased central stroma of greater than 25% of the ovarian area.[8] However, the criteria for polycystic ovaries was modified in 2004 to include greater than 12 follicles per ovary or an ovarian volume greater than 10 mL.[27] This rather specific radiologic description of the polycystic ovary should not be confused with the ultrasound appearance of the multifollicular ovary, which may reflect spontaneous ovarian follicular activity in a woman recovering from hypogonadotropic hypogonadism or ovarian stimulation as a result of ovulation induction. The multifollicular ovary has been described as being of normal size or slightly enlarged, containing six or more follicles without peripheral displacement, and having no increase in central stroma.[47]

OBESITY

Early studies of the clinical features of PCOS showed that obesity was present in slightly more than 50% of cases.[48] However, of recent note, the rate of obesity associated with PCOS has not been corroborated and there is a growing impression that the incidence may be greater, at least in the United States, than that previously described. Commonly, an increase in the upper body or central distribution of fat gives rise to an increased waist-to-hip ratio compared with obese women without PCOS.[49] This fat distribution pattern has been termed *android obesity* and can be found in other hyperandrogenic states, diabetes, and hyperlipidemia. Notably, there is a preponderance of visceral fat compared with peripheral fat, not unlike the distribution of adipose tissue in individuals with insulin

resistance.[50-52] In contrast, women with gynecoid obesity generally have an enhanced accumulation of normal fat in the hips, buttocks, and thighs. As a result, the waist-to-hip ratio in these individuals is usually less than 1.

Whether women with PCOS are predisposed to obesity has not been clarified. Obese women with PCOS tend to have great difficulty in achieving significant and permanent weight loss, despite dietary regimens and exercise. It has been shown that postprandial thermogenesis may be decreased in PCOS, thereby contributing, at least in part, to weight gain.[53] However, resting energy expenditure in PCOS appears to be equivalent to that of normal weight-matched control subjects, which suggests a relative disparity of increased caloric intake and decreased total energy expenditure.[54]

Obesity may cause functional abnormalities that ultimately affect the clinical features observed in PCOS. This is particularly true for obesity-induced insulin resistance and resultant hyperinsulinemia, which is independent of PCOS.[49] Serum insulin is inversely correlated to SHBG concentrations, which increases the clinical consequences of hyperandrogenism in affected women. Correspondingly, the effects of chronic unopposed estrogen secretion are also magnified by increased bioavailable estradiol (E_2). These reproductive–metabolic alterations may accompany the broader recognized risks of obesity that pose significant long-term health outcomes for these individuals.

INSULIN RESISTANCE

It has been well documented that women with PCOS are insulin resistant and have compensatory hyperinsulinemia as a result of their disorder.[49,55-57] The prevalence of insulin resistance in PCOS has been reported to range from 20% to 40%.[58-60] The common occurrence of insulin resistance in obesity may account, in part, for the rather wide prevalence. Nevertheless, independent of obesity, a defect in insulin action in PCOS has been clearly established.[49] Generally, the degree of insulin resistance is mild, although the prevalence of glucose intolerance and subsequent diabetes has been reported to be as high as 31% and 7.5%, respectively.[60,61] Notwithstanding the increased risk of diabetes, there is indirect evidence to indicate that insulin resistance may worsen the clinical manifestations of PCOS. Administration of insulin-lowering drugs has been shown to improve insulin sensitivity, reduce androgen levels, and restore ovulation in some, but not all, patients with this disorder.[62-72] Insulin resistance may also contribute to metabolic dysfunction in PCOS, including an increased likelihood of lipid abnormalities.[73-76] In addition, the association of insulin resistance with visceral fat distribution is underscored by the displacement of central fat to the peripheral compartment, with improvement of insulin sensitivity after administration of insulin-lowering drugs or weight reduction.[69,77,78]

The exaggeration of insulin responses in women with PCOS after a glucose load belies a distinct abnormality of beta cell function in this disorder. Early studies showed that, in PCOS, first-phase insulin secretion was equivalent to that in normal women.[79] However, first-phase insulin release is relevant to the magnitude of ambient insulin resistance in each individual. Consequently, the product of these measures can be calculated (disposition index) and related to the hyperbolic relationship of these measures established in normal women.[80] Employing this technique, it has been reported that a subset of women with PCOS with a family history of diabetes had a disposition index that was in the eighth percentile. In those without a similar family history, the index was in the 33rd percentile.[81] Other studies have confirmed these findings in obese and nonobese women with PCOS.[82] Beta cell function in PCOS has also been quantitated by assessing the insulin secretory response to graded doses of insulin infusion and the ability of the beta cell to respond to oscillations in the plasma glucose level.[81] Women with a family history of type 2 diabetes exhibit impaired responses compared with those without a family history, particularly when expressed in relation to the degree of insulin resistance.

The discovery and documentation of insulin resistance in PCOS has been achieved by time-consuming and complex procedures conducted in the course of clinical investigation. By comparison, identification of insulin resistance in the clinical setting has been difficult. Most patients exhibit normal fasting blood glucose levels, and increased circulating insulin levels are not common. As a result, effective and convenient screening tests to determine evidence-based therapeutic modalities have been limited.

ACNE AND ACANTHOSIS NIGRICANS

Women with PCOS may experience increased skin oiliness secondary to excessive stimulation of the pilosebaceous unit by increased androgen production. However, increased sebaceous gland activity in PCOS is not associated with acne, nor is acne correlated with increased ovarian androgen production. Therefore, as an isolated symptom, acne should not be considered a sign of PCOS.

Perhaps more common is the finding of acanthosis nigricans, which has been observed in 5% to 50% of hyperandrogenic women and is related to the presence and severity of hyperinsulinemia.[58,83,84] This dermatologic condition features symmetrical, darkened, velvety plaques that most commonly appear on the nape of the neck; in the intertriginous areas of the body, such as skinfolds; and on pressure-bearing surfaces, such as knuckles and elbows (Fig. 20-4).[85] In women who are hyperandrogenic and obese, the vulva is commonly affected.[86] Acanthosis nigricans originates from epidermal hyperkeratosis and dermal fibroblast proliferation. There is no evidence of an increased number of melanocytes or melanin deposition, despite apparent increased pigmentation. Whereas acanthosis nigricans is considered a potential marker for insulin resistance and diabetes in adults, a similar etiology in children remains to be established.[87,88] In PCOS, reduction of hyperinsulinemia is associated with improvement in the darkened skin areas.

INFERTILITY

A significant number of patients have infertility as a presenting feature of PCOS.[48] Clearly, anovulation would appear to be the primary defect responsible for the failure to achieve

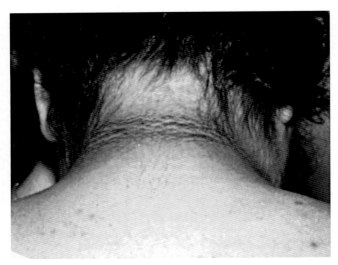

Figure 20-4. Acanthosis nigricans. Note the darkened, velvety plaque along the nape of the neck, giving the appearance of hyperpigmentation in a patient with severe insulin resistance, hirsutism, and polycystic ovaries.

pregnancy in this disorder. However, other potential considerations may preclude fertility. There is mounting evidence that women with PCOS have a higher incidence of spontaneous pregnancy loss, the mechanism of which remains unclear.[89-91] Conversely, it has been reported in a small series that the prevalence of polycystic ovaries in women with recurrent miscarriage was 56%.[92] Subsequently, in a much larger study, it was observed that polycystic ovarian morphology was not predictive of pregnancy loss among women with recurrent pregnancy loss.[93] The potential link between insulin resistance and repetitive pregnancy loss in PCOS has been suggested in studies that showed a significant reduction of first-trimester loss in women treated with metformin.[94] Clearly, additional research is necessary to determine the prevalence as well as the underlying mechanism of recurrent pregnancy loss in PCOS.

Clinical Evolution of PCOS

OVARIAN DEVELOPMENT

Early development of the ovary begins at midgestation (see Chapter 8). At this point, the gonad is replete with primitive germ cells, oogonia, and early development of the ovarian vascular network is evident. These oogonia are gradually encircled by pregranulosa cells to form primordial follicles, composed of an immature oocyte surrounded by a layer of flat granulosa cells enclosed in a basement membrane. Subsequent follicle growth occurs in utero, and the fetal ovary becomes endowed with primary, secondary, and antral follicles.[95] Intrauterine follicular development is a dynamic process, and both healthy and atretic follicles are evident on histologic examination. This pattern of follicular activity is maintained as the ovary undergoes progressive growth during the newborn period and childhood. During this interval, the ovary may be occupied by antral follicles of varying size distributed throughout the ovarian cortex. The pattern of antral follicle formation appears to coincide with that described for adult women with multifollicular ovaries shown on ultrasound imaging.[96-98] It has been reported that polycystic ovaries may accompany the clinical manifestations of PCOS in adolescent children.[99-102] However, little information exists as to whether this ovarian morphology occurred before, after, or at the same time as the reproductive–metabolic abnormalities described in these girls.

In adolescent girls with irregular menstrual cycles, the prevalence of polycystic ovaries is significant. In a study of nonobese adolescent girls with oligomenorrhea, polycystic ovaries were found in 45%.[102] Similarly, in 73 healthy girls with menstrual irregularities, the ultrasound appearance of the ovary was homogeneous in 36%, multifollicular in 23%, and polycystic in 41% of cases.[98] Subsequent examination performed 2 to 7 years later showed that the percentage of individuals with polycystic ovaries increased despite no change in the rate of anovulation. In contrast, 40% of oligomenorrheic girls with elevated LH levels and enlarged ovaries were shown to spontaneously normalize ovarian function and size during longitudinal follow-up.[101] These results point out that polycystic ovaries are a common finding in adolescent girls with abnormal menstrual cycles and suggest that the likelihood of spontaneous restoration to normal ovarian morphology is relatively small as long as menstrual irregularity persists.

ADOLESCENT PCOS

Characteristically, the symptoms of PCOS emerge insidiously, coincident with changes that accompany normal pubertal development (see Chapter 17). The events of puberty have been well documented and include acceleration of growth in height, breast budding and enlargement, appearance of sexual hair, and menstrual bleeding.[103] Once the physical changes have commenced, the temporal pattern of subsequent development is predictable. This process is gradual and may require several years to complete. The normal transition into regular menstrual function is marked by irregular bleeding as a result of anovulation, which may persist for 1 to 3 years.[104] The finding that the emergence of PCOS commonly can be traced to the events of puberty suggests that this disorder may be related to an abnormal expression of those factors that initiate and regulate the process of puberty. Because the duration of menstrual irregularity that accompanies normal puberty may be variable, it is difficult to rely solely on this historical feature as a basis for diagnosis. Moreover, with the recognition that some women with PCOS may exhibit normal ovulatory function, evidence of regular cyclic bleeding does not preclude the disorder in adolescence. Rather, early detection of PCOS in adolescent girls is predicated primarily on hyperandrogenic symptoms, such as hirsutism and acne. In the obese individual, associated metabolic–reproductive abnormalities may create uncertainty as to the mechanism of hyperandrogenism. Reduction in SHBG is directly correlated to obesity, giving rise to increased free testosterone levels. In addition, obese adolescents, particularly those with evidence of acanthosis nigricans, are highly likely to have insulin resistance

with compensatory hyperinsulinemia, which is known to suppress SHBG and probably contributes to excess ovarian androgen production. An ultrasound image of polycystic ovaries virtually confirms the diagnosis. However, the utility of ultrasonography is often limited by the necessity of an abdominal versus vaginal approach and the difficulty in securing adequate imaging in obese girls. As a result, there are no studies that have thoroughly examined the morphologic appearance of ovaries through puberty or in girls with PCOS.

It has been well documented that adolescent girls with PCOS have increased levels of circulating androgens as well as elevated LH levels and increased LH/FSH ratios.[99-102,105,106] Previous studies have shown that hyperandrogenic girls with likely PCOS exhibited changes in gonadotropin secretion patterns that were similar to those found in adults with PCOS.[98,101,102,107] Increased concentrations of serum LH are accompanied by an increase in pulse frequency and amplitude, which are significantly greater than those of normal control subjects. In addition, mean serum levels of testosterone and androstenedione were elevated. Twenty-four–hour pulsatile LH secretion studies have shown that premenarchal hyperandrogenic girls showed higher LH levels while awake, whereas the sleep-entrained increases were minimal compared with those of developmentally matched control subjects.[107] In postmenarche, there was greater LH pulse activity during waking hours, whereas pulse frequency was slowed with sleep (Fig. 20-5). By comparison, in postmenarchal normal girls, LH levels were lower and the pulse frequency reduced while awake, whereas during sleep, LH pulse frequency was significantly less than that of hyperandrogenic girls. Thus, the pattern of gonadotropin secretion in the postmenarchal normal control subject resembled that of the younger premenarchal hyperandrogenic girl. These findings suggest that the transition through neuroendocrine puberty may be accelerated in hyperandrogenic girls compared with girls who undergo normal puberty. Moreover, the data pose the question as to whether there is a chronologic difference in the onset of increased LH levels and pulse frequency between hyperandrogenic and normal pubertal girls.

Among postmenarchal girls with irregular bleeding, it has been estimated that approximately 50% of oligomenorrheic adolescent girls have increased levels of serum LH associated with mild elevations of circulating androgens.[97,105,106,108,109] In addition, these individuals exhibited an increased rate of LH release as determined from frequent sampling studies,[97] which suggested a diagnosis of PCOS. Notably, in a long-term follow-up study of oligomenorrheic girls, those with normal serum LH values eventually had regular ovulatory function compared with more than half of those with elevated LH levels. In these girls, gonadotropin abnormalities persisted along with hyperandrogenism.[101,110] These intriguing findings suggest that oligomenorrhea in early adolescence may be associated with an endocrinologic phenotype of PCOS in the absence of overt signs of hyperandrogenism. Whether the transitory nature of elevated LH and androgens represents an extension of normal hypothalamic–pituitary development remained to be determined.

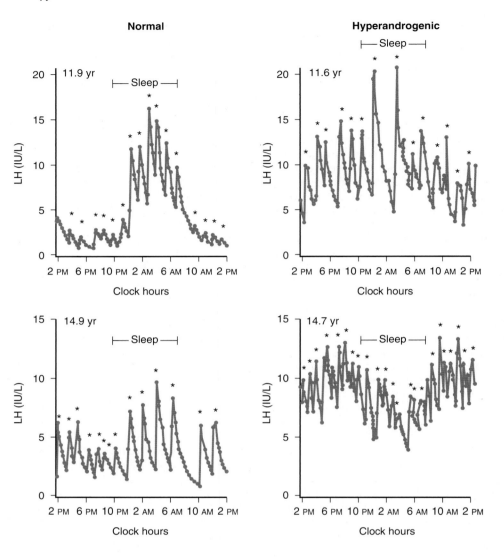

Figure 20-5. Twenty-four–hour pulsatile luteinizing hormone (LH) patterns in premenarchal and postmenarchal hyperandrogenic girls (right) and two developmentally matched healthy girls (left). Asterisks indicate significant pulses. (From Apter DA, Butzow J, Laughlin GA, el al. Accelerated 24-hour luteinizing hormone pulsatile activity in adolescent girls with ovarian hyperandrogenism: relevance to developmental phase of polycystic ovarian syndrome. J Clin Endocrinol Metab 79:119-125, 1994.)

Similar to their adult counterparts, hyperandrogenic girls, with likely adolescent PCOS, exhibit abnormal insulin responses to glucose loading.[111-113] Correspondingly, assessment of 24-hour patterns of insulin showed greater release in hyperandrogenic girls than that observed for normal girls, whereas a reciprocal relationship was found for insulin-like growth factor binding protein 1 (IGFBP-1) secretion (Fig. 20-6). Pulsatile growth hormone secretion was not altered in adolescent PCOS.[111] Lipid profiles in girls with increased androgen indices show higher ratios of low-density lipoprotein (LDL) cholesterol to high-density lipoprotein (HDL) cholesterol in conjunction with lowered SHBG levels.[113] These data suggest that any risk of long-term health consequences may be established early in reproductive life for these girls.

PREPUBERTAL DISPOSITION

Girls with premature pubarche are at increased risk for functional ovarian hyperandrogenism and polycystic ovaries after puberty.[113] This is particularly true of girls with premature pubarche and oligomenorrhea compared with those with regular cycles.[114] Moreover, with subsequent development of hyperandrogenism and hyperinsulinemia, there is a corresponding reduction in birth weight of these individuals.[113] The link between low birth weight and insulin resistance in children appears to be persistent throughout life, as indicated by studies performed in early and late adulthood.[115-117] This relationship may be of particular relevance to a possible mechanism for PCOS in this population. Low birth weight is commonly associated with hypoplasia of the fetal adrenal and correspondingly low serum DHEAS levels.[118,119] DHEAS secretion also serves as a marker for adrenarche that is independent of and precedes gonadarche by several years. In pairs of discordant siblings who achieved similar weight in childhood, DHEAS levels were higher in those of low birth weight compared with those of normal birth weight.[120] Thus, if as proposed, fetal growth modulates adrenarche, then increased DHEAS may have reflected an exaggerated adrenarche in these children. The resultant increased androgen pool may set in motion a cycle of altered physiology that is characteristic of PCOS. This notion is further reinforced by the presence of hyperinsulinemia and insulin resistance, which

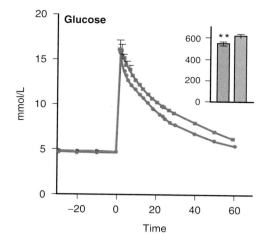

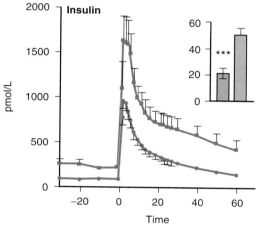

*Figure 20-6. Mean (± standard error) plasma glucose and serum insulin concentrations before and after intravenous administration of 0.3 g/kg glucose in 13 hyperandrogenic (purple lines) and 23 healthy girls (green lines). Insets represent the area under the curve: green bar for the healthy group and purple bar for the hyperandrogenic group. ***P < 0.01 and ****P < 0.001 between groups. (From Apter DA, Butzow J, Laughlin GA, et al. Metabolic features of polycystic ovary syndrome are found in adolescent girls with hyperandrogenism. J Clin Endocrinol Metab 80:2966-2973, 1995.)*

may enhance androgen production in adolescent girls at risk for PCOS.[121] In addition, elevated levels of circulating insulin coincide with a reciprocal decline of SHBG, thereby allowing for increased availability of free testosterone. Thus, the detection of hyperinsulinemia in postmenarchal girls with hyperandrogenism relates temporally to physiologic insulin resistance during puberty and may be of critical importance in the genesis of PCOS.[112]

FETAL PREDISPOSITION

It has been shown that adult female Rhesus monkeys exposed to testosterone in utero, at concentrations equivalent to those found in males, may exhibit increased LH secretion, impaired insulin secretion, hyperandrogenic anovulation, and enlarged ovaries with multiple cystic follicles.[122,123] Similar outcomes have been observed in female adult sheep after in utero exposure to high doses

of testosterone at various phases of pregnancy.[124,125] These observations have led to the hypothesis that the clinical phenotype of PCOS may be the result of intrauterine androgen exposure during pregnancy.[126] In human pregnancy, it has been reported that high maternal serum testosterone levels do not confer this clinical consequence in female offspring.[127] This is likely due to increased circulating levels of SHBG as well as the metabolic capacity of placenta aromatase to neutralize maternal androgen production. Rather, an in utero effect of hyperandrogenism may occur in the presence of abnormal steroidogenesis by the fetal ovary or adrenal gland. In support of this concept, it has been reported that in fetal ovaries, P450c17 was highly expressed in primary interstitial and theca interstitial cells during the second and third trimesters, respectively.[128] These findings indicate that the steroidogenic capacity for androgen production is present in the fetal ovary. In addition, women with 21-hydoxylase deficiency also show excessive ovarian androgen production and polycystic ovaries.[40] Therefore, androgenic programming in fetal life may predispose select individuals to the clinical features of PCOS.

Altered Physiology

HYPOTHALAMIC–PITUITARY INTERACTION

In PCOS, LH secretion is characterized by increased pulse frequency and amplitude, elevated 24-hour mean serum concentrations, and greater responses to gonadotropin-releasing hormone (GnRH) compared with normal women (Fig. 20-7).[129-131] The mechanisms responsible for this increased release of LH are not well understood. A particular characteristic of LH secretion in PCOS is increased pulse frequency, the periodicity of which is approximately 1 hour. This rapid rate of LH release does appear to be altered by experimental manipulation or physiologic change.[132-134] These observations imply that corresponding pulsatile release of hypothalamic GnRH is increased. In PCOS, the relationship between GnRH pulse frequency and gonadotrope responsiveness may be a key issue relative to inappropriate gonadotropin secretion. Previous studies in rodents have shown a preference for *LHβ* gene expression in response to rapid rates of GnRH delivery.[135-137] Not only does GnRH drive the release of LH, but in normal women it also has been shown to self-prime the pituitary. Therefore, it contributes to increased LH sensitivity to subsequent GnRH stimulation.[138] Collectively, these findings have led to the suggestion that the profound abnormality of gonadotropin secretion in PCOS may be a primary consequence of increased hypothalamic GnRH activity.[139]

In humans, progressive increases in the frequency of GnRH stimulation have resulted in corresponding increases in the rate of LH release as well as elevated basal concentrations.[139,140] In GnRH-deficient women, an increase in the rate of GnRH administration from every 90 minutes to every 60 minutes was not associated with corresponding increases in serum LH or with changes in pulse amplitude, whereas GnRH given at 30-minute intervals resulted in elevated LH levels and reduction of pulse amplitude.[139] Although consistent with the primacy of increased hypothalamic GnRH, an LH pulse frequency of 1 hour

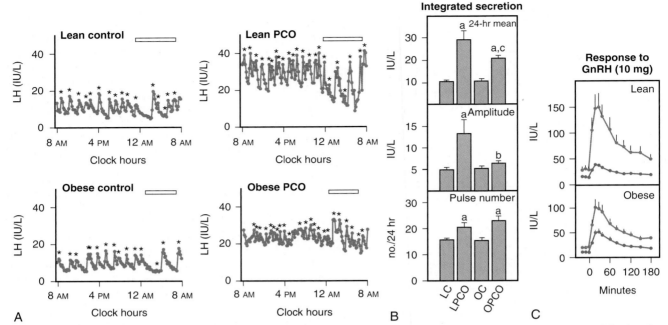

Figure 20-7. *A, Representative 24-hour luteinizing hormone (LH) pulsatile patterns in lean and obese control women during the follicular phase of the menstrual cycle and in lean and obese women with polycystic ovary syndrome (PCOS). Asterisks* indicate LH pulses. Open bars *signify sleep times. B, Twenty-four–hour mean (± standard error) LH levels, pulse amplitude, pulse frequency. C, LH responses to gonadotropin-releasing hormone (GnRH) in lean and obese women with PCOS (LPCO, OPCO) and their respective control groups (LC, OC: n = 8 for each group). a, P < 0.001 versus corresponding control group; b, P < 0.01; c, P < 0.001 versus corresponding lean group.* Green lines, *PCOS;* purple lines, *normal control subjects. (From Morales AJ Laughlin CA, Butzow T, et al. Insulin, somatotropic, and LH axes in lean and obese women with polycystic ovary syndrome: Common and distinct features. J Clin Endocrinol Metab 81:2854-2864, 1996.)*

may represent a physiologic limit beyond which more frequent pulses in women do not occur. In normal ovulatory women, during the late follicular phase and at midcycle, as well as in postmenopausal women, it has been documented that LH pulse frequency approximates 60 minutes.[141-146] In addition, previous studies have shown that GnRH release from the medial basal hypothalamus of the fetus and adult has a periodicity of approximately 1 hour.[147] Thus, in women with PCOS, the tempo and, to some degree, the magnitude of pulsatile gonadotropin secretion are probably established by hypothalamic GnRH activity. However, beyond the requisite need for GnRH, LH responsiveness to GnRH and, accordingly, maximal increases in LH pulse amplitude are probably reliant on other factors.

It has been suggested that the positive feedback effects of chronic estrogen secretion associated with this disorder may bring about an increase in LH, either by a direct effect on gonadotrope sensitivity to GnRH or indirectly by facilitating GnRH pulse frequency.[129,148,149] In vitro, estrogen has been shown to increase the fraction of individual gonadotropes responding to GnRH, which is consistent with amplification of LH responses to GnRH in normal women receiving E_2 benzoate.[150] In PCOS, baseline levels of estrone and E_2 have been correlated with LH responses to GnRH.[129] However, prolonged administration of estrone to patients with PCOS did not raise circulating levels of LH beyond baseline values or increase GnRH-stimulated LH responses.[148] Alternatively, in animals, it has been demonstrated that estrogen enhances GnRH pulse frequency, and in women with PCOS, serum GnRH levels are

increased.[151,152] The idea that estrogen may exert an effect on the hypothalamus in PCOS is supported by the strong positive correlation of mean serum E_2 levels and GnRH pulse frequency.

Hyperandrogenemia has also been implicated as a potential cause of increased LH secretion in PCOS. In vitro, it has been shown that androgen administration resulted in increased GnRH pulse generator activity.[153] Examination of LH secretion in hyperandrogenic patients with congenital adrenal hyperplasia showed that mean LH levels and LH responses to GnRH were increased and tended to normalize with the onset of treatment and a corresponding lowering of androgen levels.[40] By comparison, other studies have not been able to detect an increase in LH after the administration of androgen. Short-term infusion of androgen to both normal women and women with PCOS did not alter basal LH secretion.[154] Moreover, high-dose androgen infusion in normal women appeared to result in an acute reduction of serum LH levels.[42,155]

Notwithstanding these findings, recent studies have indicated that excess androgen production may have a profound influence on LH pulse frequency in women with PCOS. Previously, it had been shown that the administration of progesterone, either alone or in combination with estrogen (oral contraceptive), suppressed mean LH and LH pulse frequency in both women with PCOS and normal women.[156] The observation that suppression of LH release was more pronounced in normal women compared with women with PCOS suggested to the investigators that increased LH pulse frequency may reflect a fundamental

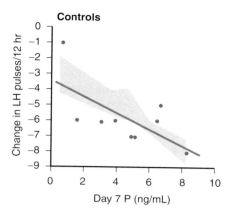

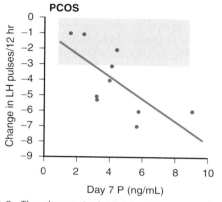

Figure 20-8. The change in luteinizing hormone pulse frequency between flutamide treatment alone and after estradiol (E_2) and progesterone (P) administration for 7 days during continued flutamide treatment. Data are shown as a function of the mean plasma P level during E_2 and P administration with flutamide for control subjects and patients with polycystic ovary syndrome (PCOS). Shaded area shows the range of responses in an identical protocol performed in the absence of flutamide. The slopes for the linear regression analysis are as follows: control subjects (with flutamide), –0.53; control subjects (without flutamide), –0.76; women with PCOS (with flutamide), –0.72; and women with PCOS (without flutamide), 0.07. (From Eagleson CA, Gingrich MB, Pastor CL, et al. Polycystic ovarian syndrome: evidence that flutamide restores sensitivity of the gonadotropin-releasing hormone pulse generator to inhibition by estradiol and progesterone. J Clin Endocrinol Metab 85:4047-4052, 2000.)

property of the hypothalamic pulse generator in PCOS.[156] In a series of elegant studies, pretreatment with an androgen-blocking agent before the administration of estrogen and progesterone in doses equivalent to midluteal concentrations resulted in restoration of LH pulse frequency to that observed in normal women[157] (Fig. 20-8). These findings suggested that in PCOS, high circulating levels of androgen prevent the negative feedback effects of estrogen and progesterone on LH pulse release, as noted in earlier studies. Moreover, the physiologic relevance in women regards a rapid rate of spontaneous hypothalamic GnRH activity, which is regulated by the feedback effects of ovarian steroids.

The potential role of hyperinsulinemia on gonadotropin secretion and, in particular, LH release has not been extensively studied. It has been previously showed in vitro that rat pituitary cells preincubated with insulin exhibit increased LH responsiveness after the administration of GnRH in a dose-dependent manner compared with those of untreated cells, which suggests a facilitative role for insulin on GnRH-stimulated LH release.[158-160] No effect of insulin was observed when these studies were performed in serum-supplemented media. Efforts to determine the effect of insulin in women with PCOS have not shown consistent alterations in LH secretion or release after GnRH stimulation.[49,161] Reduction of hyperinsulinemia by the administration of insulin-lowering drugs to patients with PCOS resulted in decreased mean serum levels of androgens and LH in some cases, whereas in others, an accompanying fall of LH was not found.[49,63,65,66,68-72,161-170] Recently, we explored the role of insulin in gonadotropin secretion in women with PCOS and normal women. Using the hyperinsulinemic–euglycemic clamp technique, we found that episodic gonadotropin secretion and LH response to multidose GnRH stimulation were not altered by insulin infusion over an interval of 12 hours in both groups. In particular, endogenous serum LH levels were unchanged before and immediately after the initiation of the insulin clamp (Fig. 20-9). These findings confirm and clarify previous studies, which have not shown consistent alterations in LH secretion or release after GnRH stimulation and insulin administration in women with PCOS.[49,161] In addition, our results may explain why changes in serum LH were not observed in women with PCOS who were treated with insulin-lowering drugs, despite significant reductions in circulating androgen levels.[49,63,65,66, 68-72, 162-164,165-170] Alternatively, interpretation of these clinical trials is potentially confounded by several factors. First, most of the patients studied were obese, and it has been shown recently that obesity is inversely correlated with LH secretion in PCOS (Fig. 20-10).[144] Second, hyperinsulinemia is positively correlated with BMI in women with this syndrome. Third, the occurrence of ovulation in PCOS is associated with a lowering of LH levels into the normal range. Although additional studies are necessary, the evidence to date has not been able to clearly demonstrate a functional interaction between insulin and LH in this disorder.

Increased LH pulse frequency and other features of PCOS have been described in women with epileptic disorders or women treated with antiepileptic drugs.[171-175] These observations have led to the intriguing consideration that epilepsy or treatment with antiepileptic drugs, in particular, sodium valproate and PCOS, are causally related. The link between epileptic and postseizure ictal states may involve stimulation of excitatory neurotransmitters, the receptors of which exist in hypothalamic nuclei that influence GnRH release. Thus, epileptic activity may result in increased GnRH activity and simulate the pattern of increased LH secretion in PCOS.[176,177] In addition to altered LH secretion, polycystic ovaries and hyperandrogenism have been reported in untreated and treated women with epileptic seizures. These findings strengthen the possible association between PCOS and epilepsy.[171,178,179] A mechanistic role for antiepileptic medication, including sodium valproate, in the development of excess androgen production or follicle cyst formation in treated subjects has not been elucidated. Unfortunately, the vast majority of reports

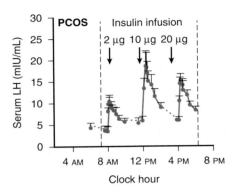

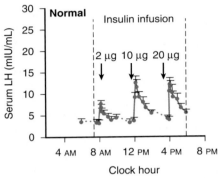

Figure 20-9. Time course of mean (± standard error) serum luteinizing hormone (LH) concentrations after intravenous administration of three successive doses of gonadotropin-releasing hormone. The doses are given at 4-hour intervals during the hyperinsulinemic–euglycemic clamp (80 mU/m²/min) in women with polycystic ovary syndrome (PCOS) and healthy women. In PCOS, significant increases in LH increment (P < 0.02) were detected compared with those of normal women. The preinfusion mean concentration of serum LH was similar to the initial preinjection mean baseline level of LH in both women with PCOS and normal women. (Patel KS, Coffler MS, Dahan MH, et al. Increased luteinizing hormone secretion in women with polycystic ovary syndrome is unaltered by prolonged insulin infusion. J Clin Endocrinol Metab 88:5456-5461, 2003.)

linking epilepsy or antiepileptic medication to PCOS have been beset by poor experimental design and insufficient rigor to determine causality.

In contrast to pituitary LH, FSH secretion in PCOS is decreased, as indicated by significantly lower serum concentrations compared with those found in normal women during the early follicular phase of the menstrual cycle.[129] In addition, FSH responses to GnRH stimulation are reduced as shown in some, but not all, studies.[180-182] The precise underlying basis for decreased FSH secretion in PCOS has not been determined, although the negative feedback effect of chronic unopposed estrogen secretion in these women has been implicated as a mechanism.[183] Support for this concept has been demonstrated by a study in which women with PCOS were treated with E_2 benzoate for 2 weeks.[148] Daily measurement of serum gonadotropin levels showed a progressive decline of circulating FSH, whereas serum LH concentrations remained unaltered, resulting in a decrease in the LH/FSH ratio. The reduction in serum FSH may also reflect the activity of hypothalamic GnRH. As mentioned earlier, increased frequency of pulsatile GnRH predisposes to a preference for *LHβ* gene expression at the expense of the *FSHβ* gene.[135-137]

THECA CELL FUNCTION

The most notable clinical feature of PCOS is hirsutism, which is the result of excessive androgen production. Both the ovary and the adrenal glands contribute to the pool of increased circulating androgens. However, in PCOS, the major serum androgens, androstenedione and testosterone, are produced by the ovary, whereas elevated concentrations of DHEAS are derived from the adrenal glands.[56] Within the polycystic ovary, numerous antral follicles are surrounded by hyperplastic theca cells that are the predominant site of androgen overproduction. There is firm evidence to indicate that excess ovarian androgen production is driven by abnormally increased secretion of pituitary LH acting on

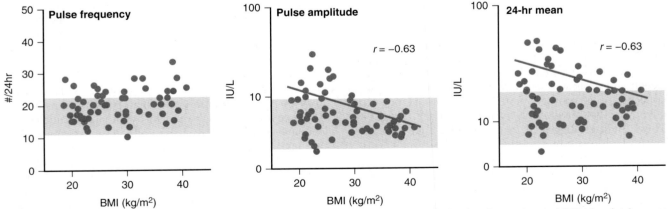

Figure 20-10. Regression of body mass index (BMI) for polycystic ovary syndrome (PCOS, purple dots) and normal control (NC, blue dots) women against luteinizing hormone (LH) pulse frequency (PCOS and NC, P = NS), LH pulse amplitude (PCOS, r = –0.63, P < 0.001; NC, P = NS), and 24-hour mean LH levels (PCOS, r = –0.63, P < 0.001; NC, P = NS). Values for LH pulse amplitude and 24-hour mean are log-transformed. Shaded area represents the 95% confidence interval for NC (frequency, 11-22 pulses/24 hr; amplitude, 2.6-9.2 IU/L; 24-hour mean, 6.1-18.2 IU/L). (From Arroyo A, Laughlin CA, Morales AJ, Yen SSC. Inappropriate gonadotropin secretion in polycystic ovary syndrome: influence of adiposity. J Clin Endocrinol Metab 82:3728-3733, 1997.)

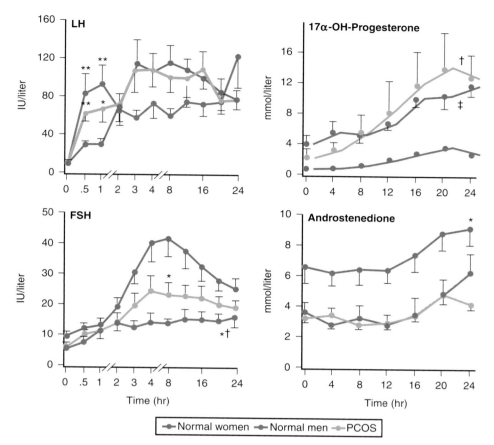

Figure 20-11. *Mean (± standard error) responses of luteinizing hormone (LH), follicle-stimulating hormone (FSH), 17α-hydroxyprogesterone, and androstenedione to gonadotropin-releasing hormone agonist (nafarelin, 100 μg) subcutaneously at time = 0 in five women with polycystic ovary syndrome (PCOS), nine healthy women, and five healthy men. **P < 0.01 and *P < 0.05, for the comparison with healthy women of the area under the response curve. †P < 0.01 and ‡P < 0.001, for the comparison with healthy women of the response at different times. (From Barnes RB, Rosenfield RL, Burstein S, et al. Pituitary-ovarian responses to nafarelin testing in the polycystic ovary syndrome. N Engl J Med 320:559-565, 1989.)*

theca cells.[184] Nonetheless, the rather broad range of LH secretion in PCOS suggests that other mechanisms may be instrumental in the excessive production of androgens, including increased theca cell sensitivity to LH and the presence of cogonadotropic growth factors.

The former notion is supported by in vitro studies that have established that theca cells from polycystic ovaries in culture produce significantly more androgen after LH stimulation than that generated by theca cells from normal ovaries.[57,185,186] In these studies, the rate of androgen production in PCOS was greater than of normal control subjects, but the magnitude of response was similar in both groups, reflecting the higher basal production of androgen in the PCOS group. Clinically, stimulation of theca cell androgen production by a GnRH agonist has shown significant increases in serum 17-hydroxyprogesterone and androstenedione concentrations in PCOS compared with those of normal women (Fig. 20-11).[180] Differences in testosterone responses between the two groups were not found. The pattern of individual steroid hormone responses indicated overexpression of the cytochrome P450c17 gene, which regulates 17-hydroxylase and C17,20-lyase activity. Moreover, these findings suggested that differential androgen production in PCOS may arise de novo within the theca cell.

It has been shown in animals that subtle increases in LH may induce cytochrome P450c17 gene expression, a mechanism that might relate to higher basal levels of androgens in women with PCOS. To further examine this issue, steroid responses to human chorionic gonadotropin (hCG) were examined in women with PCOS and in normal subjects before and after administration of a GnRH agonist that effectively suppressed and eliminated any disparity in basal LH secretion and ovarian androgen production.[187] Serum 17-hydroxyprogesterone responses to hCG were not abrogated by agonist treatment, which provided further evidence that in PCOS the magnitude of androgen responsiveness to LH is due to a primary abnormality of theca cell steroidogenesis. Despite these findings, LH may still influence selective steroid hormone production indirectly through activation of P450c17 because 17-hydroxylase and C17,20-lyase are differentially regulated.[188,189] In contrast to the stimulatory effects of low-dose LH on 17-hydroxylase, high doses of LH down-regulate the C17,20-lyase component of P450c17, which would account for the greater incremental change of 17-hydroxyprogesterone compared with androstenedione after GnRH agonist stimulation. Additionally, the relative increase in 17-hydroxyprogesterone over androstenedione may also be attributed, at least in part, to the observation that 17-hydroxyprogesterone is not a substrate for C17,20-lyase in the human ovary.[190] Collectively, these data indicate that in PCOS, to a degree, abnormal androgen production by the theca cell is an inherent defect of steroidogenesis, although the complexity of the process is evident and remains to be elucidated.

Exclusive of the direct stimulus–response dynamic of ovarian androgen production, the human theca cell is also subject to the effects of co-gonadotropic growth factors, the most notable of which are insulin and insulin-like growth factor (IGF). Receptors for insulin, IGF-I, and IGF-II have been localized to the theca compartment of ovaries from both normal women and patients with PCOS.[191] Accordingly, in vitro studies of normal human theca tissue have shown that these growth factors are capable of enhancing androgen responses to LH as well as independently stimulating androgen production.[185,192-194] In vitro, IGF-I has been shown to synergistically augment LH-stimulated androgen production from cultured theca cells.[195,196] This facilitative action of IGF-I has been attributed to increased LH receptor induction,[197] greater expression of steroidogenic enzymes,[198,199] and enhanced LH-induced cyclic AMP production.[200] However, because IGF-I mRNA and protein are not expressed in human granulosa cells, it is likely that IGF-II is the principal paracrine influence of these two proteins. In human theca cell tissue, IGF-II stimulated basal androgen release as well as enhanced LH-induced androgen production, the magnitude of which was equivalent to that of IGF-I.[192] In the same study, insulin, either alone or in combination with LH, also amplified theca cell androgen production. These findings were consistent with previously published results that also showed that the enhanced effect of insulin was dose-dependent.[193]

In contrast, studies performed on theca cells from hyperandrogenic women, including those with PCOS, have not shown a synergistic effect of LH and insulin.[194] Similarly, IGF-I did not augment LH-induced androgen formation by theca tissue obtained from women with PCOS. In vivo studies performed in Rhesus monkeys showed that IGF-I, in either the absence or the presence of human growth hormone, had no effect on gonadotropin-stimulated serum androstenedione levels.[201] The inability to show an effect of insulin on theca cell androgen production may reflect the presence of insulin resistance in the ovary similar to diminished insulin sensitivity in muscle, fat, and liver. However, recent studies have shown that insulin may increase androgen production from theca cells of women with PCOS though an alternative pathway involving inositolglycan, a downstream mediator of insulin signaling. When theca cells were incubated with insulin in the presence of antibody to inositolglycan, androgen production was inhibited, whereas hCG-stimulated androgen production was unaltered.[202] Thus, it appears that there are at least two separate signaling pathways for insulin and LH.

Clinically, the effect of hyperinsulinemia on ovarian steroidogenesis has been examined using an oral glucose tolerance test or the euglycemic hyperinsulinemic clamp technique. Most studies have not shown significant changes in androgen secretion in women with PCOS or normal women, despite considerable increases in circulating insulin levels.[49,161,203] In one study, minimal increases in androstenedione were noted during insulin infusion.[204] Whether prevailing hyperinsulinemia precluded any additional effect of superimposed insulin administration on ovarian androgen production in these patients is not clear. However, these in vivo studies may reflect insulin resistance by theca cell tissues, despite in vitro findings to the contrary. In addition, clinical evidence suggests that intact granulosa cells in women with PCOS show insulin resistance.[205] Nevertheless, a reduction in hyperinsulinemia has been associated with significant decreases in serum androgens without corresponding changes in LH in women with PCOS who are treated with insulin-lowering drugs. This observation indirectly suggests a role for insulin in LH-stimulated androgen synthesis.

GRANULOSA CELL FUNCTION

In PCOS, the mechanisms responsible for the persistence of ovulatory failure are not well understood. According to histomorphometric studies, ovarian follicle development is arrested at the midantral stage of growth, and the granulosa cells that line these follicles appear to be in various stages of degeneration.[30] Earlier studies implicated a deficiency of aromatase activity to explain the lack of follicle development because E_2 concentrations were low in follicular fluid and granulosa cells contained little measurable aromatase enzyme.[48,206-208] However, subsequent in vitro studies have demonstrated that these cells are, indeed, vital and exhibit substantial capacity for steroidogenesis.[17,29,209] We have previously shown that cultured granulosa cells obtained from women with PCOS exhibit a significantly greater rise in E_2 after FSH stimulation compared with normal granulosa cells, which indicated that the inherent capacity of these cells to respond to FSH was ample.[209] However, the time course of response was characterized by an inability to sustain peak levels, in contrast to the pattern of normal cells, which implied suboptimal granulosa cell function (Fig. 20-12). Our recent clinical studies have corroborated these in vitro findings. In women with PCOS, the capacity for E_2 production in response to the stimulatory effects of recombinant human FSH (r-hFSH) was clearly enhanced compared with that of normal women.[210] Notably, this difference was dose-dependent and only manifested at 150 IU, because increases in circulating E_2 after 37.5 IU and 75 IU r-hFSH were similar in both women with PCOS and normal women (Fig. 20-13). The amplification of E_2 responses beyond an apparent FSH threshold dose range indicated greater in vivo granulosa cell responsiveness in PCOS in the presence of an abundance of aromatase substrate because profiles of circulating FSH levels at each dose were essentially identical in both groups. This heightened E_2 response may have reflected greater follicle number in the polycystic ovary compared with the normal ovary.[30] This explanation is consistent with the recent report in which comparative E_2 responses to FSH in women with PCOS and those in normal women during ovulation induction were more likely related to the number of stimulated ovarian follicles rather than to differences in the FSH threshold.[211]

Alternatively, PCOS granulosa cells are extremely sensitive to FSH stimulation. We previously showed that, in granulosa cells obtained from 4- to 7-mm follicles of polycystic ovaries, FSH induced an approximately fourfold increase in E_2 levels compared with baseline.[212] Comparison

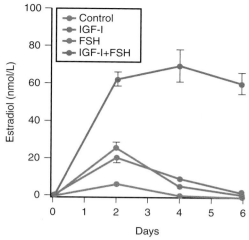

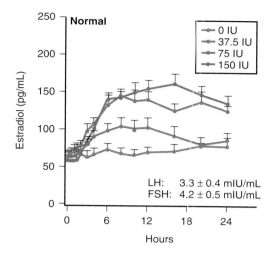

Figure 20-12. *Time course of estradiol production by cultured granulosa cells. Data are the mean (± standard error) of the pooled results from individual experiments with three patients with polycystic ovary syndrome. In each experiment, cells (20,000 viable cells) were cultured for 2, 4, and 6 days in serum-free medium containing 10^{-7} mol/L androstenedione as control subjects (androstenedione alone) with 30 ng/mL follicle-stimulating hormone (FSH) or insulin-like growth factor I (IGF-I). The medium was changed at 2-day intervals, at which time fresh hormones were added to the appropriate cultures. (From Erickson CF, Magoffin DA, Cragun JR, et al. The effects of insulin and insulin-like growth factors-I and -II on estradiol production by granulosa cells of polycystic ovaries. J Clin Endocrinol Metab 70:894-902, 1990.)*

of the effective dose 50 for FSH-stimulated E_2 production showed an eightfold higher granulosa cell sensitivity to FSH in PCOS compared with normal cells.[209] Clinically, increased granulosa cell responsiveness to 150 IU FSH in women with PCOS was nearly twofold greater than that observed in normal women. However, lower amounts of r-hFSH stimulation produced E_2 responses that were similar in women with PCOS and normal women, which raised the possibility of a putative aromatase inhibitor within the polycystic ovary microenvironment. In hyperandrogenemic women with PCOS, the abundance of aromatase substrate would have been expected to result in greater E_2 production in response to all doses of r-hFSH compared with normal women. In this regard, it is noteworthy that FSH in low pharmacologic amounts uniformly induced aromatase gene expression within 3 hours of administration, which suggests that aromatase inhibition, if present in PCOS, is relatively mild.

Whether these results reflect increased numbers of stimulated follicles, increased granulosa cell sensitivity to FSH, or both, it is evident that women with PCOS are susceptible to ovarian hyperstimulation in response to gonadotropin stimulation. It is unknown whether increased granulosa cell sensitivity arises primarily or secondarily as a result of intra- or extraovarian factors. Recent studies have shown that, in granulosa cells obtained by aspiration of follicles from unstimulated anovulatory polycystic ovaries, binding of radiolabeled FSH was significantly higher compared with that detected in cells from ovaries of ovulatory women with PCOS or from normal women (Fig. 20-14).[29] Moreover, accompanying studies showed increased E_2 release from the granulosa cells of polycystic

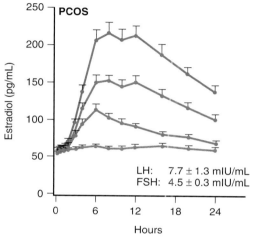

Figure 20-13. *Mean (± standard error) serum estradiol levels after intravenous administration of the indicated doses of recombinant follicle-stimulating hormone (rFSH) to subjects with polycystic ovary syndrome ([PCOS] n = 16) and normal control subjects (n = 7) at t = 0 hours. The 0-IU dose of rFSH is saline control. Mean (± standard error) baseline levels of serum luteinizing hormone (LH) and follicle-stimulating hormone (FSH) are also shown. (From Coffler MS, Patel KS, Dahan MH, et al. Evidence of abnormal granulosa cell responsiveness to follicle-stimulating hormone in women with polycystic ovary syndrome. J Clin Endocrinol Metab 88:1742-1747, 2003.)*

ovaries in response to FSH compared with cells from ovulatory ovaries, which is consistent with results from our lab and others.[209,212,213] Together, these findings link granulosa cell sensitivity to increased FSH receptor binding in granulosa cells from polycystic ovaries and provide insight into a possible mechanism for increased E_2 responsiveness to FSH stimulation. Moreover, the observation that high-dose androgen administration to nonhuman female primates increases FSH receptor expression lends credence to the possibility that androgen may facilitate granulosa cell hyperresponsiveness to FSH in women with PCOS.[46]

Among the factors that have been shown to affect granulosa cell function, insulin, and IGFs appear to act as co-gonadotropins within the ovary. When PCOS granulosa cells were co-incubated with insulin, FSH-stimulated E_2 release was mildly increased, whereas by comparison,

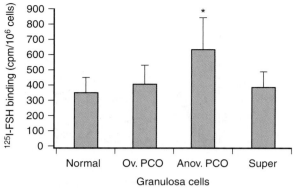

Figure 20-14. *Binding of human recombinant ^{125}I-follicle-stimulating hormone (FSH) to granulosa cells from different groups of patients. FSH binding per cell number was significantly (*P < 0.05) increased in anovulatory polycystic ovary syndrome (Anov. PCO). The values represent mean ± standard deviation obtained from different cellular preparations, each assayed at least twice in triplicate. Ov. PCO, ovulatory polycystic ovary syndrome. (From Almahbobi C, Anderiesz C, Hutchinson P, et al. Functional integrity of granulosa cells from polycystic ovaries. Clin Endocrinol 44:571-580, 1996.)*

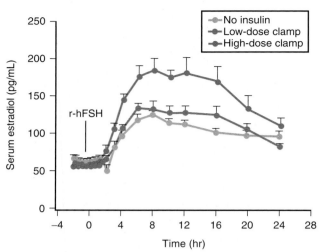

Figure 20-15. *Time course of mean (± standard error) 24-hour serum estradiol responses after injection of intravenous recombinant follicle-stimulating hormone (r-hFSH), 75 IU, to women with polycystic ovary syndrome treated with pioglitazone without insulin infusion and 2 hours after initiation of low-dose (30 mU/m^2·min) and high-dose (200 mU/m^2·min) hyperinsulinemic–euglycemic clamps administered for 10 hours. The integrated estradiol response, as determined by area under the curve, was significantly greater (P < 0.02) in subjects receiving high-dose insulin infusion compared with those observed in women without insulin or with low-dose insulin infusion (Coffler MS, Patel KS, Dahan MH, et al. Enhanced granulosa cell responsiveness to follicle stimulating hormone during insulin infusion in women with polycystic ovary syndrome treated with pioglitazone. J Clin Endocrinol Metab 88: 5624-5631, 2003.)*

addition of IGF-I amplified the response beyond that encountered with either FSH or IGF-I alone.[212] These findings suggested that in PCOS the role of insulin in granulosa cell function was minimal or, alternatively, the granulosa cell was resistant to the action of insulin. In contrast, other studies have shown that PCOS granulosa cells were extremely sensitive to insulin across a wide physiologic dose range, regardless of gonadotropin stimulation.[214] Moreover, this facilitory action of insulin appeared to be mediated through its own receptor because responsiveness was completely inhibited by insulin receptor antibody, whereas an IGF receptor–specific antibody had no effect.[215] Efforts to demonstrate a role for insulin in granulosa cell function in women with PCOS have been limited by a lack of adequate assessment of follicular activity and a preponderance of therapeutic clinical trials. After treatment with insulin-lowering drugs, women with PCOS have been shown to improve insulin sensitivity and resume ovulation, which indirectly links insulin resistance to chronic anovulation in this disorder.[62-72] In studies that evaluated granulosa cell function, measurement of serum E_2 levels did not show any particular pattern of response in women who became ovulatory or remained anovulatory. In women undergoing weight reduction, initiation of regular menses was associated with improved insulin sensitivity, as reflected by increased SHBG.[167,168] In these studies, because the rate of ovulation improved during treatment, it was unclear whether an alteration of E_2 levels was a direct result of lowered circulating insulin levels or was secondary to restoration of ovarian steroidogenesis. In addition, insulin-lowering drugs, such as thiazolidinediones and metformin, have been shown to exert direct effect on ovarian steroid enzymes.[216-219] Recently, we used FSH-stimulated E_2 responses to show potential effects of insulin resistance on granulosa cell function.[205] In women with PCOS treated with a thiazolidinedione, pioglitazone, for 5 months, granulosa cell responsiveness to FSH during a hyperinsulinemic–euglycemic clamp was significantly

increased compared with the E_2 response observed before treatment under identical experimental conditions (Fig. 20-15). The finding that amplification of the E_2 response was associated with an improvement in insulin sensitivity suggested that, in women with PCOS, the granulosa cell may be insulin-resistant. Moreover, these findings may account for the apparent paradoxical effect of insulin on granulosa cell function in that in vitro, insulin enhances E_2 production, whereas in vivo, treatment with insulin-lowering drugs induces ovulation. Whether granulosa cells in women with PCOS may be insulin-resistant on a primary basis or secondarily has not been addressed.

These findings may have relevance to clinical responses during induction of ovulation in women with PCOS. As previously mentioned, granulosa cells removed from polycystic ovaries have been shown to exhibit substantial E_2 release after incubation with insulin at doses of much less than 1 µg/ml, which simulated physiologic concentrations.[214] In vivo, this facilitory effect of insulin on PCOS granulosa cells has not been observed because initial clinical responses to FSH are characterized by reduced E_2 increments after FSH stimulation in women with PCOS compared with normal women.[129,220] The idea that PCOS granulosa cells may be insulin-resistant, could, at least in part, account for decreased E_2 responsiveness to FSH. Moreover, this reduced follicle responsiveness may be overcome with progressive increases in the dose or duration of FSH. Protracted administration of low-dose FSH has been particularly useful because the risk of ovarian hyperstimulation syndrome is considerably diminished with this method of ovulation induction.[221] The gradual accumulation of constant low-dose

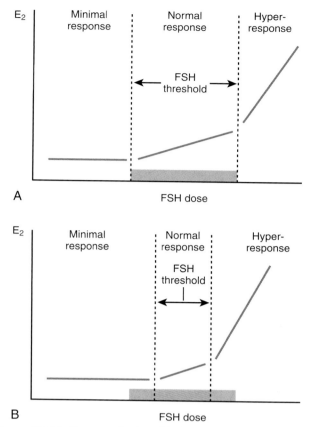

Figure 20-16. Conceptualized model of granulosa cell responses to a range of follicle-stimulating hormone (FSH) doses administered during ovulation induction in normal women (**A**) and women with polycystic ovary syndrome ([PCOS] **B**). Note the narrowed FSH threshold in women with PCOS, which may explain the minimal response to initial gonadotropin stimulation as well as the comparative hyperresponsiveness at higher threshold doses. E_2, estradiol.

FSH over time is preferred to an escalation of the daily dose because of follicular hyperresponsiveness to FSH in women with PCOS and an increased risk of ovarian hyperstimulation syndrome.[211] These observations, combined with our previous report describing greater E_2 responsiveness in women with PCOS compared with normal women at an FSH dose of 150 IU, suggests a bidirectional narrowing of the FSH threshold range in this disorder (Fig. 20-16).

The effect of insulin on FSH-stimulated follicle development may also involve the IGF system. Both IGF-I and IGF-II have been shown to enhance the response of granulosa cells to FSH.[209,222] In PCOS granulosa cells, exposure to both IGF-I and FSH resulted in significantly greater E_2 production compared with incubation with each hormone separately. The actions of IGF are likely mediated by the receptors, which have been identified on granulosa cells of both PCOS and normal follicles.[191] However, despite in vitro studies in which IGF-I clearly amplified FSH-induced aromatase activity, most studies have not detected the protein or have shown very little in human granulosa cells.[191,223,224] By comparison, IGF-II mRNA has been located in all compartments of the human ovary and is strongly expressed in granulosa cells.[191,223] A relationship between insulin and IGF-II has previously been shown by

in vitro studies of rat adipocytes in which insulin increased the expression of cell surface IGF-II receptors, probably by mobilizing internalized receptors.[225,226] Consistent with this observation are recent studies of human polycystic ovary tissue that showed that estrogen responses to IGF-II were significantly enhanced in granulosa cells preincubated with insulin compared with those without insulin.[17] Insulin also increased the response of granulosa cells to IGF-I, although the incremental change was smaller. These findings point out the potentially critical relationship between insulin and IGF-II in the regulation of granulosa cell function. In particular, in PCOS, excess insulin secretion may down-regulate insulin receptors, which would prevent translocation of subcellular IGF-II receptors to the plasma membrane and deprive granulosa cells of the stimulatory effect of a potent co-gonadotropin.

In an attempt to determine the effects of IGF-I on ovarian function in vivo, an experimental gonadotropin clamp model was developed in Rhesus monkeys that permitted assessment of steroid responses before and after IGF-I infusion.[201] E_2 responses to gonadotropin infusion were not altered in animals treated with IGF-I and human growth hormone, whereas a significant reduction in E_2 was observed in monkeys receiving IGF-I alone. These results suggested that IGF-I does not amplify gonadotropin-stimulated E_2 production, but rather implies a facilitative role for hGH in ovarian responsiveness to gonadotropin stimulation, as previously proposed.[227-229]

In PCOS, it has been reported that circulating IGF-I levels are elevated, although this is not a consistent finding. IGFs are complexed with IGFBPs, which regulate their bioactivity. In PCOS, serum IGFBP-1 is decreased as a result of hyperinsulinemia, which implies an increase in the levels of free IGF-I. This concept is supported by the finding of increased circulating levels of free IGF-I in women with PCOS.[230] Additionally, IGFBPs may be critical in regulating IGF bioactivity at the level of the ovary. Relevant to this notion, IGFBP-2 and -4 proteases have been shown to be increased in follicle fluid derived from androgenic follicles, including those of patients with PCOS.[231,232] In addition, IGFBP-4 protease was not detectable in these follicles.[233] These results are in stark distinction to those found in healthy antral follicles of normal women, in which IGFBP-2 and -4 proteases were decreased and IGF-II concentrations were increased in the follicular fluid.[234] The effect of the androgenic environment on follicular fluid IGF bioavailability has been documented in transsexuals treated with high-dose androgens. In the follicular fluid of these individuals, IGF-II levels were decreased, IGFBP levels were increased, and IGFBP-4 protease was nondetectable, thus accounting for decreased bioavilable IGF-II.[235] Whether this IGF-IGFBP profile is a consequence of follicular fluid androgen levels is not clear, although the association is compelling and suggests that hyperandrogenism of PCOS, driven in part by insulin-mediated theca cell androgen production, may be instrumental.

The recognition of abnormal follicle growth and development in women with PCOS has been derived primarily from studies involving follicle responses to gonadotropin stimulation and granulosa cell function. However, the potential role of the oocyte in this disorder has not been investigated. Recent studies have shown that oocyte-derived growth factors may be important to follicle development and function. In particular, growth differentiation factor-9 (GDF-9) and bone morphogenetic protein-15 (BMP-15)/GDF-9B appear to have major roles in folliculogenesis and female fertility.[236-238] In vitro studies have shown that these genes are selectively expressed in developing oocytes during folliculogenesis.[239-242] In addition, in GDF-9-deficient female mice, disruption of reproductive function has been associated with arrested follicle growth at the primary stage, decreased granulosa cell proliferation, inappropriate theca cell development, ovarian cyst formation, and infertility.[243-245] We have examined mRNA expression of GDF-9 and BMP-15 in ovaries obtained from women with PCOS and found that the GDF-9 signal was decreased in oocytes throughout folliculogenesis compared with GDF-9 message in oocytes from normal ovaries.[246] By comparison, there was no difference in BMP-15 mRNA expression between groups. These results suggest that the expression of GDF-9 is delayed in oocytes of developing PCOS follicles. Because of the apparent growing importance of GDF-9 in folliculogenesis and fertility, it is suggested that dysregulation of GDF-9 expression may contribute to aberrant folliculogenesis in women with PCOS.

ADRENAL FUNCTION

Approximately 50% of women with PCOS exhibit increased levels of DHEAS and 11β-hydroxyandrostenedione, indicating excess androgen production by the zona reticularis of the adrenal gland.[247-249] By comparison, basal circulating adrenocorticotropin (ACTH) levels in women with PCOS are similar to those of normal women.[250] In addition, circadian rhythms of serum dehydroepiandrosterone (DHEA) and cortisol in women with PCOS were not different from those exhibited by normal women.[56] These findings suggest that the mechanism for adrenal hyperandrogenemia may arise from either altered adrenal responsiveness to ACTH or abnormal adrenal stimulation by factors other than ACTH. Studies to address this issue have not produced consistent results. Increased 17-hydroxyprogesterone responses to ACTH, after dexamethasone, have been observed in women with PCOS and functional ovarian hyperandrogenism, which suggested dysregulation of P450c17.[251,252] However, other studies have not been able to confirm these results.[253-255] These latter studies did not employ dexamethasone suppression before ACTH stimulation, which may have accounted for the disparate results. In vitro, IGF-I and insulin have been found to enhance ACTH-stimulated P450c17 expression and adrenal androgen synthesis.[256,257] In women with PCOS, serum 17-hydroxyprogesterone and androstenedione responses to ACTH were significantly greater in those with hyperinsulinemia compared with those with normal insulin levels.[258] In the same study, circulating cortisol and DHEA responses were equivalent between groups. Subsequently, it was shown that in women with PCOS, ACTH administration during insulin infusion was associated with significantly higher 17-hydroxypregnenolone and 17-hydroxyprogesterone responses than those measured during saline infusion.[259] This facilitory effect of insulin appeared to lower the activity of C17,20-lyase, as shown by higher 17-hydroxypregnenolone/DHEA and 17-hydroxyprogesterone/androstenedione ratios. Similar results have been described in men undergoing hyperinsulinemic clamp studies.[260] These findings are consistent with reports that show a reduction in serum DHEAS in women during administration of insulin infusion or a glucose tolerance test.[161,203,261-263] Whether adrenal hyperandrogenemia contributes to the perpetuation of PCOS is not clear. However, the suggestion that an exaggerated adrenarche may be an inciting event in the pathogenesis of PCOS warrants further investigation of adrenal gland function in adolescent girls with hyperandrogenism.

INSULIN RESISTANCE

Women with PCOS exhibit insulin resistance, irrespective of obesity (Fig. 20-17).[55,56,58,264] The insulin resistance is characterized by decreased insulin-mediated glucose disposal and, in obese women with PCOS, increased hepatic glucose production.[49,265] In addition, insulin secretion by pancreatic β cells is increased as a compensatory mechanism. Increased insulin secretion has also been associated with decreased hepatic clearance in insulin-resistant conditions.[266] Although decreased clearance has not been firmly established in women with PCOS, assessment of hepatic extraction using ratios of insulin to C-peptide or model analysis is highly suggestive of impaired hepatic clearance.[267,268] Elevated fasting insulin levels may not be detected in women with PCOS, but commonly, insulin responses to a glucose load are significantly greater than those observed in normal women.[56] In contrast, first-phase insulin release in response to intravenous glucose is comparable between women with PCOS and weight-matched control subjects.[82] Nevertheless, evidence for β-cell dysfunction has been described in a series of studies that showed abnormal entrainment to oscillatory glucose infusions and diminished insulin secretory responses after ingestion of food.[81,268] Thus, despite the presence of hyperinsulinemia in women with PCOS, there is a relative defect in β-cell production and release of insulin.

In PCOS, insulin receptor binding and affinity have been shown to be normal. However, studies of adipocytes from women with PCOS have shown decreases in glucose transport and lipolysis, indicating an impairment of insulin signaling (Fig. 20-18).[269-272] Evidence of decreased tyrosine phosphorylation and increased insulin-independent serine phosphorylation have been shown in cultured skin fibroblasts removed from women with PCOS.[271] Serine phosphorylation inhibits tyrosine kinase activity of the insulin receptor and may be responsible for the observed insulin resistance in PCOS.[273-275] Notably, increased serine phosphorylation was observed in only 50% of women with PCOS who were studied. The remainder exhibited insulin-stimulated insulin receptor autophosphorylation, which was similar to that found in normal control women.[271] Thus, these findings may be applicable to a subset of women with PCOS, whereas in others, the mechanism remains unknown. Importantly, although a defect in insulin receptor phosphorylation may exist for

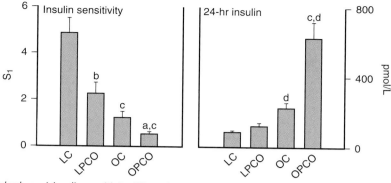

Figure 20-17. *Mean (± standard error) insulin sensitivity (S_i) as determined by the modified rapid intravenous glucose tolerance test and 24-hour mean insulin levels in lean and obese women with polycystic ovary syndrome (LPCO, OPCO) and their respective control groups (LC, OC; n = 8 for each group). a, P < 0.05; b, P < 0.01; c, P < 0.007 versus corresponding control group; d, P < 0.001 versus corresponding lean group. Eight- and 24-hour insulin levels (both log-transformed) were inversely correlated for the groups considered together (r = −0.75; P = 0.00001). (From Morales AJ, Laughlin CA, Butzow T, et al. Insulin, somatotropic, and LH axes in lean and obese women with polycystic ovary syndrome: common and distinct features. J Clin Endocrinol Metab 81:2854-2864, 1966.)*

some women with PCOS, the potential for abnormalities beyond the receptor is suggested by apparent alterations in other downstream signaling events.[276,277] Moreover, different pathways may be affected to greater or lesser degrees in various insulin-sensitive tissues, which reflects the complexity of the mechanism of insulin resistance in this disorder.

GENETICS OF PCOS

The familial predisposition to PCOS implies a disorder of inheritance, although the mode of transmission has not been established, despite a number of studies. Much of the difficulty resides with methodologic limitations due to small numbers of families and the inability to establish phenotypes among family members. The latter reflects the variable criteria used to designate individuals with PCOS.

Studies of twin sisters have not shown a substantial genetic component for polycystic ovaries, although concordance was found in affected twins relative to biochemical markers, including fasting insulin levels and serum androgen concentrations.[278-280] Similarly, efforts to detect chromosomal abnormalities among patients with PCOS have not shown alterations in number or structure.[281-283]

In pursuit of the genetics of PCOS, most studies have focused on identifying candidate genes that are linked to recognized abnormalities of steroid hormone production and action, carbohydrate and fuel metabolism, and gonadotropin secretion. Of the genes involved in steroidogenesis, *CYP17*, *CYP11A*, and *CYP21* have been examined to determine whether an association with PCOS exists. There is evidence to suggest that allelic variants of *CYP11A* may have a potential role in excess androgen production and hirsutism in PCOS,[284-287] although considerable

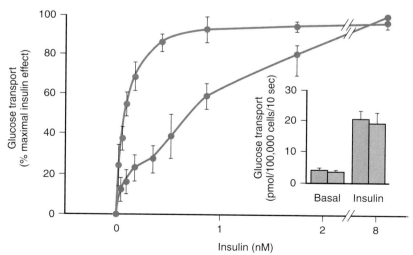

Figure 20-18. *Dose–response curve for insulin stimulation of glucose transport in isolated adipocytes form control subjects (green line) and women with polycystic ovary syndrome (purple line). Cells were incubated with insulin for 60 minutes before measurement of initial rates of 3-O-methylglucose transport. Results (mean ± standard error) are normalized against maximal activity for each subject. Inset, Absolute rates (mean ± standard error) of glucose transport in normal control subjects (green bars) and women with PCOS (purple bars). (From Ciaraldi TP, El-Roeiy A, Madar Z, et al. Cellular mechanisms of insulin resistance in polycystic ovary syndrome. J Clin Endocrinol Metab 75:577-583, 1992.)*

investigation remains. In contrast, examination of *CYP17* and *CYP21* variants and mutations has not shown associations with a phenotype that would support a role in PCOS.[288-291] The androgen receptor gene persists as a possible candidate for PCOS in light of the inverse relationship between the number of trinucleotide (CAG) repeats and androgen action.[292] In addition, the report of a missense mutation and a frameshift mutation in the SHBG allele, resulting in hyperandrogenism in a woman during pregnancy as well as four women with PCOS, warrants consideration of a genetic role for this protein.[24] Recently, it has been reported that, with microarray analysis, a cohort of genes with increased abundance of mRNA in PCOS theca cells was identified that included aldehyde dehydrogenase 6, retinol dehydrogenase 2, and the transcription factor GATA6.[293] Retinoic acid and GATA6 increased the expression of 17α-hydroxylase, providing a functional link between altered gene expression and intrinsic abnormalities in PCOS theca cells.

With respect to gonadotropin secretion, few studies have been performed to identify candidate genes for PCOS. An *Acc1* polymorphism of the *FSHβ* subunit has been described in women with PCOS,[294] whereas examination of the FSH receptor did not show sequence variants associated with PCOS.[295] Because dopamine inhibits GnRH secretion, alterations in dopamine receptor genes might account for increased LH secretion in PCOS. In Hispanic women, homozygosity for allele 2 of the D3 receptor has been associated with PCOS.[296] In a subsequent study, there was no difference in the distribution of three D3 receptor polymorphisms among non-Hispanic white women with PCOS,[297] which diminishes the likelihood of a D3 receptor candidate gene. Early screening studies suggested that the follistatin gene was overexpressed in PCOS.[286] As an activin-binding protein, increased follistatin activity might decrease FSH secretion and explain, at least in part, follicular arrest. In addition, activin inhibits ovarian androgen production and increased binding could lead to excessive androgen synthesis. However, in a large follow-up study, the follistatin gene was not observed to associate with the PCOS phenotype.[298]

Given the predisposition of women with PCOS to insulin resistance, genes that are related to carbohydrate metabolism have been the subject of considerable investigation. Of particular note is the insulin receptor gene, a mutation of which leads to severe insulin resistance, marked hyperandrogenism, and acanthosis nigricans (type A syndrome of insulin resistance). Despite the failure of the insulin receptor gene sequence to discriminate between women with PCOS with and without insulin resistance, two studies identified the region near the insulin receptor gene locus as being associated with PCOS.[286,299] As a result, this region assumes importance in that it may contain a candidate gene for PCOS. As for the insulin gene, there are conflicting reports linking this marker to PCOS.[286,300,301] Variants of the insulin receptor substrate protein genes have been shown to exhibit gene dosage effects related to fasting and postprandial plasma glucose levels in insulin-resistant women.[302] Whether these findings are manifest in women with PCOS requires further study. It has been shown that variation in the gene encoding the cysteine protease, calpain-10, influences susceptibility to type 2 diabetes.[303,304] However, two subsequent studies were unable to establish associations with multiple DNA polymorphisms in the calpain-10 gene.[305,306] The 112/121 haploid combination in African Americans and whites was associated with a twofold increase in the risk of PCOS that warrants additional investigation. Other candidate genes that have been considered for PCOS include leptin, resistin, and TNF-α, although evidence for an association with the latter two have not been found.[307-309] Recently, a PCOS susceptibility locus was mapped to chromosome 19p13.2 near the dinucleotide repeat marker D19S884.[310] Resequencing and family-based association studies were done on a large number of family members to determine the effect on reproductive and metabolic function.[311] The D19S884 allele 8 of the fibrillin-3 gene had the strongest evidence of association with PCOS. This allele was also linked to higher levels of fasting insulin and homeostatic modeling assessment for insulin resistance in women with PCOS. These results suggested that the D19S884 allele 8 is the PCOS susceptibility locus.

Pathophysiologic Concept

A clear explanation of the pathogenesis for PCOS remains elusive. Nevertheless, there are some intriguing concepts that warrant consideration. There is a growing body of evidence to suggest that excessive androgen production may be essential in the evolution of this disorder (Fig. 20-19). Notably, administration of androgen to nonhuman primates alters ovarian morphology by increasing the size of the ovary, the thickness of the capsule, and the number of preantral and antral follicles.[44] These data are consistent with the polycystic ovaries of hyperandrogenic women with 21-hydroxylase deficiency and female-to-male transsexuals administered long-term, high-dose androgen therapy.[213,223-226,231,232] The mechanism that dictates these morphologic changes has not been elucidated, although in Rhesus monkeys, androgen receptor mRNA is colocalized with that of the FSH receptor in granulosa cells and androgen treatment increases FSH expression.[46] The presence of increased FSH binding in granulosa cells of antral follicles from women with PCOS compared with normal follicles suggests that local exposure of excess androgen may drive this process and account for increased follicle number and size in this disorder.[29]

An androgen-induced increase of FSH receptors on granulosa cells of women with PCOS may also explain the robust follicular response to FSH observed in vitro and relate to heightened granulosa cell responsiveness to gonadotropin stimulation in women with this disorder.[28,209,210] It has been long recognized that androgen treatment in rodent and nonhuman primates enhances estrogen response to FSH.[57,184-186,312] In women with PCOS or those administered androgen, there is intense nuclear staining for androgen receptor in granulosa cells.[233] In rat granulosa cell culture, studies have shown that testosterone acts at a site upstream from cyclic AMP, which suggests involvement of the FSH receptor, whereas other studies have been unable to determine whether changes in cyclic AMP are

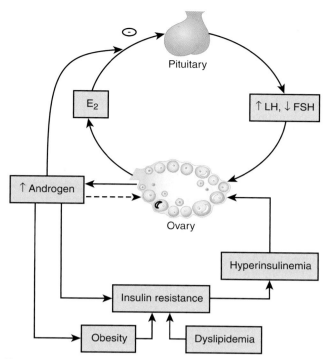

Figure 20-19. *Pathophysiologic concept of polycystic ovary syndrome (PCOS). Increased luteinizing hormone (LH) secretion, together with enhanced theca cell responsiveness, drives the production of excess ovarian androgen. Increased androgen production may inhibit steroid negative feedback effects on hypothalamic gonadotropin-releasing hormone pulse generation to account for the rapid LH pulse frequency observed in women with PCOS. In addition, increased androgens are associated with android obesity, visceral fat deposition, and dyslipidemia, all of which may contribute to insulin resistance. Independently, hyperandrogenemia, obesity, and hyperinsulinemia may decrease sex hormone–binding globulin, thereby increasing bioactive testosterone. Finally, increased androgen may have direct effects on the ovary to increase follicle number and follicle size and possibly enhance granulosa cell responsiveness to follicle-stimulating hormone (FSH). E_2, estradiol.*

induced by androgen treatment.[187,192,193] Despite these inconsistent findings, it is likely that the effect of androgen on the FSH receptor and subsequent granulosa cell function is mediated through its receptor. However, the precise mechanism for this interaction remains to be defined. Amplification of granulosa cell responsiveness to FSH is not unique to androgens because estrogens have long been known to enhance FSH-stimulated E_2 production.[313] In rodent granulosa cells, synergy between E_2 and FSH has been demonstrated with regard to increased FSH receptor binding, induction of LH receptors, increased aromatase activity, and progestin synthesis.[314-318] The mechanism for this synergy has not been completely elucidated, although estrogen-induced granulosa cell proliferation or increased FSH-binding capacity per granulosa cell has been suggested.[315,318-320] Alternatively, both processes may amplify FSH receptor number in granulosa cells of developing follicles. In nonhuman primate and human granulosa cells, studies have convincingly shown the presence of both estrogen receptor α and estrogen receptor β in the human ovary.[321-325] In particular, ERβ appears to be predominant in granulosa cells of antral follicles from both normal and polycystic ovaries. Collectively, these findings strongly

suggest that in both normal and PCOS granulosa cells, estrogen may enhance FSH-stimulated E_2 release through a mechanism that involves the FSH receptor.

Increased androgen production may have a significant effect on inappropriate gonadotropin secretion in PCOS. The critical feature of LH secretion in PCOS is increased LH pulse frequency, which remains intact in the face of physiologic and most pharmacologic manipulations. Increased pulsatile LH release implies, but by no means guarantees, increased hypothalamic GnRH activity. Until recently, it was difficult to exclude altered GnRH release as an instigating factor in PCOS. The rate of rapid LH release in women with PCOS may be normalized with administration of physiologic doses of estrogen and progesterone after treatment with an anti-androgen. This finding suggests an inhibitory effect of increased androgen bioactivity on steroid negative feedback.[157] Importantly, these results suggest that hyperandrogenism may be responsible for or, at least, contribute to increased LH pulse frequency in this disorder. The prevention of steroid negative feedback may be a unique effect of androgen because E_2 and insulin, the secretion of which are both abnormal, have not been shown to alter LH pulse frequency. Further studies are necessary to elucidate the primary and secondary mechanisms of increased GnRH pulse generator activity in PCOS.

The apparent central role of androgen excess in PCOS underscores the importance of the process by which hyperandrogenism is achieved. It is undeniable the theca cell is the primary source of hyperandrogenism in PCOS. Furthermore, evidence shows increased theca cell responsiveness to LH stimulation compared with normal theca tissue, which suggests a primary defect in this cell.[57,185,186] The precise nature of the abnormality is unclear, but it appears to involve facilitation of 17-hydroxylase, allowing for enhanced conversion of progesterone to 17-hydroxyprogesterone.[180,187] Additionally, 17-hydroxylase is encoded and regulated by the gene *CYP17*, which also encodes for 17-20 lyase, the enzyme that advances conversion of 17-hydroxyprogesterone to androstenedione. In immortalized human theca cells, including those from polycystic ovaries, the amount of androstenedione converted from 17-hydroxyprogesterone is small, indicating that Δ^5 17-20 lyase activity is correspondingly low.[190] The production of androgen is driven by pituitary LH, which has a bimodal dose effect on the enzymes regulated by *CYP17*. At low doses, LH primarily stimulates 17-hydroxylase, whereas at high doses, LH down-regulates the 17-20 lyase component of *CYP17*, which would account for the greater incremental change of 17-hydroxyprogesterone compared with androstenedione after GnRH agonist stimulation.[188,189] Thus, increased secretion of LH may be pivotal in amplifying the production of excess androgen.

Notwithstanding the physiologic effect of increased theca cell production of androgens, the bioavailability of testosterone is largely influenced by the production of SHBG, the reduction of which may lead to significant hyperandrogenism. Decreases in circulating SHBG concentrations have been observed in women with hyperinsulinemia, excessive weight gain, or hyperandrogenism, with the clinical outcome resulting in various degrees of hirsutism. In PCOS, all of these conditions may coexist simultaneously, thereby amplifying the clinical manifestations of excess androgen production. To illustrate the effect of SHBG, marked elevation of serum free testosterone levels and severe hirsutism recently have been reported during pregnancy in a woman who essentially lacked the capacity to produce bioactive SHBG. The deficiency in SHBG production was caused by a single-nucleotide polymorphism within an allele that encoded a missense mutation.[24]

In approximately 50% of cases of PCOS, adrenal androgen production is increased.[247] Despite the consistency of this finding and the contribution to the androgen pool, the precise role of adrenal hyperandrogenism has not been well established in this disorder. In women with 21-hydroxylase deficiency, the clinical manifestations may be indistinguishable from those of women with PCOS, which clearly shows the severity of hyperandrogenism in individuals with this enzyme defect. Although a milder form of androgen overproduction by the adrenal may accompany PCOS, it is the emergence of adrenal hyperactivity at or just before puberty that may be pivotal in the onset of this syndrome. The increase in steroidogenesis with puberty is characterized by an increase in the adrenal androgens DHEA and DHEAS. In girls who experience pubic hair growth before age 8 years, "premature pubarche," the risk of PCOS is increased.[326] Similarly, it has been hypothesized that exaggerated adrenarche at puberty, marked by increased production of DHEA and DHEAS, leads to abnormal androgen exposure and eventual PCOS.[327] These considerations raise the possibility that the genesis of PCOS may be critically linked to the onset of adrenal androgen production at or shortly before puberty.

The role of insulin resistance and hyperinsulinemia as a primary cause of PCOS has not been established. However, there is clear evidence to suggest that hyperinsulinemia may perpetuate the altered reproductive and metabolic physiology in this syndrome. In vitro studies have shown that insulin enhances LH-induced androgen production from normal theca cells.[185,192,193,328] Moreover, improvement in insulin sensitivity through the administration of insulin-lowering drugs has been accompanied by reduction of serum androgen levels without an effect on circulating LH concentrations.[170] In the granulosa cell, insulin has been shown to enhance E_2 responses to FSH in vitro, whereas there is indirect in vivo evidence to suggest that insulin may facilitate FSH-stimulated E_2 release.[62,63,65,66,68-72,162,214,329] Despite these findings, our recent studies have suggested that the granulosa cell may be insulin-resistant, as indicated by significantly increased E_2 responses to FSH during insulin infusion in women with PCOS treated with pioglitazone compared with responses observed before treatment.[205] Further investigation is necessary to resolve these conflicting results. At the level of gonadotropin secretion, insulin appears to exert little effect on pituitary LH and FSH release, which is in contradistinction to results obtained in vitro in the rat model. In studies employing long-term insulin infusion in normal women and those with PCOS, we were unable to detect changes in mean LH levels, LH pulse frequency and amplitude, or LH responses to GnRH compared with results obtained before insulin administration.[330] Collectively, these data suggest that the role of insulin resistance

in PCOS is directed primarily, but not exclusively, at the level of the ovary. Concomitantly, insulin resistance may also effect a reduction of serum SHBG as well as reflect a consequence of obesity. Whether insulin resistance is etiologic is unclear because not all women with this disorder exhibit abnormal insulin secretion. In addition, defining cellular defects in insulin signaling and insulin-related cell function have not been consistent within similar or different tissues of women with PCOS.[331]

Aside from the effects of increased LH secretion on theca cell androgen production, it has been suggested in PCOS that ovarian follicles undergo premature luteinization as a result of the atretogenic action of LH on the granulosa cell. This concept has been supported by the finding of increased LH-induced progesterone production from medium-sized follicles (<9 mm diameter) of granulosa cells from polycystic ovaries compared with normal granulosa cells.[332] In addition, PCOS granulosa cells have been documented to express significantly greater LH receptor mRNA than cells from normal follicles.[333] These findings, together with the increase in LH secretion, provide a compelling argument for such a process. Whether this mechanism can explain the arrest of follicle development at the midantral stage of growth in women with PCOS remains to be shown. Moreover, it is not clear how pervasive is the effect of increased LH secretion on granulosa cell viability. Most granulosa cells derived from unstimulated follicles of polycystic ovaries are extremely vital and exhibit great capacity for steroidogenesis.[29] It may be the case that only the very terminal granulosa cells become atretic quickly and suffer demise.

With several components of the altered physiology unexplained, PCOS continues to remain a pathophysiologic enigma. Although a unifying concept seems elusive, there is reason to invoke a crucial role for excess androgen exposure in the perpetuation and perhaps the pathogenesis of this disorder. This approach would account for the diversity of clinical situations that may give rise to the PCOS phenotype, including primary and secondary causes of increased androgen production as well as conditions in which androgen bioactivity is increased.

Long-Term Consequences

In PCOS, the reproductive–metabolic alterations that are responsible for the immediate concerns of hirsutism, acne, and anovulatory infertility may also pose significant long-term risks to a woman's general health and well-being. These concerns have been attributed principally to chronic anovulation, insulin resistance, and obesity, all of which are salient features of the disorder.

CANCER

Beyond the immediate problem of anovulatory infertility in PCOS, persistent stimulation of the endometrium by chronic unopposed estrogen may lead to endometrial hyperplasia or adenocarcinoma in some women. Much of this concern is derived from observations of postmenopausal women receiving estrogen replacement therapy, although untreated young women with PCOS have been known to have endometrial cancer. In a long-term follow-up study of women with PCOS based on ovarian wedge resection, the odds ratio for endometrial carcinoma was 5.3 (95% confidence interval, 1.55-18.60) compared with control subjects.[334] The relationship of endometrial cancer with PCOS was evident in a case–control study, which showed that elevated androstenedione levels were associated with 3.6- and 2.8-fold increased risks of carcinoma in premenopausal and postmenopausal women, respectively.[335] Conversely, in young women with endometrial cancer, a history of menstrual irregularities consistent with anovulation and the diagnosis of PCOS is common.[336] This problem is compounded by obesity and the associated decrease of SHBG, resulting in an increase of circulating free E_2. In PCOS, the histopathology of endometrial hyperplasia is not distinctive from that in women without hyperandrogenism. However, in the relatively few cases of endometrial cancer found in women with PCOS, the lesion is usually well differentiated compared with the poorly differentiated or undifferentiated forms seen in older postmenopausal women. It is not clear whether the histologic pattern of endometrial cancer in young women with PCOS might alter consideration of definitive therapy. However, expression of estrogen and progesterone receptors was more commonly encountered in the endometrial tissues of premenopausal versus postmenopausal women.[336] By contrast, in the same study, p53 was overexpressed by almost fourfold in older women compared with those with ovulatory function.

Studies of the association between PCOS and breast cancer generally have not revealed increased risk. However, many of these studies were limited by conditions of design or subject selection. For instance, increased risk was not found among a cohort of women with chronic anovulation from the Mayo Clinic.[337] It was presumed that these women had PCOS, and the study was retrospective. However, a subgroup analysis of postmenopausal breast cancer showed a significantly increased risk, although the affected cohort was composed of only five subjects. The Cancer and Steroid Hormone Study, involving 4730 women with breast cancer and 4688 control subjects, did not identify an increased risk of breast cancer.[338] Moreover, there was actually a 50% reduced likelihood of breast cancer. Unfortunately, the diagnosis of PCOS was self-reported and no laboratory documentation was performed. Similarly, the Iowa Women's Health Study, which did not show increased risk of breast cancer, also relied on self-reporting of PCOS.[339] In a study in which the diagnosis of PCOS was based on histologic appearance and clinical features, no association could be determined in a cohort of 786 women.[340] Recently, women with PCOS were found to have a statistically significant family history of breast cancer compared with control subjects, suggesting a familial association.[341] This study suffered from a lack of enrolled participants, because there were 41 women with PCOS and 66 control subjects. Thus, of the studies conducted to determine the relationship of PCOS to breast cancer, the vast majority have not been able to define a positive association.

A link between PCOS and ovarian cancer has been suggested from the findings of the Cancer and Steroid Hormone Study, in which women with epithelial ovarian cancer had a significantly higher likelihood of reporting a diagnosis of PCOS compared with control subjects.[342] Moreover, after adjusting for age, parity, oral contraceptive use, infertility, and education, the odds ratio, 2.4 (95% CL, 1.0-5.9), for a history of PCOS remained statistically significant. In contrast, longitudinal follow-up studies have not been able to corroborate an increased risk of ovarian cancer in women with PCOS. The Mayo Clinic cohort of 1270 subjects with presumed PCOS showed only one case in 14,499 woman-years of study.[337] Similarly, in 768 women with histologically identified polycystic ovaries followed for an average of 30 years, the mortality rate from ovarian cancer was 1 compared with an expected rate of 2.6 deaths.[340] In addition, a family history of ovarian cancer was not found in 41 women with PCOS compared with normal women.[341]

DIABETES MELLITUS

The discovery that women with PCOS have insulin resistance and are at risk for diabetes mellitus has had an enormous effect on the long-term health implications of this disorder. Although insulin resistance has been described as being relatively mild, it has been estimated that 20% to 40% of these patients will have glucose intolerance or type 2 diabetes mellitus by the fourth decade of life.[58,265,343] Conversely, premenopausal women with type 2 diabetes appear to be at increased risk for PCOS. Based on the findings of two small cross-sectional, uncontrolled studies, the prevalence of PCOS ranged from 27% to 52%.[344,345] These data are supported by a recent study that showed that postmenopausal women with a history of PCOS had a significantly higher rate of type 2 diabetes, 13%, compared with control subjects, who had a rate of 2%.[346,347] Consistent with an increased likelihood of diabetes, women with PCOS with a family history of type 2 diabetes exhibit decreased insulin secretory responses to glucose loading relative to their degree of insulin resistance.[81] Women with PCOS are at increased risk for impaired glucose tolerance and diabetes, and increased circulating concentrations of insulin have been reported to be common in first-degree relatives.[348] The combined prevalence rates for impaired glucose tolerance and diabetes in mothers and fathers of women with PCOS were 46% and 58%, respectively, considerably greater than rates in families without a history of PCOS.[21] In addition, affected sisters of women with PCOS were shown to have higher insulin-to-glucose ratios than their unaffected female siblings.[349] Collectively, these findings illuminate the trend toward abnormalities of glucose metabolism and diabetes in women with PCOS and their immediate family members.

DYSLIPIDEMIA

Lipid abnormalities in PCOS are characterized by significant increases in circulating total cholesterol, LDL cholesterol, and triglycerides compared with normal matched control subjects.[350] Conversely, serum levels of total HDL cholesterol and HDL_2 are significantly lower in women with PCOS than in normal women. Although in PCOS, this lipid profile may exist independently of several risk factors, the effect of these factors on lipid metabolism may be considerable. Previous studies have clearly shown that obesity and impaired glucose tolerance are associated with adverse lipid profiles. The effect of androgen excess on lipid metabolism is less well understood in PCOS.[351] Compared with age-matched normal women, the dyslipidemia of PCOS appeared to be less distinctive when the data were adjusted for body weight. Moreover, serum concentrations of lipoprotein-a and possibly plasmin activator inhibitor 1 were reduced by testosterone, whereas DHEA increased insulin sensitivity.

Regardless of the mechanisms that predispose patients to lipid abnormalities in PCOS, these patients should be at risk for plaque generation in coronary vessels.[352] Through the action of hepatic triglyceride lipase, very low-density lipoprotein and intermediate-density lipoprotein are converted to LDL cholesterol. LDL cholesterol appears to be the most atherogenic lipoprotein. Another lipoprotein, lipoprotein-a, is also atherogenic and has the most pronounced effect when LDL cholesterol is elevated. Hepatic triglyceride lipase is also responsible for converting HDL_2, which is rich in cholesterol, to cholesterol-poor HDL_3. Although the atherogenic properties of LDL cholesterol are well established, there is evidence to suggest that low HDL cholesterol and high triglycerides may be more predictive of coronary artery disease in women than in men.

CARDIOVASCULAR DISEASE

It is generally believed that women with PCOS are at increased risk for cardiovascular disease. This is based on the presence of several risk factors that predispose to heart disease. These include impaired glucose tolerance, android obesity, hyperandrogenism, dyslipidemia, and hypertension. Whether PCOS itself constitutes a risk factor, independent of known risk factors, is not clear. Evidence to support this association was provided by a case–control study in which 206 women with PCOS and corresponding age- and race-matched control subjects were compared.[353] The PCOS group was found to have significantly higher levels of total cholesterol, LDL cholesterol, and triglycerides than normal control subjects. With adjustment for confounding variables, such as BMI, fasting insulin, exogenous hormones, oral contraceptives, and age, by multiple regression analysis, the lipid abnormalities in women with PCOS remained highly significant. In addition, the dose–response relationship between insulin and PCOS was examined within individual cases and only approximately 20% of the variance could be attributed to insulin. Of note, androgens also did not contribute to the variance in lipids. These findings suggest that dyslipidemia in PCOS involves pathways separate from those of insulin and androgens. To determine whether the risk of cardiovascular disease may be demonstrated clinically in PCOS, a comparison of carotid ultrasonography was performed in patients with PCOS and their matched control subjects.[354] The intima media thickness, which has been directly correlated with cardiovascular disease, was significantly greater in women with PCOS than in control subjects. In addition, atherosclerotic plaque formation was found to be twofold greater in the PCOS group.

Retrospective studies have suggested that women with PCOS or at least the stigmata of PCOS have increased arterial lesions in their coronary vessels.[352,355] In premenopausal and postmenopausal women undergoing cardiac catheterization, those with coronary artery disease were more likely to have hirsutism, diabetes, and hypertension in addition to previous coronary artery disease. In another analysis that used a statistical risk factor model, women with PCOS had a significantly increased risk of myocardial infarction compared with control subjects.[356] Unfortunately, these studies were limited by their retrospective design, lack of control subjects for obesity, and insufficient categorization of patient groups. Nevertheless, the current literature clearly indicates that women with PCOS cluster risk factors for premature morbidity and mortality as a result of heart disease.[357] Despite the suggestive evidence of greater cardiovascular risk, measurement of actual death from myocardial injury has yet to be established. In two studies that examined the long-term health consequences in 786 women with PCOS, increased risk of coronary heart disease was identified, but mortality and morbidity rates did not differ from those in the age-matched control group.[334,340]

HYPERTENSION

In a retrospective study, postmenopausal women with a history of PCOS, confirmed pathologically, had an approximately fourfold increase in the rate of hypertension compared with control subjects.[346] In addition, women with PCOS tended to exhibit elevated blood pressure compared with age-matched control subjects. However, increases in blood pressure in both obese and nonobese patients with PCOS do not appear to be greater than those in control subjects, after adjusting for weight and body composition.[358] Thus, despite the presence of insulin resistance in PCOS, particularly in obese women, hypertension may not be common in affected patients. Currently, the relationship of hypertension to PCOS is under investigation.

Differential Diagnosis

The lack of a specific diagnostic test for PCOS, combined with the broad clinical spectrum resulting from anovulation and hyperandrogenism, warrants consideration of related conditions with similar presentations. These include both functional and neoplastic processes. Among the functional disorders are ovarian hyperthecosis, congenital adrenal hyperplasia, and Cushing disease. Included in the neoplastic group are androgen-producing tumors of the ovary and adrenal gland.

OVARIAN HYPERTHECOSIS

Hyperthecosis refers to an unusual proliferative condition in which the ovary contains nests of luteinized theca cells scattered throughout the stroma.[359] The extent of theca cell involvement may vary from minimal to extensive.

Severe hyperthecosis may be accompanied by extensive and dense fibroblast growth that results in an enlarged ovary of extremely firm texture, findings that are clearly distinct from those found in PCOS. Interestingly, the degree of hyperthecotic transformation in the ovary is not correlated to the severity of disease.[360] This observation would suggest that the hyperthecotic tissue may be hypersensitive to gonadotropin stimulation because serum LH levels are commonly in the normal range. Because of markedly high serum androgen concentrations, these individuals have severe hirsutism and a significant percentage of patients exhibit virilizing signs, such as clitoromegaly, temporal balding, a male body habitus, and deepening of the voice. Androgen production may be resistant to conventional forms of long-term ovarian suppression, such as oral contraceptive therapy, although administration of gonadotropin-releasing hormone agonists have been shown to dramatically decrease androgen production. There usually is marked insulin resistance, with substantially elevated circulating insulin levels. In addition, these patients are often obese and exhibit acanthosis nigricans.

CONGENITAL ADRENAL HYPERPLASIA

Among the several enzymatic defects that comprise congenital adrenal hyperplasia (CAH), the incomplete form of 21-hydroylase deficiency best simulates PCOS (see Chapters 16 and 17). This deficiency is manifested by an accumulation of 17-hyroxyprogesterone, which leads to abnormal elevations of the hormone compared with circulating values found in the follicular phase of the menstrual cycle. Because 17- hydroxyprogesterone is an androgen precursor, expression of this defect is associated with increased production of androstenedione and testosterone, with resultant hyperandrogenism. Notably, the clinical presentation may be indistinguishable from that of PCOS. However, there are several aspects of CAH 21-hydroxylase deficiency that may suggest the diagnosis. These include severe hirsutism, clitoromegaly, familial tendency, and short stature. The condition is transmitted by an autosomal recessive inheritance pattern, whereas an explanation for short stature is unknown. Morphologically, the ovaries have been reported to appear similar to those of women with PCOS. The capsule generally is dense and thickened, although peripheral cystic follicles have been an inconsistent finding. The second most common enzyme deficiency is 11β-hydroxylase, which gives rise to a mild hirsutism due to increases in 17-hydroxyprogesterone as well as 11-deoxycortisol, the immediate precursor for this enzyme. The accompanying hypertension often distinguishes this disorder from the 21-hyroxylase form of CAH.

CUSHING SYNDROME

The clinical features of Cushing syndrome primarily result from excessive cortisol production by an adrenal neoplasm or from excessive ACTH production. In most cases, ACTH overproduction is due to a pituitary tumor, although rarely, ectopic sources of ACTH may be encountered, as in adenocarcinoma of the lung. The preponderant findings are obesity, hirsutism, acne, and menstrual irregularity. These suggest the diagnosis of PCOS. However, additional evidence of moon-like facies, buffalo hump, hypertension, muscle wasting, abdominal striae, and osteoporosis indicate a primary problem of cortisol excess. Although circulating androgen levels are elevated, there is also abnormal cortisol secretion characterized by increased basal levels, loss of circadian rhythmicity, and failure of suppression in response to dexamethasone. In contrast to CAH, careful examination of the ovaries does not show changes typical of PCOS in most cases.

ANDROGEN-PRODUCING NEOPLASMS

Androgen-producing tumors may arise from the ovary and the adrenal gland. In contrast to the gradually evolving clinical presentation associated with functional hyperandrogenism, the neoplastic process can be quite dramatic. Within a matter of months, these lesions may induce severe hirsutism, a male body habitus, and virilization marked by clitoromegaly. In addition, there may be acne and lowering of the voice. Despite the severity of androgenic manifestations, in the early stages of development, these tumors can mimic PCOS or other functional hyperandrogenic syndromes. Occasionally, the hormone production may be mixed to include excess production of cortisol and progesterone.[361] Disruption of menstrual cyclicity varies from irregular bleeding to amenorrhea. The rapid onset of symptoms provides an important clue to the diagnosis. In some instances, a pelvic or abdominal mass can be palpated, which suggests an ovarian tumor.

Evaluation

LABORATORY EVALUATION

Laboratory assessment of suspected PCOS is based on clinical evidence of a functional hyperandrogenic disorder compared with a neoplastic process. In the presence of gradual and progressive hirsutism accompanied by irregular menstrual bleeding, the minimum endocrine evaluation includes serum total testosterone or free testosterone and 17-hydroxyprogesterone levels (see Chapter 32). These measurements should be performed in the morning because of diurnal variation. The rapid onset of excessive and severe hair growth, usually within months, should raise consideration of an androgen-producing tumor. In this situation, both serum total testosterone and DHEAS should be obtained; these values may suggest the source of androgen production. Threshold values beyond which a neoplasm should be considered are 200 ng/dL for testosterone and 7000 ng/dL for DHEAS. If circulating concentrations exceed these levels, then imaging studies, such as ultrasound and magnetic resonance imaging, are warranted to determine whether an ovarian or adrenal tumor exists.

Occasionally, high circulating androgen levels may not be associated with a distinct lesion, but rather with bilateral noncystic ovarian enlargement. If accompanied by gradual onset of symptoms, this presentation would suggest the diagnosis of hyperthecosis. Commonly, these patients exhibit severe insulin resistance and acanthosis nigricans.

Determination of 17-hydroxyprogesterone is useful as a screening test for CAH due to 21-hydroxylase deficiency. It has been proposed that a threshold concentration of 3 ng/mL for basal 17-hydroxyprogesterone provides the maximal cost–benefit.[362] A circulating level of less than 3 ng/mL obtained at random in anovulatory individuals or during the follicular phase in women with regular menstrual cycle excludes the diagnosis. Values in excess of 3 ng/mL warrant further evaluation with an ACTH stimulation test. After an overnight fast, 250 µg ACTH (1-24) is injected intravenously. Blood is obtained before and 1 hour afterward for measurement of serum 17-hydroxyprogesterone. Nomogram plots of baseline versus stimulated 17-hydroxyprogesterone concentrations result in three distinguishable groups: classic, nonclassic, and an overlap of heterozygotes and genetically unaffected (see Chapter 32).[363]

Women with Cushing syndrome may also present with a clinical picture consistent with PCOS. The optimal screening test is 24-hour urinary free cortisol, for which the normal value is less than 100 µg/24 hour. Abnormal values require further testing to determine the mechanism and site of excess cortisol production. These include low-dose and high-dose dexamethasone suppression tests as well as imaging studies to identify adrenal hyperplasia, Cushing disease, adrenal adenoma, or ectopic ACTH production.

As part of the assessment of oligomenorrhea due to anovulation, measurements of prolactin and TSH may be desirable. In PCOS, serum elevations of prolactin have been reported to range from 20% to 40% and probably relate to lactotrope stimulation by chronic estrogen exposure.[364-369] Coexistence of a prolactinoma and PCOS is uncommon. Disorders of thyroid secretion have been associated with irregular menstrual bleeding, although there usually are other accompanying clinical features that suggest the diagnosis.

Some comment is warranted regarding the measurement of serum gonadotropin levels. Despite the widespread practice of measuring serum LH and FSH, circulating levels of these glycoproteins really do not contribute significantly to the diagnosis of PCOS. Increased pituitary LH secretion cannot always be determined by measurement of the serum concentration, because approximately one third of patients have circulating levels of LH in the normal range. Circulating endogenous LH levels are positively correlated with BMI, which suggests that normal LH levels are not uncommon in obese women with the disorder.[133,134] Similarly, the LH/FSH ratio probably has little additive value in determining the diagnosis.

The observation that women with PCOS are insulin-resistant and have compensatory hyperinsulinemia raises the question of whether assessment of glucose metabolism and insulin secretion should be evaluated in these patients. Unfortunately, the ability to determine insulin resistance is limited by tests that lack sensitivity or are impractical for implementation. Based on fasting levels of glucose and insulin, a variety of indices have been designed to establish insulin resistance.[61,370,371] Although a reasonable correlation exists between each model and provocative glucose tolerance tests, normal values do not preclude insulin resistance (Table 20-1). However, the fasting level of glucose may be

TABLE 20-1

Measurements of Insulin Sensitivity

Test	Measurement	Normal Value*
Hyperinsulinemic clamp	M/1 (mean glucose use/mean plasma insulin concentration)	$>1.12 \times 10^{-4}$
Homeostasis model assessment of insulin resistance (HOMA IR)	Fasting insulin (µU/mL) × fasting glucose (mmol/L)	<2.77
Glucose-to-insulin ratio	Fasting glucose (mg/dL)/fasting insulin (µU/mL)	>4.5
Quantitative Insulin Sensitivity Check Index (QUICKI)	1/[log fasting insulin (µU/mL) + log fasting glucose (mg/dL)]	>0.357
Fasting insulin	—	Assay-dependent

*Normal values may vary depending on the insulin assay used.

used to distinguish glucose intolerance or diabetes and an elevated fasting insulin level will confer insulin resistance. An oral glucose tolerance test also provides valuable information, particularly if glucose measurements are accompanied by circulating insulin values. However, a reliable and reproducible assay for insulin is mandatory. It is unlikely that determination of insulin resistance is essential to the diagnosis of PCOS. Nevertheless, with the availability of insulin-lowering drugs, ascertainment of insulin resistance is warranted, particularly in high-risk individuals.

IMAGING STUDIES

In women with PCOS, ultrasound imaging of the ovaries shows bilateral enlargement, an increased number of peripheral cysts, and an increased percentage of central stroma.[8] Because this appearance is unique to the syndrome, ultrasound evidence of polycystic ovaries virtually confirms the diagnosis in women with anovulation and hyperandrogenism. However, because most cases of PCOS may be determined solely from clinical symptoms and polycystic ovaries may be found in normal women, routine use of pelvic ultrasound for the diagnosis is optional. Considerable information about the endometrial response to chronic estrogen exposure may be obtained with ultrasound.

Treatment

ORAL CONTRACEPTIVES

Notwithstanding infertility, the most problematic issue for women with PCOS is excessive hair growth. Thus, one of the primary goals of treatment includes ameliorating the clinical effects of hyperandrogenism, which may be achieved by suppression of ovarian steroidogenesis, interruption of androgen action at the target tissue, and reduction of hyperinsulinemia. Administration of an oral contraceptive containing combination estrogen–progestin has proven to be an effective treatment for hirsutism, although the range of response is variable, depending on the severity of hair growth at the time of treatment. In addition to suppression of ovarian androgen production, oral contraceptives increase SHBG and facilitate metabolic clearance of testosterone. This modality of treatment also has the advantage of instituting regular cyclic withdrawal bleeding and providing sufficient progestin to prevent excessive endometrial proliferation and hyperplasia.

ANTI-ANDROGENS

In many instances, anti-androgenic agents have been used in conjunction with oral contraceptives to maximize clinical benefit. Spironolactone is an aldosterone antagonist that, along with its major metabolite, canrenone, competes for testosterone-binding sites, thereby exerting a direct anti-androgenic effect at the pilosebaceous unit.[372] In addition, spironolactone appears to interfere with cytochrome P450, thereby inhibiting steroid enzyme action and resultant androgen production.[373] In the past, it was used to treat mild hypertension and may exert a mild diuretic effect. Because this medication opposes the action of aldosterone, serum potassium levels may increase and therefore should be monitored. Other anti-androgens include flutamide and finasteride. Flutamide competes for the androgen receptor, whereas finasteride inhibits 5α-reductase. Both agents have been shown to be effective for the treatment of hirsutism.[64,374-377] In a few cases, flutamide has been associated with liver toxicity; thus, caution should be exercised before recommending this drug.[378,379] Clinical studies have determined that these compounds exhibit comparable effectiveness in reducing hair growth.[374,375,377]

INSULIN-LOWERING DRUGS

Insulin-lowering drugs have been shown to improve insulin sensitivity in women with PCOS who have insulin resistance, which warrants their consideration in the management of this disorder. Most studies have detected a significant decrease in serum testosterone levels. However, others that included patients with severe obesity did not show a similar effect.[62,63,65,66,68-72,162,329] Metformin, a biguanide, increases insulin sensitivity in the liver to reduce gluconeogenesis and hyperinsulinemia. Clinical studies have shown that administration of metformin to women with PCOS resulted in decreased androgen levels, increased rates of spontaneous ovulation, and enhanced ovulatory response to clomiphene.[65,66,68-72] Despite these findings, the efficacy of metformin for the treatment of hirsutism remains to be established. Recent studies have shown that metformin may have a direct effect on ovarian steroidogenesis, independent of insulin action. Incubation of human ovarian theca-like tumor cells with metformin inhibited mRNA expression of steroidogenic regulatory protein and

17α-hydroxylase, whereas no effect was detected for 3β-hydroxysteroid dehydrogenase (3βHSD) or cholesterol side-chain cleavage.[380] In contrast, metformin was not associated with changes in 17α-hydroxylase or 3βHSD in studies of yeast cells.[218] The disparity between results may reflect differences in the cell systems used. Side effects of metformin include dose-related gastrointestinal symptoms that tend to resolve after several weeks. A rare adverse effect of metformin therapy is lactic acidosis. Therefore, metformin should not be prescribed to patients with renal, hepatic, or major cardiovascular disease, or hypoxia because these patients have a predisposition to elevated lactate levels. Precautionary temporal withdrawal of metformin is advised in patients undergoing radiologic procedures involving intravascular iodinated contrast materials and surgery.

Thiazolidinediones are another group of insulin-lowering drugs that include rosiglitazone and pioglitazone. These drugs act by binding to the peroxisome proliferation activator receptor γ, which forms a heterodimer with retinoic acid receptor and binds to a promoter to increase the expression of genes that regulate glucose homeostasis.[381,382] It has been well documented that thiazolidinediones decrease androgen levels in women.[63,82,329] Similar to metformin, the thiazolidinediones have not been shown to significantly lessen hirsutism in hyperandrogenemic women. In addition, in a large multicenter clinical trial, it was shown that improved insulin sensitivity was associated with resumption of ovulation after long-term treatment with troglitazone.[62] This effect was dose-dependent, as determined by the rate of ovulation and the time required to achieve ovulation. Similar to metformin, thiazolidinediones have also been shown to have a direct effect on steroidogenesis. In studies using yeast, the steroidogenic enzymes 17α-hydroxylase and 3βHSD were inhibited by troglitazone and, to a lesser extent, rosiglitazone and pioglitazone.[218] Similar results have been achieved in human granulosa cells.[216] However, studies to determine whether troglitazone influences aromatase enzyme have not produced consistent results in human granulosa cells.[217,219] Liver toxicity was associated with first-generation drugs of this class of compounds. However, both rosiglitazone and pioglitazone have been virtually devoid of liver effects. Nevertheless, thiazolidinediones should not be initiated in patients with evidence of liver disease.

OVULATION INDUCTION

See Chapters 21, 28, and 29 for a discussion of ovulation induction.

The complete reference list can be found on the companion Expert Consult Web site at www.expertconsultbook.com.

Suggested Readings

Almahbobi G, Anderiesz C, Hutchinson P, et al. Functional integrity of granulosa cells from polycystic ovaries. Clin Endocrinol 44:571-580, 1996.

Apter D, Butzow T, Laughlin GA, et al. Accelerated 24-hour luteinizing hormone pulsatile activity in adolescent girls with ovarian hyperandrogenism: relevance to the developmental phase of polycystic ovarian syndrome. J Clin Endocrinol Metab 79:119-125, 1994.

Coffler MS, Patel KS, Dahan MH, et al. Evidence for abnormal granulosa cell responsiveness to follicle stimulating hormone in women with polycystic ovary syndrome. J Clin Endocrinol Metab 88:1742-1747, 2003.

Dunaif A. Insulin resistance and the polycystic ovary syndrome: mechanism and implications for pathogenesis. Endocr Rev 18:774-800, 1997.

Eagleson CA, Gingrich MB, Pastor CL, et al. Polycystic ovarian syndrome: evidence that flutamide restores sensitivity of the gonadotropin-releasing hormone pulse generator to inhibition by estradiol and progesterone. J Clin Endocrinol Metab 85:4047-4052, 2000.

Rebar R, Judd HL, Yen SS, et al. Characterization of the inappropriate gonadotropin secretion in polycystic ovary syndrome. J Clin Invest 57:1320-1329, 1976.

Venturoli S, Porcu E, Fabbri R, et al. Longitudinal evaluation of the different gonadotropin pulsatile patterns in anovulatory cycles of young girls. J Clin Endocrinol Metab 74:836-841, 1992.

Weil S, Vendola K, Zhou J, et al. Androgen and follicle-stimulating hormone interactions in primate ovarian follicle development. J Clin Endocrinol Metab 84:2951-2956, 1999.

Willis DS, Watson H, Mason HD, et al. Premature response to luteinizing hormone of granulosa cells from anovulatory women with polycystic ovary syndrome: relevance to mechanism of anovulation. J Clin Endocrinol Metab 83:3984-3991, 1998.

CHAPTER 21

Female Infertility

Robert L. Barbieri

Fertility is defined as the capacity to conceive and produce offspring. *Infertility* is the state of a diminished capacity to conceive and bear offspring. In contrast to sterility, infertility is not an irreversible state. The current clinical definition of infertility is the inability to conceive after 12 months of frequent coitus. Infertility prevalence among women aged 15 to 44 years was 8.5% in 1982 and 7.4% in 2002. Infertility prevalence was greater in older women.[1] Because the fertility potential of the female partner decreases after 35 years of age, some authorities recommend initiating an infertility evaluation after 6 months of attempting conception in women 35 to 40 years of age and immediately in women over 40 years of age.[2,3]

A Statistical Model of Infertility

The clinical definition of infertility is relatively crude because it does not reflect the wide range of fertility potential in couples that have not conceived after 12 months. The clinical definition of infertility implies the existence of a dichotomous state, either a pregnancy is achieved in 12 months (infertility is not present) or a pregnancy is not achieved in 12 months and, by definition, infertility is present. The current clinical definition of infertility is similar to analyzing a continuous variable, such as height, by using a dichotomous variable: "short" and "tall." Height is clearly much better described by a continuous measure, such as centimeters, rather than by using the dichotomous variable of "short" and "tall."

Our clinical approach to fertility and infertility would be best advanced by the use of the concept of fecundability. *Fecundability* is the probability of achieving a pregnancy in one menstrual cycle (approximately 0.25 in healthy young couples). A related concept, *fecundity*, is the ability to achieve a pregnancy that results in a live birth in one menstrual cycle. Fecundability, a population estimate of the probability of achieving pregnancy in one menstrual cycle, is a valuable clinical and scientific concept because it creates a framework for the quantitative analysis of fertility potential. Based on the clinical characteristics of a population of infertile couples, the estimated fecundability may range from 0.00 in couples with an azoospermic male partner to approximately 0.04 in couples with a female partner who has early stage endometriosis.

In addition, fecundability provides a convenient quantitative estimate of the efficacy of various fertility treatments. An infertile couple with an estimated fecundability of 0.04, if left untreated, may have the choice of two approaches to the treatment of their fertility: a low-cost treatment (clomiphene plus intrauterine insemination) that will increase fecundability to 0.08, or an expensive treatment (in vitro fertilization) that will increase fecundability to 0.25. A clear quantitative presentation of the potential effect of each treatment on fecundability should assist the couple in choosing an optimal treatment plan. A practical problem with using fecundability as a central concept in infertility care is that the prediction models for estimating the fecundability of a couple are not yet well developed or validated. Factors that are important in estimating fecundability of a couple are age of the female partner, percentage of motile sperm, duration of subfertility, and presence of primary or secondary infertility.[4] Clinical care for infertile couples would be significantly advanced if discussions of infertility used the concept of fecundability. The "per cycle pregnancy rate" is the fecundability multiplied by 100. In this chapter, the terms "fecundability" and "per cycle pregnancy rate" are both used to mean the proportion of couples achieving pregnancy in one cycle. The concept of fecundability can be used to derive a simple statistical description of the fertility process.

Fecundability (f) is defined as the probability of conceiving during any one cycle. The probability of failing to conceive during any one cycle is $1 - f$. Over a short period of time, the fecundability of a population is often stable.[5] For a large group of couples, the probability of conception is f for the first month, $f \times (1 - f)$ for the second month, $f \times (1 - f)2$ for the third month, and $f \times (1 - f)n - 1$ for the nth month. Using this model, the mean number of months required to achieve conception is $1/f$. The cumulative probability of conception (F) through month n is calculated as follows: $F = 1 - (1 - f)n$. Based on this simple statistical model, assuming a normal menstrual cycle fecundability of 0.25 and starting with 100 couples, approximately 98 couples should conceive within 13 cycles. If each cycle is 28 days, then 98% of couples should conceive within one calendar year (13 cycles × 28 days/cycle = 364 days).

Over short periods of follow-up, a population of couples attempting pregnancy behaves in a statistically stable manner, with a fixed proportion of the cohort becoming pregnant with each additional cycle of follow-up. As the follow-up is extended, however, the fecundability of most populations appears to decline and the cumulative pregnancy rate approaches an asymptote, which is less than 100%. This pattern is likely due to heterogeneity in the fecundability of the initial population. The couples with the highest pregnancy rate are rapidly culled from the population (they became pregnant), leaving the couples with the more severe infertility problem in the residual pool. Conceptually, this issue can be managed by assuming that there is an asymptote to the cumulative pregnancy rate of the population, or by using complex mathematical modeling of the population fecundability based on the assumption that couples in the population have a range of per-cycle pregnancy rates. This issue is of special importance in the analysis of fertility rates in populations over long periods of time, such as 2 years. This issue is of less practical importance in studies where the time period for analysis is three cycles or less.

Many studies report that the observed fecundability of a population diminishes with long-term follow-up. For example, Guttmacher[6] assessed the number of months to conception in 5574 women who achieved pregnancy between 1946 and 1956. During the first 3 months of observation, the fecundability was 0.25. During the next 9 months of observation, the fecundability was 0.15. A similar observation was made by Zinaman and coworkers[7] and Wilcox and coworkers.[7,8] Zinaman and colleagues studied 200 healthy couples who desired to conceive. During the first 3 months of observation, the fecundability was 0.25. During the next 9 months of observation, the fecundability was 0.11 (Table 21-1). The drop in fecundability suggests that each large population consists of a heterogeneous mixture of couples. Some couples have completely normal fertility and achieve pregnancy at a high rate (>0.25 per cycle). The remaining couples have a lower fecundability (ranging from 0.00 to 0.15). Some of the couples in this pool will eventually present to a clinician for the treatment of infertility. At the end of 12 months of attempting conception, the couples that have not achieved conception have a fecundability in the range of 0.00 to 0.04 if left untreated (see Table 21-1). Successful interventions to improve fertility must increase the per-cycle pregnancy rate over this background pregnancy rate.

Unfortunately, not all pregnancies produce a live birth. Many pregnancies are lost soon after implantation. The terms occult pregnancy and chemical pregnancy are often used to describe these early pregnancy losses. *Occult pregnancy* was defined by Bloch[9] as a pregnancy that terminates so soon after implantation that there was no clinical suspicion of its existence. In one recent study, approximately 13% of pregnancies were occult. Unlike occult pregnancies, a *chemical pregnancy* typically occurs in the presence of a clinical suspicion that a pregnancy may exist. A blood or urine human chorionic gonadotropin (hCG) assay demonstrates the presence of a pregnancy, but no clinical evidence of the pregnancy is detectable by ultrasound. Of all clinical pregnancies, approximately 20% result in a spontaneous abortion. Of all pregnancies, approximately 30% are lost—either as occult pregnancies, chemical pregnancies, or clinical spontaneous abortions (Table 21-2).[7]

Diseases Associated with Infertility

Pregnancy is the result of the successful completion of a complex series of physiologic events occurring in both the male and female that allows for the implantation of an embryo in the endometrium (Fig. 21-1). At a minimum, pregnancy requires ovulation and the production of a competent oocyte, production of competent sperm, proximity of the sperm and oocyte in the reproductive tract, transport of the embryo into the uterine cavity, and implantation of the embryo into the endometrium. Many disease processes can result in subfertility.

Some diseases, such as those that cause azoospermia, clearly have a *cause-effect relationship* with infertility. For other disease processes, such as stage I endometriosis as defined by the revised American Society for Reproductive Medicine criteria, there is no clear cause-effect relationship between the disease and the infertile state. In these

---

TABLE 21-1

Decrease in Fecundability over Follow-up Period*

Cycle	Number of Women at Start of Cycle	Number of Pregnancies in Cycle	Per-cycle Pregnancy Rate
1	200	59	0.30
2	137	41	0.30
3	95	16	0.17
4	78	12	0.15
5	66	14	0.21
6	52	4	0.08
7	48	5	0.10
8	43	3	0.07
9	40	2	0.05
10	38	1	0.03
11	37	2	0.05
12	35	1	0.03

*Observational studies often demonstrate that the fecundability of the cohort decreases as follow-up progresses.
From Zinaman MJ, Clegg ED, Brown CC, et al. Estimates of human fertility and pregnancy loss. Fertil Steril 65:503-509, 1996.

TABLE 21-2

Pregnancy Occurrence and Outcome During Three Consecutive Menstrual Cycles in 200 Healthy Couples Desiring Pregnancy

Cycle Outcome	Cycle Numbers			
	1	2	3	Total
Not pregnant at start of cycle	200	137	95	—
Pregnant during cycle	59	41	16	116
Chemical pregnancy	7	7	1	15
Spontaneous abortion	12	5	4	21
Live births	40	29	10	79
Dropped out, not pregnant	4	1	1	6
Lost to follow-up	—	—	1	—

Age of female partner, 30.6 ± 3.3 (mean ± SD).
From Zinaman MJ, Clegg ED, Brown CC, et al. Estimates of human fertility and pregnancy loss. Fertil Steril 65:503-509, 1996.

situations it is preferable to state that there is an *association* between the disease condition and the infertile state, but that causality has not been definitively established. Because of the limits of our current understanding of fertility in humans, it is often difficult to categorize disease conditions as either causal factors (azoospermia) or associated factors (stage I endometriosis) with infertility. Consequently, a discussion of the distribution of reproductive diseases that are diagnosed in infertile couples is not necessarily based on hard scientific data, but rather comes from descriptive observations and assumptions about diseases that might *cause* or might be *associated* with infertility.

Most tabulations of the medical conditions that "cause" infertility divide the problem into male factors and female factors. The World Health Organization (WHO) task force on Diagnosis and Treatment of Infertility conducted a study of 8500 infertile couples using a standardized diagnostic protocol.[10] In developed countries, diseases that were identified as contributing to the infertile state were attributed to the female partner in 37% of couples, to the male partner in 8% of couples, and to both partners in 35% of couples. Five

percent of the couples had no identifiable cause of infertility (unexplained infertility) and 15% of the couples became pregnant during the investigation. The diseases most often identified in the female were ovulatory disorders (25%), pelvic adhesions (12%), tubal occlusion (11%), other tubal abnormalities (11%), hyperprolactinemia (7%), and endometriosis (15%); no identifiable disease was found in 20%.

In a review of 21 published reports containing 14,141 infertile couples, Collins[11] reported that the primary diagnoses in the couples were ovulatory disorders (27%), abnormal semen parameter (25%), tubal defect (22%), endometriosis (5%), unexplained (17%), and other (4%), as shown in Figure 21-2. In another data set of 2198 infertile couples the distribution of primary diagnoses was ovulatory disorders (18%), abnormal semen parameter (24%), tubal disease (23%), endometriosis (6.6%), unexplained (26%), and other (3%).[12] These observations can be broadly grouped into five major conditions that influence fecundability:

1. Abnormalities in the production of a competent oocyte (ovulatory factor or depletion of the oocyte pool)
2. Abnormalities in reproductive tract transport of the sperm, oocyte, and embryo (tubal, uterine, cervical, and peritoneal factors)
3. Abnormalities in the implantation process, including early defects in embryo development and embryo-endometrial interaction (embryo-endometrial factors)
4. Abnormalities of sperm production (male factor)
5. Other conditions, including immunologic factors that can affect multiple components of the process

The initial infertility evaluation focuses on these five major processes (Box 21-1).

The Initial Infertility Evaluation

The standard components of the infertility evaluation include a semen analysis, documentation of competent ovulation, and documentation of tubal patency—usually by hysterosalpingogram (HSG) (see Box 21-1). A repetitively

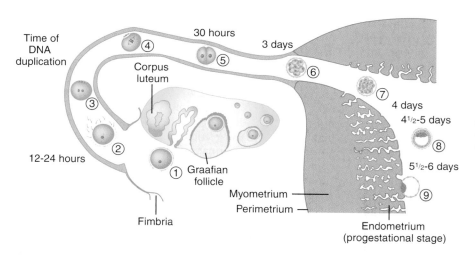

Figure 21-1. Schematic representation of the transport of the oocyte, sperm, and embryo in the female reproductive tract.

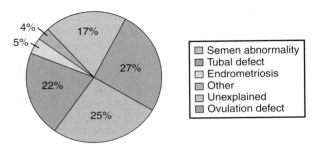

Figure 21-2. Primary clinical diagnoses in infertile couples. (From Collins JA. Unexplained infertility. In Keye WE, Chang RJ, Rebar RW, Soules MR [eds]. Infertility: Evaluation and Treatment. Philadelphia, WB Saunders, 1995, p 250, with permission.)

abnormal semen analysis is diagnostic of male factor infertility. An excellent test of tubal patency, the HSG is associated with relatively few false-negative results, but is associated with an approximately 15% false positive rate.[13] This means that if the HSG demonstrates that there is proximal tubal blockage, the finding should be confirmed by a second test (selective catheterization of each tube or laparoscopy). Infertility tests that are seldom needed as part of the initial infertility evaluation include the postcoital test, endometrial biopsy for luteal phase dysfunction, the hamster egg penetration test, routine *Mycoplasma* culture, and antisperm antibody testing.

A major problem with the postcoital test is that it has low reproducibility and low interobserver reliability, and it has not been reliably shown to help guide treatment recommendations.[14-16] In addition, there is little consensus on what constitutes an abnormal postcoital test. Given these limitations, there is little scientific rationale for performing a postcoital test. However, clinical experience suggests that clomiphene, acting as an anti-estrogen in the cervix, can cause abnormal cervical mucus production, both in quantity and quality. Some clinicians recommend performing a postcoital test to assess the impact of clomiphene on cervical mucus production in women receiving this drug for ovulation induction.

The endometrial biopsy is abnormal in many infertile women and in the past some clinicians believed that it was the gold standard for documenting ovulation and assessing endometrial preparedness for implantation. However, prospective studies demonstrate that the rates of abnormal ("out of phase") endometrial histologic findings are similar in fertile and infertile women.[17] Given the weak correlation between abnormal (out-of-phase) biopsies and fertility, most clinicians are not performing endometrial biopsy as a first-line fertility diagnostic test.

Abnormalities in Oocyte Production

Disorders of oocyte production are the most common cause of female infertility. The most common disorders of oocyte production are anovulation, oligo-ovulation, and aging of the ovarian follicle. Anovulation is typically associated with amenorrhea or severe oligomenorrhea. Oligo-ovulation is typically associated with oligomenorrhea (cycle lengths greater than 35 days).

BOX 21-1

Initial Laboratory Approach to the Infertile Couple

Primary Tests for Infertility
Documentation of competent ovulation
   Mid-luteal progesterone > 10 ng/mL
   Day 3 FSH (if female partner > 35 years old) or clomiphene challenge test
Semen analysis
   Volume 1.5-6 mL
   Concentration > 20 million/mL
   Motility > 35%
   Morphology > 30% (>14% if using "strict" criteria)
   Terminology used to describe abnormal semen analysis: low sperm concentration, oligospermia; low sperm motility, asthenospermia; sperm morphology abnormal, teratospermia; elevated white blood cells, leukocytospermia
Documentation of tubal patency
   Hysterosalpingogram
Secondary Tests for Infertility
Laparoscopy
Postcoital test
Endometrial biopsy

FSH, follicle-stimulating hormone.

Women who have monthly menses and report molimenal symptoms—such as breast tenderness and dysmenorrhea—are typically ovulatory.[18] The least expensive laboratory method for detecting ovulation is the measurement of the basal body temperature. For most women, the morning basal temperature obtained prior to rising from bed is less than 98°F before ovulation and over 98°F after ovulation. Progesterone production from the ovary appears to raise the hypothalamic set-point for basal temperature by approximately 0.6°F. The normal luteal phase is typically associated with a temperature rise, above 98°F, for at least 10 days. Occasionally basal body temperature recordings may appear monophasic even in the presence of ovulation. A biphasic pattern is almost always associated with ovulation. If the pattern is biphasic, coitus can be recommended every other day for a period including the 5 days prior to and the day of ovulation (Fig. 21-3).[19] A serum progesterone level greater than 3 ng/mL is diagnostic of ovulation. In the mid- and late-luteal phase, progesterone secretion is pulsatile due to the pulsatile nature of luteinizing hormone (LH) secretion.[20] At a conceptual level, the pulsatile nature of progesterone secretion may make it difficult to reliably use a single progesterone measurement as a marker for the adequacy of ovulation. However, in most clinical situations, a single mid-luteal progesterone measurement appears to be a useful marker of the adequacy of ovulation. Hull and colleagues have suggested that a mid-luteal progesterone concentration less than 10 ng/mL is associated with a lower per-cycle pregnancy rate than progesterone levels above 10 ng/mL.[21]

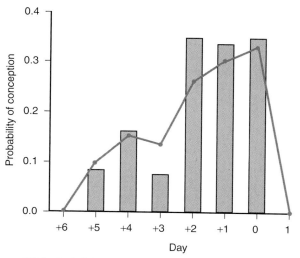

Figure 21-3. Probability of conception on specific days near the day of ovulation. The bars represent data reported by 129 women who had sexual intercourse on only 1 day in the 6-day interval ending on the day of ovulation (day 0). The green line shows the probability of conception based on a statistical analysis of data from 625 cycles. (From Wilcox AJ, Weinberg CR, Baird DD. Timing of sexual intercourse in relation to ovulation. N Engl J Med 333:1517, 1995, with permission.)

An endometrial biopsy that demonstrates secretory changes is another method of definitively diagnosing ovulation and making an estimate of the adequacy of both luteal progesterone secretion and endometrial response to progesterone. The endometrial biopsy is an invasive procedure, and therefore it is typically reserved for the diagnosis of luteal phase defect or other defects in endometrial receptivity. Endometrial proteins that can serve as clinically useful markers of endometrial receptivity will likely be identified in the future. [22]

Some authorities have suggested that a follicle may luteinize and differentiate into a corpus luteum (secreting progesterone and inducing a secretory endometrium) without rupturing and allowing the oocyte to escape the follicle.[23] The "luteinized unruptured follicle syndrome" may occur occasionally, but it is not a major cause of infertility.[24,25] Sonographic examination of the ovary and serial measurement of LH or estrone-3-glucuronide can be used to demonstrate the growth of a dominant follicle, which is often associated with ovulation.[26] During menses, the follicles in the ovary are approximately 4 mm in diameter. Prior to ovulation, the dominant follicle reaches a diameter in the range of 20 to 25 mm. Demonstration of follicle growth and rupture of the dominant follicle is presumptive evidence that ovulation has occurred. The demonstration of an LH surge is also presumptive evidence of ovulatory cycles. Ovulation typically occurs 34 to 36 hours after the onset of the LH surge and approximately 10 to 12 hours after the LH peak. In one large prospective study, the detection of a urine LH surge by patients using a home detection kit was associated with ovulation as demonstrated by a secretory endometrial biopsy in 93% of cycles.[27]

Many diseases can cause anovulation and infertility. The most common disorders are hypogonadotropic hypogonadism (WHO I), euestrogenic ovulatory dysfunction

(WHO II), and hypergonadotropic hypogonadism (WHO III). The most common causes of adult-onset anovulation are hypothalamic dysfunction (35% of cases), pituitary disease (15%), and ovarian dysfunction (50%).[28,29] The most common causes of hypothalamic dysfunction are abnormalities in weight and body composition, eating disorders, stress, and strenuous exercise. Less common causes of hypothalamic dysfunction are infiltrating diseases of the hypothalamus, such as lymphoma and histiocytosis. The pituitary disorders that cause anovulation (see Chapters 3 and 19) are prolactinoma, empty sella syndrome, Sheehan's syndrome, Cushing's disease, acromegaly, and other pituitary tumors. The most common ovarian causes of anovulation are ovarian failure (depletion of the oocyte pool) and ovarian hyperandrogenism (e.g., polycystic ovary syndrome [PCOS]). Occasionally thyroid disease can be associated with anovulation.

Evaluation of the various causes of anovulation can be complex. Typically, measurement of body weight and height, and measurement of serum follicle-stimulating hormone (FSH), prolactin, thyroid-stimulating hormone (TSH), and androgens, if indicated, can help identify the cause of the anovulation. A progestin withdrawal test may be helpful to evaluate the degree of hypogonadism present and may help guide treatment choices.[30]

Patients with anovulation have the greatest success with infertility therapy.[31] Treatment of anovulatory disorders can result in fecundability similar to that observed in normal couples (0.15 to 0.25). The choice of treatment is dependent on the cause of the anovulation. Common treatment choices include the following:

1. Interventions to modulate weight
2. Clomiphene citrate
3. Clomiphene plus other hormone adjuvants
4. Gonadotropin treatment
5. Pulsatile gonadotropin-releasing hormone (GnRH)
6. Bromocriptine
7. Glucocorticoids

WEIGHT ABNORMALITIES ASSOCIATED WITH ANOVULATION

Anovulation, oligo-ovulation, and subfertility are commonly observed in women above or below their ideal body weight (see also Chapters 18 and 19).[32] In one study of 597 cases of women with anovulatory infertility and 1695 fertile control subjects, overweight women (body mass index [BMI] greater than 27 kg/m²) had a relative risk of anovulatory infertility of 3.1 compared with women of BMI 20 to 25 kg/m². Excessively thin women with a BMI less than 17 kg/m² had a relative risk of anovulatory infertility of 1.6. The investigators concluded that the risk of ovulatory infertility is highest in overweight women but is also increased in underweight women.[33]

Anovulatory women far below their ideal body weight often have hypogonadotropic hypogonadism. Anovulatory women far above their ideal body weight often have PCOS. For women who are far below (hypogonadotropic hypogonadism) or far above (PCOS) their ideal body weight, appropriate management of dietary intake may be associated with resumption of ovulation.[34] For example, Pasquali and colleagues[35] demonstrated that anovulation in obese women with PCOS could be successfully treated with weight loss. Obese women with anovulation and PCOS were placed on a 1000- to 1500-calorie diet for 6 months. The mean weight loss was 10 kg. After weight loss there was a 45% decrease in basal LH concentration and a 35% decrease in serum testosterone. Many of the women resumed ovulation and became pregnant. Similar results were reported by Clark and colleagues.[36] Thirteen obese anovulatory infertile women were entered into a program of diet and exercise and lost on average 6.3 kg over 6 months. Fasting insulin and testosterone levels decreased, and sex hormone–binding globulin concentrations increased. Twelve of 13 subjects resumed ovulation and five became pregnant without any other intervention. Most studies of the impact of weight loss on reproductive function did not include a control group. Guzick and colleagues reported the results of a randomized, controlled trial of the impact of weight loss on reproductive function.[37] Twelve obese, hyperandrogenic, oligo-ovulatory women were randomized to either a weight reduction program or a "waiting list" observation control group. The six women randomized to the weight reduction program had a mean decrease in weight of 16 kg, a significant decrease in circulating testosterone, a decrease in fasting insulin, and no change in LH pulse frequency and amplitude. In the women who were randomized to the weight reduction program, four of six resumed ovulation. All of the women in the control group, who were anovulatory before the study, remained anovulatory during the period of study observation. Weight loss is difficult to achieve. Consultation with a nutritionist, encouragement by a physician, a hypocaloric diet, and initiation of an exercise program may be the most effective nonsurgical interventions that can help a woman lose weight. Surgical methods of weight reduction can be very effective, especially in women with a BMI over 40 kg/m^2.

Excessively lean women are at increased risk for anovulatory infertility. Energy availability in the diet that results in negative energy balance reduces LH pulse frequency and increases the risk of anovulatory infertility.[38] Some women with hypogonadotropic hypogonadism have low BMI, high-fiber or low-fat diets [39] or intense exercise regimens.[40] When these women present with anovulatory infertility, they are often reluctant to gain weight, alter their diet, or reduce their exercise regimen. However, in one study of 26 underweight women who practiced strict dieting and were infertile, the subjects were counseled by a dietician and given physician-directed advice to increase their BMI. After the intervention, the women gained a mean of 3.7 kg and 73% of the women became pregnant.[41] Interpersonal psychodynamic psychotherapy or cognitive behavior therapy may help WHO I anovulatory women resume ovulating.[42] It is important to try to achieve a normal BMI prior to initiating ovulation induction in excessively lean anovulatory women because pregnancy in women with a low BMI is associated with an increased risk of delivering infants with low birth weight, small head circumference, and microcephaly.[43]

Specific dietary factors may influence the risk of anovulatory infertility. For example, in one prospective study, women who consumed iron supplements were reported to have a 40% lower risk of anovulatory infertility.[44] In another prospective study, a dietary pattern characterized by high consumption of monounsaturated fats rather than trans fats, vegetable rather than animal protein, low glycemic carbohydrates, high-fat dairy products, and multivitamins was associated with a reduced risk of ovulatory infertility.[45]

CLOMIPHENE

Clomiphene, a nonsteroidal triphenylethylene derivative estrogen agonist-antagonist related to tamoxifen and diethylstilbestrol, was first synthesized in 1956. In 1961, Greenblatt reported clomiphene to be effective in the induction of ovulation, and the drug was approved by the Food and Drug Administration (FDA) in 1967 (see also Chapter 28).[46] Clomiphene citrate is marketed as a racemic mixture of trans (enclomiphene) and cis (zuclomiphene) isomers in a ratio of approximately 3 to 2. The cis isomer may have greater ovulation inducing properties than the trans isomer.

Clomiphene has a half-life of approximately 5 days. It is metabolized by the liver and excreted in the feces. Fecal clomiphene can be detected up to 6 weeks after discontinuing the drug. Clomiphene has both estrogen antagonist and agonist effects and is a *selective estrogen receptor modulator*. In hypoestrogenic women, clomiphene is associated with an increase in high-density lipoprotein (HDL) cholesterol concentration, an "estrogen agonist" effect. Clomiphene probably induces ovulation by binding to hypothalamic estrogen receptors, creating a hypoestrogenic state in the hypothalamus that results in an increase in GnRH secretion and, in turn, an increase in FSH and LH secretion. Tamoxifen has a similar action.[47]

In normally cycling women, the administration of clomiphene citrate, 150 mg daily for 3 days, resulted in an increase of serum concentration of LH and FSH of 40% and 50%, respectively.[48] In addition, LH pulse frequency increased from 3.3 to 6.8 pulses per 8 hours. The clomiphene-induced increase in LH pulse frequency indicates that clomiphene has an action at the hypothalamus. In women with PCOS, who already have a high LH pulse frequency, clomiphene does not further increase LH pulse frequency, but it does increase LH pulse amplitude and serum levels of LH and FSH.[49] Successful induction of ovulation with clomiphene requires an intact hypothalamic-pituitary-ovarian axis. This contrasts with exogenous gonadotropin treatment, an approach that can be effective in the absence of a functional hypothalamus or pituitary.

Evidence that clomiphene has central nervous system effects includes the observation that clomiphene induces vasomotor symptoms,[50] increases LH pulse frequency,[48] and partially blocks the contraceptive potency of estrogen.[51] Studies in laboratory animals demonstrate that clomiphene can decrease estrogen stimulated hypothalamic tyrosine hydroxylase[52] and that clomiphene increases GnRH secretion from the rat medial basal hypothalamus.[53] In addition to a hypothalamic site of action, clomiphene also has biologic effects on the pituitary, ovary, endometrium, and cervix. Adashi and coworkers[54] demonstrated that in incubations of rat pituitary cells, both estradiol and clomiphene augmented GnRH-induced release of FSH and LH. Zhuang and colleagues[55] demonstrated that clomiphene, estradiol, and diethylstilbestrol all augmented gonadotropin induction of aromatase activity in rat granulosa cells. In hypoestrogenic women receiving exogenous estrogen, clomiphene can cause endometrial atrophy.[56] Clomiphene can diminish estrogen-induced cervical mucus quantity and quality, as demonstrated by decreased ferning and spinbarkeit formation.[57,58]

The WHO classification divides women with anovulation into three major groups: WHO Group I consists of those women with anovulation, low levels of endogenous gonadotropins, and very little endogenous estrogen production (hypogonadotropic hypogonadism). WHO Group II consists of those women with anovulation or oligoovulation, a wide variety of menstrual disorders, relatively normal (or elevated) gonadotropin levels, and evidence for significant endogenous estrogen production.[59] Many women in WHO Group II have PCOS. WHO Group III are women with ovarian failure (hypergonadotropic hypogonadism). Clomiphene is most effective in inducing ovulation in women in WHO Group II. In women with severe hypoestrogenism and hypogonadotropic hypogonadism (WHO Group I), clomiphene is typically ineffective in the induction of ovulation. In contrast, women in WHO Group I respond very well to gonadotropin injections or pulsatile GnRH treatment. Failure to have a withdrawal uterine bleed following the administration of progesterone is presumptive evidence of severe hypoestrogenism in women with anovulation and an anatomically normal uterus.[60] Clomiphene is unlikely to effectively induce ovulation in this setting.[60] Clomiphene citrate is also unlikely to be effective in women with a consistently elevated FSH concentration (depletion of oocyte pool). Although clomiphene is relatively contraindicated in women with pituitary tumors, it has been reported to be effective in the induction of ovulation in women with prolactinomas who did not ovulate with bromocriptine treatment alone.[61] Many physicians prefer to document tubal patency and evaluate semen parameters before initiating ovulation induction.

The FDA-approved dosages for clomiphene are 50 or 100 mg daily for a maximum of 5 days per cycle. After spontaneous menses, or the induction of menses with a progestin withdrawal, clomiphene is started on cycle day 3, 4, or 5 at 50 mg daily for 5 days. Starting clomiphene on cycle day 3 or 5 does not appear to influence the per-cycle pregnancy rate.[62] In properly chosen women, approximately 50% will ovulate at the 50 mg daily dosage; another 25% will ovulate if the dose is increased to 100 mg daily.[63] During each cycle, determination of ovulation should be attempted. In most patients, ovulation occurs approximately 5 to 12 days after the last dose of clomiphene. Measurement of the urinary LH surge is often recommended to assist the couple in prospectively determining the periovulatory interval.

Although the FDA has approved maximal clomiphene doses of 100 mg daily, many clinicians have experience prescribing clomiphene at doses of up to 250 mg daily. A woman who does not ovulate with a clomiphene dose below 100 mg daily for 5 days may ovulate if her dose

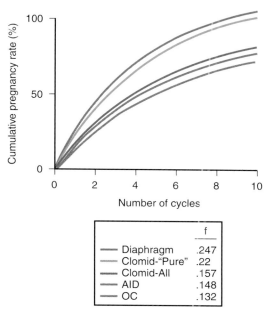

Figure 21-4. *Cumulative pregnancy rates in women treated with clomiphene for infertility, women discontinuing contraception with the diaphragm or oral contraceptives (OC), and women treated with donor insemination (AID). (From Hammond MC. Monitoring techniques for improved pregnancy rates during clomiphene ovulation induction. Fertil Steril 42:503, 1984, with permission.)*

is increased up to 250 mg daily for up to 14 days. Of the women who do not ovulate at doses below 100 mg daily, up to 70% will ovulate at higher doses, but less that 30% become pregnant.[64]

Anovulatory women in WHO Group II have a fecundability of 0.00 without treatment. Over the first three to six cycles of clomiphene treatment, the fecundability is in the range of 0.08 to 0.25. In cases in which the only fertility factor is anovulation in the female partner, fecundability with clomiphene treatment is in the range of 0.20 to 0.25[65] (Fig. 21-4). Women with hyperandrogenemia, markedly elevated BMI, amenorrhea, or advanced age are less likely to ovulate with clomiphene.[66] A unique advantage of clomiphene is that few fertility treatments are available that increase fecundability from 0.00 to 0.20 at a cost in the range of $100. After 3 to 6 months of clomiphene treatment, fecundability appears to decline.

Preliminary reports suggest that ovulation-inducing medications may be associated with ovarian tumors[67,68] and that the risk may increase with extended use of ovulation-inducing agents. My current view of this data is that nulliparity and infertility are far more important risk factors for ovarian tumors than treatment with an ovulation-inducing medication.[69-71] For example, in a cohort of 5026 women who received gonadotropin treatment as part of in vitro fertilization embryo transfer (IVF-ET) therapy there was no increase in cancer risk.[72] However, given the reduced fecundability observed in women who do not achieve pregnancy after six clomiphene cycles and the risk of ovarian tumors associated with prolonged exposure to clomiphene, limiting clomiphene treatment to fewer than 12 cycles is reasonable. Failure to achieve pregnancy after six clomiphene treatment cycles should prompt a thorough review of the potential causes of the failure and consideration of a new approach to treatment, such as gonadotropin therapy. After four ovulatory cycles induced by clomiphene without achieving a pregnancy, a diagnostic laparoscopy may reveal endometriosis or pelvic adhesions in over 50% of women.[73]

The role of hCG administration in enhancing the pregnancy rate associated with clomiphene treatment is controversial. Some authorities believe that the combination of clomiphene and a single dose of hCG may increase the efficacy of clomiphene induction of ovulation when women do not ovulate on standard doses of clomiphene.[74] However, in most trials hCG administration does not consistently improve pregnancy rate compared to women who spontaneously ovulate.[75] After administering the clomiphene, sonography can be utilized to monitor follicle size. When mean follicle diameter becomes at least 17 mm, hCG can be administered.[76] However, other authorities believe that there is little evidence to support the use of hCG in combination with clomiphene. In one small clinical trial, women receiving clomiphene from cycle days 3 to 7 to induce ovulation were randomized to receive hCG (10,000 IU) to time ovulation, or to monitor the endogenous LH surge using urinary LH testing kits. The pregnancy rate was similar in both groups.[77]

Clomiphene treatment can be associated with adverse changes in the reproductive tract, including induction of a luteal phase defect and the creation of a hostile cervical environment due to low quantity and quality of cervical mucus.[78] Some clinicians recommend endometrial biopsy in a test cycle of clomiphene treatment to assess whether or not clomiphene induces luteal phase deficiency, and many recommend that a postcoital test be performed during the first clomiphene cycle.

In one study of 2369 clomiphene-induced pregnancies, 7% were twins, 0.5% were triplets, 0.3% were quadruplets, and 0.13% were quintuplets.[79] This finding demonstrates that the absolute risk of high-order multiple gestation with clomiphene treatment is quite low. Because clomiphene is a heavily prescribed medication, however, the number of triplets resulting from clomiphene treatment is substantial. In one study that reviewed all the high-order multiple gestations at one tertiary care center, more triplets were conceived after clomiphene treatment than were conceived after treatment with exogenous gonadotropin therapy.[80] The rate of spontaneous abortion after clomiphene-induced ovulation and pregnancy is approximately 15%.[68] The most common symptoms experienced by women taking clomiphene include: vasomotor symptoms (20%), adnexal tenderness (5%), nausea (3%), headache (1%), and, rarely, blurring of vision or scotomata. Most clinicians permanently discontinue clomiphene treatment in women with clomiphene-induced visual changes.

CLOMIPHENE PLUS GLUCOCORTICOID INDUCTION OF OVULATION

Anovulatory women in WHO Group II with DHEAS (dehydroepiandrosterone sulfate) levels above the mid-normal range (approximately 2 μg/mL) appear to have reduced ovulation and pregnancy rates when treated with clomiphene. In WHO II anovulatory women, glucocorticoids appear to lower LH secretion and reduce adrenal androgen production, which may improve folliculogenesis in response to clomiphene treatment.[81,82] Daly and colleagues[83] randomized 64 anovulatory infertile women to receive either clomiphene 50 mg daily on cycle days 5 to 9, or clomiphene plus 0.5 mg dexamethasone daily. If ovulation did not occur, clomiphene was increased 50 mg daily per cycle up to 150 mg daily. The investigators observed significantly higher rates of ovulation and conception in the women who received clomiphene plus dexamethasone. The impact of the combined therapy was especially marked in the women with DHEAS concentrations above 2 μg/mL. Of the women with a DHEAS concentration greater than 2 μg/mL, 12 were randomized to receive clomiphene alone and 13 were randomized to receive clomiphene plus dexamethasone. Among the women receiving clomiphene alone, six (50%) ovulated and four (33%) conceived. Among the women receiving clomiphene plus dexamethasone, 13 (100%) ovulated and 11 (85%) conceived. Recent studies have also confirmed that women who fail to ovulate on clomiphene may respond to therapy when pretreated with glucocorticoids. In one trial, 230 women with PCOS who failed to ovulate were randomized to received clomiphene 200 mg daily for 5 days or clomiphene 200 mg daily for 5 days plus dexamethasone 2 mg daily for cycle days 5 to 14. Ovulation, as detected by serum progesterone measurement, was 88% in the clomiphene-dexamethasone group and 20% in the clomiphene-only group. Conception rates were 41% in the clomiphene-dexamethasone group and 4% in the clomiphene-only group.[84]

CLOMIPHENE AND ESTROGEN-PROGESTIN PRETREATMENT

A risk factor for failure to ovulate with clomiphene is an elevated circulating testosterone level. Estrogen-progestin pretreatment prior to a cycle of clomiphene may improve ovulation rates. In both a small case series and a randomized trial 2 months of estrogen-progestin contraceptive pill prior to treatment with clomiphene was reported to decrease circulating testosterone levels and improve ovulation and pregnancy rates in women with PCOS who had failed to ovulate with clomiphene 150 mg daily for 5 days.[85] In the randomized trial, 48 who had failed to ovulate with clomiphene 150 mg daily for 5 days were randomized with 42 to 50 days of pretreatment with estrogen-progestin contraceptive (ethinylestradiol 0.03 mg plus desogestrel 0.15 mg daily with no break) followed by clomiphene citrate (CC) 50 mg daily for 5 days, or clomiphene alone.[86] The oral contraceptive pill (OCP) regimen significantly reduced circulating testosterone prior to initiation of clomiphene. The ovulation rate in the two groups were 65% and 11%, respectively, in the OCP-CC group and the CC group. Per-cycle pregnancy rates were 54% and 4%, respectively. A regimen of OCPs followed by clomiphene may be clinically indicated in women who have failed to ovulate with clomiphene or in women known to have an elevated total testosterone. A large-scale randomized trial of this sequential regimen is warranted.

CLOMIPHENE PLUS ESTROGEN TREATMENT

In some case,[87,88] clomiphene has been reported to adversely affect cervical mucus quality and endometrial morphology. This effect is probably mediated through the anti-estrogenic properties of clomiphene. The anti-estrogenic effects of clomiphene on the cervix and endometrium possibly reduce the pregnancy rate during clomiphene treatment. A number of investigators have reported that the addition of estrogen to clomiphene treatment can increase endometrial growth compared with that observed with clomiphene alone. In a well-designed study, vaginal estradiol (0.1 mg daily) from day 8 to the LH surge and progesterone gel (90 mg daily) starting 3 days after ovulation were demonstrated to improve the number of "in-phase" endometrial biopsies in women taking clomiphene.[89] As of yet, no clinical trial has demonstrated that the combination of clomiphene plus estrogen/progesterone increases pregnancy rates compared with clomiphene without estrogen/progesterone.

An alternative approach to dealing with the anti-estrogenic effects of clomiphene is to start treatment on cycle day 1 rather than cycle day 3, 4, or 5. Conceptually, by treating with clomiphene from cycle days 1 to 4, there are more days for clomiphene to "wash out" of the body prior to ovulation. In one randomized study, 23 women with unexplained infertility were randomized to receive clomiphene (plus intrauterine insemination [IUI]) with treatment from cycle days 1 to 5 or cycle days 5 to 9. The pregnancy rate was reported to be higher in the group that received the clomiphene treatment from cycle days 1 to 4.[90]

Women with hypogonadotropic hypogonadism and low endogenous production of estrogen are resistant to induction of ovulation with clomiphene. The mechanisms responsible for the low rate of ovulation in response to clomiphene are not fully characterized. Maruo and colleagues have reported that clomiphene induction of ovulation has a low chance of success in women with triiodothyronine levels below 80 ng/mL.[91] In preliminary studies, thyroid hormone supplementation appeared to increase the efficacy of clomiphene induction of ovulation in these women.

CLOMIPHENE AND NONCLASSICAL ADRENAL HYPERPLASIA

Many authorities recommend that infertile anovulatory women with nonclassical adrenal hyperplasia (NCAH) receive glucocorticoids for induction of ovulation. However, some women with long-standing NCAH also have evidence of ovarian hyperandrogenism and polycystic ovaries by sonographic imaging. Clomiphene alone[92] or clomiphene plus glucocorticoids can be used to induce ovulation and achieve pregnancy in infertile women with NCAH.

CLOMIPHENE PLUS GONADOTROPIN INDUCTION OF OVULATION

In women who do not ovulate with standard doses of clomiphene citrate, gonadotropin injections can be added to clomiphene treatment to induce ovulation.[87] The main benefit of this approach to ovulation induction is that it tends to reduce the quantity of gonadotropins needed to induce ovulation during each cycle. The initial rise in LH and FSH induced by clomiphene increases the sensitivity of the follicles to respond to the gonadotropin injections. Typically, clomiphene at doses of 100 to 200 mg daily is administered for 5 days, followed by the initiation of FSH or LH/FSH injections. Investigators have reported that this regimen is associated with a 50% decrease in the dose of gonadotropin required to induce ovulation.[93]

CLOMIPHENE AND METFORMIN

Hyperinsulinemia is a common endocrine abnormality observed in women with PCOS (see Chapter 20). The elevated insulin levels contribute to the reproductive dysfunction by suppressing hepatic sex hormone–binding globulin production and possibly by acting as a co-gonadotropin with LH in stimulating thecal cell androgen synthesis. Thus, reducing insulin levels is a therapeutic goal in women with PCOS.

Metformin is an oral biguanide antihyperglycemic agent approved for the treatment of type 2 diabetes mellitus. Metformin decreases blood glucose by inhibiting hepatic glucose production and by enhancing peripheral glucose uptake, possibly by interacting with the Peutz-Jegher syndrome tumor suppressor gene (*LKB1*), which activates adenosine monophosphate–activated protein kinase.[94] It increases insulin sensitivity at the postreceptor level and stimulates insulin-mediated glucose disposal. A commonly used dose of metformin is 500 mg three times daily. To minimize gastrointestinal adverse effects such as nausea, many clinicians recommend that metformin should be started at 500 mg daily for 1 week, followed by an increase in the dose to 500 mg twice daily for 1 week, followed by 500 mg three times daily. Once the full dose is reached, some clinicians switch to a dosing regimen of 850 mg twice daily in order to enhance compliance. An extended-release formulation is available as a 500-mg or 750-mg tablets. When using metformin extended-release tablets, the entire daily dose is given at dinner time. The initial dose is 500 mg with dinner, with escalation to a maximum of 2000 mg once daily. Extended-release metformin may be associated with fewer adverse effects.

Progesterone levels can be measured periodically at appropriate days to determine if ovulation has occurred, or the patient can keep a basal body temperature record. If ovulation has not occurred after 5 to 10 weeks of metformin treatment, then clomiphene, 50 mg daily for 5 days, can be administered in conjunction with metformin. If the patient becomes pregnant, the metformin therapy can be discontinued. Metformin is a category B drug for pregnant women and has been used by some clinicians to treat diabetes in pregnant women.

The most common adverse effects associated with metformin are gastrointestinal disturbances, including diarrhea, nausea, vomiting, and abdominal bloating. In rare cases, metformin treatment has caused fatal lactic acidosis. In most of these cases, some degree of renal insufficiency was present. Prior to initiating treatment with metformin,

BOX 21-2

A Step-by-Step Approach to Ovulation Induction in Women with the Polycystic Ovary Syndrome

The least resource-intensive treatments are prescribed first, and the more resource-intensive treatments are prescribed in the later steps of the treatment algorithm.

Step 1. If the body mass index is greater than 30 kg/m^2, recommend weight loss of at least 10% of body weight.

Step 2. Prescribe clomiphene to induce ovulation.

Step 3. If the DHEAS (dehydroepiandrosterone sulfate) is greater than 2 μg/mL, consider combining clomiphene treatment with a glucocorticoid to induce ovulation.

Step 4. If clomiphene does not result in ovulation, consider a combination of metformin plus clomiphene.

Step 5. Initiate low-dose follicle-stimulating hormone (FSH) injections.

Step 6. Consider low-dose FSH injections plus metformin.

Step 7. Consider laparoscopic ovarian surgery.

Step 8. Consider in vitro fertilization-embryo transfer.

Adapted from Kim LH, Taylor AE, Barbieri RL. Insulin sensitizers and polycystic ovary syndrome: can a diabetes medication treat infertility? Fertil Steril 73:1097-1098, 2000.

the patient's serum creatinine concentration should be measured and demonstrated to be less than 1.4 mg/dL. Other insulin sensitizers may also be effective in induction of ovulation, either alone or in combination with clomiphene or FSH.

Clinical trials have reported conflicting results concerning the relative efficacy of metformin versus clomiphene. In general, the majority of large-scale clinical trials have reported that both metformin and clomiphene are effective at inducing ovulation in women with PCOS (Box 21-2), but clomiphene results in greater per-cycle ovulation, conception, and birth rates than metformin.[95] In one large trial, 626 women with anovulatory infertility caused by PCOS were randomized to receive clomiphene alone, metformin alone, or clomiphene plus metformin. The live birth rates were 27% in the clomiphene-metformin group, 23% in the clomiphene group, and 7% in the metformin group. In contrast, other investigators have reported that single-agent treatment with clomiphene or metformin results in similar pregnancy rates.[96]

AROMATASE INHIBITORS

Clomiphene is effective in inducing ovulation because of its anti-estrogenic properties. During clomiphene treatment, the hypothalamus and pituitary register a decrease in estradiol feedback, and consequently there is an increase in FSH and LH secretion. Aromatase inhibitors including letrozole and anastrozole block estradiol synthesis, reduce estradiol feedback, and increase production of FSH in premenopausal women. Both letrozole at doses of 2.5 mg to 7.5 mg daily for 5 days and anastrozole at a dose of 1 mg daily for 5 days have been demonstrated to induce ovulation in WHO II women. In a clinical trial comparing clomiphene 100 mg daily for 5 days versus letrozole 7.5 mg daily for 5 days in infertile couples undergoing ovarian stimulation plus IUI, the pregnancy rates per cycle were 12% in the letrozole group and 9% in the clomiphene group.[97] In a clinical trial of letrozole 2.5 mg for 5 days versus anastrozole 1 mg daily for 5 days for ovulation induction in women with PCOS, the per-cycle pregnancy rate was 19% in the women treated with letrozole and 10% in the women treated with anastrozole. Aromatase inhibitors are not approved by the Food and Drug Administration (FDA) for ovulation induction. Pregnancy and birth registries indicate that pregnancy outcome following ovulation induction with aromatase inhibitors is good.[98] In one registry, the risk of congenital cardiac malformations was greater with clomiphene-induced pregnancy than with letrozole-induced pregnancy.[99] However, concern remains about the potential adverse effects of these agents on pregnancy, especially given known adverse effects on rabbit and rodent pregnancy.

Ovulation induction and ovarian stimulation in women with estrogen-sensitive tumors, such as breast cancer, may be a special situation that warrants the use of aromatase inhibitors.[100] Aromatase inhibitors increase FSH levels but block estradiol production, resulting in folliculogenesis with relatively reduced levels of circulating estradiol. In women with a history of estrogen-sensitive tumors, inducing folliculogenesis and ovulation while maintaining relatively low levels of circulating estradiol has a theoretical advantage.[101] This effect may be especially advantageous in women with a history of breast cancer planning on undergoing an IVF cycle.[102]

GONADOTROPIN INDUCTION OF OVULATION

In 1958, Gemzell and coworkers[103] reported the efficacy of pituitary extracts of FSH to induce ovulation. In 1962, Lunenfeld and colleagues[104] described the efficacy of extracts of urinary gonadotropins (human menopausal gonadotropin [hMG]) from menopausal women to induce ovulation (see also Chapter 28). Since these two pioneering reports, the trend in the use of gonadotropin therapy for ovulation induction has been to continually improve the purity of the agents used. Advances in protein synthesis by recombinant DNA technology have resulted in the development of pure human FSH derived from yeast-expressing clones of human FSH.

The most widely used recombinant FSH preparations are Gonal-F (Serono) and Puregon (Organon). Recombinant FSH preparations have clinical efficacy similar to that observed with highly purified urinary FSH preparations.[105-107] Recombinant preparations of hCG are also available for use (Ovidrel by Serono). Recombinant preparations of LH (Luveris by Serono) have been tested in clinical trials, but their role in ovulation induction is still evolving. Purified preparations of urinary LH and FSH (Repronex by Ferring) and urinary FSH (Bravelle, also by Ferring) are also available for ovarian stimulation.

In women with ovulatory dysfunction, there is little evidence that the source of gonadotropins plays a major role in determining successful ovulation induction and pregnancy.[108] The main indications for gonadotropin induction of ovulation include the following:

1. WHO Group I patients with low levels of endogenous gonadotropins and little endogenous estrogen activity
2. Women with PCOS who fail clomiphene induction of ovulation
3. Women undergoing empirical ovarian hyperstimulation to treat unexplained infertility or early stage endometriosis
4. Women in programs of assisted reproduction, such as IVF

In anovulatory women treated with FSH, ovulation rates are greater than 80% per cycle, and pregnancy rates are in the range of 10% to 40% per cycle (Fig. 21-5). In a large group of hypoestrogenic women (WHO Group I), Lunenfeld and Eshkol[109] reported a six-cycle cumulative pregnancy rate of 91%, which reflects an average fecundability of 0.33 (Fig. 21-6). This fecundability (0.33) is higher than that seen in the normal population over six cycles. The higher fecundability achieved with gonadotropin therapy is probably due, in part, to the multifollicular development and multiple ovulations associated with gonadotropin treatment. The fecundability observed in gonadotropin treatment cycles is dependent on the age of the female partner and the underlying cause of the anovulation (see Figs. 21-5 to 21-7). Gonadotropin induction of ovulation is not recommended for women with primary ovarian failure and markedly elevated levels of FSH and

LH production. In addition, because of the expense of gonadotropin treatment, most clinicians recommend the completion of a thorough infertility evaluation prior to initiating gonadotropin therapy. Ovulation induction with gonadotropins must be individualized to the specific clinical setting. In amenorrheic WHO Group I women therapy is usually instituted 2 to 4 days after the onset of a progestin-induced menses. For most women in WHO Group I, the first treatment cycle begins with FSH or LH/FSH, 75 IU or 150 IU daily. This dosage is administered daily until cycle day 6 or 7, when serum estradiol is measured. If the estradiol level indicates an inadequate follicular response, the dose of FSH or LH/FSH can be increased to 150 IU daily. If an adequate follicular response is obtained, no further increase in gonadotropin dose is warranted. Transvaginal ovarian sonography and estradiol measurements are performed sequentially until the mean diameter of the largest follicle is in the range of 16 to 18 mm. The target range for serum estradiol is approximately 500 to 1500 pg/mL, with a serum estradiol of 150 to 250 pg/mL per large follicle (Fig. 21-8).[110,111] If estradiol levels greater than 1500 pg/mL are achieved, the risk of ovarian hyperstimulation syndrome increases. Many clinicians cancel the cycle and do not consider the addition of hCG in this situation. When appropriate follicular size has been achieved, 5000 IU of hCG is administered and ovulation is expected to occur approximately 36 hours after the injection. Some clinicians administer a second dose of hCG (2500 IU or 5000 IU) in the mid-luteal phase.[112,113] Administration of a second dose of hCG in the mid-luteal phase clearly lengthens the luteal phase compared with a single dose of hCG (11 days versus 16 days), but its impact on fecundability is not clear.[112]

In women with PCOS, induction of ovulation with low-dose FSH (50 IU) combined with small increases in dose (25 IU), if necessary, appears to result in a high pregnancy rate with a low rate of complications like high-order

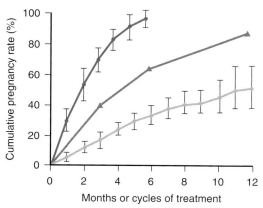

Figure 21-5. *Cumulative pregnancy rates for infertile anovulatory women treated with gonadotropins for ovulation induction. The purple line represents the cumulative pregnancy rate in women in WHO Group I. The blue line represents the cumulative pregnancy rate in women in WHO Group II who have failed induction of ovulation with clomiphene. For comparison, the green line represents the cumulative pregnancy rate in normal women. (From Dor I, Itzkowic D, Mashiach S. Cumulative pregnancy rates following gonadotropin therapy. Am J Obstet Gynecol 136:102, 1980, with permission.)*

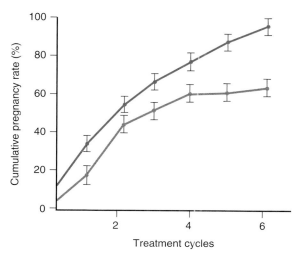

Figure 21-6. *Cumulative pregnancy rates for hypogonadotropic anovulatory women (WHO Group I) treated with gonadotropins. The purple line represents the cumulative pregnancy rate in women younger than 35 years. The green line represents the cumulative pregnancy rate in women older than 35 years. (From Lunenfeld B, Insler V. Human gonadotropins. In Wallach EE, Zacur HA [eds]. Reproductive Medicine and Surgery. St. Louis, Mosby, 1995, p 617.)*

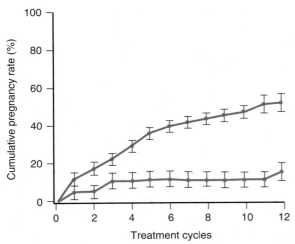

Figure 21-7. *Cumulative pregnancy rates following gonadotropin treatment for anovulatory women who did not respond to clomiphene induction of ovulation (WHO Group II). The purple line* represents *the cumulative pregnancy rate in women younger than 35 years. The green line* represents *the cumulative pregnancy rate in women older than 35 years. (From Lunenfeld B, Insler V. Human gonadotropins. In Wallach EE, Zacur HA [eds]. Reproductive Medicine and Surgery. St. Louis, Mosby, 1995, p 617.)*

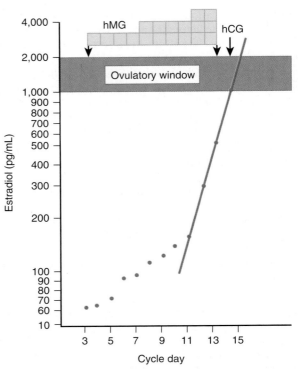

Figure 21-8. *Semilog plot of the 8 am serum estradiol concentration in response to increasing 8 pm doses of gonadotropins. In this example, human chorionic gonadotropin (hCG) was administered when the estradiol reached 1000 pg/mL. hMG, human menopausal gonadotropin. (From Stillman RJ. Ovulation induction. In DeCherney AH [ed]. Reproductive Failure. New York, Churchill Livingstone, 1986.)*

multiple gestation or ovarian hyperstimulation.[114,115] In the study reported by Homburg and colleagues, 50 women with PCOS and infertility who were unable to conceive with clomiphene were randomized to receive either conventional FSH treatment (75 IU daily and increasing by 75 IU every 5 or 6 days until follicle ripening has occurred) or low-dose FSH treatment (75 units daily for 14 days of treatment and increasing by 37.5 units every 7 days until follicular ripening was complete). The pregnancy rates were higher in the women who received chronic low-dose FSH compared with standard FSH treatment (40% versus 24%). Monofollicular development was achieved more frequently in the group that received chronic, low-dose FSH compared to standard FSH treatment (74% versus 27%). There were fewer cases of high-order multiple gestation and ovarian stimulation in the group that received low doses of FSH. Other investigators have reported similar results.[116]

For women with PCOS who do not conceive with clomiphene, low-dose FSH treatment is an effective option. Compared with women in WHO Group I, infertile anovulatory women with PCOS have low fecundability with FSH or hMG treatment. IVF has recently been demonstrated to be effective in treating infertile women with PCOS who do not become pregnant with FSH or hMG treatment.[117] In preliminary reports, IVF treatment of infertile women with PCOS is associated with a fecundability of 0.24 to 0.27.[118]

Long-acting preparations of recombinant FSH have been synthesized by combining the carboxy terminal peptide of the β subunit of human chorionic gonadotropin to the FSH β subunit. HCG has a longer half-life than FSH. These agents have the potential to reduce the number of injections of FSH required during an ovulation induction cycle.[119]

ROLE OF LH IN GONADOTROPIN OVULATION INDUCTION

An evolving area of research is the role of recombinant LH as an adjuvant in ovulation induction with recombination FSH. Most results support the idea that during the follicular phase of the cycle, LH levels can be too low, too high, or "just right."[120] In general, when LH levels are too low, thecal production of androstenedione is low and estradiol levels are low.[121] This probably prevents normal endometrial development, which can affect implantation. When LH levels are too high, thecal production of androstenedione is elevated and the follicular environment may be excessively "androgenized," resulting in suboptimal oocyte development.[122] An important goal in ovulation induction is to ensure that the LH levels are neither too low nor too high in order to optimize follicular and endometrial dynamics.

Numerous experiments demonstrate that LH levels can be too low to support optimal follicle and endometrial development. Experiments in monkeys when LH levels were reduced to extremely low levels demonstrated that the administration of FSH stimulates follicular recruitment and growth, but that estradiol production is suppressed.[123] Experiments in humans when LH was suppressed to very low levels with GnRH antagonists have demonstrated that FSH alone is not adequate to stimulate normal follicular development and pregnancy rates.[124] In clinical practice, however, apparently very few women need supplementation with exogenous recombinant LH during ovulation induction with FSH. Clearly, FSH can be used as a single agent to induce ovulation in most women with WHO Group II anovulation.[125-117]

In women with WHO I anovulation whose baseline LH concentrations are greater than 1.2 mIU/mL, FSH injections alone appear to be effective in inducing ovulation and pregnancy. For women with WHO I anovulation and a baseline serum LH level below 1.2 mIU/mL, the addition of recombinant LH injections appears to improve the efficacy of ovulation.[125,126] Some authorities believe that LH should be added to FSH regimens of ovulation induction in order to improve the consistency of ovulation and luteinization. The addition of LH activity (administered as 50 units of hCG daily) to a FSH ovulation induction regimen resulted in accelerated follicle growth, fewer days to ovulation, hastened demise of small preovulatory follicles, and decreased FSH requirements.[127] Although this is a conceptually interesting regimen that might reduce the cost of controlled ovarian stimulation and possibly the incidence of ovarian hyperstimulation syndrome, no trial has demonstrated that supplementation with LH increases pregnancy rates.[128]

For most women in WHO Group I, the LH surge will not occur spontaneously and must be triggered by the administration of an active agent (hCG, or recombinant LH or GnRH agonist) in order to cause final maturation of the follicle and trigger ovulation.

GONADOTROPIN AND GnRH AGONIST OR ANTAGONIST ANALOGUES

In women with PCOS, the elevated circulating concentration of LH may contribute to the growth of an excessive number of follicles and the production of high levels of estradiol and androgens during gonadotropin induction of ovulation.[129] The administration of a GnRH agonist or antagonist analogue can suppress pituitary LH secretion, and it may be associated with gonadotropin treatment cycles in which the basal levels of LH and androgens are suppressed and there is less premature luteinization of developing follicles.[130] In one study, 22 women with PCOS who had demonstrated premature luteinization during at least two consecutive clomiphene cycles (defined as a rise of serum progesterone greater than 1.5 ng/mL prior to hCG) were randomized to receive FSH alone or in combination with a GnRH agonist analogue (decapeptyl). In the combination FSH-GnRH analogue group, the GnRH agonist analogue was initiated 5 days before the start of the FSH injections and continued until hCG administration.[131] The women in the FSH-only group had substantially elevated follicular phase levels of progesterone compared with the women receiving the combination regimen (2.0 [1.2] versus 1.2 [0.6] ng/mL, $P = 0.03$, mean [SD]). The per-cycle pregnancy rate was lower in the FSH-only group compared with the GnRH analogue–FSH group (0% versus 33%).

Preliminary studies suggest that the combination of gonadotropin plus GnRH agonist treatment may reduce the spontaneous abortion rate compared with gonadotropin therapy alone.[132] In one study, the spontaneous abortion rate associated with gonadotropin-induced pregnancy was

TABLE 21-3

A Classification System for Ovarian Hyperstimulation Syndrome

Severity	Stage	Symptoms and Signs
Mild form	Stage A	Estradiol > 2000 pg/mL
	Stage B	Estradiol > 2000 pg/mL plus enlarged ovaries, up to 6 cm in diameter
Moderate form	Stage A	Estradiol > 4000 pg/mL; ovaries 6 to 12 cm
	Stage B	Ascites by ultrasound plus findings in Stage A
Severe form	Stage A	Estradiol > 6000 pg/mL; ovaries > 12 cm in diameter; ascites; liver function abnormalities
	Stage B	Tension ascites; ARDS; shock; renal failure; thromboembolism

ARDS, acute respiratory distress syndrome.
Adapted from Schenker JG. Ovarian hyperstimulation syndrome. *In* Wallach EE, Zacur HA (eds). Reproductive Medicine and Surgery. St. Louis, Mosby, 1995, p 650.

39%. Treatment with gonadotropin plus GnRH agonist analogue was associated with a spontaneous abortion rate of 18%.

GONADOTROPIN AND GROWTH HORMONE INDUCTION OF OVULATION

Growth hormone, a major regulator of IGF-1, may be important in sensitizing the ovary to the actions of FSH and LH.[133] Homburg reported that the combination of growth hormone (24 IU every other day) and hMG reduced the number of ampules of hMG needed to induce ovulation compared with a regimen of hMG alone (24 versus 37 ampules). There was no difference in pregnancy rates between the two groups. Because there was no change in fecundability, the high cost of growth hormone does not warrant its widespread use as an adjuvant to gonadotropin treatment.

OVARIAN HYPERSTIMULATION SYNDROME

Ovarian hyperstimulation syndrome (OHSS) is an enigmatic syndrome that occurs during ovarian stimulation resulting in cystic enlargement of the ovary, endothelial dysfunction (including increased vascular permeability), fluid accumulation in the peritoneal and pleural cavities, decreased intravascular volume, and hemoconcentration. The severity of OHSS is commonly classified as mild, moderate, or severe according to clinical criteria and, in some instances, clinical picture and ultrasound (Tables 21-3 and 21-4). In its severe form, OHSS can be associated with thromboembolism, renal failure, and death (see Tables 21-3 and 21-4). During gonadotropin induction of ovulation, mild to moderate enlargement of the ovary occurs in as many as 20% of women. Severe OHSS occurs in about 0.5% of women treated with gonadotropins.[134] Symptoms of OHSS

TABLE 21-4

Golan Classification for Ovarian Hyperstimulation Syndrome (OHSS)

Classification	Grade	Features
Mild	Grade 1	Abdominal distention and discomfort
	Grade 2	Grade 1 symptoms plus nausea, vomiting, and/or diarrhea; ovaries enlarged to 5 to 12 cm in diameter
Moderate	Grade 3	Mild OHSS plus ascites on ultrasound
Severe	Grade 4	Moderate OHSS plus clinical ascites or hydrothorax with dyspnea
	Grade 5	Grade 4 plus decreased blood volume, increased viscosity, coagulopathy, diminished renal perfusion and function

From Golan A, Ron-El R, Herman A, et al. OHSS: an update review. Obstet Gynecol Surv 44:430-440, 1989.

include abdominal pain, abdominal distention, nausea, vomiting, diarrhea, and dyspnea. Physical and laboratory findings of OHSS include weight gain, ovarian enlargement, ascites, pleural effusion, hemoconcentration, electrolyte imbalances, renal dysfunction, and thrombosis.[135] Risk factors for OHSS include age under 35 years, low BMI, high doses of FSH, high estradiol concentration, increased number and size of follicles, administration of exogenous hCG, a history of PCOS, and cycles in which conception occurs.[136,137]

The pathophysiology of OHSS is not completely defined, but during multifollicular development excessive ovarian secretion of vasoactive substances, including VEGF, is believed to trigger the syndrome. VEGF is a potent stimulator of angiogenesis and increases endothelial permeability, possibly by interfering with cellular tight junctions. Other factors that may be involved in the pathogenesis of OHSS include interleukin 6, the renin-angiotensin system, and the kinin-kallikrein system. Prevention is best achieved by limiting the dose of gonadotropin administered to young women and by withholding hCG administration if serum estradiol is greater than 1500 pg/mL. Another approach is to change the treatment plan from ovulation induction to an IVF cycle with cryopreservation of all the embryos generated.[138] Treatment includes bed rest, maintenance of intravascular volume, prophylaxis against thrombosis, and surgical correction of ovarian torsion. Physical and laboratory measurements that should be performed daily include measurement of weight and abdominal girth; complete recording of all fluid intake and urine output; measurement of electrolytes, urea nitrogen, albumin, and hemoglobin; and coagulation profile. The initial treatment of OHSS includes preservation of urine output with replacement of fluid volume. Care should be taken not to overhydrate the patient. Early reports suggest that the administration of albumin may help to reduce the risk of OHSS in women with very high estradiol concentrations (over 7000 pg/mL)

undergoing IVF.[139] Cabergoline, a dopamine receptor agonist may block VEGF activation of the endothelial VEGF receptor-2 and be an effective agent to prevent the development of OHSS. In one small clinical trial women undergoing gonadotropin stimulation for oocyte donation were treated with cabergoline 0.5 mg daily or a placebo for 8 days starting on the day of hCG administration. Compared with placebo, cabergoline was associated with lower hematocrit and less ascites as detected by sonography. The rate of moderate OHSS was 20% in the cabergoline group and 44% in the placebo group. Magnetic resonance imaging studies of endothelial function demonstrated less permeability in the cabergoline group.[140] Triggering an LH surge with a GnRH agonist rather than hCG may be associated with a lower risk of OHSS.[141-143] hCG has a half-life of approximately 30 hours and may overstimulate the production of androstenedione and estradiol by the follicle. GnRH agonist administered as a single subcutaneous or nasal dose has a short half-life and only stimulates pituitary secretion of LH and does not directly stimulate the ovary. By using GnRH agonist to trigger ovulation, the pituitary remains sensitive to feedback from estradiol, and pituitary production of LH is suppressed if estradiol levels increase to excessively elevated levels.

Prior to the utilization of repetitive estradiol measurements and sonographic evaluation of follicular development, OHSS occurred in as many as 10% of women receiving gonadotropin treatment. In recent series, where intense monitoring with estradiol measurement and sonography have been employed, approximately 1% to 2% of women treated with gonadotropins for ovulation induction have developed OHSS. OHSS is often more severe and has a longer course if a successful pregnancy occurs.

OVARIAN SURGERY FOR OVULATION INDUCTION IN PCOS

Ovarian wedge resection was one of the first treatments used to induce ovulation in women with PCOS. However, classical ovarian wedge resection was associated with ovarian and tubal adhesions. Laparoscopic ovarian drilling using insulated needle cautery has been reported to be associated with a 70% rate of ovulation and a 50% pregnancy rate.[144] The procedure can be performed by immobilizing the ovary with a probe and inserting an insulated needle electrode into the ovary. A cutting current of 100 watts can be used to ease the needle into the ovarian cortex. After the needle is inserted into the ovary, a 40-watt coagulating current is applied for 2 seconds at each point of puncture. Each ovary can be treated with 5 to 10 punctures; smaller ovaries should be treated with fewer punctures. In general, one or two punctures are not adequate to ensure ovulation postoperatively.[145] At the completion of the procedure, 1000 mL of crystalloid solution can be left in the pelvis.

In one clinical trial, 88 anovulatory, infertile women with PCOS who had not ovulated with clomiphene were randomized to ovarian surgery, FSH injections, or combination LH-FSH injections. The ovulation rate (70%) and the pregnancy rate (50%) were similar in all three groups. The spontaneous abortion rate was higher in the two groups that received gonadotropins. The investigators concluded

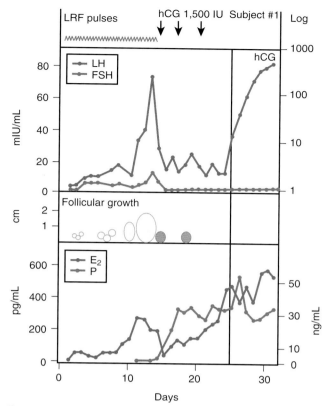

Figure 21-9. Endocrine and ovarian follicular response to induction of ovulation with luteinizing hormone releasing factor, 5 μg intravenous bolus over 2 hours. E₂, estradiol; FSH, follicle-stimulating hormone; hCC, human chorionic gonadotropin; LH, luteinizing hormone; LRF, LH-releasing factor; P, progesterone. (From Reid RL, Leopold GR, Yen SSC. Induction of ovulation and pregnancy with pulsatile luteinizing hormone releasing factor: dosage and mode of delivery. Fertil Steril 36:565, 1981, with permission.)

that ovarian surgery was as efficacious as gonadotropin injections for ovulation induction in women with PCOS who did not ovulate with clomiphene.[146] In another clinical trial women with PCOS who failed to ovulate with clomiphene 150 mg daily for 5 days were randomized to gonadotropin injections or laparoscopic ovarian diathermy. Six months after surgery cumulative spontaneous pregnancy rate was 28%. After three cycles of gonadotropin injections cumulative pregnancy rate was 33%.[147] In the opinion of the author, the risks of ovarian surgery for women with hirsutism are greater than the potential benefits. However, for women with PCOS and infertility who have been unable to become pregnant with weight loss, clomiphene, a metformin treatment, or ovarian surgery for ovulation induction may be warranted prior to induction of ovulation with FSH. Survey data indicate that many patients prefer one surgical intervention compared to ovulation with FSH injections, if the two treatments have comparable success rates.[148] Cost-benefit analyses suggest that laparoscopic surgery for ovulation induction is associated with lower health care costs than FSH injections.[149] Other authorities believe that the rare serious risks associated with surgery makes FSH injections the preferable option.[150]

GONADOTROPIN-RELEASING HORMONE INDUCTION OF OVULATION

A key feature of hypothalamic biology is the pulsatile release of the decapeptide GnRH from the arcuate nucleus into the pituitary portal circulation. The pulsatile release of GnRH stimulates the pituitary to produce LH and FSH in a pulsatile manner. In turn, pituitary gonadotropin secretion stimulates follicular development, ovulation, and progesterone secretion in the luteal phase. In women with WHO Group I anovulation (low levels of endogenous gonadotropins and decreased endogenous estrogen production), the pulsatile administration of GnRH is effective in inducing ovulation (Fig. 21-9). The advantages of GnRH induction of ovulation include a reduced need for cycle monitoring and a reduced risk of multiple gestation due, in part, to an intact pituitary feedback system. Unfortunately GnRH for ovulation induction is currently not available in the United States.

Santoro and colleagues[151] proposed eight criteria for identifying women most likely to safely achieve ovulation with pulsatile GnRH:

1. Primary or secondary amenorrhea for at least 6 months
2. Absence of hirsutism, galactorrhea, and ovarian enlargement
3. Weight not below 90% of ideal body weight
4. No excessive exercise or stress
5. Normal serum prolactin, TSH, DHEAS, and testosterone concentrations
6. Low gonadotropin concentrations
7. No evidence for a structural central nervous system lesion
8. No recent hormone treatment

GnRH is administered using a computerized pump that delivers one pulse of GnRH every 90 minutes at a dose of 75 to 100 ng/kg per pulse. Interpulse intervals as short as 1 hour[151] or as long as 2 hours[152] have been successfully utilized. GnRH doses as low as 25 ng/kg per pulse can successfully induce ovulation, but are associated with subnormal luteal phase progesterone secretion.[151] Both intravenous and subcutaneous administration of GnRH have been successfully used to induce ovulation. Intravenous administration probably results in more reliable induction of ovulation, but this route is associated with more technical problems (restarting the intravenous catheter) and risk of infection than subcutaneous administration.

The intensity of clinical monitoring can range from regular follicle monitoring with sonography and serum estradiol measurements to basal body temperature measurement with use of an ovulation predictor kit. Low-intensity monitoring is acceptable because the risk of multiple pregnancy or ovarian hyperstimulation is low with pulsatile GnRH therapy. If no response is observed after 2 to 3 weeks of treatment, the GnRH dose per pulse can be increased to the range of 10 μg to 20 μg per pulse.[153] Studies that directly compare the efficacy of gonadotropin versus pulsatile GnRH induction of ovulation report equivalent rates of ovulation and pregnancy. However, the risk of multiple gestation is probably higher with gonadotropin treatment (14%) than with pulsatile GnRH treatment (8%). This increased risk is due to a higher rate of multifollicular development with gonadotropin treatment (48% of cycles) than with pulsatile GnRH treatment (19% of cycles). Pulsatile GnRH results in a decreased risk of high-order multiple gestation when compared with gonadotropin treatment.[154]

Hyperprolactinemia

Infertile women with hyperprolactinemia and anovulation often achieve pregnancy after treatment with a dopamine agonist such as bromocriptine or cabergoline (see Chapter 3). Bromocriptine treatment at doses from 2.5 to 7.5 mg daily is usually sufficient to restore ovulatory cycles in women with anovulation due to hyperprolactinemia. For women with microprolactinomas, there is a very low likelihood that a pregnancy will be associated with growth of the prolactinoma. For women with macroprolactinomas, approximately 10% will develop clinically significant growth of the tumor during pregnancy, necessitating neurologic or neurosurgical intervention. Prior to inducing ovulation in women with a macroprolactinoma, consideration should be given to potential approaches to minimize pregnancy-associated complications (surgical treatment, radiotherapy, continuation of bromocriptine during pregnancy).[155]

LUTEAL PHASE DEFICIENCY

Historically, *luteal phase deficiency* has been defined as the delayed maturation of the endometrium, determined by histologic dating of tissue obtained by endometrial biopsy, which lags appropriate development by at least 2 days (see Chapter 8). However, most recent research indicates that delayed maturation of the endometrium is commonly observed at a similar rate in both fertile and infertile women.[156] In addition, histologic "dating the endometrium" probably does not have the accuracy or precision necessary to use it as a guide to infertility treatment.[157] Currently it is believed that endometrial maturation is "permissive" and permits embryo implantation to occur over a wider range of developmental stages than originally believed. Consequently, the role of luteal phase deficiency in female infertility has diminished.

From an endocrine perspective, follicular or luteal function that is far outside the normative range is likely associated with reduced fertility. In the most extreme example, it is known that resection of the corpus luteum, and the associated reduction in progesterone secretion, reduces fertility and causes abortion in women prior to about 49 days of pregnancy.[158] Likely, an occasional case of infertility may be caused by poor follicle development and inadequate corpus luteal secretion of progesterone or a relative resistance to progesterone effect in the endometrium.

THE AGING OVARY AND THE AGING FOLLICLE

An immutable feature of ovarian physiology is that the number of oocytes, and follicles, is fixed in utero and declines following an exponential curve (mathematically

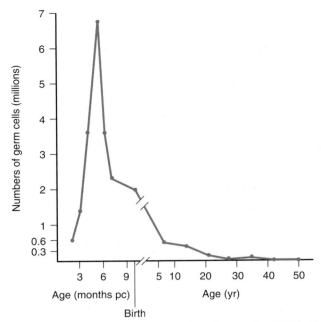

Figure 21-10. *Changes in the total number of oocytes (and follicles) in human ovaries before and after birth. The number of germ cells in the ovary peaks in utero during the second trimester. pc, postconception. (From Baker TC. Radiosensitivity of mammalian oocytes with particular reference to the human female. Am J Obstet Gynecol 110:746, 1971.)*

similar to the curve for the decay of radioactive material) from the second trimester, as shown in Figure 21-10 (also see Chapters 8 and 14). At birth, estimates of the number of oocytes and follicles in a pair of human ovaries is approximately 2 million. At the completion of puberty, the number of eggs in a pair of human ovaries is in the range of 250,000.[145] After 35 to 37 years of age, the rate of loss of oocytes and follicles appears to accelerate.[159,160] During adult reproductive life, follicles most sensitive to the growth promoting effects of FSH are apparently first selected to become the dominant follicle. As the ovary and the residual follicular pool ages, the remaining follicles appear to be relatively resistant to FSH. The aging follicles contain oocytes that are less likely to result in a successful pregnancy. The decrease in fecundability associated with aging is probably due to a decline in both the quantity and quality of the oocytes. Data to support the concept that the aging oocyte is less likely to result in a successful pregnancy come from multiple sources (see Figs. 21-6 and 21-7).

For infertile couples in whom the cause of the infertility is azoospermia in the male partner, the success of donor sperm insemination is directly related to the age of the female partner. In women under 30 years of age, the first three cycles of insemination resulted in a per-cycle pregnancy rate of 0.1. In women older than 35 years of age, the first three cycles of insemination was associated with a per-cycle pregnancy rate of 0.06.[148] Data from IVF programs also suggest that the age of the female partner is an important determinant of pregnancy rates. In women younger than 30 years of age, the clinical pregnancy rate per cycle is in the range of 0.25. In women over 40 years of age, the pregnancy rate per cycle is in the range of 0.12 with a high rate of spontaneous abortion.[161]

Many factors account for the relationship between the age of the female partner and fecundability. A major cause of the relationship appears to be the relatively poor quality of the oocytes that are in the terminal follicular pool. Biochemical correlates of the depleted follicular pool include an elevation in the FSH concentration during menses, reduced anti-müllerian hormone (AMH), and reduced inhibin B during menses. In the normal menstrual cycle, decreases in estradiol and inhibin A during menses are associated with an increase in FSH production during the first 5 days of the menstrual cycle. The increase in FSH stimulates the growth of an ovarian follicle that will be selected to achieve dominance during the cycle. As the selected follicle secretes increasing quantities of estradiol, inhibin B, and inhibin A, FSH production is suppressed. As the follicular pool ages, ever-increasing quantities of FSH are required to stimulate follicular growth, resulting in elevated serum FSH concentrations on cycle days 2, 3, and 4. An elevated serum FSH on cycle day 3 is a good marker of a depleted follicular pool and is associated with decreased fecundability and an increased rate of pregnancy loss. Particularly in infertile women older than 35 years of age, cycle day 3 FSH may be very helpful in identifying women with a reduced follicular pool.

In one study of the relationship between cycle day 3 FSH and pregnancy rate in an IVF program, Toner and co-workers[162] reported that women with a day 3 FSH concentration of less than 10 mIU/mL had an ongoing pregnancy rate of 0.18. In contrast, women with a cycle day 3 FSH level greater than 25 mIU/mL had an ongoing pregnancy rate of 0. In addition to predicting the pregnancy rate in IVF cycles, the cycle day 3 FSH also predicts the magnitude of the ovarian response to exogenous gonadotropin stimulation—including the peak estradiol concentration, the number of follicles, and the number of oocytes that are obtained at follicular aspiration. The age of the female partner clearly plays a major role in determining fecundability. Unfortunately, many clinical studies of fertility treatment have not explicitly controlled for this important variable.

Many genetic and lifestyle factors determine the rate of follicular loss and the age at which serum FSH measured during menses begins to rise. For example, cigarette smoking appears to hasten the pace at which the follicular pool is depleted. Menopause occurs significantly earlier in women who smoke.[163] In women in their mid-30s, cycle day 3 FSH also appears to be approximately 25% higher in cigarette smokers than in nonsmokers.[164] In cigarette smokers, the number of oocytes per pair of ovaries appears to be reduced.[165] Chemotherapy with alkylating agents or pelvic radiation are two important exposures that are associated with a diminished follicular pool. Women who are older than 30 years of age and have completed six courses of chemotherapy for Hodgkin's disease typically lose more than 90% of their follicles and many enter menopause immediately after the chemotherapy.[166] Radiation doses as low as 400 rads to the ovary will induce menopause in women over 35 years of age. Girls are much more resistant to the induction of menopause with chemotherapy or pelvic radiation, probably due to their large follicular pool.

As noted previously, estradiol and inhibin both exert negative feedback on FSH secretion during the early follicular phase of the cycle. Due to low levels of both estradiol and inhibin A, FSH secretion increases slightly during menses in women with a normal follicular pool and increases markedly—to elevated levels—in women with a depleted follicular pool. Some investigators have reported that the measurement of FSH after a course of clomiphene citrate is more sensitive for identifying women with diminished ovarian reserve than is the cycle day 3 FSH test.[167,168] Other investigators have reported that basal FSH and the clomiphene challenge test have similar performance in identifying women with decreased fecundity due to a depleted follicle pool.[169]

The clomiphene challenge test is performed by administering clomiphene 100 mg daily from cycle days 5 to 9. FSH levels are drawn on cycle days 3 and 10. An elevated FSH level on either cycle day 3 or 10 is associated with a diminished ovarian follicular pool and reduced fecundability. In some series, for every 100 women with an elevated day 10 FSH (post-clomiphene challenge), only 40 have an elevated day 3 FSH (pre-clomiphene challenge). Women who may be candidates for the clomiphene challenge test include those over 35 years of age, cigarette smokers, and women with unexplained infertility, stage III or IV endometriosis, previous bilateral ovarian surgery, or history of poor response to FSH stimulation. The clomiphene test is probably effective in detecting women with diminished follicular reserve because it blocks the negative feedback of estrogen, leaving only inhibin B to suppress FSH production. In women with diminished ovarian reserve, inhibin B levels appear to be very low and are incapable, on their own, of suppressing FSH production.

The pattern of secretion of the inhibins indicates that early follicular phase inhibin B may be a marker for the number of small follicles in the ovary, but inhibin A is reflective of follicle dominance. An alternative to measuring cycle day 3 FSH (or FSH response to clomiphene) is to measure inhibin B. However, studies suggest that inhibin B provides no more information for predicting the likelihood of pregnancy with IVF than that obtained by age of the female partner combined with FSH measurements.[170] In addition, inhibin B measurements are very difficult to perform with current techniques and have high interassay variation.

A new biochemical marker of the ovarian follicular pool is circulating levels of anti-müllerian hormone (AMH), also known as müllerian-inhibiting substance (MIS). AMH is secreted by granulosa cells in pre-antral and small antral follicles. Reduced concentrations of circulating AMH is associated with decreased ovarian response to stimulation. AMH levels appear to be relatively constant over the menstrual cycle, eliminating the need to time the measurement to a specific phase of the cycle.[171,172]

The number of antral follicles identified during menses by high-resolution vaginal ultrasound is also predictive of successful pregnancy in women undergoing IVF-ET.[173,174] An antral follicle (2 to 6 mm in diameter) count less than 3 to 6 is associated with poor outcomes during ovulation induction or other fertility treatments.[175,176]

Once a diminished ovarian follicular pool has been identified it is often "too late." Fertility treatments at this point have lower success than the same treatments in women with a normal follicular pool.[177] Women with diminished ovarian follicular reserve are probably best counseled to consider oocyte donation or adoption. Consequently, many authorities are recommending that infertility evaluation and treatment be initiated in women greater than 35 years of age after only 6 months of failure to conceive. Evaluation of day 3 FSH is probably warranted in infertile women older than 35 years of age. Measurement of a day 3 FSH and a day 10 FSH after a clomiphene challenge is probably warranted in infertile women older than 37 years of age. As a simple rule to guide clinicians, advancing age of the female partner is associated with poor oocyte quality, and increasing levels of basal FSH is associated with reduced oocyte number.[178]

The aging oocyte that is fertilized and implants in the endometrium appears to be associated with a markedly increased rate of spontaneous abortion. The rate of clinically detected spontaneous abortion increases 100% between 20 and 40 years of age (Fig. 21-11).[179] In IVF programs, the pregnancy loss rate is approximately 19% in women under 40 years of age and greater than 35% in women over age 40.[180] The increase in spontaneous abortion associated with the aging oocyte also contributes to the decreased fecundability apparent in aging women.

CANCER TREATMENT AND INFERTILITY

Cancer treatments, especially those involving the administration of alkylating cytotoxic agents (cyclophosphamide, busulfan, nitrogen mustard, procarbazine, bleomycin) or pelvic radiation, are associated with loss of reproductive potential in both men and women. As mentioned previously, chemotherapy reduces the number of follicles in

women.[181] Chemotherapy tends to produce "log-kill," in which a fixed proportion of sensitive cells are killed with each cycle of treatment.

Ovarian damage from cytotoxic chemotherapy is dependent on many factors, including the specific chemotherapy agent, the dose, and the age of the woman. For example, the dose of cyclophosphamide that induces amenorrhea in a 40-year-old woman is four times less than the dose needed to induce amenorrhea in a 20-year-old.[182] Numerous treatment cycles with high doses of cytotoxic agents is also likely to result in loss of ovarian function. Many specialists in oncology are focused on a primary goal of curing the patient of cancer rather than preserving future fertility. Many of these oncologists are not strongly supportive of deflecting the attention of patients to fertility issues. They would prefer that patients try to focus all their efforts and energy on curing their life-threatening disease.

Paradoxically, improvement in the successful treatment of cancer have caused many couples to focus on considering options for preserving their future fertility potential. For the male about to undergo alkylating chemotherapy, cryopreservation of sperm is a low-risk option that preserves future fertility options. For the female about to undergo pelvic radiation, transposition of the ovaries outside the radiation field may be useful.[183] For women about to receive alkylating chemotherapy, suppression of ovarian function with GnRH agonists may help to preserve follicle number.[183] In Rhesus monkeys, cyclophosphamide reduced follicle number by 65% in control animals and by 30% in animals that received a GnRH agonist.[184] In one study, 18 women between the ages of 18 and 40 who had lymphoma were given GnRH agonists prior to receiving chemotherapy. Fifteen of 16 survivors resumed spontaneous ovulation after completing chemotherapy and discontinuing the GnRH agonist. In a historical control group of women who did not receive a GnRH agonist prior to chemotherapy, only four of 16 resumed spontaneous ovulation.[185] Investigators have reported that oral contraceptives are not effective for protecting ovarian function in women receiving chemotherapy for Hodgkin's disease.[186]

Experimental treatments are beginning to expand the range of options for preserving fertility available to women and men about to undergo cancer treatment. Cryopreservation of embryos generated in an "emergency" IVF-ET cycle just before beginning chemotherapy may be one approach to preserving future fertility options for a couple. Major limitations of this approach include a delay in initiating cancer therapy and the challenge for single women and men.

Oocyte or ovarian tissue cryopreservation are two experimental techniques that are not yet routinely successful but hold considerable potential. Successful cryopreservation of unfertilized human oocytes is limited because of many technical problems—including zona hardening, digyny, and spindle disruption.[187-189] Ovarian tissue cryopreservation offers the advantage of allowing large numbers of follicles to be harvested by laparoscopic surgery. The strips of ovarian tissue that contain follicles can be cryopreserved and transplanted after chemotherapy is completed. The technology is being developed in Rhesus

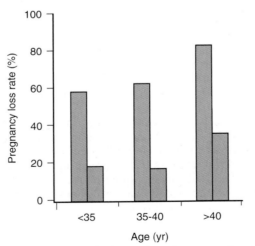

Figure 21-11. Women with abnormal ovarian reserve (basal day 3 serum FSH > 14.2 IU/L) had a significantly increased rate of reproductive loss compared with patients with normal ovarian reserve. P < 0.01 for all comparisons. Blue columns, women with abnormal ovarian reserve; purple columns, women with normal ovarian reserve. (From Levi AJ, Raynault MF, Bergh PA, et al. Reproductive outcome in patients with diminished ovarian reserve. Fertil Steril 76:666, 2001.)

monkey models and in human experiments.[190-193] In recent case reports, successful pregnancy has been reported both with grafting into the ovarian fossa and with grafting into heterotopic sites such as the abdomen or arm.[194,195] A long-term goal of fertility specialists is to generate functional oocytes from adult somatic cells by a process of gene transfer that results in reprogramming of the somatic cell. Recent research demonstrates that somatic cells can be reprogrammed to behave as embryonic stem cells by activating a small number of transcriptions factors such as OCT4, SOX2, NANOG, and LIN28.[196]

Some studies report that cancer survivors who have experienced intensive chemotherapy and radiation therapy may be at increased risk for preterm delivery and low–birth-weight babies if they become pregnant.[197]

Anatomic Factors in the Female

TUBAL FACTOR INFERTILITY

Tubal or peritoneal disease is identified in approximately 20% of the female partners of infertile couples. Pelvic inflammatory disease (PID), appendicitis, septic abortion, previous tubal surgery, and use of an intrauterine device resulting in a pelvic infection are major contributors to tubal disease. The rate of tubal infertility has been reported to be 12%, 23%, and 54% after one, two, and three episodes of PID, respectively.[198] Subclinical pelvic infections with *Chlamydia trachomatis* is a major cause of tubal disease associated with infertility. Patton and colleagues[199] studied tubal biopsy specimens from 25 women with PID and tubal infertility. *Chlamydia trachomatis* was detected in 3 out of 25 specimens by culture, 12 out of 24 specimens by in situ hybridization, 15 out of 22 specimens by immunoperoxidase staining, and 2 out of 10 specimens by transmission electron microscopy. Serum antibodies against *Chlamydia* were detected in 15 of 21 subjects. In this cohort, *Chlamydia* was identified in 19 of 24 women with PID and infertility.[199] Many subsequent studies have demonstrated that circulating high-titer *Chlamydia* antibodies are associated with tubal disease as detected at the time of laparoscopy.[200] In one large population study, the presence of *Chlamydia* antibodies was strongly associated with tubal factor infertility.[201] Approximately 1% to 4% of women of 18 to 26 years of age are infected with *Chlamydia*.[202] A history of a ruptured appendix appears to increase the risk of developing tubal factor infertility. In one case-control study, a history of ruptured appendix was associated with a 4.8-fold increase in the risk of tubal infertility. Appendicitis without rupture was not associated with an increased risk of tubal infertility.[203]

Following pelvic surgery, adhesions develop in approximately 75% of women.[204] The mechanism of postoperative adhesion formation is not fully understood, but it involves invasion of fibroblasts into the postsurgical fibrinous bridges. As a result, adhesive tissue develops, connecting two normally unconnected structures or covering the surface of a structure with de novo adhesions (Fig. 21-12). In the normal peritoneal healing process, a serosanguineous proteinaceous fluid exudes from the site of injury and coagulates into fibrin bands. In the normal healing process, endogenous fibrinolytic activity lyses these fibrin bands within 4 days. If the fibrinous bands are invaded by fibroblasts, angiogenesis occurs and a permanent bridge of tissue (an adhesion) is created. Factors that decrease fibrinolytic activity (ischemia, infection, drying of peritoneal surfaces) or increase fibroblast infiltration of the fibrin clot will increase the chance of developing adhesions.[205] Factors that increase fibrinolytic activity, such as plasmin

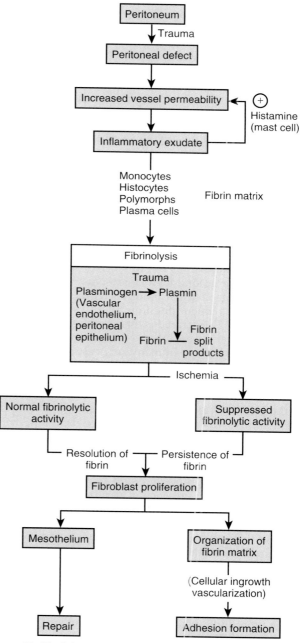

Figure 21-12. *Schematic flowchart of the normal healing response to a surgical injury in the pelvic peritoneum. (From Montz FJ, Shimanuki J, DiZerega CS. Postsurgical mesothelial re-epitheliazation. In DeCherney AH, Polan ML [eds]. Reproductive Surgery. Chicago, Mosby Year Book, 1987.)*

preparations (plasmin, actase, and fibrinolysin) or plasmin activators (streptokinase, urokinase, and tissue-type plasminogen activator), are efficacious in preventing postsurgical adhesion formation.[206]

Methods reported to minimize postoperative adhesions include the use of dextran, adhesion-prevention barriers like regenerated oxidized cellulose (Interceed) and expanded polytetrafluoroethylene (PTFE, Gore-Tex), heparin, glucocorticoids, fibrinolytic agents, hyaluronic acid–based fluid agents, polyethylene glycol hydrogel, and nonsteroidal anti-inflammatory agents. Most of these agents have been demonstrated to be effective in laboratory models of adhesion formation.[207-209] Few clinical data are available to help guide the clinical use of adhesion prevention agents.

Oxidized regenerated cellulose (Interceed), one of the best studied adhesion prevention adjuvant agents, becomes a gel shortly after placement on a surgically traumatized pelvic surface. The gel reduces the chance of formation of fibrin bridges between two opposing structures and thereby reduces the chance of adhesion formation. The material is resorbed within 1 week as it is metabolized into glucose and glucuronic acid. Oxidized regenerated cellulose has been demonstrated to reduce adhesion formation in women in well-controlled randomized prospective studies. In one study of 66 women with bilateral adnexal adhesive disease, the use of Interceed on one adnexa resulted in a 39% reduction of postoperative adhesion scores compared with the adnexa that did not receive the Interceed barrier. The use of Interceed resulted in a twofold increase in the number of adnexa without adhesions at the second-look laparoscopy.[210] Similar findings were obtained when oxidized regenerated cellulose was utilized to reduce adhesions after ovarian surgery.[211] A disadvantage of Interceed is that the surgeon must place the material over the area that is thought to be at high risk of adhesion formation. In many surgical cases, adhesions may occur at sites distant from the area where the Interceed is placed.

The two most commonly utilized tests of tubal patency are the HSG and laparoscopy. The advantages of HSG are that it utilizes few resources, produces data concerning the shape of the uterine cavity, and may increase fecundability by altering the peritoneal environment. The major disadvantages of HSG are that it causes pain during the performance of the procedure and provides no information concerning the presence of peritoneal diseases such as endometriosis and ovarian adhesions. In addition, if the HSG demonstrates proximal tubal occlusion, a confirmatory test (selective tubal catheterization or laparoscopy) is required. This additional testing is necessary because about 15% of the cases in which HSG demonstrates proximal tubal occlusion are actually due to "tubal spasm" that is spontaneously reversible. HSG is usually performed between cycle days 5 and 12. Many centers prepare women for the procedure with a short course of an antibiotic and an anti-prostaglandin agent such as ibuprofen immediately before the procedure. The risk of infection following HSG is in the range of 1%.[212] Traditional teaching is that oil-based contrast agents are associated with higher postprocedure pregnancy rates than water-based contrast agents.[213]

However, some well-designed studies do not support this conclusion.[214,215] In one trial, 175 women were randomized to undergo HSG with oil-based or water-soluble contrast agents. The oil-based contrast agent gave better resolution of the uterine cavity, the aqueous agent gave better resolution of the tubal mucosa. The postprocedure pregnancy rates were similar in the two groups. In another randomized trial of oil-based versus water-soluble contrast agents, the oil-based agent was associated with better pregnancy rates only in women with known endometriosis.[216] The main diagnostic advantage of laparoscopy over HSG is that it has better sensitivity and specificity for diagnosing tubal disease than HSG. In addition, laparoscopy can diagnose endometriosis and can be used to treat abnormalities observed at the time of the procedure.

Surgery for the treatment of infertility due to tubal disease is most successful if disease is localized in the distal portion of the tube. *Fimbrioplasty* is the lysis of fimbrial adhesions or dilatation of fimbrial strictures. *Neosalpingostomy* is the creation of a new tubal opening in a fallopian tube with a distal occlusion. Dlugi and colleagues[217] evaluated the success of unilateral versus bilateral fimbrioplasty or neosalpingostomy in 113 women with tubal factor infertility. Overall, these procedures were associated with a fecundability of 0.026. Women with major adhesions who had bilateral procedures had the lowest chance of achieving pregnancy. In contrast, in vitro fertilization treatment of tubal disease is associated with a fecundability of approximately 0.30. After tubal surgery, however, couples can attempt to achieve conception naturally over many menstrual cycles. When viewed from a cumulative perspective, approximately 20% of the patients treated with surgery became pregnant, and approximately 20% of the pregnancies achieved were ectopic pregnancies. Similar monthly pregnancy rates following fimbrioplasty or neosalpingostomy have been reported by Canis and colleagues.[218]

Poor prognostic factors for successful pregnancy following surgical treatment of tubal disease include tubal diameter greater than 20 mm, absence of visible fimbriae, dense pelvic adhesions, ovarian adhesions, advanced age of the female partner, and prolonged duration of the infertility problem (Fig. 21-13).[219] Infertile women with bilateral proximal and distal tubal disease have very low chances of conceiving following surgical treatment.[220] Treatment with IVF is much more successful than surgical treatment in this group of women.

A major advance in the treatment of proximal tubal occlusion associated with infertility is the development of flexible tip guidewire techniques to restore patency to the proximal portion of the fallopian tube (Figs. 21-14 and 21-15).[221] In one study of transcervical fluoroscopic catheter recanalization, successful recanalization was achieved in 47 of 65 tubes treated (72%). Of the 40 women with open tubes following the procedure, nine achieved live births (23%), four had ectopic pregnancies (10%), and one woman became pregnant but had an early abortion. In the 11 women in whom tubal recanalization was not successful, there were no pregnancies.[222] One of the most successful surgical procedures for infertility is the microsurgical reanastomosis of fallopian tubes that were

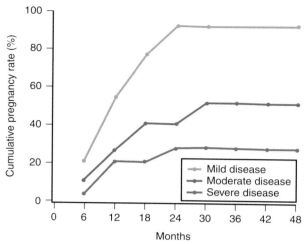

Figure 21-13. *Life table analysis of pregnancy outcome following neosalpingoneostomy, by extent of disease. (From Schlaff WE, Dassiakos D, Damewood MD, Rock JA. Neosalpingostomy for distal tubal obstruction: prognostic factors and impact of surgical technique. Fertil Steril 54:984, 1990, with permission.)*

subjected to surgical sterilization procedures. Several clinical characteristics are associated with a high success rate for surgical reanastomosis[223]:

- Patient under 40 years of age
- Tubal length greater than 4 cm
- Previous Falope ring, clip, or Pomeroy tubal ligation, and absence of associated pelvic pathology

Cumulative pregnancy rates in the year following the procedure are in the range of 50% to 80%. Recently, laparoscopic surgical reanastomosis has been proposed as an alternative to traditional laparotomy approaches to tubal reanastomosis.[224]

For infertile women with tubal disease, treatment with IVF is associated with a pregnancy rate of approximately 35% in the first cycle of treatment. Several studies indicate that hydrosalpinges decrease the pregnancy rate in IVF cycles.[225] The fluid in the hydrosalpinx may contain toxic factors that decrease the implantation rate of embryos or have direct embryotoxicity.[226] A meta-analysis of three controlled trials reported that laparoscopic salpingectomy for hydrosalpinx prior to IVF increased pregnancy rates by 75% compared with not performing the surgery.[227] In one trial,[228] 204 women were randomized to undergo salpingectomy prior to IVF or to undergo IVF without prior salpingectomy. The live birth rate was 29% in the women who had salpingectomy followed by IVF and 16% in the women who had IVF alone ($P < 0.05$). Laparoscopic salpingectomy should be consider for all women with hydrosalpinges prior to undergoing IVF. Interestingly, in infertile women with one patent tube of normal caliber, and one blocked tube with a hydrosalpinx, surgical removal of the single blocked tube is associated with a good spontaneous pregnancy rate.[229]

CERVICAL FACTOR INFERTILITY

The cervix is an active participant in shepherding sperm from the vagina to the upper reproductive tract. In the normal cervix, the secreted cervical mucus has physicochemical properties that facilitates the transport of sperm. Congenital malformation and trauma to the cervix may impair the ability of the cervix to produce normal mucus.

The postcoital test is the procedure most frequently utilized to examine the adequacy of the cervical mucus and the sperm-mucus interaction. Late in the follicular phase, the infertile couple is instructed to have sexual intercourse. The female partner is seen after intercourse and

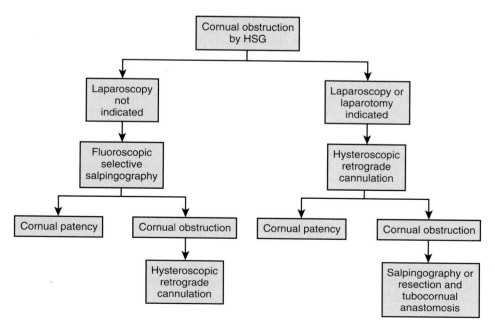

Figure 21-14. *Schematic algorithm for treatment of women with proximal tubal obstruction. If laparoscopy or laparotomy is planned because of known major pelvic disease, proximal obstruction can be evaluated and treated by a hysteroscopic procedure performed at the same operation. If the patient is not thought to require a surgical procedure for pelvic disease, proximal tubal obstruction can be evaluated and treated by fluoroscopic selective salpingography and catheter treatment. HSG, hysterosalpingogram. (From Novy MI, Thurmond AS, Patton P, et al. Diagnosis of cornual obstruction by transcervical fallopian tube cannulation. Fertil Steril 50:434, 1988, with permission.)*

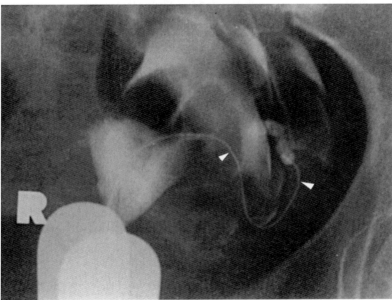

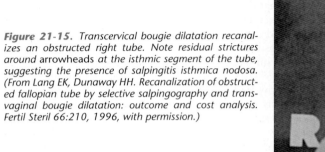

Figure 21-15. *Transcervical bougie dilatation recanalizes an obstructed right tube. Note residual strictures around arrowheads at the isthmic segment of the tube, suggesting the presence of salpingitis isthmica nodosa. (From Lang EK, Dunaway HH. Recanalization of obstructed fallopian tube by selective salpingography and transvaginal bougie dilatation: outcome and cost analysis. Fertil Steril 66:210, 1996, with permission.)*

a small amount of cervical mucus is obtained using oval forceps with a hollow aperture. The glycoproteins in the mucus support the property of *spinnbarkeit*, or stretchability of the mucus. By allowing the prongs of the forceps to separate the spinnbarkeit, the mucus can be tested. A separate aliquot is dried on a glass slide. Owing to the high concentration of salts in the normal mucus in the late follicular phase, the dried mucus will crystallize in a fernlike pattern. A third aliquot is placed on a glass slide overlaid with a coverslip and examined under the high-power microscope objective for the presence of sperm.

Two major problems with the postcoital test are that there is little consensus on the normal range, and that the test has poor predictive value for pregnancy. For example, some authorities suggest that a normal test requires more than 20 sperm per high-power field.[230] Other authorities conclude that the presence of a single sperm indicates a normal test.[231] In one study of the relationship between the postcoital test and fecundability 20% of fertile women were observed to have one sperm or less per high-power field.[230] In another study, fecundability did not seem to be altered by the presence of between 0 and 11 sperm per high-power field.[232] Further reducing the potential validity of the postcoital test is the observation that the inter- and intraobserver reproducibility is poor.[14] Dysplasia of the cervix is a common problem that is often treated with excision of cervical tissue infected with human papillomavirus. Recent epidemiologic studies have reported that loop electrosurgical excision (LEEP) of cervical tissue is associated with cervical stenosis,[233] preterm delivery, and low-birth-weight infants.[234]

ENDOMETRIOSIS

The relationship between endometriosis and infertility and the treatment of endometriosis-associated infertility are reviewed in Chapter 24.

UTERINE LEIOMYOMATA

Uterine *leiomyomata*, also known as fibroids or uterine myomata, are benign smooth muscle tumors of the uterus. The biology and pathophysiology of uterine leiomyomata are reviewed in Chapter 25. Myomata are the most common pelvic tumors of women. Uterine leiomyomata are monoclonal tumors that demonstrate nonrandom cytogenetic mutations. The most frequently reported cytogenetic abnormalities in myomata are t(12;14)(q13ql5;q23q24); del(7)(q21); and t(l;2)(p36;p24).[235] A gene at 12ql5, high-mobility group A protein gene (HMGA2), is mutated in many cases of uterine myomata.[236] HMGI-C encodes an architectural factor that binds to the minor groove of DNA and plays a role in organizing satellite chromatin. HMGA2 is a phosphoprotein and is a substrate for cell regulatory kinases, such as casein kinase and p34/cdc2. One current working hypothesis is that somatic mutations in genes such as HMGA2 in uterine myocytes results in dysregulated growth, which produces a myoma.[237] In addition, the HMGA2 mutation appears to increase the sensitivity of the mutated smooth muscle cells to the effects of estradiol.[238] The mechanisms that cause a high rate of mutations in the HMGA2 gene in uterine myocytes are unknown, but estradiol and progesterone probably play a role in regulating the rate of mitosis and mutation in the uterine myocyte.

Few well-designed clinical studies analyze the effect of uterine leiomyomata on fecundability. Farhi and colleagues[239] reported the effect of uterine leiomyomata on the results of IVF treatment. The investigators reported that among 46 women with uterine myomata treated with IVF, the pregnancy rate per transfer was 22% and the abortion rate was 36%. In a control group of women with mechanical causes of infertility, the pregnancy rate per transfer was 25% and the abortion rate was 25%. There were no statistically significant differences between the two groups. A further analysis divided the women with uterine myomata into two groups: those with a normal uterine cavity and those with an abnormal uterine cavity as assessed by hysterosalpingogram. In the 28 women with uterine myomata and a normal uterine cavity, there was a 30% pregnancy rate per embryo transfer. In the 18 women with uterine myomata and an abnormal uterine cavity, there was a 9% pregnancy rate per embryo transfer. This study suggests that uterine leiomyomata that distort the uterine cavity may be associated with a decrease in fecundability. Other investigators have also reported that leiomyomata—especially those that distort the uterine cavity—may reduce the pregnancy rate in IVF.[240,241] There are no prospective randomized studies evaluating whether removing leiomyomata improves fertility.[242] If a leiomyoma in a pregnant woman is directly under the placenta, there may be an increased risk of threatened abortion, preterm contractions, abruptio placenta, and pelvic pain.[243-245]

Immunologic Factors and Recurrent Abortion

Recurrent abortions caused by autoimmune diseases, coagulopathies, and infections are discussed in Chapter 13.

Genetic Causes of Infertility

For many decades it has been known that major chromosomal abnormalities are often associated with infertility. For example, women with 45,X (Turner's syndrome) have premature depletion of the oocyte pool and are typically sterile. Translocations and interstitial deletions of the X chromosome are associated with premature ovarian failure, although the identity of the genes in these deletions remains to be established. In infertile men, Yq11 microdeletions are observed in about 5% of cases.[246]

A major goal of reproductive scientists is to identify individual genes that are associated with infertility. Recently a few genes in women that influence fecundability have been identified.[247] Genes in which mutations affecting fertility and fecundity have been identified include galactose-1-phosphate uridyl transferase (*GALT*),[248] the FSH receptor,[249] the LH receptor,[250] pre-mutations in the *FMR1* (fragile X syndrome) gene,[251] the *FOXL2* transcription factor gene,[252] the *BMP 15* gene[253] and the ataxia-telangiectasia (*ATM*) gene[254]

Unexplained Infertility

Unexplained infertility is diagnosed when a couple has failed to achieve a pregnancy after 12 months of attempting conception and has completed a thorough evaluation without finding a cause for the infertility.[255] The diagnosis of unexplained infertility rests heavily on the definition of what constitutes a thorough fertility evaluation. For many fertility specialists, a thorough evaluation includes documentation of the following normal findings:

- Adequate ovulation, using either a mid-luteal phase serum progesterone determination of greater than 10 ng/mL or an endometrial biopsy demonstrating secretory endometrium
- Tubal patency, as determined by HSG or laparoscopy
- Normal semen analysis, demonstrating 20 million sperm/mL, greater than 50% forward motility, and greater than 40% normal morphology
- Adequate ovarian oocyte reserve, using either a cycle day 3 FSH determination (below 15 mIU/mL) or a clomiphene challenge test (both cycle day 3 and 10 FSH measurements below 15 mIU/mL)
- Absence of endometriosis or clinically significant ovarian or pelvic adhesions, as determined by laparoscopy

The benefit of laparoscopy is that it allows a complete evaluation of the pelvis for diseases such as endometriosis and pelvic adhesions. On the downside, laparoscopy is an expensive surgical procedure. Many fertility specialists argue that if laparoscopy is not performed in the evaluation of infertile couples with normal ovulation, normal semen analysis, and patent fallopian tubes, many cases of endometriosis and ovarian adhesions will be misdiagnosed as unexplained infertility. However, other fertility specialists contend that the presence of endometriosis and pelvic adhesions does not influence their approach to treatment because their practice is to move quickly to IVF, for which diseases such as endometriosis and ovarian adhesions have little impact on pregnancy success. In one large retrospective study of 495 infertile couples with normal ovulation, HSG, and male factor, when the female partner had a laparoscopy, 35% were diagnosed with either major pelvic adhesions/tubal disease (10%) or endometriosis (21%).[256]

Many cases of unexplained infertility are probably caused by the presence of multiple factors (e.g., female partner 37 years of age or older, male partner with semen parameters in the low end of the normal range). Each of these factors on their own do not substantially reduce fertility; when more than one factor is present, however, the pregnancy rate is reduced. Subtle changes in follicle development, ovulation, oocyte function, the luteal phase, and sperm function have been reported in women with unexplained infertility.[257] In some couples with unexplained infertility, the male partner has a semen analysis with sperm concentration and motility at the lower end of the normal range.[258]

When couples with unexplained infertility are treated with IVF, they demonstrate reduced oocyte fertilization and embryo cleavage rates compared with couples where tubal factor is the cause of the infertility. For example, in one study, the oocyte fertilization rate for tubal factor infertility and unexplained infertility were 60% and 52%, respectively. When couples with unexplained infertility are treated with IVF, they have a higher rate of complete fertilization failure than couples with tubal factor infertility (6% versus 3%). These results suggest that couples with unexplained infertility probably have subtle functional abnormalities in oocyte and sperm function.[259]

Empirical Treatment

The management of couples with unexplained infertility typically starts with treatments that consume few resources (lifestyle changes, expectant management, IUI, clomiphene, clomiphene plus IUI) and moves sequentially to treatments requiring proportionately greater resources (gonadotropin injections plus IUI or IVF), as shown in Figure 21-16.[260] This sequential approach to infertility, utilizing progressively more demanding interventions, can be described as a "staircase" approach to empirical infertility treatment. The rationale underlying this strategy is that treatment is initiated with low-cost, low-risk interventions; and then with each step in the program, interventions are initiated that utilize greater resources and carry more risk. This approach has been demonstrated to be cost-effective in the treatment of unexplained infertility.[261] The pace at which the staircase is climbed is dependent on many factors, including the age of the female partner and the beliefs and values of the clinicians and patients.

Lifestyle changes can enhance the fertility of couples. Epidemiologic studies indicate that for the female partner, cigarette smoking and excessive caffeine and alcohol consumption reduce fertility[262] Couples with unexplained infertility should be counseled to stop smoking cigarettes. The female partner should be counseled to reduce caffeine intake to no more than 250 mg daily (two cups of coffee) and to reduce alcohol intake to no more than four standardized drinks per week.[263] For couples with unexplained infertility and a low frequency of coitus, recommending an increase in coital frequency to at least twice per week may be associated with increased pregnancy rates.[264]

For young couples with unexplained infertility, expectant management is a reasonable approach. When couples with unexplained infertility are followed prospectively without active treatment, approximately 1% to 3% become pregnant each month. Effective fertility treatment for unexplained infertility must increase the pregnancy rate above this baseline fecundability of approximately 1% to 3%. The age of the female partner influences the pregnancy rate associated with expectant management.[265] For women over age 37, the pregnancy rate per cycle with expectant management is under 1%. Expectant management may be an option for a couple when the female partner is

under 32 years of age and the problem of oocyte depletion is not an immediate concern. For couples in which the female partner is over 37 years of age, the ovarian oocyte pool declines rapidly—inevitably causing ovarian aging to become the cause of the fertility problem. For these women, expectant management is not recommended. Many couples of all ages become frustrated with their inability to conceive. For these couples, active treatment is recommended.

INTRAUTERINE INSEMINATION

The IUI procedure consists of washing an ejaculated semen specimen to remove prostaglandins and other factors, concentrating the sperm in a small volume of culture medium that enhances capacitation and the acrosome reaction. The sperm suspension is then injected directly into the upper uterine cavity using a small catheter threaded through the cervix. In one study of various methods used to prepare the sperm for intrauterine insemination, the swim-up and Percoll gradient preparation techniques resulted in superior pregnancy rates than the simple wash, swim-down, or refrigeration/heparin techniques.[265] The intrauterine insemination is timed to take place just prior to ovulation, typically using home urine LH monitoring. In couples reporting male infertility, IUI more than doubles the pregnancy rate compared with intracervical insemination or timed natural cycles (odds ratio 2.2; 95% confidence interval, 1.4 to 3.4).[266] In one study of couples with mild male infertility, the pregnancy rate per cycle was 6.5% for IUI versus 3.1% for intracervical insemination or timed natural intercourse.[267] IUI also appears to be effective for couples with unexplained infertility.

In a large clinical trial sponsored by the National Institutes of Health, 932 infertile couples with unexplained infertility or stage I or II endometriosis were randomized to one of four treatment groups: intracervical insemination of sperm (ICI); IUI; FSH injections plus ICI; or FSH injections plus IUI. The purpose of the ICI was to be a control treatment that mimicked natural intercourse. The purpose of the IUI was to place a large number of sperm high in the reproductive tract. The purpose of the FSH injections was to stimulate multiple follicular development and ovulation, thereby increasing the number of oocytes

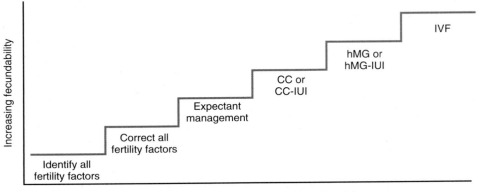

Figure 21-16. Staircase approach to empirical infertility treatment. For women over 35 years old, the first three steps in the algorithm should be rapidly completed. In women less than 30 years old, more time can be spent on the first three steps in the staircase. CC, clomiphene citrate; CC-IUI, clomiphene citrate plus intrauterine insemination; hMG, human menopausal gonadotropin; hMG-IUI, human menopausal gonadotropin plus intrauterine insemination; IVF, in vitro fertilization and embryo transfer.

available for fertilization in a single cycle (this type of treatment is explained later in this chapter). Most of the women in this study had either unexplained infertility or early stage endometriosis. The investigators reported that the per-cycle pregnancy rate in the group that received the control (ICI treatment) was 2%. This pregnancy rate is similar to expectant management. IUI treatment was associated with a 5% per-cycle pregnancy rate. The per-cycle pregnancy rates in the FSH-ICI and FSH-IUI groups were 4% and 9%, respectively. In this study, IUI was clearly effective for the treatment of unexplained infertility.[258] Multiple procedure-related factors appear to influence the effectiveness of IUI. Most recent studies report that one IUI per cycle results in a pregnancy rate similar to two IUI procedures per cycle.[268] Resting supine after the IUI procedure may also be associated with higher pregnancy rates than those in patients who ambulated soon afterward.[268]

An alternative approach to IUI is fallopian tube sperm perfusion (FSP). In this technique, pressure injection of 4 mL of sperm suspension is performed while the cervix is occluded in order to cause the infused sperm suspension to flow out through the fallopian tubes resulting in a high peritoneal concentration of sperm. In contrast to the 4 mL of sperm suspensions used in FSP, only 0.3 to 0.5 mL of sperm suspension is utilized in IUI. In a meta-analysis of six trials of FSP versus IUI, there was no difference in pregnancy or live birth rates between the two treatments. However, in a subgroup analysis, when FSP cervical occlusion techniques that used a balloon catheter were excluded, FSP was associated with an increased pregnancy rate compared to IUI. In a subgroup analysis that included only couples with unexplained infertility, FSP appear to be associated with an increased pregnancy rate compared to IUI.[270]

CLOMIPHENE CITRATE

Clomiphene has been demonstrated to be effective in the treatment of unexplained infertility. In normal ovulatory women, clomiphene treatment often results in the ovulation of two follicles and an increase in luteal phase progesterone production. These treatment-dependent changes probably increase fecundability. In a recent meta-analysis, 11 prospective trials of clomiphene treatment for women with unexplained infertility demonstrated that clomiphene was superior to placebo or no treatment. The odds ratio for clinical pregnancy per clomiphene treatment cycle was 2.5 (95% confidence interval, 1.35 to 4.62).[271] In one trial where 118 female partners from couples with unexplained infertility were randomized to treatment with placebo or clomiphene citrate (100 mg daily, cycle days 2 to 6), the per-cycle pregnancy rates were 5% and 7%, respectively ($P < 0.05$).[272]

Although the absolute treatment effectiveness is modest, the low cost and low adverse effects of clomiphene make it a useful initial treatment for unexplained infertility. The main complication of clomiphene is an increase in multiple gestation. In one study of 2369 clomiphene-induced pregnancies, 7% were twins, 0.5% were triplets, 0.3% were quadruplets, and 0.13% were quintuplets.[273] The risk of high-order multiple pregnancies with clomiphene treatment is low, but the high volume of clomiphene cycles makes this intervention an important contributor to the total number of high-order pregnancies.[80] Many normal ovulatory women undergoing empirical treatment of infertility with clomiphene have endometriosis. Many clinicians believe that clomiphene use in this setting may be associated with an increase in estradiol levels and an increase in endometriosis disease activity, including pelvic pain and the growth of ovarian endometriosis cysts.

CLOMIPHENE PLUS INTRAUTERINE INSEMINATION

The combination of clomiphene (increases the rate of double ovulation) plus IUI (places a large number of motile sperm high in the female reproductive tract) may simultaneously treat mild abnormalities of ovulation, oocyte function, and sperm function. In one study, 67 couples were randomized to treatment with clomiphene plus IUI or placebo. The pregnancy rate per cycle was 3.3% for placebo and 9.5% for clomiphene plus IUI.[274] For clomiphene-plus-IUI cycles, timing of the IUI is usually based on home urine LH measurement. Timing IUI with home urine LH measurement or exogenously administered hCG is associated with a similar pregnancy rate, but hCG administration is associated with greater cost and an increased risk of OHSS.[275] Advancing age of the female partner is associated with a decrease in success rates for IUI therapy (Fig. 21-17).[276]

GONADOTROPIN INJECTIONS AND GONADOTROPIN INJECTIONS PLUS INTRAUTERINE INSEMINATION

Both gonadotropin injections alone and gonadotropin injections plus IUI increase fecundability in women with unexplained infertility. Gonadotropin injections plus IUI also appears to increase fecundability in infertile women with stage I or II endometriosis and in infertile men with semen abnormalities (Fig. 21-18).[277] In one study, 932 infertile couples with unexplained infertility or stage I or II endometriosis were randomized to one of four treatment groups: ICI, IUI, FSH injections plus ICI, or FSH injections plus IUI. The pregnancy rate in the control, the ICI group, was 2% per cycle. In the FSH-plus-ICI and the FSH-plus-IUI groups, the pregnancy rate per cycle was 4% and 9%, respectively.[258] The main complication of the use of FSH injections in the treatment of infertility in women with unexplained infertility is an increase in the rate of multiple gestations and ovarian hyperstimulation. Of the ongoing pregnancies in this study, 3% were quadruplets, 5% were triplets, and 20% were twins. In another study of gonadotropin injections with or without IUI, Serhal[278] randomized 62 couples with unexplained infertility to receive IUI alone, gonadotropin injections alone, or gonadotropin injections plus IUI. The per-cycle pregnancy rate was 2.2% for IUI alone, 6.1% for gonadotropin injections alone, and 26% for gonadotropin injections plus IUI. Similar results have been reported by other investigators.[279,280]

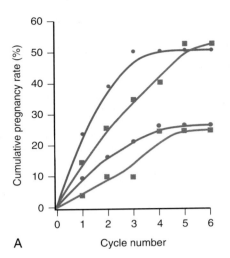

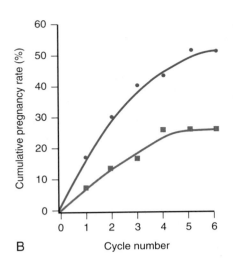

Figure 21-17. *Cumulative pregnancy rates by Kaplan Meier life-table analysis for 290 infertile couples undergoing clomiphene IUI therapy stratified by the age of the female partner. **A**, Ages of women: purple graph, under age 30; blue line, ages 31 to 35; green line, ages 36 to 40; brown line, age 41 or older. **B**, Ages of women: purple line, under 35 years; green line, over 35 years. (From Agarwal SK, Buyalos RP. Clomiphene citrate with intrauterine insemination: is it effective therapy in women above the age of 35 years? Fertil Steril 65:759, 1996, with permission.)*

Although there is evidence for the efficacy of gonadotropin with or without IUI for the treatment of unexplained infertility, many authorities highlight the increased risk of multiple gestation with these therapies, and advise that the use of gonadotropin-IUI should be very limited.[281,282] In addition, if good prognosis couples with unexplained infertility can be counseled to continue to try to get pregnant on their own, and not pursue gonadotropin therapy, many will become pregnant spontaneously.[283] In a recent trial comparing the three-step sequential treatment protocol (clomiphene-IUI, followed by gonadotropin-IUI, followed by IVF) versus a two-step sequential treatment protocol (clomiphene-IUI, followed by IVF), the clinical utility of the gonadotropin-IUI was poor.[284] In this study, the per-cycle pregnancy rate for clomiphene-IUI was 7.6%, gonadotropin-IUI 9.8%, and IVF 31%. Because gonadotropin-IUI is expensive, and much less effective

than IVF, the most cost-efficient approach was the two-step sequential treatment plan of clomiphene-IUI followed by IVF. The two-step approach was approximately 15% less expensive per live birth than the traditional three-step approach.

In IVF cycles, the addition of a GnRH agonist analogue to the gonadotropin injection regimen is known to improve pregnancy rates. However, the addition of a GnRH agonist analogue to a regimen of gonadotropin injections plus IUI does not appear to increase the pregnancy rate in couples with unexplained infertility. In one study, 91 couples with unexplained infertility were randomized to receive treatment with gonadotropin injections and IUI or GnRH agonist analogue treatment plus gonadotropin injections and IUI. The pregnancy rate per cycle was 11% and 13%, respectively.[285]

IN VITRO FERTILIZATION

IVF is effective in the treatment of unexplained infertility. One trial randomized couples with idiopathic infertility and male factor infertility to one of three treatments: IUI alone; low-dose FSH injections plus IUI; or IVF. The per-cycle pregnancy rates were 7% with IUI alone, 9% with the addition of FSH injections, and 12% with IVF ($P = 0.09$).[286] The cumulative pregnancy rate was similar in all three groups because the couples in the IUI and FSH-IUI groups were able to complete more treatment cycles than the patients in the IVF group. Severe ovarian hyperstimulation occurred in 3.5% of the women treated with IVF. Ovarian hyperstimulation did not occur in the group treated with IUI. In one randomized clinical trial comparing IVF with expectant management, there was a substantially increased pregnancy rate in the couples assigned to IVF.[287]

In a cohort study, couples with unexplained infertility were treated for up to three cycles with gonadotropin injections plus IUI. The couples who did not become pregnant were then treated with IVF.[288] The per-cycle pregnancy rate was 16% for the couples treated with gonadotropin injections plus IUI, and 37% for the couples treated with

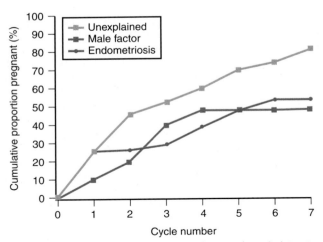

Figure 21-18. *Cumulative pregnancy rate for gonadotropin-intrauterine insemination treatment for various fertility conditions: unexplained, early stage endometriosis, and male factor. (From Nulsen JC, Walsh S, Dumez S, Metzger DA. A randomized and longitudinal study of human menopausal gonadotropin with intrauterine insemination in the treatment of infertility. Obstet Gynecol 82:780, 1993, with permission.)*

IVF. Published cohort studies with no control group report that the treatment of unexplained infertility with IVF results in per-cycle pregnancy rates in the range of 20% to 40%.[289] Some authorities have proposed that couples with unexplained infertility should be offered a "fast track" to IVF treatment, especially if the female partner is more than 37 years of age. This recommendation parallels the general trend of offering IVF treatment early in the course of infertility treatment (Fig. 21-19).

Environmental Exposures Associated with Infertility

Many environmental factors may influence fertility. Numerous studies have reported that cigarette smoking is associated with a decrease in fertility. Many studies have reported that caffeine intake of more than 250 mg daily is associated with a modest decrease in fertility. Although not consistently demonstrated in all studies, alcohol intake of more than eight drinks per week appears to be associated with a small decrease in fertility.

Approximately 12% of infertile women and 18% of infertile men smoke cigarettes.[290] Numerous studies report that cigarette smoking by the female partner decreases fertility. Smoking is associated with tubal factor infertility,[291] cervical factor infertility,[292] and ectopic gestation.[293] Cigarette smoking is also associated with premature depletion of the ovarian pool of oocytes. Polycyclic hydrocarbons activate the oocyte aromatic hydrocarbon receptor and induce *Bax*, causing apoptosis.[294] This causes premature loss of the high-quality oocytes and premature aging of the ovary.[164] Ovarian aging is thought to be a major contributor to unexplained infertility. The results from studies with a large sample size indicate that smoking by the male partner does not appear to be associated with a substantial decrease in fertility.

Population-based studies that included more than 1000 couples consistently reported that cigarette smoking by the female partner was associated with an increase in the number of couples with infertility and an increase in the waiting time to pregnancy. In one prospective study of 17,032 women using contraceptives, 4104 women stopped using contraceptives to attempt to become pregnant.[295]

In this study, the best predictor of fertility was the age of the female partner at the time she initiated attempts at conception. The older the female partner, the less likely the couple was to achieve a pregnancy. The next most important association was between the female partner smoking 20 or more cigarettes per day and an increased risk of failure to conceive. In long-term follow-up after 5 years of trying to become pregnant, 5.4% of the nonsmokers were undelivered and 10.7% of the smokers were undelivered. In a retrospective study of approximately 6630 couples in Europe, an association was observed between cigarette smoking by the female partner (more than 10 cigarettes daily) and subfecundity (odds ratio 1.7; 95% confidence interval, 1.3 to 2.1). The waiting time to conception was also dramatically increased in the couples in which the female partner smoked more than 10 cigarettes daily. Among the couples in which the female partner was a nonsmoker, 17% had not become pregnant after trying to conceive for 9.5 months. Among the couples where the female partner smoked 1 to 10 cigarettes daily, 21% of the couples had not conceived after 9.5 months of trying. When the female partner smoked more than 10 cigarettes per day, 24% of the couples had not become pregnant after attempting conception for 9.5 months.[296] The association between cigarette smoking by the female partner and subfecundity remained significant after controlling for the age of the female partner, parity, ethanol consumption, coffee intake, past history of oral contraceptive use, smoking habits of the male partner, and frequency of sexual intercourse. In this study, there was no significant relationship between cigarette smoking by the male partner and a delay in time to first conception.

Most studies with a large sample size have reported that caffeine consumption of more than 250 mg daily (a cup of coffee contains approximately 115 mg of caffeine) is associated with a modest, but statistically significant, decrease in fertility. Approximately 20% of adult Americans consume more than 300 mg of caffeine daily. Therefore, although caffeine consumption has a modest impact on fertility, the widespread consumption of caffeine at doses demonstrated to influence fertility makes it a potentially important contributor to fertility problems. In one study, caffeine consumption of more than 250 mg of caffeine daily was associated with an increased risk of

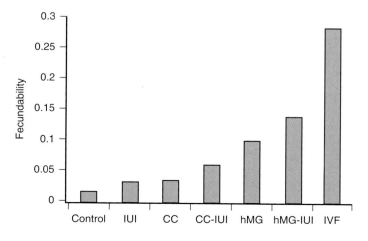

Figure 21-19. *Fecundability associated with empirical treatment of unexplained infertility. Control, no treatment; IUI, intrauterine insemination; CC, clomiphene citrate; CC-IUI, clomiphene citrate plus intrauterine insemination; hMG, human menopausal gonadotropin; hMG-IUI, human menopausal gonadotropin plus intrauterine insemination; IVF, in vitro fertilization and embryo transfer.*

tubal factor infertility and endometriosis-associated infertility.[297] In a retrospective study of 3187 couples, caffeine consumption by the female partner of more than 500 mg daily (approximately five cups of coffee daily) was associated with a delay in the time to conception—defined as the number of couples taking more than 9.5 months to conceive (odds ratio 1.45, 95% confidence interval, 1.03 to 2.04). In couples in which the woman drank no coffee, 16% of the couples had not conceived after 9.5 months of trying. In couples in which the female partner drank five or more cups of coffee daily, 23% of the couples had not conceived by 9.5 months of trying. In some countries, tea, not coffee, is the major source of dietary caffeine. The investigators also evaluated the impact of caffeine consumption from all dietary sources on fertility. In couples in which the female partner consumed 100 mg or less of caffeine daily, 16% of the couples had not conceived by 9.5 months of trying. In couples in which the female partner consumed more than 500 mg of caffeine daily, 25% of the couples had not conceived by 9.5 months of trying. These statistically significant differences in fertility persisted after controlling for age of the female partner, parity, smoking, alcohol consumption, frequency of intercourse, educational level, working status, and past use of oral contraceptives.[298] In a retrospective study of 1430 women attempting to become pregnant, caffeine intake of less than 300 mg daily was not associated with a delay in time to conception (defined as more than 12 months to conception). For nonsmoking women who consumed more than 300 mg daily of caffeine, there was an increased delay to conception, with an odds ratio of 2.65 (95% confidence interval, 1.38 to 5.07). In this study, cigarette smoking significantly delayed conception (odds ratio 1.77; 95% confidence interval, 1.33 to 2.37) but in the women who smoked, caffeine consumption did not increase time to conception.[299]

In a study of 1050 women with primary infertility, Grodstein and colleagues reported that caffeine intake greater than approximately 250 mg daily (about 2.5 cups of coffee daily) was associated with an increase in the risk of tubal factor infertility (relative risk 1.5; 95% confidence interval, 1.1 to 2) and endometriosis (relative risk 1.6; 95% confidence interval, 1.1 to 2.4).[297] Caffeine intake greater than 500 mg daily has been reported to be associated with an increased risk of spontaneous abortion. Cnattingius and colleagues explored the association in a case-control study of 562 women with spontaneous abortion between 6 and 12 weeks' gestation and 953 control women who did not have a spontaneous abortion.[300] The investigators reported a dose-response relationship between consumption of caffeine and the risk of spontaneous abortion in women who did not smoke cigarettes (Table 21-5). A caffeine intake of 500 mg daily or greater was associated with an increased risk of spontaneous abortion (adjusted odds ratio 2.2, 95% confidence interval, 1.3 to 3.8). In women who smoked, there was no relationship between caffeine intake and the risk of spontaneous abortion. When the analysis was stratified according to the results of the karyotype of the abortion specimen, the ingestion of high levels of caffeine was found to be associated with an excess risk of spontaneous abortion in pregnancies when the embryo or fetus had a normal or unknown karyotype but not when the embryo or fetal karyotype was abnormal.

Alcohol consumption by the female partner is associated with an increased risk of ovulatory infertility and endometriosis-associated infertility. Heavy alcohol use by the male partner is associated with abnormalities in gonadal function, including reduced testosterone production, impotence, and decreased spermatogenesis.[301,302] However, moderate alcohol intake by the male partner does not appear to be associated with decreased fertility. In most studies of the association between ethanol and infertility, the investigators have used the concept of a *standardized alcoholic drink*. A standardized drink is typically defined to be 12 ounces of beer, 5 ounces of wine, or 1.5 ounces of spirits. A standardized drink contains approximately 12 g of ethanol. In a study of 1050 women with infertility and 3833 fertile women, the investigators reported that alcohol consumption of more than eight standardized drinks per week was associated with an increased risk for ovulatory infertility and endometriosis-associated infertility. The odds ratio for ovulatory infertility was 1.3 in moderate drinkers (95% confidence

---

TABLE 21-5

Caffeine Intake and the Risk of Spontaneous Abortion

| Caffeine Intake | Nonsmokers* | | Smokers† | |
	Relative Risk	Confidence Interval	Relative Risk	Confidence Interval
<100 mg daily	1	1	1	1
100-299 mg daily	1.3	0.9-1.8	0.9	0.3-2.5
300-499 mg daily	1.4	0.9-2	1.7	0.6-4.6
>499 mg daily‡	2.2	1.3-3.8	0.7	0.3-1.9
P value	0.007	—	0.65	—

*Number of cases, 401; number of control subjects, 811.
†Number of cases, 115; number of control subjects, 121.
‡Caffeine intake greater than 499 mg daily (approximately four cups of coffee) in nonsmokers increased the risk of spontaneous abortion associated with normal karyotype on the products of conception.
Adapted from Cnattingius S, Signorello LB, Anneren G, et al. Caffeine intake and the risk of first-trimester spontaneous abortion. N Engl J Med 343:1839-1845. 2000.

interval, 1 to 1.7) and 1.6 in heavy drinkers (95% confidence interval, 1.1 to 2.3). The risk of endometriosis-associated infertility was approximately 1.6 in both moderate and heavy drinkers (95% confidence interval, 1.1 to 2.3 for moderate drinkers).[303] In a study of 430 Danish couples between the ages of 20 to 35 years who were attempting to conceive after discontinuing contraception, alcohol consumption of more than five drinks per week was associated with a decreased probability of conception.[304] Other studies also support a relationship between alcohol drinking by the female partner and decreased fertility.[305] Although some studies report that alcohol consumption is not associated with a decrease in fertility,[306] the weight of the evidence appears to demonstrate that alcohol consumption by the female partner is associated with a modest decrease in fertility.

Adoption

The most difficult decision in fertility treatments is deciding when to cease active interventions designed to increase fecundability. Throughout the process of fertility treatment, it is prudent to raise the issue of when to cease active intervention and to offer adoption as an alternative method of building a family. It may be useful for couples to simultaneously explore the option of adoption while they are undergoing fertility therapy. If the fertility therapy fails, adoption may help couples cope with the symbolic loss created by their infertility.

Psychosocial Aspects of Infertility

Many observational studies indicate that stress is associated with infertility; in turn, the treatment of infertility can cause stress. Reducing stress prior to initiating intensive fertility treatments may improve the ability of the couple to successfully complete the treatments recommended.[307] For example, in one study, 151 women were given a standardized test to evaluate their moods, sense of optimism, social support networks, self-perceived stress, and methods of coping prior to undergoing IVE. Elevated levels of baseline stress were associated with fewer oocytes retrieved and fertilized and fewer embryos.[308] No definitive clinical trial demonstrates that reducing stress prior to infertility treatment improves pregnancy rates. In one small clinical trial, however, Domar and colleagues reported that treatment of infertile women with a support group or a structured relaxation program was associated with better pregnancy rates with infertility treatment than those observed in a control group.[309]

Infertility, and the associated diagnostic and therapeutic procedures can produce substantial stress for both male and female partners and disrupt their relationship with each other. Inherently, diagnostic and therapeutic procedures offer hope for an imminent successful conception, but each subsequent menstrual cycle rekindles the feeling of loss. The repetitive cycles of hope and loss can be very stressful for couples with infertility.[310] Infertility may be perceived by the couple as a loss that is difficult to grieve for because the absence of fertility is somewhat intangible. Infertility may be especially stressful for couples for whom the cause of the infertility is difficult to identify.[311] The classic progression of emotions related to a loss are often expressed by the infertile couple.[312] These emotions include the feelings of disbelief and surprise, denial, anger, isolation, guilt, grief, and resolution. For many couples, the female partner bears a disproportionate degree of responsibility for the loss symbolically represented by infertility. Although infertility treatment is often perceived as extremely stressful, infertility treatment does not appear to be associated with long-term emotional distress, dysfunction, or de novo psychiatric conditions.[313] Recent preliminary findings suggest that effective management of the stress and psychosocial sequelae of infertility might decrease the cost of fertility treatments and increase the fecundability of the couple.

Patients report that it is important that they be treated with respect and dignity and have all treatment options thoroughly and fairly presented. Patients wanted their clinicians to recognize their distress and respond in an empathic manner.[314] In most surveys, patients report that they are highly satisfied with the care provided by their fertility clinicians.[315]

Social and Ethical Issues

Medicine is an ethical profession that has long adhered to basic principles of human rights: respect for the dignity of human life, the right of an individual to participate in decisions that affect his or her health, an unwavering dedication to seek good and to avoid unnecessary harm, and a commitment to treat the patient fairly. Fertility practitioners also have an ethical obligation to protect the security of the human genetic material in their custody.

Most ethicists are in agreement that the inviolability of each human precludes any medical intervention without the individual's consent. Free and informed consent is the cornerstone of ethical medical practice. Practices that are deceptive or could have the appearance of being deceptive undermine the credibility of clinicians in the fertility profession.

Embryonic development is a continuous biologic process. Current law tends to assign gradually increasing rights to the developing fetus. A human does not acquire full legal identity until birth but is offered some legal protection as a fetus in utero (e.g., restrictions on legal abortion in the third trimester). Modern society is not unified on the point in the developmental process where the developing embryo or fetus becomes a unique individual with full rights to inviolability and inalienability. This disagreement, which is most obvious in the debate over abortion, will make it difficult to reach consensus on the ethics of certain types of fertility research, such as that performed on discarded embryos. However, most practitioners and ethicists are in agreement that cloning of humans is not ethical.

The complete reference list can be found on the companion Expert Consult Web site at www.expertconsultbook.com.

Suggested Reading

Coutifaris C, Myers ER, Guzick DS, et al. Histological dating of timed endometrial biopsy tissue is not related to fertility status. Fertil Steril 82:1264, 2004.

Guzick DS, Overstreet JW, Factor-Litvak P, et al. Sperm morphology, motility and concentration in fertile and infertile men. N Engl J Med 345:1388, 2001.

Holzer H, Casper R, Tulandi T. A new era in ovulation induction. Fertil Steril 85:277, 2006.

Layman LC. BMP15—the first true ovarian determinant gene on the X-chromosome. J Clin Endocrinol Metab 91:1673, 2006.

Legro RS, Barnhart HX, Schlaff WD, et al. Clomiphene, metformin or both for infertility in the polycystic ovary syndrome. N Engl J Med 356:551, 2007.

Lobo RA. Potential options for preservation of fertility in women. N Engl J Med 353:64, 2005.

Schlechte JA. Prolactinoma. N Engl J Med 349:2035, 2003.

Wittenberger MD, Hagerman RJ, Sherman SL, et al. The FMR1 premutation and reproduction. Fertil Steril 87:456, 2007.

CHAPTER 22

Male Infertility

Paul J. Turek

Male infertility affects 15% of reproductive age men worldwide and is treatable in many cases. In the United States, 8 million couples are affected.[1] Roughly 50% of couples have causal or associated male factors.[2] In addition, 1% to 10% of male factor infertility is a result of an underlying, often treatable, but possibly life-threatening medical condition.[3] In addition to well-established etiologies, genetic causes of male infertility are now commonly diagnosed, as our knowledge of genomic medicine advances. For these reasons, the male evaluation is conducted systematically to acquire relevant information from the history, physical examination, semen analysis, and hormone assessment. The American Urological Association and the American Society for Reproductive Medicine guidelines recommend that evaluation of male and female partners occurs in parallel. Using principles of evidence-based medicine, this chapter outlines diagnostic and treatment algorithms that guide clinical management. Randomized controlled clinical trials, basic scientific studies, meta-analyses, case-controlled cohort studies, best-practice policy recommendations, and reviews from peer-reviewed literature are incorporated into algorithms that provide timely guidelines to the current management of male infertility.

The Male History and Physical Examination

A thorough history reviews past and current attempts at paternity (Fig. 22-1 and Box 22-1). Important medical problems to elucidate include fevers, systemic illnesses such as diabetes, cystic fibrosis, cancer, and infections. Prior surgery, including orchidopexy and herniorraphy; trauma; retroperitoneal, pelvic, and bladder procedures; and prostate surgery may impair fertility. A family history of cryptorchidism, midline defects, or hypogonadism is also important. A developmental history of hypospadias, congenital anomalies, prenatal DES (diethylstilbesterol) exposure, and medication use (Box 22-2) should be reviewed. A social history with the habitual use of the gonadotoxins alcohol, tobacco, recreational drugs, anabolic steroids, and wet heat exposure should be elucidated. Spermicidal lubricants and incorrect patterns of timing intercourse may be noted from a sexual history. Lastly, an occupational history determines exposure to ionizing radiation, chronic heat, benzene-based solvents, dyes, pesticides, herbicides, and heavy minerals.

The physical examination assesses body habitus including obesity, gynecomastia, and secondary sex characteristics. The phallus may reveal hypospadias, chordee, plaques, or venereal lesions. The testes should be evaluated for size, consistency, and contour irregularities suggestive of a mass. At least 80% of testis volume is determined by spermatogenesis; hence, testis atrophy is likely associated with decreased sperm production. The epididymides are palpated for induration, fullness, or nodules, which are indicative of infection or obstruction. Delineation of each vas deferens may reveal agenesis, atresia, or injury. The spermatic cords should be examined for asymmetry suggestive of lipoma or varicocele, lesions that are differentiated by an examination in both the standing and supine positions. Meaningful varicoceles are diagnosed exclusively by physical examination. Lastly, a rectal examination is important in identifying large cysts, infections, or dilated seminal vesicles, all of which can be associated with infertility.

SEMEN EVALUATION

Although not a true measure of fertility, the semen analysis, if abnormal, suggests that the probability of achieving fertility is lower than normal.[4] Two semen analyses,

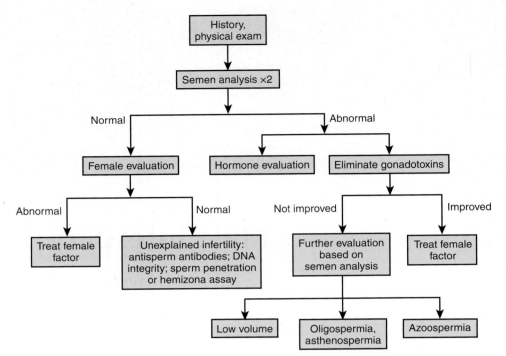

Figure 22-1. *General algorithm for the diagnostic evaluation of male infertility. (From Turek PJ. Practical approach to the diagnosis and management of male infertility. Nature Clin Pract Urol 2:1, 2005.)*

performed after 2 to 3 days of sexual abstinence, are sought owing to the large biologic variability in semen quality. Lubricants should be avoided and the specimen kept at body temperature during transport. Normal values can be found in Table 22-1,[4] however, there is recent debate concerning the precise definition of "normal" because a recent controlled study of fertile and infertile couples suggested that a threshold of 48 million sperm/mL and 63% motility best describes fertile semen.[5] Recall that human spermatogenesis takes 60 to 80 days to complete (Fig. 22-2), so that an individual semen analysis reflects biologic influences occurring 2 to 3 months prior.[6]

The formal evaluation of sperm shape is termed morphologic assessment. Several descriptive systems exist to evaluate morphology, and within each system, sperm are designated normal or abnormal based on specific size criteria. It is believed that sperm morphology may correlate with a man's fertility potential as reflected by in vitro fertilization (IVF) success.[7] Specifically, sperm morphology may correlate with the ability of sperm to successfully penetrate cervical mucus, bind to the zona pellucida, and influence embryo implantation rate. In general, the percentage of sperm with normal morphology has the greatest discriminatory power in distinguishing fertile from infertile semen, although no particular value is diagnostic of fertility.[5] However, sperm morphology provides no insight into the chromosomal complement of the cell. Morphology is usually consistent for a given patient; a change in morphology suggests stress or toxic insult to the testes. Thus, morphologic examination can complement the routine semen analysis in the male evaluation and better estimate the chances of fertility.

RESULTS OF INITIAL MALE EVALUATION

The initial male evaluation may be normal or abnormal (see Fig. 22-1). If normal, further consideration should be given to female factor evaluation, including a thorough assessment of ovulation, pelvic anatomy, and age-related fertility issues. If the initial male assessment reveals abnormalities, then further evaluation or treatment is indicated.[8] Clinicians can have a significant impact in reducing male factor infertility by simple counseling regarding coital timing, avoiding wet heat and other exposures, and lifestyle changes. For example, coital lubricants should also be avoided if possible, including Surgilube, K-Y jelly, and saliva. If necessary, vegetable oils are safe for sperm.

Likewise, androgenic steroids, often taken to increase muscle mass, act as male contraceptives.[9] Excess testosterone inhibits the pituitary-gonadal hormone axis and inhibits sperm production. The routine use of hot tubs, baths, Jacuzzis, or saunas should be discouraged, as these activities elevate intratesticular temperature and may impair sperm production.[10] Sports such as bicycling are safe unless associated with significant urinary symptoms (prostatitis) or pelvic "numbness" that may predispose to erectile dysfunction.

FURTHER MALE FACTOR EVALUATION

If lifestyle changes are unsuccessful, then further evaluation is warranted, following published best-practice policies.[8] This should include an assessment of the pituitary-gonadal axis with testosterone and follicle-stimulating hormone (FSH) levels. Hormone testing is indicated in infertile men with sperm densities below 10×10^6 sperm/mL, or with evidence of a medical endocrinopathy.[11] The chance of a clinically significant endocrinopathy presenting as

BOX 22-1

Components of the Male Infertility History

Medical History
Fevers
Systemic illness—diabetes, cancer, infection, obesity
Genetic disease—cystic fibrosis, Klinefelter syndrome

Surgical History
Orchidopexy, cryptorchidism
Herniorraphy
Trauma, torsion
Pelvic, bladder, or retroperitoneal surgery
Transurethral resection for prostatism
Pubertal onset

Fertility History
Previous pregnancies (current and with other partners)
Duration of infertility
Previous infertility treatments
Female evaluation

Sexual History
Erections
Timing and frequency
Lubricants

Family History
Cryptorchidism
Midline defects (Kartagener syndrome)
Hypospadias
Exposure to diethylstilbestrol
Other rare syndromes—prune belly, etc.

Medication History
See Table 22-2

Social History
Alcohol
Smoking/tobacco
Cocaine
Anabolic steroids
Wet heat exposure (hot tubs, baths)

Occupational History
Exposure to ionizing radiation
Chronic heat exposure (cooks, firefighter)
Aniline dyes
Pesticides
Heavy metals

BOX 22-2

Drugs with Potential Adverse Effects on Male Fertility

Competition with Androgen Receptor
Spironolactone
Cimetidine
Flutamide
Nilutamide
Bicalutamide

Direct Toxic Effect on Leydig Cells
Alkylating agents (e.g., cyclophosphamide)
Alcohol

Inhibitors of Testosterone Synthesis
Ketoconazole
Spironolactone
Cyproterone
Tetracycline
Alcohol

Stimulators of Estradiol Synthesis or Activity
DES (diethylstilbestrol)
Digoxin
Dibromochloropropane (pesticides)
Spironolactone
Medroxyprogesterone

Heavy Metal Toxins
Lead
Arsenic
Cadmium
Mercury

Pituitary Inhibition
Testosterone
Marijuana

Mitotic Inhibitors
Allopurinol
Colchicine
Sulfasalazine
Nitrofurantoin

Effects on Fertilization
Nicotine
Calcium channel blockers

Ejaculatory Dysfunction
Lithium
Antipsychotics
Tricyclic antidepressants
Valproic acid
Phenytoin

Unclear Mechanism
Monoamine oxidase inhibitors
Cocaine

infertility is approximately 2%.[11] The more common patterns of hormonal disorders observed in male infertility are found in Table 22-2.

Adjunctive sperm tests are also available to diagnose the cause of male factor infertility and are pursued based upon the predominant semen analysis finding, as discussed later. When the infertility is unexplained, several tests can be considered, the most popular of which is an assessment of sperm DNA integrity. Evidence suggests that the quality of sperm DNA-chromatin packaging is important for fertility. High levels of reactive oxygen species and oxidative stress are known to cause sperm DNA fragmentation.

The structure of sperm chromatin (the DNA-associated proteins) can be measured by several methods, including the single cell gel electrophoresis (comet) and terminal deoxynucleotidyl transferase nick end labeling (TUNEL) assays as well as by flow cytometry after acid exposure and acridine orange staining. These tests measure the degree of DNA fragmentation with chemical stress on the sperm

TABLE 22-1

Semen Analysis—WHO Minimal Standards of Adequacy

Characteristic	Standard
Ejaculate volume	1.5-5.5 mL
Sperm concentration	>20 × 10⁶ sperm/mL
Motility	>50%
Forward progression	2 (scale 1-4)
Morphology	>30% (WHO) >14% (Kruger)
Other features	No agglutination (clumping), white blood cells, or increased viscosity

WHO, World Health Organization.

TABLE 22-2

Characteristic Endocrine Profiles in Infertile Men

Condition	T	FSH	LH	PRL
Normal	NL	NL	NL	NL
Primary testis failure	Low	High	NL/high	NL
Hypogonadotropic hypogonadism	Low	Low	Low	NL
Hyperprolactinemia	Low	Low/NL	Low	High
Androgen resistance	High	High	High	NL

FSH, follicle stimulating hormone; LH, luteinizing hormone; NL, normal; PRL, prolactin; T, testosterone.

DNA-chromatin complex, and can indirectly reflect the quality of sperm DNA integrity. Abnormally fragmented sperm DNA rarely occurs in fertile men, but can be found in 5% of infertile men with normal semen analyses and 25% of infertile men with abnormal semen analyses.[12] Such testing can detect infertility that is missed on a conventional semen analysis. Often reversible, DNA fragmentation may be caused by tobacco use, medical disease, hyperthermia, air pollution, infections (leukocytospermia), chemotherapy, irradiation, sperm processing, and varicocele.

Low Volume Ejaculate

The evaluation of low ejaculate volume is almost always informative, as it is generally due to one of five problems: improper sample collection, congenital absence of the vas (and seminal vesicles), a hypoandrogenic state, retrograde ejaculation, or ejaculatory duct obstruction. These conditions can be systematically examined as outlined in Figure 22-3. A low seminal pH (<7) can replace semen fructose in this diagnosis. Importantly, classic transrectal

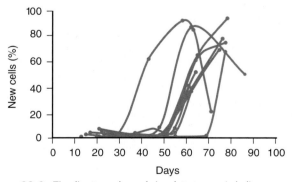

Figure 22-2. Timeline to make and ejaculate sperm. Labeling curves for 11 subjects with normal semen analyses. Subjects were given deuterated water daily for 3 weeks and semen was collected regularly for 90 days. Sperm DNA enrichment was measured and percentage of new sperm in the ejaculate was calculated. Overall, the mean time to detection of labeled sperm in the ejaculate was 64 ± 8 days (range 42 to 76), much faster than the 90 days classically ascribed to this process. (From Misell LM, Holochwost D, Boban D, et al. A stable isotope/mass spectrometric method for measuring the kinetics of human spermatogenesis in vivo. J Urol 175:242, 2006.)

ultrasound criteria to diagnose ejaculatory duct obstruction, including the presence of cysts, calcification, or dilated seminal vesicles or ducts, may "over read" the diagnosis of obstruction by 50% and should be confirmed with "functional" studies such as vasography or duct chromotubation prior to endoscopic treatment.[13] The response of retrograde ejaculation to alpha-agonist medications is best for nonsurgical nerve damage to the hypogastric plexus (e.g., diabetes mellitus).[14] Bladder harvest of sperm in nonresponders can often be used with intrauterine insemination (IUI) to overcome infertility.

Oligospermia/Asthenospermia

Low sperm motility is observed in 25% of abnormal semen analyses; an isolated low sperm concentration is much less common. Low sperm motility may be due to antisperm antibodies (>50% of sperm bound) or excessive white blood cells in the ejaculate (leukocytospermia), the latter resulting in overproduction of reactive oxygen species that can damage sperm.[15] Because "round cells" in the infertile ejaculate are more commonly immature germ cells (65%) rather than leukocytes,[16] special leukocyte stains are recommended before treatment. Semen cultures are not worthwhile in asymptomatic infertile men with leukocytospermia as 83% are normally positive with multiple organisms.[17] It is important to evaluate sexually transmitted diseases, penile discharge, prostatitis, or epididymitis. An expressed prostatic secretion is examined for leukocytes, and urethral cultures for *Chlamydia* and *Mycoplasma* can be considered. Although the findings vary by both methodology and laboratory, in general, more than 50% of sperm bound with antibodies is considered significant and merits treatment.

Low sperm concentration may be due to an endocrinopathy such as prolactinoma, varicocele, or genetic causes, as outlined in Figure 22-4. Although eternally debated, there is substantial evidence to support the role of varicocele in male infertility (Table 22-3). Increasingly, genetic abnormalities should be considered in men with sperm concentrations less than 5 million/mL.[18] Deletion of regions on the Y chromosome (microdeletions) occur in 6% of men with severely low sperm counts and in 15% of men with no sperm counts. In addition, 2% of men with low counts and 15% to 20% of men with no sperm counts will harbor

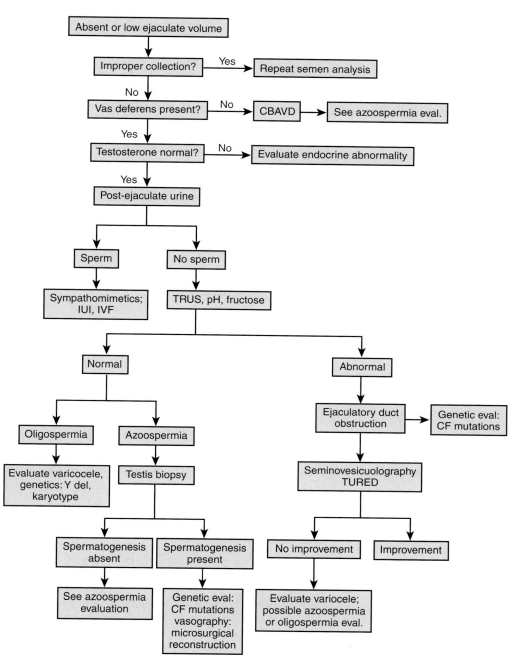

Figure 22-3. Algorithm for evaluation of absent or low ejaculate volume. CBAVD, congenital absence of vas deferens; CF, cystic fibrosis; IUI, intrauterine insemination; IVF, in vitro fertilization; TRUS, transrectal ultrasound; TURED, transurethral resection of the ejaculatory duct; Y del, Y chromosome deletion. (From Turek PJ. Practical approach to the diagnosis and management of male infertility. Nature Clin Pract Urol 2:1, 2005.)

chromosomal abnormalities detected by cytogenetic analysis (karyotype). These conditions include Klinefelter syndrome and translocations of non-sex chromosomes. Box 22-3 outlines current indications for genetic testing of infertile males. Importantly, varicocele repair for oligospermia in the setting of positive genetic findings is unlikely to improve semen quality or result in pregnancy.[19]

Azoospermia (Fig. 22-5)

If sperm are absent in a routine semen analysis, the differential diagnosis is excurrent ductal obstruction or testicular failure. The semen specimen should be centrifuged to assess for very low sperm numbers that effectively rule out complete obstruction.[20] If one or both vasa deferentia are not palpable, then a diagnosis of congenital absence of the vas deferens (CAVD) is made, and appropriate genetic testing for cystic fibrosis gene mutations is recommended prior to sperm retrieval and in vitro fertilization (IVF) and intracytoplasmic sperm injection (ICSI). Affected patients exhibit a similar spectrum of wolffian duct defects as those with cystic fibrosis, but generally lack the severe pulmonary, pancreatic, and intestinal problems. Roughly 80% of azoospermic men with CAVD and one third of men with unexplained obstruction will harbor cystic fibrosis gene mutations.[21,22] Based on FSH values and a diagnostic

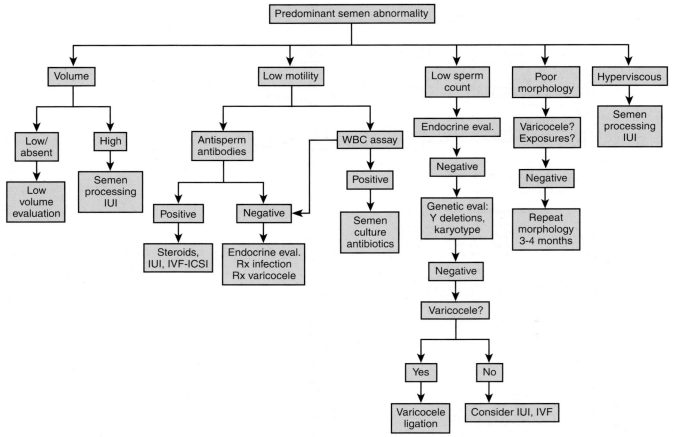

Figure 22-4. *Algorithm for evaluation of semen analysis abnormalities. ICSI, intracytoplasmic sperm injection; IUI, intrauterine insemination; IVF, in vitro fertilization; Rx, treat; WBC, white blood cell. (From Turek PJ. Practical approach to the diagnosis and management of male infertility. Nature Clin Pract Urol 2:1, 2005.)*

testis biopsy, accurate differentiation of men into nonobstructive (testis failure) or obstructive azoospermia is possible. Genetic testing for nonobstructive azoospermia with Y chromosome microdeletion and karyotype analysis is recommended, as outlined in Box 22-3. The relative frequency of the different Y chromosome microdeletions among azoospermic men is outlined in Figure 22-6. Treatment of prolactinomas with dopamine agonists or transsphenoidal resection is indicated in men with hormonal disorders.

Unexplained Infertility

Infertile couples with an unremarkable female evaluation and normal semen parameters are termed unexplained infertility (see Fig. 22-1). In such cases, further evaluation of male factor infertility is warranted, yet a precise clinical care algorithm not been defined. Antisperm antibodies and poor chromatin structure, the latter reflective of increased levels of denatured sperm DNA, are each found in 10% of semen analyses in unexplained infertility.[12,23] Tests

	Patients/Arm		Pregnancy Rate	
Study	*Control* (n)	*Treatment* (n)	*Control* (%)	*Treatment* (%)
WHO[*]	109	129	16.7	34.8
Nieschlag et al.[29]	63	62	25.4	29.7
Madgar et al.[30]	25	20	10	60

TABLE 22-3

Controlled Trials Addressing the Treatment of Clinically Palpable Varicoceles

[*]This study was conducted but never published. See Reference 29 for details.
WHO, World Health Organization.

BOX 22-3

Current Indications for Genetic Testing of Infertile Men

1. A semen analysis with sperm concentration <5 million sperm/mL in a couple considering in vitro fertilization (IVF) and intracytoplasmic sperm injection (ICSI) (Y microdeletion assay and karyotype analysis)
2. A semen analysis showing no sperm with evidence of testis atrophy in a couple considering testis sperm extraction with IVF and ICSI (Y microdeletion assay and karyotype analysis)
3. A semen analysis showing no or low sperm concentration with at least one absent vas deferens on physical examination (cystic fibrosis gene mutations)
4. A semen analysis showing no sperm with evidence of normal spermatogenesis (cystic fibrosis gene mutations)
5. A couple with other syndromes or conditions suggested by personal or family histories (e.g., Kallmann syndrome)

of sperm function such as the sperm penetration assay or the hemizona assay may also be considered. Finally, many couples proceed to intrauterine insemination at this point. As our knowledge of the genes that control sperm capacitation and fertilization grows, many cases of unexplained infertility will be more clearly defined.

Treatment of Male Infertility

Male infertility is associated with a defined cause in half of cases (Fig. 22-7). When associated with life-threatening disease, the disease should be treated (Box 22-4). Because of advances in assisted reproduction (including ICSI), there has been a concerning trend to avoid male factor treatments in favor of assisted reproduction. This is unfortunate, as many male factor treatments help infertile couples conceive without assisted reproduction.[24]

Certainly, maternal reproductive potential should be considered before correctable male factors are treated. This reasoning becomes obvious given that it takes 2 to 3 months to improve spermatogenesis after therapy. Thus, an important guiding principle in the decision to treat male infertility is to first determine whether or not the female partner has more than 1 year of stable reproductive potential. If so, then correcting male infertility is almost always warranted.

CORRECTABLE MALE FACTOR PROBLEMS

Coital Therapy

Simple counseling on issues of coital timing, frequency, and gonadotoxin avoidance can improve fertility. Coital lubricants should be avoided. Although scarcely published, hot baths, Jacuzzis and hot tubs are detrimental to sperm

production.[25] Avoidance of tobacco, marijuana, excessive alcohol, and other recreational drugs is important.

Ejaculatory Dysfunction

Retrograde ejaculation is diagnosed by finding sperm in the postejaculate bladder urine, and is treated with sympathomimetic medications or bladder harvest of sperm with assisted reproduction. Premature ejaculation occurs when men ejaculate before their partner is ready. Although not an established cause of infertility, it can produce significant relationship stress. Sexual counseling combined with serotoninergic reuptake inhibitors can be effective treatment. Ejaculatory failure or anejaculation has a variety of causes that include pelvic nerve damage from diabetes mellitus, multiple sclerosis, or abdominal-pelvic surgery; spinal cord injury; and psychosocial issues. Vibratory stimulation and rectal probe electroejaculation are common and effective techniques that help anejaculatory patients to conceive (Fig. 22-8).[14]

Leukocytospermia

Elevated leukocytes in semen (>1 million/mL) is termed pyospermia or leukocytospermia and is associated with (a) subclinical genital tract infection, (b) elevated reactive oxygen species, and (c) poor sperm function and infertility. Sperm are highly susceptible to the effects of oxidative stress induced by leukocytes because they harbor little cytoplasm and therefore little antioxidant activity. The treatment of leukocytospermia is controversial without overt bacteriologic infection. When appropriate, the limited use of broad-spectrum antibiotics such as doxycycline and trimethoprim-sulfamethoxazole in combination with frequent ejaculation has been shown in a randomized controlled study to durably reduce seminal leukocyte concentrations.[26] Generally, the female partner is also treated.

Immunologic Infertility

Antisperm antibodies are a complex problem for which available treatments include corticosteroid suppression, IUI, or IVF-ICSI. Corticosteroid suppression attempts to weaken an overactive immune system to reduce sperm antibodies and facilitate conception; however, two placebo-controlled, double-blind, crossover trials have shown conflicting findings regarding benefit of this treatment.[27,28] In addition, therapy must be undertaken for 6 to 9 months to achieve benefit. IUI places more sperm nearer to the ovulated egg to optimize the odds of fertilizaton. IVF and ICSI are very effective in overcoming infertility due to antisperm antibodies. Because the presence of antibodies is associated with obstruction in the genital tract, such lesions should be sought and corrected.

Varicocele

Although debated, there is substantial evidence to support the value of varicocele repair in male infertility. The outcomes of three controlled clinical trials that have examined treatment of palpable varicoceles generally favor varicocele repair, as summarized in Table 22-3.[29,30] Several

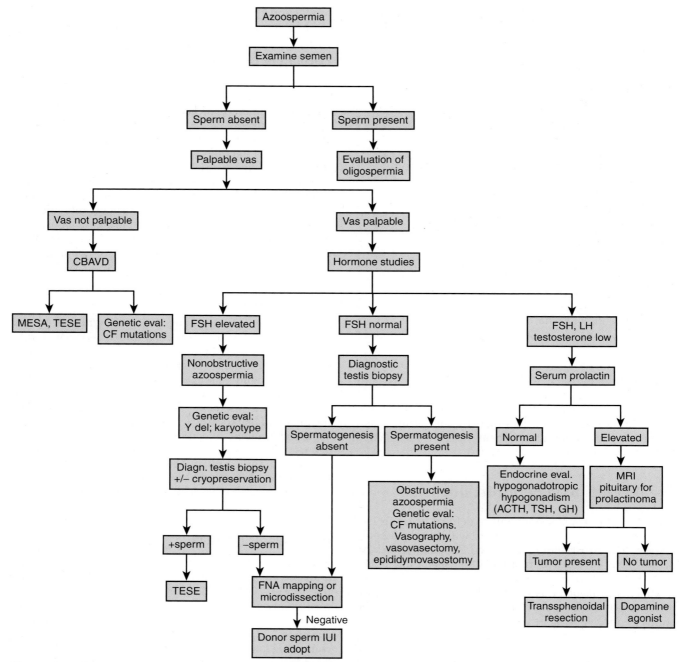

Figure 22-5. *Algorithm for evaluation of azoospermia or no sperm in the ejaculate. ACTH, adrenocorticotropic hormone; CBAVD, congenital bilateral absence of the vas deferens; CF, cystic fibrosis; FNA, fine needle aspiration; FSH, follicle-stimulating hormone; GH, growth hormone; IUI, intrauterine insemination; LH, luteinizing hormone; MESA, microscopic epididymal sperm aspiration; MRI, magnetic resonance imaging; TESE, testis sperm extraction; TSH, thyroid-stimulating hormone. (From Turek PJ. Practical approach to the diagnosis and management of male infertility. Nature Clin Pract Urol 2:1, 2005.)*

meta-analyses have also examined outcomes of varicocele treatment and did not support varicocele repair as effective treatment for male infertility.[31,32] However, one study has significant design flaws in that it examined trials that included subclinical varicoceles, the clinical relevance of which are unclear.[32] Furthermore, a controlled trial published by Madgar and colleagues[30] that showed a relative

benefit of 6 for varicocele repair was deemed an "outlier" in the meta-analysis, leaving only a single trial evaluable for clinical varicocele. Finally, the large WHO trial (238 patients) was excluded from the analysis.[32] Thus, more prospective trials are needed to prove that varicoceles improve fertility. However, clinically, semen quality will improve in 51% to 78% of men after varicocele repair; the

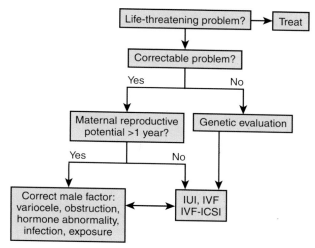

Figure 22-6. *General algorithm for treatment of male infertility. ICSI, intracytoplasmic sperm injection; IUI, intrauterine insemination; IVF, in vitro fertilization. (From Turek PJ. Practical approach to the diagnosis and management of male infertility. Nature Clin Pract Urol 2:1, 2005.)*

associated pregnancy rate is 24% to 60%, with pregnancies occurring an average of 8 months after surgery.[24,33]

In addition to clinical care arguments that suggest varicocele repair is beneficial for infertility, economic analyses also support this concept. Cost-benefit arguments demonstrate that varicocelectomy is more cost-effective than assisted reproduction[34] and "shift of care" analyses show that 30% to 50% of couples who begin as candidates for assisted reproduction due to low semen quality can be "rescued" from such procedures and conceive naturally after varicocelectomy.[24] Decision analysis research suggests that varicocele repair may have the greatest value in severe male factor cases that would otherwise require IVF-ICSI.[35] On the contrary, it is also apparent varicocele is not worthwhile in the presence of coexisting genetic infertility.[19]

Several modalities are available for varicocele treatment, including vein ligation through retroperitoneal, inguinal, or subinguinal incisions, percutaneous transvenous embolization, and laparoscopy. Success rates do not differ significantly among approaches. Complication rates range from 1% for the incisional approach to 4% for laparoscopy. The most significant complication with embolization is the 10% to 15% technical failure rate (inability to access and occlude the culprit veins).

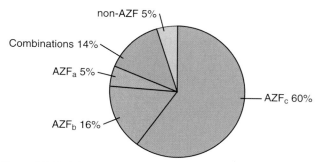

Figure 22-7. *Relative frequency of specific AZF deletions in 5000 men with Yq microdeletions. (From Shefi S, Turek PJ. Definition and current evaluation of subfertile men. Int Brazil J Urol 32:385, 2006.)*

Ejaculatory Duct Obstruction

Ejaculatory duct obstruction is observed in 5% of azoospermic men, but is often overlooked in the male evaluation. Partial obstruction is likely more common than currently diagnosed, but is more difficult to diagnose than complete obstruction, as TRUS findings are not specific for partial obstruction.[13] A 20% to 30% pregnancy rate can be expected from endoscopic treatment of the obstruction, and 70% to 80% of men will achieve significant, early, and durable improvements in semen quality.[13,36] Complications occur in 10% of cases and include hematuria, watery ejaculate, and epididymitis.

Vasovasostomy

Vasectomy reversal success depends on many factors, the most important of which are the surgeon's skill and the findings at surgery. Because of the need for superb tissue technique, experienced surgeons use a microscope. Evidence of inflammation or infection after the vasectomy,

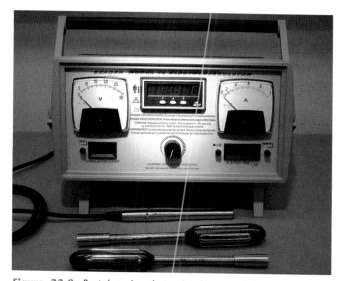

Figure 22-8. *Rectal probe electroejaculator used for patients with primary or acquired ejaculatory dysfunction. Rectal probes (foreground) of different sizes are available to accommodate differences in patient anatomy. Ejaculates can be obtained in virtually all anejaculatory patients with this technology.*

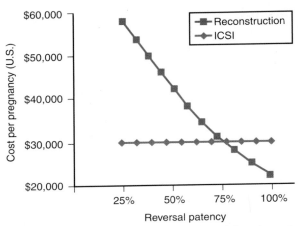

Figure 22-9. *Sensitivity analysis from decision modeling of vasectomy reversal compared with intracytoplasmic sperm injection (ICSI) and sperm retrieval. This figure shows a cost comparison of both methods over a range of reversal patency rates when the pregnancy rate is held constant at 40%. This demonstrates that a minimum threshold vasectomy reversal patency rate (78%) is important to achieve if vasectomy reversal is to remain more cost-effective than ICSI. (From Meng M, Greene K, Turek P. Surgery or assisted reproduction? A decision analysis of treatment costs in male infertility. J Urol 174:1926, 2005.)*

and a long interval from vasectomy-to-reversal are both associated with a decrease in surgical success.[37] If sperm are found at the cut edge of the vas during surgery, then 85% to 99% of patients can be expected to have a return of sperm after vasovasostomy.[38] With a healthy female partner, this is associated with a pregnancy rate of 40% to 65%.[38,39] If the vas fluid shows no sperm, the primary procedure involves connecting the vas to the epididymis in a procedure termed epididymovasostomy. In experienced hands, approximately 60% to 80% of men will have sperm in the ejaculate and a 30% to 35% pregnancy rate can be expected.[38,40]

A growing literature suggests that vasectomy reversal may be more cost-effective for pregnancy than IVF and ICSI.[40] Given the difficulty of randomizing patients to vasectomy reversal or sperm-retrieval and ICSI, decision analysis and Markov modeling research has been applied to address this issue.[35,41] Decision analytic models are methods of estimating and calculating outcomes by identifying a clinical question, disaggregating the problem into discrete units to include all reasonable choices and consequences, and assigning probabilities and costs to the various events and outcomes. Decision science has revealed that reversal surgery is often more cost-effective than sperm retrieval and ICSI, but threshold values for surgical success are required to maintain its cost-effectiveness[35] (Fig. 22-9). Markov modeling is a form of decision analysis in which hypothetical patients proceed through health states over time based on predefined probabilities and costs. As patients are cycled, outcomes, including incurred costs and events, are tracked. Markov analyses have been used to better understand the relative impact of vasectomy obstructive interval and female partner age on fertility after vasectomy. These analyses have shown that female fertility potential impacts cost-effectiveness more profoundly than does vasectomy obstructive interval[41] (Fig. 22-10). This suggests that, in the absence of randomized data

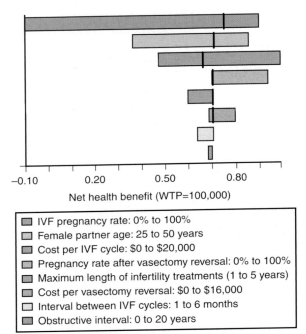

Figure 22-10. *Tornado diagram from Markov modeling for intracytoplasmic sperm injection compared with vasectomy reversal. This figure shows the relative impact of female partner age, vasectomy obstructive interval, and other clinical parameters on net health benefit (NHB) and demonstrates that female age has the largest effect on cost effectiveness. Widths of horizontal bars indicate magnitude of impact of that parameter on NHB. The wider the bar, the greater the impact on NHB. Thick vertical bars are threshold values at which reversal and assisted reproductive technology switch being more cost-effective. IVF, in vitro fertilization; WTP, willingness to pay. (From Hsieh M, Meng M, Turek PJ. Markov modeling of vasectomy reversal and ART for infertility: How do obstructive interval and female partner age influence cost-effectiveness? Fertil Steril 88:840, 2007.)*

comparing ICSI and sperm retrieval with vasectomy reversal, the primary driver of cost-effective care is the variable of female age and maternal reproductive potential. Even given this, respectable crude pregnancy rates have been reported in vasectomy reversal series in the setting of advanced maternal age.[42,43]

In addition to vasectomy, infertility can also result from idiopathic obstruction. In such cases, 65% of blockages are found within the epididymis, 30% in the vas deferens, and 5% in the ejaculatory duct.[44] In most cases of idiopathic obstruction, the blockage can be pinpointed and corrected with microsurgery. To distinguish obstructive azoospermia from that due to a sperm production problem, a testis biopsy is generally necessary.

Hormonal or Oxidative Dysfunction

Hormone therapy can and should be offered to patients with treatable diseases that predispose to infertility. Less effective treatments are those that seek to overcome ill-understood conditions or those without well-proved treatments. Examples of treatable conditions include hyperprolactinemia, hypothyroidism, congenital adrenal hyperplasia, and testosterone excess or deficiency (e.g., steroids or Kallmann syndrome). Examples of medical treatments that may not work in all men include clomiphene citrate, tamoxifen, human chorionic gonadotropin (hCG) therapy, L-acetylcarnitine, and antioxidant and herbal therapy. When given unselectively to infertile men, these measures should be considered empirical treatments for male infertility.[45] The use of aromatase inhibitors in men with elevated estradiol:testosterone ratios has shown some benefit to semen quality in a single study.[46]

ASSISTED REPRODUCTION

If neither surgery nor medical therapy is appropriate treatment for male infertility, assisted reproduction can be initiated. From a male infertility point of view, the choice of technique depends mainly on the degree of impairment in total motile sperm concentration (Fig. 22-11).

Intrauterine Insemination

Intrauterine insemination involves placement of washed ejaculated sperm within the female uterus, beyond the cervix. In this way, more motile sperm can progress to the fallopian tubes where fertilization normally occurs. The principal indication for IUI is a cervical factor, but IUI is also used for low sperm quality, immunologic infertility, and in men with mechanical problems of sperm delivery (e.g., hypospadias). There should be at least 5 million to 40 million motile sperm in the ejaculate (volume × concentration × motility) to make this procedure worth while. Success rates vary widely and are directly related to female reproductive potential; given this, pregnancy rates of 30% for four cycles can be expected.[47]

In Vitro Fertilization and Intracytoplasmic Sperm Injection

First described in 1978, IVF is more complex than IUI and removes even more obstacles to sperm in the female reproductive tract. Following ovarian hyperstimulation and ultrasound-guided transvaginal egg retrieval, oocytes are fertilized in vitro with 500,000 to 5 million motile sperm. After fertilization, embryos are placed into the uterus transcervically. This technology can bypass moderate to severe forms of male infertility in which there are low numbers of motile sperm. A revolutionary addition to IVF was described in 1992 and is referred to as sperm micromanipulation or ICSI, in which a single sperm is microinjected directly into the egg cytoplasm.[48] ICSI has lowered the sperm requirement for egg fertilization from hundreds of thousands to one viable sperm, thus allowing

treatment of the most severe forms of male infertility. In a systematic review and meta-analysis, an association was found between the degree of sperm DNA fragmentation and pregnancy rates after IVF and ICSI, but this relationship was not deemed clinically significant.[49] The current indications for IVF and ICSI for male factor diagnoses are listed in Table 22-4.

Genetic Evaluation

High-technology solutions to pregnancy, including ICSI, are now known to be a two-edged sword. On one hand, ICSI is very enabling, allowing men who would otherwise have no chance for paternity the opportunity for fatherhood. However, because man and not nature selects sperm for ICSI, how it alters natural selection is not clear. Genetic evaluation of the infertile couple is important prior to IVF and ICSI for male infertility due to oligospermia or azoospermia that is not due to acquired blockage (see Box 22-3). In addition, there is some debate about whether IVF-ICSI is as effective for men with defined genetic infertility, in particular Y chromosome microdeletions, as it is for other male factor indications[50-53] (Table 22-5). Although overall rates of major birth defects associated with ICSI (3.3%) are similar to those associated with intercourse,[54] chromosomal abnormalities are increased in offspring with ICSI[55] and increased rates of conditions such as hypospadias, and syndromes such as Angelman and Beckwith-Wiedemann have been reported.[56-58] In addition, subtle development defects and delays have been detected in children conceived with assisted reproduction.[59] For these reasons, genetic counseling is recommended for all couples considering IVF-ICSI.

SPERM RETRIEVAL TECHNIQUES

ICSI has led to the development of aggressive surgical techniques for azoospermic men to provide sperm for egg fertilization. Since 1988, epididymal sperm aspiration has been performed either microsurgically (MESA) or percutaneously (PESA). Since 1995, testis sperm retrieved by needle (TESA) or biopsy (TESE) is routinely performed

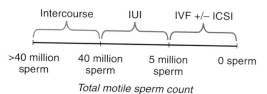

Figure 22-11. Level of assisted reproduction needed for conception based on semen quality determined by total motile count (volume × concentration × motile fraction). IUI, intrauterine insemination; IVF, in vitro fertilization; ICSI, intracytoplasmic sperm injection. (From Turek PJ. Practical approach to the diagnosis and management of male infertility. Nature Clin Pract Urol 2:1, 2005.)

TABLE 22-4

Indications for Assisted Reproduction Technologies with Male Factor Infertility

Male Factor Issue	IVF	IVF-ICSI
Retrieved sperm (testis and epididymis)	—	Yes
Low motile sperm count (<5 million)	Yes	Maybe
Poor sperm morphology (<4% strict or Kruger)	—	Yes
Failed trial of IUI	Yes	Maybe
Immunologic infertility (antisperm antibodies) and failed IUI	—	Yes
Abnormal sperm DNA integrity	?	Maybe
Correctable male factor with limited maternal reproductive potential	Yes	Maybe

ICSI, intracytoplasmic sperm injection; IUI, intrauterine insemination; IVF, in vitro fertilization.

TABLE 22-5

Summary of Studies of IVF-ICSI Outcomes in Couples with Yq Deletions

Author	Points	Yq deletions	Normal Fertilization Rate		Pregnancy/Cycle	
			Control	AZF	Control	AZF
Mulhall et al.[50]	3	AZFc	45% (n = 25 cycles)	36% (n = 6 cycles)	—	—
Van Golde et al.[52]	8	AZFc with oligospermia	71% (n = 107 pts)	55%	25%	16%
Oates et al.[51]	26	AZFc	—	47%	—	27%
Choi et al.[53]	17	AZFb and c with azoospermia and oligospermia	58%	49%	42%	33%

ICSI, intracytoplasmic sperm injection; IVF, in vitro fertilization.

BOX 22-5

Conditions Associated with Nonobstructive Azoospermia

Idiopathic primary testicular failure
Y chromosome microdeletions
Karyotype disorder
    Sex chromosomes (Klinefelter syndrome)
    Non-sex chromosomes, translocations, aneuploidy
Secondary testicular failure
    Noonan syndrome
    Kallmann syndrome
    Idiopathic gonadotropin deficiency
    Hypothalamic/pituitary tumor
    Hyperprolactinemia
    Cancer chemotherapy/radiotherapy treatment
    Varicocele effect
Gonadotropin suppression
    Drug-induced (anabolic steroids, alcohol, gluco-corticoids)
    Congenital adrenal hyperplasia
    Severe systemic illness (cancer, uremia)
Cryptorchidism
Sperm autoimmunity
Pesticide/toxin exposure

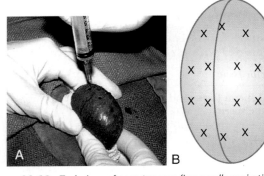

Figure 22-12. Technique of percutaneous fine-needle aspiration "mapping" for sperm in the testis. *A,* Samples are taken systematically from the testis for cytologic examination for sperm. *B,* A recent sampling template. This is done in advance of assisted reproductive technology procedures. (From Turek PJ, Cha I, Ljung B-M. Systematic fine needle aspiration of the testis: correlation to biopsy and the results of organ "mapping" for mature sperm in azoospermic men. Urology 49:743, 1997.)

in men with obstructive azoospermia. Currently, there is insufficient clinical trial evidence to recommend a preferred sperm retrieval technique in azoospermic men.[60]

Although sperm retrieval in obstructive azoospermia is not difficult, there is a failure to obtain sperm for ICSI in 25% to 50% of men with nonobstructive azoospermia (Box 22-5).[61] In addition, clinical features of testicular size, history of ejaculated sperm, serum FSH level, or histologic findings at biopsy do not accurately predict whether or not sperm will be recovered on exploration.[61] Because of this, strategies have been developed to more accurately determine which men with failing testes are candidates for ICSI, and surgical techniques have been refined to minimize the invasiveness of sperm harvest procedures. The first of these, the multi-biopsy method, involves taking as many biopsy samples as needed at the time of ICSI.[61] Another approach involves taking testis tissue by biopsy for both diagnosis (histology) and sperm retrieval simultaneously and *in advance* of ICSI to avoid cycle cancellation if sperm harvest fails.[62] Microdissection TESE uses microsurgical exploration of the widely opened testis to search for pockets of sperm.[63] Finally, diagnostic testis fine needle aspiration (FNA) "mapping" under local anesthesia literally maps out the geography of sperm production in the testis to determine patient candidacy for future sperm testis retrieval (Fig. 22-12).[64] Subsequently, at ICSI, needles or biopsies are "directed" to testis locations informed by the map. Most recently, preoperative factors such as FSH, inhibin B, and total testosterone have been used to construct formulas to predict sperm retrieval.[65] Regardless of approach, most men with nonobstructive azoospermia will have usable testis sperm by one of these methods.

Conclusions

Evaluation of male factor infertility should be conducted to uncover life-threatening conditions and correctable problems that present as infertility. Genetic causes of male infertility are assuming a greater role as our understanding of genomic medicine grows. Medical or surgical treatments should be undertaken after consideration of female partner reproductive potential. There is a need for adequately powered and well-controlled clinical trials to better understand both the value of classic male factor treatments, and the role of assisted reproduction in male infertility treatment.

The complete reference list can be found on the companion Expert Consult Web site at www.expertconsultbook.com.

Suggested Readings

Belker AM, Thomas AJ Jr, Fuchs EF, et al. Results of 1,469 microsurgical vasectomy reversals by the Vasovasostomy Study Group. J Urol 145:505-511, 1991.

Cayan S, Erdemir F, Ozbey I, et al. Can varicocelectomy significantly change the way couples use assisted reproductive technologies? J Urol 167:1749-1756, 2002.

Danziger K, Black LD, Keiles S, et al. Improved detection of cystic fibrosis mutations in infertility patients with DNA sequence analysis. Hum Reprod 19:540-546, 2004.

Evers JLH, Collins JA. Assessment of efficacy of varicocele repair for male subfertility: a systematic review. Lancet 361:1849-1852, 2003.

Guzick DS, Overstreet JW, Factor-Litvak P, et al. Sperm morphology, motility, and concentration in fertile and infertile men. N Engl J Med 345:1388-1393, 2001.

Hsieh M, Meng M, Turek PJ. Markov modeling of vasectomy reversal and ART for infertility: how do obstructive interval and female partner age influence cost-effectiveness? Fertil Steril 88:840-846, 2007.

Jarow JP, Sharlip ID, Belker AM, et al. Male infertility best practice policy committee of the American Urological Association Inc. J Urol 167:2138-2144, 2002.

Kruger TF, Acosta AA, Simmons KF, et al. Predictive value of abnormal sperm morphology in in vitro fertilization. Fertil Steril 49:112-117, 1988.

Madgar I, Weissenberg R, Lunenfeld B, et al. Controlled trial of high spermatic vein ligation for varicocele in infertile men. Fert Steril 63:120-124, 1993.

Masters V, Turek PJ. Ejaculatory physiology and dysfunction. Urol Clin North Am 28:363-375, 2001.

Turek PJ, Reijo Pera RA. Current and future genetic screening for male infertility. Urol Clin North Am 29:767-792, 2002.

Turek PJ, Cha I, Ljung B-M, et al. Diagnostic findings from testis fine needle aspiration mapping in obstructed and non-obstructed azoospermic men. J Urol 163:1709-1716, 2000.

Van Peperstraten AM, Proctor ML, Phillipson G, et al. Techniques for surgical retrieval of sperm prior to ICSI for azoospermia (Cochrane Review). The Cochrane Library, Issue 3, Chichester, UK, John Wiley and Sons, Ltd, 2004.

Yang G, Walsh T, Shefi S, et al. The kinetics of the return of motile sperm to the ejaculate after vasectomy reversal. J Urol 177:2272-2276, 2007.

Endocrine Disturbances Affecting Reproduction

Alice Y. Chang and Richard J. Auchus

The reproductive systems are vulnerable to disruption by internal and external forces including disease, malnutrition, and various forms of stress. The male and female axes are both susceptible to dysfunction from the same processes, although the female axis tends to be more sensitive. This chapter will review the influence of endocrine disorders of the pituitary, adrenal, and thyroid glands on reproduction. Each section will discuss the most important and relevant disorders of the specific gland and its effects on female reproduction first. Features specific for male reproduction will be discussed where relevant in each disease subsection.

Pituitary Disorders

OVERVIEW

As the "master gland," the anterior pituitary gland controls the secretion of several essential hormones from other major endocrine glands, including the thyroid (thyroxine and triiodothyronine), adrenal cortex (cortisol, dehydroepiandrosterone sulfate), and gonads (predominantly estradiol in females and testosterone in males). The anterior pituitary gland also produces growth hormone and prolactin, which act directly on target organs. The actions of growth hormone are largely exerted via the local or systemic production of insulin-like growth factor-1 (IGF-1). The posterior pituitary regulates water metabolism via the production of vasopressin and induces milk letdown via the production of oxytocin. Disorders of the pituitary can be partial or complete, isolated to one hormone or multiple, and related to hormone deficiency or hormone excess. The axes controlled by the pituitary gland share the following basic principles:

1. Input from higher brain centers to the hypothalamus
2. Releasing and inhibitory factors influencing pituitary hormone secretion
3. Hypothalamic factor pulsatility, leading to pulsing of pituitary and target gland hormones
4. Feedback inhibition at both the hypothalamus and pituitary by active target gland hormones
5. Peripheral metabolism of target gland products
6. Influence of diurnal rhythm

The relative importance of key regulatory components varies for each axis and is described here in more detail. These axes are shown schematically in Figure 23-1.

The thyroid axis is the simplest for several reasons. The primary product of the thyroid is thyroxine (T_4), which is a precursor of the active hormone triiodothyronine (T_3). Because T_4 is heavily protein-bound, T_4 has a long half-life of about a week, and T_4 is slowly metabolized to T_3. This scenario provides steady, well-dampened feedback, and the thyroid axis therefore shows high stability and low pulsatility. Negative feedback on thyroid-stimulating hormone (TSH) biosynthesis is tightly regulated by T_3. Therefore, hypothalamic stimulation by thyrotropin-releasing hormone (TRH) plays a minor role compared to circulating T_3 and T_4. Thus, the thyroid axis is a model endocrine feedback system because of its stability and simplicity.

In contrast, the adrenal axis is characterized by a strong diurnal rhythm, with the shorter half-life of cortisol (about 1 hour) leading to greater pulsatility. The adrenal axis is also more sensitive to factors beyond corticotropin-releasing hormone (CRH) or circulating cortisol to increase production of corticotropin (ACTH) in response to stress or illness. As a consequence, this intricate feedback system provides a more responsive axis to physiologic changes and needs. However, this level of sophistication complicates clinical testing.

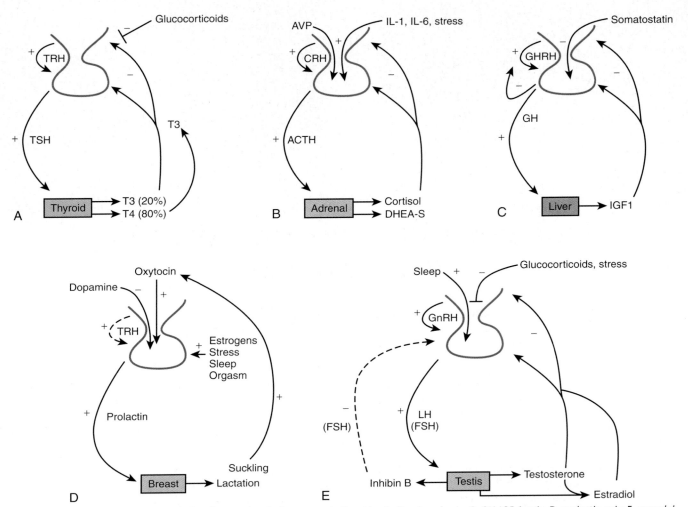

Figure 23-1. *The major factors regulating the anterior pituitary axes. A, thyroid axis; B, adrenal axis; C, GH-IGF-1 axis; D, prolactin axis; E, gonadal axis. ACTH, corticotropin; CRH, corticotropin-releasing hormone; DHEAS, dehydroepiandrosterone sulfate; FSH, follicle-stimulating hormone; GHRH, growth hormone–releasing hormone; GnRH, gonadotropin-releasing hormone; LH, luteinizing hormone; TRH, thyrotropin-releasing hormone; TSH, thyroid-stimulating hormone. (Male is shown in this figure. Female axis is discussed at length in Chapter 7.)*

The growth hormone (somatotropin, GH) axis is primarily a two-component axis regulated by the hypothalamus. Growth hormone–releasing hormone (GHRH) serves as the major positive stimulus and somatostatin (SS) as the major negative stimulus. GH stimulates the production of IGF-1 in the liver and locally in other tissues. Circulating IGF-1 derives from the liver and exerts some negative feedback on the axis, but this influence is small relative to SS. However, numerous hormonal and metabolic factors can affect GH secretion by modulating the GHRH and SS release. While the two hypothalamic hormones regulate GH pulsatility throughout the day, the greatest GH pulses are produced in deep sleep. Significant physical stressors, including hypoglycemia, also increase GH secretion.

Prolactin is the only anterior pituitary hormone that is primarily under negative control, that being by dopamine (DA). For this reason, prolactin rises whenever blood flow to the pituitary from the hypothalamus is impaired. Therefore, hyperprolactinemia may result from a non-prolactin-secreting pituitary tumor blocking blood flow from the stalk. Prolactin is also increased by stress, nipple stimulation, and TRH, so prolactin can rise transiently for several reasons and persistently for several others (Table 23-1). Prolactin acts on the breast to enable lactation, but there is no known hormonal product from the breast that exerts feedback on prolactin secretion. Estrogens can stimulate prolactotroph growth.

The gonadotropins, luteinizing hormone (LH) and follicle-stimulating hormone (FSH), and their regulation by gonadotropin-releasing hormone (GnRH) are discussed in detail for the male and female in other chapters. Here, we simply emphasize that pulsatile GnRH secretion every 90 to 120 minutes is critical to LH and FSH production. While this is true for both males and females, the influence on fertility and symptoms differs in other respects. The reproductive axis is particularly sensitive to disorders and disruptions of the pituitary-hypothalamic axes, as discussed in further detail later in the chapter.

Loss of pituitary function is most commonly caused by drugs, exogenous hormones, or tumors. Tumors affect pituitary function by overproduction of hormone that interferes with the above axes or by mass effect. Any pituitary tumor

TABLE 23-1

Causes of Hyperprolactinemia

Cause	Characteristic Features
Prolactinoma	Mass effects if macroadenoma
Acromegaly	Headaches, heavy perspiration, acral changes
Macroadenoma (not prolactin-secreting)	Peripheral vision loss, anterior pituitary defects
Other infiltrative or hypothalamic diseases	Anterior pituitary defects, maybe diabetes insipidus
Drugs	Other specific side effects of drug
Pregnancy	Positive hCG, amenorrhea
Renal failure	Comorbidities of renal failure
Chest wall stimulation	Variable prolactin
Stress	Including phlebotomy
Primary hypothyroidism	See Box 23-2

hCG, human chorionic gonadotropin.

more than 1 cm in maximal diameter is defined as a macroadenoma. The acquisition of pituitary hormone deficiencies due to tumors tends to follow the order of GH first, then LH + FSH, then TSH, and finally ACTH.[1] Consequently, the reproductive axis is fairly vulnerable to disruption by macroadenomas of any cell type. Decompression by transsphenoidal surgery can restore pituitary function, particularly for the ACTH and TSH axes,[2,3] but iatrogenic hypopituitarism is a common risk of surgery. Radiotherapy tends to cause hypopituitarism over a period of 2 to 15 years and is used judiciously in women of reproductive age.[4] In the following discussion, both the nature of the pituitary disorder and its treatment are addressed as they affect strategies for restoring reproductive function.

PITUITARY DISORDERS THAT AFFECT REPRODUCTION

Prolactinoma and Hyperprolactinemia

The combination of amenorrhea and galactorrhea in a young woman is a classic presentation of prolactinoma; however, these two symptoms may occur individually or not at all.[5] Why menstrual function and lactation in response to prolactin vary greatly among women is not known. Hyperprolactinemia should be considered as part of any evaluation for menstrual irregularity and certainly for galactorrhea. Another common symptom is a decrease in libido, which is less often reported on presentation in women than men, but it is helpful to ascertain during the evaluation and treatment of hyperprolactinemia. Although women are less likely than men to present with mass effects, macroprolactinomas may result in vision loss.

Hyperprolactinemia has many potential causes (see Table 23-1). The mechanisms of reproductive dysfunction in hyperprolactinemia may vary somewhat with the cause, but in all cases, prolactin disrupts the pulses of GnRH and also directly reduces the production of LH and FSH.[6-8] Prolactin exerts direct effects on the gonads as well, but in the female, the effects on the hypothalamus and pituitary dominate.

The diagnosis of hyperprolactinemia is established by measuring a serum prolactin at any time of day without dynamic testing. The normal range for prolactin is less than about 20 ng/mL but varies by laboratory and assay. Slight elevations of less than twofold could simply reflect the stress of phlebotomy and should be repeated before further evaluation.[9] If the prolactin is clearly elevated, causes other than pituitary tumors should be considered first (Table 23-1). If no other cause is identified, a dedicated magnetic resonance imaging (MRI) study of the sella with gadolinium contrast agent should be performed.

Microprolactinomas (tumors <1 cm in greatest diameter) are common, found in about 1% of women age 20 to 40.[10] The degree of prolactin elevation is roughly proportional to the size of the tumor.[11] If a prolactinoma is more than 1 cm in diameter (macroprolactinoma), the prolactin secretion is usually more than 200 ng/mL. The prolactin rarely, if ever, rises above 250 ng/mL if a non-prolactin-secreting tumor is causing stalk compression and impaired dopamine delivery.[12] For example, a patient with a 3-cm pituitary mass and a prolactin level of 150 ng/mL probably does not have a prolactinoma. However, in cases of large pituitary tumors with mild prolactin elevations, the prolactin measurement should be repeated with dilutions to identify the "high-dose hook effect," which artifactually lowers the assayed value.[13] In these cases, it is also important to exclude the diagnosis of acromegaly. GH is a full prolactogen in humans; consequently, galactorrhea with mildly elevated prolactin and a pituitary tumor could be secondary to a somatotropinoma rather than prolactinoma.[14] Dopamine agonist therapy could lower prolactin but would not prevent growth of a somatotropinoma. These considerations avoid the danger of undiagnosed acromegaly and the risk of irreversible damage from unrestrained tumor growth.

On T_1-weighted MRI, microprolactinomas tend to be hypointense relative to the normally bright pituitary and usually do not distort the architecture of the gland (Fig. 23-2). Frequently, small microprolactinomas are not seen on MRI if the enhancement of the normal pituitary and the adenoma are similar or if imaging is delayed too long after administration of gadolinium. Therefore, the diagnosis of suspected microprolactinoma can be made if symptomatic hyperprolactinemia is present and secondary causes have been excluded. Although the larger macroprolactinomas tend to enhance with gadolinium, the pattern is quite variable, ranging from homogeneous or heterogeneous, and greater, lower, or comparable to the normal pituitary. Macroprolactinomas tend to distort the architecture of the gland (Fig. 23-3B), and the inferior portion of the pituitary stalk often deviates away from the tumor.

Prolactinomas, regardless of size and magnitude of prolactin elevation, are generally very responsive to medical therapy with dopamine agonists (bromocriptine and cabergoline).[15] These drugs rapidly lower prolactin secretion and cause absorption of the cell cytoplasm, which results in tumor shrinkage. Even for large and invasive macroprolactinomas with visual changes, tumor shrinkage by dopamine agonists can be immediate and effective. Figure 23-3 shows an example of drug therapy relieving compression

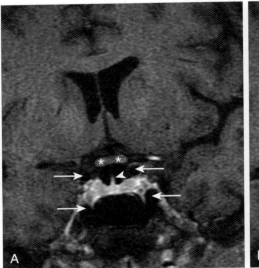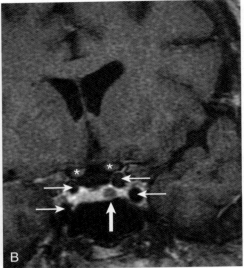

Figure 23-2. **A,** *Normal pituitary gland. In this T₁-weighted coronal image with gadolinium contrast agent, the pituitary gland is seen in the area of high-signal below the pituitary stalk (indicated by chevron arrowhead). The carotid arteries are indicated by thin arrows, and the optic nerves are labeled with asterisks.* **B,** *Pituitary microadenoma. The thick arrow shows the tumor as a hypointensity within the high-signal pituitary gland.*

of the optic nerve. Visual symptoms were relieved within 6 weeks, and MRI changes are shown after 3 months (see Fig. 23-3B).

Treatment options are selected based on symptoms, tumor size, and patient goals. Indications for treatment include infertility, amenorrhea, galactorrhea (particularly if spontaneous and bothersome), hypopituitarism, and mass effect. A woman with a 5-mm microprolactinoma, serum prolactin of 60 ng/mL, regular menses, and only trace expressible galactorrhea does not require treatment. In contrast, the same woman with infertility would be treated if she desires pregnancy. Patients with microprolactinomas and irregular menses but without galactorrhea who do not desire pregnancy can receive cyclic estrogen and progestin for endometrial protection or estrogen deficiency. A few small studies failed to see significant tumor growth in microprolactinomas after cyclic estrogen and progestin treatment.[16-18]

Bromocriptine is administered in two or three divided doses with a total of 2.5 to 40 mg/day, depending on tumor size and serum prolactin. The main side effects of bromocriptine are nausea, lightheadedness, and nasal stuffiness. To improve tolerability, the first dose is administered at 1.25 mg with a snack before bedtime. The dose

is slowly advanced every 4 to 10 days as tolerated until the serum prolactin is normalized and the symptoms are relieved. Cabergoline, administered at 0.25 to 2 mg once or twice weekly, is much more potent and better tolerated than bromocriptine.[19] Bromocriptine is generally preferred if pregnancy is desired, and the medication is stopped upon conception.[20] Recent data on cabergoline early in pregnancy found no increase in the risk for miscarriage or fetal malformations.[21] Visual fields and serum prolactin should be monitored throughout pregnancy and during lactation, more closely for macroprolactinomas.

Women with microprolactinomas who are treated with dopamine agonists for infertility do not need to be treated indefinitely. They may be cycled on and off treatment to allow for subsequent pregnancies. Macroprolactinomas often require chronic therapy and may be cured with these drugs if treated for at least 2 to 5 years. In one study, dopamine agonists could be discontinued in greater than 20% of patients with prolactinomas who received over 2 years of therapy, irrespective of initial tumor size and serum prolactin.[22] Predictive factors for apparent cure include a normal serum prolactin off therapy and a lack of visible tumor on MRI scan. Thus, patients who meet these criteria after 2 to 5 years of treatment should have a trial without drug.

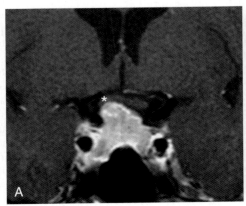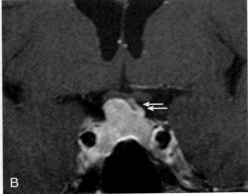

Figure 23-3. *Macroprolactinoma and response to cabergoline.* **A,** *T₁-weighted coronal image after gadolinium contrast at diagnosis with a serum prolactin of 350 ng/mL. The tumor is pressing against the optic nerve on the left (asterisk).* **B,** *After 3 months of treatment with cabergoline at 0.5 mg twice weekly, the serum prolactin had fallen to 10 ng/mL. The stalk is now visible (arrows), and the tumor no longer abuts the optic nerve (black space separating the tumor from the optic nerve).*

Chronic treatment with high doses of cabergoline has rarely been associated with cardiac valve disease, and patients should be warned of this complication. Most of these cases received high doses around 3 mg/day for the treatment of Parkinson's disease.[23,24] Only rare reports have suggested this complication in patients treated for prolactinomas. The valvulopathy is due to the serotonin receptor agonism by cabergoline, which is not a property of bromocriptine. Periodic cardiac examination is therefore necessary in patients treated with cabergoline, and echocardiography is indicated if a murmur is appreciated or if high doses are required.

Occasionally, patients present with normoprolactinemic galactorrhea and regular menses. These patients may have a tiny prolactinoma or may have had transient hyperprolactinemia that has spontaneously remitted. If the galactorrhea is bothersome, treatment with bromocriptine or cabergoline to lower the prolactin to less than 2 ng/mL is effective in stopping the galactorrhea.[25] The duration of therapy required is roughly proportional to the duration of time that the galactorrhea has been present. Patients should be counseled to wear a tight bra or breast binder and to avoid both nipple stimulation and checking for expressible milk production during the course of therapy.

Surgery and radiotherapy are reserved primarily for rare tumors unresponsive to dopamine agonists and for patients intolerant to these drugs.[26] Surgery is most effective for microadenomas, with success rates approaching 90% for microadenomas but only about 60% for macroprolactinomas.[26,27] An immediate postoperative prolactin of less than 2 ng/mL is reliable evidence of cure. Radiotherapy takes at least a year to lower the prolactin significantly and to stop tumor growth. Higher doses of radiation are required to impair hormone secretion than the doses used to slow tumor growth.

In men, prolactinomas present more indolently, and in contrast to women, the majority that come to medical attention are macroprolactinomas with markedly elevated prolactin values.[28] It is likely that the majority of microprolactinomas in men are clinically silent. Previously, the predominance of macroprolactinomas in men was attributed to greater delays in diagnosis, but microprolactinomas rarely transition to macroprolactinomas.[29] Men present with symptoms attributable either to mass effect, such as vision loss and diplopia, or to hypogonadism, including fatigue, loss of libido, and erectile dysfunction.[28] Galactorrhea is rare but does occur, particularly if gynecomastia is present and hyperprolactinemia is severe. Sperm count is rarely affected and usually only after many years of hyperprolactinemia.

Prolactinomas in men are managed by the same treatments used for women. Indications for treatment include mass effects and hypopituitarism. In particular, the hypogonadism associated with prolactinomas in men often responds well to dopamine agonist therapy, unless the duration of hypogonadism is prolonged. The erectile dysfunction of hyperprolactinemia does not always improve with testosterone replacement unless the prolactin is normalized.[30] Sperm count is not immediately restored by dopamine agonist therapy and may not return to normal after several months of therapy. In these cases, human chorionic gonadotropin may be used.

Acromegaly

Acromegaly results from overproduction of GH and IGF-1 accompanied by acral and soft tissue growth. Because symptoms are subtle and gradual in onset, the diagnosis may be delayed for several years. The majority of patients with acromegaly have a GH-secreting pituitary tumor (somatotropinomas), and less than 10% have GHRH-producing tumors. Menstrual abnormalities may result from tumor mass effect and consequent impaired delivery of hypothalamic releasing factors to the anterior pituitary or from hyperprolactinemia.

As noted in the previous section, galactorrhea can occur in acromegaly from the direct action of GH. However, less differentiated tumors that co-secrete GH and prolactin also exist, which complicates the evaluation.[31] Prolactin co-secretion does not predict an improved response to medical therapy.[32]

A serum IGF-1 is a good screening test for acromegaly if performed in a reliable laboratory and reported in normal ranges corrected for gender and age or Tanner stage in children. The diagnosis of acromegaly formally requires failure of GH suppression to less than 0.1 ng/mL in males or less than 1 ng/mL in females after an oral glucose load of 100 g.[33] However, an elevated IGF-1 in the presence of acral changes in a patient with a pituitary tumor is usually sufficient evidence to make the diagnosis.

Combined modality therapy is the norm in acromegaly. Surgery is usually the treatment of choice, particularly for microadenomas, for which cure rates are high and the risk of hypopituitarism is low by experienced pituitary neurosurgeons.[34] However, somatotropinomas are often advanced and invasive macroadenomas (Fig. 23-4). Patients may require both transsphenoidal surgery and craniotomy to debulk the tumor sufficiently for drug or radiotherapy.[35] Many somatotropinomas express somatostatin receptors and remain responsive to somatostatin agonists such as octreotide or lanreotide, given as monthly long-acting intramuscular injections of 10 to 40 mg or 60 to 120 mg, respectively. These agents lower GH secretion and normalize IGF-1 in about two thirds of patients. Some tumor shrinkage occurs in over half of somatotropinomas treated with somatostatin analog agents, but the degree of regression is not as dramatic as for prolactinomas treated with dopamine agonists. Nevertheless, moderate tumor shrinkage over many months may restore gonadal function and fertility when mass effect impairs gonadotrope function.

Pegvisomant, a growth hormone receptor antagonist that is modified with polyethylene glycol, normalizes IGF-1 in up to 95% of patients.[36] The drug is given by subcutaneous injection of 10 to 40 mg/day, and it is generally well tolerated except for transaminase elevation in rare cases. The drug is quite expensive and rarely causes tumor shrinkage or restoration of gonadal function, so this drug is generally reserved for patients in whom somatostatin agonists are contraindicated, not tolerated, or ineffective.

Pure somatotropinomas occasionally respond to dopamine agonists with reduced GH secretion or tumor

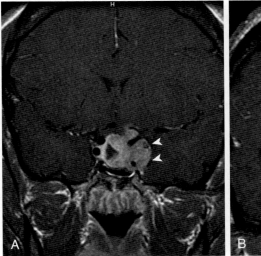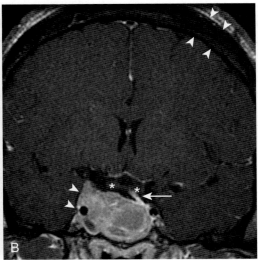

*Figure 23-4. Magnetic resonance imaging of invasive somatotropinomas. The tumor on the left (**A**) invades the carotid sinus on the right (arrowheads) and obliterates the optic nerve on that side. The tumor on the right (**B**) has heterogeneous intensity from internal hemorrhage, and this tumor invades the carotid sinus on the left (arrowheads). The stalk (arrow) is visible on the right but the normal pituitary is not discernable, and the optic nerves (asterisks) are not compromised. Also note widened diploic space on the right (between arrowheads).*

shrinkage, but typically at high doses.[37] Medical management with dopamine agonists is rarely successful and limited by side effects at the high doses needed.

GH normally rises in pregnancy owing to the secretion of placental GH, which is the product of a separate gene from pituitary GH. Consequently, GH elevation does not interfere with fertility, nor is elevated GH during pregnancy per se harmful to the fetus. Consequently, medical treatment is normally withheld during pregnancy. Octreotide, lanreotide, and pegvisomant are all pregnancy category B drugs, although they are generally avoided unless absolutely necessary.

Cushing's Disease

Pituitary tumors that secrete ACTH cause Cushing's disease. Hypercortisolism causes infertility both from the effects of glucocorticoids on the hypothalamic-pituitary-gonadal axis and from mass effect if it is caused by a macroadenoma. This topic will be covered later in the adrenal section, and the principles of hypopituitarism from macroadenomas are the same as discussed earlier.

Other Macroadenomas

Functional pituitary tumors (discussed in this section) that secrete prolactin, GH, ACTH, or very rarely TSH or functional LH tend to be detected earlier in women. However, many pituitary adenomas are "nonfunctional," meaning that they do not produce significant amounts of biologically active hormones. Most of these "nonfunctional" tumors derive from the glycoprotein hormone cell lineage, and messenger RNA for the common alpha subunit or the beta subunits of LH, FSH, or TSH is found in these cells.[38] For the most part, the glycoprotein products of these cells are not biologically active owing to improper glycosylation, dimerization, and assembly.[39] In general, these tumors present with symptoms due to mass effect (vision loss, headache) or hypopituitarism.

Unlike prolactinomas, these tumors tend to be resistant to medical therapy, and surgery with hormone replacement is the general treatment approach. Indications for surgery include vision compromise or other mass effect, hormone hypersecretion, and severe hypopituitarism, which usually means ACTH deficiency or panhypopituitarism. For the woman with panhypopituitarism and infertility, ovulation induction with gonadotropins is discussed in detail in other chapters. For men, when fertility is desired, human chorionic gonadotropin (hCG) is administered at 1000 to 2000 units intramuscularly, two to three times weekly, to normalize testosterone levels. Sperm production can take 84 days, so semen analysis should not be analyzed before 3 months. If azoospermia persists after 9 to 12 months, FSH, 25 to 75 IU subcutaneously three times a week, can be added.

Lymphocytic Hypophysitis

Acute and chronic autoimmune diseases with lymphocytic infiltration affect all the endocrine glands, most commonly the thyroid. Lymphocytic infiltration of the pituitary is a relatively rare disorder, which most commonly occurs in postpartum women.[40] The disease is also called "infundibulohypophysitis" because the stalk and posterior pituitary can also be affected. Patients may present with inability to lactate post partum due to impaired prolactin production or with polyuria and polydipsia from diabetes insipidus.[41] Others are relatively asymptomatic but develop amenorrhea or nonspecific symptoms of hypopituitarism over time. During the active phase, MRI shows a symmetrically enlarged pituitary and stalk that enhances markedly with gadolinium. After the damage has occurred and the disease has subsided, the MRI can show an empty sella, with a variable amount of residual normal tissue that may or may not be seen at the base of the pituitary.

In some cases, pharmacologic doses of potent glucocorticoids such as methylprednisolone in the acute phase have been effective.[42] Comprehensive hormone assessment is mandatory in all patients. The pattern of pituitary deficiencies is highly variable and often follows a pattern much different from that observed with macroadenomas. The gonadotropin function, if lost, rarely recovers. Ovulation induction with injectable gonadotropins is performed as with any other condition causing hypopituitarism.

OTHER DISORDERS AFFECTING THE PITUITARY

Granulomatous diseases such as sarcoidosis[43] and tuberculosis can involve the hypothalamus and pituitary, also causing central hypogonadism. Most patients with hypopituitarism from sarcoidosis have neurosarcoidosis with other manifestations such as optic neuritis and meningial enhancement on MRI scans. Nonetheless, hypopituitarism can be the initial manifestation of sarcoidosis, and hypothalamic or pituitary abnormalities on MRI may be absent.

Hemochromatosis (primary or secondary) and amyloidosis are infiltrative diseases that cause hypopituitarism.[44] Hemochromatosis is an iron storage disease with severe juvenile forms, secondary forms mainly resulting from chronic blood transfusions (thalassemias), and the most common hereditary form due to mutations in the *HFE* gene with manifestations in adulthood. Menstrual blood loss protects females from iron overload in hereditary hemochromatosis, so the disease is often ascertained only in males. The classic triad includes liver dysfunction, skin bronzing, and diabetes mellitus ("bronze diabetes"), but arthropathy, cardiomyopathy, and various endocrinopathies including adrenal insufficiency[45] and hypogonadotropic hypogonadism[46] are common as well. Iron deposition in the hypothalamus has predilection for impairing GnRH production among the releasing hormones, explaining the high prevalence of hypogonadism without central hypothyroidism or adrenal insufficiency. Hemochromatosis is one of the few disorders in which the male reproductive axis is more vulnerable to disruption than in the female.

Nonpituitary tumors may arise in the hypothalamus and pituitary, including germinomas and lymphomas. Carcinomas may metastasize to the pituitary and the stalk. Diabetes insipidus is often a presenting manifestation of primary neoplasms and metastases involving the pituitary stalk. Hypogonadism is one of the most frequent manifestations of hypopituitarism in these neoplastic disorders.

Adrenal Disorders

OVERVIEW

The adrenal gland consists of a cortex, with three distinct zones, and a medulla. The medulla is an extension of the sympathetic nervous system and produces epinephrine. The steroid-producing cells of the cortex are arranged into the outermost zona glomerulosa, which produces aldosterone; the zona fasciculata, which produces cortisol; and the zona reticularis, which produces the androgen precursor dehydroepiandrosterone sulfate (DHEAS). DHEAS is metabolized to testosterone in peripheral tissues. Cortisol and DHEAS production is regulated primarily by ACTH (see Fig. 23-1B), whereas aldosterone synthesis is mainly stimulated by the renin-angiotensin system and by potassium.

> **BOX 23-1**
>
> ### *Causes of Cushing Syndrome*
>
> Exogenous glucocorticoids (oral, intravenous, injected, inhaled, topical)
> Endogenous
>   ACTH-independent
>   Adrenocortical adenoma
>   Adrenocortical carcinoma
>   Macronodular hyperplasia
>   Micronodular hyperplasia
>   ACTH-dependent
>   Corticotropic tumor (Cushing's disease)
>   Corticotropic hyperplasia
>   Ectopic ACTH syndrome
>   Ectopic CRH syndrome
>
> ACTH, corticotropin; CRH, corticotropin-releasing hormone.

Diseases of the adrenal gland causing hormone deficiency rarely interfere with reproduction, but certain hormone excess states may contribute to infertility, particularly for women. In the male, the contribution of adrenal DHEAS to circulating testosterone concentrations is normally small, but in women, the majority of testosterone normally derives from adrenal DHEAS. Consequently, disorders that increase adrenal DHEAS production cause hyperandrogenemia in women, which may impair fertility. Hypercortisolism may suppress gonadotropin production in women and, to a lesser extent, in men. Because they rarely affect the reproductive axis, we will not discuss primary aldosteronism, adrenal insufficiency, or pheochromocytomas in this chapter.

ADRENAL DISORDERS THAT AFFECT REPRODUCTION

Cushing Syndrome

The Cushing syndrome may be characterized as iatrogenic or endogenous, and endogenous Cushing syndrome is dichotomized as being ACTH-dependent or ACTH-independent (Box 23-1). The majority of Cushing syndrome is ACTH-dependent, the most common cause being ACTH-producing pituitary tumors, which is called Cushing's disease. The differential diagnosis of ACTH-dependent Cushing syndrome also includes ectopic production of ACTH or CRH by carcinomas, pheochromocytomas, and bronchial carcinoids.[47] ACTH-independent Cushing syndrome is caused by unilateral adenomas or carcinomas and by bilateral micronodular or macronodular hyperplasia. Cushing's disease occurs most commonly in young women, and DHEAS production is more commonly elevated in ACTH-dependent Cushing syndrome. Consequently, Cushing's disease in women is the most relevant form of hypercortisolism that influences reproduction.

The clinical manifestations of cortisol excess can be subtle in the early stage when the diagnosis is most difficult but the benefits of treatment the greatest. Cortisol is a catabolic hormone that causes lipolysis and fat

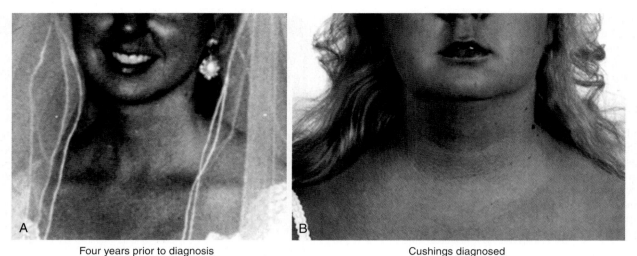

Four years prior to diagnosis   Cushings diagnosed

Figure 23-5. *Subtle clinical signs of Cushing syndrome. This woman is shown 4 years before diagnosis (**A**) and at the time of diagnosis (**B**). In part **B**, she demonstrates facial plethora and loss of clavicular silhouettes due to supraclavicular fat.*

redistribution, as well as breakdown of body tissues, including muscle, skin, and bone. Central obesity is a prominent and common feature, with disproportionate fat accumulation around the face and neck. The dorso-cervical fat pad ("buffalo hump") is a well-known feature of Cushing syndrome, but supraclavicular fat pads are more specific for this disorder, especially in an otherwise nonobese individual (Fig. 23-5). Facial and upper chest plethora is observed (see Fig. 23-5), and women often develop hirsutism.

Proximal muscle weakness and skin thinning are two very specific features of Cushing syndrome, and osteoporo-sis in an obese individual should raise suspicion as well.[47] Patients will complain of difficulty arising from a chair or getting out of a car, combing their hair, or changing an over-head light bulb. Skin thinning and capillary fragility causes easy bruising, and if weight gain is rapid, the striae formed are violaceous and nonblanching, reflecting hemorrhage into the new skin by fragile blood vessels. These striae are found on the abdomen and flanks, near the axillae, and sometimes on the thighs. If more than 1 cm, purple striae are very specific for hypercortisolism, but these findings are a late development in severe disease.

The most important scenario in which Cushing syn-drome should be considered is in the young woman with oligomenorrhea and hirsutism who could be mistaken for having simple polycystic ovary syndrome (PCOS). A his-tory of hirsutism onset after age 25 or specific findings for hypercortisolism, such as easy bruising, thin skin, proxi-mal muscle weakness, and osteoporosis, should prompt screening for Cushing syndrome.

The diagnosis of hypercortisolism can be difficult early in the disease because of the large overlap with nor-mal findings. Testing is based on the principles that the cortisol production rate is increased,[48] that the normal diurnal rhythm is disrupted, and that cortisol is not sup-pressible. These principles are employed by the 24-hour urinary free cortisol,[49] late-night saliva,[50] or serum cor-tisol measurements[51] and overnight dexamethasone

suppression testing,[52] respectively. The caveats of testing are beyond the scope of the chapter, but the reader should be aware that both false positive and false nega-tive results are common. Consequently, tests often must be repeated several times before a diagnosis can be made or excluded.

Once hypercortisolism is confirmed, an ACTH measure-ment will determine if the disease is ACTH-dependent or ACTH-independent. If ACTH-independent (ACTH < 5 pg/mL), an abdominal computed tomography scan of the adrenal glands is obtained. If the ACTH is normal or elevated, the next step is an MRI scan of the pituitary with gadolinium contrast material. The caveat of pitu-itary imaging is that small abnormalities of the pituitary are common, and about half of patients with Cushing's disease do not have a visible tumor by MRI. To conclu-sively exclude the ectopic ACTH syndrome, inferior pe-trosal sinus sampling is performed.[53] Blood draining both sides of the pituitary is sampled from the inferior petrosal sinuses under CRH stimulation, and the ACTH values in these specimens is compared with those obtained in peripheral blood drawn simultaneously. An ACTH step-up greater than 3 from peripheral blood to the inferior petrosal sinus is reliable evidence for a pituitary source of ACTH.

Treatment of Cushing syndrome is primarily surgical. Cushing's disease is treated with transsphenoidal pituitary adenomectomy, yet even in the hands of an experienced surgeon, long-term cure rates are not above 80%. Repeat surgery, radiotherapy, and even bilateral adrenalectomy may be recommended if disease persists. Medical manage-ment with metyrapone, ketoconazole, and triolstane has been employed, but these drugs are seldom very effective in severe disease. Cabergoline is effective in reducing hy-percortisolism for a subset of tumors that express dopa-mine type 2 receptors.[54] In contrast, ACTH-independent Cushing syndrome is normally cured by adrenalectomy, except in the case of adrenocortical carcinomas with inop-erable or metastatic disease.

TABLE 23-2

21-Hydroxylase Deficiency

Form	Common Mutations
Classical	
Salt-wasting	Large deletions, 656A/C-G*, G110del8nt, Q318X R356W*, R483P, I236N + V237E + M239K
Simple virilizing	656A/C-G*, I172N, R356W*
Nonclassical	P30L, V281L, R339H, P453S

*Can be associated with either salt-wasting or simple virilizing disease.

Congenital Adrenal Hyperplasia: 21-Hydroxylase Deficiency

The manifestations of 21-hydroxylase deficiency (21-OHD) in the infant as an intersex disorder were discussed in Chapter 16, so this discussion will be restricted to adults with classical and nonclassical forms of 21-OHD. Among the forms of congenital adrenal hyperplasia (CAH), 21-OHD is by far the most common form, accounting for over 90% of cases.[55] Classical 21-OHD is caused by mutations in the *CYP21A2* gene encoding P450c21 that severely impair enzyme activity to less than 2% of the wild-type enzyme.[56] Nearly all these patients have clinical manifestations and require therapy with glucocorticoid and mineralocorticoid replacement. Milder mutations, particularly the V281L allele, cause nonclassical 21-OHD (Table 23-2).[57] Males with nonclassical 21-OHD are usually asymptomatic, whereas females present variably with hyperandrogenism.[58] Occasionally, patients with intermediate severity are not diagnosed until adulthood (Fig. 23-6).

The diagnosis of 21-OHD is based on elevated circulating concentrations of 21-deoxysteroids, in particular 17-hydroxyprogesterone (17-OHP). In the case of nonclassical disease, serum 17-OHP should be measured 30 to 60 minutes after administration of cosyntropin (250 μg IV or IM).[59,60] A random 17-OHP greater than 10,000 ng/dL establishes the diagnosis of classical 21-OHD, and post-cosyntropin 17-OHP values in the 1500 to 3000 ng/dL range are typical of nonclassical 21-OHD.[61] If laboratory data are equivocal, genetic testing for mutations in the *CYP21A2* gene on DNA from peripheral blood cells is now commercially available.

The repertoire of mutations commonly found in 21-OHD is limited due to the molecular mechanism responsible for most cases. The *CYP21A2* gene is located in a duplicated locus within the HLA region on chromosome 6p that includes the genes for the fourth component of complement. In the duplicated region, the DNA corresponding to the *CYP21A2* gene is replaced by the *CYP21A1* pseudogene.[62,63] This pseudogene contains several mutations that render the cognate mRNA and protein nonfunctional. Most cases of 21-OHD derive from gene conversion events, in which some or all of the *CYP21A2* gene is replaced by the corresponding region of the *CYP21A1* pseudogene.[64] Consequently, the spectrum of mutations and the worldwide prevalence of 21-OHD is fairly consistent,

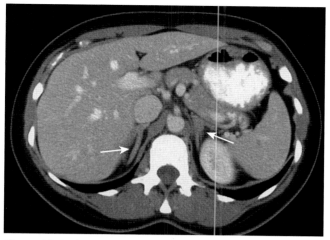

Figure 23-6. *Computed tomography of adrenal glands in a woman with nonclassical 21-hydroxylase deficiency (21-OHD) diagnosed at age 50. She had both severe hirsutism and rapid somatic growth in childhood with normal external genitalia. She menstruated regularly during her reproductive years and gave birth to 3 children. Screening laboratory values included a testosterone of 179 ng/dL, sex hormone–binding globulin of 52 nmol/L, dehydroepiandrosterone sulfate of 427 μg/dL, cortisol of 16 pg/mL, and 17-hydroxyprogesterone (17-OHP) of 1100-2500 ng/dL. The 17-OHP rose to >17,000 ng/dL with cosyntropin stimulation, establishing the diagnosis of 21-OHD. The enlarged but normally shaped adrenal glands are indicated by* arrows.

but certain mutations are particularly common in specific populations, such as V281L in Yupik Eskimos.[65] Occasionally, true point mutations are found instead.[66] Heterozygous carriers may be identified with confidence by genetic testing, whereas 17-OHP values, even after cosyntropin stimulation, show broad overlap with normal individuals of either gender.

The mechanisms of reduced fertility in women with classical 21-OHD are complex, although affected women have given birth to normal female infants.[67] Chronic hyperandrogenemia, even though largely adrenal in origin, causes chronic oligoanovulation. In addition, many women with 21-OHD develop a secondary PCOS, with characteristic ovarian morphologic picture, thecal hyperplasia, and ovarian androgen excess as well.[68] The block in 17-OHP metabolism causes accumulation of adrenal-derived progesterone as well, and high circulating progesterone concentrations impair endometrial maturation and implantation.[69] Overtreatment with synthetic glucocorticoids may both suppress gonadotropins and cause glucose intolerance with its attendant reproductive disturbances.[70]

Women with virilization of the external genitalia face additional difficulties related to anatomic changes. An inadequate vaginal opening, due to either lack of repair or unsuccessful surgery or dilation, may cause dyspareunia, which is an impediment to coitus.[71,72] Vaginal anomalies may interfere with the optimal deposition of sperm, and high circulating progesterone concentrations impair sperm penetration and fertilization. Psychosocial influences should not be underestimated. The fact that 21-OHD is a genetic disorder associated with masculinization contributes to difficulties in finding a partner and has been associated with high prevalence of lesbian behavior.[73]

Women with nonclassical 21-OHD are sometimes identified during an evaluation of hirsutism, oligomenorrhea, or infertility mimicking PCOS. It is difficult to distinguish nonclassical 21-OHD from idiopathic PCOS on clinical grounds.[58,74] More careful studies suggest that the frequency of PCOS in women with nonclassical 21-OHD is not much higher than in the general population. Nevertheless, if infertility and chronic anovulation are present in a woman with nonclassical 21-OHD, these women may benefit from glucocorticoid replacement.

Little data exist to guide the optimal management of adults with 21-OHD, either for long-term glucocorticoid replacement or for improving fertility.[70] The minimum amount of glucocorticoid replacement to maintain testosterone and 17-OHP in an acceptable range is recommended for chronic therapy, although this dose and target steroid values vary among women. Hydrocortisone (20-40 mg/day) is preferable for chronic therapy, although prednisone and dexamethasone may be required for short-term treatment, particularly to enable ovulation. Fludrocortisone acetate (0.05-2 mg/day) in doses sufficient to suppress plasma renin activity, is added to minimize the dose of glucocorticoid required, whether salt-wasting is present or not. Ovulation induction with standard methods and agents may be necessary despite optimal adrenal replacement regimens. Despite clinical features of PCOS shared with 21-OHD, metformin and other insulin sensitizers have not been studied adequately in women with 21-OHD.

Almost all men with nonclassical 21-OHD are asymptomatic and can be identified only with genetic testing. Men with classical 21-OHD, in contrast, may suffer from infertility, particularly if poorly controlled. Severe adrenal androgen excess rarely causes gonadotropin suppression with subsequent Leydig cell atrophy, reduced testicular testosterone production, and impaired spermatogenesis.[75] Glucocorticoid replacement often normalizes testicular function, although high doses may be required initially.

More commonly, adrenal rests are the cause of male infertility in 21-OHD.[76] The steroid-producing cells of the adrenal cortex and the gonads derive from the same pool of precursors during embryogenesis. The migration of adrenal cells to the suprarenal space can be imperfect, and adrenal cortex cells may be found in the testis or within the groin and abdomen. ACTH is trophic for these adrenal rest cells as well, and when ACTH is high, as in poorly controlled 21-OHD, these cells will form masses, most often in the testis itself. These tumors are present in most men with 21-OHD, and testicular ultrasonography is the most sensitive method of diagnosis.[77] Because the testis is confined to a rigid capsule, the growth of intratesticular adrenal rests impairs testicular blood flow and efflux of sperm into the ejaculate. Treatment of adrenal rests requires potent glucocorticoids, such as dexamethasone, 2 mg at night, although even this therapy is not always successful in reducing tumor size and restoring fertility. Surgical resection of the adrenal rests by a competent urologist is associated with a low risk of recurrence but with little improvement in spermatogenesis.[78] However, this outcome may reflect a selection bias in reserving surgery for the most severely affected men.

Other Forms of Congenital Adrenal Hyperplasia

The other forms of CAH associated with androgen excess in women are 11-hydroxylase deficiency (11-OHD) and 3β-hydroxysteroid dehydrogenase/isomerase deficiency (3βHSDD). In 11-OHD, caused by mutations in the *CYP11B1* gene, the 11-deoxysteroids 11-deoxycorticosterone (DOC) and 11-deoxycortisol are markedly elevated, and excess DOC causes hypertension, unlike 21-OHD.[79] Serum 17-OHP may be elevated in 11-OHD, but much less than in 21-OHD with similar hyperandrogenemia. In 3βHSDD, caused by mutations in the *HSD3B2* gene, the diagnostic steroid ratios are those of Δ^5 to Δ^4 steroids, such as pregnenolone-to-progesterone ratios greater than 6 standard deviations above normal.[80] Note that circulating testosterone concentrations are paradoxically elevated in women with 3βHSDD. The Δ^5 steroid DHEAS is metabolized to active androgens in the periphery and converted to Δ^4 steroids by 3βHSD type 1, which is abundant in liver and skin, explaining this phenomenon.

The mechanisms responsible for infertility in men and women with 11-OHD are similar to those in 21-OHD. Treatments are similar, except that aldosterone antagonists (spironolactone, eplerenone) are useful to control hypertension during chronic therapy. Note that spironolactone is also an androgen antagonist and is contraindicated in women who may become pregnant. Women with 3βHSDD, even in the most severe cases, have mild clitoromegaly and little labioscrotal fusion, so anatomic impediments to pregnancy are less important, and high progesterone is less of a factor than in 21-OHD and 11-OHD.[80]

Forms of CAH that impair both androgen and estrogen production include combined 17-hydroxylase/17,20-lyase deficiency[81] or isolated 17,20-lyase deficiency,[82,83] both caused by mutations in the *CYP17A1* gene encoding P450c17[84]; lipoid CAH, due to mutations in the *STAR* gene encoding the steroidogenic acute regulatory protein (StAR)[85] or rarely the *CYP11A1* gene encoding P450scc[86]; and cytochrome P450-oxidoreductase deficiency, due to mutations in the *POR* gene and associated with a spectrum of phenotypes[87] from primary amenorrhea in phenotypically normal women to the Antley-Bixler syndrome, with skeletal dysmorphologies.[88,89] The discussion of these diseases is beyond the scope of this chapter, and fertility is very rare in these patients despite the optimal therapy.

Thyroid Disorders

OVERVIEW

Before discussing the specific effects of thyroid disorders on reproductive function, it is important to understand some basic principles and potential areas of interaction between elements of thyroid hormone physiology and reproductive function.

Within the thyroid gland, millions of follicles are the factories and storage silos for all the circulating T_4 and 20% of the active T_3 thyroid hormone. The thyroid follicle is composed of simple secretory epithelial cells surrounding

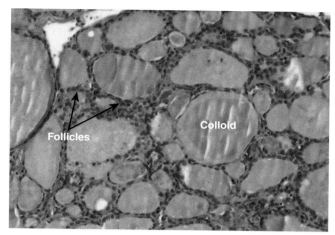

Figure 23-7. *Histologic appearance of a normal thyroid gland (100×, hematoxylin and eosin). Single-layer, epithelial-lined follicles of variable sizes are filled with pink colloid where thyroglobulin, T_3, and T_4 are stored.*

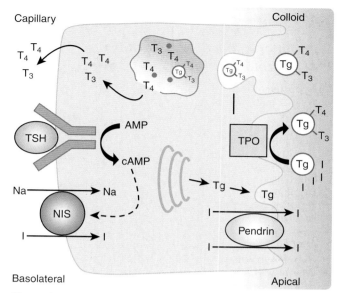

Figure 23-8. *Production of thyroid hormone in the follicular epithelial cell. This schematic illustrates the variety of functions carried out in the follicular epithelial cell from iodine (I) transport via the sodium (Na) iodide symporter (NIS), thyroglobulin (Tg) synthesis, iodination and T_4 production by thyroid peroxidase (TPO) at the apical membrane where Tg and Tg complexed with T_3 and T_4 are stored. Reuptake and Tg digestion of the complexes allows for secretion of T_3 and T_4 through the basolateral membrane into the abundant capillary network. Stimulation by thyrotropin (TSH) of the TSH receptor results in cyclic AMP (cAMP) production, which can exert effects on many functions of the cell.*

a lumen containing colloid—a gelatinous substance composed primarily of thyroglobulin and T_4 (Fig. 23-7). The unique aspect of the thyroid gland is its ability to store enormous quantities of thyroid hormone in the follicular colloid. Iodide imported from the circulation and concentrated in colloid is used for iodination of the thyroglobulin backbone by thyroid peroxidase (TPO) to produce inactive precursor mono- and diiodotyrosines. Synthesis of T_4 and T_3 using these precursors is also catalyzed by TPO. Reuptake and Tg digestion of the stored T_3 and T_4 from the colloid allows for secretion through the basolateral membrane into the abundant capillary network (Fig. 23-8).

As described in the pituitary section overview, the hypothalamic-pituitary-thyroid axis is a straightforward model of an endocrine feedback system. The anterior pituitary secretes TSH, which regulates multiple steps in thyroid hormone production: (1) growth of the follicles, (2) iodine uptake, and (3) iodination of thyroid hormone by the secretory epithelial cells. Control of TSH secretion, and therefore, ultimate control of all elements required for thyroid hormone production, is tightly regulated by negative feedback of circulating T_4 and T_3, suppressing production of both TRH from the hypothalamus and TSH by the anterior pituitary (see Fig. 23-1A).

Outside the hypothalamic-pituitary-thyroid axis, the major regulator of thyroid hormone production is the concentration of thyroid hormone globulin (TBG). Circulating T_4 is almost entirely (99%) bound to plasma proteins: approximately 70% bound to TBG, 20% to transthyretin (prealbumin), and 10% to albumin. In women, significant changes in TBG glycosylation in the liver are induced by rises in estradiol during pregnancy or exogenous estrogens, prolonging TBG half-life and increasing circulating TBG concentrations.[90] The rise in TBG can transiently decrease free T_4 concentrations, leading to an increase in the TSH and total T_4 to maintain normal free T_4. During pregnancy, this may also lead to a visible enlargement of the thyroid gland or goiter. Peripheral conversion of T_4 to T_3 is mediated by deiodinases types 1 and 2 located in different locations both at the tissue and cellular

level. Interestingly, type 3 deiodinase is almost exclusively expressed in the placenta, where it is tightly regulated by thyroid hormone concentrations.

THYROID DISORDERS THAT AFFECT REPRODUCTION

Diseases of the thyroid are 5 to 10 times more common in females than males, and peak incidence occurs during the reproductive years. The most common conditions are Hashimoto's thyroiditis and Graves' disease, both autoimmune diseases of the thyroid. Despite its central role in maintaining normal organ and endocrine function throughout the body, the exact mechanisms for thyroid hormone's effects are not well understood. Notably, it is the absence of thyroid hormone (hypothyroidism) and the multitude of accompanying symptoms that demonstrates its importance throughout the body. Similarly, for reproduction, hypothyroidism has more significant effects on menstrual cycles and fertility than hyperthyroidism, or more generally, thyrotoxicosis.

Hypothyroidism

Women with hypothyroidism present with any of numerous symptoms and signs (Box 23-2). The reproductive age woman may experience irregular menses, anovulatory cycles, or menorrhagia or may present only with infertility.[91] The mechanism for significant alterations in the reproductive system is likely through the hypothalamic-pituitary

Common Clinical Presentations of Thyroid Disorders

Hypothyroidism
Weight gain
Fatigue
Constipation
Cold intolerance
Hair loss
Menorrhagia
Infertility
Dry skin
Periorbital edema
Hoarseness
Delayed reflexes
Anemia

Hyperthyroidism
Weight loss
Fatigue
Increased frequency of bowel movements
Heat intolerance
Anxiety
Dyspnea on exertion
Palpitations
Diaphoresis
Lid lag or "stare"
Tremor
Hyperreflexia
Supraventricular tachyarrhythmias

Common Causes of Thyroid Disorders

Primary Hypothyroidism
Chronic autoimmune thyroiditis (Hashimoto's)
Radioiodine ablation
Thyroidectomy
Silent/postpartum thyroiditis (hypothyroid phase)
Subacute thyroiditis (hypothyroid phase)
Iodine deficiency
Drugs (thionamides, lithium)

Primary Hyperthyroidism
Graves' disease
Toxic multinodular goiter
Solitary toxic nodule
Silent/postpartum thyroiditis (lymphocytic)
Subacute thyroiditis (granulomatous)
Iodine-induced (e.g., amiodarone)
Exogenous thyroid hormone ingestion

axis. Even though basal gonadotropins are normal, elevated TRH can stimulate lactotrophs to produce prolactin, which interferes with GnRH pulsatility, as described earlier in the pituitary section. Outside of effects on the hypothalamic-pituitary axis, hypothyroidism may interfere with ovarian function. Experimentally, T_4 has been shown to stimulate ovarian steroidogenesis in granulosa cells cultured in vitro.[92] In women and men, hypothyroidism may also increase the free fractions of androgens and estrogens by reducing sex hormone–binding globulin (SHBG) binding affinity through altered sialic acid content[93]; conversely, hyperthyroidism increases SHBG.[94] In men, hypothyroidism has been associated with decreased libido, impotence, and oligospermia. The hypogonadism can correct after thyroxine replacement,[95] and abnormalities of sperm count and motility and poor testosterone response to hCG injections also improve after T_4 replacement.[96] As opposed to women, the hypogonadotropic hypogonadism associated with hypothyroidism is not associated with hyperprolactinemia.[95]

While more severe hypothyroidism clearly interferes with successful ovulation and fertility, more subtle abnormalities of the pituitary-thyroid axis or the underlying disease rather than abnormal T_4 hormone concentrations may also affect fertility. In one study of women presenting to an infertility clinic with normal thyroid function tests, women with lower or higher than normal responses to TRH stimulation had lower pregnancy rates than women with normal responses.[97] The most common cause of hypothyroidism is chronic autoimmune thyroiditis (Hashimoto's thyroiditis). In a study that tested for the autoantibodies associated with Hashimoto's thyroiditis (anti-TPO and anti-thyroglobulin), there was a higher prevalence of antibody-positive women presenting with infertility than age-matched control subjects. Despite normal thyroid function tests, these women had twice the rate of miscarriage than the antibody-negative group.[98] Therefore, a more generalized autoimmune state may contribute significantly and independently to the infertility associated with hypothyroidism.

In addition to Hashimoto's thyroiditis, hypothyroidism may also be seen in patients with acute (silent) and subacute thyroiditis (Box 23-3). Postpartum thyroiditis is an acute thyroiditis that occurs within 6 months of delivery and is usually self-limited. Thyroiditis typically has an acute thyrotoxic phase followed by a recovery hypothyroid and eventually a euthyroid phase. Postpartum thyroiditis typically presents with symptoms in the hypothyroid phase, whereas subacute thyroiditis presents with pain during the hyperthyroid phase. Although most return to a euthyroid state in the short-term, 20% to 64% of these women will develop chronic hypothyroidism over the next few years.[99] An important secondary cause of hypothyroidism is radioactive iodine ablation or thyroidectomy for definitive treatment of Graves' disease, thyroid nodules, or thyroid cancer.

The diagnosis of hypothyroidism itself is easily made with modern immunoassays. Clinical hypothyroidism is defined by both higher than normal TSH and lower than normal free T_4 concentrations. Subclinical hypothyroidism describes the mild or early changes when the TSH rises before the free T_4 falls below normal. The mild elevation in TSH compensates for the early decline in T_4 production by the thyroid gland. Although not necessary for the diagnosis of hypothyroidism, additional tests of anti-TPO and anti-thyroglobulin antibodies can influence treatment decisions by establishing underlying Hashimoto's thyroiditis. The presence of anti-TPO antibodies increases the risk for developing clinical hypothyroidism from 2.1% to 4.3% per year.[100] Age and female gender also increase the risk of progression to overt hypothyroidism. In addition, antithyroid antibodies have been associated with infertility and risk for miscarriage.[101]

During pregnancy, there are subtleties to the diagnosis of thyroid disease with a low TSH in early pregnancy, but an elevated TSH is a clear indicator of hypothyroidism. Widespread screening of pregnant women with TSH and antibody testing is not routinely recommended because of the low prevalence of clinical thyroid disease (1%). However, the prevalence of subclinical hypothyroidism is as high as 5%, and 10% to 15% of reproductive age women have detectable antithyroid antibodies.[102] Hypothyroidism and subclinical hypothyroidism are associated with a higher risk for spontaneous miscarriage,[103] hypertension, preeclampsia, and eclampsia, along with low birth weight from premature delivery.[104]

Multiple studies have reported an association of antithyroid antibodies and miscarriage in euthyroid women. However, it is not clear whether this association represents a more generalized autoimmunity. Others have not found an association between antithyroid antibodies and infertility.[101] Only one study reported that treatment of antibody-positive euthyroid women with T_4 decreases miscarriage rate and preterm delivery.[105] Until there is stronger and consistent evidence of a treatment effect, routine antithyroid antibody screening is debatable, though it may be considered in any woman with symptoms being tested for thyroid disease, with a strong family history, or with other autoimmune disease.

The treatment of hypothyroidism involves replacement of thyroid hormone with synthetic T_4 (levothyroxine). A general guide for replacement is a weight-based dose of 1.6 µg/kg once daily, but actual requirements may vary. After initiation or dose adjustment, follow-up tests should be ordered after at least 6 to 8 weeks. To minimize problems with absorption, levothyroxine should be taken without other drugs, especially calcium or iron-containing tablets.

For the woman known to have hypothyroidism prior to pregnancy, very close monitoring of the TSH is required to maintain a euthyroid state given the increase in TBG and therefore total T_4 requirements. This is particularly important for the fetus, with strong evidence that maternal hypothyroidism during the first trimester may affect fetal intellectual development.[106] Another reason to optimize treatment before and early in pregnancy is the association of first trimester hypothyroidism with fetal distress and cesarean section despite adequate replacement at delivery.[107] Guidelines suggest achieving a target of TSH less than 2.5 µU/mL before pregnancy.[108] The T_4 dose usually needs to be increased by a total of 30% to 50% within the first month of gestation and should be monitored 4 weeks after any adjustment.[109]

Generally, screening for and treating subclinical hypothyroidism is somewhat controversial without well-established treatment benefit. For women trying to conceive and pregnant women, treatment is advised when subclinical hypothyroidism is diagnosed given the potential risks of miscarriage and preterm labor, and risks to the fetus in terms of neuropsychological development.[108]

Although there is no literature supporting that treatment with thyroxine will improve fertility, it is still warranted to attain euthyroid status for women with infertility and subclinical hypothyroidism to improve outcomes when pregnancy is achieved. For men, one study did find an association of subclinical hypothyroidism with low testosterone.[110] However, subclinical hypothyroidism has not been associated with changes in sperm quality.

Hyperthyroidism

Women and men with hyperthyroidism present with typical findings of weight loss, palpitations, anxiety, and increased frequency of bowel movements. For women, menstrual cycles are affected to a lesser degree than hypothyroidism. Although abnormalities in basal and stimulated gonadotropins have been observed in women with hyperthyroidism, ovulation is maintained.[91] Therefore, hyperthyroidism is less of a concern in terms of fertility but presents more of a problem in the management and diagnosis during pregnancy. During pregnancy, there can be subtleties to the diagnosis of thyrotoxicosis and distinguishing hyperthyroidism from normal physiologic changes, hyperemesis gravidarum, and gestational trophoblastic disease. As opposed to association of antithyroid antibodies with fertility and miscarriage rates, the thyroid receptor stimulating antibodies of Graves' disease have more of an impact on the fetus and the risk for neonatal thyrotoxicosis.

In men with Graves' disease, symptomatic hypogonadism and bioavailable testosterone lower than normal control subjects have been observed despite the overall increase in total testosterone and SHBG. These findings have been associated with impaired gonadotropic response to hCG and significant abnormalities in semen quality. Changes in semen parameters could be reversed with antithyroid treatment.[111,112] Older men are more likely to be clinically affected because of a lower gonadal reserve to compensate for the increases in SHBG. Elevated estradiol may result in gynecomastia and also likely explains the normal gonadotropin concentrations with low free testosterone.

Graves' disease is the most common cause of hyperthyroidism. In addition to the symptoms of thyrotoxicosis and goiter, patients may present with the typical stare and extraocular muscle paralysis resulting from infiltrative orbitopathy and ophthalmopathy. Graves' disease is an autoimmune disease with the thyroid-stimulating immunoglobulin (TSI) or anti-TSH receptor antibody resulting in unregulated stimulation of thyroid hormone production.

Thyroiditis refers to any inflammatory state of the thyroid. The thyrotoxicosis of thyroiditis results from release of stored thyroid hormone which may persist for up to 2 months. As discussed earlier, the usual course is then transient hypothyroidism followed by recovery of thyroid function, although chronic hypothyroidism may also develop. Subacute (de Quervain's) thyroiditis is distinguishable by a history of neck pain and recent viral infection and physical findings of fever and exquisitely tender thyroid.

	↓ TSH	Normal TSH	↑ TSH
↓ Free T$_4$	Central hypothyroidism Nonthyroidal illness Drug effect		Primary hypothyroidism
Normal Free T$_4$	Subclinical thyrotoxicosis Nonthyroidal illness T$_3$ thyrotoxicosis	Normal	Subclinical hypothyroidism
↑ Free T$_4$	Thyrotoxicosis	TSH-secreting pituitary adenoma Thyroid hormone resistance syndrome Familial dysalbuminemic hyperthyroxinemia	

Figure 23-9. Differential diagnosis based on thyroid-stimulating hormone (TSH) and free T$_4$ results.

Other potential causes of thyrotoxicosis include an autonomous thyroid nodule and multinodular goiter. Toxic adenoma, which is less common than Graves' disease or toxic multinodular goiter, is usually a benign, solitary tumor with autonomous T$_4$ and T$_3$ production. In a large proportion of toxic adenomas, a somatic or germline mutation in the TSH receptor or G protein genes results in constitutive activation of the TSH receptor.[113] Multinodular goiter is less likely to cause hyperthyroidism in reproductive age women and is more common in older patients. Growth and the development of autonomous function take years to manifest as hyperthyroidism, and most toxic adenomas are greater than 3 cm in diameter.

The diagnosis of thyrotoxicosis is clear with an elevated free T$_4$ and low TSH. However, a low TSH with a low or normal free T$_4$ suggests several additional diagnoses to consider other than subclinical hyperthyroidism (Fig. 23-9). Diagnosis of thyrotoxicosis during pregnancy should be made more cautiously than hypothyroidism because the TSH level can be low in the first trimester due to hCG-mediated thyroid stimulation. Although total T$_4$ is elevated because of the increased TBG during a normal pregnancy, a free T$_4$ concentration will be normal.

Radioactive iodine scans are not necessary to make the diagnosis of hyperthyroidism and are most useful for distinguishing Graves' disease from toxic adenoma (Fig. 23-10), thyroiditis, and factitious disorder. Usually, clinical factors obviate the need for diagnostic scans. Especially since radioactive iodine scans are contraindicated during pregnancy, another useful test is the thyroid-stimulating immunoglobulin (TSI). Elevated TSI supports the diagnosis of Graves' disease, but the test is not very sensitive though it is very specific. Measurement of TSI in the third trimester has utility in predicting the risk of developing neonatal Graves' disease.[114] In pregnancy, during breastfeeding, or in women trying to conceive, ultrasonography with Doppler blood flow may be useful for distinguishing Graves' disease from thyroiditis in experienced hands.[115,116]

The pharmacologic treatment of Graves' disease is antithyroid treatment with a thionamide – propylthiouracil from 50 mg tid to 100 mg qid or methimazole 5 to 40 mg daily. The goal of therapy initially is a free T$_4$ in the normal range as the TSH rise may lag behind. Elevated free T$_4$ from thyroiditis is transient and will not respond to antithyroid treatment. Symptoms of palpitations, anxiety, and tremor can be managed with a beta-blocker such as propranolol or metoprolol. Patients may experience a sustained remission after 12 to 18 months of therapy. In the case of subacute painful thyroiditis, pain responds to nonsteroidal anti-inflammatory drugs or a course of corticosteroid therapy. Thionamides are useful for restoration of euthyroidism in patients with toxic adenomas and multinodular goiters, but usually definitive therapy (see later discussion) is required.

Radioactive iodine-131 ablation is an alternative to antithyroid agents for hyperthyroidism (aside from thyroiditis). For women desiring pregnancy, there is no evidence that previous radioactive iodine ablation at even the high doses used for thyroid cancer remnant ablation will affect subsequent fertility or increase the risk for congenital abnormalities. Although a subset of women treated with radioactive iodine for thyroid cancer may experience temporary amenorrhea with symptoms and high FSH values, menses returned in less than 6 months in most women, and certainly within 12 months as for any other women with temporary ovarian failure.[91] However, it is generally advised that a woman wait at least 1 year before trying to conceive because of the potential increased risk for miscarriage.[117]

Women being treated with antithyroid drugs generally are switched to propylthiouracil before trying to conceive. Propylthiouracil (PTU) has been preferred over methimazole for treatment of Graves' disease in pregnancy for two reasons: it is less likely to cross the placenta and methimazole has been rarely associated with congenital abnormalities. In practice, methimazole is often used if PTU is unable to successfully control free T$_4$ concentrations due to tolerability and efficacy issues. The goal for therapy prior to conception or while pregnant is a free T$_4$ value in the upper limit of the normal range to avoid hypothyroidism.

Surgery—thyroidectomy or resection of a toxic adenoma—is generally reserved for treating hyperthyroidism in disease refractory to medical therapy, for glands that are producing obstructive symptoms, for large nodules, and when radioactive iodine is contraindicated or refused. In pregnancy, surgery is reserved for cases when disease is severe and refractory to medical therapy, or when antithyroid agents cannot be used because of the side effect of agranulocytosis or liver damage.

The complete reference list can be found on the companion Expert Consult Web site at www.expertconsultbook.com.

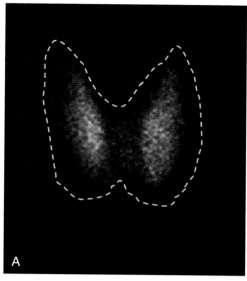 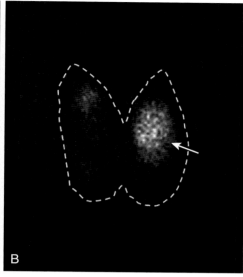

Figure 23-10. Radioactive iodine-123 scans for Graves' disease versus toxic adenoma. *A,* Increased radioactive iodine uptake seen symmetrically throughout a thyroid gland with Graves' disease. *B,* Increased uptake by a toxic adenoma indicated by arrow with little uptake elsewhere. The dotted lines approximate the outline of the thyroid gland with minimal uptake in comparison to the adenoma.

Suggested Readings

Abalovich M, Amino N, Barbour LA, et al. Management of thyroid dysfunction during pregnancy and postpartum: an Endocrine Society Clinical Practice Guideline. J Clin Endocrinol Metab 92:S1-47, 2007.

Claahsen-van der Grinten HL, Otten BJ, Takahashi S, et al. Testicular adrenal rest tumors in adult males with congenital adrenal hyperplasia: evaluation of pituitary-gonadal function before and after successful testis-sparing surgery in eight patients. J Clin Endocrinol Metab 92:612-615, 2007.

Colao A, Abs R, Barcena DG, et al. Pregnancy outcomes following cabergoline treatment: extended results from a 12-year observational study. Clin Endocrinol (Oxf) 68:66-71, 2008.

Colao A, Di Sarno A, Cappabianca P, et al. Withdrawal of long-term cabergoline therapy for tumoral and nontumoral hyperprolactinemia. N Engl J Med 349:2023-2033, 2003.

Cozzi R, Attanasio R, Lodrini S, et al. Cabergoline addition to depot somatostatin analogues in resistant acromegalic patients: efficacy and lack of predictive value of prolactin status. Clin Endocrinol (Oxf) 61:209-215, 2004.

Falhammar H, Filipsson H, Holmdahl G, et al. Metabolic profile and body composition in adult women with congenital adrenal hyperplasia due to 21-hydroxylase deficiency. J Clin Endocrinol Metab 92:110-116, 2007.

Fluck CE, Tajima T, Pandey AV, et al. Mutant P450 oxidoreductase causes disordered steroidogenesis with and without Antley-Bixler syndrome. Nat Genet 36:228-230, 2004.

Lo JC, Schwitzgebel VM, Tyrrell JB, et al. Normal female infants born of mothers with classic congenital adrenal hyperplasia due to 21-hydroxylase deficiency. J Clin Endocrinol Metab 84:930-936, 1999.

McDermott JH, Walsh CH. Hypogonadism in hereditary hemochromatosis. J Clin Endocrinol Metab 90:2451-2455, 2005.

Pivonello R, Ferone D, de Herder WW, et al. Dopamine receptor expression and function in corticotroph pituitary tumors. J Clin Endocrinol Metab 89:2452-2462, 2004.

Singh A, Dantas ZN, Stone SC, et al. Presence of thyroid antibodies in early reproductive failure: biochemical versus clinical pregnancies. Fertil Steril 63:277-281, 1995.

Speiser PW, Knochenhauer ES, Dewailly D, et al. A multicenter study of women with nonclassical congenital adrenal hyperplasia: relationship between genotype and phenotype. Mol Genet Metab 71:527-534, 2000.

Testa G, Vegetti W, Motta T, et al. Two-year treatment with oral contraceptives in hyperprolactinemic patients. Contraception 58:69-73, 1998.

Trainer PJ, Drake WM, Katznelson L, et al. Treatment of acromegaly with the growth hormone-receptor antagonist pegvisomant. N Engl J Med 342:1171-1177, 2000.

Tyrrell JB, Lamborn KR, Hannegan LT, et al. Transsphenoidal microsurgical therapy of prolactinomas: initial outcomes and long-term results. Neurosurgery 44:254-261. discussion 261-253, 1999.

CHAPTER 24

Endometriosis

Robert N. Taylor and Dan I. Lebovic

Endometriosis is a chronic condition characterized by the growth of hormone-responsive endometrial tissue outside the uterine cavity. Typically, ectopic endometriotic implants are found on the peritoneal surface, within the ovary or invading the rectovaginal septum; however, many examples of more widely distributed lesions have been described. Several studies suggest that the overall prevalence of endometriosis among reproductive-age women is around 10%.[1] This disease is accompanied by pelvic pain or infertility in up to 90 million women worldwide. Its symptoms are associated with work absenteeism, social isolation, and high costs of therapy. In addition, endometriosis is the third most common indication for hysterectomy in the United States.[2] This outcome can be particularly devastating in women who undergo hysterectomy for endometriosis before the age of 30, because they are likely to have residual somatic symptoms and a psychological sense of loss.[3] Careful estimates of health care costs for endometriosis in 2002 in the United States were $22 million.[4]

History and Histogenesis

CLASSICAL THEORIES OF THE ORIGINS OF ENDOMETRIOSIS

Scholars of this disease have traced original sources that describe the pathologic features of endometriosis in Dutch and Belgian women of the late 1600s.[5] Curiously, the prevalence of endometriosis remains high in that part of the world.[6] The great German pathologists von Rokitansky and Meyer wrote extensively about this disorder in the latter part of the 19th century. In the United States, the first clear pathologic description of an ovarian endometrioma was reported to the Johns Hopkins Medical Society in 1899.[7] Dr. John A. Sampson graduated from Johns Hopkins that same year. After more than 25 years in the practice of gynecologic surgery, he put forward the hypothesis that endometriosis lesions arose from endometrial tissue that escaped through the fallopian tubes at the time of menstruation. This tissue, he postulated, implanted on peritoneal surfaces and regenerated an endometrial epithelial lining.[8] Contemporaneously, Halban proposed that viable endometrial cells might travel via hematogenous or lymphatogenous vascular transport.[9] Although this metastatic theory explains rare manifestations of distant, extraperitoneal lesions (e.g., endometriosis in the brain[10] or nose[11]), it does not explain the gravity-dependent, intraperitoneal location of most foci of endometriosis.

RETROGRADE MENSTRUATION AND IMPLANTATION

Even today, the prevailing theory concerning the etiology of endometriosis is the implantation hypothesis set forth by Sampson.[8] This theory has been supported by the documentation of reflux menstruation[12] and intraperitoneal spillage of viable endometrial cells[13] in ovulating women (Fig. 24-1).[14] Furthermore, the incidence is increased in cases of menstrual outflow obstruction; in women with known endometriosis, ablation of the eutopic endometrium dramatically reduced the risk of recurrence.[15] That more than 60% of unilateral lesions occur in the left hemipelvis also is consistent with accumulation of refluxed cells in this location, due to the position of the mesentery of the sigmoid colon.[16]

The adhesion of shed endometrial cells to peritoneal and subperitoneal surfaces involves the expression of extracellular membrane adhesion molecules and their coreceptors. Although some researchers have argued that implants of endometrium have never been clearly visualized microscopically in the process of attaching to the peritoneum,[17] the in vitro findings of Witz and colleagues[18] indicate that the process of implant invasion into the

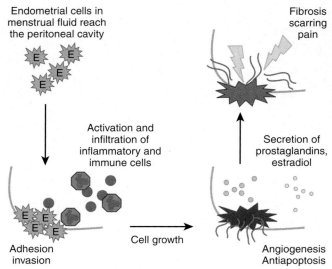

Figure 24-1. *Proposed establishment of peritoneal endometriotic implants via retrograde menstruation, attachment, proliferation, migration, neovascularization, inflammation, and fibrosis. E, endometrial cell. (From Flores I, Rivera E, Ruiz LA, et al. Molecular profiling of experimental endometriosis identified gene expression patterns in common with human disease. Fertil Steril 87[5]:1180-1199, 2007.)*

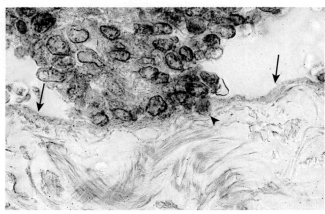

Figure 24-2. *Early invasion of an endometrial implant through the mesothelium. The mesothelium is labeled with monoclonal antibody to cytokeratin and stained with diaminobenzidine (arrows). An endometrial stromal cell (arrowhead) passing through the mesothelium is thought to represent the initial step of invasion into the stroma of the peritoneum. Original magnification, ×31,000. Counterstained with hematoxylin. (From Witz CA, Monotoya-Rodriguez IA, Schenken RS. Whole explants of peritoneum and endometrium: a novel model of the early endometriosis lesion. Fertil Steril 71[1]:56-60, 1999.)*

subperitoneal space is so rapid that one would not expect to observe adherent fragments of endometrium (Fig. 24-2).[19] This origin has been proposed by Nisolle et al.[20] to be the most likely source of intraperitoneal lesions in vivo.

COELOMIC METAPLASIA

An alternative hypothesis, historically attributed to Meyer,[21] suggests that metaplasia of the coelomic epithelium is the origin of endometriosis. This theory is logical, because cells from both the peritoneum and endometrium derive from a common embryologic precursor: the coelomic cell. However, this theory has been difficult to support scientifically. If the postulate were correct, one would expect much higher rates of pleural endometriosis because that mesothelium is the same as that which lines the abdominal cavity. Furthermore, investigators have been unable to show that peritoneal cells can be experimentally differentiated into endometrial cell types. Lastly, metaplasia is an age-related process. Endometriosis occurs early in reproductive-age women, and its incidence peaks in the third decade. This pattern would not be predicted by a linear, progressive likelihood of metaplasia. Nevertheless, this has been postulated as the most likely source of deep, adenomyotic nodules of endometriosis in the rectovaginal septum[20] and in some cases of endometrioma.[22]

NEOCLASSICAL THEORIES OF ENDOMETRIOSIS HISTOGENESIS

In the past decade, scholars of endometriosis have considered integrated models for the etiology of this disorder. We currently recognize that genetic, anatomic, endocrine, immunologic, and possibly environmental factors influence the risk of developing endometriosis. Hence, the neoclassical view of this syndrome requires a broader conceptualization of its etiology and the mechanisms whereby endometriosis produces its clinical symptoms. Based on histologic and biochemical similarities of endometriosis lesions with the basalis layer of the endometrium, Leyendecker and colleagues suggested that endometriosis is derived from the subendometrial zone that they refer to as "archimetra."[23] More recently, authors have posited that endometriosis may arise from rare adult stem cells residing within the uterus.[24,25] Proof of the latter hypothesis is complicated by the physiologic recruitment of bone marrow–derived immune cells into the endometrium and will require identification of specific stem cell markers that represent these endometrioid side populations.

Epidemiology

Endometriosis has been found in women between the ages of 12 and 80, with the average age being approximately 28. Exposure to ovarian hormones appears to be essential to fostering lesion growth, with the vast majority of the cases found in women aged 20 to 50. The estrogen dependency of this condition led Barbieri to propose the hypothesis that concentrations of estradiol over 50 pg/mL were needed to support the growth of endometriosis lesions (Fig. 24-3).[26] This hypothesis will be discussed in more detail when the medical treatment of endometriosis is considered.

In severe disease there seems to be a familial correlation; however, no clear mendelian genetic trait has been identified and most researchers believe it to be complex and multifactorial.[27] These points will be discussed more fully later in this chapter. Retrograde menstruation and increased exposure to menstrual flow (reduced parity,

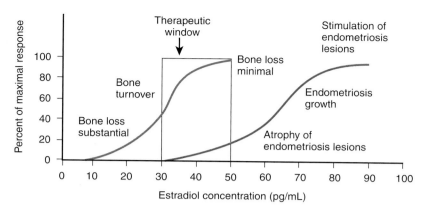

Figure 24-3. The estrogen threshold hypothesis postulates that different estrogen target tissues have differential hormone sensitivity. In this model, a therapeutic window of serum estradiol concentration, between 30 and 50 pg/mL, should protect against bone mineral loss and prevent stimulation of endometriosis lesion growth. (From Barbieri R. Hormone treatment of endometriosis: the estrogen threshold hypothesis. Am J Obstet Gynecol 166:740-745, 1992.)

longer duration of menstrual periods, and shorter cycle length) have been identified as risk factors for endometriosis.[28] Recently, environmental factors, such as dioxin[29,30] and other presumed endocrine disrupters have been implicated.[31]

DEMOGRAPHY

The prevalence of endometriosis ranges from 2% to 50% of reproductive-age women. Unfortunately, this number is widely disparate, depending upon the study. In women with infertility, the prevalence ranges from 21% to 47%. This high frequency may be due to the fact that endometriosis plays a causative role in infertility, but it also may be due to a diagnostic selection bias. Women with infertility are more likely to undergo laparoscopy as part of their clinical evaluation, thereby confirming the diagnosis.

Observations of a high prevalence of endometriosis in primate colonies exposed to dioxin,[29] a particularly potent polychlorinated biphenyl (PCB) industrial contaminant, have suggested that this compound might influence the risk of endometriosis in women. Recent case-control studies revealed increased adjusted odds ratios for endometriosis in women exposed to dioxins and other PCB chemicals of this type.[32,33] In utero exposure to PCBs was shown to induce an endometriosis-like uterine phenotype (e.g., reduced progesterone recetor levels) in females of the F1 generation.[34]

Genomics, Genetics, and Epigenetics

Genes seem to influence susceptibility for endometriosis[35]; however, as previously noted, the mode of hereditary transmission appears to be polygenic and likely to involve multiple loci.[27] Several lines of evidence implicate genetics as a risk factor. In one study, first-degree female relatives (mothers and sisters) of women with severe endometriosis had a 7% incidence, whereas primary female relatives of their partners (who typically have similar ethnic and socioeconomic status) had less than 1% incidence of endometriosis.[36] Consistent with this observation is the finding of Kennedy and colleagues that familial cases of

endometriosis tend to be more severe and have an earlier onset of symptoms than sporadic cases.[37] Large population studies based in Iceland and Australia and the United Kingdom identified loci on chromosome 9q and 10q, respectively, significantly associated with endometriosis, but retrospective sib-pair analyses of this type can be complicated by diagnostic misclassification.[38,39]

Over the past several years, cDNA microarray methods have been used to identify endometriosis-related genes. Giudice and colleagues[40] were among the first to use Affymetrix chips with arrayed oligonucleotides and observed that many progesterone-regulated genes are relatively down-regulated in eutopic (intrauterine) endometrium of women with endometriosis. This effect appears to be most dramatic for gene expression in the early secretory phase of the cycle (Fig. 24-4).[41] Genes involved in oxidative stress, and the Wnt and MAP (mitogen-activated protein) kinase signaling pathways have been consistently reported.[42] Our group[43] focused on the reduced expression of glycodelin mRNA, which encodes a progesterone-regulated, secreted glycoprotein associated with immunologic tolerance of the semiallogeneic blastocyst. These findings are consistent with a comprehensive meta-analysis showing lower embryonic implantation rates in women with advanced endometriosis undergoing in vitro fertilization. This study is discussed in more detail later.

Another powerful genomic screening technique was introduced by Liang and Pardee in 1992.[44] Differential display–polymerase chain reaction (dd-PCR), in a fashion akin to subtraction hybridization, employs random sets of oligonucleotide primers and PCR to amplify fragments of differentially expressed cDNAs from two different tissues. Endometriotic implants and biopsies of eutopic endometrium from normal and endometriosis cases were obtained in the mid-proliferative phase of the ovulatory cycle and analyzed by Lundeen et al.[45] using this technique. One interesting PCR product was observed to be consistently up-regulated in ectopic and eutopic endometriotic tissue relative to normal eutopic endometrium. The cDNA was shown to correspond to the zinc-finger transcription factor, early growth response-1 (EGR-1). EGR-1 is an interesting candidate because it can be activated by a variety of upstream signaling molecules that are known to be associated with endometriosis, including

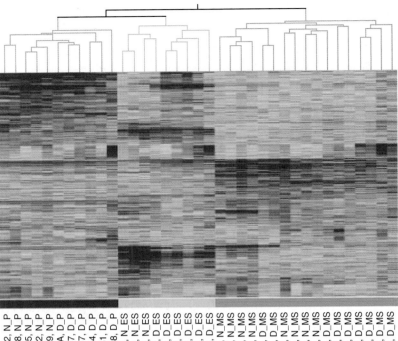

Figure 24-4. *Hierarchical clustering analysis of endometrial gene expression from subjects with moderate/severe endometriosis (D) and subjects without disease (N) in the proliferative (P, red), early secretory (ES, gold), and mid-secretory (MS, light blue) phases. (From Burney RO, Talbi S, Hamilton AE, et al. Gene expression analysis of endometrium reveals progesterone resistance and candidate susceptibility genes in women with endometriosis. Endocrinology 148[8]:3814-3826, 2007.)*

estradiol, interleukin (IL) lβ, IL-6, and tumor necrosis factor-α (TNF-α).[43]

Lebovic et al.[46] compared cDNAs expressed in normal endometrial stromal cells with those derived from endometriotic implants, with and without pretreatment with the inflammatory cytokine IL-lβ. Endometriotic stromal cells substantially down-regulated a tumor suppressor gene (*TOB1*) in response to IL-1β treatment, whereas normal endometrial stromal cells showed no effect of IL-1β. *TOB1* is an endogenous inhibitor of the *ERBB2* receptor, a member of the epidermal growth factor receptor family that is overexpressed in many human cancers. Monoclonal antibodies directed against this receptor, such as trastuzumab, and other inhibitors of *ERBB2* have been shown to reduce the progression of metastatic breast cancer.[47] In a similar study of normal endometrial stromal cells, Rossi et al. found angiogenic and extracellular matrix remodeling genes were up-regulated by IL-1β.[48] The significance of these findings in endometriosis is that endometriotic stromal cells appear to have a growth advantage in an inflammatory environment, mediated by the attenuation of a natural inhibitor of mitotic activity induced through the *ERBB2* receptor pathway.

A new development in the genetics of endometriosis is the identification of micro-RNA expression. These small RNAs hybridize with mRNA transcripts and induce their degradation, functionally repressing gene actions. Micro-RNAs have been identified that would be expected to reduce production of steroid receptors known to be down-regulated in endometriosis. These may become interesting new targets for endometriosis therapeutics.[49]

CYTOGENETICS OF ENDOMETRIOSIS

Cytogenetic methods that assess gene content in intact or microdissected endometriotic tissues include chromosome satellite painting and comparative genomic hybridization. Kosugi et al.[50] used fluorescence in situ hybridization (FISH) to find substantially increased aneuploidy and loss of heterozygosity of chromosome 17 in endometriotic lesions. Interestingly, this chromosomal region is the location of several tumor suppressor genes important in the normal regulation of the mitotic cycle. Among these is the *p53* locus, which is lost in cases of severe endometriosis,[51] and the *TOB1* tumor suppressor, noted to be preferentially down-regulated in endometriotic cells treated with IL-1β.[46] A 50% loss of heterozygosity (LoH) for chromosomes 1p and 22q was noted by Gogusev et al.[52] in endometriotic implants. Lower levels of LoH also have been reported for chromosomes 9p and 11q.[53] These findings suggest that genomic instability is a feature of endometriosis.

Comparative genomic hybridization is a technique based on the competitive in situ hybridization of differentially labeled DNA from endometriosis and normal endometrial tissue to human metaphase spreads. Regions of gain of DNA sequences are seen as an increased color ratio of the two fluorochromes labeling the respective DNAs. Using this method, Gogusev and colleagues in Paris identified chromosomal regions in which gene copy numbers are altered in endometriosis.[52] In an established endometriosis cell line (FbEM-1), these investigators observed that the *c-ERBB2* proto-oncogene was overexpressed.[54] This result complements the finding that *TOB1* is reduced in endometriosis and suggests that *ERBB2* signaling is important in endometriosis.

GENETIC POLYMORPHISMS IN ENDOMETRIOSIS

Several candidate gene polymorphisms have been evaluated in women with endometriosis. In general, these have fallen into three major classes, each representing presumed pathogenetic abnormalities:

1. Genes involved in xenobiotic metabolism
2. Genes that mediate inflammatory responses
3. Genes regulating steroid action

An *N*-acetyltransferase 2 allele (*NAT2*4/*6*) was significantly more common among affected women (35.2%) than population control subjects (8.1%) or unaffected women (4.2%; *P* = 0.02). More affected women (57.4%) were found to be "fast acetylators" than were population control subjects (32.3%) or unaffected women (33.3%; *P* < 0.05). Altered NAT2 enzyme activity, which would enhance the rate of xenobiotic acetylation, may be a predisposing factor in endometriosis.[55]

Based on the observation that women with vaginal agenesis carried N314D mutations in the *GALT* gene regulating galactose metabolism (galactose-1-phosphate uridyl transferase [GALT] activity),[56] Cramer et al.[57] speculated that this defect also might be associated with increased retrograde menstruation and may predispose to endometriosis.

In the latter study they observed that women with endometriosis were more likely to carry at least one N314D allele of the *GALT* gene versus control subjects (30% compared with 14% in their initial study). This association, however, has not been confirmed in other populations.[58]

Viganò et al. reported a polymorphism of the intercellular adhesion molecule-1 (*ICAM-1*) in women with severe endometriosis.[59] The implication of such a protein, where abnormal cellular adhesion is suspected, deserves further investigation. Despite the hypothesis that dioxins and other environmental toxicants might play an etiologic role in endometriosis,[29] Japanese women with this condition were not observed to have an increased incidence of polymorphisms in the aryl hydrocarbon receptor gene or associated factors studied to date.[29] Variants in the glutathione S transferase genes were reported by Baranova et al.[60] in a group of French and Slavic women with endometriosis, but the same polymorphisms were not identified in subjects from the United Kingdom.[61] A polymorphism in the 5′ untranslated region of the human *VEGF* (vascular endothelial growth factor) gene (+405G>C) also has been correlated with an increased risk of endometriosis development in Italian Caucasian, South Indian, and Korean populations.[62]

Inconsistent observations reflect some of the inherent methodologic problems with genetic association studies. In particular, the recruitment of relatively small numbers of preexisting cases and the willingness of these subjects to participate in research can bias the results. There also are pitfalls in control recruitment, including the use of patients who have other diseases as control subjects. Failure to replicate findings in a different ethnic group may not mean that the original study is flawed, but could reflect differences in allele frequency between populations. Finally, if gene-environment interactions affect the magnitude of a genetic risk factor, another population may not be exposed to the same environmental factor as in the original study.

NUCLEAR RECEPTOR GENES AS BIOMARKERS OF ENDOMETRIOSIS RISK

Homozygosity for a *Pvu II* polymorphism in the estrogen receptor *(ER)-α* gene was found less frequently in women with endometriosis when compared with a disease-free group.[63] A variant progesterone receptor *(PR)* allele, called *PROGINS*, is characterized by an *Alu* insertion in intron G and two additional mutations in exons 4 and 5. The *PROGINS* allele codes for a progesterone receptor with increased stability and augmented hormone-induced transcriptional activity. Homozygosity for this allele was present in 3.2% of women with endometriosis and 0.9% of control subjects.[64] This result is at odds with the evidence that progesterone action is decreased in endometriotic tissue, due to a relative decrease in the ratio of PR-B (which generally activates gene transcription) to PR-A (which generally suppresses transcription) isoforms.[65]

Bulun and colleagues observed that ERβ mRNA is overexpressed approximately 40-fold and PR-B is underexpressed by 88% in endometriotic tissue. The apparent mechanism in the former case involves hypomethylation of CpG islands in the ERβ gene promoter, indicating that epigenetic regulation may, in part, explain this observation.[66]

Familial aggregation of endometriosis also could be attributed to epigenetic factors, and although sparse, recent evidence supports this interesting hypothesis. Another pertinent gene that was found to be hypomethylated in endometriosis is the homeobox transcription factor HOXA10. This protein also is expressed in midsecretory phase endometrium and its expression is reduced in clinical endometriosis and in an induced baboon model of the disorder.[67,68]

Clinical Presentation

SYMPTOMS AND SIGNS

The most common symptom in women with endometriosis is progressive, secondary dysmenorrhea. The pain usually begins before menses and continues throughout the duration of menstrual flow. It may be accompanied by dyspareunia, dysuria, or dyschezia. The pain also may be referred to musculoskeletal regions, such as the flank or low back. Cyclic in situ menstruation at the site of an endometriotic lesion is believed to result in a chronic inflammatory nidus. Cytokine release and activation of prostaglandin-mediated pain perception, or direct infiltration of endometriotic cells into afferent nerves have been proposed.[69] Furthermore, the enhanced inflammatory milieu may result in sensitization of nociceptors and central neurons.[70]

The second most common symptom is infertility with monthly fecundity rates similar to unexplained infertility patients at 0.02 to 0.10. It has long been accepted that women with moderate and severe endometriosis have fertility problems due to the mechanical interference with sperm-egg union or zygote transport, as a result of pelvic adhesions and disruption of normal anatomy. Interestingly, women with minimal or mild endometriosis also have decreased fertility outcomes when compared with those patients without clinical evidence of disease. The exact causes remain elusive to date, but several postulated mechanisms are addressed later in this chapter.

Unfortunately, due to the diffuse and pusillanimous nature of endometriotic lesions, the physical examination is commonly unrevealing. The bimanual examination is of limited precision in either localization or diagnosis of endometriosis. However, the astute clinician can appreciate pain or induration in the vicinity of otherwise nonpalpable lesions, most commonly in the cul-de-sac or rectovaginal septum. Tender nodules may be palpable along the uterosacral ligaments or within the cul-de-sac, especially if the examination is done just before the menses. Rarely, impaired renal function and azotemia can develop in women with retroperitoneal ureteric fibrosis.

Ectopic endometrium within the uterine corpus is termed adenomyosis, and although this entity is not covered in this chapter, there seems to be an association between adenomyosis and endometriosis. Utilizing junctional zone measurements from magnetic resonance imaging (MRI) to diagnose adenomyosis in patients with endometriosis, the prevalence of adenomyosis was 90% in one recent study.[71] Interstitial cystitis is another comorbidity in at least 60% of women with endometriosis.[72]

DIAGNOSIS

Direct visualization of endometriotic implants is the current gold standard for diagnosis. Although endometriosis is associated with certain biochemical characteristics (described later in this section), none of these features have adequate sensitivity or specificity for clinical application. Hence, laparoscopy, and rarely laparotomy, are the most common means to establish a firm diagnosis. The histopathologic confirmation of endometriosis is established on the microscopic identification of ectopic endometrial epithelium and stroma, often with fibrosis and the infiltration of hemosiderin-laden macrophages. These pathognomonic features are documented in only approximately 70% of clinically suspicious cases.

Radiologic imaging techniques have been evaluated as noninvasive approaches to endometriosis diagnosis, but these methods have not replaced surgical verification of lesions. The diagnostic sensitivity and specificity of imaging modalities are reviewed later in this chapter.

Because disease is found in the dependent areas of the pelvis, performance of a systematic rectovaginal examination is critical. Some authors have advocated the use of needle biopsy to confirm the histologic features of the nodular rectovaginal lesion.[73]

VARIABLE LESION APPEARANCE

Visually, peritoneal endometriosis can take on a variety of appearances. Classically, physicians were taught that endometriosis implants were blue-black "powder burns" or "mulberry lesions" of the peritoneum. In recent years, several stages of implant development have been appreciated, each with a corresponding appearance. Early, active lesions can appear as papular excrescences or vesicles, and can range in color from clear to bright red.[74] About one third of lesions are in phase with the eutopic endometrium and have a tendency to spontaneously grow and regress. This characteristic suggests a fluctuating proliferation in association with hormone production during the menstrual cycle.[75]

Advanced, active lesions are associated with inflammation, fibrosis, and hemorrhage, and they take on the more classic pigmented appearance (Fig. 24-5). These lesions can express myriad colors—black, brown, purple, red, or green—due to the presence of heme degradation products as the foci undergo periodic hemorrhage and fibrosis. Dormant and healing lesions appear white or calcified, reflecting remnants of glands embedded in fibrous tissue.[74] In one recent histologic study, visually white and mixed-color lesions were more likely to contain histologic evidence of endometriosis than were black or red lesions.[76]

Although difficult to prove in cross-sectional clinical studies, endometriosis appears to be a progressive disease, as evidenced by longitudinal laparoscopies in female baboons.[77] At least eight studies were reported of repeat laparoscopy in women assigned placebo treatment.[78-85] Combining these placebo participants yields a total of 163 women that confirm that endometriosis is a disease in flux. There was a nearly equal distribution among women whose disease stage deteriorated (31%), was unchanged

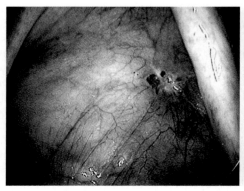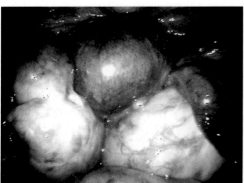

Figure 24-5. Laparoscopic photographs of pigmented peritoneal implant (left) and bilateral ovarian endometriomas, or so-called "kissing ovaries" (right). *(Images courtesy of Dr. Michael D. Mueller, University of Bern, Switzerland.)*

(32%), or improved (38%). In fact, all but one study noted that 23% of placebo patients had complete regression of disease over intervals of 4 to 39 months (Table 24-1). Regrettably, this means for over two thirds of women the disease will either persist or progress, and this situation must be addressed with postoperative medical management.

An evolution of the visual appearance of the lesions from clear to red to black to white has been suggested to correlate with the subject's age.[86] This observation implies that the appearance of endometriotic lesions may correlate with their biology. Deeply invasive lesions of the rectovaginal septum have the histologic characteristic of smooth muscle hyperplasia, so-called *adenomyotic nodular endometriosis*. Some argue that this reflects a unique histogenesis from müllerian remnants,[20] but other authors accept that these lesions also may be manifestations of retrograde menstruation and implantation.[87,88]

A specific manifestation is the *endometrioma*, or *chocolate cyst* (see Fig. 24-5). These ovarian cysts gained their moniker by the characteristic chocolate syrup appearance of their contents, often seen at rupture. These cysts arise after implantation of ectopic endometrial tissue and subsequent invasion into the ovarian cortex or alternatively as a result of metaplasia (Fig. 24-6).[22] The cell types present in these cysts include endometrial epithelium (both as glands and flattened cells), endometrial stroma, and hemosiderin-laden macrophages. In some cases ciliated cells, similar to those of oviduct epithelium, have been observed.[89] It is reported that pelvic pain associated with endometrioma is positively correlated with ovarian blood flow and microvascular density, suggesting that enhanced angiogenesis may relate to symptoms.[90] Techniques to culture the endometriotic lining of these cysts[91] have been widely adapted and allow a reliable and reproducible source of primary endometriosis cells for in vitro research.

Under scanning electron microscopy, microscopic lesions have been found in the normal-appearing peritoneum of women with and without endometriosis.[92] The clinical significance of these findings is a matter of controversy at present, but researchers argue that the prevalence of histologic endometriosis may be underestimated.

CLASSIFICATION

The system most widely used to classify the extent of endometriosis was promulgated by the American Fertility Society in 1985.[93] This scheme designates disease extent based upon total three-dimensional volume of endometriosis. Importance is placed upon depth of invasion, bilaterality, and ovarian involvement, as well as density of associated adhesions and extent of cul-de-sac involvement. Using this classification, scores are tallied to objectify and compare natural history and treatment outcomes among different centers and surgeons. Scores of 1 to 15 reflect minimal or

TABLE 24-1

Natural Course of Endometriosis

Study	Increase in Disease	No Change	Decrease in Disease [Elimination]
Thomas EJ, 1987[79]*			
Stage I-III, n = 17 6 mo follow-up L/S	47% (8)	24% (4)	29% (5) [18% (3)]
Telimaa S, 1987[78]*			
Stage I-II, n = 17 6 mo follow-up L/S	25% (4)	63% (10)	19% (3) [13% (2)]
Cooke ID, 1989[80]*			
Stage I-II, n = 17 6 mo follow-up L/S	47% (8)	24% (4)	29% (5) [18% (3)]
Mahmood TA, 1990[81]*			
Stage I-III, n = 11 9-18 mo follow-up L/S	64% (7)	9% (1)	27% (3) [9% (1)]
Overton CE, 1994[82]*			
Stage I-II, n = 15 6-9 mo follow-up L/S	27% (4)	20% (3)	53% (8) [NR]
Sutton CJ, 1997[83]			
Stage I-III, n = 24 6-39 mo follow-up L/S	29% (7)	42% (10)	29% (7) [4% (1)]
Harrison RF, 2000[84]*			
All stages, n = 43 4-6 mo follow-up L/S	9% (4)	28% (12)	63% (27) [44% (19)]
Abbott J, 2004[85]			
Stage II-IV, n = 19 6 mo follow-up L/S	42% (8)	42% (10)	29% (7) [4% (1)]
Totals (n = 163)	31% (50)	32% (50)	38% (62) [23% (29)]

*Infertile patients.
L/S, laparoscopy; NR, not reported.

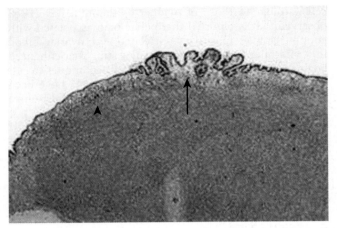

Figure 24-6. *Presumptive development of ovarian endometrioma via surface epithelial metaplasia. Low-power view of an endometriotic lesion arising in ovarian surface epithelium. The typical or well-developed area of endometriosis is seen in the center of the lesion (arrow), with transition from minimal epithelial changes from normal ovarian surface epithelium on the sides of the focal lesion (arrowhead). (From Zheng W, Li N, Wang J, et al. Initial endometriosis showing direct morphologic evidence of metaplasia in the pathogenesis of ovarian endometriosis. Int J Gynecol Pathol 24[2]:164-172, 2005.)*

mild disease; 16 to 40, moderate; and over 40, severe. It is important to note that this staging system was established to predict fertility outcomes, and it has not been shown to correlate with the more common symptom of pelvic pain.[94] Some authors have suggested the incorporation of objective biochemical markers of inflammation as a means to assess disease parameters beyond laparoscopically visible lesions.[95,96] Future studies will evaluate the utility of the latter recommendations.

RADIOLOGIC IMAGING

Economic pressures and perioperative risks associated with surgical staging have stimulated attempts to develop noninvasive tests for endometriosis. Radiologic evaluation by MRI and ultrasonography show some promise.

Compared with other imaging modalities, MRI is the best technique to identify endometriosis. It lacks, however, sufficient sensitivity and specificity, especially in the detection of small implants and adhesions. MRI also may have a role in evaluating treatment response with endometriosis patients receiving medical therapies such as danazol, progestins, or gonadotropin-releasing hormone analogs.[97, 98]

Overall sensitivity of MRI in the detection of endometrial implants is 77%, with a specificity of 78%.[99] MRI identification of endometriomas is more satisfactory and has high sensitivity (90% to 92%) and specificity (91% to 98%) rates.[97] MRI scans of endometriomas are characteristically identified by "shading," with homogeneous hyperintensity on T_1-weighted images and relative hypointensity on T_2-weighted images. The signal intensity pattern is consistent with the presence of intracellular methemoglobin (Fig. 24-7). Endometriomas may have a complex appearance, usually related to the presence of blood clots or debris within the cyst, and in this setting use of intravenous contrast material may be helpful in distinguishing these products from more worrisome ovarian neoplasms.

ULTRASONOGRAPHY

Endometriomas may be difficult to differentiate from ovarian neoplasms by ultrasonographic features alone. Recurrent episodes of bleeding and surrounding inflammation sometimes result in a heterogeneous internal appearance (suggesting solid components), a thickened wall, or apparent septations. Apparent septations may be particularly misleading because they can reflect compressed ovarian parenchyma intervening between the endometrioma and a satellite cyst. Endometriomas tend to be well vascularized and Doppler blood flow may erroneously suggest a neoplastic mass.

Although endometriomas may mimic neoplasms, they typically demonstrate a characteristic sonographic appearance. Because of ease of use, cost-effectiveness, and accessibility, transvaginal ultrasonography has become the imaging modality of choice when evaluating the ovary for an endometrioma.[100] The classic endometrioma has diffuse low-amplitude internal echoes, enhanced sound transmission, and a visible uniform wall, sometimes containing bright reflectors (see Fig. 24-7).[101,102] The reflectors have been postulated to represent red blood cell breakdown

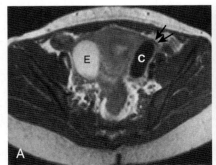
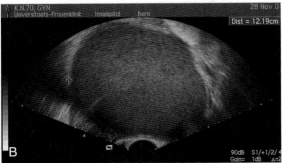

Figure 24-7. *A, Magnetic resonance imaging of the pelvis reveals characteristic high signal intensity in the right ovarian lesion suggesting an endometrioma (E). The low signal intensity lesion of the left ovary is consistent with a simple ovarian cyst (C). Note enhancement of the periphery of the cyst (arrows). B, Transvaginal ultrasonography reveals a cystic adnexal mass with diffuse, homogenous moderate-level echoes consistent with an endometrioma. (Part A from Jaffe R, Pierson RA, Abramowicz JS (eds). Imaging in Infertility and Reproductive Endocrinology. Philadelphia, Lippincott, 1994; part B courtesy of Dr. Michael D. Mueller, University of Bern, Switzerland.)*

products. About 50% of ovarian masses that are histologically confirmed endometriomas demonstrate this characteristic sonographic appearance.[103] Although the same appearance may occur in an acutely hemorrhagic cyst, the latter will evolve or resolve over time but an endometrioma usually remains stable or enlarges. Serial sonograms are often necessary before the physician may reliably assume that a mass is an endometrioma.

SERUM MARKERS OF ENDOMETRIOSIS

Although they might provide great clinical value, serum markers of endometriosis have proved to be elusive. The best studied of these is the tumor marker CA-125. This transmembrane glycoprotein, initially identified in serous ovarian carcinomas, was noted by Barbieri and colleagues to circulate at elevated concentrations in women with endometriosis.[104] The CA-125 gene has yet to be fully characterized, but it encodes a 4-megadalton product with repetitive peptide motifs and O-linked polysaccharides, which is synthesized and secreted by cells of coelomic origin.[105] Some authors have found this marker to be a better correlate of active endometriotic lesions than peritoneal adhesions, and it may have utility in monitoring the progression of disease or recurrence during therapy.[106] Although the sensitivity of preoperative CA-125 for the detection of endometriosis is too low for a screening test, high concentrations may be predictive of advanced disease.[107] The addition of serum soluble ICAM-1 only modestly improved the sensitivity of concomitant CA-125 screening for endometriosis.[108]

Two recent papers have addressed the use of serum biomarkers in the identification of women with endometriosis. Othman and colleagues reported significantly elevated levels of IL-6, monocyte chemoattractant protein-1 (MCP-1), and interferon-γ (IFN-γ) in the serum of women with endometriosis relative to infertile controls without laparoscopic evidence of endometriosis.[109] Among these, IL-6 was the most predictive biomarker. An algorithm including several of the same cytokines was found to perform better than any individual analyte in separating endometriosis and control subjects in a similar study.[110] Zhang et al. used two-dimensional gel electrophoresis and serum proteomics to identify elevated levels of actin, heat shock, and complement-associated proteins in cases of endometriosis.[111] This unbiased strategy may be a fruitful approach to discover new biomarkers.

Pathogenesis

HORMONE RESPONSIVENESS (STEROIDS AND NUCLEAR RECEPTORS)

One of the defining characteristics of endometriosis is its endocrine responsiveness. Typically endometriosis only becomes symptomatic after the onset of menses[112] and, in the majority of cases, resolves spontaneously with menopause. An unusual case of persistent postmenopausal endometriosis led investigators to the discovery that aromatase expression and estradiol biosynthesis occurred

within the endometriotic implant per se.[113] Aromatase activity is particularly high in ovarian endometrioma (Fig. 24-8).[114] Relative overexpression of the orphan nuclear receptor SF-1 in endometriotic cells appears to be a major reason for increased aromatase activity in these lesions.[115] Steroid biosynthesis and metabolism are clearly intrinsic activities within these lesions. Also identified in ectopic endometrial tissues were messenger RNA transcripts encoding steroid acute regulatory (StAR) protein,[116] which controls the delivery of cholesterol to the inner membrane of mitochondria, cholesterol P450 side chain cleavage (SCC) enzyme, 3β-hydroxysteroid dehydrogenase type 2, and 17α-hydroxylase. Further, oxidative metabolism of estradiol to the less biologically active estrone by 17β-hydroxysteroid dehydrogenase type 2 is decreased in endometriosis, aggravating local estrogen action.[117] Thus, endometriotic lesions appear to have co-opted the ability to generate their own estrogenic milieu (Fig. 24-9).

Like their derivative eutopic endometrium, endometriotic lesions express estrogen and progesterone receptors. Over the years, however, several authors have indicated that concentrations of these steroid receptor proteins may be altered in endometriotic implants.[118-120] In cultured stromal cells from these lesions, both estrogen[121] and progesterone receptor[65] isoform expression appear to differ from those in normal endometrium. These differences may impart a growth advantage to endometriotic implant cells. Estrogen receptor β is highly expressed in endometriosis and is an emerging target for new therapeutics.[122] The roles of androgen action in endometriosis are as yet poorly defined; however, androgen receptors are expressed

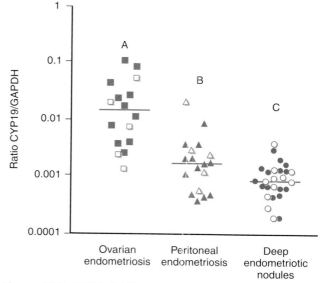

Figure 24-8. *CYP19 (P450 aromatase) expression in ovarian endometriosis (A), peritoneal endometriosis (B), and deeply invasive endometriosis (C) of the rectovaginal septum. Data are expressed relative to glyceraldehyde-3-phosphate dehydrogenase (GAPDH) mRNA. Filled symbols represent patients under medical treatment; scatters with different letters are significantly different at a level of $P = 0.05$ (bar indicates median, note log scale along abscissa). (From Heilier JF, Donnez O, Van Kerckhove V, et al. Expression of aromatase [P450 aromatase/CYP19] in peritoneal and ovarian endometriotic tissues and deep endometriotic [adenomyotic] nodules of the rectovaginal septum. Fertil Steril 85[5]:1516-1518, 2006.)*

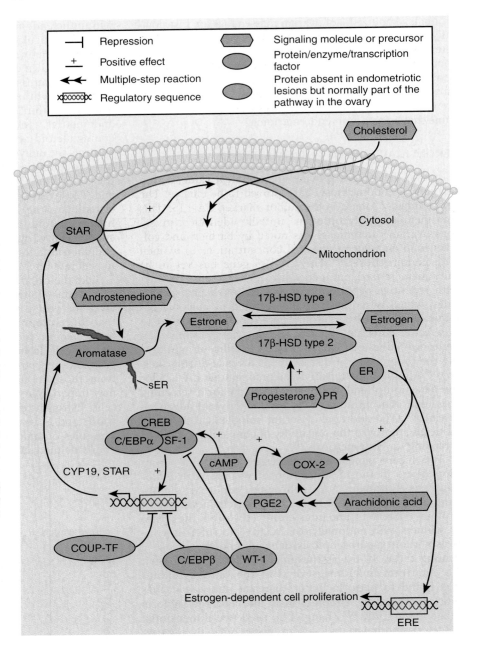

Figure 24-9. *Steroid biosynthesis and metabolism in endometriotic lesions and their effects on inflammation and growth. All the enzymes necessary for de novo steroid biosynthesis from cholesterol are expressed in stromal cells isolated from endometriotic implants. Among these, the steroid acute regulatory (StAR) protein, aromatase P450, and 17β-HSD type 1 appear to be the most highly regulated in this cell type. StAR and aromatase activities are modulated via the cAMP pathway and the transcription of these genes is activated by the aberrant expression of steroidogenic factor-1 (SF-1), resulting in estradiol synthesis and lesion proliferation. Cyclic AMP response element binding protein (CREB) and CCAT/enhancer binding protein alpha (C/EBPα) also participate in the regulation of these genes, whereas chicken ovalbumin upstream promoter-transcription factor (COUP-TF) and C/EBPβ can interfere with steroidogenesis. Prostaglandin synthesis and metabolism via the intermediates prostaglandin H_2 and prostaglandin E_2 are regulated by cyclooxygenase-2 (COX-2), which in turn is controlled by estradiol and cytokines, contributing to inflammation and a feedforward effect on local estradiol production. (From Simsa P, Mihalyi A, Kyama CM, et al. Selective estrogen-receptor modulators and aromatase inhibitors: promising new medical therapies for endometriosis? Women's Health 3:617-628, 2007.)*

in normal endometrium and endometriosis lesions,[123] and clinical evidence supports the efficacy of danazol therapy for relief of pain associated with endometriosis.[124]

LESION ESTABLISHMENT (ADHESION, PROTEOLYSIS, INVASION)

As discussed previously, the Sampson hypothesis[8] posits that viable endometrial cells spill into the peritoneal cavity apposing the peritoneal surface and adhere to the mesothelial monolayer. Although some controversy exists as to whether or not such invasion requires an a priori breach in the mesothelial surface[125] or if the cells are capable of invading intact mesothelium,[18] this is a necessary step in lesion establishment. The expression

of hyaluronic acid (peritoneum) and its receptor, CD44 (endometrium), have been proposed to play a role in this early attachment step.[126] Enhanced cytokine (e.g., IL-lβ, IL-6, and TNF-α) expression and action in the eutopic endometrium of women with endometriosis[127] may predispose the adhesion of shed endometrial fragments in these cases. The ability of endometriotic cells to invade the peritoneal surface has stimulated extensive research into their cancer-like proteolytic properties.[128] The identification of specific matrix metalloproteinases (MMPs), which themselves are regulated by cytokines and ovarian steroid hormones, has been a particularly active area of investigation.[129,130] In the eutopic endometrium, these enzymes and their endogenous inhibitors (TIMPs), are activated and repressed, respectively, following hormone

TABLE 24-2

**Cytokines and Growth Factors
in Peritoneal Fluid**

Concentrations Increased in Endometriosis

Complement	Badawy et al., 1984[131]
Eotaxin	Hornung et al., 2000[132]
Glycodelin	Koninckx et al., 1992[133]
Interleukins (IL)	
IL-1	Anderson and Hill, 1987[134]
IL-6	Rier et al., 1994[135]
IL-8	Ryan et al., 1995[136]
Monocyte chemoattractant protein 1 (MCP-1)	Akoum et al., 1996[137]
Platelet-derived growth factor (PDGF)	Halme et al., 1988[138]
RANTES (regulated upon activation, normal T cell expressed and secreted)	Khorram et al., 1993[139]
Soluble intercellular adhesion molecule-1 (ICAM-1)	Daniel et al., 2000[140]
Transforming growth factor β (TGF-β)	Oosterlynck et al., 1994[141]
Vascular endothelial growth factor (VEGF)	Shifren et al., 1996[142]

Concentrations Unchanged in Endometriosis

Epidermal growth factor (EGF)	De Leon et al., 1986[143]
Basic fibroblast growth factor (FGF)	Huang et al., 1996[144]
Interferon-γ (IFN-γ), Interleukins	Khorram et al., 1993[139]
IL-2	Keenan et al., 1995[145]
IL-4	Gazvani et al., 2001[146]
IL-12	Mazzeo et al., 1998[147]

Concentrations Decreased in Endometriosis

IL-13	McLaren et al., 1997[148]
IL-1RA	Zhang et al., 2007[149]

withdrawal in the late luteal phase of the cycle. Implications of this work suggest that hormonal medications, particularly progestins, may inhibit invasive behavior. However, relative steroid hormone insensitivity and increased cytokine activity observed in endometriotic tissues may enhance MMP action in endometriosis, facilitating peritoneal invasion.

PROLIFERATION AND APOPTOSIS

A variety of human growth factors stimulate endometrial cell mitogenic activity. Many of these factors also have been identified in endometriotic tissues and in the peritoneal fluid of women with endometriosis. Although their precise roles in endometriosis are not well known, these factors are potential regulators of endometriosis implant proliferation. Table 24-2 summarizes the principal mitogens detected in the pelvic fluid of women with endometriosis and compares their concentrations with women without evidence of this disorder. The table provides reference sources for more detailed information.

Programmed cell death (apoptosis) is also an important mechanism for the cyclical remodeling of the endometrium.[150] Eutopic endometrial apoptosis was found to be decreased in women with endometriosis[151] and in endometriotic epithelium.[152] These findings indicate another potential selective advantage for the persistence of endometriotic lesions within the peritoneal cavity.[153]

ANGIOGENIC FACTORS

Given the ubiquity of retrograde menstruation, it is not clear why endometriosis only develops in a subset of women. Using the analogy of tumor metastasis[154,155] some authors have postulated that the angiogenic potential of the intraperitoneal environment may predict the likelihood that lesions become established.[156,157] Indeed, on visualization, endometriotic implants are often surrounded by exaggerated vascularity; extrapelvic endometriosis, while rare, typically occurs in well-vascularized sites.[158] This concept is consistent with other analogous aspects of endometriosis pathogenesis and cancer biology. In addition to increased angiogenesis, endometriotic lesions manifest enhanced proliferative, adhesive, and invasive capacity; more LoH and genomic instability; and decreased apoptosis.

The sprouting of new blood vessels from preexisting vessels is complex and includes the proteolytic degradation of extracellular matrix, proliferation and migration of endothelial cells, and ultimately the formation of patent capillary tubules supplying the angiogenic stimulus. Many different growth factors and cytokines have been shown to exert chemotactic, mitogenic, or inhibitory activities on endothelial cells, smooth muscle cells, and pericytes. Increased IL-1β sensitivity increases the angiogenic potential of endometriosis lesions.[159] An attractive interpretation of this finding (assuming the Sampson hypothesis is accepted) is that the endometrial lining of women destined to develop endometriosis already manifests an "activated" angiogenic phenotype. As an analogy to Knudson's "two-hit" hypothesis of oncogenesis,[160] women susceptible to the development of endometriosis may carry a "first hit" genetic trait that enhances endometrial cell angiogenic factor production. This proposal is in keeping with the familial trends observed in cases of endometriosis.[27,36,161] Angiogenic activity within advanced stage endometriomas appears to be particularly robust.[162]

Although pelvic fluid is a complex medium containing and influenced by multiple cell types, we and other investigators have found this to be a useful biologic medium to define intercellular mediators of the local reactions associated with endometriosis.[136,139,163] Peritoneal fluid seems to play an important role in the process of neovascularization. Oosterlynck et al.[163] used the chick chorioallantoic membrane bioassay to show that pelvic fluid from women with endometriosis had more angiogenic activity than pelvic fluid from healthy control subjects. We confirmed this observation using an in vitro model of human endothelial cell proliferation. Thymidine incorporation into nascent cellular DNA demonstrated that peritoneal fluid from women with endometriosis contains substantially more angiogenic activity than pelvic fluid from normal control subjects.[156]

A vast array of angiogenic principles are synthesized by human endometrium and endometriosis. Among these are basic fibroblast growth factor, IL-6, IL-8, platelet-derived growth factor, and vascular endothelial growth factor (VEGF), which is the most potent of these (see Table 24-2). We initially reported that endometrial VEGF levels were expressed highest in the midsecretory phase of the cycle, a time when estradiol and progesterone levels were elevated, and confirmed VEGF expression in endometriotic implants.[142] Other studies using immunohistochemistry and endometrial cultures corroborate these findings.[164] These two ovarian steroid hormones have direct transcriptional effects on the human VEGF gene promoter.[165,166] VEGF, IL-6, and IL-8 mRNA were noted to be substantially up-regulated in endometriomas in relation to normal ovarian tissue.[167,168] In totality, these findings suggest that the local expression of angiogenic cytokines in endometriosis implants contributes to implant neovascularization and may correlate with symptoms.[90]

FIBROSIS

Biochemical principles secreted by endometriotic lesions (perhaps in response to apoptosis) or their neighboring cells may contribute to the fibrosis and adhesions that classically surround the implants and adjoining pelvic organs.[169,170] Indeed, TGF-β, a growth factor associated with other types of intraperitoneal adhesion formation,[171] was noted to be elevated in peritoneal fluid of women with endometriosis.[141]

OXIDATIVE STRESS AND ENDOMETRIOSIS

The role of oxygen free radicals as mediators of the cellular pathology associated with endometriosis has been postulated in recent years. *Free radicals* are highly reactive molecules that transiently contain one or two unpaired electrons. The transfer of electrons to other structural or regulatory molecules can induce cell damage. Most free radicals of biologic significance are referred to as *reactive oxygen species* (ROS), such as hydroxyl (HO•), peroxyl (ROO•) or superoxide (O_2•−) radicals. Oxidative stress implies a homeostatic deviation, wherein the pro-oxidant environment exceeds the defensive ability of antioxidant vitamins and enzymes in a physiologic system. Endometrial stromal cells in vitro have a mitogenic response to oxidative stress[172] and free radicals may contribute to lesion proliferation and invasion.

Murphy et al. found that peritoneal fluid levels of the antioxidant vitamin E were decreased and the ratio of lysophosphatidylcholine to phosphatidylcholine increased in women with endometriosis.[173] These findings were interpreted to reflect increased lipid peroxidation in endometriosis. However, attempts by others to directly assay lipid peroxidation by measurements of malondialdehyde[174] or 2,2′-azino-di-3-ethylbenzthiazoline sulfonate reduction[175] failed to detect differences between endometriosis subjects and control subjects. Nevertheless, this novel hypothesis is an excellent focus of further investigation.[176]

INFLAMMATION (IMMUNE CELLS, CHEMOKINES, CYTOKINES, PROSTAGLANDINS)

The accumulation of immune cells within the peritoneal cavity and endometriotic lesions has been recognized in women with this disorder for over 15 years.[177-179] This phenomenon is thought to be initiated via the innate immune system, which is not antigen-specific and has no memory. Granulocytes, natural killer (NK) cells, and macrophages are the major cells providing this type of defense and they are recruited into tissues via the expression of soluble chemoattractant proteins referred to as *chemokines*. Given the predominant monocytic inflammatory response in endometriosis, chemokines specific for this cell lineage have been evaluated and identified in peritoneal fluid and endometriotic lesions. In particular, IL-8, MCP-1, and RANTES (regulated upon activation, normal T cell expressed and secreted) have been studied intensively. Specific references to these important chemokines are provided in Table 24-2, and the general topic of peritoneal chemokines has been reviewed in recent literature in detail.[180]

We have postulated that the accumulation of peritoneal macrophages initiates a rather complex network of chemokines, cytokines, and growth factors that contribute to the pathophysiology of endometriosis.[181] This hypothesis is summarized in Figure 24-10. The activation of autoregulatory loops may contribute to a feedforward amplification of local inflammation within endometriotic implants.

Adaptive immunity, by contrast, refers to that "learned" by experience and induces an enhanced anamnestic response with repeated antigen exposure. T and B lymphocytes and antibody-producing plasma cells are the primary cell types providing adaptive immunity. Weed and Arquembourg[182] first observed IgG and complement deposits in the eutopic endometrium of women with endometriosis and proposed that development of endometrial autoantibodies might explain poor reproductive outcomes in some women with this syndrome. Elevated levels of complement component C3 also were noted in peritoneal fluid of women with endometriosis.[131] Increased concentrations of T cells were observed in baboons with spontaneous endometriosis but not in those with surgically induced disease. This observation led the authors to suggest that an underlying immunocyte abnormality might precede, rather than reflect a response to, intraperitoneal endometrial implants.[183]

In the 1980s, serum of women with endometriosis was used to identify endometrial autoantigens by Western blotting methods. Similar findings were confirmed with enzyme-linked immunosorption assays against solubilized endometrial antigens and endometrial cell monolayers.[184] It has been suggested that a generalized adaptive immune response, manifested by polyclonal B-cell activation, occurs in some cases of endometriosis.[185]

Leukocytes recruited and activated by endometriosis-derived chemokines secrete a variety of soluble inflammatory mediators. Particularly potent among these are proinflammatory cytokines (reviewed in Table 24-2) and prostaglandins. These mediators also have intrinsic vasoactive and pain-activating properties and are thought to lie along a critical common pathway involved in the symptoms of endometriosis.[181]

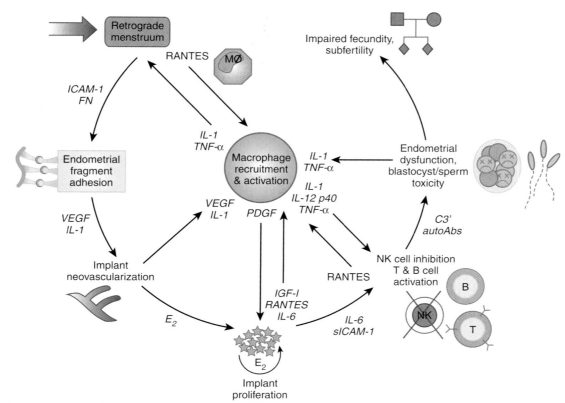

Figure 24-10. *Schematogram depicting the network of chemokines, cytokines, and growth factors in the pathophysiology of endometriosis. autoAbs, autoantibodies; C3', complement 3; E_2, estradiol; FN, fibronectin; sICAM, soluble intercellular adhesion molecule; IGF-1, insulin-like growth factor-1; IL, interleukin; MØ, macrophage; NK cell, natural killer cell; PDGF, platelet-derived growth factor; RANTES, regulated on activation, normal T cell expressed and secreted; TNF, tumor necrosis factor; VEGF, vascular endothelial growth factor.*

Although no clear associations were found in early genotyping studies assessing the major histocompatibility type I and II loci (HLA-A, -B, and -DR),[186,187] more recent immunohistochemical analyses of tissues from women with endometriosis suggest an increased expression of HLA-DR antigen in endometrial and endometriotic epithelial cells than what is seen in other infertile control subjects.[188] Moreover, the coincidence of surgically confirmed endometriosis with other autoimmune disorders, including systemic lupus erythematosus, Sjögren's syndrome, rheumatoid arthritis, and multiple sclerosis, was documented in a self-reported, cross-sectional survey of more than 3500 members of the North American Endometriosis Association.[189] In a recent histochemical and microarray study of ovarian endometriosis, macrophages, plasma cells, complement proteins, and a B-lymphocyte stimulating cytokine (BLyS), all were found to be markedly upregulated relative to matched eutopic endometrium. These same markers are elevated in other autoimmune diseases, including systemic lupus erythematosus, Sjögren's syndrome, and rheumatoid arthritis.[190]

IMMUNOSURVEILLANCE

An intriguing concept in the etiology of endometriosis is defective immunosurveillance in susceptible women. If normal eutopic endometrium elicited an immune response, antiendometrial autoantibodies would be prevalent

in all women rather than a subset of cases with endometriosis.[191] Hence, adaptive immunity toward these cells seems to occur as a result of their ectopic location. As an overwhelming majority of cycling women regurgitate menstrual endometrium into the peritoneal cavity, why does endometriosis occur in only 10% to 15% of these individuals?

In normal women, intraperitoneal menstrual debris appears to be eliminated without loss of immune tolerance, presumably mediated by CD8+ T cells and immunosuppressive cytokines (e.g., IL-13, IL-1RA). However, as noted in other autoimmune disorders, immune tolerance might break down in endometriosis, resulting in the recognition of ectopic implants by a chronic inflammatory response. Induction of so-called "blocking antibodies" or tolerance to endometrial antigens[192] have been postulated but never confirmed. Nevertheless, defects in NK cell activity and reduced production of immunosuppressive cytokines have been reported in cases of endometriosis. For example, ICAM-1 may interfere with peritoneal immunosurveillance and allow refluxed endometrium to escape clearance from the peritoneal cavity.[193] Increased concentrations of this protein have been noted in pelvic fluid of women with endometriosis.[140] Endometrial cells also are inherently resistant to apoptosis and phagocytosis,[194] yet endometriosis only occurs in a minority of menstruating women, as previously noted. Some researchers have suggested that mediators of the innate immune system, particularly macrophages and

NK cells, clear regurgitated endometrial cells from the peritoneal cavity. Oosterlynck et al. first described decreased NK cell cytotoxicity against endometrial and hematopoietic cells in women with endometriosis.[195] The same group showed that peritoneal fluid from women with endometriosis contained more soluble NK cell suppressive activity than peritoneal fluid from fertile control subjects.

We postulated that expression or secretion of the nonclassical major histocompatibility antigen HLA-G by endometriotic cells might inhibit NK cell function in this setting, but were unable to detect this protein in ectopic or eutopic endometrial stromal cells or tissues by Western blotting, and no soluble HLA-G protein was detectable in peritoneal fluid.[196] However, using in situ methods, Barrier and colleagues observed HLA-G in endometriotic glands.[197] Interestingly, reduced expression of other anti-inflammatory cytokines (i.e., IL-13 and IL-1RA) was reported in the peritoneal fluid of women with endometriosis.[148,149]

POSSIBLE MECHANISMS OF ENDOMETRIOSIS-ASSOCIATED INFERTILITY

How mild to moderate endometriosis reduces fertility is among the most controversial aspects of research in this field. In addition to mechanical effects of lesions and adhesions on the adnexa, evidence supports the hypothesis that endometriosis causes an immunologically hostile environment within the pelvis. Evidence from oocyte donor programs indicates that egg or early embryonic development are disturbed in women with endometriosis[198,199] and specific chemokine concentrations are elevated in the follicular fluid of affected women undergoing in vitro fertilization (IVF).[200] The resolution of this critical issue will advance our understanding of endometriosis-associated infertility and should pave the way to improved therapies.

In general, inflammatory responses in the vicinity of the ectopic endometrial implants are thought to impair sperm transport,[201] tubal motility,[202] and oocyte development.[203] In situ menstruation within endometriotic lesions has been proposed to cause adhesion formation, fibrosis, and proximal tubal obstruction.[204,205] Moreover, the eutopic endometrium of women with endometriosis manifests a variety of histologic and biochemical perturbations, including increased immune cell infiltration[178] and increased cytokine and chemokine expression.[127,206,207] Increased concentrations of complement component C3[177] and decreased $\alpha v \beta 3$ integrin,[208] glycodelin,[209] HOX-A10, and HOX-A11[210] have been reported. Based on our current knowledge of their functions, down-regulation of the latter four gene products would be predicted to cause impaired implantation.

High peritoneal fluid concentrations of prostaglandins have been noted by some authors but not by others. As these are rapidly acting autocrine and paracrine substances, circulating levels may not be revealing. Prostanoids offer an attractive mechanism for endometriosis-associated pain and also may affect fertility via interference with tubal motility and ovum pick-up.[211]

Some data indicate that the spontaneous abortion rate is increased in women with endometriosis,[212] although this finding has been disputed in other studies.[213] In a meta-analysis of IVF outcomes, women with advanced endometriosis had substantially lower fertilization and implantation rates compared with other indications.[214] These observations are discussed in further detail later in this chapter.

ENDOMETRIOSIS AND GENITAL TRACT CARCINOMA

Endometriosis is identified concurrently in approximately 17% of ovarian carcinoma cases, and the diagnosis of endometriosis is reported to carry a 7.4-fold increased risk for ovarian cancer (most commonly endometrioid and clear cell) even when controlling for parity.[215] The majority of cases are associated with unopposed estrogen replacement therapy in postmenopausal women. A new murine model that combined an oncogenic K-ras allele activation with a tissue-specific conditional knock-out of the tumor suppressor Pten resulted in aggressive and widely metastatic endometrioid ovarian adenocarcinoma, recapitulating the histomorphologic appearance seen in the human disease (Fig. 24-11).[216]

A rare but serious complication of cervical endometriosis is the misclassification of cervicovaginal cytologic smears as harboring a high-grade intraepithelial lesion, atypical glandular cells of undetermined significance, or even an adenocarcinoma in situ.[217]

Treatment

SURGICAL THERAPY FOR PAIN ASSOCIATED WITH ENDOMETRIOSIS

Owing to their peritoneal location, most endometriotic lesions are amenable to laparoscopic extirpation. Techniques involving aggressive implant excision, electrofulguration, or laser vaporization have been adapted through endoscopic ports and these procedures have been taught widely to gynecologic surgeons. It is relatively rare that laparotomy or hysterectomy is necessary in the treatment of women who wish to preserve their uterus.

Figure 24-11. *Combined K-ras^{G12D} activation and conditional deletion of Pten lead to endometrioid ovarian cancer. **A**, A single intrabursal injection of adenoviral vector expressing Cre recombinase (AdCre) in LSL-K-ras$^{G12D/+}$ Pten$^{loxP/loxP}$ mice on one side results in hemorrhagic ascites and a large, cystic ovarian tumor (T, arrow) normal (N, arrowhead). **B**, Histopathologic appearance of endometrioid ovarian carcinomas. Areas of solid growth with squamous differentiation (black arrow), confluent glandular pattern areas (black arrowhead), and hemorrhage (red arrow) are shown. The remaining normal ovary is depicted by the white contour and arrow. **C**, AdCre-infected Pten$^{loxP/loxP}$ ovaries show normal ovarian surface epithelium (arrow) at 12 weeks after injection. **D** and **E**, Peritoneal tumor implants with a cribriform glandular architecture (**D**) or a villoglandular growth pattern (**E**, arrowhead). **F** and **G**, Peritoneal tumor implants (arrowhead) infiltrate the pancreas (**F**) and liver (**G**). **H**, Tumor cells circulating through a lymphovascular channel (arrow) are seen near the lung metastasis (arrowhead). (From Dinulescu DM, Ince TA, Quade BJ, et al. Role of K-ras and Pten in the development of mouse models of endometriosis and endometrioid ovarian cancer. Nat Med 11[1]:63-70, 2005.)*

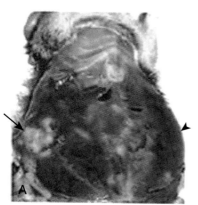

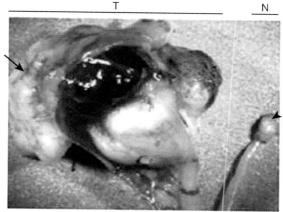

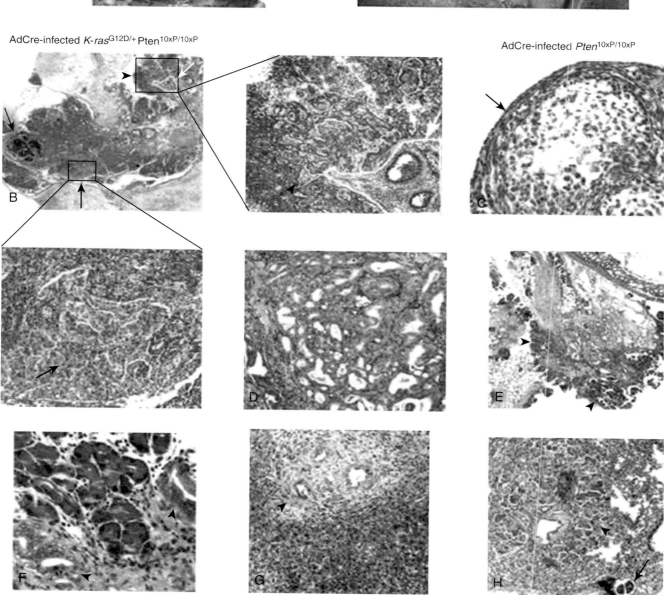

One of the first evidence-based evaluations of laparoscopic treatment of endometriosis-associated pelvic pain was carried out in the United Kingdom in the early 1990s. Sutton and colleagues conducted a randomized, prospective, double-blind trial in 63 patients with minimal to moderate endometriosis. Half of the subjects underwent laser ablation of endometriotic deposits and laparoscopic uterine nerve ablation, and the others received a diagnostic laparoscopy and expectant management. Pain symptoms quantified by a visual analog scale were significantly improved in 62.5% of those receiving laser ablation, compared with 22.6% in the expectant group at 6 months after surgery.[218] In a long-term follow-up study of the laser-treated cohort (approximately 72 months after surgery), continued symptom relief was reported in 55.3% of the respondents.[219] In a more recent randomized, blinded, crossover pain study, Abbott et al. demonstrated an 80% success rate in excisional endometriosis surgery compared to an approximately 30% response to sham surgery. The effects were independent of extent of disease.[85] These reports substantiate a therapeutic role for laser laparoscopy in the management of endometriosis pain and indicate that the median time to pain recurrence after surgical treatment was 20 months. Future innovations in endoscopic surgery for endometriosis may include targeted energy absorption, such as photosensitization of the lesions using hematoporphyrin derivatives[220] or autofluorescence to detect nonpigmented endometriotic lesions.[221]

Treatment of ovarian endometriomas (chocolate cysts) can be particularly challenging. These respond very poorly to medical therapy, and hence, operative extirpation is the preferred approach. Jones and Sutton treated 73 consecutive cases of endometrioma larger than 2 cm by laser or bipolar diathermy. After 1 year, 16.4% of subjects had recurrences. This prognosis was noted to be particularly more likely if the cysts were bilateral.[222] According to a recent Cochrane Review, excision was better than drainage and ablation for (1) recurrence of the endometrioma, (2) recurrence of symptoms, and (3) fertility outcome.[223]

Definitive treatment for endometriosis consisting of a hysterectomy with removal of both ovaries leads to the dilemma of postoperative hormonal therapy (for hypoestrogenemia) in the face of exacerbating residual endometriosis. The recurrence rate with hormonal therapy is 3.5% or 0.9% per year and there is no greater risk of recurrence of pain if estrogen is started immediately after surgery compared with a 6-month delay.[224]

MEDICAL THERAPY FOR PAIN ASSOCIATED WITH ENDOMETRIOSIS

Hormonal treatments approved for endometriosis treatment by the U.S. Food and Drug Administration (FDA) include gonadotropin-releasing hormone analogue (GnRHa), depot medroxyprogesterone acetate, and the androgen danazol. In addition, continuous oral contraceptives have been evaluated and are widely used.[225] The majority of evidence supporting medical therapy for endometriosis is observational; however, some randomized clinical trials have been evaluated.[226] An evidence-based assessment of treatment of endometriosis-associated pelvic pain in two randomized, placebo-controlled trials indicated that medroxyprogesterone acetate, danazol, or GnRHa were all more effective than placebo. Pain relief of more than 6 months' duration was noted in 40% to 70% of women.[227]

Although highly effective in the management of chronic pain with endometriosis, GnRHa treatment has been limited to 6 months by the FDA because of the hypoestrogenic effects induced by ovarian suppression. The previously mentioned principle of an estrogen threshold (see Fig. 24-4)[26] has been used to overcome this limitation. Suppression of the hypothalamic-pituitary axis with GnRHa is now accompanied with "add-back" of exogenous ovarian steroids. Dose-seeking trials have identified "add-back" regimens that reverse vasomotor symptoms and bone mineral loss. The combination of GnRHa with progestins alone did not prove to be protective for bone.[228] Add-back regimens consisting of norethindrone acetate combined with low-dose estrogen can safely extend pain relief and bone preservation for at least 1 year, and one trial with a limited number of participants found no ill effect after 10 years of add-back therapy.[229,230] Three months of the nasal spray formulation of GnRHa seemed to be as effective as a 6-month course.[231] Another option is subcutaneous depot medroxyprogesterone. Two randomized, clinical trials demonstrated that the 6 months of subcutaneous progestin was as effective as leuprolide acetate in diminishing endometriosis-associated pain.[232,233] Drop-out rates were significant for both groups, however. The purported benefits of the subcutaneous progestin are decreased cost, easier administration, and more favorable effect on bone mineral density.

In a double-blind, placebo-controlled, crossover study, a nonsteroidal anti-inflammatory drug (naproxen) was twice as effective as placebo in relief of secondary dysmenorrhea associated with endometriosis.[234] High levels of cyclooxygenase-2 (COX-2) are expressed in endometriotic lesions,[235] implying that selective COX-2 inhibitors might also be of clinical benefit. Although this class of drugs is effective in the treatment of primary dysmenorrhea,[236] the limited data available from endometriosis trials were inconclusive.[237]

EXPERIMENTAL MEDICAL THERAPY

Like COX-2 inhibitors, a variety of evolving new medical treatments hold theoretical promise for the treatment of endometriosis-associated pain and inflammation. GnRH antagonists, which induce an immediate suppression of gonadotropin production without the initial "flare" effect of the GnRH superagonists,[238] may be advantageous in this setting.[239] Selective estrogen receptor modulators (SERMs) also may be of theoretical benefit. Due to its partial agonist activity within the endometrium, tamoxifen can exacerbate endometriosis.[240] Although raloxifene was shown to reduce endometriosis in murine and rhesus models of this disease,[241] a preliminary clinical trial unexpectedly showed exacerbation of this SERM on pain symptoms.[242] Through their effects on estrogen production and action, aromatase inhibitors[113] have been proposed as new therapeutics in endometriosis.[243] Acceptance must await larger clinical trials. Although there is no randomized controlled trial, an

TABLE 24-3

Effects of Medicinal Herbs Used for Treatment of Endometriosis

Medicinal Herbs	Anti-proliferative	Anti-nociceptive	Anti-oxidant	COX-2↓	Cytokines↓	NF-κB↓
Bupleurum	+					
Chinese angelica	+	+	+		+	+
Dahurian angelica	+	+			+	
Cattail pollen				+	+	+
Cinnamon twigs		+		+	+	
Cnidium fruit	+	+				
Corydalis		+				
Curcuma	+	+		+	+	
Cyperus	+		+	+	+	+
Frankincense	+	+				
Licorice root	+	+			+	+
Myrrh		+		+	+	+
Persica			+		+	
Poria	+	+		+	+	
Red peony root			+			
Rhubarb	+	+			+	+
Salvia root		+	+			+
Scutellaria	+					+
Sparganium		+			+	
Tortoise shell					+	+
White peony root				+	+	

From Wieser F, Cohen M, Gaeddert A, et al. Evolution of medical treatment for endometriosis: back to the roots? Hum Reprod Update 13:487-499, 2007.

early open-label, nonrandomized proof-of-concept study suggests a benefit in the treatment of rectovaginal endometriosis.[244] Endometriosis in this anatomic location also expresses the aromatase enzyme (see Fig. 24-8).[114]

Progesterone receptor modulators also have also been investigated.[245] Early experiences with high and low doses of the antiprogestin mifepristone showed an improvement in pelvic pain without ostensible regression of peritoneal implants.[246,247] The antiglucocorticoid effects of this class of compounds, and their ability to create a hyperestrogenic endometrial milieu,[248] are likely to limit clinical applicability. Interesting recent in vitro studies suggest that part of the effectiveness of mifepristone might be due to its antioxidant properties.[249] Ligands for another nuclear receptor, peroxisome proliferator-activated receptor (PPAR)-γ, were shown to reduce RANTES and IL-8 secretion and the proliferation of endometriotic stromal cells; inhibit macrophage activation and migration in in vitro and murine models of endometriosis;[250-252] and to reduce endometriotic lesion volume in rat and baboon models of the disease.[253-256]

Therapeutic agents that target cytokine production and action also are under investigation as possible clinical adjuncts for endometriosis treatment. Using a rat model of endometriosis there was efficacy shown with imiquimod (toll-like receptor agonist), recombinant human INF-α-2b, leflunomide, and levamisole.[257-260] Administration of recombinant TNF-binding protein-1 or anti-TNF-α monoclonal antibody c5N inhibited the development of endometriosis in a baboon model[261,262] and blockade of VEGF action in mouse endometrium can be achieved using soluble VEGF-R1 (sflt-1).[263] Future applications of the same strategies may possibly be useful in clinical endometriosis.

A novel approach to the treatment of pain associated with deep, rectovaginal endometriosis was introduced[264] in a prospective, self-controlled trial of 11 symptomatic patients with rectovaginal endometriosis. Use of a levonorgestrel-releasing intrauterine device for 12 months resulted in significant improvement in dysmenorrhea, pelvic pain, and deep dyspareunia, and objective resolution of the size of rectovaginal endometriotic lesions by ultrasonography was noted. Another trial found similar pain relief after 6 months of therapy comparing the levonorgestrel intrauterine device with GnRHa.[265] Other agents that may have some potential if confirmed in larger clinical trials include, etonogestrel nonbiodegradable contraceptive implant, bufalin, BAY 11-7085, (a soluble inhibitor of NK-κB activation), French maritime pine bark extract, yiweining, rapamycin, metformin, human chorionic gonadotropins, melatonin, genistein, atorvastatin, trichostatin A, and vaginal danazol.[266-274]

Evidence is accumulating to suggest that medicinal botanicals with anti-inflammatory and pain-alleviating properties hold promise for treatment of endometriosis. Although their safety remains untested formally, in general these additives are not thought to impair ovulation or fertilization and hence may be taken by women attempting conception. Medicinal herbs and their active components exhibit cytokine-suppressive, COX-2-inhibiting, antioxidant, sedative, and pain-alleviating properties, which would be predicted to have salutary effects in endometriosis. Although controlled, randomized clinical trials are rare, phytotherapies with a long tradition of safe use (e.g., curcumin and its analogs) have multiple beneficial characteristics and should be evaluated more thoroughly (Table 24-3).[275]

SURGICAL THERAPY FOR INFERTILITY ASSOCIATED WITH ENDOMETRIOSIS

The role of laparoscopic surgery in the amelioration of infertility in women with minimal to mild endometriosis has long been an accepted dictum. This question was objectively addressed in a recent meta-analysis of two randomized controlled trials: the multicenter Canadian trial[276] and a smaller Italian study.[277] In this analysis, destruction of lesions—even in early-stage disease with infertility—led to improved pregnancy rates in women attempting spontaneous conception. One of the criticisms of the Canadian study is that adhesiolysis was performed preferentially in the surgical treatment group and that this intervention, rather than lesion ablation per se, may have accounted for the higher pregnancy rate. Based upon the larger (and more positive) of the two studies,[273] an additional pregnancy was achieved for every eight operative laparoscopies performed (Fig. 24-12). Given an estimated prevalence of 30% endometriosis in an otherwise undiagnosed infertile population, the total number of laparoscopic cases to yield a single additional pregnancy would jump to 24. Hence, although a place exists for surgical treatment of endometriosis-associated infertility, it carries a relatively high cost.

No published trials compare surgical treatment versus no treatment in women with moderate to severe endometriosis; however, many publications cite a near-zero pregnancy rate for women with extensive disease. Uncontrolled trials show increased pregnancy rates for these women if normal pelvic anatomy is restored.[278]

When considering surgical extirpation of endometriomas, the data are limited and conflicting. Some studies indicate that cystectomy may be deleterious to residual oocyte and hormone function,[279,280] whereas another showed no differences in fertility outcomes between those women with resected endometriomas, those with endometriosis, and those with tubal infertility.[281] The study of Beretta et al.[282] demonstrated better pain and fertility outcomes after cystectomy compared with drainage and coagulation. A recent Cochrane review of the published literature supports this recommendation.[223] Further studies will be needed to clarify the risk-to-benefit ratio of endometrioma excision in women with endometriosis-associated infertility.

In cases of infertility due to moderate-to-severe endometriosis, some authors have advocated combined medical and surgical therapy.[283] The current medical treatments are described later in this section, but due to their anovulatory side effects, these treatments impair fertility in the short term.

MEDICAL THERAPY FOR INFERTILITY ASSOCIATED WITH ENDOMETRIOSIS

Most established medical therapies are aimed at inhibition of ovulation as a means of interrupting hormonal stimulation of endometriotic implants. Therefore, these approaches are used only for short periods of time to decrease the size or activation state of endometriotic lesions prior to attempted conception. Five trials using six different treatments were compared with placebo or no treatment. Another eight randomized trials were performed in which danazol was compared with a second medication. A meta-analysis[284] of several trials showed no differences between the treatment and control arms with respect to fertility outcomes (odds ratio = 0.85; 95% confidence interval, 0.45-1.22). However, when one considers the time from diagnosis, commencement of medical treatment, and interruption of ovulation versus no treatment, patients undergoing medical treatment had a substantially lower monthly fecundity rate than control subjects because of the loss of opportunities for conception.[277] Conventional hormonal regimens, therefore, have no place in the treatment of endometriosis-associated infertility.

Superovulation has been studied in three randomized trials and led to an improved clinical pregnancy rate in women with endometriosis.[285-287] Whether or not intrauterine insemination is of any added benefit remains to be determined.

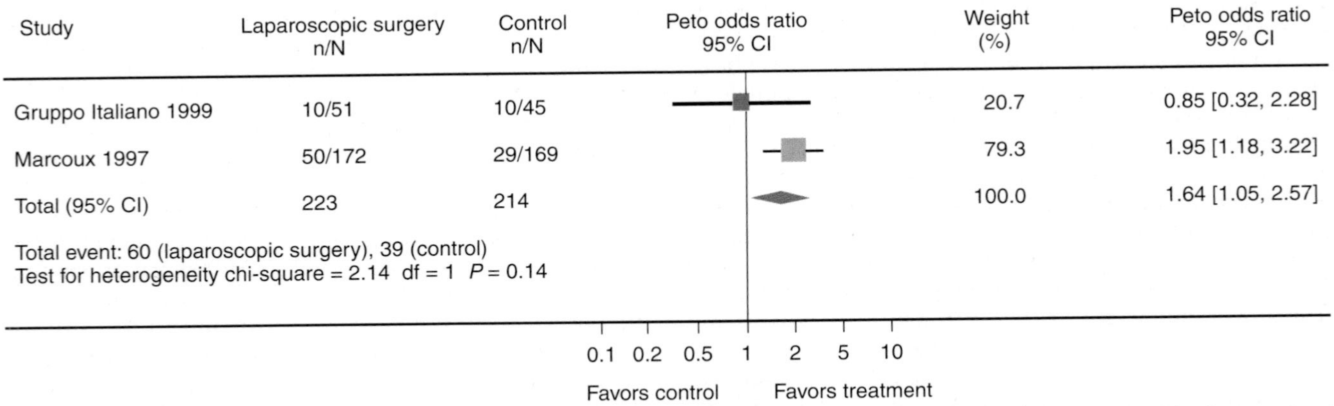

Study	Laparoscopic surgery n/N	Control n/N	Peto odds ratio 95% CI	Weight (%)	Peto odds ratio 95% CI
Gruppo Italiano 1999	10/51	10/45		20.7	0.85 [0.32, 2.28]
Marcoux 1997	50/172	29/169		79.3	1.95 [1.18, 3.22]
Total (95% CI)	223	214		100.0	1.64 [1.05, 2.57]

Total event: 60 (laparoscopic surgery), 39 (control)
Test for heterogeneity chi-square = 2.14 df = 1 $P = 0.14$

0.1 0.2 0.5 1 2 5 10

Favors control   Favors treatment

Figure 24-12. Meta-analysis of the two randomized trials assessing the efficacy of laparoscopic surgery in the treatment of subfertility associated with minimal-to-mild endometriosis. Combining live birth and ongoing pregnancy data from the two studies shows an improvement with laparoscopic surgical treatment (OR 1.64, 95%; CI 1.05-2.57). (From Jacobson TZ, Barlow DH, Koninckx PR, et al. Laparoscopic surgery for subfertility associated with endometriosis. df, degrees of freedom. Cochrane Database Syst Rev 4:CD001398, 2002.)

ASSISTED REPRODUCTIVE TECHNOLOGY

Three randomized trials have been done comparing ovulation induction[287] and ovulation induction combined with intrauterine insemination in women with endometriosis.[285,286] It was clearly shown in these studies that these treatments enhanced fertility relative to timed coitus alone.

A single randomized controlled IVF trial was reported, but only 15 patients underwent IVF and six had no treatment. These numbers are too small to derive meaningful conclusions.[288] In a retrospective study, no differences were found in women undergoing IVF versus expectant management over a 3-year period.[289] Although it seems that IVF may reduce the time to pregnancy, it is unknown whether it actually increases the absolute pregnancy rate. Further trials will be needed before recommendations can be made.

In a meta-analysis of 22 independent studies, Barnhart and colleagues[214] determined that the overall likelihood of achieving pregnancy was significantly lower for stage III-IV endometriosis patients (adjusted odds ratio, 0.56; 95% confidence interval, 0.44-0.70) compared with tubal factor control subjects. Multivariate analysis demonstrated a decrease in fertilization and implantation rates and fewer oocytes in the endometriosis subjects.

Summary

Although recognized for centuries, the etiology and pathogenesis of endometriosis remain topics of intense debate and investigation. The classical theories of histogenesis have been replaced by a neoclassical concept that this is a complex, multigenic disorder influenced by epigenetic and environmental factors. Definitive establishment of a clinical diagnosis requires direct observation, and ideally histopathologic confirmation of ectopic endometriotic implants. However, a presumptive clinical impression (supported by physical findings and confirmatory radiologic imaging) is adequate for most clinicians to initiate therapy.[290] Future confirmatory biochemical tests, based on endometrial biopsy findings, and possibly by serum analytes may reduce the necessity of laparoscopic evaluation for diagnosis. However, surgical treatment of endometriosis, perhaps with improved means of endoscopic lesion ablation, will likely retain a prominent place in endometriosis therapy.

The development of new medical treatments for endometriosis will parallel our further understanding of its underlying pathophysiology. Increased concentrations of activated pelvic macrophages and lymphocytes and elevated levels of specific cytokines and growth factors support the hypothesis that the immune response is activated in endometriosis. Angiogenesis inhibitors may play a more prominent therapeutic role in the future, but care must be taken to avoid the potential teratogenic side effects of this drug class. Medicinal herbs, despite millennia of clinical use, remain untested formally and

potentially harbor untoward effects on ovulation, fertilization, or embryonic development. Whether components of the innate and adaptive immune systems play primary, causative roles, or merely reflect a reaction to the presence of ectopic implants, is unknown at present. A complex network of locally produced chemokines, cytokines, and prostaglandins is proposed to modulate the growth and inflammatory behavior of endometriosis—affecting implant proliferation and invasion, the recruitment of capillaries to the growing lesions, and further attraction of leukocytes to foci of peritoneal inflammation. Future endometriosis therapeutics will need to exploit our identification of relatively specific targets within pathways that regulate the growth and invasion of endometriotic lesions, ideally sparing or correcting the function of a woman's eutopic endometrium.

The complete reference list can be found on the companion Expert Consult Web site at www.expertconsultbook.com.

Suggested Readings

Attar E, Bulun SE. Aromatase inhibitors: the next generation of therapeutics for endometriosis? Fertil Steril 85(5):1307-1318, 2006.

Brosens I, Puttemans P, Campo R, et al. Non-invasive methods of diagnosis of endometriosis. Curr Opin Obstet Gynecol 15(6):519-522, 2003.

Buchweitz O, Staebler A, Tio J, Kiesel L. Detection of peritoneal endometriotic lesions by autofluorescence laparoscopy. Am J Obstet Gynecol 195(4):949-954, 2006.

De Hondt A, Meuleman C, Tomassetti C, et al. Endometriosis and assisted reproduction: the role for reproductive surgery? Curr Opin Obstet Gynecol 18(4):374-379, 2006.

DiZerega GS, Barber DL, Hodgen GD. Endometriosis the role of ovarian steroids in initiation, maintenance and suppression. Fertil Steril 33:649-653, 1980.

Giudice LC, Kao LC. Endometriosis. Lancet 364(9447):1789-1799, 2004.

Halme J, Becker S, Haskell S. Altered maturation and function of peritoneal macrophages possible role of pathogenesis of endometriosis. Am J Obstet Gynecol 56:783-789, 1987.

Jacobson TZ, Barlow DH, Koninckx PR, et al. Laparoscopic surgery for subfertility associated with endometriosis. Cochrane Database Syst Rev. CD001398, 2002.

Jaffe R, Pierson RA, Abramowicz JS. Imaging in infertility and reproductive endocrinology. Philadelphia, Lippincott, 1994.

Kao LC, Germeyer A, Tulac S, et al. Expression profiling of endometrium from women with endometriosis reveals candidate genes for disease-based implantation failure and infertility. Endocrinology 144(7):2870-2881, 2003.

Lebovic DI, Mueller MD, Taylor RN. Immunobiology of endometriosis. Fertil Steril 75(1):1-10, 2001.

Marcoux S, Maheux R, Berube S, et al. Canadian Collaboration Group on Endometriosis. Laparoscopic surgery in infertile women with minimal or mild endometriosis. N Engl J Med 377:212-222, 1997.

Sampson JA. Peritoneal endometriosis due to menstrual dissemination of endometrial tissue into the peritoneal cavity. Am J Obstet Gynecol 71:422-469, 1927.

Simsa P, Mihalyi A, Kyama CM, et al. Selective estrogen-receptor modulators and aromatase inhibitors: promising new medical therapies for endometriosis? Women's Health 3:617-628, 2007.

Somigliana E, Vigano P, Parazzini F, et al. Association between endometriosis and cancer: a comprehensive review and a critical analysis of clinical and epidemiological evidence. Gynecol Oncol 101(2):331-341, 2006.

Vercellini P, Abbiati A, Daguati R, et al. Endometriosis: current and future medical therapies. Best Pract Res Clin Obstet Gynaecol 22(2):275-306, 2008.

CHAPTER 25

Benign Uterine Disorders

Elizabeth A. Stewart

The traditional concept of the uterus is that the endometrium is the dynamic tissue, providing an intricate set of functions throughout the menstrual cycle that rarely culminates in implantation and pregnancy. The myometrium has been viewed as an inert tissue chiefly important during pregnancy and, when abnormal, being a major cause of gynecologic surgical procedures.

However, to understand both the physiology of menstruation and the pathophysiology of abnormal uterine bleeding, both the myometrial and the endometrial layers of the uterus are important. First, both myometrial processes (adenomyosis and leiomyomas) and endometrial processes (polyps) can result in abnormal uterine bleeding. Second, on the molecular level, because the mass of the myometrial layer is so much greater than that of the endometrial layer, the myometrium can act as a reservoir of growth factors or immune cells that then may act on the endometrium in a paracrine or local endocrine fashion.

The study of uterine molecular mechanisms is in its infancy. Study of the human uterus is difficult because all the surgical specimens available for in vitro study are by definition abnormal. Additionally, many of the disorders that cause abnormal uterine bleeding (such as leiomyomas) appear to be heterogeneous in their molecular mechanisms. Just as the clinical phenotype of polycystic ovaries can result from various molecular defects, leiomyomas likely have many underlying genetic etiologies and environmental stimuli.

Nevertheless, basic investigation is beginning to reveal a number of common molecular mechanisms shared by phenotypically different diseases such as leiomyomas, adenomyosis, and endometrial polyps. We can speculate that in the future these diseases may be classified on the basis of molecular defects rather than on microscopy. This would allow us to understand the genotype/phenotype relationships that we currently find puzzling: for example, why some women have profound menorrhagia with these diseases and others are asymptomatic. Understanding new elements of the biology of these diseases will lead to innovative therapy.[1]

Our lack of understanding of molecular physiology and pathophysiology has left us with extirpative surgical treatment as our therapeutic mainstay. Although we have become more elegent in our surgical approach, the high risk of recurrent disease following conservative surgeries indicates that understanding the underlying mechanism and moving toward prevention are likely to be more successful.

The fact that modern women spend a larger percentage of their lifespan menstruating compared with women in previous centuries and females of other species may also contribute to many pathologic conditions. Many genes are differentially regulated at specific parts of the menstrual cycle. Thus, constantly turning the same molecular switches on and off may have the same effect as constantly turning a light switch on and off: the system becomes disrupted. This fact, as well as physiologic differences between species, has made it difficult to use animal models to study the function of uterine tissue.

Finally, the economic implications of these diseases are significant. The cost of leiomyomas alone in the United States has been estimated at $2.1 billion annually.[2] Lost productivity due to clinically significant leiomyomas is also a substantial cost, accounting for over 40% of total costs which average in excess of $4800 per woman per year in a commercially insured population.[3] Neither of these figures takes into account the cost of sanitary protection, alternative and complementary remedies, or the costs of women who are symptomatic but not seeking care.

Uterine Leiomyomata

EPIDEMIOLOGY

Uterine leiomyomas, frequently termed myomas or fibroids, are benign clonal smooth muscle cell tumors ranging in size from several millimeters to many centimeters (Fig. 25-1). Clinically, they are appreciated in approximately 25% of all women and in black women appear to have a threefold increased incidence and relative risk.[4] Careful pathologic study of surgical specimens suggests approximately 77% of women have detectable leiomyomas, a proportion that parallels the lifetime incidence of clinical disease.[5,6] Thus, in black women, it appears there is little occult disease, suggesting that in this group, growth acceleration of transformed myocytes into clinical fibroids may be ubiquitous.[5,7] Black women are significantly more likely to have leiomyomas than white, Latina, or Asian women and to be younger at the time of diagnosis and hysterectomy.[4,8-10] They also have more severe diseases.[8,10]

Known risk factors don't adequately explain this racial disparity.[11] However, a recent study has suggested that the experience of racism may have an influence on fibroid risk.[12] Understanding the unique genetic and environmental factors leading to increased risk for black women is a key part of the research agenda for leiomyomas.

Reproductive factors also affect the risk of leiomyomas. Numerous studies have shown that parity decreases the chance of fibroid formation.[11,13,14] One hypothesis is that the remodeling of the postpartum uterus can clear nascent fibroids.[15] Although clinical dogma traditionally suggested that oral contraceptive pills (OCPs) were contraindicated

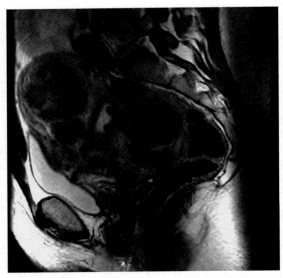

Figure 25-1. *A T₂-weighted fast-spin echo (FSE) sagittal image of the leiomyomatous uterus. The sagittal image allows the endometrial cavity to be seen in continuity with the cervix and is often the easiest image to visualize the clinically important submucous fibroids. Two small submucous lesions are seen in the posterior portion of the endometrial cavity in this image but may be less clinically important than the larger intramural myoma abutting the posterior part of the endometrial cavity. The visualization of the sacrum and coccyx allows assessment of the bulk effects of the leiomyoma in the pelvis.*

for women with myomas, OCPs instead protect against clinically evident fibroids with the caveat that timing of use may be important.[11,13,14] Exposure to OCPs between ages 13 and 16 for women in the Nurses' Health Study led to an increased relative risk of leiomyomas, but later OCP use was protective in direct proportion to duration of use.[11] Progestin-only injectable contraceptives also appear to decrease risk of fibroid formation.[16] Thus, a more acyclic environment may be more important than specific steroid levels.

Environmental factors also influence the risk of fibroid formation. Dietary habits appear to influence risk of myoma formation. Significant consumption of red meats was associated with an increased relative risk of fibroids and consumption of green vegetables with a decreased risk of myomas.[17] Also, increased intake of alcohol, especially beer, appears to increase risk in black women.[18] However, no one has demonstrated that dietary intervention leads to changes in fibroid incidence or symptomatology. Increased body mass index (BMI) or weight gain since age 18 also appears to influence myoma risk in some cohorts.[9,19,20] Finally, women with leiomyomas appear to be more likely to have hypertensive disease than control women.[21] It is unclear whether this commonality is due to a common underlying mechanism.

PATHOPHYSIOLOGY: ESTROGEN AND PROGESTERONE

The standard explanation for leiomyomas is that they are estrogen-sensitive tumors. A number of clinical scenarios suggest this: their absence before menarche, their growth during pregnancy, and their regression at menopause or with gonadotropin-releasing hormone (GnRH)-agonist therapy. However, with each of these states, the level of progesterone moves in concert with the estrogen level; either both are elevated or both are dramatically suppressed. Additionally, there are specific clinical scenarios that suggest that progesterone may be more important.[7]

There are substantial in vitro data supporting major roles for both estrogen and progesterone in the biology of uterine leiomyomas. Recent work suggests that the clinical evidence that progesterone promotes myoma growth via increasing mitosis may be less important than by inhibiting the apoptosis pathway via *Bcl2* induction.[22] Likewise, regarding estrogen action, local action is likely key via an up-regulation of the enzyme aromatase P450 and its gene *CYP19*.

Modulation of steroid receptors is also important. Leiomyomas have increased amounts of both estrogen and progesterone receptor mRNA compared with normal myometrial tissue.[23,24] Both the A- and the N-terminally truncated B-isoforms of the progesterone receptor appear to be present in both leiomyomas and myometrium. However, the A-isoform appears to predominate in both tissues.[25] Similarly, estrogen receptor (ER)α rather than ERβ appears to be the predominant form in leiomyomas.[26]

In addition to the direct action of ovarian steroids on the uterus, it is possible that the reproductive axis may also influence uterine metabolism through the direct action of pituitary gonadotropins on the uterus. The placental glycoprotein human chorionic gonadotropin (hCG) has been shown by several laboratories to have direct actions on myometrial metabolism.[27-29] Additionally, our work has shown that follicle-stimulating hormone (FSH), luteinizing hormone (LH), thyroid-stimulating hormone (TSH), and their common α subunit can all have stimulatory effects on uterine prolactin production.[28,30] There appears to be a variant LH/hCG receptor present in human uterine tissue that may modulate this action.[31,32]

There is also indirect evidence for a uterine FSH receptor.[33] Support for the physiologic importance of this putative receptor comes from an animal model in which FSH receptor-haploinsufficent mice developed uterine abnormalities with aging characteristic of adenomyosis and with evidence of abnormal angiogenesis.[34] These pathologic changes were also associated with changes in the expression pattern of the A- and B-subtypes of the progesterone receptor.[34]

Fibrotic Factors

Leiomyomas can also be viewed as fibrotic tumors with a dynamic extracellular matrix (ECM) playing an important role in pathophysiology.[35] This hypothesis dates back to the 1990s when experiments demonstrated that the ECM characterizing fibroids contains significant amounts of collagen types I and III protein, and up-regulation of mRNA levels occurs during the proliferative phase of the menstrual cycle in leiomyomas but not myometrium (Fig. 25-2).[36] Other matrix components including matrix metalloprotease stromelysin 3 (MMP 11) and dermatopontin have also been shown to be dysregulated in leiomyomas.[37,38]

The fibrotic growth factor transforming growth factor-β (TGF-β), its subtypes, homologues, receptors, and downstream agents also appear to be involved in the pathophysiology of leiomyomas, as in other fibrotic processes. A complete review of this topic is beyond the scope of this chapter.

Leiomyomas appear to have higher levels of TGF-β, particularly TGF-β3 mRNA and protein, and this in turn affects cellular proliferation.[39,40] Additionally, granulocyte macrophage colony-stimulating factor (GM-CSF), connective tissue growth factor (CTGF), TGF-β4 (also known as lefty or ebaf, endometrial bleeding-associated factor), the SMAD family of transcriptions factors and the mitogen-activated protein (MAP) kinase signaling pathway appear to be part of the fibrotic pathway dysregulated in myomas, or the myometrium or endometrium of the uterus in women with leiomyomas or abnormal uterine bleeding.[41-46]

Angiogenesis

Angiogenesis, the formation of new blood vessels, is physiologic in the female reproductive tract, as opposed to most other tissues, where it is pathologic. Abnormalities in uterine blood vessels and angiogenic growth factors also appear to play a role in the pathobiology of myoma formation and function. The myomatous uterus shows increased numbers of arterioles and venules as well as venule ectasia.[47] These changes should be thought of as not confined to the leiomyoma itself but a global uterine problem

with involvement of the myometrium and the endometrium.[48,49] Although such venous abnormalities were originally postulated to be the result of physical compression of the vascular structures by bulky myomas, it is likely that molecular alterations are actually responsible for increased vessel number or abnormal function[1,50] (Table 25-1).

Several of the stages of angiogenesis involve interactions with specific components of the ECM that are dysregulated in fibroids such as collagens type I and III.[51] There is also some preliminary data that the resident immune cells may contribute to myoma physiology by modulating angiogenesis.[52]

The basic fibroblast growth factor (bFGF) receptor/ligand system appears to be a significant factor in leiomyoma pathophysiology. In addition to promoting angiogenesis, bFGF is a smooth muscle cell mitogen and acts similarly to estradiol on leiomyoma smooth muscle cells.[53-55] Leiomyomas have increased levels of bFGF mRNA compared to matched myometrium and a reservoir of bFGF protein in the extracellular matrix that characterizes myomas as well as dysregulation of the type I bFGF receptor in the endometrium.[56,57]

Genetic Influences: Clinical

As with many complex diseases, there are several lines of evidence that suggest that fibroids have a genetic component. First, monozygotic twins have twice the rate of concordance for hysterectomy of dizygotic twins.[58,59] There is also familial clustering; there is a two- to sixfold increased risk of a woman having fibroids if she has affected first-degree relatives.[60,61] Finally, there are also specific syndromes that have a demonstrated genetic component and whose phenotype includes uterine leiomyomas in association with other specific lesions:

Hereditary Leiomyomatosis and Renal Cell Cancer (HLRCC, MIM 605839). * This syndrome is autosomal dominant, and affected families manifest cutaneous leiomyomas and papillary renal cell carcinoma (RCC).[62-64] Affected women can have uterine leiomyomas as well as uterine leiomyosarcomas.[62] Both malignancies (sarcomas and RCC) are atypical in their presentation compared to their sporadic counterparts; uterine sarcomas can appear in young premenopausal women, and the papillary RCC is often metastatic at presentation and more likely to be seen in women.[62] Two other syndromes had described only the association of cutaneous and uterine leiomyomas, but lessons from molecular genetics suggest these are incomplete forms of the HLRCC syndrome and should be of historical interest only [Reed's syndrome or multiple cutaneous and uterine leiomyomas (MCUL), MIM 150800].[65,66]

Bannayan-Zonana syndrome (MIM 153480) and Cowden disease (MIM 158350). Both types of hamartomatous polyposis syndromes are characterized by leiomyomas as well as other benign tumors, including lipomas and hamartomas. Both these syndroms are also autosomal dominant in their inheritance and have the same candidate gene *phosphatase and tensin homologue (PTEN).*[67,68]

---

*The Web site www3.ncbi.nlm.nih.gov/omim/contains the full online catalog of these genetic disorders.

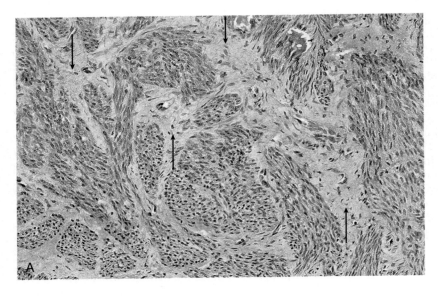

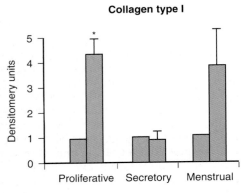

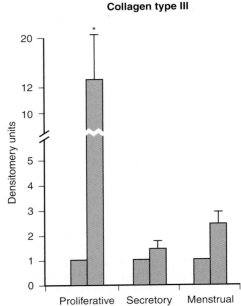

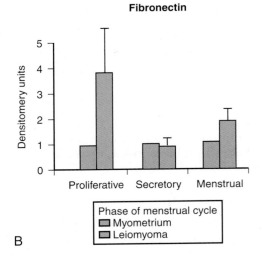

Figure 25-2. *Extracellular matrix in uterine leiomyomas. **A**, The large tracts of acellular extracellular matrix (arrows), such as seen in this hematoxylin and eosin section, not only contain significant amounts of collagen type I and III but can act as a significant reservoir for growth factors such as basic fibroblast growth factor (bFGF). **B**, The mRNA for collagens type I and III have significant menstrual cycle stage-specific regulation, suggesting the active remodeling of this tissue. (Part B from Stewart EA, Friedman AJ, Peck K, Nowak RA. Relative overexpression of collagen type I and collagen type III messenger ribonucleic acids by uterine leiomyomas during the proliferative phase of the menstrual cycle. J Clin Endocrinol Metab 79:900-906, 1994.)*

TABLE 25-1

TABLE 25-1

Postulated Factors Which Influence Angiogenesis in the Myomatous Uterus*

Factor	Potential Mechanisms
Basic fibroblast growth factor (bFGF)	Induction of endothelial proliferation
	Production of extracellular matrix remodeling enzymes
	Vascular and leiomyoma smooth muscle cell mitogen
Vascular endothelial growth factor (VEGF)	Mitogen for endothelial cells
Heparin-binding epidemial growth factor (HBEGF)	Mitogen for smooth muscle cells and fibroblasts
Platelet-derived growth factor (PDGF)	Mitogen for smooth muscle cells
Transforming growth factor-β (TGF-β)	Regulator of smooth muscle cellular proliferation and extracellular matrix production
Parathyroid hormone related peptide (PTHrP)	Vasodilator and smooth muscle cell relaxant
	Regulation of extracellular matrix production
Prolactin	Smooth muscle cell mitogen

*Molecular alterations, which lead to an increased number, increased caliber, or altered function of blood vessels, have been hypothesized to play an important role in leiomyoma-related menorrhagia.

Cytogenetic and Molecular Genetics

There is also cytogenetic and molecular genetic evidence for the role of genetics in leiomyomas. Leiomyomas are monoclonal, and each tumor is an independent clonal event. Although this fact was originally investigated using G6PD (glucose-6-phosphate dehydrogenase) polymorphisms, androgen receptor polymorphism studies concur.[69,70] This later study also suggests that karyotypic evolution is a late event in the pathogenesis of leiomyomas.[70]

Also, certain cytogenetic rearrangements characterize leiomyomas. Although 40% of fibroids are 46,XX there are specific karyotypic abnormalities that have been consistent in a number of studies:

- Translocations between chromosomes 12 and 14, t(12;14)
- Trisomy 12, rearrangements of 6p, 10q, and 13q
- Deletion of 3q and 7q[71,72]

There is also some evidence that genotype is related to both fibroid size and location.[72,73] Thus, many of the characteristics we attribute to submucous fibroids, as an example, may be related to genotype, and thus, the clinical heterogeneity we see may be more intelligible when genotypic information is available.[74]

Most, but not all, candidate genes identified for uterine fibroids map to the regions involved in the karotypic groups noted. *HMGA2* (formerly called *HMGI-C*) is an architectural transcription factor located on chromosome 12 that is involved in the pathogenesis of fibroids with t(12;14).[75,76] The *HMGA2* gene is very large (13 kb with 5 exons) and most translocations involving leiomyomas map to the 5' region of the gene.[75] However, recent evidence

suggests that unique transcripts from the opposite DNA strand may also play a role in pathogenesis.[77] *HMGA1* [*HMGI(Y)*] codes for a related HMG protein whose gene resides on chromosome 6p.[78,79] Interestingly, abnormalities in expression of *HMGA2* in a murine model produce abnormalities of fat deposition and metabolism.[80,81]

Rad51L1, also known as *hREC2*, is a gene encoding an enzyme which repairs double-stranded DNA breaks. The gene is on chromosome 14, and there are reports that in some myomas with t(12;14) fusion transcripts are produced with 5'*HMGA2* and 3'*Rad51L1*.[82] However, it does appear that a fusion transcript is a rare event with this translocation.[83]

Fumarate hydratase (FH), an enzyme that is part of the Krebs tricarboxylic acid cycle, is the gene mutation at 1q 42-43 responsible for HLRCC syndrome.[62,63] Germline mutations appear to result in absent or nonfunctional proteins, and thus, *FH* appears to act as a tumor suppressor.[64,84,85] *FH* appears to play a role in a small percentage of nonsyndromic leiomyomas and in a racially diverse cohort only to be linked to myomas in white women.[86,87]

Although work on elucidating the pathogenesis of HLRCC syndrome continues, *FH* mutations appear to induce a change toward a hypoxic phenotype.[88,89] Thus, the hypothesized relationship between hypoxia and myoma pathogenesis appears linked for this subset of leiomyomas.[90]

Inactivation of tumor suppressor genes appears to be a common mechanism for leiomyomas. In addition to *FH*, *PTEN* has been shown in individuals with Bannayan-Zonana syndrome to have a germline mutation.[67] A third tumor suppressor gene, cut-like homeobox gene (*CUTL1*), acts in some myomas to suppress transcription of the *C-Myc* oncogene[91] Finally, the Eker rat model for leiomyomas has a germline defect in the *tuberous sclerosis complex 2* (*Tsc-2*) tumor suppressor gene.[92] In this model, recent work suggests that there is a developmental window where the expression of disease is modulated by the effect of interaction of the tumor suppressor and the steroidal mileu.[92] The high incidence of myomas may be explained in part by the predominance of tumor suppressor mechanisms.

A significant limitation of genetic studies is that they have largely been conducted in areas where whites predominate and may not accurately reflect the karyotypes seen in black women. Given the different clinical behavior of myomas in black women, it is reasonable to believe that unique genes may be contributing to this risk. Linkage analysis for *FH* in nonsyndromic leiomyomas demonstrated a significant effect of race with linkage only seen in white women and a negative relation in African-American patients.[87]

Additionally, association of a polymorphism in the *catechol-O-methyltransferase* (*COMT*) gene seen more frequently in African-American women was linked to leiomyoma risk.[93] In vitro work also suggests there may be differences in growth factor regulation in leiomyomas from African-America women.[94] Work is under way to identify susceptibility genes for fibroids in a racially diverse cohort using a genome-wide scan, which will likely identify new candidate genes specifically for African-American women.[10]

Currently, identifying women at higher risk of malignancy due to HLRCC syndrome is an important clinical task, just as is identifying women whose families carry the BRCA mutations.[95] However, in the future, individualized therapy will likely be possible based on genotype and underlying predisposition genes.[95]

Other Influences

Epidermal growth factor (EGF) is a growth factor mitogenic for smooth muscle cells and EGF mRNA is up-regulated in leiomyomas only in the secretory phase of the cycle.[96] Receptor levels appear to be similar in leiomyomas and myometrium.[97]

Heparin-binding growth factors are important biologic regulators in leiomyomas because they can be secreted and bound to the reservoir of heparin sulfate proteoglycans filling the leiomyomatous ECM. Heparin-binding epidermal growth factor (HBEGF), vascular endothelial growth factor (VEGF), platelet-derived growth factor (PDGF), hepatoma-derived growth factor (HDGF), and the previously described basic FGF are all found in myomas.[56,98,99] Many have also been documented to be stored in the ECM.

Insulin-like growth factors (IGFs) can act as smooth muscle cell mitogens and were originally shown to have increased binding to leiomyomas compared to myometrium.[97] However, assessment of mRNA levels suggests that gene expression differed among studies.[100-102] Later studies suggested specific modulation of the IGF-binding proteins.[103] Regulation of these factors following GnRH-agonist treatment has also been reported.[104] There may also be increased prevalence of leiomyomas in women with acromegaly.[105]

The apoptotic inhibitor BCL2 is present in leiomyomas but is largely undetectable in myometrium; BCL2 is increased in leiomyomas taken from women in the secretory phase of the menstrual cycle.[105] In vitro experiments show that BCL2 expression is up-regulated in response to progesterone via the action of the progesterone receptor.[22,106]

Prolactin also appears to play an important role in myoma pathogenesis. In vitro studies suggest that it is mitogenic for leiomyoma and myometrial smooth muscle cells and that the prolactin receptor is present in these tissues, setting up an autocrine or local endocrine system.[107] Additionally, agents that appear to cause clinical regression of uterine leiomyoma also appear to decrease prolactin production in vitro.[25,30]

The resident immune cells also appear to influence leiomyoma biology. Mast cells have been implicated in leiomyoma pathobiology given that they are generally uniformly distributed in myometrium but highly variable in leiomyomas.[108] Recent work has suggested a correlation of mast cell number with vasculature.[52] A number of cytokines have also been shown to be differentially regulated in leiomyomas and myometrium. Interleukin 8 (IL-8) has decreased expression of both the ligand and its receptor in myometrium compared to leiomyomas.[109] The functional significance of this is shown by the fact that neutralizing antibody to IL-8 decreases cellular proliferation in vitro.[109] Monocyte chemotactic protein-1 (mcp1)

is largely undetectable in normal samples of leiomyoma and myometrium but is increased significantly following GnRH-agonist therapy.[110]

Wnt 7a, the human homologue of the wingless *Drosophila* genes involved in anterior–posterior axis formation and smooth muscle cell patterning, appears to be suppressed in leiomyomas compared to normal myometrium and to be inversely related to ERα expression.[111] In contrast, secreted frizzled related protein-1 (*sFRP1*), a modulator of *Wnt* signaling, is increased in leiomyomas (particularly in the late proliferative phase) and increased by estradiol treatment and hypoxia.[112] *HOX* gene expression does not appear to differ between leiomyomas and myometrium.[113] The mRNA for proto-oncogenes *cfos* and *cjun* is also overexpressed in leiomyomas compared to normal myometrium.[114]

Parathyroid hormone-related peptide (PTHrP) mRNA is also overexpressed in leiomyomas compared with normal myometrium.[115] In at least one patient, there appears to have been serum overexpression of the protein originating from a fibroid simulating the hypercalcemia of malignancy.[116]

PRINCIPLES OF TREATMENT

Uterine leiomyomas do not always necessitate treatment. Generally, expectant management is appropriate until the woman develops enough symptoms that she requests treatment. There are two important caveats to this generalization. First, although bleeding symptoms are usually evident, bulk symptoms can be insidious in their onset and often may be attributed to other processes such as aging. Second, women not electing therapy cannot reflexively be termed asymptomatic; they may have substantial symptoms but view the therapies they are offered as worse than the disease.[117]

A number of factors influence treatment decisions, including the size, number, and location(s) of the myomas; the symptoms, the age, and proximity to menopause; the reproductive desires of the patient; and the skill of her surgeon or other treating individuals. Unfortunately, there has been little evidence-based assessment of myoma therapies. The U.S. Agency for Healthcare Research and Quality, after performing a comprehensive survey of evidence-based treatment for myomas, concluded there is little high-quality evidence regarding myoma treatments.[118] The report cited evidence supporting hysterectomy for symptom relief but found data insufficient to support the efficacy of other interventions. The full report is available via the Internet at www.ahrq.gov/clinic/tp/uteruptp.htm.

Hysterectomy provides the only cure for fibroids and will remain a viable treatment option for the near term. Additionally, outcome studies suggest that women with myomas experience improved quality of life following hysterectomy, and hysterectomy also eliminates concomitant conditions including adenomyosis, endometrial polyps and abnormal Pap smears.[117,119,120] Unlike the case in hysterectomy for endometriosis, the ovaries can be retained at the time of hysterectomy for fibroids without losing efficacy. Generally, women weigh the risk of menopausal symptoms against the risk of ovarian tumors in making this decision. The attention paid to the ovary's production of androgens postmenopausally and their possible importance in mood and libido appear to be leading to an increase in the number of women who retain their ovaries even if they are perimenopausal.[121] The fact that hysterectomy, even without oophorectomy, decreases the risk of ovarian cancer may also affect decision making on this issue.[122,123]

Finally, the use of supracervical or subtotal hysterectomy in women with leiomyomas is debated. The fact that 7% of women in an unselected population have cyclic bleeding following this type of hysterectomy deserves further study to see whether these women had bleeding complaints or fibroids prior to hysterectomy.[124] Women may also run the theoretical risk of the formation of cervical fibroids following supracervical hysterectomy. Finally, accumulating data suggest that, at least in the short term, sexual functioning is not improved with supracervical hysterectomy.[125,126]

Menopause can also be a cure for women with myomas. Clearly, menorrhagia ceases with the cessation of menses. However, not all women have enough volume reduction to alleviate their symptoms. In addition, bleeding symptoms may continue for women who elect postmenopausal hormone replacement therapy (HRT), and one study has suggested that there may be some growth of myomas for women who take HRT.[127]

Nonetheless, as women seek less invasive options and the health care system seeks less costly options, hysterectomy is seldom performed these days without first pursuing at least one alternative. All surgical alternatives to hysterectomy, however, share the risk of what is termed fibroid "recurrence." Unlike the similar phenomenon after surgery in malignant disease, this is unlikely to be persistence of the same tumor but instead growth acceleration of additional tumors that may have been missed, not treated, resistant to treatment, or not yet present at the time of the prior therapy. Thus, following a variety of techniques, including abdominal myomectomy and uterine artery embolization, the risk of subsequent procedures is significant (Table 25-2).[128,129]

An initial assessment of whether bleeding, bulk-related symptoms, or both are prompting therapy helps to guide appropriate therapeutic options. As a second step, assessing the patient's desire regarding reproduction helps refine the available options. In general, women with complaints of menorrhagia alone tend to have more options for therapy (e.g., endometrial ablation, hysteroscopic myomectomy, and hormonal therapy including progestin-containing intrauterine device) than women with concurrent bulk-related symptomatology.

Surgical Therapies

Since the 1930s abdominal myomectomy has been the traditional alternative to hysterectomy because it preserves the uterus and allows childbearing.[130] However, it does have a morbidity rate similar to that of hysterectomy and has significant risk of subsequent surgery.[131,132] It is increasingly used primarily for women attempting childbearing because myomectomy has led to good pregnancy outcomes over many decades of experience.

TABLE 25-2

Multivariate Hazard Ratios (HR) for Variables Leading to Significantly Altered Risk of a Second Surgery Following Abdominal Myomectomy*

	Multivariate HR	95% Confidence Interval
Preoperative uterine size in excess of 12 menstrual weeks	0.1	0.01-0.4
Weight gain in excess of 30 pounds since age 18	4.8	1.2-18.5
History of endometriosis	5.2	1.3-20.2
Presence of menorrhagia	1.4	1.4-4.7
At least one birth (parity)	5.0	1.1-22.5

*A cohort of women followed for a mean of 84 months demonstrated that 15% of women had a second abdominal myomectomy or hysterectomy and 35% of women had a second surgery when less invasive techniques were also assessed. This table shows multivariate hazard ratios for recurrent surgery.

Modified and reprinted with permission from Stewart EA, Faur AV, Wise LA, et al. Predictors of subsequent surgery for uterine leiomyomata after abdominal myomectomy. Obstet Gynecol 99:426-432, 2002.

Abdominal myomectomy permits healthy pregnancies after surgery. Uterine rupture is very rare following myomectomy when compared to risk following classical cesarean section (0.002% versus 0.1%).[132] The common clinical practice of counseling women who have had a myomectomy with a transmural uterine incision to undergo an elective cesarean section is based on this risk comparison; however, there is no evidence they are analogous situations.[133]

Although laparoscopic myomectomy involves much smaller incisions and a quicker recovery time, it does require a surgeon skilled in laparoscopic suturing and not all women have the size and number of fibroids amenable to this technique. Updated series suggest that the risk of uterine rupture is low following laparoscopic myomectomy, but rare cases continue to be reported.[134-138] Because these uterine ruptures typically occur remote from term, appropriate counseling for patients contemplating pregnancy is important, especially if devascularization with cautery occurs intraoperatively. The use of robotic myomectomy closure is one attempt to decrease this concern.[139]

Myolysis is a variation on the technique of laparoscopic myomectomy in which the leiomyoma tissue is coagulated rather than removed.[140] Although this technique is easier to master than laparoscopic morcellation or suturing, localized destruction without repair may also increase the chance of uterine rupture and adhesion formation.[141]

For women with submucous myomas, the use of hysteroscopic myomectomy has distinct advantages. With their accessible location, type 0 and I (European Society of Hysteroscopy classification) myomas can be resected with an operative endoscope placed through the cervix with good long-term results.[142] Although this procedure requires highly skilled practitioners, it can be done as outpatient surgery, often with a regional or local anesthetic and sedation that eases recuperation. Symptomatic relief is good with fewer than 16% of women in one large series

TABLE 25-3

Complication Rates Following Uterine Artery Embolization*

Morbidity	% of Patients	Confidence Interval
Readmission	3.5	1.9-5.8
Unintended procedure	2.5	1.2-4.5
Allergic reaction/rash	2.5	1.2-4.5
Leiomyoma passage per vagina†	2.5	1.2-4.5
Febrile morbidity (including initiation of antibiotics more than 24 hours after surgery)	2	0.9-3.9
Recurrent or prolonged pain	1.25	0.4-2.9
Urinary tract infection	1	0.3-2.5
Femoral nerve injury	0.75	0.2-2.7
Hemorrhage	0.75	0.2-2.2
Life-threatening event	0.5	0.1-1.8
Endometriosis	0.5	0.1-1.8
Vessel injury	0.5	0.1-1.8
Urinary retention	0.5	0.1-1.8

*A compilation of complications in a cohort of 400 consecutive women undergoing UAE in a single institution. Complications are based on criteria from either the American College of Obstetricians and Gynecologists (ACOG) or the Society of Cardiovascular and Interventional Radiology (SCIVR). Thus, some complications may be reported twice in this table.
†This complication was as likely to occur 91 days to 1 year following procedure as in first 30 days following discharge.
Modified from Spies JB, Spectar A, Roth AR, et al. Complications after uterine artery embolization for leiomyomas. Obstet Gynecol 100: 873-880, 2002.

who were treated for menorrhagia reporting second surgeries after 9 years.[142,143] Fertility rates appear excellent after hysteroscopic myomectomy, and there have been no case reports of uterine rupture after uncomplicated hysteroscopic myomectomy.[144]

For women who have completed childbearing and for whom bleeding is the primary problem, endometrial ablation, either alone or in combination with hysteroscopic myomectomy, may give relief with minimal invasiveness. Increasingly, a levonorgestrel intrauterine device (IUD) is used for a "reversible endometrial ablation."[145,146] In addition to providing effective control of bleeding, it provides contraception for women in this premenopausal age group.

Uterine Artery Embolization. Transcatheter arterial embolization has long been an effective percutaneous technique for controlling bleeding in a wide variety of obstetric and gynecologic disorders. Its use for the treatment of leiomyomas was first reported in 1995.[147] Although initially used as an alternative for patients who were felt to be poor surgical candidates, the resolution of symptoms in the initial cohort encouraged the use of this technique as a primary therapy.

Uterine artery embolization (UAE) is increasingly the first-line alternative to hysterectomy for women with bulk-related symptoms and no desire for future pregnancy.[148,149] It provides a decrease in menorrhagia and bulk-related symptoms in 75% to 85% of women and a volume reduction similar to that seen with GnRH-agonist therapy. A series of randomized clinical trials conducted in Europe comparing UAE and hysterectomy suggest that women undergoing UAE have shorter hospital stay and a quicker return to work.[149] Complications are different with the two procedures, but the rate of complications is similar (Table 25-3). Outcomes at 1 year appear to be similar; however, in the single reported study, the rate of subsequent procedures in the UAE group was 9%.[150] It will be important to discover whether these failures represent poor patient selection or if there is a high continuing risk of treatment failure.

It is relatively common for submucous myomas to be expelled vaginally after treatment,[149] and thus, most hysteroscopically resectable fibroids are still approached surgically. Although greater volume reduction is achieved, there is not a predictable time course. Similarly, the presence of pedunculated subserosal fibroids is considered a relative contraindication to UAE therapy, although no cases have been reported of intraperitoneal expulsion. Studies also suggest that high T_2 signals predict greater volume reduction and complete devascularization predicts outcome at 5 years.[151-153]

Most patients develop significant pain following the procedure and usually require intravenous narcotics for pain control. However, randomized clinical trials report this pain is less than that seen following surgery.[150] "Postembolization syndrome," defined as the combination of diffuse abdominal pain, mild fever, and mild leukocytosis, is common and can occur in 30% to 40% of patients in some series.

Pregnancy Following Uterine Artery Embolization. It is important to assess the effects of UAE on the ability of women to become pregnant subsequently or to carry a pregnancy to term. Thus far, there are reports of several series of patients who became pregnant following UAE.[154-157]

Pregnancy clearly can and does occur following UAE, but there are two major areas of caution for women wishing to optimize their fertility potential: effects on ovarian function and myometrial wall integrity. Most of the data on ovarian damage examines amenorrhea as the indicator of perturbed ovarian function.[155,158] It is clear that amenorrhea risk is age related, with women under 40 having a 3% risk and women over 50 a 41% risk.

However, for women desiring fertility more subtle forms of damage may lead to impaired ovarian reserve and subfertility or infertility. A recent report examining anti-müllerian hormone (AMH) in women participating in a randomized clinical trial of UAE versus hysterectomy does suggest that UAE causes more of a decrement in AMH levels than following hysterectomy or age-related predicted decline.[159] A putative mechanism is suggested by a second study which indicated significantly increased

FSH levels following UAE in patients with utero-ovarian vascular anastomoses.[160]

Focused Ultrasound: Noninvasive Treatment

High-intensity focused ultrasound (HIFU or FUS) provides a noninvasive ablation method that is FDA-approved for the treatment of uterine fibroids. Although pioneered for the treatment of uterine fibroids, this modality can be used to treat multiple diseases and may prove to be the next step in surgical innovation from open to minimally invasive to noninvasive approaches.

Just as a laser amplifies and collates light into a therapeutic modality, FUS can deliver a large amount of energy to target tissues in a noninvasive way. Treatment may be accomplished by placing a transducer against the abdomen as is currently done for diagnostic ultrasound, targeting an intra-abdominal myoma without breaching the skin. The intensity of FUS used for treatment is significantly higher than that used in diagnostic ultrasound and can rapidly increase temperature at the focal point in excess of 70°C. At this temperature, coagulative necrosis will occur.

Multiple reports of outcomes following magnetic resonance imaging (MRI)-guided focused ultrasound surgery (MRgFUS) have now been reported.[161-164] In the initial feasibility study of 55 women, all were successively treated as outpatients with either oral diazepam or IV-conscious sedation.[161] Complications from FUS were minimal compared with those experienced after uterine artery ablation with no hyperstimulation syndrome. The targeting accuracy of the image-guided component was confirmed in a subset of the patients going to hysterectomy.[161] The feasibility studies additionally demonstrated that avoiding treatment through abdominal wall scars and careful assessment of structures being the ultrasound focus are critical to avoid complications.[162]

Further studies show that with more extensive treatment, symptomatology is decreased with fewer adverse events.[162] Although all early studies primarily examined symptomatology using the Uterine Fibroid Symptom Quality of Life tool (UFSQOL)[162,163] more recent work demonstrated that shrinkage occurred over time with reciprocal decreases in the nonperfused area (that devascularized by successful treatment).[164] Additionally, optimal patient outcomes, both in symptom reduction on the UFSQOL but also in the use of alternative treatments and the time to additional treatment, is correlated with the extent of treatment with more aggressive treatments producing optimal results.[163,164]

Ultrasound-guided focused ultrasound (typically referred to as high-intensity focused ultrasound, HIFU) has been used to treat several human diseases, including breast fibroadenomas and benign prostatic hypertrophy. Vaezy and colleagues initially tested the efficacy of HIFU for ablation of uterine fibroids in a nude mouse model, which develops subcutaneous tumors after injection of an Eker rat cell line ELT-3.[165] There are two reports of feasibility studies of ultrasound-guided HIFU, one utilizing a transvaginal approach and the other a transabdominal approach.[166,167]

Medical Therapies

Although many algorithms for the management of uterine leiomyomas suggest initial treatment with the modulation of steroid hormones, there is little evidence to support this practice.[118] Oral contraceptive pills, progestins, nonsteroidal anti-inflammatory drugs, antifibrinolytic agents, and androgenic compounds, all of which are useful in the treatment of idiopathic menorrhagia, have not been studied with leiomyoma-related menorrhagia. Nonetheless, they are widely used and are likely effective in at least a subset of women with myomas.

GnRH-Agonists. Gonadotropin-releasing hormone (GnRH) has pulsatile release from the arcuate nucleus of the hypothalamus, which stimulates synthesis and secretion of the gonadotropins luteinizing hormone (LH) and follicle-stimulating hormone (FSH), which in turn stimulate the ovary to produce mature eggs and secrete both estrogen and progesterone. In the treatment of uterine leiomyomas, these steroid hormones act not only upon the endometrium but also upon the leiomyomas themselves.

Because the action of native GnRH depends on its pulsatile release, the effects of GnRH-agonists depend upon their continuous presence. They first cause a time-limited increase in gonadotropin release, termed the flare. This subsequently leads to receptor down-regulation, followed 1 to 3 weeks later by a hypogonadotropic hypogonadal state. This state, often incorrectly termed a "medical menopause," is similar to menopause in its low steroid levels yet differs in having low, rather than high, gonadotropin levels. It is this down-regulated phase that is useful clinically in the treatment of myomas. Alterations of the GnRH molecule, typically at amino acids 6 and 10, produce a longer half-life and are more useful for clinical purposes.[168]

In 1983, Filicori and colleagues were the first to report the administration of a GnRH-agonist for the treatment of leiomyomas.[169] Since then, many studies have focused on the efficacy and benefits of GnRH-agonist treatment for women with fibroids. Most women experience a substantial reduction in mean uterine volume of 30% to 60% over 3 to 6 months of therapy. However, there is a wide range of responsiveness, with rare individuals achieving no volume reduction. Both the estradiol levels at week 12 and the weight of the woman are correlated with the degree of uterine shrinkage.[170]

The other primary benefit of GnRH-agonist treatment is the induction of amenorrhea. Most women will achieve cessation of menstrual flow within 4 weeks, although there are rare reports of vaginal hemorrhage that occur during the flare phase. Menses typically return 4 to 10 weeks following the end of GnRH-agonist treatment. Fibroid and uterine volume usually returns to pretreatment size within 3 to 4 months. The rapid return of ovarian steroidogenesis, coupled with an increase in the concentration of estrogen receptors in fibroids recently treated with GnRH-agonists, may contribute to the rapid regrowth of these tumors.[171]

GnRH-agonists can have significant adverse effects, the most important of which is bone loss. Six months of

GnRH-agonist treatment can cause a 6% loss in trabecular bone, not all of which is reversible on discontinuation of therapy. Symptomatic side effects of GnRH-agonist therapy are common. Hot flashes are universal in women undergoing treatment. Other less common side effects include sleep disturbance, irregular vaginal bleeding, vaginal dryness, headache, depression, hair loss, and musculoskeletal symptoms. Animal studies show no evidence of teratogenic effects with GnRH-agonist treatment, though women are typically advised to use barrier contraception during GnRH-agonist therapy.

Because of the concerns regarding bone loss with GnRH-agonists, clinical use of these drugs is typically confined to use as preoperative therapy or in women for whom a short period of treatment will be effective. The GnRH-agonist Lupron is FDA-approved for the presurgical treatment of uterine fibroids to correct anemia in conjunction with iron administration. This is the only medical treatment approved by the FDA for treatment of this disease.

Administration prior to either hysterectomy or myomectomy is the most common current use of these agents. Length of therapy varies from 1 to 6 months depending on the surgical and hematologic goals and the planned procedure. The amenorrhea induced by GnRH therapy leads to improved hemoglobin concentrations, which permit women who are anemic to correct this problem and potentially to donate their own blood for transfusion. However, studies have demonstrated that 40% of anemic women improve on iron supplements alone.[172] Preoperative GnRH therapy also has been shown to reduce intraoperative blood loss significantly. Although current guidelines from the American College of Obstetricians and Gynecologists suggest that use of GnRH-agonists is beneficial preoperatively, they also state that for each individual the benefit must be weighed against the cost and the side effects.[133]

GnRH-Agonist Therapy with Estrogen/Progestin Add-Back Regimens. For many women, 3 to 6 months of symptomatic relief from leiomyomas does not allow them to avoid surgery but does afford them the opportunity to prepare themselves optimally for an operation. Therefore, the concept of adding additional therapy to minimize the side effects of prolonged therapy was developed: the so-called add-back regimens.[173,174] The goal of add-back regimens was to achieve a window of therapeutic efficacy during which side effects would be lessened or eliminated, yet no regrowth of the myomas would occur.

Studies have utilized one of two treatment strategies: simultaneous and sequential administration. With simultaneous treatment regimens, both the GnRH-agonist and the add-back regimens are started at the same time. In sequential treatment regimens, the GnRH-agonist is given alone for up to 6 months before steroid hormone treatment is added, reducing the period of hypoestrogenism before steroid add-back therapy is started. Early studies suggested that sequential treatment was essential for therapeutic efficacy in the treatment of fibroids.

Initially, a simultaneous add-back regimen was tested utilizing leuprolide acetate and oral medroxyprogesterone acetate (MPA).[175] Although MPA significantly reduced hot flashes, it inhibited the decrease in uterine volume normally seen with GnRH-agonist therapy. Patients receiving placebo experienced a mean reduction in uterine volume of 51% at 24 weeks compared with only a 14% reduction in patients receiving MPA. A second study utilizing the same drugs but with a crossover trial design noted a similar phenomenon.[176]

A subsequent study of five women utilized a sequential regimen using leuprolide acetate alone for 3 months, followed by the addition of conjugated equine estrogens (0.625 mg daily, days 1 to 25) and MPA (10 mg daily, days 16 to 25) to leuprolide for an additional 24 months.[174] Using this regimen, a reduction in uterine volume of 49% was achieved at 3 months and was maintained for the additional 24 months of combination drug therapy. There was no significant decline in bone density loss over the study period, and women had significant symptomatic improvement. Since publication of these results, most studies have utilized sequential add-back regimens for leiomyomas with estrogen and progestin.

Innovative GnRH-Agonist Add-Back Therapies. The estrogen receptor antagonist tamoxifen (20 mg daily) was used in a randomized prospective 6-month study in a simultaneous add-back study design with the GnRH agonist goserelin.[177] Despite significantly lower estradiol concentrations and significant suppression of FSH and LH levels compared with the goserelin-only group, uterine volume was not significantly reduced in the combined goserelin and tamoxifen group. In this study, a single patient received sequential goserelin and tamoxifen therapy; goserelin was administered alone for 12 weeks and tamoxifen was added to goserelin for 12 additional weeks. In this individual, the reduction in uterine volume of 59% at 12 weeks was maintained during the 24-week study period.

More recent studies used raloxifene therapy in postmenopausal women with leiomyomas and were able to cause a reduction in size.[178] However, in the more clinically relevant group of premenopausal women, raloxifene has only been able to have measurable effect when combined with GnRH-agonist. In this group, there is a reported reduction in the size of the uterus compared to women receiving GnRH-agonist plus placebo. However, symptoms were equivalent in the two groups.

Tibolone, a synthetic steroid, has been used as a single agent for menopausal HRT for its combination of estrogenic and progestational actions in the same molecule. In menopausal women, it alleviates climacteric symptoms and prevents osteoporosis without stimulating endometrial proliferation, resulting in less vaginal bleeding than traditional HRT regimens. In a study of postmenopausal women with leiomyomas who were receiving tibolone for HRT, it was noted women were more likely to achieve amenorrhea than with conventional HRT.[179] Subsequently, it was studied in premenopausal women receiving GnRH-agonists for the treatment of myomas.[180] There was no inhibition of uterine shrinkage with tibolone, and patients showed preservation of bone density as well as symptomatic improvement. Thus, tibolone may be used as a single-agent add-back in the future.

Ipriflavone, an isoflavone that is a weak estrogen modulator, has been studied in add-back regimens.[181] Although originally studied to determine its effect on bone, it appears effective in slowing bone loss and decreasing symptoms without impeding the volume reduction of GnRH-agonist therapy.

Innovative Steroidal Therapy. Novel strategies for the manipulation of steroid hormone action may also be employed as direct therapy in the future, just as GnRH-agonists are currently employed. However, more specificity of action may be attainable through the use of hormone antagonists or receptor blockade.

GnRH-Antagonists. GnRH-antagonists have also been studied in the treatment of uterine leiomyomas.[182-184] Although they are not FDA-approved for this indication, they have several significant advantages over GnRH-agonists. First, they have no flare effect, so the rare instances of heavy bleeding that can be provoked at the start of therapy are not an issue. Second, they have a much more rapid onset of action; a decrease in steroidal levels has been documented within 48 hours and significant clinical effects can be seen in less than 1 month. Thus, GnRH-antagonists could be used preoperatively for volume reduction; however, currently marketed doses for other indications are not similar to the doses used for leiomyoma treatment. In addition, because of differences in mechanisms of action, sequential treatment with a GnRH-antagonist followed by a GnRH-agonist is not beneficial.

Progesterone Antagonists. Mifepristone (RU486) is a steroidal derivative of norethindrone, which acts primarily as an antiprogestin. Pilot studies of mifepristone have been conducted in normally cycling premenopausal women with symptomatic leiomyomas with good results.[185-187] In the first study, 50 mg/day of mifepristone was administered for 3 months to 10 women with leiomyomas. The reduction in myoma volume was equivalent to that seen with GnRH-agonist (49% at 12 weeks), and all patients achieved amenorrhea. Thus, the clinical benefit was equivalent to that seen with GnRH-agonists, yet follicular levels of estradiol were maintained to support bone mass and provide symptomatic relief. Identical results were found with a reduction in dose to 25 mg/day; however, with a 5 mg/day dose, although acyclicity was maintained, volume reduction was less than 30%. More recent studies suggest that doses of 5 and 10 mg produce volume reduction equivalent to those elicited by the higher doses, but produced amenorrhea in only 60% to 65% of women.[186,187] Nonetheless, this provides significant symptomatic improvement.

Mifepristone has mild side effects compared with GnRH-agonists. Adverse effects included mild and infrequent hot flashes in approximately 20% of patients during the first month of treatment only with higher doses; however, more persistent symptoms appeared in another study.[185,186] Simple hyperplasia without evidence of atypia has been observed with high-dose mifepristone therapy.[188]

A new class of selective progesterone-receptor modulators (SPRMs) are being studied for the treatment of uterine leiomyomas.[189,190] These drugs appear to have efficacy similar to mifepristone but decreased side effects and increased specificity when interacting with the progesterone receptor.

Serum Estrogen-Receptor Modulators. Selective estrogen-receptor modulators (SERMs), which exhibit tissue-specific agonist or antagonist activity, may prove as useful for the treatment of leiomyomas as they have been for HRT. Studies have examined both tamoxifen and raloxifene. Clomiphene has not been studied and has been reported to cause growth of myomas in a single case report.[191] Raloxifene differs from tamoxifen in its lack of agonist activity in the uterine endometrium. In preclinical studies in the Eker rat model, both tamoxifen and raloxifene caused a significant reduction (40% to 60%) in tumor incidence.[192,193] Tumors that were exposed to tamoxifen or raloxifene also exhibited decreased proliferative capacity compared with untreated tumors.

Clinical studies have had less impressive results. In a study of postmenopausal women receiving raloxifene, there was a decrease in uterine and leiomyoma size after short-term treatment but no change in bleeding patterns.[178] However, in premenopausal women raloxifene alone or when combined with GnRH-agonists demonstrated little efficacy despite use at three times the conventional dose.[194,195]

Androgens. Danazol, an androgenic steroid most commonly used for the medical treatment of endometriosis, can be used to induce amenorrhea in order to control anemia due to fibroid-related menorrhagia. A second androgenic steroid, gestrinone, has been shown to cause volume reduction and amenorrhea in women with myomas.[196] A great advantage of this drug is that, after it is discontinued, there is a carry-over effect; in one study, 89% of the women maintained a decreased uterine volume 18 months after cessation of therapy.[196]

Growth Factor–Directed Treatments. Particular factors which appear to be relevant to leiomyoma biology include the angiogenic factor basic fibroblast growth factor (bFGF), the fibrotic growth factor transforming growth factor-beta (TGF-β), and insulin-like growth factors I and II (IGF-I and -II), which mediate the effects of growth hormone (GH).[1,90,99] These molecules, as well as other growth factors, are likely to be targets for leiomyoma treatment in the future.

GH- and IGF-Directed Therapy. Both GH and the IGFs appear to have metabolic effects on uterine leiomyomas and the surrounding myometrium.[103] Because women with acromegaly (an excess of growth hormone) have a high incidence of leiomyomas, researchers decided to test the hypothesis that interfering with the growth hormone axis might work as a treatment for leiomyomas.[105]

Lanreotide is a long-acting somatostatin analog that has been used to treat acromegaly. Seven premenopausal women with uterine myomas were treated with this analog in a pilot study in Italy.[197] Over the 3 months of treatment, both uterine volume and the volume of the largest leiomyoma were significantly reduced by 24% and 42%, respectively. Three months following the discontinuation of therapy there was some regrowth, but a significant reduction in uterine volume persisted at 17% and 29%, respectively. Levels of estradiol were not affected by this treatment, though both plasma GH and IGF-I levels were significantly reduced and additional pathologic modulators may be effective.[198]

Anti-angiogenic Therapies. There is significant evidence that the angiogenic factor bFGF and its type I receptor are important in the pathogenesis of leiomyoma-related bleeding.[56,57] Based on the hypothesis that leiomyoma smooth muscle cells are targets for the angiogenic factor bFGF, factors that decrease bFGF production or prevent its action might be clinically useful in the treatment of leiomyoma-related bleeding.[1] In a variety of systems, interferons (INFs) IFN-α or INF-β antagonize the effects of bFGF and have proved clinically useful in the treatment of a variety of vascular tumors. In vitro studies of leiomyomas demonstrate that IFN-α is an effective inhibitor of serum-stimulated and bFGF-stimulated DNA synthesis in both leiomyoma and normal myometrial cells, as well as in endometrial cells.[55]

A case report also raises the possibility that IFNs may provide effective treatment for fibroids. A premenopausal woman who was treated with IFN-α for hepatitis C was noted to have significant shrinkage of a leiomyoma after 7 months of interferon therapy.[199] Prior to treatment, a magnetic resonance image showed an intramural myoma of 202 cm³. Five months after her treatment was completed, the myoma volume was noted to have substantially decreased (to 29 cm³) and 17 months after therapy, the volume reduction persisted at 21 cm³; she continued to have regular menses throughout treatment.

Tranilast [N-(3′4′-dimethoxycinnamonyl) anthranilic acid (N-5′)], a drug currently used in the treatment of a variety of allergic conditions, has been shown in vitro to decrease leiomyoma cellular proliferation by arresting cells at the transition from G0 to G1 phase.[200] While it acts as an angiogenesis inhibitor, it also works as a mast cell stabilizer and a fibrosis inhibitor, which may have relevance for leiomyomas.[200]

Investigational Image-Guided Surgical Therapy

The gold standard for assessing both the safety and accuracy of surgical techniques has been direct visualization, which in open procedures can be augmented by palpation. With minimally invasive surgeries, this latter component is completely absent and often the options for visualization are restricted by limitations of the equipment, such as the angle of the endoscope.

Image-guided therapy offers several advantages for the treatment of leiomyomas. First, it can allow you to "see" from serosal surface to mucosal surface as well as the intramural portion of the uterus while a traditional surgical approach allows only one view. Second, it can image other relevant tissues, such as bowel or bladder. Both ultrasound and MRI can direct image-guided therapy.

While ultrasound clearly has the advantage of ease, there are instances in which MRI may be more useful. First, the ability of MRI to delineate and characterize lesions in the uterine wall is superior. Therefore, this technique may be preferable in instances in which it is important to distinguish between three small intramural fibroids and one large myoma, or where the lesion is suggestive of adenomyosis instead of a myoma.

Also, with the increasing use of thermally ablative therapies, the capacity of MRI to measure temperature shifts in real time allows for both accuracy in targeting and complete tissue destruction. Using assessment of the proton shift capacity, very small temperature shifts can be detected. This allows the initial use of energy too low to cause tissue destruction to be delivered and detected to confirm targeting accuracy.

Additionally, by monitoring peak temperature during treatment, it allows confirmation of the completeness of the tissue destruction without concern about injury to surrounding tissue. It is this combination of accuracy and safety that may cause image-guided therapy to become far more cost-effective than surgical therapy.

Percutaneous Laser Ablation. Thermal ablation using percutaneously placed laser fibers has been studied for the treatment of uterine fibroids. The procedure was performed under real-time magnetic resonance (MR) guidance to allow proper insertion of laser fibers and to record the extent of uterine fibroid necrosis during treatment.[201] Three months after laser ablation, treated fibroid volume had decreased by a mean of 37.5% (range, 25% to 49%). Follow-up at 12 months suggests that women have a significant decrease in menstrual blood loss and continue to extend their volume reduction from 6 to 12 months.[202]

Cryomyolysis. Cryomyolysis is a thermal ablation technique that freezes the tissue in order to destroy it.[203,204] Initially, the technique was studied using laparoscopic guidance. A small series of image-guided cryomyolysis have been reported using MRI as the imaging modality.[205,206] These series showed a mean reduction in the fibroid size at 8 weeks of 65% and 53%, respectively. Symptom decrease was reported at 2 weeks.

Adenomyosis

Adenomyosis, formerly termed endometriosis interna, is another benign uterine disease characterized by the presence of ectopic endometrial glands and stroma within the myometrium (Fig. 25-3). Furthermore, the surrounding myometrium is usually altered revealing hypertrophy. Disease ranges from grossly visible nodules termed adenomyomas, which can initially resemble leiomyomas, to disease that is only detectable by microscopy. Various sources choose different definitions for the abnormal presence of gland within the stroma, with most settling on a definition of one to three low-power fields from the endomyometrial junction. Clearly, differences in definition will lead to differences in perceived rates. Additionally, much like leiomyomas, rigorous microscopic analysis suggests an incidence as high as 65%.[207]

Classically, the typical uterus with adenomyosis is termed boggy, globular, and symmetrically enlarged. However, this disease coexists with many other uterine conditions. In a series of hysterectomies, adenomyosis appears in about one quarter of all uterine specimens but is no more likely to coexist with symptomatic leiomyomas (23.3%) than with endometrial cancer (28.2%) or ovarian cancer (28.1%).[208]

Unlike leiomyomas, adenomyosis is associated with increasing parity.[208,209] It is estimated that at least 80% of women with this disorder are parous. However, this may be a confounding variable because women with a history of multiple pregnancies may simply have had more indications or inclination to proceed to hysterectomy during which the diagnosis could be made.

Clinically, adenomyosis is similar to leiomyomas in that its peak incidence is in women ages 40 and 50 years with approximately 60% of women reporting abnormal uterine bleeding, chiefly menorrhagia. Dysmenorrhea is the other frequent symptom in women with adenomyosis, occurring in approximately one quarter of all cases.[207] Dysmenorrhea has been correlated with deep penetration and a high density of endometrial glands within the myometrium.[210]

The most widely quoted hypothesis regarding the pathogenesis of this disease is that invasion of the myometrium by the endometrium induces hypertrophy and hyperplasia of the myometrium. Proponents of this theory often quote the association of parity with adenomyosis to suggest that disruption of the layers of the uterus at the time of pregnancy and cesarean section may predispose to this condition. However, evidence indicates instead that adenomyosis is a metaplastic process or a developmental defect. First, adenomyosis has been diagnosed in a woman with Rokitansky-Kuster-Hauser syndrome, who lacked eutopic endometrium.[211] Additionally, studies comparing the molecular expression of growth factors show distinct differences between ectopic and eutopic endometrium.[212,213] Factors that appear common to the pathogenesis of leiomyomas and adenomyosis include angiogenic factors such as bFGF, fibrotic factors including GM-CSF, the gonadotropin receptor LH, and resident immune cells.[43,214,215] Microvessel density is also increased in adenomyosis, suggesting increased angiogenesis.[216]

Interestingly, a murine model of adenomyosis has been developed by placing a graft of pituitary tissue in a uterine horn.[217] Prolactin appears to be the key pathogenic agent in this model: the mice have elevated levels of plasma prolactin, and administration of bromocriptine prevents the development of adenomyosis.[217,218] In this model, there does appear to be endometrial cell invasion due to degeneration of myometrial cells.[217] A second model using the FORKO (follitropin receptor knockout) mouse suggests that the rising levels of FSH seen with aging may also play an important pathogenic role in this disease.[34]

Although definitive diagnosis of adenomyosis requires histologic examination, imaging techniques are increasingly able to suggest the appropriate diagnosis. Both transvaginal ultrasonography (TVS) and MRI are used for this purpose. Overall, the techniques appear to have similar sensitivity (0.68 for TVS and 0.70 for MRI) with MRI showing significantly greater specificity (0.65 versus 0.86).[219]

The only definitive treatment for adenomyosis is total hysterectomy. GnRH-agonist treatment has been shown to produce a transient decrease in uterine size, in amenorrhea, and even in the ability to conceive.[220-222] Unfortunately, resumption of pretreatment uterine size and recurrence of symptoms are usually documented within 6 months of cessation of therapy.

Both UAE and MRgFUS have been reported for the treatment of adenomyosis. With UAE, success rates of approximately 50% can be achieved over 36 months of follow-up.[223,224] For MRgFUS, long-term follow-up is not available but in a single case, subsequent pregnancy did occur.[225] A single case, report suggests local treatment with a danazol-containing IUD was successful in achieving symptom control.[226]

Endometrial Polyps

Endometrial polyps, as their name suggests, arise from the endometrial layer of the uterus. They are characterized by glandular proliferation surrounding a central core of prominent blood vessels in the stroma. Disregarding speculation surrounding an increased surface area of the mucosal lining, the mechanism whereby polyps cause abnormal uterine bleeding has not been articulated. However, unpublished data from our laboratory suggest that polyps share the molecular alterations of bFGF seen in leiomyomas and adenomyosis (Fig. 25-4).

The prevalence of polyps has been estimated at 10% to 24% among women undergoing endometrial biopsy

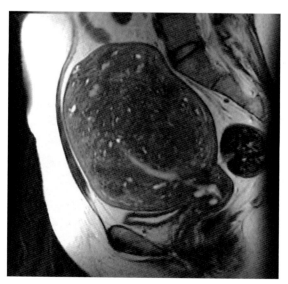

Figure 25-3. *A T₂-weighted fast-spin echo (FSE) image of the adenomyotic uterus. Adenomyosis is characterized by proliferation of glandular elements of the uterus so that bright (white) areas similar in intensity to the endometrial cavity are seen deep into the uterine wall. The wall also appears to be thickened, and in this image, the posterior wall is markedly thicker than the anterior wall.*

or hysterectomy.[227] Endometrial polyps are rare among women under 20 years of age. The incidence of polyps peaks in the fifth decade of life, and approximately 60% of polyps are found in premenopausal women. Despite significantly changed methods of diagnosis and treatment, the epidemiologic characteristics of polyps have remained constant over the last decade.[228]

The most frequent symptom in women with endometrial polyps is metrorrhagia, reported in 50% of symptomatic cases.[227] Of women who have abnormal bleeding, approximately 30% have evidence of endometrial polyps.[229] Polyps can also be found in approximately 10% of asymptomatic women but tend to be smaller than polyps associated with bleeding and also are more likely to regress with time.[229,230] However, overall there is no relationship between symptoms and the size and number of endometrial polyps.[231]

Endometrial polyps are still diagnosed in specimens obtained after a dilation and curettage (D&C) or hysterectomy, though new methods of diagnosis and treatment are being utilized more frequently.[228] Increasingly, the use of saline-infusion sonography, also termed sonohysterograms, or less commonly, office hysteroscopy, diagnoses polyps. Some polyps can also be diagnosed by hysterosalpingogram if the uterine cavity is also visualized. The majority of cases of endometrial polyps are now treated with hysteroscopic resection or hysteroscopically guided D&C rather than the traditional D&C.

Research shows little data on the effects of polyps on infertility. One small study suggested that miscarriage rates were increased, although pregnancy rates were similar in women with polyps managed expectantly during in vitro fertilization compared to women having embryos frozen and transferred after polyp removal.[232]

It appears that polyps may share common pathophysiologic mechanism with leiomyomas and adenomyosis. Polyps share common cytogenetic rearrangements with leiomyomas including rearrangements of 6p,12q, and 7q.[233] Additionally, both spontaneous and tamoxifen-stimulated polyps manifest rearrangements of *HMGI-C* and *HMGI(Y)*.[234]

Abnormal Uterine Bleeding

Abnormal uterine bleeding affects up to one third of women of reproductive age and can occur in conjunction with the pathologic processes we have discussed or in their absence. Menorrhagia may occur in 10% to 30% of women and in up to 50% of women in the perimenopause.[235,236] However, the self-reporting of menstrual regularity and flow is highly variable. For example, less than 50% of women presenting with a complaint of menorrhagia will have this confirmed on objective analysis. Change in pattern of flow is probably the most important sign. Menorrhagia is the type of abnormal bleeding frequently associated with benign uterine disease, including leiomyomas, adenomyosis, endometrial polyps, and use of certain intrauterine devices. Fragile, large thin-walled vessels and an aglandular endometrium appear to underlie the menorrhagia associated with submucous myomas.[237] These vessels may arise from abnormalities in angiogenesis associated with growth factors released by myomas (e.g., basic fibroblast growth factor, vascular endothelial growth factor).[1] Systemic disease is a rare cause of menorrhagia except in adolescents in whom coagulopathies including thrombocytopenia, von Willebrand disease or other coagulopathies, or leukemia may be the underlying cause.[238]

Dysfunctional uterine bleeding is another common cause of menorrhagia. This term has different meanings in different parts of the world, and this discrepancy creates some confusion in the literature. Although efforts are under way to lead toward simple descriptive terminology, the literature still reflects this issue.[239]

In the United States, dysfunctional uterine bleeding is commonly equated with anovulatory bleeding, whereas in Europe it is a diagnosis of exclusion of excessive bleeding not due to demonstrable pelvic disease, complications of pregnancy, or systemic disease. Anovulatory dysfunctional uterine bleeding is characterized by irregular and prolonged bleeding secondary to disturbances in the hypothalamic-pituitary-ovarian axis. It is most common in the extremes of reproductive life and in association

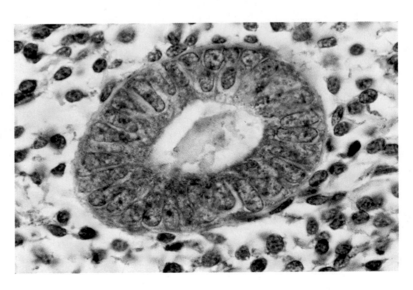

Figure 25-4. Immunohistochemical staining for the type I basic fibroblast growth factor receptor (bFGFR1). A high-power (100×) view of a single endometrial gland from an endometrial polyp shows the significant deposition of bFGFR1 protein (brown stain) in the apical region of the glandular cells. This protein expression was significantly reduced in autologous endometrium from the postmenopausal women studied. (Photomicrograph courtesy of AR Gargiulo, MD.)

with polycystic ovary syndrome. The unopposed action of estrogen on the uterus, resulting in dilated veins and the suppression of spiral arteriole development, represents the underlying pathophysiology.[235,236,240] Large, thin walled tortuous vessels can be demonstrated on the surface of the hyperplastic endometrium. Unopposed estrogen reduces vascular tone either through direct effects of estrogen on vascular smooth muscle cells or increased production of nitric oxide, leading to vasodilatation. The endometrium often breaks down unevenly in these circumstances. Scattered patches of thrombotic foci and necrotic degeneration are found adjacent to abnormally proliferated endometrium.

Ovulatory dysfunctional uterine bleeding is characterized by regular episodes of heavy menstrual flow, usually with the heaviest loss during the first 3 days of menstruation. The underlying abnormality appears to be defects in processes that regulate loss of blood during menstruation, primarily angiogenesis, vasoconstriction, and hemostasis. In contrast to anovulatory dysfunctional uterine bleeding, the surface vessels of the endometrium appear to be grossly normal and only minor abnormalities have been described in endometrial and myometrial veins.

The expression of genes governing the stability of the endometrial extracellular matrix and angiogenesis is dysregulated in menorrhagia.[235,236,240] Endometrial bleeding associated factor (i.e., TGF-β4 and lefty), a member of the TGF-β family of growth factors, suppresses production of collagen and promotes expression of collagenolytic and elastinolytic enzymes by antagonizing the normal signaling pathway activated by TGF-β growth factors. Abnormal expression of lefty, which in a normal cycle occurs only in the late secretory and menstrual phases, has been reported in the endometrium of women with menorrhagia.[41] An altered ratio of Ang-1 to Ang-2 in the endometrium due to down-regulation of Ang-1 expression is also associated with menorrhagia.[241] This would favor vessel destabilization and contribute to increased blood loss.

Increased fibrinolytic activity resulting from elevated endometrial tissue plasminogen activator levels exacerbates blood loss. In addition, vascular smooth muscle cell proliferation is reduced in the spiral arterioles in the mid- and late secretory stages in women with menorrhagia, possibly contributing to vessel instability.

Alterations in levels of regulators of vascular tone have been suggested to promote excessive uterine bleeding.[235,236,240] Diminished expression of endothelin in endometrial glands and luminal epithelium may lead to reduced myometrial contraction and greater blood loss. In addition, increased prostaglandin release and a disproportionate rise in prostaglandin E_2 (PGE_2), and increased PGI_2 (prostacyclin) and PGE_2 receptors predispose to vasodilatation. Augmented PGI production by the myometrium may contribute to the vasodilatation and prevention of platelet activation.

These pathophysiologic mechanisms proposed to underlie dysfunctional uterine bleeding are targets for novel therapeutic interventions (Fig. 25-5). Options would include the use of progestin-releasing intrauterine devices,[242] of antiprogestins or selective progesterone receptor modulators to suppress endometrial growth and stabilize the endometrial vasculature; MMP inhibitors to prevent extracellular matrix catabolism, including the matrix of the vessel walls; and selective COX-2 inhibitors to suppress prostanoid synthesis. Surgical destruction or removal of endometrium via endometrial ablation is also a less directed option.

Intrauterine Adhesions

The formation of intracavitary synechiae in an organ that routinely undergoes sloughing and regrowth without scarring is not well understood.[243] The clinical literature consistently reports that pregnancy frequently precedes the formation of intrauterine adhesions. The relationship between intrauterine adhesions and pregnancy is thought to be the result of defects in the regeneration of the endometrium after delivery, especially the area underlying the placenta. The placental site takes up to 6 weeks to repair with the thrombosed vessels and superficial necrotic tissue exfoliated as growing endometrial tissue undermines the area. Trauma to the regenerating endometrium involved in restoring stroma and epithelium at this site, for example, as a consequence of curettage performed 1 to 4 weeks after delivery, may result in a permanent scar with adhesions. Another cause of synechiae is intrauterine infection, particularly involving *Mycobacterium tuberculosis*, which is not uncommon outside the United States.

Women with intrauterine adhesions may have no symptoms or a variety of menstrual disorders including hypomenorrhea, oligomenorrhea, amenorrhea, and dysmenorrhea. Infertility, amenorrhea, and hypomenorrhea are the most common presenting complaints. Hysterosalpingography performed with a short catheter and hysteroscopy reveals the intrauterine lesions. Ultrasonography, sonohysterography, and MRI can be valuable in certain cases.

There is no consensus regarding the optimal methods to treat and prevent intrauterine adhesions. Surgical removal with blunt dissection, scissors, electrocautery, and laser ablation have all been recommended. Insertion of an intrauterine device or balloon catheter after lysis of adhesions is commonly employed to prevent recurrence. Stimulation of endometrial proliferation with exogenous estrogens alone or in combination with a progestin has been advocated, although there is debate as to the efficacy of this treatment as well as the administration of antibiotics and anti-inflammatory steroids.

Dysmenorrhea

Primary dysmenorrhea, menstrual pain not associated with recognizable pelvic disease, is due to intrinsic uterine dysfunction. Occurring only in ovulatory cycles, the symptoms of dysmenorrhea usually commence a few hours before the onset of the menstrual flow. Pain is greatest when the endometrium is shedding rapidly, approximately 12 hours after flow begins. The diagnosis of primary dysmenorrhea is based on medical history and normal findings on pelvic and rectovaginal examination.

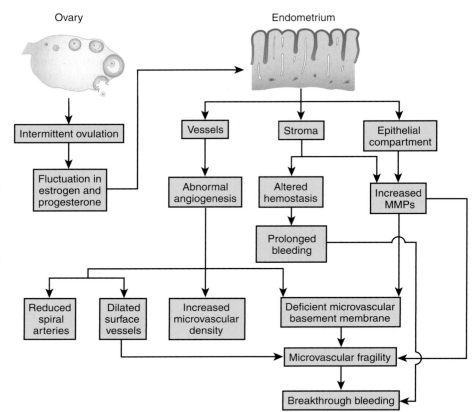

Figure 25-5. *Ovarian and uterine mechanisms underlying breakthrough bleeding. A schematic drawing detailing the interaction between ovarian steroids and local endometrial factors leading to abnormal uterine bleeding. MMPs, matrix metalloproteinases. (Modified and reprinted with permission from Gargett CE, Weston G, Rogers PA. Mechanisms and regulation of endometrial angiogenesis. Reprod Med Rev 10:45-61, 2002.)*

The painful cramps of dysmenorrhea are associated with uterine contractions; in women with dysmenorrhea, uterine contractile activity is heightened during menses, and basal myometrial tone and amplitude of contractions are increased. During intense contractions, there is a reduction in blood flow to the endometrium suggesting that ischemia, in part, causes the pain of dysmenorrhea.

The uterine contractions are prompted by prostaglandins, which are potent uterotonic agents both in vitro and in vivo acting through cell surface prostaglandin receptors (see Chapter 6).[244] Prostanoids may also directly sensitize uterine pain fibers. The notion that prostanoids are central to the pathogenesis of dysmenorrhea is supported by the observations that eicosanoids, most prominently $PGF_{2\alpha}$, are found in high concentrations in menstrual fluid and that $PGF_{2\alpha}$ levels are higher in the endometrium and menstrual fluid of women complaining of dysmenorrhea than in women with pain-free menses.[245] All drugs effective in inhibiting prostaglandin synthesis, including the potent nonsteroidal anti-inflammatory drugs ibuprofen, naproxen, and mefenamic acid alleviate symptoms of dysmenorrhea.[246] Calcium antagonists, such as nifedipine, are also effective because they prevent uterine contraction. Combination-type oral contraceptives, which reduce endometrial mass and thus total endometrial prostaglandin synthesis, prevent dysmenorrhea in 90% of cases.

In addition to prostanoids, other uterotonic substances including lipoxygenase products, vasopressin, and oxytocin may have a role in dysmenorrhea. Thus, antagonists of the V_1 receptor and oxytocin receptor have a therapeutic effect in dysmenorrheic subjects. Reductions in nitric oxide (NO), which relaxes uterine smooth muscle, may also contribute to the intensified contractions associated with dysmenorrhea.[247]

ACKNOWLEDGEMENT. The author acknowledges the contributions of Jerome F. Strauss III, MD, PhD, in the fifth edition.

The complete reference list can be found on the companion Expert Consult Web site at www.expertconsultbook.com.

Suggested Readings

Agency for Healthcare Research and Quality. Evidence Based Practice for Uterine Fibroids. Available at www.ahrq.gov/clinic/tp/uteruptp.htm. Accessed Dec. 19, 2008.

Gupta J, Sinha A, Lumsden M, Hickey M. Uterine artery embolization for symptomatic uterine fibroids. Cochrane Database Syst Rev 1: CD005073, 2006.

Lefebvre G, Vilos G, Allaire C, et al. The management of uterine leiomyomas. J Obstet Gynaecol Can 25(5):396-418. quiz 419-22, 2003.

Marjoribanks J, Lethaby A, Farquhar C. Surgery versus medical therapy for heavy menstrual bleeding. Cochrane Database Syst Rev 2: CD003855, 2006.

Pritts EA. Fibroids and infertility: a systematic review of the evidence. Obstet Gynecol Surv 56(8):483-491, 2001.

Pron G, Bennett J, Common A, et al. The Ontario Uterine Fibroid Embolization Trial. Part 2. Uterine fibroid reduction and symptom relief after uterine artery embolization for fibroids. Fertil Steril 79(1):120-127, 2003.

Pron G, Mocarski E, Bennett J, et al. Pregnancy after uterine artery embolization for leiomyomata: the Ontario multicenter trial. Obstet Gynecol 105(1):67-76, 2005.

Spies JB, Bruno J, Czeyda-Pommersheim F, et al. Long-term outcome of uterine artery embolization of leiomyomata. Obstet Gynecol 106(5):933-939, 2005.

Spies JB, Pelage J-P, (eds). Uterine Artery Embolization and Gynecologic Embolotherapy, Philadelphia, Lippincott Williams & Wilkins, 2005.

Stewart EA. Uterine Fibroids: The Complete Guide. Baltimore, Johns Hopkins University Press, 2007.

Stewart EA, Gostout B, Rabinovici J, et al. Sustained relief of leiomyoma symptoms by using focused ultrasound surgery. Obstet Gynecol 110 (2 Pt 1):279-287, 2007.

Stewart EA, Morton CC. The genetics of uterine leiomyomata: what clinicians need to know. Obstet Gynecol 107(4):917-921, 2006.

Stewart EA, Nowak RA. Leiomyoma-related bleeding: a classic hypothesis updated for the molecular era. Hum Reprod Update 2(4):295-306, 1996.

Stewart EA, Nowak RA. New concepts in the treatment of uterine leiomyomas. Obstet Gynecol 92(4 Pt 1):624-627, 1998.

Walker CL, Stewart EA. Uterine fibroids: the elephant in the room. Science 308(5728):1589-1592, 2005.

CHAPTER 26

Endocrine Diseases of Pregnancy

Stephen F. Thung and Errol R. Norwitz

Physiologic and endocrine adaptations occur in the mother in response to the demands of pregnancy. These demands include support of the fetus (volume support, nutritional and oxygen supply, and clearance of fetal waste), protection of the fetus (from starvation, drugs, toxins), preparation of the uterus for labor, and protection of the mother from potential cardiovascular injury at delivery. The presence of a preexisting endocrine disorder is likely to affect the ability of the mother to adapt to the demands of pregnancy and, as a result, may influence fetal growth and development. Drugs used to treat such disorders may also affect perinatal outcome. The most common preexisting endocrine disorders that can complicate pregnancy are diabetes mellitus, thyroid dysfunction, and obesity. Less common preexisting maternal endocrine disorders include pituitary tumors, diabetes insipidus, and hyperparathyroidism.

The physiologic and endocrine adaptations that characterize pregnancy can also lead to the development of pregnancy-specific diseases in previously healthy women, the most common of which are gestational diabetes and disorders of the endocrine and sympathetic nervous systems associated with preeclampsia and preterm labor. This chapter is designed to review in detail the underlying pathophysiology of these pregnancy-specific diseases, as well as the effects of pregnancy on preexisting endocrine disorders. A better understanding of these conditions will improve the ability of clinicians to optimize maternal and perinatal outcome in such pregnancies.

Diabetes Mellitus

EFFECTS OF PREGNANCY ON MATERNAL GLUCOSE METABOLISM

Normal pregnancy can be regarded as a diabetogenic (pro-diabetic) state with evidence of insulin resistance, maternal hyperinsulinism, and reduced peripheral uptake of glucose. These endocrine alterations, which result primarily from the production of anti-insulin hormones from the placenta (see Chapter 11), are designed to ensure a continuous supply of glucose for the developing and growing fetus. In pregnancy, therefore, the control of maternal glucose metabolism is shared by the mother and the fetoplacental unit. The endocrine and molecular mechanisms by which the fetoplacental unit is able to reset the carbohydrate homeostatic equilibrium in the mother are not clear, but likely involve the action of several placental hormones. These hormones include growth hormone (GH), human chorionic somatomammotropins (hCS, placental lactogens), corticotropin-releasing hormone (CRH), cortisol, and progesterone.

INSULIN PRODUCTION AND ACTION CHANGES DURING PREGNANCY

Major functional changes occur in insulin production and action during pregnancy. β cells in the islets of Langerhans within the pancreas—the cells responsible for insulin production—undergo hyperplasia, leading to insulin hypersecretion and an increase in circulating insulin levels throughout pregnancy.[1-3] It is this mechanism, along with the hemodilution of pregnancy and the initial enhanced responsiveness of cells to circulating levels of insulin,[4-6] that is likely responsible for the fasting hypoglycemia seen in early pregnancy. However, as pregnancy progresses, peripheral resistance to insulin increases.[4-6] In an attempt to overcome this resistance, the pancreas further increases insulin secretion. This compensatory response serves to return circulating maternal glucose levels to the normal range, but results also in chronically elevated insulin levels (both in the fasting and fed state), in the postprandial hyperglycemia that characterizes normal pregnancy,[7] and in islet cell hyperplasia.

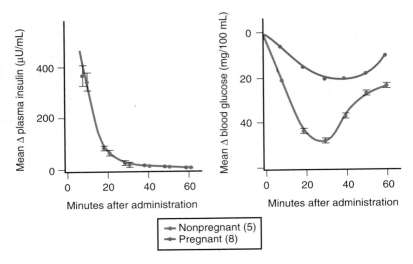

Figure 26-1. *Effect of pregnancy on insulin clearance and insulin sensitivity. Left, Intravenous injection of insulin (0.1 unit/kg) results in identical clearance curves for circulating insulin in nonpregnant and pregnant subjects (closed circles). Right, In pregnant subjects, the intravenous injection of insulin results in a smaller decline in circulating glucose than that seen in nonpregnant subjects. The blunted biologic effect of insulin in pregnancy suggests that pregnancy is a state of insulin resistance. (From Burt RL, Davidson WF. Insulin half-life and utilization in normal pregnancy. Obstet Gynecol 43:161, 1974, with permission from the American College of Obstetricians and Gynecologists.)*

Insulin resistance refers to a decrease in the ability of a fixed concentration of circulating insulin to stimulate peripheral glucose uptake in adipocytes and muscle cells. The condition can be demonstrated either by the insulin tolerance test or by glucose loading tests. An insulin tolerance test involves the injection of a standard dose of insulin followed by serial blood glucose measurements. The clearance of insulin from the circulation is not altered by pregnancy (Fig. 26-1).[8] The half-life of insulin is approximately 7 minutes both before and during pregnancy.[8] However, in pregnant subjects, the administration of insulin results in a smaller decline in circulating glucose than that seen in nonpregnant subjects (see Fig. 26-1). Furthermore, in pregnancy, intravenous (Fig. 26-2) or oral (Fig. 26-3) administration of glucose causes significant hyperinsulinemia as compared with the nonpregnant state,[4] resulting in relative hyperinsulinemia after meals. Taken together, these data provide evidence in support of pregnancy being an insulin-resistant state.

The molecular mechanisms responsible for the insulin resistance in pregnancy are not well understood, but several factors are likely involved. Although insulin receptor kinase activity does not appear to be affected by pregnancy, the numbers of high-affinity insulin receptors on the surface of adipocytes are threefold lower in pregnancy than in nonpregnant women.[2,9] The glucose transport system also appears to be perturbed in pregnancy, with a threefold reduction in insulin-stimulated glucose transport as compared with nonpregnant control subjects.[9]

The movement of glucose into adipocytes and skeletal muscle cells is mediated by the glucose transport proteins, GLUT-1 and GLUT-4. GLUT-1 is responsible for basal glucose transport and is not responsive to insulin. Insulin increases glucose uptake in cells by stimulating the translocation of GLUT-4 from intracellular sites to the cell surface.[10,11] Up to 75% of insulin-dependent glucose disposal occurs in skeletal muscle, whereas adipose tissue accounts for only a small fraction.[12] In some pregnancies complicated by gestational diabetes, GLUT-4 is markedly reduced and fails to translocate to the cell surface with insulin stimulation, leading to a reduction in glucose transport in both the basal and insulin-stimulated states.[13] Taken together,

these data suggest that the peripheral insulin resistance that characterizes pregnancy likely results from several integrated mechanisms, including a decrease in insulin receptor number, a "post-receptor" defect in insulin action, and alterations in glucose transport systems.[12-15]

Although the molecular mechanisms have yet to be fully elucidated, the fetoplacental unit is clearly responsible for the pregnancy-induced insulin resistance. Indeed, the insulin-glucose dynamics typically return to normal within hours to days of delivery.[5] The fetoplacental unit exerts its effect, in large part, through the production of counterregulatory (anti-insulin) hormones.

FETOPLACENTAL COUNTERREGULATORY HORMONES

Insulin promotes the uptake of glucose by adipocytes and muscle cells. Counterregulatory hormones inhibit insulin-mediated glucose uptake by adipocytes and muscle cells, acting largely at a postreceptor level. Such hormones include, among others, GH, hCS, cortisol, and progesterone.

Placental Growth Hormone and Human Chorionic Somatomammotropin

Placental GH differs from pituitary GH by 13 amino acid (191 nucleotide) substitutions[16] and circulates in at least three isoforms: 22, 24, and 26 kDa.[17] Human chorionic somatomammotropins are single-chain proteins produced largely by the syncytiotrophoblast with a high degree of sequence homology to both GH and prolactin. In primates, hCS genes appear to have evolved from a precursor GH gene; in nonprimate species, on the other hand, the placental lactogens appear to have evolved from a precursor prolactin gene. Because of these differences in evolution, we have chosen to use the term "human chorionic somatomammotropins" to refer to these genes collectively.[18] The dominant isoform of hCS is 191 amino acids in length, with a molecular mass of 23 kDa.[16,19]

The factors that regulate GH and hCS synthesis and secretion are not fully understood, but somatostatin and

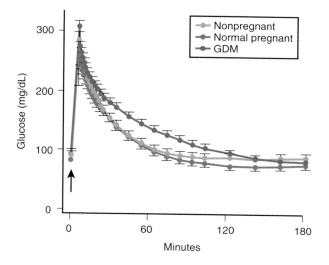

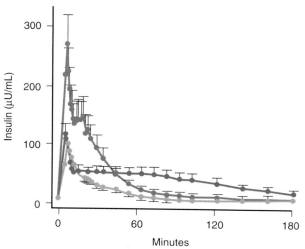

Figure 26-2. Insulin and glucose response to an intravenous glucose challenge. Comparison of insulin and glucose responses to a rapid intra-venous infusion of glucose (300 mg/kg) in nonpregnant women, preg-nant women, and pregnant women with gestational diabetes mellitus (GDM). In GDM, there are both elevated glucose and insulin concentra-tions, suggesting that the condition is an insulin-resistant state. The arrow indicates injection of glucose. (From Buchanan TA, Metzger BE, Freinkel N, Bergman B. Insulin sensitivity and B-cell responsiveness to glucose during late pregnancy in lean and moderately obese women with normal glucose tolerance or mild gestational diabetes. Am J Obstet Gynecol 162:1008, 1990.)

GH-releasing hormone produced by the cytotrophoblast may play inhibitory and stimulatory roles, respectively.[20-22] Additional regulation of hCS may be provided by insulin and angiotensin II, which both stimulate hCS release,[23,24] as well as by dynorphin (Fig. 26-4).[25] This placental endo-crine and paracrine/autocrine regulatory system is similar to that observed in the hypothalamic-pituitary axis, which has led Dr. Samuel Yen to refer to the placenta as "the third brain."[26]

The genes coding for GH and hCS are clustered to-gether in a single region of chromosome 17 in the follow-ing order (5′ to 3′): hGH-N (pituitary GH gene), hCSL, hCS-A, hGH-V (placental GH gene), and hCS-B.[27] The

pattern of expression of these genes is tissue-specific and changes throughout gestation. For example, the placenta does not express the hGH-N (pituitary GH) gene. Pituitary GH is secreted in a pulsatile fashion from the maternal anterior pituitary gland, and can be measured in the ma-ternal serum throughout the first trimester of pregnancy.[28] Thereafter, however, pituitary GH secretion progressively declines. By the third trimester of pregnancy, pituitary GH secretion is effectively suppressed and cannot be rescued by induction of a hypoglycemic stimulus or by amino acid infusions (which will be discussed later in this chapter).[29,30] In contrast, circulating concentrations of pla-cental GH—encoded by the hGH-V (placental GH) gene and expressed exclusively in the placenta—increase pro-gressively throughout the second and third trimesters of pregnancy.[28,31] Similar differences are seen in the expres-sion of the hCS genes. For example, at 8 weeks' gestation, the hCS-A and hCS-B genes are expressed equally in the placenta; however, at term, expression of hCS-A is five times greater than that of hCS-B. Results of radioreceptor assay studies suggest that the relative contributions to circulating GH-like activity in pregnancy at term are 85% from hGH-V (placental GH), 12% from hCS, and less than 3% from hGH-N (pituitary GH).[32] Multiple genes, multiple mRNA species (as in the hCS-L and hGH-V genes, which generate two distinct mRNA transcripts on the basis of alternative splice-acceptor sites for each gene[33]), and heterogeneity in post-translational processing result in many isoforms of these key placental hormones. The potential teleologic advantages of having multiple placental GH-like genes are to ensure that the placenta can generate sufficient quan-tities of GH-like hormone to regulate maternal and fetal metabolism, and to minimize the risk of pregnancy failure due to a functional "knockout" of any single gene.

During pregnancy, there is a major transition in the locus of control of the GH axis from the maternal hypothalamic-pituitary unit to the placenta. Circulating levels of pla-cental GH and hCS increase throughout pregnancy. These proteins act through cell surface receptors (GH and pro-lactin receptors belong to a superfamily of cytokine recep-tors that share a high degree of sequence homology[18]) to stimulate the production of insulin-like growth factor-1 (IGF-1). Circulating concentrations of IGF-1 in the ma-ternal serum increase throughout pregnancy, reaching a peak near term.[34,35] This increase in IGF-1 has also been observed in a pregnant dwarf with complete pituitary GH deficiency,[29] suggesting that placental hormones may me-diate this effect. Concentrations of IGF-binding protein-1 (IGFBP-1) rise in the first trimester, reach a peak at ap-proximately 12 to 14 weeks of gestation, and thereafter remain stable for the remainder of pregnancy.[36] The level of unbound (bioavailable) IGF-1 therefore increases as pregnancy progresses, and likely contributes to the sup-pression of hGH-N (pituitary GH) gene expression in the latter half of gestation.

In the circulation, GH can exist in a free form or bound to a GH-binding protein (GHBP). Approximately 30% of circulating GH is bound to GHBP and therefore not bio-logically active.[37] Veldhuis and colleagues[38] proposed that GHBP may serve as a buffer to prevent the level of free (bioavailable) GH from falling too low between secretory

Glucose

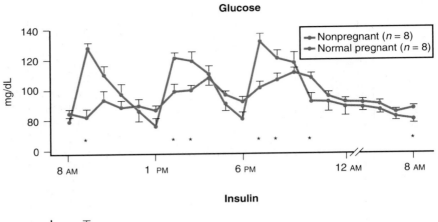

Insulin

Figure 26-3. Effect of pregnancy on carbohydrate and lipid metabolism in the fed and fasting state. Comparison of glucose, insulin, free fatty acid, and triglyceride responses to 24 hours of feeding and fasting in nonpregnant and normal pregnant women in the third trimester. In the fed state (asterisks), pregnancy is associated with elevated levels of circulating glucose and insulin. In the fasting state, pregnancy is associated with decreases in glucose below those that are seen in the nonpregnant state. The arrows indicate timing of meals. FFA, free fatty acids. (From Phelps RL, Metzger BE, Freinkel N. Carbohydrate metabolism in pregnancy. Am Obstet Gynecol 140:730, 1981.)

FFA

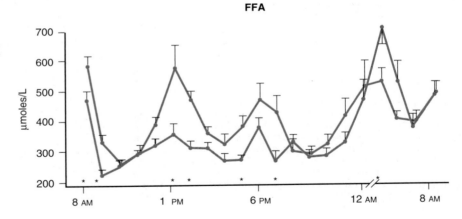

Triglyceride

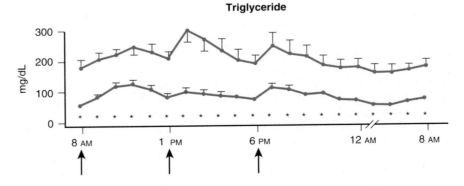

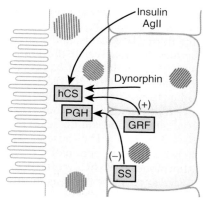

Syncytiotrophoblast   Cytotrophoblast

Figure 26-4. *Regulation of placental counterregulatory hormones. Diagrammatic depiction of a potential placental regulatory system involving growth hormone–releasing factor (GRF), somatostatin (SS), human chorionic somatomammotropin (hCS), and placental growth hormone (PGH). The modulating roles of dynorphin, insulin, and angiotensin II (AgII) are also shown. The placenta has endocrine regulatory systems that parallel those in the maternal and fetal hypothalamic-pituitary units. Yen has proposed that the placenta is a "third brain."*

pulses. GHBP is the ectodomain of a larger cellular GH receptor and is released into the circulation after proteolytic cleavage of the parent molecule. It is likely, therefore, that circulating concentrations of GHBP parallel that of the cellular GH receptor in important target organs such as the liver. This relationship allows for a balance between GH action (mediated through the GH receptor) and inactivation (by binding to the GHBP). The greater the levels of circulating GHBP, the greater the concentration of cellular GH receptors and the greater the sensitivity of cells to the actions of GH. GHBP concentrations tend to decline as gestation advances,[39] although the reason for this change and its physiologic significance remain unclear.

This system is not a prerequisite for pregnancy success, because a normal pregnancy is possible in women with Laron dwarfism in which both the GH receptor and GHBP are absent.[40] However, aberrations in this system may be associated with pregnancy-related complications. For example, GHBP levels have been shown to be significantly higher in women with gestational diabetes compared with nondiabetic pregnant women.[41] This observation suggests that the concentration of GH receptors is also increased in women with gestational diabetes, leading to a degree of sensitization to the effects of GH and hCS. An increased sensitivity to the effects of circulating GH could explain many of the endocrine changes observed in gestational diabetes, including insulin resistance, higher serum glucose levels, and an increased incidence of fetal macrosomia.

Circulating levels of placental GH (hGH-V), IGF-1, and the IGFBPs appear to correlate with birth weight. For example, a decrease in both placental GH and IGF-1 levels has been associated with intrauterine growth restriction (IUGR).[42] The decrease in placental GH levels is due both to a decrease in placental mass and a decrease in the density of placental GH-secreting cells.[43] There is also a strong inverse correlation between maternal IGFBP-1 concentrations and

birth weight in both term and preterm pregnancies.[44,45] The higher the IGFBP-1 concentration, the lower the circulating level of unbound (bioavailable) IGF-1 and the lower the birth weight. Moreover, several investigators have reported a positive correlation between birth weight and circulating concentrations of IGF-1 in the fetus and neonate.[46,47] Reece and colleagues[47] reported that IGF-1 concentrations were significantly lower in neonates below the mean birth weight for gestational age than levels in neonates above the mean (mean ± SEM: 40 ± 11 versus 86 ± 6 ng/mL, respectively), with no differences in IGF-2 concentrations. Similar findings were reported by Lassarre and colleagues.[46] Taken together, these data suggest that GH, hCS, and IGF-1, as well as their binding proteins (GHBP and the IGFBPs), may play an important role in governing fetal growth and pregnancy outcome, and that these endocrine factors may be regulated by both the mother and the fetoplacental unit.

Cortisol

Cortisol is a potent diabetogenic hormone. It promotes lipolysis in adipocytes and protein breakdown in muscle, leading to an increase in circulating free fatty acids and amino acids.[48] Levels of adrenocorticotropic hormone (ACTH) and cortisol increase in pregnancy.[49] The increase in ACTH is due, at least in part, to an increase in CRH production by the placenta (discussed later in this chapter). Much of the increase in total cortisol concentration in pregnancy is due to the excessive production of corticosteroid-binding globulin by the liver under the influence of estrogen. However, there is also a significant increase in urinary free cortisol excretion during pregnancy, suggesting that circulating levels of free cortisol may also be increased.[50] The relative contribution of an increase in circulating free cortisol to the insulin resistance of pregnancy is unclear.

Progesterone

High concentrations of progesterone have been shown to cause insulin resistance in cells in culture and in laboratory animals by decreasing insulin receptor number and causing a post-receptor defect in insulin action, which has yet to be fully elucidated.[51-53] High circulating concentrations of progesterone may likely contribute to the pregnancy-related insulin resistance.

FASTING STATE

In nonpregnant women, there is a constant need to maintain circulating glucose concentrations for use by the brain. During an overnight fast, glucose is released from the liver by both glycogenolysis (breakdown of glycogen stores [75%]) and gluconeogenesis (production of glucose from circulating metabolic precursors [25%]). The precursors for gluconeogenesis include pyruvate, alanine (from muscle), glycerol (from the breakdown of triglycerides in adipose tissue), and lactate (from anaerobic metabolism).

Pregnancy is associated with an increased demand for glucose and alanine, both of which are required by the developing fetus. As such, the fasting state in pregnancy is characterized by a rapid and often severe decrease in

TABLE 26-1

Fasting Maternal Glucose, Insulin, Glucagon, Amino Acid, Alanine, Free Fatty Acid, and Cholesterol Concentrations in Late Pregnancy Compared With the Nonpregnant State

	Measurement (mean ± SEM)	
	Nonpregnant State	Late Pregnancy
Glucose (mg/dL)	79 ± 2.4	68 ± 1.5*
Insulin (μ/mL)	9.8 ± 1.1	16.2 ± 2*
Glucagon (pg/mL)	126 ± 6.1	130 ± 5.2
Amino acids (μM)	3.82 ± 0.13	3.18 ± 0.11*
Alanine (μM)	286 ± 15	225 ± 9*
Free fatty acids (mg/dL)	76 ± 7	181 ± 10*
Cholesterol (mg/dL)	163 ± 8.7	205 ± 5.7*

*$P < 0.05$

From Freinkel N, Metzger BE, Nitzan M, et al. Facilitated anabolism in late pregnancy: some novel maternal compensations for accelerated starvation. *In* Malaisse WJ, Pirart J (eds). Diabetes International Series 312. Amsterdam, Excerpta Medica, 1973, p 474.

maternal serum glucose and alanine concentrations. Associated with these changes is an increase in the circulating levels of free fatty acids (derived from triglyceride breakdown in adipose cells) and ketone bodies (Table 26-1; see Fig. 26-3).[54,55] The hyperketonemia that characterizes late pregnancy is the result of enhanced lipolysis, which is likely due, in turn, to the insulin resistance in adipocytes caused primarily by the placental counterregulatory hormones.

In pregnancy, the acceleration of lipid catabolism during fasting helps the mother to rely on fat as a major energy source, thereby minimizing protein catabolism (preserving muscle mass) and allowing both glucose and amino acids to be used preferentially by the fetus.[7] These metabolic adaptations have been termed "accelerated starvation" by Freinkel.[56] Although a useful descriptive term, this characterization of pregnancy is largely inaccurate because fat mass is known to increase significantly during pregnancy.[57]

FED STATE

The fetus is a thief! Many of the metabolic and endocrine adaptations associated with pregnancy are designed to maintain a preferential and uninterrupted supply of metabolic fuel from mother to fetus as dictated by the progressively increasing demands of the growing fetus. The placenta is relatively impermeable to fat, but readily transports glucose, amino acids, and ketone bodies from the maternal to the fetal circulation.

Pregnancy is associated with hyperlipemia, both in the fasting and the fed states. Total plasma lipid concentrations increase progressively after 24 weeks of gestation. Increases in triglycerides, cholesterol, and free fatty acids are significant (Figs. 26-5 and 26-6; see Table 26-1).[7,55,58,59] High-density lipoprotein cholesterol levels rise during early pregnancy, and low-density lipoprotein cholesterol concentrations increase in later pregnancy.[58,59]

In pregnancy, an oral glucose load is associated with a greater increase in circulating glucose concentration, a smaller decline in free fatty acids, and a larger increase in serum triglycerides than that seen in the non-pregnant state (see Fig. 26-5).[7,55] A similar effect has been observed in pregnancy after meals (see Fig. 26-3).[7] These adaptations allow the mother to use primarily available triglycerides, glycerol, and free fatty acids for metabolic fuel after meals, and to preserve glucose and amino acids for preferential use by the fetus (Fig. 26-7). The cause of these metabolic changes is likely the lipolytic action of the placental counterregulatory hormones (GH, hCS, cortisol, and progesterone), which serve to promote lipolysis during fasting and hypertriglyceridemia in the fed state.

Gestational Diabetes

The American Diabetes Association (ADA) classification of diabetes mellitus is summarized in Box 26-1.[60,61] Gestational diabetes mellitus (GDM) is defined as any degree of glucose intolerance with the onset of pregnancy or first recognized during pregnancy.[62] In light of this definition, GDM may include a small group of women with previously unrecognized type 1 or type 2 diabetes. True gestational diabetes, however, is associated with a normal glycosylated hemoglobin level and a normal glucose tolerance test after delivery. Depending on the patients screened and the diagnostic criteria used, GDM complicates approximately 3% to 12% of all pregnancies, resulting in approximately 140,000 cases annually in the United States alone.[63-65] Women with GDM far exceed the number of pregnant women with pregestational diabetes, the ratio being approximately 10 to 1.

GDM poses little immediate risk to the mother. Indeed, such women are not at risk of diabetic ketoacidosis (DKA), which is primarily a disease of absolute insulin deficiency. However, GDM has been associated with increased rates of birth trauma and perinatal mortality[65,66] making diagnosis very important. Patients with GDM are typically asymptomatic. Some experts and organizations—including the ADA[60] and the Fourth International Workshop Conference on Gestational Diabetes[67]—have recommended screening all pregnant women for GDM. Not all organizations are in agreement, however.[65,66,68] Universal screening is probably not cost-effective in women at low risk for GDM. Falling into this low-risk category are women under age 25 who have normal body mass index (BMI), who have no first-degree relatives with the condition, and who are not members of ethnic or racial groups with a high prevalence of diabetes (Hispanic, Native American, Asian, and African American). Identifying and deferring screening in these low-risk women will decrease the overall number of patients screened by approximately 10% and will overlook only 3% of all women with GDM.[69]

For all other women, screening for GDM is recommended between 24 and 28 weeks of gestation.[65] For women at particularly high risk (such as women with a history of gestational diabetes or polycystic ovary syndrome, a high BMI, persistent glycosuria, a strong family history of diabetes, a prior macrosomic infant, or a prior

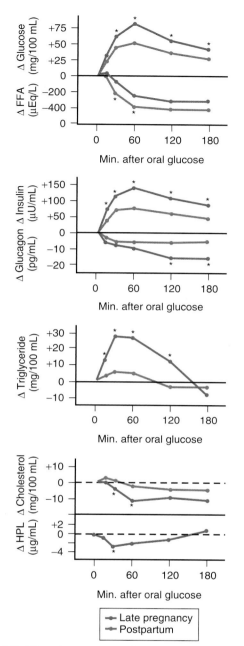

Figure 26-5. *Effect of pregnancy on short-term carbohydrate and lipid metabolism following an oral glucose challenge. Differences in the central metabolic response to an oral glucose load in pregnant and postpartum subjects. FFA, free fatty acids; HPL, human placental lactogen (chorionic somatomammotropin). (From Freinkel N, Metzger BE, Nitzan M, et al. Facilitated anabolism in late pregnancy: Some novel maternal compensations for accelerated starvation. In Malaisse WJ, Pirart J [eds]. Diabetes International Series 312. Amsterdam, Excerpta Medica, 1973, p 474.)*

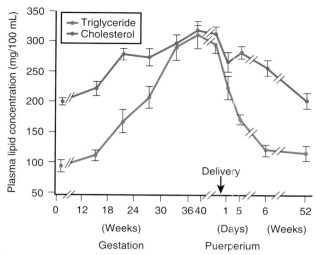

Figure 26-6. *Changes in plasma cholesterol and triglyceride concentrations during pregnancy and in the puerperium. Fasting lipid concentrations were measured serially throughout pregnancy, at delivery, in the puerperium, and at 12 months postpartum. The results are the mean + SEM. (From Potter JM, Nestel PJ. The hyperlipidemia of pregnancy in normal and complicated pregnancies. Am J Obstet Gynecol 133:165, 1979.)*

O'Sullivan et al in 1973,[70] the GLT is a nonfasting 50-g oral glucose challenge followed by a venous plasma glucose measurement at 1 hour.[62-65] The GLT is considered positive if the 1-hour glucose measurement is greater than a previously agreed-upon threshold. Both 130 mg/dL and 140 mg/dL have been suggested.[65,71] Use of a lower cutoff will increase the detection rate of women with GDM, but will result in a substantial increase in the false-positive rate (Table 26-2).[71,72] Which threshold is more cost-effective has yet to be determined.

A definitive diagnosis of GDM requires a 3-hour *glucose tolerance test* (GTT). There is no absolute GLT cutoff that should be regarded as diagnostic of GDM,[65,71-74] although a fasting glucose measurement of at least 105 mg/dL in the setting of a positive GLT is highly predictive of an abnormal GTT.[74] In pregnancy, the GTT involves an overnight fast and subsequent 100-g oral glucose challenge. Venous plasma glucose is measured fasting and at 1 hour, 2 hours, and 3 hours after the glucose load.

Although there is general agreement that two or more abnormal values are required to confirm the diagnosis,[65,71] there is little consensus about the glucose values that define the upper range of normal in pregnancy and no threshold that perfectly predicts adverse pregnancy outcome. Even one elevated value has been associated with an increased incidence of macrosomia and birth injury. The recommendations of the ADA and those proposed by other authorities are presented in Table 26-3.[75-77] The ADA recommends the Carpenter and Coustan values and the American College of Obstetricians and Gynecologists (ACOG) recommends using either the Carpenter and Coustan criteria or the National Diabetes Data Group criteria.[65] The gestational 3-hour GTT should not be confused with the 2-hour GTT used to diagnose diabetes outside of pregnancy, which is a 75-g oral glucose challenge performed in nonpregnant women and uses different serum glucose cutoff

unexplained late fetal demise), early screening for GDM is recommended between 16 and 20 weeks' gestation.[65] If the early screen is negative, the screen should be repeated at 24 to 28 weeks.

The most commonly used screening test for GDM is the *glucose load test* (GLT), also known as the *glucose challenge test* (GCT). First proposed as a screening test for GDM by

Mother

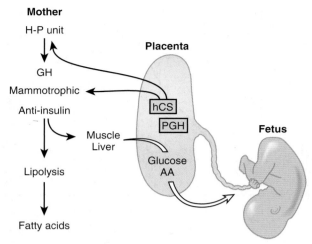

Figure 26-7. Effect of pregnancy on maternal carbohydrate metabolism. The proposed functional role of human chorionic somatomammotropin (hCS) and placental growth hormone (PGH) in the adjustment of maternal metabolic homeostasis with preferential transfer of amino acid (AA) and glucose to the fetus. Maternal metabolism relies on triglycerides and fatty acids. GH, growth hormone; H-P, hypothalamic-pituitary.

BOX 26-1

American Diabetes Association (ADA) Classification of Diabetes Mellitus

Type 1 diabetes mellitus: Caused by β-cell dysfunction, usually leading to absolute insulin deficiency

Type 2 diabetes mellitus: Typically associated with peripheral insulin resistance and varying degrees of abnormalities in insulin secretion

Gestational diabetes mellitus: Characterized by peripheral insulin resistance resulting from counterregulatory (anti-insulin) hormones produced by the placenta

Other types: Genetic defects in carbohydrate metabolism, drug-induced diabetes

---

measurements. Glycosylated hemoglobin estimation is of no value in making the diagnosis of GDM,[65,71] although it may be useful in the diagnosis of pregestational diabetes.

Transplacental glucose transport is a facilitated process that is mediated by the glucose transporter isoform GLUT-1.[78,79] Some researchers have hypothesized that maternal hyperglycemia in diabetes increases placental glucose transfer, resulting in fetal hyperglycemia and increased fetal insulin concentration that in turn stimulates fetal growth.[80] However, even in diabetic pregnancies with evidence of strict glycemic control, fetal macrosomia (defined as an estimated fetal weight of at least 4500g[81]) is not uncommon,[82-84] which suggests a complex relationship between metabolic derangement and fetal growth in diabetes.[85] Other factors that may contribute to fetal macrosomia include obesity and high circulating levels of amino acids and lipids.[71]

TABLE 26-2

Glucose Screening for Gestational Diabetes*

Glucose Cutoff	Proportion of Women With a Positive Test	Sensitivity for Gestational Diabetes Mellitus
≥140 mg/dL (≥7.8 mmol/L)	14-18%	≈80%
≥130 mg/dL (≥7.2 mmol/L)	20-25%	≈90%

*Using the 50-g oral glucose load screening test.
From Kjos SL, Buchanan TA. Gestational diabetes mellitus. N Engl J Med 341:1749, 1999.

Many of the complications of GDM are due to fetal macrosomia. Increased birth weight is associated with an increased risk of cesarean delivery, operative vaginal delivery, and birth injury to both the mother (vaginal, perineal, and rectal trauma) and fetus (including orthopedic and neurologic injury).[65,66,68,70,71,86,87] Shoulder dystocia with resultant brachial plexus injury are serious consequences of fetal macrosomia, and are further increased in the setting of GDM because the macrosomia of diabetes is associated with increased diameters in the upper thorax of the fetus.

Interventions that definitively decrease the risk of macrosomia and subsequent adverse outcomes are limited. A recent randomized trial comparing women whose GDM was diagnosed and treated to those with untreated GDM[88] demonstrated that good glycemic control achieved through a combination of dietary counseling, four times daily home blood glucose monitoring (maintaining fasting glucose levels <99 mg/dL and 2-hour postprandial levels <126 mg/dL),and insulin for persistent hyperglycemia resulted in a significant improvement in perinatal outcome, specifically shoulder dystocia, orthopedic injury, nerve palsy, and death (from 4% to 1%). There was also a reduction in the diagnosis of macrosomia (21% to 10%), but an increase in ICU admissions (61% to 71%). Induction of labor was increased in the intervention groups (from 29% to 39%) with no increase in the cesarean delivery rate, which was stable at 31% to 32%.

GDM cannot be prevented. The goal of antepartum management is to prevent fetal macrosomia and its resultant complications by maintaining maternal blood glucose at desirable levels throughout gestation (fasting, below 95 mg/dL; 1 hour postprandial, below 140 mg/dL; or 2 hours postprandial, below 120 mg/dL).[65] Initial recommendations should include a diabetic diet consisting of 30 to 35 kcal/kg of ideal body weight given as 40% to 50% carbohydrate, 20% protein, and 30% to 40% fat to avoid protein catabolism. Daily home glucose monitoring and weekly antepartum visits to monitor glycemic control should also be instituted. If diet alone does not maintain blood glucose at desirable levels, insulin administration may be required.[89] If initial fasting glucose levels are consistently greater than 95 mg/dL and 2-hour postprandial values are over 120 mg/dL, insulin therapy can be started right away with every effort made to avoid iatrogenic hypoglycemia.[90,91] The Fourth International Workshop on Gestational

TABLE 26-3

Diagnostic Thresholds for Gestational Diabetes During 100-g Glucose Tolerance Test

	Plasma Glucose Values, mg/dL (mmol/L)		
	National Diabetes Data Group	*Sacks et al.*	*Carpenter and Coustan*
Fasting	105 (5.8)	96 (5.3)	95 (5.2)
1-hour	190 (10.6)	172 (9.4)	180 (9.9)
2-hour	165 (9.2)	152 (8.3)	155 (8.6)
3-hour	145 (8.1)	131 (7.2)	140 (7.7)

Data from National Diabetes Data Group. Classification and diagnosis of diabetes and other categories of glucose intolerance. Diabetes 28:1039, 1979; Sacks DA, Abu-Fadil S, Greenspoon JS, Fotheringham N. Do the current standards for glucose tolerance testing in pregnancy represent a valid conversion of O'Sullivan's original criteria? Am J Obstet Gynecol 161:638, 1989; Carpenter MW, Coustan DR. Criteria for screening tests for gestational diabetes. Am J Obstet Gynecol 144:768, 1982.

Diabetes[67] recommended exercise as an adjunct to diet for the treatment of GDM, although randomized studies have failed to demonstrate a beneficial effect of exercise on glycemic control in women with GDM.[92]

In the United States, oral hypoglycemic agents (such as sulfonylureas) have not been recommended for use during pregnancy because of the possibility of fetal teratogenesis and prolonged neonatal hypoglycemia. This class of drugs works by stimulating pancreatic β-cells to synthesize and release insulin. Because the adverse fetal consequences of GDM are likely related to fetal hyperinsulinemia, any agent that could cross the placenta and increase fetal insulin production should be used with caution in pregnancy. First-generation sulfonylureas have been shown to cross the placenta and, as such, are contraindicated in pregnancy. However, there are conflicting data regarding the transplacental passage of second-generation sulfonylurea agents (glyburide and glipizide), though human studies to date have demonstrated minimal fetal exposure.[93-95]

Congenital malformations associated with the use of oral sulfonylurea drugs in pregnancy have been described,[96] but most of these reports failed to take into account maternal glycemic control. More recent studies have shown that the risk of malformations correlates strongly with the degree of glycemic control at the time of conception and is unrelated to the type of antidiabetic therapy.[97] Moreover, such reports refer to oral hypoglycemic treatment in early pregnancy, whereas treatment for GDM only begins after the period of fetal organogenesis thereby eliminating any concern regarding malformations due to treatment alone.

Between 1974 and 1983, Coetzee and Jackson[98] treated more than 150 women with GDM with oral hypoglycemic agents and found no cases of serious neonatal hypoglycemia and no increase in perinatal mortality rate. A clinical trial by Langer et al[99] randomized 404 women with singleton pregnancies and GDM requiring treatment to either glyburide or insulin therapy. Results showed no difference in glycemic control or neonatal outcome (including congenital malformations, macrosomia, neonatal hypoglycemia, and admission to neonatal intensive care). Eight women (4%) in the glyburide group required insulin therapy. Glyburide was not detected in the cord blood of any of the infants in the glyburide group. Although the limited data currently available do not permit firm conclusions to be drawn about the efficacy and safety of oral hypoglycemic drugs in pregnancy, these agents are being used more frequently by obstetric care providers.[100]

Unlike glyburide, metformin is known to cross the human placenta,[101] which has reduced enthusiasm for its use during pregnancy. Metformin acts to reduce peripheral insulin resistance. Because insulin acts as a potent growth factor, there is a theoretical concern that metformin passage across the placenta may lead to excessive fetal growth. Despite these concerns, metformin is now commonly being used by reproductive endocrinologists to achieve pregnancy in women with polycystic ovary syndrome (PCOS).[102] Although in vitro models[103,104] and in vivo studies[101] have shown that metformin does cross from the maternal to the fetal compartment, multiple small retrospective studies have failed to show any significant adverse outcome with first trimester metformin exposure.[102,105,106] There are as yet no randomized studies comparing metformin with either glyburide or insulin therapy in the management of GDM.

The risk of stillbirth is increased in women with poorly controlled GDM,[65,71,87] although it is not clear whether this is true also of pregnancies with mild disease.[107,108] For this reason, many centers recommend weekly fetal testing starting at 32 weeks and early delivery (typically at 38 to 40 weeks) for women with GDM who require oral or insulin therapy and those with a pregnancy complication (macrosomia, polyhydramnios, or hypertension). Whether weekly fetal testing and early delivery are necessary in pregnancies complicated only by diet-controlled GDM is not clear. Sonographic estimation of fetal weight should be considered at around 36 to 38 weeks' gestation. The use of prophylactic elective cesarean delivery to reduce the risk of maternal and fetal birth injury in the setting of fetal macrosomia remains controversial.[65] It is clear, however, that induction of labor for so-called *impending macrosomia* does not decrease the risk of cesarean delivery or intrapartum complications.[109,110] In labor, maternal glucose levels in pregnancies complicated by GDM should be maintained at 100 to 120 mg/dL to minimize the risk of fetal hypoxic injury. For the same reason, neonatal blood glucose levels should be measured within 1 hour of birth, and early feeding should be encouraged. Delivery of the fetus and placenta effectively removes the source of the anti-insulin hormones that cause GDM.

TABLE 26-4

White Classification of Diabetes in Pregnancy

White Class	Age of Onset (yr)		Duration (yr)	Vascular Disease	Therapy
A	Only in pregnancy		Only in pregnancy	No	A1: Diet controlled A2: Insulin requiring
B	>20	or	<10	No	Insulin
C	10-19	or	10-19	No	Insulin
D	<10	or	>20	Benign retinopathy hypertension	Insulin
F	Any		Any	Nephropathy	Insulin
R	Any		Any	Proliferative retinopathy	Insulin
H	Any		Any	Atherosclerotic heart disease	Insulin
T	Any		Any	Renal transplant	Insulin

As such, no further management is required in the immediate postpartum period.

GDM frequently indicates underlying insulin resistance. Fifty percent of women with GDM will experience GDM in subsequent pregnancies, and 30% to 65% will develop type 2 diabetes later in life.[71,111-113] All women with GDM should, therefore, have a standard (nonpregnant) 75-g GTT at approximately 6 weeks post partum and should consider preventive and early diagnostic strategies such as weight reduction, increased exercise, and regular screening for diabetes.

Pregnancy in Women with Type 1 or Type 2 Diabetes Mellitus

Pregestational diabetes, which affects approximately 1% of women of childbearing age, can be due either to absolute insulin deficiency (type 1, insulin-dependent diabetes mellitus [IDDM]) or to increased peripheral resistance to insulin action (type 2, non-insulin-dependent diabetes mellitus [NIDDM]), as shown in Box 26-1. The fasting glucose cutoff for diagnosing pregestational diabetes was recently reduced from 140 mg/dL to 126 mg/dL.[60] On the basis of this change, there are approximately 21 million people with pregestational diabetes in the United States alone.[114]

The White classification of diabetes in pregnancy (Table 26-4) was developed by Dr. Priscilla White at the Joslin Diabetic Center in Boston, Massachusetts, in an attempt to correlate severity of diabetes with pregnancy outcome.[115] Although this classification is commonly used, any direct correlation between White class and prognosis remains unclear. Features known to be associated with poor pregnancy outcome include DKA, poor compliance, hypertension, pyelonephritis, and vasculopathy.

In contrast to GDM, pregestational diabetes is associated with significant rates of maternal and perinatal mortality and morbidity (summarized in Box 26-2).[116,117] One of the more important complications is the increased risk of congenital malformations associated with hyperglycemia at the time of fertilization and embryo development. The incidence of congenital anomalies and spontaneous

BOX 26-2

Pregnancy-Related Complications of Pregestational Diabetes

Maternal
Spontaneous abortion
Diabetic ketoacidosis
Hypertension
Preeclampsia/eclampsia
Preterm birth
Cesarean delivery
Severe perineal injury
Infectious morbidity (chorioamnionitis, endometritis, wound infection)

Fetal
Congenital anomalies
Macrosomia
Intrauterine growth restriction
Late fetal demise
Nonreassuring fetal testing (previously referred to as "fetal distress")

Neonatal
Birth trauma (e.g., hypoxic ischemic cerebral injury; skull, clavicular, and long bone fractures; shoulder dystocia and brachial plexus injury)
Hypoglycemia
Neonatal sepsis
Delayed organ maturation (respiratory distress syndrome, hyperbilirubinemia)

abortions in such patients correlates directly with the degree of glycemic control at conception, as measured by circulating maternal glycosylated hemoglobin levels.[118-120] Overall, approximately 30% to 50% of the perinatal deaths in diabetic pregnancy are due to fetal malformations.[121] Structural anomalies commonly seen in association with diabetes include cardiac defects (ventricular septal defects, transposition of the great vessels), renal agenesis, and neural tube defects (anencephaly, open spina bifida).[122] Some congenital defects—specifically sacral agenesis and caudal dysplasia—are as much as 400 times more common in the offspring of women with diabetes than in women with normal glucose metabolism[123] and, as such, are considered characteristic of diabetic embryopathy; the overall prevalence of these anomalies, however, is low.

The factors responsible for diabetic embryopathy are not well defined, but glucose[124,125] and ketone bodies such as β-hydroxybutyrate[126,127] have both been implicated. Recently, oxidative stress[128,129] and apoptosis dysregulation[130,131] have been identified as potential mechanisms for diabetic embryopathy in animal models. Moreover, in a rat model of oxidative stress-induced diabetic embryopathy, the abnormal phenotype can be rescued by the use of antioxidants.[132,133] Several prospective randomized studies have shown that strict glycemic control around the time of conception is effective in reducing the risk of congenital malformations in women with established diabetes.[117,122,134-138] In one trial, intensive preconception management of diabetic women with vascular disease reduced the malformation rate from 19% to 8.5%.[138] Unfortunately, most women with diabetes do not seek care prior to conception.[139,140] Maternal serum α-fetoprotein estimation at 15 to 20 weeks' gestation and a detailed sonographic fetal anatomic survey (with or without a fetal echocardiogram) at 18 to 22 weeks can be useful in screening for fetal malformations.

Intensive antepartum management should be initiated as early as possible and continued throughout gestation with a view to maintaining maternal blood glucose at desirable levels (fasting, below 95 mg/dL; 1 hour postprandial, below 140 mg/dL; or 2 hours postprandial, below 120 mg/dL). Initial recommendations should include a strict diabetic diet, regular exercise, daily home glucose monitoring, insulin treatment, and weekly antepartum visits to monitor glycemic control.[116] Such an approach has been shown to decrease perinatal mortality rate from a baseline of 20% to 30% to approximately 3% to 5%.[83,117,134,136,138] Insulin should be administered subcutaneously at 0.7 to 1 unit/kg/day in divided doses: two thirds in the morning (60% NPH, 40% regular/rapid acting) and one third in the evening (50% NPH, 50% regular/rapid acting). Care should be taken to avoid iatrogenic hypoglycemia due to excessive insulin administration.[90] As discussed previously, oral hypoglycemic agents are best avoided in early pregnancy.

Assessment of thyroid function is recommended (6% of diabetic women have coexisting thyroid disease), and baseline liver and renal function tests should be performed in the second trimester (including 24-hour urinary protein quantification and creatinine clearance determination). An ophthalmologic examination should also be carried out every trimester. Glycosylated hemoglobin levels should be determined every 4 to 6 weeks throughout gestation.[116,118,119] At any one time, approximately 5% of maternal hemoglobin is glycosylated, known as hemoglobin A_1 (HbA$_1$). HbA$_{1c}$ refers to the 80% to 85% of HbA$_1$ that is irreversibly glycosylated and is therefore a more accurate measure of glycemic control. Because red blood cells have a life span of around 120 days, HbA$_{1c}$ measurements reflect the degree of glycemic control over the past 3 months.

Hypertension, prematurity, and late fetal demise are the most common complications of pregnancy in diabetic women.[83,116,121,141] Approximately 30% of diabetic women will develop hypertension in the third trimester. Pregnancy-induced hypertension often results in labor induction and is a major contributor to premature delivery in diabetic women. Sustained maternal hyperglycemia results in fetal hyperglycemia that leads, in turn, to fetal hyperinsulinemia and increased oxygen demand. As such, fetuses of diabetic mothers are at increased risk of antepartum hypoxic ischemic cerebral injury and late fetal demise.[141,142] For this reason, weekly antepartum fetal testing (fetal cardiotocography) is usually recommended starting at 32 weeks' gestation.[143] After 36 weeks, testing is usually performed twice weekly. If the fetal heart rate tracing is abnormal, further testing (either a biophysical profile or contraction stress test) is mandatory.

A major issue in the care of the pregnant diabetic women is the proper timing of delivery. No pregnant diabetic woman should be delivered later than 40 weeks because of the increased risk of late fetal demise. If metabolic control is good, spontaneous labor at term should be awaited. Women with poorly controlled diabetes or with complications (worsening hypertension, IUGR, oligohydramnios), on the other hand, should probably be delivered at around 37 to 38 weeks. Early delivery in pregnancies complicated by pregestational diabetes is associated with an increased risk of fetal respiratory distress syndrome, and consideration should be given to validation of fetal lung maturity prior to elective induction. Fetal lung maturation is inhibited by insulin and testosterone, and enhanced by endogenous cortisol, thyroxine, prolactin, and estradiol-17β. In infants of diabetic mothers, hyperinsulinemia and hyperandrogenemia are common findings and may contribute to the delay in lung maturation observed in diabetic pregnancies.[144-146] The increased testosterone observed in male infants of diabetic mothers may be due to elevated concentrations of human chorionic gonadotropin (hCG), which stimulates testosterone synthesis in fetal Leydig cells.

As many as 25% of infants of diabetic mothers are macrosomic.[116,147] If the estimated fetal weight is at least 4500 g, many authorities would recommend elective cesarean delivery at or beyond 39 weeks to minimize the risk of birth trauma, primarily shoulder dystocia and resultant brachial plexus injury. Elective cesarean delivery in women with pregestational diabetes should always be scheduled early in the morning, and the patient's morning insulin dose should be withheld.

During labor, patients are starved. Intravenous glucose should therefore be administered (typically 5% dextrose at a rate of 75 to 100 mL per hour) to all women with pregestational diabetes, and blood glucose levels should be checked every 1 to 2 hours. Regular insulin should be given as needed either by intravenous infusion (starting at 0.5 to 1 unit per hour) or subcutaneous injection to maintain maternal glucose levels at around 100 to 120 mg/dL. Strict maternal glycemic control in labor is critical to preventing fetal hyperglycemia and hyperinsulinemia, both of which increase fetal oxygen demand and thereby predispose to fetal cerebral hypoxic ischemic injury.[141]

During the first 48 hours post partum, women may have a "honeymoon period" during which their insulin requirement is decreased. Moreover, the need for strict glycemic control is reduced, and circulating glucose levels of 150 to 200 mg/dL can be comfortably tolerated during this period pending discharge from the hospital and regulation of glucose levels in the home environment. Once a woman is able to eat, she can return to her prepregnancy insulin regimen.

OBESITY AND PREGNANCY

Obesity is one of the greatest public health challenges in the United States.[148] The prevalence of obesity has steadily risen since the 1980s.[149] In 2003-2004, 61.8% of U.S. women were overweight and 33.2% were obese.[150] Even more concerning, U.S. female children/adolescents (age < 20 years) had a 16% overweight prevalence, suggesting that this public health issue will worsen rather than improve in the near future. As expected, the increased obesity prevalence is now evident also in the obstetric population.[151,152]

The preferred method of weight assessment is the body mass index (BMI). BMI is calculated as the body weight in kilograms divided by the square of the height in meters. Normal weight is defined as a BMI between 18.5 and 24.9 kg/m^2.Overweight refers to a BMI between 25 and 29.9 kg/m^2. Obesity is a BMI greater than 30 kg/m^2. Obesity is further divided into Class I (30-34.9 kg/m^2), Class II (35-39.9 kg/m^2), and Class III (BMI > 40 kg/m^2), also known as "morbid obesity" or "extreme obesity." The advantage of using BMI for defining obesity is that no adjustments need to be made for gender or height, and no tables are required for determining the normal range.[153]

Obesity is a complex neuroendocrine and metabolic disorder that has been implicated in a large number of fetal and maternal complications, including spontaneous abortion, congenital malformations, stillbirth, preeclampsia, GDM, fetal macrosomia, cesarean delivery, venous thromboembolic disease, surgical complications, and urinary tract infections.

Congenital malformations associated with obesity include neural tube defects, ventral wall defects, and abnormalities of the great vessels.[154-156] In one study, obese women weighing more than 110 kg had a fourfold increased risk of having a fetus with a neural tube defect as compared with a control population weighing 50 to 59 kg. For women weighing 80 to 89 kg, the risk was increased 1.9-fold.[156] Interestingly, folic acid supplementation (0.4 mg daily) did not appear to reduce the risk of neural tube defects in this cohort of obese women.[156] These data are consistent with other studies showing that a BMI greater than 29 kg/m^2 is associated with a 1.9-fold increase in the risk for neural tube defects.[154] The mechanism by which obesity causes congenital anomalies is not known. It is conceivable that, in obese women, subtle abnormalities in glucose metabolism contribute to the increased risk of congenital malformations, similar to that of pregestational diabetes.

Perinatal mortality rate is increased with progressive obesity.[157-159] In a cohort of 167,750 Swedish women, Cnattingius et al.[159] demonstrated a 1.7-fold increased risk in late fetal death for overweight women (BMI, 25-29.9 kg/m^2) and a 2.7-fold increase for obese women

(BMI > 30 kg/m^2) when compared to women with a prepregnancy BMI less than 20 kg/m^2.[158,160]

Obesity has consistently been associated with hypertensive disorders of pregnancy.[161,162] For example, one large prospective multicenter cohort study of more than 20,000 women demonstrated that obese women with a BMI between 30 and 34.9 kg/m^2 had a 2.5- and 1.6-fold relative risk for gestational nonproteinuric hypertension and preeclampsia, respectively. For obese women with a BMI greater than 35 kg/m^2, a similar association was found with a relative risk of 3-fold and 3.3-fold, respectively.[163] In a systematic review of 13 studies including over 1.4 million women, O'Brien et al (2003) calculated a 2-fold increased risk of developing preeclampsia with every 5 to 7 kg/m^2 increase in BMI.[164]

Other well-documented risks of obesity include an increased incidence of GDM and fetal macrosomia,[152,163,165] birth injury, maternal perineal trauma, and cesarean delivery.[152,163,165] In a study of 20,130 births, a BMI greater than 39 kg/m^2 was associated with a 46% cesarean delivery rate compared with 20% in a control group of women with a BMI less than 29 kg/m^2.[166] In obese women, limiting total pregnancy weight gain to no more than 15 to 25 pounds appears to decrease the risk of fetal macrosomia without increasing the risk of low birth weight or IUGR.[167] The increased cesarean delivery rate is associated also with increased surgical morbidity in obese women, including anesthestic complications, wound separation and infection, and venous thromboembolic events.[168-170]

Obstetric management of the obese patient should include calculation of BMI, careful attention to blood pressure, a nutrition consultation, institution of a daily exercise program, and early screening for GDM. A careful sonographic anatomy survey (with or without fetal echocardiogram) at 18 to 22 weeks' gestation is indicated in obese women given the increased risk of fetal structural anomalies, although body habitus may result in suboptimal imaging. Serial growth scans should also be considered given the limitations of other methods of fetal growth assessment. Anesthesia consultation in the third trimester should also be considered prior to the onset of labor. If cesarean section is required, every effort should be made to reduce the risk of wound separation and infection, including prophylactic antibiotics, and closure of the subcutaneous layer.[171]

For women in developed countries, obesity has become one of the leading endocrine causes of morbidity and death. Effective treatments for obesity have so far eluded medical science. Bariatric surgery, which includes a multitude of procedures to reduce gastric capacity or bypass the stomach, has been shown to promote weight loss and reduce mortality.[172,173] Its use as a weight loss tool has increased in popularity,[174] and the resultant weight loss often leads to improved fertility. The safety of pregnancy after these procedures is unclear. Early case reports suggested an increased risk of adverse pregnancy outcomes.[175-177] However, more recent studies have suggested no significant increased risks during pregnancy but a number of potential benefits, including reduced risks of diabetes and hypertension.[178-181] Such women should all be given vitamin and mineral supplementation, especially iron, folate, and vitamin B_{12}.[171]

Leptin is a hormone secreted primarily by adipocytes and acts to suppress appetite while increasing energy expenditure, thereby regulating body weight. Mice lacking the leptin gene (*ob/ob* mice) are obese and anovulatory. Administration of human leptin to *ob/ob* mice increases energy expenditure, reduces weight and fat mass, and restores ovulation and fertility.[182,183] In humans, absolute leptin deficiency is rare and supplemental recombinant leptin has not been shown to promote weight loss. During pregnancy, leptin is produced by maternal and fetal adipocytes as well as syncytiotrophoblast cells.[184] Circulating leptin levels rise rapidly in the first trimester, maintain high levels throughout pregnancy, and drop precipitously after delivery, suggesting a major contribution from the placenta.[185,186] Leptin levels in the maternal circulation correlate with maternal body mass, but not with levels in umbilical cord blood at birth or birth weight. However, leptin levels in umbilical cord blood do correlate directly with both birth weight[187,188] and fetal adiposity.[189] The significance of the increased leptin levels in the maternal circulation during pregnancy are unclear, although it has been suggested that leptin may act to mobilize maternal fat stores and increase the availability of substrates to the fetus.[190] In diabetic pregnancies, alterations in maternal and fetal leptin levels have not been particularly informative.[189] In pregnancies complicated by preeclampsia, umbilical cord leptin levels are decreased and reflect the reduction in fetal growth and fat stores.[191] Interestingly, maternal leptin levels are increased in preeclampsia and appear to correlate with the severity of the disease.[192,193] The significance of this observation remains unclear. Although the regulation and mechanisms of action of leptin are not fully understood, it is possible that manipulation of the leptin-leptin receptor system may ultimately prove to be a safe and effective treatment for adult obesity and fetal macrosomia.

Hypothalamic-Pituitary Diseases

PREGNANCY-ASSOCIATED CHANGES IN PITUITARY STRUCTURE AND FUNCTION

The pituitary gland is composed of three parts: the anterior lobe (adenohypophysis), the intermediate lobe (prominent in the fetus but attenuated in the adult), and a posterior lobe (neurohypophysis). During pregnancy, the structure and function of the pituitary gland are significantly altered.[194] In the nonpregnant state, the pituitary gland weighs between 0.5 and 1 g. One autopsy study of 118 pregnant women demonstrated a 30% increase in the weight of the pituitary gland compared with nonpregnant control subjects (1070 versus 820 mg, respectively).[195] This increase in weight is associated also with an increase in volume (Table 26-5)[196,197] and a change in shape. In pregnancy, the pituitary gland develops a convex, dome-shaped superior surface,[198] which may impinge on the optic chiasm and account, in part, for the bitemporal hemianopia observed in some apparently healthy pregnant women.[199,200] Pregnancy is *not* associated with an increased incidence of pituitary adenoma.

TABLE 26-5

Volume of the Pituitary Gland Throughout Pregnancy as Determined by Magnetic Resonance Imaging

Gestational Age (wk)	Number of Subjects	Pituitary Volume (mm³), Mean ± SEM
Nonpregnant	20	300 ± 60
9	10	437 ± 90
21	11	534 ± 124
37	11	708 ± 123

Data from Gonzalez JG, Elizondo G, Saldivar D, et al. Pituitary gland growth during normal pregnancy: an in vivo study using magnetic resonance imaging. Am J Med 85:217, 1988.

On the basis of the hormones they produce, the adenohypophysis contains at least five different cell types: lactotropes (that primarily secrete prolactin), corticotropes (adrenocorticotropic hormone [ACTH]), somatotropes (GH), gonadotropes (luteinizing hormone [LH] and follicle-stimulating hormone [FSH]), and thyrotropes (thyroid-stimulating hormone [TSH]). The cellular composition of the adenohypophysis, however, changes throughout pregnancy. This is especially true of the lactotrope cell population. Immunohistochemical studies have shown that, in the nonpregnant state, approximately 20% of cells in the adenohypophysis are lactotropes.[201,202] This number increases in pregnancy such that, by the third trimester, approximately 60% are lactotropes. Moreover, the increase in lactotropes is most pronounced in the lateral portions of the adenohypophysis. By 1 month post partum, the number of lactotropes in the anterior pituitary of nonlactating women is decreased. However, postpartum resolution of lactotrope hyperplasia is incomplete, and nonpregnant multiparas have on average more lactotrope cells than do nulligravid women.

In contrast to lactotropes, the numbers of somatotropes, gonadotropes, and α-subunit–secreting cells in the adenohypophysis decrease in pregnancy and the number of thyrotropes does not change. These changes in cellular composition are associated with changes in circulating hormone levels.

PROLACTIN

Levels of prolactin in the maternal circulation increase throughout pregnancy, reaching concentrations of approximately 140 ng/mL at term (Fig. 26-8).[203] Although the maternal decidua is a major site of prolactin production during pregnancy, prolactin in the maternal circulation originates primarily from the maternal pituitary with small contributions from the maternal decidua and fetal pituitary. The observation that circulating levels of prolactin in pregnant women with preexisting hypopituitarism remain low throughout pregnancy supports the hypothesis that very little decidual prolactin enters the maternal circulation.[204,205] Decidual production of prolactin leads to elevated levels in the amniotic fluid, which peaks at approximately 6000 ng/mL at the end of the second trimester.[202]

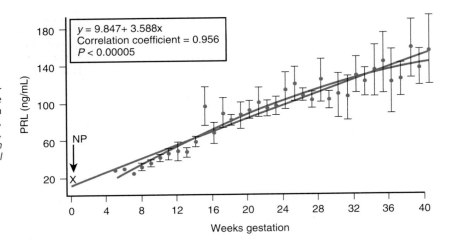

Figure 26-8. *Prolactin (PRL) concentration in maternal circulation throughout gestation. The* purple line *represents the linear regression, and the* green line *represents the second-order regression. NP, nonpregnant PRL value. (From Rigg LA, Lein A, Yen SSC. Pattern of increase in circulating prolactin levels during human gestation. Am J Obstet Gynecol 129:454, 1977.)*

The hyperprolactinemia of pregnancy is likely due to increased circulating levels of estradiol-17β. Aside from this increase in basal levels, prolactin secretion by the maternal pituitary is stimulated by thyrotropin-releasing hormone (TRH),[206] arginine,[207] meals,[207] and sleep[208] in a manner similar to that seen in nonpregnant women. After delivery, maternal prolactin concentrations in non-lactating women decrease to prepregnancy levels within 3 months.[209] In lactating women, basal circulating prolactin levels decrease slowly to nonpregnant levels over a period of several months with intermittent episodes of hyperprolactinemia in conjunction with nursing.

Pregnancy is also associated with a shift in prolactin isoforms. In the nonpregnant state, the N-linked glycosylated isoform of prolactin (G-PRL) predominates in the circulation. As pregnancy progresses, increasing amounts of nonglycosylated prolactin appear in the circulation.[210] In the third trimester, the concentration of circulating nonglycosylated prolactin exceeds that of G-PRL. Nonglycosylated prolactin appears to be more biologically active than G-PRL.[211] The precise function of the elevated circulating levels of prolactin in pregnancy is not clear, but it appears to be important in preparing breast tissue for lactation by stimulating glandular epithelial cell mitosis and increasing production of lactose, lipids, and certain proteins.[210-212] The role of prolactin in amniotic fluid is not known.

Pregnancy produces changes in prolactin secretion that persist long after delivery. Musey and colleagues[213] reported that the basal serum prolactin level and the prolactin response to perphenazine stimulation was lower after pregnancy than before pregnancy. They also found that the serum prolactin concentration was significantly lower in the parous women (mean, 4.8 ng/mL) than in the nulliparous women (8.9 ng/mL).[213] These and other studies[214,215] suggest that pregnancy permanently suppresses the secretion of prolactin by the maternal pituitary.

ADRENOCORTICOTROPIC HORMONE

ACTH levels in the maternal circulation increase from approximately 10 pg/mL in the nonpregnant state to 50 pg/mL at term,[49] and increase further to approximately 300 pg/mL in labor (Fig. 26-9).[49] Although the placenta can produce ACTH,[216] the majority of circulating ACTH appears to come from the maternal pituitary.[217] Placental production of corticotropin-releasing hormone (CRH) may be a major cause of the elevated levels of ACTH in the maternal circulation.[218-220] In nonpregnant women, serum CRH levels range from approximately 10 to 100 pg/mL. In the third trimester of pregnancy, these concentrations increase to 500 to 3000 pg/mL but then decrease precipitously after delivery.[220,221]

In addition to increasing pituitary ACTH secretion, chronically elevated levels of CRH in the maternal circulation reduce the ability of exogenous glucocorticoids to suppress the maternal ACTH-cortisol axis,[222-224] enhance the ability of vasopressin to induce an ACTH response, and diminish the effect of exogenous CRH.[218,219] CRH binding protein (CRH-BP) inactivates CRH, thereby preventing its action on the maternal or fetal pituitary. CRH-BP levels in the maternal circulation decrease during the last few weeks of pregnancy, resulting in an increase in free (biologically active) CRH.[225]

Although the maternal adrenal glands do not change in size, pregnancy is associated with significant changes in the circulating concentrations of adrenal hormones. For example, serum cortisol levels increase substantially in pregnancy. The majority of circulating cortisol is bound to cortisol-binding globulin (CBG), which is produced by the liver. Circulating levels of CBG increase during pregnancy in response to elevated levels of estrogen, and CBG may retard the clearance of these hormones. It is not surprising, therefore, that levels of total cortisol increase in pregnancy. However, levels of *free* cortisol in the circulation[222,223]—as well as in saliva[226] and urine[50,222,223]—are also increased, which is likely due the increased levels of ACTH in the maternal circulation. Maternal hypercortisolemia is also observed in complete molar pregnancy, suggesting that the increased cortisol is not derived from a fetal source. Other changes in adrenal hormone levels that occur in association with pregnancy include an increase in circulating levels of aldosterone[227] and adrenal androgens, primarily androstenedione and testosterone.

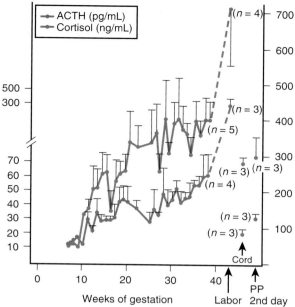

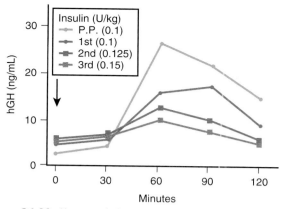

Figure 26-9. Adrenocorticotropic hormone (ACTH) and total cortisol concentration in the maternal circulation throughout gestation. PP, postpartum. (From Carr BR, Parker CR, Madden J D, et al. Maternal plasma adrenocorticotropin and cortisol relationships throughout human pregnancy. Am J Obstet Gynecol 139:416, 1981.)

Figure 26-10. Human pituitary growth hormone (hGH) response to insulin hypoglycemia in pregnancy. In pregnancy, pituitary growth hormone response to hypoglycemia is blunted. Arrow, insulin infusion; PP, postpartum. (From Yen SSC, Vela P, Tsai CC. Impairment of growth hormone secretion in response to hypoglycemia during early and late pregnancy. J Clin Endocrinol Metab 31:29, 1970.)

GROWTH HORMONE

Maternal serum GH levels begin to increase at around 10 weeks' gestation, plateau at approximately 28 weeks, and can remain elevated for several months post partum.[228] The majority of this GH is derived from the placenta (GH-V), with a marked reduction in basal somatotropin (GH-N) production by the maternal pituitary.[32] Moreover, the release of GH-N in response to either insulin-induced hypoglycemia (Fig. 26-10)[30] or arginine stimulation[229] is markedly attenuated, suggesting that maternal pituitary GH secretory reserve is diminished in pregnancy.

THYROID-STIMULATING HORMONE

In general, the concentration of TSH (thyrotropin) in the maternal circulation remains within the normal range during pregnancy.[230,231] At 9 to 13 weeks of gestation, there is a modest decline in circulating TSH levels (Fig. 26-11).[232,233] This coincides with the peak placental production of hCG, and some authorities have suggested that the decrease in TSH may be due to the weak thyrotropic properties of hCG.[234-236] An alternative hypothesis is that the placenta may secrete a hormone with TRH or TSH-like properties, but this hypothesis is not supported by most data.[237]

Enlargement of the thyroid gland is a common finding during pregnancy. This growth is not due to any deficiency in the hypothalamic-pituitary-thyroid axis, but rather a result of relative iodide deficiency and increased demand for thyroid hormone (because of elevated levels of thyroid-binding globulin[232]) leading to increased vascularity, cellular hyperplasia, and ultimately glandular hypertrophy.[232] Indeed, the TSH response to exogenous TRH

stimulation remains normal throughout pregnancy.[230,231] An appreciation of the physiologic changes in thyroid hormone levels is important to accurately assess thyroid status in pregnancy. As a rule, total thyroxine (T4) and triiodothyronine (T3) levels are not helpful in evaluating thyroid status during pregnancy. The most appropriate test to detect thyroid dysfunction during pregnancy is the TSH assay. If this assay is abnormal, free T4 and free T3 levels should be measured.

GONADOTROPINS

Maternal serum LH and FSH levels are decreased by 6 to 7 weeks of pregnancy and are below the limits of detection of many radioimmunoassays by the second trimester.[238-240] The marked decrease in gonadotropin immunoreactivity in the pituitary glands of pregnant women[202,241] coupled with the blunted LH and FSH response to exogenous gonadotropin-releasing hormone (GnRH) stimulation (Fig. 26-12)[238-240] suggests that this effect is localized primarily to the pituitary. The suppression of pituitary LH and FSH synthesis and secretion likely results from elevated circulating levels of sex steroids (estradiol-17β, progesterone) and regulatory peptides (such as inhibin) during pregnancy.

Pituitary Tumors in Pregnancy

Mutations are the primary cause of pituitary tumors. Most pituitary tumors are monoclonal, indicating that a somatic mutation in a single progenitor cell is the cause of the tumor. In one study, 100% of GH-producing tumors and 75% of ACTH-producing tumors were found to be monoclonal.[242] In one series of GH-secreting tumors, mutations in the gene coding for the Gs protein were reported in 10 of 25 tumors, resulting in a constitutively active mutant Gs protein.[243] Other endocrine factors (such as the levels of estradiol-17β, progesterone, and dopamine) can influence tumor phenotype, and changes in these hormones during pregnancy may affect

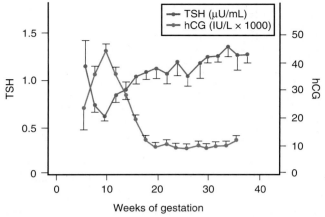

Figure 26-11. *Maternal concentration of serum thyroid-stimulating hormone (TSH) and human chorionic gonadotropin (hCG) as a function of gestational age. The decrease in serum TSH at approximately 10 weeks' gestation may be due to thyrotropic effects of hCG. (From Glinoer D, de Nayer P, Bourdoux P, et al. Regulation of maternal thyroid during pregnancy. J Clin Endocrinol Metab 71:276, 1990.)*

tumor growth. In general, pituitary tumors are benign and slow growing.

Pituitary tumors are commonly classified according to size as either microadenomas (<10 mm in diameter) or macroadenomas (>10 mm). The clinical behavior of microadenomas and macroadenomas vary considerably during pregnancy. Macroadenomas may be associated with extrasellar extension, local invasion, or compression of the optic chiasm with resultant bitemporal hemianopia, and such conditions may become exacerbated in pregnancy. In one series of 60 pregnant women with

macroadenomas, for example, 20% showed evidence of worsening visual field defects, significant enlargement on serial imaging studies, or neurologic signs.[194] Urgent neurosurgical decompression may be required during pregnancy if the tumor enlarges markedly or causes neurologic sequelae.

In contrast, microadenomas tend to behave in a relatively benign manner in pregnancy, with no evidence of functional pituitary deficiency and a low risk of neurologic complications. In a longitudinal observational study of 215 pregnant women with microadenomas, for example, approximately 5% of women developed headaches, and less than 1% experienced worsening of visual field defects or demonstrated neurologic signs.[194]

PROLACTINOMA

Prolactinoma refers to a tumor of prolactin-secreting lactotrope cells, and is typically associated with elevated levels of prolactin in the maternal circulation (see Chapter 3). In the initial evaluation of a suspected prolactinoma, measurement of circulating levels of thyroxine, TSH, and IGF-1 is important. This evaluation will exclude secondary causes of hyperprolactinemia, specifically hypothyroidism (thyroxine, TSH) and acromegaly (IGF-1). An imaging study of the hypothalamus and pituitary is also indicated, and computerized evaluation of the visual fields is recommended if compression of the optic chiasm is suspected.

Women with marked hyperprolactinemia are usually anovulatory and, as such, infertile. If such a patient does not desire pregnancy, treatment with combination estrogen-progestin therapy will reduce the risk of osteoporosis and regulate the menstrual cycle. This approach appears to be safe and is associated with few tumor-related

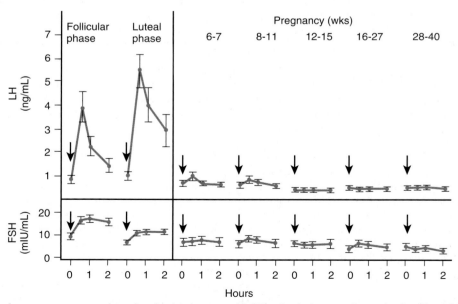

Figure 26-12. *Effect of pregnancy on gonadotropin-releasing hormone (GnRH) stimulation test. Serum levels of luteinizing hormone (LH) and follicle-stimulating hormone (FSH) before and after a 100-µg bolus of GnRH (arrows) in pregnant women and normal menstruating women. During pregnancy, LH and FSH levels are markedly suppressed. (From Miyake A, Tanizawa O, Aono T, Kurachi K. Pituitary responses in LH secretion to GnRH during pregnancy. Obstet Gynecol 49:549-551, 1977, with permission from the American College of Obstetricians and Gynecologists.)*

complications, including minimal risk of tumor growth.[244] For infertile women with significant hyperprolactinemia who wish to conceive, treatment is usually required to induce ovulation. Controversy continues as to whether surgery or dopamine-agonist treatment represents the best first-line therapy for such women. Some authorities would recommend surgical treatment prior to conception to reduce both the need for dopamine-agonist treatment and the incidence of neurologic complications during pregnancy.[245] However, microsurgical resection of a prolactinoma can result in death (in 0.3% of cases) or serious morbidity, such as a cerebrospinal fluid leak (0.4%).[246] Moreover, a long-term cure can be expected in only approximately 60% of women treated surgically. For these reasons, the weight of evidence in the literature suggests that medical treatment should be regarded as the best first-line therapy for infertile women with significant hyperprolactinemia.[247,248]

Having confirmed the diagnosis of a pituitary microprolactinoma, the goals of treatment are fourfold:

1. Suppress prolactin production and induce ovulation
2. Decrease tumor size
3. Preserve pituitary reserve
4. Prevent tumor recurrence

Treatment with a dopamine agonist can normalize circulating prolactin levels, establish regular ovulation, decrease tumor size, and preserve pituitary reserve.[249,250] A disadvantage of dopamine-agonist treatment is that it is not effective in preventing tumor recurrence once treatment is discontinued. Four dopamine agonists have been demonstrated to be effective in the treatment of hyperprolactinemia: bromocriptine, pergolide, quinagolide, and cabergoline. Cabergoline is administered once weekly and may be more effective than bromocriptine in the treatment of microadenomas.[251]

Little information is available concerning the effects of pergolide, quinagolide, and cabergoline on pregnancy, though increasing experience with cabergoline suggests that it is safe.[252] In contrast, there is substantial experience that bromocriptine is safe in pregnancy, with no significant increase in the overall rate of fetal congenital abnormalities.[253] The most common adverse effects associated with bromocriptine therapy are nausea, vomiting, and postural hypotension. Starting with low-dose therapy (0.625 mg daily) and increasing the dose slowly over a period of a few weeks can minimize these side effects. In some patients, doses as low as 2.5 mg daily may be effective. Prolactin levels should initially be checked every month for 3 months and thereafter every 3 months until the levels have returned to normal.

In women with microprolactinomas, bromocriptine can be discontinued once pregnancy is established. The majority of such women will have no further complications during pregnancy. For those women who do experience neurologic sequelae such as headache or cranial nerve dysfunction, bromocriptine therapy can be immediately reinstituted. Marked enlargement of a microprolactinoma or persistence of neurologic sequelae despite medical treatment may be an indication for urgent neurosurgical intervention, but such complications are rare. In contrast,

pituitary insufficiency and neurosurgical complications are far more common in women with macroadenomas. Such women should therefore be evaluated for panhypopituitarism before dopamine-agonist treatment is initiated. Women with macroprolactinomas are also more likely to develop complications in pregnancy.[194] One approach to the management of such women is to discontinue bromocriptine treatment once pregnancy is established, and to reinstitute therapy if symptoms or signs of increasing tumor volume develop.[254] An alternative plan, which is equally appropriate, is to continue bromocriptine treatment throughout pregnancy.[255,256] Lactation does not appear to worsen the clinical course of women with prolactinomas, and such women should be encouraged to breastfeed.[257]

CUSHING'S DISEASE

Cushing's disease refers to the clinical syndrome resulting from excessive pituitary ACTH production. It is typically associated with depressed gonadotropin secretion, and spontaneous pregnancy is rare in women with untreated Cushing's disease. Most cases of Cushing's disease are due to pituitary microadenomas. As such, neurosurgical complications are rarely seen in pregnancy. However, the metabolic derangements associated with Cushing's disease have been implicated as the cause of the observed increases in pregnancy-related complications, including premature labor, pregnancy-induced hypertension, and GDM.

ACROMEGALY

Acromegaly refers to the clinical syndrome associated with elevated circulating levels of GH. Acromegaly is often associated with anovulation, but spontaneous pregnancy can occur.[258,259] Except for complications associated with pituitary enlargement, acromegaly does not appear to adversely affect pregnancy outcome.[260] Because GH is an insulin antagonist, pregnancies complicated by excess circulating GH are at increased risk of hyperglycemia and diabetes.[261] In most women, definitive treatment for acromegaly can be deferred until after delivery. Bromocriptine, transsphenoidal surgery, and more recently octreotide, a somatostatin agonist, have been used successfully to treat acromegaly during pregnancy.[260]

Pituitary Insufficiency

SHEEHAN'S SYNDROME

Sheehan's syndrome (pituitary apoplexy) refers to the onset of acute hypothalamic-pituitary dysfunction that typically occurs after severe obstetric hemorrhage and resultant maternal hypotension at delivery. It is the most common cause of hypopituitarism worldwide, though the syndrome is not commonly seen in the United States.[262] During pregnancy, the pituitary volume increases by approximately 100%. This increase in pituitary size, coupled with the low-flow, low-pressure nature of the portal circulation, appears to make the pituitary and parts of the hypothalamus particularly susceptible to ischemia caused by obstetric hemorrhage and hypotension. The majority of cases of Sheehan's syndrome occur in developing countries where deliveries are not performed in health care facilities by skilled attendants, increasing the risk of complications from obstetric hemorrhage.

The hallmark of this syndrome is a loss of anterior pituitary hormone reserve, which may be complete or partial. Prolactin and GH deficiency are the most common abnormalities observed in Sheehan's syndrome, but every imaginable pattern of pituitary hormone deficiency has been described. In a study of 10 African women with Sheehan's syndrome, Jialal and co-workers[263] described the pituitary hormone response to a combined intravenous insulin (0.1 unit/kg), TRH (200 mg), and GnRH (100 mg) challenge test. The pattern of pituitary hormone response revealed the following loss of secretory reserve: 100% of these women had both prolactin and GH deficiency, 90% had cortisol deficiency, 80% had TSH deficiency, 70% had LH deficiency, and 40% had FSH deficiency.

The initial clinical manifestations of Sheehan's syndrome include failure of lactation, failure of hair regrowth over areas shaved for delivery, poor wound healing after cesarean delivery, and generalized weakness. The best single test to confirm the diagnosis of Sheehan's syndrome is to administer intravenous TRH (100 mg) and measure serum prolactin levels at 0 and 30 minutes. The ratio of prolactin measured at 30 minutes to that before TRH treatment (time 0) should be greater than 3.[264] If the ratio is abnormal, a complete evaluation for panhypopituitarism should be initiated.

In addition to loss of anterior pituitary hormone reserve, mild hypothalamic and posterior pituitary dysfunction is also frequently seen in women with Sheehan's syndrome. Detailed neuropathologic reports of autopsy specimens by Sheehan and Whitehead[265] have shown that 90% of women with postpartum hypopituitarism have evidence of atrophy and scarring of the neurohypophysis. Subsequent studies have also demonstrated atrophy of the supraoptic and paraventricular nuclei in such patients.[266] These observations have been confirmed in several clinical studies demonstrating that most women with Sheehan's syndrome have mild functional defects in both vasopressin secretion and maximal urinary concentrating capability.[267,268]

LYMPHOCYTIC HYPOPHYSITIS

Lymphocytic hypophysitis is a rare disorder caused by infiltration of the adenohypophysis with lymphocytes and plasma cells. Most cases of lymphocytic hypophysitis occur in women in the third trimester of pregnancy or immediately post partum.[269] In some cases, circulating antipituitary antinuclear or antimitochondrial antibodies have been detected. Pituitary enlargement can result in neurologic complications (headache, visual field defects, cranial nerve palsy) requiring surgical intervention,[270] and pituitary cell damage may result in hyperprolactinemia, hypothyroidism, or adrenal insufficiency.[271] High-dose glucocorticoid therapy may be effective in treating some cases of lymphocytic hypophysitis when neurologic sequelae are present.[272]

DIABETES INSIPIDUS

Arginine vasopressin-antidiuretic hormone (AVP-ADH) is a cyclic nonapeptide secreted by the axonal terminals of the neurohypophysis emanating from neurosecretory neurons located in the supraoptic and paraventricular nuclei of the hypothalamus. Blood osmolality is carefully monitored by sensitive osmoreceptors in the anterior hypothalamus. AVP-ADH is released in response to increasing osmotic pressures or decreasing hydrostatic pressures and act on the kidney to increase water retention. This system is designed to adjust blood osmolality over a relatively narrow range (±1.8%) with a mean of 285 mOsm/kg in nonpregnant women.[273] Pregnancy is associated with a decrease in plasma osmolality of approximately 9 to 10 mOsm/kg, which is evident early in the first trimester and persists throughout gestation[274] and appears to mirror changes in maternal hCG levels.[275] However, circulating AVP-ADH levels do not change in pregnancy.[276] These data suggest that pregnancy is associated with a modest resetting of the osmostat, leading to a 9 to 10 mOsm/kg decrease in the osmotic threshold for AVP-ADH release.

Diabetes insipidus (DI) involves the inappropriate loss of water resulting from failure of adequate tubular reabsorption by the kidney. The condition is characterized by polyuria (defined as more than 3 L of urine in 24 hours), polydipsia, and plasma hyperosmolarity. The causes of DI can be divided into two groups: central and peripheral.

Central (hypothalamic) DI refers to lesions of the hypothalamus or posterior pituitary that lead to inadequate production of AVP-ADH. The differential diagnosis of central DI includes pituitary surgery, trauma, infection, and infiltration of the neurohypophysis by tumors or inflammatory cells. Central DI is typically characterized by the acute onset of massive polyuria of 4 to 15 L per day. *Peripheral (nephrogenic) DI* refers to peripheral resistance to AVP-ADH action. Measurement of plasma AVP-ADH levels may be able to distinguish these two groups (levels are low in central DI and elevated in nephrogenic DI).

Transient nephrogenic DI can occur in pregnancy, usually in association with preeclampsia, HELLP (hemolysis, elevated liver enzymes, low platelet count) syndrome, or acute fatty liver of pregnancy.[277] High levels of placental vasopressinase may contribute to pregnancy-associated DI by degrading endogenous AVP-ADH. This increase in vasopressinase activity may also cause women with partial hypothalamic AVP-ADH deficiency to develop overt DI in pregnancy. D-arginine vasopressin (DDAVP) is resistant to degradation by placental vasopressinase. As such, DDAVP may be more effective than native AVP-ADH in the treatment of women with DI. In most cases, DI improves after delivery.[278]

DI is a rare disease in pregnancy. If suspected, the diagnosis of DI should be confirmed by performing a water-deprivation test. After an overnight fast, the patient is denied water until 3% of body weight is lost or urine osmolarity shows no increment in three successive hourly specimens. In women with DI, urine osmolarity remains low while plasma osmolarity increases significantly. This test is best performed by an endocrinologist because of the risks associated with dehydration and hypernatremia.[279] To help identify the cause, 10 μg of DDAVP can be administered immediately after the completion of the water-deprivation test. In women with central DI, there will be a decrease in urine output and an increase in urine osmolarity. In women with nephrogenic DI, on the other hand, there will be only a minimal change in urine output and osmolarity.[280]

Disorders of Thyroid Function

For reasons that are not fully understood, thyroid disease is 5 to 10 times more common in females than in males at all ages. Moreover, many of these conditions are autoimmune in nature with a peak incidence during the childbearing years. For these reasons, thyroid disease is one of the most common endocrine diseases affecting women of reproductive age and—despite the adverse effect of thyroid disease on fertility—such disorders are commonly encountered in pregnancy. Thyroid disease may also present for the first time during pregnancy. Pregnancy may complicate the management of functional thyroid disorders by affecting their clinical manifestations and limiting the approaches commonly used for diagnosis and treatment. The approach to other thyroid conditions such as nodular disease must also be modified during pregnancy because of concern over the safety of the fetus.

THYROID PHYSIOLOGY

Normal Thyroid Function

Thyroid hormone production is dependent in large part on the supply of iodine, which is derived solely from dietary sources and actively transported into the thyroid gland. The functional unit of the thyroid gland is the thyroid follicle, which is composed of a spherical alignment of cuboid epithelial cells surrounding a core of colloid. Colloid consists primarily of thyroglobulin, which provides tyrosine residues for serial iodination that results, through a complex series of biochemical and biophysical alterations, in the production of the thyroid hormones T_4 and T_3.[281] The thyroid gland is responsible for the production of all circulating T_4 and approximately 20% of T_3. Most of the body's supply of T_3 results from peripheral conversion of T_4 through a variety of tissue-specific deiodinase enzymes.

The thyroid hormones T_4 and T_3—whose total serum concentrations in nonpregnant women are approximately 4 to 12 μg/dL and 90 to 200 ng/mL, respectively (Table 26-6)—circulate in a mostly bound form, such that less than 1% circulates as free hormone.[282] Thyroid hormone is bound primarily to a specific serum-binding protein known as thyroid-binding globulin (TBG), with lesser amounts bound to albumin and prealbumin. As in most endocrine systems, it is the *free* fraction of these hormones, not the total concentration, that is physiologically important.

Regulation of Thyroid Hormone Secretion

Under normal circumstances, the circulating concentration of T_4, the most abundant and commonly measured thyroid hormone, is maintained within a narrow range that varies little from day to day. The follicular cell within the thyroid gland is responsible for the uptake of inorganic iodide from the circulation, its organification into iodinated thyronine compounds, storage of thyroid prohormone in the form of thyroglobulin, and reuptake of formed thyroid hormone and its ultimate release into the systemic circulation.

Follicular cell activity is under the direct control of the hypothalamic-pituitary-thyroid axis (Fig. 26-13). The hypothalamus produces the tripeptide TRH, which enters the portal circulation of the infundibular stalk and travels to the anterior lobe of the pituitary where it stimulates specific cells (thyrotropes) to produce TSH. TSH secretion varies diurnally, with a peak secretion occurring between 11 PM and 4 AM.[283] TSH enters the systemic circulation and interacts with specific heptahelical, G-protein-coupled receptors on the surface of thyroid follicular cells, which triggers a series of signal transduction cascades culminating in the synthesis and release of thyroid hormones. Through a classical endocrine negative feedback loop, decreased circulating levels of thyroid hormones lead to a decrease in TRH and TSH secretion (see Fig. 26-13), which in turn leads to increased thyroid growth and activity.

TABLE 26-6

Changes in Thyroid Function Test Results in Normal Pregnancy and Thyroid Disease

Thyroid Function Test	Units	Normal Nonpregnant Values	Normal Pregnant Values		Hyperthyroidism	Hypothyroidism
Thyroid-stimulating hormone (TSH)	mU/L	0.2-4	0.8-1.3	No change	Markedly decreased	Markedly increased
Thyroid-binding globulin (TBG)	mg/L	11-21	23-25	Increased	No change	No change
Total levothyroxine (T_4)	μg/dL	3.9-11.6	10.7-11.5	Increased	Increased	Decreased
Free levothyroxine (T_4)	ng/dL	0.8-2	1-1.4	No change	Increased	Decreased
Total L-triiodothyronine (T_3)	ng/dL	91-208	205-233	Increased	Normal to increased	Normal to decreased
Free L-triiodothyronine (T_3)	pg/dL	190-710	250-330	No change	Increased	Decreased

Data from Nissim M, Giorda G, Bailable M, et al. Maternal thyroid function in early and late pregnancy. Horm Res 36:196, 1991; O'Leary PC, Boyne P, Atkinson G, et al. Longitudinal study of serum thyroid hormone levels during normal pregnancy. Int J Gynaecol Obstet 38:171, 1992; Burrow GN, Lisher DA, Larsen PR. Maternal and fetal thyroid function. N Engl J Med 331:1072, 1994; American College of Obstetricians and Gynecologists. Thyroid disease in pregnancy. ACOG Practice Bulletin No. 37. Washington, DC, ACOG, 2002.

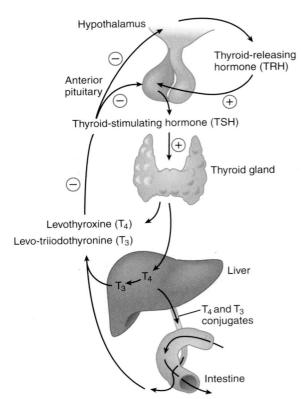

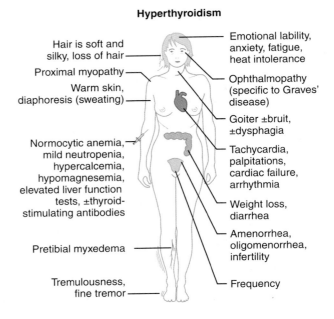

Figure 26-13. *Diagrammatic representation of the hypothalamic-pituitary-thyroid axis. The hypothalamic-pituitary-thyroid axis and factors responsible for the regulation of thyroid hormone production and metabolism are shown.*

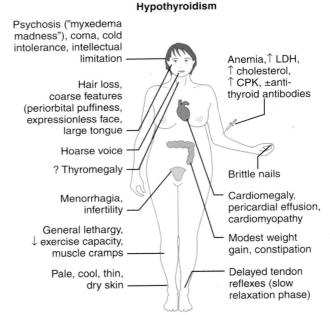

Figure 26-14. *Diagnosis of maternal thyroid dysfunction in pregnancy. Common symptoms and signs associated with maternal hyperthyroidism and hypothyroidism. CPK, creatine phosphokinase; LDH, lactic dehydrogenase. (From Norwitz ER, Schorge JO. Obstetrics and Gynecology at a Glance. Oxford, Blackwell Science, 2001, p 96.)*

Physiologic Role of Thyroid Hormone

The precise role of thyroid hormone remains incompletely understood, although it clearly interacts with numerous biologic systems. This fact is underscored by the complex series of symptoms and signs that are evident in patients with thyroid dysfunction (Fig. 26-14). At a cellular level, the active hormone (T_3) is transported into cells where it interacts with specific nuclear receptors. The T_3-receptor complex binds to specific thyroid hormone response elements within the promoter sequences of target genes and functions as a transcription factor, working along with other nuclear proteins to regulate gene expression.[284] In addition to these genomic effects, thyroid hormone also appears to have important extranuclear actions. These actions include regulation of deiodinase activity and, possibly, mitochondrial function.

EFFECT OF PREGNANCY ON THYROID FUNCTION

Maternal Thyroid Function in Pregnancy

In pregnancy, renal clearance of iodide increases (because of an increase in the glomerular filtration rate) and substantial amounts of iodide and iodothyronines are transferred to the fetus. As pregnancy progresses and fetal thyroid hormone production increases, the fetus needs increasing amounts of iodide.[285,286] To meet this demand, the placenta is able to rapidly and efficiently transport available iodide from the maternal to the fetal circulation. The placenta is also capable of mono-deiodination of iodothyronines, thereby making more iodide available for transport. The net result of these pregnancy-related physiologic alterations is a decrease in the circulating concentration of inorganic iodide during pregnancy and a resultant increase in volume of the thyroid gland by 10% to 20% during pregnancy.[232] In light of this relative iodide deficiency during pregnancy, the recommended daily intake of iodine is increased from a baseline of 100 to 150 µg/day to approximately 200 µg/day.

Serum concentrations of TBG increase in pregnant women by 75% to 100% (the T_4 resin uptake decreases proportionally). Moreover, much of the increase in circulating TBG levels occurs during the first trimester and results from the effects of the hyperestrogenemic state on hepatocytes, with stimulation of TBG synthesis and reduced hepatic clearance due to estrogen-induced TBG sialylation.[287,288] The concentration of TBG plateaus at around 12 to 14 weeks' gestation and is associated with a concomitant increase in circulating total thyroid hormone concentrations (Fig. 26-15).

Indeed, mean concentrations of both total T_4 and T_3 in the maternal circulation increase by 10% to 30% in most longitudinal studies,[232,289,290] usually into a range that is considered elevated in the general population. In the first trimester, the increase in total T_4 exceeds the rise in TBG, resulting in a slight increase in free T_4, although free hormone levels typically return to normal by the early second trimester (see Fig. 26-15). However, these changes are so subtle that serum free T_4 concentrations in most pregnant women remain within the normal range for nonpregnant women.[232,288-291] The negative-feedback control system of the hypothalamic-pituitary-thyroid axis functions normally in pregnant women.[288]

The pregnancy-specific glycoprotein hormone hCG is structurally similar to TSH and has some weak thyrotropic activity, which is estimated at approximately 0.025% that of TSH.[236,292] The production of hCG begins during the first week after fertilization and is highest near the end of the first trimester, after which it declines. This increase causes a transient increase in serum free T_4 concentrations, which in turn decreases serum TSH concentrations during the first trimester [236,293] (see Fig. 26-15). This cross-reactivity only becomes clinically significant if circulating levels of hCG are markedly elevated, such as that seen in complete molar pregnancies.

Fetal Thyroid Function in Pregnancy

The fetal thyroid gland and pituitary-thyroid axis becomes functional late in the first trimester. Before that time, any thyroid hormone in the fetus must come from the maternal circulation. By 9 to 10 weeks of gestation, the fetal thyroid begins to concentrate iodine, thyroid follicles become visible, and T_4 synthesis can be demonstrated. TBG and T_4 are first detected in fetal serum at approximately 10 to 12 weeks of gestation and increase thereafter, reaching a plateau at 35 to 37 weeks.[288,294] At term, the T_4 concentration in the fetal circulation is similar to that seen in adults, with a mean level of approximately 8 to 10 µg/dL (see Table 26-6).[294-298] The progressive increase in serum TBG concentrations with increasing gestational age presumably reflects maturation of the fetal liver and its responsiveness to estrogen stimulation. Increases in pituitary and serum concentrations of TSH during the second trimester coincide with the development of the hypothalamic-pituitary-portal circulation, which facilitates the regulation of pituitary TSH secretion by hypothalamic TRH. The increased secretion of TRH despite higher serum free T_4 concentrations implies immaturity of the negative-feedback system that regulates the secretion of TSH and TRH in utero.[288,297,298]

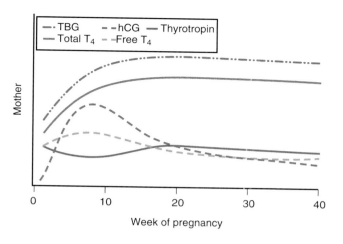

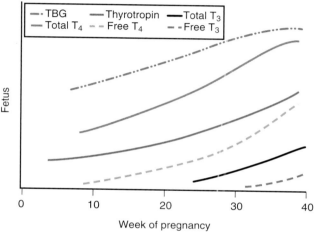

Figure 26-15. *Relative changes in maternal and fetal thyroid function during pregnancy. The effects of pregnancy on the mother include a marked and early increase in hepatic production of thyroxine-binding globulin (TBG) and placental production of human chorionic gonadotropin (hCG). The increase in serum TBG, in turn, increases serum T_4 concentrations; hCG has thyrotropin-like activity and stimulates T_4 secretion. The transient hCG-induced increase in serum free T_4 inhibits maternal secretion of thyrotropin. T_3, triiodothyronine. (From Burrow CN, Fisher DA, Larsen PR. Maternal and fetal thyroid function. N Engl J Med 331:1072, 1994.)*

Transplacental passage of thyroid hormones (T_4 and T_3) from the mother to the fetus does occur but is minimal, estimated at less than 0.1%. This is likely due to the large amount of type III deiodinase enzyme in the placenta, which serves to maintain low serum T_3 concentrations in the fetus while protecting decidual cells from hypothyroidism.[288,297-300] As such, tests of fetal thyroid function—although rarely, if ever, indicated in clinical practice—accurately reflect functioning of the fetal thyroid and are largely unrelated to maternal thyroid status.[288] That said, however, in neonates with congenital hypothyroidism, enough maternal thyroid hormone is able to cross the placenta to prevent the overt stigmas of hypothyroidism at birth and maintain cord blood thyroid hormone levels at approximately 25% to 50% of normal.[301] Iodine, TRH, and TSH receptor immunoglobulins do cross the placenta,[302] as does TSH, but to a far lesser extent.[303] Fetal

Etiology of Thyrotoxicosis in Pregnancy

Graves' disease: The most common cause (95%) of maternal thyrotoxicosis in pregnancy.
Results from the circulating thyroid-stimulating IgG autoantibodies, which can cross the placenta, leading to fetal thyroid dysfunction.
Thyroiditis (silent/postpartum [lymphocytic], subacute [granulomatous], suppurative [bacterial]): Characterized by hyperthyroidism and the presence of a large, palpable thyroid gland. An acute enlarged, painful, and tender thyroid is suggestive of subacute (De Quervain's) thyroiditis.
Toxic multinodular goiter
Solitary toxic nodule (also referred to as a hyperfunctioning thyroid adenoma)
Gestational trophoblastic neoplasia: Probably secondary to elevated levels of hCG
Struma ovarii: Refers to thyroid tissue in a mature ovarian teratoma
Exogenous thyroid hormone: Most commonly due to inadvertent ingestion of thyroid hormone
Iodine-induced thyrotoxicosis
TSH-secreting pituitary adenoma
Hyperemesis gravidarum: Associated with elevated levels of hCG in the first trimester; 50% to 70% of women will have high circulating levels of free T_4 and decreased levels of TSH. Other symptoms and signs of hyperthyroidism are often absent.

HCG, human chorionic gonadotropin; T_4, thyroxine; TSH, thyroid-stimulating hormone.

Effects of Drugs on Thyroid Hormone Synthesis and Metabolism

Inhibition of thyroid hormone synthesis by thyroid gland: Iodine, sulfonylureas, lithium
Increase in thyroid-stimulating hormone (TSH): Iodine, cimetidine, dopamine agonists, lithium
Decrease in TSH: Glucocorticoids, dopamine agonists, somatostatin
Inhibition of thyroid hormone binding to TBG (thyroid-binding globulin): Phenytoin, diazepam, sulfonylureas, furosemide, salicylates
Inhibition of conversion of T_4 to T_3 in peripheral tissues (liver): Glucocorticoids, Propylthiouracil (PTU), ipodate, propranolol, amiodarone
Inhibition of gastrointestinal resorption of thyroid hormones: Cholestyramine, cholestipol, ferrous sulfate

thyroid function is completely dependent on the supply of iodine from the mother.

Thyroid hormone is also present in measurable quantities in amniotic fluid. At term, total T_4 concentrations in the amniotic fluid are about 0.6 µg/dL, much lower than in maternal or fetal serum. Because protein and TBG concentrations are low in amniotic fluid, however, the free T_4 and T_3 concentrations are slightly higher than in maternal or fetal serum.[304] The source of this thyroid hormone is not known, but studies in fetuses with congenital hypothyroidism suggest that it may come from the maternal circulation.[305] Late in gestation, fetal swallowing appears to allow for the transfer of thyroid hormones from amniotic fluid to the fetal circulation. The physiologic role of thyroid hormone in the amniotic fluid is not known.

FUNCTIONAL THYROID DISORDERS IN PREGNANCY

Maternal Thyrotoxicosis

Thyrotoxicosis is the clinical and biochemical state that results from an excess production of and exposure to thyroid hormone from any cause. In contrast, *hyperthyroidism* refers to thyrotoxicosis caused by hyperfunctioning of the thyroid gland.[295] Hyperthyroidism occurs in 0.05% to 0.2% of pregnancies. Graves' disease is the most common

cause of maternal hyperthyroidism in pregnancy, accounting for 95% of cases.[294,295,299-301,304-306] Other causes of thyrotoxicosis in pregnancy are summarized in Box 26-3. In addition, numerous drugs are known to interfere with thyroid hormone synthesis and metabolism (Box 26-4). Symptoms and signs may suggest the diagnosis (see Fig. 26-14). For example, ophthalmopathy (lid lag, lid retraction) and dermopathy (localized or pretibial edema) are clinical signs that are specific to Graves' disease. However, as in nonpregnant patients, confirmation of maternal hyperthyroidism in pregnancy requires thyroid function testing (see Table 26-6).

As compared with well-controlled disease, inadequately treated maternal hyperthyroidism is associated with infertility and adverse perinatal outcome. Maternal complications in pregnancy include an increased risk of preeclampsia, cardiac failure, thyroid storm, and possibly spontaneous pregnancy loss.[294,295,299-301,304-307] Fetal and neonatal risks associated with poorly controlled hyperthyroidism include preterm delivery, low birth weight, IUGR, and increased perinatal mortality rate. Because a large proportion of hyperthyroidism in pregnancy is mediated by IgG antibodies that cross the placenta (Graves' disease and chronic autoimmune thyroiditis), the fetus is at risk of immune-mediated thyroid dysfunction. This is true also of women with a history of Graves' disease treated with thyroidectomy or radioactive iodine. Fetal sinus tachycardia (greater than 160 beats per minute) is a sensitive index of fetal hyperthyroidism. Although the majority of women with Graves' disease will have anti-TSH receptor, antimicrosomal antibodies, or antithyroid peroxidase antibodies, measurement of such antibodies in the maternal circulation is neither required nor recommended to establish the diagnosis.[295] Moreover, circulating antibody levels do not correlate with either pregnancy outcome or risk of fetal or neonatal hyperthyroidism. Only 1% to 5% of neonates born to women with poorly controlled thyrotoxicosis will develop transient hyperthyroidism or neonatal Graves' disease caused by the transplacental passage of maternal antithyroid antibodies.[308]

In order to minimize complications, hyperthyroidism is best diagnosed and treated prior to conception. The goal of therapy during pregnancy is to control thyrotoxicosis while avoiding fetal and transient neonatal hypothyroidism. Hyperthyroidism in pregnancy is best treated with thioamide drugs, specifically propylthiouracil (PTU) and methimazole, which decrease thyroid hormone synthesis by blocking the organification of iodide. PTU also reduces the peripheral conversion of T_4 to T_3, and may therefore have a quicker suppressive effect than methimazole.

Traditionally, PTU has been preferred in pregnant patients because methimazole was believed to pass the placenta more easily and was associated with fetal aplasia cutis congenita, a rare congenital skin defect of the scalp.[294,295,299-301,304-309] Recent data, however, have refuted both of these assertions. No difference in free T_4 and TSH concentrations has been demonstrated in the umbilical cord blood of fetuses delivered to women treated with PTU or methimazole,[310] and no increase in the incidence of aplasia cutis or structural anomalies over healthy control subjects has been shown.[309-311] PTU treatment is usually initiated at 100 to 150 mg three times daily. The goal is to utilize the least amount of drugs to maintain maternal free T_4 at the upper limits of normal.[295] TSH and T_4 levels should be checked monthly and treatment adjusted accordingly. Clinicians should remember that stored hormone may not be depleted for 3 to 4 weeks, therefore delaying a clinical response. Complete blood counts should be monitored monthly because of the risk of drug-induced agranulocytosis.[295]

Radioactive iodine (^{131}I) administration to ablate the thyroid gland is absolutely contraindicated in pregnancy. Moreover, breastfeeding should be avoided for at least 120 days after ^{131}I treatment.[312] Surgery is best avoided, but may be performed in the second trimester if indicated for failed medical therapy.

Subclinical hyperthyroidism, defined as low TSH with normal free T_4 and T_3 in an asymptomatic patient, is not associated with adverse perinatal outcome.[313] Long-term subclinical hyperthyroidism is associated with osteoporosis, atrial fibrillation, and increased mortality rate and, as such, should be treated. However, there is little data on the appropriate course of action during pregnancy. Many cases resolve spontaneously.

Thyroid Storm

Thyroid storm (thyrotoxic crisis) is a medical emergency characterized by a severe acute exacerbation of the signs and symptoms of hyperthyroidism. It is a rare complication, occurring in approximately 1% of pregnant patients with hyperthyroidism, but is associated with a high rate of maternal mortality and morbidity.[65] Thyroid storm is diagnosed by a combination of the following symptoms and signs in patients with thyrotoxicosis: fever, tachycardia out of proportion to the fever, altered mental status (restlessness, nervousness, confusion, seizures), diarrhea, vomiting, and cardiac arrhythmia.[65] An inciting event (infection,

surgery, or labor and delivery) can be identified in many instances. The diagnosis can be difficult to make, however, and requires expeditious treatment to avoid severe consequences such as shock, stupor, coma, and death.

If thyroid storm is suspected, serum TSH and free T_4 and T_3 levels should be evaluated to help confirm the diagnosis. If the clinical index of suspicion is high, however, *treatment should not be withheld pending the results of the biochemical tests.* The treatment of thyroid storm is summarized in Box 26-5. The goals of treatment are as follows:

- Reduce synthesis and release of hormone from the thyroid gland (using thioamides such as PTU or methimazole, supplemental iodide, and glucocorticoids)
- Block the peripheral actions of thyroid hormones (using glucocorticoids, PTU, and high-dose beta blockers)
- Treat complications and support physiologic functions (supplemental oxygen, fluid and caloric replacement)
- Identify and treat precipitating events (such as hypoglycemia, thromboembolic events, and diabetic ketoacidosis)

As with other acute maternal illnesses, fetal well-being should be evaluated and consideration given to delivery, if appropriate.

Maternal Hypothyroidism

Hypothyroidism is caused by inadequate thyroid hormone production. It complicates approximately 0.6% of all pregnancies but is more common in women with other autoimmune diseases, such as type 1 diabetes.[314] The classic signs and symptoms of hypothyroidism (summarized in Fig. 26-14) may suggest the diagnosis. Again, however, thyroid function testing is required for a definitive diagnosis (see Table 26-6). The causes of hypothyroidism in pregnancy are summarized in Box 26-6. In developed countries, chronic autoimmune thyroiditis (Hashimoto's disease) is the most common cause.[294,295,299-301,304-312,314,315] Worldwide, however, the most common cause of hypothyroidism is iodine deficiency.[294,295,299-301,304-306,315] Women previously treated for Graves' disease (by radioactive iodine or surgery) may manifest with post-therapy hypothyroidism. Although such women may themselves be asymptomatic, their fetuses remain at risk for thyroid dysfunction as circulating antithyroid antibodies are still present. In women with preexisting Hashimoto's disease, pregnancy may actually result in a transient improvement of symptoms.

Untreated or inadequately treated maternal hypothyroidism in pregnancy is associated with an increased risk of adverse pregnancy outcome, including preeclampsia, low birth weight, placental abruption, preterm birth, and stillbirth.[294,295,299-301,304-306,315] It is not clear whether untreated hypothyroidism is a risk factor for IUGR independent of other complications. Thyroid hormones also have important roles in embryogenesis and fetal maturation. Maternal hypothyroxemia is associated with neonatal hypothyroidism and with defects in IQ and long-term neurologic function in the offspring.[295,316,317] Women with iodine-deficient hypothyroidism are at particularly high risk of having a child with congenital cretinism (growth failure, mental retardation, and other neuropsychologic deficits).

BOX 26-5

Treatment of Thyroid Storm in Pregnant Women

Propylthiouracil (PTU), 600-800 mg orally stat, then 150-200 mg orally every 4-6 hours. If oral administration is not possible, use methimazole rectal suppositories.

Starting 1-2 hours after PTU, administer **saturated solution of potassium iodide (SSKI),** 2-5 drops orally every 8 hours, or **sodium iodide,** 0.5-1 g intravenously every 8 hours, or **Lugol's solution,** 8 drops every 6 hours, or **lithium carbonate,** 300 mg orally every 6 hours.

Dexamethazone, 2 mg intravenously or intramuscularly every 6 hours for four doses.

Propranolol, 20-80 mg orally every 4-6 hours or 1-2 mg intravenously every 5 minutes for a total of 6 mg, then 1-10 mg intravenously every 4 hours. If the patient has a history of severe bronchospasm, **reserpine** (1-5 mg intramuscularly every 4-6 hours), **guanethidine** (1 mg/kg orally every 12 hours), or **diltiazem** (60 mg orally every 6-8 hours) should be given.

Phenobarbital, 30-60 mg orally every 6-8 hours as needed for extreme restlessness.

Data from Ecker JL, Musci TJ. Thyroid function and disease in pregnancy. Curr Probl Obstet Gynecol Fertil 23:109, 2000.

BOX 26-6

Etiology of Hypothyroidism in Pregnancy

Primary Hypothyroidism

Iodine deficiency (the most common cause of hypothyroidism worldwide)

Chronic autoimmune thyroiditis (Hashimoto's): Characterized by hypothyroidism, a firm goiter, and the presence of circulating antithyroglobulin and/or antimicrosomal autoantibodies.

Silent/postpartum thyroiditis (hypothyroid phase)

Prior treatment for hyperthyroidism (includes women previously treated with radioactive iodine or surgery [thyroidectomy] leading to post-therapy hypothyroidism)

Prior high-dose external beam irradiation of the neck

Infectious (suppurative) thyroiditis: Characterized by fever and a painful, swollen thyroid gland. Common infections include *Staphylococcus aureus, S. hemolyticus,* and fungi.

Subacute thyroiditis (hypothyroid phase): Similar to suppurative thyroiditis, but it is usually the result of a viral infection and is self-limiting.

Thyroid agenesis/dysgenesis

Drug-induced hypothyroidism

Dietary goitrogens (includes such drugs as thioamides and lithium)

Organification enzyme defects

Secondary Hypothyroidism

Pituitary adenoma

Pituitary necrosis/hemorrhage

Lymphocytic hypophysitis

Central nervous system sarcoidosis

Prior hypophysectomy

Cranial irradiation

Suprasellar/parasellar

Traumatic injury to pituitary/hypothalamus

Early diagnosis and treatment of maternal hypothyroidism is essential to avoid antepartum pregnancy complications and impaired neonatal and childhood development. Indeed, in an iodine-deficient population, treatment with iodine in the first and second trimesters of pregnancy has been shown to significantly reduce the incidence of congenital cretinism.[318] With the advent of routine newborn screening for congenital hypothyroidism, it has become clear that size, weight, appearance, behavior, extrauterine adaptation, and immediate postnatal development are usually normal in infants with hypothyroidism, even those with thyroid agenesis.[319]

Although untreated hypothyroidism is associated with adverse perinatal outcome, growing evidence suggests that subclinical hypothyroidism during pregnancy (defined as an elevated TSH with normal free T_4 and T_3 in an asymptomatic patient) carries an increased perinatal risk.[295,316,317,320,321] For example, one retrospective cohort study of over 17,000 women demonstrated that subclincal hypothyroidism was associated with a threefold risk of placental abruption and a 1.8-fold risk of preterm birth before 34 weeks.[321] Most controversial, however, is the association between subclincal hypothyroidism and neurologic impairment in the offspring.[315,322,323] To date, there is no consistent evidence that screening for asymptomatic hypothyroidism and treatment will abrogate this association. As such, ACOG does not currently recommend universal screening of all pregnant women for subclinical hypothyroidism.[295] However, targeted screening for thyroid dysfunction is indicated in women with a personal history of thyroid disease or symptoms suggestive of thyroid dysfunction, and such an approach will identify approximately two thirds of women with asymptomatic hypothyroidism.[324] Screening is not indicated in asymptomatic pregnant women who have a mildly enlarged thyroid.[295]

Levothyroxine (Synthroid) is the treatment of choice for pregnant and nonpregnant women with hypothyroidism. Treatment should be initiated at an oral dose of 100 to 150 µg daily. TSH levels should be measured serially every 4 to 6 weeks, and the dose of levothyroxine adjusted accordingly. As thyroid hormone production is increased during pregnancy, most women will need an increase in their daily dose by approximately 30% to 50% during pregnancy.[325,326]

Postpartum Thyroiditis

Postpartum thyroiditis is an autoimmune inflammation of the thyroid gland that presents as new-onset, painless hypothyroidism, transient thyrotoxicosis, or thyrotoxicosis followed by hypothyroidism within 1 year post partum. The condition occurs in approximately 5% (range, 4% to 10%) of women without preexisting thyroid disease[327,328] and may also occur after early pregnancy loss. Studies have found that approximately 44% of women with postpartum thyroiditis have hypothyroidism (with fatigue, weight gain, and depression), and the remaining women are evenly split between thyrotoxicosis (characterized by dizziness, fatigue, weight loss, and palpitations) and thyrotoxicosis followed by hypothyroidism.[327,329]

The diagnosis of postpartum thyroiditis requires a high clinical index of suspicion. The diagnosis is confirmed by documenting abnormal serum levels of TSH and T$_4$ in a previously euthyroid patient. The need for treatment in women with postpartum thyroiditis is not clear, although it may be warranted to control symptoms.[295,329] In one prospective study of 605 asymptomatic pregnant and postpartum women, none of the women with thyrotoxicosis and only 40% of women with hypothyroidism required treatment.[329] If treatment is required, it can usually be tapered within 1 year. Only around 10% of women with postpartum thyroiditis will require long-term treatment.[329] Women with the highest levels of TSH and antithyroid antibodies have the highest risk for developing permanent hypothyroidism.[295,329] Even in women whose thyroid function returns to normal, the risk of recurrent postpartum thyroiditis in a subsequent pregnancy is approximately 70%.[330,331]

STRUCTURAL THYROID DISORDERS IN PREGNANCY

Goiter

Goiter refers to enlargement of the entire thyroid gland. Goiters can be classified into several categories according to the functional status of the gland (hypothyroid, hyperthyroid, or euthyroid) or to its clinical or scintigraphic appearance (diffuse or multinodular). The most common causes of goiter are summarized in Box 26-7.

Treatment is rarely necessary for diffuse goiter if the patient is asymptomatic and thyroid function testing is normal. With time, however, diffuse enlargement of the thyroid gland typically evolves into multinodular goiter, with progressive autonomous functioning of one or more follicles and occasional progression to thyrotoxicosis. This progression is seen most often in the largest goiters, those with nodules greater than 2.5 cm in size, and in older patients.[332] Large, dominant nodules should undergo fine-needle aspiration because malignant neoplasms can coexist with this typically benign condition. A trial of thyroid hormone suppression is reasonable in most patients, although fewer than 50% of nodules will respond to medical therapy by decreasing in size.[333] The approach to therapy in the patient with a toxic multinodular goiter includes thyroid ablation with radioactive iodine, thioamides, or thyroidectomy.

Thyroid Nodules

Nodules of the thyroid are common; they are palpable in 5% of the general population and may be even more common in areas of relative iodine deficiency. Careful

---

BOX 26-7

Most Common Causes of Goiter

Endemic goiter (iodine deficiency)
Sporadic goiter (diffuse nontoxic goiter; multinodular goiter)
Diffuse toxic goiter (Graves' disease)
Thyroiditis (chronic autoimmune [Hashimoto's disease]; subacute; silent/postpartum; suppurative)
Drugs (thioamides, iodides, lithium)
Dietary/environmental goitrogens
Organification enzyme defects
Diffuse malignant disease (lymphoma, anaplastic carcinoma)
Infiltrative diseases (Riedel's thyroiditis, sarcoidosis, amyloidosis)

---

attention must be taken to examination of the thyroid nodule and surrounding tissues because of the small but real potential of malignancy. Malignant transformation is more common in the largest nodules, in those with progressive growth, in older women, and in women with other risk factors for malignancy (such as prior neck irradiation).

The majority of thyroid nodules are found on pathologic examination to be either hyperplastic or adenomatous in origin. Benign and malignant neoplasms of the thyroid are listed in Box 26-8. Papillary and follicular carcinomas represent the majority of the cancers. The incidence of thyroid cancer in pregnancy is 1 per 1000.[334] Pregnancy itself does not appear to increase the risk of malignant transformation[312,314-317] or alter the course of thyroid cancer.[334,335] Moreover, treatment for thyroid cancer does not appear to increase the risk of congenital anomalies, low birth weight, or stillbirths.[336]

Any thyroid nodule discovered during pregnancy should be further evaluated, because malignancy may be found in up to 40% of these nodules.[332,334-337] Fine-needle aspiration coupled with careful cytopathologic examination of the aspirate is the technique of choice for evaluation of a thyroid nodule. Ultrasound examination may be helpful in distinguishing simple cysts from solitary nodules, in the evaluation of a multinodular goiter, or in the follow-up of known thyroid lesions. However, ultrasonography is a purely anatomic study and does not provide any functional or histologic information. Similarly, scintigraphy (with either technetium or radioiodine) can provide functional information that may be important, because functional ("hot") nodules are rarely malignant and almost all carcinomas are nonfunctional ("cold"). However, such testing cannot definitively exclude malignancy. As such, neither of these diagnostic tests can replace fine-needle aspiration for the initial evaluation of a thyroid nodule.

If a diagnosis of thyroid cancer is made, a multidisciplinary treatment plan should be established. Management options include pregnancy termination, treatment during pregnancy, and preterm or term delivery with definitive treatment after pregnancy. The decision will be affected by the gestational age at diagnosis and by the tumor characteristics.[295] Definitive treatment for thyroid cancer is thyroidectomy and radiation. If necessary, thyroidectomy can be performed during pregnancy, preferably in the second trimester. However, given the slow progression of most thyroid cancers, surgery can often be delayed until after delivery.[334] Radiation is best deferred until after pregnancy.

Disorders of Calcium Metabolism

Total calcium stores in the mother are distributed between a large skeletal pool of "inert" calcium (1 kg) and a small extracellular pool of bioavailable calcium. These two pools of calcium are maintained in a state of dynamic equilibrium, controlled on the one hand by parathyroid hormone (PTH) and by calcitonin on the other. PTH stimulates release of calcium from bone and promotes calcium uptake from the gastrointestinal tract, and calcitonin suppresses calcium release from bone. Calcium uptake from the gastrointestinal tract is also regulated by vitamin D metabolites. Calcium is excreted by the kidneys and is sequestered by the fetoplacental unit to build the fetal skeleton.

Pregnancy is associated with a net accumulation of calcium. At term, the total accumulation of calcium in the mother is approximately 25 to 30 g, most of which is sequestered in the fetal skeleton. This is due primarily to elevated circulating levels of biologically active 1,25-hydroxyvitamin D (cholecalciferol) leading to an increase in calcium absorption from the gastrointestinal tract.[338-340] The decidua may be a major source of 1,25-hydroxyvitamin D in pregnancy.[341] Calcitonin levels do not change in pregnancy. Although initial studies suggested that serum PTH levels increase during pregnancy,[342] subsequent studies using more sensitive dual-antibody assays have shown that PTH levels are lower throughout gestation.[343,344] Urinary excretion of calcium increases during pregnancy,[345] but the ratio of urinary calcium to creatinine decreases,[346] suggesting an attempt by the kidneys to reabsorb and conserve calcium even in the face of an increased glomerular filtration rate. In general, bone density remains relatively constant during pregnancy, although some investigators have reported a slight decrease in bone density in the third trimester.[347] Pregnancy is also associated with a decrease in serum albumin and a concomitant decrease in total calcium concentrations (Fig. 26-16).[342,343] The upper limit of normal for total serum calcium in pregnancy is approximately 9.5 mg/dL. However, ionized calcium concentrations do not change significantly during pregnancy.[343]

Calcium from the maternal compartment is actively transported across the placenta against a concentration gradient to the fetal compartment. This process is regulated, at least in part, by the production of PTH-related protein (PTHrP), a PTH homologue, by the fetal parathyroid glands.[348] PTHrP levels rise in maternal serum throughout gestation.[344,349] In mice lacking the gene coding for PTH-related protein, calcium transport from the maternal to the fetal compartment is markedly impaired but can be rescued completely by administration of exogenous PTH-related

protein.[350] Compared with the mother, the human fetus is relatively hypercalcemic, hypercalcitonemic, and hypoparathyroid. Separation of the fetus from the mother is associated with a fall in serum calcium and a compensatory rise in serum PTH and a fall in calcitonin levels.

HYPERPARATHYROIDISM

Primary hyperparathyroidism in pregnancy is rare; only a few hundred cases have been reported. Causes of hyperparathyroidism include a solitary parathyroid adenoma (80% of cases), generalized hyperplasia (15%), multiple adenomas (3%), and carcinoma (less than 2%). Maternal complications of untreated or poorly controlled hyperparathyroidism include hyperemesis gravidarum, generalized weakness, headache, confusion, emotional lability, nephrolithiasis, pancreatitis, and hypertension.[351] Spontaneous abortion and perinatal mortality rates are also increased in pregnancies complicated by hyperparathyroidism[352]; however, improved diagnosis and treatment have led to a substantial decrease in perinatal mortality rate.[353] Most authorities recommend surgical excision of the parathyroid adenoma in symptomatic women,[351,354,355] but controversy persists as to the optimal management for asymptomatic women and women with mild hyperparathyroidism. At birth, neonatal hypocalcemic tetany is common and typically occurs in the first 2 weeks of life.[356,357]

Unusual causes of hypercalcemia in pregnancy include familial hypocalciuric hypercalcemia (FHH) and sporadic cases of inappropriate secretion of PTH-related protein.[358] Women with FHH typically present with mild hypercalcemia, mild elevations in circulating PTH concentrations, and low urinary calcium. Because of the autosomal dominant nature of the disease and high penetrance, infants can present with either hypercalcemia (if the neonate has FHH) or hypocalcemia (if the neonate does not have FHH but is responding to maternal hypercalcemia).[358]

BOX 26-8

Most Common Causes of Thyroid Nodules

Benign
Follicular adenoma
Colloid nodule
Hürthle cell adenoma
Multinodular goiter
Simple cyst
Nodular autoimmune thyroiditis
Marine-Lenhart nodule (in Graves' disease)

Malignant
Papillary carcinoma
Follicular carcinoma
Hürthle cell carcinoma
Medullary carcinoma
Anaplastic carcinoma
Lymphoma
Metastases to the thyroid

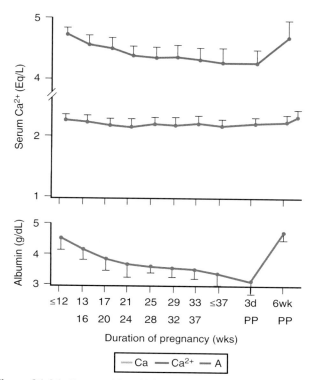

Figure 26-16. *Serum calcium (Ca), ionized calcium (Ca²⁺), and albumin (A) concentrations during pregnancy. During pregnancy, there is a marked decrease in circulating albumin concentration; this results in a decrease in total calcium. There is no change in ionized calcium. PP, postpartum. (From Pitkin RM, Reynolds WA, Williams CA, Hargis CK. Calcium metabolism in normal pregnancy: a longitudinal study. Am J Obstet Gynecol 133:781, 1979.)*

HYPOPARATHYROIDISM

The most common cause of maternal hypoparathyroidism is incidental resection of the parathyroid glands at the time of thyroidectomy. This complication occurs in approximately 1% of thyroidectomy cases. Symptoms of hypocalcemia include numbness and tingling of the fingers and orofacial area. Chvostek's sign (twitching of the facial muscles when the facial nerve is tapped) and Trousseau's sign (induction of carpopedal spasm by applying pressure to the upper arm with a blood pressure cuff) are often present.

If untreated, maternal hypocalcemia can lead to compensatory hyperparathyroidism in the fetus, leading to bone demineralization. The treatment of maternal hypoparathyroidism is calcium (1.2 g daily) and either vitamin D (50,000 to 150,000 IU daily) or the active metabolite calcitriol (0.25 to 3 μg daily).[359] If circulating calcium levels can be maintained at or near the normal range, pregnancy outcome will not be adversely affected.[360] In women with hypocalcemia, labor may be complicated by generalized tetany that requires intravenous calcium administration. Vitamin D is secreted into breast milk and may lead to hypercalcemia in the newborn.[361] As such, breastfeeding may not be advisable in women receiving high-dose vitamin D therapy.

Adrenal Diseases

ADRENAL INSUFFICIENCY

Adrenal insufficiency may be either primary or secondary. *Primary adrenal insufficiency* (Addison's disease) results from destruction of both adrenal cortices. The most common cause of primary adrenal insufficiency is autoimmune destruction of the adrenal glands, which can occur in isolation or in association with other autoimmune endocrinopathies such as autoimmune polyglandular diseases, type I and type II (Box 26-9).[362] The presence of circulating antibodies against cytochrome P450 mono-oxygenases involved in steroidogenesis may suggest the diagnosis of autoimmune adrenal insufficiency.[363] Other causes of primary adrenal insufficiency include human immunodeficiency virus (HIV) infection, tuberculosis, sarcoidosis, and adrenal leukodystrophy.

Secondary adrenal insufficiency, on the other hand, results from an abnormality in the hypothalamic-pituitary-adrenal axis that leads to ACTH deficiency and resultant adrenocortical atrophy. In secondary adrenal insufficiency, the zona glomerulosa of the adrenal gland (and thus mineralocorticoid production) are preserved, because they are under the control of the renin-angiotensin system.[364,365]

Regardless of the cause, the most common symptoms of adrenal insufficiency are generalized weakness, fatigue, nausea, anorexia, diarrhea, and weight loss. Pigmentation in the creases of the palms of the hands, knuckles, and knees can be seen in some patients with primary adrenal insufficiency (Addison's disease) due to an increase in secretion of melanocyte-stimulating hormone from an overactive adenohypophysis. Laboratory features of Addison's disease include hyponatremia, hyperkalemia, and an increase in plasma blood urea nitrogen. The diagnosis of Addison's disease can be confirmed using the ACTH stimulation test, in which a serum cortisol level is measured 60 minutes after an intravenous bolus of 0.25 mg synthetic[1,24] ACTH (cosyntropin). A normal ACTH stimulation test result is associated with a serum cortisol measurement greater than 18 μg/dL.[365] The absence of an adequate cortisol response is highly suggestive of primary adrenal insufficiency. Secondary adrenal insufficiency should be suspected if there is a suboptimal cortisol response to the ACTH stimulation test but a normal serum aldosterone concentration.[366]

Adrenal insufficiency in pregnancy has been described, and initial reports suggested a high perinatal mortality rate. More recent experience suggests good outcomes with the use of glucocorticoid therapy,[367,368] although fetal growth restriction has been described.[369]

Treatment of Addison's disease should include physiologic replacement of cortisol as well as mineralocorticoid, if necessary. Endogenous cortisol production rates are typically in the range of 20 to 30 mg daily, but may be as high as 300 mg daily. Hydrocortisone (cortisol) at a dose of 20 to 30 mg daily (two thirds in the morning and one third in the late afternoon or early evening) is typically prescribed as replacement for both pregnant and nonpregnant women. An alternative is oral prednisone at 2.5 to 7.5 mg daily. Fluorohydrocortisone (Florinef) at a dose of 0.1 mg daily should adequately treat mineralocorticoid

BOX 26-9

Autoimmune Polyglandular Syndromes

Common Type 1*
Addison's disease
Hypoparathyroidism
Mucocutaneous candidiasis

Less Common Type 1
Hypogonadism
Malabsorption
Vitiligo
Pernicious anemia
Alopecia
Hypothyroidism

Common Type 2
Addison's disease
Thyroid dysfunction
Type 1 diabetes mellitus

Less Common Type 2
Hypogonadism
Myasthenia gravis
Vitiligo
Pernicious anemia
Alopecia

---

*Type 1 is also known as autoimmune polyendocrinopathy-candidiasis-ectodermal dystrophy syndrome.
Data from Neufeld M, MacLaren NK, Blizzard RM. Two types of autoimmune Addison's disease associated with different polyglandular autoimmune syndromes. Medicine (Baltimore) 60:355, 1981.

deficiency. Mineralocorticoid therapy is not necessary for secondary adrenal insufficiency.

Addisonian crisis (adrenal crisis) refers to a state of acute adrenal insufficiency. This condition is rarely seen during pregnancy but frequently develops in the immediate postpartum period.[370] This timing is likely because, in pregnancy, the kidney synthesizes large amounts of deoxycorticosterone (a weak glucocorticoid and mineralocorticoid) from progesterone.[371] The immediate treatment of adrenal crisis should include intravenous hydration with normal saline, glucose replacement, and high doses of cortisol given either intramuscularly or intravenously (100 mg bolus every 6 to 8 hours for the first 24 hours).

Women with Addison's disease undergoing surgery should be given stress doses of cortisol. On the day of surgery, 100 mg of cortisol can be administered either intramuscularly or intravenously and repeated every 6 to 8 hours during surgery and in the immediate postoperative period. This dose can be reduced by 50 mg daily until oral glucocorticoid replacement can be reinstated. Consideration should also be given to administering stress doses of cortisol in labor. By the second trimester, very little cortisol crosses the placenta intact owing to high placental type 2 11β-hydroxysteroid dehydrogenase activity that converts cortisol to cortisone. As such, the fetus is highly resistant to adrenal suppression caused by maternal ingestion of glucocorticoids.[372]

CUSHING'S SYNDROME

Cushing's syndrome results from exposure to excessive circulating levels of cortisol. The condition may be ACTH-dependent, as in ACTH-secreting pituitary adenoma (Cushing's disease) and ACTH- or CRH-secreting tumors such as bronchial carcinoids. Cushing's syndrome can also be ACTH-independent, resulting from exogenous glucocorticoids, adrenal adenoma, or carcinoma. In nonpregnant women, Cushing's disease is threefold more common than adrenal adenomas. In pregnancy, however, adrenal adenomas are the most common cause of Cushing's syndrome (Table 26-7).[373]

The most common clinical features of Cushing's disease include proximal muscle weakness, centripetal obesity ("potato stick" person with thick trunk and thin limbs), facial plethora, supraclavicular and dorsal ("buffalo hump") fat pads, violaceous striae, hirsutism, personality changes, and hypokalemia. In nonpregnant women, significant and persistent elevation in urinary free cortisol excretion (greater than 200 µg/day) confirms the diagnosis.

Cushing's syndrome can be difficult to recognize and diagnose during pregnancy, however, because normal pregnancy is associated with physiologic hypercortisolism and increased urinary free cortisol excretion. Initial studies suggested that urinary free cortisol excretion was significantly increased in pregnancy, with a mean of 130 (range, 60 to 250) µg/day.[374] However, more recent studies using high-performance liquid chromatography have shown that normal pregnant subjects have a 24-hour urinary free cortisol excretion of approximately 23 µg, which is increased to 165 to 3360 µg daily in the setting of Cushing's syndrome.[375] As such, urinary free cortisone and cortisol as determined by high-performance chromatography may have greater sensitivity and specificity in the diagnosis of Cushing's syndrome than does the measurement of urinary free cortisol by standard assay techniques.[376]

Once diagnosis has been confirmed, every effort should be made to identify the cause. Given the high incidence of adrenal adenomas and carcinomas in pregnant women with Cushing's syndrome (see Table 26-7), it may be appropriate to first perform a high-resolution imaging study of the adrenal glands, either with computed tomography or magnetic resonance imaging. If the imaging study is negative, then tests should be performed to identify an ACTH-secreting pituitary tumor (CRH stimulation followed by petrosal sinus sampling for ACTH) or an extrapituitary source of ACTH or CRH (computed tomography of the chest).[377]

Cushing's syndrome is associated with an increased risk of pregnancy-related complications, including hypertension (65%), diabetes (32%), preeclampsia (10%), congestive heart failure, and maternal death.[378] Perinatal morbidity and mortality rates are also increased in such pregnancies. Adverse perinatal outcomes include an increased risk of prematurity (65%), IUGR (26%), and perinatal death (16%).[378]

Cushing's syndrome is a rare condition in pregnancy owing to the high frequency of ovulation dysfunction. As such, it has not been possible to systematically examine and compare treatment strategies for this condition. Given the

Etiology of Cushing's Syndrome in Nonpregnant and Pregnant Populations

Etiology	Nonpregnant (n = 108)	Pregnant (n = 58)
ACTH-secreting pituitary tumor leading to bilateral adrenal hyperplasia	64 (59%)	19 (33%)
Adrenal adenoma	17 (16%)	29 (50%)
Adrenal carcinoma	10 (9%)	6 (10%)
Ectopic ACTH	17 (16%)	1 (2%)
Unknown	0 (0%)	3 (5%)

ACTH, adrenocorticotropic hormone.
Data from Buescher MA, McClamrock HD, Adashi EY. Cushing's syndrome in pregnancy. Obstet Gynecol 79:130, 1992. Reprinted with permission from the American College of Obstetricians and Gynecologists.

high rates of maternal and perinatal morbidity associated with this condition, aggressive antepartum and intrapartum management is indicated. Surgery (unilateral adrenalectomy) should be considered if a functional adrenal adenoma is identified. In the case of an ACTH-secreting pituitary tumor, transsphenoidal resection can be performed during pregnancy.[379] Medical treatment options include antiglucocorticoids and inhibitors of adrenal steroidogenesis. Metyrapone,[380,381] aminoglutethimide,[382] and ketoconazole[378,383] have all been used to treat Cushing's syndrome in pregnancy. However, the efficacy or safety of these agents during pregnancy has yet to be established.

CONGENITAL ADRENAL HYPERPLASIA

Congenital adrenal hyperplasia (CAH) refers to a group of genetic disorders of steroidogenesis. It occurs in approximately 1 in 14,000 live births but is more common in certain populations. In the Yupik Inuit, for example, CAH occurs at a frequency of 1 in 300 live births.[384] The most common cause of CAH is a deficiency of 21-hydroxylase enzyme activity, which leads, in turn, to a decrease in circulating cortisol levels, a compensatory increase in ACTH production, and an increase in adrenal androgen production.

The exposure of a female fetus to high levels of androgens during early embryonic development can lead to clitorimegaly, labioscrotal fusion, ambiguous genitalia, abnormal course of the urethra, and virilization. In severe forms of 21-hydroxylase deficiency, the conversion of progesterone to mineralocorticoids (deoxycorticosterone, corticosterone, and aldosterone) is reduced, resulting in "salt wasting." If undetected and untreated, the saltwasting form of the disease may be associated with neonatal hyponatremia, hyperkalemia, and death. In CAH due to 21-hydroxylase deficiency, 75% of cases are associated with salt wasting and 25% present with virilization but no salt wasting. For the obstetrician evaluating a newborn with ambiguous genitalia, the most important disease to exclude is 21-hydroxylase deficiency associated with salt wasting. Failure to recognize this condition can lead to

discharge of the newborn resulting in neonatal dehydration and death.

If a mother has previously delivered a child with CAH, or if either she or the father has CAH, then appropriate recommendations include antenatal genetic counseling, prenatal glucocorticoid treatment, and genetic testing of the neonate after delivery. Women with nonclassical 21-hydroxylase deficiency who have not previously delivered a child with CAH do not require prenatal intervention because the probability that the fetus is severely affected is low (less than 1%) in most cases.

For parents wishing to pursue glucocorticoid therapy to reduce the risk of virilization of a female fetus, the suggested management of these pregnancies is summarized in Figure 26-17.[385] In such cases, the mother should be treated with dexamethasone (20 μg/kg daily in three divided doses) as soon as the pregnancy is confirmed. This dose has been shown to normalize 17-hydroxyprogesterone levels in the amniotic fluid of affected fetuses.[386] Chorionic villus sampling should be offered at 9 to 11 weeks' gestation. If a male fetus is identified, steroid therapy can be discontinued. If the fetus is a female, prenatal diagnosis can be achieved by CYP2 genotyping. If an affected female fetus is identified, glucocorticoid treatment should be continued for the entire pregnancy. The goal of this protocol is to suppress endogenous androgen production by the fetal adrenal and thereby prevent virilization of an affected female fetus. If dexamethasone therapy is initiated too late in gestation (typically regarded as later than 9 weeks' gestation), clitorimegaly and labioscrotal fusion may already have occurred.

Because estriol in the maternal circulation is derived almost exclusively from placental metabolism of fetal androgens (primarily 16-hydroxydehydroepiandrosterone sulfate [16-OH-DHEAS]), estriol levels can be used to monitor the efficacy of maternal glucocorticoid therapy to suppress fetal adrenal steroidogenesis. An estriol level of less than 0.2 nM in the maternal circulation is associated with marked suppression of fetal adrenal steroidogenesis, whereas a level of greater than 10 nM is associated with inadequate suppression of the fetal adrenal.[387]

Exactly how effective this protocol is in preventing virilization is not clear. In one study, implication of this protocol in 14 pregnancies at risk resulted in the treatment of two affected female fetuses, one of whom was virilized.[388] A subsequent report described the effects of antenatal glucocorticoid treatment on 15 female fetuses found to have CAH on the basis of antepartum genetic testing. Of the 15 female infants, 5 responded completely and 10 responded partially.[388] In the largest experience to date of 61 affected female fetuses, New et al demonstrated that, for affected females, the average Prader score (an objective scoring system of virilization graded on a scale from 1 [mild] to 5 [severe]) for those treated prenatally at or before 9 weeks' gestation was 0.96, whereas those with no prenatal treatment had an average Prader score of 3.75.[389] Taken together, these data suggest that approximately 85% of affected female fetuses who receive glucocorticoid therapy will have either no or mild virilization.[385]

Potential complications of long-term antepartum dexamethasone treatment include the development of

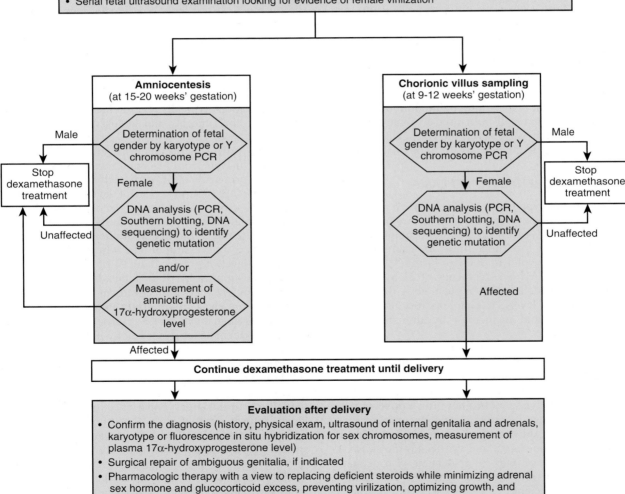

Prepregnancy assessment
- Indicated in all patients with an affected sibling, first-degree relative, and/or child with known genetic mutations causing classic CAH, proven by DNA analysis
- Components of prenatal treatment program should include prepregnancy genetic counseling and genotyping of the proband and both parents
- Patients at high risk should be managed by a multidisciplinary team, including a pediatric endocrinologist, an expert in high-risk obstetrics, a genetic counselor, a reliable molecular genetics laboratory, and a pediatric surgeon, if indicated

Start dexamethasone therapy
- Dexamethasone therapy should start as soon as pregnancy is confirmed and no later than 9 weeks after the first day of LMP
- The optimal dosage and timing is 20 µg/kg maternal body weight per day in divided oral doses t.i.d.
- Consider written informed consent for treatment

Routine antenatal follow-up
- Maternal blood pressure, weight, glycosuria, HbA$_{1c}$, plasma cortisol, dehydroepiandrostenedione sulfate (DHEA-S), and androstenedione should be measured initially and then every 2 months
- Measurement of plasma or urinary estriol should be added after 15-20 weeks' gestation
- Serial fetal ultrasound examination looking for evidence of female virilization

Amniocentesis (at 15-20 weeks' gestation)

Male

Stop dexamethasone treatment

Determination of fetal gender by karyotype or Y chromosome PCR

Female

Unaffected

DNA analysis (PCR, Southern blotting, DNA sequencing) to identify genetic mutation

and/or

Measurement of amniotic fluid 17α-hydroxyprogesterone level

Affected

Chorionic villus sampling (at 9-12 weeks' gestation)

Determination of fetal gender by karyotype or Y chromosome PCR

Male

Stop dexamethasone treatment

Female

Unaffected

DNA analysis (PCR, Southern blotting, DNA sequencing) to identify genetic mutation

Affected

Continue dexamethasone treatment until delivery

Evaluation after delivery
- Confirm the diagnosis (history, physical exam, ultrasound of internal genitalia and adrenals, karyotype or fluorescence in situ hybridization for sex chromosomes, measurement of plasma 17α-hydroxyprogesterone level)
- Surgical repair of ambiguous genitalia, if indicated
- Pharmacologic therapy with a view to replacing deficient steroids while minimizing adrenal sex hormone and glucocorticoid excess, preventing virilization, optimizing growth, and protecting potential fertility

Figure 26-17. Proposed algorithm for the management of pregnant women at risk for congenital adrenal hyperplasia (CAH). CVS, chorionic villus sampling; LMP, last menstrual period; PCR, polymerase chain reaction. (From LWPES/ESPE CAH Working Group. Consensus statement on 21-hydroxylase deficiency from the Lawson Wilkins Pediatric Endocrine Society and the European Society for Pediatric Endocrinology. J Clin Endocrinol Metab 87:4048, 2002.)

iatrogenic Cushing's syndrome in the mother[387] and subtle cognitive and motor deficits in the child,[390,391] although not all studies have confirmed this association.[392]

PHEOCHROMOCYTOMA

Pheochromocytomas are catecholamine-secreting tumors that arise from chromaffin cells. Although the majority (90%) occur in the adrenal gland, these tumors can also be found outside the adrenal, primarily at the base of the bladder and at the aortic bifurcation (organ of Zuckerkandl). Of all cases, 10% are bilateral and 10% are malignant. In a minority of cases (10%), pheochromocytomas may occur in association with other systemic disorders such as neurofibromatosis (von Recklinghausen's disease), multiple endocrine neoplasia type IIA (Sipple's syndrome), and von Hippel-Lindau disease.

Pheochromocytomas account for 0.1% of hypertension in adults. These tumors are rare in pregnancy, and only a few hundred cases have been reported in the literature. However, they pose a very high risk for both mother and fetus. Anesthesia, vaginal delivery, uterine contractions, or even vigorous fetal movements can precipitate fatal maternal hypertension. Fetal growth restriction is a common finding due primarily to uteroplacental insufficiency. If untreated, the overall maternal mortality rate ranges from 4% to 17%, with a fetal loss rate of 11% to 26%.[393-395] Antenatal diagnosis reduces the maternal mortality rate to zero to 2% and the fetal loss rate to 1% to 15%[393-395]; however, only half of such cases are diagnosed prior to conception.[393] Delay in diagnosis is, therefore, associated with considerable rates of morbidity and mortality. Any pregnant woman with paroxysms ("spells") of labile hypertension, headaches, palpitations, sweating, flushing, blurred vision, anxiety, emesis, dyspnea, or convulsions should prompt an investigation to exclude the diagnosis. It should be remembered, however, that 50% of women with pheochromocytoma will present with sustained hypertension.

Maternal and fetal survival depends on early diagnosis, aggressive medical therapy, and correct timing of delivery and surgery. Confirmation of the diagnosis requires documentation of elevated circulating levels of metanephrines and catecholamines in either urine or blood. Although testing for fractionated plasma free metanephrines appears to be the most sensitive, it is not as specific as the standard 24-hour urine catecholamines and metanephrines measurements.[396] Given the ease of a random plasma test over a 24-hour urine collection, some authorities have advocated the former as a first-line test, especially in women with a high clinical suspicion for pheochromocytoma.[397] Plasma catecholamines and urinary vanillylmandelic acid (VMA) are used less commonly because of their poor accuracy.[397] Catecholamine levels are not affected by pregnancy. Localization of the tumor can be achieved by radiologic imaging (magnetic resonance imaging is the modality of choice) or, rarely, by selective sampling of the adrenal veins. Scintigraphy (^{131}I) is contraindicated in pregnancy.

Initial treatment should include pharmacologic control of hypertension and tachycardia. Alpha-adrenergic blockage should be initiated immediately, preferably with phenoxybenzamine (starting at 10 mg every 8 hours

and increasing gradually until orthostatic hypotension is achieved). Alternative agents include prazosin or labetalol. Beta-blockade should be reserved for women with persistent tachycardia or arrhythmias and selective and short-acting agents are preferred (such as metoprolol or atenolol). Optimal management of a pregnant patient with pheochromocytoma involves collaboration between obstetricians, endocrinologists, anesthesiologists, and general surgeons. The decision of whether or not to proceed with surgical resection depends on the success of medical treatment, the size of the tumor, estimated risk of malignancy, and gestational age.[393-395] In the first and second trimesters, surgical resection of the tumor is associated with good fetal outcome. More recently, laparoscopic tumor resection has been described in pregnancy.[398] In later pregnancy, delivery by elective cesarean followed by tumor resection is commonly recommended.

Ovarian Endocrine Tumors

The precise incidence of adnexal masses in pregnancy is not known. Increasing use of ultrasonography during pregnancy suggests that sizable adnexal masses complicate as many as 1 in 200 pregnancies.[399-401] These data are consistent with a large retrospective study that showed significant adnexal neoplasms were identified in 1 of 197 cesarean deliveries.[402] The majority of adnexal masses occurring in pregnant women are simple cysts less than 5 cm in diameter, which carry a small risk of complications such as malignancy (less than 5%), torsion, rupture, or hemorrhage.[400,401,403] Some of these adnexal masses will be functional endocrine tumors of the ovary.

The major risk of an ovarian endocrine tumor during pregnancy is virilization of a female fetus. Levels of testosterone[404,405] and androstenedione[405] increase in the maternal circulation throughout gestation, peaking in the third trimester. However, circulating levels of free testosterone remain relatively unchanged prior to 28 weeks' gestation, suggesting that the increase in total testosterone is due in large part to increases in sex hormone–binding globulin.[406] These data are consistent with the observation that the clearance of testosterone decreases during pregnancy.[407] After 28 weeks, however, levels of both total and free testosterone appear to increase in the maternal circulation. In contrast, DHEA and DHEAS concentrations decrease precipitously in pregnancy.[408] This decrease occurs despite an increase in maternal DHEAS production[409] and is likely due to increased metabolic clearance by the placenta.[408,409]

These endocrine changes serve to protect a female fetus from virilization. Other protective mechanisms include a high capacity of the placenta to aromatize androgens such as testosterone and androstenedione to estrogens (estrone, estradiol-17β, and estriol).[410] In this way, the placenta is able, at least in part, to protect a female fetus from exposure to excessive concentrations of testosterone and androstenedione. Dihydrotestosterone, on the other hand, is not a substrate for aromatization. As such, the placenta may be less effective in preventing this steroid from crossing into the fetal compartment and causing virilization.

Some female fetuses appear to be uniquely resistant to the virilizing effects of androgens, especially in the second and third trimesters of pregnancy. Although the mechanism is not clear, there are several cases in which markedly elevated levels of androgens have been demonstrated in the umbilical cord blood of female infants without evidence of virilization.[411]

Three ovarian endocrine tumors can cause virilization: luteomas, gestational theca-lutein cysts (hyperreactio luteinalis), and Sertoli-Leydig cell tumors (arrhenoblastomas),[412] all of which are associated with markedly elevated levels of testosterone, dihydrotestosterone, and androstenedione. Luteomas are derived from luteinization and hyperplasia of theca interna cells,[413,414] and are bilateral in approximately 45% of cases.[412] Maternal virilization or hirsutism occurs in approximately 35% of such women, and the risk of virilization of a female fetus is high.

In contrast, theca-lutein cysts are associated with a lower risk of virilization of a female fetus. This disorder occurs typically in conditions with elevated circulating levels of hCG (such as gestational trophoblastic tumors, diabetes, and Rh isoimmunization), which directly stimulates ovarian steroid production. In the majority of cases, the cysts are bilateral.

The risk of both maternal and fetal virilization is highest with Sertoli-Leydig cell tumors. These tumors are usually unilateral. Fortunately, such tumors are usually associated with chronic anovulation and infertility and are therefore rarely seen in pregnancy.

Preeclampsia

Preeclampsia (gestational proteinuric hypertension) complicates 6% to 8% of all pregnancies.[415,416] The second most common cause of maternal death in the United States (after thromboembolic disease), preeclampsia accounts for 12% to 18% of all pregnancy-related maternal deaths (around 70 maternal deaths per year in the United States and an estimated 50,000 maternal deaths per year worldwide).[416-419] It is also associated with a high rate of perinatal mortality and morbidity, due primarily to iatrogenic prematurity.[420]

Preeclampsia is an idiopathic multisystem disorder specific to human pregnancy and the puerperium.[415] More precisely, it is a disease of the placenta because it has also been described in pregnancies where there is trophoblast but no fetal tissue (complete molar pregnancies).[421] Similarly, in the rare situation of an advanced extrauterine intra-abdominal ectopic pregnancy complicated by preeclampsia, removal of the placenta is not possible at the time of delivery of the fetus and, as such, preeclampsia persists post partum instead of resolving.[422]

Despite aggressive research efforts, the pathogenesis of preeclampsia remains poorly understood. Pathologic and physiologic observations as well as examination of epidemiologic studies and biochemical aberrations (summarized in Table 26-8) have led to a number of theories to explain preeclampsia. At present, four major hypotheses are under intense investigation[423,424]:

1. Genetic imprinting
2. Immune maladaptation
3. Placental ischemia
4. Generalized endothelial dysfunction

The data in support of each theory are summarized in Box 26-10.[425-462] In addition to endocrine changes, preeclampsia is also associated with abnormalities in the nervous system. For example, Schobel and colleagues[463] have shown that postganglionic sympathetic nerve activity is increased in women with preeclampsia compared with pregnant women without hypertension. This finding suggests that the increase in peripheral vascular resistance and blood pressure that characterize preeclampsia may be due, at least in part, to increased firing of sympathetic neurons. Interestingly, heart rate was not increased in the women with preeclampsia, implying either that increased vagal tone suppressed sympathetic activity in the heart or that the increase in peripheral sympathetic activity is a secondary compensation to plasma volume contraction.

Despite a plethora of hypotheses, there is as yet no single unifying theory that can account for all the findings in preeclampsia. It is clear, however, that the blueprint for its development is laid down early in pregnancy. Researchers have suggested that the pathologic hallmark of preeclampsia is a complete or partial failure of the second wave of trophoblast invasion from 16 to 20 weeks' gestation, which is responsible in normal pregnancies for destruction of the muscularis layer of the spiral arterioles.[448-450,464] As pregnancy progresses, the metabolic demands of the fetoplacental unit increase. Because of the abnormally shallow invasion of the placenta, however, the spiral arterioles are unable to dilate to accommodate the required increase in blood flow, resulting in "placental dysfunction" that manifests clinically as preeclampsia.

A number of recent studies have provided an improved understanding of the pathophysiology of preeclampsia, suggesting that aberrant expression of angiogenic factors may be the elusive "toxemia" factors leading to widespread maternal endothelial injury.[465] VEGF is an important mitogen involved in angiogenesis and the maintenance of vascular integrity. VEGF acts by binding to two cell surface receptors, VEGF receptors type 1 (flt1) and type 2 (KDR). The flt1 receptor exists in two major isoforms: a functional transmembrane isoform and a soluble truncated isoform known as soluble fms-like tyrosine kinase-1 (sFlt-l). sFlt-1 lacks a membrane-binding domain and thus exists free in the maternal circulation where it binds and functionally inactivates VEGF and placental growth factor (PlGF) leading to increased vascular permeability.[466] Levels of sFlt-1 in the maternal circulation increase during pregnancy but increase earlier and to higher levels in pregnancies destined to develop preeclampsia as compared with normotensive control subjects. The source and molecular mechanisms responsible for the increase in circulating sFlt-1 levels in preeclampsia remain unclear. Interestingly, anti-VEGF antibodies have been used as pharmacologic therapy in nonpregnant individuals for conditions resulting from inappropriate or excessive angiogenesis, such as neoplastic disorders and macular degenerative disease. Common side effects associated with this therapy include hypertension and proteinuria.[467]

More recently, another anti-angiogenic factor, known as soluble endoglin (sEng), has been implicated in the

TABLE 26-8

Biochemical Aberrations Associated with Preeclampsia

Elevated*	Diminished*	Unchanged†
Vasoactive Agents		
Endothelin-1	Prostacyclin (PGI₂)	
Thromboxane A₂ (TXA₂)	Prostaglandin E₂ (PGE₂)	
Nitric oxide synthase activity	Antithrombin III activity	
Nitric oxide production	Placental endothelin-1 production	
	Endothelin A and B receptors	
	Urinary excretion of nitric oxide metabolites (including nitrate and nitrite)	
	? Plasma levels of nitric oxide metabolites	
Markers of Endothelial Cell Dysfunction and/or Injury		
Fibronectin and fibronectin degradation products	PGI₂	Total cholesterol
Endothelin-1	Low-density lipoprotein-1 (LDL-I), LDL-II, and high-density lipoprotein (HDL)	Intermediate-density lipoprotein
Elastase		Total LDL
Triglycerides, very low density lipoprotein (VLDL), LDL-III	VLDL and LDL receptors	
Lipid peroxidases	Nitric oxide	
Malonydialdehyde (metabolite of lipid peroxidation)		
Urinary protein excretion		
Markers of Neutrophil Activation		
Neutrophil elastase		
Neutrophil defensins		
Soluble L-selectin		
Leukocyte adhesion molecules, including E-selectin, vascular cell adhesion molecule-1 (VCAM-1), intercellular adhesion molecule-1 (ICAM-1)		
Neutrophil reactive oxygen species (ionized oxygen, hydrogen peroxide, hydroxyl radical)		
Markers of Platelet Activation		
Platelet endothelial cell adhesion molecule-1		
Cytokines/Growth Factors		
Interleukin 6 (IL-6)	Insulin-like growth factor-1 (IGF)	Interleukin 8 (IL-8)
Tumor necrosis factor-α (TNF-α)	IGF-binding proteins (IGFBP-1 and placental protein 12)	Interleukin 4 (IL-4)
TNF-α soluble receptors	? Granulocyte-macrophage colony- stimulating factor (GM-CSF)	Interleukin 10 (IL-10)
Platelet-derived growth factor		
Vascular endothelial growth factor (VEGF)		
VEGF receptor (flt1)	Placental growth factor	
Soluble endoglin		
Interferon-γ (IFN-γ)		
IL-6 and IL-1 receptor antagonists		
Activin A		
Inhibin A		

Continued

647

TABLE 26-8

Biochemical Aberrations Associated with Preeclampsia—Cont'd

Elevated*	Diminished*	Unchanged†
Hormones		
Testosterone		Estradiol-17β
β-Human chorionic gonadotropin (β-hCG)		Dehydroepiandrosterone sulfate (DHEAS)
Corticotropin-releasing factor		Sex hormone–binding globulin (SHBG)
Leptin		
Coagulation Factors		
Von Willebrand factor	Platelets	Soluble fibrin
Thrombomodulin	Thrombopoietin	Thrombin–antithrombin III complexes
		Fibrin degradation products
Tissue plasminogen activator		
Plasminogen activator inhibitor I		
Miscellaneous		
Uric acid	Albumin	Sodium
Free fatty acids (oleic, linoleic, and palmitic acids)	Antioxidant vitamins (vitamins C and E)	Glucose
Urinary albumin excretion	Urinary calcium excretion	Lactoferrin
Free radical superoxide formation	Magnesium	C-type natriuretic peptide
Homocysteine	Zinc	α-Fetoprotein
Ceruloplasmin	Calcium	
Haptoglobin	β-Carotene	
α₁-Antitrypsin	Transferrin	
Serotonin (5-hydroxytryptamine)	Vitamin B$_{12}$	
Atrial and brain natriuretic peptide		
Circulating fetal erythroblasts		
Circulating syncytiotrophoblast microvilli fragments		

*Data reflect an overall summary of published literature by the author. Unless otherwise indicated, measurements refer to maternal serum concentrations.

†Relative to measurements in pregnancies not complicated by preeclampsia.

BOX 26-10

Theories of Etiology of Preeclampsia and Their Supportive Evidence

Genetic

Familial inheritance pattern (increased incidence in women with a positive family history of preeclampsia[425] and in pregnancies conceived by men born themselves of preeclamptic pregnancies[426])

Increased incidence in African-American race[427]

Increased incidence in women with a prior history of preeclampsia[428]

Association with Factor V Leiden mutation[429]

Association with angiotensinogen gene variant[430]

Association with protein C and/or protein S deficiency[431]

Association between fetal 3-hydroxyacyl-coenzyme A dehydrogenase deficiency and HELLP (hemolysis, elevated liver enzymes, low platelets) syndrome[432]

Immunologic Maladaptation

Increased incidence in first pregnancies (nulliparity)[433]

Increased incidence with changed paternity (new partner)[434,435]

Advanced maternal age > 40 years)[436]

Association with maternal-fetal HLA-DR discordance[437]

Association with reduced in vitro lymphocyte activity[438]

Lower plasma levels of T lymphocytes[439]

Higher plasma levels of immune complexes and complement[440,441]

Lower level of HLA-G mRNA expression in chorionic tissue[442]

Elevated end-organ deposition of immune complexes and immunoglobulins[443,444]

Lower incidence of preeclampsia in women who have received a blood transfusion[445]

Lower incidence of preeclampsia with an extended duration of sexual cohabitation prior to conception[435]

Higher incidence of preeclampsia in women using contraception that prevents exposure to sperm[446]

Higher incidence of preeclampsia in women impregnated by men from a different racial group[447]

Association with autoimmune disease (such as systemic lupus erythematosus)[448]

Placental Ischemia

Association with abnormal placentation[449-451]

Association with excessive placental mass (increased incidence with increasing gestational age, in molar and multifetal pregnancies,[452] in nonimmune hydrops fetalis,[453] and in women with malaria)[454]

Association with intrauterine fetal growth restriction[455]

Pathologic evidence of placental thrombosis and infarction

Generalized Endothelial Injury

Increased incidence in women with chronic hypertension[456,457]

Increased incidence in women with chronic renal disease[458]

Increased incidence in women with antiphospholipid antibody syndrome[459]

Increased incidence in women with diabetes mellitus[460]

Association with imbalance in prostaglandin synthesis (elevated thromboxane A_2/prostacyclin ratio)[461]

Association with coagulopathy

Association with abnormalities in free fatty acid, lipoprotein, and lipid peroxidase metabolism[462]

---

pathogenesis of preeclampsia. This factor serves as a co-receptor for transforming growth factor-β (TGF-β), and its use in rats leads to a syndrome similar to severe preeclampsia.[468] Like sFlt-1, levels of sEng are elevated in the circulation of women with preeclampsia several weeks before the disease becomes evident clinically.[469]

Although an attractive hypothesis, the role of the anti-angiogenic factors (sFlt-1 and sEng) in the pathogenesis of preeclampsia and the ability to use these factors to predict, diagnose, and potentially treat this disorder remains to be validated. It is likely that preeclampsia is not a single disease entity, but rather a clinical syndrome encompassing three distinct elements:

1. New-onset hypertension (defined as a sustained sitting blood pressure of at least 140/90 mm Hg in a previously normotensive woman)

2. New-onset proteinuria (defined as greater than 300 mg/24 hours or at least 1+ on a clean-catch urinalysis in the absence of urinary infection)

3. New-onset significant nondependent edema,[415] although more recent consensus reports have eliminated edema as a criterion for the diagnosis[470]

The diagnosis of preeclampsia can only reliably be made after 20 weeks' gestation. Evidence of proteinuric hypertension prior to 20 weeks' gestation should raise the possibility of an underlying molar pregnancy,[421] multiple pregnancy,[452] drug withdrawal, antiphospholipid antibody syndrome, uniparental disomy in the placenta, or rarely, a chromosomal abnormality (trisomy) in the fetus.[471]

Although numerous risk factors for the development of preeclampsia have now been defined (Table 26-9),[415,452,472,473] it is not possible to predict with any certainty which pregnancies are going to be complicated by this disease.[473,474] Moreover, despite intensive research efforts, there is no effective way at this juncture in time to prevent the development of preeclampsia in women at high risk.[475,476] As such, the current focus of obstetric care providers is regular prenatal visits with routine blood pressure and urinary protein screening with a view to early identification of preeclampsia followed by aggressive and gestational age-appropriate management.

Preeclampsia is classified as either mild or severe. A diagnosis of severe preeclampsia should be entertained in women with new-onset proteinuric hypertension accompanied by one or more of a series of complications

TABLE 26-9

Epidemiologic Risk Factors for Preeclampsia

Factor	Risk Ratio
Nulliparity[433]	2.9:1
African-American race[427]	1.2:1
Advanced maternal age > 40 years[433]	2:1
Interval between pregnancies (<1 year)[472]	1.2:1
Body mass index[163]	
26-35 kg/m^2	1.6:1
≥35 kg/m^2	3.3:1
Blood pressure[161]	
Initial systolic blood pressure 120-136 mm Hg	4:1
Initial diastolic blood pressure 60-84 mm Hg	2:1
Multiple gestation[433]	2.9:1
Family history of preeclampsia (first-degree relative)[433]	2.9:1
History of preeclampsia[429]	
History of mild preeclampsia	10:1
History of severe preeclampsia	7:1
History of eclampsia	3:1
History of preeclampsia ≤ 30 weeks' gestation	5:1
Chronic hypertension[456]	10:1
Chronic renal disease[458]	20:1
Antiphospholipid antibody syndrome[459]	10:1
Diabetes mellitus[460]	2:1
Factor V Leiden mutation[473]	
Homozygous	?
Heterozygous	1.8:1
Maternal-fetal HLA-DR discordance[437]	3:1
Angiotensinogen gene T235[430]	
Homozygous	20:1
Heterozygous	4:1

BOX 26-11

Features of Severe Preeclampsia

Symptoms
Symptoms of central nervous system dysfunction (headache, blurred vision, scotomas, altered mental status)
Symptoms of liver capsule distention or rupture (right upper quadrant and/or epigastric pain)

Signs
Severe elevation in blood pressure (defined as >160/110 mm Hg on two separate occasions at least 6 hours apart)
Pulmonary edema
Eclampsia (generalized seizures and/or unexplained coma in the setting of preeclampsia and in the absence of other neurologic conditions)
Cerebrovascular accident
Cortical blindness
Fetal intrauterine growth restriction (IUGR)

Laboratory Findings
Proteinuria (>5 g/24 hours)
Renal failure (rise in serum creatinine concentration by 1 mg/dL over baseline) or oliguria (<500 mL/24 hours)
Hepatocellular injury (serum transaminase levels ≥ 2× normal)
Thrombocytopenia (<100,000 platelets/mm^3)
Coagulopathy
HELLP syndrome (hemolysis, elevated liver enzymes, low platelets)

(Box 26-11). It should be emphasized that only *one* such criterion is required for the diagnosis of severe preeclampsia. Fetal IUGR was excluded from the criteria in 2000 by the National High Blood Pressure in Pregnancy Working Group[470] because of inconsistencies in its definition, but was still included as a criterion for the diagnosis of severe preeclampsia by ACOG in 2002.[415] Mild preeclampsia includes all women with preeclampsia who do not have any features of severe disease.

The only definitive treatment of preeclampsia is delivery of the fetus and placenta to prevent potential maternal complications. Delivery is recommended for women with mild preeclampsia at or near term. In contrast, delivery should be recommended for all women with severe preeclampsia, regardless of gestational age.[415] That said, there are three situations in which expectant management of women with severe preeclampsia may be appropriate:

1. Severe proteinuria (>5 g in 24 hours), because this finding alone is not associated with serious maternal or fetal sequelae[477]

2. Mild IUGR (fifth to tenth percentile) remote from term, as long as antepartum fetal testing remains reassuring, oligohydramnios is not severe, umbilical artery diastolic flow is not reversed on Doppler velocimetry, and there is progressive fetal growth

3. Severe preeclampsia by blood pressure criteria alone before 32 weeks' gestation that is managed with antihypertensive therapy[478,479]

The rationale for delaying delivery in these pregnancies is to reduce risk of perinatal morbidity and death by delivery of a more mature fetus and, to a lesser degree, to achieve a more favorable cervix for vaginal birth. The risk of prolonging pregnancy is continued poor perfusion of major organs in both the mother and fetus, with the potential for severe end organ damage to the brain, liver, kidneys, placenta/fetus, and hematologic and vascular systems. Delivery should be initiated—after a course of antenatal corticosteroid therapy, if possible—when there is poorly controlled severe hypertension, thrombocytopenia, eclampsia, elevated liver function tests with epigastric or right upper quadrant pain, pulmonary edema, renal insufficiency, placental abruption, or persistent symptoms (severe headache or visual changes) (see Box 26-11). Fetal indications for immediate delivery include nonreassuring fetal testing ("fetal distress"), severe oligohydramnios, or severe fetal growth restriction (less than the fifth percentile).[415]

Delivery is usually by the vaginal route, with cesarean delivery reserved for appropriate obstetric indications. Severe preeclampsia does not mandate immediate cesarean birth.[480] The decision to proceed with cesarean or induction of labor and attempted vaginal delivery should be individualized based on such factors as parity, gestational age, cervical examination (Bishop score), maternal desire for vaginal delivery, and fetal status and presentation. Cervical ripening agents may be used if the cervix is not favorable prior to induction, but prolonged inductions should be avoided.[415] The rate of vaginal delivery after labor induction decreases to about 33% at less than 34 weeks, primarily because of nonreassuring fetal testing and failure to progress in labor.[481,482]

The use of antihypertensive agents to control mildly elevated blood pressure in the setting of preeclampsia has not been shown to alter the course of the disease or diminish perinatal morbidity or mortality rate.[483] Indeed, such therapy may adversely affect uteroplacental perfusion, leading to reduced birth weight.[484] Moreover, the use of antihypertensive agents in preeclampsia may provide a false sense of security by masking an increase in blood pressure as a sensitive measure of worsening disease, and is therefore not generally recommended. These studies serve to confirm that hypertension is a clinical feature—and not the underlying cause—of preeclampsia.

The cause of the blood pressure elevation in preeclampsia is not clear. It has been suggested that it may represent an attempt of the body to maintain perfusion through an underperfused (ischemic) placenta, and may be triggered by a distress signal from the fetoplacental unit.[485] Although treatment of mild to moderate hypertension has not been shown to improve maternal or perinatal outcome, antihypertensive agents should be administered to prevent a maternal cerebrovascular accident from severe hypertension, which accounts for 15% to 20% of deaths from preeclampsia. The risk of hemorrhagic stroke correlates directly with the degree of elevation in systolic blood pressure (and is less related to the diastolic pressure), but there is no clear threshold systolic pressure above which emergent therapy should be instituted.[486] The National High Blood Pressure Education Program Working Group on High Blood Pressure in Pregnancy has recommended initiating therapy when systolic blood pressure exceeds 150 to 160 mm Hg and diastolic pressure exceeds 100 to 110 mm Hg.[470] However, this threshold has not been tested prospectively and the cerebral vasculature of women with underlying chronic hypertension can probably tolerate higher systolic pressures without injury.

The traditional drug of choice for the antepartum management of chronic hypertension is the central acting agent, methyldopa, primarily because of the extensive experience with its use during pregnancy. However, other agents have been increasing in popularity including β-blockers (primarily labetalol) and calcium channel blockers (nifedipine). Hydralazine, labetalol, and nifedipine have all been used for the management of acute hypertensive episodes in pregnancy.[415,470,483]

In term nulliparous women, the duration of labor is not affected by either preeclampsia or magnesium sulfate seizure prophylaxis.[415,487] Close and continuous monitoring of both the mother and fetus is indicated during labor to identify worsening hypertension or deteriorating maternal hepatic, renal, cardiopulmonary, or hematologic function as well as uteroplacental insufficiency with evidence of nonreassuring fetal testing. Anticonvulsant therapy is generally initiated during labor or while administering corticosteroids or prostaglandins prior to a planned delivery and continued until 24 to 48 hours post partum, when the risk of seizures is decreased.

Magnesium sulfate is the drug of choice for seizure prevention.[415,487-490] The safety and efficacy of magnesium sulfate seizure prophylaxis was illustrated in the largest study performed on preeclamptic women, the Magpie (Magnesium Sulfate for Prevention of Eclampsia) Trial.[490] The trial followed over 10,000 pregnant women with preeclampsia (defined as blood pressures of at least 140/90 mm Hg on two occasions and proteinuria of 1+ or more) in whom the obstetric care provider was uncertain about the benefit of starting magnesium sulfate therapy. The women were randomly assigned to receive magnesium sulfate (4 g intravenous loading dose, then 1 g per hour, or 5 g intramuscularly into each buttock followed by 5 g intramuscularly every 4 hours) or placebo for 24 hours. The maintenance dose was given only if a patellar reflex was present (loss of reflexes being the first manifestation of symptomatic hypermagnesemia), respirations exceeded 12 per minute, and the urine output exceeded 100 mL per 4 hours. Approximately 25% of patients met criteria for severe preeclampsia.

The major finding from this trial was that magnesium sulfate significantly reduced the risk of eclampsia as compared with nonhypertensive control subjects (0.8% versus 1.9%, respectively). This reduction in eclamptic seizures was observed regardless of the severity of preeclampsia, gestational age, and parity. The data also demonstrated a reduction in maternal mortality rate (0.2% versus 0.4%, respectively), but no difference in maternal morbidity, perinatal mortality, and neonatal morbidity rates (except for a lower rate of abruption in treated women [2% versus 3.2%, respectively]). The study concludes that, to prevent one convulsion, 63 women with severe preeclampsia or 109 women with mild preeclampsia would need to be treated. Magnesium sulfate therapy should therefore be considered for prevention of eclampsia in all women with preeclampsia, including those with mild disease.[490-492] However, some authors have questioned the value of treating all preeclamptic women to prevent seizures in only 0.6% to 3.2% of patients.[493] The incidence of seizures is much lower (approximately 0.1%) in women with nonproteinuric hypertension.[489] For this reason, it may be safe to withhold seizure prophylaxis in such women.

Hypertension due to preeclampsia resolves post partum, often within a few days, but sometimes takes a few weeks. Elevated blood pressures that persist beyond 12 weeks post partum are unlikely to be related to preeclampsia.

Parturition

Labor is the physiologic process by which the products of conception are passed from the uterus to the outside world (see also Chapter 11). The definition of labor includes an increase in myometrial activity or, more precisely, a switch in the myometrial contractility pattern from irregular *contractures* (long-lasting, low-frequency activity) to regular *contractions* (high-intensity, high-frequency activity),[494] leading to effacement and dilatation of the uterine cervix. An initial cervical examination of at least 2 cm dilatation or at least 80% effacement in the setting of regular phasic uterine contractions is also accepted as being sufficient for the diagnosis of labor in nulliparous women. A bloody discharge ("show") is often included in the description of labor, but is not a prerequisite for the diagnosis.

Considerable evidence suggests that, in most viviparous animals, the fetus is in control of the timing of labor.[495-502] Horse-donkey crossbreeding experiments performed in the 1950s, for example, resulted in a gestational length intermediate between that of horses (340 days) and that of donkeys (365 days), suggesting a role for the fetal genotype in the initiation of labor.[497,500] However, the factors responsible for the initiation and maintenance of labor in humans remain poorly defined. The slow progress in our understanding of the biochemical mechanisms involved in the process of labor in humans reflects, in large part, the difficulty in extrapolating from the endocrine control mechanisms in various animals to the paracrine/autocrine mechanisms of parturition in humans—processes which, in humans, preclude direct investigation.

Regardless of whether the trigger for labor begins within the fetus or outside the fetus, the final common pathway for labor ends in the maternal tissues of the uterus and is characterized by the development of regular phasic uterine contractions. As in other smooth muscles, myometrial contractions are mediated through the ATP-dependent binding of myosin to actin. This process is dependent in large part on the phosphorylation of myosin light chain by a calcium-dependent enzyme, myosin light chain kinase. In contrast to vascular smooth muscle, however, myometrial cells have a sparse innervation that is further reduced during pregnancy.[503] The regulation of the contractile mechanism of the uterus is therefore largely humoral and dependent on intrinsic factors within myometrial cells.

A "parturition cascade" likely exists in the human (Fig. 26-18), responsible for the removal of mechanisms maintaining uterine quiescence and for the recruitment of factors acting to promote uterine activity.[502] Given its teleologic importance, such a cascade would likely have multiple redundant loops to ensure a fail-safe system of securing pregnancy success and ultimately the preservation of the species. In such a model, each element is connected to the next in a sequential fashion, and many of the elements demonstrate positive feedforward characteristics typical of a cascade mechanism. A comprehensive analysis of each of the individual paracrine/autocrine pathways

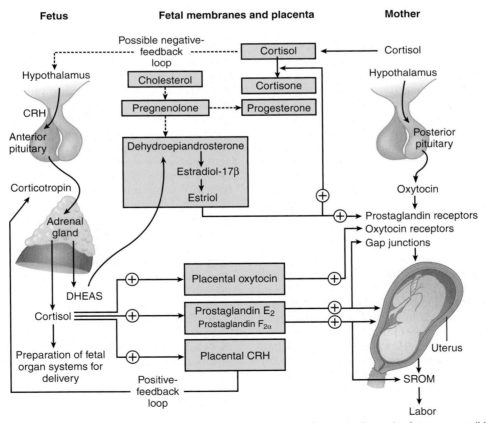

Figure 26-18. *Proposed mechanism of labor induction at term. The major hormones and paracrine/autocrine factors responsible for promoting uterine contractions at term in an integrated parturition cascade are shown. Plus signs indicate activation or up-regulation. CRH, corticotropin-releasing hormone; DHEAS, dehydroepiandrosterone sulfate; SROM, spontaneous rupture of fetal membranes. (From Norwitz ER, Robinson JN, Challis JRC. The control of labor. N Engl J Med 341:660, 1999.)*

implicated in the process of labor has been reviewed in detailed elsewhere [495,497,499,504]

In brief, human labor is a multifactorial physiologic event involving an integrated set of changes within the maternal tissues of the uterus (myometrium, decidua, and uterine cervix) that occur gradually over a period of days to weeks. Such changes include, but are not limited to, an increase in prostaglandin synthesis and release within the uterus, an increase in myometrial gap junction formation, and up-regulation of myometrial oxytocin receptors (uterine activation). Once the myometrium and cervix are prepared, endocrine or paracrine/autocrine factors from the fetoplacental unit bring about a switch in the pattern of myometrial activity from irregular contractures to regular contractions (uterine stimulation). The fetus may coordinate this switch in myometrial activity through its influence on placental steroid hormone production, through mechanical distention of the uterus, and through secretion of neurohypophyseal hormones and other stimulators of prostaglandin synthesis.

The final common pathway for the initiation of labor appears to be activation of the fetal hypothalamic-pituitary-adrenal axis, resulting in an increase in C19 steroid (DHEA) production from the intermediate (fetal) zone of the fetal adrenal, the primary substrate for estrogen synthesis in the placenta. This activity is necessary because the human placenta is an incomplete steroidogenic organ, and estrogen synthesis by the placenta has an obligate need for C19 steroid precursor from the fetus.[499] In the Rhesus monkey, infusion of C19 precursor (androstenedione) leads to preterm delivery.[505] This effect is blocked by concurrent infusion of an aromatase inhibitor,[506] demonstrating that conversion to estrogen is important. However, systemic infusion of estrogen failed to induce delivery, suggesting that the action of estrogen is likely paracrine/autocrine.[505,507,508]

In humans, activation of the fetal HPA axis results in increased estrogen production, which is responsible for up-regulating myometrial gap junctions and preparing the myometrium for contractions and labor.[509] The major estrogen produced in the human placenta is estriol, which is found in concentrations 10 to 20 times higher than other estrogens. Unlike other estrogens that are made primarily by maternal tissues, estriol is produced almost exclusively by fetal and placental tissues. Because estriol passes easily from the placenta to the maternal circulation, its relative concentrations in serum and saliva have been used as a direct marker of the activity of the fetal HPA axis.[510] Estriol is detectable as early as 9 weeks' gestation, and increases gradually after 30 weeks with a rapid rise prior to the onset of labor.[511,512] This surge in circulating estriol levels occurs approximately 3 to 5 weeks prior to the onset of labor, both at term and preterm,[512,513] but does not occur in patients requiring induction of labor or whose pregnancies are complicated by premature rupture of membranes in the absence of labor.[514] Although critical for the maintenance of early pregnancy, the role of progesterone in the latter half of pregnancy and in labor is less clear. Unlike most other mammalian species, systemic progesterone withdrawal is not a prerequisite for labor in humans[515] and the administration of a progesterone antagonist at term does not result in labor.[516,517]

The exact mechanism responsible for activation of the fetal HPA axis at term remains unclear, although changes in corticotropin-releasing hormone (CRH) seem to be important. MacLean et al suggested that CRH may serve as a "placental clock" that controls the length of gestation, and that elevated levels of CRH in the maternal circulation may predict the timing of labor and delivery.[518] Unlike total CRH levels, CRH bioactivity does not increase throughout gestation owing to increased production of CRH binding protein (CRH-BP) by the liver. Approximately 3 to 5 weeks before the onset of labor, levels of CRH-BP in the maternal circulation fall precipitously leading to an increase in free (biologically active) circulating CRH.[518]

The CRH gene is expressed in the human placenta. CRH is found in low concentrations in nonpregnant women, rises in the second and third trimesters of pregnancy, and rises exponentially in the last 3 to 5 weeks of pregnancy for both term and preterm births.[220,519,520] Fetal and maternal glucocorticoids, such as cortisol, stimulate placental CRH production.[521,522] In response, CRH stimulates the production of corticotropin (ACTH) in the mother and fetus resulting in further cortisol release. Thus, a positive feedforward system is initiated that results ultimately in the onset of labor.[523]

The mean duration of human singleton pregnancy is 280 days (40 weeks), dated from the first day of the last normal menstrual period. A term pregnancy is defined as the period from 37 weeks (259 days) to 41 weeks, 6 days (293 days). Preterm (premature) labor is defined as labor occurring prior to 37 weeks of gestation.

PRETERM LABOR

Preterm birth occurs in 7% to 12% of all deliveries, but accounts for over 85% of all perinatal morbidity and death.[524,525] Preterm labor likely represents a syndrome rather than a diagnosis because the causes are varied. Approximately 20% of preterm deliveries are iatrogenic and are performed for maternal or fetal indications, including IUGR, preeclampsia, placenta previa, and nonreassuring fetal testing.[526] Of the remaining cases, approximately 30% occur in the setting of preterm premature rupture of the membranes, 20% to 25% result from intra-amniotic inflammation or infection, and the remaining 25% to 30% are due to spontaneous (unexplained) preterm labor.

Spontaneous preterm labor may reflect a breakdown in the normal mechanisms responsible for maintaining uterine quiescence[495] or a short-circuiting or overwhelming of the normal parturition cascade.[502] An important feature of the proposed parturition cascade would be the ability of the fetoplacental unit to trigger labor prematurely if the intrauterine environment became hostile and threatened the well-being of the fetus. For example, up to 25% of preterm births are thought to result from intra-amniotic infection.[526-528] In many patients with infection, elevated levels of lipoxygenase and cyclooxygenase pathway products can be demonstrated.[527,529,530] There are also increased concentrations of cytokines in the amniotic fluid of such women. Cytokines and eicosanoids appear to interact and to accelerate each other's production in a cascade-like fashion, which may act to overwhelm the

BOX 26-12

Risk Factors for Preterm Delivery

Nonmodifiable Risk Factors
Prior preterm birth
African-American race
Age <18 years or >40 years
Poor nutrition
Low prepregnancy weight
Low socioeconomic status
Absent prenatal care
Cervical injury or anomaly
Uterine anomaly or fibroid
Excessive uterine activity
Premature cervical dilatation (>2 cm) or
    effacement (>80%)
Overdistended uterus (twins, polyhydramnios)
Vaginal bleeding

Modifiable Risk Factors
Cigarette smoking
Illicit drug use
Anemia
Bacteriuria/urinary tract infection
Lower genital tract infections (including bacterial vaginosis, *Neisseria gonorrhoeae, Chlamydia trachomatis,* group B streptococcus, *Ureaplasma urealyticum,* and *Trichomonas vaginalis*)
Gingival disease
Strenuous work
High personal stress

normal parturition cascade and result in preterm labor. Recently, thrombin has been shown to be a powerful uterotonic agent,[531,532] providing a physiologic mechanism for preterm labor secondary to placental abruption.

Numerous risk factors for preterm birth have been identified (Box 26-12), and several tests have been developed in an attempt to predict women at risk of preterm delivery (summarized in Box 26-13).[517,533-548] Prevention of preterm labor, however, has been largely unsuccessful (Box 26-14).[549-553] Improvements in perinatal outcome during this same time period have resulted primarily from antepartum corticosteroid administration and from advances in neonatal care.

Guidelines for the management of preterm labor are summarized in Box 26-15. In many instances, premature labor represents a necessary escape of the fetus from a hostile intrauterine environment and, as such, aggressive intervention to stop labor may be counterproductive. Every effort should be made to exclude contraindications to expectant management and tocolysis, including, among others, intrauterine infection, unexplained vaginal bleeding, nonreassuring fetal testing, and intrauterine fetal demise. Bed rest and hydration are commonly recommended for the treatment of preterm labor, but without confirmed efficacy.[549,554] Although there is substantial data that broad-spectrum antibiotic therapy can prolong latency in the setting of preterm premature rupture of the membranes remote from term, there is no consistent evidence that such an approach

can delay delivery in women with preterm labor and intact membranes.[555]

Pharmacologic tocolytic therapy remains the cornerstone of management for acute preterm labor. Although a number of alternative agents are now available (Table 26-10),[502,556-559] there are no reliable data to suggest that any of these agents are able to delay delivery in women presenting with preterm labor for longer than 48 hours. Because no single agent has a clear therapeutic advantage, the adverse effect profile of each of the drugs will often determine which to use in a given clinical setting.

Maintenance tocolytic therapy beyond 48 hours has not been shown to confer any therapeutic benefit, but does pose a substantial risk of adverse effects.[348,560,561] As such, maintenance tocolytic therapy is not generally recommended. Similarly, the concurrent use of two or more tocolytic agents has not been shown to be more effective than a single agent alone, and the cumulative risk of adverse effects generally precludes this course of management.[562] In the setting of preterm premature rupture of the fetal membranes, tocolysis has not been shown to be effective and is best avoided.[563]

There is increasing evidence that prophylactic supplemental progesterone may reduce the rate of preterm birth in women at high risk. For example, one randomized, double-blind, placebo-controlled clinical trial of 463 women at high risk for preterm birth because of a prior preterm delivery demonstrated a significant reduction in recurrent preterm birth in those women randomized to weekly injections of 17α-hydroxyprogesterone caproate from 16 to 20 weeks through 36 weeks of gestation.[564] Subsequent randomized studies using vaginal preparations of progesterone have had mixed results.[565,566] A recent meta-analysis of 10 placebo controlled trials involving progesterone supplementation suggested a significant reduction in the overall frequency of recurrent preterm birth from 35.9% to 26.2% (OR 0.45; 95% CI, 0.25-0.80).[567] However, enthusiasm for progesterone supplementation should be tempered until there is evidence of long-term benefit.[568] The use of progesterone supplementation in women at high risk for preterm birth for reasons other than a prior preterm delivery remains controversial. Recent studies showed a benefit of vaginal progesterone suppositories in the prevention of preterm birth in asymptomatic women with cervical shortening,[569] but no benefit of progesterone supplementation to prevent preterm birth in women with multiple pregnancies.[570] Further investigations are needed to confirm the effectiveness of progesterone supplementation in various high-risk populations and to understand its mechanism of action.

POST-TERM PREGNANCY

Post-term (prolonged) pregnancy refers to a pregnancy that has extended to or beyond 42 weeks (294 days) of gestation. Approximately 10% (range, 3% to 14%) of all singleton pregnancies continue beyond 42 weeks of gestation and 4% (2% to 7%) continue beyond 43 completed weeks in the absence of obstetric intervention.[571] Accurate pregnancy dating is critical to the diagnosis. The lowest incidence of postterm pregnancy is reported in studies using routine sonography for confirmation of gestational age.[572]

BOX 26-13

Efficacy of Screening Tests Used to Identify Women at High Risk for Preterm Delivery

Risk Factor Scoring

Risk factor scoring systems based on historical factors, epidemiologic factors, and daily habits have been developed in an attempt to predict women at risk of preterm birth. However, reliance on risk factor–based screening protocols alone will fail to identify over 50% of pregnancies that deliver preterm (low sensitivity) and the majority of women who screen positive will ultimately deliver at term (low positive predictive value).[533,534]

Home Uterine Activity Monitoring (HUAM)

HUAM of women at high risk of preterm delivery has not been shown to reduce the incidence of preterm birth.[535] Such an approach, however, does increase antepartum visits, obstetric intervention, and the cost of antepartum care.[535] There is no role for HUAM in preventing preterm birth.

Cervical Assessment (Digital and Sonographic Examinations)

Serial digital evaluation of the cervix in women at risk for preterm delivery is useful if the result remains normal. However, an abnormal cervical examination (shortening and/or dilatation) is associated with preterm delivery in only 4% of low-risk women and 12% to 20% of high-risk women.[536]

Ultrasound has demonstrated a strong inverse correlation between cervical length and preterm birth.[537,538] If the cervical length is below the 10th percentile for gestational age, the pregnancy is at a sixfold increased risk of delivery prior to 35 weeks.[538] A cervical length of <15 mm at 23 weeks occurs in under 2% of low-risk women, but is predictive of delivery prior to 28 weeks and 32 weeks in 60% and 90% of cases, respectively.[537]

Biochemical Markers (Fetal Fibronectin)

Elevated level of fetal fibronectin (fFN) in cervicovaginal secretions is associated with preterm delivery.[539] However, in a low-risk population, the positive predictive value of a positive fFN test at 22 to 24 weeks' gestation for spontaneous preterm delivery prior to 28 weeks and 37 weeks is only 13% and 36%, respectively.[540] The value of this test lies in its negative predictive value (99% of patients with a negative fFN test will not deliver within 7 days[541]), which may prevent unnecessary hospitalization.

Endocrine Markers (Salivary Estriol, Corticotropin-Releasing Hormone)

Salivary estriol accurately mirrors the level of biologically active (unconjugated) estriol in the maternal circulation.[510] Elevated levels of estriol in maternal saliva (>2.1 ng/mL) is predictive of delivery prior to 37 weeks in a high-risk population with a sensitivity of 68% to 87%, a specificity of 77%, and a false-positive rate of 23%.[542,543]

Corticotropin-releasing hormone (CRH) can stimulate prostaglandin production from the decidua and fetal membranes,[544] and can potentiate the contractile effects of oxytocin and prostaglandins on the myometrium.[545] Maternal plasma CRH levels increase and CRH-binding protein levels decrease prior to the onset of labor, both at term and preterm, resulting in a marked increase in bioactive CRH. Some authorities have proposed that CRH may serve as a "placental clock" that controls the duration of pregnancy, and that measurement of plasma CRH levels in the late second trimester may predict the onset of labor.[517] However, recent studies have shown that such tests are not clinically useful.[465,467,546-548] In light of these data, the use of plasma CRH as a predictor of preterm labor—as well as other serum markers such as activin A—remains investigational.[547]

BOX 26-14

Guidelines for the Prevention of Preterm Delivery

Strategies That Have No Proven Efficacy

Bed rest[549]
Regular prenatal care[550]
Treatment of asymptomatic lower genital tract infection[551]
Treatment of gingival disease[552]

Strategies That May Have Some Efficacy

Prevention and early diagnosis of sexually transmitted diseases and genitourinary infections
Treatment of symptomatic lower genital tract infection[553]
Cessation of smoking and illicit substance use
Prevention of multifetal pregnancies
Cervical cerclage, if indicated
Progesterone supplementation[567]

BOX 26-15

Guidelines for the Management of Preterm Delivery

Confirm the diagnosis of preterm labor
Exclude contraindications to expectant management and tocolysis
Administer antenatal corticosteroids, if indicated
Group B β-hemolytic streptococcus (GBS) chemoprophylaxis, if indicated
Pharmacologic tocolysis
Consider transfer to tertiary care center

TABLE 26-10

Management of Acute Preterm Labor

Tocolytic Agent	Route of Administration (Dosage)	Efficacy*	Maternal Adverse Effects	Fetal Adverse Effects
Magnesium sulfate	IV (4-6 g bolus, then 2-3 g/hr infusion)	Effective	Nausea, ileus, headache, weakness Hypotension Pulmonary edema Cardiorespiratory arrest ? Hypocalcemia	Decreased beat-to-beat variability Neonatal drowsiness, hypotonia ? Ileus ? Congenital ricketic syndrome (with treatment >3 wk)
β-Adrenergic agonists Terbutaline sulfate	IV (2 μg/min infusion to a maximum of 80 μg/min) SC (0.25 mg q 20 min)	Effective Effective	Jitteriness, anxiety, restlessness, nausea, vomiting, rash Cardiac dysrhythmias, myocardial ischemia, palpitations, chest pain	Fetal tachycardia Hypotension Ileus Hyperinsulinemia, hypoglycemia (more common with isoxsuprine)
Ritodrine hydrochloride†	IV (50 μg/min infusion to a maximum of 350 μg/min) IM (50-10 mg q 2-4 hr)	Effective Effective	Hypotension, tachycardia (more common with isoxsuprine) Pulmonary edema Paralytic ileus Hypokalemia Hyperglycemia, acidosis	Hyperbilirubinemia hypocalcemia ? Hydrops fetalis
Prostaglandin inhibitors Indomethacin	Oral (25-50 mg q 4-6 hr) Rectal (100 mg q 12 hr)	Effective	Gastrointestinal effects (nausea, heartburn), headache, rash Interstitial nephritis Increased bleeding time	Transient oliguria, oligohydramnios Premature closure of the neonatal ductus arteriosus and persistent pulmonary hypertension ? Necrotizing enterocolitis, intraventricular hemorrhage
Calcium channel blockers Nifedipine	Oral (20-30 mg q 4-8 hr)	Effective	Hypotension, reflex tachycardia (especially with verapamil) Headache, nausea, flushing Potentiates the cardiac depressive effect of magnesium sulfate Hepatotoxicity	
Oxytocin antagonists Atosiban	IV (1 μM/min infusion to a maximum of 32 μM/min)	Effective	Nausea, vomiting, headache, chest pain, arthralgias	? Inhibit lactation
Phosphodiesterase inhibitor Aminophylline	Oral (200 mg q 6-8 hr) IV (0.5-0.7 mg/kg/hr)	? Effective ? Effective	Tachycardia	Fetal tachycardia
Nitric oxide donor Nitroglycerine	TD (10-50 mg q day) IV (100 μg bolus, then 1-10 μg/kg/min infusion)	Unproven Unproven	Hypotension, headache	Fetal tachycardia

*Efficacy is defined as proven benefit in delaying delivery by 24-48 hr compared with placebo or standard control.
†The only tocolytic agent approved by the Food and Drug Administration.
IM, intramuscular; IV, intravenous; SC, subcutaneous; TD, transdermal.

Although the majority of postterm pregnancies have no known cause, an explanation may be found in a minority of cases. Primiparity and prior postterm pregnancy are the most common identifiable risk factors for prolongation of pregnancy.[571,573,574] Genetic predisposition may also play a role,[573,574] as concordance for postterm pregnancy is higher in monozygotic twins than in dizygotic twins.[575] Women who themselves are a product of a prolonged pregnancy are at 1.3-fold increased risk of having a prolonged pregnancy, and recurrence for prolonged pregnancy is increased two- to threefold in women who previously delivered after 42 weeks.[576,577] Rarely, postterm pregnancy may be associated with placental sulfatase deficiency or fetal anencephaly (in the absence of polyhydramnios) or CAH.[578]

Perinatal mortality rate after 42 weeks of gestation is twice that at term (4 to 7 versus 2 to 3 deaths per 1000 deliveries) and is increased fourfold at 43 weeks and five- to sevenfold at 44 weeks compared with 40 weeks.[578-580] Uteroplacental insufficiency, asphyxia (with and without meconium), intrauterine infection, and "fetal dysmaturity (postmaturity) syndrome" (which refers to chronic IUGR due to uteroplacental insufficiency) all contribute to the excess perinatal deaths. Postterm infants are larger than term infants, with a higher incidence of macrosomia (2.5% to 10% versus 0.8% to 1%).[581-582] Complications associated with fetal macrosomia include prolonged labor, cephalopelvic disproportion, and shoulder dystocia with resultant risks of orthopedic or neurologic injury. Prolonged pregnancy does not appear to be associated with any long-term neurologic or behavioral sequelae.[583]

Postterm pregnancy is also associated with risks to the mother, including an increase in labor dystocia (9% to 12% versus 2% to 7% at term), an increase in severe perineal injury related to macrosomia (3.3% versus 2.6% at term), and a doubling in the rate of cesarean delivery.[568,584,585] The latter is associated with higher risks of complications such as endometritis, hemorrhage, and thromboembolic disease.

The management of postterm pregnancy should include confirmation of gestational age, antepartum fetal surveillance, and induction of labor if spontaneous labor does not occur. Postterm pregnancy is a universally accepted indication for antenatal fetal monitoring.[571,572,586] However, the efficacy of this approach has not been validated by prospective randomized trials.[572] No single method of antepartum fetal testing has been shown to be superior.[572,587] ACOG has recommended that antepartum fetal surveillance be initiated between 41 and 42 weeks of gestation, without a specific recommendation regarding type of test or frequency.[571,584] Many investigators would advise twice-weekly testing with some evaluation of amniotic fluid volume.

Delivery is typically recommended when the risks to the fetus by continuing the pregnancy are greater than those faced by the neonate after birth. In high-risk pregnancies, the balance appears to shift in favor of delivery at around 38 to 39 weeks of gestation. Management of low-risk pregnancies is more controversial. Factors that need to be considered include results of antepartum fetal assessment, favorability of the cervix, gestational age, and

maternal preference after discussion of the risks, benefits, and alternatives to expectant management with antepartum monitoring versus labor induction. Delivery should be affected immediately if there is evidence of fetal compromise or oligohydramnios.[588,589]

In low-risk postterm gravida, both expectant management and labor induction are associated with low complication rates. However, the risk of unexplained intrauterine fetal demise—which, in one large series, was 1 in 926 at 40 weeks, 1 in 826 at 41 weeks, 1 in 769 at 42 weeks, and 1 in 633 at 43 weeks[590]—disappears after a fetus is delivered. Hannah et al[591] randomly assigned 3407 low-risk women with uncomplicated singleton pregnancies at 41 weeks of gestation to induction of labor (with or without cervical ripening) within 4 days of randomization or expectant management until 44 weeks. Elective induction resulted in a lower cesarean delivery rate (21.2% versus 24.5%, respectively), primarily related to fewer surgeries performed for nonreassuring fetal testing. These findings have been confirmed by a subsequent large randomized clinical trial.[592] In addition, a meta-analysis of 26 trials of routine versus selective induction of labor in postterm patients found that routine induction after 41 weeks was associated with a lower rate of perinatal mortality (OR 0.20; 95% CI, 0.06-0.70) and no increase in the cesarean delivery rate.[587,593] Taken together, these data suggest that there does appear to be an advantage to routine induction of labor at 41 weeks of gestation using cervical ripening agents, when indicated, regardless of parity or method of induction.

The complete reference list can be found on the companion Expert Consult Web site at www.expertconsultbook.com.

Suggested Readings

Cnattingius S, Bergstrom R, Lipworth L, Kramer MS. Prepregnancy weight and the risk of adverse pregnancy outcomes. N Engl J Med 338(3):147-152, 1998.

Consensus statement on 21-hydroxylase deficiency from the Lawson Wilkins Pediatric Endocrine Society and the European Society for Paediatric Endocrinology. J Clin Endocrinol Metab 87(9):4048-4053, 2002.

Crowther CA, Hiller JE, Moss JR, et al. Effect of treatment of gestational diabetes mellitus on pregnancy outcomes. N Engl J Med 352(24):2477-2486, 2005.

Gabbe SG, Gregory RP, Power ML, et al. Management of diabetes mellitus by obstetrician-gynecologists. Obstet Gynecol 103(6):1229-1234, 2004.

Haddow JE, Palomaki GE, Allan WC, et al. Maternal thyroid deficiency during pregnancy and subsequent neuropsychological development of the child. N Engl J Med 341(8):549-555, 1999.

Highman TJ, Friedman JE, Huston LP, et al. Longitudinal changes in maternal serum leptin concentrations, body composition, and resting metabolic rate in pregnancy. Am J Obstet Gynecol 178(5):1010-1015, 1998.

Levine RJ, Maynard SE, Qian C, et al. Circulating angiogenic factors and the risk of preeclampsia. N Engl J Med 350(7):672-683, 2004.

McLean M, Bisits A, Davies J, et al. A placental clock controlling the length of human pregnancy. Nat Med 1(5):460-463, 1995.

Meis PJ, Klebanoff M, Thom E, et al. Prevention of recurrent preterm delivery by 17 alpha-hydroxyprogesterone caproate. N Engl J Med 348(24):2379-2385, 2003.

Miller E, Hare JW, Cloherty JP, et al. Elevated maternal hemoglobin A1c in early pregnancy and major congenital anomalies in infants of diabetic mothers. N Engl J Med 304(22):1331-1334, 1981.

Norwitz ER, Robinson JN, Challis JR. The control of labor. N Engl J Med 341(9):660-666, 1995.

Pop VJ, Kuijpens JL, van Baar AL, et al. Low maternal free thyroxine concentrations during early pregnancy are associated with impaired psychomotor development in infancy. Clin Endocrinol (Oxf) 50(2):149-155, 1999.

Thorpe-Beeston JG, Nicolaides KH, Felton CV, et al. Maturation of the secretion of thyroid hormone and thyroid-stimulating hormone in the fetus. N Engl J Med 324(8):532-536, 1991.

Venkatesha S, Toporsian M, Lam C, et al. Soluble endoglin contributes to the pathogenesis of preeclampsia. Nat Med 12(6):642-649, 2006.

Weiss JL, Malone FD, Emig D, et al. Obesity, obstetric complications and cesarean delivery rate: a population-based screening study. Am J Obstet Gynecol 190(4):1091-1097, 2004.

CHAPTER 27

Breast Cancer

Richard J. Santen

Etiology

Mutations of key genes involved in cell proliferation, DNA repair, vasculogenesis, invasion, metastasis, and apoptosis must accumulate to produce cancer. These attributes allow "cancer cells to generate their own mitogenic signals, to resist exogenous growth-inhibitory signals, to evade apoptosis, to proliferate without limits (i.e., to undergo immortalization), to acquire vasculature (i.e., to undergo angiogenesis), and in more advanced cancers, to invade and metastasize."[1] Recent whole genome analyses provide major new insight into this process.[2] These studies suggest that multiple mutations are present in breast cancers to allow these tumor capabilities to emerge.

Tumor mutations can be subdivided into causative "driver" mutations that occur frequently and associative "passenger mutations" that occur uncommonly.[2,3] Based upon these concepts, the specific signaling pathways altered by mutations are considered more important for emphasis than identification of individual mutations. With whole genomic analysis, Wood et al identified 167 mutated genes in the breast cancers examined, with 14 considered to be candidate "driver" cancer genes when examined by sophisticated statistical methods. These mutations probably alter no more than 20 key signaling pathways.[3] "This new view of cancer is consistent with the idea that a large number of mutations, each associated with a small fitness advantage, drive tumor progression."[4] These landmark studies suggest that at least 14 key mutations are required to convert benign into malignant breast tissue.[2,3]

A number of specific mutations have been associated with a high incidence of breast cancer.[5] The most common include *BRCA1, BRCA2, MLH1, MSH2, FGFR2, CHEK2, IKBKE, ATM, BRIP1, STK11, BR1P1, TP53,* and *PTEN* genes.[6-12] The *BRCA1* and *BRCA2* genes cause approximately 5% of breast cancer cases.[13] Rarer genetic syndromes include mutations of the *TP53* gene in the Li-Fraumeni syndrome; impaired cell cycle checkpoint surveillance in the ataxia-telangiectasia syndrome (*ATM*); mutations in the *PTEN* gene in the Cowden syndrome; the *MLH1/MSH2* genes in the Muir-Torre syndrome; a *STK11* mutation the Peutz-Jeghers syndrome, and *CHEK2* mutations.[5] Studies in identical twins suggest that approximately 27% of breast cancers are associated with genetic factors, but the specific genes are unknown in 22% of these.[14]

Dietary, environmental, and lifestyle factors play a key role in breast cancer etiology and contribute to the four-fold differences in incidence between Japan with a rate of 23 women per 100,000 per year and the United States at 90 women per 100,000 per year.[15-19] Epidemiologic observations suggest a role for high-fat diet, alcohol, exercise, and obesity in the genesis of breast cancer. In Japan, the rate of breast cancer peaks at the age of menopause, but in the United States, incidence continues to increase until age 90. The difference in postmenopausal patterns may result from the increase in obesity and associated aromatase increments in women in the United States compared to those in Japan. This differential postmenopausal rate does not appear genetic because Japanese women who move to the United States experience an increased rate of breast cancer that later approaches that of North American women.

A variety of data suggest that hormonal factors and particularly estrogens contribute to the development of breast cancer. Administration of exogenous estrogens to various animal species results in breast cancer. Spontaneous development of breast cancer in aging rats can be prevented by oophorectomy or administration of aromatase inhibitors to block estrogen production. As outlined in Figure 27-1, epidemiologic studies implicate several hormonal factors in the genesis of breast cancer. In women, oophorectomy before the age of 35 lowers the risk of breast cancer by 75%

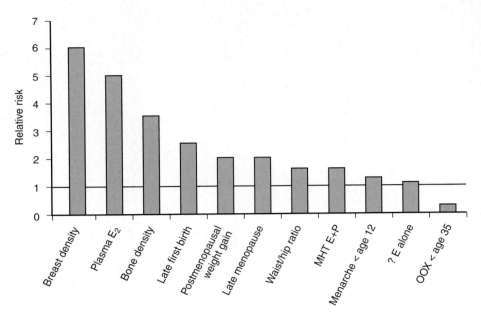

Figure 27-1. Relative risk of breast cancer as a function of several factors which relate to the long-term exposure to estradiol (E₂). The question mark indicates data are conflicting, but the bar represents majority opinion. E, estrogen; MHT, menopausal hormone therapy; OOX, oophorectomy; P, progesterone. (From Santen R. Endocrine-responsive cancer. In Kronenberg HM, Melmed S, Polonsky KS, Larsen PR [eds]. Williams Textbook of Endocrinology, 11th ed. Philadelphia, WB Saunders, 2008, Fig. 42-2.)

over a 25-year period. The ages of menarche and menopause also correlate with breast cancer risk. Administration of anti-estrogens to women at high risk of developing breast cancer results in a 50% reduction in tumor development.

SOURCES OF ESTROGEN

The estradiol present in breast tissue is synthesized in three sites: the ovary, extraglandular tissues, and the breast itself. Direct glandular secretion by the ovary results in delivery of estradiol to the breast through an endocrine mechanism in premenopausal women. After the menopause, extraglandular production of estrogen from ovarian and adrenal androgens in fat and muscle provides the second source of estradiol. Third, the breast itself can synthesize estradiol via aromatization of androgens to estrogens or cleavage of estrone sulfate to free estrone via the enzyme sulfatase. Estradiol acts through paracrine, autocrine, and intracrine mechanisms on cells in the breast. Several factors regulate in situ estradiol synthesis but the most important is the degree of obesity, which increases the amount of aromatase in breast and consequently estradiol production.

ESTROGEN-INDUCED CARCINOGENESIS

It is likely that mitogenic as well as mutagenic effects of estradiol act in concert to initiate and promote the development of breast cancer.[20,21] As a general rule, the frequency of mutations increases in parallel with the number of mitotic divisions in a proliferating tissue. Accordingly, estrogens may *initiate* mutations leading to neoplastic transformation by increasing the rate of cell proliferation. As cells divide more rapidly, less time is available for DNA repair. Estrogens may also enhance tumor *promotion* by increasing the rate of cell division with propagation of the mutations already present.

Metabolites of estradiol may be directly mutagenic through a pathway involving the CYP 1B1 cytochrome P450 enzyme.[20] This catalyzes conversion of estradiol to 4-OH-estradiol, a catechol estrogen which is then further metabolized to 3,4-estradiol quinone. This highly reactive species binds covalently to guanine or adenine molecules in the DNA helix and forms an unstable complex, which results in removal of purine from the DNA backbone. Error-prone or replicative repair of the depurinated sites leads to point mutations.[20] The 3,4-estrogen quinones can also be back-converted to 4-OH-estradiol, forming a redox cycle, which generates reactive oxygen species. These in turn may directly damage DNA. The mutagenic hypothesis involving estrogen metabolites is supported experimentally by studies demonstrating the mutagenic potential of estradiol on estrogen receptor negative (ER–) MCF-10 breast cancer cells in vitro and the transformation of these cells to cancer in vivo.[22] Additional evidence derives from experiments in castrated estrogen receptor knockout animals bearing the Wnt-1 oncogene. In these animals, estradiol can also increase the rapidity of onset and absolute number of breast cancers.[23]

HORMONAL RISK FACTORS FOR BREAST CANCER

The majority of risk factors for breast cancer relate to the duration or intensity of a woman's exposure to endogenous or exogenous estrogens (see Fig. 27-1). Early menarche and late menopause increase breast cancer risk.[24] Elevations in circulating estradiol levels predict the risk of developing breast cancer over the ensuing years in postmenopausal women (Fig. 27-2).[25,26] A recent analysis concluded that estrogen levels provide information independent of other known risk factors.[27] An estradiol level in the top quintile increases the relative risk of breast cancer by as much as fivefold.[25,26,28]

Putative markers of long-term estrogen exposure such as bone density are also predictive. Women in the top quartile of bone density have a threefold increased risk of breast cancer; a history of fracture or height loss lowers the

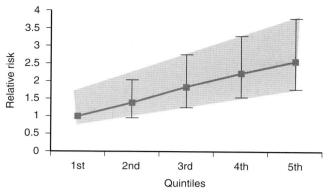

Figure 27-2. *Risk of breast cancer related to levels of plasma estradiol in postmenopausal women. (From Key T, Appleby P, Barnes I, Reeves G, Endogenous Hormones and Breast Cancer Collaborative Group. Endogenous sex hormones and breast cancer in postmenopausal women: reanalysis of nine prospective studies. J Natl Cancer Inst 94[8]:606-616, 2002.)*

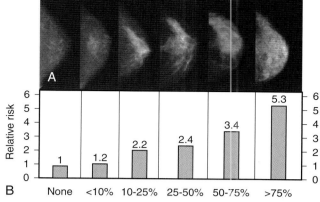

Figure 27-3. *Relative risk of breast cancer as a function of the degree of mammographic density.* **A,** *Six categories of breast density as illustrated by mammograms. (From Boyd NF, Byng JW, Jong RA, et al. Quantitative classification of mammographic densities and breast cancer risk: results from the Canadian National Breast Screening Study. J Natl Cancer Inst 87[9]:670-675, 1995.)*

risk.[29,30] Late first birth increases the risk 2.8-fold and is believed to relate to the lack of the differentiating effect of pregnancy on type of breast lobule present. Gain of at least 20 kg as an adult increases breast cancer risk twofold[31] and weight loss reduces the risk.[15] Increased waist-hip ratio exerts a similar increase in risk.[16] Several but not all studies suggest that alcohol intake can increase the risk of breast cancer, perhaps by decreasing the clearance of estradiol.[32] Increased exposure to estradiol in utero, as shown by twin studies, may increase risk of breast cancer by as much as twofold. Early pregnancy and prolonged duration of breastfeeding diminish the risk. More dramatic is the 75% reduction in risk caused by bilateral oophorectomy before age 35.[33]

Mammographic density represents the most powerful risk factor for breast cancer[34,35] (Fig. 27-3). Increased breast density probably reflects either an increase in exposure to estrogen or a sensitivity to it. Exogenous estrogens increase and anti-estrogens reduce breast density. Because of these effects, menopausal hormone therapy (MHT) alters the sensitivity and specificity of reading standard film screen mammograms.[35] Increase in breast cancer risk from lowest to highest breast density category is on the order of fivefold, depending upon the age of the patient (see Fig. 27-3), with greater relative risk in older women. Recent data indicate that mammographic density, when added to the factors used in the Gail predictive model, increases the power of prediction substantially and thus is independent of several other risk factors.[36,37]

EXOGENOUS ESTROGENS AND BREAST CANCER RISK

In premenopausal women, use of oral contraceptives for 10 or more years increases the relative risk of breast cancer by approximately 10%.[38,39] However, this increase in relative risk affects very few women because the age-related incidence of breast cancer is quite low in women taking oral contraceptives. Controversy previously surrounded the concept that MHT in postmenopausal women increases

the risk of breast cancer. More than 50 observational studies have examined this question but reported conflicting results.[40] However, several recent key studies clarified the factors responsible for the differing conclusions among the various observational reports. One study, the meta-analysis from the Collaborative Group on Hormonal Factors in Breast Cancer (CGHFBC)[40] examined data from 52,705 women with breast cancer and 108,411 without. Five objective factors that had confounded interpretation of prior studies were identified:

1. The relative risk of breast cancer from MHT appears to be quite small and large studies with a long duration of follow-up are required to minimize type I and type II statistical errors.
2. The risk of breast cancer appears to increase linearly with duration of MHT use. Accordingly, comparisons of "ever users" with "never users" are invalid because duration of estrogen use is not considered.
3. The increased risk of breast cancer imparted by MHT appears to dissipate within 4 years of cessation of therapy. Therefore, only women using MHT within 4 years of study might be found to be at increased risk.
4. Breast cancer risk diminishes over a 4-year period following the menopause, presumably as a reflection of decreased estrogen levels. As a result, analyses of observational studies need to match users against nonusers as to time following menopause.
5. The increased risk of breast cancer appears to be limited predominantly to nonobese women (i.e., body mass index [BMI] < 25 kg/m^2). Inclusion of a large proportion of obese women in a single study might then obscure an association between MHT use and breast cancer risk.

Taking into account these five factors, the CGHFBC meta-analysis concluded that the relative risk of breast cancer increases linearly by 2.3% per year of MHT for up to 25 years.[40] The slope of the line correlating relative risk with duration of use of MHT was statistically significant,

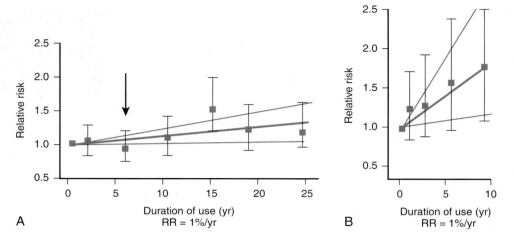

Figure 27-4. **A,** *Observational data on the risk of breast cancer in women taking estrogen alone.* **B,** *Observational data on the risk of breast cancer in women taking estrogen plus a progestin. The* squares *and* error bars *show the mean and confidence intervals of relative risk at each time point. The* solid line *represents the linear trend, and the* shaded area *represents the confidence intervals. The* arrow *draws attention to the decreased risk at the early time point. (From Schairer C, Lubin J, Troisi R, et al. Menopausal estrogen and estrogen-progestin replacement therapy and breast cancer risk. JAMA 283[4]:485-491, 2000.)*

indicating an effect of duration of MHT use. The overall risk of breast cancer among MHT users, independent of duration of use, was also highly statistically significant. This study detected no increased risk of breast cancer with MHT use in obese women (i.e., BMI > 25 kg/m²). A hypothetical explanation for the differences between obese and thin women relates to the degree of in situ estrogen production. Obese women may have an increase in breast tissue estrogen as a result of increased aromatase activity, whereas lean women would have lower levels. Exogenous estrogen might then produce a greater percentage increase in breast tissue estradiol levels in thin than in obese women.

Another large observational database, the Million Women Study, supported the CGHFBC findings and extended them by comparing the use of estrogen alone to estrogen plus a progestin.[41] The relative risk (RR) of breast cancer from estrogen alone used for more than 10 years was increased (RR 1.37, 95% confidence interval [CI] 1.22-1.54) but use of estrogen plus a progestin for longer than 10 years was associated with an even greater relative risk (RR 2.31, 95% CI 2.08-2.56). Other observational studies report a linear increase in risk of breast cancer first appearing after 10 years of use and continuing to increase in a linear fashion for up to 25 years of use[42] (Fig. 27-4A and B).

Until recently, only observational studies were available to assess breast cancer risk and unidentified biases could have confounded data interpretation. However, the large, prospective, randomized Women's Health Initiative (WHI) trial in postmenopausal women recently provided compelling evidence for an adverse effect of an estrogen/progestin combination on breast cancer incidence.[43] Nearly 16,000 postmenopausal women with an average age of 63 enrolled in the estrogen plus progestin arm of the Women's Health Initiative study and received either placebo or conjugated estrogens (0.625 mg) plus medroxyprogesterone acetate (MPA) (2.5 mg) for 5 years. The study was terminated early because of an increased incidence of breast cancer in the MHT group with a relative risk of 1.26 and 95% confidence interval of 1-1.59 (Fig. 27-5). The absolute excess of cases was small with only 4 more invasive breast cancers per 1000 women over 5 years of therapy in the MHT group. Nonetheless, these data confirm the prior observational

studies and indicate a relative risk increase of 5.5% per year in those receiving MHT. This is similar to the 8% per year reported in the observational studies.[42]

Many authors have criticized the WHI conjugated estrogen plus MPA study because of the frequency of dropouts, occurrence of drop-ins (i.e., patients randomized to placebo and then deciding to take MHT during the study), the exclusive use of MPA as the progestin, and the fact that the average age of participants was 63 and no attention was given to menopausal symptoms. In addition, the increase in risk was limited to women who had previously used MHT and then stopped before randomization. Finally, the placebo group appeared to have a lower risk of breast cancer than expected from the placebo group in the estrogen-alone study.[44] Even with these criticisms, the majority of properly conducted studies indicate an increased risk from estrogen plus a progestin, as shown by a recent meta-analysis.[45]

Another arm of the Women's Health Initiative study compared placebo with conjugated equine estrogen alone in women who had previously undergone a total abdominal hysterectomy.[46] This study did not demonstrate an increased risk of breast cancer after 5 years of hormonal therapy. Surprisingly, the risk of breast cancer (RR = 0.77)

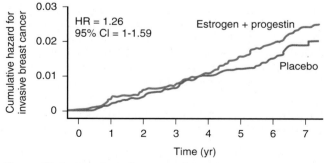

Figure 27-5. Data from the Women's Health Initiative relating risk of breast cancer to use of conjugated equine estrogen plus medroxyprogesterone acetate. CI, confidence interval; HR, hazard ratio. (From Rossouw JE, Anderson GL, Prentice RL, et al. Risks and benefits of estrogen plus progestin in healthy postmenopausal women: principal results from the Women's Health Initiative randomized controlled trial. JAMA 288[3]:321-333, 2002.)

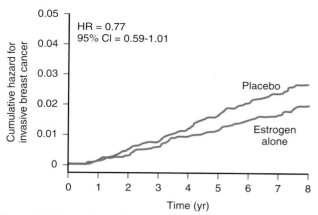

Figure 27-6. *Randomized controlled trial data from the Women's Health Initiative relating risk of breast cancer to use of estrogen alone. CI, confidence interval; HR, hazard ratio. (From Anderson GL, Limacher M, Assaf AR, et al. Effects of conjugated equine estrogen in postmenopausal women with hysterectomy: the Women's Health Initiative randomized, controlled study. JAMA 291:1701-1712, 2004.)*

TABLE 27-1

Occult Breast Cancers Found at Autopsy

Report	Number of Cases	Incidence (%)
1962 Ryan	200	0
1973 Kramer	70	4.3
1975 Wellings	67	1.9
1984 Nielsen	77	14.3
1985 Alpers	101	8.9
1985 Bhathal	207	12.1
1987 Bartow	221	0
1988 Nielsen	109	14.7
Total cases	**1052**	**6**

Data from Ryan JA, Coady CJ. Intraductal epithelial proliferation in the human breast—a comparative study. Can J Surg 5:12-19, 1962; Kramer WM, Rush BF Jr. Mammary duct proliferation in the elderly. A histopathologic study. Cancer 31:130-137, 1973; Wellings SR, Jensen HM, Marcum RG. An atlas of subgross pathology of the human breast with special reference to possible precancerous lesions. J Natl Cancer Inst 55:231-273, 1975; Nielsen M, Jensen J, Andersen J. Precancerous and cancerous breast lesions during lifetime and at autopsy. A study of 83 women. Cancer 54:612-615, 1984; Alpers CE, Wellings SR. The prevalence of carcinoma in situ in normal and cancer-associated breasts. Hum Pathol 16:796-807, 1985; Bhathal PD, Brown RW, Lesueur GC, Russell IS. Frequency of benign and malignant breast lesions in 207 consecutive autopsies in Australian women. Br J Cancer 51:271-278, 1985; Bartow SA, Pathak DR, Black WC, et al. Prevalence of benign, atypical, and malignant breast lesions in populations at different risk for breast cancer. A forensic autopsy study. Cancer 60:2751-2760, 1987; and Nielsen M, Thomsen JL, Primdahl S, et al. Breast cancer and atypia among young and middle-aged women: a study of 110 medicolegal autopsies. Br J Cancer 56:814-819, 1987.

Table prepared by D. Craig Allred, Baylor College of Medicine, Houston, TX.

was reduced, although not statistically significantly (95% CI 0.59-1.01), at 5 years in those in the hormonal arm (Fig. 27-6). A post hoc subset analysis reported a statistically significant reduction in risk in three subgroups: those with localized tumors (hazard ratio [HR] 0.69, 95% CI 0.51-0.95), invasive ductal carcinoma (HR 0.71, 95% CI 0.52-0.99), and women adherent to the study protocol and not dropping out (HR 0.67, 95% CI 0.47-0.97).[46] The Nurses' Health observational study reported a similar, statistically significant reduction in risk in women with a BMI greater than 25 who took estrogen alone for 5 to 9 years (HR 0.74, 95% CI 0.55-1).[47] The reduction in risk at 5 years in the observational study of Shairer et al also supports a potential beneficial effect of short-term estrogen[42] (Fig. 27-6, see data at 6 years). The studies of Lyytinen et al, the Mission Study, and the Million Women study also suggest reductions of breast cancer risk with short-term use of estrogens alone (7%, 43%, and 19%, respectively, with short-term use).[41,48,49] Observational data regarding long-term use of estrogen alone indicate the opposite effect, namely, a 41% to 77% increase in relative risk, of breast cancer at 25 years as observed in both the Schairer et al, Million Women, and Nurses' Health Studies.[41,42,47,50]

Comparison of short-term estrogen use (which may decrease breast cancer risk by 30%) with long-term administration (which appears to increase risk by 41% to 77%) suggests an "estrogen paradox." One potential explanation for the "estrogen paradox" is that estradiol can exert two separate mechanistic effects: estradiol-induced apoptosis in the short term and initiation/promotion of new cancers over the long term. Recent studies demonstrate that estradiol can induce apoptosis in breast tumors that have been deprived of estradiol over a prolonged period.[51] In addition, high-dose estrogen administration to women with advanced breast cancer induces tumor regressions in approximately 40% of ER-positive (ER+) patients.[52,53] At entry to the WHI estrogen-alone study, the average age of the women was 63 years, 12 years beyond

the average age of menopause. Accordingly, women who never previously took hormone therapy were in a state of long-term estradiol deprivation, 12 years on average. If these patients had occult undiagnosed tumors (see later discussion), estrogen alone might have caused apoptotic cell death in them.

One hypothesis to explain these finding is that a reservoir of undiagnosed breast cancer is present in women starting on estrogen alone as MHT. Estrogen could decrease the size of these tumor by apoptosis and result in a decreased frequency of diagnosis 5 years later.[54] How common are undiagnosed breast cancers in the population? A review of eight studies which examined 1052 breasts at autopsy revealed a 5% prevalence of undiagnosed ductal carcinoma in situ and 1% prevalence of invasive breast cancer (Table 27-1). Two of the more recent studies describe the meticulous methodology needed to detect occult tumors.[55,56] What effect would estrogen have on those small undiagnosed lesions? A pro-apoptotic effect of estradiol would be expected to reduce the size of those tumors such that they would not be detected over the 5 years of follow-up. This could explain the significant reductions of breast cancer in subgroups of women in the WHI and Nurses' Health studies. This short-term estrogen effect might then be superseded by a pro-carcinogenic effect of estradiol if the patients received this hormone over a prolonged period of up to 25 years[42,47] (see Fig. 27-4A).

The "estrogen paradox" hypothesis is speculative and will require prospective, randomized, controlled trials over a longer period of time for confirmation. At the present time, only observational studies with long-term follow-up are available, and these findings suggest a 1% increase in relative risk of breast cancer with estrogen alone which is only apparent after 10 to 15 years of exposure[42,47] (Fig. 27-4A).

Critical review of the WHI data suggests that the adverse effects on breast cancer risk over the 5-year period resulted from the addition of a progestin to the administered estrogen. It is unclear if this is a progestin class effect or unique to the progestin used, medroxyprogesterone acetate. Several observational studies examined the effects of various types of progestin as well as differences between combined continuous and sequential regimens.[41,43] The Million Women Study suggested that all types of progestin are associated with an increased risk of breast cancer and that a class effect of progestins is responsible. Another large observational study, the EPN-3/EPIC study, on the other hand, reported no increased risk of breast cancer from use of crystalline progesterone, whereas it found increased risks similar to those in the Million Women Study with other types of progestin.[57] The Mission Study, while smaller, reported a similar trend.[49] More data will be necessary to confirm this finding regarding crystalline progesterone, which if valid has major implications regarding which progestin should be used clinically.

An understanding of the physiologic basis for the association of progestins with breast cancer rests on data indicating that progestins are mitogenic on breast tissue in contrast to their antimitogenic effects on the uterus.[58] Although data from cell cultures and animal studies are conflicting, the weight of evidence from patients suggests that progestins are mitogenic in breast. Mammographic studies demonstrate that estrogen/progestin combinations increase breast density to a greater extent than estrogen alone or placebo.[59] Histologic examination demonstrates enhanced cell proliferation and percentage of the breast containing glandular tissue as a function of duration of progestin usage.[58] Increased proliferation would be expected to increase both *initiation* and *promotion* of breast cancer in a manner similar to that thought to occur with estrogens.[20]

Decreasing Breast Cancer Incidence in the United States

Breast cancer incidence decreased by 6.7% as documented by SEER population data in 2003.[60] With respect to ER+ tumors, the decrease was 14.7% (95% CI 11.6-17.4) and for ER− 1.7% (95% CI −46 to +8). This finding was surprising because breast cancer incidence had been gradually increasing until 1999 and then plateaued until 2003. Ravdin et al[60] suggested that this might reflect the substantial cessation of use of MHT in women noted in 2002 and 2003 after publication of the WHI study. A county-by-county analysis from California indicated that the steepest decline in breast cancer incidence (22.6%) occurred in counties with the greatest drop in MHT use, whereas the smallest decrease (8.8%) was observed in those with the lowest

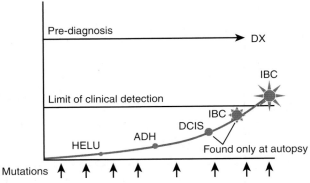

Figure 27-7. Diagram representing the sequential development of breast cancer. The first predisposing lesion is called a hyperplastic elongated lobule unfolded (HELU), which progresses to atypical ductal hyperplasia (ADH) and then ductal carcinoma in situ (DCIS), and finally to invasive breast cancer (IBC). It has been recently estimated that 14 mutations on average are found in established breast cancers (see text). A lesion must reach 1 cm before it is clinically detectable. Accordingly there is a large reservoir of undiagnosed tumors too small to be detected by palpation or imaging techniques (see text). DX, diagnosis.

fall-off in use.[61] Although decreased screening mammography could possibly explain these results, such a confounder would not be expected to result in a decline in incidence in ER+ tumors exclusively. One mechanistic explanation for these findings is that a subset of the occult breast cancers might regress in response to cessation of estrogen plus progestin use and therefore not grow to the threshold of diagnosis over the next 2 to 3 years (Fig. 27-7). If this explanation proves correct, one might expect a rebound in breast cancer incidence over the ensuing years.

RELATIVE, ABSOLUTE, AND ATTRIBUTABLE RISKS FROM MHT

A full understanding of the magnitude of risk from MHT requires knowledge of the precise meaning of statistical terms. Epidemiologists use *relative risk analysis* as a tool that provides substantial power to determine statistical significance of differences between groups. However, the term "relative risk" is misleading to patients because absolute or actual risk may be quite small in magnitude when relative risk is high. The lay press, patients, and many physicians confuse the terms relative, absolute, and attributable risk.

Relative risk is defined as the ratio of risk under one condition compared to risk under another and does not take into account the frequency of occurrence of that condition. *Absolute risk* is determined by multiplying the underlying incidence rate in the group being considered by relative risk. For example, an average 50-year-old woman in the United States has an absolute risk of developing breast cancer of 1.26 per 100 women over a 5-year period. A 35% increase in relative risk resulting from an estrogen/progestin combination would increase her absolute chances of getting a breast cancer to 1.7 per 100 women. *Attributable* risk (alternatively called "excess risk") is defined as the number of women who would develop a breast cancer that would not have otherwise occurred unless they had used estrogen/progestin therapy. Using the preceding example, the difference between breast cancer risk of 1.26 per 100 and 1.7 per 100 represents the increased (or excess) risk *attributable* to estrogen of 0.44 per 100 women (or 4.4 per 1000 women). This increase is interpreted by patients to be less than that conveyed by an increase in relative risk of 26%.

BENIGN BREAST DISEASE AND RISK OF BREAST CANCER

A large recent study from the Mayo Clinic confirmed prior observations that benign breast lesions with an enhanced rate of proliferation predict an increased incidence of breast cancer over time (Fig. 27-8).[62] Hyperplastic ductal lesions are often multicentric, suggesting that some type of underlying abnormality is present which predisposes to such lesions. This has been called a "field defect" or, more recently, a "mutator phenotype."[63] The multifocal nature of the associated benign hyperplastic lesions is most apparent in breast tissue from women with cancer. Examination of tissue adjacent to an invasive breast cancer or in the contralateral breast reveals one or more additional hyperplastic lesions in approximately 40% of patients.[64]

The nature of the *field defect* or mutator phenotype has not been specifically identified but hypothetically could represent a single mutation of a gene controlling local estrogen production, cellular proliferation, DNA repair, metabolism of pro-carcinogens to carcinogens, or other cellular events. Preliminary data suggest progression from adenomas to frank neoplasms. From 80% to 90% of hyperplastic lesions contain DNA mutations similar to those in the contiguous tumors. Extensive molecular genetic studies have now described progression of abnormalities in the spectrum of breast lesions.[63]

A major consideration for women who present with breast problems is whether they have a higher than normal risk of developing breast cancer. Certain breast lesions such as fibrocystic changes are associated with no increased risk of subsequent breast cancer (see Fig. 27-8) unless a strong family history is present. Other lesions, characterized by the presence of increased cellular proliferation such as usual ductal hyperplasia, hyperplastic elongated lobular units, and solitary or multiple papillomas impart a small (i.e., less than twofold) relative increase in risk.[62,63,65] With atypical ductal hyperplasia (ADH), the relative risk is 3.88 overall and 10.35 in those with multifocal (i.e., three or more) lesions with calcifications. In younger women, ADH imparts a 6.75 RR (i.e., women younger than 45).[65] The relative risk of development of invasive cancer is increased 10- to 12-fold when ductal carcinoma in situ (DCIS) and lobar carcinoma in situ (LCIS) are present.

Proliferative lesions can progress to invasive cancer as evidenced by the increase in ipsilateral breast cancer in women harboring these lesions. However, the presence of proliferative lesions also reflects a "field defect" or "mutator phenotype" because risk of contralateral breast cancer is also increased when the period of observation extends over more than 10 years. The Mayo Clinic study of nearly 15,000 women confirmed the concept that only lesions with increased proliferation impart an increased risk of breast cancer unless a strong family history is

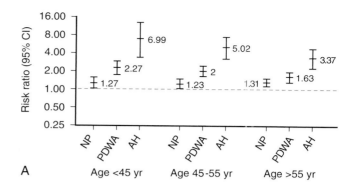

A

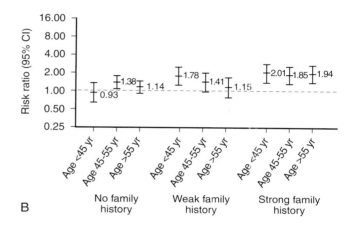

B

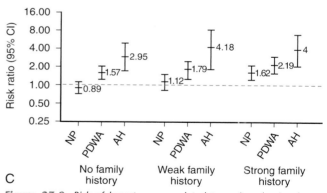

C

Figure 27-8. Risk of breast cancer related to various benign breast lesions and family history of breast cancer. AH, atypical hyperplasia; NP, nonproliferating; PDWA, proliferating duct without atypia. (From Hartmann LC, Sellers TA, Frost MH, et al. Benign breast disease and the risk of breast cancer. N Engl J Med 353[3]:229-237, 2005.)

present.[62] This finding clarified a prior study which did not distinguish proliferative from nonproliferative and concluded that low category breast disease, including fibrocystic changes, conveys an increased risk.[66]

ESTIMATING BREAST CANCER RISK

To aid in assessing breast cancer risk, a questionnaire developed by Gail utilizes answers to seven questions to calculate the 5-year and lifetime risk of developing breast cancer.[67] This model has recognized deficiencies in that it does not consider breast density, plasma estradiol levels, bone density, body mass index, weight gain in adulthood, second-degree relatives with breast cancer, proliferative lesions of breast other than ADH, alcohol intake, or birth control pill and MHT use.[7] Nonetheless, two major prospective studies validated the Gail model in a high-risk (NSABP prevention study) and in an average-risk population of women (the Nurses' Health Study). The ratio of observed to expected cancers using this tool was 1.03 (95% CI 0.88-1.21) in the high-risk patients and 0.94 (95% CI 0.89-0.99) in average-risk women, and both were highly statistically significant. This risk tool is available as the "RISK DISK" from the National Cancer Institute. When second-degree relatives with breast cancer predominate, the Claus model provides a more valid risk assessment tool.

Newer models are being developed to enhance the power of risk prediction. Although only validated in one prospective study, the Tyrer/Cuzick model appeared to outperform the Gail and Claus models in a population with a high familial breast cancer component.[68] This new model combines the factors utilized in the Claus and Gail models as well as a history of MHT use, and appears quite promising as a new risk prediction tool. As mentioned before, addition of mammographic density to the Gail model improves risk prediction.[37] However, precise quantitation of breast density is infrequently utilized and a practical method (such as the "Risk Disk") is not yet available to integrate breast density into the Gail model to make the necessary calculations.

BREAST CANCER RISK AND CLINICAL DECISIONS

Knowledge about underlying breast cancer risk influences advice given by health care providers and choices made by patients. Women known to be at high risk of breast cancer will frequently choose a surrogate for MHT (see later discussion) to treat menopausal symptoms. Those at low risk will usually chose estrogen or an estrogen/progestin combination to relieve symptoms of estrogen deficiency. Those at intermediate risk of breast cancer have several options including use of a selective estrogen receptor modulator (SERM), other alternatives to estrogen, watchful waiting, or MHT.

As a working guide, we arbitrarily define risk categories based upon use of risk prediction models: high risk is 3% or greater chance of breast cancer in 5 years; intermediate risk is 1.5% to 3% chance; and low risk is 1.5% or less chance. Those classified as high risk include patients with a strong family history of breast cancer (particularly if associated with ovarian cancer), prior history of ADH or lobular carcinoma in situ, and age over 60 when combined with early menarche, late menopause, or first live birth. Intermediate-risk patients have some risk factors but not others. Low-risk patients are under 60 years of age; have a late onset of menarche, early menopause, early age of first live birth, and no family history of breast cancer; and lack predisposing breast lesions. Because no formal risk tool incorporates breast density, bone density, and plasma estradiol levels into its assessment, a physician must take these factors into account in advising patients.

Prevention of Breast Cancer

Depending upon risk category, women may wish to take tamoxifen or raloxifene to prevent breast cancer. Both raloxifene and tamoxifen are now approved for this use in the United States. Evidence supporting anti-estrogens for prevention is substantial. A meta-analysis of the five large prevention trials demonstrated a 50% reduction in breast cancer risk with tamoxifen when compared to placebo.[69] The most definitive trial, NSABP (National Surgical Adjuvant Breast and Bowel Project) P-1, involved 13,388 women randomized to receive either placebo or 20 mg of tamoxifen daily[70] (Fig. 27-9). Eligibility into the study required an intermediate or high risk of developing breast cancer, defined in the study as a 1.67% or greater chance of developing a new breast cancer over a 5-year period. The rate of breast cancers in the placebo group was 9.4 per 1000 women-years versus 4.7 in the tamoxifen group, a relative risk reduction of 50% (RR 0.5) (see Fig. 27-9). Considered separately, the risk of invasive breast cancer was reduced by 49% and noninvasive breast cancer was reduced by 50%. This effect occurred in women of all ages studied (≤49, 50-59, 60-69, and >70) and in those with LCIS, ADH, and a family history of breast cancer. The benefits of tamoxifen related to the underlying risk of breast cancer and the specific risk factor present (Fig. 27-10). These results led a panel of experts commissioned by the American Society of Clinical Oncology (ASCO) to conclude that tamoxifen does reduce the incidence of newly diagnosed breast cancer in high-risk women.[71]

Tamoxifen for treatment of breast cancer is considered well tolerated and safe. However, for use in otherwise normal women, infrequent side effects and toxicity become more important. Up to 40% of women starting on tamoxifen do not continue it because of perceived side effects including depression and mood changes.[72-76] Tamoxifen belongs to the class of agents called selective

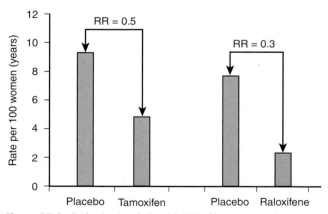

Figure 27-9. *Reduction in relative risk (RR) of breast cancer in response to the administration of tamoxifen or to raloxifene for a mean duration of 5 years. (Data from Fisher B, Costantino JP, Wickerham DL, et al. Tamoxifen for prevention of breast cancer: report of the National Surgical Adjuvant Breast and Bowel Project P-1 Study [see comment]. J Natl Cancer Inst 90(18):1371-1388, 1998; and Cummings SR, Eckert S, Krueger KA, et al. The effect of raloxifene on risk of breast cancer in postmenopausal women: results from the MORE randomized trial. Multiple Outcomes of Raloxifene Evaluation [see comment] [erratum appears in JAMA 282(22):2124, 1999]. JAMA 281[23]:2189-2197, 1999.)*

estrogen receptor modulators (SERMs). Agents in this class exert anti-estrogenic effects on tissues such as breast but estrogenic effects on others such as uterus and liver. These various actions of the SERMs must be factored in when estimating risks and benefits in the setting of breast cancer prevention.

To compare risks and benefits in a meaningful way, the NSABP data are expressed as the number of women per 100 with a specific benefit or adverse event after 5 years of study. With respect to benefits, new invasive breast cancers were prevented in 1.7 of 100 women, noninvasive cancers in 0.67, and bone fractures in 0.50 for a total of 2.87 in 100 women benefited after 5 years. Risks of tamoxifen are primarily related to its estrogenic effects on uterus, a prothrombotic effect, and adverse effects on the lens of the eye. To validly estimate actual risks to a patient, one must correct for the underlying risks in the population under study. For that reason, analysis of adverse events includes determination of *attributable risk* and involves subtracting the underlying rate from the total observed on tamoxifen. This indicates an excess of 1.5 of 100 women who developed cataracts, 0.69 with endometrial cancer (nearly exclusively in postmenopausal women), 0.27 with stroke, 0.25 with deep venous thrombosis, and 0.23 with pulmonary embolus, or a total of 2.94 per 100.[77] The new endometrial cancers were predominantly stage I and pulmonary emboli nonfatal. Neither risk nor benefit was observed regarding cardiovascular effects, but the number of patients was not sufficient for statistical significance.

The increased incidence of uterine cancer in patients on tamoxifen presents a clinical management problem. Substantial study has examined how best to detect this cancer early.[78] Transvaginal ultrasound was initially proposed as a means of assessing both endometrial hyperplasia, as a precursor lesion, and early cancer. A prospective study demonstrated a mean increase in endometrial thickness from 3.5 ± 1.1 to 9.2 ± 5.1 mm in response to 5 years of tamoxifen. In 20% of women, endometrial thickness exceeded

10 mm or appeared suspicious for neoplasm. In this subset of women, biopsies revealed atrophy in 73%, polyps in 17%, hyperplasia in 7.7%, but endometrial cancer in only one patient.[79] This and other studies conclude that endometrial thickness does not usually indicate hyperplasia but, rather, the presence of edema and dilated myometrial glands. It should be noted that nonprospective studies report a higher prevalence of benign polyps (5% to 55%) and hyperplasia (8% to 16%)[80,81] but these numbers are likely to be overestimates from selection bias. Based upon these studies, recommendations for screening include yearly gynecologic examination and endometrial sampling and ultrasound only for those with signs of abnormal vaginal bleeding.[78,79]

Another SERM, raloxifene, appears to prevent breast cancer in postmenopausal women without increasing the risk of endometrial cancer. The MORE trial and its follow-on extension, the Core Trial, compared raloxifene with placebo in osteoporotic women and demonstrated a 75% reduction in breast cancer risk over an 8-year period in women with an average or reduced risk of breast cancer (see Fig. 27-9A). The STAR trial then compared raloxifene with tamoxifen in a "head-to-head" prevention trial in 18,000 postmenopausal women with a predicted risk greater than 1.67% at 5 years. Both agents prevented invasive breast cancer similarly (by an estimated 50%) but raloxifene exhibited a superior toxicity profile with 30% fewer thromboembolic events (P = 0.01); 38% fewer endometrial cancers (P = 0.07); 21% fewer cataracts (P = 0.002); an 84% reduction in uterine hyperplasia (P < 0.01), and 55% fewer unplanned hysterectomies. No differences between agents were observed in cardiovascular events, strokes, and fracture rates. A surprising finding was that raloxifene did not appear to prevent noninvasive breast cancer, whereas tamoxifen has previously been shown to do so.[82] These effects of raloxifene were confirmed in a randomized comparison to placebo in the Ruth trial.[83] The STAR and Ruth trials suggest that raloxifene provides a reasonable preventive option for postmenopausal women at increased risk of breast cancer, particularly if they have low bone density or an intact uterus.

GUIDELINES FOR BREAST CANCER PREVENTION

Premenopausal women with a 5-year risk of breast cancer greater than 1.67% over 5 years are candidates for tamoxifen unless they are at increased risk for deep venous thrombosis (DVT) or pulmonary emboli. Postmenopausal women with similar breast cancer risk are candidates for tamoxifen if they no longer have a uterus and lack a predisposing risk for DVT or pulmonary emboli. Raloxifene may be preferred over tamoxifen in postmenopausal women with a uterus. The decision to take tamoxifen or raloxifene should be made by the patient in partnership with her health care provider and based upon a full discussion of individual risks and benefits expressed in absolute and not relative terms.[71] Prevention strategies for women carrying BRCA1 or BRCA2 mutations often involve more aggressive steps such as bilateral oophorectomy or mastectomy, but tamoxifen may also be effective in these patients.[13,84]

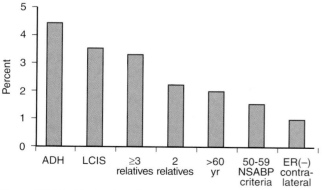

Figure 27-10. *Absolute benefit from tamoxifen expressed as percentage of women whose breast cancer was prevented as a function of the underlying risk factor present. ADH, atypical ductal hyperplasia; ER, estrogen receptor; LCIS, lobar carcinoma in situ; NSABP, National Surgical Adjuvant Breast and Bowel Project. (From Santen R. Endocrine-response cancer. In Kronenberg HM, Melmed S, Polonsky KS, Larsen PR [eds]. Williams Textbook of Endocrinology, 11th ed. Philadelphia, WB Saunders, 2008, Fig. 42-8B.)*

CRITICAL ASSESSMENT OF BREAST CANCER PREVENTION STRATEGIES

Estimates indicate that between 20 and 100 women (depending upon underlying risk) need to be treated to prevent one breast cancer. Clinical decisions depend upon analysis of risk/benefit ratios and should be made after full discussion between health care provider and patient. Regarding efficacy, available data demonstrate only a reduction in newly diagnosed breast cancers but effects on overall survival are not yet known. Whether tamoxifen actually prevents breast cancer, cures some preexisting subclinical cancers (reservoir tumors), or delays the onset of diagnosis of small tumors remains to be determined. Mathematical modeling techniques suggest that the "preventive effects" of tamoxifen are equally divided between blockade of growth of occult tumors and prevention of new ones.[85] Tumors whose growth was blocked by tamoxifen during its 5 years of administration might be expected to regrow later. For this reason, data on overall survival (to be available from the ongoing IBIS 1 trial) will be critically important.[69]

Future studies will need to utilize additional factors to select women at higher risk of developing breast cancer.[7] A study of raloxifene examined women with factors suggesting high long-term exposure to estrogen (i.e., increased bone mineral density, high BMI, and high plasma estradiol levels). Results indicated that raloxifene was more effective in preventing breast cancer in women with high than with low long-term estrogen exposure. For example, for those with high versus low bone mineral density, the prevention rates were 94% versus 56%; for the high versus low BMI groups, 82% versus 64%; and for the high versus low plasma E_2 groups, 77% versus 55% ($P < 0.005$).[86] A critical need at present is to develop a more powerful breast cancer risk model that incorporates breast density, plasma estrogen levels, history of fracture, waist-hip ratio, and obesity as well as the factors utilized in the Gail and Claus risks prediction models.[7]

Trials of the aromatase inhibitors (AIs) in the adjuvant setting uniformly demonstrate a greater reduction of contralateral cancers with the aromatase inhibitors than with tamoxifen.[87-90] The crossover study from tamoxifen to letrozole or placebo at 5 years also demonstrated a reduction of contralateral breast cancer incidence with the AI.[91] These data provide strong indirect evidence that aromatase inhibitors will be more effective than tamoxifen in breast cancer prevention. Two trials (IBIS II and MAP 3) have been initiated to examine this issue, and data should be forthcoming in approximately 4 years.

Treatment of Established Breast Cancers

The American Cancer Society statistics documented that 279,900 new cases of breast cancer were diagnosed in the United States in 2006 and 40,970 died of this disease.[92] One approach to effective treatment is early diagnosis. Use of digital mammography and magnetic resonance imaging (MRI) have increased the sensitivity of detecting early disease.[93] As a result of early screening and use of adjuvant therapy, the death rate from breast cancer over the past 10 years has declined by 12% in the United States as well as in Western Europe.

Hormonal treatment provides effective and well-tolerated therapy for women with hormone-dependent tumors. The mechanisms whereby estradiol stimulates breast cancer growth are complex and involve direct regulation of genes involved in control of proliferation and apoptosis, induction of growth factors through secondary actions, and cross-talk between growth factor and estrogen pathways at both upstream and downstream levels.[94] Membrane-initiated (extranuclear) effects of estradiol on growth factor–mediated mitogenic pathways may also be involved.[95,96] Treatment strategies utilize agents which abrogate the effects of estrogen on these pathways and thus inhibit growth and induce apoptosis. Emerging evidence suggests that tumor stem cells may be the most important target for therapy.[97]

Common approaches involve anti-estrogens or blockade of estrogen synthesis with aromatase inhibitors or GnRH superagonist analogs.[98] Patients who initially respond to hormonal therapy eventually relapse. A standard strategy for responders to first-line treatment is to administer secondary and tertiary hormonal therapies upon relapse. The sequential responses to hormonal therapies suggest an adaptive process whereby tumors do not become totally resistant to hormonal therapy but develop a transitional state during which alternative means of blocking hormonal pathways cause tumor regression. Patients relapsing following oophorectomy or tamoxifen treatment commonly respond secondarily to inhibitors of estrogen production (aromatase inhibitors) or rarely to the withdrawal of tamoxifen.[98]

DEVELOPMENT OF HORMONAL RESISTANCE

Women respond to each hormonal therapy on average for 12 to 18 months and then relapse.[98] At some time in the course of treatment, tumors become totally resistant to further hormonal therapy. Several explanations for development of secondary resistance have been suggested[94,99-104]:

1. Changes in metabolism of tamoxifen with production of estrogenic metabolites
2. A constitutive increase in growth factor production as a result of additional oncogene mutations
3. Enhanced growth factor receptor functionality
4. Increased use of extranuclear estrogen receptor pathways
5. Down-regulation of transcriptional co-repressors;
6. Outgrowth or selection of hormone-resistant clones of tumor cells.
7. Up-regulation of nuclear receptor co-activators
8. Other adaptive mechanisms

An additional hypothesis to explain resistance is that tumors adapting to hormonal therapy become hypersensitive to lower amounts of circulating estrogen or to the estrogen-agonist properties of tamoxifen.[105] Experimental support for this concept emanates from observations in xenograft models and in vitro studies. Breast tumor xenografts adapt to long-term exposure to tamoxifen by responding to it as an estrogen, rather than as an anti-estrogen. Under these circumstances, the pure anti-estrogen, fulvestrant, blocks the stimulatory effect of tamoxifen, causing tumor regression. In cell culture systems, long-term deprivation of estradiol renders breast cancer cells hypersensitive to the proliferative effects of this sex steroid.[106] This adaptive process is associated with increments in ERα and *HER2/neu* (now more often designated as erbB-2) as well as in MAP (mitogen-activated protein) kinase, an enzyme which stimulates cell proliferation, and in growth factor pathways involving PI3 (phosphoinositide 3) kinase and mTOR (mammalian target of rapamycin).[107,108] The hypersensitivity concept could explain secondary responses to aromatase inhibitors in patients relapsing after oophorectomy or tamoxifen and secondary responses to the pure anti-estrogen, fulvestrant.

Data from several laboratories have demonstrated a variety of events that occur commonly in vitro in cells exposed to long-term estrogen deprivation or tamoxifen. These events include up-regulation of the MAP kinase pathway; increased phosphorylation of *AKT*; enhancement of mTOR; increased activation of IGF-1 (insulin-like growth factor 1), EGF (epidermal growth factor), and *HER2/neu* receptors; up-regulation of adaptor proteins, such as CAS 130; and increased activation of ER-mediated transcription.[94,99,100] One theory is that the growth factor–activated kinases phosphorylate the estrogen receptor to render it transcriptionally more active and, at the same time, phosphorylate co-activators such as AIB1 (activated in breast cancer 1). Another is that cells adapt to the pressure exerted by hormonal therapy to enhance utilization of membrane-initiated signaling pathways involving the estrogen receptor.[94,109] Under these circumstances tamoxifen becomes an estrogen agonist at the level of the cell membrane and cells are stimulated to grow in its presence.

Clinical data support these concepts in that *HER2/neu* and *AIB1* overexpressing tumors exhibit resistance to tamoxifen.[94] Secondary responses to aromatase inhibitors in patients resistant to tamoxifen may also reflect hypersensitivity to estrogen because the third-generation aromatase inhibitors lower estradiol levels by more than 99%. De novo or primary resistance to endocrine therapy may also involve many of the mechanisms occurring during development of secondary resistance. As an example, primary tumors overexpressing *HER2/neu* appear to be relatively resistant to tamoxifen therapy.

PROGNOSTIC FACTORS

Clinical decision making requires knowledge of the degree of aggressiveness and natural history of the type of breast cancer present. Much attention has been directed toward multivariant and neural network analysis to calculate the precise prognosis in individual women. Investigators previously developed means of pooling various risk factors in order to improve prognostication. The Nottingham index is an example of a method that integrates the findings of tumor size, nodal status, and histologic grade of the tumor. In general, these methods have not been particularly useful

in practical decision making and individual factors are used in treatment algorithms. However, a recently developed Web-based tool (www.adjuvantonline.com) has been very useful to calculate prognosis in individual women and to guide patients and their physicians in the choice of various therapeutic options.

Figure 27-11 illustrates the prognostic power of various biologic factors by comparing the effects of individual parameters on 5-year survival rates. The most powerful clinical and pathologically based prognostic parameters include nodal status, tumor grade and size, proliferative indices, and ER status. Other prognostic characteristics include *HER2/neu* positivity by fluorescence in situ hybridization (FISH) analysis, degree of aneuploidy, and overexpression of certain oncogenes or co-activators (e.g., D-cyclin, A1B1, MAP kinase, Ras, HER3 and HER4, heregulin, c-Src, and ODC levels).[110] Finally, based upon data from the Women's Health Initiative study, tumors diagnosed in postmenopausal women while receiving conjugated equine estrogen plus medroxyprogesterone acetate are associated with larger size and more frequently involve lymph nodes.[43] These new findings contradict conclusions from observational studies that such tumors have lower histologic grade and a 10% better prognosis than those in women not receiving MHT.

Recent studies detected circulating tumor cells in the blood of patients with breast cancer as well as micrometastases in lymph nodes and bone marrow.[110,111] This information clearly provides prognostic information, but no data are as yet available on how these findings should be used to influence therapeutic decisions.[112]

cDNA Array Analysis: New Biologic Subtypes

A major recent advance is the performance of cDNA array analysis to assess the effect of a particular tumor signature on prognosis.[113] This type of analysis has allowed a new biologic classification of breast cancer based upon the degree of expression of key discriminant genes. Five subtypes of breast cancer are defined: luminal A, luminal B, basal epithelial, erbB-2+, and normal breast tissue–like subtype.[113] As shown in Figure 27-12, each subtype has a different prognosis. Of interest is the fact that all *BRCA1*-positive tumors fall into the basal subtype category.[113] Data from five separate molecular signature methods are largely concordant.[114-119] Studies are currently ongoing to validate these molecular techniques in subsets of patients categorized by tumor size, nodal status, tumor grade, age, and type of treatment. Such information will be necessary before routine common clinical application of this methodology is implemented.

Predictive Factors

Other biologic parameters allow assessment of the potential effectiveness of certain therapies. Older age, long disease-free survival, high degree of tumor differentiation, and prior response to endocrine therapy predict a higher likelihood of responses to hormonal therapy.[98] The ability to measure receptors markedly improves the process of selection of patients for hormonal therapy. Absence of ER in the

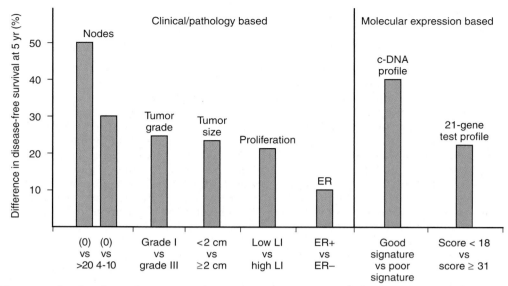

Figure 27-11. *The prognostic value of several parameters related to patients with an initial diagnosis of breast cancer. All values are presented as the percent difference in disease-free survival at the 5-year interval. This method of presentation allows one to determine the increased number of women per 100 who would be alive without recurrence at 5 years if they have a favorable prognostic factor compared with those with an unfavorable factor. ER, estrogen receptor; LI, labeling index. (From Santen R. Endocrine-response cancer. In Kronenberg HM, Melmed S, Polonsky KS, Larsen PR [eds]. Williams Textbook of Endocrinology, 11th ed. Philadelphia, WB Saunders, 2008, Fig. 42-9.)*

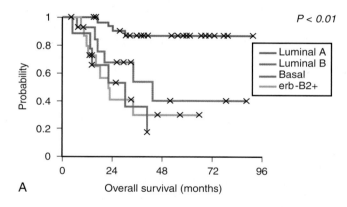

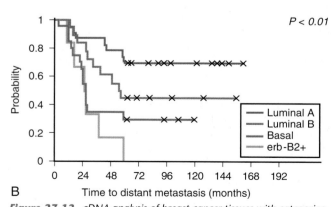

Figure 27-12. *cDNA analysis of breast cancer tissues with categorization into Luminal A, Luminal B, Basal, and erb-B2 and the probability of overall survival and time to distant metastasis. The normal subtype is not shown. (Data reproduced from Sotiriou C, Neo SY, McShane LM, et al. Breast cancer classification and prognosis based on gene expression profiles from a population-based study. ProcNatl Acad Sci U S A 100(18):10393-10398, 2003, with the permission of the authors and publisher.)*

tumor predicts that fewer than 5% to 10% of women will respond to hormonal therapy. If both ER and progesterone receptor (PR) are negative, an even lower percentage will respond. Patients with both ER+ and PR+ tumors respond to hormonal therapy 50% to 75% of the time, but 30% to 50% of ER+ but PR– tumors are responsive.[98,120] Emerging data suggest that patients with ER+ and PR+ tumors respond to tamoxifen therapy less frequently if *HER2/neu* is positive.[121] However, *HER2/neu*-positive tumors respond similarly to aromatase inhibitors as do *HER2/neu*-negative lesions. It should be noted that new data confirm the old observations of Lippman and Allegra that low ER levels, in addition to predicting nonresponsiveness to hormonal therapy, also predict a high likelihood of responding to chemotherapy.[122,123]

Receptor measurements are commonly performed by immunohistochemical (IHC) analysis, which correlates well with the ligand-binding assays. An increasing trend is to semiquantitate the level of ER positivity in tumors using the Allred scoring system, which classifies tumors on the basis of the proportion of cells that are positive and the intensity of staining on a scale of 0 to 8.[124] With routinely utilized IHC techniques, only ERα is measured, but about half of breast tumors also contain ERβ. A recent study suggests that low levels of ERβ predict resistance to tamoxifen therapy[125] and that isoforms of ERβ may provide additional predictive information.[126,127] Recent data suggest that certain tumors make ERβ variant proteins which can heterodimerize with full-length ERα or ERβ and exert dominant negative effects.[128] This concept suggests that further refinement of receptor assays may improve their predictive value. However, insufficient data are currently available to know the precise clinical value of ERβ variants.

An FDA approved assay utilizing quantitative polymerase chain reaction (PCR) of selected genes has been

TABLE 27-2

Definition of Risk Categories for Patients with Postoperative Breast Cancer

Risk Category	Description
Low risk	Node negative AND all of the following features: pT ≤ 2 cm, AND Grade 1, AND Absence of peritumoral vascular invasion, AND ER and/or PR overexpressed AND HER2/neu gene neither overexpressed nor amplified, AND Age ≥ 35 years
Intermediate risk	Node negative AND at least one of the following features: pT > 2 cm, OR Grade 2-3, OR Presence of peritumoral vascular invasion, OR HER2/neu gene overexpressed or amplified, OR Age < 35 yr Node positive (1-3 involved nodes) AND ER and/or PR expressed AND HER2/neu gene neither overexpressed nor amplified
High risk	Node positive (1-3 involved nodes) AND ER and PR absent, OR HER2/neu gene overexpressed or amplified Node positive (4 or more involved nodes)

Endocrine Response Category	Description
Highly endocrine responsive	High expression of both ER and PR in a majority of cells
Incompletely endocrine responsive	Lower expression of ER and/or PR
Endocrine nonresponsive	Complete absence of both ER and PR

ER, estrogen receptor; PR, progesterone receptor; pT, primary tumor.
From Santen R. Endocrine-response cancer. In Kronenberg HM, Melmed S, Polonsky KS, Larsen PR (eds). Williams Textbook of Endocrinology, 11th ed. Philadelphia, WB Saunders, 2008, Table 42-1.

validated in a prospective study to determine which patients with node-negative, ER+ disease will experience distant disease recurrence while on tamoxifen.[116,117] This method, the Oncotype DX assay, measures 16 informative genes and 5 housekeeping genes as controls. On this basis, women with node-negative, ER+ breast cancers are categorized into groups with low, intermediate, or high risk of recurrence. The low-risk group had a 6.8% recurrence at 10 years versus a rate of 30.5% in the high-risk group. When patient age and tumor size were added to the model, only the cDNA score remained statistically significant upon multivariate analysis. These data provide prognostic information as well as predictive information as to the treatment of women with ER+, node-negative disease. Emerging data from the Oncotype DX assay suggest that

the absolute level of ER mRNA, which varies by more than a 300-fold range, may be a better predictor of responses to hormonal therapy than qualitative IHC assessment of ER protein content. The Oncotype Dx assay is gradually gaining usage in the United States. A cDNA array assay utilizing a 70-gene profile is being used in Europe (MammaPrint) on an investigational basis and was recently FDA approved for use in the United States. Both methods are currently being studied in prospective trials.[129,130]

New Prognostic and Predictive Classification System

Investigators at the 2005 St. Gallen meeting devised a new, logical method for both prognostic and predictive use[112] and it was slightly modified and updated in 2007[131] (Table 27-2). This provides a practical means of choosing specific therapies. The first level of categorization places patients into one of three predictive groups: highly endocrine responsive (high receptor content), incompletely endocrine responsive (low receptor content), and endocrine nonresponsive (no receptor present). The second level of categorization places patients into prognostic groups including high risk, intermediate risk, and low risk as defined in Table 27-2.

HORMONAL THERAPIES FOR BREAST CANCER: BASIC MECHANISTIC PRINCIPLES

Surgical Ablative Therapies

Historically, the initial approach to hormonal therapy involved surgical removal of endocrine glands responsible for synthesis of estrogen or its precursors. Beatson in 1896 first demonstrated that oophorectomy caused regression of breast cancer in premenopausal women, and comprehensive studies later documented responses in one third of patients not selected with ER measurements.[98] The availability of glucocorticoid replacement therapy in the 1940s enabled the use of adrenalectomy or hypophysectomy. More recently, development of medical means to block hormone synthesis or action has replaced adrenalectomy and hypophysectomy, although surgical oophorectomy is still used.[98]

HORMONE ADDITIVE THERAPIES

Clinicians learned from empirical observations that high doses of estrogen, androgen, or progestins caused tumor regression.[53,98] High-dose estrogen therapy is most effective in women who had experienced menopause several years previously. A series of recent studies suggests a possible mechanism to explain this paradoxic effect, estrogen-induced apoptotic cell death.[51] With prolonged deprivation of estradiol, tumors up-regulate the estrogen-responsive Fas/Fas ligand death receptor system and down-regulate the anti-apoptotic factor, NFκB. With respect to androgens, a variety of observations suggest that an increased ratio of androgens to estrogens exerts an antagonistic effect on breast tissue. Progestins exert glucocorticoid actions which suppress circulating estrogen levels and could also act via progestational mechanisms.

Medical Ablative Therapies

GnRH Agonist Analogs. Medical means of "ablating hormone secretion or action" avoid the need for surgical oophorectomy and can effectively replicate the hormonal and clinical effects of these procedures. High doses of GnRH agonist analogs suppress ovarian function to the same extent as surgical oophorectomy, and this strategy is referred to as medical oophorectomy (Med OOX) in this chapter. As the pituitary requires pulsatile exposure to GnRH to maintain gonadotropin secretion, GnRH agonists suppress LH and FSH by exposing the pituitary to a continuous GnRH stimulus which causes a paradoxic gonadotropin inhibition. Preparations lasting 3 to 12 months can be given by intramuscular injection. For the first several days after initiation of therapy, an increase in LH, FSH, and estradiol occurs but thereafter suppression ensues.

Selective Estrogen Receptor Modulators. In premenopausal women, these agents exert anti-estrogenic effects on breast which are similar to those of surgical oophorectomy and in postmenopausal women, hypophysectomy or adrenalectomy. Tamoxifen, the initial anti-estrogen of this type, was introduced for use in the United States in the mid-1970s.[98] Early clinical observations noted that this drug is an anti-estrogen on breast tissue but an estrogen agonist on uterus, vagina, bone, pituitary, and liver.[98]

Attempts to determine the divergent actions of tamoxifen led to an understanding of the complexity of ER-mediated transcriptional regulation and actions of the anti-estrogens (reviewed briefly here and covered in detail in Chapter 5). Tamoxifen binds to both ERα and ERβ in the ligand-binding domain (activation function [AF] 2 region) of the receptor which then facilitates the binding of the anti-estrogen-ER complex to specific estrogen response elements (EREs) on DNA. Conformational changes in the ER binding pocket at helix 12 induced by anti-estrogens hinder binding of co-activators to the ER and facilitate binding of co-repressors. The continued presence of co-repressor in the complex is thought to explain the anti-estrogenic properties of tamoxifen. The relative amounts of co-repressor and co-activator in certain tissues and the presence of other unknown factors regulate whether tamoxifen acts as an agonist or antagonist. As one example, up-regulation of *HER2/neu* and *AIB1* appears to enhance the estrogen agonistic properties of tamoxifen.[104] Additional estrogenic effects are mediated by membrane initiated (extra-nuclear) actions at the cell membrane as well as by tethering to ER and binding sites on c-Jun, SP-1, IGF-R, PI3 kinase, HER2/neu, c-Src and potentially other factors.[95,96,109,132]

Based upon the SERM concept, other agents have been introduced or are being developed to enhance breast antagonistic and bone agonistic properties. One of these, toremiphene, is quite similar to tamoxifen, albeit slightly less effective as an agonist on bone. Raloxifene, on the other hand, appears not to stimulate uterus or cause endometrial cancer, and yet is an anti-estrogen on breast. The STAR and Ruth trials[82,83] established the efficacy of raloxifene as a breast cancer preventive drug, but minimal data are available regarding its efficacy for treatment.

Pure Antagonist Anti-estrogens. Clinical and experimental data suggested that long-term exposure to tamoxifen might induce tumors to undergo adaptive mechanisms to cause the agonistic properties of this SERM to predominate.[104] Based upon these observations, anti-estrogens were developed that were relatively devoid of agonist properties. Fulvestrant, the FDA-approved drug in this class, increases the rate of degradation of the ER and also inhibits E_2-mediated transcription by favoring binding of co-repressors to the ER complex.[133] Because of its effect to reduce the concentration of the ER, fulvestrant has been termed a selective estrogen receptor down–regulator, or SERD.

Inhibitors of Estradiol Synthesis. Aromatase catalyzes the rate-limiting step in the conversion of androgens to estrogens.[134] Aromatase has been a key target for development of inhibitors over the past 25 years. The first-generation inhibitor, aminoglutethimide, blocks aromatase by 90% in postmenopausal women and is as effective as tamoxifen in causing breast tumor regressions. The substantial side effect profile and lack of specificity of amino-glutethimide served as an impetus to develop second- and third-generation inhibitors.[98]

Three third-generation agents (anastrozole, letrozole, and exemestane) are now approved drugs in the United States and Europe. These agents are 100- to 10,000-fold more potent than aminoglutethide and are called selective aromatase inhibitors (SAI) because they do not inhibit other enzymatic steps. The two major subclasses include nonsteroidal competitive inhibitors and steroidal enzyme inactivators.[134] The competitive inhibitors bind to the active site of the enzyme with high affinity and compete with substrate. Aromatase inactivators bind covalently to the enzyme and permanently destroy its activity. Theoretically, the inactivators could have advantages over the competitive aromatase inhibitors because inhibition might continue if a patient missed one or more doses of medication. However, no experimental proof of this advantage is as yet available in patients.

Both subclasses of inhibitor reduce aromatase to 1% to 2.5% of baseline activity,[135] substantially reduce plasma estradiol levels, and suppress tissue concentrations of this steroid in breast tumors (Fig. 27-13). The greater degree of suppression with the third-generation than with first-generation inhibitors may explain their enhanced efficacy in causing tumor regression. As the AIs are devoid of estrogen agonistic properties, these agents do not increase the incidence of endometrial cancer, as occurs with tamoxifen. However, as expected from the known effects of estrogen deprivation on bone, the aromatase inhibitors do accelerate the rate of bone loss and fracture incidence.[136] Although a trend toward an increased incidence of cardiac events has been reported, these adverse findings are inconsistent among studies and not yet statistically significant (Table 27-3).[137] Cholesterol levels are slightly higher in patients taking aomatase inhibitors as opposed to tamoxifen, but this may reflect the lipid-lowering properties of tamoxifen. If cholesterol levels do rise in response to the AIs, the increase is minor.[137]

Chemical Castration. Chemotherapeutic agents destroy granulosa cells in the ovary and may result in transient or

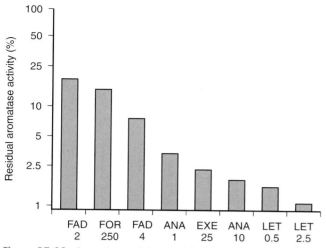

Figure 27-13. Aromatase activity remaining during the administration of first-, second-, and third-generation aromatase inhibitors and inactivators. Data are expressed on a log scale to emphasize the expected log dose response characteristics of hormone actions. With the most potent inhibitor, only 1% of aromatase activity persists during therapy. Degree of aromatase suppression determined by an isotopic kinetic method using ^{3}H-androstenedione and ^{14}C-estrone to assess the Rho value before and during therapy. The Rho value represents the percent conversion of androgens to estrogens under equilibrium conditions. ANA, anastrozole; EXE, exemestane; FAD, fadrazole; FOR, formestane; LET, letrozole. (From Geisler J, Lonning PE. Endocrine effects of aromatase inhibitors and inactivators in vivo: review of data and method limitations [review] [57 refs]. J Steroid Biochem Mol Biol 95[1-5]:75-81, 2005.)

permanent amenorrhea in premenopausal women.[138] Accordingly, practical clinical issues of infertility and menopausal symptoms ensue. Complete ovarian destruction, as evidenced by the onset of amenorrhea, is more common in women over age 40 as opposed to those younger (Fig. 27-14). Of interest is the return of menses in up to 20% of women over 40 when an aromatase inhibitor is started.[139] Incomplete information is available regarding estradiol levels under these circumstances. The effect of chemical castration was not initially felt to be clinically important. However, recent data suggest that adjuvant chemotherapy in premenopausal women exerts its antitumor effects on neoplasms with high ER levels through an ovarian ablative effect to a substantial degree.[140]

Radiation Castration. Radiation treatment (RT) of the ovaries in premenopausal women has been used as adjuvant treatment of breast cancer for many years, but the majority of studies do not adequately document the degree of suppression of estradiol levels. An Eastern Cooperative Oncology Group study examined 22 women receiving RT to induce ovarian ablation. Only 75% experienced complete ablation based upon estradiol or FSH levels. In one quarter of patients, the effect was delayed until 7 to 28 months after RT was completed. These data suggest that surgical or medical oophorectomy with GnRH agonists should be used in preference to RT to induce ovarian ablation.[141]

Complete versus Partial Estradiol Ablation. Removal of the ovaries causes a marked decrease in estradiol production, but adrenal precursors remain and are aromatized

TABLE 27-3

Cardiovascular Events Reported in Trials of Adjuvant Aromatase Inhibitors

Events (%)	Placebo	Tam	Ana	Let	Exem
ATAC					
Ischemic, cardiac		3.4	4.1		
Ischemic, CNS		2.8	2.0		
Thromboembolism		4.5	2.8		
BIG 1-98					
Ischemic, cardiac		1.2		1.4	
Ischemic, CNS		1.0		1.0	
Thromboembolism		3.5		1.5	
CHF		0.4		0.8	
ARNO/ABCSG					
Ischemic, cardiac		<1.0	<1.0		
Thromboembolism		<1.0	<1.0		
IES					
Cardiovascular		39.0*			42.0*
Thromboembolism		2.4			1.3
MA.17					
Ischemic, cardiac	2.1			1.5	
Ischemic, CNS	0.6			0.7	
Thromboembolism	0.2			0.4	

*Stratification by grade not reported.

CHF, congestive heart failure; CNS, central nervous system.

Trials: ATAC, Anastrozole, Tamoxifen Alone or in Combination; IES, Intergroup Exemestane Study; ABCSG/ARNO, Austrian Breast Cancer and Colorectal Cancer Study Group/Arimidex-Nolvadex; ITA, Italian Tamoxifen Anastrozole.

Drugs: Ana, anastrozole; Tam, tamoxifen; Let, letrozole; Exem, exemestane.

to estrogens in peripheral tissues or in the breast cancer itself. Accordingly, partial estrogen deprivation involves surgical or medical oophorectomy and complete deprivation consists of addition of either tamoxifen or an aromatase inhibitor to the oophorectomy regimen. A major focus

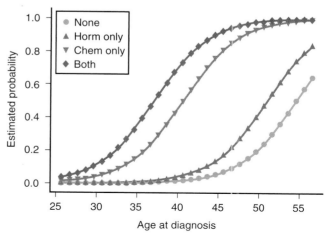

Figure 27-14. Cumulative frequency analysis of development of amenorrhea as a function of age in response to chemotherapy, hormonal therapy, or both in women with breast cancer in comparison with no treatment. The effect of chemotherapy on ovarian function reduces the age of menopause by an average of nearly 20 years. (Taken from the data of Goodwin PJ, Ennis M, Pritchard KI, et al. Risk of menopause during the first year after breast cancer diagnosis. J Clin Oncol 17[8]:2365-2370, 1999.)

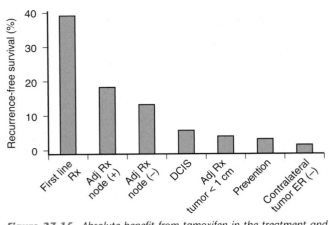

Figure 27-15. *Absolute benefit from tamoxifen in the treatment and prevention setting. Absolute benefit is defined as the number of women per 100 who will benefit from the use of tamoxifen. In the adjuvant or treatment settings, tamoxifen was used for a period of 5 years. DCIS, ductal carcinoma in situ; ER, estrogen receptor. (From Santen R. Endocrine-response cancer. In Kronenberg HM, Melmed S, Polonsky KS, Larsen PR eds). Williams Textbook of Endocrinology, 11th ed. Philadelphia, WB Saunders, 2008, Fig. 42-13.)*

of investigation currently is to determine if complete estrogen deprivation is superior to partial deprivation and if aromatase inhibitors are superior to tamoxifen to produce complete estrogen deprivation.

HORMONAL THERAPIES FOR BREAST CANCER: OVERVIEW OF CLINICAL EFFICACY

Background

Nearly all patients with breast cancer undergo lumpectomy or mastectomy and, if warranted, radiotherapy. Most patients then receive adjuvant therapy to destroy occult cancer cells at local-regional and distant metastatic sites. Upon tumor recurrence, first-, second-, and third-line hormonal or chemotherapies are then utilized in sequence for advanced disease. A recently introduced approach, called neoadjuvant hormonal therapy, involves use of hormonal therapy for 3 to 4 months prior to surgery for patients with large tumors.[142] The goal is to reduce the size of the lesion so as to make lumpectomy a feasible alternative to mastectomy.

Selective Estrogen Receptor Modulators

Tamoxifen was the first anti-estrogen approved for treatment of breast cancer. Until recently, the overall benefit of tamoxifen was usually reported as the relative improvement in frequency of defined events such as tumor recurrence or survival. In the neoadjuvant, adjuvant, and advanced disease settings, tamoxifen results in a *relative benefit* of approximately 50%. However, a more useful parameter, the absolute benefit rate, has now been widely accepted. The absolute benefit rate is defined as the number of women per 100 women treated who benefit from taking tamoxifen. As illustrated in Figure 27-15, the absolute benefit increases as the event becomes more common, even though the relative percentage benefit remains

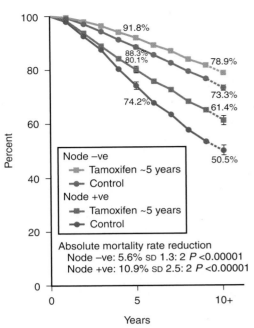

Figure 27-16. *Disease specific survival rate (percentage) in women receiving tamoxifen or placebo as adjuvant therapy for node negative (–ve) or node positive (+ve) disease. (Data taken from Early Breast Cancer Trialists' Collaborative Group. Tamoxifen for early breast cancer: an overview of the randomized trials. Lancet 351[9114]:1451-1467, 1998.)*

approximately 50%. The effects of tamoxifen on disease-specific survival rate can also be expressed as an absolute benefit rate, which is shown on Figure 27-16.

Adjuvant Therapy. When tamoxifen is used as adjuvant therapy, pre- or postmenopausal women with positive lymph nodes at the time of diagnosis experience approximately a 10.9% absolute increase of recurrence-free survival at 5 years, and for those with negative nodes, the rate is 5.6%[143] (see Fig. 27-16). Tamoxifen causes an absolute reduction of contralateral breast cancers of 1% to 5% at 5 years depending upon underlying risk factors. Tamoxifen is active in both pre- and postmenopausal women with breast cancer but only in those whose tumors are ER+ or PR+. The optimal duration of use is 5 years. Direct comparative studies indicate superiority of 5 years versus 1 or 2 years of tamoxifen therapy, whereas 10 years of therapy provides no additional benefit over 5 years.[144] In two studies, tamoxifen for 10 years, as opposed to 5 years, slightly reduced disease-free and overall survival rates.[145,146] This finding may perhaps be explained by tumor adaptation and emergence of a predominant estrogen agonistic effect of tamoxifen, as initially suggested in animal studies.[147] Although tamoxifen is only administered for 5 years, benefit persists for the long term ("carry over effect") because disease-specific survival rate increases from approximately 6% at 5 years to 10% at 10 years in node-positive patients.[143] In premenopausal women, tamoxifen is used as the preferred hormonal agent either alone in low-risk patients or after chemotherapy in those at high risk. In postmenopausal women, the role of tamoxifen is undergoing reconsideration in light of the greater efficacy of aromatase inhibitors in this setting.[148]

Advanced Disease. Approximately 40% of women with advanced disease benefit from tamoxifen. Responses last 12 to 18 months on average before relapse.[98] Efficacy is limited to those with ER+ or PR+ tumors.[143] The presence of *HER2/neu* appears to be associated with a decreased response to tamoxifen.[121,149] One large study (ATAC) also suggested that ER+/PR− tumors also respond less well to tamoxifen, but a similar trial (BIG-FEMTA) did not confirm this observation.[87,88] Central laboratory analysis of receptors in a subset of the ATAC study patients also failed to confirm the original observation.[150] Women with disease in soft tissue, bone, or viscera are the best candidates for tamoxifen, whereas chemotherapy is indicated when extensive liver metastases, brain metastases, or lymphangitic spread to lung is present.[98] The other SERM, toremifene, appears to exert clinical effects similar to those of tamoxifen.

Pure Antagonistic Anti-estrogens

Fulvestrant is an agent that exhibits primarily anti-estrogenic effects and acts both by down-regulating the ER molecule itself and by interfering with estradiol-induced transcription. A comparative study in 458 women with advanced disease demonstrated similar efficacy in patients treated with fulvestrant as with the aromatase inhibitor anastrozole in patients progressing after prior endocrine treatment. Clinical benefit (i.e., complete objective response, partial objective response, and stable disease for 6 months) occurred in 44.5% receiving fulvestrant versus 45% receiving the AI anastrozole. Another study compared tamoxifen with fulvestrant as first-line therapy of advanced breast cancer and found similar efficacy with respect to all parameters examined.[151] Finally, patients initially treated with fulvestrant and relapsing continue to maintain responsiveness to aromatase inhibitors or to tamoxifen. Based upon these data, the appropriate role of fulvestrant in the clinical armamentarium remains to be fully defined.

Aromatase Inhibitors

Only postmenopausal patients benefit from aromatase inhibitors because interruption of estradiol-negative feedback results in override of aromatase blockade in premenopausal women. Until recently, tamoxifen was considered the preferred agent for the initial treatment of breast cancer in both the adjuvant and advanced disease settings. However, the third-generation aromatase inhibitors (AIs) anastrozole, letrozole, and exemestane have now been proved superior to tamoxifen in direct head-to-head trials.[87,88]

Advanced Disease. Five large, multicenter, multinational, randomized trials directly compared the AIs with tamoxifen (Fig. 27-17).[152-158] All followed similar trial designs and included postmenopausal patients with locally advanced or metastatic breast cancer. No women had received adjuvant tamoxifen within 12 months and

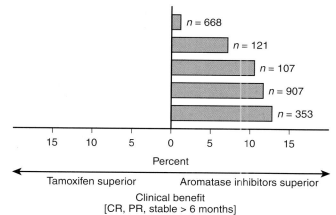

Figure 27-17. *Comparison of tamoxifen versus aromatase inhibitors in five randomized, controlled studies in advanced disease. CR, complete objective tumor regression; PR, partial objective tumor regression. (Data taken from Bonneterre J, Thurlimann B, Robertson JF, et al. Anastrozole versus tamoxifen as first-line therapy for advanced breast cancer in 668 postmenopausal women: results of the Tamoxifen or Arimidex Randomized Group Efficacy and Tolerability study [see comment]. J Clin Oncol 18[22]:3748-3757, 2000; Nabholtz JM, Buzdar A, Pollak M, et al. Anastrozole is superior to tamoxifen as first-line therapy for advanced breast cancer in postmenopausal women: results of a North American multicenter randomized trial. Arimidex Study Group [see comment]. J Clin Oncol 18[22]:3758-3767, 2000; Mouridsen H, Gershanovich M, Sun Y, et al. Phase III study of letrozole versus tamoxifen as first-line therapy of advanced breast cancer in postmenopausal women: analysis of survival and update of efficacy from the International Letrozole Breast Cancer Group [see comment]. J Clin Oncol 21[11]:2101-2109, 2003; Milla-Santos A, Milla L, Portella J, et al. Anastrozole versus tamoxifen as first-line therapy in postmenopausal patients with hormone-dependent advanced breast cancer: a prospective, randomized, phase III study. Am J Clin Oncol 26[3]:317-322, 2003; Mouridsen H, Gershanovich M, Sun Y, et al. Superior efficacy of letrozole versus tamoxifen as first-line therapy for postmenopausal women with advanced breast cancer: results of a phase III study of the International Letrozole Breast Cancer Group [see comment] [erratum appears in J Clin Oncol 19[13]:3302, 2001]. J Clin Oncol 19[10]:2596-2606, 2001; and Smith R, Sun Y, Barin A, et al. Femara showed significant improvement in efficacy over tamoxifen as first line treatment in postmenopausal women with advanced breast cancer. Proceedings of the 23d Annual San Antonio Breast Cancer Symposium. Breast Cancer Res Treat 64:27, 2000.)*

none were known to be ER−. All trials demonstrated the superiority of the AIs in clinical efficacy with incremental responses ranging from 2% to 13% (see Fig. 27-17). The differences were statistically significant in all but one trial in which the receptor status was unknown in 55% of patients.[152]

Pooled data indicate that tamoxifen was associated with DVT and pulmonary emboli (7.6% versus 4.5%) significantly more frequently than the AI anastrozole.[156,158,159] If one combines observations from all trials, it appears that nausea, hot flashes, and gastrointestinal distress were comparable with tamoxifen or an AI. Comparisons of aromatase inhibitors with placebo (or with tamoxifen) reveal an increase in hot flashes, arthritis, osteoporosis, arthralgia, and myalgia with aromatase inhibitors. Surprisingly, women receiving placebo or tamoxifen also experience these same side effects quite commonly (Table 27-4).

Taken together, these trials provide evidence that the third-generation aromatase inhibitors are superior in efficacy and toxicity to tamoxifen in the advanced disease

TABLE 27-4

Side Effects from Aromatase Inhibitors versus Tamoxifen or Placebo

Side Effect	Exemestane (%)	Letrozole (%)	Placebo		Tamoxifen	
			Percentage	*Probability*	*Percentage*	*Probability*
Arthralgia	5.4	21.3	16.6	$P < 0.001$	3.6	$P = 0.01$
Arthritis	—	5.6	3.5	$P < 0.001$	—	—
Hot flushes	42	47.2	40.5	$P < 0.001$	39.6	$P = 0.28$
Myalgia	—	11.8	9.5	$P = 0.02$	—	—
Osteoporosis	7.4	5.8	4.5	$P = 0.07$	5.7	$P = 0.05$

From Santen R. Endocrine-response cancer. *In* Kronenberg HM, Melmed S, Polonsky KS, Larsen PR (eds). Williams Textbook of Endocrinology, 11th ed. Philadelphia, WB Saunders, 2008, Table 42-2.

setting. Letrozole, anastrozole, and exemestane have now been approved in the United States and Europe as first-line therapy for advanced breast cancer. It should be noted that these trials showed for the first time that one endocrine therapy could be superior to another. Prior to these studies, dogma held that each available endocrine therapy produced similar rates of response and could be distinguished only on the basis of side effects and cost.

Comprehensive, direct head-to-head comparisons of the three approved AIs—letrozole anastrozole, and exemestane—are now needed to determine if one agent is superior to the other. This is particularly important because hormonal data suggest that letrozole may be more potent as an aromatase inhibitor than anastrozole.[160] At the present time, only one such direct comparison is available in which anastrozole and letrozole were used in 713 women with advanced breast cancer. Letrozole was superior with respect to objective response rate (19.1% versus 12.3%, $P = 0.013$), but no differences in time to progression, time to treatment failure, or duration of response were observed. Additional studies are considered necessary before clinical decisions can be made regarding equivalency or superiority of one agent over the other .

The choice of aromatase inhibitors over tamoxifen as first-line therapy for advanced disease at the present time is considered reasonable[148] but based upon incomplete data. Prior comparisons of tamoxifen with the first-generation aromatase inhibitor aminoglutethimide demonstrated equal efficacy but a different pattern of cross resistance.[98] The aromatase inhibitors were efficacious if used after tamoxifen, but tamoxifen appeared less effective when used after the aromatase inhibitors. If this were true for the third-generation aromatase inhibitors, tamoxifen might remain as the first-line agent. However, preliminary data suggest that tamoxifen is effective after crossover from the aromatase inhibitor anastrozole. In a crossover comparison, 48.7% of 119 patients experienced clinical benefit from tamoxifen when used as a second-line agent after initial use of letrozole. By comparison, second-line letrozole following initial tamoxifen produced clinical benefit in 56.8% of 95 patients.[161] The issue of choosing the proper sequence between the AIs and tamoxifen is currently being tested in a four-arm study, the BIG-FEMTA trial.

Adjuvant Therapy. Aromatase inhibitors provide a means to block estrogen effectively without the emergence of estrogen agonistic effects in the adjuvant setting. On the other hand, detrimental effects could result from deprivation of estradiol on vaginal mucosa, bone density, and cholesterol levels. A summary of the clinical efficacy of AIs versus tamoxifen and their relative safety profiles are shown in Table 27-5. Two similar large trials, the ATAC (Anastrazole and Tamoxifen Alone and in Combination) and the BIG-FEMTA trial, compared the effects of either agent on time to progression of disease, time to treatment failure, and overall survival.[87,88] At 5 years of follow-up, both trials demonstrated an absolute superiority of the AI of approximately 3% (Figs. 27-18 and 27-19). The results from exemestane were similar.[162] In one study, the aromatase inhibitor increased overall survival in a subset of women with positive nodes.[163] A meta-analysis also demonstrated and increase in overall survival.[164] In this setting, tamoxifen caused an increase in endometrial cancer and in veno-thrombotic episodes (VTEs). AIs were associated with accelerated bone loss, symptoms of urogenital atrophy, and arthralgias. Cholesterol levels appear slightly higher in women receiving AIs rather than tamoxifen, but this increase may be partially due to the low-density lipoprotein (LDL) cholesterol-lowering properties of tamoxifen AI[88,137] (see Tables 27-3 to 27-5). On the basis of these data, the AIs have now been approved in the United States for use in the adjuvant setting. Published guidelines still suggest initial use of tamoxifen unless patients are at risk of VTEs.[112,148] Use of an AI should be also considered in patients with *HER2/neu* or ER+/PR– tumors (who in one trial appeared to respond less well to tamoxifen[87]) or in high-risk patients.

Recent data suggest a hypothesis explaining why the AIs might be superior to tamoxifen. The enzyme, cytochrome P450 2D6 (CYP 2D6) is required to convert tamoxifen to its active metabolite, endoxifen. Six percent to 8% of women taking tamoxifen harbor relatively inactive alleles of this enzyme and selective serotonin reuptake inhibitors (SSRIs) (or selective serotonin-norepinephrine reuptake inhibitors, SNRIs) such as paroxetine, fluoxetene, sertraline, and citalopram can inhibit CYP 2D6. Individuals with reduced activity of CYP 2D6 on a genetic or drug/drug interaction basis exhibit lower plasma levels of endoxifen. In a large recent study, women with defective CYP 2D6 experienced a shortened disease-free and overall survival compared to those with normal function.[165] Accordingly, the lack of activating metabolism of tamoxifen to endoxifen may at least partially explain the inferiority of tamoxifen to the AIs.[166]

TABLE 27-5

Efficacy of Aromatase Inhibitors in Substitution and Sequential Regimens in the Adjuvant Setting—Risk Reduction in Disease-Free Survival Event Rate

Treatment Strategy	Trial	Trial Protocol	Follow-up (months)	Relative Risk Reduction (%)	Absolute Risk Reduction (%[Time from Randomization in Years])
Substitution	ATAC	Ana vs. Tam	68	13	3.3
	BIG 1-98	Let vs. Tam	25.8	19	2.6
Sequential (switch)	IES	Tam → Exem vs. Tam	31	32	4.7
	ABCSG/ARNO*	Tam → Ana vs. Tam	28	40	3.1
	ITA	Tam → Ana vs. Tam	36	65	5.8
Extended adjuvant	MA-17	Tam → Let vs. Tam → Placebo	30	42	4.6

*Event-free survival.

Trials: ATAC, Anastrozole, Tamoxifen Alone or in Combination; IES, Intergroup Exemestane Study; ABCSG/ARNO, Austrian Breast Cancer and Colorectal Cancer Study Group/Arimidex-Nolvadex; ITA, Italian Tamoxifen Anastrozole; MA-17, MA-17 trial of the NCI of Canada Clinical Trial Group.

Drugs: Ana, anastrozole; Tam, tamoxifen; Let, letrozole; Exem, exemestane.

Several studies are currently comparing the sequential use of AIs after initial adjuvant therapy with tamoxifen (see Table 27-5). The MA-17 trial compared placebo to letrozole in women who had received tamoxifen for 5 years (Fig. 27-20).[91] The results demonstrate a 35% greater relative reduction in new events and an absolute reduction of 4% in women receiving the AI. Overall survival was improved only in the node-positive group. As shown in Table 27-4, the AI was associated with an increase in hot flashes, bone loss, and arthralgias. The increase in arthralgias attributable to the AI was less than expected because of the high rate in the placebo group (i.e., 16.6% placebo, 21.3% letrozole). The IES study (International Exemestane Study) compared the effect of 5 years of tamoxifen with 2 to 3 years of tamoxifen with crossover to exemestane at 2 to 3 years (Fig. 27-21).[90] This study also showed a reduction in new cancer events in the AI compared to the tamoxifen group. The ABCSG/ARNO trial was similar but used anastrozole rather than exemestane. Switch to the AI resulted in a 3% improvement in event-free survival.[167]

These crossover data demonstrate that women with breast cancer can experience additional benefit by the sequential addition of an AI after tamoxifen. Based upon these three studies, the American Society of Clinical Oncology (ASCO) guidelines recommend that appropriate therapy is now to use an AI somewhere in the course of adjuvant therapy.[148]

Hormone Additive Therapy

Androgens or estrogens are generally considered inferior to use of tamoxifen and aromatase inhibitors.[98] Until recently, high-dose estrogen had been used sparingly because of the increased side effect profile versus tamoxifen. However, a 20-year follow-up of a randomized comparison of tamoxifen with DES (diethylstilbestrol) reported a significant survival advantage in patients receiving the estrogen and lack of cross-resistance between these two therapeutic approaches.[53] This surprising study suggests reconsideration of use of high-dose estrogen in selected patients.[52]

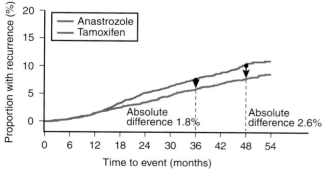

Figure 27-18. *Comparison of tamoxifen with anastrozole in the ATAC trial of breast cancer treatment in the adjuvant setting. (From The ATAC Trialists' Group. Anastrozole alone or in combination with tamoxifen versus tamoxifen alone for adjuvant treatment of postmenopausal women with early breast cancer: first results of the ATAC randomised trial [see comments]. Lancet 359[9324]:2131-2139, 2002.)*

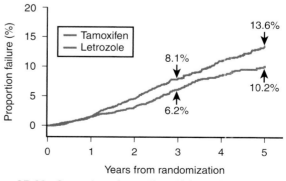

Figure 27-19. *Comparison of tamoxifen with letrozole in the BIG-FEMTA trial of breast cancer treatment in the adjuvant setting. (From Roeberle D, Thuerlimann B. Letrozole as upfront endocrine therapy for postmenopausal hormone-sensitive breast cancer: Pausal hormone-sensitive breast cancer: BIG 1-98. Breast Cancer Res Treat 105(Suppl 1):55-66, 2007.)*

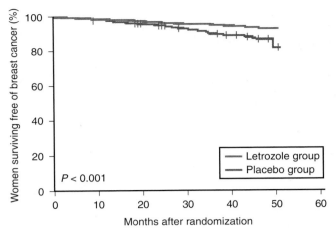

Figure 27-20. *Comparison of placebo with letrozole in patients with breast cancer treated initially with tamoxifen in the adjuvant setting and randomized to receive with therapy after 5 years of tamoxifen. P < 0.001 indicates statistical difference between effects of placebo and aromatase inhibitor. (From Goss PE, Ingle JN, Martino S, et al. A randomized trial of letrozole in postmenopausal women after five years of tamoxifen therapy for early-stage breast cancer [see comment]. N Engl J Med 349[19]:1793-1802, 2003.)*

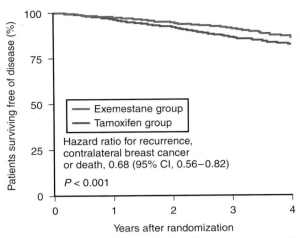

Figure 27-21. *Comparison of tamoxifen with exemestane in patients with breast cancer treated initially with tamoxifen and then randomized to exemestane or continued tamoxifen after 2 to 3 years of tamoxifen. (From Coombes RC, Hall E, Gibson LJ, et al. A randomized trial of exemestane after two to three years of tamoxifen therapy in postmenopausal women with primary breast cancer [see comment] [erratum appears in N Engl J Med 351(23):2461, 2004]. N Engl J Med 350[11]:1081-1092, 2004.)*

A series of preclinical studies demonstrated the likely mechanism for the beneficial effects of estradiol, namely, the stimulation of apoptotic tumor cell death by estrogens.[51,168] A recent review reports a 30% response to use of high-dose estrogen in women refractory to multiple hormonal agents.[52] Clinical trials to assess its place in the therapeutic armamentarium are under way (personal communication from V. C. Jordan and M. Ellis).

Surgical Oophorectomy. Prophylactic oophorectomy represented the first adjuvant endocrine therapy for breast cancer. Although initially thought to be ineffective, recent meta-analyses demonstrate clear benefit with a 6% absolute survival advantage at 15 years for patients younger than 50 years of age who are lymph node negative and a 12.5% survival advantage for node-positive patients (Fig. 27-22). Because receptor status was unknown in patients in these trials, a large fraction of receptor-negative patients was likely included. Accordingly, one would have expected even better results if hormone receptor–positive patients only were so treated. In the advanced disease setting, surgical oophorectomy induces clinical benefit in approximately 50% of ER+ or PR+ patients.[98]

Medical Oophorectomy. Emerging data support the use of GnRH-induced medical oophorectomy (Med OOX) in the adjuvant setting and recent research emphasis has focused upon this strategy.[169] In the opinion of some experts, this approach may soon replace surgical oophorectomy while others believe that laparoscopic oophorectomy may still be a more attractive approach. Demonstration of the effectiveness of prophylactic oophorectomy (see Fig. 27-22) was surprising to the medical community and led to a reconsideration of this approach, albeit with use of GnRH agonists rather than surgery. The goal of these studies was to determine the efficacy of Med OOX in patients who are

exclusively ER+. Two studies in the *advanced* setting indicate that the GnRH analogs produce clinical effects similar to those induced by surgical oophorectomy.[170,171] No data are available to compare Med OOX alone versus no treatment or versus surgical oophorectomy in the adjuvant setting.

Rather than comparing Med OOX to no treatment, studies examined the effects of chemotherapy versus Med OOX in the adjuvant setting. The Zoladex Early Breast Cancer Research Association Study (ZEBRA) demonstrated equivalence of goserelin to standard CMF (cytoxan, methotrexate, 5-fluorouracil) chemotherapy on overall survival

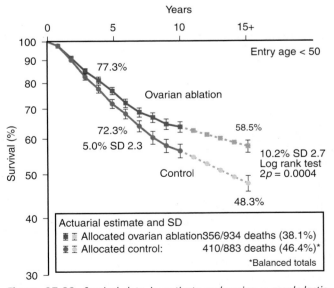

Figure 27-22. *Survival data in patients undergoing a prophylactic oophorectomy in comparison with a group of women not receiving this therapy. (From Santen R. Endocrine-response cancer. In Kronenberg HM, Melmed S, Polonsky KS, Larsen PR [eds]. Williams Textbook of Endocrinology, 11th ed. Philadelphia, WB Saunders, 2008, Fig. 42-18.)*

but only in ER+ patients.[172] This study has been criticized on the basis that CMF is not as effective as anthracycline-based regimens such as FAC (5-fluorouracil, Adriamycin, and Cytoxan) and the latter might be more effective than Med OOX. Tamoxifen can also be considered a form of Med OOX and studies demonstrate similar efficacy of this approach when compared with surgical oophorectomy.

Complete Estrogen Blockade. Recent trials have compared Med OOX alone (partial estrogen deprivation) versus Med OOX plus tamoxifen or an AI in the *advanced* disease setting. Complete estrogen blockade (Med OOX plus tamoxifen) appeared superior to tamoxifen alone in a single large trial and in a meta-analysis of four similar studies.[173] The combined approach resulted in more frequent objective response rates and improved progression-free and overall patient survival. In the adjuvant setting, use of MED OOX plus an AI or tamoxifen is the subject of the ongoing SOFT, TEXT, and PERCHE studies.[112]

Chemical Castration. Chemotherapy generally causes permanent amenorrhea in women over 40 and temporary cessation of menses in younger women (see Fig. 27-14).[138] Studies are ongoing to determine whether chemotherapy exerts some if its actions via suppression of estrogen production in premenopausal women. At least three possibilities for tumor regression exist:

1. Hormonal effects resulting from chemotherapeutic destruction of the ovary
2. Direct cytotoxic effects on the tumor
3. A combination of these two effects

Several trials have compared adjuvant chemotherapy to Med OOX with and without tamoxifen in premenopausal women.[174-176] The chemotherapy and hormonal therapies appear to produce comparable antitumor effects in women with moderate or high levels of estrogen receptor (ZEBRA trial).[174] The International Breast Cancer Study Group (IBCSG) trial VII compared CMF with goserelin as adjuvant therapy in premenopausal women. In those with ER+ tumors, disease-free survival rate was 81% in both groups at 5 years.[177] However, trends suggest that in ER− patents, chemotherapy is more effective than Med OOX.[112,174] These results suggest that at least part of the benefit of chemotherapy in premenopausal women results from "chemical castration."

Further support of the chemotherapy castration hypothesis comes from studies showing that chemotherapy is less effective in patients without complete cessation of menses[178,179] and that addition of Med OOX is this setting provides improved responses.[178] Although effects of varying chemotherapeutic regimens on ovarian function differ, nearly 100% of women over 40 develop permanent amenorrhea following adjuvant chemotherapy (see Fig. 27-14). However, it was recently observed that use of AIs in this setting can induce return of menses, a potentially problematic phenomenon, and careful monitoring according to written guidelines should be followed.[139]

It would appear, then, that in women younger than age 40, addition of medical oophorectomy to chemotherapy would be beneficial. On the other hand, addition of Med OOX to chemotherapy in women older than 40 with ER+ tumors might not be beneficial because chemical castration will be complete. In younger women at high risk of recurrence, chemotherapy followed by hormonal therapy is more efficacious than chemotherapy alone. These and other observations suggest that effects of chemotherapy are partially due to a reduction of hormone secretion and partially to cytotoxic effects.

Use of Hormonal Therapy Alone in Premenopausal Women

Nearly all premenopausal women are treated with chemotherapy in the adjuvant setting and the evidence for this in women in high-risk groups is substantial. However, for patients in the low- or intermediate-risk/endocrine-responsive categories, current data support equivalent efficacy of hormonal therapy and chemotherapy. On this basis, the new St. Gallen guidelines favor the use of hormone therapy without chemotherapy in low- and intermediate-risk/hormone-responsive premenopausal patients[131] (Fig. 27-23A and B).

Use of Chemotherapy Followed by Hormonal Therapy

Based upon the meta-analysis recently published, the combination of surgical or Med OOX (GnRH agonists or tamoxifen) plus chemotherapy provides additional benefit over chemotherapy alone in the adjuvant setting in premenopausal women.[180] The addition of the GnRH agonists might be particularly important for women younger than age 40 in whom estradiol remained in the premenopausal range after chemotherapy, as suggested by a recent trial.[169,181] In postmenopausal women, addition of tamoxifen after six courses of CAF chemotherapy improved disease-free survival compared to tamoxifen alone,[182] but the chemotherapy provided little benefit in the subgroup with very high ER levels.[183] Recent data indicate that chemotherapy should be given first, followed by endocrine therapy later to allow maximal effectiveness of the chemotherapy.

Use of Chemotherapy Followed by Complete Estrogen Deprivation

Ongoing studies are addressing two questions. The first is whether chemotherapy followed by complete ovarian deprivation is superior to chemotherapy followed by partial ovarian deprivation. Davidson et al showed the superiority of CAF (cytoxan, Adriamycin [doxorubicin], fluorouracil) followed by Med OOX plus tamoxifen versus CAF alone or CAF plus Med OOX.[169] The complete estrogen blockade strategy (Med OOX plus tamoxifen) improved time to treatment failure and disease-free survival but not overall survival when compared to Med OOX without tamoxifen. One component of the SOFT trial is also addressing this point by comparing tamoxifen alone versus medical oophorectomy plus tamoxifen, versus medical oophorectomy plus an AI in patients who had received standard chemotherapy.[174]

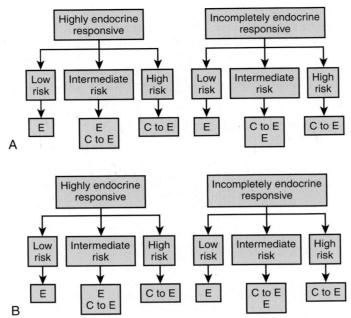

Figure 27-23. *Decision-making algorithm for breast cancer. The approach to adjuvant hormonal therapy in premenopausal (**A**) and postmenopausal (**B**) women is illustrated here. This is adapted from the published guidelines from the 2007 St. Gallen Conference on treatment of early breast cancer and divides women into highly endocrine responsive and endocrine response uncertain categories as well as low, intermediate, and high risk. Tamoxifen (Tam) is considered the preferred endocrine therapy based upon level I evidence. Medical oophorectomy (Med OOX) is preferred if tamoxifen is contraindicated. Sequences using combinations of tamoxifen and Med OOX or Med OOX plus an aromatase inhibitor (AI) are currently undergoing study and are considered acceptable alternatives. Chemotherapy (C) is often recommended prior to endocrine therapy (E), and the various types of chemotherapy are outlined in the National Comprehensive Cancer Network guidelines. The sequence of therapies for advanced disease in women still considered to be anti-estrogen responsive (see text) is shown. This algorithm is applicable for patients who have never received an anti-estrogen or who have taken this therapy but have been off for at least 1 year. In patients thought to have very aggressive disease, chemotherapy may be chosen prior to hormonal therapy. The only currently available selective estrogen receptor down-regulator (SERD) is fulvestrant. Note: Herceptin (trastuzumab) should be added in patients who are HER2-positive. Endocrine therapy is effective for prevention and ductal carcinoma in situ and therefore might be considered even for very low risk invasive breast cancer.*

The second question addresses whether AIs are superior to tamoxifen for complete ovarian deprivation when given following chemotherapy and Med OOX. The TEXT Trial is addressing this issue by comparing Med OOX plus tamoxifen with Med OOX plus exemestane. Finally, to determine if chemotherapy is required at all when using complete estrogen deprivation, the PERCHE study will compare a chemotherapy/complete estrogen deprivation arm with one using only complete estrogen deprivation. Complete analyses of these various approaches and trials are beyond the scope of this review and can be found in a recent review.[174,184] Very young patients with cancer have a worse prognosis than older premenopausal women. The ongoing trials (SOFT, TEXT, PERCHE) which examine the individual roles of Med OOX, an AI, chemotherapy, and the combination of these agents should provide information regarding this subset of patients.

Emerging Therapies

Neoadjuvant therapy represents the use of an antitumor agent prior to surgery in an attempt to shrink the tumor sufficiently to allow lumpectomy rather than mastectomy.[142] The concept of neoadjuvant chemotherapy has been adopted into clinical practice, whereas neoadjuvant hormonal therapy is now undergoing clinical trial.

A nonrandomized trial demonstrated an 81% reduction on tumor volume with letrozole versus 75% with anastrozole and 48% with tamoxifen.[185] More recently, a randomized trial involving 324 patients compared letrozole 2.5 mg daily with tamoxifen 20 mg daily in women with ER+ tumors larger than 2 cm.[186] Letrozole caused a 55% rate of objective response (complete objective tumor response [CR] and partial objective tumor response [PR]) versus 36% for tamoxifen (P < 0.001). Breast-conserving surgery was chosen in 45% of patients receiving letrozole and 35% receiving tamoxifen (P < 0.001). Approximately 50% of women had a sufficient reduction in size of tumor to allow lumpectomy. Of interest is the fact that *HER2/neu*-positive tumors responded better to the AI (i.e., 88% response) than to tamoxifen (i.e., 21%).[121]

A similar trial (IMPACT) confirmed the greater ability to perform lumpectomy in women receiving the AI (46% versus 22%, P = 0.03), but objective tumor responses in the AI and tamoxifen arms were similar.[187] Current guidelines consider neoadjuvant endocrine therapy still to be experimental, but this approach is becoming more widely used with emergence of these two studies. Nonetheless, comparison of groups of patients treated conventionally and with neoadjuvant endocrine therapy with analysis of survival will be required to confirm the major utility of this approach.

Responses to neoadjuvant therapy might provide predictive information regarding long-term hormonal responsiveness or even overall survival. Emerging evidence suggests that a reduction of the Ki67 proliferation index might provide the best parameter to predict long-term outcome, whereas apoptotic indices appear not to be informative.[188] cDNA array changes might also provide useful predictive information, but verification of this possibility requires additional study.[189]

Preclinical data suggest that tumors exposed to tamoxifen or to aromatase inhibitors adapt by up-regulating growth factor pathways. A compelling hypothesis is to administer growth factor pathway inhibitors concomitantly with endocrine therapies to inhibit the development of resistance. Several studies in xenograft models have proved the principle that this strategy can work and several clinical trials of this concept are under way. Use of the monoclonal antibody against *HER2/neu* (trastuzumab) in combination with or after adjuvant chemotherapy in women with breast cancer has been highly successful in delaying recurrence and perhaps implementing cure.[190] Pertinent studies included women with estrogen receptor-positive tumors. The tandem study examined the efficacy of adding trastuzumab (Herceptin) to an aromatase inhibitor.[191] Although the clinical benefit was increased from 27.9% to 42.9% with addition of Herceptin, it is not clear whether all of the added benefit was from Herceptin alone.

RECOMMENDED APPROACHES TO HORMONAL TREATMENT OF BREAST CANCER

Several highly specific guidelines base recommendations on nine subgroups of patients categorized as to low-, intermediate-, and high-risk prognostic categories and highly endocrine responsive, incompletely endocrine responsive, and endocrine nonresponsive[112] (see Fig. 27-23A and B). Level I evidence supports the use of tamoxifen as adjuvant hormonal therapy for both pre- and postmenopausal women. Med OOX provides an acceptable alternative for premenopausal women in whom tamoxifen is contraindicated. Conclusive data regarding the superior efficacy of complete estrogen deprivation with Med OOX plus tamoxifen or an AI are lacking and the subject of ongoing study. Nonetheless, the St. Gallen Panel accepted the concept of complete estrogen suppression as reasonable for very young patients, especially in the intermediate- and high-risk groups. This approach was also considered appropriate alternative therapy for premenopausal women at any age at high risk, especially if chemotherapy did not induce complete ovarian failure. The Panel did not recommend GnRH analogs plus aromatase inhibitors outside clinical trials. The St. Gallen Guidelines are more specific than those of the National Comprehensive Cancer Center Network, but in general the two sets of guidelines do not substantially conflict.[131]

Adjuvant Therapy

Premenopausal Women. Current opinion recommends initial chemotherapy for most premenopausal women with ER+ tumors greater than 1 cm in diameter followed by the addition of tamoxifen for 5 years after completion of chemotherapy (see Fig. 27-23A). Those considered to have low-risk disease may benefit from tamoxifen alone. Evidence regarding combined therapy comes from a recent meta-analysis that demonstrated statistically significant prolongation of survival with a combination of tamoxifen plus chemotherapy versus chemotherapy alone.[180] Clinical data have established that the chemotherapy must be given first and completed before initiating tamoxifen. Med OOX with tamoxifen could be considered as an alternative for women averse to chemotherapy, particularly those at low risk of recurrence and with a high level of ER.[112] The use of Med OOX and an AI is suggested only if tamoxifen is contraindicated.

Current recommendations suggest tamoxifen after chemotherapy but Med OOX in combination with an AI may later be proved to be superior to tamoxifen alone in young women with aggressive disease. It should be noted that this is the subject of the ongoing studies in the TEXT and PERCHE trials.[174] Some women who develop amenorrhea after chemotherapy may be candidates for aromatase inhibitors. However, Med OOX is considered necessary in women under 40 years old whose amenorrhea may only be temporary following chemotherapy and in women over 40 with return of menses.[139] The use of aromatase inhibitors in women over 40 who are rendered amenorrheic after chemotherapy may pose an unexpected problem regarding return of menses. This clinical scenario is being encountered by oncologists and requires hormonal monitoring.[139] By interrupting estradiol-negative feedback, the AI might trigger return of ovulation and overcome the AI effects.

Postmenopausal Women. Tamoxifen is the preferred initial adjuvant therapy for postmenopausal women with ER+ or PR+ tumors larger than 1 cm unless there are contraindications. If the tumor is *HER2/neu*-positive or ER+/PR−[112] or the patient has a propensity for thromboembolism, an AI would generally be considered preferable according to recent guidelines. Crossover to an AI after either 2 to 3 years or 5 years of tamoxifen is now recommended in responding patients.[148,180] Several trials have now shown that crossover to an AI after 2 to 5 years of tamoxifen results in prolongation of disease-free survival[90,91,192] (see Fig. 27-17A and B). Only in the MA-17 trial was overall survival improved and this occurred only in the node-positive subgroup.[163] It is likely that a longer time of follow-up will be necessary to demonstrate a potential survival advantage for the AIs in this setting. In women considered to have aggressive disease, particularly those who are younger, chemotherapy followed by tamoxifen may be chosen.[193,194] Information obtained from meta-analyses suggests that chemotherapy followed by tamoxifen may be preferable to use of tamoxifen alone in postmenopausal women.

Recommendations regarding the initial use of an AI rather than tamoxifen are rapidly evolving. The most recent ASCO guidelines stated that "optimal hormonal therapy for postmenopausal women with ER+ breast cancer should include an AI."[148] An AI should probably be used initially (replacing tamoxifen) based upon preliminary results of the BIG-FEMTA trial.[195] For patients at low risk of relapse or with co-morbidity raising concern about the safety of an AI, adjuvant tamoxifen alone remains a reasonable alternative and may be the only economically viable option in many situations.

The major problems with the AIs in the extended adjuvant setting may be an increased risk of cardiovascular and cerebrovascular events, although this has not yet been shown to be statistically significant in randomized trials.[137] An increased rate of fracture has been demonstrated, but this can be compensated for by concomitant use of a bisphosphonate.[136] Quality of life issues may be deleterious in the AI-treated patients with respect to an increase in arthralgia, vaginal dryness, dyspareunia, decreased libido, and an increase in hot flashes. On the other hand, the major problems with tamoxifen are the increased risk of VTEs and the increased incidence of endometrial carcinoma.

Small Tumors in Pre- and Postmenopausal Women

No randomized trial has examined use of tamoxifen in women with tumors of 1 cm or less. However, pooled data from four NSABP[193] trials indicates a 4% absolute benefit regarding disease-free recurrence and 5% survival benefit for this group of women when given tamoxifen. Individual decisions are made based upon risk/benefit analysis and not all women are offered this therapy. With availability of the Oncotype DX test, one can stratify risk and offer tamoxifen to those at high or intermediate risk of recurrence but use of this test is not yet widely accepted.[131]

Ductal Carcinoma in Situ

Tamoxifen appears to provide benefit for ER+ women with DCIS.[196] In a large NSABP clinical trial, 13% of women treated with lumpectomy, irradiation, and placebo experienced a new tumor event over 5 years.[196] One third of these new events involved appearance of a contralateral breast cancer; one third a new ipsilateral tumor, and one third local recurrence of the original tumor. Tamoxifen reduced these events in absolute terms by 5% with equal benefit in reducing new contralateral, ipsilateral, and original tumor events. A later post hoc analysis reported that only women with ER+ tumors benefited from this approach.[197] Risk benefit analysis regarding tamoxifen is required to advise patients appropriately.

Decision Making

An overview of these data suggests that all women with ER+ or PR+ tumors are potential candidates for tamoxifen as adjuvant therapy. In postmenopausal women, an aromatase inhibitor can be considered initially.[195] In order to guide informed decision making, one must determine whether the benefits of tamoxifen outweigh the risks in individual patients. From the NSABP prevention trial, the absolute risks of tamoxifen are known and include uterine cancer, cataracts, DVT, pulmonary emboli, and CVA.[77] Presence of a uterus, past history of DVT or pulmonary embolus, or existent cataract would enhance these risks. Presence of larger or invasive tumors would enhance the absolute benefits of tamoxifen. In general, most women

with invasive tumors larger than 1 cm should be advised to take tamoxifen or an aromatase inhibitor. Those with small or noninvasive tumors should be counseled based upon risk/benefit ratios. Those without prior history of thromboembolic event or cataract and with prior hysterectomy might be advised to take tamoxifen, particularly if they also have osteopenia. Raloxifene has not been used in the adjuvant setting and would not be advised for the patients discussed here.

With the demonstrated superiority of the AIs in postmenopausal women in this setting, the risks and benefits of these agents versus tamoxifen should be considered. Regarding the AIs, risk of development of osteoporosis and heart disease should be weighed against the risks associated with tamoxifen. Based upon current guidelines, all postmenopausal women with lesions over 1 cm should receive an AI at some point in the adjuvant treatment sequence.

TREATMENT OF ADVANCED DISEASE

The majority of women who develop advanced disease had previously received tamoxifen as adjuvant therapy. Those experiencing tumor recurrence while receiving tamoxifen or within 1 year of its cessation are considered resistant to this anti-estrogen. For them, other hormonal therapies are chosen. The women whose tumors recur more than 1 year after stopping tamoxifen are candidates for an additional course of tamoxifen. An algorithm can then be used to choose hormonal therapy in women considered candidates for tamoxifen (Fig. 27-24). In those resistant to tamoxifen, the next therapy in the sequential approach can be utilized.

Premenopausal Women

Initial therapy would usually consist of a course of chemotherapy followed by hormonal therapy. However, this trend may be changing for low-risk, hormonally responsive patients in whom endocrine therapy alone may be chosen. It should be emphasized that aromatase inhibitors do not effectively inhibit ovarian estrogen production in premenopausal women who have not experienced amenorrhea from chemotherapy. In those women under 40 with chemotherapy-induced amenorrhea, tamoxifen (or toremifene) is usually considered first-line therapy for recurrent tumors. Based upon current data, this might be combined with a GnRH analog to induce a Med OOX in high-risk patients. If the initial therapy is tamoxifen alone, Med OOX with use of a GnRH agonist analog as second-line therapy would be recommended. Surgical oophorectomy could be substituted for the GnRH analog.[112] Ovarian ablation with radiation is not recommended (see St. Gallen 2007 Guidelines[131]). Aromatase inhibitors could then be used if the GnRH analog is continued. Megestrol acetate is then advised as additional therapy.

Postmenopausal Women

Data from trials comparing aromatase inhibitors with tamoxifen as first-line therapy for advanced disease suggest that aromatase inhibitors be considered the first

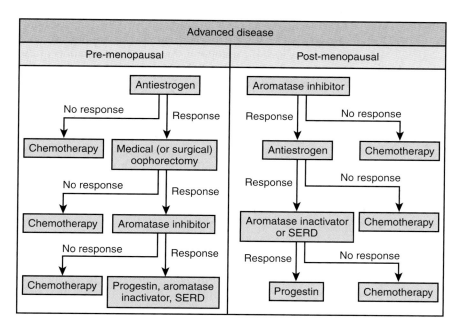

Figure 27-24. Decision algorithm for women with advanced breast cancer. SERD, selective estrogen receptor down-regulator.

choice of endocrine therapy.[152,157,159,198] Responders would then be treated with tamoxifen as second-line therapy upon relapse but nonresponders would receive chemotherapy. Third-line therapy would utilize meges-trol acetate and fourth line, the aromatase inactivator, exemestane. After this, high-dose estrogen or androgens might be chosen. The use of the pure anti-estrogen ful-vestrant could be substituted for tamoxifen. If the patient develops rapidly progressive disease at any time in this sequence, chemotherapy may be chosen instead of the next endocrine therapy.

Chemotherapy

Discussion of the current choices of chemotherapy is beyond the scope of this chapter. The interested reader is referred to the book on management of breast diseases by Lippman et al.[199]

Long-Term Quality of Life in Breast Cancer Survivors

With earlier diagnosis of breast cancer, an increasing percentage of women survive breast cancer in the long term. Two thirds of these women are menopausal at the time of diagnosis and half of the premenopausal women undergo permanent ovarian failure as a result of chemotherapy. Menopausal hormone therapy (MHT) is generally thought to be contraindicated in these women because estrogens may cause regrowth of residual tumor tissue after surgery or cause a second primary tumor.[200] Data from *observational* studies, however, do not provide evidence of a deleterious effect. *Prospective* studies of the safety of MHT in this setting are conflicting: the HABITS trial[201] reports an increase in risk of recurrent breast cancer with MHT whereas the Stockholm trial does not.[202] The differences in

results may relate to the increased use of tamoxifen (51%) in the Stockholm trial versus the HABITS trial (22%), but this conclusion requires experimental confirmation. Until this issue is more definitively resolved, it is prudent to avoid estrogens in breast cancer survivors if alternatives to estrogen are effective.[200]

As reviewed previously, effective agents are available to substitute for estrogen. These include bisphosphonates to prevent or treat osteoporosis, statins to prevent heart disease, venlafaxine (see earlier discussion regarding CYP 2D6 and tamoxifen) and gabapentin[203-205] to diminish the number and severity of hot flashes, vaginal moisturizers and lubricants without estrogen for symptoms of urogenital atrophy, and SSRIs for depression thought to be related to estrogen deficiency. This approach does not protect against Alzheimer's disease or improve cognitive function, but the recent WHI study demonstrated that MHT increased rather than decreased the risk of dementia.[206] Low-dose vaginal estrogens should only be used with caution and informed consent of the patient because of systemic absorption.[207] If alternatives to estrogen are not satisfactory, women might choose to receive MHT after a full discussion of the risks and benefits and with informed consent.

Breast Cancer in Men

The incidence of breast cancer in men is 100-fold lower than in women, with 1450 new cases in 2004 and 470 deaths. The incidence of male breast cancer increased over the past 26 years from 0.86 per 100,000 population to 1.08. Median age at diagnosis is 65 years and 35% occur in men 70 and older.[208] Known risk factors include family history, clinical disorders associated with reduced testosterone production or estrogen excess such as orchitis, orchiectomy, undescended testes, testicular injury, Klinefelter's syndrome, radiation exposure, *BRCA2* carrier, family history, obesity, and exogenous estrogen.[209] Suggestive risk factors include Cowden syndrome and cirrhosis. Inconclusive factors reported in the literature to be possibly associated include mutations of the androgen receptor gene, the *CHEK2* gene, prostate cancer, gynecomastia, occupational exposures, electromagnetic frequency exposure, high temperatures, diet, and alcohol.[209]

A painful retroareolar lump is the most frequent symptom and serosanguineous discharge is not uncommon. At presentation of breast cancer, 37.5% of men have regional lymph node involvement versus only 29.2% of women with this disease. Tumors are larger at diagnosis in men than in women, and 41.7% of men have tumors localized to their breast versus 50.5% of women. The percent ER+ and PR+ is higher in men (90.6% and 81.2%) than in women (76% and 66.7%, respectively). The 5-year survival rate is 63%, and 10-year survival rate is 41%.[208,210]

Breast cancer is suspected when a subareolar or upper outer quadrant, firm, painless or painful lesion is palpated and a diagnosis is then made by mammography and biopsy of the lesion. Most patients are then treated by mastectomy, radiotherapy, and adjuvant tamoxifen. Later therapy could include orchiectomy followed by aromatase inhibitors or progestins and chemotherapy upon relapse. No randomized controlled trials are available to accurately assess relative efficacies of various therapies.[210]

Endometrial Cancer

Approximately 40,800 new cases of endometrial cancer occur annually in the United States and 3710 die of this disease each year. Genetic factors such as those underlying the HNPCC (hereditary nonpolyposis colorectal cancer) syndrome, probably related to one or more polymorphic alleles, are related to uterine cancer. Other risk factors relate to conditions causing overexposure to endogenous or exogenous estrogen. Enhanced tumor initiation and promotion mediated by the proliferative effects of estrogen occur, as with breast cancer.[211] Progestins are antimitogenic on the endometrium as opposed to breast tissue and result in a decreased rate of cell proliferation. Thus, unopposed estrogen increases the risk of endometrial cancer and progestins reduce that risk.[212,213] Continued stimulation of the endometrium without progestin-induced endometrial shedding causes an increase in cell proliferation rate and a concomitant increase in genetic mutations. Those mutations which are not repaired accumulate and ultimately result in neoplastic growth. With prolonged stimulation of the endometrial lining, typical hyperplasia occurs first, followed by atypical adenomatous hyperplasia, a premalignant lesion. It is thought that 30% of such lesions later progress to frank cancer.

Several clinical conditions are characterized by increased estradiol production and anovulation, a state in which the proliferative effects of estrogen are not opposed by the antimitotic effects of progesterone. One of these involves exogenous obesity. As the number of adipocytes

increases, the amount of aromatase enzyme increases proportionately. With a normal amount of androgenic substrate, estradiol production increases as a function of the amount of enzyme present and in proportion to the degree of obesity. Polycystic ovary syndrome is associated with increases in estrone levels and lack of cyclic increments in progesterone as a result of absence of the luteal phase of the cycle. The polycystic ovary syndrome is associated with decreased sex hormone–binding globulin (SHBG) and presumably an increase in the free fraction of estradiol and an increased rate of conversion of androgens to estrogens (i.e., aromatase excess). Exercise and cigarette smoking appear to decrease the risk, perhaps related to decreased obesity and enhanced hepatic metabolism of estrogens, respectively.[214,215]

Estrogen-producing ovarian and adrenal tumors are also conditions of unopposed estrogen and increased incidence of endometrial cancer. Other risk factors for endometrial cancer include nulliparity, late menopause, increasing age, metabolic syndrome, history of breast cancer, long-term use of tamoxifen, HNPCC family syndrome, first-degree relative with endometrial cancer, radiation to the pelvis, diabetes, and hypertension.[216]

A large body of observational data reported the risks of endometrial carcinoma in women receiving MHT.[217] Estrogen, unopposed by a progestin, increases the relative risk of endometrial cancer by two- to fourfold, depending upon duration of use.[212,213,218] This risk increases over time with a relative risk of 1.30 for 2 years of use of unopposed estrogen, 2.22 for 2 to 5 years, and 4.49 for 5 to 10 years.[219] Progestins reduce this risk by opposing the mitogenic effects of estrogen on the endometrium and reducing the proliferative stimulus.

Four estrogen/progestin regimens are commonly used:

1. Combined continuous estrogen plus progestin
2. Sequential addition of a progestin to an estrogen for 10 or more days each month
3. Sequential addition of a progestin to an estrogen for less than 10 days, usually 5 to 7 days
4. The so-called "long cycle" with progestin added to an estrogen for 14 days every 3 to 4 months

The combined continuous regimen reduces endometrial cancer risk substantially, if not completely. Pike et al.[218] report a relative risk of 1.07 (95% CI 0.8-1.43) for combined continuous estrogen plus progesterone but a nonsignificant trend of increased risk for more than 5 years of use (RR 1.34—no confidence limits given). The large, randomized, controlled WHI study now provides level I evidence regarding MHT use and risk of endometrial cancer. This study compared women receiving continuous conjugated equine estrogen plus medroxyprogesterone acetate with women taking placebo. After an average follow-up of 5.6 years the hazard ratio for endometrial cancer was 0.81 (95% CI 0.48-1.36). There were no differences in tumor histologic type, stage, or grade between the women receiving MHT and those receiving placebo.

For sequential use of a progestin for 10 or more days each month and use for less than 5 years, there is no increase in endometrial cancer risk[219] (Pike et al. study, RR

1.07, 95% CI 0.82-1.41; Beresford, RR 0.7, 95% CI 0.4-1.4). There was a trend, however, for an increase in endometrial cancer with longer term use of this continuous regimen. Beresford et al.[213] report a relative risk of 2.7 (95% CI 1.2-6) for current users of this regimen for more than 5 years, whereas Pike et al report a relative risk of 1.09 (nonsignificant).[219] Caution should then be advised for long-term use of such regimens.

Sequential regimens that administer a progestin for less than 10 days are associated with an increase in risk of endometrial cancer. Pike et al report an increase in relative risk of 1.87 per 5 years of use (95% CI 1.33-2.65),[219] and Beresford reports RR 2.2 (95% CI 0.9-5.2)[213] for less than 5 years of use and 4.8 (95% CI 2-11) for more than 5 years of use. Use of the long cycle approach also may not be not associated with an increased risk of endometrial cancer but additional data are needed for confirmation.[220]

Taken together, these data suggest that progestins protect against estrogen-induced endometrial cancer when taken continuously with an estrogen. In premenopausal women, oral contraceptives containing both estrogen and a progestin decrease the risk of endometrial cancer. Multiple pregnancies also increase the duration of exposure to large amounts of progesterone and decrease the risk.

Tibolone is a hormonal agent used in Europe for more than two decades for treatment of menopausal symptoms. The relative risk of endometrial cancer in women using this agent was reported as 1.79 in the Million Women Study (95% CI 1.43-2.25).[217] Although the overall data analysis in the Million Women Study has been criticized, the other results reported regarding use of estrogen alone (RR 1.45, 95% CI 1.02-2.06) and cyclic progestin with estrogen (RR 1.05, 95% CI 0.91-1.22) appear to confirm other reports regarding MHT and breast cancer risk. Data from prospective trials regarding endometrial cancer are now needed before a clear conclusion regarding tibolone can be drawn.

Use of tamoxifen as adjuvant therapy for breast cancer or prevention is associated with an increased risk of endometrial cancer as well as hyperplasia and polyps (see earlier discussion). Of interest is that raloxifene, another selective estrogen receptor modulator (SERM), did not cause an increase in endometrial cancer in a large study monitoring this as a safety parameter.[221] Animal studies with raloxifene suggest that this SERM does not exert estrogen agonistic effects on uterus whereas tamoxifen does.

ENDOCRINOLOGY OF ENDOMETRIAL CANCER

Endometrial carcinoma is divided into two general types: endometrioid (type I, low-grade lesions) which accounts for 90% and nonendometrioid cancers (type II, high-grade lesions). The latter tumors are not estrogen driven and most are associated with endometrial atrophy. Serous carcinoma is the most aggressive type of nonendometrioid tumor. Accordingly, only the type I lesions retain some degree of hormonal responsiveness. Most endometrial cancers contain appreciable levels of estrogen receptor, whereas only differentiated ones generally have progesterone receptors.[222] Tumors resulting from estrogen

replacement therapy are generally well differentiated, have estrogen and progesterone receptors, and are of low grade and stage. The diagnosis is suspected when unexplained vaginal bleeding is detected. Instillation of saline into the uterine cavity followed by ultrasound can reveal an area of focal thickening which on biopsy is cancer. An associated finding is generalized thickening of the endometrial stripe to greater than 6 mm as a sign of concomitant endometrial hyperplasia. Any unexplained vaginal bleeding in a postmenopausal woman requires such evaluation to rule out endometrial cancer.

Treatment requires initial hysterectomy and bilateral oophorectomy in all patients. The use of preoperative radiotherapy has been abandoned because it interferes with adequate surgical staging and there is no proven benefit over postoperative radiotherapy. Those with a poor prognosis (approximately 25% of patients) are treated postoperatively with external beam radiotherapy or with implants. Upon recurrence, one may use high doses of systemic progestagens.[223] Response to therapy is independent of age, site of metastasis, or previous or concurrent therapy. Two large, gynecologic oncology studies reported that objective responses to a progestin occurred in 24% to 25% of patients.[224,225] The exact mechanism causing tumor regression is unknown but could involve direct effects on tumor cells; stimulation of the inactivating 17β-hydroxylsteroid dehydrogenase type I enzyme, which converts estradiol to estrone; inhibition of the production by the adrenals of androgenic estrogen precursors; down-regulation of estrogen receptors by progestagen; or suppression of gonadotropin production in premenopausal women. Experimental trials are ongoing to test the efficacy of aromatase inhibitors, anti-estrogens, GnRH analogs, and combinations of these agents. Various chemotherapeutic regimens are also available for such patients.

HRT IN ENDOMETRIAL CANCER SURVIVORS

Patients with an excellent prognosis and disease-free survival for at least 1 year can be treated with MHT to relieve menopausal symptoms. This recommendation is based upon several nonrandomized studies as well as a large randomized Gynecologic-Oncology Group (GOG) study.[226]

The complete reference list can be found on the companion Expert Consult Web site at www.expertconsultbook.com.

Suggested Readings

Chen J, Pee D, Ayyagari R, et al. Projecting absolute invasive breast cancer risk in white women with a model that includes mammographic density. J Natl Cancer Inst 98(17):1215-1226, 2006.

Collaborative Group on Hormonal Factors in Breast Cancer. Breast cancer and hormone replacement therapy: collaborative reanalysis of data from 51 epidemiological studies of 52,705 women with breast cancer and 108,411 women without breast cancer. Lancet 350(9084):1047-1059, 1997; erratum appears in Lancet 350(9089):1484;1997.

Eastell R, Hannon R. Long-term effects of aromatase inhibitors on bone. J Steroid Biochem Mol Biol 95(1-5):151-154, 2005.

Goss PE, Ingle JN, Martino S, et al. A randomized trial of letrozole in postmenopausal women after five years of tamoxifen therapy for early-stage breast cancer. N Engl J Med 349(19):1793-1802, 2003.

Hahn WC, Weinberg RA. Rules for making human tumor cells. N Engl J Med 347(20):1593-1603, 2002.

Key T, Appleby P, Barnes I, Reeves G. Endogenous Hormones and Breast Cancer Collaborative Group. Endogenous sex hormones and breast cancer in postmenopausal women: reanalysis of nine prospective studies. J Natl Cancer Inst 94(8):606-616, 2002.

Robbins AS, Clarke CA. Regional changes in hormone therapy use and breast cancer incidence in California from 2001 to 2004. J Clin Oncol 25(23):3437-3439, 2007.

Santen RJ, Boyd NF, Chlebowski RT, et al. Critical assessment of new risk factors for breast cancer: considerations for development of an improved risk prediction model. Endocr Rel Cancer 14(2):169-187, 2007.

Sorlie T. Molecular portraits of breast cancer: tumour subtypes as distinct disease entities. Eur J Cancer 40(18):2667-2675, 2004.

Vogel VG, Costantino JP, Wickerham DL, et al. Effects of tamoxifen vs raloxifene on the risk of developing invasive breast cancer and other disease outcomes: the NSABP Study of Tamoxifen and Raloxifene (STAR) P-2 trial. JAMA 295(23):2727-2741, 2006.

Yager JD, Davidson NE. Estrogen carcinogenesis in breast cancer. N Engl J Med 354(3):270-282, 2006.

PART III

Reproductive Technologies

CHAPTER 28

Medical Approaches to Ovarian Stimulation for Infertility

Nicholas S. Macklon and Bart C. J. M. Fauser

Introduction

CONCEPTS OF OVARIAN STIMULATION

Ovarian stimulation is a central component of many infertility therapies. At the outset of this chapter, it is important to emphasize that two different concepts of ovarian stimulation exist. These approaches differ in both the starting point (i.e., the type of patients) and end points (i.e., the aim of the medical intervention).

Ovulation Induction

In the strict sense of the term, ovulation induction refers to the triggering of ovulation, that is, the rupture of the preovulatory follicle and release of the oocyte. In the clinical context however, this term refers to the type of ovarian stimulation for anovulatory women aimed at restoring normal fertility by generating normo-ovulatory cycles (i.e., to mimic physiology and induce single dominant follicle selection and ovulation). Ovulation induction represents one of the most common interventions for the treatment of infertility.[1] Anovulation represents one of the few states of absolute infertility, but excellent cumulative pregnancy rates can be achieved if normal menstrual cyclicity is restored.

After the exclusion of intrinsic ovarian abnormalities (such as premature ovarian failure) follicle development can be stimulated by various pharmacologic compounds and normo-ovulatory cycles can usually be obtained. This can be achieved with appropriate monitoring of ovarian response and in the hands of skillful clinicians. Because of various more subtle inherent ovarian abnormalities in most of these women, especially in patients suffering from polycystic ovary syndrome (PCOS), the risks of multiple pregnancy and ovarian hyperstimulation syndrome (OHSS)

are considerable. However, the occurrence of these complications can be reduced to an acceptable level, especially with low-dose gonadotropin protocols.[2] The therapeutic window for an acceptable ovarian response is small, with a major individual (and to some extent cycle-to-cycle) variability in response. Approaches for gonadotropin ovulation induction include slowly and prudently surpassing the individual follicle-stimulating hormone (FSH) threshold for ongoing follicle development, as will be discussed later in this chapter.

Many other approaches for ovulation induction are available. These approaches include interfering with negative estrogen feedback, the use of insulin-sensitizing agents, and laparoscopic surgical methods.

Ovarian Hyperstimulation

This treatment modality has become an integral part of assisted reproductive technologies (ART). The aim is to bring more male and female gametes closer together and thereby increase the chances of pregnancy. The goal of ovarian hyperstimulation is to induce ongoing development of multiple dominant follicles and to mature many oocytes in order to improve chances for conception either in vivo (empirical ovarian hyperstimulation with or without intrauterine insemination, IUI) or in vitro with in vitro fertilization (IVF). This approach of interfering with physiologic mechanisms underlying single dominant follicle selection is usually applied in normo-ovulatory women. Although ovarian hyperstimulation can also be performed in anovulatory women, this approach should be clearly differentiated from ovulation induction. The physiologic concepts which underlie current approaches to ovulation induction and ovarian hyperstimulation are described later in this chapter.

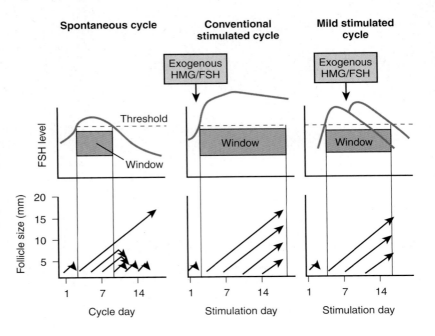

Figure 28-1. *The follicle-stimulating hormone (FSH) threshold and window concept for monofollicular selection* (left panel), *as conventionally applied to achieve multifollicular development* (middle panel). *Each arrow represents a developing follicle. The* right panel *represents the concept of extending the FSH window by administering exogenous FSH in the midfollicular phase to maintain FSH levels above the threshold allowing multifollicular development. HMG, human menopausal gonadotropin. (From Macklon NS, Stouffer RL, Giudice LC, Fauser BC. The science behind 25 years of ovarian stimulation for in vitro fertilization. Endocr Rev 27[2]:170-207, 2006.)*

CONCEPTS OF FOLLICLE DEVELOPMENT REGULATION RELEVANT TO OVARIAN STIMULATION

Initiation of growth of primordial follicles, also referred to as primary recruitment, occurs continuously and in a random fashion and development from the primordial up to the preovulatory stage takes several months.[3,4] The great majority of primordial follicles which enter this development phase undergo atresia prior to reaching the antral follicle stage. The regulation of early follicle development and atresia and the degree to which early stages of follicle development are influenced by FSH remain unclear, but evidence suggests that the transforming growth factor β superfamily and factors regulating apoptosis (i.e., programmed cell death) are involved.[5] Only at more advanced stages of development do follicles become responsive to FSH and obtain the capacity to convert the theca cell–derived substrate androstenedione (AD) to estradiol (E_2) by the induction of the aromatase enzyme.

Owing to demise of the corpus luteum during the late luteal phase of the menstrual cycle, E_2, inhibin A, and progesterone levels fall. This results in an increased frequency of pulsatile gonadotropin-releasing hormone (GnRH) secretion inducing rising FSH levels at the end of the luteal phase.[6,7] Although each growing follicle may initially have an equal potential to reach full maturation, only those follicles that happen to be at a more advanced stage of maturation during this intercycle rise in FSH (levels surpassing the so-called *threshold* for ovarian stimulation) gain gonadotropin dependence and continue to grow[2] (Fig. 28-1). This process is referred to as cyclic, gonadotropin-dependent recruitment as opposed to the above-mentioned initial, gonadotropin-independent recruitment of primordial follicles.[4] Based on indirect observations it is believed that the cohort size of healthy early antral follicles recruited during the luteofollicular transition is around 10 per ovary.[3,8,9] During the subsequent

follicular phase, FSH levels plateau during initial days[10,11] and are gradually suppressed thereafter by ovarian inhibin B[12] and E_2[13] negative feedback. A rise in inhibin B occurs just after the intercycle rise in FSH. It may therefore be proposed that inhibin B limits the duration of the FSH rise. Decremental follicular phase FSH levels (effectively restricting the time when FSH levels remain above the threshold, referred to as the FSH *window*) (see Fig. 28-1) appear to be crucial for selection of a single dominant follicle from the recruited cohort.[10] Only one follicle escapes from atresia by increased sensitivity for stimulation by FSH and luteinizing hormone (LH).[2] The important concept of increased sensitivity of the dominant follicle for FSH has been confirmed by human studies showing developing follicles to exhibit a variable tolerance for GnRH antagonists-induced gonadotropin withdrawal.[14,15] On the other hand, early stages of follicle development being independent from gonadotropins is confirmed in hypophysectomized women presenting with preovulatory graafian follicles within 2 weeks after the initiation of ovarian stimulation with exogenous gonadotropins.[16]

A central role has also been demonstrated for LH in monofollicular selection and dominance in the normal ovulatory cycle.[17,18] Although granulosa cells from early antral follicles respond only to FSH, those from mature follicles also contain LH receptors and therefore become responsive to both FSH and LH. The maturing dominant follicle may become less dependent on FSH because of the ability to respond to LH. It is suggested that the leading follicle continues its development owing to LH responsiveness, whereas smaller follicles enter atresia because of insufficient support by decreasing FSH concentrations during the late follicle phase. The dominant follicle can be distinguished by ultrasound from other cohort follicles by a size greater than 10 mm diameter.[9] The concept of both endocrine and autocrine up-regulation is supported by several other observations that characterize the dominant follicle, including the in vitro induction of aromatase enzyme activity,[19] ovarian morphology,[20] and endocrine changes in follicle fluid[21] and serum. These observations all show that enhanced E_2 biosynthesis is closely linked to preovulatory follicle development.

These concepts of follicular development and selection have come to underlie contemporary approaches to therapeutic ovulation induction in women suffering from anovulatory infertility. Moreover, our increasing understanding of the processes underlying monofollicular selection has enabled the development of new approaches to ovarian hyperstimulation for assisted reproduction treatments.

PREPARATIONS USED FOR OVARIAN STIMULATION

Evidence of the endocrine pituitary-gonadal axis arose early in the 20th century, when it was observed that lesions of the anterior pituitary resulted in atrophy of the genitals. The first convincing evidence supporting the existence of two separate gonadotropins (initially referred to as Prolan A and Prolan B) was provided by Fevold and Hisaw in 1931, and both LH and FSH were subsequently isolated and purified. In 1928 Aschheim and Zondek described the capacity of urine from pregnant women to stimulate gonadal function. The concept of stimulating ovarian function by the exogenous administration of gonadotropin preparations has intrigued investigators for many decades. As early as 1938, Davis and Koff had already described the ability of purified pregnant mare serum to induce ovulation in humans by intravenous administration. However, these initial attempts had to be stopped due to species differences and resulting antibody formation impacting on efficacy and safety. Not until 1958 did Gemzell describe the first successful use for ovulation induction of gonadotropin preparations derived from human pituitaries. Shortly thereafter, Lunenfeld reported the clinical use of gonadotropin extracts from urine of postmenopausal women (for an historical overview, see Gruhn and Kazer[22] and Lunenfeld[23]).

A second important development allowing for ovarian stimulation on a large scale was a fine example of medical serendipity. The first estrogen antagonist tested in cancer patients was found to induce ovulation.

Clomiphene Citrate

In the late 1950s the first nonsteroidal estrogen antagonist (MER-25) was tested in patients to assess the efficacy of the compound in women with cystic mastitis, breast cancer, endometrial hyperplasia, or endometriosis. Some of these women with endometrial hyperplasia were of reproductive age and suffering from long-standing amenorrhea due to the Stein-Leventhal syndrome. To the great surprise of the investigators, the initiation of the medication in these women was followed by the recommencement of menstrual cycles.[24] Shortly thereafter, the ovulation-inducing capacity of the next generation of closely related anti-estrogens (MRL/41; clomiphene citrate, CC) (Fig. 28-2) was recognized.[25] More than 30 years later, CC is still the most applied drug for infertility

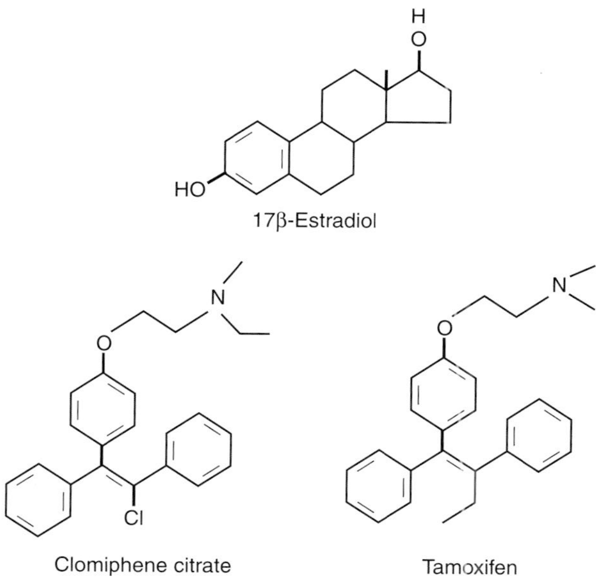

Figure 28-2. *Structure of 17β-estradiol and the anti-estrogenic triphenylethylene derivates clomiphene citrate and tamoxifen.*

therapies worldwide, accounting for around two thirds of all prescriptions.

CC is a racemic mixture of two stereoisomers. The enclomiphene isomer has a relatively short half-life, whereas the zuclomiphene isomer has an extended clearance. The two isomers demonstrate different patterns of agonistic and antagonistic activity in vitro.[26] Stimulation of ovarian function is elicited by raised pituitary FSH secretion due to blockage of E_2 steroid feedback by CC. Overall a 50% to 60% increase of serum FSH levels above baseline has been described.[27] The exact nature of the mechanism of action of CC is still uncertain.[28] Induced changes in other systems, like insulin-like growth factor (IGF) may partly explain the capacity of CC to stimulate the ovary.[27] However, anti-estrogenic effects at the uterine level (cervical mucus production and endometrial receptivity) are believed to underlie the observed discrepancy between achieved ovulation and pregnancy rates. The impact of a concomitant rise in LH on ovarian response to CC is also uncertain. CC for ovulation induction is considered to be relatively safe because steroid negative feedback remains intact. The oral route of administration and low costs represent additional advantages of this preparation. CC was originally developed for clinical use by the Merrel company in 1956, and it is still considered to represent the first-line treatment strategy in most anovulatory infertility. In addition, this compound was a central component in the early days of IVF[29,30] and is still often applied for the empirical treatment of unexplained infertility, alone or in combination with IVF.

Gonadotropin Preparations

Clinical experiments in the late 1950s demonstrated that extracts derived from the human pituitary could be used to stimulate gonadal function.[31] Subsequently, experiments involving the extraction of both the gonadotropic hormones LH and FSH from urine of postmenopausal women led to the development of human menopausal gonadotropin (hMG) preparations. From the early 1960s these preparations were used for the stimulation of gonadal function in the human.[32] It soon became clear that hMG was a very potent compound. Its ability to directly stimulate the ovaries was accompanied by the inherent risks of ovarian hyperstimulation. Initial use in the treatment of anovulation was associated with high rates of multiple pregnancy and OHSS. The potential for dangerous complications induced the need for monitoring of ovarian response and dose adjustment. More recently introduced low-dose protocols applied in conjunction with intense ovarian response monitoring have substantially contributed to improved treatment outcomes.

Initial attempts in the 1970s by Edwards and Steptoe to enable the conception of a baby through IVF also involved hMG stimulation protocols. Because of a lack of pregnancies (presumed due to abnormal luteal function) it was decided to switch to natural cycle IVF. It was an unstimulated cycle that led to the conception of the first IVF baby Louise Brown, who was born on July 25, 1978.[33] Subsequent IVF pregnancies were reported from Australia to occur after ovarian stimulation with CC.[29] The more widespread use of hMG for successful IVF was developed thereafter in the United States.[34] For over two decades, gonadotropin preparations have also been extensively applied for ovarian stimulation in ovulatory women for empirical treatment of unexplained subfertility. Here the aim is to increase monthly fecundity rates by increasing the number of oocytes available for fertilization in vivo (with or without the additional use of IUI). These trends, and the rapid expansion in the use of IVF treatment, underlie the enormous increase in worldwide demand and sales for gonadotropin preparations.

The early extraction techniques were very crude, requiring around 30 L of urine to manufacture enough hMG needed for a single treatment cycle. The FSH to LH bioactivity ratio of these early preparations was 1:1. As purity improved, it was necessary to add human chorionic gonadotropin (hCG) in order to maintain this ratio of bioactivity.[35] These initial preparations were very impure with many contaminating proteins; only less than 5% of the proteins present were bioactive. Bioactivity of gonadotropin preparations continues to be assessed by the crude in vivo rat ovarian weight gain Steehlman and Pohley assay. This rather anachronistic technique has the disadvantage of allowing considerable batch-to-batch inconsistency in bioactivity. However, improved protein purification technology allowed for the production of hMG with reduced amounts of contaminating nonactive proteins and eventually the development of purified urinary FSH (uFSH) preparations by using monoclonal antibodies since the late 1980s. The currently available pure products allow for less hypersensitivity reactions, and less painful subcutaneous administration. Because of the worldwide increased need for gonadotropin preparations, demands for postmenopausal urine increased tremendously and adequate supplies could no longer be guaranteed. In addition, concern regarding the limited batch-to-batch consistency along with possibilities of urine contaminants emerged.[26]

Through recombinant DNA technology and the transfection of human genes encoding for the common α subunit and hormone-specific β subunit of the glycoprotein hormone (Fig. 28-3) into Chinese hamster ovary cell lines,[36] the large-scale in vitro production of human recombinant FSH (recFSH) has been realized.[37] The first pregnancies using this novel preparation in ovulation induction[38] and in IVF[39] were reported in 1992. Since then, numerous large-scale, multicenter studies have been undertaken, demonstrating their efficacy and safety. The recombinant products offer improved purity, consistency, and large-scale availability. Because of its purity, recFSH can now be administered by protein weight rather than

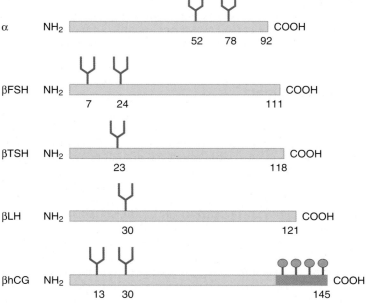

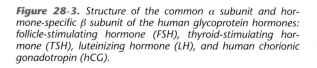

Figure 28-3. Structure of the common α subunit and hormone-specific β subunit of the human glycoprotein hormones: follicle-stimulating hormone (FSH), thyroid-stimulating hormone (TSH), luteinizing hormone (LH), and human chorionic gonadotropin (hCG).

bioactivity, and so-called "filled-by-mass" preparations[40] are now available for clinical use. During recent years, recLH and rechCG have also been introduced for clinical application.[26] Finally, a long-acting recFSH agonist (a chimeric hormone generated by the fusion of the carboxy-terminal peptide of hCG to the FSH β chain) is undergoing clinical IVF trials, and the birth of the first healthy child using this preparation was reported in 2003.[41]

GnRH Analogs

In 1971, the small decapeptide gonadotropin-releasing hormone (GnRH) was isolated and its structure elucidated by Schally and Guillemin (Fig. 28-4). Some years later, both investigators jointly received the Nobel prize for this discovery. Amino acid substitutions have revealed the significance of specific regions for its stability, receptor binding, and activation of the gonadotrope cells. This decapeptide is secreted by the hypothalamus into the portal circulation in an intermittent fashion, stimulating the pituitary gonadotropes to synthesize and secrete LH and FSH. Early studies demonstrated that pituitary down-regulation could be induced by the continued administration of GnRH.[42] Clinically safe GnRH agonists were developed relatively easily by replacing one or two amino acids. An increased potency could be achieved by replacing glycine for D-amino acids at position 6 and by replacing Gly-NH$_2$ at position 10 by ethylamide.[43] Such simple structural changes render these compounds more hydrophobic and more resistant to enzymatic degradation. The administration of GnRH agonists induces an initial stimulation of gonadotropin release for 2 to 3 weeks (the so-called "flare effect") followed by a down-regulation (or desensitization) due to the clustering and internalization of pituitary GnRH receptors.

GnRH agonists have been used clinically since 1981 to induce a "chemical castration" for steroid-dependent disease states such as fibroids and endometriosis in females and prostate cancer in males. The first paper concerning its use in IVF for the prevention of a premature LH rise also appeared in the early 1980s.[44] Shortly thereafter, the

use of GnRH agonists such as buserelin, triptorelin, or leuprorelin to down-regulate the pituitary prior to administration of gonadotropins (a combination that became known as the "long protocol") became the standard of care. The recent clinical introduction of GnRH antagonists may ultimately lead to a new standard of care in IVF practice.

It has taken almost three decades to develop GnRH antagonists with acceptable safety and pharmacokinetic characteristics. The first-generation antagonists were developed by replacing amino acids histidine at position 2 and tryptophan at position 3, but these compounds suffered from low potency. In second-generation compounds, the activity was increased by incorporating a D-amino acid at position 6. However, the widespread clinical application of these compounds was hampered by frequent anaphylactic responses due to histamine release. By introducing further replacements at position 10, third-generation compounds were developed.[45,46] Subsequently both the compounds ganirelix and cetrotide were shown to be safe and efficacious in IVF. These third-generation GnRH antagonist were registered in 2001 for use in IVF. The immediate suppression and recovery of pituitary function renders these compounds appropriate for short-term use in IVF. Commencing administration in the late follicular phase of the stimulation cycle still prevents premature luteinization. Further extended use of GnRH antagonist in steroid-dependent disease states such as endometriosis or myomas will depend on the development of depot or slow release formulations.

OUTCOMES OF OVARIAN STIMULATION

Ovulation Induction

Amenorrheic women with anovulation exhibit virtually no chance of spontaneous conception and ovulation induction may restore normal fertility. However, the aim of mimicking normo-ovulatory cycles cannot always be achieved, and therefore, the chances of complications such as multiple pregnancy or OHSS should be taken seriously, especially in PCOS patients. Oligomenorrheic women may

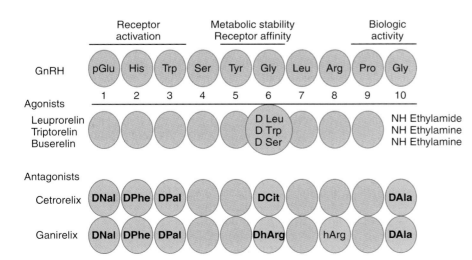

Figure 28-4. Structure of the native decapeptide gonadotropin-releasing hormone (GnRH), as well as the modified, commercially available GnRH agonists and antagonists. Arg, arginine; D, dextro; DAla, D-alanine; DCit, D-citroline; DhArg, D-homoarginine; DNal, D-naphthylalanine; DPal, D-pyridylalanine; DPhe, D-phenylalanine; Gly, glycine; hArg, homoarginine; His, histidine; Leu, leucine; pGlu, pyroglutamate; Pro, proline; Ser, serine; Trp, tryptophan; Try, tyrosine.

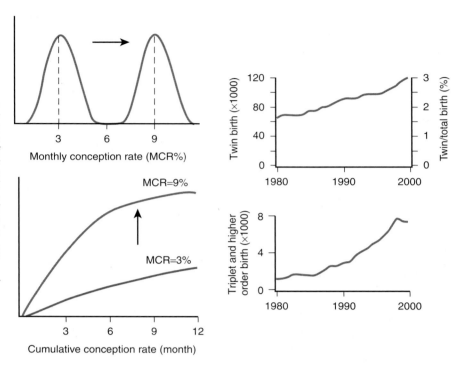

Figure 28-5. *Monthly conception rate in unexplained infertility increasing from 3% to 9% per cycle due to ovarian stimulation and resulting increase in cumulative conception rates over a 12-month period* (left); *increased occurrence of multiple pregnancies (twin, triplet, and higher order) between 1980 and 2000 associated with ovarian stimulation* (right). *(Left from Stovall DW, Guzick DS. Current management of unexplained infertility. Curr Opin Obstet Gynaecol 5:228-233,1993; right from Rowland Hogue CJ. Successful assisted reproduction technology: the beauty of one. Obstet Gynecol 100:1017, 2002; Jones HW. Multiple births: how are we doing? Fertil Steril 79:17-21, 2003.)*

or may not have incidental spontaneous ovulations, and therefore, spontaneous pregnancies may occur. For obvious reasons, fertility specialists see only oligomenorrheic women who have failed to conceive, and these patients will usually respond well to ovulation induction. The balance between success and complications resulting from ovulation induction is dependent on many factors, including patient characteristics, gonadotropin preparations and dose regimens used, the intensity of monitoring ovarian response to stimulation, and willingness to cancel the cycle in case of hyper-response. Cumulative success rates of ovulation induction are reported to be around 75%,[47] with a coinciding incidence of multiple pregnancies of more than 10% and of OHSS of less than 2%.

OHSS is a potentially life-threatening complication characterized by ovarian enlargement, high serum sex steroids, and extravascular fluid accumulation, primarily in the peritoneal cavity. In severe cases, hypotension, increased coagubility, reduced renal perfusion, and oliguria may occur. Deranged liver function tests, venous and arterial thrombosis, renal failure, and adult respiratory distress syndrome can ensue, and fatalities have been reported.[48] Moderate to critical OHSS is very rare with CC but constitutes an important complication of gonadotropin use.[49] The incidences of mild, moderate, and severe OHSS following gonadotropin ovulation induction have been reported to be 20%, 6% to 7%, and 1% to 2%, respectively.[26] In addition to PCOS, risk factors for the development of OHSS include young age and low body weight.[49] The risk is further increased when adjuvant GnRH agonist treatment is employed.[50]

The contribution of ovulation induction treatment to the number of triplet and higher order pregnancies is considerable.[51,52] It has been calculated that 40% of higher order multiple births in the United States could be attributed to the use of ovulation-inducing drugs without assisted reproduction.[51]

Ovarian Stimulation

As previously outlined, the aim of ovarian hyperstimulation alone or in combination with assisted reproductive techniques is to bring an increased number of gametes (oocytes and sperm) together in order to augment pregnancy chances. Hyperstimulation may give rise to a two- to fourfold increase in pregnancy rates. The associated risk of OHSS and the occurrence of twin and higher order multiple births is dependent on the magnitude of ovarian stimulation, the intensity of ovarian response monitoring, and the criteria applied for cycle cancellation should too many follicles develop. The overall incidence of severe ovarian OHSS associated with ovarian hyperstimulation is less than 5%.[53]

Initial studies suggested that a threefold increase in monthly probability of pregnancy can be achieved with empirical ovarian hyperstimulation in the treatment of unexplained infertility[54] (Fig. 28-5). Subsequently, a large multicenter study showed that ovarian hyperstimulation with gonadotropins and IUI both exhibit an independent additive effect on pregnancy chances. Moreover, overall cumulative pregnancy rates with this combined therapy was reported to be 33% within three cycles, but at the price of an unacceptably high multiple pregnancy rate of 20% for twins and 10% for higher-order multiple pregnancy.[55] It has been proposed that a similar cumulative pregnancy rate could be achieved by expectant management over a 6-month period, obviously with much lower chances of multiple pregnancy.[56] In an analysis from one

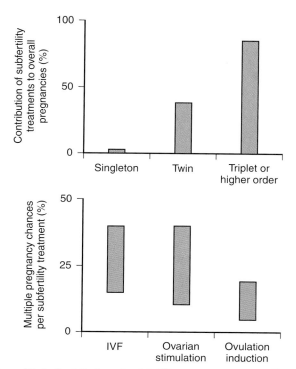

Figure 28-6. *Contribution of subfertility treatments to overall pregnancies* (upper) *and reported frequency of multiple pregnancy in relation to in vitro fertilization (IVF), ovarian stimulation, and ovulation induction* (lower). *(From Fauser BC, Devroey P, Macklon NS. Multiple birth resulting from ovarian stimulation for subfertility treatment. Lancet 365[9473]:1807-1816, 2005.)*

hyperstimulation for IVF is merely the factor allowing for the generation of multiples, but not the sole determining factor like in IUI. Unsurprisingly, the incidence of twin pregnancies following IVF without stimulation[61] or with hyperstimulation combined with single embryo transfer is close to normal.[62,63] Over the years, the number of embryos transferred in IVF has decreased, but larger numbers continue to be transferred in the United States compared to Europe. On the basis of a large nationwide data set from the United Kingdom, it was reported that the number of embryos transferred could be reduced from three to two without a concomitant drop in overall pregnancy chances.[64] The policy of two embryo transfer was adopted by many major European IVF centers during the 1990s. Subsequently it was demonstrated that in young women in whom two high-quality embryos are transferred, the chances of a twin pregnancy are actually higher than for a singleton pregnancy.[65,66] An increasing number of leading centers in Europe are currently moving toward a policy of single embryo transfer in selected women. The number of embryos transferred in the United States is substantially higher, with current revised guidelines still recommending the number for transfer to be between two and five, depending on patient's age and prognosis.[67]

This trend to reduce the numbers of embryos transferred is beginning to be reflected in birth statistics. After many years of rising multiple births, a decline in the reported percentage of higher-order multiple births after IVF are beginning to appear. IVF registries for 1999 from the United States involving 88,000 initiated ART cycles indicate a continued slight overall improvement in pregnancy chances (currently 25% delivery rate per started cycle), with overall 32% twin pregnancies and 4.9% ($n = 1024$ deliveries) triplet and higher-order multiple birth.[68] In young women below 35 years of age, the overall multiple birth rate was 42%. Data from the European IVF-Monitoring Consortium show a continuing trend toward transferring fewer embryos. Whereas in 1999, in 49% of embryo transfer cycles three or more embryos were still being transferred,[69] in 2003, a similar analysis of over 280,000 cycles showed this figure to have fallen to 28%.[60] Single embryo transfer accounted for 16%.[60] Despite these trends, overall clinical pregnancy rate per retrieval of 24% rose in the same period from 24% to 26%. Twin deliveries accounted for 22% of pregnancies and triplet or higher order deliveries were 1.1%.[60] In general, overall IVF results in Europe are slightly lower compared to the United States, but with an overall reduced incidence of multiple and premature birth (Fig. 28-7).

Given the risks associated with ovarian stimulation, couples should be well counseled regarding their spontaneous chances for pregnancy prior to commencing therapy (Table 28-1). These chances are often underestimated[70] both by the doctor and by the patient and the price to be paid for interventions (the increased incidence of multiple pregnancies) may frequently be underemphasized. How should the increased chances for pregnancy on the one hand be balanced with the high complication rates inevitably associated with ovarian hyperstimulation? Until recently, fertility specialists tended to lean heavily in the direction of increasing pregnancy rates at all costs. In

large European fertility center of 1878 pregnancies obtained from IUI cycles stimulated with gonadotropins, 16% were twins and 6% were triplets or higher order.[57] Less intense ovarian stimulation may reduce the incidence of higher order multiple pregnancies, but probably at the expense of a reduction in overall conception rate. On the basis of a 2-year experience in a large U.S. infertility clinic involving 3347 consecutive ovarian stimulation cycles (ovulation induction and ovarian hyperstimulation combined) in approximately 1500 women, a 30% pregnancy rate was described. Twenty percent of these pregnancies were twins, along with 5% triplets and 5% quadruplets or higher order.[58] The most worrying conclusion of this analysis was that the number of large antral follicles or serum E_2 levels during the late follicular phase had only limited value in predicting higher order multiple gestations. The true rate of multiple pregnancies arising from ovarian stimulation with or without IUI remains uncertain, however,[59] as few national registers record the outcome of ovarian stimulation. The European IVF Monitoring consortium reported twin rates among women under 40 years of age as 11.4% and triplet rates as 2.2% in 2003.[60] Although these data included natural cycle IUI treatments, the triplet rate was higher than that reported for IVF. It is estimated that ovarian stimulation with or without IUI is responsible for around 30% of multiple births (Fig. 28-6). It is easier to influence chances for multiple gestations after IVF, because the occurrence is primarily dependent on the number of embryos transferred. Therefore, ovarian

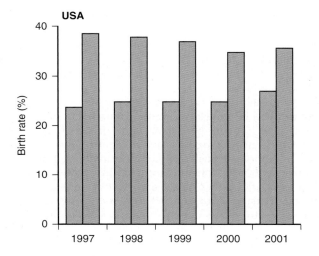

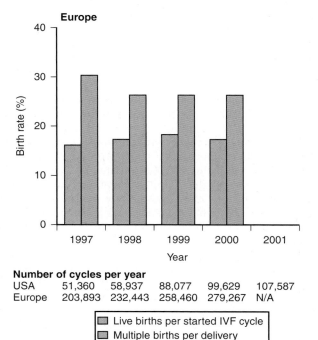

Number of cycles per year

	1997	1998	1999	2000	2001
USA	51,360	58,937	88,077	99,629	107,587
Europe	203,893	232,443	258,460	279,267	N/A

☐ Live births per started IVF cycle
☐ Multiple births per delivery

Figure 28-7. Rates of live births per started in vitro fertilization (IVF) cycle and multiple births. N/A, not available. (From Fauser BC, Devroey P, Macklon NS. Multiple birth resulting from ovarian stimulation for subfertility treatment. Lancet 365[9473]:1807-1816, 2005.)

doing so, an iatrogenic epidemic of multigestation came about, with major health, psychosocial, and financial consequences.

Higher order multiple pregnancies have a major adverse impact on perinatal morbidity and mortality rates. Mortality rate is increased four- to sevenfold in twins and up to 20-fold in triplets.[52] Children born from multiple pregnancies have more chances for perinatal complications and subsequent health problems, chiefly associated with prematurity and low birth weight.[52] Chances for cerebral palsy are increased almost 50-fold in children from triplet pregnancies.[71] Even the second child from a twin pregnancy delivered at term presents with a significant

increased risk for death due to complications of vaginal delivery.[72] Besides the medical and emotional burden, the financial costs associated with multiple pregnancies should be taken into account by policy makers. Obstetric and neonatal costs are increased five- to sevenfold in higher order multiples, and by the age of 8 costs for low-birth-weight children are increased eightfold.[52] Finally, possibilities of more subtle health risks which may be revealed only later in life should also be taken seriously.

Perhaps one strategy that may help improve the situation would be to agree to a new way of defining success from infertility therapy. The appropriate outcome measure should be shifted from pregnancy rate per treatment cycle toward live birth or preferably, healthy singleton child per started course of treatment.[63,73]

Ultimately, however, the risk/benefit ratio of ovulation induction and ovarian hyperstimulation is determined by the practice of the clinician. In the following sections we provide an overview of the medical approaches applied in contemporary practice.

Induction of Ovulation in Anovulatory Women

PRINCIPLES OF OVULATION INDUCTION

The aim of induction of ovulation in anovulatory women is to stimulate a single follicle to develop up to the preovulatory stage and subsequently ovulate. As stated before, this therapeutic goal should be clearly distinguished from two other forms of ovarian stimulation. First, ovulatory women with unexplained infertility may undergo a mild form of ovarian stimulation aimed at producing two or three follicles and an increased chance of fertilization in a given cycle. This treatment, which is frequently combined with IUI, is discussed later in the chapter. Second, ovarian hyperstimulation may be applied in ovulatory women undergoing IVF treatment, where multifollicular development is required to produce multiple oocytes. In contrast to these two therapeutic approaches, which produce a superphysiologic situation, ovulation induction aims to mimic the normal physiologic monofollicular ovulatory cycle. Ovulation induction is characterized therefore by tighter therapeutic margins and a need for careful monitoring and skilled management if success without complications is to be achieved. Ovarian surgical techniques such as laparoscopic drilling offer an alternative to medical therapies in this context. Again, the aim of this treatment paradigm is to institute monofollicular ovulatory cycles.

Anovulatory disorders account for around 25% of causes of infertility.[74] This proportion may increase with the rising prevalence of obesity. Anovulation is usually manifested as the absence (amenorrhea) or infrequent occurrence (oligomenorrhoea) of menstrual periods. Although oligomenorrhoea may be associated with occasional ovulation, the chance of a woman conceiving within a year of unprotected intercourse is clearly diminished unless therapeutic steps are taken. Many medical approaches have been developed to achieve the goal of inducing the monthly development of a single dominant follicle and

TABLE 28-1

Hypothetical Model of Cumulative Spontaneous Pregnancy Rates in Five Categories, According to Duration of Subfertility

Category	MFR (%)	Cumulative Pregnancy Rate After (%)			
		6 mo	12 mo	24 mo	60 mo
Superfertile	60	100	—	—	—
Normally fertile	20	74	93	100	—
Moderately subfertile	5	26	46	71	95
Severly subfertile	1	6	11	21	45
Infertile	0	0	0	0	0

MFR, monthly fecundity rate.
From Evers JLH. Female subfertility. Lancet 360:151-159, 2002.

subsequent ovulation. In recent years, increased understanding of the pathophysiology of ovarian dysfunction have enabled the development of clinical strategies which aim to mimic the endocrine control of normo-ovulatory cycles. Achieving this within the narrow therapeutic margins of stimulating single rather than multiple follicular developments remains a challenge to clinicians.

CLASSIFICATION OF ANOVULATION

Ovarian dysfunction can be readily classified in everyday clinical practice on the basis of the assessment of serum gonadotropin and estrogen levels in peripheral blood. This concise approach, currently known as the World Health Organization (WHO) classification of anovulation, was developed by Insler.[75] Amenorrhea may coincide with either low or normal E_2, whereas oligomenorrhea is associated with normal estrogens only. Low estrogens combined with low gonadotropin levels suggest a central origin of the disease at the hypothalamic-pituitary level.[76] This cause of anovulation occurs in less than 10% of infertile women and is termed WHO class 1. Low estrogens in combination with high gonadotropins suggest defective ovarian function per se, usually on the basis of premature ovarian failure (POF) or ovarian dysgenesis. This cause of anovulation, termed WHO class 3, occurs in around 5% of infertile women. The majority (80% to 90%) of anovulatory women present with estrogen and FSH levels within normal limits. LH levels may be increased in these women. Polycystic ovary syndrome (PCOS), exhibiting FSH and E_2 concentrations within the normal range, represents the great majority of these women. Recently, new criteria for the diagnosis of PCOS have been supported by the ASRM (American Society for Reproductive Medicine) and ESHRE (European Society of Human Reproduction and Embryology). The so-called Rotterdam consensus criteria are broader than the NIH (National Institutes of Health) criteria primarily because polycystic ovaries are now included. The incidence of PCOS as defined by the Rotterdam criteria is therefore higher.[77]

An additional cause of anovulation with an endocrine etiology is hyperprolactinemia which may present with normal or reduced gonadotropin and E_2 concentrations. This may be considered as a variant of WHO class 1 anovulation because high serum prolactin levels suppress GnRH release by the hypothalamus by altering opioid receptor stimulation. Hyperprolactinemia may also present with normal gonadotropin and E_2 concentrations, and may then be considered as a variant of WHO class 2. The pathophysiology and treatment of hyperprolactinemia are dealt with in Chapter 3.

PREPARATIONS FOR TREATING ANOVULATION

Anti-Estrogens

Background. The most widely used anti-estrogen for treating anovulation is CC, the development and pharmacology of which are addressed in the introduction to this chapter. In terms of its relative efficacy, safety, cost, and ease of use, it remains some 40 years after its introduction into clinical practice the most important therapeutic agent in use. The principal indication for CC is the treatment of anovulatory infertility in women with an intact hypophyseal-pituitary-ovarian axis. In this role it remains the first-line therapy. Given orally in the early to midfollicular phase, it causes a 50% rise in the endogenous serum FSH level,[78] thus stimulating follicle growth. This rise in FSH is accompanied by a similar rise in serum LH levels. Limitation of the duration of administration to 5 days is aimed at allowing FSH levels to fall in the late follicular phase and the mechanisms for monofollicular development and ovulation to operate. However, elevated gonadotropin levels may persist into the late follicular phase in some women.[79] The long half-life zuclomiphene isomer (which exhibits predominant estrogen agonist activity) has been shown to persist and accumulate across consecutive cycles of treatment.[80] However, the resulting concentrations are well below those demonstrated to have any effects in vitro and are unlikely to be of clinical significance.

Preparations and Regimens. The conventional starting dose of CC is 50 mg/day, starting from day 2 until day 5 of the menstrual cycle, for 5 consecutive days. In normogonadotropic amenorrheic women, treatment can be initiated following a progesterone-induced withdrawal bleeding. Whether CC is commenced on cycle day 1 or 5 does not appear to affect outcomes.[81] Should 50 mg/day fail to elicit follicle growth, the dose should be increased to 100 mg/day in the subsequent cycle, followed by

150 mg/day, which is usually considered to be the maximum dose beyond which alternative treatments are indicated. The LH surge occurs between 5 and 12 days following the last day of CC administration. Intercourse is therefore advised for a week from the fifth day after the last day of CC administration. Some advocate hCG administration as a surrogate for the LH surge to trigger ovulation and to time intercourse. However, recent studies showed no improvement in outcomes, despite the increased monitoring required to time hCG administration.[82,83]

Clinical Outcome. Between 60% and 85% of anovulatory women will become ovulatory with CC, and 30% to 40% will become pregnant.[84] In a meta-analysis based on four placebo-controlled studies in oligomenorrheic patients, the odds ratio with CC was 6.8 for ovulation and 4.2 for pregnancy.[85]

Why some women with WHO class 2 anovulation do not respond to CC is not fully understood. Altered individual requirements for FSH at the ovarian level, the local intraovarian effect of autocrine or paracrine factors, and variations in FSH receptor expression or FSH receptor polymorphisms may contribute. A number of studies have pointed to overweight as a factor.[84] In a multivariate analysis of factors found to predict outcome of CC ovulation indication, the free androgen index (FAI), body mass index (BMI), presence of amenorrhea (as opposed to oligomenorrhea), and ovarian volume were found to be independent predictors of ovulation.[86] The possibility of using clinical data to individualize treatment and optimize outcomes is discussed later in this chapter.

The occurrence of ovulation can be identified by the use of temperature charts and midluteal urinary pregnanediol or serum progesterone measurements.[84] Although results of large trials indicate that monitoring by ultrasound is not mandatory to ensure good outcomes,[87] the practice in many centers is to monitor the first cycle to allow adjustment of dose where necessary. The cumulative pregnancy rate in ovulatory women with CC in 6 to 12 months of treatment is around 70%,[86] with conception rates per cycle around 22%.[84]

Why do some women who become ovulatory with CC not conceive? Reasons include patient selection, the regimen used, and the presence of other causes of subfertility. The anti-estrogenic effects of CC on the reproductive tract have been particularly implicated. Negative effects on tubal transport, quantity and quality of cervical mucus,[26] and the endometrium[88] have all been reported.

Miscarriage rates of 13% to 25% are reported. Although these numbers appear high, they are similar to the spontaneous miscarriage rate[89] and those observed in infertile women undergoing IVF. In general, it does not appear that the miscarriage rate is significantly increased in anovulatory women treated with CC.

Side Effects and Complications. Apart from hot flushes, which may occur in up to 10% of women taking CC, side effects are rare. Nausea, vomiting, mild skin reactions, breast tenderness, dizziness, and reversible hair loss have been reported, but less than 2% of women are affected. The mydriatic action of CC may cause reversible blurred vision in a similar number.[24]

The multiple pregnancy rate is less than 10%, and OHSS is rare.[84] The putative increased risk of ovarian cancer reported to be associated with the use of CC for more than 12 months[90] has led CC to be licensed for just 6 months of use in some countries.

Tamoxifen is, like CC, a nonsteroidal selective estrogen receptor modulator (SERM). In contrast to CC, tamoxifen contains only the zu-isomer and appears to be less anti-estrogenic at the uterine level. The possible advantages of tamoxifen over CC include an agonistic effect at the endometrium. Many uncontrolled studies in the area of ovulation induction have suggested that tamoxifen may be a safe and efficacious alternative to CC. A meta-analysis of four randomized controlled studies revealed tamoxifen to be as effective as CC in inducing ovulation. However, despite the theoretical benefits, no significant improvement in pregnancy rates was observed compared with CC.[91] Clinicians should therefore base their choice of treatment on familiarity with the given regimen.

Insulin-Sensitizing Agents

Background. The role of insulin-resistance in the pathogenesis of ovarian dysfunction in many PCOS patients has led to the introduction of insulin-sensitizing agents as adjuvant or sole treatment regimens for the induction of ovulation. The most extensively studied insulin-sensitizing drug in the treatment of anovulation is metformin. Metformin (dimethylbiguanide) is an orally administered drug used to lower blood glucose concentrations in patients with non-insulin-dependent diabetes mellitus (NIDDM).[92] It is antihyperglycemic in action, and increases sensitivity to insulin by inhibiting hepatic glucose production and by increasing glucose uptake and utilization in muscle. These actions result in reduced insulin resistance, lower insulin secretion, and reduced serum insulin levels.

Many papers have been published in recent years advocating the clinical usefulness of this compound for ovulation induction. The absence of well designed and properly powered studies did not dampen enthusiasm for metformin in this context, and it has been widely introduced into clinical practice. Recently, however, two large, placebo-controlled randomized studies comparing metformin to CC and metformin as adjunctive therapy to CC have shown no benefit of metformin.[87,93]

Preparations and Regimens. The first studies reporting the use of metformin as an ovulation induction agent suggested that metformin improved insulin sensitivity; lowered LH and total and free testosterone concentrations; and increased FSH and sex hormone–binding globulin levels.[94,95] This, and subsequent uncontrolled studies, indicated that correction of hyperinsulinemia has a beneficial effect in anovulatory women, by increasing menstrual cyclicity, improving spontaneous ovulation, and thus promoting fertility.[94,96,97] It is recommended that metformin be commenced at 500 mg/day orally, rising to 500 mg three times a day over 7 to 10 days.[96] Depending on response, this may be increased to 1000 mg twice a day. The optimal duration of treatment remains unclear. However, most studies reporting a beneficial effect from metformin have shown this within 2 to 4 months.[98,99] Given the side effects of metformin (see later discussion), should the patient remain anovulatory, it is recommended by some that alternative therapy be instituted after 3 months.[98] In those who respond to treatment, metformin should be continued for 6 to 12 months once ovulatory cycles are established.

Clinical Outcome. The majority of studies on the outcome following metformin therapy are small and uncontrolled or simply case series.[100] Most of the available data on restoration of menses following metformin therapy are on predominantly obese hyperinsulinemic women with PCOS. Similarly, studies of the ability of metformin to induce ovulation have been primarily carried out in obese women. In a meta-analysis of 15 studies involving 543 participants with PCOS, metformin was found to be effective in achieving ovulation with odds ratios of 3.88 (CI 2.25-6.69) for metformin versus placebo and 4.41 (CI 2.37-8.22) for metformin and clomiphene versus clomiphene alone.[101] Metformin was also shown to have a significant effect on pregnancy rates in combination with clomiphene (OR 4.4, CI 1.96-9.85). This meta-analysis suggested that women with PCOS who failed to ovulate with CC should receive combination therapy with metformin ahead of moving to gonadotropin therapy, particularly obese women. However, a recent large multicenter study has clarified the role of metformin as an alternative first-line ovulation induction agent in women with PCOS.[87] In this study, 626 women with PCOS were randomized to receive 50 to 150 mg CC plus placebo from cycle day 3 to 7, 500 to 2000 mg daily doses of extended release metformin plus placebo, or a combination of metformin and CC. Treatment was continued for up to 6 months. Obesity was not an exclusion criterion. The results of this study are summarized in Figure 28-8. The primary end point of live birth rate was 22.5% after treatment with CC, compared with a significantly lower rate of just 7.2% following metformin treatment. Combination therapy with both metformin and CC yielded a live birth rate of 26.8%, which did not differ significantly from that achieved with CC treatment alone. The relatively poor performance of metformin in terms of live birth rates was partly explained by a low conception rate, which was just 21.7% following metformin, compared with 39.5% in the CC group. In terms of ovulation rates alone, the combination of metformin and CC was superior to either individual therapy. However, in a study of 228 women randomized to receive CC plus metformin or CC plus placebo, no significant difference in ovulation rates was observed (64% versus 72%, respectively).[93] A significantly larger proportion of women in the metformin group discontinued treatment because of side effects (16% versus 5%).

It has been suggested that metformin may reduce the rate of miscarriage compared with CC-derived pregnancies. However, in the study of Legro et al., the rate of first trimester loss did not differ significantly between the treatment groups, although the study was not powered to detect this.[87] Regarding side effects, gastrointestinal complaints were more common in those receiving metformin. However, no multiple pregnancies arose after metformin treatment, compared with a 6% twinning rate following CC. Metformin was also shown to have a positive effect on

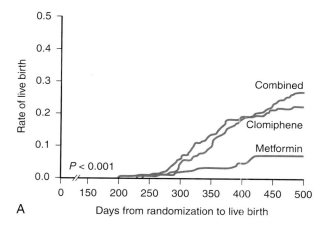

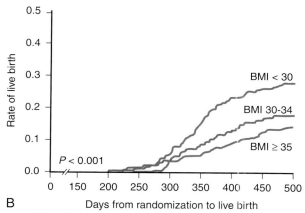

Figure 28-8. *Kaplan-Meier curves for live births following ovulation induction with clomiphene, metformin, or both treatments combined (A) and body mass index (BMI) (B). (From Legro RS, Barnhart HX, Schlaff WD, et al. Clomiphene, metformin, or both for infertility in the polycystic ovary syndrome. N Engl J Med 356:551-566, 2007.)*

insulin sensitivity and BMI. However, these benefits were not translated into higher pregnancy rates.

Since women with WHO type 2 anovulatory infertility frequently demonstrate a hyper-response to FSH, it has been proposed that metformin may also have an adjuvant role to gonadotropin ovulation induction by correcting hypersinsulinemia and reducing hyperandrogenism, and hence normalizing the response of the patient to gonadotropin stimulation.[96] In a study of CC-resistant women with PCOS who were randomized to pretreatment with metformin or no pretreatment prior to ovulation induction with FSH, the incidence of multiple follicular development was reduced in those receiving metformin beforehand.[102] In a randomized trial comparing metformin co-administration versus placebo during rFSH treatment in 32 CC-resistant women with PCOS no differences were observed in indices of insulin sensitivity or ovarian response during rFSH treatment.[103] In another similar randomized study, metformin co-administration was observed to normalize the endocrine profile and increase the rate of monofollicular cycles.[104] More adequately powered studies are now required to further elucidate the role of metformin as an adjunctive therapy to ovulation induction with gonadotropins.

Metformin therapy has also been proposed to aid weight loss in obese women with PCOS. Many studies have now examined the effect of metformin on BMI, and the evidence is conflicting. However, the majority of observational studies addressing weight loss with metformin have revealed a reduction in the BMI of 1% to 4.3%.[98] More recently, a double-blinded randomized trial compared metformin 850 mg twice daily treatment with placebo in 143 PCOS women with a BMI greater than 30. After 6 months' treatment no significant difference in weight loss or menstrual frequency was observed.[105] In contrast, lifestyle modification was to improve cycle regularity by improving weight loss.

Attention has turned in recent years to the possible benefits and safety of metformin administration during pregnancy. PCOS pregnancies demonstrate a greater incidence of perinatal and maternal complications such as gestational diabetes, preeclampsia, and premature delivery[106] (Box 28-1. A number of studies have appeared suggesting a role for metformin to ameliorate these complications. However, most of these studies are not randomized or suffer from small numbers and surrogate outcomes. Although metformin crosses the placenta, there is no clear evidence of toxicity when taken during pregnancy.[84] Larger well-designed studies are still required to address the possible therapeutic benefits of metformin during pregnancy in women with PCOS.

Side Effects and Complications. Metformin has been used for many years for the treatment of diabetic patients and appears to be safe for long-term use, with few side effects reported. Rarely, lactic acidosis may occur[96] if hepatic or renal disease is present, and these patients should be excluded before commencing therapy. The main side effects of metformin are nausea and diarrhea, which may occur in 10% to 25% of patients and contribute to the weight loss effects observed with metformin. If these symptoms persist despite lowering the dose, alternative therapy should be

given. For this reason, metformin should be started at a low dose that gradually rises (see earlier discussion).

Gonadotropins

Background. Women with WHO class 2 anovulation who fail to ovulate or conceive following ovulation induction with anti-estrogens can be successfully treated with exogenous gonadotropins. Exogenous gonadotropins have been widely used for the treatment of anovulatory infertile women since 1958.[2,23] Improvements in purification techniques led to increasing relative amounts of the active ingredients and the first urine-derived preparation containing only FSH (uFSH) became available in 1983. The development and application of production techniques based on immunoaffinity chromatography with monoclonal antibodies enabled the production of highly purified uFSH. In the 1980s, recombinant DNA technology led to the development and, later, the clinical introduction of human recombinant FSH (recFSH). This advance promised not only unlimited availability, but improved purity and batch-to-batch consistency compared to urinary derived products.

The development of recombinant gonadotropins also provided the opportunity to elucidate more clearly the physiology of ovarian E_2 synthesis. During further follicular development, LH has a synergistic action with FSH. Theca cells are stimulated by LH to convert cholesterol into androstenedione (AD) and testosterone (T) by cytochrome P450 side chain cleavage oxidases and 3β-hydroxysteroid dehydrogenase. Aromatase activity in the granulosa cells is induced by FSH and converts AD and T into estrone and E_2. The involvement of two cell types (granulosa and theca cells) and two hormones (LH and FSH) to produce estrogens from cholesterol has led to the concept of the "two cell, two gonadotropin" theory. In addition to stimulating aromatase activity, FSH also induces LH receptors and further increases FSH receptor formation while stimulating DNA and protein synthesis by the cell.[107] Clinical observations in the treatment of anovulatory women have supported this concept.

In the treatment of WHO class 1 (hypogonadotropic hypogonadal) anovulation, women with intact pituitary function can be treated with pulsatile GnRH therapy to restore the periodic release of FSH and LH. The treatment of hypogonadotropic women with FSH alone leads to follicular development but not pregnancy.[16] Exogenous LH is therefore required to treat this form of anovulatory infertility. Until recently, hMG was the only source of exogenous LH for this group of patients. Now recLH offers the possibility for a more sophisticated and individualized approach to treatment.

Recent studies have demonstrated the safety and appropriate dose required to effect follicle development and subsequent pregnancy. It has been established that resting levels of at least 0.5 to 1 IU should be sufficient to provide maximal stimulation to thecal cells.[108] In a study of hypogonadotropic women undergoing treatment with recFSH and recLH, a dose of 75 IU per day of recLH was observed to result in follicular development and pregnancy. However, further increases in LH levels above the threshold

---

BOX 28-1

Maternal and Perinatal Risks Associated with Polycystic Ovary Syndrome

Maternal
  Gestational diabetes*
  Pregnancy-induced hypertension*
  Preeclampsia
  Delivery by cesarean section
Neonatal
  Admission to a neonatal intensive care unit
  Perinatal mortality
  Premature deliveries

*Outcome confirmed by subgroup analysis of higher validity studies.
From Boomsma CM, Eijkemans MJ, Hughes EG, et al. A meta-analysis of pregnancy outcomes in women with polycystic ovary syndrome. Hum Reprod update 12:673-683, 2006.

level needed to gain a response did not appear to induce a greater degree of ovarian stimulation.[109]

Preparations and Regimens. In addition to urinary derived FSH products, recFSH has been clinically available since 1996 in the form of follitropin alpha and follitropin beta. More recently, a long-acting recFSH, an LH, and an hCG have been added to the clinical arsenal for ovarian stimulation.

In order to achieve development of a single dominant follicle with exogenous gonadotropins, specific treatment and monitoring protocols are needed. The two most frequently encountered in the literature and in clinical practice are the low-dose step-up and, more recently, step-down protocols (Fig. 28-9). The initially described standard step-up protocol had a starting dose of FSH 150 IU/day.[110] However, this regimen was associated with a high complication rate. Multiple pregnancy rates of up to 36% were reported, and ovarian hyperstimulation occurred in up to 14% of treatment cycles.[2] As a result, this protocol has been largely abandoned.

The concept of the FSH threshold proposed by Brown[111] postulated that FSH concentrations must exceed a certain level before follicular development will proceed (see Fig. 28-1). Once this level is reached, normal follicular growth requires only a minor further increase above this threshold. Exposure to excessive FSH serum concentrations may lead to excessive follicular development. This concept formed the theoretical basis for low-dose step-up regimens for ovulation induction. A low-dose, step-up protocol designed to allow the FSH threshold to be reached gradually has now become the most widely used regimen, reducing the risk of excessive stimulation and development of multiple preovulatory follicles. The initial starting dose of FSH is 37.5 to 50 IU/day.[84] The dose is increased by 50% if after 14 days, no response is observed on ultrasonography (and serum estradiol monitoring).[84] The detection of an

ovarian response is an indication to continue the current dose until hCG can be given to trigger ovulation. If equal daily doses of FSH are given from the beginning of the follicular phase, steady-state serum FSH concentrations are reached after 5 to 7 days.[112] During step-up regimens elevated FSH serum concentrations may occur during the late follicular phase which may, in a similar manner, interfere with selection of a single dominant follicle. Previous suppositions that steroid negative feedback remained intact during low-dose step-up regimens have not been substantiated by scientific data.

In contrast to the concept of the FSH threshold on which the low-dose step-up protocol is based, the concept of the FSH "window" stresses the significance of the duration of FSH elevation above the threshold level, rather than the magnitude of elevation of FSH for single dominant selection.[13,113] This concept was substantiated by the demonstration that elevating FSH levels high above the threshold level for a short period of time in the early follicular phase does not increase the number of dominant follicles[114] (Fig. 28-10). Conversely, when the physiologic decrease of FSH in a normal cycle is prevented by administration of FSH in the late follicular phase, the augmented sensitivity for FSH allows several follicles to gain dominance[115] (Fig. 28-11). As demonstrated previously in the monkey model, when the negative feedback effect of estradiol on gonadotropin production is suppressed by administration of anti-estrogens, selection of the preovulatory follicle is overridden.[116] Further studies regarding the process of selection of the dominant follicle in the normal cycle have indicated that throughout the cycle up to 10 nondominant follicles (measuring between 2 and 10 mm in diameter) can be visualized by transvaginal ultrasound. The dominant follicle itself can be identified once it has reached a diameter beyond 9 mm.[9] Endocrine studies have confirmed that E_2 levels in the serum[10] and follicle fluid[21] begin to rise only after a dominant follicle is present. The above-mentioned initial research findings provided the theoretical basis for developing and monitoring a step-down regimen of ovulation induction.

It was subsequently demonstrated that the late follicular phase FSH profile during a step-down regimen closely resembled serum FSH levels in the spontaneous cycle.[117] Moreover, a median daily fall of 5% to 10% in serum FSH levels was observed in women treated with the step-down regimen, and in those treated with a low-dose step-up regimen a reduction was observed in just 39% of treated women.[118] In the majority of women, the FSH levels remained stable in the late follicular phase.

With the aim of rapidly achieving the FSH threshold for stimulating follicle development, step-down regimens normally begin therapy with 150 IU/day, started shortly after a spontaneous or progesterone-induced bleed. This dose is continued until a dominant follicle (≥10 mm) is observed. The dose is then decreased to 112.5 IU/day followed by a further decrease to 75 IU/day 3 days later, which is continued until hCG is administered to induce ovulation.[119] Should no ovarian response be observed after 3 to 5 days, the FSH starting dose should be continued.

For some patients an initial dose of 150 IU/day is too high, reflecting major individual differences in the FSH

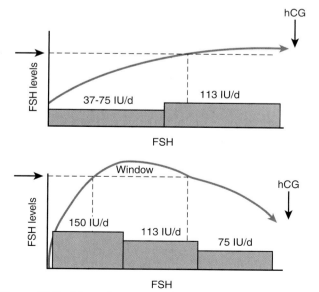

Figure 28-9. *Schematic representation of serum follicle-stimulating hormone (FSH) levels and daily dose of exogenous FSH during low-dose step-up or step-down regimens for ovulation induction.*

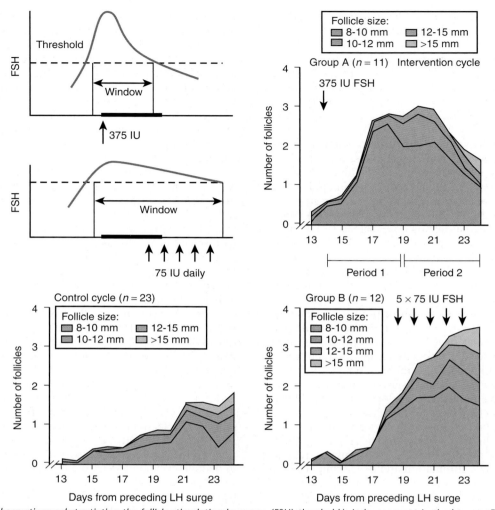

Figure 28-10. *Observations substantiating the follicle-stimulating hormone (FSH) threshold/window concept in the human. Differences in follicle growth response in normo-ovulatory women can be observed to be dependent on whether exogenous FSH is administered either as a single bolus during the early follicular phase (top left) or as daily low doses during the mid-late follicular phase. LH, luteinizing hormone. (From Schipper I, Hop WC, Fauser BC. The follicle-stimulating hormone [FSH] threshold/window concept examined by different interventions with exogenous FSH during the follicular phase of the normal menstrual cycle: duration, rather than magnitude, of FSH increase affects follicle development. J Clin Endocrinol Metab 83:1292-1298, 1998.)*

threshold. The appropriate starting dose may be determined by using the low-dose step-up regimen for the first treatment cycle in order to assess the individual FSH response dose.[120] Patients who demonstrate good follicular growth with a fixed regimen of 75 IU/day, (the "good responders" who might have been at risk of OHSS with the normal starting dose of the step-down regimen) can thus be identified. Conversely, those who do not respond with ongoing follicle growth to the initial dose should have the daily dosage increased. The second cycle may then be initiated as a step-down regimen with a starting dose 37.5 IU above the effective dose in the preceding low-dose step-up cycle.[119]

Experience to date has indicated that the major drawback of the step-down regimen is the risk that the initial starting dose is too high for some patients. In an effort to overcome this problem, sequential low-dose step-up and step-down regimens have been proposed.[121] Starting with a step-up regimen, the FSH dose is reduced when the leading follicle has reached 14 mm diameter. Comparisons with

a group treated with a low-dose step-up regimen showed the incidence of monofollicular cycles to be similar. This approach requires further evaluation and the problem of the large individual variability in the dose of exogenous FSH required for monofollicular development remains to be properly addressed.

Clinical Outcomes. In what remains one of the largest series describing outcomes using the low-dose step-up regimen, 225 women with PCOS, with ovulation and pregnancy rates of 72% and 45%, respectively, were reported.[122] Studies focusing on further reducing the starting dose have reported the feasibility of commencing with 50 IU or 37.5 IU.[119]

In a randomized trial comparing outcomes following the low-dose step-up versus step-down protocol, the clinical benefits of a more physiologic means of stimulating follicle development were reflected in an incidence of monofollicular cycles of 88% compared to 56% observed in women

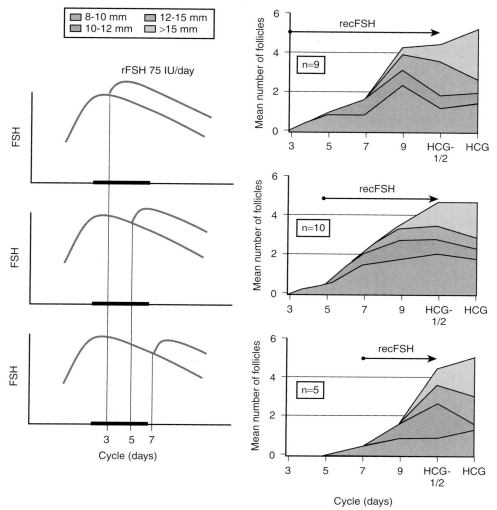

Figure 28-11. *Observations substantiating the follicle-stimulating hormone (FSH) window concept in the human. Multiple dominant follicle growth can be observed in normo-ovulatory women receiving daily low doses of exogenous FSH, starting on cycle day 3, 5, or 7. (From Hohmann FP, Laven JS, de Jong FH, et al. Low dose exogenous FSH initiated during the early, mid or late follicular phase can induce multiple dominant follicle development. Hum Reprod 16:846-854, 2001.)*

treated with the step-up regimen, presumably reducing the risk of multiple pregnancy and hyperstimulation[118] (Table 28-2). Potential health and economic benefits were also apparent because those treated with the step-down regimen required a mean duration of treatment of just 9 days, as opposed to 18 days in women treated with the low-dose step-up regimen.

A multicenter randomized study comparing the step-up versus step-down protocol using recFSH reported a shorter duration of stimulation when the step-down protocol was used.[123] The cumulative rate of clinical gestations did not differ between the two groups, but in contrast to the findings of an earlier single-center study,[118] the step-up protocol was associated with a higher rate of monofollicular development and a lower rate of ovarian hyperstimulation (see Table 28-2). These differences may reflect the necessity for increased skill and care in monitoring step-down stimulation cycles, which is easier to ensure in a single-center setting. Largely for this reason, low-dose step-up protocols remain the most widely used approach.

The degree to which the type of FSH compound employed may influence outcomes in ovulation induction continues to be subject of some controversy. Two meta-analyses comparing the effectiveness of daily uFSH to daily hMG for inducing ovulation in women with PCOS who had not responded to CC demonstrated no difference in pregnancy rate per treatment cycle. However, the women given FSH were less likely to have moderately severe or severe ovarian hyperstimulation syndrome.[50] The total dose of recFSH needed and duration of treatment was less, and the complication rates were similar. In a later meta-analysis of randomized controlled trials comparing recFSH with uFSH for ovulation induction in women with CC-resistant PCOS, no significant differences were demonstrated for the ovulation rate (OR 1.19, 95% CI 0.78-1.8). Furthermore, the odds ratios for pregnancy rate (0.95, 95% CI 0.64-1.41), miscarriage rate (1.26, 95% CI 0.59-2.7), multiple pregnancy rate (0.44, 95% CI 0.16-1.21), and ovarian hyperstimulation syndrome (1.55, 95% CI 0.5-4.84) showed no significant difference between recFSH and uFSH.[124] In terms of

TABLE 28-2

Comparison of Ovarian Response and Clinical Outcome Following the Low-Dose Step-Up and the Step-Down Regimens for Gonadotropin Induction of Ovulation

	Low-Dose Step-Up			Step-Down	
Response and Outcome	Hamilton (1991)	Hull (1991)	Christin-Maitre (2003)	Christin-Maitre (2003)	van Santbrink (1995)
Number of patients	100	144	44	39	82
Number of cycles	401	459	85	72	234
Duration treatment (days)	14	NR	15	10	11
Ampules per cycle	19	NR	13	13	14
Ovulation rate (%)	72	74	70	61	91
Monofollicular cycles					
% of ovulatory cycles	73	NR	77	35	62
% of all started cycles	55	NR	68	32	56
Pregnancy rate (%)					
Per started cycle	11	11	19	16	16
Per ovulatory cycle	16	15	NR	NR	17
Cumulative pregnancy rate (%)	55	NR	37	31	47
Multiple pregnancy rate (%)	4	11	12	25	8
Ongoing singleton pregnancy rate (%)	7	10	NR	NR	12
Ovarian hyperstimulation syndrome rate (%)	1	NR	2	11	2

NR, not recorded.

cost-effectiveness, a recent randomized study showed that a lower total dose of recFSH than highly purified urinary FSH was required to achieve the same outcomes. This translated into a 9.4% cost reduction in favor of recFSH.[125]

The success in early clinical studies of pure FSH preparations, increasingly devoid of LH, has served to enhance the impression that excess LH is detrimental to oocyte development and chances of pregnancy following therapeutic intervention. However, a number of recent clinical studies, together with an increasing understanding of the function played by LH in oocyte maturation, have begun to redefine the role of LH as a therapeutic agent in anovulatory fertility. In normogonadotropic anovulation, endogenous LH does not normally require supplementation. Indeed, the focus on LH in this group of patients has been primarily directed at reducing the potential detrimental effects associated with excessive LH.[126] More recently, however, the demonstration of the importance of late follicular LH in optimizing dominant follicle development oocyte quality has reopened the debate as to the role of LH in ovulation induction.[18] Supplementation of LH activity may offer advantages in some patients by hastening large follicle development and therefore shortening the duration of treatment.[127] Moreover, the work of Zeleznik and co-workers[17] referred to a potential therapeutic role for LH in effecting monofollicular stimulation as part of a sequential ovarian stimulation protocol following initiation with recFSH. This concept has been supported in a study in which anovulatory women with a hyper-reponse to recFSH were randomized to continue treatment with the addition of either placebo or recLH.[128] In those in whom LH was administered, a trend toward fewer preovulatory follicles was observed. As the availability of recombinant gonadotropins leads to increasing knowledge of the processes of

follicular development and selection, further refinements in the efficacy and safety of ovulation induction are likely.

Adverse Effects and Complications. The complications of ovulation induction with gonadotropins are primarily related to excessive ovarian stimulation. Although the aim of therapy is monofollicular growth, multiple follicular developments may occur, causing symptoms of OHSS. Moreover, the development of multiple follicles raises the real risk of multiple pregnancies. In order to increase the chance of therapeutic success and reduce the risks of complications, careful monitoring of treatment is required. Ovarian response to gonadotropin therapy is monitored using ultrasound to measure follicular diameter. The scans, usually performed every 2 or 4 days, should be focused on identifying follicles of intermediate size; hCG (5000-10,000 IU subcutaneously or intramuscularly) is given on the day that at least one follicle measures more than 18 mm. If more than three follicles larger than 15 mm are present, stimulation should be stopped, hCG withheld, and use of a barrier contraceptive advised in order to prevent multiple pregnancies and OHSS. Measurements of serum E_2 may also be useful.[119] Ovarian stimulation with gonadotropins has not been shown to be associated with long-term risks. Urinary derived FSH is associated with a theoretical risk of transmission of prion proteins. However, the risk of infection is considered to be minimal and not in itself a reason to prescribe recFSH over uFSH.[129]

Pulsatile GnRH

In the normo-ovulatory woman, the pattern of GnRH pulse stimulation alters with the phase of the menstrual cycle, effecting differential gonadotropin synthesis and secretion.[130]

During the luteal-follicular transition, pulses occur every 90 to 120 minutes. This slow pulse frequency, in the presence of low E_2 and inhibin A levels, favors FSH production. In the mid- or late follicular phase GnRH frequency increases, favoring LH secretion.[131] In the luteal phase, the production of progesterone increases hypothalamic opioid activity, thus slowing GnRH pulse secretion. This again favors FSH secretion in the luteofollicular transition.

The application of pulsatile GnRH therapy has been demonstrated to be an effective reliable and safe alternative to gonadotropin therapy for treating this form of anovulation.[132] Due to the intact ovarian-pituitary feedback system during pulsatile GnRH treatment, the resulting serum FSH and LH concentrations remain within the normal range and the chances of multifollicular development and ovarian hyperstimulation are therefore low. Little ovarian response monitoring is therefore needed during treatment.

The intravenous route appears superior to the subcutaneous route.[133] In order to mimic the normal pulsatile release of GnRH, a pulse interval of 60 to 90 minutes is used with a dose of 2.5 to 10 μg per pulse.[133] The lower dose should be used initially in order to minimize the likelihood of multiple pregnancies.[134] The dose should then be increased to the minimum dose required to induce ovulation. Pulsatile GnRH administration may be continued throughout the luteal phase until menses or a positive pregnancy test. Alternatively, it may be discontinued after ovulation, and the corpus luteum supported by hCG.[43]

Clinical Outcomes. Pulsatile GnRH administration is primarily indicated for women with hypogonadotropic hypogonadal anovulation (WHO class 1) who have normal pituitary function.[135] In these patients cumulative pregnancy rates of 83% to 95% after six cycles have been reported, with multiple pregnancies accounting for 3% to 8% of pregnancies.[134,136] Lower ovulation and pregnancy rates have been observed in women with WHO type 2 anovulation, including PCOS.[137] This may be because anovulation in PCOS in part reflects the effects of a persistant, rapid frequency of GnRH stimulation of the pituitary, causing increased LH and T levels.[131] In a recent meta-analysis of four trials comparing pulsatile GnRH with gonadotropins for ovulation induction in women with PCOS, the small size and short follow-up of the studies meant that the authors were unable to draw conclusions on their relative effectiveness.[138]

Regular menstruation occurring approximately every 4 weeks indicates that the woman is having ovulatory cycles. Ultrasonography and measurements of serum progesterone are not usually needed for monitoring therapy. Local complications such as phlebitis may occasionally be encountered when intravenous administration is used. To avoid this, pulsatile GnRH can be administered subcutaneously. This route is certainly simpler than the intravenous approach. However, pharmakinetic studies comparing the two routes have shown that the plasma GnRH profiles are damped after subcutaneous administration, and that bioavailability is reduced.[139] However, the increased convenience offered by the subcutaneous route has led to this approach being in favored by many.

Aromatase Inhibitors

In recent years the concept of using aromatase inhibitors to mimic the action of CC has been proposed.[140] Rather than antagonizing estrogen feedback activity at the hypothalamic-pituitary axis, this approach aims at reducing the amount of estogens being synthesized. Aromatase inhibitors block the conversion of AD and T to estriol (E_3) and estrodiol (E_2), respectively.[141] This increases gonadotropin secretion, resulting in stimulation of ovarian follicles.[140] Aromatase inhibitors have been in clinical use for more than 20 years, primarily in the treatment of postmenopausal patients with advanced breast cancer. The more recently developed third generation of aromatase inhibitors are characterized by their potency in inhibiting the aromatase enzyme without significantly inhibiting inhibition of other steroidogenesis enzymes. One of the third generation compounds, letrazole, has been the focus of study as a potential therapeutic agent for inducing ovulation.

Clinical Outcomes. When given in the early follicular phase, letrozole reduces estrogenic feedback at the pituitary-hypothalamic axis, causing a subsequent increase in gonadotropin secretion. This was shown in monkeys to stimulate follicle development.[142] Subsequent small clinical studies employing a dose of 2.5 mg/day from day 3 to day 7 of the menstrual cycle have suggested that it may be an effective ovulatory agent in CC-resistant women.[140] A local effect at the ovary to increase sensitivity to FSH by blocking the conversions of androgens to estrogens has also been proposed, because accumulating intraovarian androgens may increase FSH receptor gene expression.[143] On the other hand, significantly increased intraovarian androgen/estrogen ratios may also induce follicle atresia.

Although the concept of applying aromatase inhibitors as an alternative to CC or as adjuvant therapy to CC or gonadotropins is attractive, and preliminary data on pregnancy outcome were encouraging,[140,144] adequately powered comparative controlled randomized studies are still awaited.

Adverse Effects and Complications. Although letrozole has a half-life that allows rapid disappearance following cessation of treatment in the midfollicular phase, the possible effects of this drug on ensuing pregnancy remain to be clarified. The performance of further clinical studies has been inhibited because an association was reported between letrozole and fetal toxicity. However, a recent analysis of outcomes in 911 newborns following conceived by CC or letrozole showed no difference in the overall rates of major and minor congenital malformations.[145] In the absence of sufficiently powered, randomized controlled trials establishing efficacy and safety, the routine clinical use of aromatase inhibitors is not advocated.[84]

Opioid Antagonists

Background. Endogenous opioid peptides have been shown to play an important role in regulating the pulsatile secretion of gonadotropins by inhibiting the hypothalamic pulse generator that directs GnRH secretion.[146] Infusion of the opiate receptor antagonist naloxone was shown to increase serum LH levels when administered during the late follicular and luteal phase of the cycle.[147]

Clinical Outcomes. Several groups have used naltrexone, an orally active opioid receptor antagonist, to treat ovulatory disorders, with varying degrees of success. The earlier observation that gonadal steroids enhance opioid modulation of gonadotropin secretion was postulated to explain the inability of two groups to demonstrate an increase in gonadotropin secretion or resumption of ovulation in women with WHO class 1 anovulation.[148] However, others have observed restoration of the menstrual cycle.[149] In an uncontrolled study, 19 of 22 women with CC-resistant anovulation were observed to become ovulatory under naltrexone treatment (sometimes in combination with CC), with 12 conceiving.[150] Treatment with 25 mg twice daily was commenced on the first day of a spontaneous or progesterone-induced cycle and continued until a positive pregnancy test occurred or, if no response was observed, for 21 days of treatment. Others have employed doses of up to 100 mg/day.[151] Conclusions as to the efficacy, optimal regimen, and safety of opiate antagonists for inducing ovulation cannot yet be made, however. No randomized controlled studies demonstrating their value for this condition have yet been published, and opiate anatagonists remain at best second-line, alternative therapy.

Dopamine Agonists

These agents are primarily used in the treatment of anovulation secondary to hyperprolactinemia. The treatment of hyperprolactinemia and the agents available for treatment are covered in detail elsewhere (see Chapter 3).

ADJUNCTIVE THERAPIES

Dexamethasone

Glucocorticoids have been proposed as a useful adjuvant to both CC and gonadotropin ovulation induction in women with PCOS with a therapeutic rationale based on reducing ovarian androgen levels, improving ovulatory function, and reducing resistance to ovulation induction agents.[152] Although the source of high androgen secretion in anovulatory women with PCOS is primarily ovarian, 50% to 70% also demonstrate excessive adrenal androgen levels.[152]

In order to normalize (without suppressing) adrenal steroid production, daily oral doses of dexamethasone (0.25-0.5 mg) or prednisone (5-10 mg) have been employed in a continuous regimen. Although widely used, the value of adjuvant corticosteroid administration with CC or gonadotropins for ovulation induction remains uncertain. In a study of women with PCOS, the chance of ovulation after glucocorticoid suppression of adrenal androgens was not predicted by either basal DHEAS (dehydroepiandrosterone sulfate) levels or suppressed levels, and limited effects on ovulation were observed.[153] A randomized controlled study in 80 women with CC resistance and normal

serum DHEAS levels showed significantly higher ovulation and pregnancy rates when 2 mg/day dexamethasone was added from cycle day 2 to 12 to CC 100 mg.[154]

While major complications from the adjuvant use of low-dose glucocorticoids are rare, weight gain is a common problem. Other reported side effects include glucose intolerance and osteoporosis. Given possible side effects, their use should remain as a second-line therapy subject to further research.

Gonadotropin-Releasing Hormone Agonists

Adjuvant GnRH agonist treatment has also been proposed to improve outcomes and reduce complications of ovulation induction. Early uncontrolled studies indicated that the concomitant use of GnRH agonist with ovarian stimulation regimens in women with PCOS was safe and improved treatment outcome.[155] Further studies indicated that premature luteinization could be prevented by employing GnRH agonists, but no clear difference in pregnancy rates was demonstrated.[156] Although, a meta-analysis of five prospective studies[157] suggested that improved pregnancy rates could be achieved at similar ovulation rates when GnRH agonists were also employed, a later systematic review concluded that GnRH agonist as an adjunct to FSH/hMG does not improve pregnancy and OHSS rates, and should therefore not be recommended as a standard treatment for this patient group.[158]

Conflicting data on the effects on ovulation and pregnancy rates, combined with reports of severe OHSS with adjuvent GnRH agonist therapy and the additional burden for the patient of prolonged treatment cycles, mean that adjuvant GnRH agonists remain a second-line therapy in conjunction with FSH stimulation.

The availability of GnRH antagonists provides new opportunities to modify ovulation induction regimens. Particular attributes of GnRH antagonists which might be of value in this context include their competitive binding properties, immediate suppression of the pituitary without a flare-up effect, and rapid resumption of gonadal function on discontinuation. However, few studies have appeared which further explore its role in this clinical context.

ADDITIONAL TREATABLE FACTORS INFLUENCING THE BALANCE OF EFFICACY AND RISKS

Obesity

Among women with WHO class 2 anovulation, obesity may be present in up to 50%. In addition to enhancing the features of insulin resistance mentioned earlier, overweight (BMI > 32) is also associated with reproductive dysfunction, despite regular menstrual cycles.[159] In recent years, considerable attention has been given to the role of lifestyle factors and management in improving outcomes in obese anovulatory women. Even a small (2% to 5%) reduction in weight has been shown to improve metabolic indices including insulin resistance.[160] In addition, weight loss can lead to a rise in sex hormone–binding globulin (SHBG) concentrations, a decrease in FAI and T levels, and improvement in cyclicity.[161-163] A relatively modest reduction in weight has been shown to increase the frequency of ovulation in obese anovulatory women to more than 70%.[164] Energy restriction acting to temporarily improve insulin senstivity may be important,[163] because improvements in endocrine and clinical parameters occurred maximally during the period of energy restriction. During subsequent weight maintenance, many benefits were reversed.[163]

The evidence for the benefits of weight loss, combined with recent data confirming BMI to be a major factor influencing outcome of ovulation induction,[165] make the treatment of obesity an important adjuvant treatment that should precede ovulation induction.[84] Given the baseline risks of ovulation induction, and the possible risks of obesity for subsequent pregnancy and general health, weight loss in cases of obesity should be considered as a prerequisite to medical ovulation induction treatment.[166-168]

Tobacco Smoking

Epidemiologic data provide strong evidence for a causal association between cigarette smoking and decreased fertility. For a recent review of the impact of smoking and other lifestyle factors on fertility treatment outcomes, see Homan et al.[168] Dose-dependent effects of smoking have been reported in relation to the duration to conception.[169] Moreover, there is evidence of increased risk of early pregnancy loss in smokers[170] and a reduced mean age at menopause.[171] Although properly designed studies of the effect of smoking on outcomes of ovulation induction are scarce, data from studies in assisted conception point to detrimental effects on ovarian function and oocyte quality, which are likely to be applicable to the situation concerning ovulation induction.[172] In any discussion of infertility therapy, the clinician should emphasize the risks of smoking for outcome of treatment. Indeed, preconceptional care and lifestyle advice should be an integral part of the modern fertility clinic.[168]

Ovarian Stimulation in the Empirical Treatment of Unexplained Infertility

PRINCIPLES OF OVARIAN STIMULATION

The aim of ovarian stimulation is to intervene in the mechanisms regulating single dominant follicle selection in order to mature multiple follicles and obtain multiple oocytes for fertilization in vivo (either after timed intercourse or IUI) or in vitro (IVF). Ovarian stimulation is usually performed in normo-ovulatory infertile women in order to increase chances for pregnancy. However, the development of multiple follicles inherently also increases the undesired risk of (higher order) multiple pregnancies and OHSS. In IVF OHSS risks are reduced because of the puncture of all visible large follicles to retrieve the oocytes, and the incidence of multiple pregnancies can be controlled by limiting the number of embryos transferred.

Obviously, oligo/anovulatory women may also qualify for either IUI or IVF after failed ovulation induction.

Hyperstimulation may also be performed in these women, aiming at multiple follicle development. It should again be emphasized that this condition of hyperstimulation in these patients is distinctly different from ovulation induction in which the aim is to mimic physiology and stimulate ongoing growth and ovulation of a single dominant follicle. However, these patients are usually difficult to manage because of an unpredictable major individual variability in response and a tendency to hyper-respond to stimulation protocols.[173]

Although daily administration of ovary stimulating agents allows for dose adjustments based on individual ovarian response monitoring, the clinical evidence for the efficacy of such an approach is scant. A hyper-response may be counteracted by a dose decrease or the complete cessation of exogenous gonadotropins for some days (the latter strategy is referred to as "coasting").[174] An excessive number of follicles for ovulation induction or hyperstimulation for IUI may be reduced by follicle puncture[175] or cycle cancellation. When, in contrast, low ovarian response to standard stimulation is observed, recent evidence indicates that a gonadotropin dose increase does not result in improved outcome.[176] This is not surprising if the pathophysiologic background of low response is taken into consideration. Low response to ovarian hyperstimulation may be the first sign of advanced ovarian aging.[177] Women with a previous low response to hyperstimulation have been shown to enter menopause at an earlier age.[178]

During the normal menstrual cycle the mid-cycle LH surge represents the trigger for inducing final oocyte maturation, the rupture of the follicle and release of the oocyte, and finally luteinization of granulosa and theca cells allowing for the formation of the corpus luteum. As mentioned before, the synchrony of endocrine events inducing the LH surge is disrupted in ovarian hyperstimulation. Therefore, the endogenous LH surge is replaced by an exogenous hCG bolus injection, timed by the visualization of large graafian follicles upon ultrasound. Finally, these follicular phase interventions result in luteal phase abnormalities[179] requiring luteal phase supplementation by either hCG or exogenous progestins.

THERAPEUTIC APPROACHES

Unexplained infertility is usually diagnosed by exclusion, when standard infertility investigation shows no abnormalities. However, no agreement exists with regard to the preferred extent of standard investigation as well as the interpretation and prognostic value of many of these tests. Usually, ovulation is assessed by a mid-luteal phase serum progesterone assay, tubal patency is established by hysterosalpingogram, and male factor infertility excluded by semen analysis. Again, the interpretation of any of these tests is not without difficulty and many clinicians perform additional tests to further explore possible causes of infertility.[53] Hence, the term *unexplained infertility* is notoriously ambiguous and may mean anything in between undiagnosed infertility and normal fertility in which a pregnancy did not occur merely by chance. This may especially be the case in young women who have been attempting to conceive for a relatively short time.[56]

It should be realized that many biologically relevant processes important for obtaining a pregnancy—such as oocyte chromosomal constitution, subtle sperm abnormalities, in vivo conception, embryo transport and nidation, and finally endometrial receptivity—cannot be studied accurately as yet. It is to be expected that with the advancement of our understanding of these processes, the percentage of couples diagnosed with unexplained infertility, and therefore potential need for empirical ovarian hyperstimulation, will decrease.

When a couple presents with unexplained infertility, it is extremely important to assess chances of spontaneous pregnancy before commencing on any kind of empirical therapy. As mentioned before, ovarian hyperstimulation (with or without additional interventions such as IUI) may enhance pregnancy chances per cycle, but at the cost of patient stress and discomfort, chances for side effects such as multiple gestation and OHSS, and high costs[180,181] (see also Fig. 28-5). Similar cumulative pregnancy rates may be achieved with expectant management for 6 to 12 months.[56] Expectant management may represent the most favorable approach in young women with a short duration of infertility.

Results are frequently reported from combined interventions such as ovarian hyperstimulation and IUI. These studies are often uncontrolled, and few are sufficiently powered to differentiate between the independent effects of hyperstimulation and IUI and the potential additive effects of combining both interventions. In recent years, the picture has become clearer. Although the absolute treatment effect appears relatively limited, given the low cost and ease of administration, CC can be recommended as first choice medication for the treatment of unexplained infertility. In terms of pure efficacy, however, a meta-analysis of five trials indicated that gonadotropins may be superior to CC as ovarian stimulation agents for the treatment of unexplained infertility.[182] Treatment with CC was associated with significantly reduced odds ratios of pregnancy per woman compared to gonadotropins (OR 0.41; 95% CI 0.17-0.8). As far as complications are concerned, no significant differences could be found for miscarriage (OR 0.61; 95% CI 0.09-4) or multiple birth (OR 1.1; 95% CI 0.2-7). The incidence of OHSS or cycle cancellation rates could not be assessed.

For unexplained infertility, the combination of IUI with ovarian hyperstimulation potentially bypasses several possible barriers to fertility, including minor sperm abnormalities, sperm-cervical mucus interactions, timing of sperm delivery problems, and a possible beneficial effect of ovarian stimulation on endometrial receptivity. The most important benefit is likely to be the stimulation of multiple follicles. Although a meta-analysis by Hughes[183] has addressed questions relating to the benefits of FSH and IUI alone compared with combined therapy, less than a third of the studies included in the analysis make use of treated control subjects. Moreover, the conclusions that both FSH and IUI improve fecundity are derived from regression analysis and are open to discussion.[59,184] Other studies have indicated that ovarian hyperstimulation with both CC and gonadotropins improve the fecundity rate compared to IUI alone.[59] However, a study comparing intracervical insemination alone with FSH in combination

with IUI showed a statistically higher pregnancy rate with the latter treatment combination.[55] The number needed to treat was 31 cycles. This implies that it would take 31 cycles of treatment before there would be one more singleton live birth with FSH/IUI than with intracervical insemination alone.[185] The number needed to treat of FSH in combination with IUI in order to obtain an extra pregnancy above that obtained with IUI alone is even greater.[185] When the costs of multiple pregnancies arising from multiple follicle development are taken into account, the cost effectiveness of FSH/IUI combined therapy for this indication may be limited. Cost-effectiveness analyses have led to the conclusion that IUI with or without hyperstimulation should precede IVF.[186] In clinical practice the benefits of ovarian hypertimulation in combination with IUI need to be weighed against the additional discomfort and costs of monitoring applied, often unsuccessfully,[58] to avoid multiple pregnancy. Clearly, more studies are needed to elucidate the optimal approach to treating unexplained infertility, and the role ovarian hyperstimulation should play. Although it is increasingly recognized that treatment success should be defined in terms of cumulative multiple cycles, at present cumulative live birth rates remain poorly reported, and comparisons with expectant management after multiple cycles have not been made.

PREPARATIONS FOR OVARIAN STIMULATION

Clomiphene Citrate

Preparations and Regimens. Daily doses of 50 to 100 mg are applied usually from days 5 until 9[26] and ovulation is triggered by exogenous hCG. Little ovarian response monitoring is required, and luteal support is probably not necessary.

Clinical Outcome. A retrospective analysis of 45 published reports conclude that the adjusted pregnancy rate per initiated cycle is 5.6% for CC alone, versus 8.3% for CC plus IUI compared to an estimated pregnancy rate from expectant management of 1.3%.[187] A meta-analysis on the basis of six randomized trials[188] concluded that CC administration was superior to no treatment, with an odds ratio for clinical pregnancies of 2.4 (95% CI 1.2-4.6) per patient and 2.5 (1.4-4.6) per cycle. As stated before, an earlier meta-analysis[183] indicated an independent significant improvement in pregnancy rates for clomiphene, exogenous FSH, and IUI.

Adverse Effects and Complications. Adverse effects include hot flushes, mood swings, headache, and visual disturbances. The principal complication remains multiple pregnancy, which occurs in around 10% of pregnancies, and a slightly increased chance for OHSS. Long-term use of CC (>12 months) may be associated with a slight increase in the risk of ovarian epithelial cancer.[90]

Gonadotropins

Preparations and Regimens. Usually exogenous gonadotropin administration is started around cycle day 3 to 5 at daily doses of 75 to 225 IU for several days in fixed dose regimens. Thereafter, doses may be adjusted on the basis of ovarian response monitoring by ultrasound and or E_2 assays. The therapeutic window for gonadotropins achieving the desired goal (two to three preovulatory follicles) is rather small, and a considerable proportion of treatment cycles are canceled because of hyper-response (and the related increased chance of higher order multiple pregnancy) or because they fail to achieve multiple dominant follicle development. The need for cancellation is highly dependent on the stimulation protocol applied and the rigidity of cancellation criteria applied. This in turn depends on whether higher order multiple pregnancies are considered an acceptable side effect of treatment, or whether this should be seen as a failure of treatment to be prevented at any price. Moreover, premature luteinization during ovarian hyperstimulation for IUI may occur more frequently than generally assumed. This may have a detrimental impact on treatment outcome. Recent studies of GnRH antagonist co-treatment during gonadotropin hyperstimulation have demonstrated a reduced incidence of a premature LH rise but no significant improvement in pregnancy rates.[189] However, this approach renders ovarian stimulation protocols more complicated and expensive, increasing the frequency of hospital visits required for monitoring.

Clinical Outcome. A meta-analysis based on 5214 cycles reported in 22 trials concluded an odds ratio for pregnancies associated with FSH compared to expectant management of 2.35 (95% CI 1.9-2.9).[183] A retrospective analysis based on 45 previous papers concluded a significantly increased pregnancy rate occurred after either hMG alone (7.7%) or hMG plus IUI (17.1%).[187] A subsequent large multicenter study[55] confirmed that ovarian hyperstimulation with gonadotropins and IUI both exhibit an independent additive effect on pregnancy chances. The applied treatment regimen for ovarian hyperstimulation (150 IU/day FSH from cycle day 3 to 7) resulted in high frequency of conception. Overall cumulative pregnancy rates when this was combined with IUI therapy were reported to be 33% within three cycles, but at the price of an unacceptable high multiple pregnancy rate of 20% twins and 10% higher-order multiple pregnancy.[55] Women undergoing combined hyperstimulation and IUI were 1.7 times more likely to achieve a pregnancy in a given cycle compared to those receiving IUI alone. However, only 53% of these pregnancies resulted in a live birth with a substantial number of triplet and quadruplet births, despite the fact that fetal reduction has been applied in some of these women. Indeed, 30% of occurring pregnancies were multiples, including 9% triplets and quadruplets. No information was provided regarding perinatal mortality and morbidity rates.

Adverse Effects and Complications. Those effects relating to gonadotropins in general are discussed earlier. In the context of ovarian stimulation for the treatment of unexplained infertility, we again stress the risk of multiple pregnancy associated with the use of these drugs. The ability of careful monitoring to allow prevention of this complication is limited even in highly skilled hands,[58]

and the decision to employ gonadotropins in the context of treating ovulatory women for unexplained infertility should be preceded by an open and informed discussion with the couple over the risks of treatment and the limitations of monitoring. It is clear that an individual approach is required when addessing these issues, and that there is a need to individualize treatment in order to ensure optimal outcomes.

Ovarian Stimulation for in Vitro Fertilization

THERAPEUTIC APPROACHES

The general aim of ovarian stimulation in this clinical context is to induce the development of multiple dominant follicles in order to be able to retrieve many oocytes to allow for inefficiencies in subsequent fertilization in vitro, embryo culture, and embryo selection for transfer and implantation (Fig. 28-12).[26] Hence, multiple embryos can be transferred in the great majority of patients and often spare embryos can be cryopreserved to allow for subsequent chances of pregnancy without the need for repeated ovarian stimulation and oocyte retrieval.[26] The paradigm of so-called "controlled" ovarian stimulation by high doses of exogenous gonadotropins and GnRH agonist long protocol co-treatment for IVF has constituted the gold standard for clinicians throughout the world since the early 1990s. It appears that large numbers of developing follicles is still considered a useful surrogate marker of successful IVF, whereas its significance in relation to the chance of achieving a pregnancy resulting in a healthy baby born is in doubt.[63,73,190] The ovarian stimulation protocols required to produce a large number of follicles have become extremely complex and costly over the years,[26,46] creating considerable side effects, risks of complications, and the need for intense monitoring of ovarian response.[191]

Physicians appear to be in control of ovarian stimulation owing to their ability to adjust the gonadotropin doses or the type of preparation on the basis of ovarian response monitoring. However, the major individual variability in response is out of the doctor's control and is an extremely important determining factor for both success and complications of IVF treatment.[192] A good ovarian response to standard stimulation indicates normal ovarian function and a good prognosis for successful IVF. A low ovarian response suggests ovarian aging and is therefore associated with poor IVF outcome. A low response can to some extent be predicted by chronological age and endocrine and ultrasound aging parameters assessed before the initiation of treatment, as will be discussed later.[178,193] However, the widely applied approach to increase gonadotropin doses administered in case of insufficient ovarian response has very little scientific foundation.[176] The occurrence of a severe hyper-response comes as a surprise in most cases and therefore cannot be predicted.[49,174] Severe OHSS is induced by hCG and is therefore associated with pregnancy. This can be prevented from happening by refraining from embryo transfer in the cycle at risk and cryopreserving all available embryos for transfer in another cycle.

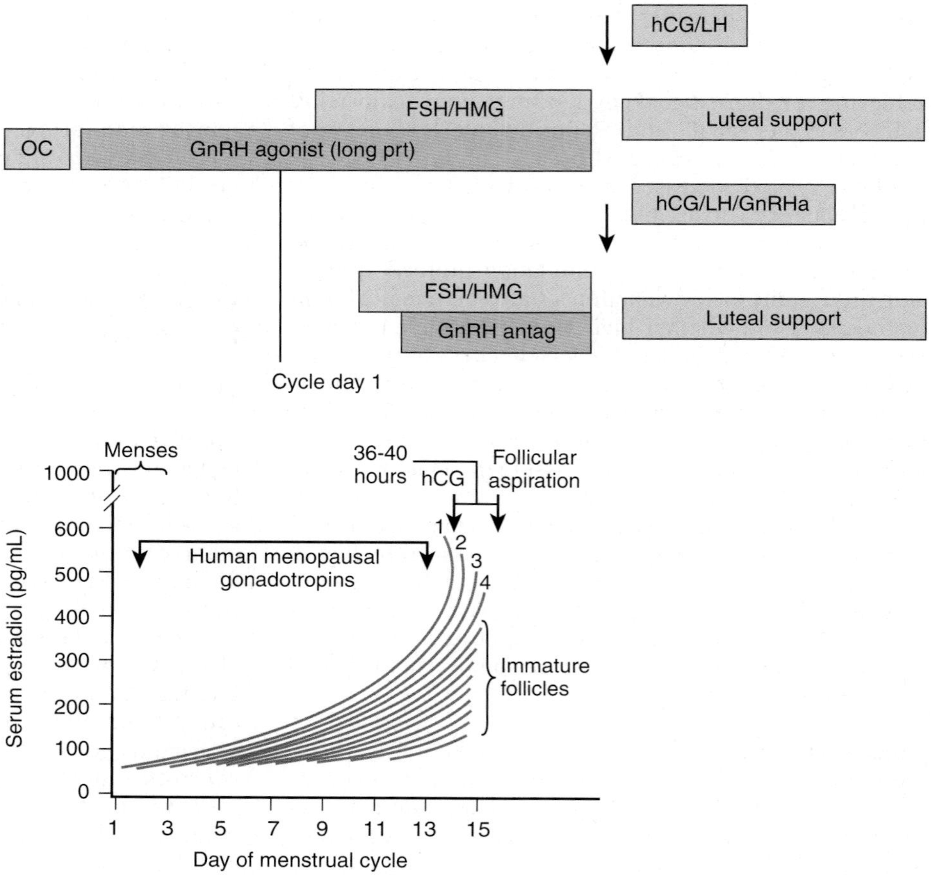

Figure 28-12. Schematic representation of complex medication regimens involved in ovarian hyperstimulation for in vitro fertilization (top), and the heterogeneous cohort of recruited and selected follicles (bottom). antag, antagonist; FSH, follicle-stimulating hormone; GnRH, gonadotropin-releasing hormone; HMG, human menopausal gonadotropin; LH, luteinizing hormone; OC, oral contraceptives; prt, protocol. (Graph from Oehninger S, Hodgen GD. Introduction of ovulation for assisted reproduction programmes. *Baillieres Clin Obstet Gynecol* 4:451-573, 1990.)

Slowly, ovarian stimulation protocols have shifted from the use of hMG to uFSH to recFSH.[194] In recent years several groups have focused on the potential significance of late follicular phase LH levels for clinical IVF outcome. Indeed, it has been shown that dominant follicle development can be stimulated exclusively by LH rather than FSH, opening new possibilities for therapeutic interventions,[18] as discussed in more detail later.

Despite the fact that the first child born after IVF was conceived in a spontaneous menstrual cycle, natural cycle IVF received little attention. The major focus has been the improvement of complex ovarian stimulation regimens. Natural cycle IVF offers major advantages such as negligible complications (arising from multiple pregnancy or OHSS), reduced patient discomfort, and a low cost. The efficacy of natural cycle IVF is hampered, however, by high cancellation rates due to premature ovulation or luteinization. A systematic review of 20 selected studies involving a total of 1800 cycles showed a 7.2% overall pregnancy rate per started cycle, and 16% per embryo transfer.[61] Cumulative pregnancy and live birth rates over four cycles of 42% and 32%, respectively, have been reported.[195] Despite the relatively high failure rate, the approach of natural cycle may still be cost effective. In one study, it was calculated that natural cycle IVF could be offered at 23% of the cost of a stimulated cycle.[195]

More recently a modified natural cycle[196] has been proposed, in which GnRH antagonists are instituted to prevent premature ovulation, and low-dose exogenous gonadotropin co-treatment is given as add-back to prevent a GnRH antagonist induced involution of follicle development. Using this approach, which (like natural cycle IVF) aims to achieve monofollicular development, cumulative pregnancy rates of 44% have been reported over 9 cycles of treatment.[197]

PREPARATIONS

Clomiphene Citrate

Background. After the first baby born following IVF in a natural cycle[33] four normal IVF pregnancies were reported following ovarian stimulation with CC.[29] In subsequent years, many groups reported IVF results following CC, with or without gonadotropin co-treatment.[198] Combined CC/hMG regimens were considered the standard of care before GnRH agonist co-treatment to induce pituitary downregulation came into use. (For a comprehensive historical overview see reference 198.) The advantages of these combined regimens included reduced requirements for hMG and higher luteal phase progesterone levels alleviating the need for luteal phase supplementation.[26] Recent studies have reported clinical outcomes of combined regimens applying CC, gonadotropins, and GnRH antagonist.[26]

CC usually induces the development of at least two follicles, which may sometimes elicit a premature LH rise. By virtue of the fact that CC is therapeutically active through interference with estrogen feedback, this compound cannot be combined with GnRH agonist co-treatment for prevention of a premature LH surge. Moreover, undesired anti-estrogenic effects of CC at the level of the endometrium have been implicated by some in the observed discrepancy between relatively low embryo implantation rates coinciding with successful ovarian hyperstimulation.

Preparations and Regimens. CC administration is usually initiated on cycle day 2, 3, or 5, and given daily for 5 subsequent days with doses varying between 100 and 150 mg/day. In most applied regimens exogenous gonadotropin medication (150 IU/day) is initiated after cessation of CC. It seems that CC alone induces a limited but dose-dependent increase in the number of developing follicles. However, the addition of gonadotropins elicits a more intense ovarian response. Sufficiently powered randomized comparative trials to support one approach over the other are lacking.

Clinical Outcome. Reported outcome is variable in the literature, but in general pregnancy rates appear higher compared to natural cycle IVF, but lower compared to conventional gonadotropin/GnRH agonist protocols. Again, most studies are uncontrolled but an extensive summary of almost 40,000 cycles reported in the literature suggests an overall pregnancy rate per embryo transfer of 20.5%.[199]

Adverse Effects and Complications. Because of the relatively mild stimulation, the incidence of side effects or complications of CC treatment for IVF is low, as discussed earlier. Overall side effects are CC dose related and are completely reversible once medication is stopped.

Gonadotropins

Background. Gonadotropin preparations have been used for ovarian stimulation since the early days of IVF and were originally developed in the United States.[198] The daily administration of these preparations is usually efficacious in the induction and maintenance of growth of multiple dominant follicles, allowing for the retrieval of many oocytes for IVF. Preparations initially used were hMG (containing both LH and FSH bioactivity), followed by purified uFSH and more recently recFSH. No general consensus exists with regard to starting day and doses of gonadotropins. An overview of published randomized studies is given in Table 28-3. In conclusion, based on seven randomized controlled trials (RCTs) involving a total of 2563 cycles, although higher gonadotropin doses may result in the retrieval of 1 or 2 more oocytes, improved clinical outcomes in terms of pregnancy rates could not be demonstrated.

A chimeric FSH agonist (so-called recFSH-CTP), generated by the fusion of the carboxy-terminal peptide (CTP) of hCG (responsible for its prolonged metabolic clearance compared to LH) with the FSH-β chain has recently been underoing phase 3 studies in IVF. The birth of a first healthy baby was reported in 2003 following the single injection of this novel compound in the early follicular phase of the cycle and a 7-day medication-free period (see Fig. 28-5).[41] Phase 2[200] and phase 3 studies are establishing the optimal dose and the clinical efficacy of this preparation in comparision to recFSH. It is anticipated that this latter development is going to represent a step forward in rendering stimulation regimens more patient friendly, but it is not to be expected that clinical outcome will improve.

The type, duration, and dosing of GnRH analog co-treatment to suppress endogenous pituitary gonadotropin release (as will be discussed later) may also affect the preferred gonadotropin preparation. Classical principles teach us that both LH and FSH are required for adequate ovarian estrogen biosynthesis and follicle development. Theca cell–derived androgen production (which is under LH control) is mandatory as a substrate for the conversion to estrogens by FSH-induced aromatase activity of granulosa cells.[26] A number of studies have indicated that excessively suppressed late follicular phase LH concentrations may be detrimental for clinical IVF outcome.[201,202] Under these circumstances the use of urinary preparations containing both LH and FSH activity or the addition of recLH or rechCG next to exogenous FSH may be useful.[26] It is uncertain as yet, however, for which patients this approach may be beneficial. Recent meta-analyses failed to show clinically relevant differences in relation to late follicular phase LH concentrations,[203] or when cycles with or without the addition of exogenous LH are compared.[204]

Recently the concept that exogenous LH is capable of selectively stimulating the development of the more mature dominant follicles has been developed. A shift from FSH to LH preparations during stimulation may therefore be useful in order to stimulate a more homogeneous cohort of follicles for IVF.[17,18]

Preparations and Regimens. To allow for the clinical introduction of recombinant FSH, large-scale, multicenter, comparative trials in IVF were published from 1995 onward.[205] It should be noted, however, that these studies, including several hundreds of women, were sponsored by pharmaceutical companies. The results should therefore be interpreted with an appropriate degree of caution. For instance, it was arbitrarily chosen for all initial studies that recFSH would only be compared with uFSH and not hMG, although the latter preparation was still considered to be the gold standard by the majority of clinicians. Several independent comparative trials have been published since then, but sample size of these single-center studies was usually insufficient to allow for the detection of relatively small differences. An early meta-analysis[206] as well as health economics studies[207,208] indicate a slightly improved outcome for recFSH compared to uFSH. In addition, a meta-analysis involving a limited number of IVF studies comparing recFSH versus hMG suggested comparable outcomes.[209] However, recently published multicenter, company-sponsored trials reported similar clinical outcomes comparing uFSH versus recFSH, or hMG versus recFSH.[210]

Many different regimens are applied with little if any proof of their efficacy and safety. Different starting days and doses are applied worldwide along with incremental or decremental doses. In case of imminent OHSS resulting from the development of too many follicles, the possibility of complete cessation of gonadotropin administration (coasting) has been advocated by several investigators.[174] Studies of the efficacy of this approach thus far undertaken have been limited and inconclusive. Adequate doses

TABLE 28-3

Randomized Controlled Trials Comparing Different Gonadotropin Doses for Ovarian Stimulation for in Vitro Fertilization

Reference	Patients	n	Study Design	Conclusion (High- vs Low-Dose Regimen)
van Hooff, HR '93	Low response after 5 d 225 IU/d hMG	64	225 vs 450 IU/d from day 5 of stimulation GnRH ag, long prt	No difference E_2, follicle #
Hoomans, HR '99	<39 yr, nl cycle, nl indic, BMI < 29 kg/m^2	165	150 IU rFSH vs 225 IU/d uFSH, fixed GnRH ag, long prt	Same oocyte #, same ongoing PR
Out, HR '99	30-39 yr, nl cycle, nl indic, BMI < 29 kg/m^2	199	100 vs 200 IU/d rFSH, fixed GnRH ag, long prt	More oocytes, same clinical PR
Out, HR '00	30-39 yr, nl cycle, nl indic, BMI < 29 kg/m^2	205	150 vs 250 IU/d rFSH, fixed GnRH ag, long prt	Similar oocyte # (also in older age!)
De Jong, FS '00	<38 yr, nl cycle, nl indic	15	100 vs 150 IU/d rFSH, fixed, late start GnRH antagonist	Reduced cycle cancellations in high-dose group
Latin-Am, FS '01	30-39 yr, nl cycle, nl indic, BMI < 29 kg/m^2	201	150 vs 250 IU/d rFSH, fixed GnRH ag, long prt	same oocyte #, same vital PR, 2 cases OHSS in high-dose group
Out, HR '01	<38 yr, nl cycle, male factor	91	100 vs 200 IU/d rFSH, fixed GnRH ag, long prt	More oocytes, same vital PR, 4 cases OHSS in high-dose group
Wikland, HR '01	<39 yr, nl cycle, nl indic, BMI < 30 kg/m^2	60	150 vs 225 IU/d rFSH, fixed GnRH antagonist	More oocytes (9 vs 11), same ongoing PR in high-dose group
Yong, FS '03	<40 yr, nl cycle, nl FSH, BMI < 34 kg/m^2	120	150 vs 225 IU/d rFSH, fixed GnRHa, long prt	Same oocyte #, same embryo, same PR, 4 cases OHSS in high-dose group
Popovic, HR '03	<39 yr, nl cycle, nl indic, first cycle, nl FSH	267	individual (100-250)* vs fixed 150 IU/d rFSH GnRHa, long prt	More nl response (5-14 oocytes), higher ongoing PR in individual dose group
Hohmann, JCEM '03	20-38 yr, nl cycle, nl indic, BMI 19-29 kg/m^2	142	cycle day 2 vs day 5 start 150 IU/d rFSH GnRH antagonist, flexible start	Shorter stimulation, higher cancellations, similar ongoing PR in late start group
Out, HR '04	<39 yr, nl cycle, nl FSH, BMI < 29 kg/m^2	257	150 vs 200 IU/d rFSH GnRH antagonist	Same oocyte #, same embryo #, same vital PR
Aboulghar, HR '04	< 40 yr, nl cycle, nl indic	150	150-300 IU/d hMG: same dose vs 75 IU/d increase on day start GnRH antagonist	Same oocyte #, same embryo #, same clinical PR
Klinkert, HR '05	Expected low response (low AFC), nl cycle	52	150 vs 300 IU/d rFSH, fixed GnRHa, long prt	Same oocyte #
Propst, FS '06	< 38 yr, nl indic, nl FSH, BMI < 33 kg/m^2	60	150-300 IU/d rFSH, same dose vs 75 IU/d increase on day start GnRH antagonist	Same E_2 levels, same implantation #, same PR, same live birth #
Baart, HR '07	< 38 yr, nl cycle, nl indic, BMI 19-29 kg/m^2	111	150 IU/d rFSH (late start), GnRH antag vs 225 IU/d rFSH, GnRHa long prt	Fewer oocytes, fewer embryos, fewer aneuploid embryos in late-start GnRH antagonist group
Heijnen, Lancet '07	<38 yr, nl cycle, nl indic, BMI < 29 kg/m^2	404	150 IU/d rFSH (late start), GnRH antag vs 150 IU/d rFSH, GnRHa long prt	Fewer oocytes, fewer embryos in late-start GnRH antagonist group†

*Based on prediction model (including follicle number, ovarian volume, age, smoking, and Doppler).
†Pregnancy rates are not given because ovarian stimulation protocols were combined, with differences in embryo transfer policies.
AFC, antral follicle count; ag, agonist; antag, antagonist; BMI, body mass index; E_2, estrodiol; FSH, follicle-stimulating hormone; GnRH, gonadotropin-releasing hormone; GNRHa, GNRH analog; hMG, human menopausal gonadotropin; indic, indications; nl, normal; OHSS, ovarian hyperstimulation syndrome; PR, pregnancy rate; prt, protocol; rFSH, recombinant FSH; uFSH, urinary FSH.

for gonadotropin preparations may also vary, depending on whether GnRH agonist or antagonist co-treatment is used.[211] Major individual differences in body weight may also determine response.[212] Because endogenous gonadotropins are suppressed by GnRH antagonists for a limited period of time (as will be discussed later), less exogenous FSH is required. The ideal day of initiation of gonadotropin therapy is another variable which has been poorly characterized so far, and may also vary dependent on GnRH agonist or antagonist co-treatment. It is surprising to conclude that very few of the above-mentioned questions with regard to applied dose regimens can be answered on the basis of scientific evidence by properly designed studies.

Usually starting doses vary between 100 and 300 IU/day and doses are often altered depending on the observed individual ovarian response. A typical daily starting dose would currently be 150 to 225 IU in Europe and 225 to 300 IU in the United States. Only few randomized studies regarding dose regimens can be found in the literature. A single-center RCT from Rotterdam showed that a doubling of the hMG dose in low responders after a 225 IU/day dose for 5 days is not efficacious compared to continued similar doses.[213] Moreover, an RCT in which higher versus standard dose of FSH was administered to expected poor responders showed no difference in pregnancy rates.[214] Table 28-3 summarizes further comparative studies, which taken together fail to show a difference in favor of high-dose regimens, indicating that the widely applied practice of a gonadotropin dose increase in case of low response is not efficacious.

The approach of starting exogenous FSH early during the luteal phase of the preceding cycle recognizes the physiologic principle of early recruitment of a cohort of follicles for the next cycle.[2] However, this protocol did not result in improved ovarian response in women with a low oocyte yield during previous IVF attempts.[215]

The perceived need to allow programming of oocyte retrieval led to a number of studies addressing the role of oral contraceptives (OCs) for this indication. Fixed schedule protocols were developed by a number of groups in which OCs were administered in advance of ovarian stimulation and planned follicle aspiration. Despite their apparent efficacy, ease of administration, and fewer side effects, subsequent randomized studies comparing OCs to GnRH agonists as a means of preventing premature luteinization showed the superiority of the latter and because of this, OCs are no longer widely used for this indication. To facilitate the planning of the initiation of exogenous gonadotropins in a GnRH antagonist cycle, independent of the menstrual period, OC pretreatment has been evaluated in a number of small studies and a recent meta-analysis.[216] Although there is evidence that OC pretreatment may aid in the scheduling of IVF cycles when GnRH anatagonists are used, at present there is no evidence that they improve live birth rates.[216]

Gonadotropin-Releasing Hormone Agonist Co-treatment

During initial studies with hMG stimulation of multiple follicle development for IVF it became apparent that a premature LH peak occurred in around 20% to 25% of cycles, due to positive feedback activity by high serum E_2 levels during the midfollicular phase of the stimulation cycle.[26] This advanced exposure to high LH resulted in premature luteinization of follicles and either cycle cancellation due to follicle maturation arrest or severely compromised IVF outcome. The clinical development of GnRH agonists in the early 1980s[45] allowed for the complete suppression of pituitary gonadotropin release during ovarian stimulation protocols for IVF.[26] Induced pituitary down-regulation indeed resulted in significantly reduced cancellation rates and improved overall IVF outcome.[217,218] Moreover, the approach of GnRH agonist co-treatment did facilitate scheduling of IVF and timing of oocyte retrieval. Frequently used preparations include buserelin, triptorelin, nafarelin, and leuprorelin. To some degree, the extent and duration of pituitary suppression are dose related, but surprisingly few dose finding studies have been performed. In addition, randomized studies comparing different GnRH agonists are scarce.

Due to the intrinsic agonist activity of the compound, pituitary down-regulation is preceded by an initial stimulatory phase (referred to as the "flare" effect) which lasts for around 2 weeks. In this long protocol, GnRH agonist treatment therefore usually commences in the luteal phase in the preceding cycle and is continued until hCG administration. Stimulation with gonadotropins is started when pituitary and ovarian quiesence has been achieved. Moreover, it is uncertain whether ovarian response to exogenous stimulation is affected by GnRH agonist co-treatment.[219] Some women suffer from serious hypoestrogenic side effects, such as mood changes, sweating, and flushes. Alternative approaches include the short (and sometimes ultrashort) protocols in which the initial flare effect of GnRH agonist treatment is used to stimulate the ovaries. Attempts to discontinue GnRH agonist administration during the ovarian stimulation phase[220,221] have not shown beneficial effects. Reported clinical results of these alternative clinical protocols remain variable, and the GnRH agonist long protocol has remained the standard of care for over a decade.[26]

Gonadotropin-Releasing Hormone Antagonist Co-treatment

Two third-generation GnRH antagonists (cetrorelix and ganirelix) became available for large-scale clinical studies around 1995. Previous generations of the antagonist suffered from problems with pharmaceutical formulation and related bioavailability along with the local or systemic induction of histamine release. The potential advantage of a GnRH antagonist is that pituitary gonadotropin secretion is suppressed immediately after initiation of therapy. Therefore the co-treatment with GnRH antagonist can be restricted to the time in the cycle at risk for a premature rise in LH (i.e., the mid- to late follicular phase of the cycle).[26]

Both single, high-dose and multiple, low-dose GnRH antagonist regimens have been described. Multiple, daily dose regimens are most widely used at present. Initial dose finding studies suggested that a daily injection of 0.25 mg represents the minimal effective dose to suppress a premature LH rise in most patients. In all phase 3 comparative trials of the daily GnRH antagonist co-treatment regimen, it was initiated on cycle day 6. However,

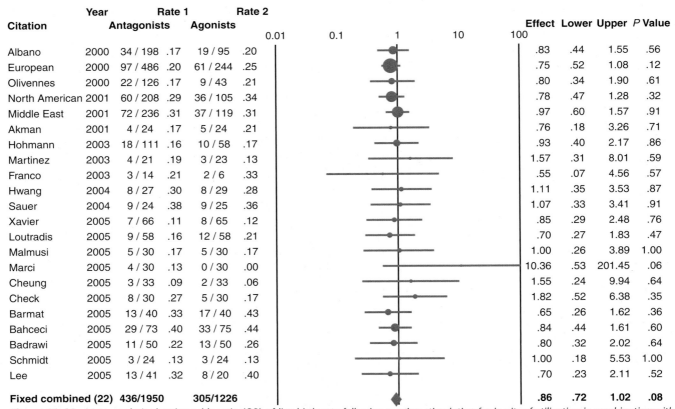

Citation	Year	Rate 1 Antagonists		Rate 2 Agonists		Effect	Lower	Upper	P Value
Albano	2000	34 / 198	.17	19 / 95	.20	.83	.44	1.55	.56
European	2000	97 / 486	.20	61 / 244	.25	.75	.52	1.08	.12
Olivennes	2000	22 / 126	.17	9 / 43	.21	.80	.34	1.90	.61
North American	2001	60 / 208	.29	36 / 105	.34	.78	.47	1.28	.32
Middle East	2001	72 / 236	.31	37 / 119	.31	.97	.60	1.57	.91
Akman	2001	4 / 24	.17	5 / 24	.21	.76	.18	3.26	.71
Hohmann	2003	18 / 111	.16	10 / 58	.17	.93	.40	2.17	.86
Martinez	2003	4 / 21	.19	3 / 23	.13	1.57	.31	8.01	.59
Franco	2003	3 / 14	.21	2 / 6	.33	.55	.07	4.56	.57
Hwang	2004	8 / 27	.30	8 / 29	.28	1.11	.35	3.53	.87
Sauer	2004	9 / 24	.38	9 / 25	.36	1.07	.33	3.41	.91
Xavier	2005	7 / 66	.11	8 / 65	.12	.85	.29	2.48	.76
Loutradis	2005	9 / 58	.16	12 / 58	.21	.70	.27	1.83	.47
Malmusi	2005	5 / 30	.17	5 / 30	.17	1.00	.26	3.89	1.00
Marci	2005	4 / 30	.13	0 / 30	.00	10.36	.53	201.45	.06
Cheung	2005	3 / 33	.09	2 / 33	.06	1.55	.24	9.94	.64
Check	2005	8 / 30	.27	5 / 30	.17	1.82	.52	6.38	.35
Barmat	2005	13 / 40	.33	17 / 40	.43	.65	.26	1.62	.36
Bahceci	2005	29 / 73	.40	33 / 75	.44	.84	.44	1.61	.60
Badrawi	2005	11 / 50	.22	13 / 50	.26	.80	.32	2.02	.64
Schmidt	2005	3 / 24	.13	3 / 24	.13	1.00	.18	5.53	1.00
Lee	2005	13 / 41	.32	8 / 20	.40	.70	.23	2.11	.52
Fixed combined (22)		**436/1950**		**305/1226**		**.86**	**.72**	**1.02**	**.08**

Figure 28-13. Meta-analysis showing odds ratio (OR) of live birth rate following ovarian stimulation for in vitro fertilization in combination with either a GnRH agonist or a GnRH antagonist. The probability of live birth between GnRH agonists and GnRH antagonists was not significantly different (OR, 0.86; 95% CI 0.72-1.02; P = 0.085; heterogeneity, P = 0.99; fixed effect model). (From Kolibianakis EM, Collins J, Tarlatzis BC, et al. Among patients treated for IVF with gonadotrophins and GnRH analogues, is the probability of live birth dependent on the type of analogue used? A systematic review and meta-analysis. Hum Reprod Update 12:651-671, 2006.)

in principle, GnRH antagonists need only be given when there is folliclular development and rising E_2 levels which might give rise to a premature elevation in pituitary LH release due to positive feedback mechanisms. However, a meta-analysis of four studies comparing fixed with flexible regimens showed a trend toward lower pregnancy rates following the flexible protocol (OR 0.7, 95% CI 0.47-1.05).[222] The first meta-analysis published comparing outcomes following co-treatment with GnRH antagonist versus GnRH agonist[211] based on five multicenter RCTs concluded that the GnRH antagonist is as efficient as GnRH agonist in preventing a premature LH surge in IVF (OR 1.76, 95% CI 0.75-4.16). However, a small but significant reduction in pregnancies was observed per started cycle (OR 0.79, 95% CI 0.63-0.99). Since then, protocols have been refined, and a recent meta-analysis of later studies has shown no difference in live birth rates[223] (Fig. 28-13).

Concerns have been raised regarding the possibility of direct effects of GnRH antagonists on the embryo. However, no adverse effects were observed on the freeze–thaw embryos of GnRH antagonist cycles.[224] Possible detrimental effects of GnRH antagonists at the endometrial level and on follicle development have not been confirmed.[26] Moreover, recent studies have indicated that gonadotropin regimens do not need to be adjusted

when GnRH antagonists are commenced.[225,226] Furthermore, exogenous LH is probably not required next to FSH.[203,204,227]

Despite improving outcomes the debate regarding the advantages and disadvantages compared with GnRH agonists continues.[228] A summary of the advantages and disadvantages for the use of GnRH antagonists in IVF is given in Box 28-2.

APPROACHES FOR INDUCTION OF FINAL OOCYTE MATURATION

In the natural normo-ovulatory cycle, rupture of the dominant follicle and release of the oocyte are triggered by the mid-cycle surge of LH. This sudden enhancement of pituitary synthesis and release of LH (and FSH) is elicited by high late-follicular phase E_2 levels in combination with slightly elevated progesterone levels.[229] In stimulated cycles for IVF, estrogen levels are prematurely elevated, which may induce unpredictable but advanced LH rises. As mentioned before, GnRH agonist co-treatment is required in order to prevent this from happening. Consequently, exogenous hCG should be used during the late follicular phase under these circumstances to replace the endogenous LH surge. This approach has been considered the standard of care for the induction of final

BOX 28-2

Advantages and Disadvantages for the Use of GnRH Antagonists in IVF

Advantages

Prevention of premature LH increase is easier and takes less time.

GnRH antagonists are not associated with an acute stimulation of gonadotropins and steroid hormones.

The initial stimulation by GnRH agonists can induce cyst formation, which is avoided with GnRH antagonists.

No hot flushes are observed with GnRH antagonists.

Inadvertent administration of the GnRH analog in early pregnancy can be avoided as GnRH antagonist is administered in the midfollicular phase.

Requirements for exogenous gonadotropins are reduced, rendering ovarian stimulation less costly.

Duration of ovarian stimulation protocols is shortened, improving patient discomfort.

Disadvantages

GnRH antagonist co-treatment represents a novel approach and more knowledge is necessary for its optimization.

GnRH antagonists offer less flexibility regarding cycle programming as compared with the long GnRH agonist protocol.

Reduced ability to gain an orderly daily volume of oocyte retrievals compared with GnRH agonist, although this can be improved by using the oral contraceptive pill.

GnRH, gonadotropin-releasing hormone; IVF, in vitro fertilization; LH, luteinizing hormone.
*Adapted from Tarlatzis B, Fauser BCJM, Kolibianakis EM, et al. GnRH antagonists in ovarian stimulation for IVF. Hum Reprod Update 12:333-340, 2006.

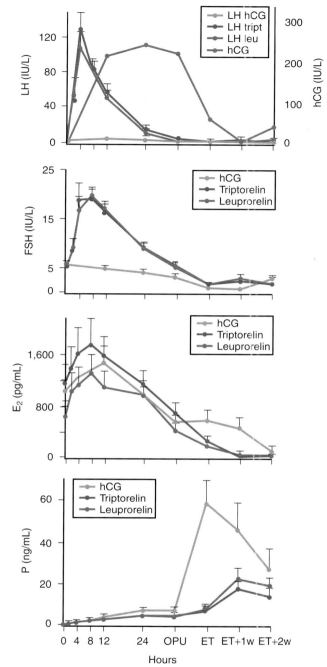

Figure 28-14. Endocrine characteristics of the supplemented luteal phase following ovarian hyperstimulation for in vitro fertilization using exogenous follicle-stimulating hormone and gonadotropin-releasing hormone (GnRH) antagonist co-treatment, where oocyte maturation is induced by either human chorionic gonadotropin or the GnRH agonists triptorelin or leuprorelin. E_2, estradiol; ET, embryo transfer; FSH, follicle-stimulating hormone; hCG, human chorionic gonadotropin; LH, luteinizing hormone; OPU, ovum pickup; P, progesterone; w, week. (From Fauser BC, de Jong D, Olivennes F, et al. Endocrine profiles after triggering of final oocyte maturation with GnRH agonist after cotreatment with the GnRH antagonist ganirelix during ovarian stimulation for in vitro fertilization. J Clin Endocrinol Metab 87:709-715, 2002.)

stages of oocyte maturation before oocyte retrieval along with corpus luteum formation in IVF.[26] Exogenous hCG is also implicated in sustained luteotropic activity[220] due its prolonged circulating half-life.[230] Unfortunately, hCG is therefore also believed to contribute to chances of developing OHSS.[174]

Initial studies during ovarian hyperstimulation for IVF (before the widespread use of GnRH agonist co-treatment) showed that an endogenous LH surge could be induced reliably by the administration of GnRH or a bolus injection of GnRH agonist.[231] The induction of an endogenous LH (and FSH) surge is more physiologic compared to exogenous hCG because of the much shorter half-life.[232] Moreover, luteal phase steroid concentrations seem closer to the physiologic range[233] (Fig. 28-14), which may improve endometrial receptivity.[234] As the follicular phase co-treatment with GnRH agonist has been the standard of care for over a decade, alternative approaches for the induction of oocyte maturation has received little attention in recent years. However, the suppressive effect of follicular phase GnRH antagonist administration can be reversed immediately by administering native GnRH or GnRH agonist.[14,234] Indeed, a randomized trial confirmed that the triggering of final stages of oocyte maturation can be induced effectively by a single bolus injection of GnRH agonist even after the follicular phase co-treatment with a GnRH antagonist. This was demonstrated by the observed gonadotropin surge and quality and fertilization rate of recovered oocytes.[233]

Recombinant LH and recombinant hCG have recently become available for clinical use. An early large randomized trial comparing 250 μg rechCG versus 5000 IU uhCG for the induction of oocyte maturation in a total of 190 women undergoing IVF showed that the number of mature oocytes retrieved and luteal phase serum concentrations of progesterone and hCG concentrations were significantly higher.[235] Considering the short half-life of recLH two injections with a 1- to 3-day interval may be considered.

The introduction of GnRH antagonists into clinical practice now makes it possible to employ a bolus injection of GnRH agonist to induce an endogenous LH surge. Although previously shown to be effective in achieving this,[233] randomized studies comparing this approach to hCG administration showed lower implantation and ongoing pregnancy rates.[236] Recent data indicate that standard luteal support regimens may be insufficient in this setting, and improved results may be achieved when this is addressed. In a meta-analysis of 23 randomized studies, the use of GnRH agonist to trigger final oocyte maturation in IVF yielded a number of oocytes capable to undergo fertilization and subsequent embryonic cleavage comparable to that achieved with hCG.[237] However, the likelihood of an ongoing clinical pregnancy after GnRH agonist triggering was significantly lower as compared to standard hCG treatment. For women at risk of developing OHSS who have been co-treated with GnRH antagonists, replacing hCG with a GnRH agonist bolus has been shown in a randomized study to reduce the risk.[238]

LUTEAL PHASE SUPPLEMENTATION

Since the early days of IVF it has been described that the luteal phase of stimulated IVF cycles is abnormal. In fact, it was already stated in the first extended report on IVF by Edwards and Steptoe[33] that "the luteal phase of virtually all patients was shortened considerably after treatment with gonadotropins" and it was suggested that high follicular phase estrogen levels due to ovarian hyperstimulation might be involved. Initial studies in the United States in 1983 concerning hMG-stimulated IVF cycles also confirmed the occurrence of an abnormal luteal phase in IVF cycles with characteristic features of elevated progesterone levels along with a significantly reduced luteal phase length[239] (Fig. 28-15).

As mentioned earlier, GnRH agonist co-treatment became the standard of care for the prevention of a premature rise in LH. Typically, GnRH agonist treatment is initiated in the luteal phase of the preceding cycle and continued until the late follicular phase. It became apparent, however, that

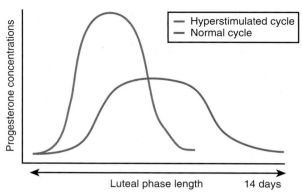

Figure 28-15. *Schematic representation of changes in luteal phase length and endocrine profile induced by ovarian hyperstimulation for in vitro fertilization (From Jones HWJ. What happened? Where are we? Hum Reprod 11[Suppl 1]:7-21, 1996.)*

prolonged pituitary recovery from down-regulation during the luteal phase[240] resulted in lack of support of the corpus luteum by endogenous LH and advanced luteolysis.[241] It was observed shortly thereafter that the corpus luteum can be rescued by the administration of hCG,[26] and this treatment modality became the standard of care for luteal support during the late 1980s. Outcome was better compared to progesterone supplementation, but 5% of hCG-supplemented patients developed OHSS. Because of this association between hCG and OHSS,[174] luteal phase hCG support has been largely replaced over the years by luteal phase progesterone supplementation.[242] In a recent meta-analysis of luteal support in stimulated IVF cycles, both hCG (OR 2.72; 95% CI 1.56-4.9, P < 0.05) and progesterone (OR 1.57; CI 1.13-2.17, P < 0.05) were confirmed to result in an increased pregnancy rate compared with placebo.[243] However, hCG was clearly associated with an increased risk of OHSS. Natural micronized progesterone was not efficient if taken orally, but both the vaginal and intramuscular routes were effective and demonstrated comparable outcomes. With respect to the addition of estradiol, while it showed some benefit in long GnRH agonist protocols, there was no evidence to support its use in short GnRH agonist or GnRH antagonist protocols.

Attempts to secure pituitary recovery during the luteal phase by the early follicular phase cessation of GnRH agonist co-treatment all failed, because it takes at least 2 to 3 weeks for LH secretion to recover.[26] Because of the rapid recovery of pituitary gonadotropin release after discontinuation of GnRH antagonist it has been speculated that luteal phase supplementation may not be required following the late follicular phase administration of antagonist.[244] Preliminary observations related to ovarian stimulation and GnRH antagonist co-treatment for IUI seem to favor this contention.[245] However, various studies in IVF applying GnRH antagonist co-treatment have now clearly shown that luteolysis is also initiated prematurely resulting in a significant reduction in the length of the luteal phase along with greatly compromised chances for pregnancy.[246-248] More detailed studies could confirm that early and midluteal phase LH levels remained suppressed following the follicular phase administration of GnRH antagonist.[248,249]

Moreover, luteolysis is advanced in the nonsupplemented luteal phase after either hCG or GnRH agonist triggering of oocyte maturation.[248] Collectively, this indicates that high early luteal phase steroid production is primarily responsible for advanced luteolysis, due to massive negative feedback resulting in greatly suppressed LH secretion.[179] Mild stimulation regimens resulting in lower serum steroid levels have therefore been advocated as a means of benefiting the luteal phase.[243]

CLINICAL OUTCOME OF IVF

ESHRE IVF data for the year 2003 from 28 European countries involving a total of 725 clinics and over 360,000 IVF and ICSI cycles report major differences between countries, with an overall clinical pregnancy rate of 26.1% per retrieval and 29.6% per transfer for IVF (26.5% and 28.7%, respectively, for ICSI). Singleton deliveries involved 76.7% of pregnancies.[60] The most recent report of U.S. centers involving a total of 92,389 cycles performed in 2005 (www.cdc.gov/ART/index.htm) continue to indicate higher clinical pregnancy rates per retrieval, reaching 41% in women under 35 years. Respective live birth rates per cycle are also highly age dependent, ranging from 37% in women under 35 years, to 11% in women of 41 to 42 years of age. Respective twinning rates are 33% and 13%, while triplets or more constitute 4% to 5% of pregnancies. The percentage of miscarriages, fetal reduction procedures, or immature births following IVF are largely unknown. Next to differences in quality of fertility laboratories, this discrepancy in success rates may depend on how success is defined. Currently, live birth is defined as delivery of a fetus with a heartbeat from 20 weeks onward, and may also be associated with differences in indications for IVF, smoking habits, and the age of patients treated, along with the number of embryos transferred. In the United States, up to five embryos can be transferred, and in 2005 a mean of 2.5 embryos were transferred per cycle (www.cdc.gov/ART/index.htm).

ADVERSE EFFECTS AND COMPLICATIONS

Complications related to invasive IVF procedures such as oocyte retrieval and embryo transfer, predominantly involve infection and bleeding along with anesthesia problems.[250] The drawbacks associated with profound ovarian stimulation for IVF include considerable patient discomfort such as weight gain, headache, mood swings, breast tenderness, abdominal pain, and sometimes diarrhea and nausea. In this respect it is important to comprehend that after a first unsuccessful IVF attempt around 25% of patients refrain from a second cycle, even in countries where costs are covered by health insurance companies.[251]

OHSS is a potentially life-threatening complication characterized by ovarian enlargement, high serum sex steroids, and extravascular fluid accumulation, primarily in the peritoneal cavity. Mild forms of OHSS constitute around 20% to 35% of IVF cycles, moderate forms 3% to 6% of cycles, along with 0.1% to 0.2% severe forms.[48,174] To some extent, patients at risk of developing OHSS may be recognized by the following features: young age, PCOS,

profound hyperstimulation protocols with GnRH agonist long protocol co-treatment, large numbers of preovulatory graafian follicles, high serum E_2 levels, high (>5000 IU) bolus doses of hCG to induce final oocyte maturation, the use of hCG for luteal phase supplementation, and finally the occurrence of pregnancy. In fact, the incidence of OHSS is directly related to hCG concentrations with a two- to fivefold increased incidence in case of multiple pregnancy.

Preventive strategies in case of imminent OHSS include cessation of exogenous gonadotropins for several days (coasting), follicular aspiration, prevention of pregnancy during the stimulation cycle by cryopreserving all embryos, or the prophylactic infusion of glucocorticoids or albumin. The risk of OHSS may also be lowered by using alternative strategies to induce oocyte maturation, such as inducing an endogenous LH surge by administration of a single bolus dose of GnRH agonist or the short half-life preparation of recLH instead of hCG.

The most important complication related to IVF treatment is multiple pregnancy. The magnitude of the problem has been discussed previously in this chapter (see Fig. 28-5). (For recent reviews see Fauser et al.[51] and Verberg et al.[52]) Between the years of 1980 and 2000, twin birth rates in the United States increased by 75%, and currently represent around 3% of total births.[51] Similar trends have been reported in European countries.[52] Although an association between increased female age and multiple gestation is clearly established, the delay in childbearing accounts for no more than 30% of the observed overall increase in multiple pregnancies.[51] Although the available data indicate that the majority of twin births are still unrelated to infertility therapies[51] up to 80% of higher order multiple births are considered to be due to ovarian stimulation and ART. Births resulting from infertility therapies account for around 1% to 3% of all singleton live births, 30% to 50% of twin births, and more than 75% of higher order multiples.

Pregnancy complications include increased risk of miscarriage, preeclampsia, growth retardation, and preterm delivery. Perinatal mortality rates are at least fourfold higher in twin, and at least sixfold higher in triplet, births compared with singleton births. Moreover, the risks of prematurity in twin and higher order multiple birth are increased 7- to 40-fold, and for low-birth-weight infants 10- to 75-fold, respectively. Adverse outcomes among children conceived through IVF are largely associated with multiple gestation.

Recent data are reassuring with respect to possible long-term health consequences such as ovarian cancer, breast cancer, and advanced menopausal age.[252]

NEW APPROACHES TO MILD OVARIAN STIMULATION FOR IVF

After the initial years of IVF, profound ovarian stimulation became the rule for more than two decades. The stimulation of growth of large numbers of follicles and the retrieval of many oocytes has been viewed as an acceptable marker of successful IVF treatment. Medication regimens to achieve profound ovarian stimulation are extremely complex and expensive, take many weeks of frequent injections, and require intense monitoring. Moreover, patient discomfort and chances for serious side effects and complications are considerable. In addition, this profound stimulation gives rise to greatly abnormal luteal phase endocrinology, and its impact on endometrial receptivity and therefore IVF success is mostly unknown.

Attitudes toward profound ovarian stimulation are changing,[191,253] particularly given the growing tendency to transfer a reduced number of embryos. It has previously been demonstrated on the basis of the U.K. national database that reducing the number of embryos tranferred from three to two does not diminish chances of birth despite a reduction in risk of multiple birth.[64] In Europe, an increasing number of centers are carrying out single transfer in younger women. Emphasis may therefore now be directed toward the development of more simple mild stimulation protocols[26,191,196,254] or the improvement of natural cycle IVF outcomes.[61,195,197] The increasing quality of embryo cryopreservation programs will serve to encourage the transfer of one embryo at a time.[255]

Previous studies in normo-ovulatory female volunteers[114,115] confirmed that the development of multiple dominant follicles can be induced by interfering with decremental FSH concentrations during the mid- to late follicular phase. As shown previously, this decrease is required for the selection of a single dominant follicle.[9,10] These observations are in agreement with previous findings in the monkey model.[116,256] We were subsequently able to demonstrate that the initiation of exogenous FSH (fixed dose, 150 IU/day, GnRH antagonist co-treatment) as late as cycle day 5 results in a comparable clinical IVF outcome, despite a reduced duration of stimulation (number of ampules used) and increased cancellation rates[257] (Fig. 28-16).

To test the efficacy of this mild stimulation protocol in standard practice, a large randomized effectiveness study has been performed to analyze whether a strategy including the mild stimulation protocol in combination with single embryo transfer (SET) would lead to a similar outcome assessed over a 1-year interval after initiation of treatment, while reducing patients' discomfort, multiple pregnancies, and costs compared with standard treatment.[63] The study included a total of 404 patients and observed that because of the shorter duration of treatment per cycle, less medication needed, and a reduction in twin pregnancies, the mild approach led to an equal chance of live birth after a year of treatment while reducing the total costs (Fig. 28-17).

Apart from clinical efficacy and costs (see later), emotional stress should be considered an important negative side effect associated with IVF treatment. Following mild stimulation, patients reported fewer side effects and stress related to hormone treatment and cycle cancellation compared with conventional stimulation.[258] Treatment-related stress has been found to be the most important reason patients drop out of IVF treatment.[259] The early drop-out of treatment deprives the couple of an optimal cumulative chance of achieving pregnancy, and therefore also impacts on the success of the respective IVF program. Mild stimulation might therefore have a positive impact on cumulative treatment success rates as it positively affects the

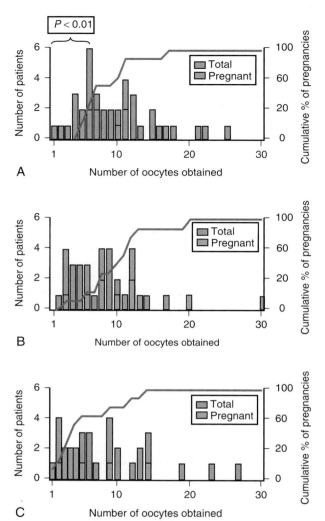

Figure 28-16. *Number of women undergoing in vitro fertilization who did or did not achieve a pregnancy in relation to the amount of oocytes retrieved, comparing conventional hyperstimulation with gonadotropin-releasing hormone (GnRH) agonist long protocol (A) with two mild stimulation protocols employing GnRH antagonist co-treatment (B and C). (From Hohmann FP, Macklon NS, Fauser BC. A randomized comparison of two ovarian stimulation protocols with gonadotropin-releasing hormone [GnRH] antagonist cotreatment for in vitro fertilization commencing recombinant follicle-stimulating hormone on cycle day 2 or 5 with the standard long GnRH agonist protocol. J Clin Endocrinol Metab 88:166-117, 2003.)*

chance that patients are willing to continue treatment following a failed attempt.

Other novel protocols under investigation include the replacement of FSH by LH, an approach based on the acquired LH responsiveness of granulosa cells of dominant follicles. Besides the expected reduction of gonadotropin usage, this ovarian stimulation approach might also reduce the number of small, less mature follicles, possibly reducing the chance of OHSS, because smaller ovarian follicles are unlikely to be responsive to LH.[127] Three randomized controlled trials[260-262] have shown that this approach can result in a significant reduction in FSH needed and in the number of small follicles at final oocyte maturation. Pregnancy rates do not appear to be compromised. More

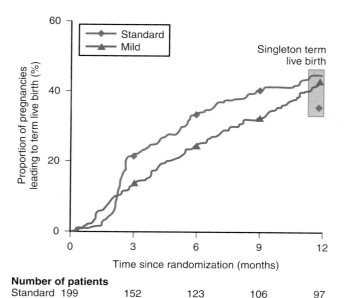

Number of patients

Standard	199	152	123	106	97
Mild	205	174	149	130	109

Figure 28-17. Proportions of pregnancies leading to cumulative term live birth within 12 months after starting in vitro fertilization. Mild: mild ovarian stimulation with GnRH antagonist and single embryo transfer. Standard: standard ovarian stimulation with GnRH antagonist and dual embryo transfer. The shaded area represents the singleton live birth rate after 12 months. (From Heijnen EM, Eijkemans MJ, De Klerk C, et al. A mild treatment strategy for in-vitro fertilisation: a randomised non-inferiority trial. Lancet 369[9563]:743-749, 2007.)

extensive studies are required to determine the critical threshold for FSH replacement by LH stimulation and the most appropriate dosage of LH or hCG.

There are indications that the degree of ovarian stimulation affects both the morphologic embryo quality and the chromosomal constitution of the developed embryos.[263,264] This phenomenon could be the result of interference with the natural selection of good quality oocytes or the exposure of growing follicles to the potentially negative effects of ovarian stimulation. A randomized trial concerning the chromosomal analysis of human embryos following mild ovarian stimulation for IVF showed a significantly higher proportion of euploid embryos compared to conventional ovarian stimulation, suggesting that through maximal stimulation the surplus of obtained oocytes results in chromosomally abnormal embryos.[265]

Toward Individualized Treatment Algorithms

As previously highlighted, the chance of achieving a spontaneous pregnancy is frequently underestimated by couples and their physicians.[70] An increasingly assertive patient population, who continue to delay childbearing for career, social, or other reasons is putting physicians under greater pressure to intervene in order to aid the couple in achieving their goal quickly and with minimal disruption to busy lives. Time is increasingly an issue for couples seeking to conceive, and the commercial pressures and competition between IVF centers can lead to couples being accepted

into IVF programs without a sound indication. Yet the virtue of patience can pay dividends for many who are now subject to premature and unnecessary intervention. Most couples seeking help will present with subfertility rather than absolute infertility. On the basis of a modest range of investigations and certain individual characteristics, the chances of an individual couple conceiving spontaneously over a given period of time can be calculated. It is known for instance that the spontaneous monthly fecundity rate declines with increasing duration of subfertility. After 3 years the residual likelihood of spontaneous pregnancy in untreated couples with unexplained infertility falls to 40% and after 5 years to 20%.[70]

In recent years a number of prediction models for calculating individual chances of spontaneous conception in subfertile couples have been published.[266-268] The chance of conception over a given time frame can be calculated from the results of a number of fertility investigations and patient parameters such as age and duration of infertility. Caution is, however, required when applying a prediction model developed elsewhere to one's own patient population. Before a prediction model can be introduced into everyday clinical practice, prospective external validation is required. Furthermore, knowledge of the development cohort is important when selecting a model for application in one's own setting. The mean duration and degree of subfertility in a primary care population is less than in a tertiary population. As a result, the conclusions derived from model developed in academic centers may have limited relevance for primary subfertility management and vice versa.[70]

The majority of women undergoing ovulation induction have WHO class 2 anovulation. Although this is a highly heterogeneous group, the treatment for these women is the same.[269] The identification of patient characteristics predictive of ovulation induction outcome would allow the design of individual treatment regimens, and would provide useful information regarding the factors that determine the extent of ovarian dysfunction.[269] In recent years a number of studies addressing these issues have been published. In one study the criteria that could predict the response of women with WHO class 2 anovulation to treatment with CC were identified.[86] Following multivariate analysis, the free androgen index (FAI), body mass index (BMI), presence of amenorrhea (as opposed to oligomenorrhea), and ovarian volume were found to be independent predictors of ovulation. The area under the receiver operating curve in a prediction model using these factors was 0.82. By adding additional endocrine factors, the area under the curve increased to 0.86.[270] In a subsequent study, those factors which could predict conception following ovulation were studied. Multivariate analysis of a number of clinical, endocrine, and ultrasound characteristics revealed lower age and the presence of amenorrhea to be the only significant parameters for predicting conception. Initial LH levels were not found to be important. From these data, a nomogram was constructed[165] (Fig. 28-18) which may assist in the selection of patients for clomiphene therapy, and those for whom this first-line treatment will be of little value. In this latter group, early recourse to gonadotropin therapy is indicated.[271,272]

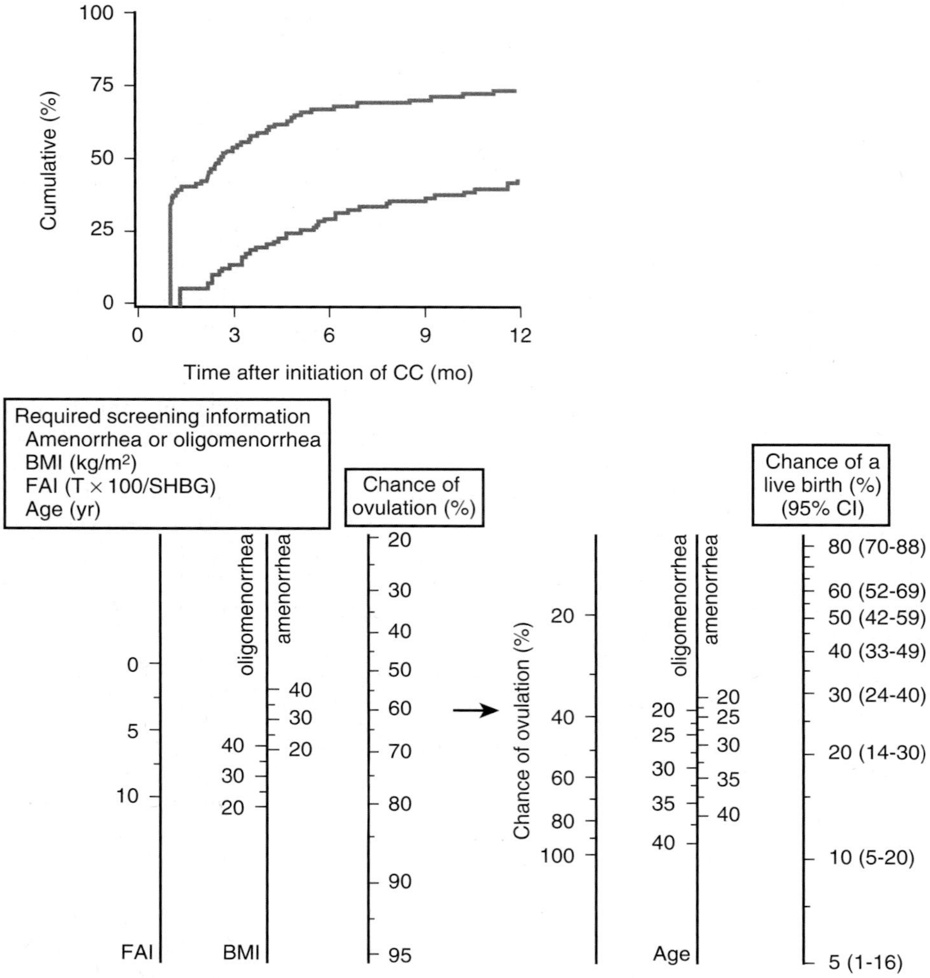

Figure 28-18. *Cumulative percentage of patients who ovulate or conceive following the initiation of clomiphene citrate, CC (top), and a two-step nomogram predicting chances of live birth following clomiphene citrate on the basis of initial screening characteristics (bottom). BMI, body mass index; FAI, free androgen index. (From Imani B, Eijkemans MJ, te Velde ER, et al. A nomogram to predict the probability of live birth after clomiphene citrate induction of ovulation in normogonadotropic oligoamenorrheic infertility. Fertil Steril 77:91-97, 2002.)*

When gonadotropin therapy for ovulation induction is selected, the duration of treatment, the amount of gonadotropins administered, the associated risks of cycle-to-cycle variability, multifollicular development, OHSS, and multiple pregnancy might all be reduced if the starting dose were individualized. This would require the means to reliably predict the dose of FSH at which a given individual will respond by way of monofollicular selection to dominance—in other words, their individual FSH threshold for stimulation. A prediction model has recently been developed which may be used to determine the individual FSH response dose (which is presumably closely related to the FSH threshold).[120] Women about to undergo low-dose step-up ovulation induction with recFSH, were subject to a standard clinical, sonographic, and endocrine screening. The measured parameters were analyzed for predictors of the FSH dose on the day of ovarian response. In multivariate analysis, BMI, ovarian response to preceding CC medication (CC-resistant anovulation [CRA], or failure to conceive despite ovulatory cycles), initial free insulin-like growth factor-I (free IGF-I), and serum FSH levels were included in the final model.[120] In a subsequent analysis of women with PCOS who had undergone ovulation induction with the step-down regimen, a correlation was

observed between the predicted individual FSH response dose and the number of treatment days before dominance was observed.[273] Application of this model may enable the administration of the lowest possible daily dose of exogenous gonadotropins to surpass the individual FSH threshold of a given patient and achieve follicular development and subsequent ovulation. Refining ovulation induction therapy in this way offers the prospect of improving safety, reducing the risk of multiple pregnancies, and improving the efficiency of gonadotropin ovulation induction.

The ability to predict clinical outcome from ovulation induction with gonadotropins would also be of value in the individualization of treatment regimens. In a prediction model for outcome after FSH ovulation induction[173] simple patient characteristics combined with endocrine factors were again shown to enable (limited) prediction of outcome following FSH ovulation induction. The most important end point for ovulation induction is overall singleton live birth. Data are now available to allow the prediction of a given couple achieving this from conventional ovulation induction strategies over an extended period of time (Fig. 28-19).[47]

Regarding IVF treatment, it appears that the most prominent factor determining outcome is the individual

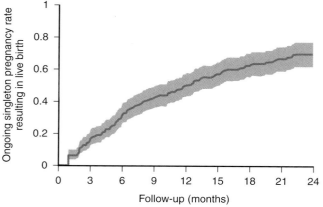

Figure 28-19. *Cumulative singleton live birth rate of 72% within 2 years after the initiation of a conventional ovulation induction algorithm (using clomiphene citrate as first-line and gonadotropins as second-line therapy) for the medical treatment of anovulatory infertility. (From Eijkemans MJ, Imani B, Mulders AG, et al. High ongoing single-ton live birth rate following classical ovulation induction in anovulatory infertility. Hum Reprod 18:2357-2362, 2003.)*

variability in ovarian response to stimulation. Rather than exhibiting the desired response, women can present with either a hyporesponse or a hyper-response to stimulation. Studies undertaken so far have been unable to demonstrate a beneficial effect of gonadotropin dose increase in patients who exhibit a poor response to standard dose regimens.[176,213] This may help in counseling the patient, because the chances of successful IVF in these women will be extremely low.

Poor ovarian response appears to be related to ovarian aging[177] and early menopause[178] (Fig. 28-20). In IVF, the association between poor ovarian response due to diminished ovarian reserve with cycle cancellation and poor success rates is well established.[274] Age is an important predictor of IVF outcome.[275] However, chronological age is poorly correlated with ovarian aging. A major individual variability exists in follicle pool depletion within the

normal range of menopausal age, as complete follicle pool exhaustion may occur between 40 and 60 years. The quantity and quality of the primordial follicle pool diminishes with age, reducing ovarian reserve.[276] This results in a decline in both therapy-induced and spontaneous pregnancies.[277] However, some women above 40 years of age will show a good response to ovarian stimulation and subsequently conceive with IVF, yet other women under 40 may fail to respond as a result of accelerated ovarian aging. In recent years attention has been given to the identification of sensitive and specific markers for ovarian aging which may enable prediction of poor or good response. This would open the way to improved counseling and patient selection for IVF.

The first and still most widely used endocrine marker for ovarian reserve is the early follicular phase FSH level,[278] which has been shown to be an independent predictor to age of IVF outcome.[279] More recent studies have indicated that while FSH level is a stronger predictor of cycle cancellation due to poor response and the number of oocytes collected at pick-up, age is more closely related to the chance of pregnancy.[279] In current practice, women with raised baseline FSH levels are usually advised against IVF treatment due to the anticipated poor outcome. However, although young women with high FSH levels demonstrate lower numbers of growing follicles and a high probability of cycle cancellation, normal ongoing pregnancy rates may be observed if oocytes and embryos are obtained.[279] Older women (>40 years) with normal baseline FSH levels may demonstrate lower cancellation rates, but the implantation rate per embryo and the ongoing pregnancy rates are lower than those observed in young women with elevated FSH.[279] FSH has been suggested to be of greater value in predicting ovarian reserve than other ovarian markers such as inhibin B. However, in a meta-analysis, baseline FSH levels showed only a moderate predictive performance for poor response and a low predictive performance for nonpregnancy was observed.[280] Other markers may therefore have an adjunctive value when diagnosing diminished ovarian reserve. The ultrasound measurement

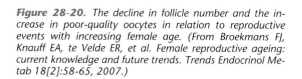

Figure 28-20. *The decline in follicle number and the increase in poor-quality oocytes in relation to reproductive events with increasing female age. (From Broekmans FJ, Knauff EA, te Velde ER, et al. Female reproductive ageing: current knowledge and future trends. Trends Endocrinol Metab 18[2]:58-65, 2007.)*

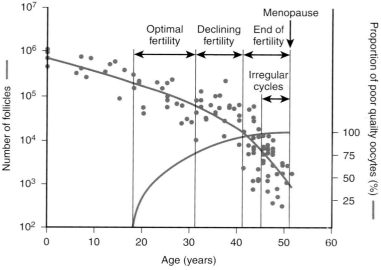

of the number of antral follicles present on cycle day 3 has been shown in a number of studies to predict poor ovarian reponse. Addition of basal FSH and inhibin B levels to a logistic model with the antral follicle count appears to further improve the performance of this marker.[281] At present no single reliable marker for ovarian reserve has been identified.[279] Anti-müllerian hormone (AMH), a member of the transforming growth factor-β superfamily, has been proposed as a novel candidate in this context. It is produced by granulosa cells of growing preantral and small antral follicles and is directly involved in primordial follicle pool depletion in the rat. Serum levels decline with age[282] and recent studies have shown that poor reponse to IVF can be predicted by reduced baseline serum AMH concentrations.[279] Although this hormone is a promising marker, additional prospective studies and multivariate analyses of potential factors are required in order to improve predictive potential.

To some extent, women likely to present with a reduced response to ovarian stimulation can be predicted, but hyper-response (and the threat of OHSS) comes as a surprise in the great majority of cases. It is uncertain, as yet, which patients are likely to present with hyper-response (at risk for OHSS).[192] Early recognition of women at risk may give rise to effective, altered stimulation protocols and improved safety.[174]

The use of normograms for individualising FSH dose for ovarian stimulation in IVF may optimize the risk/benefit dose of FSH in IVF. In recent years, several models have been developed based on multiple regression analysis.[283,284] Factors consistently observed to be predictive of the number of oocytes obtained were age, the total number of antral follicles, and smoking status.[285] Others have suggested that ovarian volume and and blood flow as measured by Doppler ultrasound are predictive factors. A model combining all these factors has been developed to prescribe the optimal dose of rFSH that will yield 5 to 14 oocytes.[283] In a prospective randomized study, the application of this model increased the proportion of "appropriate ovarian responses" and decreased the need for dose adjustments during ovarian stimulation.[284]

In those who do respond to ovarian hyperstimulation for IVF and for whom embryos are available for transfer, individualizing treatment in order to optimize outcomes should involve consideration of the number of embryos to be transferred. As stated earlier, although a trend toward the transfer of fewer embryos is now clear, fear of a lower chance of pregnancy may discourage couples and their physicians from transferring two embryos or less. This applies particularly when single embryo transfer is being considered. The ability to identify those treatment cycles in which single embryo transfer would avoid the risk of twin pregnancy without reducing the chance of achieving a singleton pregnancy would certainly encourage the adoption of single embryo transfer into clinical practice. In recent years, a number of authors have tried to identify those factors that may predict the chance of birth and of multiple birth on the basis of key characteristics of the patient, the cycle, and the embryos available for transfer.[57,286] Important determining factors thus far identified include the age of the woman, the duration of infertility, and the

number of oocytes obtained following ovarian hyperstimulation. We have previously developed a prediction model to allow the chance of pregnancy and twin pregnancy to be assessed in a given transfer cycle should one or two embryos be transferred.[65] Application of this model allows a subgroup of young patients with good quality embryos to be identified for whom applying single embryo transfer could drastically diminish the twin rate without compromising singleton pregnancy rates.

As with models designed to predict spontaneous pregnancy, untested models for predicting IVF outcome can show a disappointing performance when used on patients from a different but plausibly similar population.[287] Therefore, before such a model can be applied in clinical practice, its reliability in predicting the selected outcomes should be validated on a different population to that on which it was developed. External validation of our model has demonstrated that it may be applied in different populations following a simple calibration process to adjust for local success rates.[66]

Health Economics of Ovarian Stimulation

Although a tendency to increased IVF consumption can be observed every year, IVF or IUI should not be routinely applied for all kinds of infertility problems. Assisted reproduction should not replace a proper infertility workup. Moreover, the economic implications of a more widespread use of assisted reproduction should be considered seriously when making decisions regarding treatment.[288,289]

The diagnosis by exclusion of unexplained infertility/subfertility is made in around 30% of couples in whom conventional diagnostic tests are normal. The prognosis for conception significantly decreases when the duration of infertility is at least 3 years along with an advanced female age beyond 35.[267] Again, chances of spontaneous conception are usually underestimated both by the doctor and the patient.[70] It appears that high costs prevent many couples with an indication for this treatment modality from undergoing IVF (i.e., undertreatment due to insufficient access to ART services). Data from the United States suggest that in states where IVF is not covered, only one third of couples with a valid indication for IVF actually undergo treatment.[290] Moreover, IVF is available in only 25% of the countries worldwide.[289] On the other hand, in a commercial environment couples may be exposed to risks associated with assisted reproduction too early (i.e., overtreatment under conditions in which expectant management might have been more appropriate). Indeed, in various European countries such as France, The Netherlands, and Sweden where IVF is covered by health insurance, a threefold higher use of IVF per capita compared to the United States can be observed.[289]

Cost-effective health care involves the achievement of a desired treatment goal at the lowest possible expenditure. IVF cost effectiveness should assess costs per live birth. So far, calculations of costs per live birth have only included direct costs related to neonatal care. The inclusion of indirect costs (i.e., including mid- and long-term health sequelae such as mental retardation, cerebral palsy, and learning disabilities) would presumably double the overall costs.

The financial consequences of multiple pregnancies are substantial for both parents and health care providers. However, the economic impact of a multiple pregnancy is not limited to increased costs of maternal hospitalization and obstetric and neonatal (intensive) care. Lifetime costs for chronic medical care, rehabilitation, and special education related to extreme prematurity must also be taken into account. For a low-birth-weight child, the average cost of health care and education up to the age of 8 years is 17-fold higher than the costs for a normal birth weight child.[291] It has also been shown that multiple births contribute disproportionately to hospital inpatient costs, especially during the child's first year of life.[292]

Because of the limited use of ovarian stimulating medication, the per cycle costs of mild stimulation IVF cycles will be lower than conventional stimulation approaches. However, to analyze the cost effectiveness of mild stimulation, the total cost per live birth should be analyzed. Besides the costs for medication, medical consultations and visits, laboratory charges (general, hormone and embryology), ultrasound procedures, IVF procedures (oocyte retrieval and embryo transfer), hospital charges, nurse coordinator costs, administrative charges, fees for anesthesia, costs for complications, travel expenses, and lost wages should be taken into account.[289]

Those who advocate milder strategies in IVF point to recent studies that show that the costs for IVF per year of treatment are comparable with conventional stimulation approaches, and the costs for the pregnancy and neonatal period are significantly lower following mild stimulation and single embryo transfer.[293]

Conclusions and Future Perspective

Any form of ovarian stimulation increases chances of pregnancy per cycle but at the expense of increased complication rates, most importantly multiple pregnancies (see Fig. 28-8) and OHSS. This holds especially true for ovarian hyperstimulation aiming at maturing multiple dominant follicles for fertilization either in vivo (following intercourse or IUI) or in vitro by IVF. With IVF, the incidence of occurring multiple pregnancies can be controlled by the number of embryos transferred. Moreover, various strategies may significantly reduce chances for OHSS. In skillful hands and with proper ovarian response monitoring, chances for complications are lowest for ovulation induction. The aim of this intervention is to mimic physiologic circumstances in anovulatory women, hence, single dominant follicle development and ovulation.

Special care should also be taken to carry out a proper infertility workup in order to diagnose other treatable infertility factors. This will also allow a proper assessment to be made of pregnancy chances for a given couple, either spontaneously or after infertility therapies. Along these lines, only patients with a proper indication will be exposed to the discomfort, risks, and costs associated with assisted reproduction and ovarian hyperstimulation.

Milder forms of ovarian hyperstimulation (or indeed none at all) may be considered for empirical treatment of unknown infertility (with or without IUI) due to the inherent risk of higher order multiple pregnancies. In general, however, the price to pay is a slightly lower pregnancy rate per cycle. Overall, assessment of cumulative pregnancy rates over a given period of time (which may involve multiple cycles) may be similar.

A trend can be observed toward hyperstimulation and assisted reproduction as first-line treatment in anovulatory infertility, especially PCOS. This shift in clinical practice is not based on sound scientific evidence. In fact, healthy live birth rates from conventional ovulation induction strategies are good, with acceptable rate of multiple pregnancies and OHSS.[47] Newly introduced compounds to the field of ovulation induction such as insulin sensitizers and aromatase inhibitors may further improve outcomes.

With regard to IVF, many new treatment modalities have been introduced over the years without proper preceding evaluation for efficacy and safety. The current most profound clinical challenge is to find the right balance between improving chances for success coinciding with an acceptable complication rate. The paradigm of so-called "controlled" ovarian hyperstimulation using maximum stimulation by exogenous gonadotropins together with the GnRH agonist long protocol has been taken for granted for more than a decade. Potential detrimental effects of this approach with regard to patient discomfort and safety, oocyte quality, corpus luteum function, and endometrial receptivity have been largely ignored. Large numbers of preovulatory follicles and oocytes subsequently retrieved have been applied as useful surrogate outcome parameters for successul IVF.[253] Maximum ovarian stimulation along with the transfer of large numbers of embryos in an attempt to maximize pregnancy rates per IVF cycle may by itself have a major impact on patient dropout rates, costs, and overall IVF outcome and should therefore be considered seriously. The introduction of GnRH antagonists allows for a careful reevaluation of current IVF strategies. We can now render stimulation protocols simpler, starting with a spontaneous menstrual cycle, allowing for more subtle interference with dominant follicle selection. Final stages of oocyte maturation can now also be stimulated, applying different drugs and strategies for the induction of an endogenous LH surge. Finally, effects of these altered follicular phase interventions on corpus luteum function and endometrial development (important for embryo implantation) should be assessed.

Especially in the light of a continued trend worldwide to reduce the number of embryos transferred, novel approaches of mild ovarian stimulation or even natural cycle IVF deserve reevaluation. It does not seem logical to stimulate the ovary profoundly in order to generate numerous embryos in case the aim is to transfer only one or two of them. Moreover, the possible relationship between quantity of oocytes stimulated and quality (i.e., genetic competence) of embryos obtained[265] should be studied in greater detail. Finally, in the light of a reduced number of fresh embryos being transferred, the continuing improvement of techniques to cryopreserve supernumerary embryos such as vitrification (allowing couples additional pregnancy chances without having to go through ovarian stimulation and oocyte retrieval) seems of pivotal significance.

Individualizing ovarian stimulation in order to optimize outcomes between risks and desired outcomes is likely to improve in the future with the development of pharmacogenetics. Clinical studies have shown that FSH receptor gene polymorphisms can influence the ovarian response to stimulation in women undergoing IVF.[294] Genotyping of patients prior to treatment may therefore aid in tailoring FSH doses dependent on individual ovarian sensitivity.[272]

Choosing the "best" embryo for transfer is still problematic, because the assessment of embryo morphology is still crude and inaccurate. More information is urgently needed regarding randomized controlled trials replacing a single embryo with or without preimplantation genetic aneuploidy screening. The paradigm of measuring success in terms of positive pregnancy test per IVF retrieval or transfer treatment should shift in future studies to take into account the balance between the chance of a healthy live (singleton) birth per started IVF treatment, which may involve multiple cycles in relation to risks and complications, patient discomfort, and costs.[73] The health economics evaluation of IVF should be no different from other complex medical interventions. In this context, the impact of ovarian stimulation on embryo quality (applying aneuploidy blastomere screening through fluorescence in situ hybridization [FISH] procedures), corpus luteum function, and endometrial receptivity should be studied in greater detail.

The complete reference list can be found on the companion Expert Consult Web site at www.expertconsultbook.com.

Suggested Reading

Fauser BC, Devroey P, Macklon NS. Multiple birth resulting from ovarian stimulation for subfertility treatment. Lancet 365:1807-1816, 2005.

Fauser BC, Van Heusden AM. Manipulation of human ovarian function: physiological concepts and clinical consequences. Endocr Rev 18(1):71-106, 1997.

Macklon NS, Stouffer RL, Giudice LC, Fauser BC. The science behind 25 years of ovarian stimulation for in vitro fertilization. Endocr Rev 27(2):170-207, 2006.

The Thessaloniki ESHRE/ASRM Sponsored PCOS Consensus Workshop Group. Consensus on infertility treatment related to polycystic ovary syndrome. Human Reprod 23(3):462-477, 2008.

CHAPTER 29

Assisted Reproduction

Mark D. Hornstein and Catherine Racowsky

The essence of mammalian reproduction is the fusion of a sperm and an egg resulting in a conceptus, which can grow and differentiate into a new organism. Mammalian reproduction is an efficient process that typically occurs entirely within the bodies of the male and female partners and requires no intervention or assistance from a third party. The essence of *assisted reproduction* is that a third party, the reproductive biologist, directly handles the oocyte and sperm to enhance the probability of achieving a pregnancy. In general, at least part of the manipulation of the sperm and oocyte occurs outside the body of the male and female partners. Assisted reproductive technologies refer to a large number of techniques, including in vitro fertilization and embryo transfer (IVF-ET), gamete intrafallopian tube transfer (GIFT), zygote intrafallopian tube transfer (ZIFT), intracytoplasmic sperm injection (ICSI), use of donor gametes, gestational carriers, and cryopreservation of embryos. Collectively these techniques are referred to as the assisted reproductive technologies (ART).

Assisted reproduction is more than 110 years old, beginning with the attempts of Schenck to achieve fertilization in vitro and the successful transfer of embryos from a donor to a recipient rabbit by Heape.[1] In 1959, Chang[2] successfully fertilized a rabbit oocyte in vitro. In the human, successful capacitation of sperm in vitro and the fertilization of human oocytes matured in vitro[3] were followed by the insight that preovulatory oocytes were optimal for in vitro fertilization.[4] These exploratory steps culminated in 1978 with a term birth resulting from the in vitro fertilization of a single preovulatory human oocyte obtained from a natural menstrual cycle, transferred to the uterus at the eight-cell stage.[5]

Assisted reproduction is the jewel in the crown of reproductive medicine. It is one of the best examples in reproductive medicine of the transfer of knowledge obtained by laboratory scientists to an application that treats human disease. Assisted reproduction is a vast field encompassing both the sublime secrets of how two haploid cells combine to create a diploid zygote that contains all the information necessary to grow and develop into a complex mammal, and the pragmatically empirical application of the technology to treat infertility. As assisted reproduction becomes the standard treatment for infertility, the pace of the transfer of knowledge from bench to bedside is increasing, challenging our concepts of self, family, and society.

The Gametes

Sex is not necessary for successful reproduction. Single cell organisms propagate directly by mitotic division. Some species of reptiles are all female and reproduce without mating. However, the majority of fish, birds, reptiles, and mammals reproduce sexually. The key feature of sexual reproduction is that unique haploid cells fuse at fertilization to form a diploid cell that can divide, with the daughter cells undergoing differentiation to develop into an entire organism. In turn, some diploid progenitor cells divide by the process of meiosis to produce unique haploid cells that can fuse to yield a new, totally unique diploid organism.

Sexual reproduction has two processes that maximize diversity in a species. One crucial process is that diploid cells give rise to unique haploid cells through genetic recombination between homologous chromosomes during meiosis (see Chapter 31). Exchange of genetic material between maternally and paternally derived chromosomes markedly increases the genetic diversity of the resultant haploid cells (Figs. 29-1 and 29-2). One theoretical advantage of sexual reproduction is that the process of meiosis permits the random recombination of genetic material, thereby increasing the range of traits displayed by members of the species. This diversity increases the chances of success of the species in adapting to an ever-changing

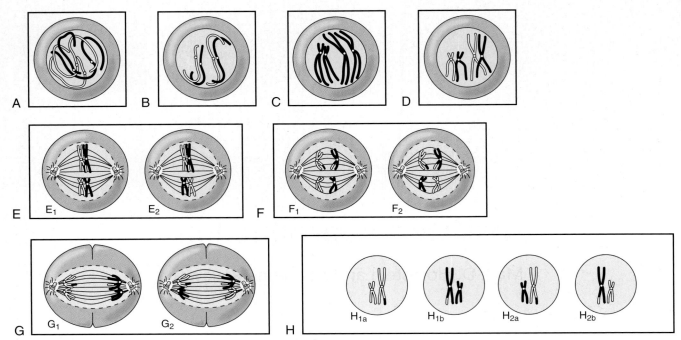

Figure 29-1. *The first meiotic division. Two of the 23 chromosome pairs are shown to simplify the presentation. Chromosomes from the maternal source are shown in outline, chromosomes from the paternal source are shown in solid color. **A**, Leptotene. **B**, Zygotene. **C**, Pachytene. **D**, Diplotene. **E**, Metaphase (E$_1$, and E$_2$). **F**, Early anaphase (F$_1$, and F$_2$). **G**, Late anaphase (G$_1$ and G$_2$). **H**, Telophase (H$_1$ and H$_2$). One set of distributions of chromosome pairs is delineated in E$_1$ through H$_1$, an alternative combination in E$_2$ through H$_2$. Homologous recombination and random segregation increase the diversity of genetic material passed to the gametes. (From Thompson JS, Thompson MW. Genetics in Medicine. Philadelphia, WB Saunders, 1986, p 19.)*

environment. A second process of sexual reproduction is that the haploid cells fuse during fertilization to form a new and unique diploid cell. The single-cell diploid zygote has all the genetic information necessary to grow and develop into an adult organism.

The generation of the germ cells is achieved through meiosis (see Figs. 29-1 and 29-2). During meiosis, duplication of diploid deoxyribonucleic acid (DNA) in the progenitor cell is followed by two successive cell divisions, which result in derivative packets of haploid DNA. As the progenitor cell enters prophase I, each duplicated chromosome consists of two joined sister chromatids; homologous chromosomes align in bivalents and genetic recombination occurs. In the first meiotic division, one homologue (consisting of linked sister chromatids) of each chromosome pair is distributed to each daughter cell (see Fig. 29-1). No DNA replication occurs in the second meiotic division, and the strands of the sister chromatids are separated to the derivative haploid cells (see Fig. 29-2).

In most species that reproduce by sexual reproduction, two types of gametes are produced. The egg, or ovum, is large and nonmotile. The developing egg is referred to as an *oocyte*. The sperm or spermatozoa are small and motile. In some species, the oocyte is totipotent; once stimulated by artificial means, it can give rise to an entire adult organism. Such an artifical stimulus can occur by mechanical activation or chemical stimulation (parthenogenesis).

The process of formation of female gametes (known as *oogenesis*) begins when the primordial germ cells migrate into the embryonic gonad and become *oogonia* (see Chapter 8). The oogonia proliferate by mitotic division, become invested with a single layer of granulosa cells, and differentiate

into primary oocytes. The primary oocyte enters the meiotic process, duplicates its complement of DNA, reaches diplotene of prophase I of meiosis, and then enters a state of prolonged meiotic arrest or "hibernation." The primary oocyte synthesizes a coat of glycoproteins, the *zona pellucida*.

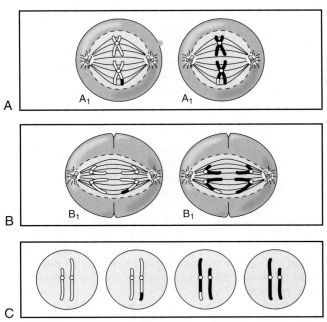

Figure 29-2. *The second meiotic division. **A**, Metaphase. **B**, Anaphase. **C**, Telophase. A$_1$ and A$_2$ represent H$_{1a}$ and H$_{1b}$ from Figure 29-1. (From Thompson JS, Thompson MW. Genetics in Medicine. Philadelphia, WB Saunders, 1986, p 20.)*

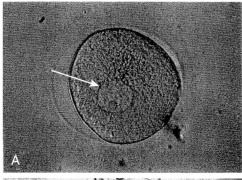

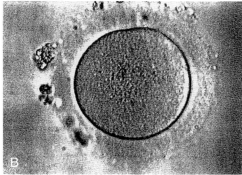

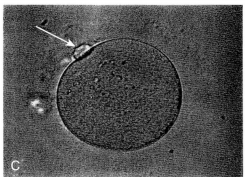

Figure 29-3. *Oocytes at the three most commonly observed stages of meiotic maturation.* **A,** *Oocyte at the germinal vesicle (GV) stage; note the nucleus with its characteristic single nucleolus (arrow) and granular cytoplasm.* **B,** *Oocyte at metaphase I; note the absence of both a nucleus and a polar body and less granular cytoplasm compared with the GV-stage oocyte.* **C,** *Oocyte at metaphase II; note the presence of the first polar body (arrow) and the smooth cytoplasm. (All photos courtesy of Dr. Gena Ratiu, Brigham and Women's Hospital ART Laboratory, Boston, MA.)*

The oocyte is one of the largest cells in the body through mechanisms that are not fully characterized. However, one possibility is that the extra copies of genes that are present in prophase I (diploid chromosome complement in duplicate) allow the oocyte to increase the rate of ribonucleic acid and protein synthesis. The primary oocyte remains arrested at this so-called germinal vesicle (GV) stage of prophase I (Fig. 29-3A) until the follicle in which it is enclosed either undergoes degeneration (atresia) or is recruited into a pool of developing follicles. Upon recruitment, under the influence of luteinizing hormone (LH) surge, the fully grown GV-stage oocyte resumes meiosis to progress through metaphase I (Fig. 29-3B) and anaphase I, to reach telophase I. Upon extrusion of the first polar body at telophase I, the oocyte completes meiosis I to become a secondary oocyte. The secondary oocyte then rapidly proceeds to metaphase II of meiosis (Fig. 29-3C) to complete the so-called process of "meiotic maturation." The oocyte is ovulated at metaphase II, the stage at which it awaits subsequent fertilization. The progression through meiotic maturation from prophase I to metaphase II, and then to telophase II following fertilization, is shown diagrammatically in Figure 29-4.

A normal mature haploid human oocyte has a complement of 23 chromosomes. However, meiotic errors occur resulting in a high incidence of aneuploid oocytes. Such errors typically occur during the first meiotic division and involve a variety of mis-segregations including nondysjunction of homologous chromosomes and predivision of sister chromatids.[6] Resulting oocytes either possess too few chromosome copies and are referred to as hypohaploid, or have too many copies and are termed hyperhaploid. Maternal age is the main factor associated with the occurrence of aneuploidy[7,8] which, in turn, accounts for the majority of failed conceptions (reviewed by Hassold et al.[9]). The root cause of such age-related aneuploidy appears to be abnormalities in morphology of the meiotic spindle.[10]

In contrast to the egg, sperm are among the smallest cells in mammals. Sperm are highly specialized for the sole purpose of transporting DNA to an oocyte. Sperm consist of four key functional components:

1. The acrosomal vesicle
2. The nucleus containing highly compacted DNA
3. A midpiece enriched in mitochondria
4. The tail, which contains the axoneme and the dynein motor proteins

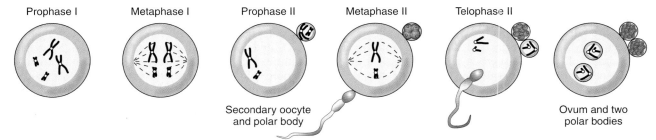

Figure 29-4. *Stages of meiotic maturation and completion of the second meiotic division after fertilization. (From Thompson JS, Thompson MW. Genetics in Medicine. Philadelphia, WB Saunders, 1986, p 23.)*

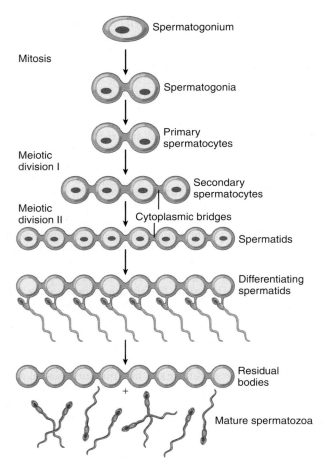

Mitosis

Spermatogonium

Spermatogonia

Primary spermatocytes

Meiotic division I

Secondary spermatocytes

Meiotic division II

Cytoplasmic bridges

Spermatids

Differentiating spermatids

Residual bodies

+

Mature spermatozoa

Figure 29-5. The progeny of a single maturing spermatogonium remain connected to each other by cytoplasmic bridges. The cytoplasmic bridges allow the spermatids to receive proteins from the parent cell apparatus without bearing the burden of protein machinery (e.g., endoplasmic reticulum). (Redrawn from Alberts B, Bray D, Lewis J, et al. Molecular Biology of the Cell. New York, Garland Publishing, 1994, p W31.)

To maximize transport efficiency, the sperm has no ribosomes, endoplasmic reticulum, or Golgi apparatus.

Spermatogenesis differs significantly from oogenesis (Fig. 29-5) (see Chapter 12). In the embryo, primordial germ cells migrate to the testis and enter a state of arrest until puberty. Under the influence of testosterone and other hormones, the spermatogonia divide mitotically and generate two pools of derivative cells. The cells of one pool continue to divide mitotically and serve as the spermatogonial stem cells. The second pool of cells will enter meiosis and become primary spermatocytes (46 duplicated chromosomes). The primary spermatocytes proceed through the first meiotic division and then become secondary spermatocytes (22 duplicated autosomal chromosomes, plus a duplicated X chromosome or a duplicated Y chromosome). After the second meiotic division, the secondary spermatocytes become spermatids (haploid number of single chromosomes), which then differentiate into mature sperm. The process of meiotic maturation of the spermatogonia occurs inside the seminiferous tubule, with the precursor cells located at the outer border of the tubule and the mature sperm in the lumen of the tubule. The

developing sperm cells undergo nuclear division but do not complete cytoplasmic division until near the end of sperm differentiation (see Fig. 29-5). Consequently, the developing germ cells are connected by cytoplasmic bridges in a syncytium, which allows the diploid spermatogonium to produce proteins and cellular materials for the haploid sperm.

The sperm then enters the epididymis, where its surface is reorganized both by absorbing secretions from the epididymis and by internal processes.[11] When sperm enter the female reproductive tract, they undergo the process of capacitation. During capacitation, the proteins and lipids of the sperm membrane change, including a significant efflux of membrane cholesterol, in preparation for interaction with the oocyte.[12] Sperm penetrate the cumulus cell layer surrounding the egg through their hyperactivated motility, a consequence of capacitation and hyaluronidase tethered to the sperm surface by a glycosylphosphatidylinositol anchor. The sperm motility and hyaluronidase secretion allow the sperm to move through the cumulus extracellular matrix to reach the zona pellucida. On reaching the zona pellucida, the capacitated sperm then undergo the *acrosome reaction*, a process that is essential for fertilization. The acrosome is a large secretory granule that contains proteases and hyaluronidases. In the acrosome reaction, the outer acrosome membrane fuses with the plasma membrane of the sperm and the contents of the acrosome are emptied. In many species, the acrosome reaction is initiated by the proteins of the zona pellucida and can be accelerated by progesterone.[13]

Fertilization

The process of fertilization involves at least two key initial steps: interaction and penetration of the zona pellucida by the sperm, and fusion of the sperm and oocyte membranes (Fig. 29-6). Although the mechanisms that allow the human sperm and zona pellucida of the oocyte to interact are not fully characterized, use of antibodies and antagonists to candidate molecules has greatly advanced understanding in this area (reviewed by Nixon et al.[14]). Prevailing data suggest that a complex glycoprotein on the zona pellucida interacts with lectin-like proteins on the sperm head.[15,16] In mouse, the zona pellucida contains three glycoproteins (ZP1, ZP2, and ZP3)[17] but in humans there is evidence for a fourth glycoprotein, ZP4/B.[18] ZP2 and ZP3 have a filament structure, and ZP1 appears to link ZP2 and ZP3 in a complex three-dimensional array, for the absence of either ZP2 or ZP3 prevents assembly of the zona matrix. In a dose-dependent manner, purified ZP3 blocks the ability of sperm to bind to the oocyte zona pellucida. This implies that ZP3 is the zona pellucida sperm receptor,[19] although it appears that O-linked carbohydrate moieties such as N-acetylglucosamine,[20] mannose and N-acetylgalactosamine (reviewed in Benoff[21]) in ZP3 underly the interaction of ZP3 and the sperm receptor.[22,23] Nevertheless, the biologic complexity of the sperm-egg recognition process appears to reflect participation by a series of sperm proteins (see Nixon et al.[14]). The interaction of the sperm with ZP3 induces the acrosome reaction. ZP3 cross-links the sperm receptors on the sperm membrane, inducing an influx of calcium that causes

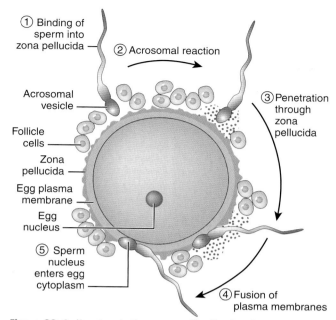

① Binding of sperm into zona pellucida
② Acrosomal reaction
Acrosomal vesicle
③ Penetration through zona pellucida
Follicle cells
Zona pellucida
Egg plasma membrane
Egg nucleus
⑤ Sperm nucleus enters egg cytoplasm
④ Fusion of plasma membranes

Figure 29-6. Key steps in the process of fertilization. Step 1, binding of sperm to zona pellucida involves zona protein ZP3 and a sperm protein, probably a carbohydrate-binding protein such as 1,4-galactosidase. Step 2, acrosome reaction. Step 3, penetration of sperm through zona pellucida. Step 4, fusion of plasma membranes of sperm and oocyte. Depolarization of oocyte membrane and secretion of cortical granules—the primary and secondary blocks to polyspermy. Step 5, sperm nucleus enters egg cytoplasm. (Redrawn from Alberts B, Bray D, Lewis J, et al. Molecular Biology of the Cell. New York, Garland Publishing, 1994, p 1031.)

the exocytotic release of proteases and hyaluronidases from the acrosome. Induction of the acrosome reaction can be inhibited by pertussis toxin, implying that a G protein complex is necessary for the acrosome reaction.[24]

After completion of the acrosome reaction, the sperm lose their affinity for ZP3,[25] and the continued attachment of the sperm to the oocyte appears to be dependent on ZP2.[26] The sperm penetrates the zona pellucida, in part, by the forward mechanical thrust provided by the flagellum and by the hydrolytic enzymes secreted by the acrosome that cause disruption of the continuity of the zona pellucida.

A small number of proteins on the sperm surface appear to be responsible for interaction with ZP3. These proteins include fertilin,[27] galactosyltransferase, and cyritestin. β1,4-Galactosyltransferase on the sperm surface appears to be important for the ZP3-induced acrosome reaction.[28] Fertilin and cyritestin are members of the ADAM (a *dis*integrin *a*nd *m*etalloprotease) family of proteins, which can bind to integrins but also have proteolytic activity. The sperm of mice lacking cyritestin (ADAM3) have defective binding to the zona pellucida.[29] Fertilin, a heterodimeric sperm surface protein composed of α and β subunits, was originally thought to be involved in fusion of sperm with the egg plasma membrane (the oolemma). However, mice lacking fertilin β (ADAM2) show defects in zona binding.[30] More recent studies have implicated involvement of a new candidate enzyme, mouse sperm lysozyme-like protein (mSLLP1), in sperm-oolemmal binding.[31] This protein is located in the equatorial segment of acrosome-reacted

sperm in both mouse and human, and appears to bind to the entire oolemma except in that region where sperm normally do not bind, overlying the meiotic spindle.[31]

The role of ZP3 and the galactosyltransferase and ADAM proteins in fertilization in the human is not fully characterized. Studies suggest that some metaphase II oocytes that fail to be fertilized have reduced ZP3 levels in the zona pellucida as determined by immunohistochemistry.[31] Another egg protein that is essential for successful fertilization is CD9, a member of the tetraspanin family. In mouse eggs lacking this oolemma protein, sperm-egg fusion fails to occur, resulting in infertility.[32]

Once the sperm fuses with the oolemma, a depolarization of the oolemma occurs that acts as the primary block to polyspermy. Shortly thereafter, the inositol phospholipid cell-signaling pathway is activated, resulting in an increase in cytosolic calcium, which induces the submembrane cortical granules to release their contents. The contents of the cortical granules change the glycoprotein coat of the zona pellucida, preventing sperm binding by hydrolyzing the oligosaccharides of ZP3 and by the proteolytic cleavage of ZP2. This process creates a secondary block to polyspermy.

The Early Conceptus and Implantation

Sperm penetration into the oocyte triggers the oocyte to complete meiosis by rapid progression from metaphase II to telophase II. Telophase II is characterized by elimination of one of the sister chromatids of each chromosome through extrusion of the second polar body. The retained set of oocyte chromatids undergoes decondensation, followed by decondensation of the set of sperm chromatids, each to form a pronucleus. The pre-zygote is therefore characterized by the presence of two pronuclei and two polar bodies (Fig. 29-7A). Following migration to the center of the oocyte, and then apposition of the two pronuclei, pronuclear membrane breakdown occurs, the maternal and paternal chromosomes intermingle at syngamy, and the diploid zygote is formed. Shortly thereafter, the chromosomes undergo condensation and the paired homologues (one maternal and one paternal) align on the metaphase plate of the first mitotic spindle, in preparation for the first cleavage division. The pre-embryo then progresses through several cleavage divisions (see Fig. 29-7B through D), giving rise to an embryo comprising multiple cells or blastomeres.

In human pre-embryos, the blastomeres are totipotent up to around the eight-cell stage[33] and removal of one, or even two, blastomeres from eight-cell embryos does not necessarily disrupt embryo development (see Chapter 30). Beyond the eight-cell stage, the cells clearly begin to undergo differentiation. Compaction ensues to form the morula stage as blastomeres adhere because of secretion of cell adhesion molecules such as E-cadherin.[34] Tight junctions form between blastomere membranes, and pockets of fluid begin to accumulate among the blastomeres (Fig. 29-8A). Concomitant with onset of coalescence of these small fluid collections to form a fluid-filled cavity

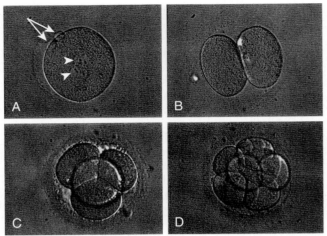

Figure 29-7. Development of human embryos during the first 72 hours after insemination. **A,** A zygote at 18 hours, showing two polar bodies (arrows) and two pronuclei in apposition (arrowheads) with several distinct nucleoli polarized toward the juxtaposed nuclear membranes. **B,** A two-cell embryo at 28 hours. **C,** A four-cell embryo at 44 hours. **D,** An eight-cell embryo at 68 hours.

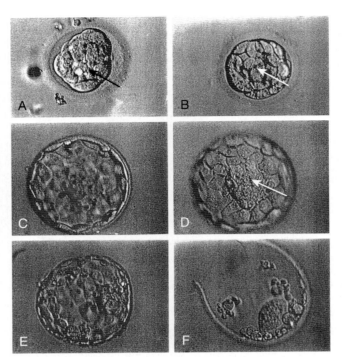

Figure 29-8. Development of human embryos between 90 and 120 hours after insemination. **A,** A morula transitioning to a very early blastocyst at 92 hours; note the characteristically compacted cells of a morula, yet the accumulation of small pockets of fluid accumulation (arrow), and the first signs of cellular differentiation as reflected by the epithelial cells forming at the periphery that will develop into the trophectoderm cells. **B,** An early blastocyst at 100 hours; note the increasing size of fluid pockets, further differentiation of the trophectoderm cells, and the appearance of a small cluster of spherical cells that will form the inner cell mass (arrow). **C** and **D,** A fully expanded blastocyst at 116 hours in two focal planes to show the trophectoderm layer surrounding the blastocoelic cavity (**C**) and the innercell mass (**D**). **E,** A hatched blastocyst at 118 hours and, **F,** its corresponding zona pellucida containing discarded cytoplasmic fragments.

(the blastocoele), the first signs of overt cellular differentiation occur; the surface cells begin to undergo a change in shape from spherical to squamous epithelial-like to form trophectoderm cells, while a small cluster of inner cells retain their spherical appearance, ultimately to form the inner cell mass (Fig. 29-8B). The trophectoderm cells form the trophoblast, which gives rise to the extra-embryonic structures, such as the placenta, and the inner cell mass gives rise to the embryo. Following enlargement of the blastocoelic cavity, which causes expansion of the blastocyst (see Fig. 29-8C and D), the blastocyst ultimately escapes from the zona pellucida in preparation for implantation (see Fig. 29-8E and F).

Strictly speaking, the embryonic stage consists of the period from the development of the primitive streak through the initial steps in the development of all the major organs. In the human, the embryonic stage begins approximately 14 days after fertilization. In assisted reproduction, most authorities use the term "embryo" to describe the conceptus from the first cleavage through the initial stages of organ development. This convention will be followed in the remainder of this chapter.

The molecular events underlying the process of implantation in humans are not completely understood (see Chapter 9). The human embryo enters the uterus approximately 4 days after fertilization at the *morula stage.* Within 5 to 6 days of fertilization, the embryo reaches the *blastocyst stage* and begins the hatching process, thereby allowing the outer covering of syncytial trophoblast cells to interact with the endometrial surface. The trophectoderm nearest the inner cell mass probably plays an important role in the interaction of the blastocyst and the endometrium.[35] The interaction of the blastocyst with the endometrium involves phases of apposition, stable adhesion, and invasion. The blastocyst can attach to the endometrium only during a critical window of implantation

corresponding to menstrual cycle days 19 to 24.[36] Although the molecules that control the attachment of the blastocyst to the uterine epithelium are not well characterized, the integrins, fetal fibronectin, laminin, heparin-binding epidermal growth factor, leukemia inhibitory factor, and interleukin 11 have been proposed as playing important roles.[37] After attachment, the conceptus enters the endometrium, and by 12 days after fertilization is completely embedded in the endometrial stroma. Once this contact is established, human chorionic gonadotropin (hCG) can be detected in the maternal circulation.[38] At the same time, the trophoblast invades the maternal endothelium, establishing a hemochorial placentation.

Assisted Reproductive Technologies

Many techniques are currently utilized that involve manipulation of oocytes, sperm, and conceptuses to improve the probability of a successful outcome. In vitro fertilization and embryo transfer (IVF-ET) is the most commonly performed procedure, involving the laboratory

TABLE 29-1

In Vitro Fertilization Outcome as Reported by Those Programs Participating in the Society for Reproductive Technology/American Society for Assisted Reproductive Medicine Registry 1986, 1994, 1998, and 2005[*]

Results	1986	1994	1998	2005
Cycles initiated	4867	26,555	58,937	92,405
Clinical pregnancies	485	6089	17,943	32,682
Deliveries	NR	4896	14,789	26,872
Delivery per cycle initiated (%)	<9[†]	18.4	25.1	29.1

[*]Fresh cycles, non-donor egg.

[†]Assumes an abortion and ectopic rate of at least 10%.

Adapted from Society for Reproductive Technology/American Society for Assisted Reproductive Medicine. Fertil Steril 49:212-215, 1988; Fertil Steril 66:697, 1996; Fertil Steril 71:798-8907, 1999; Fertil Steril 77:18-31, 2002; Society for Assisted Reproductive Technology and Centers for Disease Control and Prevention Web sites, 2005 (www.sart.org and www.cdc.gov/art).

culture of aspirated oocytes and spermatozoa in vitro, followed by the transcervical replacement of the resulting embryo(s) into the uterine cavity. One variation of IVF-ET is intracytoplasmic sperm injection (ICSI), in which fertilization is achieved by injection of a sperm into the oocyte. In contrast, GIFT is the direct placement of aspirated oocytes and prepared spermatozoa into the fallopian tube, and ZIFT entails the laboratory culture of aspirated oocytes with spermatozoa followed by the direct placement of fertilized zygotes into the fallopian tubes. This chapter focuses on IVF-ET, its indications, implementation, and outcomes. ICSI and manipulation of gametes and embryos is the focus of Chapter 30.

A major deficiency in the field of assisted reproduction is that there are few randomized studies demonstrating the superiority of assisted reproductive techniques over other forms of fertility treatment, such as pelvic reconstructive surgery or empirical ovarian stimulation with gonadotropins. Consequently, much of the discussion of clinical assisted reproductive technologies is limited to data from descriptive studies, often without adequate control groups. Furthermore, many new assisted reproductive technologies are introduced into clinical practice without adequate clinical trials to demonstrate their utility in relation to "standard" methods of treatment. Notwithstanding these deficiencies, there has been consistent improvement in the success of IVF during the past two decades (Table 29-1).

IN VITRO FERTILIZATION

Indications for in Vitro Fertilization

In current clinical practice, the standard indications for IVF are tubal factor infertility, endometriosis, mild to moderate cases of male factor infertility, and idiopathic or unexplained infertility. The most recent national report for the United States shows that among couples who underwent ART using autologous oocytes, only 10.6% had tubal factor, with 5.6% having endometriosis, 18.9% having male factor, and 12.2% diagnosed with unexplained infertility, with the remainder diagnosed with such conditions as ovulatory dysfunction, polycystic ovary syndrome, and uterine conditions.[39] Indeed, as the technology has

improved, the application of IVF has broadened; it now is recommended for essentially all infertility conditions that have not been successfully treated by other modalities. For example, IVF has recently been advocated for the treatment of polycystic ovary syndrome (PCOS). However, IVF is likely to be less successful if the female partner has diminished ovarian reserve (a depleted ovarian follicular pool). In this situation, donor egg has been demonstrated to be effective. Likewise, IVF is not likely to be successful in cases of severe male factor infertility. In this situation, ICSI is very effective (see Chapters 22 and 30).

Tubal Factor Infertility. For women with infertility and complete distal fallopian tube occlusion, expectant management is unlikely to be successful. Rather, surgical treatment and IVF are possible therapeutic options, although no prospective trials have been reported comparing their relative efficacies. Nevertheless, one randomized study did demonstrate that IVF was more effective than expectant management in this setting,[40] and a retrospective analysis revealed a 70% cumulative live birth rate after up to four cycles of IVF in patients with tubal factor infertility.[41] This cumulative success compared favorably with surgical treatment of tubal disease causing infertility. Women who have failed to conceive after 6 to 12 months following tubal surgery should undergo IVF. Notwithstanding the absence of clinical trials, as IVF success increases and its cost remains stable, the procedure is likely to become the preferred treatment of tubal factor infertility.

Endometriosis. For women presenting with infertility and early-stage endometriosis, IVF has not been definitively documented by a randomized clinical trial to be superior to other available treatments, such as expectant management, human menopausal gonadotropin (hMG) with intrauterine insemination (IUI), or surgical treatment (see Chapter 24).[42] However, some studies suggest that IVF treatment results in a higher pregnancy rate per cycle than after surgical treatment, hMG with IUI, clomiphene treatment with IUI, or expectant management. For example, in one retrospective study of infertile women with advanced endometriosis, surgical treatment was associated with a cumulative pregnancy rate of 24% at

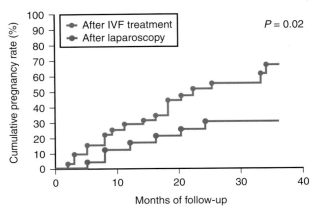

Figure 29-9. Cumulative conception rate curves during 36 months for women older than 32 years of age with infertility and endometriosis. Top curve, Cumulative conception rate after in vitro fertilization (IVF) treatment. Bottom curve, Cumulative conception rate with expectant management after laparoscopy. (From Kodama H, Fukuda J. Karube H, et al. Benefit of in vitro fertilization treatment for endometriosis-associated infertility. Fertil Steril 66:974-979, 1996, with permission of the American Society for Reproductive Medicine.)

9 months after surgery. In a similar group of infertile women with advanced endometriosis, two cycles of IVF treatment were associated with a 70% pregnancy rate.[43]

The preceding study demonstrates the time-effectiveness of IVF treatment. For infertile couples, the older the female partner, the more important is timely treatment with IVF. For example, Kodama and associates[44] demonstrated that in women 32 years of age or older with endometriosis, treatment with IVF resulted in a significantly higher pregnancy rate than that observed in the control group (Fig. 29-9). In women 32 years of age or older, the cumulative pregnancy rate was 59% in those women treated with IVF and 29% in women treated with expectant management. In contrast, in women under 32, the cumulative pregnancy rate during the 3 years of the study was 64% in the women treated with IVF and 53% in the control group. Because IVF is often more expensive per cycle than other treatments (such as hMG/IUI), it is usually reserved for couples who have failed to conceive after trials of these other forms of treatment (see Chapter 28).

IVF was originally developed as a method to treat tubal factor infertility. However, retrospective analyses from many IVF centers indicate that IVF treatment of infertility associated with endometriosis is associated with a pregnancy rate similar to that observed with IVF treatment of tubal factor infertility. Olivennes and colleagues[45] reported that IVF treatment resulted in a live birth rate per cycle of 31% for women with endometriosis and 32% for women with tubal factor infertility. When the results were analyzed by surgical stage of the endometriosis (revised American Society for Reproductive Medicine classification), the live birth rate per cycle was stage I, 27%; stage II, 31%; stage III, 36%; and stage IV, 33%. However, some women with advanced endometriosis (stage III and IV) have undergone oophorectomy plus a contralateral ovarian cystectomy (for endometriomas); these women appear to have reduced success with IVF due to premature depletion of the oocyte pool.[46-49]

Male Factor. Male factor infertility is a broad category that ranges from minimally abnormal semen parameters to total sperm counts of less than 5 million per ejaculate. In general, men with severe semen abnormalities are probably best treated with ICSI (see Chapters 22 and 30). Prior to undergoing ICSI, men with severe male factor infertility should have a karyotype assessment because the incidence of karyotypic abnormalities is in the range of 10% in this group.[50] In men with minimally to moderately abnormal semen parameters, the incidence of chromosomal abnormalities increases with decreasing sperm count.[51] Nevertheless, such men are good candidates for IVF. Though male factor infertility is associated with reduced fertilization rates in IVF, ICSI in these cases provides fertilization and pregnancy rates comparable to those seen in standard IVF. Severe decreases in the number of motile sperm per ejaculate (less than 1.5 million) and decreases in the number of sperm with normal morphology are associated with poor pregnancy rates in standard IVF.[52]

Idiopathic Infertility. For 10% to 17% of infertile couples, thorough evaluation reveals no identifiable cause of infertility. "Unexplained," or idiopathic, infertility is a term applied to those couples who have completed an infertility evaluation that includes laparoscopy. For the purposes of this chapter, however, idiopathic infertility refers to couples who have completed the basic steps of the infertility evaluation (semen analysis, documentation of ovulation and tubal patency), but who may not have had laparoscopy.

Many couples with idiopathic infertility achieve successful pregnancies after a stepwise treatment approach (see Chapter 28), which includes empirical clomiphene treatment followed by empirical gonadotropin ovarian stimulation, with or without IUI treatment.[53] If the couple fails to conceive after empirical gonadotropin ovarian stimulation with IUI, IVF often results in a successful pregnancy. In one study of 117 couples with idiopathic infertility,[54] the clinical pregnancy rate per cycle of IVF was similar to that observed for couples with tubal factor infertility (21% and 22%, respectively). However, those couples with idiopathic infertility had a lower fertilization rate than couples with tubal factor infertility (44% versus 56%, $P < 0.005$), and complete fertilization failure was more frequent in the group with idiopathic infertility (20% versus 8%, $P < 0.001$). The cumulative pregnancy rate after three cycles of IVF was similar in both groups (45% versus 44%). These results indicate that IVF can be effective for the treatment of unexplained infertility in many patients, when ovarian stimulation with gonadotropins has failed.[54]

Complete fertilization failure suggests that some couples with idiopathic infertility have subtle defects in oocyte and sperm function that are not identified with routine laboratory testing. Such defects may include the abnormal release of sperm proteasomes resulting in inhibition of sperm binding to the zona pellucida,[55] or impairment of microtubule nucleation in the ooplasm and subsequent disruption of pronuclear formation.[56]

Polycystic Ovary Syndrome and Anovulation. Until recently, infertile women with polycystic ovary syndrome

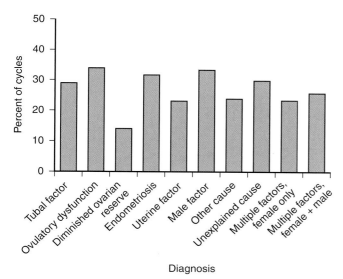

Figure 29-10. *Percentages of ART (assisted reproductive technology) cycles using fresh nondonor eggs or embryos that resulted in live births, by diagnosis, 2005. (From CDC Assisted Reproductive Technology [ART] Report 2005. Available at www.cdc.gov/art/ART2005. Accessed Dec. 21, 2008.)*

(PCOS) in whom both clomiphene and gonadotropin ovulation induction failed had few remaining treatment options except surgical procedures to reduce thecal and stromal androgen production. However, evidence has accumulated that IVF can be effective for such patients. In one study, the effects of IVF were compared between a group of 68 infertile women with PCOS who did not become pregnant after six ovulatory cycles of gonadotropin treatment and 68 age-matched women with tubal factor infertility. The women with PCOS had more oocytes retrieved (14 versus 11) but a lower fertilization rate (57% versus 66%) than women with tubal factor infertility. The clinical pregnancy rate per embryo transfer (23% versus 26%) and the multiple gestation rate (19% versus 16%) were similar for the PCOS and the tubal factor infertility groups.[57] It may be concluded that for women with PCOS who do not conceive with standard ovulation induction, IVF is effective.

Multiple Infertility Factors. Many couples have multiple factors contributing to their low fecundability. In general, the greater the number of infertility factors, the lower the success with IVF treatment. For example, in one study of the efficacy of IVF on couples for whom the only identifiable infertility factor was endometriosis, the live birth rate per cycle was 31%. In women with endometriosis and a male partner with an abnormal semen analysis, the live birth rate per cycle was 16%. For women with both endometriosis and tubal disease, the live birth rate per cycle was 8%.[45] Similarly, in a study of the effectiveness of IVF on women presenting with tubal disease with or without other infertility diagnoses, the live birth rate per transfer was 30% in women with tubal disease alone, 25% in women when tubal factor occurred in combination with male factor, and 20% and 19%, respectively, in cases of previous diethylstilbestrol exposure or immunologic infertility.[41]

TABLE 29-2

Assisted Reproductive Technology (ART) Report 2005: National Summary*

Cycle Data	Age of Woman			
	<35	*35-37*	*38-40*	*41-42*
Number of cycles	41,302	22,624	19,482	8997
Cycles resulting in live births (%)	37.3	29.5	19.7	10.5

*Using fresh embryos from nondonor eggs.
From CDC Assisted Reproductive Technology [ART] Report 2005. Available at www.cdc.gov/art/ART2005. Accessed Dec. 21, 2008.

Overview of in Vitro Fertilization Statistics

As IVF has evolved as a scientific field, the reporting of outcomes associated with IVF procedures has continued to change and improve. Currently, most authorities recognize that the live delivery rate per IVF cycle initiated (i.e., per cycle in which gonadotropin therapy was begun) provides the most realistic estimate of the likely outcome of an IVF cycle. For the calculation of the delivery rate, multiple gestations are counted as one delivery, not two deliveries in the case of twins or three deliveries in the case of triplets. Unfortunately, many investigators use other numerators (clinical pregnancy, ongoing pregnancy) and denominators (transfer cycles, retrieval cycles) in calculating IVF success rates. Many critics believe that these rates are overly optimistic and are not a realistic estimate of the success of IVF. One of the most remarkable features of IVF is the continuous improvement in its efficacy. From 1986 to 2005, there has been a significant increase in the deliveries per IVF cycle initiated, from less than 9% to more than 29% (see Table 29-1).[58,59]

IVF is a great equalizer. Unlike other treatments for infertility whose success is highly dependent on the diagnosis, IVF yields similar pregnancy rates with most infertility diagnoses (Fig. 29-10). The exception is diminished ovarian reserve, a condition that produces a live birth rate per cycle initiated of only 13%.

The live birth rate is highly dependent on the ovarian reserve. Not surprisingly, advancing female age correlates inversely with successful IVF outcome (Table 29-2). As a woman ages, her follicular numbers are depleted and her chances to achieve a pregnancy with IVF diminish. As seen in Figure 29-11, live birth rates in IVF are relatively stable between the age of 25 and 31, when they gradually decline to 35. The decline becomes steeper after age 35, and by age 45, the live birth rate approaches 0%.

Selection of Patients

As results continue to improve, it has become increasingly clear that IVF-ET is most successful for infertile couples when the female partner has an adequate ovarian follicular pool. As a woman ages, there is a decline in her ovarian follicular pool.[60] Some reports suggest that the decline in the oocyte pool accelerates after age 37 (Fig. 29-12). In addition to the chronologic age of the female partner, the biologic age of the ovary (a measure of the remaining

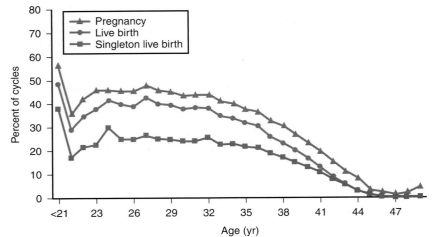

Figure 29-11. Percentages of ART (assisted reproductive technology) cycles using fresh, nondonor eggs or embryos that resulted in pregnancies, live births, and singleton live births by age of woman in 2005. (From CDC Assisted Reproductive Technology [ART] Report 2005. Available at www.cdc.gov/art/ ART2005. Accessed Dec. 21, 2008.)

ovarian follicular pool) as determined by follicular phase cycle day 3 follicle-stimulating hormone (FSH) concentration[61] or the FSH response to clomiphene citrate is also an excellent predictor of IVF outcome.

In one study of the relationship between cycle day 3 FSH concentration and IVF pregnancy and delivery rates, investigators determined that a day 3 FSH level greater than 25 mIU/mL was associated with a clinical pregnancy rate in the range of 5% per cycle, and the delivery rate was about 2% per cycle (Fig. 29-13). In contrast, for a cycle day 3 FSH level under 15 mIU/mL, the clinical pregnancy rate was approximately 23%, and the delivery rate was approximately 16% per cycle.[62] When the interaction of age and the results of a clomiphene challenge test were examined, in women with a normal clomiphene citrate challenge test response (suggesting an adequate follicular pool), the age of the female partner remained an important prognostic variable.[62] Similar results have been observed in a general infertility population (Fig. 29-14).

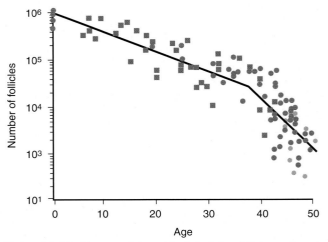

Figure 29-12. Biexponential model of declining follicle numbers in women up to 51 years of age. Accelerated rate of follicle loss appears to occur after age 37. Circles and squares represent data from various authors. (From Faddy MI, Cosden R, Cougeon A, et al. Accelerated disappearance of ovarian follicles in mid-life: implications for forecasting menopause. Hum Reprod 7:1342-1346, 1992.)

Recently, several investigators have proposed that the ovarian antral follicle count (the number of ovarian antral follicles between 2 and 10 mm in diameter) is a good predictor of ovarian reserve. Women with fewer than 10 total antral follicles have diminished ovarian reserve and have generally poorer outcomes in IVF.[63] In addition, ovarian volume also appears to correlate with IVF success. Women with small ovarian volumes also suffer lower pregnancy rates with ART.[64,65] Inhibin B, a hormone secreted by granulosa cells in the follicles, has also been studied as a marker of ovarian reserve. Inhibin B directly inhibits pituitary secretion of FSH in a manner similar to that of estradiol, and thus was thought to be a marker of ovarian health.[66,67] The utility of inhibin B as a marker of ovarian reserve is limited by the lack of a uniform commercial assay. Müllerian inhibiting substance (MIS), also known as anti-müllerian hormone (AMH), is a glycoprotein growth factor synthesized in granulosa cells. A number of studies have demonstrated that AMH is reduced with increasing age and, as such, could potentially be used as a marker of ovarian reserve. Seifer et al. were the first to demonstrate that MIS/AMH is significantly reduced in women who responded poorly to ovarian stimulation in IVF cycles.[68] Pregnancy rates are also lower in ART in women with low serum levels of MIS/AMH.[69] Although MIS/AMH has the advantages of minimal cycle-to-cycle variation, and its levels do not change across the menstrual cycle, its clinical utilization in ART is currently limited by the lack of a commercially available assay.

As demonstrated in Figure 29-15, in assisted reproduction cycles the proportion of pregnancies that end in spontaneous abortion increases with age of the female partner. Many authorities advise that women with a depleted oocyte pool and women over age 40 who have a poor response to gonadotropin stimulation should instead consider either treatment with donor oocytes or adoption.

For men with severely abnormal semen parameters, standard IVF therapy is associated with low success rates. These men may be counseled to consider treatment with ICSI rather than standard IVF. For men with fewer than 5 million sperm per ejaculate, ICSI may be indicated as primary treatment.

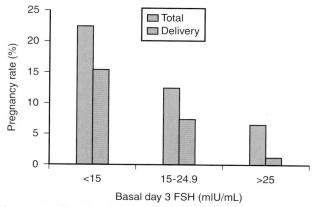

Figure 29-13. *Clinical pregnancy and delivery rates after IVF (in vitro fertilization) treatment as a function of the cycle day 3 follicle-stimulating hormone (FSH) concentration of the female partner. Note the decrease in live birth rates with day 3 FSH levels greater than 25 mIU/mL. Data based on 758 couples. (From Scott RT, Hofmann CE. Prognostic assessment of ovarian reserve. Fertil Steril 63:1-11, 1995, with permission of the American Society for Reproductive Medicine.)*

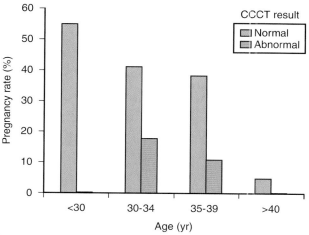

Figure 29-14. *Clinical pregnancy rates as a function of both age and the response to a clomiphene citrate challenge test (CCCT) in a general infertility population observed prospectively. The illustration is based on data from 236 couples. In women with an abnormal CCCT result (suggestive of a depleted oocyte pool), pregnancy rates are low regardless of the age of the female partner. In women older than 40 years of age, pregnancy rates are low with in vitro fertilization even if the CCCT result is normal. (From Scott RT, Hofmann CE. Prognostic assessment of ovarian reserve. Fertil Steril 63:1-11, 1995, with permission of the American Society for Reproductive Medicine.)*

Ovarian Stimulation

The number of oocytes retrieved is positively correlated with the live birth rate per cycle. Consequently, success is critically dependent on generating an adequate number of mature follicles that contain developmentally competent oocytes. Many techniques and medications for stimulating multiple follicle maturation for oocyte retrieval have been developed (see also Chapter 28). Medications include clomiphene, clomiphene-hMG; clomiphene-rhFSH (recombinant human FSH); hMG alone; immunopurified urinary human FSH (hFSH) alone; rhFSH alone; combinations of hMG, hFSH, and rhFSH; and pulsatile gonadotropin-releasing hormone (GnRH). One common regimen involves the long GnRH-agonist protocol with step-down gonadotropin stimulation (Fig. 29-16).

Careful monitoring of the menstrual cycle with serum hormones and pelvic sonography can identify the time in the natural cycle when the dominant follicle can be aspirated to yield a fertilizable oocyte. Although conceptually appealing, natural cycle IVF is associated with low pregnancy rates. In one study of 74 such cycles, oocytes were harvested in approximately 50% of the cycles, and the pregnancy rate per cycle initiated was 3%.[70] In another study of 114 natural IVF cycles, the pregnancy rate per cycle initiated was 4%.[71] IVF is a resource-intensive treatment, and pregnancy rates in the range of 3% to 4% per IVF cycle initiated are not cost effective. In the near term, natural-cycle IVF is unlikely to play a central role in infertility treatment.

Clomiphene citrate, at a dose of 100 mg daily for 5 days, induces one to three follicles to grow in normally cycling women. In IVF cycles stimulated with clomiphene, one or two oocytes are retrieved and the pregnancy rate per cycle initiated is in the range of 10%. For example, in one randomized study comparing IVF using a natural cycle to clomiphene stimulation, the mean number of oocytes retrieved was 0.3 in the natural cycle and 1.8 in the clomiphene groups. The clinical pregnancy rates per cycle initiated were 0% and 12%, respectively.[72] In IVF cycles where clomiphene is used for ovarian stimulation, support of the luteal phase with both estradiol and progesterone may improve the clinical pregnancy rate by overcoming the anti-estrogenic effect of clomiphene on the endometrium.[73] Compared to clomiphene alone, the combination of clomiphene plus human gonadotropins (FSH or hMG) increases the number of follicles stimulated to grow, the number of oocytes retrieved, and the pregnancy rate.[74] However, in terms of the expected live birth rate, the ovarian stimulation regimen of clomiphene plus gonadotropin is not clearly superior to gonadotropins alone.

Pulsatile, native GnRH, at the proper doses (approximately 14 µg per pulse every 90 minutes), can induce the growth of one to three follicles in normally cycling women. When stimulation with clomiphene citrate is followed by pulsatile GnRH, up to seven mature follicles can be obtained.[75] Use of pulsatile GnRH requires a programmable infusion pump and continuous parenteral access. These factors have limited its application in IVF.

Exogenous gonadotropins override the mechanisms that produce mono-ovulation. At the proper doses, clomiphene-hMG, hMG, and hFSH ovarian stimulation regimens produce numerous follicles containing fertilizable oocytes and a pregnancy rate in the range of at least 20% per cycle initiated in favorable patients. However, a number of studies demonstrate that the combination of GnRH agonist plus gonadotropin stimulation is more effective for ovarian stimulation in IVF-ET cycles than gonadotropin alone.[76] The addition of a GnRH agonist analog to a gonadotropin stimulation regimen appears to suppress premature LH surges, lowers the chance of premature luteinization of granulosa cells, and reduces cycle cancellation due to premature luteinization or ovulation. The

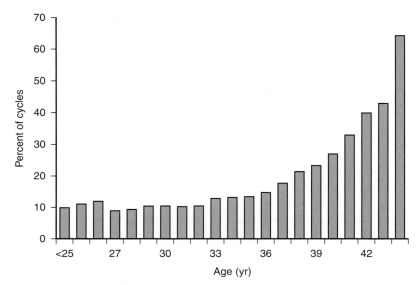

Figure 29-15. *Percentage of ART (assisted reproductive technology) cycles using fresh nondonor eggs or embryos that resulted in spontaneous abortion, by age of woman in 2005. (From CDC Assisted Reproductive Technology [ART] Report 2005. Available at www.cdc.gov/art/ART2005. Accessed Dec. 21, 2008.)*

introduction of GnRH antagonists has complemented the established GnRH-agonist regimens. The combination of a GnRH analog, either agonist or antagonist, plus gonadotropins is currently the gold standard for controlled ovarian stimulation in IVF. There are three main contemporary regimens for controlled ovarian stimulation in IVF:

1. GnRH-agonist down-regulation (Figs. 29-16 and 29-17)
2. GnRH-agonist flare regimens (Fig. 29-17)
3. GnRH-antagonist regimens (Fig. 29-18)

GnRH-Agonist Down-Regulation Regimens. In ovarian stimulation for IVF, the main purpose of a GnRH-agonist analog or antagonist is to prevent a premature LH surge (triggered by the high concentrations of estradiol) while follicles are still immature. GnRH-agonist analogs differ from the native decapeptide GnRH in amino acid positions 6 and 10. They are resistant to degradation, giving them long half-lives and prolonged receptor occupancy. The initial administration of a GnRH-agonist analog is associated with an increase in LH and FSH secretion (agonist phase). Long-term administration causes down-regulation

and partial desensitization of the pituitary GnRH receptor, resulting in the suppression of pituitary secretion of LH and FSH. The addition of a GnRH-agonist analog to regimens of ovarian stimulation for IVF-ET appears to be associated with an increase in the number of oocytes retrieved, the number of embryos transferred, and the clinical pregnancy rate.[77,78]

For example, one study demonstrated that treatment with a GnRH agonist (buserelin) plus hMG resulted in more oocytes retrieved (9.3 versus 6.2), more embryos (4.3 versus 2.8), and a higher clinical pregnancy rate (20% versus 14%) than did stimulation with clomiphene plus hMG.[79] In another study, comparison of a stimulation regimen using the same medications also demonstrated that buserelin-hMG stimulation resulted in a higher pregnancy rate than that observed with clomiphene-hMG (36% versus 18%).[80] The type of GnRH-agonist analog used appears not to be crucial to obtaining the improved outcomes. Studies with D-Trp6 GnRH-agonist analog also demonstrate improved pregnancy rates (21% versus 12%) compared with ovarian stimulation regimens that do not use GnRH agonists for IVF-ET.[81] The addition of a GnRH-agonist analog to a gonadotropin-stimulation regimen appears to suppress premature LH surges, reduces the chance of premature luteinization of granulosa cells, and reduces cycle cancellation due to premature luteinization or ovulation.

Among a smaller number of women, GnRH-agonist down-regulation protocols may excessively suppress endogenous pituitary LH secretion in a small number of women. If rhFSH is the only exogenous gonadotropin used, LH stimulation may be suboptimal, and low serum levels of estradiol may result.[82] When LH levels are too high, premature ovarian luteinization occurs. When LH levels are too low, both estradiol production and endometrial development are suboptimal. During ovarian stimulation, LH levels need to be within a range that optimizes follicle development and estradiol production but minimizes premature luteinization.

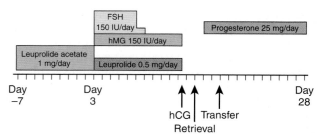

Figure 29-16. *Schematic representation of the long gonadotropin-releasing hormone-agonist analog protocol (using leuprolide acetate) with step-down gonadotropin stimulation. Note the decrease in FSH dose. FSH, follicle-stimulating hormone; hCG, human chorionic gonadotropin; hMG, human menopausal gonadotropin. (From Davis OK, Rosenwaks Z. In vitro fertilization. In Keye WR, Chang RJ, Rebar RW, Soules MR [eds]. Infertility: Evaluation and Treatment. Philadelphia, WB Saunders, 1995, p 763.)*

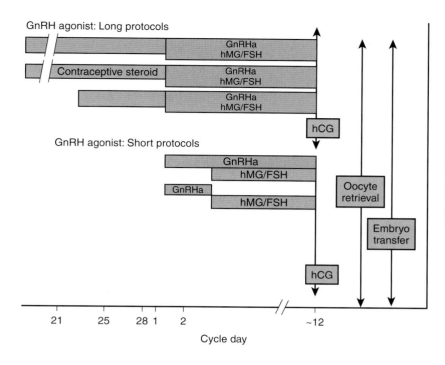

Figure 29-17. Schematic representation of the different approaches to ovarian stimulation that have been used in in vitro fertilization programs. FSH, follicle-stimulating hormone; GnRHa, gonadotropin-releasing hormone-agonist analogs; hMG, human menopausal gonadotropin; FSH, follicle-stimulating hormone; hCG, human chorionic gonadotropin.

GnRH-Agonist Flare or Short-Course Regimen. In the down-regulation protocol, GnRH-agonist analogs are usually started in the luteal phase of the cycle preceding the IVF-ET cycle (long protocol). In the GnRH-agonist flare regimen, the GnRH agonist is begun in the early follicular phase of the IVF-ET cycle (see Fig. 29-17). Basically, the flare regimens take advantage of both the agonist and down-regulation properties of GnRH-agonist analogs. In the first few days of treatment, the GnRH agonist stimulates endogenous LH (and FSH) secretion from the pituitary during the early follicular phase of ovarian stimulation. The increased LH secretion stimulates more

ovarian androstenedione production, which increases the substrate available for aromatization. This results in higher estradiol levels, especially among "poor responders" to ovarian stimulation. With continuing administration of the GnRH-agonist analog, the down-regulation effects of the analog begin and premature LH surges are prevented.

In one study, women with a poor response to standard long-protocol GnRH-agonist down-regulation plus gonadotropin stimulation were treated with a flare regimen using microdose leuprolide acetate (20 µg every 12 hours), initiated in the follicular phase of the treatment cycle,

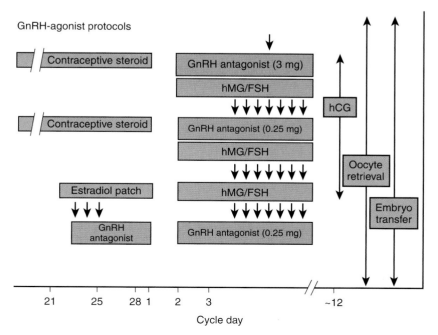

Figure 29-18. Schematic representation of different approaches to ovarian stimulation for in vitro fertilization utilizing GnRH-antagonists. FSH, follicle stimulating hormone; GnRH, gonadotropin-releasing hormone; hCG, human chorionic gonadotropin; hMG, human menopausal gonadotropin.

plus gonadotropin. Compared with a previous cycle of down-regulation, microdose GnRH agonist plus gonadotropin resulted in greater ovarian stimulation, higher serum estradiol concentration, and increased numbers of follicles and oocytes retrieved.[83]

A popular flare protocol for poor responders involves use of an oral contraceptive in the cycle preceding the IVF cycle, followed by a microdose leuprolide flare regimen during the IVF cycle. In this regimen, an estrogen-progestin oral contraceptive is given until cycle day 0 of the IVF-ET cycle and then, on cycle day 3, leuprolide acetate is initiated at a dose of 20 µg subcutaneously every 12 hours. On cycle day 5, FSH is started at a dose of 150 IU intramuscularly every 12 hours until the administration of hCG.[84] As an alternative for poor responders, more LH activity can be given during ovarian stimulation by using hMG or rhLH.[85]

The GnRH flare regimens are associated with increased secretion of both LH and ovarian androstenedione. In one study of women treated with a GnRH-agonist down-regulation or a GnRH flare regimen, follicular fluid androstenedione concentrations were 27 ng/mL versus 57.3 ng/mL ($P < 0.05$), respectively.[86] Numerous studies suggest that elevated circulating LH and intrafollicular androgen levels are not associated with optimal oocyte function.[87] GnRH flare regimens are also associated with an increased cycle cancellation rate compared with GnRH-agonist down-regulation regimens.[88] In one large cohort study of women under 40 with normal baseline FSH levels, the GnRH flare regimen was associated with a lower delivery rate per cycle compared with the GnRH-agonist down-regulation regimen (15.1% versus 21.3%, $P < 0.05$).[89] Other investigators have reported similar trends.[90] The GnRH flare probably should not be the first choice of ovarian stimulation regimens in women undergoing their first cycle of IVF and who have a good prognosis. GnRH flare regimens are best suited to women with a poor response to the down-regulation regimen.

GnRH-Antagonist Regimens. A major problem with the GnRH-agonist analogs is that LH secretion is stimulated at the initiation of treatment. The GnRH antagonists offer the possibility of acutely suppressing LH secretion without an initial increase in LH release.[91,92] Thus, pituitary LH secretion can be controlled within the stimulation cycle itself; such control is not possible with the GnRH agonists, which must be begun during the previous menstrual cycle to achieve full down-regulation. GnRH antagonists have been administered as a small daily dose (cetrorelix or ganirelix, 0.25 mg daily by subcutaneous injection), usually starting on cycle day 6 to 8 or when the lead follicle reaches 14 mm in diameter,[93] or as a single large dose (cetrorelix, 3 mg subcutaneously) on approximately cycle day 8[94] (see Fig. 29-18). Both protocols block a spontaneous LH surge.

The impact of a GnRH antagonist on ovarian stimulation for IVF is heavily dependent on the dose of GnRH antagonist administered. At small doses, the suppression of LH is minimal. With large doses, near complete suppression of LH is achieved. In one study, the impact of six doses of the GnRH antagonist ganirelix on LH secretion and IVF outcomes was studied.[95] A fixed daily dose of recombinant FSH was administered. Ganirelix produced a dose-dependent suppression not only of LH (Table 29-3) but also of serum androstenedione and estradiol. Larger doses of Ganirelix were associated with low levels of LH, androstenedione, and estradiol, and a markedly reduced pregnancy rate. These data support the use of at least a minimal concentration of LH to foster proper follicle development, steroidogenesis, and endometrial growth in preparation for IVF. With the GnRH antagonists, the challenge is to administer a dose sufficient to prevent an LH surge, but not so large that it will oversuppress LH secretion.

A variation of GnRH antagonist use in IVF utilizes a luteal estradiol patch followed by GnRH-antagonist suppression. Following a menstrual period, gonadotropin

---

TABLE 29-3

Efficacy of Gonadotropin-Releasing Hormone in Preventing Premature Luteinizing Hormone Surges in Women Undergoing Ovarian Stimulation

Group	Dose of Ganirelix (mg)	Number of Women	FSH (IU/L)	LH (IU/L)	Androstenedione (ng/mL)	Estradiol (pg/mL)	Pregnancy Rate per Cycle (%)
1	0.0625	30	9.1	3.6	2.6	1475	23.3
2	0.125	65	9	2.5	2.6	1130	23.1
3	0.25	68	9.1	1.7	2.4	160	33.8
4	0.5	69	10.2	1	2.2	823	10.1
5	1	64	9.8	0.6	2	703	14.1
6	2	26	8.8	0.4	1.5	430	0

Note: Women undergoing in vitro fertilization received recombinant follicle-stimulating hormone (FSH) (Puregon) starting on cycle day 2 and continuing daily until three follicles with a mean diameter > 17 mm (as determined) were achieved when human chorionic gonadotropin (hCG) was given to initiate the ovulatory process. The women were randomized to receive the gonadotropin-releasing hormone antagonist ganirelix on a daily basis starting on cycle day 7 at one of six doses (0.0625 mg, 0.125 mg, 0.25 mg, 0.5 mg, 1 mg, 2 mg). Serum FSH, luteinizing hormone (LH) androstenedione, and estradiol concentration were measured on the day of hCG administration. Large doses of ganirelix markedly suppressed serum LH, androstenedione, and estradiol concentrations. Pregnancy rate per cycle was maximal with a dose of ganirelix of 0.25 mg.
Adapted from the Ganirelix Dose Finding Study Group. A double-blind randomized dose-finding study to assess the efficacy of the gonadotropin-releasing hormone antagonist ganirelix [org 37462] to prevent premature luteinizing hormone surges in women undergoing ovarian stimulation with recombinant follicle stimulating hormone [Puregon]. Hum Reprod 13:3023-3031, 1998.

stimulation with GnRH antagonist support is utilized. The hypothetical advantage of this approach is to improve the synchrony of the developing follicles by reducing antral follicle sizes and follicular phase heterogeneity,[96] making it best suited for use in poor responders. In one report, patients using the "patch" protocol had a lower cycle cancellation rate, more oocytes retrieved and more embryos transferred than in a prior cycle.[97] Most studies of IVF have demonstrated that both GnRH agonists in a down-regulation protocol and GnRH antagonists are associated with similar rates of cycle cancellation due to a premature LH surge and similar rates of ovarian hyperstimulation syndrome (OHSS). However, the clinical pregnancy rate appears to be slightly lower in cycles using GnRH antagonists. In a Cochrane review of five randomized controlled trials comparing GnRH antagonist ($n = 1211$) to GnRH agonists in a down-regulation protocol ($n = 585$) for IVF, the odds ratio (OR) for becoming pregnant in the GnRH antagonist group was 0.79 (95% confidence interval [CI], 0.63-0.99) compared with the GnRH agonist group.[98] GnRH agonists used in a down-regulation protocol remain the gold standard for prevention of a premature LH surge in IVF programs.

Selection of Gonadotropin: hMG or uFSH or rFSH. For the stimulation of multiple ovarian follicle growth, exogenous gonadotropins are essential to override the endogenous negative feedback loop involving ovarian follicle secretion of estradiol and inhibins, and pituitary secretion of FSH.[99] FSH is the key hormone required to stimulate ovarian follicle development. LH stimulates secretion of ovarian thecal androgen secretion, which is the substrate for granulosa cell aromatase, an FSH inducible enzyme. FSH is available for administration as human menopausal urinary gonadotropins (hMG) in combination with LH, as highly immunopurified urinary FSH (uFSH), and as recombinant FSH (rFSH). All three forms are highly effective for ovarian stimulation in IVF-ET. In one prospective study, compared with other forms of FSH, rFSH use resulted in more oocytes retrieved and slightly higher cumulative pregnancy rates.[100] However, a meta-analysis of randomized controlled trials comparing rFSH and uFSH failed to demonstrate any difference in pregnancy rate between the two FSH preparations.[101] Moreover, the highly purified preparations of hMG appear to have clinical efficacy similar to rFSH when used for IVF.[102] Because the various FSH preparations appear equally efficacious in the treatment of IVF, additional factors such as patient acceptability, cost, and drug availability should be part of the choice of FSH.[103-107]

Final Follicle Maturation: hCG or rhLH or GnRH Agonist. Final follicle and oocyte maturation prior to retrieval requires stimulation by high concentrations of LH. Prior to the availability of recombinant hormones, the most accessible source of LH-like material was urinary chorionic gonadotropin (hCG). Recently, recombinant hCG (rhCG) has become available.[108] Typically hCG is administered as 5000 or 10,000 units (250 µg of rhCG is approximately equivalent to 10,000 units of hCG) to stimulate final follicle maturation. In a clinical trial, hCG was

compared with recombinant human LH (rhLH) for final follicle maturation. The investigators reported that hCG and rhLH had similar efficacy for maturing follicles and oocytes and performed similarly in terms of pregnancy rates. However, the rhLH was associated with slightly lower rates of OHSS, probably due to its short half-life, in contrast to the long half-life of hCG.[109] It should be noted that the rate of OHSS is highly dependent on the dose of FSH administered during follicle stimulation.[110]

When ovarian stimulation is performed using a combination of GnRH antagonist plus rhFSH, it is possible to use a single dose of a GnRH agonist to stimulate the pituitary to release a surge of LH that will initiate final follicle maturation. For example, in one small clinical trial, women undergoing IVF were stimulated with rhFSH and the GnRH antagonist ganirelix, and then randomized to receive either hCG (10,000 IU), triptorelin (0.2 mg), or leuprolide (0.5 mg) to initiate final follicle maturation. In the GnRH agonist groups (triptorelin and leuprolide), the endogenous secretion of LH peaked at 4 hours after the injection and LH levels returned to baseline by 24 hours. After the hCG injection, circulating hCG peaked at 24 hours and remained elevated for 5 days. Estradiol and progesterone levels were similar up until the day of oocyte retrieval in all three groups. In the luteal phase, estradiol and progesterone levels were greater in the hCG group than in the triptorelin or leuprolide groups. Similar numbers of oocytes and mature oocytes were retrieved in all three groups, and fertilization rates were also similar.[111] Stimulation of an endogenous LH surge with a GnRH agonist will likely be associated with a lower rate of OHSS.

Adverse Effects of Ovarian Stimulation for IVF. Current regimens of ovarian stimulation for IVF produce major increases in circulating estradiol, with estradiol concentrations reached being routinely in the range of 1200 pg/mL. The intensive stimulation of ovarian follicle growth increases the risk of OHSS (see Chapter 28). Circulating androgen levels also increase substantially in women undergoing ovarian stimulation for IVF (Fig. 29-19),[112] though the impact on the ovary and endometrium remains to be fully characterized. However, in many model systems, excessive follicular androgen secretion is associated with suboptimal follicle and oocyte function.

Although GnRH-agonist analogs have few adverse effects in ovarian stimulation protocols for IVF-ET, a few cases of OHSS caused by the administration of the GnRH agonist alone have been reported.[113]

Oocyte Retrieval

Oocyte retrieval is typically performed 35 to 36 hours after hCG administration by a transvaginal sonography-guided technique. Reports of oocytes in the human fallopian tube after hCG administration suggest that a time interval between hCG administration and oocyte retrieval of about 36 hours maximizes oocyte maturation and minimizes the chance of spontaneous ovulation (Fig. 29-20). Before 30 hours, oocytes in the lead follicles may not be mature. After 38 hours following hCG administration, ovulation begins and oocytes are lost into the peritoneal cavity. The

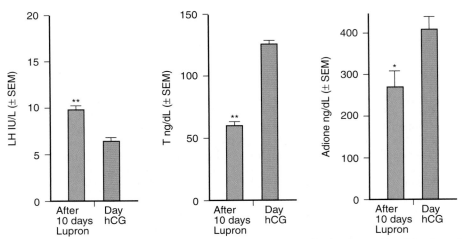

Figure 29-19. *Androgen levels in normal ovulatory infertile women undergoing in vitro fertilization and receiving leuprolide (Lupron) and hMG (human menopausal gonadotropin) for ovarian stimulation in preparation for oocyte retrieval. Luteinizing hormone (LH), testosterone (T), and androstenedione (Adione) were measured after 10 days of leuprolide acetate treatment, 1 mg daily by subcutaneous injection, and then again after leuprolide plus hMG stimulation, just before the administration of human chorionic gonadotropin (hCG). After 10 days of leuprolide treatment, LH concentrations were in the normal follicular phase range. Testosterone and androstenedione concentrations increase significantly with ovarian stimulation. Mean, SEM; *P < 0.05; **P < 0.001. (From Martin KA, Hornstein MD, Taylor AE, et al. Exogenous gonadotropin stimulation is associated with increases in serum androgens in IVF-ET cycles. Fertil Steril 68:1011-1016, 1997, with permission of the American Society for Reproductive Medicine.)*

number of oocytes retrieved is largely dependent on the number of large follicles present at the time of retrieval. In general, oocytes can be harvested with a high rate of success from follicles with a mean diameter greater than 12 mm (Fig. 29-21).[114]

Oocyte Meiotic Stage

Current techniques for evaluating the meiotic stage and quality of oocytes obtained by ovarian follicle aspiration remain rudimentary, although molecular screening approaches are currently under development (reviewed by Patrizio[115]). Routine assessment of meiotic stage continues to rely on visual inspection of the morphologic appearance of the surrounding cumulus oophorus with a light microscope. During the periovulatory period in response to the midcycle surge of LH or exogenous hCG, the cumulus cells secrete glycosaminoglycans,[116,117] resulting in expansion of the cumulus oophorus, and a radiating

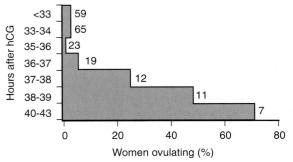

Figure 29-20. *Interval between an injection of human chorionic gonadotropin (hCG) and the percentage of women in whom follicular rupture has occurred. The number of women studied is indicated to the right of the bar. (From Edwards RG. Physiological aspects of human ovulation. J Reprod Fertil 18[suppl]:87-101, 1973.)*

appearance of the inner corona radiata cells. Therefore, the disposition of the surrounding cumulus-corona cells may provide some guide to meiotic maturity of the enclosed oocyte.[118] However, the meiotic stage is most accurately assessed by visualization of the oocyte itself (see Fig. 29-3). As discussed earlier, immature oocytes at prophase I exhibit a germinal vesicle, maturing oocytes at metaphase I have no GV evident, and mature oocytes at metaphase II exhibit a smooth cytoplasm and an extruded first polar body. Typically, 70% to 80% of retrieved oocytes are in metaphase II, with 20% to 30% being at metaphase I.

An oocyte that has reached metaphase II (i.e., completed nuclear maturation) has not necessarily achieved cytoplasmic maturation. In the case of cytoplasmic immaturity, the oocyte is unable to undergo normal fertilization and to support syngamy and subsequent early developmental events. Only about 70% of metaphase II oocytes fertilize. Although more than 90% of zygotes proceed through syngamy and the first cleavage division, the majority of these zygotes subsequently exhibit aberrant development in culture. Techniques to assess oocyte quality and developmental competency are therefore needed. Preimplantation genetic screening of the first polar body enables, by extrapolation, assessment of the oocyte chromosomal complement[119] (see Chapter 30). However, this approach fails to provide information regarding oocyte cytoplasmic maturity and the subsequent ability of the oocyte to support normal embryonic development. To this end, alternative strategies are being developed to assess oocyte quality. Cumulus cell apoptosis[120] and expression of genes expressed during cumulus expansion (such as *PTGS2*, *HAS2*, and *GREM1*)[121,122] have all been found to have some predictive value. Alternatively, visualization of the size and shape of the meiotic spindle using polarized light has been correlated with outcome.[123,124] However, because of the cost of the polarizing system and the sensitivity of the results to

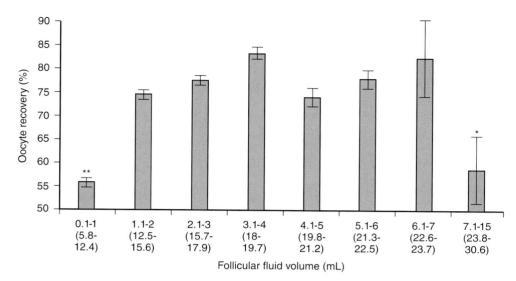

Figure 29-21. *Percentage of follicles from which an oocyte was obtained at the time of retrieval as a function of follicle size. Mean, SEM; *P < 0.01; **P < 0.001. Numbers in parentheses represent corresponding follicular diameter in millimeters as determined by sonography. (From Wittmaack FM, Kreger DO, Blasco L, et al. Effect of follicular size on oocyte retrieval, fertilization, cleavage, and embryo quality in in vitro fertilization cycles: a 6-year data collection. Fertil Steril 62:1205-1210, 1994, with permission of the American Society for Reproductive Medicine.)*

oocyte positioning it is unlikely that this approach will be routinely adopted in the IVF laboratory.

Incubation of Oocytes and Sperm

Semen is collected by masturbation or occasionally by sexual intercourse using a condom lacking spermicide. The semen specimens are processed for sperm collection by a variety of techniques, including swim-up and centrifugation techniques using a density gradient comprising a polymer (e.g., Percoll or Isolate). For normal semen specimens, both techniques generate high-motility sperm for oocyte insemination.[125] For semen with abnormal sperm characteristics (e.g., low sperm concentration), however, most studies demonstrate that sperm prepared by the gradient centrifugation technique have a greater fertilization capacity than sperm prepared by the swim-up technique. For example, in one study on semen with sperm concentration under 15 million/mL, the swim-up technique resulted in the collection of more sperm with higher motility, but the

sperm obtained by gradient centrifugation were associated with a higher fertilization rate.[126] The superiority of the gradient centrifugation technique when semen characteristics are abnormal has been reported by other investigators.[127]

Sperm prepared by either the swim-up or gradient centrifugation technique are then incubated in a protein-supplemented medium for up to 4 hours to initiate the process of capacitation before their co-incubation with the oocytes. For standard IVF, many laboratories incubate 25,000 to 50,000 capacitated sperm with a single oocyte. Preliminary studies suggest that for men with normal semen parameters, higher concentrations of sperm do not significantly improve the fertilization rate. Insemination is typically performed 4 to 6 hours after oocyte retrieval. Approximately 18 hours later, the oocytes are examined for fertilization. A pre-zygote with two pronuclei and two polar bodies is morphologic evidence of fertilization. For couples using IVF, if the male partner has abnormal semen parameters, the number of sperm harvested from the semen specimen is related to both the fertilization and pregnancy rate (Table 29-4). As the number of sperm in the unwashed specimen decreases below 10 to 20×10^6/mL, the incidence of chromosomal abnormalities increases (Table 29-5). Interestingly, the incidence of aneuploidy in sperm appears to increase with increased incidence of sperm DNA fragmentation.[128]

For men with markedly abnormal semen parameters, ICSI (see Chapters 22 and 30) is recommended.

Evaluating Embryo Quality

The key goal of evaluating embryo quality is identification of an embryo marker that predicts pregnancy rate more accurately than the age of the female partner and the number of embryos transferred.[129] Such a marker should lead to the development of highly successful single embryo transfer protocols and reduce the risk of multiple gestations.[130]

Several recent studies have investigated possible marker candidates in the medium used to culture the embryos.

TABLE 29-4

Results of In Vitro Fertilization in Couples With Severe Male Factor, Analyzed by Number of Total Motile Sperm Harvested After Semen Preparation by Swim-Up Technique

Total Motile Sperm After Swim-Up ($\times 10^6$)	Fertilization Rate (%)	Clinical Pregnancy Rate per Oocyte Retrieval (%)
<0.5	22 ± 5	8
0.51 to 1	40 ± 4	15
1.01 to 1.5	60 ± 5	21
>1.5	64 ± 1	22

Adapted from Ben-Chetrit A, Senoz S, Greenblatt EM, Casper RM. In vitro fertilization outcome in the presence of severe male factor infertility. Fertil Steril 63:1032–1037, 1995, with permission of the American Society for Reproductive Medicine.

TABLE 29-5

Incidence of Chromosomal Abnormalities According to Sperm Concentration

Sperm Concentration in Unwashed Semen	Incidence of Chromosomal Abnormalities
>20 × 10⁶/mL	2.2%
10-20 × 10⁶/mL	2.7%
5-10 × 10⁶/mL	4.9%
0-5 × 10⁶/mL	6.9%
Azoospermia	13.1%

From Yoshida J, Miura K, Shirai M. Chromosome abnormalities and male infertility. Assisted Reprod Rev 6:93-99, 1996.

TABLE 29-6

The Timeline for the Development of the Conceptus from Pre-Zygote (Fertilized Egg) to Implanting Blastocyst and the Location of the Conceptus in the Reproductive Tract

Stage of Conceptus	Days after Fertilization	Location of Conceptus in the Reproductive Tract
Pre-zygote fertilized	0	Fallopian tube (oocyte)
Two-cell embryo	1	Fallopian tube
Four-cell embryo	2	Fallopian tube
Eight-cell embryo	3	Fallopian tube
Morula	4-5	Uterotubal junction
Blastocyst	5	Intrauterine
Implanting, hatched blastocyst	5-6	Intrauterine

These markers include soluble human leukocyte antigen (sHLA-G),[131] markers for amino acid metabolism,[132,133] and specific protein peaks associated either with implantation failure or success using proteomic profiling.[134] Each of these approaches hold some promise for identifying a marker(s) for embryonic developmental competency, but their standard application in the IVF laboratory awaits further research and confirmation of efficacy.

Despite limitations to determining embryo quality using the light microscope, such morphologic evaluation remains the first-line approach for assessing viability. Human embryos follow a specific developmental timeline,[135] during which milestones are reached in a coordinated sequence that are typified by characteristic morphologic features (Table 29-6). Therefore, utilization of the darwinian concept of "survival of the fittest" has proved useful. Historically, evaluation has been performed only once, within a few hours of transferring cleavage stage embryos on either day 2 or day 3. In this setting, evaluations have included assessment of cell number, degree of fragmentation (typically assessed as percentage of the volume of the embryo fragmented), cytoplasmic pitting, compaction, symmetry of blastomeres with respect to size and shape, and absence of vacuoles and multinucleation. Each of these parameters has been shown to have some value in predicting quality and pregnancy rate,[136-138] although cell number, fragmentation, and symmetry remain the most commonly assessed characteristics for day 3 embryos. Compared with eight-cell embryos lacking fragments and having perfect to near-perfect symmetry (i.e., blastomeres of uniform size and shape; Fig. 29-22A), those exhibiting low cell number and fragmentation, but with severe asymmetry (Fig. 29-22B), have significantly lower implantation rates,[138] which are further compromised when fragmentation is very high (Fig. 29-22C).

In addition to evaluations performed on day 3, assessments on day 1 have revealed a relationship between implantation potential and pre-zygote morphology at 16 to 18 hours after insemination (pronuclear size, size and number of nucleolar precursor bodies, and cytoplasmic appearance),[139-141] as well as the ability of embryos to complete the first mitotic division by 27 hours after insemination.[142,143] Moreover, embryos are typically considered of high quality if they are able to reach the blastocyst stage by 120 hours after insemination, exhibit a complete trophectoderm surrounding an expanded fluid-filled cavity, and have a tightly packed cluster of inner cell mass cells.[144]

In view of the reported benefit of independent morphologic evaluations on specific days of culture, numerous studies have investigated the possible additional value of undertaking morphologic evaluations on sequential days in culture. This approach enables a developmental library of morphologic information to be built on each embryo that might improve embryo selection. Compared with evaluations performed exclusively on day 3, available evidence indicates that multiscoring systems may enable improved embryo assessment.[145] However, further research is required in this area, and the ultimate combination of morphologic features required for optimum evaluation of developmental competence remains to be identified.

Embryo Transfer

Mechanical aspects of embryo transfer appear to influence implantation and pregnancy rates. For example, traumatic embryo transfers resulting in blood on the catheter are associated with a decreased rate of embryo implantation and clinical pregnancy.[146] In addition, transfers made in the presence of high-frequency uterine contractions (as detected by ultrasound) appear to be associated with lower pregnancy rates.[147] On the other hand, certain types of catheters are associated with higher pregnancy rates.[148] Several investigators have reported that ultrasound guidance of the catheter during embryo transfer slightly improves implantation rate and may improve pregnancy rates.[149-151] In one of these studies, the goal was to position the tip of the transfer catheter 6 cm from the external cervical os, leaving at least 1 cm between the tip of the catheter and the uterine fundus.[152] Other investigators have reported that a distance of 1.5 cm or 2.0 cm from the tip of the catheter to the fundus results in better pregnancy rates than transfers where the distance was only 1.0 cm.[153] A recent meta-analysis of 20 prospective randomized trial studies including 5968 embryo transfer cycles, concluded

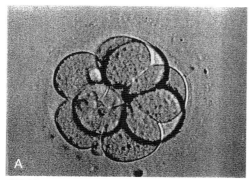

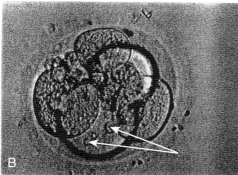

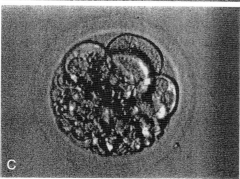

Figure 29-22. Day 3 embryos showing various degrees of asymmetry and fragmentation. *A,* An eight-cell embryo with minimal fragmentation but having blastomeres somewhat discordant for size and shape (i.e., exhibiting moderate asymmetry). *B,* A six-cell embryo with severely asymmetrical blastomeres but exhibiting slight fragmentation, with a few fragments interspersed among the blastomeres (arrows). *C,* A five-cell embryo showing moderately asymmetrical blastomeres and a high degree of fragmentation, with more than half the volume of the embryo fragmented, likely resulting from the fragmentation of several blastomeres.

that ultrasound-guided embryo transfer significantly increased the chance of a clinical pregnancy (OR = 1.5, 95% CI = 1.34 to 167) and a live birth (OR = 1.78, CI = 1.19 to 2.67) compared to the clinical touch technique.[154] In this large review there was no increase in multiple pregnancy, ectopic pregnancy, or spontaneous abortion rates in the ultrasound-guided group.

Number of Embryos to Transfer. The issue of multiple gestations, particularly high-order multiple gestations (triplets and above), is a significant problem in assisted reproduction, associated with poorer obstetric outcomes and the neonatal complications of prematurity and low birth weight. The

TABLE 29-7

ASRM/SART Recommended Limits on Number of Embryos to Transfer

Prognosis	Age (yr)			
	<35	35-37	38-40	>40
Cleavage-Stage Embryos				
Favorable*	1-2	2	3	5
All others	2	3	4	5
Blastocysts				
Favorable*	1	2	2	3
All others	2	2	3	3

*Favorable = first cycle of IVF, good embryo quality, excess embryos available for cryopreservation, or previous successful IVF cycle.
ASRM, American Society for Reproductive Medicine; SART, Society for Assisted Reproductive Technologies.
From ASRM Practice Committee. Guidelines on number of embryos transferred Fertil Steril 86:S51-S52, 2006.

social and economic impact of such gestations on the families involved and on society in general cannot be underestimated. As a result numerous approaches have been tried to reduce the rate of multiple gestations. In some Western European countries a legislative approach has severely restricted the number of embryos transferred in IVF cycles. Several countries have included significant disincentives for physicians who exceed the mandated number of transferred embryos. For example, such physicians face loss of license in Sweden and the United Kingdom and potential imprisonment in Germany and Switzerland. The United States has taken a largely voluntary approach, with a series of published guidelines on the number of embryos transferred by the Society for Assisted Reproductive Technologies (SART) of the American Society for Reproductive Medicine (ASRM) (Table 29-7). These guidelines, based on age and prognosis, have gradually reduced the acceptable number of transferred embryos particularly in women age 37 and younger.[155] The result has been a decline in the percentage of triplet births from ART from 11.4% to 7.4%, a 35% decline between 1995 and 2001, with the largest decrease (20.8%) from 1998 and 1999, the year following the publication of the first SART guidelines (reviewed in Jain et al.[156]).

To date the most significant impact on reducing multiple gestations, not only high-order multiples but also twins, has come from the use of elective single embryo transfer (SET). This practice has been more widely accepted in Europe; single embryo transfer represented only 6.7% of U.S. cycles versus 13.7% of European cycles in 2002,[157] with only a modest increase to 9.3% of cycles in the United States in 2005 (Fig. 29-23).

Over the last several years, several groups have investigated the use of SET in women undergoing IVF. In the first randomized clinical trial, Gerris et al. randomized patients younger than 34 years old undergoing their first IVF cycle with at least two "top-quality" embryos to either SET or double embryo transfer (DET). Within this group with excellent prognosis, those women with a DET achieved a higher ongoing pregnancy rate than those with a SET (74.0% versus 38.5%, *P* = 0.013); however, the multiple

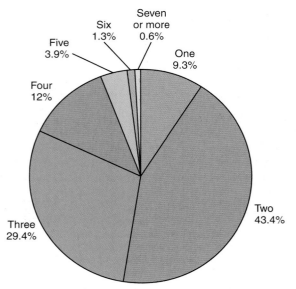

Figure 29-23. *Distribution of assisted reproductive technology (ART) cycles using fresh nondonor egg or embryos, according to the number of embryos transferred. (From CDC Assisted Reproductive Technology [ART] Report 2005. Available at www.cdc.gov/art/ART2005. Accessed Dec. 21, 2008.)*

important question remains: How many embryos should be transferred to maximize the live birth rate and minimize the number of high-order multiple gestations? Overall, there are correlations among the number of embryos transferred and both the pregnancy rate and the high-order multiple gestation rate,[161] with the quality of the embryos transferred an important determinant in both. As discussed earlier, most centers take advantage of this relationship by stringent morphologic grading to assess embryo quality. However, in general, scoring of cleavage-stage embryos is not a foolproof predictor of implantation rate. The pregnancy and multiple gestation rates are also dependent on the age of the female partner. For women older than 36, more embryos must be transferred to produce the pregnancy rates achieved in younger women,[162,163] a trend that is even more pronounced in women over the age of 39.[164]

A major contributor to the high-order multiple pregnancy rate may be patients' pressure on physicians to transfer more than two embryos to increase the probability of a successful cycle.[165] This pressure is especially strong when patients pay for their IVF treatment.[166] Where patients pay for their IVF therapy, the rate of triplet pregnancies is higher than in areas where insurance pays for IVF therapy.

Blastocyst Transfer. Early attempts to culture human embryos to the blastocyst stage required the use of feeder cells to support embryo development.[167] However, improvements in human IVF culture media in the late 1990s provided the opportunity to perform routine blastocyst transfer without the use of feeder cells; two different approaches to media development were adopted: the so-called "back to nature" approach and the "let the embryo choose" approach.[168]

The "back to nature" approach drew upon assessment of the energy substrate profiles in fallopian tube and uterine fluids. The results indicated that, in contrast to the fallopian tube, the glucose concentration in uterine fluid was relatively high, but the lactate and pyruvate concentrations were relatively low.[169] These observations led to development of a pair of media, reflecting these differences in energy substrate concentration, that are used in sequence for support of human blastocyst formation: the first medium, relatively high in lactate and pyruvate, is used from days 1 to 3 of culture, and the second medium, relatively high in glucose, is used from days 3 to 5.[170,171]

The "let the embryo choose" approach is based on determination of blastocyst formation rates following systematic changes in medium composition using the simplex optimization approach.[172] This paradigm involves use of a single medium to culture human embryos to the blastocyst stage. Available data show no differences in efficacy of this single step medium as compared with sequential media.[173,174]

Culturing human embryos to the blastocyst stage offers several theoretical advantages: (a) improved synchronization between embryonic development and uterine receptivity at the time of transfer; cleavage-stage embryos typically undergo development in the fallopian tube with traversal of the uterotubal junction being at the morula stage, 4 to 5 days after fertilization (see Table 29-6); (b) the possibility of selecting developmentally more competent embryos, because blastocyst stage embryos have proved their ability

gestation rate of 30% was higher in the DET group than in the SET group (30% versus 4%).[158]

A large Scandinavian multicenter study randomized 661 women under 36 years of age undergoing IVF treatment to either a single cycle of DET or a cycle with SET, followed by cryoembryo transfer for those patients who failed to conceive in their SET cycle. The live birth rate was 38.8% in the SET group versus 42.9% in the DET group (*P* > 0.05).[159] The authors concluded that the live birth rate was not substantially lower in the SET group. That conclusion, however, was based on the fact that to achieve such a pregnancy rate, two cycles (one fresh and one frozen) were necessary in 158 patients (48%), and the live birth rate for SET-only patients was 27.6%, substantially lower than that in the DET group (42.9%, *P* < 0.001). It is not clear how acceptable to patients two cycles of ART would be to achieve similar results to those in a single DET cycle.

The challenge in balancing the risks of multiple gestations and the lower pregnancy rate with elective SET may lie in defining an appropriate patient population for SET. The studies to date show that SET may be a viable option for women younger than 36, undergoing their first or second IVF cycle who have at least two excellent-quality embryos. Of note, the SART/ASRM guidelines recommend that consideration be given to SET for patients younger than 35 years having the most favorable prognosis, defined as the first IVF attempt with good-quality embryos and excess embryos for cryopreservation.

Since the 1950s, the incidence of twin gestations has doubled and the number of triplet gestations has tripled. Currently, approximately 40% of twin gestations and 80% of triplet gestations are the result of infertility therapy; however, only 8% of twins and 14% of triplets result from ART.[160] Moreover, since 1998, the percentage of triplets resulting from IVF has progressively decreased.[156] Nevertheless, an to progress through normal developmental milestones in vitro, and there may be some selection against aneuploid embryos progressing to blastulation[175]; and (c) the rationale to transfer fewer embryos with higher implantation potential, thereby reducing the risk of multiple gestations.[170,176]

Despite these theoretical advantages to blastocyst transfer, there are several potential disadvantages. In some centers, blastocyst transfer is associated with lower pregnancy rates compared with embryo transfer at 72 hours,[177] leading some to question the benefit of blastocyst transfer. Extending culture to the blastocyst stage appears to result in attrition of some embryos that otherwise would support viable pregnancies following cleavage-stage transfer. In one study of blastocyst transfer, when there was no eight-cell embryo present at 72 hours of culture, the pregnancy rate was higher with transfer at 72 hours (33%) than with transfer at 120 hours (0%).[178] Moreover, for some patients with healthy-appearing embryos at 72 hours of culture, all of the embryos undergo developmental arrest or degeneration before 120 hours of culture, leaving no embryos for transfer.[178] The inability to predict which cleavage-stage embryos will develop into blastocysts in vitro has led to a significantly higher incidence of canceled embryo transfers in patients randomized to day 3 versus day 5 culture.[179] Finally, blastocyst transfer has been associated with an increased risk of monozygotic twinning[180,181] and the obstetrically more serious condition of monochorionic twinning.[182]

Comparison of the efficacy of blastocyst transfer with cleavage-stage transfer has led to conflicting results. In a meta-analysis of 16 trials involving 1068 day 2 or 3 transfers and 1048 day 5 to 7 transfers, no differences were observed in the clinical pregnancy rates (15 studies; OR, 1.05; 95% CI, 0.88-1.26) or the live birth rate (7 studies; OR, 1.03; 95% CI, 0.74-1.44). Similar results were obtained when restricting the analysis to the six randomized controlled trials involving only women younger than 34 years having a good prognosis for success. In contrast, a subsequent trial with similarly good prognosis patients revealed that blastocyst transfer resulted in higher pregnancy rates and delivery rates than cleavage-stage embryos when a single embryo was transferred (32% versus 21.6%, OR 1.48; 95% CI, 1.04-2.11.[183] However, fewer surplus embryos were frozen in the blastocyst cycles (2.2 ± 2.7 versus 4.2 ± 4.1), raising the possibility that overall cumulative pregnancy rates from all transfers of fresh and frozen embryos may not be different after cleavage stage or blastocyst transfer.[183]

Collectively, available data indicate that the best candidates for blastocyst transfer are those women with good prognosis (based on age, number and quality of embryos). Indeed, the first IVF human pregnancy occurred after the transfer of a single blastocyst-stage embryo to the uterus, although it resulted in an ectopic implantation.[184] It is possible that for patients with good prognosis, the IVF technique will eventually go full circle, returning to the transfer of a single, blastocyst-stage embryo.

Luteal Phase Support

In IVF cycles, the ovary and endometrium are buffeted by numerous countervailing forces that are not controlled by normal feedback mechanisms. The endometrium, for example, is exposed to extremely high levels of estradiol and abnormally high levels of androgen. These high hormone levels may result in abnormal epithelial and stromal maturation, especially if luteal progesterone does not adequately balance the estrogen effect. Because oocyte retrieval is associated with the removal of a large number of granulosa cells, the adequacy of ovarian progesterone production after oocyte retrieval has been a major concern since the inception of IVF.[185] Two major methods of luteal-phase support have been used in IVF cycles: progesterone supplementation, usually by injection at doses of 25 or 50 mg daily[186]; and intramuscular hCG at doses ranging from 1500 to 10,000 IU administered once or more during the luteal phase.[187] Both hCG and progesterone appear to be associated with an increased pregnancy rate compared with no luteal support.[185] In general, hCG appears to be associated with a slightly higher pregnancy rate than progesterone, but it also appears to cause a higher rate of OHSS.[185]

The timing of the initiation of luteal phase support with progesterone affects the pregnancy rate. In a well-designed clinical trial, women undergoing IVF were randomized to receive progesterone supplementation starting either after oocyte retrieval or 12 hours before oocyte retrieval. The pregnancy rate with progesterone supplementation after oocyte retrieval was significantly better than with progesterone 12 hours before oocyte retrieval (24.6% versus 12.9%, P < 0.011).[188] In another well-designed study, women were randomized to start luteal phase support with vaginal progesterone either 3 days after oocyte retrieval or 6 days after oocyte retrieval. The clinical pregnancy rate per transfer was significantly better in the group that started luteal phase support at 3 days rather than 6 days after oocyte retrieval.[189] These studies demonstrate that the optimal window for initiating luteal phase support begins after oocyte retrieval but ends by the third day after oocyte retrieval, though the length of time necessary for luteal phase support has not been clearly delineated. Most centers continue support until it is clear whether the patient is pregnant. In one study, discontinuing progesterone support after a positive hCG resulted in pregnancy outcomes similar to continuing progesterone for an additional 3 weeks after a positive hCG.[190]

A major problem with the use of progesterone for luteal phase support is the pain and sterile abscesses associated with numerous daily intramuscular injections. Alternative routes have been explored, although oral administration does not appear to be as effective as intramuscular injection.[191] Early studies with a vaginal progesterone administered in a polycarbophil gel preparation appeared to hold promise as an alternative to intramuscular progesterone.[192] Although more recent studies indicated that the pregnancy rate with IVF was decreased with the vaginal progesterone Crinone, compared with intramuscular progesterone luteal phase support,[193,194] a more recent prospective trial has revealed that this negative effect of vaginal progesterone was due to the day that support was initiated.[195] When gel administration was delayed until day 2 after retrieval, there was no decrease in pregnancy rate compared with that associated with intramuscular administration initiated day 1 after retrieval. A vaginal progesterone-releasing polysyloxane ring has been tested in pilot studies for application in IVF cycles.[196]

Another controversy regarding luteal phase support concerns estrogen. Though the importance of luteal progesterone's effect on the endometrium in implantation and early pregnancy maintenance is well established, the role of supplemental estrogen is less clear. In cycles utilizing GnRH agonists or GnRH antagonists, the profound suppression of gonadotropins in the follicular phase may carry over to the luteal phase. Several groups have investigated the benefit of the addition of estrogen in the luteal phase in IVF. A prospective randomized study involving 166 women undergoing 231 IVF cycles with long-protocol GnRH-agonist suppression examined the effect of luteal phase estrogen support. Participants were given 0 mg, 2 mg, or 6 mg estradiol over the entire luteal phase. Pregnancy rates were improved by estrogen supplementation in a dose-related manner, with the highest rates in the 6 mg group (23.1% versus 32.8% versus 51.3%, $P < 0.001$).[197] A similar result was recently reported from a group from Greece,[198] with neither group reporting any adverse effects with the addition of estrogen.

Another area of controversy concerns the utilization of low-dose (baby) aspirin as an adjunct to IVF-ICSI treatment. Aspirin inhibits cyclooxygenase in platelets as well as thromboxane A_2 (a potent vasoconstrictor) and prostacyclin (a vasodilator). However, in low doses the vasoconstrictor inhibition predominates. Therefore, use of low-dose aspirin has been proposed to increase ovarian blood flow, improving folliculogenesis and promoting implantation. Some practitioners begin aspirin during ovarian stimulation, while others utilize it only in the luteal phase, believing that it may contribute to excessive bleeding during oocyte retrieval. A recent meta-analysis of seven trials included 1241 women undergoing ovarian stimulation for IVF or ICSI.[199] There was no significant improvement in IVF/ICSI outcome for women taking aspirin in terms of clinical pregnancy (relative risk [RR] 1.11, 95% CI 0.95-1.31) or live birth (RR 0.96, 95% CI 0.64-1.39). There were no differences between the groups with respect to miscarriage or ectopic pregnancies. The authors concluded that the currently available data do not support the use of aspirin in IVF cycles.

Repeat in Vitro Fertilization Cycles

Because the majority of couples completing a single IVF cycle do not become pregnant, many will request a repeat IVF cycle. A specific cause of the IVF cycle failure may be identified (e.g., elevated cycle day 3 FSH concentrations). In most cases, however, a specific cause cannot be identified. At many centers, repeat IVF cycles up to cycle 8 appear to have a per-cycle pregnancy rate similar to the first cycle.[200] At some centers, repeated IVF cycles after cycle 3 are associated with lower per-cycle pregnancy rates (Fig. 29-24).[201] For example, in one study, the delivery rate per oocyte retrieval was 27% in the first and second cycles but decreased to 23% in cycle 3, 16% in cycle 4, and 15% in subsequent cycles.[202] Data concerning the pregnancy rate in repeat IVF cycles are confounded by decisions made by clinicians and patients. For example, when a patient has

had a poor response to ovarian stimulation, the clinician may suggest discontinuation of IVF treatments. This would select patients with a "better prognosis" to repeat IVF. In fact, according to 2005 data from the CDC, 57.2% of U.S. ART cycles were in women undergoing their first cycle, 19.7% in women undergoing their second cycle, 10.7% in women undergoing their third cycle, and 12.3% in women who had four or more previous treatments. These data suggest a selection bias in who receives prolonged ART treatment.[203] In every age bracket, women with prior ART cycles but no live births have a lower pregnancy rate than women undergoing their first ART cycle.[204]

Risks of in Vitro Fertilization

Ovarian stimulation with gonadotropins for IVF is associated with up to 5% risk of severe OHSS. Risk factors seem to be peak estradiol concentrations greater than 2000 pg/mL, more than 15 follicles greater than 12 mm in diameter, and the establishment of a successful pregnancy.[205] OHSS that develops during IVF cycles typically resolves with conservative management (see Chapter 28).

A number of strategies have been proposed to prevent OHSS. Withholding hCG and cancellation of the cycle is effective but fails to achieve a pregnancy. Continuing the cycle and freezing all embryos created is largely effective but requires a second cycle (albeit a simpler, cryoembryo transfer) to achieve a pregnancy. As previously noted, some reduction in the incidence of OHSS has been achieved in non-GnRH-agonist cycles by giving an ovulatory dose of a GnRH-agonist.[113]

Another strategy involves "coasting," in which the doses of gonadotropins are withheld (sometimes for several days) until estradiol levels decline to safer levels and ovulatory doses of hCG may be given.[206] The practice seems effective in many cases but appears to be associated with a lower pregnancy rate.[207] A number of investigators have proposed that administration of albumin may have a protective effect against development of OHSS.[208]

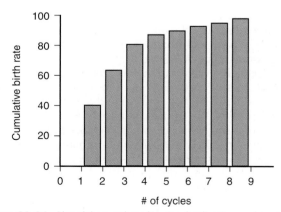

Figure 29-24. Plot of the number of in vitro fertilization–embryo transfer cycles and the cumulative clinical live birth rate. (From Copperman AB, Selick CE, Crunfeld L, et al. Cumulative number and morphological score of embryos resulting in success: realistic expectations from in vitro fertilization embryo transfer. Fertil Steril 64:88-92, 1995, with permission of the American Society for Reproductive Medicine.)

Alvarez et al. have recently proposed a novel treatment for the prevention of OHSS: administration of the dopamine agonist cabergoline to at-risk patients.[209] These authors previously observed that the enzyme tyrosine hydroxylose, critical in the production of dopamine, was down-regulated eightfold in OHSS.[210] By adding the dopamine agonist cabergoline they hoped to restore dopamine and at the same time reduce vascular permeability through the vascular endothelial growth factor (VEGF) pathway. They randomized 82 oocyte donors at risk of developing OHSS to 0.5 mg daily cabergoline for 8 days or placebo. The incidence of moderate OHSS was reduced to 20% in the cabergoline group compared with 44% in the placebo group ($P = 0.04$). Hematocrit, hemoglobin, and ascites were all significantly lower in the group treated with cabergoline compared to placebo.

Another promising strategy is the continuation of GnRH-agonist therapy following hCG injection. Though this approach requires cryopreservation of the embryos, such a regimen could work nicely in egg donation patients.[211]

IVF is known to carry the risk of ectopic pregnancy with the incidence double to triple that in the general population. The Bourne Hall Clinic, site of the first successful human IVF treatment, reported an ectopic pregnancy rate of 4.5% in IVF patients.[212] Presumably the high prevalence of tubal disease in women undergoing IVF may contribute to this increased rate. However, factors intrinsic to the IVF process may also contribute, such as high volumes of culture medium used during embryo transfer or an elevated progesterone/estradiol ratio on the day of transfer.[212] There

does not seem to be a difference in the incidence of ectopic pregnancies between women undergoing a day 3 or day 5 blastocyst embryo transfer.[213]

Heterotopic pregnancies, involving a concomitant intrauterine and extrauterine gestation, occur in approximately 1 in 100 pregnancies after IVF. This is due to both the transfer of multiple embryos and the underlying fertility problems of the IVF population, including tubal disease. In the general population, the rate of heterotopic pregnancies is approximately 1 in 3500 conceptions.[214,215] The ectopic pregnancy can be treated either by surgical removal or by the selective injection of potassium chloride or hyperosmolar glucose.[216,217] If the ectopic pregnancy is to be treated surgically, most clinicians prefer to remove the entire tube rather than perform a salpingostomy. In a heterotopic pregnancy, it is not possible to determine whether the salpingostomy has been successful, because the intrauterine pregnancy maintains the elevated hCG levels. If the ectopic pregnancy is to be removed surgically, sutures or staples are preferred to electrocautery or vasopressin to minimize the chance of diminished blood flow to the intrauterine pregnancy.[218,219]

Although some epidemiologists have suggested that drugs used to induce ovulation may be associated with an increased risk of ovarian cancer, the data are very weak. Most recent studies have reported no relationship between cancer and ovarian stimulation in women who have had IVF or in the offspring derived from IVF pregnancies.[220] A recent meta-analysis of infertile patients concluded that the risk of ovarian cancer does not appear to be increased by treatment with ART compared to nontreatment.[221] There is some association between ovarian cancer and having no children, whether because of infertility or by choice. Oocyte retrieval can be associated with pelvic bleeding that requires transfusion or surgical exploration, or pelvic infection. Both complications are rare, occurring in fewer than 1 per 500 cases.

Many couples treated with IVF experience significant stress. In one study that assessed stress scores for the female partner of the couple across an entire IVF cycle (Fig. 29-25),[222] ovarian stimulation was associated with an increase in self-reported stress. Stress levels increased markedly when couples were informed that the result of a pregnancy test obtained 2 weeks after embryo transfer was negative. When couples were told that the pregnancy test result was positive, there was no significant increase in the self-report of stress. This observation supports the theory that failure to conceive in an IVF cycle is similar to a significant loss and that the couple must grieve for that loss. Support, counseling, and relaxation techniques can all help reduce the stress associated with IVF.

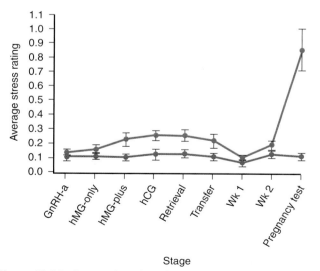

Figure 29-25. Stress ratings throughout an in vitro fertilization cycle. The upper line represents self-reported scores from women who did not become pregnant. The lower line represents self-reported scores from women who did become pregnant. Note the large increase in stress rating at the time the woman learns that her pregnancy test result is negative. GnRH-a, gonadotropin-releasing hormone-agonist analogs; hMG, human menopausal gonadotropin; hCG, human chorionic gonadotropin. (From Boivi J, Takefman IE. Stress level across stages of in vitro fertilization in subsequently pregnant and nonpregnant women. Fertil Steril 64:802-810, 1995, with permission of the American Society for Reproductive Medicine.)

Pregnancy Outcome

Among women who achieve pregnancy after IVF, approximately 20% will experience a spontaneous abortion, and up to 5% will have an ectopic pregnancy. Early pregnancy can be monitored both by transvaginal sonography and by serial hCG levels (Figs. 29-26 and 29-27). The issue of IVF and the risk of birth defects is complex and the analysis of this subject has been limited by additional testing

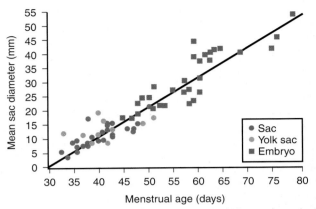

Figure 29-26. *Relationship between pregnancy dating as determined by menstrual age and gestational sac size as measured by the mean sac diameter. (From Nyberg DA, Mack LA, Liang FC, Patten RM. Distinguishing normal from abnormal gestational sac growth in early pregnancy J Ultrasound Med 6:23-27, 1987.)*

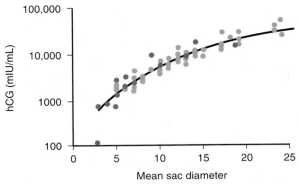

Figure 29-27. *Relationship between mean gestational sac diameter as measured by the mean sac diameter and the serum human chorionic gonadotropin (hCG) concentration. Green dots represent present series; gray dots represent previously published data. (From Nyberg DA, Mack LA, Liang FC, Jeffrey RB. Early pregnancy complications: Endovaginal sonographic findings correlated with human chorionic gonadotropin levels. Radiology 167:619-622, 1988.)*

performed on ICSI offspring, underreporting of malformations in national birth registries, the effect of maternal age, the effect of multiple gestations, and the inclusion of severe male factor patients, whose children may be subject to an increased rate of chromosomal anomalies.[223] Nonetheless, IVF and ICSI appear to be associated with a small increase in the rate of offspring with congenital malformations.

The picture is further complicated by the fact that congenital malformations are more common in offspring from multiple pregnancies than from singleton pregnancies and are more common in children of women of advanced reproductive age. Because multiple gestations in older gravida are more common in IVF pregnancies, a potential bias may be introduced. Therefore, analyses restricted exclusively to singleton births in age-matched women make sense. In a review of some such studies, Van Voorhis found a general trend toward more malformations, though the effect was small.[224] One of the difficulties in designing such studies is that pregnancies resulting from IVF are often scrutinized more carefully than other pregnancies. For example, the frequency and intensity of ultrasound testing might be higher in such pregnancies. In one of the larger and better-controlled matched cohort studies, Hansen et al. reported a twofold increase in major malformations from IVF (8.6%) compared to normal control subjects (4.2%) from a birth registry in Western Australia.[225] One strength of this particular study was that a single-blinded pediatrician determined which anomalies would have been detected independent of the surveillance method used. However, even this approach has been criticized on the presumption that a pediatrician could hypothesize which malformation might be ICSI-induced.[226]

There have been several meta-analyses examining the question of congenital malformations in IVF and ICSI offspring. One examined 19 IVF and ICSI studies and found a modest increase in malformations overall (OR = 1.29, 95% CI 1.01-1.67).[227] A second and larger meta-analysis reviewed 25 studies comparing birth defects in ART and non-ART offspring.[228] The overall OR of malformations was 1.29 (95% CI 1.21-1.37) and reached statistical

significance. The statistical significance remained in subgroup analysis of singleton births and major malformations. The authors concluded that there is an overall 30% to 40% increased risk of birth defects associated with ART.

Another way to consider birth defect data is to analyze the specific malformations. For example, if IVF offspring have a minimally increased risk of birth defects, but the vast majority of defects were clustered within a single organ system, it would be a greater cause for concern than if the defects were found to involve multiple organ systems. Although cardiovascular, musculoskeletal, and urogenital malformations seem more common in IVF offspring than non-IVF offspring, no single defect seems to predominate.[224]

The interpretation of all the data on birth defects and ART hinges on the appropriateness of the control groups. It is possible that infertile couples by the nature of their infertility are at risk of having children with congenital malformations. In fact, one might argue that the correct control group is not naturally conceived children but rather children from previously infertile couples who conceived, but without IVF.

A study from the Danish national birth cohort examined the incidence of congenital malformations in children born of fertile couples compared to (a) children born of infertile couples who conceived without treatment and (b) children of infertile couples who required treatment to conceive.[229] Compared to children conceived by fertile couples, singletons conceived by infertile couples without treatment had a higher rate of malformations, hazard ratio (HR) 1.70 (95% CI 1.07-1.35); with treatment, the HR was 1.39 (95% CI 1.23-1.57). Although this study did not specifically examine the type of infertility treatment and thus did not address the effect of IVF on birth defects, it did demonstrate that infertility in and of itself confers a higher risk of birth defects, even without treatment.

In the largest U.S. study to examine congenital malformations associated with infertility treatments, Olson et al. compared offspring from naturally conceived pregnancies, IVF, and intrauterine inseminations (IUI).[230] The malformation rate among the IVF children (6.2%; OR 1.44, 95% CI 1.12-1.85) was higher than among control subjects (4.4%), though the rate among IUI children was not statistically higher than the control group (5.0%; OR 1.14, 95% CI 0.7-1.87). The authors speculated that they were not able to show an increase in malformations among the IUI-conceived children because the number of infants was so small (*n* = 343) compared to that in the IVF group (*n* = 1462) or the control group (*n* = 8422).

It has recently been postulated that reproductive technologies may be associated with epigenetic abnormalities known as genomic imprinting, which produce an increase in rare congenital disorders such as Beckwith-Wiedemann and Angelman syndromes. Epigenetic defects involve stable alterations in DNA other than the nucleotide sequence itself, and differential DNA methylation causing expression of only one of the two inherited alleles for a particular gene results in genomic imprinting.[231] In 2003, De Baun et al. were the first to report an association between an imprinting disorder and ART.[232] Among ART offspring, they found a 4.6% prevalence of Beckwith-Wiedemann syndrome, a congenital disorder involving growth and neoplasia, compared with a background rate of 0.8% in the U.S. population. An increased incidence of several imprinting syndromes has been reported in children conceived through assisted reproductive technologies.[233]

Although one study from the Netherlands reported five cases of retinoblastoma in children from IVF, a much higher prevalence than seen in the general Dutch population,[234] the Boston Collaborative Drug Surveillance Program identified no children born from IVF with retinoblastoma compared with 6.7 cases per 100,000 births in the general population.[235] A very large study from the Swedish national health registry involving more than 16,000 children born after ART failed to find an increase in childhood cancers or infant tumors in either IVF or ICSI offspring.[236]

Taken together, this series of studies suggests a slight increase in the risk of congenital malformations, perhaps 3% to 4% associated with the assisted reproduction technologies. However, it is not clear whether this presumed increased incidence is due to IVF, or ICSI, or characteristics of the infertile couples themselves. Although there appears to be an association between IVF and some rare imprinting disorders, the overall risk of such disease is low. The available evidence does not suggest an increase in childhood cancers in children conceived through IVF.

The outcome of pregnancies produced by IVF is directly related to the number of fetuses established. Of the live births resulting from IVF in 2005, 28.8% were twins, and 4.5% were triplets or higher-order gestations. Pregnancies complicated by multiple gestations are associated with increased prematurity, low birth weight, gestational hypertension, diabetes, and increased perinatal mortality rate. Early studies proposing an association between IVF and poor obstetric and perinatal outcomes often did not adequately control for the increased rate of multiple gestations associated with IVF treatment. Several recent large studies and meta-analyses have reviewed the obstetric outcomes associated with ART. The FASTER (First and Second Trimester Evolution of Risk) Research Consortium, sponsored by the National Institute of Child Health and Human Development (NICHHD) prospectively investigated singleton pregnancies from an unselected obstetric population between 1999 and 2002.[237] A total of 36,062 pregnancies, including 1222 that used ovulation induction and 554 that used ART, were evaluated. Ovulation induction was associated with a greater risk of placental abruption, total loss after 24 weeks, and gestational diabetes, and IVF was associated with an increase in preeclampsia, gestational hypertension, placental abruption, placenta previa, and risk of cesarean delivery compared with naturally established pregnancies. There was no association between IVF and total growth restriction or aneuploidy for fetal anomalies. Significantly, this study adjusted for age, race, marital status, years of education, prior preterm delivery, prior total anomaly, body mass index, and bleeding with the recent pregnancy. A meta-analysis of 15 studies comprising 12,283 IVF and 1.9 million spontaneously conceived singletons concluded that IVF singleton pregnancies were associated with increased rates of perinatal mortality (OR 2.2; 95% CI 1.6-3), preterm delivery (OR 2, 95% CI 1.4-2.2), low birth weight (OR 1.8, 95% CI 1.4-2.2), very low birth weight (OR 2.7, 95% CI 2.3-3.1), and small size for gestational age (OR 1.6, 95% CI 1.3-2).[238] A recent systematic review of controlled studies concluded that IVF singleton pregnancies were at elevated risk for very preterm and preterm births as well as very low birth weight, low birth weight, and small-for-gestational-age infants. The IVF pregnancies were associated with more neonatal intensive care unit (NICU) admissions, cesarean delivery, and increased perinatal mortality rate.[239] These differences largely held when IVF twin gestations were compared to natural twin pregnancies. Finally, a large meta-analysis examining 27 studies resulting in singleton births concluded that the risk of preterm births in singleton pregnancies resulting from IVF-ET/GIFT was twice that of naturally conceived pregnancies.[240]

A NICHID workshop on infertility, assisted reproductive technology, and adverse pregnancy outcome summarized the areas of increased risk as follows: Increased perinatal risks included preterm birth, low birth weight (<2500 g), very low birth weight (<1500 g), small size for gestational age, NICU admissions, stillbirths, neonatal mortality, and cerebral palsy. Maternal risks identified were preeclampsia, placenta previa, placental abruption, gestational diabetes, and cesarean delivery.[241] An American College of Obstetricians and Gynecologists Committee opinion concluded that "a growing body of evidence suggests an association between pregnancies resulting from ART and perinatal morbidity (possibly independent of multiple births), although the absolute risk to children conceived through ART is low."[242]

Some have argued, however, that it is not possible to separate the ART-associated perinatal risks from those due to the underlying reproductive disease.[241] Infertile couples may also be at risk for a wide range of adverse reproductive outcomes not necessarily related to their treatment. A large cohort study from Belgium examined the perinatal outcome of 12,011 singleton and 3108 twin births from non-IVF assisted reproduction treatments compared with outcomes from natural conceptions.[243] The treatments consisted of controlled ovarian stimulation with and without intrauterine insemination. Among singletons resulting from infertility treatment, there was a higher incidence of prematurity, low and very low birth weight, and transfer to the NICU; among twin pregnancies resulting from infertility treatment they found an increased rate of neonatal mortality, assisted ventilation, and respiratory distress syndrome. The study demonstrated that both singleton and twin pregnancies resulting from non-IVF fertility treatment have worse perinatal outcomes than naturally conceived children.

Another clue as to why IVF pregnancy outcomes may fare worse than naturally conceived pregnancies comes from a recent Danish study examining the effect of vanishing twins on pregnancy outcomes from IVF.[244] This study included 642 survivors of a vanished co-twin, 5237 primary singletons, and 3678 primary twins. The rate of small-for-gestational-age infants was significantly higher in survivors than in singletons (OR 1.5, 95% CI 1.03-2.2), as was the risk of low birth weight (OR 1.71, 95% CI 1.06-2.74). Because ART cycles produce more multiple gestations than naturally conceived pregnancies, it is likely that they also produce more vanishing twins. This study implies that the survivor of a vanishing co-twin has a worse obstetric prognosis than an otherwise normal singleton fetus. Whether or not the vanishing twin phenomenon accounts for all or some of the increased perinatal risk requires future investigation.

Another concern regarding pregnancies resulting from ART is the neurologic development of children conceived through IVF. Although the majority of such studies are reassuring, several studies have demonstrated an increased incidence of cerebral palsy in children born through ART. One study found an increased risk for cerebral palsy in IVF children (OR 3.7, 95% CI 2-6.6); some of the increased risk was associated with multiple gestations, but the higher risk persisted when singletons alone were analyzed (OR 2.8, 95% CI 1.3-5.8). No difference in neurologic development was seen between IVF twins and control twins.[245]

A second study also showed an increased risk of cerebral palsy among IVF offspring even after accounting for maternal age, educational level, parity, gender of offspring, and small size for gestational age. Importantly, however, the differences disappeared with adjustment for multiple gestations and prematurity.[246]

Long-term developmental, psychological, and cognitive studies on offspring of ART pregnancies are now available and generally show normal cognitive and motor development, as well as appropriate neurologic function up to age 8.[247-249] Cognitive and psychological development each have also been demonstrated to be normal in children conceived via ART up to age 5.[249,250] However, IVF offspring appear to be at elevated risk of hospitalization in childhood, perhaps reflecting their higher rate of medical problems in the neonatal period.[251,252] Interestingly, recent work suggests that metabolic parameters and body composition may differ between children conceived via IVF and spontaneous conception. From 8 to 18 years of age, IVF children appear to have altered body fat composition,

though they also appear to have a more favorable lipid profile and higher IGF-I and IGF-II levels than non-IVF children.[253,254]

Despite attempts to reduce the number of multiple gestations, they remain the single greatest risk of assisted reproduction. Women with triplet pregnancies are at risk for both maternal and fetal complications.

Couples who achieve triplet pregnancy are faced with two major options: expectant management or reduction of the triplet pregnancy to a twin or singleton gestation. The most widely used method of pregnancy reduction is transvaginal or transabdominal injection of potassium chloride into the fetal heart. The transabdominal approach is usually performed at 10 to 13 weeks of gestation; the transvaginal approach is typically used earlier. For couples choosing expectant management, approximately 15% will spontaneously lose one embryo-fetus, resulting in a twin pregnancy.[255] About 10% of multifetal pregnancies are completely lost after reduction.[256] Some studies demonstrate that reduction of a triplet gestation to a twin gestation may decrease the risk of preeclampsia, increase the gestational age at birth, and increase the mean birth weights.[257-260] An alternative to embryo reduction for triplet pregnancy due to IVF is to reduce the number of embryos transferred to the woman.

Some researchers maintain that it is "fairly well established" that multifetal reduction for quadruplet pregnancy improves pregnancy outcomes.[261] Although no randomized studies have been reported, some series observe an increase in the length of gestation from 31 weeks to 35 weeks, in quadruplet pregnancies that have been successfully reduced to twins. Reduction in the number of quadruplet pregnancies after IVF treatment is undoubtedly best achieved by transferring no more than two high-quality embryos in those women at highest risk for multifetal pregnancy.

Embryo Cryopreservation

IVF often generates substantial numbers of excess embryos that cannot be safely transferred in the cycle of oocyte retrieval because of the risk of high-order multiple gestation. The development of successful embryo cryopreservation techniques allows multiple transfer cycles after just one ovarian stimulation and oocyte retrieval, as first reported by Zeilmaker and colleagues in 1984.[262] An important issue in embryo cryopreservation is use of the optimal cryoprotectant and freezing protocol. In one randomized prospective study, dimethyl sulfoxide (DMSO) was found superior to 1,2-propanediol as a cryoprotectant for multicellular human embryos.[263] Embryos were randomized to freezing with DMSO (n = 232) or 1,2-propanediol (n = 250). The live birth rates per embryo thawed were 3.5% for DMSO and 0.8% for 1,2-propanediol. Preliminary results suggest that embryos can be successfully frozen for at least 7 years (Fig. 29-28).[264] Interestingly, embryos that were cryopreserved for only 2 to 10 months did not result in as many pregnancies as did embryos cryopreserved longer than 12 months. This is probably due to the fact that women who became pregnant with the initial embryo transfer (suggesting that many

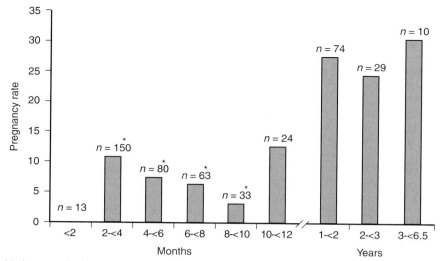

Figure 29-28. *Relationship between the length of time that embryos were preserved in cryostorage and the clinical pregnancy rate resulting from the thawing and transfer of the cryopreserved embryos. The embryos that were stored for 1 to 6.5 years had a high rate of establishing pregnancy when they were thawed and transferred. One explanation of this result is that women who became pregnant on the initial in vitro fertilization— embryo transfer cycle kept their embryos cryopreserved for a long time before accessing them. (From Lin YP, Cassidenti DL, Chacon RR, et al. Successful implantation of frozen sibling embryos is influenced by the outcome of the cycle from which they were derived. Fertil Steril 63:262-267, 1995, with permission of the American Society for Reproductive Medicine.)*

high-quality embryos were present) did not need to access their cryopreserved embryos until after they completed their first pregnancy.

The challenges associated with freezing blastocysts are different from those associated with freezing multicellular embryos due to the large fluid-filled blastocoelic cavity that presents an increased risk of intracellular ice crystal formation. Success of blastocyst freezing has varied widely,[265] and can be achieved either with slow-freezing[265] or vitrification protocols.[266] Further studies are required to determine which cryopreservation is superior.

A typical protocol for the transfer of cryopreserved embryos during a natural cycle is as follows:

1. Start transvaginal ultrasound (TVS) on cycle day 12 for measurement of endometrial stripe and follicle diameter.
2. Measure serum progesterone to ensure ovulation has not occurred.
3. Begin testing for the urine LH surge when the endometrial stripe is greater than 7 mm and the dominant follicle is greater than 15 mm.
4. Perform TVS 24 to 48 hours after the urine LH surge is detected and recheck serum progesterone to ensure it is greater than 3 ng/mL.
5. Perform transfer 72 hours after the day of ovulation for multicellular embryos, and 100 to 120 hours for blastocysts.

Predictors of in Vitro Fertilization Success

The number and quality of the follicles developing, and the number and quality of oocytes obtained at retrieval are critical in the success of IVF. Relevant biologic markers include the following:

1. Cycle day 3 baseline FSH and estradiol concentration[267,268]
2. FSH response to a clomiphene challenge[269,270]
3. Ovarian antral follicle number and volume as determined by high-resolution transvaginal sonography[271,272]
4. Chronologic age of the female partner (see Fig. 29-11)
5. Inhibin B concentration[273]

Also correlated with IVF success are markers of follicle development, which include serum estradiol[274] and inhibin A.[275] To some extent, the same is true of markers of endometrial development, such as endometrial thickness (a biomarker of both follicle development and endometrial responsiveness) as determined by sonography and uterine artery impedance (see Chapters 9 and 33).[276]

Women who experience an early pregnancy loss after IVF have a greater likelihood of pregnancy in a subsequent IVF cycle than women who do not conceive with their first cycle of IVF.[277]

Other factors have been proposed to influence IVF outcome, but on further study were discovered to have no impact. For example, many investigators once believed that antiphospholipid antibodies were associated with decreased pregnancy rates with IVF. However, a review of the available trials demonstrated no relationship.[278,279]

Impact of Gynecologic Diseases on in Vitro Fertilization Outcome

Many gynecologic diseases appear to influence the outcome of IVF. For example, numerous investigators have reported that fallopian tube hydrosalpinges decrease the pregnancy rate in IVF (see also Chapter 9).[280,282] Tubal hydrosalpinges may cause the accumulation within the uterine cavity of pathologic quantities of fluid[283] that may contain proteins and other factors that inhibit embryo interaction with the endometrium.[284] In one randomized trial of the clinical benefit of laparoscopic salpingectomy prior to IVF, 204 women with hydrosalpinges who were planning IVF treatment were randomized to pre-IVF laparoscopic salpingectomy or no salpingectomy. The delivery rates per cycle were 28.6% and 16.3%, respectively (P < 0.05). In this study, hydrosalpinx was defined as a distally occluded fallopian tube that was pathologically dilated or became pathologically dilated when patency was tested with a hysterosalpingogram or at laparoscopy.[285] A later follow-up of this study extending the results past the first treatment cycle showed an improvement in birth rate with salpingectomy (HR 2.1, 95% CI 1.6-3.6). The subgroups of patients with ultrasound-visible hydrosalpinges showed an even greater improvement in birth rate with salpingectomy (HR 3.8, 95% CI 1.5-9.2).[286] Based on these and other studies, the American Society for Reproductive Medicine recommends removal of a hydrosalpinx prior to an IVF cycle when possible.

Many investigators have reported that submucosal leiomyomas are associated with decreased pregnancy rates with IVF (see Chapter 25). In addition, a number of studies suggest that hysteroscopic myomectomy of submucosal myomas improves pregnancy rate with IVF.[287-289]

The effect of intramural myomas on IVF outcome is less certain. Some investigators found that intramural myomas are associated with decreased pregnancy rates in IVF. In one report, 112 women with intramural myomas (the largest of which had a mean diameter of 2.3 cm) and 322 women without myomas undergoing IVF were prospectively studied.[290] The ongoing pregnancy rate was 15.1% in the women with myomas and 28.3% in the women without myomas (P < 0.003). Logistic regression demonstrated that intramural myomas were associated with a reduced OR for pregnancy (OR 0.46, 95% CI 0.24-0.88, P < 0.02) after controlling for age of the female partner and number of embryos available for transfer. Other investigators have reported that intramural myomas up to 7 cm in diameter that do not distort the uterine cavity do not substantially influence IVF outcome. The impact of myomas on IVF was studied in 141 patients with myomas and 406 women without myomas. The OR for pregnancy was 0.73 in the myoma group (95% CI 0.49-1.19, P = 0.21) after controlling for the age of the female partner.[291] Additional large-scale studies will be needed to determine if intramural myomas reduce IVF success rates.

Surry et al. examined consecutive IVF cycles in 399 women undergoing IVF with and without leiomyomas. They found that the live birth rate was not affected by the presence of intramural leiomyomas provided that the endometrial cavity was hysteroscopically normal. They did not recommend prophylactic surgical intervention for intramural fibroids.[292]

Endometrial polyps may also decrease live birth rates with IVF.[293] Cervical stenosis can cause infertility and can impair effective embryo transfer, lowering pregnancy rates with IVF. Placing a Malecot catheter after hysteroscopic evaluation in preparation for IVF appears to improve the efficacy of embryo transfer in women with cervical stenosis.[294]

Müllerian anomalies appear to be associated with a reduced pregnancy rate in IVF. In a study of 37 women with müllerian anomalies undergoing IVF, the live birth rate per initiated cycle was 8%, compared with 25% in a control group without müllerian anomalies. Women with in utero exposure to diethylstilbestrol and uterine anomalies had very low pregnancy rates when treated with IVF.[295]

Cost-Benefit Analysis of in Vitro Fertilization

In today's medical care environment, where resource constraints assume ever-greater importance in medical decision making, the costs and benefits of IVF have been keenly debated. In the early 1990s, the cost of an IVF birth was estimated to be in the range of $44,000 to $211,940.[296] However, this analysis assumed a live birth rate in the range of 10% per cycle, far below what is actually achieved at most centers. A more contemporary estimate would be about $30,000 per delivery, taking into account the use of cryopreserved embryos.[297] In a report from the Brigham and Women's Hospital IVF program, actual charges and live births for calendar year 1993 were analyzed.[298] Couples were assigned to one of three groups on the basis of their clinical characteristics. Group A consisted of couples in which the woman was younger than 32 years of age and the male partner had a normal semen analysis. Group B consisted of women younger than age 40 who had a male partner with an abnormal semen analysis. Group C consisted of women 40 to 42 years of age who had a male partner with a normal semen analysis. The live birth rates in the three groups were 35%, 24%, and 19%, respectively. For group A, the cost of a live birth was $23,000. For group B, the cost of a live birth was $34,000. For group C, the cost of a live birth after the first cycle of IVF was $43,000. Because the live birth rate was lower in group C, many of these couples had multiple cycles of IVF. When the analysis was restricted to couples in group C who completed three cycles of IVF, the cost of a live birth was $75,000.

Even though the cost of IVF is high, it may be the most cost-effective therapy for certain infertility conditions. A retrospective analysis found the cost per delivery for tubal surgery by laparotomy to be double that of IVF.[299] The cost of laparoscopic tubal surgery would be expected to be lower than laparotomy. In particular, male factor patients may benefit from initial treatment with IVF/ICSI. Even in cases of mild male or unexplained infertility it may be more cost effective to utilize IVF as a first-line therapy. An English mathematical model concluded that, for such patients, direct retrieval to IVF was associated with lower total costs than unstimulated IUI followed by IVF for treatment failures or stimulated IUI followed by IVF.[300]

Important considerations when estimating the cost of IVF include both the hospital costs and the lifetime costs of multiple gestations. Although the lifetime costs have not been specifically analyzed, several high-quality studies from Europe, Canada, and the United States have enabled some strong conclusions to be drawn[301]; known costs associated with consequences of twin births and their sequelae are four times higher than singleton births, and costs for triplets are ten times higher than singleton births. Clearly, the leaders in assisted reproductive technology must reduce the rate of multifetal pregnancy to balance the costs and benefits of IVF. As noted previously, one approach to this problem is to transfer no more than two cleavage-stage embryos in good-prognosis couples. Another approach is to culture all embryos to the blastocyst stage prior to transfer on day 5. As discussed earlier, transferring blastocyst-stage embryos improves identification of the embryos with the greatest chance for implantation and hence may reduce the need to transfer more than two embryos. In some programs, the use of blastocyst transfer reduces the rates of multifetal pregnancy without reducing the overall pregnancy rate.[302] However, these potential benefits must be weighed against the reduced cumulative pregnancy rates due to fewer embryos being cryopreserved, and the increased risk of monozygotic/monchorionic twinning following blastocyst transfer.

In Vitro Fertilization with Oocyte Donation

A venerable question in reproduction is, "Which factor has the greater impact on fertility, oocyte age or uterine age?" On the basis of results from IVF with oocyte donation, both affect pregnancy and its outcome, but oocyte age appears to have a far greater impact on fecundability than uterine age. Early studies of IVF with oocyte donation clearly established the feasibility of the technique and reported pregnancy rates in the range of 25% per cycle.[303,304] Studies suggest that oocyte age and uterine age both influence pregnancy rates in programs of IVF with oocyte donation. For example, one study of 114 compared implantation and pregnancy rates for women younger than 40 and women between 40 and 49.[305] The clinical pregnancy rates per embryo transfer were 47% and 25%, respectively. In another study of IVF with oocyte donation, the pregnancy losses were substantially higher in women older than 40 compared with women under 40.[306] A comparison of live birth rates per transfer using fresh embryos from infertility patients' eggs and donor eggs shows the dramatic effects of the egg age on IVF outcome (Fig. 29-29). While there is a dramatic and unrelenting decline in pregnancy rates with increasing age in women using their own oocytes, this decline is not seen in women using donor (and presumably younger) eggs.

The reproductive options for women with ovarian failure are limited. For women with depletion of the oocyte pool, IVF with donor oocytes is the only method that currently allows these women to carry a pregnancy. IVF with oocyte donation was originally intended for women with premature ovarian failure. As the technique developed, it has been applied more frequently to women older than 40 years.[307] An important ethical issue is the age at which women should be advised not to pursue IVF with oocyte donation. Some centers have treated women over 60 years of age; other centers restrict the application of this technique to women younger than 50.

IVF with oocyte donation requires the coordination of the reproductive tracts of the donor and recipient (Fig. 29-30). An important insight provided by this technique is that for women with ovarian failure, steroid replacement with estradiol and progesterone is adequate to prepare the endometrium for successful pregnancy. No other ovarian hormone is required to achieve a successful pregnancy. Most oocyte donation programs use "fresh" oocytes, and the problem of possible transmission of infection from oocyte donor to recipient has not been fully solved.

In Vitro Fertilization with Gestational Carrier

Another form of third-party reproduction involves the use of a gestational carrier in which a woman other than the infertile woman conceives a pregnancy for her. In this scenario, the infertile woman undergoes ovulation induction and egg retrieval and her oocytes are fertilized in vitro, but the resulting embryo(s) are implanted into the uterus of a gestational carrier. The carrier's endometrium is prepared and the synchronization of the cycles of the two women is similar to that of our egg donor and recipient.

Indications for the use of a gestational carrier include congenital absence of the uterus, müllerian congenital malformations, hysterectomy, or surgically uncorrectable anatomic abnormalities such as intrauterine adhesions. Another indication involves women who have a serious medical illness that precludes a safe pregnancy.

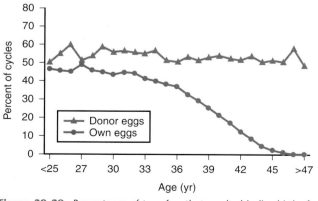

Figure 29-29. Percentages of transfers that resulted in live births for 2005 assisted reproductive technology (ART) cycles using fresh embryos from own or donor eggs, by patient's age. (From CDC Assisted Reproductive Technology [ART] Report 2005. Available at www.cdc.gov/art/ART2005. Accessed Dec. 21, 2008.)

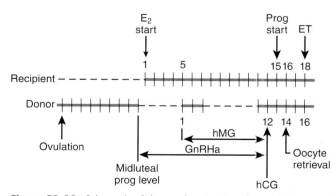

Figure 29-30. Schematic of the synchronization of oocyte donor and embryo recipient on a gonadotropin-releasing hormone-agonist analog (GnRHa) with exogenous estrogen (E₂) and progesterone (Prog) protocol. hMG, human menopausal gonadotropin; hCG, human chorionic gonadotropin; ET, embryo transfer. (From Schmidt-Sarosi CL. In vitro fertilization with donor oocytes. In Keye WR, Chang RJ, Rebar RW, Soules MR [eds]. Infertility: Evaluation and Treatment. Philadelphia, WB Saunders, 1995, p 781.)

Although the mechanics of a gestational carrier cycle are relatively straightforward and routine, this type of third-party reproduction involves complex legal, psychological, and sometimes ethical issues. Potential carriers should have undergone prior uncomplicated pregnancies and completed psychological as well as medical screening. A signed contract between the parties is necessary and laws pertaining to the legal status of the baby vary according to state. Pregnancy rates are dependent on the reproductive prognosis of the oocyte source. Despite its many medical and social complexities, gestational carriers offer some infertile women the opportunity to reproduce using their own and their partner's gametes who otherwise would not be able to have a genetic child.

EXPERIMENTAL PROCEDURES IN THE IVF LABORATORY

In Vitro Oocyte Maturation

An alternate approach to the retrieval of mature oocytes following ovarian stimulation is the aspiration of immature oocytes and their subsequent maturation in vitro. In the setting of in vitro maturation (IVM), GV-stage oocytes are retrieved when the follicles reach a diameter of 6 to 12 mm, and are subsequently cultured for 28 to 36 hours to allow time for progression to metaphase II,[308] thereby simulating the timing from the LH surge in vivo.[309] A specialized, larger needle (19 or 20 gauge) is needed to remove the more adherent immature oocyte-cumulus complex from the membrana granulosa cells lining the follicle, and a lower pressure on the aspiration pump (180 mm Hg versus the typical 300 mm Hg used to aspirate mature oocytes) is desirable to a higher yield of oocytes.[310]

The efficiency of IVM varies depending upon whether the oocytes arise from polycystic ovaries, naturally cycling ovaries, or ovaries primed with low doses of gonadotropin. Regardless, the majority of studies indicate that while more than 60% of IVM oocytes achieve nuclear maturation by progressing to metaphase II,[311] a low percentage successfully acquire cytoplasmic maturation and exhibit the ability to support pronuclear formation and early embryonic development. Only 40% to 80% of fertilized IVM oocytes progress through early cleavage,[312,313] and of those that do cleave and that are transferred, only 7% to 12% form a viable fetus.[314]

Several challenges remain before IVM can be reliably applied in ART. The IVM system requires optimization; the culture medium requires further refinement beyond the reported benefits of supplementation with meiosis-activating sterol[315]; and use of a three-dimensional culture system to support the structural integrity of the oocyte-cumulus complex[316,317] requires further investigation. Moreover, the optimal duration of IVM remains to be determined, and the optimal protocols for preparation of a receptive endometrium need to be identified. Research targeting these gaps in our knowledge is worthwhile. IVM is associated with lower costs due to use of less gonadotropin and the technique eliminates the possibility of OHSS, thereby having particular application in women at increased risk for this syndrome such as those with PCOS. Furthermore, available data, albeit with relatively small numbers of children born, indicate that obstetric, perinatal, and neonatal outcomes after IVM are comparable to those resulting from IVF and ICSI.[318] Finally, an efficacious IVM protocol is required when oocytes are cryopreserved at the GV stage for subsequent attempts to achieve pregnancy.

Oocyte and Ovarian Tissue Cryopreservation

Despite improvements in survival following cancer therapy, the aggressive regimens used for treatment frequently induce premature ovarian failure, rendering the patient infertile. For women facing cancer therapy, there is frequently insufficient time before treatment to undergo ovarian stimulation and IVF. Currently, oocyte or ovarian tissue cryopreservation provides the only hope of preserving fertility for these patients.

Early experience with cryopreservation of oocytes resulted in disappointingly low overall efficiency with poor survival rates, and low fertilization and implantation rates of those oocytes that did successfully survive the freeze/thaw procedures.[319,320] Gook et al.[319] reported that use of ICSI partially overcame damage caused by cryopreservation. They observed that cryopreserved-thawed oocytes failed to demonstrate normal embryo development after being fertilized with standard insemination-incubation techniques. In contrast, some of the cryopreserved-thawed oocytes demonstrated normal embryo development up to the blastocyst stage after being fertilized by ICSI. Subsequent studies showed that hardening of the zona induced by the freezing procedure may interfere with the normal fertilization process per se.[321] Accordingly, it is now routine practice to achieve fertilization of thawed oocytes with ICSI rather than with standard insemination.

More recent studies have reported fertilization rates of thawed oocytes comparable to those of fresh oocytes.[322,323] These improvements have been achieved by adopting earlier refinements in temperature profiles of the freezing programs,[324,325] and adjustments to the concentration of sodium in the freezing solutions.[326] Advancements in vitrification procedures have also been achieved with births being reported following thaw and IVF of vitrified mature oocytes.[322]

Despite these improvements in oocyte cryopreservation, the technique is still considered experimental and further research is required to improve efficiency and optimize protocols. Although the survival of thawed GV-stage oocytes is increased compared with that of mature oocytes,[327] the inefficiency of current in vitro maturation protocols results in comparable numbers of usable oocytes following cryopreservation of immature versus mature oocytes. Vulnerability of the meiotic spindle to damage during the freeze/thaw procedures[328] exposes the mature oocyte to an increased theoretical risk of aneuploidy. However, the limited available data indicate no increased incidence of chromosomal abnormalities in children born from cryopreserved oocytes.[320] A recent meta-analysis indicates that success rates with oocyte cryopreservation technology are increasing, and that vitrification may provide improved implantation rates per thawed oocyte as compared with slow frozen oocytes (8.8% versus 4.9%).[329] Although the ASRM considers oocyte cryopreservation to still be experimental, a handful of anonymous oocyte donor banks exist. In order to meet FDA eligibility requirements for gamete donation,[330] an oocyte (or sperm) donor must undergo medical chart review for risk assessment and be clear of infectious diseases including HIV, hepatitis B, and hepatitis C. Disease testing must be performed within 30 days of the oocyte retrieval.

Another approach for preservation of female fertility involves cryopreservation of ultra-thin slices of ovarian cortical tissue and subsequent transplantation of thawed explants to either an orthotopic or heterotopic site for follicular stimulation.

While this approach obviates the need for a reliable in vitro maturation system, it has several potential risks including poor follicle survival after thaw, unsuccessful transplantation of the autograft, and the possibility for reseeding tumor cells following the transplantation.[331] Nevertheless, a birth has been reported following orthotopic transplantation of cryopreserved tissue,[332] although there is a slim chance that this resulted from ovulation from one of the ovaries that remained in situ before cancer treatment. Ovarian function has been restored after heterotopic transplantation of thawed cortex to the forearm, but no pregnancy was achieved following successful percutaneous aspiration and fertilization of an oocyte.[333]

Environmental Exposures and Life Style Factors in Assisted Rerproductive Techniques

Assisted reproduction procedures provide a unique opportunity to explore the effects of environmental exposures on fecundability. The effect of cigarette smoking has been studied both for IVF and GIFT cycles. In IVF cycles,

cigarette smoking is associated with no major change in peak estradiol concentration or number of oocytes retrieved. However, cigarette smoking appears to decrease the pregnancy and live birth rates in IVF if the female partner smokes but not if the male partner smokes (Fig. 29-31).[334] The effect of smoking on IVF outcome may be dose-dependent. Smoking produces the greatest effects on IVF delivery rates when the female partner smokes more than 20 cigarettes daily (Fig. 29-32).[335]

A clue to the link between cigarette smoking and reduced pregnancy rates in IVF and GIFT is the observation that smoking accelerates the rate of oocyte loss. Smoking appears to increase prematurely a woman's cycle day 3 FSH concentrations.[336] In addition, women between 35 and 39 years of age have a post-clomiphene FSH level more than twice as high as that of women who do not smoke.[337] Both the elevated cycle day 3 FSH, and the elevated FSH level in response to clomiphene suggest that women who smoke have a depleted oocyte pool and may have prematurely aged follicles. Alternatively, the mechanism may involve uterine receptivity. An egg donation model assessing smoking in the recipient found a dose-dependent effect. Recipients smoking more than 10 cigarettes a day had a lower pregnancy rate (52.2% versus 34.1%) than recipients smoking 0 to 10 cigarettes per day.[338] Components of cigarette smoke may increase the rate of oocyte loss. Although the effects of smoking on ovarian function may be irreversible, women who smoke cigarettes should discontinue smoking before undergoing an IVF cycle.

The effects of other life style factors on IVF outcome have not been well studied and the results should be interpreted with caution; however, they may offer insight into "modifiable" factors" in infertility patients undergoing IVF. A prospective study of 221 couples undergoing ART in Southern California reported a reduced pregnancy

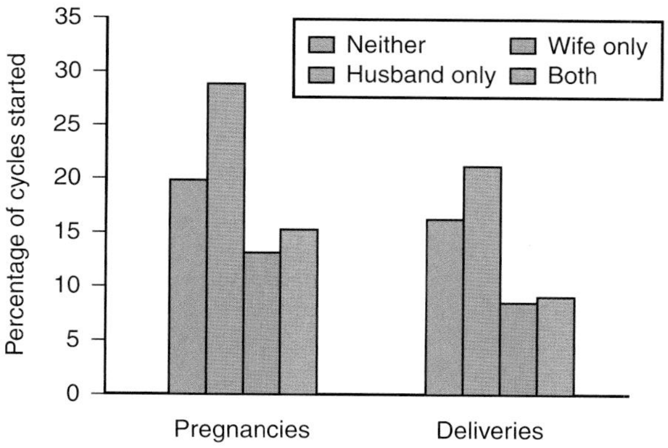

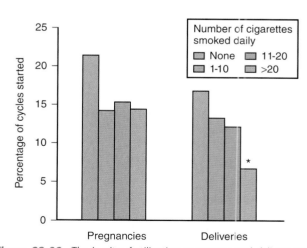

Figure 29-31. *The pregnancy and delivery rates per cycle intiated after in vitro fertilization, stratified by the smoking habits of the male and female partners. Smoking by the female partner substantially decreased the delivery rate per cycle initiated. Smoking by the male partner did not decrease the pregnancy rate. (From Pattinson HA, Taylor PJ, Pattinson MH. The effect of cigarette smoking on ovarian function and early pregnancy outcome of in vitro fertilization treatment. Fertil Steril 55:780-784, 1991, with permission of the American Society for Reproductive Medicine.)*

Figure 29-32. *The in vitro fertilization pregnancy and delivery rates per cycle initiated, stratified by the magnitude of the exposure of the female partner to cigarette smoke. When the female partner smoked more than 20 cigarettes per day, there was a substantial decrease in the delivery rate per cycle initiated. (From Pattinson HA, Taylor PJ, Pattinson MH. The effect of cigarette smoking on ovarian function and early pregnancy outcome of in vitro fertilization treatment. Fertil Steril 55:780-784, 1991, with permission of the American Society for Reproductive Medicine.)*

rate for women consuming 2 to 50 mg caffeine/day (50 mg is roughly the amount of caffeine in half a cup of coffee), compared with women consuming 0 to 2 mg per day during the week of their initial visit (OR 3.1, 95% CI, 1.1-9.7). Caffeine intake the week before the procedure or the week after the procedure was not associated with a reduction in IVF success.[339]

The same dataset was also used to examine the effect of alcohol consumption on ART success rates. The addition of one drink per day increased a woman's risk of not becoming pregnant and significantly increased her risk of miscarriage (OR 2.21, 95% CI 1.09-4.99).[340]

There are only minimal data on marijuana use and IVF, but a single study reported that women who used marijuana more than 90 times in their lifetime had fewer eggs retrieved and one fewer embryo transferred than nonusers. Moreover, women smoking marijuana more than 10 times in their lives also had smaller infants at birth compared to nonusers.[341]

There has been only one study examining the effect of exercise on IVF outcome. Three large IVF programs in the Boston area prospectively enrolled 2232 patients undergoing their first IVF cycle in a study of predictors of successful outcome. All patients filled out a questionnaire that included the amount, type, and frequency of exercise. Women who reported exercising 4 or more hours per week for 1 to 9 years were almost three times more likely to experience cycle cancellation (OR 2.8, 95% CI, 1.5-5.3), twice as likely to experience pregnancy loss (OR 2, 95% CI, 1.2-3.4), and 40% less likely to have a live birth (OR 0.6, 95% CI, 0.4-0.8) than women who reported not exercising.[342] In this same study, women reporting cardiovascular exercise had a 30% lower chance of a successful live birth than those reporting no cardiovascular exercise.

Although one should be cautious about drawing conclusions based on single studies, several modifiable lifestyle behaviors seem to influence successful outcomes in assisted reproduction. As with other questions in this field, well-designed clinical trials are sorely needed.

Nuclear Cloning and Stem Cells

The genomic DNA, and its linear sequence of A, G, C, and T nucleotides, contains all the information necessary to produce an organism. The diploid cells in the body inherit the DNA that was present in the fertilized egg. It is theoretically possible to harvest the DNA from a diploid adult cell, inject it into an oocyte that has had its DNA removed, and stimulate the development of the oocyte into an adult organism. Successful nuclear transplantation of DNA from an adult cell into an oocyte was first accomplished in an amphibian. In the frog, cloning can be accomplished by first destroying the DNA in an oocyte by ultraviolet radiation and then injecting a nucleus from an adult skin cell or an erythrocyte into the oocyte. The trauma of the injection activates the egg, and a swimming tadpole is the product.[343-345]

Similar techniques have recently been used to clone mammals.[346,347] Oocytes were recovered from Scottish Blackface ewes 28 to 33 hours after the injection of GnRH.

The oocytes were enucleated and then fused with donor cells by use of electrical pulses. Before fusion with the enucleated oocyte, the donor cells were forced into quiescence (G_0 stage of the cell cycle) by culturing in media with low serum concentration. Live-born sheep were obtained with the use of donor cells derived from adult mammary tissue, fetal tissue, and an embryonic cell line. These results demonstrate that reproduction of some mammalian species is possible without the use of sperm.

The aspect of these experiments that drew the attention of the public was the possibility of generating a large number of genetically identical clones. The investigators suggest that nuclear transfer from the cells of elite animals to recipient oocytes may enhance the replication of animals with preferred performance characteristics. Although nuclear cloning may be supported by some experts in animal husbandry, many scientists are concerned about the potential misuse of cloning technology. Ironically, one major advantage of sexual reproduction is that it increases the genetic diversity of the species; excessive use of cloning would have exactly the opposite result. Public awareness of the technical advances achieved with nuclear cloning resulted in a call for either a moratorium or ban on all work whose goal was to clone a human. The potential of this technology may be too threatening to our societal concepts of self, family, and society to ever allow widespread application of these techniques to humans.

Embryonic stem cells offer the possibility of treating many human diseases. Human embryos from IVF provide a source of embryonic stem cells that might aid researchers in developing effective disease treatments by allowing growth in the laboratory of functional cell lines, tissues, and organs. Typically, embryonic stem cells are derived from the inner cell mass of the blastocyst-stage embryo. Technical, ethical, and legal problems need to be overcome to make this technology a therapeutic reality. Many scientists believe that the use of embryonic stem cells derived from embryos that would otherwise have been discarded is ethical and should be both allowed and encouraged. Recent work shows that while early-arrested or highly fragmented embryos only rarely yield cell lines, those otherwise discarded poor quality cleavage-stage embryos that undergo blastulation are a robust source of human embryonic stem cell lines.[348] It is likely that with further development of the technology of stem cell derivation, protocols will be perfected and society will strongly support the use of embryonic stem cells for therapeutic purposes. This advancement will bring IVF full circle, from a specialized treatment of tubal factor infertility to a new method for addressing common lethal diseases in humans.

The complete reference list can be found on the companion Expert Consult Web site at www.expertconsultbook.com.

Suggested Readings

Ingerslev HJ, Hojgaard A, Hindkjaer J, et al. A randomized study comparing IVF in the unstimulated cycle with IVF following clomiphene citrate. Hum Reprod 16:696-702, 2001.

Jurema MW, Nogueira D. In vitro maturation of human oocytes for assisted reproduction. Fertil Steril 86:1277-1291, 2006.

Mannaertis B, Devroey P, Abyholm T, et al. A double-blind randomized dose finding study to assess the efficacy of the gonadotropin releasing hormone antagonist ganirelix to prevent premature luteinizing hormone surges in women undergoing ovarian stimulation with recombinant follicle stimulating hormone. Hum Reprod 13:3023-3031, 1998.

Oktay K, Cil AP, Bang H. Efficiency of oocyte cryopreservation: a meta-analysis. Fertil Steril 86:70-80, 2006.

Scott RT, Navot D. Enhancement of ovarian responsiveness with microdoses of gonadotropin releasing hormone agonist during ovulation induction for in vitro fertilization. Fertil Steril 61:880-885, 1994.

Skiadas CC, Racowsky C. Development rate, cumulative scoring and embryonic viability. *In* Elder K, Cohen J (eds): Human Preimplantation Embryo Selection, Colchester, UK, Taylor & Francis, 2007, pp 101-121.

Society for Assisted Reproductive Technology and the American Society for Reproductive Medicine. Assisted reproductive technology in the United States; results generated from the American Society for Reproductive Medicine/Society for Assisted Reproductive Technology Registry, 2005 (www.SART.org)

Steptoe PC, Edwards RG. Birth after the reimplantation of a human embryo. Lancet 2:366, 1978.

Thurin A, Hausken J, Hillensjo T, et al. Elective single-embryo transfer versus double-embryo transfer in in vitro fertilization. N Engl J Med 351:2392-2402, 2004.

Toner JP, Philput CB, Jones GS, et al. Basal follicle stimulating hormone level is a better predictor of in vitro fertilization performance than age. Fertil Steril 55:784-791, 1991.

CHAPTER 30

Gamete and Embryo Manipulation

Anick De Vos and André Van Steirteghem

Since the birth of the first test tube baby in 1978,[1] in vitro fertilization (IVF) has become a well-established treatment procedure for certain types of infertility, including long-standing infertility due to tubal disease, endometriosis, unexplained infertility, or infertility involving a male factor. However, soon it became obvious that certain couples with severe male factor infertility could not be helped by conventional IVF. Extremely low sperm counts, impaired motility, and poor morphology represent the main causes of failed fertilization in conventional IVF.

To tackle this problem, several procedures of assisted fertilization based on micromanipulation of oocytes and spermatozoa have been established. These strategies have culminated in intracytoplasmic sperm injection (ICSI), in which a single spermatozoon is directly injected into the ooplasma. In 1992, our group reported the first human pregnancies and births after replacement of embryos generated by this novel procedure of assisted fertilization.[2] Since then, the number of worldwide centers offering ICSI has increased tremendously, as have the number of treatment cycles per year.[3] Because of the widespread use of ICSI as the ultimate and only option for successful treatment of severe male infertility due to impaired testicular function or obstruction of the excretory ducts, concern about its efficacy and safety is appropriate.

Whereas ICSI represents the major breakthrough for male infertility treatment, preimplantation genetic diagnosis (PGD) would be inconceivable without the establishment of embryo biopsy procedures. Initial attempts to penetrate or open the zona pellucida were undertaken to assist oocyte fertilization[4-6] or increase embryo implantation by facilitating the hatching process.[7,8] This very close access to oocytes or embryos soon resulted in the removal of cellular material (polar bodies or blastomeres, respectively), which allowed genetic testing in this very early developmental stage.[9-12]

As much as PGD relies on embryo biopsy, equally indispensable was the progress in molecular genetics leading to the development of diagnostic procedures at the single-cell level[13-15] (see Chapter 31). These procedures include gene amplification using polymerase chain reaction (PCR) for monogenic diseases and fluorescence in situ hybridization (FISH) for the evaluation of numeric and structural chromosome aberrations or for sex determination in cases of sex-linked diseases. Since the first pregnancy report from the clinical application of PGD,[12] there has been a steady increase in the number of PGD cycles and also in the number of centers performing PGD worldwide.[16] More recently, aneuploidy screening (PGD-AS) has been introduced in an attempt to increase the implantation rate in older women, in couples with previous assisted reproduction failures, and in couples with recurrent abortions.[17,18] Embryos resulting from the injection of testicular spermatozoa in cases of nonobstructive azoospermia can also undergo PGD-AS to evaluate their genetic content.[19]

This chapter surveys the current status of ICSI, emphasizing patient selection, oocyte and sperm handling before microinjection, the procedure and outcome parameters, clinical application, and overall results, including follow-up of the pregnancies and children. The clinical relevance of assisted hatching before embryo transfer is discussed. Embryo biopsy procedures and single-cell analysis (at the chromosomal level by FISH; at the monogenic level by PCR) as diagnostic tools for PGD and PGD-AS are described. Indications for PGD and PGD-AS are summarized, and the clinical outcome of PGD is presented.

Intracytoplasmic Sperm Injection

HISTORY OF ICSI

Extremely low sperm counts, impaired motility, and abnormal morphologic features are the main causes of failed fertilization in conventional IVF. Today, ICSI is the ultimate option to treat these cases of severe male factor infertility (see Chapter 22). One single viable spermatozoon, preferably with good morphologic characteristics, is selected by the embryologist and injected into each oocyte available.

The ICSI procedure is based on micromanipulation of oocytes and spermatozoa. Initially, *partial zona dissection* (PZD) was established to facilitate sperm penetration.[4,5,20,21] The barrier to fertilization represented by the zona pellucida was disrupted mechanically to allow the inseminated sperm cells direct access to the perivitelline space of the oocyte. *Subzonal insemination* (SUZI) was the next step in micromanipulation techniques.[22-25] SUZI enabled the immediate delivery of several motile sperm cells into the perivitelline space by means of an injection pipette.[26] ICSI is even more invasive because a single spermatozoon is directly injected into the ooplasma, thereby crossing not only the zona pellucida but also the oolemma.

The first successful use of ICSI was to obtain live offspring in rabbits and cattle.[27] The first human pregnancies and births resulting from this novel assisted fertilization procedure were reported in 1992.[2] Shortly thereafter, ICSI was found to be superior to SUZI in terms of oocyte fertilization rate,[28-31] number of embryos produced, and embryo implantation rate.[28-31] As a result, ICSI has been used successfully worldwide to treat infertility due to severe oligo-astheno-teratozoospermia or azoospermia caused by impaired testicular function or obstructed excretory ducts.[32,33]

Since the first publication describing the ICSI procedure,[2,25,28,30,31] minor modifications have contributed to reduced rates of oocyte degeneration, oocyte activation (one-pronuclear [1-PN]), and abnormal fertilization (three-pronuclear [3-PN]).[34] Hyaluronidase may be responsible for oocyte activation; therefore, the concentration used during oocyte denudation and the exposure time of oocytes to the enzyme has been reduced.[35] The timing of denudation relative to oocyte pickup (immediately or 4 hours later) does not influence the ICSI results.[36] The orientation of the polar body during injection does, however, influence embryo quality.[37] Motile sperm cells are selected and immobilized before injection.[38] Cytoplasm aspiration to ensure oolemma rupture is critical to the success of the ICSI procedure, because the method of rupture has been correlated with oocyte degeneration.[37] Furthermore, the morphologic features of the injected spermatozoon are related to the fertilization outcome of the procedure as well as to the pregnancy outcome.[39]

The outcome of the ICSI procedure may benefit from the introduction of some new technical improvements. Noninvasive spindle imaging in human oocytes on the basis of its birefringence with a computer-assisted polarization microscopy system (PolScope, Cambridge Research & Instrumentation, Woburn, MA) may serve as an accurate indicator of oocyte maturity, quality, and developmental potential.[40-48] High-magnification ICSI, on the other hand, would provide a better morphologic selection of spermatozoa to be used for fertilization.[49-54]

The presence of a birefringent spindle in human oocytes can predict not only a higher fertilization rate, but also greater embryo developmental competence.[41,42] Meiotic spindles can be detected in up to 91% of human metaphase II oocytes at the time of ICSI.[43] Because most oocytes possess spindles, the mere presence of a spindle is of limited value. High degrees of misalignment between the meiotic spindle and the first polar body have been described,[43] probably due to polar body displacement during manipulations for cumulus corona removal.[46] The relative position of the spindle within the oocyte, however, has little influence on the developmental potential of the resulting embryos.[42,43] Whether quantitative spindle analysis (estimating the density of tubules within the spindle) offers added value needs to be seen.[45,47] So far, spindle imaging, in addition to the appearance of the first polar body, is an accurate indicator of oocyte maturity[44] and can help to determine the timing of ICSI.[48,55] Additionally, meiotic spindle dynamics[55] and possible meiotic spindle destruction due to cryopreservation can be monitored.[46]

Conventional ICSI involves sperm selection at an optical magnification of approximately ×400.[39] However, spermatozoa appearing morphologically normal at this magnification may carry various structural abnormalities at the subcellular level, which then remain undetected by the embryologist. This limitation was alleviated by the use of higher optical magnifications and resulted in a new method of motile sperm organellar morphologic examination.[50] Real-time fine morphologic examination of motile human sperm cells showed that the morphologic state of the sperm nucleus is a relevant and crucial factor for successful ICSI.[50,52] The possible advantage of intracytoplasmic morphologically selected sperm injection in terms of pregnancy has been shown in several matched control comparisons[49,50,54]; however, a prospective randomized trial would be welcome. High-magnification ICSI might be especially useful in cases of paternally caused repeated ICSI failure.[53]

In contrast to visually selected spermatozoa, hyaluronic acid–mediated sperm selection is a novel and efficient technique that may alleviate potential problems related to ICSI fertilization with sperm of diminished maturity.[56-58] The presence of hyaluronic acid receptor on the plasma membrane of mature sperm, coupled with hyaluronic acid–coated glass or plastic surfaces, facilitates testing of sperm function and selection of single mature sperm for ICSI.

CURRENT INDICATIONS FOR ICSI

Before the era of ICSI, attempts were made to modify and refine conventional IVF to achieve increased rates of conception in cases of male infertility. Today, ICSI has clearly overshadowed the use of modified IVF procedures (including high insemination concentration) for the treatment of severe male factor infertility. ICSI requires only one spermatozoon with a functional genome and centrosome for the fertilization of each oocyte. Indications for ICSI are not restricted to morphologically impaired spermatozoa and include low sperm count and impaired kinetic quality of the sperm cells. ICSI can also be used with spermatozoa from the epididymis or testis when there is an obstruction in the excretory ducts. Azoospermia caused by testicular failure can be treated by ICSI if enough spermatozoa can be retrieved in testicular tissue samples. Box 30-1 gives an overview of the current indications for ICSI.

The ICSI procedure with ejaculated spermatozoa can be used successfully in patients with fertilization failures after conventional IVF, and also in patients with too few morphologically normal and progressive motile spermatozoa present in the ejaculate (<500,000). High fertilization and pregnancy rates can be obtained when a motile spermatozoon is injected.[31] Injection of only immotile or probably nonvital spermatozoa results in lower fertilization rates.[59] When only nonvital sperm cells are present in the ejaculate, the use of testicular sperm is indicated.[60] Other semen parameters, such as concentration, morphologic features (except for globozoospermia),[61] and high titers of antisperm antibodies,[62] do not influence success rates.[61] Successful ICSI has also been described in patients with acrosomeless spermatozoa.[63,64]

Any form of infertility due to obstruction of the excretory ducts can be treated by ICSI with spermatozoa microsurgically recovered from either the epididymis[65-67] or the testis.[68-70] Obstructive azoospermia can result from congenital bilateral absence of the vas deferens, failed

vasectomy reversal, or vasoepididymostomy. When no motile spermatozoa can be retrieved from the epididymis due to epididymal fibrosis, testicular spermatozoa can be isolated from a testicular biopsy specimen.

Testicular biopsy has also proven useful in some cases of nonobstructive azoospermia.[71-74] In patients with severely impaired testicular function as a result of incomplete germ cell aplasia (Sertoli cell–only syndrome), hypospermatogenesis, or incomplete maturation arrest, spermatozoa may be recovered, sometimes only after multiple biopsy specimens are obtained. Testicular sperm recovery may not be successful in all azoospermic patients. Cryopreservation of supernumerary spermatozoa recovered from the epididymis[75] or the testis[76] is an important issue because microinjection of cryothawed sperm cells can avoid repeated surgery in future ICSI cycles.

The ICSI procedure cannot be carried out in approximately 3% of scheduled cycles. Most cancellations occur because no cumulus–oocyte complexes or metaphase II oocytes are available or because no spermatozoa are found in testicular biopsy specimens of patients with nonobstructive azoospermia.

OOCYTE HANDLING AND SPERM PREPARATION BEFORE ICSI

A successful ICSI program depends on ovarian stimulation, which is essentially similar to methods used for conventional IVF (see Chapters 28 and 29). Current ovarian stimulation regimens use a combination of gonadotropin-releasing hormone (GnRH) agonists, human menopausal gonadotropin, or recombinant follicle-stimulating hormone (FSH) and human chorionic gonadotropin (hCG). This treatment allows the retrieval of a high number of cumulus–oocyte complexes.[77,78] Administration of GnRH agonists allows pituitary down-regulation to occur before the initiation of exogenous FSH. A gonadotropin preparation or recombinant FSH is administered to stimulate multiple follicle development. Ovulation is usually induced with hCG (10,000 IU), which is administered when the serum estradiol level exceeds 1000 pg/mL and when at least three follicles 18 mm or more in diameter are observed on ultrasound examination. The optimal time for ultrasound-guided transvaginal oocyte aspiration is 36 hours after hCG administration.[79] On average, 11 cumulus–oocyte complexes per cycle can be retrieved.[80] After cumulus and corona cell removal, approximately nine metaphase II oocytes per cycle are available for microinjection.[80]

Although hCG may be used for luteal-phase supplementation, exogenous progesterone (administered intravaginally) is frequently applied in an attempt to avoid the risk of hCG stimulation of the remaining growing follicles. The clinical introduction of GnRH antagonists[81-83] allowed a powerful and immediate suppression of pituitary gonadotropin release and a rapid recovery of normal secretion of endogenous luteinizing hormone and FSH.[84] By making optimal use of endogenous FSH, the amount of exogenous FSH required for follicular growth could be substantially reduced. A rapid recovery of pituitary luteinizing hormone and FSH release after cessation of GnRH

BOX 30-1

Current Indications for Intracytoplasmic Sperm Injection

Ejaculated Spermatozoa
Oligozoospermia
Asthenozoospermia (caveat for 100% immotile spermatozoa)
Teratozoospermia (≤4% normal morphology using strict criteria—caveat for globozoospermia)
High titers of antisperm antibodies
Repeated fertilization failure after conventional in vitro fertilization and embryo transfer
Autoconserved frozen sperm from patients with cancer in remission
Ejaculatory disorders (e.g., electroejaculation, retrograde ejaculation)

Epididymal Spermatozoa
Congenital bilateral absence of the vas deferens
Young syndrome
Failed vasoepididymostomy
Failed vasovasostomy
Obstruction of both ejaculatory ducts

Testicular Spermatozoa
All indications for epididymal sperm
Failure of epididymal sperm recovery because of fibrosis
Azoospermia caused by testicular failure (maturation arrest, germ cell aplasia)
Necrozoospermia

antagonist administration might eliminate the need for additional luteal-phase support.

Fertilization with micromanipulation requires denudation of oocytes (i.e., removal of the surrounding cumulus and corona cells). This strategy allows not only precise injection of the oocytes, but also assessment of their maturity, which is of critical importance for ICSI. Cumulus and corona cells are removed with a combination of enzymatic and mechanical procedures.[35] Hyaluronidase-purified preparations of bovine origin digest the hyaluronic acid interspersed between the cumulus cells, liberating the oocyte for maturity grading and microinjection. Both the enzyme concentration and the duration of exposure to the enzyme should be limited because they can result in parthenogenetic activation of the oocytes.[85] Because of its purity, a recently developed recombinant human hyaluronidase Cumulase (Halozyme Therapeutics), may be used at higher concentrations; as a result, the incubation time becomes less critical.[86] For these reasons, this product may reduce, if not eliminate, the risk of damage or trauma to the oocytes by the mechanical denudation step. Additionally, the risk of animal pathogen contamination is alleviated. Microscopic observations of the denuded oocytes include assessment of the zona pellucida and oocyte and determination of the presence or absence of a germinal vesicle or first polar body. In 95% of cases, the retrieved cumulus–oocyte complexes usually contain an intact oocyte. The remaining 5% are empty zonae, cracked zonae, or morphologically abnormal oocytes.

Figure 30-1 shows three stages of oocyte maturation. On average, 3.9% of the intact oocytes are at the metaphase I stage, having undergone breakdown of the germinal vesicle, but not yet extrusion of the first polar body.[80] Approximately 10.3% of the intact oocytes are at the germinal vesicle stage, and approximately 85.8% are in the metaphase II stage, showing the presence of the first polar body.[80] ICSI is carried out only on metaphase II oocytes, because only such oocytes have reached the haploid state and thus can be fertilized normally. Frequently, metaphase I oocytes achieve meiosis after a few hours in vitro and are available for ICSI on the day of oocyte retrieval. Despite somewhat lower fertilization rates (52.7% versus 70.8%), injection of matured metaphase I oocytes results in embryos of similar quality to metaphase II oocytes at the moment of oocyte retrieval.[87] Denuded and rinsed oocytes are incubated until the time of microinjection.

For microinjection, spermatozoa from three different origins are processed: ejaculated sperm and surgically retrieved sperm from either the epididymis or the testis. For all three categories, ICSI, in combination with sperm cryopreservation, is currently used successfully.[75,88,89] All patients selected for ICSI with ejaculated semen undergo a preliminary semen assessment before treatment to verify whether enough spermatozoa (preferably motile) are present to perform ICSI.

Routinely, sperm samples for ICSI are processed by density-gradient centrifugation (using silane-coated silica particle colloid solutions[90]), enriching the number of motile and morphologically normal sperm cells needed for assisted reproduction. Only in cases of extreme oligozoospermia (i.e., when gradient centrifugation results in an insufficient yield of sperm cells for ICSI) is simple washing of the sperm sample performed to reduce the loss of sperm cells for injection. Immediate injection of the oocytes is then indicated because sperm cells lose their initial motility and often die when the sample is simply washed. This consequence can be ascribed to the presence of reactive oxygen species and other damaging substances.[91,92]

During microsurgical epididymal sperm aspiration,[93,94] several sperm fractions are collected into separate tubes. Sperm fractions with similar concentration and motility are pooled, and a density-gradient centrifugation is performed. Microdroplets of the resuspended pellet are placed in separate medium droplets adjacent to a central polyvinylpyrrolidone (PVP) droplet in the injection dish. This facilitates the search for and selection of single motile spermatozoa. Spermatozoa are collected using a testicular sperm extraction pipette, which is larger in diameter than an injection pipette (outer diameter 8-10 μm instead of 6-7 μm). The spermatozoa are then transferred to the PVP droplet and immobilized before injection. Whenever possible, some of the freshly recovered sperm should be frozen for later use in subsequent ICSI cycles, thereby avoiding the need for repeated surgical procedures.[93]

Testicular biopsy specimens, usually obtained with surgical excisional biopsy,[69] are shredded into small pieces with sterile microscope slides[95] on the heated stage of a stereomicroscope. The presence of spermatozoa is assessed with an inverted microscope, which determines whether the surgical procedure can be stopped or whether extra biopsy specimens must be taken. The pieces of biopsy tissue are removed, and the medium is centrifuged at 300 × g for 5 minutes. The pellet is then resuspended for

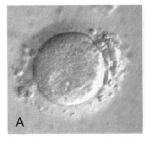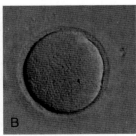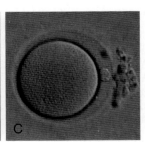

Figure 30-1. *Oocyte maturity after cumulus and corona cell removal. **A,** A germinal vesicle–stage oocyte is recognized by the presence of a typical germinal vesicle. **B,** Oocytes that have undergone germinal vesicle breakdown but have not yet extruded the first polar body are called "metaphase I oocytes." **C,** A typical metaphase II oocyte shows a first polar body, which indicates that the ooycte is mature and has reached the haploid state. Only metaphase II oocytes are submitted to intracytoplasmic sperm injection.*

the ICSI procedure. Single motile spermatozoa are collected in a manner similar to that used for epididymal sperm, using separate medium droplets that contain fractions of the testicular sperm suspension. If no sperm cells can be found, the tissue pieces can be treated with red blood cell lysis buffer[96] or an enzymatic collagen digestion medium.[97] Lysis of excess red blood cells may facilitate the search for sperm cells, and the use of enzymes may result in the recovery of otherwise inaccessible sperm cells that are initially attached to the tissue. It is not always possible to retrieve testicular spermatozoa from biopsy specimens in patients with nonobstructive azoospermia due to germ cell aplasia or maturation arrest.[98] When testicular spermatozoa are retrieved under local anesthesia with fine-needle aspiration,[99] the aspirated fractions are immediately collected in the injection dish. No further sample processing, except collecting the single motile spermatozoa with a microneedle (testicular sperm extraction pipette), is needed before ICSI.

ICSI PROCEDURE

For the ICSI procedure itself, an inverted microscope equipped with micromanipulators and microinjectors should be available.[34] Magnification capability of ×200 and ×400 is a prerequisite for precise procedures such as ICSI. High-magnification ICSI involves a digitally enhanced magnification of ×6000.[52] A heating stage on the inverted microscope maintains the temperature at 37°C. Ambient temperature control is of vital importance for the survival of oocytes, which are very sensitive to a decrease in temperature that can cause irreversible damage to the meiotic spindle.[100] The micromanipulators allow three-dimensional manipulation (coarse and fine movements) of the holding and injection pipette on the left-hand and right-hand sides, respectively. The microinjectors are used to either fix or release the oocyte with the holding pipette, or to aspirate and inject a spermatozoon with the injection pipette. The injectors can be filled with air or mineral oil. A micrometer controls the plunger. The whole setup is placed on a vibration-proof table to avoid possible interfering motion. Several companies supply microtools for holding and injection; however, some centers still prepare their own microtools, which demands extra effort, time, and specialized equipment.[34]

The ICSI procedure involves the injection of a single motile spermatozoon into the oocyte. The procedure is carried out in a plastic microinjection dish containing microdroplets covered with mineral oil. A fraction (±1 µL) of the sperm suspension is added to the periphery of the central PVP droplet. Separate medium droplets are used in cases of epididymal or testicular sperm. The oocytes, denuded from their surrounding cumulus and corona cells, are placed in the eight surrounding medium droplets. The viscous character of the PVP solution slows the motility of sperm cells, thereby facilitating manipulation. It also allows for better control of the fluid in the injection needle and prevents sperm cells from sticking to the pipette.

During ICSI, the following steps can be distinguished: selection and immobilization of a viable sperm cell, correct

positioning of the oocyte before injection, and rupture of the oolemma before the release of the sperm cell into the oocyte.

Figure 30-2 shows the whole injection procedure. In the injection pipette, which is filled with PVP, a single living, morphologically normal spermatozoon is aspirated. Viability is evidenced by the motility of the sperm cell, even if it is only a slight twitching of the tail. The sperm cell is then released in a perpendicular position to the injection pipette, which facilitates immobilization. Immobilization of a sperm cell involves rubbing the tail with the pipette against the bottom of the dish, which results in a breakage at one point, preferably below the midpiece. Immobilization of spermatozoa has been proven to be important for oocyte activation, which is achieved by release of sperm cytosolic factors via the ruptured membrane. Increased fertilization rates with ICSI have been reported after aggressive damage to the sperm tail plasma membrane.[38,101] Changes in the sperm plasma membrane and acrosome after immobilization before ICSI have been confirmed by transmission electron microscopy[102] and scanning electron microscopy.[103] Although sperm immobilization is usually performed mechanically with the ICSI needle, laser-induced immobilization has also been described,[104-106] resulting in identical fertilization rates.[105,106]

After immobilization, the sperm cell is again aspirated (now tail-first) to allow the injection of a minimal volume of medium together with the sperm cell. The oocyte is held in position with minimal suction by the holding pipette. The polar body is located at the 6 o'clock position, which avoids damage to the spindle.[37] Experiments in our laboratory using Hoechst dye–stained oocytes for microinjection clearly showed no interference with the spindle

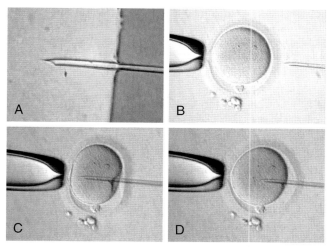

Figure 30-2. *Intracytoplasmic sperm injection procedure. A, A single motile spermatozoon is selected and immobilized by pressing its tail between the microneedle and the bottom of the dish. The sperm cell is then aspirated tail-first into the injection pipette. B, Using the holding pipette, the mature oocyte is fixed with the polar body at the 6 o'clock position. The sperm cell is brought to the tip of the injection pipette. C, The injection pipette is introduced at the 3 o'clock position and rupture of the oolemma is ascertained by slight suction. Then the sperm cell is delivered into the oocyte with a minimal volume of medium; afterward, the pipette can be carefully withdrawn. D, A single sperm cell can be appreciated in the center of the ooplasma.*

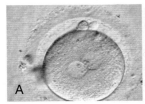 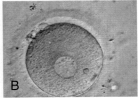 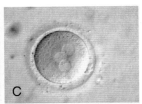

Figure 30-3. *Fertilization outcome after intracytoplasmic sperm injection.* **A,** *Oocytes are considered normally fertilized when two individualized or fragmented polar bodies are present, together with two clearly visible pronuclei that contain nucleoli.* **B,** *Abnormal fertilization may occur as one pronuclear oocyte, probably due to parthenogenic activation.* **C,** *The occasional finding of three pronuclear oocytes after injection of a single spermatozoon into the ooplasm is probably caused by nonextrusion of the second polar body at the time of fertilization.*

if oocytes are injected with the polar body at the 6 o'clock position. Although the first polar body does not always coincide with spindle localization, no reports so far describe spindle monitoring during ICSI to reduce spindle damage and increase the chance of fertilization. If both the holding pipette and the oocyte are in perfect focus, the injection needle, containing the immobilized sperm cell near the tip, can be introduced in the equatorial plane of the oocyte at the 3 o'clock position. Permanent focus of the injection pipette tip ensures that the needle remains in the equatorial plane of the oocyte. Passing through the zona pellucida is fairly easy and is achieved by simply advancing the injection pipette. In contrast, the oolemma is not always immediately pierced by simple injection of the needle, and often, minimal suction must be applied. The ooplasm then enters the injection pipette, and sudden acceleration of the flow indicates membrane rupture. Aspiration is immediately stopped, the sperm cell is slowly released into the oocyte with a minimal volume of medium, and the pipette is withdrawn carefully.

Different patterns of oolemma breakage have been described, depending on whether the ooplasm breaks during insertion of the pipette, whether slight or stronger aspiration of the ooplasm is needed, or whether breakage of the oolemma in another place must be attempted.[37,101] Immediate rupture of the oolemma without aspiration has been associated with lower oocyte survival rates.[37,101]

OUTCOME PARAMETERS OF ICSI: FERTILIZATION AND EMBRYO CLEAVAGE

After the injection procedure, oocytes are rinsed and cultured in microdroplets covered with lightweight paraffin oil. The conditions are similar to those used for IVF-inseminated oocytes. The oocytes are kept at 37°C in an atmosphere of 5% O_2, 5% CO_2, and 90% N_2. Injected oocytes are examined for integrity and fertilization approximately 16 to 18 hours after ICSI.[107] An average damage rate of approximately 9% of injected oocytes can be expected, regardless of the origin of the sperm used.[80] Oocytes are considered normally fertilized when two individualized or fragmented polar bodies are present together with two clearly visible pronuclei (2-PN) that contain nucleoli (Fig. 30-3).

The fertilization rate after ICSI is usually expressed per number of injected oocytes and ranges from 57% to 67%, according to the sperm origin.[80] As shown in Figure 30-3, abnormal fertilization may occur, reflected by 1-PN oocytes (approximately 3% of injected oocytes).[80] These oocytes are likely to be parthenogenetically activated as a result of mechanical or chemical factors.[108,109] The occasional finding of 3-PN oocytes (approximately 4%)[80] after injection of a single spermatozoon into the ooplasm is probably caused by failure of extrusion of the second polar body at the time of fertilization.[109] Neither type of embryo resulting from 1-PN or 3-PN oocytes is transferred to patients.

As early as the pronuclear stage, morphologic scoring, including alignment and size of pronuclei, alignment and number of nucleoli, and halo effect of the cytoplasm, can serve as a valuable noninvasive selection method in addition to the morphologic characteristics on the day of transfer. The morphologic features of the pronuclear zygote are related to implantation and pregnancy rates.[110-112] Pronuclear evaluation, therefore, is considered useful in determining the most suitable embryos for transfer, thus achieving an optimal chance of conception.[113,114]

Postfertilization, approximately 90% of 2-PN oocytes obtained by ICSI enter cleavage, resulting in multicellular embryos. Cleavage characteristics of the fertilized oocytes are evaluated daily. Early cleavage into the two-cell stage approximately 25 to 27 hours after ICSI seems to be a strong biologic indicator of embryonic potential, and may be used as an additional criterion for embryo selection.[115-117] Normally developing, good-quality embryos reach the four-cell and eight-cell stages, respectively, on day 2 and on the morning of day 3 postmicroinjection (Fig. 30-4). Numbers and sizes of blastomeres and the presence of anucleate cytoplasmic fragments are recorded. The cleaving embryos are scored according to equality of size of the blastomeres and proportion of anucleate fragments.[118,119] Type A (excellent) embryos do not contain anuclear fragments. Type B (good-quality) embryos have a maximum of 20% of the volume of the embryo filled with anucleate fragments. In type C (fair-quality) embryos, anucleate fragments represent 21% to 50% of the volume of the embryo. Type D (poor-quality) embryos have anucleate fragments present in more than 50% of the volume of the embryo. These embryos cannot be used for transfer to patients. Embryos of types A, B, and C are eligible for transfer. Because embryos with uneven cell cleavage have a lower developmental capacity in comparison with evenly cleaved embryos, emphasis on blastomere size within embryo scoring systems seems appropriate.[120,121] Assessing the degree of compaction is valuable as well because early compaction on day 3 may be associated with increased implantation potential.[122] Multinucleation is a frequently observed phenomenon in cleavage-stage embryos.[123] It may occur

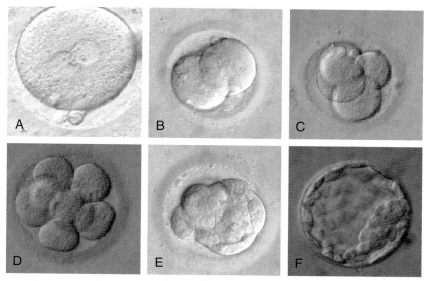

Figure 30-4. *Embryo cleavage after intracytoplasmic sperm injection. Only embryos resulting from normally fertilized oocytes (A) will be transferred to patients. Embryo cleavage is evaluated daily. Two-cell embryos (B), four-cell embryos (C), and eight-cell embryos (D) are usually obtained on day 1 (late afternoon), on day 2, and on the morning of day 3, respectively. The blastomere number is recorded and the embryos are scored according to equality of size of the blastomeres and the presence of anucleate cytoplasmic fragments. On day 4 (sometimes on day 3), a certain degree of compaction can be observed (E). For blastocyst (F) scoring, the classification system introduced by Gardner and Schoolcraft is used. Embryo transfer is usually done on day 3 (eight-cell stage) or day 5 (blastocyst stage). (From Staessen C, Camus M, Khan I, et al. An 18-month survey of infertility treatment by in vitro fertilization, gamete and zygote intrafallopian transfer, and replacement of frozen-thawed embryos. In Vitro Fertil Embryo Transfer 6:22,1989; and Gardner DK, Lane M, Stevens I, et al. Blastocyst score affects implantation and pregnancy outcome: towards a single blastocyst transfer. Fertil Steril 73:1155, 2000.)*

as early as the two-cell stage,[124] but has also been observed on days 2 and 3 of preimplantation development.[125,126] Of course, the proportion of multinucleated blastomeres within one embryo is an important parameter. Embryos presenting more than 50% of their blastomeres with multinucleation are not considered for transfer, regardless of the developmental stage at first detection. The presence of one or more multinucleated blastomeres ($\leq$50%) has been associated with impaired cleavage and increased fragmentation,[123] a poor prognosis for blastocyst formation,[126] and is compromising the ongoing implantation rate,[123] probably due to chromosomal abnormalities.[127] Excluding these embryos for transfer (if other mononucleated embryos are available) seems prudent practice.

Currently, most centers perform embryo transfers on day 3 after oocyte retrieval. At that time, the embryos are expected to be at the eight-cell stage. Because the embryonic genome is fully activated after the eight-cell stage,[128] it may be beneficial to continue to evaluate embryos at least until after the transition from the maternal to the embryonic genome, making it possible to identify embryos with better developmental potential. The number of embryos transferred depends on the age of the woman and the rank of trial. The only possible strategy to prevent multiple pregnancies in IVF and ICSI is to transfer a single embryo, especially in young women in their first or second attempt.[129-133] In women older than 36 years of age who are undergoing a first or second ICSI attempt, the preference is to transfer two excellent or good-quality embryos. In other cases, three or more embryos may be placed into the uterus. Higher pregnancy rates can be obtained when elective transfer of two or three embryos is possible.[80,134]

A new generation of commercially available sequential culture media allows the culture of human embryos up to the blastocyst stage (day 5 or day 6).[135] On day 4 (sometimes on day 3), a certain degree of compaction can be observed. Compaction in the mammalian pre-embryo is a fundamental event that leads to the formation of the trophectoderm, the inner cell mass, and the blastocoele. Full compaction (16-cell to 32-cell stage) is followed by immediate cavitation and blastocoele expansion.[136] For blastocyst scoring, the classification system introduced by Gardner and Schoolcraft can be used.[137] A distinction between early and expanded blastocysts is made, and the latter category is further scored according to the quality of the inner cell mass and the trophectoderm. The possibility of prolonged human embryo culture allows for day 5 or blastocyst transfers. Preferably, expanded blastocysts with a cohesive trophectoderm and a clear inner cell mass are transferred.

Possible advantages of blastocyst transfer are better embryo selection and better synchronization between embryo and endometrium, which may result in higher implantation rates per blastocyst transferred.[138,139] This, in turn, would allow transfer of fewer embryos, thereby decreasing the number of multiple pregnancies.[140-142] However, the superiority of blastocyst transfer over early embryo transfer remains to be proven. A limited number of randomized controlled studies are available. Some show the benefit of blastocyst transfer, whereas others show no advantage of day 5 transfers over day 3 transfers.[139-150]

The cumulative success of a single embryo transfer policy, either on day 3 or on day 5, depends on a good cryopreservation program of cleavage-stage embryos or blastocysts. Supernumerary embryos with less than 20% of anucleate fragments (types A and B) can be cryopreserved on day 2 or day 3 after oocyte retrieval by means of a slow-freezing protocol with dimethylsulfoxide.[151] Alternatively, embryos are frozen at the blastocyst stage on day 5 or day 6, with glycerol and sucrose used as cryoprotectant agents.[152] Vitrification with ethylene glycol has been proposed recently.[153-156]

CLINICAL APPLICATION AND RESULTS

The results of 7 years of ICSI practice (1991-1997) have been reported previously.[80] Here we present the results from 2000 and 2001, involving 2431 ICSI cycles in which 21,572 metaphase II oocytes were injected. The ICSI procedure could not be carried out in 50 cycles (2%) because there were no cumulus–oocyte complexes or metaphase II oocytes (22 cycles) or because no spermatozoa were available for the microinjection procedure (28 cycles, mainly testicular biopsy cases). The majority of cycles involved injection with ejaculated sperm (88.9%). Epididymal sperm was used in only 1.8% of the cycles, and in 9.4% of the cycles, spermatozoa were retrieved from the testis.

In total, 25,721 cumulus–oocyte complexes were retrieved (i.e., a mean of 10.6 per treatment cycle). Of the retrieved cumulus–oocyte complexes, 95% contained an intact oocyte. Of these, 8.7% were in the germinal vesicle stage, 2.7% were in the metaphase I stage, and 88.6%

represented mature metaphase II oocytes. ICSI was performed on most of the mature oocytes (99.8%), and an oocyte survival rate of 92.6% was obtained. The oocyte survival rate was similar in the four categories of sperm cell origin (Table 30-1).

Normal fertilization (2 PN) was obtained in 80.1% of the intact oocytes or in 74.2% of the injected oocytes (see Table 30-1). Normal fertilization rates with ejaculated sperm (75.7% per injected oocyte) were higher than with epididymal (72.1%) or testicular sperm (60% and 63.8% with fresh and frozen-thawed testicular sperm, respectively). Abnormal fertilization (1 PN or at least 3 PN) occurred in 5.1% and 3.5% of the injected oocytes, respectively.

Embryo cleavage was evaluated daily. The percentages of 2-PN oocytes developing into excellent, good-quality, and fair-quality embryos, according to the different types of spermatozoa used for ICSI, are summarized in Table 30-1. On day 2, 80.3% of the 2-PN oocytes resulted in excellent and good-quality embryos. On day 3, this percentage was 72.9%. More excellent and good-quality embryos were obtained in the group using ejaculated spermatozoa than in the groups with epididymal and testicular sperm cells. The percentage of eight-cell embryos on day 3 (including compacting and compact embryos and those with more than eight cells) varied between 34.8% and 47.5%. The total blastocyst formation rate per 2-PN oocyte was 44.7%. However, when only good-quality blastocysts were included (i.e., expanded blastocysts with a cohesive

TABLE 30-1

Sperm Origin, Oocyte Damage and Pronuclear Status, and Embryo Development After Intracytoplasmic Sperm Injection

	Ejaculated Sperm	Epididymal Sperm	Testicular Sperm		Total
			Fresh	Frozen-Thawed	
Cycles	2160	43	122	106	2431
Oocytes undergoing intracytoplasmic sperm injection	19,027	373	1215	957	21,572
Intact oocytes (%)	92.5	93.8	92.1	94.1	92.6
Injected oocytes (%) with:					
One pronucleus	4.8	9.1	8.3	5.9	5.1
Two pronuclei	75.7	72.1	60.0	63.8	74.2
Three or more pronuclei	3.5	2.1	3.3	3.9	3.5
Two-pronuclear oocytes	14,396	269	729	611	16,005
Embryonic development (day 2)					
Excellent embryos (%)	18.8	10	14.5	14.2	18.3
Good-quality embryos (%)	62.1	62.8	58	64	62
Fair-quality embryos (%)	10.6	13.4	12.2	12.1	10.8
Embryonic development (day 3)					
Excellent embryos (%)	15	5.3	11.5	9.9	14.5
Good-quality embryos (%)	58.7	58.4	53.2	57.3	58.4
Fair-quality embryos (%)	12.4	15.5	13.6	13.1	12.5
Embryonic development (day 5)					
Blastocysts (%)	45.6	43.5	32.7	37.6	44.7
Good-quality blastocysts (%)	27.1	27.7	14.1	26.2	26.6
Transfer and cryopreservation					
Transferred embryos (%)	34.2	32	38	38.8	34.5
Frozen embryos (%)	19.9	19	11.2	11.9	19.2

trophectoderm and a clear inner cell mass), this formation rate was limited to 26.6%. More good-quality blastocysts were obtained when ejaculated (27.1%), epididymal (27.7%), and frozen testicular (26.2%) sperm cells were used for ICSI than when fresh testicular sperm cells were used for microinjection (14.1%).

The percentages of embryos actually transferred were similar for the four types of spermatozoa, varying from 32.0% to 38.8%. Cryopreservation of supernumerary embryos was postponed until day 5 or day 6, allowing a better selection of embryos actually frozen. More blastocysts were frozen when ejaculated (19.9%) or epididymal (19%) sperm cells were used for ICSI than when testicular sperm cells were used (11.2% and 11.9%, respectively, with fresh and frozen-thawed testicular sperm). Overall, approximately half of the 2-PN oocytes (53.7%) result in embryos available for transfer or cryopreservation. This percentage does not differ between the different sperm categories (see Table 30-1).

Transfer of at least one embryo was possible in 2293 of the 2431 ICSI treatment cycles (94.3%). As shown in Table 30-2, the transfer rate was similar across the four sperm groups used for ICSI, varying from 92.5% to 95.3%. In 2000, mainly day 2 transfers were performed, whereas in 2001, we switched from day 2 to day 3 transfers. Of the 2293 embryo replacement cycles, 822 occurred on day 2, 1100 occurred on day 3, and 360 occurred on day 5. Day 4 transfers were performed only occasionally (10 cycles), and one transfer involved a day 6 transfer. On average, 2.4 embryos (± 0.8; range, 1-8 embryos) were replaced per treatment cycle. Fourteen transfer cycles remained with an unknown serum hCG outcome, whereas for all other transfer cycles (n = 2279), the outcome was known. The overall pregnancy rates per transfer with known hCG outcome were similar for the four types of spermatozoa, varying from 32.4% to 35.7%. The overall pregnancy rate per treatment cycle was 32.8%. The implantation rate per embryo transferred was 15.1%, similar in all four sperm

groups, except for the higher implantation rate obtained with embryos resulting from ICSI with epididymal sperm cells. Of the embryo replacements with positive serum hCG, all but 35 (27 in the ejaculated semen group, 1 in the epididymal spermatozoa group, 4 in the freshly collected testicular spermatozoa group, and 3 in the frozen-thawed testicular spermatozoa group) resulted in a known outcome until delivery. Delivery rates per transfer varied from 23.4% to 28.2%.

Assisted Hatching

It is generally accepted that human embryos generated by IVF have a low implantation potential: a 10% to 15% rate of implantation per embryo is routinely reported in the literature.[157] Some researchers have suggested that premature transfer of the human embryo into the uterus may account for these low implantation rates. Data on the transfer of human cavitating morulae or blastocysts on day 4 or day 5 of development indicate that such embryos have a higher implantation rate.[138,158] In the case of blastocysts, implantation rates that are twice those of cleavage-stage embryos have been reported.[139] However, many cleavage-stage embryos do not reach the blastocyst stage in in vitro culture conditions, and it is not clear how many of these embryos would have implanted had they been transferred at the cleavage stage.[159]

Consequently, a remaining challenge in assisted reproduction is to overcome the obstacle of low implantation rates. Several factors, apart from synchronization between the endometrium and replaced embryos, are responsible. On one hand, endometrial receptivity is a factor in successful embryo implantation[160]; on the other hand, two embryonic factors play a major role in the implantation process. First, implantation failure may result from developmental arrest due to aneuploidy observed in

TABLE 30-2

Sperm Origin and Outcome of Embryo Transfers after Intracytoplasmic Sperm Injection

			Testicular Sperm		
	Ejaculated Sperm	Epididymal Sperm	Fresh	Frozen-Thawed	Total
Cycles	2160	43	122	106	2431
Transfers	2040	41	114	98	2293
Transfer rate (%)	94.4	95.3	93.4	92.5	94.3
Embryos transferred					
Mean ± standard deviation	2.4 ± 0.9	2.1 ± 0.5	2.4 ± 0.8	2.4 ± 0.8	2.4 ± 0.8
Range	(1-8)	(1-3)	(1-5)	(1-4)	(1-8)
Pregnancies	708	14	36	35	793
Transfers (known human chorionic gonadotropin outcome)*	2030	40	111	98	2279
Pregnancy rate per transfer*	34.9	35	32.4	35.7	34.8
Pregnancy rate per cycle*	32.9	33	30.3	33	32.8
Implantation rate (%)†	15	21.4	14	15.1	15.1
Delivery rate per transfer‡	23.8	28.2	23.4	25.3	24.2

*With known human chorionic gonadotropin.outcome.
†Number of fetal heartbeats (at seven weeks) as a percentage of the number of embryos replaced.
‡With known outcome until delivery.

human preimplantation embryos.[161,162] PGD-AS programs, especially in older patients, have been proposed and are undertaken to address this issue (described in more detail later). Second, to implant, the preimplantation embryo must escape from its zona pellucida by means of a process called *hatching*. The zona pellucida containing the preimplantation embryo acts as a protective shell-like structure. Developing embryos show a gradual thinning of the zona pellucida during culture. The mammalian late blastocyst both expands and thins its zona pellucida through alternating expansion and contraction.[163] Intrinsic processes allowing this thinning before successful hatching include pressure of the blastocyst as it expands against the zona and a lytic mechanism mediated by zona lysins.[164-166] Finally, the zona pellucida ruptures, allowing the embryo to hatch and implant itself into the endometrium.

Many embryos may not succeed in hatching from the zona for different reasons. A naturally thick zona pellucida or hardening of the zona pellucida due to prolonged (suboptimal) in vitro culture conditions may interfere with (and prevent) the natural hatching process,[7] leading to implantation failure. Suboptimal culture conditions may cause trophectoderm lysin production to fall below the threshold level needed to promote zona thinning before successful hatching and subsequent implantation.[166] Alternatively, intrinsic lysin production failure unrelated to culture conditions may inhibit normal hatching.[166]

To overcome hatching failure, three different micromanipulation procedures—mechanical, chemical, and more recently, laser-induced hatching—have been used to produce holes in the zona pellucida of cleavage-stage embryos or to thin the zona pellucida superficially. Partial zona dissection[5] allows mechanical incision of the zona. The zona pellucida is pierced twice with a microneedle, leaving a small part of the zona trapped against the microneedle. Rubbing this part of the zona against a holding pipette leaves a narrow incision in the zona.

Chemical-assisted hatching involves the use of acidic Tyrode's solution (pH 2.35) to "drill" the zona pellucida.[8] A microneedle filled with acidic Tyrode's solution is used to produce an opening at the 3 o'clock position, facing either empty perivitelline space or extracellular anucleate fragments. The acidic solution is expelled gently over a small area (30 μm), with the tip of the needle held very close to the zona until an opening is obtained. The mean diameter of the gap thus created is 20 ± 6.7 μm (range, 10-36 μm). It should be noted that the acidic Tyrode's solution is embryotoxic and may alter the viability of the embryos.

Chemical-assisted hatching may be carried out with extracellular fragment removal.[167,168] However, the real benefit of this procedure must be shown in controlled randomized studies, which are lacking. Cruciate thinning of the zona pellucida using acidic Tyrode's solution has been described, but chemical removal of the outside of the zona pellucida of day 3 human embryos has no effect on the implantation rate,[169] whereas the creation of a hole in the zona pellucida does increase embryo implantation.[8] The limiting factor for successful hatching is, therefore, not the overall thickness, but the resilience of the thin inner layer of the double-layered human zona pellucida.[169]

Occasionally, complete removal of the zona pellucida from cleavage-stage embryos is performed.[170]

More recently, laser-assisted zona pellucida drilling has been introduced and has been shown to be a suitable alternative to the use of acidic Tyrode's solution for zona drilling.[171,172] Several types of laser sources have been investigated. In a most convenient setup, the laser beam is guided through an optical lens and focused on the biologic specimen. There is no need for holding and cutting tools. Lasers with different wavelengths have been proposed to operate in this nontouch mode; however, infrared radiation is the most appropriate, especially when mutagenic risks are taken into account. The 1.48-μm diode laser allows rapid, precise, and easily controlled lysis of the zona pellucida.[173-176] The hole size can be chosen by varying the irradiation time; typically, a hole with a diameter of 20 μm is produced within 12 to 30 msec irradiation time. Larger hole diameters are obtained by increasing the irradiation time.

Piezo technology, an alternative to laser technology, also produces a precise and controllable defect in the zona, without chemicals that are potentially embryotoxic.[177] The vibration produced by the piezoelectric pulse is used for the assisted hatching. The zona pellucida is carved easily in a limited area that is conical and approximately 30 μm in diameter. Five to eight applications in adjacent areas are needed to treat approximately one third of the visible circumference of the zona pellucida. Thereafter, weaker vibrations are used to create a hole 20 μm in diameter in the thinned zona at the junction between blastomeres.

Assisted hatching techniques, designed to facilitate embryo escape from the zona pellucida, have been used in IVF centers since 1992. The initial indications for assisted hatching were patient age, zona pellucida thickness, high basal FSH value, and repeated IVF failure. Several retrospective and prospective studies assessing assisted hatching in these cases have given disparate results. Therefore, the clinical relevance of assisted hatching in cleavage-stage embryos within an assisted reproduction program is debated. Some of the controversy may be due to the different methods used for assisted hatching and, consequently, the irreproducibility of the hole sizes obtained. Patient selection may also be an important origin of conflicting findings. Moreover, many studies are uncontrolled and retrospective. In summarizing the existing randomized studies, several conclusions can be drawn.

Assisted hatching might be beneficial in women with a poor prognosis for IVF or ICSI, particularly those with repeated implantation failure.[170,178-180] However, there is no further evidence of an age-related benefit of assisted hatching in patients with advanced maternal age.[181,182] In an unselected population of patients, assisted hatching did not increase pregnancy and implantation rates.[183-186] A recent meta-analysis that included randomized controlled trials of assisted hatching versus no assisted hatching and reported live births, clinical pregnancies, or implantation rates, concluded that insufficient evidence exists to recommend assisted hatching.[187]

Recently, there has been tremendous interest in improving the results of assisted reproduction through transfer of blastocysts after extended culture. Although human blastocysts expand readily in vitro, most blastocysts have hatching problems or cannot completely hatch out of the zona pellucida, and subsequently degenerate by day 6 or day 7. If the zona pellucida is softened enzymatically and zona-free blastocysts can be replaced, better cell–cell interactions and anchoring of the embryo to the endometrium may be expected, hopefully with improved implantation rates, reduced embryonic losses, and fewer embryos replaced.[188] Before transfer, blastocysts are exposed to pronase (10 IU at 37°C) for no longer than 90 seconds, which is the optimal time for softening or complete removal of the zona.[189]

The safety of this procedure was evaluated by light microscopy and transmission electron microscopy, showing that the human embryonic trophectoderm is a very hardy, robust epithelium that withstands pronase treatment.[189] Initial reports are promising, in that improved pregnancy and implantation results were shown with zona-free blastocyst transfers.[188,190-192] In the first randomized controlled study,[193] no statistically significant differences were found in clinical pregnancy, ongoing pregnancy, and implantation rates between zona-intact, blastocyst-stage transfers and zona-manipulated (enzymatic treatment), blastocyst-stage transfers. However, further studies with larger groups of patients are needed to clarify the real effect of this zona manipulation on pregnancy outcome. Whether a possible benefit may be differential for good-quality or poor-quality blastocysts, as reported by Urman et al.,[194] also must be confirmed.

Embryo Biopsy

THEORETICAL BACKGROUND

Genetic analysis of preimplantation developmental stages before transfer into the uterus inevitably involves removal of some cellular material at one of these stages. Theoretically, cells can be removed for diagnosis at any stage between the two-cell stage and the blastocyst stage. Even earlier, polar bodies can be removed from the oocyte (first polar body, preconceptionally, before injection of the oocyte; second polar body, from the zygote stage, after insemination and fertilization). Both polar bodies represent extraembryonic material and are expected to have no biologic role in the development of the future embryo. However, a major limitation of polar body analysis is that only the maternal genetic contribution to the future embryo can be evaluated. When the paternal contribution must be evaluated, biopsy at preimplantation developmental stages is therefore inevitable.

It seems essential to determine the developmental stage, to allow maximum retrieval of cells at biopsy with minimum reduction in the pregnancy potential of the embryos after the procedure. In humans, the best time for embryo biopsy would be the eight-cell stage, which is normally on the morning of day 3. At this stage, all of the cells are still totipotent (as confirmed by lineage tracing[195]) and the embryos are not yet compacting. It is believed that allocation to the two lineages of the blastocyst is initiated in the early eight-cell stage. Cells then become polarized at both the membrane and cytoplasmic levels.

It appears that removal of cells after the initiation of polarization does not compromise allocation to the inner cell mass.[196] However, cellular totipotency wanes with further embryonic development and may not be an all-or-none property (i.e., sister blastomeres could express it to different degrees).[197] Blastomeres of cleaving mammalian embryos can replace the loss of one or two blastomeres; this property presumably lasts, whereas blastomeres are allocated to, but not committed to, specific pathways. Apart from the reduction in cellular mass, the development of human embryos to the blastocyst stage in vitro is unaffected by biopsy and removal of one or two cells at the eight-cell stage.[198] This means that up to one fourth of the embryo can be removed without impairment of its further in vitro development. Similar results were obtained in a mouse model.[199]

When Handyside et al.[12] reported the first pregnancies from the clinical application of PGD, it became clear that in vivo development was not impaired by the biopsy procedure either. In 1994, 32 pregnancies worldwide were reported after all types of preimplantation diagnosis using cleavage-stage biopsy, with 29 infants born and no evidence of adverse effects on development.[200] Moreover, it became clear that pregnancy rates after PGD were comparable to those obtained after standard IVF.[201,202] Despite the reassuring clinical results so far, however, the discussion remains as to whether the removal of two cells from a seven-cell–stage embryo (or larger) reduces its capacity to implant more than if only one cell were removed.[203] A recent randomized controlled trial showed that removal of two blastomeres significantly decreases the likelihood of blastocyst formation compared with removal of one blastomere, although this did not translate into a significant difference in implantation rate (23.5% versus 17.3% for one-cell and two-cell biopsy, respectively, $P = 0.216$).[204] Taking live births per started cycle as an end point of this study (including 592 biopsy cycles), no significant difference was obtained between one-cell (20.2%) and two-cell biopsy (17.2%, $P = 0.358$). The recommendation is the removal of only one blastomere, provided that diagnostic safety measures are in place to ensure a correct diagnosis on one cell. If these are not available, two cells are needed for diagnosis.

The advantage of biopsy at later developmental stages, such as the morula or blastocyst stage, is that relatively more cells can be collected than with biopsy at earlier developmental stages. However, the morula stage is an inappropriate stage for embryo biopsy because of extensive compaction, which occurs at the 16-cell to 32-cell stage in human embryos.[136] The blastocyst stage, on the other hand, offers the advantage that extraembryonic trophectoderm cells can be removed, leaving the inner cell mass (representing the future fetus) fully intact. A major limitation of PGD at the blastocyst stage is our lack of knowledge of whether the trophectoderm cells are representative of the embryo proper. The degree of blastocyst mosaicism seems lower than in cleavage-stage embryos[205,206]; however, no evidence exists to support the hypothesis of a preferential allocation of euploid cells to the inner cell mass and aneuploid cells to the trophectoderm.[205,207] No single study has compared the genetic constitution of the

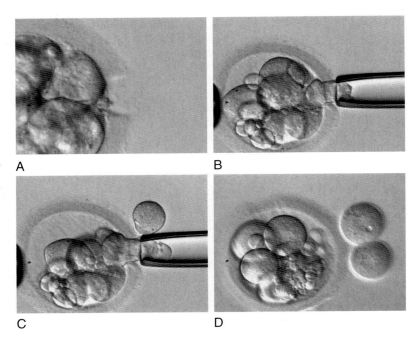

Figure 30-5. *Cleavage-stage embryo biopsy.* **A,** *Laser-assisted zona drilling results in an opening in the zona pellucida with an average size of 20 to 30 μm.* **B,** *A biopsy pipette is introduced through the hole and a first blastomere is aspirated.* **C,** *Aspiration of a second blastomere can be done in a similar way.* **D,** *Preferentially, blastomeres with a clearly visible nucleus are aspirated.*

trophectoderm and that of the inner cell mass of single human blastocysts, which could finally help to clarify the uncertainty about the representation of a trophectoderm cell sample. Another disadvantage of blastocyst biopsy is the time limitation to obtain the diagnostic result if a fresh transfer is attempted.

EMBRYO BIOPSY PROCEDURES

According to the developmental stage, three different biopsy procedures are well established: polar body removal from oocytes and zygotes, cleavage-stage embryo biopsy, and biopsy at the blastocyst stage (reviewed in De Vos and Van Steirteghem[208]). The biopsy procedure always involves two steps: opening of the zona pellucida and removal of the cellular material. Opening of the zona pellucida can be done in three ways:

1. Mechanically by direct puncture,[209] conventional PZD,[11,210] or three-dimensional PZD[211]
2. Chemically, using acidic Tyrode's solution[212]
3. Recently introduced laser technology[173,174,213]

Polar body removal has, so far, been exclusively linked with mechanical opening of the zona pellucida.[209] Cleavage-stage biopsy mainly involves the use of acidic Tyrode's solution or drilling or laser opening of the zona pellucida[16]; for blastocyst biopsy, both mechanical PZD[214] and laser drilling[215] have been described. Removal of polar bodies and biopsy of blastomeres is performed mainly by aspiration.[209] Extraembryonic trophectoderm cells are often removed by needle dissection at the moment of herniation through the slit created in the zona pellucida.[214,215] Animal models have been used to evaluate the efficacy and safety of most, if not all, of these procedures. Experimental work with human embryos donated for research has

confirmed the feasibility and efficacy of the procedures; however, safety evaluation has been limited to in vitro development.

As indicated by Handyside et al.,[216] cleavage-stage biopsy remains the main approach to the removal of genomic DNA for genetic analysis at preimplantation stages. Cleavage-stage biopsy is performed in the morning of day 3 after oocyte retrieval (Fig. 30-5). Unfortunately, not all human embryos reach the seven-cell or eight-cell stage by that time. Six-cell–stage embryos may, therefore, be included for one- or two-cell removal, although they are suspected of being of inferior quality because of delayed cleavage.[217] Embryos for PGD are ideally obtained by microinjection of a single sperm cell to avoid contamination with naked sperm DNA.

At the moment of oocyte denudation, care is taken to remove all of the remaining cumulus and corona cells, which can also represent a source of DNA contamination. Chemical zona drilling, followed by blastomere aspiration, is normally done with separate pipettes, using a double-holder setup: one drilling pipette with an inner diameter of approximately 5 to 7 μm and one aspiration or biopsy pipette with an inner diameter of 35 to 40 μm. The target site for drilling is chosen between two blastomeres or in front of anucleate fragments to minimize the deleterious effect of the acidic medium on the cells. Zona drilling for embryo biopsy[212] is not different from the zona drilling technique described earlier for assisted hatching.[8]

Chemical zona drilling is in itself an extremely simple procedure in terms of equipment, but some technical skill may be required when exposing the embryo to an acidified solution. The opening should be of appropriate size, while limiting the extent and duration of exposure of the embryo. The mean diameter of the gap thus created is approximately 20 μm (range, 10-36 μm).[8] The rate of dissolution of the zona may vary, and the time taken to complete this process varies accordingly (30 seconds to 2 minutes). Acidic drilling, despite its toxicity and cytoplasmic acidification, is considered safe on the basis of the pregnancies and births reported in the literature.[16]

As an alternative to chemical zona opening, laser-assisted zona pellucida drilling has been introduced for cleavage-stage biopsy[213] (which is similar to the laser drilling technique previously described for assisted hatching). Using the X-Y microscope stage, the embryo is positioned to place a region of the zona pellucida on the aiming spot. Typically, a trench-like hole with a diameter of 5 to 10 μm is produced in 10 to 15 msec.[174] For embryo biopsy, on average, two to three pulses of 7 msec are applied, resulting in 20- to 30-μm openings. It is important to perforate the zona completely without harming the embryonic cells with the laser. The holes obtained with a laser are more precise than the ones obtained with acidic Tyrode's solution. Laser zona opening results in more intact blastomeres compared with the use of acidic Tyrode's solution, and because similar pregnancy rates were obtained, it seems advantageous to use a laser for zona drilling.[218]

Blastomere removal involves the introduction of the biopsy pipette into the perivitelline space through the hole in the zona, allowing one or two blastomeres to be removed by gentle aspiration. Cells can be aspirated completely and then removed; alternatively, cells are only partially aspirated and pulled out (given full decompaction and thus no adherence to other blastomeres). Whereas full compaction does not occur before the 16- to 32-cell stage,[136] relatively early assembly of tight junctions occurs between human blastomeres, as shown by ultrastructural studies.[219,220] Because of these membrane adhesions, the biopsy procedure at the seven-cell to eight-cell stage may be difficult to perform because the blastomeres show a strong tendency to adhere to each other. Manipulating the embryos as such may result in a high lysis rate of cells.

A calcium- and magnesium-free medium has been used to loosen the membrane adhesions between blastomeres,[221,222] which allows easier removal of cells and results in less lysis. Embryo biopsy can be performed completely in this medium or, to limit exposure time, embryos can be preincubated for 5 to 10 minutes (normally sufficient for full decompaction) before biopsy in calcium- and magnesium-containing medium. Whether the implantation rate or postimplantation development is affected by the use of calcium- and magnesium-free medium for biopsy remains to be assessed. Therefore, the long-term safety of its clinical application should be further substantiated.

Biopsy of the first and second polar bodies has been successfully used to screen for maternal mutations in cases of several single-gene defects.[223-226] However, the method appeared to be of particular relevance to patients who undergo IVF because of advanced maternal age, and the reduced pregnancy rates may be due to the increased incidence of age-related aneuploidies.[227-229] In addition to numeric chromosome anomalies, analysis of the first polar body can be used to analyze the meiotic segregation of maternal structural abnormalities.[230-233] A beveled pipette is used for mechanical perforation of the zona pellucida, and once inside the perivitelline space, the first and second polar bodies can be drawn out simultaneously by aspiration into the pipette.[223]

Polar body analysis is an indirect method in which the genotype or chromosomal constitution of the oocyte is derived from the complement present in the polar bodies. Both first and second maternal meiotic errors can be excluded only if information on the two polar bodies is obtained.[234] Currently, this can be expected for approximately 70% of oocytes.[229] For single-gene disorders, occasional recombination of homologous chromosomes also requires information on both polar bodies. Today, great accuracy in PGD of single-gene disorders is achieved by application of sequential analysis of the first and second polar bodies in combination with multiplex PCR to detect possible allele dropout and contamination.[235,236]

The clinical application of biopsy at the blastocyst stage in view of PGD is still limited.[16] However, two recent studies report promising clinical results with trophectoderm biopsy.[237,238] The technique of zona slitting (similar to partial zona dissection) can be used to open the zona pellucida with a microneedle,[214] although laser zona opening in the blastocyst stage has been described by Veiga et al.[215] Care is taken to avoid touching the trophectoderm cells, and the slit or opening is made opposite the inner cell mass. After definite herniation, trophectoderm cell removal is performed by excision using a glass needle[214,239] or laser energy.[215] Serial biopsy specimens can even be taken from the same blastocyst[240,241] to maximize the number of cells available for PCR or FISH analysis.

FISH AND PCR PROCEDURES

Two major methods are currently used for diagnostic purposes in PGD: FISH and PCR. FISH allows the visualization of chromosomal regions and is used in sexing and PGD-AS and in PGD for translocations. PCR, which allows the exponential amplification of a short DNA fragment, is widely used for diagnosis in monogenic diseases (see Chapter 31).[242]

In FISH, fluorochrome-labeled DNA probes are used that are complementary to DNA sequences specific to individual chromosomes. Simultaneous analysis of several chromosomes is possible, even in interphase cells.[243-245] Polar bodies or blastomeres obtained for biopsy are spread on a glass slide and fixed.[244-246] The labeled probes are added and allowed to hybridize to the chromosomes. Excess probe is removed, and the result can be analyzed using fluorescence microscopy with different filters for different fluorochromes.

At least one FISH probe is now available for every chromosome, although the limited number of fluorochromes available restricts the number of probes that can be simultaneously applied to a single interphase nucleus. Additionally, misdiagnosis due to overlapping signals would become a problem. Commercially available kits containing five chromosome-specific probes are often used in a first round; after probe removal, a second round of hybridization for even more chromosomes can be performed.[245] With this expansion of probe sets, sexing of early human embryos[247] could soon be combined with PGD-AS.[248,249]

For robertsonian translocations (in which a whole chromosome is translocated), simple enumeration of the chromosomes leads to a reliable diagnosis,[250,251] but the situation is more complex for reciprocal translocations (exchange of fragments between chromosomes). A generally adopted practice is the simultaneous use of two differentially labeled subtelomeric probes distal to the breakpoint (one for each chromosome), together with a centromeric probe (to one of the chromosomes involved). This strategy allows for the distinction between normal, balanced genotypes and unbalanced genotypes.[252]

The obvious limitation of FISH is that a restricted number of chromosomes can be tested in a single cell. Aneuploidies at the level of chromosomes that have not been analyzed—undoubtedly existing—are overlooked.[253] If more chromosomes could be analyzed, the value of PGD-AS could likely be increased. Ideally, it would be possible to identify every chromosome in single blastomeres for PGD. The most successful technique for complete karyotyping of single cells is comparative genomic hybridization (CGH).[254] Differentially labeled test DNA (green) and normal reference DNA (red), obtained by whole-genome amplification, are hybridized simultaneously to normal metaphase chromosomes. The relative green-to-red ratio for each chromosome is measured using a cooled charge-coupled device camera and image analysis. Deviations from a 1:1 ratio (which in itself lights up as yellow) are indicative of loss (red) or gain (green) of chromosomal material in the tested cell. The obvious advantage of CGH over FISH is that the copy number of all chromosomes can be determined. In addition, CGH provides a more detailed picture of the entire length of each chromosome. Although FISH is routinely used to determine the ploidy of particular chromosomes, all that it really shows is that the target sequence of the probe (often located in the centromere) is present. It does not provide information about the rest of the chromosome. CGH has been successfully applied to single cells[255,256] and interphase blastomeres.[257,258] The early clinical applications[259-261] in view of aneuploidy testing are promising, and CGH seems to hold promise for translocation carriers as well.[262] However, further technical modification will be required before CGH can be offered to a larger population of infertile patients. CGH is a relatively labor-intensive procedure, and it takes several days to obtain a result. This is longer than 3-day-old embryos can be maintained in culture, and so embryos undergoing biopsy must be frozen until results become available. The necessity to cryopreserve embryos undergoing biopsy while CGH results are obtained is not ideal, and there is probably a loss of implantation potential.

The use of metaphase CGH to screen all human chromosomes for aneuploidy in preimplantation embryos is hindered by the time required to perform the analysis. Microarray CGH could alleviate this time constraint.[263,264] These microarrays are made up of DNA sequences specific to human chromosomes spotted onto a glass slide. The principle is the same as metaphase chromosome CGH in that differentially labeled reference DNA and test DNA are hybridized to the slide and differences in the fluorescence ratio are indicative of changes in DNA copy number. Array CGH takes less time, primarily because less than 24 hours is required for hybridization. The benefit of complete karyotyping for PGD is that all CGH studies on blastomeres have

identified chromosome errors that would not have been detected if the cells had been analyzed by FISH; however, the procedure remains technically challenging.[254]

The PCR procedure involves exponential amplification of short DNA fragments using two short, single-stranded DNA pieces (primers) that are complementary to the boundaries of the sequence to be amplified. A standard PCR protocol involves 20 to 45 cycles of repeated denaturation (of the double-stranded template DNA) at high temperature, annealing (of the primers to the template DNA) at a lower temperature, and elongation using Taq DNA polymerase. PCR allows analysis of the genetic content of a single cell.[265] In PGD, DNA amplification is used to detect single-gene defects (so-called *monogenic diseases*).

However, PCR protocols are subject to a variety of pitfalls, such as variable amplification efficiency, contamination, and allele dropout.[266] Fluorescent single-cell PCR has not only a higher sensitivity, but also a higher resolution.[14,267] Different measures are taken to avoid—or at least detect—contamination from genomic DNA (patient or operator) or carry-over contamination (from PCR products amplified earlier).[242] To show contaminating DNA, an increasing number of PCR-based tests now include amplification of hypervariable fragments of DNA in addition to the loci used for diagnosis. These hypervariable polymorphisms are essentially the same as those used for DNA fingerprinting. The presence of more than the expected two alleles indicates contamination (either from an external source or from parental origin). Contamination with parental DNA can occur as a result of inadvertent sampling of a sperm or cumulus cell at the time of embryo biopsy. The management of amplification failure and allele dropout (i.e., nonamplification of one of the two alleles in a single cell) is of extreme importance because it may result in misdiagnosis. Multiplex PCR with linked markers, with or without fluorescent detection,[235,268] is a straightforward strategy. Today, multiplex PCR (i.e., simultaneous amplification of two or more DNA sequences) is used extensively in PGD, especially for more frequently occurring diseases.[269,270] Usually, attempts are made to combine a specific mutation with ideally linked markers or otherwise unlinked markers.[235,270] Allowing simultaneous testing of linked markers alongside the mutation test significantly increases the accuracy of single-cell PCR.[271,272]

The more recent advent of highly effective whole-genome amplification methods, generating abundant assay-ready DNA from single cells for diagnosis of any known single-gene defect, marks a new era for preimplantation genetic testing.[273] The ideal whole-genome amplification technique should have high yield, faithful representation of the original template, and complete coverage of the genome.[274] The use of whole-genome amplification as a universal first step allows subsequent simultaneous analysis of more than one mutation by standard PCR protocols[275-277] or microarrays.[278] The inclusion of several polymorphic markers allows haplotype analysis.[279,280] Preimplantation genetic haplotyping definitely widens the scope and availability of preimplantation testing because one panel of markers can be used for all carriers of the same monogenic disease, bypassing the need for the development of mutation-specific tests.[280]

INDICATIONS FOR PREIMPLANTATION GENETIC DIAGNOSIS

The PGD procedure is a very early form of prenatal diagnosis for patients with a preexisting genetic risk. Oocytes or embryos obtained in vitro through assisted reproductive techniques, in particular, ICSI, undergo biopsy and the cells obtained (polar bodies, blastomeres, or trophectoderm cells) are used for genetic diagnosis. In principle, the indications for PGD are similar to those for prenatal diagnosis after chorionic villus sampling or amniocentesis, given that PGD at the single-cell level is technically possible. The main reasons for PGD (in addition to the genetic risk) are previous termination of pregnancy and objection to pregnancy termination. The genetic risk can also be combined with subfertility or infertility.

The PGD-FISH procedure is performed for couples at risk for chromosomal disorders, which can be divided into two groups: structural and numeric abnormalities. Structural aberrations involve reciprocal translocations, robertsonian translocations, inversions, deletions, and microdeletions. PGD-AS is performed for multiple reasons (discussed later). Patients with Klinefelter syndrome can benefit from PGD-FISH because the normal sex chromosome content of the embryos is determined before transfer.

A main disadvantage of sexing for X-linked disease is that half of the male embryos are healthy and will not be transferred, and the transfer of female carrier embryos cannot be avoided. Given that the mutation is known or can be analyzed through linked markers, couples may opt for a specific DNA diagnosis rather than simple sexing. For PGD-FISH, feasibility testing involves a search for the appropriate probes, which are then tested on lymphocytes of the couple.

The PGD-PCR procedure is used for couples at risk for monogenic disorders. Three disease groups can be distinguished according to the mode of inheritance: X-linked disorders (e.g., Duchenne and Becker muscular dystrophy, fragile X syndrome, hemophilia); autosomal recessive disorders (e.g., cystic fibrosis, thalassemia, spinal muscular atrophy, sickle cell anaemia); and autosomal dominant disorders (e.g., myotonic dystrophy, Huntington disease, Charcot-Marie-Tooth disease, Marfan syndrome).[16] Several laboratories offer patients custom-made PGD tests for monogenic disease, so the exact number of indications for which PGD is offered would be difficult to establish. A prerequisite for PGD-PCR is that the mutation is known or otherwise can be analyzed through linked markers. Appropriate primer sets are designed and tested on genomic DNA of the couple and family members. Lymphoblasts of the couple or an affected child allow determination of the amplification efficiency as well as the contamination and allele dropout rate for each PCR protocol.

More recently, combined PGD and human leukocyte antigen (HLA) matching has been reported,[281] representing a novel way to preselect an unaffected potential donor for an affected sibling requiring stem cell transplantation. Transplantation of hematopoietic stem cells from an HLA-identical sibling donor may be the best treatment option for children with neoplastic and congenital diseases affecting hematopoiesis, such as Fanconi anemia,[282] leukemia,

Wiskott-Aldrich syndrome, and β-thalassemia. Cord blood collected at birth is an established source of hematopoietic stem cells. In contrast to individual establishment of protocols for each requesting couple, indirect HLA typing using markers evenly distributed in the HLA polymorphic region is a more elegant and time-saving approach.[283]

PREIMPLANTATION GENETIC SCREENING

In PGD-AS, embryos are screened for chromosomal abnormalities in patients with impaired fertility—patients of advanced maternal age, patients with several failed IVF cycles (i.e., recurrent implantation failure), patients with recurrent miscarriages, or male patients with nonobstructive azoospermia. Selecting chromosomally normal embryos for replacement should increase implantation rates, reduce spontaneous miscarriage rates, reduce aneuploid conceptions, and improve delivery rates in assisted reproductive technology cycles.[17,18,283,284] The number of referrals for PGD-AS has only increased since its first clinical application,[285] as evidenced by the European Society of Human Reproduction and Embryology PGD Consortium data collection,[16] but the benefit of PGD-AS is still under debate.[16] It should be emphasized that there is a need for large randomized controlled trials to investigate the effectiveness of PGS for well-defined indications. Currently, there are insufficient data that determine whether PGS is an effective intervention in IVF/ICSI for improving live birth rates.[286-288] Until such trials are performed, PGS should not be used in routine patient care.[287]

CLINICAL APPLICATION AND RESULTS

Our experience with more than 5 years of clinical PGD has been reported previously.[202] In total, 183 PGD cycles (performed between February 1993 and October 1998) were summarized: specific diagnosis was carried out by PCR ($n = 108$), and FISH was used for sexing ($n = 64$) and determination of structural aberrations ($n = 11$). The ongoing pregnancy rate was 16.4% per cycle and 19.9% per transfer.

Here we present the results of 2 years of clinical PGD practice (2000 and 2001), involving 472 PGD cycles (Tables 30-3 and 30-4). Of the 472 cycles, 214 were PGD *stricto sensu* cycles (143 with PCR for monogenic diseases and 71 with FISH for sexing and structural aberrations), whereas 258 were PGD-AS cycles. Within the group of monogenic diseases, 84 were autosomal dominant (mainly Charcot-Marie-Tooth disease, Huntington disease, and myotonic dystrophy), 34 were autosomal recessive (mainly cystic fibrosis and spinal muscular atrophy), and 25 were X-linked (mainly fragile X syndrome and Duchenne muscular dystrophy). FISH was performed for sex chromosome aberrations ($n = 21$), for autosomal structural aberrations ($n = 22$), and for sexing for X-linked diseases ($n = 28$). Additionally, FISH was used for 258 PGD-AS cycles, in which the indications were advanced maternal age ($n = 156$), recurrent abortions or repeated IVF failure ($n = 78$), and nonobstructive azoospermia ($n = 24$).

In total, 5627 cumulus–oocyte complexes were retrieved (i.e., a mean of 11.9 per started cycle), with little

TABLE 30-3

Results of Two Years of Preimplantation Genetic Diagnosis Practice: Oocyte Damage, Pronuclear Status, and Embryo Development

	Monogenic Diseases	Sexing and Structural Aneuploidy	PGD Aneuploidy Screening	Total
PGD cycles	143	71	258	472
Oocytes undergoing ICSI	1483	731	2625	4839
Intact oocytes (%)	91.8	91	92.7	92.1
Injected oocytes (%) with:				
One pronucleus	3.6	5.6	5.3	4.8
Two pronuclei	77.1	73.1	75	75.4
Three or more pronuclei	3.4	3.7	4	3.8
Two-pronuclear oocytes	1143	534	1970	3647
Embryonic development (day 3)				
Excellent embryos (%)	13.6	11.2	12.5	12.7
Good-quality embryos (%)	57.6	59.2	60.8	59.5
Fair-quality embryos (%)	12.7	15.2	14.3	13.9
Eight-cell embryos or larger (%)*	32.2	45.5	38.4	37.5
Cycles with biopsy	129	66	244	439
Embryos subjected to biopsy	677	409	1523	2609
Blastomeres removed	1396	808	2971	5175
Blastomere lysis rate (%)	3.9	2.7	3.4	3.4
Postbiopsy development (day 5)†				
Early blastocysts (% of those undergoing biopsy)	17.9	23.9	20.3	20.3
EGQ blastocysts (% of those undergoing biopsy)	21.9	19.2	15	16.6

*Including compacting and compact embryos.
†Only in 342 cycles where day 5 evaluation of the embryos undergoing biopsy was available.
EGQ, expanded good quality, ICSI; intracytoplasmic sperm injection; PGD, preimplantation genetic diagnosis.

variance for the three groups (PCR, FISH, or PGD-AS). The distribution of oocyte maturity was not different from that of the overall population treated with ICSI (i.e., 96.2% of the cumulus–oocyte complexes containing an intact oocyte, of which 89.5% were metaphase II oocytes). In five cycles, no ICSI was performed. In two cycles (planned for PCR), no cumulus–oocyte complexes were retrieved. Another two cycles (one PCR cycle and one PGD-AS cycle) remained without mature oocytes, and in one cycle, no

spermatozoa were found in the testicular biopsy specimen of a patient with Klinefelter syndrome.

The ICSI procedure was performed on 4839 mature metaphase II oocytes (i.e., 10.3 per started cycle, similar for the three groups). An oocyte survival rate of 92.1% was obtained and did not differ for the three groups. Normal fertilization was obtained in 81.8% of the intact oocytes and 75.4% of the injected oocytes. Normal fertilization rates were highest in the PCR group (77.1% of the

TABLE 30-4

Results of Two Years of PGD Practice: Outcome of Embryo Transfers after PGD

	Monogenic Diseases	Sexing and Structural Aneuploidy	PGD Aneuploidy Screening	Total
PGD cycles with transfer	106	57	189	352
Transfer rate per started cycle (%)	74.1	80.3	73.3	74.6
Transfer rate per cycle with biopsy (%)	82.2	86.4	77.5	80.2
Embryos transferred				
Mean ± standard deviation	1.9 ± 0.7	1.9 ± 0.7	2.2 ± 1.1	2.1 ± 0.9
Range	(1-4)	(1-3)	(1-5)	(1-5)
Pregnancies	28	17	57	102
Pregnacy rate per transfer*	26.7	29.8	30.3	29.1
Pregnacy rate per cycle*	19.7	23.9	22.2	21.7
Implantation rate (%)†	13.7	18.9	12.5	13.7
Delivery rate per transfer*	21	17.5	20.7	20.3

*With known human chorionic gonadotropin outcome (two cycles remained with an unknown human chorionic gonadotropin outcome: one polymerase chain reaction, and one preimplantation genetic diagnosis aneuploidy screening cycle).
†Number of fetal heartbeats (at seven weeks) as a percentage of the number of embryos replaced.
PGD, preimplantaion genetic diagnosis.

injected oocytes) and lowest in the FISH group (73.1% of the injected oocytes). In the PGD-AS group, 75.0% of the injected oocytes were normally fertilized. Abnormal fertilization (1 PN or at least 3 PN) occurred in 4.8% and 3.8% of the injected oocytes, respectively. The 3-PN rate was similar for the three groups, and more 1-PN oocytes were observed in the PGD-AS group and FISH group (5.3% and 5.6%, respectively) than in the PCR group (3.6%).

The percentages of 2-PN oocytes developing into excellent, good-quality, and fair-quality embryos on day 3 were similar for the three groups and did not differ from those of the overall population undergoing ICSI (12.7%, 59.5%, and 13.9%, respectively). The percentage of eight-cell embryos on day 3 (including those with more than eight cells, those compacting, and compact embryos) was 38.4% in the PGD-AS group, 45.5% in the FISH group, and 32.2% in the PCR group (overall rate, 37.5%). The percentages of seven-cell embryos and six-cell embryos were 13.5% and 13.4%, respectively, and were not different for the three groups. Embryo biopsy on at least one embryo was possible in all but 28 of the 467 PGD cycles where ICSI was performed. In 10 cycles, no fertilization occurred (6 PGD-AS cycles and 4 PCR cycles); in 18 cycles (7 PGD-AS cycles, 4 FISH cycles, and 7 PCR cycles), embryo development was insufficient for embryo biopsy.

In total, 2609 embryos underwent biopsy: a mean of 5.6 embryos per PGD cycle when ICSI was performed (n = 467), or a mean of 5.9 embryos per PGD cycle with biopsy (n = 439). This latter number was higher in the PGD-AS group and the FISH group (6.2 in both groups) than in the PCR group (5.2). For the PGD-AS group, this elevation is related to the fact that sometimes only one cell was used for testing (occasionally from four-cell and five-cell embryos). In the FISH group, more eight-cell embryos were available than in the PCR group. As a percentage of 2-PN oocytes, the biopsy rates were 77.3%, 76.6%, and 59.2% in the PGD-AS group, the FISH group, and the PCR group, respectively (overall rate, 71.5%).

In total, 5175 blastomeres were removed from 2609 embryos (i.e., a mean of 1.98 cells per embryo obtained for biopsy). Care was taken to remove cells containing a single, clearly visible nucleus. The overall lysis rate was limited to 3.4% and was similar for the three groups. In cases of blastomere lysis (n = 177), only 85 extra cells were removed. No extra cell was removed when the nucleus of the lysed cell was still available for FISH analysis or when diagnosis or analysis was possible on one cell. In 78 blastomeres, no nucleus was found at fixation for FISH (i.e., 2.1%), for which one extra cell needed to be removed. The loss of blastomeres at transfer into PCR tubes was limited to 12 cells (i.e., only 0.9%).

Mainly embryos of at least eight cells, with or without compaction, underwent biopsy (55.6%). Seven-cell embryos (20.7%) and six-cell embryos (16.3%) were also included for biopsy. Four-cell and five-cell embryos (only 7.4%) were included only in FISH or PGD-AS cycles. In most cases, two cells were removed from embryos of six or more cells, whereas only one cell was removed from four-cell and five-cell embryos.

An important aspect of successful embryo biopsy is the critical evaluation of post-biopsy development. Further preimplantation development should not be impaired as a result of the biopsy procedure. In 342 PGD cycles with biopsy, day 5 evaluation of the embryos obtained for biopsy (n = 2093) was available. In total, 425 early blastocysts (20.3%) and 348 good-quality blastocysts (16.6%) were obtained. Taking into account that only 71.5% of the 2-PN zygotes yielded embryos that actually underwent biopsy, a total blastocyst formation rate (including both early and expanded blastocysts) of 26.4% can be calculated.

Transfer of at least one embryo was possible in 352 of the 472 started cycles (i.e., 74.6% per started cycle or 80.2% per cycle with biopsy). The transfer rate per cycle with biopsy was highest for the FISH group (86.4%) and lowest for the PGD-AS group (77.5%). The transfer rate per cycle with biopsy for the PCR group was 82.2%. No transfer was possible in 120 started cycles for the following reasons: 33 cycles did not reach the stage of embryo biopsy; in 63 cycles, no genetically normal embryos were available; and in 24 cycles, despite the presence of genetically normal embryos, post-biopsy development did not allow embryo transfer.

Mainly day 5 transfers were performed (n = 265). Eighty-four transfers occurred on day 4, and only occasionally, day 3 (n = 1) or day 6 transfers (n = 2) were performed. On average, 2.1 embryos (± 0.9; range, 1-5) were transferred per treatment cycle. In the PGD-AS group, more embryos were transferred (average, 2.2 ± 1.1). Similar numbers of embryos were transferred in the FISH group and the PCR group (1.9 ± 0.7). Two cycles remained with an unknown serum hCG outcome (one PCR cycle and one PGD-AS cycle). The outcome was known for all other transfer cycles (n = 350).

The overall pregnancy rate per transfer with known hCG outcome was 29.1%, with little difference among the three groups, varying from 26.7% (PCR group) to 30.3% (PGD-AS group). The pregnancy rate per transfer in the FISH group was 29.8%. The overall pregnancy rate per treatment cycle was 21.7%. The implantation rate (positive fetal heartbeat at 7 weeks) per number of embryos transferred was 13.7%. This percentage was highest in the FISH group (18.9%) and similar in the PGS-AS group (12.3%) and the PCR group (13.8%). All but six (three PGD-AS cycles and three PCR cycles) embryo transfers with positive serum hCG values resulted in a known outcome until delivery. The overall delivery rate per transfer was 20.3% and was similar for the three groups, varying from 17.5% to 21.0%.

ACKNOWLEDGMENTS: The authors thank the clinical, scientific, nursing, and technical staff of the Centers for Reproductive Medicine and Medical Genetics at the University Hospital, Brussels, Belgium. The work was supported by grants from the Fund for Scientific Research (Flanders).

The complete reference list can be found on the companion Expert Consult Web site at www.expertconsultbook.com.

Suggested Reading

Bartoov B, Berkovitz A, Eltes F. Selection of spermatozoa with normal nuclei to improve the pregnancy rate with intracytoplasmic sperm injection. N Engl J Med 345:1067, 2001.

Cohen Y, Malcov M, Schwartz T, et al. Spindle imaging: a new marker for optimal timing of ICSI? Hum Reprod 19:649, 2004.

Edwards RG, Beard HK. Oocyte polarity and cell determination in early mammalian embryos. Mol Hum Reprod 3:863, 1997.

Gerris J, De Neubourg D, Mangelschots K, et al. Elective single day 3 embryo transfer halves the twinning rate without decrease in the ongoing pregnancy rate of an IVF/ICSI programme. Hum Reprod 17:2626, 2002.

Handyside AH, Scriven PN, Ogilvie CM. The future of preimplantation genetic diagnosis. Hum Reprod 13(Suppl 4):249, 1998.

Hardarson T, Hanson C, Sjögren A, et al. Human embryos with unevenly sized blastomeres have lower pregnancy and implantation rates: indications for aneuploidy and multinucleation. Hum Reprod 16:313, 2001.

Joris H, Nagy Z, Van de Velde H, et al. Intracytoplasmic sperm injection: laboratory set-up and injection procedure. Hum Reprod 13(Suppl 1):76, 1998.

Los FJ, Van Opstal D, van den Berg C. The development of cytogenetically normal, abnormal and mosaic embryos: a theoretic model. Hum Reprod Update 10:79, 2004.

Twisk M, Mastenbroek S, van Wely M, et al. Preimplantation genetic screening for abnormal number of chromosomes (aneuploidies) in in vitro fertilisation or intracytoplasmic sperm injection. Cochrane Database Syst Rev CD005291, 2006.

Wilton L. Preimplantation genetic diagnosis and chromosome analysis of blastomeres using comparative genomic hybridization. Hum Reprod Update 11:33, 2005.

CHAPTER 31

Cytogenetics in Reproduction

Cynthia C. Morton and Charles Lee

Cytogenetics is the area of biology that deals with the study of chromosomes. Classic cytogenetics provides both an overview of the genome and the ability to identify chromosome rearrangements and numeric abnormalities. Molecular cytogenetics permits a finer examination of specific areas of the genome and has been a powerful tool in gene mapping. Application of molecular cytogenetic techniques, particularly fluorescence in situ hybridization (FISH) and array-based comparative genomic hybridization (array CGH), now makes possible routine diagnosis of microdeletion syndromes and cryptic chromosome rearrangements in the clinical laboratory. Furthermore, FISH provides a means to assess ploidy of any chromosome both in uncultured cells (largely for rapid diagnosis of trisomy) and in archival materials, which previously were not easily evaluated. The use of FISH with uncultured cells also allows assessment of a single blastomere, permitting genetic screening of preimplantation embryos in a procedure commonly termed *preimplantation genetic diagnosis* (see Chapter 30).

Cytogenetics is a critical component of reproductive endocrinology. Chromosome abnormalities are a common cause of infertility and pregnancy loss, as well as of sexual dysmorphology. Most chromosomally abnormal conceptions arise de novo after a meiotic nondisjunction event, but chromosomal anomalies in some conceptuses are inherited from a chromosomally abnormal parent. The chromosome abnormality in these conceptuses may or may not be identical to that of the parent, depending on recombination and segregation of chromosomes during gametogenesis. Although some chromosome aberrations cause overt phenotypic abnormalities, other aberrations have no apparent phenotypic effect. Carriers of these apparently phenotypically neutral chromosome aberrations may still produce chromosomally unbalanced gametes and, as such, may be identified after multiple pregnancy losses or the birth of an abnormal child.

Organization of Human Chromosomes and Methods of Study

The human chromosome is a complex structure that consists of deoxyribonucleic acid (DNA), ribonucleic acid (RNA), and protein. Each normal human chromosome has one *centromere*, the site at which the kinetochore forms, allowing for attachment of the mitotic spindle and proper segregation of the chromosome during cell division. The centromere also divides the chromosome into two arms that are identified as p (petit) for the short arm and q for the long arm. In human chromosomes, the position of the centromere can be central (metacentric), distal (acrocentric), or somewhere in between (submetacentric), providing a useful landmark in the identification of a particular chromosome. At the tip of the short arms of the acrocentric chromosomes (chromosomes 13, 14, 15, 21, and 22) are *satellites*, variably sized structures composed of heterochromatin. Satellites are attached to the chromosome through a secondary constriction known as a *satellite stalk*, which contains the genes for 18S, 5.8S, and 28S ribosomal RNA. At each end of every chromosome arm is a *telomere*, a structure composed of tandemly repeated, short nucleotide sequences (Fig. 31-1).

Human chromosomes vary in size, with the largest chromosome designated as chromosome 1. In 1956, Tjio and Levan[1] determined the total normal number of chromosomes in each human somatic cell to be 46, with 22 pairs of autosomes and 1 pair of sex chromosomes. For each chromosome pair, one chromosome is inherited from the father and one chromosome is inherited from the mother. With the exception of chromosome pairs 21 and 22, the numeric designation reflects the size of the chromosome (e.g., chromosome 4 is the fourth largest chromosome in the human complement). Although chromosome 21 is smaller than chromosome 22,

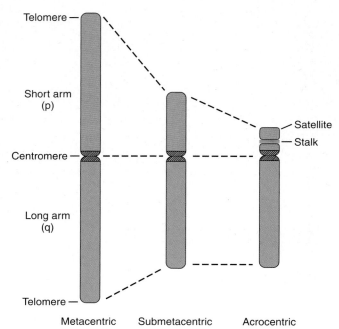

Telomere —

Short arm
(p)

Centromere —

Long arm
(q)

Telomere —

— Satellite
— Stalk

Metacentric   Submetacentric   Acrocentric

Figure 31-1. Schematic diagram of human metacentric, submetacentric, and acrocentric chromosomes. The locations of the telomere, centromere, short arm, and long arm are shown, as are the locations of the satellite and stalk on the acrocentric chromosome.

this inconsistency in nomenclature has been perpetuated to avoid confusion due to historical references to Down syndrome as trisomy 21.

A *karyotype* is a display of chromosomes in numeric order, with the chromosomes oriented such that the p arm is on top (Fig. 31-2). In humans, the female is the homogametic sex, with a normal female karyotype being designated as 46,XX. The male is the heterogametic sex,

with a normal male karyotype being described as 46,XY. Excluding chromosome abnormalities and variants, the karyotypes of two unrelated males or females may appear virtually identical. Furthermore, excluding sex chromosomes, karyotypes of males and females are usually microscopically indistinguishable. However, there are submicroscopic differences that will be discussed later.

METHODS IN CLASSIC CYTOGENETICS

Metaphase Preparations of Cultured Cells

Most cytogenetic analyses are performed on chromosomes that are in mitotic metaphase. The metaphase cell can show both numeric and structural chromosomal abnormalities. At this stage of the cell cycle, condensation of chromosomal DNA results in distinguishable entities (i.e., that can ultimately be visualized as specific patterns of alternating dark and light bands, characteristic for each species). To examine a particular chromosomal region at higher resolution, less condensed chromosomes (e.g., those found at prometaphase) may be useful.

The most frequently used tissues for cytogenetic evaluation, primarily because of their accessibility, are peripheral blood lymphocytes, amniotic fluid cells, chorionic villi, skin fibroblasts, bone marrow, lymph nodes, and solid tumors. The process of preparing chromosomes for analysis is known as a *harvest*. Chromosomes are harvested either after culture of the tissue or after direct harvest of mitotic cells, as in the cases of bone marrow, some solid tumors, cytotrophoblasts, and cord blood. The harvest itself may be performed in solution, as is commonly done for lymphocyte cultures and for other cultures in which attached cells have been released from the tissue culture vessel, or it may be performed in situ, that is, attached to the tissue culture surface. The in situ procedure is frequently used for amniotic

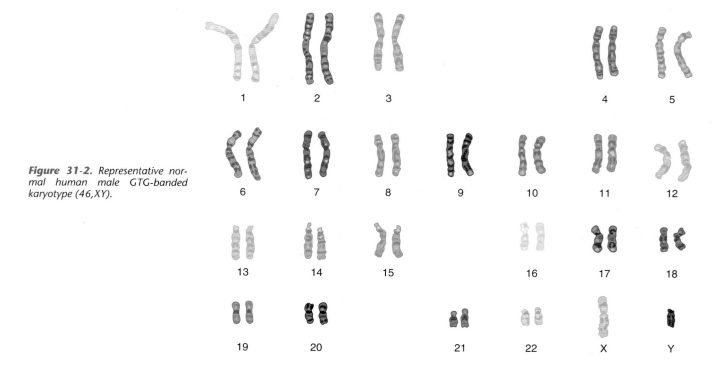

Figure 31-2. Representative normal human male GTG-banded karyotype (46,XY).

1   2   3   4   5

6   7   8   9   10   11   12

13   14   15   16   17   18

19   20   21   22   X   Y

fluid cultures when it is desirable to evaluate colonies of cells to ascertain possible chromosomal mosaicism.

In all cases, dividing cells must be arrested during mitosis. This is accomplished by the addition of colchicine (or colcemid), which destroys the mitotic spindle and thus arrests cells in metaphase. After incubation, the harvest continues with a hypotonic treatment that swells the cells. Several rounds of fixation (usually methanol/glacial acetic acid in a 3:1 ratio) complete the harvest. Metaphases will now be either dropped onto slides if they have been harvested in solution or spread on a coverslip or slide if they have been harvested in situ. Preparation of slides or coverslips after the harvest is one of the most crucial steps in obtaining quality material for analysis. Factors that influence surface tension, such as temperature and humidity, are doubtless critical variables in slide making.

Banding Techniques

Before the development of banding techniques, not all chromosomes could be distinguished, and they were grouped according to their size and centromere position. Today, several different banding techniques are used routinely in cytogenetics to allow the unequivocal identification of each chromosome. The most popular banding techniques are GTG- and reverse-banding (Fig. 31-3).

In the United States, GTG-banding, also known as *G-banding*, is the most commonly used method. This method of banding produces a pattern of alternating light and dark bands that allows identification of each chromosome pair by bright-field microscopy. Investigations of chromosome banding patterns with antinucleotide antibodies indicate that light G-bands are predominantly GC-rich and that dark G-bands are AT-rich.[2] More recently, sequence analysis of the human genome confirmed suggestions that large GC-poor regions are strongly correlated with dark G-bands.[3] Light G-bands are believed to contain more euchromatin, DNA that is replicated early in S-phase of the cell cycle and is transcribed. In contrast, dark G-bands are believed to be composed of a larger percentage of heterochromatin, DNA that is more condensed and late replicating. Housekeeping genes reside in the light G-bands, and most tissue-specific genes appear to be situated in the dark G-bands.[4-6]

Q-banding, a fluorescent staining procedure, produces a pattern similar to that of G-banding. Brightly fluorescent bands correspond to G-dark bands, and dull Q-bands correspond to G-light bands. Q-banding was one of the most commonly used techniques, historically, for identifying chromosomal heteromorphisms associated with the centromeres of chromosomes 3, 4, 13, and 22; the short arms and satellites of acrocentric chromosomes 13, 14, 15, 21, and 22; and the distal region of the Y chromosome. In general, these polymorphisms are stable heritable markers without clinical significance.[7-9] In the past, they were valuable tools in the determination of both paternity[10] and the parental origin of the extra chromosome in a trisomy,[11,12] but much more informative molecular markers are now used to make these determinations. Nonetheless, chromosome polymorphisms are still useful, particularly because they may indicate maternal cell admixture in a culture of amniotic fluid cells or a tissue sample from an abortus.[13]

Reverse banding, also known as *R-banding*, produces a banding pattern that is essentially the opposite of that seen with G-banding or Q-banding. In other words, a light G-band will be a dark R-band, and vice versa. Terminal regions of many chromosomes tend to be pale by G-banding or Q-banding, and small deletions or rearrangements in these regions may be difficult to detect. In such cases, an R-banded preparation may make such an aberration visible, but molecular methods have largely replaced this use of R-banding in the analysis of telomeric regions (described in the section "Molecular Cytogenetic Methods"). Protocols exist for both bright-field and fluorescent R-banding.[14]

Special Stains

Special staining techniques have been used to assist in the analysis of particular chromosomes or regions of particular chromosomes. For example, C-banding (also referred to as *constitutive heterochromatin* or *centromere banding*) has been useful in the analysis of centromeres.[15] This technique involves acid treatment of metaphase chromosomes, followed by incubation in alkali (e.g., barium hydroxide) and then staining in Giemsa. The basis of C-banding is that a different type of chromatin, known as *constitutive heterochromatin*, is present in the centromeric regions of all normal chromosomes and the distal portion of the Y chromosome. Constitutive heterochromatin consists of DNA that is believed to remain condensed and genetically inactive. On the other hand, facultative heterochromatin (such as on the inactive X chromosome) is specifically inactivated in certain cell types or at certain phases of development, but still has the potential to decondense and become genetically active. Chromosomes 1, 9, and 16 tend to have larger amounts of C-banded material in the pericentromeric region, which can vary considerably in size among the human population.[16] C-banding may also be used to show an inversion in the pericentromeric region of chromosome 9, a common polymorphism limited to heterochromatin.[17] Although C-banding was used in the past to elucidate the origin of unidentified marker chromosomes or derivative chromosomes, molecular methods using centromere-specific DNA probes are less subjective and are now the preferred method (described in the section "Molecular Cytogenetic Methods").

Other special stains include silver staining, also known as *NOR staining*,[18] which identifies active nucleolar organizer regions (i.e., sites of the ribosomal RNA genes) on acrocentric chromosomes, and distamycin A/diamidinophenylindole (DA/DAPI) staining,[19] which reacts with

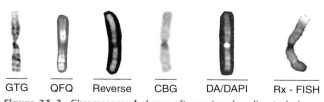

| GTG | QFQ | Reverse | CBG | DA/DAPI | Rx - FISH |

Figure 31-3. Chromosome 1 shown after various banding techniques: GTG, QFQ, reverse, CBG, DA/DAPI (distamycin A/diamidinophenylindole), and Rx-FISH (cross-species color banding). The three-letter code banding designations refer to the type of banding, the method used, and the stain employed (e.g., GTG = G-banding by trypsin with Giemsa). (From Shaffer LG, Tommerup N (eds). ISCN 2005: An International System for Human Cytogenetic Nomenclature. Basel, S. Karger, 1995.)

centromeres of chromosomes 1, 9, and 16; the short arm of chromosome 15; and the distal end of the Y chromosome. More recently, banding patterns have been produced with a combination of molecular genetic and cytogenetic techniques. Chromosomes can also be enzymatically digested and stained[20] or hybridized with specific repetitive DNA sequences[21] to produce banding patterns reminiscent of G- and C-bands and R-bands, respectively.

High-Resolution Banding

In general, clinical laboratories perform banding techniques on chromosomes in midmetaphase, at which time 400 to 550 bands can be resolved. Other techniques that enrich for chromosomes in earlier stages of metaphase, or in prophase, provide higher-resolution banding methods and are useful with targeted analysis of a particular region of a chromosome. High-resolution methods in practice include amethopterin synchronization of cell cultures with thymidine release[22] and addition of actinomycin D (dactinomycin)[23,24] or ethidium bromide[25] during the final hours of culturing, before harvest.

Idiograms and Chromosome Nomenclature

An idiogram is a schematic standardized karyotype that is derived from measured band sizes (Fig. 31-4). Chromosome idiograms and nomenclature have been designed by an international committee that has met periodically since 1960 to establish uniform language for describing chromosome bands and chromosome aberrations.[26] Chromosome regions are subdivided into bands and, at higher resolution, into sub-bands. For example, the designation 14q24 indicates chromosome 14, the long arm, region 2, band 4. On the idiogram, chromosome bands are numbered in an ascending manner from the centromere and toward the telomere of each chromosome arm.

A fairly sophisticated set of rules governs the description of chromosome abnormalities. These rules are set out in the *ISCN 2005: An International System for Human Cytogenetic Nomenclature.*[27] Basically, the total number of chromosomes is specified first, followed by the sex chromosomes (e.g., the normal male karyotype is given as 46,XY). Chromosome aberrations are listed with sex chromosome aberrations first (in the position of the normal sex chromosome), followed by abnormalities of the autosomes in numeric order, irrespective of aberration type. For each chromosome, numeric abnormalities are listed before structural changes. Multiple structural changes of homologous chromosomes are presented in alphabetical order, according to the abbreviated term of the abnormality.

MOLECULAR CYTOGENETIC METHODS

Molecular biologic methods have revolutionized cytogenetic studies and will continue to change the discipline. Chromosomal in situ hybridization was first used to determine the map location of particular DNA sequences and is employed routinely in the clinical cytogenetics laboratory. It has become an invaluable method to screen rapidly for aneuploidy in uncultured, interphase cells and to detect

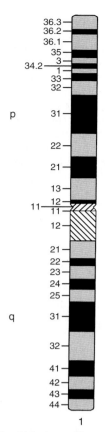

Figure 31-4. *Standardized idiogram of human chromosome 1 at the 400-band stage. p, short arm; q, long arm.*

a growing number of microdeletion and microduplication syndromes on interphase and metaphase cells. This method is also applied regularly on metaphase chromosomes to characterize subtle chromosome rearrangements and identify marker chromosomes, which are by definition unidentifiable by classic cytogenetics (Fig. 31-5).

Although in situ hybridization was first developed with isotopic probes, clinical laboratories now use commercially available nonisotopic fluorescent probes. This method has become widely known as FISH (fluorescence in situ hybridization). In contrast to conventional cytogenetic analysis, in which chromosomal abnormalities are globally assessed directly with a microscope, most FISH assays are considered targeted approaches that require a priori knowledge of a suspected aberration (Table 31-1). Probes may be labeled with biotin or digoxigenin, which requires fluorochrome-conjugated antibodies for detection, or with fluorochromes directly conjugated to the DNA. Multicolor FISH methods (e.g., spectral karyotyping [SKY], multiplex FISH [M-FISH], and cross-species color banding [Rx-FISH]), are genome-wide, FISH-based technologies that can readily show complex chromosomal rearrangements in a single hybridization experiment. Chromosomal CGH is classically a variation of the FISH method that is used to identify imbalances in cells being tested at a resolution of approximately 5 to 10 Mb for one-copy gains or losses. More recent applications of CGH on a microarray platform (array CGH) containing spotted genomic clones

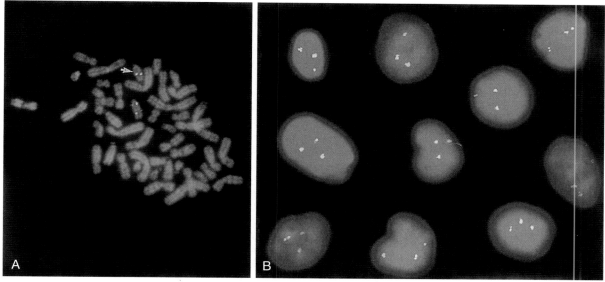

Figure 31-5. *A, Metaphase chromosome spread showing a microdeletion in one chromosome 15 in the Prader-Willi/Angelman syndrome region. Metaphase chromosomes were hybridized with a fluorescently labeled gamma-aminobutyric acid A receptor, beta 3 (GABRB3) probe and, as a control for chromosome 15, a fluorescently labeled promyelocytic leukemia (PML) probe. After hybridization, chromosomes were counterstained with diamidinophenylindole (DAPI). Chromosome 15 showing hybridization with only the PML probe has a deletion of the GABRB3 probe, which maps to the Prader-Willi/Angelman syndrome region (arrow). B, Interphase amniotic fluid cells with trisomy 21. Cells were hybridized with a fluorescently labeled probe to chromosome 21 and counterstained with DAPI. Three signals indicate the presence of three copies of chromosome 21, consistent with a clinical diagnosis of Down syndrome.*

(e.g., bacterial artificial chromosomes [BACs]) or short DNA sequences (oligonucleotides) permit identification of genomic gains and losses at as much as 30- to 40-kb resolution. Array CGH is becoming a significant technologic improvement in clinical cytogenetics, and implementation of this technology in studies of human disease is bringing new insights into the pathogenesis of disease.

A variety of types of probes are used to detect chromosomal abnormalities by FISH.[28] Repetitive DNA probes, whole-chromosome–painting probes, and unique sequence probes can be visualized. In general, repetitive DNA probes (e.g., alpha-satellite and beta-satellite sequences) hybridizing to particular centromere sequences are usually used in chromosome enumeration, whereas whole-chromosome paints are applied to show cryptic rearrangements and decipher the origin of marker chromosomes. Unique sequence probes are employed to detect microdeletions, certain microduplications, and other chromosomal rearrangements.

Chromosome-specific centromeric probes are available for most chromosomes. However, the centromeric sequences of chromosome pairs 13 and 21 and pairs 14 and 22 are similar, and a commercially available centromeric probe has not yet been developed that selectively hybridizes to only one of the two chromosomes. Thus, to detect aneuploidy of these chromosomes, unique sequence probes are used. The major disadvantage of these probes relative to the centromeric repetitive probes is that the intensity of the signal is generally weaker and some marker chromosomes may be missing distally located unique sequences, making these probes less informative in certain clinical cases.

Chromosome-painting probes may be developed from DNA libraries from flow-sorted human chromosomes or DNA amplified from human monochromosomal somatic cell hybrids.[29] Hybridization with these DNA probes results in fluorescent staining of the entire chromosome (hence, the term "chromosome painting"). These probes are available for each human chromosome, and are particularly useful for determining interchromosomal rearrangements (i.e., chromosomal rearrangements that involve nonhomologous chromosomes) that cannot be interpreted by conventional chromosome banding analyses. Painting probes are not particularly useful in interphase analysis because the hybridization signals are large and diffuse, compared with probes developed for specific chromosomal regions (e.g., alpha-satellite centromeric probes or unique sequence probes).

A third type of FISH probe hybridizes to unique locus-specific DNA sequences. These probes are usually genomic clones and typically vary in size from approximately 40 kb to hundreds of kb. These probes have become the standard in evaluating clinical specimens for microdeletion disorders (e.g., Prader-Willi and X-linked Kallmann syndrome).

Array-Based Comparative Genomic Hybridization

As mentioned earlier, array CGH is becoming an extremely important molecular cytogenetic method for clinical cytogenetic diagnostics.[30] This technique is a modification of a procedure initially introduced in 1992[31] for surveying genomic DNA imbalances (i.e., DNA gains and losses) in cancer specimens, but it is now being applied to all areas of cytogenetic diagnostics and research. In this procedure, thousands (or even millions) of DNA fragments, each representing a specific region of the human genome, are first attached to a glass slide. Then, a patient's DNA is labeled with one fluorescent color/dye, combined with

TABLE 31-1

Reasons to Request a Patient's Karyotype or Fluorescence in Situ Hybridization

Clinical Indication	Test	Possible Chromosome Abnormality
Couple with ≥3 spontaneous abortions	K	Balanced structural rearrangement
Parent of child with structural chromosome abnormality	K	Balanced structural rearrangement
First-degree relative with structural chromosome abnormality	K	Balanced structural rearrangement
Female expressing X-linked disorder	K	X-autosome translocation or 45,X
Female <10th percentile in height	K	45,X; possibly mosaic
Female with elevated gonadotropins	K	45,X; possibly mosaic
Female with infertility/ovarian dysgenesis	K	Structural rearrangement of X
Male with elevated gonadotropins, whether		
Tall	K	47,XXY
Short	K	45,X/46,XY
Normal height	K	46,XX (follow up with PCR for *SRY*)
Gynecomastia	K	47,XXY
azoospermia or oligospermia	K	Balanced structural rearrangements, particularly involving sex chromosomes; deletions in Yq (PCR for Yq microdeletions)
Sexual ambiguity	K	
associated with Wilms' tumor, aniridia	F	11p13 deletion
Hypogonadism and other features of Prader-Willi syndrome	F	15q11q13 deletion

F, fluorescence in situ hybridization; K, karyotype; PCR, polymerase chain reaction.

genomic DNA from a normal control subject labeled with a different fluorescent color/dye, and then applied to the glass slide containing the DNA fragments that recapitulate the human genome at a certain resolution. The fluorescence intensity ratio of the two labeled dyes at each DNA fragment "spot" on the glass slide reflects the copy number ratio of that DNA sequence in the patient's DNA compared with the normal control subject. For example, if the patient's DNA is labeled with cy5 fluorescence and the control DNA is labeled with cy3 fluorescence, a significant increase in cy5 fluorescence, compared with cy3 fluorescence, for a particular DNA fragment may be indicative of a gain of that DNA sequence in the patient, compared with the control subject. Conversely, a significant decrease in cy5 fluorescence, compared with cy3 fluorescence, for the same DNA fragment, may be indicative of a loss of that DNA sequence in the patient.

Array CGH platforms that are now typically used in cytogenetic diagnostics have an effective genome-wide resolution of as low as 30,000 bp (30 kb) to 40,000 bp (40 kb). This is a substantial improvement over the 3,000,000-bp (3 Mb) to 5,000,000-bp (5 Mb) resolution associated with detecting gains and losses by GTG-banded karyotypic analysis, and is associated with less subjective interpretation. Some of the array CGH platforms used for cytogenetic diagnostics also have an increased number of probes at clinically informative sites of the human genome (including the pericentromeric regions, subtelomeric regions, and known critical regions for microduplication and microdeletion syndromes).

Array CGH offers a less subjective and cost-effective way to detect DNA gains and losses in a patient's genome at unprecedented high resolution. Therefore, it is possible to detect whole-chromosome aneuploidy, subtelomeric imbalances, microdeletions/microduplications, and the origin of marker chromosomes (e.g., Fig. 31-6). However, as with any technology, array CGH also has specific limitations. First, it is not possible for current array CGH strategies to detect truly balanced chromosomal rearrangements, such as inversions, insertions, and translocations. However, recent higher-resolution analyses are finding that as many as 30% to 40% of these chromosomal rearrangements that were previously believed to be balanced at the GTG-banded resolution are actually unbalanced.[32] Second, because array CGH specifically detects genomic imbalances, it is unable to identify "copy-neutral" chromosomal aberrations (e.g., uniparental disomy [UPD]). For detecting such aberrations, single-nucleotide polymorphism–detecting arrays may be informative (e.g., Affymetrix 6.0 arrays [Affymetrix, Santa Clara, CA]; Illumina 1 million feature arrays [Illumina, San Diego, CA]). Third, the level of mosaicism that is detectable can be less than that of classic cytogenetic analysis. Current estimates are that whole-chromosome mosaicism of less than 10% and segmental genomic imbalances of less than 30% could go undetected by array CGH.

Along with the increased resolution of array CGH testing comes another level of complexity in the clinical interpretation of the data obtained. Much of this complexity stems from the recent realization that healthy individuals harbor hundreds to thousands of genomic imbalances that do not appear to cause early-onset, highly penetrant diseases or genomic disorders.[33,34] These copy number variants can range in size from 1000 bases (1 kb) to more than 2,000,000 bases (2 Mb).[35] Several criteria have been proposed for differentiating a "benign" copy number variant from a genomic imbalance that is pathogenic,[36] but the most significant criterion appears to be whether the imbalance is de novo (i.e., both healthy parents do not carry the specific copy number variant detected in the affected offspring).

Chromosome Aberrations and Reproduction

Chromosome aberrations are common in humans and account for a large proportion of pregnancy loss and congenital malformations. Chromosome aberrations, especially

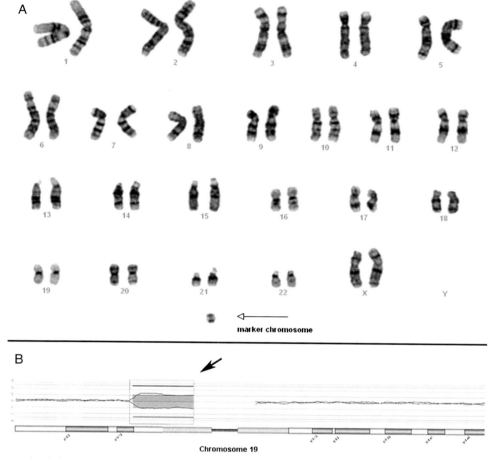

Figure 31-6. *An example of the utility of array comparative genomic hybridization (CGH) in clinical cytogenetic diagnostics. **A,** A GTG-banded karyotype obtained from amniotic fluid taken at 15 weeks' gestation from a 39-year-old woman carrying a pregnancy achieved through in vitro fertilization. Of 49 cells examined, 13 carried a marker chromosome of unknown origin. GTG-banded karyotype analysis from cord blood taken at 21 weeks' gestation showed similar results. **B,** Array CGH testing, using a 244K oligo-based platform (Agilent, Santa Clara, CA) with an approximately 10-kb effective resolution, showed a significant gain of genomic DNA from an approximate nucleotide position of 15,927,891 to 24,158,055, at the proximal short arm of chromosome 19. Taken together, these results suggest that the marker chromosome is composed of approximately 8.2 million bases of DNA from the proximal short arm of chromosome 19. (Images kindly provided by Chun Hwa Ihm, MD, PhD, of Eulji University Hospital [Daejeon, South Korea], and Ji Hyeon Park, MD, of CHA General Hospital [Seoul, South Korea]).*

aberrations of the X and Y chromosomes, can also be a cause of infertility. Common clinical practice for couples who have experienced three or more spontaneous abortions includes full cytogenetic analysis. For the reproductive specialist, chromosome abnormalities can be divided into two clinically distinct groups: (1) normal findings on G-banded karyotypic analysis, in which a reproductive error results in a chromosomally abnormal conceptus; and (2) a recognized de novo or inherited constitutional chromosome anomaly associated with reproductive implications and perhaps other phenotypic effects.

Chromosome abnormalities arising during reproduction are fairly common. An estimated 8% of conceptuses possess a chromosome abnormality.[37-39] Most of these chromosomally abnormal products of conception are not viable, but an estimated 0.7% of liveborn infants are chromosomally abnormal.[40] Errors in gametogenesis are the most common cause of chromosomally abnormal conceptuses, but fertilization and postfertilization errors also occur.

GAMETOGENESIS ERRORS

Review of Oogenesis and Spermatogenesis

Meiosis, the cell division process that produces haploid germ cells from diploid germ cell precursors, is the fundamental event in both oogenesis and spermatogenesis. The overall sequence of meiotic events is the same in oogenesis and spermatogenesis, but several key differences exist.

In both female and male gametogenesis, the chromosome number is reduced by half, producing haploid gametes with 23 chromosomes through a process in which diploid germ cell precursor cells replicate their DNA and then undergo two successive cell divisions. The first cell division, meiosis I, is termed the *reduction division*, because it is here that the number of chromosomes is halved. Homologous chromosomes pair or synapse and then exchange material by recombination or crossing over. Recombination greatly increases the genetic diversity in gametes by reassorting paternally and maternally inherited genetic information. After recombination, homologous chromosomes, whose chromatids now contain segments of both paternally and maternally derived DNA, segregate to opposite poles and form two cells with 23 chromosomes. At this point, each chromosome is composed of two sister chromatids that remain together until meiosis II, during which time they separate in a manner analogous to a mitotic division. The result of meiosis in both spermatogenesis and oogenesis is the production of haploid germ cells with 23 chromosomes composed of one chromatid each.

Although meiosis produces haploid germ cells in both female and male gametogenesis, these two processes differ in several critical ways. One crucial difference is in the timing of events in gametogenesis. In spermatogenesis, the production of mature haploid sperm from diploid spermatogonia does not begin until puberty, but continues throughout life. Production of haploid sperm from diploid spermatogonia requires approximately 64 days and involves a continuing series of both mitotic and meiotic divisions. In oogenesis, the mitotic divisions that precede meiosis are completed during fetal development and do not continue throughout life, as in spermatogenesis. The onset of meiosis in females occurs during fetal development, but is arrested before birth, at the end of prophase I. Meiosis does not proceed again until ovulation, at which time one oocyte completes meiosis I and proceeds to meiosis II. Meiosis II is completed only if fertilization occurs.

The difference in the timing of both mitotic and meiotic divisions is believed to play a significant role in the susceptibility of oocytes and spermatocytes to mutation and reproductive errors. Spermatogenesis, which involves continual cell division and hence replication of DNA, is more vulnerable to DNA damage and replication errors. Thus, de novo point mutations are more commonly of paternal than maternal origin. Conversely, the protracted meiotic arrest in oogenesis is believed to contribute to nondisjunction, and the extra chromosome in trisomies is usually of maternal origin.

The manner in which cytoplasm is divided during meiosis also differs in female and male gametogenesis. In spermatogenesis, a primary spermatocyte divides its cytoplasm equally to produce four functionally equivalent sperm. By contrast, a primary oocyte divides its cytoplasm unequally in the first meiotic division, producing one polar body and one secondary oocyte that retains most of the cytoplasm. If the secondary oocyte is fertilized, it will complete meiosis II, generating a second polar body and a fertilized ovum that again retains most of the cytoplasm. This unequal division of cytoplasmic contents is important because the ovum contributes most of the non-nuclear cytoplasmic contents to the fertilized product. Thus, mitochondria and other cytoplasmic components are essentially exclusively of maternal origin.

A third important difference between oogenesis and spermatogenesis is the synapsis configuration of sex chromosomes during meiosis. In female meiosis, the two X chromosomes pair and recombine over the entire length of the chromosomes.[41,42] In male meiosis, by comparison, the morphologically dissimilar X and Y chromosomes pair and recombine in only two regions.[43-47] The first of these regions identified is located on the distal short arms of the X and Y chromosomes and is known as *pseudoautosomal*

region 1 (PAR1). DNA in this region can be transferred from one sex chromosome to the other,[44,45,48,49] and none of the at least 24 genes mapped to this region appears to be required for specific male or female sexual differentiation.[50-53] This region is probably important for initiating chromosome pairing and forming a synaptonemal complex in male meiosis, and it appears that one recombination event is required in this region for proper disjunction of the XY bivalent.[54,55] The X and Y chromosomes also occasionally pair and recombine at a second region on the long arm of each chromosome containing at least five genes, at a region termed *pseudoautosomal region 2* (PAR2).[46,47,53]

Meiotic Nondisjunction

Meiotic nondisjunction errors are common in humans, resulting in *aneuploidy,* a term used when the total number of chromosomes in a cell is not an exact multiple of the haploid number. Aneuploidy usually involves a single chromosome, but in rare circumstances, may involve more than one. Aneuploidy is present in approximately 0.6% of newborns[56] and nearly 70% of spontaneous abortions.[57] Trisomy for all chromosomes has been observed in spontaneous abortions, indicating that nondisjunction for each chromosome does occur.[58-60]

Meiotic nondisjunction can involve only one chromosome or the whole chromosome set. Nondisjunction of a single chromosome will produce germ cells that have either two (disomy) or zero (nullisomy) copies of the specific chromosome. If a germ cell with an extra chromosome is combined with a chromosomally normal germ cell, the product will be trisomic (i.e., having 47 chromosomes). If a germ cell missing a chromosome is combined with a chromosomally normal germ cell, the product will be monosomic (i.e., having 45 chromosomes). Nondisjunction of the entire chromosome set will lead to either germ cells with two copies of every chromosome or germ cells with no chromosomes. The clinical phenotype and the histopathology of conceptuses that can result from numerically abnormal gametes depend on both the total number of chromosomes and the relative number of paternal versus maternal chromosomes.

Nondisjunction can take place in either meiosis I or meiosis II. If nondisjunction occurs in meiosis I, all four products of meiosis will be chromosomally abnormal. Two of the four products of meiosis will have two copies of the chromosome involved in the nondisjunction event, and two of the four products of meiosis will have no copies of that particular chromosome. Of further note, in germ cells with two copies of the chromosome, the copies, although homologous, will not be identical. Homologous chromosomes do not separate in nondisjunction errors in meiosis I, but sister chromatids separate properly in meiosis II. Thus, each of the germ cells with an extra chromosome will have a maternally derived chromosome and a paternally derived chromosome. In the absence of recombination, one chromosome would be entirely of maternal origin and the other entirely paternal.

If nondisjunction occurs in meiosis II, two of the four products will be unaffected by the event and two of the products will be abnormal. One abnormal product will

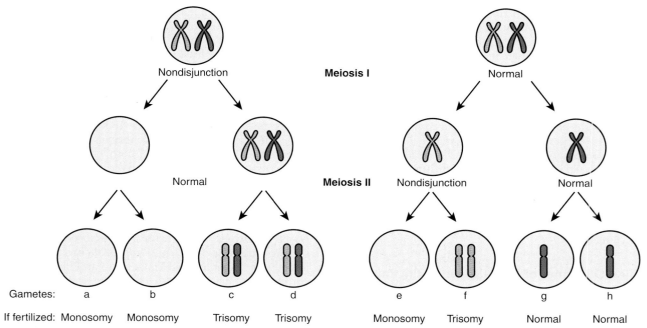

Figure 31-7. *Comparison of nondisjunction in meiosis I and meiosis II. With an error in meiosis I, all four gametes (a, b, c, and d) are aneuploid. Two gametes (a and b) are nullisomic, potentially resulting in a monosomic conceptus. Two gametes (c and d) are disomic, potentially resulting in a trisomic conceptus. The two homologous chromosomes in the disomic gametes (c and d) are heterodisomic. With an error in meiosis II, only two gametes (e and f) are aneuploid. One gamete (e) is nullisomic, and the other aneuploid gamete (f) is disomic. The two homologous chromosomes in the nonreduced gamete (f) are isodisomic.*

have an extra chromosome, and the other abnormal product will be missing that chromosome. With nondisjunction errors in meiosis II, homologous chromosomes separate properly in meiosis I, but sister chromatids do not separate in meiosis II. Thus, in contrast to meiosis I nondisjunction errors, the two nondisjoined chromosomes would be genetically identical in the absence of recombination (Fig. 31-7). This apparently trivial difference between errors in meiosis I and errors in meiosis II can have important clinical consequences that are discussed later. Furthermore, the study of the parental origin of chromosomes involved in aneuploidies has led to important observations about the origin and meiotic stage of nondisjunction.

It is difficult to study meiotic nondisjunction for all chromosomes directly in gametes and even indirectly in products of conception because many aneuploid products of conception are lost early in pregnancy and are never brought to clinical attention. However, conceptuses with trisomies for some chromosomes survive long enough to be clinically recognized, and several studies have used DNA polymorphisms to analyze the parental origin of the extra chromosome in these cases of trisomy. These studies have shown that maternal nondisjunction accounts for significantly more cases of autosomal trisomy than does paternal nondisjunction. For trisomies 13, 14, 15, 16, 18, 21, and 22, maternal nondisjunction accounted for 88%, 83%, 88%, 100%, 93%, 91%, and 89% of cases, respectively.[54,61-65] Direct studies of aneuploidy in gametes give estimates of 2% to 4% meiotic nondisjunction in sperm[58,66,67] and 13% to 18% meiotic I nondisjunction in oocytes.[68,69] These findings indicate that the excess of maternal nondisjunction relative to paternal

nondisjunction seen in trisomic conceptuses does indeed reflect differences in the rate of nondisjunction in oocytes and spermatocytes. It is still possible, however, that selection against aneuploid sperm occurs after spermatogenesis as well.

The rate of aneuploidy is higher in oocytes than in spermatocytes, and it also increases markedly with maternal (but not paternal) age.[69,70] Although the relationship between increased maternal age and Down syndrome was first described in 1933,[71] the mechanism for this aging effect remains to be fully elucidated. Most nondisjunction errors in oocytes occur in meiosis I, and it has been hypothesized that the prolonged arrest in meiosis I contributes to these errors.[72]

Paternal nondisjunction is more common in cases of aneuploidy involving sex chromosomes than in cases involving autosomes. It has been hypothesized that the XY bivalent is more susceptible to nondisjunction than are the homologous bivalents. FISH studies on sperm have supported this hypothesis, showing rates of sex chromosome disomy to be two to four times higher than disomy for particular autosomes.[66,73] Eighty percent of 45,X karyotypes can be attributed to paternal nondisjunction, although some of these cases may be caused by early loss of the Y chromosome through mitotic nondisjunction in the zygote.[74,75] Cases of 47,XXY are divided approximately equally between maternal and paternal nondisjunction.[76,77] However, as with the autosomal trisomies, the extra X chromosome is of maternal origin in 90% of cases of 47,XXX.[77]

Studies have shown that recombination is crucial for proper segregation of homologous chromosomes. Yeast experiments have shown that recombination is required for formation of the synaptonemal complex and for complete pairing of homologous chromosomes. From this, it has been suggested that, in the absence of pairing and recombination, nondisjunction would be increased.[78] In humans, studies of trisomies 15, 16, 18, and 21, as well as of XXY and XXX, have shown that, on average, the particular chromosomes involved in a specific nondisjunction event participated in fewer recombinations than usual.[54,79-83] Presumably, the limited region of homology in which recombination occurs in the XY bivalent accounts for its increased susceptibility to nondisjunction. Interestingly, the overall rate of recombination is higher in female gametogenesis than in male gametogenesis, although some specific chromosomal regions, including the telomeric regions of many chromosomes, have higher recombination rates in males.[84,85]

Clinical Outcomes of Meiotic Nondisjunction

Most numeric chromosome abnormalities caused by meiotic nondisjunction errors result in spontaneous abortion. As a group, chromosome abnormalities are the most common cause of pregnancy loss, accounting for 50% to 60% of spontaneous losses. Triploidy, tetraploidy, trisomy, and monosomy have all been reported in spontaneous abortions. The most common chromosome abnormalities in chromosomally abnormal spontaneous abortions are 45,X (20%), trisomy 16 (16%), and triploidy (16%). Trisomy 21 accounts for approximately 5% of chromosomally abnormal spontaneous abortions.[39]

The overall incidence and distribution of numeric chromosome abnormalities differ in newborns and spontaneous abortions, reflecting the differential viabilities of the abnormalities. Trisomies 13, 18, and 21 are compatible with life, although most of these conceptuses result in spontaneous abortion (Table 31-2). No other nonmosaic autosomal trisomy or autosomal monosomy (with the exception of monosomy 21[86]) has ever been reported in a liveborn infant. In newborn surveys, trisomy 21 is the most common autosomal aneuploidy, with an overall

incidence of approximately 1:800. Estimates of trisomy 18 range from 1:3500 to 1:7000 newborns, and estimates of trisomy 13 range from 1:7000 to 1:21,000.[87-89]

Trisomy 21, the least severe of the autosomal trisomies, results in Down syndrome, a well-defined and familiar disorder. Down syndrome was first described by Langdon Down in 1866 and is the single most common cause of moderate mental retardation. In addition to mental impairment, individuals with Down syndrome frequently have other serious clinical phenotypes, including cardiac defects and increased risk of both childhood leukemia and early-onset Alzheimer disease. Approximately 95% of cases of Down syndrome result from the presence of three separate copies of chromosome 21 (i.e., 47,XX,+21 or 47,XY,+21), reflecting a parental nondisjunction event involving chromosome 21. Approximately 3% of cases of Down syndrome result from a chromosomal translocation in which one of the three copies of chromosome 21 is joined in a "head-to-head" manner to another acrocentric chromosome, usually through repetitive sequences in the p arms. Such chromosomal rearrangements are referred to as *robertsonian translocations*. The remaining 2% result from a mosaic chromosome constitution in which one normal cell line has 46 chromosomes and a second abnormal cell line carries an additional copy of chromosome 21. In these cases, the original conceptus may have been trisomic for chromosome 21 with a postzygotic mitotic nondisjunction event, resulting in an additional cell line disomic for chromosome 21. Another possibility is that the original conceptus may have been disomic for chromosome 21 with a postzygotic mitotic nondisjunction event, resulting in an additional cell line trisomic for chromosome 21.

Trisomy 18, described by John Edwards in 1960, also has a severe clinical phenotype. Only 10% of these individuals survive beyond the first year of life.[90] Failure to thrive and mental retardation are seen in all individuals who are trisomic for chromosome 18. Prominent occiput, recessed jaw, short sternum, low-set and malformed ears, clenched fists with a characteristic overlapping of the fingers, and rocker-bottom feet are features of this syndrome. Approximately 80% of cases of trisomy 18 result from the presence of three separate copies of chromosome 18, approximately 10% are mosaic, and the remaining cases primarily involve a chromosomal translocation.[91]

Trisomy 13, first described by Klaus Patau in 1960, is much less common than trisomy 21 and is clinically much more severe. Approximately 45% of liveborn infants die within the first month after birth and 90% die by the age of 6 months. The phenotype of trisomy 13 involves severe central nervous system malformations, including severe mental retardation, holoprosencephaly, and arrhinencephaly. Cleft lip and cleft palate are frequently seen. Eye anomalies, ranging from microphthalmia to anophthalmia, are also common. Postaxial polydactyly, clenched fists, and rocker-bottom feet are further features of this syndrome. As with trisomy 21, trisomy 13 occurs as a result of the presence of three separate copies of a chromosome (chromosome 13) or in conjunction with a robertsonian translocation.

Recurrence risks in cases of trisomy in which there are three separate copies of a given autosome (i.e., not due to a

TABLE 31-2

Probability of Survival to Birth for Viable Aneusomic Conceptuses

Karyotype	Probability of Survival to Birth (%)*
47,+13	2.8
47,+18	5.4
47,+21	22.1
45,X	0.3
47,XXX	70.0
47,XXY	55.3
47,XYY	100.0

*Based on the incidence of chromosome abnormalities in spontaneous abortions, stillbirths, and livebirths, assuming an overall 15% rate of spontaneous abortion and 1% rate of stillbirth in the population.
Adapted from Jacobs PA, Hassold TJ. The origin of numerical chromosome abnormalities. Adv Genet 33:101-133, 1995.

chromosomal translocation) can be calculated on the basis of empirical data for trisomy 21. However, minimal empirical data exist for trisomies 13 and 18 because of the rarity of these conditions. For mothers younger than 35 years, the recurrence risk is approximately 0.5% for a subsequent trisomy 21 and 1% for any chromosome abnormality. For mothers older than 35 years, in whom the age-related risk of trisomy 21 is equal to or greater than 0.5%, the recurrence risks are equivalent to the general population age-related risks.[92] The reasons for the additional risk in younger mothers are not entirely clear and may be due to individual differences in rates of nondisjunction or to cases of parental gonadal mosaicism (discussed in further detail later) for trisomy 21. In such instances, a phenotypically normal individual has a cell line that is trisomic for chromosome 21 in gonadal tissue, but not somatic tissue.

Recurrence for trisomies 13 and 18 is rare, but the risk of trisomy 21 may be increased after the occurrence of one of these other trisomies. All of these recurrence risks are based on a liveborn index case. As already mentioned, nonviable autosomal trisomies are common in spontaneous abortions, and it is unclear whether such an event increases the risk of trisomy in subsequent pregnancies. If a trisomy is detected in a late abortion or in a stillbirth, it is probably prudent to use the same risk figures as for a live birth.[92] Finally, recurrence risks after a chromosomal translocation-based trisomy (i.e., not a result of meiotic nondisjunction) depend on several factors, including whether the translocation was inherited or occurred de novo, the particular chromosomal translocation involved, and the sex of the carrier parent (discussed later; see also Table 31-4).

Trisomies of the sex chromosomes resulting in XXX, XXY, and XYY are viable and have a much lower rate of spontaneous abortion than do the autosomal trisomies (see Table 31-2). In newborn surveys, 47,XXX, 47,XXY, and 47,XYY are all found at an approximate incidence of 1:1000.[40] Monosomy for the X chromosome, unlike autosomal monosomy, can be viable. However, more than 99% of conceptuses with monosomy X result in spontaneous abortion, and its frequency of approximately 1 affected newborn in 10,000 is much lower than that of the other numeric sex chromosome abnormalities.[40] In general, phenotypes of sex chromosome aneuploidies are more subtle than those of the autosomal aneuploidies (discussed further in the section on sex chromosome abnormalities). Recurrence of any of the sex chromosome abnormalities is exceedingly rare.[92]

Infrequently, meiotic nondisjunction for the complete chromosome set can occur. One outcome of such an event is a benign cystic teratoma. In the absence of fertilization, an unreduced egg with 46 chromosomes can develop into a benign cystic teratoma. Benign cystic teratomas represent a duplication of the maternal genome with no contribution from a paternal genome. These teratomas can also arise after endoreduplication of a haploid egg.

As with benign cystic teratomas, complete hydatidiform moles are diploid. However, with rare exceptions, they are composed of chromosomal DNA solely of paternal origin,[93,94] although the mitochondrial DNA is of maternal origin. Studies of molecular polymorphisms have shown that 75% to 85% of complete moles are homozygous at every

locus and thus developed from duplication of the haploid paternal genome in an egg containing no maternal chromosomes.[94-96] Duplication of the haploid paternal genome must be caused either by nondisjunction in meiosis II or by endoreduplication of a haploid sperm after fertilization.

The mechanism by which an egg becomes devoid of maternal chromosomes is unclear. Possibilities include meiotic nondisjunction, enucleation of the oocyte, and exclusion of the maternal chromosomes after fertilization.[97] An estimated 4% to 15% of complete moles are 46,XY and are believed to arise from fertilization of a chromosomally empty egg with two sperm.[95,98] This same mechanism is believed to account for the 5% of complete moles that are 46,XX, but are not genetically identical at every locus.[95] Note that 46,YY moles are not seen, presumably because this chromosomal constitution is not compatible with development.

Comparing the pathophysiology of benign cystic teratomas and complete hydatidiform moles provided some of the first evidence for *imprinting,* the differential effect of genetic material depending on whether the inheritance is of maternal or paternal origin. Although both benign cystic teratomas and complete hydatidiform moles are diploid entities with genetic contribution from only one parent, their development is dissimilar. Benign cystic teratomas have little trophoblast development, but do have some embryonic development. In contrast, complete moles have no embryonic development, but do have placental trophoblast development, albeit abnormal.

Another outcome involving unreduced gametes is triploidy. Although dispermy is believed to be the most common cause of triploidy, fertilization with an unreduced (diploid) egg or sperm also leads to triploidy. Triploidy almost always results in spontaneous abortion, although it is seen in approximately 1:57,000 births. Most of these newborns die within the first day. However, in some isolated cases, patients reportedly have survived for several months.[99,100]

The phenotype of triploidy differs, depending on whether the origin of the extra chromosome set is paternal (diandric) or maternal (digynic). Although both diandric and digynic triploid products can be associated with a fetus, the diandric triploid is associated with a less developed fetus, and no diandric triploid surviving to term has ever been reported. Diandric triploids are associated with excessive placental growth and partial hydatidiform moles. Digynic triploids are associated with smaller, nonmolar placentas. Thus, diandric triploids have increased placental growth but decreased fetal development compared with digynic triploids.[101] These differences in placental and fetal development between diandric and digynic triploids are similar to the developmental differences between complete moles and benign cystic teratomas, in which paternal chromosomes are associated with placental development, but no embryonic development. In contrast, maternal chromosomes are associated with embryonic development, but little placental development.

Errors of Recombination

As already mentioned, not only is meiotic recombination crucial for genetic diversity, but its frequency also appears to influence rates of meiotic nondisjunction. Accuracy of

TABLE 31-3

Microdeletions and Microduplications: Chromosomal Location and Availability of Commercial Fluorescence in Situ Hybridization Probes

Syndrome	Location	Deletion or Duplication	Commercially Available FISH Probe[*]
Monosomy 1p36	1p36	Deletion	Yes
Sotos	5q35	Deletion	Yes
Williams	7q11.23	Deletion	Yes
Langer-Giedion/trichorhinophalangeal 2	8q24.1	Deletion	No
DiGeorge/velocardiofacial (DGS2)	10p14	Deletion	Yes
WAGR[†]	11p13	Deletion	No
Retinoblastoma	13q14	Deletion	Yes
Angelman	15q11q13	Deletion	Yes
Prader-Willi	15q11q13	Deletion	Yes
15q13.3	15q13.3	Deletion	No
α-Thalassemia/mental retardation	16p13.3	Deletion	No
Rubinstein-Taybi	16p13.3	Deletion	No
Smith-Magenis	17p11.2	Deletion	Yes
Miller-Dieker	17p13.3	Deletion	Yes
Neurofibromatosis type 1	17q11.2	Deletion	No
17q21.3	17q21.3	Deletion	No
Alagille	20p11.23p12.2	Deletion	Yes
DiGeorge/velocardiofacial (DGS1)	22q11.2	Deletion	Yes
Steroid sulfatase deficiency	Xp22.32	Deletion	Yes
Duplication 1p36	1p36	Duplication	Yes
Beckwith-Wiedemann	11p15	Duplication	No
Charcot-Marie-Tooth 1A	17p11.2p12	Duplication	No
Cat-eye	22q11	Duplication	No

[*]Also available are fluorescence in situ hybridization probes for the usually classically detectable deletions associated with cri du chat (5p15) and Wolf-Hirschhorn (4p16) syndromes.

[†]Wilms' tumor, aniridia, genital abnormalities, and mental retardation.

FISH, fluorescence in situ hybridization.

recombination is no less important and is critical in maintaining the fidelity of genetic information. Recombination between mispaired chromosomes or misaligned chromatids, known as *unequal crossing over,* can lead to duplication or deletion of genetic material. On occasion, the resulting rearrangements are large enough to be detectable through conventional cytogenetic studies, but more commonly, they can be detected only through high-resolution cytogenetic methods, such as FISH or array CGH. The number of genetic diseases known to be caused by microdeletions or microduplications is growing, as is the number of commercially available probes used for their detection. Currently commercially available FISH probes include those for the detection of Prader-Willi syndrome, Angelman syndrome, DiGeorge/velocardiofacial syndrome, and Williams syndrome (Table 31-3).

FERTILIZATION AND POSTFERTILIZATION ERRORS

In addition to meiotic errors of gametogenesis, a variety of errors can occur at the time of fertilization. Normally, penetration of the zona pellucida by one sperm triggers a series of events leading to prevention of penetration by other sperm, resumption of meiosis II in the egg, and extrusion of the second polar body. Failure of any of these processes can lead to numeric chromosome aberrations,

most notably, triploidy. As previously mentioned, fertilization of one egg by two sperm is the most common cause of triploidy and results in a partial hydatidiform mole. Fertilization of the first polar body or retention of the second polar body may also result in triploidy.

Postfertilization errors occur as well. Cleavage errors, resulting in chromosome duplication without subsequent cell division, produce tetraploidy. If a cleavage error occurs during the first division, the result is nonmosaic tetraploidy. With rare reported exceptions,[102,103] this condition is incompatible with life. A cleavage error at a later, multicellular stage produces mosaicism for tetraploid and diploid cell lines, which can be observed in spontaneous abortuses and rarely in liveborn infants.

Mosaicism

Just as cleavage errors at a multicellular stage produce mosaicism for tetraploidy and diploidy, mitotic nondisjunction errors at a multicellular stage produce mosaicism for individual chromosomes. Theoretically, mitotic nondisjunction should create two new cell lines, one monosomic for the chromosome that underwent nondisjunction and one trisomic for the same chromosome. However, not all cell lines are compatible with development; therefore, the monosomic cell lines, which are frequently inviable, are not usually observed.

The three autosomal trisomies, trisomies 13, 18, and 21, which can result in liveborn infants, are also observed as mosaics in conjunction with a diploid cell line. Two additional autosomal trisomies, trisomies 8 and 9, are only viable as mosaics. The presence of a normal cell line can allow the otherwise lethal trisomies 8 and 9 to be viable, and may, in some cases, improve the phenotype for trisomies 13, 18, and 21. However, in the setting of prenatal diagnosis, a mosaic result for trisomy 13, 18, or 21 is usually given a prognosis equivalent to that for a complete trisomy. Mosaic trisomy for the other autosomes, such as the respective complete trisomy, almost always results in spontaneous abortion, although rare cases of trisomy mosaicism have been confirmed postnatally for all autosomes except chromosomes 1 and 11.[89,104-109] The prognosis for mosaicism involving sex chromosomes, particularly 45,X/46,XY, is more variable (discussed in the section on sex chromosome abnormalities).

Tissue-Limited Mosaicism and Uniparental Disomy

Tissue-limited mosaicism is a specialized form of mosaicism in which some but not all tissues in an individual have two or more cell lines. This type of mosaicism arises when mitotic nondisjunction occurs in a cell type that is a precursor for a subset of tissues. Gonadal mosaicism occurs when the abnormal cell line is present in the gonadal tissue. This type of mosaicism becomes apparent only when an individual has multiple offspring with the same chromosome abnormality, and it is one reason why recurrence risks are increased after diagnosis of an abnormality. Confined placental mosaicism (CPM) occurs when the abnormal cell line is confined to the placenta, with the fetus being karyotypically normal. CPM is suspected most often after cytogenetic studies of tissue obtained from chorionic villus sampling indicate a mosaic karyotype, possibly reflective of an abnormal placenta and a normal fetus. Subsequent chromosome studies of amniotic fluid cells may be performed to confirm that the abnormal cell line is most likely confined to the placenta.

Theoretically, CPM could arise through at least two possible mechanisms. Because the embryo derives from a relatively small number of progenitor cells,[110,111] one possibility is that CPM could occur after a postzygotic nondisjunction event in a cell lineage that contributes only to extraembryonic tissues. Alternatively, CPM may arise through a mechanism in which the original conceptus is trisomic, but then undergoes a nondisjunction event, leading to loss of the aneuploid chromosome in some but not all daughter cells. Those pregnancies with a resulting diploid fetal karyotype may be more likely to progress; this mechanism is known as *trisomy rescue*.

To complicate matters further, CPM resulting from trisomy rescue places the fetus at risk for UPD, a condition in which both homologues of a given chromosome are inherited from one parent. This risk of UPD arises because the three chromosomes involved in the original trisomy are not equivalent. Two of the three chromosomes are inherited from one parent, and one of the three chromosomes

is inherited from the other parent. Thus, if one of the three chromosomes is randomly lost in the mitotic nondisjunction event, the remaining chromosomes will be of biparental inheritance two thirds of the time, but of uniparental inheritance one third of the time.

Two types of UPD occur: heterodisomy, in which the two chromosomes, although homologous, are not genetically identical, and isodisomy, in which the two chromosomes are identical. Because of recombination, both heterodisomic and isodisomic regions may be present. Centromeric heterodisomy results when the nondisjunction error occurs in meiosis I, and centromeric isodisomy results when the error occurs in meiosis II.

Clinical Outcomes of Confined Placental Mosaicism and Uniparental Disomy

A wide range of clinical phenotypes of CPM occur, depending on the extent of aneuploidy in the placenta, the particular chromosome involved in the aneuploidy, the presence or absence of UPD, and the type of UPD. Isodisomic UPD always carries the risk of "unmasking" a recessive gene and in fact was first identified in an individual with cystic fibrosis and short stature who had inherited two identical maternal copies of chromosome 7.[112] Both heterodisomic UPD and isodisomic UPD are problems for chromosomes with imprinted regions, areas in which gene expression is not equivalent for maternally and paternally inherited genes.

Uniparental disomy for chromosome 15 has been studied extensively. Maternal disomy results in Angelman syndrome, and paternal disomy results in Prader-Willi syndrome. Imprinted genes also exist on chromosomes 6, 7, 11, and 14. Established phenotypic effects result from maternal UPD for chromosomes 7 and 14 and from paternal UPD for chromosomes 6 and 11.[113] Paternal UPD for chromosome 21 and maternal UPD for chromosome 22 do not appear to have any phenotypic effect. Additional information on human imprinted regions and genes has been published.[114,115]

Constitutional Chromosome Anomalies Affecting Reproduction

Constitutional chromosome anomalies affecting reproduction can be divided into two classes: abnormalities involving autosomes and abnormalities involving one or more of the sex chromosomes. Within each of these groups, chromosome abnormalities can be numeric or structural.

In practice, numeric abnormalities affecting reproduction are limited to sex chromosome abnormalities, although issues of reproduction do affect individuals with trisomy 21. Males with trisomy 21 are usually subfertile or sterile and rarely reproduce, although exceptions have been reported.[116,117] Females with trisomy 21 are fertile, but they also rarely reproduce. Therefore, data on the risk of trisomy 21 in offspring are limited. According to Harper,[92] a risk of 1:3 is most likely.

A variety of structural chromosome rearrangements can affect reproductive outcome. Structural chromosome

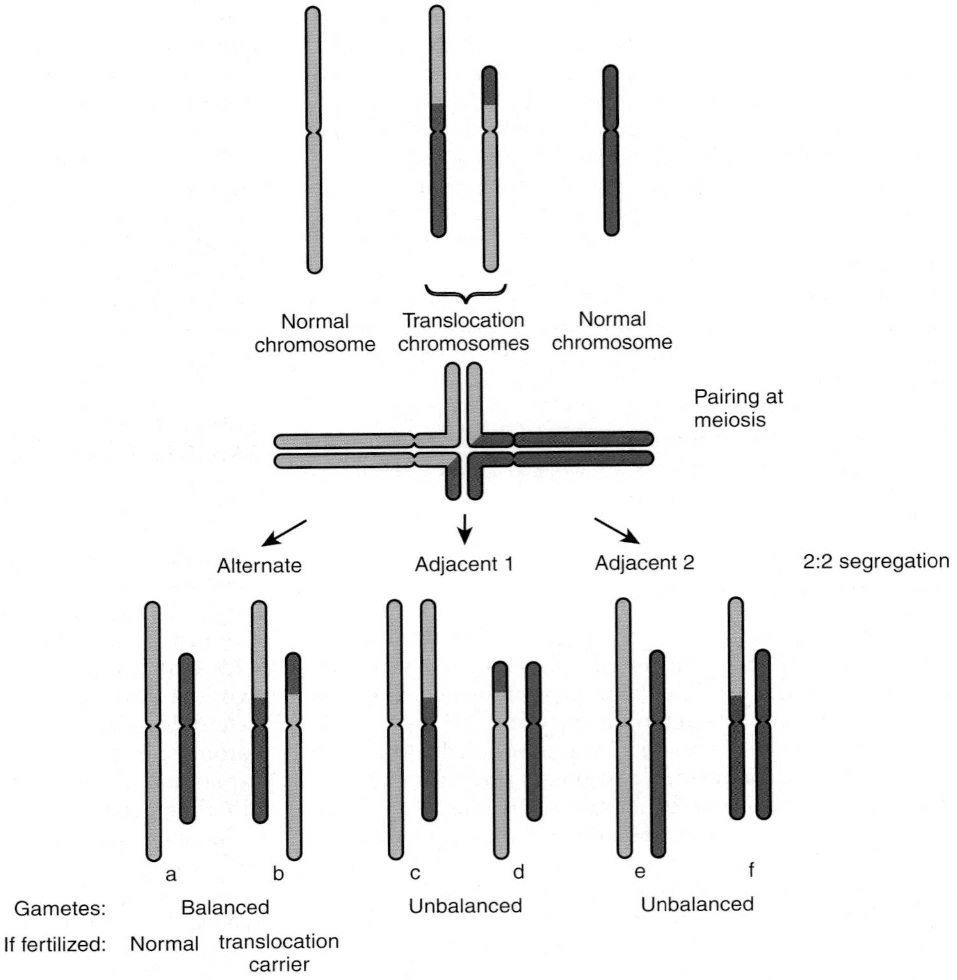

Figure 31-8. *Meiotic segregation with a reciprocal translocation. Of six possible gametes after 2:2 segregation, two will be balanced (a and b) and four will be unbalanced (c, d, e, and f). After fertilization with a normal haploid gamete, gamete a will produce a chromosomally normal conceptus and gamete b will produce a balanced carrier of the translocation.*

rearrangements can be considered either balanced or unbalanced. In balanced rearrangements, chromosomes contain the normal complement of genetic information. In unbalanced rearrangements, genetic information is either duplicated or missing. As with numeric abnormalities, unbalanced rearrangements with significant reproductive concerns are basically limited to sex chromosome rearrangements because unbalanced autosomal rearrangements produce fairly severe phenotypes or are nonviable. Balanced chromosome rearrangements usually do not have a phenotypic effect because essentially all of the genetic information is present, although the rearrangement may occasionally disrupt a gene or result in a cryptic duplication or deletion. Recent studies have shown that a substantial number (reported to be as large as approximately 40% of cases) of apparently balanced chromosomal rearrangements (as defined by G-banded karyotypic analysis) actually have gains or losses at or near the breakpoints or elsewhere in the genome.[31] However, even in the absence of any associated phenotype, carriers of presumably balanced structural rearrangements can produce unbalanced gametes, that is, gametes in which genetic information is duplicated or deleted. Because of this, carriers of balanced rearrangements are at increased risk for having abnormal offspring with unbalanced karyotypes. Balanced rearrangements also increase

the risk of both spontaneous abortions, which are presumably chromosomally unbalanced, and male infertility.[118-120]

STRUCTURAL CHROMOSOME REARRANGEMENTS

Translocations

Translocations (an exchange of chromatin between two or more chromosomes) are classified as reciprocal and robertsonian. Reciprocal translocations, as the name implies, involve presumably reciprocal exchange of a segment of one chromosome with a segment of another chromosome. Robertsonian translocations, the most common chromosome rearrangements in humans, involve essentially whole-arm exchange of the acrocentric chromosomes. More specifically, most robertsonian translocations involve two nonhomologous chromosomes and appear to result from recombination between homologous DNA sequences present in the proximal short arms of the acrocentric chromosomes.[121-123] The resulting rearrangement is a dicentric chromosome composed of the two long arms of the acrocentric chromosomes, with loss of most of the short arm material. One of the two centromeres is inactivated, allowing the robertsonian fusion to be stable throughout

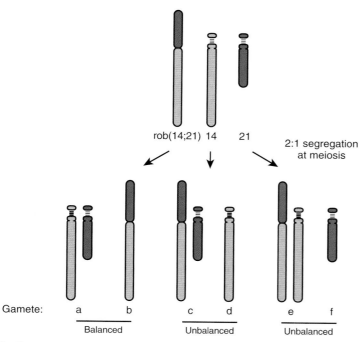

rob(14;21)   14   21

2:1 segregation
at meiosis

Gamete: a   b   c   d   e   f

            Balanced   Unbalanced   Unbalanced

If fertilized: Normal   rob(14;21) Trisomy 21 Monosomy 21 Trisomy 14 Monosomy 14
                         carrier

Figure 31-9. *Meiotic segregation in a robertsonian t(14;21)(q10;q10) carrier. Of six possible gametes after 2:1 segregation, two (a and b) will be balanced and four (c, d, e, and f) will be unbalanced. Of the unbalanced gametes, only one (c) has the potential to result in a live-born offspring.*

the cell cycle. Homologous robertsonian translocations are much less common than nonhomologous robertsonian translocations and, in fact, are usually isochromosomes, cytogenetically indistinguishable from homologous translocations.[124-127] Carriers of either homologous or non-homologous robertsonian translocations have a balanced karyotype containing 45 chromosomes.

Carriers of reciprocal translocations can produce both balanced and unbalanced gametes. Because homologous chromosome segments pair in meiosis, the two translocated chromosomes and the two normal chromosomes form a quadrivalent figure (Fig. 31-8). If the chromosomes segregate in such a way as to keep the two normal chromosomes together and the two translocation chromosomes together, the resulting gametes are either karyotypically normal or balanced. Of normal offspring, 50% will be karyotypically normal and 50% will be translocation carriers. On the other hand, if a normal chromosome segregates with a translocation chromosome, the resulting gametes will be unbalanced. Chromosomes from these quadrivalent figures can also undergo abnormal 3:1 segregation, which always produces unbalanced gametes.

In reciprocal translocation carriers, the risk of having an unbalanced liveborn offspring depends on several factors. Clearly, some unbalanced conceptuses are viable, whereas others are not. As a result, the risk of having a chromosomally abnormal offspring is different for carriers identified by chance and for those identified through a previous unbalanced liveborn offspring. In general, viability is more likely if the chromosome duplication or deletion is small, and duplicated material is usually more easily tolerated than deleted material. If the imbalance is a subset of a known viable imbalance, for example, duplication of a chromosome 21 segment, viability is a possibility and the phenotype

is likely to include some, if not all, of the features of the complete trisomy. Some translocations undergo 3:1 segregation more often than others; one common translocation, t(11;22)(q23;q22), frequently segregates in a 3:1 manner. Finally, for reasons that remain to be elucidated, female carriers of chromosome rearrangements are more likely than male carriers to have unbalanced offspring.

In carriers of robertsonian translocations, the risk of having unbalanced offspring depends both on the specific translocation and on the sex of the carrier. Presumably, unbalanced gametes produced by carriers of robertsonian translocations lead to conceptuses that are either monosomic or trisomic for one of the acrocentric chromosomes involved in the translocation. However, in assessing the risk of unbalanced offspring, only viable outcomes need to be considered. For example, carriers of the most common robertsonian translocation involving chromosome 21, rob(14;21), theoretically would produce, in equal proportion, six types of gametes, two of which would be balanced. Of the other four gametes, two would be nullisomic for either chromosome 14 or 21, and two would be disomic for one of these chromosomes. The two nullisomic gametes would lead to nonviable monosomy, whereas the two disomic gametes would lead to trisomy for either chromosome 14 or 21. Because trisomy 14 is nonviable, only three of the gametes could develop into viable offspring, and the risk of Down syndrome might be assumed to be approximately 1:3 (Fig. 31-9). In actuality, empirical risks to carriers of rob(14;21) and other nonhomologous robertsonian translocations are much lower (Table 31-4). The risks of unbalanced offspring are greater for female carriers of robertsonian translocations than for male carriers.

The risk of an abnormal trisomic conceptus increases to virtually 100% when a translocation involves whole-arm

TABLE 31-4

Empiric Probabilities of Unbalanced and Balanced Carrier Offspring for Robertsonian Carriers

Translocation	Sex of Carrier	Empiric Probability (Risk) of Unbalanced Offspring (%)	Empiric Probability of Balanced Carrier Offspring (%)
rob(13;14)*	Female	<1	50
	Male	Very low	50
rob(13;13)	Either sex	100	0
rob(14;21)*	Female	10	50
	Male	2.5	50
rob(21;22)	Female	6.8	50
	Male	<2.9	50
rob(21;21)	Either sex	100	0

*The risks for rob(13;15) are probably similar to those for rob(13;14); the risks for rob(13;21) and rob(15;21) are probably similar to those for rob(14;21). These translocations are much less common, so risk data are less extensive.

Adapted from Therman E, Susman M. Human Chromosomes: Structure, Behavior, and Effects, 3rd ed. New York, Springer-Verlag, 1993, p 295.

exchanges between two homologous acrocentric chromosomes. Most of these conceptuses end in spontaneous abortion. However, because trisomies 13 and 21 are viable, carriers of rob(13;13) and rob(21;21) can have liveborn offspring with trisomy. Thus, for genetic counseling purposes, a carrier of a homologous robertsonian translocation will have only spontaneous abortions or abnormal offspring with rare exceptions of trisomy rescue.

Rare exceptions include offspring carrying the same homologous robertsonian translocation without an additional copy of the chromosome inherited from the other parent. These exceptions arise either from fertilization with a nullisomic gamete or from a postzygotic loss of the normal, nontranslocated chromosome. These rare individuals, although karyotypically identical to the phenotypically normal carrier parent, have UPD because both copies of the chromosome have been inherited from the parent with the robertsonian translocation. Some of these individuals are phenotypically normal. Maternal UPD for chromosome 22 and paternal UPD for chromosome 21 appear to have no unusual phenotype.[124] However, UPD for chromosome 15, whether maternally or paternally inherited, has severe phenotypic consequences, resulting in either Prader-Willi syndrome or Angelman syndrome, respectively.

In addition to the risk of producing unbalanced gametes, male carriers of balanced translocations are at increased risk for infertility. The incidence of balanced autosomal translocations is approximately sixfold higher in infertile men than in the general population,[119] and translocations involving the X or Y chromosome frequently cause sterility.[128-130]

Inversions

Apparently balanced inversions, similar to apparently balanced translocations, most often have no phenotypic effect. However, like translocations, they are associated with an increased risk of abnormal gametes in the carrier. Two types of inversions exist: paracentric inversions, in which the inverted segment does not include the centromere, and pericentric inversions, in which the inverted segment includes the centromere. These two types of inversions carry different risks for chromosomally unbalanced offspring. In both types of inversions, the risk of chromosome imbalance is the result of meiotic recombination within the inverted segment. For a paracentric inversion, structural rearrangement resulting from recombination will lead to a dicentric chromosome and an acentric chromosome fragment. With rare exceptions, these recombinant chromosomes are not stable and will not lead to viable offspring. Pericentric inversions are more problematic. Recombination can produce monocentric chromosomes with duplicated and deleted material. These recombinant chromosomes are stable and can be found in unbalanced offspring. For two reasons, carriers of large pericentric inversions are at higher risk for having unbalanced offspring than are carriers of small pericentric inversions. First, a larger inverted chromosome segment is more likely than a small inverted segment to be involved in a recombination event. Second, the resulting duplication and deletion will be smaller if the inverted segment is larger, and thus, the offspring is more likely to be viable.

Insertions

Balanced insertions, another type of rearrangement, rarely have a phenotypic effect on the carrier, but portend an increased risk of abnormal gametes. If the two chromosomes involved in the insertion do not segregate together in meiosis, gametes with duplication or deletion of the inserted segment will result. Meiotic recombination can also produce recombinant chromosomes by crossing over between a specific region of a rearranged chromosome with the normal homologue. The risk of unbalanced liveborn offspring depends on the viability of the duplication or deletion.

SEX CHROMOSOME ABNORMALITIES

In humans, as in all mammals, the Y chromosome is the key determinant of sex. In the embryo, the human gonad is undifferentiated until approximately 6 to 7 weeks of development. The presence of a normal Y chromosome causes the indifferent gonad to develop into a testis. Testes produce two effectors responsible for subsequent male sexual differentiation, testosterone and anti-müllerian hormone. In the absence of a Y chromosome, the male differentiation pathway is not initiated, the indifferent gonad develops into an ovary, and female differentiation ensues. The Y-encoded gene critical for testes development, the SRY gene, has been cloned and characterized,[110-113,131-134] but the complete story of sexual differentiation remains to be elucidated. Clearly, additional gene products are required for normal sexual differentiation in both males and females. This observation has been evident for a long time on the basis of phenotypes of individuals with sex reversal and individuals whose chromosomes differ from the normal 46,XX or 46,XY.

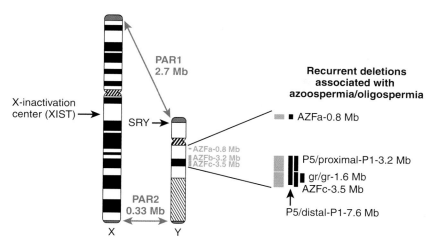

Figure 31-10. Idiograms of G-banded human X and Y chromosomes at the 450-band stage. Approximate locations of the two pseudoautosomal regions (PAR1 and PAR2) are indicated on the X and Y chromosomes. On the X chromosome, the location of the X-inactivation center that contains the XIST gene is also indicated. On the Y chromosome, the locations of the heterochromatic region (diagonally hatched lines), the azoospermic factors AZFa-c, and the testis-determining gene SRY, and the locations of recurrent deletions associated with either azoospermia or oligospermia (black vertical bars) are indicated.

The Y Chromosome

The structure of the Y chromosome has been studied extensively at both cytogenetic and molecular levels (Fig. 31-10). The Y chromosome is easy to distinguish cytogenetically on the basis of its small size and its extraordinarily bright fluorescence with quinacrine staining. This bright staining represents a heterochromatic region present in the distal segment of the long arm, which varies greatly in size in the human population without any apparent phenotypic effect. An essentially complete physical map of the Y chromosome was constructed in 1992 and estimated that the chromosome contains 58 to 60 Mb DNA.[3,135] More recently, an almost complete sequence of the euchromatic region of one Y chromosome was reported. This report shows the euchromatic region to be approximately 23 Mb, including 8 Mb on the short arm and 14.5 Mb on the long arm.[136] Euchromatin in the Y chromosome is derived from several million base pairs of DNA from autosomes, and represents a majority of noncoding genes and a minority of coding gene families predominantly expressed in testis.[137] Large palindromic repeats in this region maintained by intrachromosomal gene conversion lead to predictable patterns of DNA loss and spermatogenic failure.[138] More than 100 Y-linked, testis-specific transcripts have been identified.

Two regions on the Y chromosome can pair and recombine with the X chromosome during male meiosis. These two homologous regions are known as *pseudoautosomal regions* because DNA sequences in these regions undergo homologous recombination and hence do not show strictly sex-linked inheritance.[53] These two regions, PAR1 and PAR2, are found at the tips of the short and long arms, respectively. PAR1 is the major pseudoautosomal region and the site of an obligate crossing over between X and Y chromosomes during male meiosis. PAR2 is the minor pseudoautosomal region. Crossing over in this chromosome segment is neither necessary nor sufficient for successful male meiosis.

Genes within PAR1 have homologous copies on the X chromosome and escape X-inactivation in females. The 24 PAR1 genes have no known sex-specific functions. *SHOX*, located in PAR1, is the only known disease gene within PAR1 and PAR2 and plays a role in various short stature conditions and disturbed bone development.[139-143] Of the five genes mapped to PAR2, the two most proximal, *SPRY3* and *SYBL1*, undergo X-inactivation.[144]

Just proximal to PAR1 on Yp, the short arm of the Y chromosome, is the *SRY* gene. In rare cases, recombination outside of PAR1 occurs and can produce XX males and XY females. XX males carry *SRY* on one of their X chromosomes, whereas XY females have a Y chromosome deleted for *SRY*. DNA analysis of these sex-reversed individuals was instrumental in mapping *SRY* to an approximately 140-kb segment of the Y chromosome.[145] The *SRY* gene was cloned several years later.[131] Its identity was verified by molecular analysis of female 46,XY individuals with point mutations in *SRY*.[146,147]

Between the two PAR regions is the bulk of the Y chromosome, termed the *male-specific region,* or MSY.[136] An essentially complete sequence of the Y chromosome, with discussion of its salient features, has been published.[136] This region accounts for 95% of the chromosome and contains a combination of heterochromatic sequences plus three categories of euchromatic sequences: X-degenerate, X-transposed, and ampliconic. The X-degenerate sequences reflect a common autosomal ancestor from which the X and Y chromosomes have diverged, whereas the X-transposed sequences are the result of a more recent transposition event that occurred after the divergence of humans and chimpanzees.[136,148] The ampliconic sequences are composed of long repeat units with greater than 99.9% identity between repeat pairs, which is hypothesized to be maintained by gene conversion. The ampliconic sequences contain 64 of the 83 MSY genes.

The ampliconic and X-degenerate sequences represent most of the genes on the Y chromosome. Genes within the ampliconic sequences have testis-specific expression. Most are members of Y chromosome gene families and do not have homologous copies on the X chromosome. Genes within the X-degenerate sequences have homologous X chromosome copies, and most have ubiquitous tissue expression. One notable exception is *SRY*, which has predominantly testis-specific expression.

The idea that genes involved in spermatogenesis and growth control are present in the euchromatic portion of the long arm of chromosome Y was first hypothesized more than 30 years ago because of the association of cytogenetically visible Yq deletions with azoospermia and short stature.[149-151] Seven recurrent deletions in Yq have been defined, AZFa (azoospermic factor a), P5-proximal P1 (AZFb), P5-distal P1, AZFc (b2/b4), gr/gr, b1/b3, and b2/b3, and several are known to affect spermatogenesis.[152] Y chromosome microdeletions can lead to azoospermia or severe oligospermia, with an estimated incidence of a minimum of 15% of cases of idiopathic male infertility.[153-155] AZFc deletions are the most commonly diagnosed molecular cause of spermatogenic failure and are associated with a variable phenotype. Furthermore, gr/gr deletions (sometimes referred to as "DAZ1/DAZ2"—deleted in azoospermia), a subset of AZFc (b2/b4) deletions, have an even more variable spermatogenic failure phenotype and have been associated with susceptibility to testicular germ cell tumors.[156] Diagnostic testing includes screening for deletions in AZFa, P5/P1, and AZFc, and in some cases, for gr/gr.[152] There is extremely little chance of finding sperm during a testicular sperm extraction procedure in the presence of either an AZFa or a P1/P5 deletion, whereas men with AZFc deletions may have sperm in their testis.

Genes within AZF regions have been identified and include *USP9Y* (ubiquitin-specific peptidase 9, Y-linked) and *DDX3Y* (DEAD [Asp-Glu-Ala-Asp] box polypeptide 3, Y-linked) in AZFa and *RBMY* (RNA-binding motif protein on the Y chromosome) in AZFb. The *DAZ* genes, present in a cluster of four copies within AZFc, are predicted to be RNA-binding proteins by DNA sequence[153,157] and have been shown to have testis-limited expression.[153] Although no point mutations have been identified within these genes, approximately 6% to 13% of men with oligospermia or azoospermia have deletions of most or all of this gene cluster. No deletions have been seen in men with normal sperm counts.[153,157-159]

In both *Drosophila* and mice, loss of function of the *DAZ* gene homologues leads to infertility, further supporting a critical role for the human *DAZ* genes in spermatogenesis. Similar to the *DAZ* genes, *RBMY* is a member of a multicopy gene family.[160,161] Its gene product localizes to the nucleus of spermatogenic cells, and deletions of this gene have been documented in infertile males.[162,163] A point mutation in *USP9Y*, one of two genes located within AZFa, has been associated with spermatogenic failure.[164] Unlike *DAZ* and *RBMY*, which are members of multigene families residing in ampliconic sequences with testis-limited expression, *USP9Y* is a single-copy gene, with an X-linked homologous gene and tissue-ubiquitous expression.[136]

In addition to sterility, structural aberrations of the Y chromosome can have other phenotypic effects, including intersex and females with symptoms of Turner syndrome. Correlations between specific structural aberrations and phenotypes have been difficult to make because the abnormal Y chromosome is frequently present in one of multiple cell lines within an individual. The second cell line may be normal male, normal female, or 45,X, or may have an additional abnormal sex chromosome. Whenever the possibility of Y chromosome material in a phenotypic female exists, molecular testing to determine the presence

of Y material is important because these females are at increased risk for gonadoblastoma.

Structural aberrations of the Y chromosome with no phenotypic effect exist as well. Large portions of the heterochromatic region can be deleted without any phenotypic effect, and large variations in the size of this region are common polymorphisms. Also fairly prevalent is a pericentric inversion that is present in approximately 1:200 males and moves the centromere to the border of the heterochromatic region. More rare (but still considered a normal variant) is the presence of satellites on the long arm of the Y chromosome, resulting from a translocation between the Y chromosome and an acrocentric chromosome (usually chromosome 15).

The X Chromosome

The structure of the X chromosome has also been studied extensively at the cytogenetic and molecular levels. The X chromosome is estimated to be 185 cM[165] and contains approximately 152 Mb of DNA.[3,137] Approximately 1100 genes are annotated on the X chromosome, and at least 800 encode proteins.[166]

The presence of two X chromosomes in normal mammalian females compared with a single X chromosome in normal mammalian males demands a mechanism for dosage compensation of X-linked genes. This is accomplished through inactivation of essentially one X chromosome in females. The theory of X-inactivation[167] was developed from studies in cats in which condensed chromatin (Barr body) was detected in females, but not in males. Subsequently, it was shown that humans with numeric sex chromosome abnormalities always had one fewer Barr body than the number of X chromosomes, resulting in a single active X chromosome.

The process of X-inactivation is believed to involve three mechanisms: a counting mechanism that determines X chromosome number, a choice mechanism that randomly selects an active and an inactive X chromosome, and a silencing mechanism that causes transcriptional inactivation of most of the genes along the inactive X chromosome. The silencing mechanism is further subdivided into three separate processes: initiation of inactivation, spreading of inactivation along the length of the X chromosome, and lastly, maintenance of inactivation throughout subsequent cell divisions. Inactivation requires, in *cis*, the X-inactivation center (XIC), which maps to chromosome region Xq13.[168,169] *XIST*, the critical gene within the X-inactivation center that initiates inactivation, encodes a functional, non–protein-encoding RNA that is transcribed from the inactive X chromosome.[170-174] This RNA coats the inactive X chromosome, which also acquires other features associated with transcriptional inactivation (e.g., late replication, hypoacetylation, and hypermethylation). The product of *XIST*, although critical for initiation of X-inactivation, does not appear to be required for maintenance of inactivation.[175] X chromosome inactivation is opposed by *TSIX*, an anti-sense transcript of *XIST* that regulates *XIST* in *cis* and determines X chromosome choice without affecting silencing.[176] Recently, it has been determined that murine (and presumably human) *Xist* and *Tsix* form duplexes in vivo that are processed to small RNAs, most likely on the active X chromosome in a Dicer-dependent manner, implicating RNA interference (RNAi) in X chromosome inactivation.[177]

X-inactivation occurs early in development and is considered random for maternal and paternal X chromosomes. However, nonrandom X-inactivation is seen in females with structural abnormalities and with single-gene disorders of the X chromosome (e.g., Duchenne muscular dystrophy). In females carrying a structurally abnormal X chromosome, cells with the normal active X may survive preferentially. Conversely, in females with balanced translocations between an X chromosome and an autosome, the normal X chromosome may appear to be inactivated preferentially. Presumably, this reflects survival of cells with active autosomal material because inactivation can spread into autosomal material in X-autosome rearrangements. Once X-inactivation occurs, it appears to be irreversible, except in oogenesis, during which time reactivation of the inactive X chromosome occurs at some point before meiosis.

Inactivation does not abrogate transcription of all genes on the X chromosome. The first genes discovered to escape X-inactivation were located within PAR1, and it was once believed that all genes escaping inactivation would be located in this region, thus maintaining equal dosage between males and females for genes with functional copies on the Y chromosome. Now genes escaping inactivation have been identified throughout the X chromosome. Some of these genes have functional copies on the Y chromosome outside the pseudoautosomal regions (e.g., ZFX and RPS4X), and thus, as with genes in the pseudoautosomal region, equal dosage between males and females is maintained by the absence of X-inactivation in females. However, some of the genes escaping X-inactivation do not have homologues on the Y chromosome (e.g., UBA1 and SMC1A). These genes may have higher expression in females than in males. Most likely, the activity of genes escaping X-inactivation leads to some of the abnormalities seen in individuals with an abnormal number of X chromosomes.[178] The mechanism whereby specific genes escape X-inactivation remains enigmatic and is an area of intense research.

Numerous aberrations of the X chromosome have been identified and used to define regions of the chromosome. Just distal to XIC is the "critical region" that appears to be required on both X chromosomes for normal ovarian function.[179] Although many balanced rearrangements of the X chromosome have no phenotype, this critical region must remain intact for normal female sexual development. In addition to this critical region, specific ovarian maintenance determinants may exist on both arms of the X chromosome because a variety of deletions in either the short or the long arm are associated with ovarian dysgenesis in Turner syndrome. However, it is also possible that the ovarian dysgenesis seen with deletions or translocations of the X chromosome is caused, not by deletion of specific critical genes, but by an alteration of chromosome structure or dynamics, perhaps affecting the ability of the X chromosomes to pair completely during meiosis.[180,181] Several genes along the X chromosome contribute to ovarian

function, and both X-linked and non–X-linked factors are likely to contribute to premature ovarian failure. The most common cause of premature ovarian failure is an FMR1 premutation. Unlike fragile X syndrome, in which full mutations of FMR1 result in the absence of FMR1 protein, in cells with premutation alleles, FMR1 messenger RNA levels are elevated and reduced translational efficiency of the premutated alleles results in decreased FMR1 protein.[182]

X-autosome translocations have a variety of phenotypes. They may occasionally disrupt an X-linked gene, resulting in X-linked recessive diseases both in males and in females. Males manifest the recessive disease because they are hemizygous for the X chromosome. Females may be affected because of preferential inactivation of the normal X chromosome. X-autosome translocations may also impair fertility in both sexes, and as with any translocation, they may segregate improperly and result in unbalanced offspring. Individuals with translocations between an X and a Y chromosome can be phenotypically female or male, depending on the breakpoints of the translocation, the pattern of X-inactivation, and the remaining chromosome constitution.

Numeric Abnormalities of Sex Chromosomes

Numeric abnormalities of sex chromosomes are much more prevalent than numeric abnormalities of autosomes, with an overall frequency of 1:500 births. Individuals with as many as five sex chromosomes (penta-X syndrome) have been identified, but the most common sex chromosome abnormalities are the trisomies XXX, XXY, and XYY. The viability of those affected by these abnormalities is good, as evidenced by the fairly high frequency among liveborn infants and the low frequency among spontaneous abortions. Conversely, monosomy for the X chromosome is significantly less common among liveborn infants, but is the most frequent chromosomal abnormality in spontaneous abortions.[39,74] For all sex chromosome abnormalities, mosaicism with normal and abnormal cell lines is often observed.

Turner Syndrome and Variants. Turner syndrome is widely known as 45,X, although approximately 50% of individuals with Turner syndrome have a variation of this karyotype (see Chapters 16 and 17). Approximately 15% of patients have one normal X chromosome and one structurally aberrant X chromosome. These structural abnormalities of the X chromosome include deletions of portions of the short and long arms as well as isochromosomes. Approximately 25% to 30% of patients are mosaic, with one 45,X cell line and a second cell line that might contain, among others, either two normal X chromosomes (i.e., 45,X/46,XX), one normal and one abnormal X chromosome (i.e., 45,X/46,X,i[Xq]), or one X and one Y chromosome (i.e., 45,X/46,XY).

In apparent nonmosaic 45,X individuals, the single X chromosome is maternal in origin 80% of the time. In other words, the meiotic error is usually paternal.[183,184] The basis for the unusually high frequency of X or Y chromosome nondisjunction in paternal meiosis is unknown, but may relate to limited meiotic recombination between the X and Y chromosomes. Of note, the X–Y bivalent is estimated to have the highest rate of nondisjunction in paternal meiosis I among all chromosome pairs.[185] Whether paternal age is a risk factor for Turner syndrome is unclear. Advanced maternal age, however, is not correlated with this disorder. An alternative mechanism is postfertilization loss of either the X or the Y chromosome, based on the high frequency of 45,X (1% to 2% of clinically recognized pregnancies) compared with the reciprocal products of 47,XXY, 47,XYY, and 47,XXX. Random loss of an X or a Y chromosome in a normal XX or XY embryo would result in an excess of 45,X of paternal origin and the 45,Y embryo would not be viable.[185]

A number of phenotypic abnormalities are characteristic of Turner syndrome. The most common findings are short stature (<5 feet or 150 cm) and gonadal dysgenesis (usually streak gonads). Fetal cystic hygroma, resulting from lymphedema and leading to postnatal webbed neck, is also common. Other associated anomalies include low posterior hairline, shield chest with widely spaced nipples, cubitus valgus, cardiac anomalies (frequently coarctation of the aorta), and renal anomalies. Although mental retardation is not more common in individuals with Turner syndrome than in females with two X chromosomes, deficiencies in spatial perception, perceptual motor organization, and fine motor skills are more frequent. Turner syndrome is fully compatible with life. It is therefore puzzling why 45,X is usually lethal in utero. Furthermore, 45,X is the most common chromosomal abnormality in spontaneous abortions, with more than 99% of 45,X conceptuses being spontaneously aborted.[74]

Another phenotype of Turner syndrome is infertility, resulting from increased germ cell attrition. In the absence of a Y chromosome, the gonad develops into an ovary in which germ cells are initially present. However, germ cells rapidly degenerate during the fetal period and the resulting lack of oocytes leads to streak gonads and amenorrhea. Most patients carrying deletions of either the short or the long arm of the X chromosome have ovarian dysgenesis.[179] Thus, two complete X chromosomes are necessary for normal ovarian development and function.

Obtaining the karyotype of individuals with Turner syndrome is clinically important, because although many of the distinct symptoms of Turner syndrome seem to be randomly distributed with respect to different deletions throughout the X chromosome, some correlations with phenotype can be made.[180] Most individuals with breakpoints distal to Xq25 have few abnormalities except occasional secondary amenorrhea or premature menopause. Short stature is almost always associated with deletions of the distal portion of the short arm, and less often with long arm deletions. Determination of the presence of Y chromosomal material is of critical medical importance because it leads to an increased risk of gonadoblastoma in sex-reversed individuals, as mentioned earlier. Routine cytogenetic testing for individuals with a suspected sex chromosome disorder often includes a count of 30 metaphase preparations, which rules out greater than 10% mosaicism at a 95% confidence level.[186]

Even with this stringent level of classic cytogenetic workup, some individuals with a nonmosaic 45,X karyotype may have an undetected cell line with Y chromosomal material. As such, molecular studies for the detection of Y chromosomal DNA should be considered. In addition, rare patients with features of Turner syndrome are determined to have a 46,XY karyotype missing a portion of the Y chromosome.[187] These individuals also have an increased risk of gonadoblastoma.

Mosaicism for 45,X and a second cell line is not uncommon. In addition, 45,X/46,XX mosaicism is the most common sex chromosome mosaicism diagnosed from genetic amniocentesis. Of 114 cases reviewed,[89] approximately 10% had some features of Turner syndrome and approximately 4% had other anomalies. Although the majority of these cases were phenotypically normal at either birth or termination, many of the features of Turner syndrome might not be recognized until puberty, and prenatal counseling remains difficult. For 45,X/46,XY individuals, the phenotype ranges from normal fertile males to individuals with ambiguous genitalia to females with Turner syndrome. Presumably, different phenotypes reflect different tissue distributions of the various cell lines. In a compilation of prenatally diagnosed cases,[89] 90% to 95% of cases of 45,X/46,XY resulted in a normal male phenotype. When a karyotype of 45,X/46,XY is detected at prenatal diagnosis, detailed ultrasonography of the genitalia is recommended. If the genitalia appear to be normal male, the prognosis is fairly reliable for a phenotypically normal male. If the genitalia appear to be female, Turner syndrome or ambiguous genitalia are more likely to be present at birth.

In normal females and males, loss of a sex chromosome in peripheral blood cells can occur, leading to apparent mosaicism for 45,X. Although this type of X chromosome aneuploidy was once thought to be more frequent in women with multiple pregnancy losses, it is now recognized that 45,X aneuploidy in peripheral blood increases with age and that this age-related phenomenon is not associated with reproductive loss.[188,189]

47,XXX. Individuals with three X chromosomes, or triple X syndrome, appear physically normal, although by adolescence, many are taller than average. Despite the expectation that 50% of offspring would carry an extra X chromosome, the actual empirical risk to offspring is low. Prospective studies with long-term follow-up of 47,XXX individuals indicate that although mental retardation is not present, the IQ of many of these patients is 10 to 15 points below that of their siblings. Language delay, learning disabilities, and impaired gross motor skills are also common, as are psychosocial disorders, particularly depression.[190-193]

In females with three X chromosomes, approximately 90% have two maternal X chromosomes and 10% have two paternal X chromosomes. When there are two maternal X chromosomes, 66% of cases are due to meiosis I errors, 18% are due to meiosis II errors, and 16% are due to postzygotic errors. In two of the informative cases describing two paternally derived X chromosomes, both were due to postzygotic errors.[183] Increased maternal age is a risk factor for 47,XXX.

Klinefelter Syndrome/47,XXY. Males with the 47,XXY karyotype have a fairly well-defined phenotype known as Klinefelter syndrome. They are tall and thin, with long legs (see Chapters 16 and 17). Physical appearance is fairly normal until puberty, when a characteristic eunuchoid habitus presentation develops. Secondary sexual characteristics are underdeveloped and testes remain small, with azoospermia and subsequent infertility. Gynecomastia may occur. IQ is reduced in this patient population, and two thirds of patients have educational problems, particularly dyslexia.

Approximately 50% of 47,XXY individuals have two paternally derived sex chromosomes, and approximately 50% have two maternally inherited X chromosomes.[77,183] In all cases, when there are two paternally derived sex chromosomes (i.e., one X and one Y chromosome), the error must have occurred in meiosis I. When there are two maternal sex chromosomes (i.e., two X chromosomes), approximately 70% of cases are due to a meiosis I error, 25% to a meiosis II error, and 5% to postzygotic nondisjunction.[183] Increased maternal age appears to be associated only with maternal meiosis I errors.

47,XYY. The most consistent phenotype in 47,XYY individuals is increased height. Increased risk of behavioral problems and perhaps some decrease in intelligence may be associated with this karyotype. Fertility is normal, and these individuals are not found to be at increased risk for having a chromosomally abnormal child. All 47,XYY cases result from either a paternal meiosis II error or a postzygotic error.

Sex Chromosome Tetrasomy and Pentasomy. Although studies of the phenotype of sex chromosome tetrasomy and pentasomy do not exist from unbiased ascertainment (i.e., all information is based on case reports of postnatally identified individuals), it is generally assumed that with an increasing number of supernumerary sex chromosomes comes an increasingly severe phenotype. Supernumerary X chromosomes are clinically more severe than supernumerary Y chromosomes, presumably because the Y chromosome encodes so few genes. Even though supernumerary X chromosomes are inactivated essentially, some genes escape X-inactivation, and increased dosage of these gene products presumably leads to the clinical phenotype. Mental capacity is increasingly diminished with each supernumerary X chromosome, with an estimated decrease of 15 IQ points for each additional X chromosome. In males, supernumerary X chromosomes lead not only to infertility but also to malformed genitalia. The effect on fertility in females with supernumerary X chromosomes is unclear. Fewer cases of supernumerary Y chromosomes have been reported, but additional Y chromosomes also appear to cause decreased mental capacity, although the effect is less pronounced than with supernumerary X chromosomes (reviewed by Linden et al.[192]).

Chromosome Abnormalities and Sex Reversal

Although the testis-determining factor on the Y chromosome has been identified for almost two decades, elucidation of the human sex determination pathway is far from complete (see Chapter 16). SRY itself is expressed in a temporal and tissue-specific manner, indicating interaction of upstream regulatory genes, such as GATA4, FOG2, and WT1.[131,194] Although no direct target gene for SRY has been conclusively identified, indirect observations suggest that SOX9 (SRY HMG box–related gene 9) is one molecular target. The SRY gene product binds DNA sequences in vitro, indicating that the SRY protein exerts its effect in vivo by regulating transcription of other genes.[131] Loss-of-function mutations in SRY account for approximately 10% to 15% of XY sex reversal through gonadal dysgenesis after birth.[195]

The existence of several chromosome abnormalities associated with sex reversal has played an integral role in the identification of additional genes involved in sex determination. Both deletions of 9p24 and duplications of Xp21 have been associated with XY sex reversal.[196,197] DMRT1 has emerged as a likely gene within 9p24 to be involved in male sex determination.[198,199] DMRT1 contains a zinc finger DNA-binding domain (termed "DM") that is also present in two genes involved in invertebrate sex determination, the Drosophila doublesex (dsx) gene and the Caenorhabditis elegans mab-3 gene. In the mouse, DMRT1 was also shown to be required for testis formation.[200,201] Within Xp21, NROB1 was identified as encoding another critical component of the male sex determination pathway. NROB1, an orphan nuclear hormone receptor, exerts an antagonistic effect in the male sex determination pathway. Overexpression of the gene prevents testes development, despite the presence of an intact SRY gene.[197,202] Because duplications of NROB1 lead to XY sex reversal, whereas supernumerary X chromosomes do not, NROB1 is presumably subject to X-inactivation.

Other transcription factors implicated in male sex determination include SOX9, SF1 (steroidogenic factor-1), WT1 (Wilms tumor 1), and GATA4 (a zinc finger transcription factor). SOX9 was first mapped to 17q24-q25 in patients with apparently balanced translocations and campomelic dysplasia.[203] A portion of the SOX9 gene has significant homology to the DNA-binding domain (high-mobility group box) of SRY and has been shown to bind to the same DNA sequences in vitro.[204] SOX9 is likely to be a critical component of sex determination in all vertebrates. In mammals, SRY may act directly through SOX9.[205]

Any phenotypic female with the SRY gene is susceptible to gonadoblastoma. At risk are not only patients with Turner syndrome, but also XY individuals with gonadal dysgenesis or an androgen insensitivity syndrome. As more of the genes involved in sex determination are identified, it will remain important to identify all phenotypic females carrying the SRY gene.

Preimplantation Genetic Diagnosis

Over the last decade, multicolor FISH has contributed to the field of preimplantation genetic diagnosis ([PGD] see Chapter 30). By combining assisted reproductive technologies with genetic analysis of single cells, PGD allows the screening of pre-embryos before their transfer, with the goal of transferring only those embryos that would not develop into an individual with a specific genetic disease or condition. However, because the genetic analyses of PGD are performed on only one or two cells per embryo, it is critical to view these tests as screening tests only.

To obtain material for genetic analysis, most centers performing PGD employ embryo biopsy.[206] Blastomeres removed from pre-embryos are tested for specific gene defects using single-cell PCR, followed by a variety of molecular diagnostic techniques or FISH screening for specific chromosomal aberrations. PGD with FISH has been used in the following three ways: sex identification for carriers of X-linked recessive disorders[207,208]; chromosome imbalance screening for couples in which one member is a carrier of an apparently balanced chromosome rearrangement (e.g., chromosome translocation carriers)[209-211]; and aneuploidy screening for patients with advanced maternal age, a history of multiple spontaneous abortions, or repeated in vitro fertilization failures.[212-215]

Among these three applications of FISH, identification of presumptive fetal sex is the most straightforward because it requires analysis of only two chromosomal regions, one Y-specific region and one X-specific region. Commercial probes producing bright hybridization signals are available for both the X and Y chromosomes in a variety of colors. With just two probes labeled in different colors, hybridization patterns for normal male, normal female, and sex chromosome aneuploidy can be distinguished. FISH analysis is the method of choice for sex identification because 45,X and 47,XXY embryos have been misdiagnosed as normal by PCR.[216]

When the indication for PGD is the presence of a balanced chromosomal rearrangement in one member of a couple, testing is complicated by the need to distinguish the two balanced chromosomal configurations (balanced carrier and normal noncarrier) from the numerous possible unbalanced segregation products. Probe strategies that detect all possible unbalanced products may not be as good as strategies that miss some of the unbalanced products, especially if the undetected products are unlikely to occur or unlikely to be viable. The addition of extra probes required to detect all possible segregation products will reduce the overall efficiency of hybridization and increase the likelihood of visualizing overlap of the probe signals, thus reducing the diagnostic accuracy of the test.[217] For this reason, when devising the detection strategy, it is important to balance the risks of occurrence and potential viability for any specific abnormal segregation product against the decreased accuracy created by the addition of any probe. Similarly, the use of each additional color can increase the information provided (e.g., discriminate between a balanced carrier and a normal noncarrier), but simultaneously can increase the difficulty of interpretation.

A limited number of centers have offered preimplantation genetic screening for aneuploidy for indications of advanced maternal age, history of multiple in vitro fertilization failures, and repeat spontaneous abortions.[212-215] With the commercial availability of probe sets designed to enumerate five chromosomes simultaneously (either 13, 18, 21, X, and Y or 13, 16, 18, 21, and 22), additional laboratories may begin to offer preimplantation genetic diagnosis–based aneuploidy screening. Although the data support a high rate of aneuploidy in the embryos from these patient populations, it is controversial whether this type of aneuploidy screen actually increases the likelihood of a successful pregnancy (reviewed by Handyside and Ogilvie[218]). Recent guidelines from the British Fertility Society show no robust evidence that the use of preimplantation genetic screening for advanced maternal age improves the live birth rate.[219]

The complete reference list can be found on the companion Expert Consult Web site at www.expertconsultbook.com.

Cytogenetics Web Resources

www.biologia.uniba.it/rmc/
This site from the Cytogenetics Unit at the University of Bari, Italy, provides information on probes, protocols, and chromosome idiograms.

www.bwhpathology.org/dgap
This site represents the Developmental Genome Anatomy Project (DGAP) at Harvard University. The DGAP posts balanced chromosome rearrangements in individuals with congenital anomalies with the goal of identifying genes critical to human development that are disrupted or dysregulated at the breakpoints.

www.hcforum.net
The Human Cytogenetics Forum provides a database of chromosome rearrangements and their references. Chromosomal rearrangements can be queried for their previous description and for their potential to result in liveborn infants, based on their genetic content, as assessed by R-banding. This site provides a useful resource for genetic counseling for couples with chromosomal rearrangements.

www.mcndb.org
This site represents a network of cytogenetic laboratories, Mendelian Cytogenetics Network (MCN), for the systematic identification and mapping of disease-associated balanced chromosome rearrangements (DBCRs) that truncate or inactivate specific genes. The online database, MCNdb, serves as a resource for genotype–phenotype delineation in humans.

www.molgen.mpg.de/~cytogen
This site at the Max-Planck-Institute for Molecular Genetics includes the YAC/BAC FISH mapping resource for the Mendelian Cytogenetics Network (MCN Reference Center).

Suggested Readings

Anderson RA, Pickering S. The current status of preimplantation genetic screening: British Fertility Society Policy and Practice Guidelines. Hum Fertil (Camb) 11(2):71-75, 2008.

Blaschke RJ, Rappold G. The pseudoautosomal regions, SHOX and disease. Curr Opin Genet Dev 16(3):233-239, 2006.

Camerino G, Parma P, Radi O, Valentini S. Sex determination and sex reversal. Curr Opin Genet Dev 16(3):289-292, 2006.

Disteche CM. Escape from X inactivation in human and mouse. Trends Genet 11:17-22, 1995.

Hall H, Hunt P, Hassold T. Meiosis and sex chromosome aneuploidy: how meiotic errors cause aneuploidy; how aneuploidy causes meiotic errors. Curr Opin Genet Dev 16(3):323-329, 2006.

Higgins AW, Alkuraya FS, Bosco AF, et al. Characterization of apparently balanced chromosomal rearrangements from the developmental genome anatomy project. Am J Hum Genet 82(3):712-722, 2008.

Iafrate AJ, Feuk L, Rivera MN, et al. Detection of large-scale variation in the human genome. Nat Genet 36(9):949-951, 2004.

Kallioniemi A, Kallioniemi OP, Sudar D, et al. Comparative genomic hybridization for molecular cytogenetic analysis of solid tumors. Science 258(5083):818-821, 1992.

Lee C, Iafrate AJ, Brothman AR. Copy number variations and clinical cytogenetic diagnosis of constitutional disorders. Nat Genet 39(7 Suppl):S48-S54, 2007.

Ogawa Y, Sun BK, Lee JT. Intersection of the RNA interference and X-inactivation pathways. Science 320(5881):1336-1341, 2008.

Ross MT, Bentley DR, Tyler-Smith C. The sequences of the human sex chromosomes. Curr Opin Genet Dev 16(3):213-218, 2006.

Schreck RR, Disteche CM. Chromosome banding techniques. Curr Protoc Hum Genet Chapter 4:Unit 4.2, 2001.

Schreck RR, Warburton D, Miller OJ, et al. Chromosome structure as revealed by a combined chemical and immunochemical procedure. Proc Natl Acad Sci U S A 70(3):804-807, 1973.

Shaffer LG, Agan N, Goldberg JD, et al. American College of Medical Genetics statement of diagnostic testing for uniparental disomy. Genet Med 3(3):206-211, 2001.

Shaffer LG, Tommerup N (eds). ISCN 2005: An International System for Human Cytogenetic Nomenclature. Basel, S. Karger, 2005.

CHAPTER 32

Evaluation of Hormonal Status

Enrico Carmina and Rogerio A. Lobo

This chapter reviews the assessment of hormonal status in the practice of reproductive endocrinology. The patient will often provide useful biologic information, such as changes induced by hypoestrogenism, skin changes with androgen excess, and galactorrhea in hyperprolactinemia. The clinically relevant symptoms and signs associated with various disorders are discussed in other chapters. This chapter describes various types of hormonal assays and dynamic tests used in the evaluation of reproductive disorders, as well as diagnostic radiographic techniques. This new edition includes several hormones and substances that are produced in adipose tissue and describes the methods used to measure fat quantity and distribution. It also offers several algorithms for diagnosis with hormonal assessments.

Principles of Hormonal Assays

Most hormone assays are based on immunologic methods. Antibodies are particularly useful for measuring hormones because they are able to detect very small quantities of the target antigen (picomolar range in biologic fluids). The immunologic reaction between the antibody and the antigen allows the process of competitive binding of the labeled hormone or antibody with hormone in the biologic fluid, showing the concentration of the hormone in question through comparison with a standard curve generated with known quantities of hormone. Two main immunologic methods exist: immunoassays and immunometric assays.[1] Immunoassays use small quantities of antibodies that can bind either labeled (added reagents) or unlabeled antigen (hormone present in the specimen). Because the labeled reagent will compete with the unlabeled hormone for binding, the higher the concentration of the natural hormone in the patient's fluid (usually serum), the less labeled reagent will bind to antibody.

Immunometric assays are useful for larger hormones, such as peptide hormones, and consist of labeled antibodies (generally two different antibodies that recognize two different parts of the hormone). This immunologic reaction forms a "sandwich" with the antigen in the middle. The label is placed on the second antibody.

The more common labels are radioactive isotopes (usually iodine or tritium), but enzymes, fluorescent compounds, and chemiluminescent molecules are increasingly used. Most laboratories use radioimmunoassays (RIAs), in which the label is radioactive; immunoradiometric assays (IRMAs); enzyme-linked immunosorbent assays (ELISA); or chemoluminescent assays (ICMA). The latter methods have gained popularity, both because of their flexibility and because they do not require radioactive material. In Figure 32-1, a scheme of the most common methods is shown.[2] In general, RIAs, IRMAs, and chemiluminescent immunometric assays are more sensitive and may be needed to measure very low concentrations of hormones.

In recent years, there also has been a trend toward the use of immunoassay systems that are able to analyze multiple analytes and process multiple samples rapidly. An example of this technology is the Immulite system (Siemens Healthcare Diagnostics, Deerfield IL; described in greater detail later in this chapter), which uses a chemiluminescent label and can simultaneously perform several immunometric assays.

The major issues in evaluating a hormonal assay are sensitivity (i.e., the capacity to accurately measure the lowest possible value) and specificity (i.e., the capacity to accurately measure only the hormone in question, without cross-reacting with other hormones or substances). Another possible problem is that some protein hormones are produced in different isoforms that may have different biologic activities. The specificity of the various antibodies used will determine to what extent these isoforms will be detected. Assay specificity problems may occur with a particular hormone, or they may be common to a general

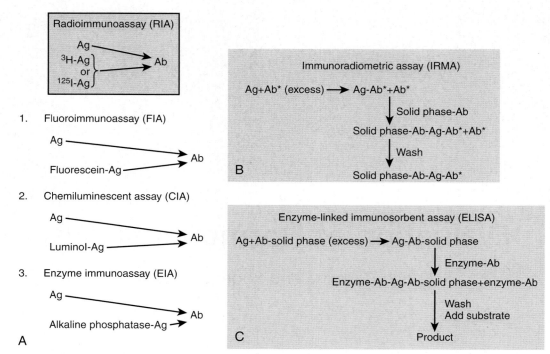

Figure 32-1. *A, Competition between excess antigen (Ag, analyte or standard) and excess radioactive or nonradioactive antigen (marker) for a limited amount of antibody (Ab). B, Principle of the immunoradiometric assay. C, Principle of the enzyme-linked immunosorbent assay. (Adapted from Nakamura RM, Stanczyk FZ. Immunoassays. In Lobo RA, Mishell DR, Paulson RJ, Shoupe D [eds]. Mishell's Textbook of Infertility, Contraception, and Reproductive Endocrinology, 4th ed. Oxford, Blackwell Science, 1997.)*

class of hormones. For example, steroid hormones have the problem of specificity, because there are many different molecules with very small structural differences. To avoid cross-reactivity, it is preferable to separate the steroid of interest from similar compounds before measuring it by RIA. This separation can be achieved by extraction and chromatography, a technique that separates compounds on the basis of polarity. Unless very specific antibodies are used, completely different values are often obtained if a steroid is measured directly by RIA rather than with RIA after extraction and separation with chromatography. In women who have low circulating levels of certain hormones, this remains a problem with commercial assays. Examples include testosterone levels in normal women[3] and estradiol, which is in the picogram per milliliter range and is notoriously measured inaccurately by direct clinical assays.

The assay of peptide hormones has the generic problem of the presence of different circulating isoforms or different peptide subunits that have differing biologic activities. Certain immunoassays of peptide hormones measure particular ratios of biologic to immunologic activity, depending on the epitopes detected by the antibody. Accordingly, at times it is important to measure biologic activity. Several bioassays have been described and are mainly used for research purposes.

VALIDATION AND QUALITY CONTROL OF IMMUNOASSAYS

Assay Validation

Before an immunoassay can be used to measure a compound, it must first be validated with respect to accuracy, precision, specificity, and sensitivity.

Accuracy

Assay *accuracy* defines the extent to which a given measurement agrees with the actual value. One commonly used method to establish the accuracy of an immunoassay is based on the finding of parallelism between the assay standard curve and serial dilutions (using assay buffer) of several samples containing known high concentrations of the analyte. Another method for establishing immunoassay accuracy is based on the recovery of added standard, at different levels, from patient samples. This method is often used for assays that require an extraction or a chromatographic step (e.g., steroid hormone assays). Both the parallelism and the "spiked" sample methods are limited by the precision of carrying out the dilutions or "spiking."

Precision

The *precision* of an assay refers to the variability that exists when multiple measurements of the compound are made on the same sample. In practice, both intra-assay precision and interassay precision are determined and are usually expressed as the coefficient of variation of replicate measures. The coefficient of variation (expressed as a percentage) is calculated by dividing the standard deviation (*SD*) by the mean of replicate determinations of an analyte, and then multiplying by 100. *Intra-assay precision* is assessed by measuring the analyte in replicate samples (usually 7-10) within the same assay. *Interassay precision* is determined by measuring the analyte in replicate samples (at least five), each of which is included in a different assay. Both intra-assay and interassay precision should be determined in three different concentrations of the analyte (high, midrange, and low).

The intra-assay and interassay coefficients of variation are usually 5% to 10% and 10% to 15%, respectively.

Specificity

Assay *specificity* refers to the degree of interference from cross-reaction that is encountered from substances other than the target analyte. The specificity of an immunoassay is usually assessed in two different ways. First, the cross-reactivity (expressed as a percentage) of the antibody is determined by comparing the dose–response standard curve of the substance being measured with dose–response curves obtained for compounds that may be present in the same sample as the analyte and that may bind to the antibody. The percent cross-reaction of an antiserum with a substance is calculated from the mass of standard that yields 50% inhibition of binding of assay marker to the antibody, divided by the mass of the cross-reacting substance that gives the same percentage of inhibition (50%), and multiplied by 100%.

A second approach for defining immunoassay specificity is to compare the analyte values of a group of samples measured by a specific immunoassay method with those obtained by a classic method, such as gas chromatography–mass spectrometry. If this is not possible and the analytes are being measured in an immunoassay without chromatography, the analyte values should be compared with the values obtained by an immunoassay that uses a chromatographic step to separate the analyte in question before assay (e.g., celite or dextran gel [Sephadex, Sigma-Aldrich, St. Louis, MO] column chromatography or high-performance liquid chromatography).

Sensitivity

The *sensitivity* of an assay is defined as the smallest amount of the substance being measured that can be distinguished from zero. In practice, assay sensitivity depends on the precision of the standard curve, which can be measured by assaying 10 replicates of each concentration of standard and the "zero" standard. This allows calculation of the mean amount ($\pm SD$) of the antibody-bound marker, corresponding to each concentration of standard. The sensitivity of an assay is the lowest standard concentration that yields a mean amount (e.g., counts per minute bound) of antibody-bound marker differing by 2 SDs from the mean amount of antibody-bound marker associated with the zero standard.

Assay sensitivity expressed in this manner, in practical terms, refers to the sensitivity of the standard curve. However, it is important to know the assay sensitivity in terms of the lowest amount of analyte that can be measured per milliliter of sample. This can be determined by calculating the product of the lowest standard concentration (based on standard curve sensitivity) and dilution factors, as well as the factor accounting for procedural loss (in assays using an extraction or chromatographic step).

Assay Quality Control

Parameters used to monitor the reliability of an immunoassay include internal quality control and external quality control. The internal quality control parameters can be subdivided into those related to the standard curve and those related to the analyte being measured in samples. The parameters related to the standard curve include the following: total counts, nonspecific binding, zero-standard binding (Ba), slope, *y*-intercept, and the doses of the standard at which the percentage of label-bound (B/Bo) substance is equal to 20%, 50%, and 80%. Parameters related to the analyte include the results of measuring the analyte in quality control samples and the performance characteristics of pipettes and instruments. Before evaluating the quality control characteristics of an assay, it is important to reject any replicate values that are outside of the laboratory's accepted limits of reproducibility (e.g., ±10%). The single most important quality control parameters are the results of repeated measurements on quality control samples. These samples should contain the analyte at low, medium, and high concentrations.

External quality control monitoring involves the measurement of quality control samples obtained from a designated center or company that is responsible for monitoring such samples in a number of laboratories. The basic methods used by the external scheme are similar to those used for internal monitoring, except that external monitoring allows a laboratory to compare results with other laboratories.

COMMERCIALIZED ASSAY SYSTEMS

Dissociation-Enhanced Lanthanide Fluorescence Immunoassay

A number of complex and nonsymmetrical compounds called *fluorochromes* emit characteristic visible light during relaxation when they are excited by radiation, such as ultraviolet light. One of the best known fluorochromes is fluorescein isothiocyanate. However, use of this compound and related fluorochromes was not adopted as a replacement for radioisotopes in immunoassays because high background activity was encountered because of light scattering and interference by serum constituents.

These problems have now been resolved by the use of a fluorochrome that consists of europium, an element of the lanthanide series, chelated to a suitable compound (e.g., a benzyl derivative of ethylenediaminetetraacetic acid). To enhance fluorescence, the chelated europium is dissociated from the complex by lowering the pH and forming a new chelator with an enhancement solution that also prevents quenching.

The dissociation-enhanced lanthanide fluorescence immunoassay (DELFIA), a solid-phase, two-site fluoroimmunometric assay based on the direct sandwich technique using two monoclonal antibodies, has been used widely. The antibodies are directed against two separate antigenic determinants on the luteinizing hormone (LH) molecule. Standards, controls, and samples containing LH are first reacted with immobilized (on a microtiter plate) monoclonal antibodies directed against a specific antigenic site on the LH β subunit. Europium-labeled antibodies directed against a specific antigenic site on the LH β-subunit are then reacted with the LH already bound to the solid-phase antibody. An enhancement solution dissociates europium ions from the labeled antibody into solution, where they form tightly fluorescent chelates with components of the enhancement solution. The fluorescence is proportional to the concentration of LH in the sample. Use of the enhancement solution in the DELFIA system allows analytes to be measured with great sensitivity as a result of the chelate's long fluorescence decay time and large Stoke's shift, which dramatically reduces the background signal.

Immulite System

The Immulite system uses enzyme-amplified chemiluminescent technology. The mechanism involves hydrolysis of a stable chemiluminescent substrate, adamantyl dioxetane phosphate, through the action of the enzyme alkaline phosphatase. This process results in the constant production of the unstable adamantly dioxetane anion. Constant production of the anion gives rise to sustained emission of light that provides a longer window for more numerous and precise readings than can be performed with other luminescent methods, which rely on their characteristic "flash" of light. The emitted light is quantified by use of the Immulite luminometer.

The Immulite LH assay, a solid-phase, two-site IRMA, is an example of this system. The solid phase consists of a polystyrene bead that is coated with a polyclonal antibody directed against LH. The bead is sealed into an Immulite test unit; the LH standard or serum sample and the monoclonal antibody conjugated to alkaline phosphatase are then added simultaneously. During a 30-minute incubation period at 37ºC, LH is bound to the polyclonal antibody coating the bead and to the monoclonal antibody–enzyme conjugate in the form of a sandwich complex. After unbound antibody is removed by a wash and centrifugation, the amount of bound complex, which is directly proportional to the LH (standard or sample), is quantified by use of the chemiluminescent substrate described earlier. The new Immulite system (Immulite 1000) is used by many laboratories and permits the simultaneous assay of more than 10 different hormones.

IMx System

The IMx System (Abbott Diagnostics, Santa Clara, CA) is an automated immunoassay analyzer that incorporates the microparticle enzyme immunoassay (MEIA) technology for high–molecular-weight analytes and fluorescence polarization immunoassay (FPIA) technology for lower–molecular-weight analytes. The two methods are complementary. In general, the FPIA is the method of choice for measurement of steroid hormones, whereas the MEIA is used for quantifying protein hormone levels. The FPIA uses a fluorescence polarization optical system to quantify the extent of marker binding to the antibody. In contrast, the MEIA uses a fluorometer to quantify a fluorescent product that is generated enzymatically.

The IMx LH assay, based on the MEIA system, is an example of this assay technology. A probe–electrode assembly delivers sample or standard and anti–βLH-coated microparticles into an incubation well of a reaction cell; an antibody–LH complex is formed. An aliquot of the complex bound to the microparticles is transferred to a glass fiber matrix, resulting in irreversible binding of the microparticles to the glass fiber matrix. The matrix is washed to remove unbound materials, and anti α subunit conjugated to alkaline phosphatase is added. This conjugate binds to the LH of the initial antigen–antibody complex. After the matrix is washed to remove unbound reagents, the substrate, 4-methylumbelliferyl phosphate, is added to the matrix and the fluorescent product is measured by the MEIA optical assembly. The amount of fluorescent bound complex is directly proportionate to the LH concentration.

RADIOIMMUNOASSAY COMBINED WITH BIOASSAY

Assays that combine features of both RIA (immunologic) and bioassay (biologic) properties have been developed. These more refined bioassays are different from the original crude bioassays that were first used to measure gonadotropins by their effect on a target organ (e.g., an increase in mouse uterine weight). The first bioassay–RIA method was first described by Dufau et al.[4] who measured production of testosterone by dispersed Leydig cells under the influence of LH or human chorionic gonadotropin (hCG).

A similar method to that previously described has been used to measure the effect of follicle-stimulating hormone (FSH) on estradiol production by granulosa cells or on aromatase activity in Sertoli cells.[5] The advantage of these bioassays is that only the biologic activity of LH or FSH may vary under certain conditions, and not the immunologic activity, depending on the immunoassay used (e.g., use of a gonadotropin-releasing hormone agonist or antagonist). Bioassays may be the method of choice for similar situations in the absence of a very specific immunoassay that reflects biologic activity.

Measurement of Gonadotropins

Serum concentrations of LH and FSH are expressed in international units, using as a reference partially purified pituitary hormone preparations, such as LER-907 or urinary gonadotropins (Second International Reference Preparation–human menopausal gonadotropin [2nd IRP-HMG]). The use of different hormone reference preparations complicates comparisons between different assays.

Classic RIAs of gonadotropins have low specificity and sensitivity and often cannot distinguish low levels from low-normal values. This difficulty is compounded by the pulsatile nature of gonadotropin secretion. Immunometric assays are more sensitive and have improved the measurement of gonadotropins.[6] As previously described, IRMA, immunofluorometric assay (IFMA), or ICMA should be used when low levels of gonadotropins are expected, but these methods may not offer advantages when elevated or normal levels are anticipated. The ELISA for gonadotropins is considered less sensitive and exhibits higher nonspecific binding.

Additional problems that may arise in LH measurements include significant cross-reactivity with hCG and the pulsatile secretion pattern (pulses approximately every 60-90 minutes).[7] The requirement of precision in values would necessitate that samples, taken 15 to 20 minutes apart, be pooled for analysis. In the clinical setting, however, this is not necessary because low levels usually remain low and high values are not usually within the normal range. The concern about pulsatility is more for research purposes and is far less pronounced for FSH samples, where pulses are less frequent, occurring approximately every 3 hours.

Apart from alterations in FSH and LH associated with various disorders and physiologic states, FSH levels are increased by levodopa and ketocanozole and decreased by the administration of estrogens and phenothiazines. LH is increased by ketoconazole and decreased by administration of sex steroids, phenothiazines, digoxin, and propranolol.

A special issue exists with measurement of low levels of βhCG in normal women. When low levels are found (usually in the range of 5-20 mIU/mL), possibilities include pregnancy, an hCG-producing tumor (including choriocarcinoma), normal pituitary secretion (usually in a postmenopausal woman), and interference in the assay (often encountered with "sandwich"-type assays.) The first approach is to repeat the value with a different assay system. Other, more specific types of hCG assays may be helpful in the differential diagnosis.

BLOOD LEVELS OF LH AND FSH IN WOMEN

In adult women, during the follicular phase, serum levels of LH and FSH by RIA range from 4 to 15 mIU/mL (2nd IRP-HMG standard), although individual laboratory ranges vary somewhat. In our laboratory, the mean level for LH is 8.2 ± 2.1 mIU/mL (*SD*), with a range of 4 to 12.4 mIU/mL; the mean level for FSH is 8 ± 1.8 mIU/mL, with a range of 4.4 to 11.6 mIU/mL. Many commercial assays, including ICMA, report lower normal ranges of LH (1.9-12.5 mUI/mL). Also, with these systems, it is impossible to detect the low levels of gonadotropins that would occur in cases of hypothalamic or pituitary failure or before puberty. Consequently, the more sensitive assays described later (third-generation assays) should be used in the evaluation of patients suspected of having hypogonadotropic hypogonadism and in pediatric patients.

During midcycle, serum LH levels increase four- to sixfold, whereas serum FSH levels increase two- to threefold. The midcycle increase of gonadotropins lasts approximately 2 days.

During the luteal phase, serum LH and FSH levels are similar to or slightly lower than their respective levels during the follicular phase. Therefore, in healthy women, the *LH/FSH ratio* is approximately 1.0 during the follicular phase, but increases during ovulation.

Before puberty, gonadotropin levels are lower than in adult women, and the LH/FSH ratio is less than 1.0 because of the relative predominance of FSH secretion. At this age, classic RIAs have not been helpful in distinguishing patients with low gonadotropin secretion from healthy children; therefore, third-generation LH IRMA or ICMA is used.[8,9] These assays are also useful for measuring changes in LH and FSH during the pubertal progression. From Tanner stages P1 to P5, LH concentrations using IRMA

increase more than 30-fold, but increase only two- to fourfold when measured by RIA. Therefore, IRMA and fluorescence immunoassay third-generation LH assays are the preferred techniques in all prepubertal patients, in patients with suspected precocious puberty, and in those with suspected hypogonadotropic hypogonadism. It has been reported that, using a third-generation fluorometric assay, values of LH higher than 0.6 mUI/mL are sufficient to suggest the diagnosis of gonadotropin-dependent precocious puberty and may permit this diagnosis to be made in two thirds of such patients.[10]

During the perimenopausal period, serum FSH levels increase substantially, whereas LH levels remain within the normal range. After menopause, levels of both gonadotropins are high, but serum FSH levels are higher than LH levels. In older women, LH levels progressively decrease, approaching premenopausal levels.[11]

High values of LH, with increased LH/FSH ratios, are found in 50% of women with polycystic ovary syndrome (PCOS).[12] In the past, some clinicians based the diagnosis of PCOS on the finding of elevated LH levels and LH/FSH ratios higher than 2 or 3. Although an increased LH level or LH/FSH ratio may be useful for confirming the diagnosis of PCOS, many patients with PCOS have normal serum LH levels and LH/FSH ratios.[12,13]

High levels of serum LH and FSH are typical of ovarian failure and may be found in patients with gonadal dysgenesis. Rarely, pituitary tumors may produce FSH or LH.[14] Measurement of α subunits and determination of the gonadotropin responses to thyrotropin-releasing hormone (TRH) may be useful for the diagnosis of gonadotropin adenomas.

DYNAMIC TESTS FOR GONADOTROPIN EVALUATION

Gonadotropin-Releasing Hormone Test

Synthetic gonadotropin-releasing hormone (GnRH), the hypothalamic decapeptide, has been used to stimulate LH and FSH secretion to identify abnormalities that cannot be diagnosed with baseline determinations. This test is primarily used to differentiate between hypothalamic and pituitary causes of gonadotropin deficiency and to uncover a maturational delay in secretion at the time of puberty. Otherwise, the test largely reflects baseline measurements.[15] For example, in patients with PCOS and women with ovarian failure, GnRH stimulation results in exaggerated increases in LH in the setting of PCOS and in FSH elevations in women with ovarian failure.

When differentiating hypothalamic from pituitary defects in gonadotropin secretion, the test requires initial GnRH priming. The priming may be accomplished by daily intramuscular administration of 100 μg GnRH for 1 week before testing. With this approach, an absent or low response distinguishes the more common patient with a hypothalamic problem from a rare patient with a congenital or acquired pituitary defect of gonadotropin secretion.

The GnRH test is also used to probe the maturational state of the hypothalamic–pituitary–gonadal axis. Pubertal LH and FSH responses are observed in patients with gonadotropin-dependent precocious puberty (GDPP), and this test is needed when no third-generation assays are available. The test may be performed in many ways, but requires at least two baseline samples obtained 15 minutes apart before GnRH administration. Intravenous doses of 25 or 100 μg are then administered, and blood samples are obtained at 20, 30, 60, 90, and 120 minutes. For practical purposes, samples obtained at 30 minutes and 60 minutes are sufficient for clinical interpretation. Using conventional RIA methods, after administration of 100 μg GnRH, an LH peak of more than 15 mIU/mL in girls and greater than 25mIU/mL in boys is suggestive of GDPP.[8] Using ICMA LH assay, after the same dose of GnRH, the cutoff value is greater than 8.0 mIU/mL.[16] Similar cutoff values are observed when using LH IFMA (>6.9 mIU/mL in girls and >9.6 mIU/mL in boys).[10]

Another approach is to use LH responses 2 hours after a long-acting GnRH analog is administered. LH values of greater than 10 mIU/mL (by IFMA) suggest GDPP.[17]

The only validated method to assess hypothalamic GnRH release is by measuring the *spontaneous pulsatility of gonadotropins,* which is generally reserved for research purposes. Blood samples are obtained at 10- to 15-minute intervals for 6 to 24 hours, depending on whether diurnal changes are being assessed.

Clomiphene Citrate Test

In the past, the ability of the hypothalamic–pituitary axis to respond to negative feedback of estrogen was assessed with clomiphene. Clomiphene (50-100 mg daily) is given orally for 5 days, and LH and FSH levels are measured before and at the end of the test. A normal response is an LH response of greater than 50%. This test lacks sensitivity and specificity and should be abandoned for this purpose.

The clomiphene citrate test is actually used in the assessment of ovarian reserve. It used to be considered more valuable than a single measurement of FSH and estradiol on day 3 of the cycle.[18,19] Clomiphene (100 mg) is administered on days 5 through 9 of the cycle, and the FSH level is measured initially on day 3 and again on day 10. Any value (day 3 or 10) above the threshold for the laboratory is considered a positive test result. Generally, an abnormal FSH level in this setting is a value of more than 10 to 12 mIU/mL; however, it is important that each laboratory define its own abnormal cutoff point because of the considerable variability among the different FSH assays.[20] Some recent data, however, suggest that this test may not be more valuable than baseline FSH assessments.[21]

Measurement of Prolactin

Serum prolactin (PRL) is generally measured by RIA or IRMA. The upper limit of the normal range is generally reported as 15 to 20 ng/mL in men and 20 to 25 ng/mL in women, although the true normal levels are usually lower (up to 18 ng/mL in women). Serum PRL values are influenced by estrogens, drugs (e.g., phenothiazines, metoclopramide), stress, food consumption, breast stimulation,

and even venipuncture. Because of diurnal changes and transient increases after meals, samples should routinely be obtained at midmorning.

The presence in blood of macroprolactin (monomeric PRL + PRL autoantibody)[22] or dimeric forms of PRL (so-called *big-PRL forms*)[23] may lead to elevated PRL levels that are not associated with biologic activity. In particular, macroprolactinemia may be an important clinical problem resulting in up to 10% of cases of misdiagnosed hyperprolactinemia.[22,24] When macroprolactinemia is suspected (e.g., in patients with autoimmune diseases), polyethylene glycol precipitation should be carried out before the immunoassay. Recently, new commercial methods for the measurement of PRL that involve ultrafiltration have been introduced and may be useful to detect macroprolactin or big prolactin in clinical practice.[25]

In pregnancy, serum PRL begins to increase by 6 weeks' gestation and rises progressively to reach approximately 200 ng/mL at term. In nonlactating women, PRL levels return to normal 2 to 3 weeks postpartum.[26] With menopause, serum PRL declines slightly as a result of the reduction of estrogen.[27]

Serum PRL levels greater than 200 ng/mL are diagnostic of pituitary adenoma, but patients with microadenomas often have levels that are considerably lower.[28] Levels between 50 and 200 ng/mL may be found in patients with non–PRL-secreting adenomas compressing the pituitary stalk. If moderately elevated PRL levels are found, evaluation of thyroid function is necessary because hypothyroidism results in elevations in serum PRL.

DYNAMIC TESTS FOR PROLACTIN EVALUATION

Dynamic tests for the evaluation of PRL secretion are seldom used and were popular when brain imaging was less sophisticated. Computed tomography (CT) or magnetic resonance imaging (MRI) is much more valuable for the diagnosis and assessment of a pituitary microadenoma or macroadenoma.[28]

Thyrotropin-releasing hormone, the hypothalamic peptide that stimulates the secretion of thyroid-stimulating hormone (TSH), may be used to evaluate the pituitary secretion of PRL.[29] In general, patients with a prolactinoma do not experience further increases in serum PRL after TRH stimulation. Therefore, this test has been used to differentiate between functional forms of hyperprolactinemia and PRL-secreting pituitary adenomas. However, the utility of the TRH test has been questioned because the PRL response largely depends on basal PRL levels. The test is carried out after an overnight fast, with TRH (200 μg) being administered intravenously. Blood samples for PRL are taken at the initiation of the test and again at 30, 60, and 90 minutes. A normal PRL response is an increase of at least 100% of basal levels. Psychiatric disorders and ingestion of thyroid hormone, corticosteroids, and tranquilizers may affect the PRL response.

The TRH test is still used to diagnose pituitary thyroid disorders and for subtle forms of hypothyroidism; for these purposes, TSH levels are measured.

An alternative to the TRH test for the assessment of PRL disorders is the use of metoclopramide (10 mg intravenously). A blood sample is obtained immediately after metoclopramide administration, and again at 30, 60, 90, and 120 minutes.[30] A PRL increment of 100 ng/mL at 60 to 120 minutes is considered normal.

Measurement of Estradiol and Other Estrogens

Most assays for estradiol involve RIA. Commercial RIA kits are optimized for measuring normal to high levels; therefore, low levels are usually not measured accurately. For measuring low levels, samples should be extracted with organic solvents and subjected to chromatographic separation to remove interfering steroids, particularly estrogen conjugates. Several commercial laboratories perform an extraction procedure alone. Although the premise is that accurate values will be obtained with highly specific antibodies, this is not always the case. Extraction before RIA is most important in women receiving oral estrogen because high levels of conjugates (in the nanogram per nanoliter range) will be present in blood. Serum estrone levels are higher than values of estradiol in women receiving any oral estrogen, and its measurement is sometimes useful for the assessment of absorption and metabolism problems with estrogen therapy. Although not frequently measured, estrone sulfate reflects the circulating reservoir of estrogen and is quantitatively the greatest circulating estrogen.[31]

Estriol may be measured by RIA in serum or by spectrophotometric methods or RIA in urine. In the past, estriol measurements were used for prenatal genetic testing for fetal aneuploidy and in late pregnancy for the assessment of fetal well-being.

BLOOD LEVELS OF ESTRADIOL

In most laboratories, serum estradiol levels range from 20 to 80 pg/mL during the early to midfollicular phase of the menstrual cycle and peak at 200 to 500 pg/mL during the preovulatory LH surge. During the midluteal phase, serum estradiol levels range from 60 to 200 pg/mL.[32]

Before puberty, serum estradiol levels are less than 20 pg/mL, indistinguishable from cases of hypogonadism. After menopause, estradiol levels fall to prepubertal levels; the mean serum estradiol level is typically 10 to 20 pg/mL, and levels are lower than 10 pg/mL in women who have undergone oophorectomy.

In men, serum estradiol levels should be less than 40 pg/mL, but may be increased in several testicular and nontesticular diseases. Serum estradiol levels are relatively constant and, unlike testosterone, are unchanged with age.[33] In men, it is important to measure serum estradiol with assays that are able to distinguish between low values.

Male serum estrone levels should be less than 60 pg/mL. The measurement of serum estradiol and estrone may be useful in the clinical evaluation of hypogonadism and gynecomastia. However, obesity is the most common cause of mildly increased levels of circulating estrogens in men.[33]

Measurement of Progesterone

Serum progesterone may be measured by a variety of immunoassays. The specificity of the assay is highly dependent on lack of cross-reactivity with 17α-hydroxyprogesterone (17α-OHP).

BLOOD LEVELS OF PROGESTERONE AND EVALUATION OF OVULATION

Serum progesterone is low during the follicular phase, less than 1.5 ng/mL. Levels begin to increase just before the onset of the LH surge and then increase progressively to peak 6 to 8 days after ovulation. After menopause, serum progesterone of adrenal origin is less than 0.5 ng/mL.

The measurement of serum progesterone during the midluteal phase (days 21 and 22) is most frequently used to assess ovulatory status. Although single samples are acceptable in clinical practice, progesterone levels exhibit a pulsatile pattern[34] as well as some diurnal variation.

During the midluteal phase, serum progesterone levels are usually higher than 7 ng/mL. Some physicians have proposed using three luteal determinations with a total serum value of 15 ng/mL or more to indicate normal luteal function.[35] For patients being monitored for fertility, other assessments may be used, including basal body temperature charts, urinary LH kits, and timed endometrial biopsy. In conception cycles, properly timed midluteal progesterone levels are more than 10 ng/mL.[36] Progesterone is also often used to assess ovulation after induction of ovulation. In clomiphene cycles, midluteal progesterone levels should be higher than 15 ng/mL.[37]

During pregnancy, serum progesterone may be useful to assess corpus luteum and placental function.[38] Maternal serum progesterone levels rise slowly to 40 ng/mL near the end of the first trimester and then increase progressively to reach 150 ng/mL at term. Low levels of progesterone (<10 ng/mL) at 6 to 8 weeks signify an abnormal intrauterine pregnancy or an ectopic pregnancy.

Measurement of Androgens

Androgens in women arise from three different sources: the ovaries, the adrenal glands, and the peripheral compartment. Most androgens are produced or metabolized by more than one compartment and, in evaluating women with androgen excess, several androgens are usually measured.[39] In the past, the measurement of urinary 17-ketosteroids was the most common method used to evaluate androgen production in women. However, 17-ketosteroid measurements reflect adrenal androgen production, poorly reflect testosterone production,[40] and are nonspecific; therefore, they have been abandoned for use in current practice.

Most commonly, serum testosterone and dehydroepiandrosterone sulfate levels are measured. These levels largely reflect ovarian and adrenal contributions, respectively.[41] Serum testosterone reflects mostly ovarian androgen production, with two thirds of circulating levels resulting from the peripheral conversion of androstenedione; therefore, increases in either ovarian or adrenal androstenedione production results in elevated serum testosterone levels. On the other hand, whereas serum dehydroepiandrosterone sulfate (DHEAS) reflects adrenal androgen secretion well, levels may be normal in certain cases of adrenal androgen hypersecretion (as in 21-hydroxylase deficiency).[42] The pathway of adrenal enzymatic blockade (affecting the Δ^4 pathway) explains this discrepancy. Conversely, serum DHEAS may be elevated in many patients with a prevalent ovarian source of hyperandrogenemia (as in PCOS).[43] Accordingly, increased levels of serum DHEAS do not predict androgen responses to dexamethasone suppression,[44] which has been used as a test to determine adrenal responsivity to suppression.

Serum testosterone should be measured by RIA or ICMA, after extraction and chromatography. These assays are cumbersome, time-consuming, and relatively costly, and accordingly, many laboratories use direct assays without purification. However, these methods have some major disadvantages, including overestimation of the values and low specificity. It has been reported that these direct testosterone assays have poor or no validity in females.[3,45]

Unbound testosterone may be measured as bioavailable testosterone[46] or as free testosterone.[47,48] The first method, which is also referred to as *non–sex hormone–binding hormone globulin-bound testosterone*, relies on sex hormone–binding hormone (SHBG) to assess the percentage that is "free." In healthy women, up to 75% of testosterone is bound to SHBG; the percentage that is unbound includes testosterone that is entirely "free" and the moiety associated with albumin that is available to the target cells.

Free testosterone is measured by equilibrium dialysis and has remained the gold standard for assessing the amount of testosterone that is neither bound to SHBG nor associated with albumin. Variations in incubation temperature significantly affect results in the dialysis method.[49] Some laboratories measure unbound testosterone by a direct method using a ^{125}I-labeled testosterone analog as tracer. This analog method gives 75% lower values than equilibrium dialysis assays[40-42] and, although it is easy to perform, its clinical utility is questionable.[49] It has been reported that direct assays of free testosterone result in unacceptably spurious values with high random variability and, therefore, should not be used in clinical practice.[50] It is most practical, for clinical purposes, to calculate a free testosterone index (free androgen index [FAI]) using levels of testosterone and SHBG. The calculation is made using the ratio between testosterone and SHBG (in units of nanomole per liter): (T [ng/mL] × 3.467/SHBG × 100).[51] At least in females, FAI values correlate well with free testosterone determined by equilibrium dialysis.[52] However, FAI values have low validity in men[53] and are strongly dependent on the accuracy of testosterone and SHBG assays. In general, FAI should be used primarily for clinical rather than research purposes, when testosterone assays using chromatography and purification techniques are not available.

There are other androgens that may be useful to measure under different circumstances. These include 11β-hydroxyandrostenedione,[54] which reflects adrenal production of androstenedione because 11β-hydroxylase activity is usually absent in the ovary.

Assessment of peripheral androgen production requires the measurement of products of 5α-reductase activity. Although serum dihydrotestosterone (DHT) does not appropriately reflect increases in peripheral 5α-reductase activity, more distal metabolites may be helpful. Serum 3α-androstanediol glucuronide best reflects peripheral testosterone metabolism in hirsutism,[55] and androsterone glucuronide best reflects the state in androgenic acne.[56]

In assessing androgen excess in women, it is preferable to obtain blood samples in the morning because of diurnal variation from the adrenal. Values are often reduced during the afternoon or evening.

BLOOD LEVELS OF ANDROGENS IN WOMEN

In women of reproductive age, an accurate range for serum testosterone is 20 to 50 ng/dL. With direct immunoassays, the upper end of the normal range is approximately 70 to 80 ng/dL, or even higher. Serum testosterone levels higher than 200 ng/dL are suggestive of ovarian neoplasms, but some tumors may present with lower levels.[57] Because upper normal ranges vary, a rule of thumb is to be concerned about a tumor in women whose values exceed 2.5 times the upper normal range of a particular assay. Patients with PCOS have mildly increased serum testosterone (usually <100 ng/dL), whereas markedly increased levels may be found in patients with hyperthecosis and in those who have adrenal enzymatic deficiencies.

The normal range of serum DHEAS is 0.8 to 2.8 μg/mL. Values greater than 8 μg/mL are suggestive of an adrenal neoplasm; if the adrenal tumor produces testosterone, however, only modestly elevated values (3-4 μg/mL) may be found.[58]

Serum androstenedione levels range from 1 to 2.5 ng/mL.

The range for unbound testosterone is 0.6 to 5 ng/dL, whereas free testosterone levels are between 1 and 8.5 pg/mL. Normal ranges for SHBG are between 30 and 90 nmol/L.

Serum androgens are low before puberty, with adrenal androgen levels beginning to increase 1 or 2 years before the onset of puberty. Serum DHEAS values higher than 0.8 μg/mL indicate the presence of adrenarche.[59] After menopause, serum androgens decline slightly.[60] Aging is the principal determinant of this decline. Serum DHEAS levels have been suggested to be useful in excluding adrenal deficiency in young women with autoimmune ovarian failure.[61]

MEASUREMENT OF CIRCULATING ANDROGEN PRECURSORS IN WOMEN

Measurements of intermediates in steroid metabolism are useful for the diagnosis of adrenal enzymatic deficiencies. Serum 17α-OHP is used in the diagnosis of 21-hydroxylase deficiency.[62] Because 17α-OHP is secreted by the corpus luteum, the measurement should be carried out in the morning during the follicular phase. In healthy women, serum 17α-OHP is generally lower than 1 ng/mL, but hyperandrogenic patients (mostly those with PCOS) generally have slightly higher levels. Therefore, values up to

2 to 3 ng/mL are not indicative of an adrenal enzymatic eficiency. Patients with classic neonatal forms of 21-hydroxylase deficiency have very high levels of 17α-OHP (50-200 ng/mL), whereas most patients with nonclassic, late-onset 21-hydroxylase deficiency have serum 17α-OHP levels between 10 and 20 ng/mL. The adrenocorticotropin hormone (ACTH) stimulation test, described later in this chapter, can be used to diagnose 21-hydroxylase deficiency. From a practical standpoint, most patients can now have genotyping for the various mutations in the CYP21β gene, particularly when there is pertinent family history.

The measurement of serum 11-deoxycortisol may be used to diagnose 11β-hydroxylase deficiency when 17α-OHP is elevated. This less common condition may be associated with hypertension. The measurement of serum 17α-hydroxypregnenolone (and the ratio of 17α-OHP to 17α-hydroxypregnelone), as well as the ratio of dehydroepiandrosterone to androstenedione, is useful in the diagnosis of 3β-hydroxysteroid deficiency.[63] In adults, this latter diagnosis is controversial in that no genetic mutations in the 3βol gene have been identified and most patients seem to have a variant of PCOS.[64]

TESTS TO ESTABLISH THE SOURCE OF HYPERANDROGENISM

Because serum androgens may arise from different sources in women, several tests have been established to distinguish adrenal from ovarian hyperandrogenism. However, most tests are not specific and their use is generally limited.[41]

The tests may be divided into two groups: tests that assess adrenal androgen secretion and those that assess ovarian androgen secretion. The first group of tests includes the dexamethasone suppression test and the ACTH stimulation test.

Dexamethasone Suppression Test

For evaluation of hyperandrogenism, a prolonged test is used in which dexamethasone (0.5 mg) is given orally every 6 hours for 3 to 7 days. Evaluation of the suppression of serum DHEAS requires 7 days because of the prolonged half-life of this steroid; for the evaluation of the suppression of testosterone and free testosterone, however, 3 days of dexamethasone administration is sufficient. For practical reasons, measurement of testosterone and free testosterone is sufficient because DHEAS is always profoundly suppressed by dexamethasone unless an adrenal tumor is present. Therefore, the prolonged test (7 days) is used only if DHEAS levels are very high (>8 μg/mL) and an androgen-secreting adrenal tumor is suspected. This testing is not recommended to diagnose a neoplasm because the sensitive imaging techniques now available are more efficient and specific. In most common forms of hyperandrogenism, a decrease of total and unbound testosterone of at least 60% of basal values suggests an adrenal cause of hyperandrogenism.[65] The test is not specific, but has been useful to suggest women who would be sensitive to dexamethasone for the treatment of

hyperandrogenism.[65] However, dexamethasone is rarely used to treat hyperandrogenism.

Adrenocorticotropic Hormone Stimulation Test

The ACTH stimulation test is generally used for the diagnosis of cortisol deficiency or to identify mild adrenal enzymatic deficiencies. Also, it has been used to distinguish between adrenal and ovarian sources of hyperandrogenism, but is not generally used for this purpose because of its lack of specificity. ACTH stimulation is not recommended for uncovering subtle defects in hyperandrogenism unless there is a strong suggestion that 21-hydroxylase deficiency (congenital adrenal hyperplasia) may be present. For example, the ACTH stimulation test would be indicated in adult women with hyperandrogenism who have baseline levels of 17α-OHP of more than 3 mg/mL but less than 10 mg/mL, the 17α-OHP level above which the diagnosis of 21-hydroxylase deficiency would be obvious.[66] Some authors have suggested a baseline 17α-OHP value cutoff of greater than 2 ng/mL as a threshold for ACTH stimulation testing. The index of suspicion should be higher in certain ethnic groups, including Yupik Eskimos, Ashkenazi Jews, and certain Southern European groups.[67] As stated earlier, many patients now undergo genotyping.

The test is best performed between 8 AM and 9 AM, with 0.25 mg cosyntropin injected intravenously. Although the test may also be accomplished by intramuscular injection, more consistent results have been obtained with intravenous administration. Blood samples are generally obtained at 30 minutes and 60 minutes, but the 60-minute value suffices as a single time point for practical purposes. For the diagnosis of nonclassic 21-hydroxylase deficiency, serum cortisol and 17α-OHP are measured. Serum 11-deoxycortisol may be evaluated if the rare 11-hydroxylase defect is suspected.

Nonclassic 21-hydroxylase deficiency may be diagnosed using the New nomogram (Fig. 32-2),[68] in which the log of the baseline 17α-OHP level is plotted against the log of the 17α-OHP level 60 minutes after ACTH administration. However, most laboratories diagnose 21-hydroxylase deficiency if the peak 17α-OHP level is higher than 10 ng/mL, with an increase from baseline of at least 5 ng/mL.[62]

After ACTH stimulation, Δ^5 and Δ^4 intermediate steroid measurements may be used to confirm a diagnosis of 3-beta-hydroxysteroid deficiency.[63]

Gonadotropin-Releasing Hormone Agonist Test

A GnRH agonist (GnRH-A) is generally used to downregulate the secretion of pituitary gonadotropins and inhibit ovarian steroid secretion. However, before downregulation, the early agonistic action of a GnRH-A causes prolonged stimulation of gonadotropin secretion, which in turn, stimulates the ovary. The test has been used in the setting of PCOS[69]; however, in our view, it does not add clinical information beyond that obtained by combining clinical and baseline hormonal data. Nevertheless, we have observed a strong association between increased

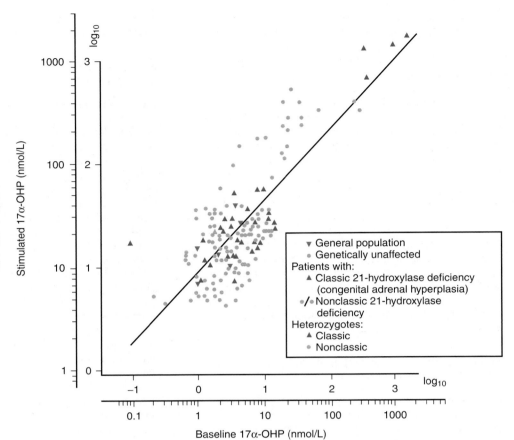

Figure 32-2. *Nomogram of 17α-hydroxyprogesterone (17α-OHP) in different types of patients with congenital adrenal hyperplasia. (Adapted from New MI, Lorenzen F, Lamer AJ, et al. Genotyping steroid 21-hydroxylase deficiency: hormonal reference data. J Clin Endocrinol Metab 57:320-326, 1983.)*

responses to a GnRH-A and the finding of polycystic ovaries on ultrasound.[70]

The original test was performed using nafarelin,[69] but buserelin[71] or, more commonly, leuprolide,[72] may be used with no substantial differences. Generally, leuprolide (500 or 1000 µg) is given subcutaneously in the morning between days 5 and 8 of the cycle. Blood samples are taken at 0 minutes and after 8 and 24 hours. Serum androstenedione and 17α-OHP are measured, but the more discriminating response is with serum 17α-OHP. A delta (increase from baseline) in serum 17α-OHP greater than 2.6 ng/mL suggests an increased or exaggerated response that is characteristic of women with PCOS (Fig. 32-3).

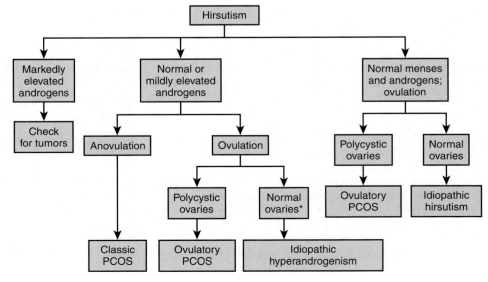

Figure 32-3. *Diagnosis of hirsutism. *Note that the ultrasound diagnosis of polycystic ovaries is somewhat subjective. Therefore, the diagnostic distinction between ovulatory polycystic ovary syndrome (PCOS) and idiopathic hyperandrogenism is fluid.*

HORMONAL EVALUATION OF HIRSUTISM

Hirsutism is excessive hair growth in women where it is not normally found, usually with a central body distribution. When this biologic signal is manifest, laboratory tests may be indicated to pinpoint the abnormality. Most commonly, total testosterone, DHEAS, and SHBG are measured (as well as 17α-OHP to exclude nonclassic congenital adrenal hyperplasia). In approximately 10% to 15% of hirsute women, all of these hormone levels are within the normal range and a diagnosis of "idiopathic hirsutism" is made.[12,73] Although it is not our intent to discuss the differential diagnosis of hirsutism, a simple algorithm is provided in Figure 32-3.

BLOOD LEVELS OF ANDROGENS IN MEN

In adult men, total testosterone and unbound testosterone are the only androgens measured in the evaluation of testicular function. Serum testosterone levels range from 300 to 1000 ng/dL. Serum testosterone decreases during the day, and in the evening, levels are approximately 15% lower.

The normal range for bioavailable testosterone is 66 to 417 ng/dL; for free testosterone, normal values are between 50 and 210 pg/mL. These assays may be useful in patients with low testosterone values. Serum DHT values range from 30 to 86 ng/dL, but this assay is not recommended on a routine basis. In evaluating children and neonates for 5α-reductase deficiency, serum DHT assays have been useful.

Measurement of Inhibins

Serum inhibin A and B levels may be measured by specific RIAs, ELISA, or enzyme-linked immunoassay, and reflect the secretion from various populations of granulosa cells. As previously noted, a characteristic of peptide assays is that multiple subunits make assays difficult. This is particularly true in the case of inhibin assays, which have been highly variable and imprecise. Serum values vary in adult women during the menstrual cycle, with inhibin A being lowest during the follicular phase and peaking during the midluteal phase; inhibin B exhibits an opposite pattern (Fig. 32-4).[74,75] During pregnancy, inhibin A decreases during the second trimester, whereas inhibin B rises from the third trimester to peak at term.[76,77] After menopause, levels of both inhibins decline markedly.[78]

The measurement of inhibin may be useful in several conditions.[79] Some granulosa cell tumors produce high quantities of inhibin B, which may be useful for postoperative surveillance, because it may detect tumor recurrence.[80] Measurement of inhibin B also has been proposed for monitoring certain complications of pregnancy[77] and for evaluating the number of small follicles present in the ovary in the early follicular phase.[79] The measurement may be useful in assessing reproductive aging because a low level of inhibin B on day 3 may indicate a declining ovarian reserve.[78]

In men, inhibin B is produced by Sertoli cells and has been considered a good marker of spermatogenesis.[81] It has also been used in the differential diagnosis of cryptorchidim versus anorchia.[82]

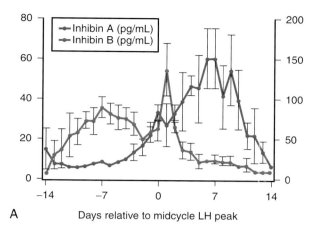

A

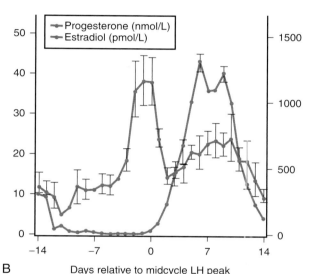

B

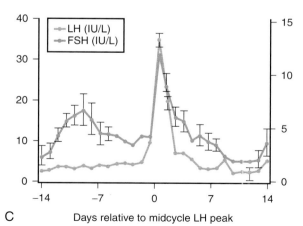

C

Figure 32-4. *Plasma concentrations of inhibin A and inhibin B (**A**), estradiol and progesterone (**B**), and luteinizing hormone (LH) and follicle-stimulating hormone (FSH) (**C**), during the female menstrual cycle. Data displayed with respect to the day of midcycle LH peak. Mean concentrations are shown ± standard error of the mean. (Adapted from Groome NP, Illingworth PJ, O'Brien M, et al. Measurement of dimeric inhibin B throughout the human menstrual cycle. J Clin Endocrinol Metab 81:1401-1405, 1996.)*

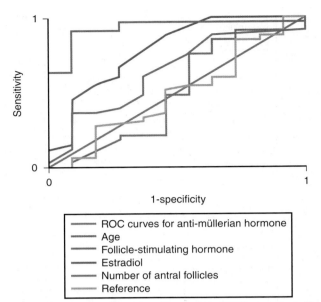

Figure 32-5. *Receiver operating characteristic (ROC) curve for müllerian inhibiting substance predicting ovarian reserve. (From Ficicioglu C, Kutlu T, Baglam E, BaKacak Z. Early follicular antimullerian hormone as an indicator of ovarian reserve. Fertil Steril 85:592-596, 2006.)*

Measurement of Anti-Müllerian Hormone and Assessment of Ovarian Reserve

Assessing ovarian reserve has become an extremely important part of the management of women with reproductive disorders. Whereas ovarian aging becomes accelerated in the late 30s, even younger women, particularly those who have undergone cancer treatment, may have diminished ovarian reserve.[83]

Although measurement of serum FSH and estradiol levels on day 2 to 3 has been used widely, other tests include the clomiphene challenge test (described earlier), counting antral follicles on ultrasound, measuring levels of inhibin B, and measuring anti-müllerian hormone (AMH).[83,84] Although some have suggested using a combination of these to provide a composite score criterion of ovarian reserve, in our hands, AMH level has proved to be the most useful, as suggested by others (Fig. 32-5).[83] Levels of AMH are cycle-dependent and tend not to fluctuate as much as FSH levels. Receiver operating characteristic curves have been constructed to assess the probability of pregnancy. Our experience suggests that a value of less than 0.35 ng/mL carries a poor prognosis.[83]

Measurement of βhCG

Many tissues, including the pituitary, produce hCG at very low levels, whereas the placenta produces it in large quantities. Most assays are standardized to measure only the large quantities produced by the placenta or by hCG-secreting tumors.[84]

During pregnancy, hCG levels increase rapidly, doubling approximately every 2 days until 12 weeks. After the third month of pregnancy, hCG levels decrease and plateau at a constant level until term. Measurements of hCG are used widely to confirm pregnancy and monitor trophoblastic function in complications of pregnancy, such as spontaneous abortion and ectopic pregnancy.[85,86] Measurements of β-hCG during pregnancy, when combined with other tests (nuchal translucency, pregnancy-associated plasma protein A, or inhibin A), may be useful for screening for trisomies, such as Down syndrome.[87]

High quantities of hCG are produced in trophoblastic disease and by nongestational trophoblastic tumors,[88] and in men by germ cell tumors.[89] In general, all of these tumors may produce the intact hormone, but most produce only βhCG. Patients with elevated βhCG levels should be evaluated extensively to exclude an underlying malignant process. Measurement of βhCG levels by sensitive assays is also useful for monitoring for a recurrence after tumor extirpation and may aid in the diagnosis of the tumor and reflect disease prognosis.[89]

Measurement and Blood Levels of Insulin

Serum insulin is most frequently measured by RIA. Use of heparin causes falsely elevated values, whereas hemolysis of the blood may result in falsely low values. Insulin antibodies in blood result in low levels in some assays and high levels in others. Insulin exhibits day-to-day variability of up to 15% to 25%.[90] Pulsatile secretion[91] is greatest in the portal circulation, but only contributes to small changes in the general circulation.

In most laboratories, normal fasting insulin levels range from 5 to 15 µU/mL. Obese subjects have increased values, whereas very high circulating levels are found in patients with severe insulin resistance. Approximately 40% to 50% of women with a normal body mass index who have classic PCOS have slightly increased insulin levels.[92,93] Higher levels are observed in obese women with PCOS.[93]

EVALUATION OF INSULIN RESISTANCE

Insulin resistance is considered extremely important in health and disease and is a pivotal aspect of the pathophysiology of PCOS. There are several ways to assess peripheral insulin sensitivity.[94] The most precise methods involve the use of glycemic clamps. However, these methods are very cumbersome and should be reserved for research purposes. Use of the minimal model of Bergman applied to a frequently sampled intravenous glucose tolerance (FSIGT) test is considered the gold standard for assessing insulin resistance. This method is as sensitive as the euglycemic insulin clamp.[95] An insulin tolerance test (ITT) is a good alternative for use in clinical practice. Methods based on the oral glucose tolerance test (OGTT), or on fasting blood concentrations for glucose and insulin with the use of various calculations, show only a partial correlation with the FSIGT test.[96]

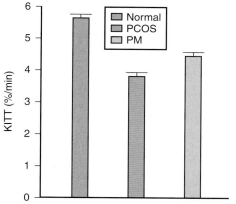

Figure 32-6. *Insulin tolerance test to evaluate insulin sensitivity. PCOS, polycystic ovary syndrome; PM, postmenopausal women. (Adapted from Carmina E, Lobo RA. Dynamic tests for hormone evaluation. In Lobo RA, Mishell DR, Paulson Rj, Shoupe D [eds]. Mishell's Textbook of Infertility, Contraception, and Reproductive Endocrinology, 4th ed. Oxford, Blackwell Science, 1997.)*

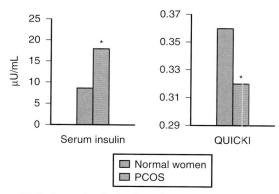

Figure 32-7. *Serum insulin levels and quantitative insulin sensitivity check index (QUICKI) values in normal women and women with polycystic ovaries. QUICKI values less than 0.33 are suggestive of insulin resistance. PCOS, polycystic ovary syndrome. (Data from Carmina E, Longo RA, Rini GB, Lobo RA. Phenotypic variation in hyperandrogenic women influences the finding of abnormal metabolic and cardiovascular risk parameters. J Clin Endocrinol Metab 90:2545-2549, 2005.)*

Frequently Sampled Intravenous Glucose Test

Two different catheters (one for glucose and insulin administration and one for blood samples) are placed in two antecubital veins. Glucose (0.3 g/kg) is injected over a period of 1 minute intravenously, followed 20 minutes later by an intravenous insulin bolus (0.03 U/kg). In the original method,[97] blood samples were taken 15, 10, and 5 minutes, and then 1 minute before the glucose load; additional samples were taken every minute for 10 minutes after loading, and again at 12, 14, 16, 20, 22, 23, 24, 25, 27, 30, 40, 50, 60, 70, 80, 90, 100, 120, 150, and 180 minutes. Because of the great number of blood samples required ($n = 33$), the test has been modified[98] to require only 12 samples: one taken 5 minutes before the glucose load, and then additional samples taken 2, 4, 8, 20, 22, 30, 40, 50, 70, 100, and 180 minutes afterward. In all samples, glucose and insulin are measured and insulin sensitivity (S_I), which is reciprocally inversely related to insulin resistance, is calculated with the minimal model method[99] by using a computerized algorithm. According to the American Diabetes Association, this test and the euglycemic insulin clamp are the only two methods that accurately estimate peripheral resistance to insulin.[95]

Insulin Tolerance Test

The ITT also has been used to assess insulin resistance[100] and has shown a good correlation with both the FSIGT test and the clamp studies. After an overnight fast, regular insulin (0.1 U/kg) is infused intravenously over 1 minute. Blood glucose is measured 0, 2, 5, 8, 10, and 15 minutes after insulin administration. Hypoglycemia generally occurs after 15 minutes; therefore, a solution of dextrose 50% in water ($D_{50}W$) is injected at 15 minutes to block this reaction. Because the test is so rapid (15 minutes), the usual counterregulatory factors (growth hormone [GH], cortisol, catecholamine release) that can affect insulin sensitivity are not yet in play. The linear slope of the declining blood glucose concentrations (2-15 minutes after insulin administration) is calculated and expressed as KITT percentage per minute. Young, healthy women have KITT

values of 5 to 6, whereas patients with PCOS generally have values lower than 4 (Figs. 32-6 and 32-7).[15] Although the ADA considers the ITT less sensitive than the FSIGT test, several researchers have reported that it gives comparable results.[100-101] We have used this test widely[93,102] because it requires only six blood samples for blood glucose determinations, thus reducing time and cost, particularly for repeated testing in clinical research (see Fig. 32-6).

Oral Glucose Tolerance Test

The OGTT is generally used to evaluate glucose tolerance, but the test has also been used to obtain a contemporaneous estimate of insulin resistance. Several calculations have been proposed:

- Area under the curve of glucose ÷ area under the curve of insulin[103]
- Area under the curve of glucose × area under the curve of insulin[104]
- S_I 2 hours after OGTT (calculated as 10^8/glucose at 2 hours × insulin at 2 hours × 150 × kg[105]
- Cederholm equation (a complex calculation considering total and mean glucose and insulin levels)[106]

Among these calculations, only the S_I 2 hours after an OGTT and the Cederholm equation show some correlation with the most precise methods.[95]

Fasting Glucose and Insulin Calculations

Several authors have proposed to evaluate insulin resistance using mathematical calculations applied to simultaneously obtained fasting glucose and insulin values. The most frequently used methods are:

- Glucose-to-insulin ratio[107]
- Fasting insulin resistance index[108] = (glucose × insulin) ÷ 25
- Homeostasis model assessment of insulin resistance (HOMA-IR)[109] = (glucose × insulin) ÷ 22.5

- Logarithm of the HOMA-IR[110]
- Quantitative insulin sensitivity check index (QUICKI)[111] = 1 ÷ (log glucose + log insulin)

Some of these methods, in particular, HOMA-IR, have gained popularity and are often used for a rapid assessment of insulin resistance in clinical practice. However, the relationships between the insulin level and direct glucose–insulin correlations are hyperbolic rather than linear. Therefore, the use of logarithmic or reciprocal transformation of these mathematical calculations is needed. In fact, the logarithm of the HOMA-IR and QUICKI correlate well with the results of clamp studies and should be the preferred calculations over other fasting measures of insulin sensitivity as long as there is no major impairment of glucose tolerance, as in diabetes.[112] The correlation, however, is better in patients with more marked insulin resistance, as in obesity, than in patients with mild insulin resistance (lean PCOS). We generally prefer to use the QUICKI method because it correlates reasonably well with the euglycemic clamp study. Values lower than 0.335 suggest insulin resistance and may be found in most women with PCOS[93] (see Fig. 32-7).

Measurement of Adipose Hormones

Adipose tissue is a complex endocrine organ that secretes hormones, cytokines, free fatty acids, and various proteins that have profound effects on metabolism and the cardiovascular system.[113] In recent years, many of these factors have been characterized and measured in various endocrine disorders, including PCOS.[114] Although most assays are useful only for research purposes, the measurement of two adipose hormones, leptin and adiponectin, also may be useful in clinical practice.

Leptin is a 146–amino acid protein that acts mostly as a signaling factor from adipose tissue to the central nervous system to serve as a metabolic indicator of energy sufficiency.[115] It may be measured by RIA or ELISA, and in our laboratory, in adult women with normal body weight, leptin values are 10 to 30 pg/mL. Serum levels of leptin increase in obese subjects, probably because in obesity there is a condition of leptin resistance. However, some massively obese subjects have a genetically determined leptin deficiency and the finding of low leptin levels in severe obesity suggested the possibility of using leptin in the treatment of these subjects. In PCOS, the levels of leptin are strictly related to body weight,[116] and are not different compared with weight-matched normal women. Finally leptin levels are lower in children than in adults and increase progressively during puberty.[117]

Adiponectin is a large protein composed of 244 aminoacids that has a major role in preventing or counteracting the development of diet-induced insulin resistance.[118] Moreover, adiponectin has been reported to have an important function in protecting endothelial cells from injury.[119] Adiponectin may be measured by RIA or ELISA, and in our laboratory, in adult women with normal body weight, adiponectin values are between 8 and 18 μg/mL. Adiponectin is decreased in obesity,[120] probably because of a negative feedback driven by hyperinsulinemia, and this reduction may contribute to the effects of obesity on insulin resistance, endothelial disease, and cardiovascular risks.

In PCOS, adiponectin levels are lower than those in weight-matched control subjects and may represent a major mechanism for the development of early endothelial disease in these patients.[116,121] We have hypothesized that the adiponectin assay may be useful to evaluate individual risk profiles for atherosclerosis; however, this is unproven. In our experience, 30% of women with PCOS have serum levels of adiponectin of less than 8 μg/mL, suggesting a particular risk of early endothelial disease.

EVALUATION OF FAT QUANTITY AND DISTRIBUTION

Because excess fat and altered fat distribution represent very important factors in determining insulin resistance and metabolic and cardiovascular risk,[122,123] many methods have been developed to assess these parameters.

The simplest way to assess fat quantity is to calculate the body mass index by the following formula: body weight (kg)/height^2 (cm). Values of 30 or higher indicate obesity, with values greater than 40 indicating severe obesity. Values between 25 and 30 suggest an overweight status, whereas values between 19 and 25 indicate normal body mass. However, body mass index does not take into account differences in lean body mass and, in some patients, it may be useful to measure fat quantity directly by total body dual x-ray absorptiometry (DEXA).[124,125] This method permits the measurement of fat quantity in the total body and in several different areas. Particularly important is the measurement of fat quantity in the trunk because this represents a way to assess abdominal fat mass. An increase in abdominal fat, mainly visceral fat, has been suggested to be the main cause of cardiovascular and metabolic risks of obesity.[113,125]

Because of the role of abdominal fat, it has been suggested that the measurement of waist circumference is more important than the evaluation of body weight in assessing the health problems linked to obesity. In women, values of 88 cm or greater indicate excessive abdominal fat accumulation and increased metabolic and cardiovascular risks. However, in young women, a normal waist circumference is less than 80 cm, and values greater than 80 and less than 88 cm may indicate some abdominal fat increase (Fig. 32-8).

To assess abdominal fat more accurately, other methods may be useful. Abdominal CT and MRI are very sensitive tests, but cannot be used routinely in clinical practice for this purpose. Therefore, abdominal ultrasound and DEXA are generally the preferred methods.[126] Ultrasound is a simple method to assess abdominal fat, but its accuracy is highly dependent on the operator's skill level. With this method, omental thickness in centimeters is assessed by using the distance between the posterior surface of the aponeurosis of the rectus abdominal muscle and the anterior wall of the aorta, 5 cm above the umbilicus.

Although DEXA scans are simple and sensitive, the software used generally measures fat in the trunk, which includes the thorax. The sensitivity of this method may therefore be enhanced by measuring abdominal fat in a 50-cm^2 area around the central point of the midline, between the lateral iliac crests and the lowest rib margins at the end of a normal

TABLE 32-1

Evaluation of Abdominal Fat by Dual X-Ray Absorptiometry (DEXA)

	Mean	Upper Normal Limits	
Trunk fat (g)	5200	8000	High values indicate abdominal fat accumulation
Trunk fat (%)	31.4	38	High values indicate abnormal fat distribution (abdominal obesity)
Central abdominal fat (g)	300	520	High values indicate abdominal fat accumulation; more sensitive index than trunk fat

Modified from Friedman JM, Halaas JL. Leptin and the regulation of body weight in mammals. Nature 395:763-770, 1998.

expiration.[125] This point generally corresponds to the umbilicus (but may not) and is located in the midline. Other authors have preferred to measure fat quantity between L1 and L4. Because DEXA measures total body fat and trunk (or central abdominal) fat, it is possible to calculate with the same examination the percentage of abdominal fat.

We recently determined normal values and the upper limits (Table 32-1) of fat parameters (measured by DEXA) in young women of normal weight. In general, values of more than 40% of trunk fat indicate abdominal obesity.[125]

Depending on the population studied, 30% to 60% of women with PCOS may be considered obese and most of them have abdominal obesity.[125] However, 60% of overweight women with PCOS and 30% of women of normal weight with PCOS exhibit an increase in abdominal fat.[125]

METABOLIC SYNDROME

In recent years, the term *metabolic syndrome* has become popular to denote a condition of increased atherosclerosis and cardiovascular risk. This is based primarily on the findings of insulin resistance or abdominal obesity.[127] According to National Cholesterol Education Program Adult treatment guidelines,[128] the syndrome is present if an individual has altered values of at least three of five parameters (blood glucose, blood triglycerides, blood high-density lipoprotein cholesterol, waist circumference, and blood pressure; Fig. 32-9). The concept of metabolic syndrome has been

debated because the health risk may be merely the sum of the single risks. However, the diagnosis of metabolic syndrome may be useful in that it helps to identify women and men who have a particularly high metabolic and cardiovascular risk. In PCOS, metabolic syndrome is very common and its prevalence ranges from 10% to 50%, depending on body weight, age, and lifestyle variables.[129,130]

Measurement of Growth Hormone and Growth Factors

Circulating GH may be measured by conventional RIA or IRMAs. With any method, because of very low basal values and pulsatile secretion, the measurement of an unstimulated random GH value is usually not very meaningful.[131] Measurement of overnight urinary GH may be useful,[132] but urinary concentrations of GH are also very low and may not be detectable in some assays. There is also a high degree of variability in renal excretion of GH.

Insulin-like growth factor 1 (IGF-1) is measured by specific immunoassays and, because these values reflect the integrated 24-hour concentrations of serum GH, IGF-1 may be used for the screening of GH deficiency.[133,134] Circulating IGF-1 levels are low in prepubertal children, making differentiation between healthy and GH-deficient children difficult. Moreover, several conditions result in low IGF-1 concentrations, including malnutrition, hypothyroidism, renal failure, and diabetes mellitus. Therefore, confirmation of the diagnosis requires at least two GH provocative tests.[134]

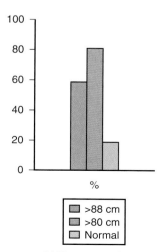

Risk factor	Defining level
Waist circumference	>88 cm
HDL cholesterol	<50 mg/dL
Triglycerides	≥150 mg/dL
Blood pressure	≥130/>85 mm Hg
Glucose	Fasting ≥100 mg/dL

Figure 32-9. *Criteria for metabolic syndrome in women. The syndrome is present if an individual has any three of the five criteria shown. HDL, high-density lipoprotein. (Data from executive summary of the third report of National Cholesterol Education Program [NECP] Expert Panel on Detection, Evaluation and Treatment of High Blood Cholesterol in Adults [Adult Treatment Panel III]. JAMA; 285:2486-2497, 2001; Grundy SM, Cleeman JI, Daniels SR, et al. Diagnosis and management of the metabolic syndrome: an American Heart Association/National Heart, Lung, and Blood Institute scientific statement. Circulation 112:2735, 2005.)*

Figure 32-8. *Percentage of 170 women with polycystic ovary syndrome with various waist circumferences.*

Serum IGF-1 is also useful in the screening evaluation of GH hypersecretion.[135] Persistently elevated serum IGF-1 levels can identify acromegaly better than several random GH serum measurements and overnight urinary GH tests; however, some acromegalic patients may have normal IGF-1 levels, requiring other investigations if acromegaly is suspected. Serum IGF-1 assessment is particularly useful in evaluating the effects of treatment in acromegalic subjects; the finding of increased levels of IGF-1 indicates that the disease is not well controlled. Finally, because IGF-1 is low in malnutrition, this assay also may be useful in assessing the general nutritional status of patients.

Insulin-like growth factor 2 (IGF-2) may be evaluated by specific IRMAs, but this level is less dependent on GH secretion. The measurement of IGF-2 is useful only in islet cell tumor hypoglycemia, an uncommon syndrome caused by some tumors (generally mesenchimal tumors) and associated with low levels of insulin, IGF-1, and IGF binding protein 3 (IGFBP-3).[136]

There are six IGF binding proteins. Among these, circulating IGFBP-1, IGFBP-2, and IGFBP-3 have been the subject of evaluation for clinical purposes. IGFBP-3 is GH-dependent and reflects changes in GH levels. Because of its long half-life and nonpulsatile secretion, IGFBP-3 measurement is an alternative to IGF-1 measurement for the screening of perturbations in GH.[134]

Levels of serum IGFBP-1 are significantly influenced by hyperinsulinemia, with low levels found in insulin resistance[137]; in PCOS, where IGF-1 levels are normal, "free" IGF-1 is increased because of a reduced level of IGFBP-1. Serum IGFBP-1 may be measured in diabetes to evaluate whether hyperglycemia is due to inadequate insulin dosage or to other factors.

Serum IGFBP-2 correlates inversely with GH secretion and the IGFBP-2/IGFBP-3 ratio is a marker of GH action. Serum IGFBP-2 also increases in patients with some tumors (mostly gliomas and prostate cancers) and may be used to assess the growth of these tumors and in conjunction with prostate-specific antigen in the management of certain patients with prostatic carcinoma.[138]

DYNAMIC TESTS FOR EVALUATION OF GROWTH HORMONE SECRETION

Many provocative or inhibitory tests to diagnose GH deficiency or excess have been described.[139] Reduced responses to at least two provocative tests are diagnostic of GH deficiency. The cutoff for a normal peak GH level in response to provocative tests is generally 10 ng/mL using a conventional polyclonal assay and 2.5 to 3.5 ng/mL with a monoclonal assay.

Insulin Tolerance Test

The ITT is the first choice for the diagnosis of GH deficiency. Blood samples are taken at 0, 15, 30, 60, and 90 minutes, and glucose and GH levels are measured. The measurement of glucose is required for validation of hypoglycemia (<40 mg/dL), which is necessary to evoke a GH response. An increase in serum GH levels to 10 ng/mL or greater excludes GH deficiency. A peak serum GH value of less than 3 ng/mL (by polyclonal assay) has been considered indicative of severe GH deficiency, according to the Growth Hormone Research Society.[140]

Clonidine Stimulation Test

Clonidine, a well-known antihypertensive drug, may be used for the diagnosis of GH deficiency. Oral clonidine (0.15 mg/m^2) is administered after an overnight fast. Blood pressure must be monitored during the test because a modest decrease in blood pressure is often observed.

Growth Hormone–Releasing Hormone and Arginine Test

The GH-releasing hormone (GnRH) and arginine test is considered an alternative to the ITT for the diagnosis of adult GH deficiency in patients for whom insulin hypoglycemia is contraindicated. GH-releasing hormone (1 µg/kg) and arginine (0.5 g/kg to a maximum of 30 g in 30 minutes) are combined in the same stimulation test.[141]

Oral Glucose Tolerance Test

The OGTT is the primary test used for the diagnosis of GH hypersecretion. After an overnight fast, administration of 75 to 100 g oral glucose will cause a suppression of serum GH. Blood samples are taken every 30 minutes for 2 hours. With the usual polyclonal RIAs, a decrease in GH to less than 2 ng/mL is found in normal subjects, whereas 80% of subjects with acromegaly do not suppress GH to this level. The monoclonal assays are much more sensitive for testing, and failure of GH to suppress to less than 1 ng/mL is diagnostic of acromegaly.[142]

Measurement of Calcium-Regulating Hormones and Bone Markers

In humans, the main calcium-regulating hormones are parathyroid hormone (PTH) and 1,25-dihydroxyvitamin D. The measurement of PTH is difficult because of the complex metabolism of this hormone, which results in a multiplicity of circulating molecular forms with different bioactivities as well as the presence in blood of PTH fragments. The bioactive forms (intact PTH molecule and the aminoterminal fragment) circulate in small quantities because of their shorter half-lives. Therefore, immunoassays using antibodies that recognize the mid- or carboxyterminal regions of PTH may be useful in subjects with primary hyperparathyroidism because they provide an index of integrated secretory function of the parathyroid gland. On the contrary, assays that use antibodies against the intact molecule or aminoterminal fragment should be used in patients with renal failure, or when studying physiologic changes associated with PTH function.

An important advance has been the development of two-site IRMAs for intact PTH. This assay uses antibodies directed against the aminoterminal and midregion (or carboxyterminal) fragments.[143] Because intact PTH is labile at room temperature, specimens should be frozen within 2 to 4 hours of collection. Normal PTH values range from

10 to 65 pg/mL, but must be correlated with circulating calcium levels. The finding of increased serum PTH and calcium is diagnostic of hyperparathyroidism, although some patients may have normocalcemic hyperparathyroidism that results in a form of osteoporosis that is often clinically indistinguishable from postmenopausal osteoporosis. This condition must be differentiated from the more common mild deficiency of vitamin D, in which PTH levels are moderately increased but calcium blood values are normal. In these patients, the administration of vitamin D normalizes serum PTH values.

Clinical assay techniques for circulating monohydroxylated (25-OH) and dihydroxylated (1,25-OH) vitamin D have progressed from competitive protein-binding assays to RIAs that use both ^{125}I and chemiluminescent reporters. These methods are used in the screening of osteoporotic women for underlying vitamin D deficiency.[144] Depending on the assay, different ranges of values have been reported, but serum 25-hydroxyvitamin D levels of less than 10 µg/L indicate severe vitamin D deficiency. Levels between 10 and 20 µg/L suggest partial vitamin D deficiency.[145] It has been suggested that a large percentage of the female population, particularly in the northern hemisphere, is vitamin D–deficient.

Several biochemical markers of bone turnover are measurable and may be useful in assessing bone formation and resorption (see Table 14-3).[146] These include RIAs and ELISA measurements of serum bone alkaline phospahatase (BAP) and osteocalcin as markers of bone formation, and of serum or urinary pyridolines cross-links and N-collagen or C-collagen telopeptides (aminotelopeptide or carboxytelopeptide) as markers of bone resorption. Carboxyterminal propeptide and aminoterminal propeptide also are produced by skin and are less useful than BAP (one alkaline phosphatase) or osteocalcin in distinguishing normal from disease states. Tartrate-resistant acid phosphatase is not specific for the osteoclast (as was hoped), and is relatively unstable. Urinary hydroxyproline is not specific for bone collagen and is influenced by dietary proteins.

The clinical utility of markers of bone turnover in assessing osteoporosis, in spite of their popularity, is still debated. Serum markers are usually preferred because they are less variable. The variability is on the order of 20% to 30% for urinary markers and 10% to 15% for blood markers. Although bone resorption markers and bone mineral density (BMD) are correlated, markers cannot be used to predict BMD, which is used to monitor the effectiveness of antiresorptive therapy.[146] However, high levels of resorption markers may provide additional important information about fracture risk because, independent of BMD alone, fracture risk may depend more on bone strength, for which the microarchitectural deterioration of bone[147] is important, and this cannot be determined by measurements of the density of bone alone.

METHODS FOR MEASUREMENT OF BONE DENSITY

Measurement of bone density is essential for the diagnosis of osteopenia and osteoporosis. Although many methods have been widely used, including ultrasound evaluation of the calcaneus, a precise determination of bone density requires DEXA. The lumbar spine, hip, and femoral and neck areas are the most important regions to be evaluated. The data are expressed as a T score, which provides the number of standard deviations below the mean peak bone density of a normal adult. Values between −1 and −2.5 are indicative of osteopenia, and values less than −2.5 indicate osteoporosis. DEXA of peripheral bones (e.g., forearm) is possible and is sometimes used as an additional assessment, particularly in metabolic disease. Osteoarthritis and other degenerative bone diseases may result in artificially higher T scores; therefore, this condition is suspected when there is a discrepancy in T scores between different lumbar vertebrae.

Measurement and Blood Levels of Thyroid Hormones

Circulating TSH is measured by two-site noncompetitive immunometric assays using enzymes, luminescent compounds, or ^{125}I as labels.[148] These assays have completely replaced the original RIAs because of the need for greater sensitivity to distinguish the low levels in hyperthyroid individuals from suppressed levels carrying some other significance (Fig. 32-10).

Normal serum TSH levels range from 0.5 to 4 µU/mL. Values between 0.1 and 0.45 µU/mL and 4.5 and 10 µU/mL are generally associated with normal levels of thyroid hormones and suggest subclinical thyroid disease.[149] Some authors have suggested that the normal upper cutoff level for TSH is as low as 2.5 µU/ml,[150] but there is no agreement about this.[151] During pregnancy, it is particularly important to maintain serum levels of TSH in the strict normal range because subclinical maternal hypothyroidism is also associated with complications of pregnancy and adverse effects on the fetus.[152,153]

For a more complete evaluation of thyroid function, the measurement of thyroid hormones is necessary. Circulating total thyroxine (T_4) and triiodothyronine (T_3) and their free fractions may be measured. Many laboratories prefer to measure only total T_4, but in some conditions (such as pregnancy), free thyroid hormones must be evaluated. Any condition that increases levels of circulating thyroxine-binding globulin, as occurs in pregnancy and with estrogen treatment, also increases total thyroid hormone. During pregnancy, thyroxine-binding globulin increases approximately 2.5 times, with peak levels occurring at 15 to 20 weeks' gestation.[152] Normal T_4 levels are higher than 7.8 µg/dL.[154] Free thyroid hormone levels remain within the normal range; the only exception occurs late in the first trimester, when a transient increase may occur.

The most precise determination of free T_4 is obtained by equilibrium dialysis, whereas some commercial RIA kits—which use a T_4 analog—may give inaccurate results.[155]

Because the most common causes of thyroid disorders are autoimmune disorders, assay of thyroid autoantibodies is often useful.[156] Several autoantibodies may be measured, but the most used in clinical practice are thyroid peroxidase antibody and thyroid-stimulating immunoglobulins (thyroid receptor antibodies or thyroid-stimulating immunoglobulin [TSI]). Measurement of thyroid peroxidase antibody is useful for diagnosing autoimmune chronic thyroiditis, but levels also may be increased in Graves' disease.

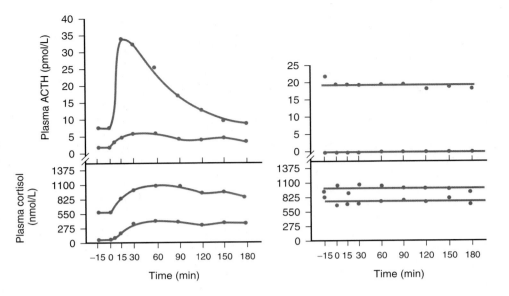

Figure 32-10. *Adrenocorticotropin hormone (ACTH) response to corticotropin-releasing hormone Colored lines represent different patients. (Adapted from Kaye TB, Crapo L. Cushing's syndrome: an update on diagnostic tests. Ann Intern Med 112:435-444, 1990.)*

TSI levels are increased in 80% to 90% of patients with Graves' disease and, during pregnancy, measurement of TSI levels may be useful to predict neonatal Graves disease.

THYROTROPIN-RELEASING HORMONE STIMULATION TEST

With the improvement and sensitivity of TSH assays, a TRH stimulation test is not required in the evaluation of primary hypothyroidism or hyperthyroidism in patients with low TSH levels. The test is still useful in the evaluation of central hypothyroidism, in rare patients with TSH-dependent hyperthyroidism, and in patients with pituitary tumors.

After an overnight fast, a 200-μg dose of TRH is administered intravenously. Blood samples for TSH are then taken at 0, 30, and 60 minutes. The mean peak TSH response is a value 8 to 9.5 times the basal values; however, the range in euthyroid subjects is large (3-23 times baseline).[157]

Evaluation of Glucocorticoids and Adrenal Function

Traditionally, cortisol, the main glucocorticoid produced by the adrenal, is conveniently measured by immunoassay. Several corticosteroids, including prednisone, prednisolone, and cortisone, cross-react in the assay.[158] Because cortisol secretion is highly pulsatile, a single random serum cortisol determination is usually not diagnostic for adrenal disorders.[159] Moreover, blood cortisol levels have a circadian variation, with the highest values occurring in the morning and the lowest levels in the late evening. Nevertheless, a midnight cortisol level of less than 50 nmol/L (<1.8 μg/mL) excludes Cushing syndrome.[160]

Because of the diurnal variability in levels, it is useful to measure 24-hour urinary free cortisol, which provides an index of cortisol secretion during the day. Although the upper normal range of urinary cortisol is 50 to 60 μg/day, some commercial assays report normal ranges of as high

as 100 to 130 μg/day. Urinary free cortisol should be measured by high-performance liquid chromatography combined with RIA or a competetive binding assay. This assay is valuable for diagnosing excessive cortisol secretion, not diminished secretion. In general, three to four completely normal 24-hour collections exclude the diagnosis, whereas a value more than four times the upper limit of normal is diagnostic of Cushing syndrome. Unfortunately, many patients, especially individuals with psychiatric disease, obesity, or alcohol abuse, have intermediate values and other diagnostic tests are needed.[160]

Plasma ACTH may be measured to help interpret values of serum or urinary cortisol. ACTH is measured by IRMAs. Plasma ACTH levels of more than 100 pg/mL in the presence of low serum cortisol are suggestive of primary adrenal insufficiency (Addison syndrome).[161] A plasma ACTH level of greater than 20 pg/mL at 9 AM is highly indicative of ACTH-dependent Cushing syndrome. A level of less than 10 pg/mL suggests ACTH independence and a primary adrenal cause of Cushing syndrome.[160,162] However, in many individuals, evaluation of blood ACTH and cortisol is not sufficient to diagnose adrenal disorders; therefore, dynamic tests must be performed.

DEXAMETHASONE SUPPRESSION TEST

As a simple screening test for hypercortisolism, overnight dexamethasone suppression may be used. Dexamethasone (1 mg) is given at 11 PM and serum cortisol is measured the next morning. Although we previously considered a serum cortisol level of less than 5 μg/dL suggestive of a normal response, 18% of patients with Cushing syndrome have been shown to suppress serum cortisol to these levels after overnight dexamethasone. A lower cutoff of less than 1.8 μg/dL is more effective for excluding Cushing syndrome, but the specificity of this test remains low.[160,162]

The classic low-dose dexamethasone suppression test has greater diagnostic accuracy.[160] The test may be performed reliably, even in outpatients, and involves the administration of dexamethasone, 0.5 mg every 6 hours for 2 days, followed by collection of blood for cortisol measurement on the morning of the third day. Serum cortisol levels of greater than 1.8 µg/dL are a sensitive indicator of Cushing syndrome. Some drugs that increase the hepatic clearance of dexamethasone, such as carbamazepine, phenytoin, nifedipine, rifampicin, and phenobarbital, may interfere with dexamethasone tests and should be discontinued before investigation. Estrogens may give falsely elevated cortisol levels (increasing corticosteroid-binding globulin) and should be discontinued at least 6 weeks before testing.

The high-dose dexamethasone suppression test (2 mg dexamethasone every 6 hours for 2 days) has been used to differentiate between the sources of hypercortisolism. A decrease in serum cortisol of at least 50% may suggest pituitary Cushing disease. However, the use of this test has been questioned because of its very low sensitivity, specificity, and accuracy.[163]

CORTICOTROPIN-RELEASING HORMONE STIMULATION TEST

Corticotropin-releasing hormone (CRH) is a 41–amino acid hypothalamic peptide that stimulates the secretion of ACTH and related peptides. After an overnight fast, 1 µg/kg human CRH is given intravenously; ACTH and cortisol are then measured in blood samples obtained at 0, 15, 30, and 60 minutes (Fig. 32-11). ACTH values peak at 15 minutes, whereas cortisol levels peak between 30 and 60 minutes. In healthy patients, plasma ACTH levels increase by 100% or more and serum cortisol levels increase by more than 50%. The test is generally used in patients with ACTH-dependent Cushing syndrome to differentiate the pituitary form from an ectopic source.[160,162]

In patients with Cushing disease (pituitary form), 85% have an increase in serum cortisol of 20% or more. However, 15% of patients with Cushing disease do not respond to CRH at all. In patients with an ectopic ACTH source, 10% may show some response to the test. Inferior petrosal vein sampling after CRH stimulation may be used to increase the sensitivity and specificity of the test. A basal central-to-peripheral gradient of ACTH of more than 2 or a stimulated gradient of 3 is indicative of Cushing disease.[164] The test may be used to determine the location of the pituitary adenoma, but the results should be interpreted cautiously because, in up to 30% of cases, the adenoma is localized incorrectly.[165]

The CRH test also has been used to differentiate between pituitary and hypothalamic ACTH insufficiency.[166] A low ACTH level (<10 pg/mL) that increases to no more than 10 pg/mL after CRH suggests a hypothalamic defect.

DEXAMETHASONE–CORTICOTROPIN-RELEASING HORMONE TEST

Dexamethasone and CRH have been combined to more accurately diagnose hypercortisolism.[167,168] Low-dose dexamethasone suppression (starting at noon on the first day, with the last dose given at 6 AM on the third day) is followed by CRH (1 µg/kg intravenously) at 8 AM. A plasma cortisol level of greater than 1.4 µg/dL 15 minutes after CRH administration suggests Cushing syndrome. However, some

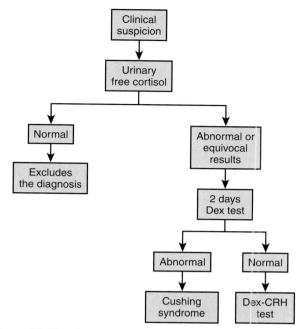

Figure 32-11. *Diagnostic algorithm for Cushing syndrome. Dex-CRH, dexamethasone–corticotropin-hormone.*

false-positive results have been reported, and most assays of serum cortisol do not have the sensitivity to distinguish between very low levels of cortisol. Therefore, it has been suggested that higher sensitivity and specificity may be obtained using a 15-minute cortisol threshold of 2.5 µg/dL.[169]

IMAGING STUDIES IN CUSHING SYNDROME

Because ACTH-secreting pituitary adenomas are often small, with standard MRI protocols, 40% of these microadenomas are not visualized. With the development of dynamic pituitary MRI, which uses multiple coronal dynamic sequences after the administration of gadolinium intravenous contrast, most pituitary corticotroph adenomas may be visualized, although in one study, in 16% of individuals, false-positive results were observed.[170]

For visualization of adrenal tumors, CT scanning is preferred. In general, large tumors (>6 cm) should be considered malignant.

Chest CT scan (high-definition spiral CT) is useful for identifying ectopic ACTH secretion because the most common source is a small cell lung cancer or a bronchial carcinoid tumor.[160,162] Some ACTH-secreting carcinoid tumors are visualized by somatostatin receptor scintigraphy, only, but 30% to 50% of ectopic ACTH-secreting lesions remain occult[171] and need careful follow-up.

DIAGNOSTIC PROCEDURE IN SUSPECTED CUSHING SYNDROME

The diagnosis of Cushing syndrome is suspected in many patients on the basis of clinical findings. The first step is to establish the status of hypercortisolism (see Fig. 32-11);

measurement of urinary free cortisol is preferred over the overnight dexamethasone suppression test for this purpose. More than one measurement should be considered. Urinary free cortisol levels of greater than 240 µg/24 hours are consistent with hypercortisolism, whereas values of up to 60 µg/24 hours are normal. If the results are abnormal or equivocal, a 2-day dexamethasone test should be performed. If sufficient cortisol suppression is not achieved, Cushing syndrome is established and the patient should be evaluated by a specialized center to determine the source of the increased cortisol secretion. If the results of the dexamethasone test are not consistent with the level of free urinary cortisol, a dexamethasone–corticotropin-hormone (Dex-CRH) test should be performed.

TESTS FOR ADRENAL INSUFFICIENCY

ACTH Test

Stimulation with ACTH (250 µg), administered intravenously with measurements of cortisol at 0, 30, and 60 minutes, is an excellent test for primary adrenocortical insufficiency.[161] Serum cortisol levels lower than 13 µg/dL after ACTH administration ensure the diagnosis of adrenal glucocorticoid insufficiency. Levels between 13 and 18 µg/dL are intermediate and require additional diagnostic evaluation. A serum cortisol level higher than 18 µg/dL after ACTH stimulation excludes the diagnosis. Low-dose ACTH (1 µg intravenously) may also be used, and researchers have suggested that this protocol identifies milder forms of adrenal insufficiency that are not diagnosed with the classic ACTH stimulation test.

The following tests are used for the diagnosis of secondary adrenal insufficiency.[161]

Insulin Tolerance Test

After an overnight fast, regular insulin (0.1 U/kg) is infused intravenously over 1 minute. Blood glucose and cortisol levels are measured at 0, 15, 30, 45, 60, 75, and 90 minutes. Once hypoglycemia (blood glucose < 40 mg/dL) is documented, serum cortisol levels of more than 18 g/dL exclude adrenal insufficiency. The test is contraindicated in elderly patients and those with cardiovascular, psychiatric, or seizure disorders.

Metyrapone Test

Metyrapone, which blocks 11β-hydroxylation, is used to test the adrenal response to endogenous ACTH.[161] This agent further reduces serum cortisol, however, and may induce adrenal insufficiency. For this reason, many endocrinologists prefer to perform an ITT. Metyrapone is generally used when an ITT test is contraindicated. Metyrapone, 30 mg/kg, is given orally at midnight with a snack; blood samples for cortisol and 11-deoxycortisol are obtained at 8 AM the next morning. After the blood samples are obtained, a prophylactic dose of prednisone or hydrocortisone is usually given. For the test result to be valid, cortisol has to decrease to less than 5 µg/dL. Peak values of 11-deoxycortisol of less than 7 µg/dL suggest reduced activity of the pituitary adrenal axis (see Fig. 32-11).

Diagnostic Procedure in Suspected Pituitary Tumors

Patients with pituitary tumors seek evaluation because of the symptoms (e.g., headache, diabetes insipidus, visual field alterations) or because of the finding of increased hormone secretion (e.g., acromegaly Cushing syndrome, amenorrhea with or without galactorrhea). Once a pituitary lesion is suspected, radiographic investigation is required.

The preferred technique to evaluate hypothalamic-pituitary lesions is MRI with gadolinium enhancement[172,173]; however, CT scanning with intravenous contrast and thin coronal sections may be also used. Examples of MRI and CT techniques may be found in Figures 32-12 and 32-13. Table 32-2 lists the major MRI characteristics of the more common hypothalamic–pituitary lesions. Dynamic pituitary MRI may increase the number of microadenomas that may be visualized.[170]

If hypothalamic or pituitary lesions are found, detailed evaluation of all pituitary hormones should be performed.[174] Regardless of the size of the lesion, patients should initially be evaluated for hormone hypersecretion. Serum PRL, GH with IGF-1, and 24-hour urinary free cortisol could be used for the initial screening. In selected patients, basal and TRH-stimulated gonadotropins and α subunits should be measured for the evaluation of possible

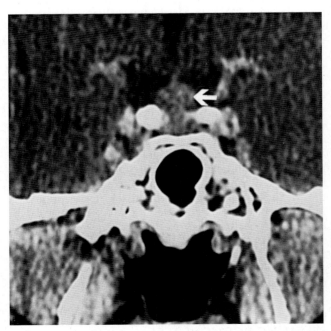

Figure 32-12. Typical close-up coronal view of a pituitary microadenoma by computed tomography (CT). The neoplasm cannot be distinguished from normal pituitary. Thus, the arrow indicates an enlarged abnormal pituitary bulging superiorly. The stalk is seen superior to the gland in the midline. The bone appears white on CT scan. Magnetic resonance imaging may allow better resolution of neoplasms from normal pituitary. (Adapted from Rebar RW. Practical evaluation of hormonal status. In Yen SC, Jaffe RB, Barbieri RL [eds]. Reproductive Endocrinology, Physiology, Pathophysiology, and Clinical Management, 4th ed. Philadelphia, WB Saunders, 1999, p 709.)

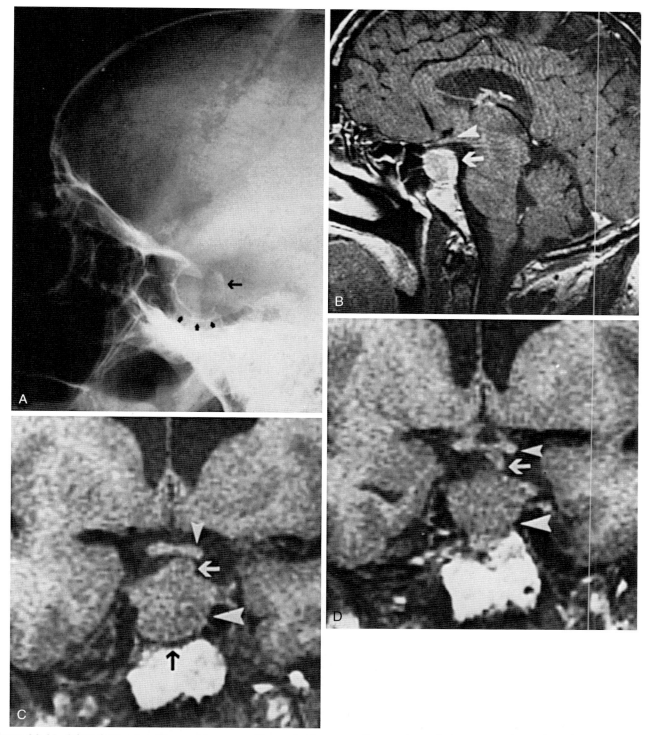

Figure 32-13. *Selected views in a 39-year-old woman with a probable nonsecreting neoplasm who has amenorrhea, galactorrhea, and prolactin levels of approximately 50 ng/mL. The radiographs suggest that the mild hyperprolactinemia is due to stalk compression.* **A,** *Lateral skull film showing ballooning of the sella turcica with a thin double floor (small arrows) and erosion of the clinoid processes posteriorly (large arrow).* **B,** *Sagittal view of magnetic resonance imaging with contrast material showing the large pituitary tumor (arrow) and normally positioned optic chiasm (arrowhead).* **C,** *Coronal view showing the large neoplasm (large arrowhead) bulging superiorly (white arrow) toward the optic chaism (small arrowhead). The* black arrow *shows the diaphragm sella.* **D,** *Another view of the neoplasm shows displacement of the optic chiasm (arrow) below the optic nerves and chiasm (small arrowhead). The* large arrowhead *indicates the lesion. The diaphragm is indistinct and there is the suggestion of bony erosion. (Adapted from Rebar RW. Practical evaluation of hormonal status. In* Yen SC, Jaffe RB, Barbieri RL [eds]. Reproductive Endocrinology, Physiology, Pathophysiology, and Clinical Management, *4th ed. Philadelphia: WB Saunders, 1999, p 709.)*

TABLE 32-2

Magnetic Resonance Imaging Characteristics of Some Hypothalamic-Pituitary Lesions

Type of Mass	MRI Images	MRI with Contrast Images	Particular Features
Pituitary adenoma	Hypointense	Hypointense	Hyperintense with hemorrhage
Pituitary cyst	Hyperintense	No change	Cystic; may be hypointense if CSF is in the cyst
Craniopharyngioma	Hyperintense	No change	Cystic with isohypointense solid portions
Meningioma	Isointense	Hyperintense	Hyperostosis of adjacent bone

CSF, cerebrospinal fluid; MRI, magnetic resonance imaging.

gonadotroph adenomas. Hyperthyroid patients should be screened for rare TSH adenomas. In a large series of 1043 pituitary tumors,[175] the most common pituitary hormone–secreting adenomas were prolactinomas (27.2%), followed by GH-secreting adenomas (14%), GH- and PRL-secreting adenomas (8.4%), and ACTH-secreting adenomas (8%).

Some pituitary adenomas produce only α subunit, a component of glycoprotein pituitary hormones (LH, FSH, TSH). Therefore, in patients with pituitary tumors and no increase in levels of pituitary hormones, assay of α subunit may be used. The subunit is measured by RIA, and in young adults, the circulating values are less than 1 ng/ml. Some gonadotropin-secreting pituitary tumors produce high quantities of α subunit, and this assay may be useful in postmenopausal women with pituitary adenomas. However, normal values of α subunit are higher in postmenopausal women (<3.6 ng/mL) than in young women.

Pituitary microadenomas do not generally cause disruption of pituitary function[174]; therefore, pituitary hypofunction should be assessed only in patients with large sellar masses that do not have increased secretion. Tests for GnRH, TRH, GH-releasing hormone, and CRH (all four releasing factors) may be performed together for contemporaneous evaluation of gonadotropins TSH, PRL, GH, and ACTH.[176]

Pelvic Evaluation

Pelvic ultrasound has become an extremely important tool for the reproductive endocrinologist. Assessment of ovarian function and monitoring for endometrial development are useful for clinical management and have been discussed elsewhere (see Chapters 8, 9, 20, 21, and 33). The finding of polycystic ovaries on ultrasound has been included as a criterion for the diagnosis of PCOS[177]; therefore, pelvic ultrasound evaluation should be performed in all patients with androgen excess, as well as those with persistently irregular cycles.

The ultrasound diagnosis of polycystic ovaries has shifted somewhat from the classic criteria to the newer Rotterdam criteria,[178] in which ovarian size alone is sufficient for the diagnosis. The size also has been scaled back recently from 10 cc to 7.5 cc.[179,180] Figure 32-14 shows the transvaginal ultrasound appearance of a polycystic ovary, with assessment of ovarian blood flow, which is increased in PCOS.[181]

If androgen excess is the central issue in PCOS, then a more meaningful criterion is the ratio of ovarian stroma to total surface area. As shown in Figure 32-15, some authors have suggested that a cutoff value of 0.32 correlates well with androgen excess (with values greater than this being significant).[182]

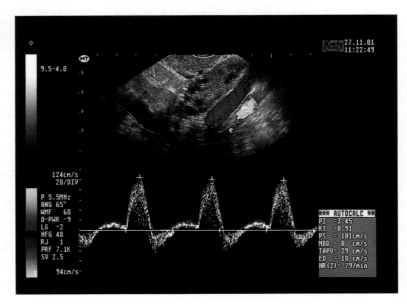

Figure 32-14. Typical color Doppler ultrasound of a polycystic ovary showing increased blood flow.

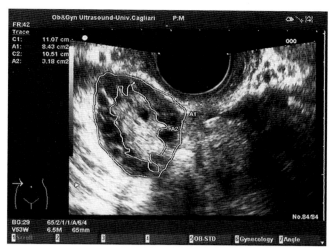

Figure 32-15. *Example of median ovarian section with outlined ovarian and stroma areas. A1 is the total area and A2 is the stroma area. (From Fulghesu AM, Angioni S, Frau E, et al. Ultrasound in polycystic ovary syndrome--the measuring of ovarian stroma and relationship with circulating androgens: results of a multicentric study. Hum Reprod 22:2501-2508, 2007.)*

Using three-dimensional ultrasound, which has also been found to be useful for the diagnosis of PCOS, müllerian anomalies can be detected. Whereas routine two-dimensional ultrasound is not able to distinguish between various müllerian anomalies, three-dimensional ultrasound is as sensitive as MRI in this regard. Nevertheless,

MRI may still have an advantage over ultrasound when differentiating between fibroids and adenomyosis.

The complete reference list can be found on the companion Expert Consult Web site at www.expertconsultbook.com.

Suggested Readings

Carmina E, Bucchieri S, Esposito A, et al. Abdominal fat quantity and distribution in women with polycystic ovary syndrome and extent of its relation to insulin resistance. J Clin Endocrinol Metab 92:2500, 2007.

Carmina E, Lobo RA. Use of fasting blood to assess the prevalence of insulin resistance in women with polycystic ovary syndrome. Fertil Steril 82:661, 2004.

Carmina E, Rosato F, Janni A, et al. Relative prevalence of different androgen excess disorders in 950 women referred because of clinical hyperandrogenism. J Clin Endocrinol Metab 91:2, 2006.

Casey BM, Leveno KJ. Thyroid disease in pregnancy. Obstet Gynecol 108:1283, 2006.

Chetty M, Elson J. Biochemistry in the diagnosis and management of abnormal early pregnancy. Clin Obstet Gynecol 50:55, 2007.

Macklin NS, Fauser BC. Ovarian reserve. Semin Reprod Med 23:248, 2005.

Newell-Price JNP, Bertagna X, Grossman AB, Nieman LK. Cushing's syndrome. Lancet 367:1605, 2006.

Rennert J, Doerfler A. Imaging of sellar and parasellar lesions. Clin Neurol Neurosurg 109:111, 2007.

Roberts B, Katzenlson N. Approach to the evaluation of the GH/IGF-axis in patients with pituitary disease: which test to order? Pituitary 10:205, 2007.

Rosner W, Auchus RJ, Azziz R, et al. Position statement: utility, limitations, and pitfalls in measuring testosterone: an Endocrine Society position statement. J Clin Endocrinol Metab 92:405, 2007.

CHAPTER 33

Pelvic Imaging in Reproductive Endocrinology

Dominique de Ziegler, Timothée Fraisse, Anne Elodie Millischer-Belaïche, and Charles Chapron

Introduction

VAGINAL ULTRASOUND AND IN VITRO FERTILIZATION

The advent of vaginal ultrasound approximately two decades ago revolutionized imaging of pelvic organs, particularly imaging of the ovaries and uterus. Originally, vaginal ultrasound was developed with the intent of simplifying the then-emerging technique of ultrasound-guided oocyte aspiration for in vitro fertilization (IVF).[1] A short-lived initiative proposed conducting transvaginal oocyte retrievals under transabdominal ultrasound guidance.[2] It readily became evident, however, that the future lay in oocyte retrievals conducted under vaginal ultrasound vision, using probes that were specially designed for vaginal use and equipped with needle holders.[3-5] The practical advantages of vaginal ultrasound for oocyte retrieval were so obvious that it nearly overnight became the primary mode of oocyte retrieval.

The development of ultrasound probes specially designed for vaginal use rapidly opened the way for diagnostic applications beyond the narrow context of monitoring assisted reproductive techniques (ART).[6] For diagnostic purposes, the advantage of vaginal ultrasound primarily rested in the possibility of using high-frequency high-resolution probes, which was made possible by the short distance between the probe (vaginal) and the organ scanned (uterus, ovaries). The improvements in image resolution that resulted from using high-frequency probes were soon recognized, leading to instant interest in the use of vaginal ultrasound in general gynecology.[7-9] Subsequently, all the technologic improvements incorporated in general ultrasound equipment, such as pulsed, color, and power Doppler functions[10,11] and later three-dimensional (3D) capabilities,[12,13] also became available on vaginal probes. Ultimately, the increase in image resolution provided by vaginal ultrasound and its multiple refinements (3D, Doppler, etc.) allowed the capability to meticulously assess parameters that reflect not only the anatomic characteristics of pelvic organs but also their functional status. These parameters include, for example, the descriptive benchmarks of the hormone-sensitive endometrium, which provides an indication about the integrated hormonal environment. Likewise, the count of small antral follicles (AFC) stands today as a cornerstone for assessing the functional state of the ovaries or *ovarian reserve*. Over the years, the relevance of these echographic parameters has been extensively validated so that they now complement classic hormonal measurements.

VAGINAL ULTRASOUND AND PELVIC EXAMINATION

Beyond improving image resolution and quality, it rapidly became evident that vaginal ultrasound studies could also provide further information about functional interactions that exist between pelvic organs and nearby structures, which could not be assessed previously. This advantage stems from the fact that vaginal ultrasound examinations do not require a full bladder. Consequently, it is possible to freely slide pelvic organs against one another and move them about the pelvic cavity under direct ultrasound vision by gentle pressure applied to the vaginal probe. This approach offers glimpses of the functional status of the pelvic cavity not available with static images. Practically speaking, assessing dynamic interactions between pelvic organs offers two distinct advantages:

1. It can precisely determine the limits of pathologic structures, such as those of an ovarian cyst, for example. It is thus possible to determine how the identified structure (i.e., the cyst in our example) can move with respect to other nearby organs when pelvic structures are mobilized by the vaginal probe. At times, positioning by an "abdominal hand" may be necessary to better mobilize the organ(s) under study.
2. The ability to slide organs also provides clues about the possible presence of pelvic adhesions otherwise unidentified on ultrasound images by analyzing how different structures move with respect to one another. For example, the ovary and nearby loops of bowel may move together when mobilized by the probe.

The ability to not only study the static appearance of pelvic organs but also to analyze their functional interactions within the pelvic cavity when moved about introduced a functional dimension to the clinical information that ultrasound provides. This *functional dimension* of vaginal ultrasound studies rapidly expanded their role for studying the pathophysiology of the pelvic cavity and reproductive function in general, therefore allowing ultrasound to reach beyond the realm of static imagery. In expert hands, vaginal ultrasound actually provides a true *pelvic examination with a view,* which literally revolutionized diagnostic explorations of the female pelvis. More specifically, the concept of *pelvic examination with a view* aims at conveying the message that vaginal ultrasound studies offer the possibility of integrating images of pelvic structures and clinical parameters of nonimaging nature. These parameters include data such as pain and tenderness that may be electively triggered by mobilizing specific organs or touching specific sites identified on imagery and ultimately, assessing the mobility of pelvic organs, and the like. Vaginal ultrasound, therefore, can fuse various forms of information to provide a global assessment of the pelvic status, in a process that remains the essence of clinical examination, yet with the added benefit of viewing internal organs.

Taken together, the improvements that vaginal ultrasound techniques have benefited from over the past 20 years have contributed to make ultrasound the primary and key diagnostic tool, not just for specialized explorations of reproductive function, but also in everyday gynecology. In this context, vaginal ultrasound pursues two primary aims:

1. Assessing the morphologic characteristics of pelvic organs and specific parameters that are pertinent to the hormonal environment.
2. Exploring the dynamic interactions of the studied organ with other pelvic structures and fusing this information with functional characteristics such as pain and tenderness and free mobility.

Therefore, functional exploration of pelvic organs by vaginal ultrasound, including its extensions to Doppler analysis, contrast enhancement, and 3D reconstruction, will be given the lion's share of attention in this chapter. As discussed in the section dedicated to the exploration of endometriosis, we will see that the boundaries of the clinical competence of vaginal ultrasound are constantly expanding. This leads us to predict that in expert hands vaginal ultrasound will soon become the first-line diagnostic tool for exploring and staging all facets of nonovarian endometriosis, thereby overtaking the current lead position that magnetic resonance imaging has been holding for staging endometriosis.

TECHNICAL REFINEMENTS OF VAGINAL ULTRASOUND: DOPPLER AND 3D RECONSTRUCTION

As vaginal ultrasound progressively became the primary diagnostic tool in gynecology over the past 20 years, two distinct technical refinements have come to enrich its capabilities and scope. These are the Doppler-based analyses of organ perfusion offered by ever more complex technical applications and the *off-line* and later *built-in* 3D image reconstruction systems. Both techniques carry the potential for further enhancing the descriptive and functional capabilities of vaginal ultrasound. In the case of 3D image reconstruction from saved 3D volumes, the technical novelty also offers new possibilities for improving the quality control of diagnostic ultrasound through secondary explorations of saved 3D volumes, previously a clear weakness of ultrasound studies at large. Both techniques have become ever more widely available over the years, with Doppler now being offered in all but the simplest entry-level equipment. Likewise, 3D is becoming more readily available, with most manufacturers offering some 3D option starting with their mid-level machines. Yet the respective advantages of either Doppler or 3D functions will vary depending on the organ (the uterus or ovaries) studied. Therefore, we will review the role and respective advantages of Doppler and 3D ultrasound studies and their clinical usefulness at enhancing the benefit of regular vaginal ultrasound in the respective sections dedicated to the uterus and ovaries.

CONTRAST-ENHANCED VISION OF THE UTERUS AND TUBES: SALINE INFUSION SONOGRAPHY

It struck many that the ultrasound images of the uterine cavity obtained in early pregnancy largely surpass in quality those of the nonpregnant uterus. Because of the sharpness with which fetal parts are depicted in early pregnancy, ultrasound-based prenatal diagnosis has made a formidable forward leap in use over the last decade. The explanation for the difference in quality between images of the pregnant and nonpregnant uterus was attributed to the presence of amniotic fluid in early pregnancy, which plays the role of a contrast enhancer that facilitates the visualization the developing embryo. Being sono-transparent like water, amniotic fluid creates a *black* interphase between the walls of the gestational sac and the developing embryo, a phenomenon that enhances image resolution.

Therefore, there was interest in reproducing the conditions that prevail in early pregnancy by infusing isotonic saline (NaCl) or other solutions in the uterine cavity of the nonpregnant uterus in order to create an artificial interphase, providing contrast enhancement. This procedure, given several designations such as sonohysterography,[14] is more commonly referred to today as saline infusion sonography (SIS). Following pioneering work in this field, numerous variants of the original procedure have been proposed that use either sono-transparent[15,16] or sono-refractory contrast media, such as Echovist, Levovist, or Albumex,[17,18] which provide *black* contrast and *white* contrast effects, respectively. The former, *black* contrast, is superior for exploring the uterine cavity, and *white* contrast SIS offers the added advantage of being able to explore the fallopian tubes on ultrasound.

SIS using negative or *black* contrast medium will be addressed in the section of this chapter dedicated to the uterus, as it stands as a helpful extension of regular ultrasound when screening for intrauterine disease, notably polyps and fibroids. Black contrast SIS of the uterine cavity has been found to be so helpful for exploring uterine malformations that it is now the primary tool for exploring uterine malformations. This is because SIS offers a combined vision of the intrauterine cavity(ies) and uterine muscle.

Conversely, SIS using positive or *white* contrast is mainly of interest for studying the fallopian tubes, which are not otherwise readily visible on ultrasound images. Uterine images are of lesser quality, however, when positive rather than negative contrast is used because some degree of shadowing is generated by the *white* contrast material.

IMAGING IN EVALUATING ENDOMETRIOSIS AND ADENOMYOSIS

We believe that the preeminent gynecologic disease of the pelvic cavity, endometriosis, deserves a separate section in this chapter on pelvic imaging in reproductive endocrinology. Endometriosis is capable of affecting all the pelvic organs, where it may undergo various degrees of extension and infiltration. In order to avoid fragmenting the descriptions of the imaging characteristics of endometriosis among the various organs discussed in this chapter, we will consolidate our discussion of endometriosis in one place.

Endometriosis is likely to extend to or invade organs such the uterine ligaments, vaginal wall, bladder, bowel, and other structures that are not readily identifiable on ultrasound. Exploring endometriosis, therefore, often requires "nonechographic" imaging, particularly magnetic resonance imaging (MRI). Hence, for many practical reasons, all aspects pertinent to MRI of the pelvic cavity will be concentrated and addressed in the discussion of endometriosis later in this chapter. Likewise, a variant of endometriosis, adenomyosis, both the diffuse and focal forms, can be reliably diagnosed on MRI with good correlation with anatomic findings. Thus, imaging of adenomyosis will be included in the

discussion of endometriosis rather than the section on uterine imaging.

FUNCTIONAL PELVIC IMAGING WITHIN THE SCOPE OF REPRODUCTIVE ENDOCRINOLOGY AND INFERTILITY

The primary emphasis of this chapter on pelvic imaging will parallel that of the textbook itself, providing a functional perspective about reproductive endocrinology and infertility. In considering all the pertinent issues of pelvic imaging, a clear emphasis has been put on those aspects that are at the core of the primary interest of the book, reproductive physiology and infertility. In addition, we restricted the concept of pelvic imaging to nonendoscopic images of pelvic organs, the latter stemming from the realm of surgical exploration.

Functional Imaging of the Uterus

ANATOMY AND MORPHOLOGIC MEASUREMENTS

The different nature of endometrial and myometrial tissues provides an easily identifiable interphase at the point of junction of the two uterine constituents. The lower extension of the endometrium delineates the internal os of the cervix, which serves as a landmark for individually measuring the cervix and uterine corpus. Specifically, the total length of the cervical canal is measured after identifying the external os of the cervix. The endometrium, which is hormonally sensitive, undergoes changes in thickness, volume, and aspect (echogenicity) during the various phases of the menstrual cycle. Similar and parallel changes are seen following various hormonal treatments, as discussed later in this chapter.

Anatomically speaking, the myometrium is composed of 3 layers.[19] The inner or sub endometrial layer of the myometrium is of müllerian origin. It is endowed with estrogen receptors (ERs) and progesterone receptors (PRs) showing cyclic changes that mimic those encountered in the endometrium.[20] In contrast, the two outer non-müllerian layers of the myometrium have stable concentrations of ERs and PRs throughout the menstrual cycle, which do not display the changes seen during the menstrual cycle in the endometrium.[21] The outer layer of the myometrium or stratum supravasculare offers extramuscular fibers that serve the needs of parturition in larger mammals. In the nonpregnant uterus, the outer layer participates in the uterine contractions encountered at the time of menses in response to progesterone withdrawal, but not in other forms of contractility encountered at other times in the menstrual cycle. As discussed later, disruptions of the contractile process taking place at the time of menses may cause dysmenorrhea and endometriosis.

Current imaging is capable of identifying the subendometrial layer of the myometrium where the peristaltic contractions that culminate in the late follicular phase are initiated. High-resolution vaginal ultrasound can describe this myometrial segment, the intermediate layer of lighter echogenic appearance, or *subendometrial halo*. It lies between the echoic basal layer of the endometrium and the underlying myometrium. Similarly, but using a different terminology, MRI identifies the subendometrial layer of the myometrium as a hypointense layer that separates the endometrium from the myometrium on T_2-weighted images; this layer is the *junctional zone* (JZ) (see section on endometriosis and adenomyosis).

Video recordings have identified that uterine contractions during the late follicular phase under the stimulus of rising estradiol (E_2) levels originate from the *subendometrial halo* or JZ area.[22,23] In an ex vivo trial, Tetlow et al.[24] studied six uteri obtained from fertile women aged 32.9 to 48.5 years. Following hysterectomy, all uteri were needle-biopsied in the subendometrial halo under ultrasound guidance. The results indicate that the subendometrial halo or JZ area is a distinct section of the myometrium with increased vascularitiy and more tightly packed myometrial cells. As discussed in a later section of this chapter, endometriosis and adenomyosis are considered to be associated with dysfunctions of the endometrial-subendometrial unit.[19]

Because the boundaries between the cervix and the uterine corpus and between the endometrium and myometrium are easily identifiable, the uterus can easily be measured on noninvasive ultrasound scans that depict the functionally distinct constituents of the uterus (Fig. 33-1). In adult women, uterine corpus length ranges from 5 to 8 cm[25] following a fairly abrupt growth period at the time of puberty. In a prospective trial looking at 139 girls between the ages of 1 and 13 years and addressing radiologic bone age measurement, uterine volume was calculated from transabdominal scan images taking the measured values of length, width, and depth and using the ellipse formula.[26] Uterine measurements and volume were markedly smaller in pretelarchial girls at 1.8 ± 1.2 cm^3 as compared to 8.1 ± 6.6 cm^3 after telarche.[27] In a large prospective trial conducted in 380 school girls aged 6 to 18 years, Holm et al. observed no age-related differences in uterine and ovarian size in 44 prepubertal girls, whereas a direct correlation with Tanner stages was observed in 163 prepubertal girls.[28] A further enlargement of the uterus was observed between Tanner stage 3 and adult girls (mean age 19).

Looking at 114 premenarchial girls, Orsini et al. observed that until the age of 7 the uterus and cervix were of similar size, with the corpus gradually becoming larger than the cervix thereafter.[29] These authors observed that the uterus continued to grow after menarche for several years with uterine size correlating with the number of postmenarchial years but not with height, a finding that is being challenged by others, however.[28]

In some clinical conditions the uterus was believed to be smaller than normal, but this finding was not always verified by actual measurements. Doerr et al. reported on a series of 75 women affected by Turner syndrome. Of 50 women with a karyotype 45,X0 who had received estrogen replacement, 42 (84%) had a normal size uterus, whereas it was smaller (length < 5 cm) in the remaining 8 women (16%) who received no estrogen treatment.[30] In this study, uterine size might have been affected by the age at which estrogen therapy had been started but showed no

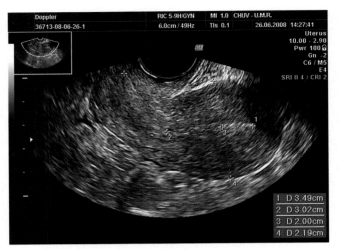

Figure 33-1. *Uterine size. Interphase between endometrium and myometrium is clearly identifiable on ultrasound images. The lower end of endometrial development identifies the internal os of the cervix, which delineates the limits of the uterine corpus and cervix.*

correlation with other factors, notably the final height.[30] The impact of growth hormone (GH) treatment on uterine size remains a matter for debate, with Sampaolo et al.[31] showing a positive effect, whereas Snajderova et al. found none.[32]

We know from the report of Herbst et al.[33,34] that in utero exposure to diethylstilbestrol (DES) may affect the genitalia. These authors were the first to blow the whistle on possible adverse effects of in utero exposure to DES when linking seven cases of adenocarcinoma of the vagina, an otherwise excessively rare tumor, with in utero DES exposure. Puzzlingly, all these cases had occurred at a single hospital in DES-exposed women between the ages of 7 and 22,[34] a finding later confirmed by others.[35] Further studies of DES-exposed women also revealed many benign morphologic abnormalities of the genital tract, including transverse ridges in the vagina, vaginal adenosis, and morphologic anomalies of the uterus, such as the characteristic T-shaped uterus (Fig. 33-2).[36] Viscomi et al. analyzed the echographic appearance of the uterus in cases of DES exposure.[37] An abnormal T-shaped uterus was found in 3 of 18 (16%) women exposed to DES, a number in agreement with an incidence of 12% observed on hysterosalpingography (HSG).[38,39] Furthermore, Viscomi et al. reported a reduced uterine size with a mean uterine length of 6.8 ± 0.4 cm in 18 DES-exposed women as compared to 8.1 ± 0.8 cm in 20 age-matched control subjects, even in the absence of gross morphologic anomalies.[38] Calculated uterine volume was of 49.4 and 90 cm^3 in DES-exposed and control subjects, respectively. Salle et al. have reported altered uterine vascularity in women exposed to DES with higher uterine artery pulsatility index and resistance index and an absence of the cycle-related changes in these women.[40] As discussed in a later section of this chapter, uterine artery Doppler flow indices have been extensively studied with the hope of finding markers of endometrial receptivity. Yet in spite of hopes sparked by early studies, none of the differences between receptive and nonreceptive endometrium proposed as predictors of either good

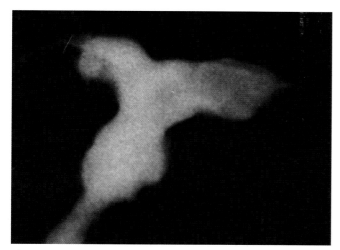

Figure 33-2. Effects of in utero exposure to diethylstilbestrol (DES): T-shaped uterus with characteristic miduterine ridges.

or poor ART outcome ended up being verified. As a result, today there is overwhelming agreement that Doppler does not predict endometrial receptivity, thus casting serious doubts about any predictive value of Doppler results for reproductive outcome in DES-exposed women.

Several authors have proposed surgical correction (metroplasty) of uterine anomalies related to DES exposure, including T-shaped distortion[41] or simple overall reduction of uterine size.[42] Although authors reporting on small series recount positive impressions about the impact of surgery on subsequent reproductive outcome,[43] formal studies on the efficacy of these procedures are strikingly missing.

THE UTERINE CERVIX

Vaginal ultrasound studies can precisely delineate the anatomic limits of the cervix, which extends downward from the internal os of the cervix identified as the outer (or lower) tip of the hormonally sensitive endometrium. This point constitutes the inner end of the cervical canal from which the total length of the uterine cervix can be calculated by reference to the external os of the cervix normally seen on ultrasound. The cervical canal can easily be identified, either as a hyperechoic line or as a sono-transparent hypoechoic canal when cervical mucus is being produced and accumulates in the cervical lumen, as during the follicular phase of the menstrual cycle or when women are exposed to exogenous E_2. We use a semi-quantitative system in which the mucus is graded +, ++, and +++ when a sono-transparent dilatation of the cervical canal can be measured at less than 1 mm, 1 to 2 mm, and more than 2 mm, respectively—an approach that is close, if not similar, to that of others.[44]

The presence of cervical mucus visible on ultrasound serves as a biomarker for estrogen exposure as well as a reflection of the absence of progesterone bioeffects. This latter parameter is particularly helpful when following ART treatments. Indeed, exposure to progesterone readily modifies the acoustic properties of cervical mucus,

which loses its sono-transparency and therefore stops being visible on ultrasound. Conversely, identifying that cervical mucus is present on ultrasound allows us to disregard possible increases in plasma progesterone levels. This finding has been used for assessing the hormonal environment of the later stages of the follicular phase either in the menstrual cycle or in controlled ovarian hyperstimulation (COH). When cervical mucus is present on ultrasound we tend to not measure plasma progesterone. Conversely, an abrupt disappearance of cervical mucus observed concomitantly with plasma progesterone elevation in late stages of COH, as is sometimes encountered in poor ovarian responders, is an ominous sign.[45] In our opinion, the sudden disappearance of cervical mucus on ultrasound associated with pre-hCG progesterone elevation constitutes grounds for canceling the ART cycle or simply freezing embryos and deferring transfer.[46]

Changes in echographic characteristics of the cervix have received little attention.[47] As expected from visual examination of the outer cervix, 3D assessment of the whole cervix reveals size differences between nulliparus and multiparous women.[48]

Links between cervical length and the risk of preterm labor (PTL) and delivery were monitored before and throughout pregnancy with mounting successes, thus offering new imaging-based approaches for screening for PTL.[49-54] Screening for PTL by cervical assessment on ultrasound is, however, beyond the scope of this chapter. More pertinent to infertility is the early identification of cervical incompetence and its corollary, clinical indications for preemptive cervical cerclage. This clinical issue remains confused, however, in spite of the high-quality cervical length measurements and the number of well-designed studies. The persistence of queries stems from the notoriously poor efficacy of cervical cerclage in preventing premature delivery from cervical incompetence. In the current context, the sole well-established indication for cervical length measurement is during the middle trimester in women with a history of pregnancy losses due to cervical incompetence and prior short cervix measurements detected on ultrasound.[55] Various technical refinements may help in assessing cervical length using sonoelastography[56] or harmonic imaging.[57]

THE ENDOMETRIUM: A BIOMARKER OF THE HORMONAL ENVIRONMENT

Endometrial Thickness: A Biomarker for Estrogen Action

By convention, the endometrial thickness is measured on ultrasound from one myometrial-endometrial interphase to the next, on the thickest point of the endometrium (Fig. 33-3). This widely accepted practice really amounts to measuring a double endometrial thickness, something that has become a universally accepted convention.

From being relatively thin at the time of menses, the endometrium progressively thickens during the proliferative phase of the menstrual cycle, commonly peaking at 7 to 9 mm on the day of luteinizing hormone (LH) surge.[58-60] Prior to ovulation the endometrium takes a typical multilayered or three-line appearance formed by echogenic layers: the two hypoechoic functional layers separated by the hyperechoic interphase of the virtual uterine cavity (Fig. 33-4). The increase in endometrial thickness seen throughout the follicular phase represents the endometrial proliferation identified on histologic slides that occurred under the influence of E_2. This effect of estrogen leads to the deployment of estrogen receptors (ERs) and progesterone receptors (PRs) in endometrial glands and stroma. Collectively, these changes in endometrial tissue are called endometrial priming, as they reflect a critical step for the subsequent response of the endometrium to progesterone. At the histologic level, estrogenic effects of the follicular phase lead to proliferation and growth of endometrial glands, which develop vertically with straight lumens. Data from donor egg IVF and endometrial receptivity induced in donor egg recipients with the sole help of exogenous hormones are used to experimentally sort out the respective roles of E_2 and progesterone on various endometrial characteristics and receptivity. Astonishingly, donor egg data revealed an exceptional leeway in the duration and amplitude of the endometrium E_2 priming phase, which can range from 10 to 100 days without consequences on ART outcome.[61,62] This large range for the possible duration of the E_2 priming phase that remains compatible with optimal receptivity dwarfs the possible differences in E_2 exposure that results from duplicating or not the preovulatory rise in E_2 levels encountered in the menstrual cycle. Interestingly, the large range along which E_2 priming duration can vary without affecting ART outcome also has none or little impact on endometrial thickness or other endometrial parameters of estrogen effects on the uterus such as contractility,[63] provided that E_2 priming is sufficient.[46] As discussed later in this chapter, an endometrial thickness of 7 mm or greater is seen as reflecting sufficient endometrial priming by E_2. Therefore, we are led to accept that within the limits of physiologic endometrial priming by E_2, other factors such as growth factors have a primary impact on endometrial

thickness. Differences in endometrial thickness, however, do not modify the endometrial responsiveness to progesterone. The relationship between endometrial thickness and other endometrial markers of estrogen effects on one hand and pregnancy rates in ART on the other are addressed in the section "Imaging Markers of Endometrial Receptivity."

McWilliams and Frattarelli took an original perspective for looking at endometrial thickness in ART in that they studied the dynamic changes rather than mustering mere static data, that is, endometrial thickness at a single given point.[64] For this, fresh IVF cycles were studied in which the changes in endometrial thickness were analyzed from baseline to day 6 and from there to the day of human chorionic gonadotropin (hCG). Increments in endometrial thickness from baseline to day 6 and from day 6 to day of hCG were of 3.6 ± 2.4 and 2 ± 2.2 and of 2.3 ± 2.6 and 2.5 ± 2.1 in women who became pregnant ($n = 70$) and those who did not ($n = 62$), respectively. This dynamic comparison revealed that increments in endometrial thickness from baseline to day 6 were more important in women who became pregnant, whereas there were no differences in the further increment taking place from day 6 to day of hCG. Subset analyses indicated that the early increment in endometrial thickness was substantially less in women suffering from diminished ovarian reserve, as compared to the rest of the women having different causes of infertility. In our opinion, these characteristics of the dynamic changes in endometrial thickness stress the positive bias that exists between endometrial thickness and the quality of the ovarian response to COH, explaining how endometrial thickness can be wrongly interpreted as reflecting endometrial receptivity. Supporting the concept

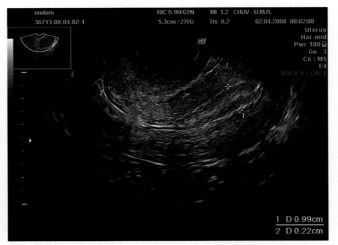

Figure 33-4. *Hypoechogenic or type I endometrium: Echographic appearance of the endometrium during the follicular phase. Between the hyperechogenic layer of the endometrial basalis and the echogenic line of the virtual endometrial cavity lies a characteristically hypogenic endometrium. Taken together, this constitutes the characteristic three-layer pattern of the proliferative endometrium. On this figure one can also identify mucus present in the cervical canal. On our semiquantitative grading system, this correspond to a +++ score for the quantity of mucus because the mean diameter of the dilated cervical canal is dilated at 2.2 mm.*

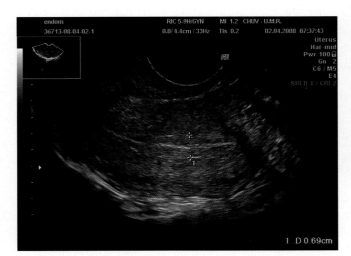

Figure 33-3. *Endometrial thickness. Measurements are made from one endometrial to myometrial interphase to the one on the opposite side, therefore amounting to a true dual endometrial thickness measurement.*

that endometrial thickness reflects hormonal exposure but not endometrial receptivity per se, Ng et al. found no differences in endometrial thickness between women who became pregnant after frozen embryo transfers (FET) and those who did not.[65] In this study, all the participants received a standardized E_2 and progesterone regimen amounting to similar hormonal exposure for all.[65]

Comparisons of endometrial thickness in the late follicular phase of the menstrual cycle, following physiologic E_2 and progesterone replacement or mild ovarian stimulation for FET, revealed similar findings.[66,67] This suggests that similar forms of hormonal priming have similar effects on endometrial thickness. Furthermore, exposure of the endometrium to E_2 levels that are more than 10 times higher than menstrual cycle values, as encountered in ART[68] and following the vaginal administration of 2 mg of E_2 per day,[69] barely resulted in a 20% thicker endometrium. This suggests that E_2 priming that results from menstrual cycle levels of E_2 is nearly maximum. As noted earlier, the same leeway that exists for the amount of E_2 that is used for endometrial priming is also seen for the duration during which this priming is applied. In a retrospective analysis of their donor egg data, Pellicer's group showed that extending the E_2 priming phase for up to 100 days had no significant impact on ART outcome[70] and endometrial thickness,[62] a finding confirmed by others.[71,72] The minimal effects of increased or prolonged E_2 priming on endometrial thickness contrasts with reports indicating that excessive ovarian responses to COH with markedly elevated E_2 levels have a negative impact on pregnancy and embryo implantation rates.[73,74] To account for these divergent findings, we proposed that in strong responses to COH, it is the excessive production of ovarian factors other than E_2 that is responsible for the adverse effects seen on the endometrium, not an action of the high E_2 levels per se.[46,75]

There is consensus that women whose endometrium is less than 7 mm in ART have markedly decreased chances of becoming pregnant.[76,77] In rare cases, albeit disturbing ones, this condition may persist and can be found in menstrual, stimulated, and E_2-supplemented cycles,[78] and is typically resistant to markedly elevated estrogenic exposure.[69] This may be encountered in the aftermath of total body irradiation or other cancer treatments,[79] or in the absence of a readily available explanation. The treatments that have been proposed for these women include low-dose aspirin,[80] E_2 challenge test,[81] locally active vasodilators,[82] and the combination of pentoxifylline and tocopherol (vitamin E).[78,83] The latter products, pentoxifylline and tocopherol, were tested on the grounds that they had been reported to be effective at reducing fibrosis induced by radiation therapy.[84] Unfortunately no proof of efficacy exists for these products, as the encouraging case reports that sparked interest for these treatments were not followed by prospective trials.

Issues regarding the possible poor predictive value of thickened endometrium in ART reported by Casper's team[85] remains a matter for debate. While confirmed by some,[76] a larger group of publications failed to confirm that a thicker endometrium has an overt negative impact on ART outcome.[86-89]

Endometrial Echogenicity: A Biomarker for Progesterone Action

Echogenicity is the physical property by which a tissue interacts with ultrasound, either letting ultrasound waves penetrate or reflecting the beam aimed in its direction. Hence, tissue echogenicity ranges from absolute sonotransparent properties, as encountered in certain constituents of the body, notably water, to high echogenic properties offered by air (as encountered in the bowel) through which ultrasound waves do not penetrate and bounce back. On gray scale image reconstruction, low echogenicity, as that of water, is commonly depicted in black, while high echogenicity appears in white. Typically, solid tissues of the body have echogenic characteristics that range between those of water (lowest) and air (highest), and are depicted by various degrees of gray. The final echogenicity of a given tissue or organ therefore results in part from that given tissue's water and air content and, in part, from the number of interphases between tissue constituents of different nature within the organ, which will each reflect sound waves and, thus, also contribute to increasing overall tissue echogenicity.

In the uterus, we recognize that the echogenicity of the myometrium is constant throughout the menstrual cycle and following various hormonal treatments. It is likely to be modified, however, by the presence of pathologic structures such as leiomyomas or adenomyosis as well as being affected by the overall size of the organ. On the contrary, the echogenicity of the endometrium and, to a lesser extent, that of the subendometrial layer of the myometrium vary between the follicular and luteal phases of the menstrual cycle and in response to exogenous hormones.

We know from an early prospective trial conducted in 80 infertile patients by Forrest et al.[90] that endometrial echogenicity increases after ovulation under the influence of progesterone produced by the corpus luteum (CL). These authors were first to recognize the hypoechoic characteristics of follicular phase endometrium (see Fig. 33-4), which were found in 80% of women scanned by these authors during the follicular phase. The endometrium is characterized by a hypoechoic aspect of the functional layer of the endometrium bordered by the hyperechoic basal layers of the endometrium with the center hyperechoic line provided by the interphase generated by the virtual endometrial cavity. Together, the hypoechoic functional layer of the endometrium and its outer limits, the two basal layers and the center line of the endometrial cavity offer the so-called *three-line pattern*.

Changes in endometrial echogenicity are seen soon after ovulation when the endometrium progressively acquires a characteristic hyperechoic aspect spreading from the endometrium basalis layer upward to be fully deployed starting in the midluteal phase. In their trial, Forrest et al.[90] observed a hyperechoic endometrium in 78% of women scanned during the luteal phase. Likewise, Templeton's group identified a similar sequence of changes from hypoechogenic endometrium in the follicular phase to a primarily hyperechogenic pattern in the luteal phase of stimulated cycles.[58] The sonographic changes from the estrogenic pattern seen in the follicular phase to that characteristic of the luteal

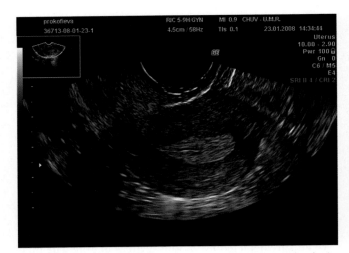

Figure 33-5. *Hyperechogenic or type III endometrium: Under the influence of progesterone, the endometrium becomes hyperechogenic in relation to the surrounding myometrium during the luteal phase. From studies conducted in estradiol (E2) and progesterone substitution cycles, it has been determined that the endometrium becomes fully hyperechogenic after 4 days of exposure to luteal phase levels of progesterone. The hyperechogenic characteristics of the secretory endometrium are believed to result from the abundance of mucus-filled tortuous glands, which generate as many sound interphases and therefore increase the overall echogenicity of the endometrium.*

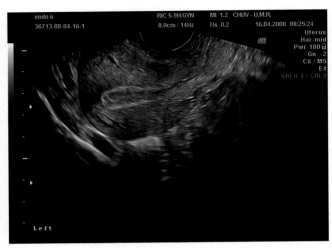

Figure 33-6. *Intermediate or type II endometrium: During the first days of the luteal phase there is a characteristic thickening of the endometrial basalis, which progressively spreads upward to ultimately reach the hyperechogenic interphase of the virtual endometrial cavity. The condition encountered after 2 days of exposure to progesterone when the hyperechogenic endometrial basalis layer extends over approximately 50% of the whole endometrium is described as type II endometrium.*

phase starts to be visible within 48 hours of ovulation with a progressive hyperechoic transformation of the functional layer spreading from the endometrium basalis upward. From the various publications available, we know that the hyperechoic transformation of the functional layer of the endometrium takes 4 to 7 days to complete.

Grunfeld et al. studied the changes in endometrial echogenicity that took place in 18 women receiving sequential E2 (0.2-0.4 mg/day, transdermally) and progesterone (50 mg/day IM) in preparation for donor egg IVF.[91] Vaginal ultrasound scans were performed starting before the onset of progesterone administration and every 3 days thereafter until the eighth day of progesterone, when an endometrial biopsy was performed. Endometrial echogenicity was scored as ranging from pattern I, showing a triple line pattern before the start of progesterone treatment, to pattern III, showing full hyperechoic transformation of the fucntionalis layer from the lamina basalis all the way to the endometrial lumen (Fig. 33-5). In these authors' hands, endometrial thickness was a poor discriminator between advanced and retarded stromal changes on endometrial biopsies. Conversely, the degree of hyperechogenic changes on ultrasound scans (complete or partial) correlated with the degree of advancement of luteal changes (condensation, predecidualization) in the endometrial stroma. All women whose endometrial biopsy revealed delayed secretory changes in endometrial glands and stroma had ultrasound scans showing partial hypoechogenic images (pattern II) (Fig. 33-6).

Analyzing endometrial echogenicity on the day after hCG administration in ART, Gonen and Casper observed a typical hypoechogenic triple-line pattern in 60/123 (49%) women.[92] In this subgroup of ART partic-

ipants, the pregnancy rate was 30% (18/60), which was significantly higher than the figure obtained in the whole cohort (19.5%). Conversely, a full and partially hyperechogenic endometrium was found in 33% (41/123) and 18% (22/123) women in whom pregnancy rates at 9% and 9.1%, respectively, were markedly lower than in their hypoechogenic counterparts. The original data of Casper and Gonen on the poor prognosis value of a hyperechoic endometrium in the late follicular phase of ART[92] were subsequently largely confirmed by many publications[93-98] with yet others that failed to find this relationship.[99,100]

In an effort to analyze how ultrasound data and, specifically, echogenicity, could reflect endometrial receptivity, we further studied the endometrial appearance on ultrasound on the day of hCG administration in 228 consecutive COH cycles.[101] In this study, we retained only women younger than 38 years whose uteri were morphologically normal and in a position that offered optimal visualization on ultrasound (anterior or posterior, to the exclusion of intermediate uteri). Ultrasound images were digitized and analyzed using a computer-assisted system designed for measuring the degree of endometrial echogenicity (Fig. 33-7). Specifically, we studied the extent of the hyperechogenic changes that develop from the basal endometrium upward during the follicular-luteal transition, as described in E2 and progesterone cycles,[91] but at times reported in ART before exposure to progesterone, at the time of hCG administration.[92] Our results indicated that in the selected population of IVF candidates 14% of women (34/228) had a fully hypoechoic *triple-line* endometrium (<30% hyperechoic at the base of the endometrium) while 12% (28/228) had a fully hyperechoic endometrium (>70% of hyperechoic invasion of the functionalis layer).[101] The remaining 166 women had four degrees of progressive hyperechoic changes that extended from 31% to 40% to 61% to 70% of the full functionalis layer of the endometrium. Demographic,

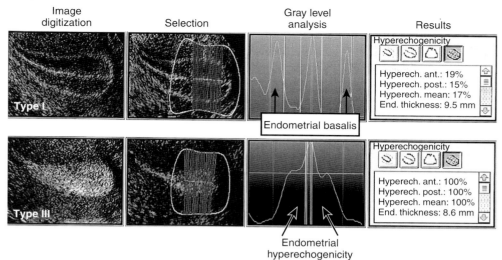

Figure 33-7. *Computer-assisted measurement of endometrial echogenicity. Endometrial echogenicity was studied on transverse slices of endometrium. In the follicular phase (type I endometrium), one recognizes the characteristic hyperechogenicity of proximal and distal endometrial basalis and that generated by the virtual endometrial cavity. In the luteal phase (type III endometrium), the thickness of the hyperechogenic basalis has developed to ultimately reach that of the virtual endometrial cavity, thus providing the characteristic global hyperechogenic appearance to the endometrium. (From Fanchin R, Righini C, Ayoubi JM, et al. New look at endometrial echogenicity: objective computer-assisted measurements predict endometrial receptivity in in vitro fertilization-embryo transfer. Fertil Steril 74:274, 2000.)*

hormonal, and biologic characteristics of each of these groups were similar, including endometrial thickness and plasma progesterone levels, which remained less than 1 ng/mL in each group. This latter observation indicates that the *premature* increase in echogenicity seen in certain IVF patients is not the result of premature luteinization with increased progesterone production. Finally, the number of embryos transferred was also similar in all six groups with in each case two to four embryos transferred (as commonly done in the 1990s). Pregnancy and embryo implantation rates varied greatly, however, between the different echogenicity-based groups. From a highest value of 59% and 16%, respectively, for the hypoechogenic group, it decreased to 23% and 3%, respectively, for the hyperechoic group with progressively diminishing results for increasing echogenicity in the intermediate groups (Fig. 33-8).

In a different study we assessed endometrial echogenicity on the day of hCG administration, oocyte retrieval, and embryo transfer (ET) (day 2) in patients whose plasma progesterone was below or above the cut-off value of 0.9 ng/mL.[102] On the day of hCG, the mean hyperechoic transformation of the functionalis layer of the endometrium was similar in the two groups at 40% and 41%, respectively. During the 4 days that followed hCG administration, the hyperechoic transformation was much faster, however, in the high progesterone group, with values of 70% versus 63% at oocyte retrieval and 90% versus 79% at ET, respectively.

The histologic basis for the hyperechogenic transformation seen in certain IVF women remain unclear to this date. During the follicular-luteal transition, it has been hypothesized that it is the development of spiral arteries and the coiling of the glands taking place under the influence of progesterone that causes the increase in echogenicity. Yet, the fact that progesterone remained low (<1 ng/mL) in all the echogenicity groups excludes this

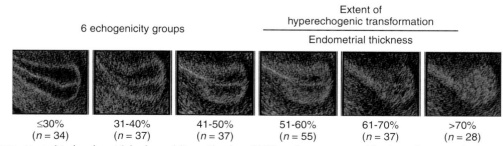

Figure 33-8. *Computer-assisted endometrial echogenicity on the day of hCG and pregnancy and implantation rates. Pregnancy and implantation rates (59%, 57%, 35%, 20%, 16%, and 11%, respectively) and implantation rates declined from 59% to 11% and 35% to 3%, respectively, when hyperechogenicity ranged from <30% to >70% of endometrial thickness. (From Fanchin R, Righini C, Ayoubi JM, et al. New look at endometrial echogenicity: objective computer-assisted measurements predict endometrial receptivity in in vitro fertilization-embryo transfer. Fertil Steril 74:274, 2000.)*

explanation. Moreover, the explanations are not found in morphologic differences that might exist between certain ART patients on the day of hCG administration. Recent work from Devroey's team[103] examined the issue through a provocative approach in which IVF patients underwent endometrial biopsies in the very cycle of their embryo transfer. These findings, which stressed the fact that the sequence of morphologic changes in the endometrium was hastened early in the luteal phases in ART, indicated that none of these changes existed at the end of the follicular phase, on the day of hCG administration.[103,104] This leaves us at a loss for finding a plausible explanation for the increase in echogenicity found in certain women on the day of hCG administration in ART, which largely bears ominous predictive values for ART outcome.

The considerable interstudy differences as to the predictive value of various echogenic patterns on the day of hCG administration, oocyte retrieval, and embryo transfer are puzzling. We do not hold a definitive explanation for these diverging findings. Yet, we believe that at least some of the differences reported by various teams about the predictive value for ART outcome of the various ultrasound patterns are likely to stem from methodologic as well as population factors. The endometrium of women whose uteri are in an intermediate position is likely to appear hyperechoic because sound waves will hit endometrial glands at an angle rather than entering the organ along an axis that parallels the axis of the glands, as when the uterus is in a marked ante- or retroverted position. Hence, rather than providing their classical hypoechoic appearance, straight glands of a normal proliferative endometrium are likely to generate increased sonic returns when hit by the sound wave at an angle. This will generate a hyperechoic appearance, but not linked to any secretory transformation of the endometrium. In an unpublished trial, we performed manual rotations of freshly removed uteri before an ultrasound probe and confirmed that the hypoechoic pattern obtained when the uterus is held in ante- or retroverted position before the probe becomes hyperechoic when the intermediate position is mimicked.[105] Artifacts of measurement may also occur in case of uterine fibroid, adenomyosis, and overall enlarged uteri. In our opinion, therefore, endometrial echogenicity should not be interpreted when the uterus is in an intermediate position or other factors interfere with the quality of endometrial readings. We restricted our studies to cases that satisfied these requirements,[101,102] but this issue is often not mentioned, if not ignored, in most published reports on the clinical value of endometrial echogenicity in ART.

THREE-DIMENSIONAL VOLUME RECONSTRUCTION OF THE ENDOMETRIUM

Interest in measuring endometrial volume rather than its mere thickness stems from the belief that volume represents a more global and more encompassing parameter for assessing the primary issues at stake: endometrial proliferation or priming in response to estrogens.[12] From a clinical standpoint, there are two issues: (i) determining endometrial receptivity in infertile patients and (ii) assessing the

risk of endometrial hyperplasia or cancer in women who present with dysfunctional uterine bleeding (DUB). Early assessments of endometrial volume estimated from two-dimensional (2D) ultrasound images by simple formulas, such as the prolate ellipsoid,[106,107] were of little help in assessing the uterus probably because the irregular shapes of this organ made volume calculation based on theoretical formulas too inaccurate. The advent of off-line and, later, the more convenient and precise built-in 3D volume reconstruction systems that are incorporated in the ultrasound machines offered genuinely new approaches for volume measurement. The 3D-based volume calculation of territories such as the endometrium uses either of the two following methods:

1. The simplest or *multiplanar approach* consists in scrolling through multiple serial slices, which allows more measurements of less regularly shaped objects.[108]
2. A more elaborate yet direct precise approach is based on using a virtual organ computer-aided analysis (VOCAL) imaging program developed by a 3D ultrasound manufacturer, GE-Kretz in Zipf, Austria.

A detailed description is provided by Raine-Fenning et al.[13] Briefly, 3D reconstruction encompasses two primary steps. First, the relevant boundaries of the volume to be studied are identified on 2D gray-scale images in order to delineate the limits of the 3D reconstruction, using a computer mouse. For the endometrium volume, the endometrial to myometrial interface is either manually or semiautomatically identified by the examiner on 2D images, using the B (transverse) or C (coronal) plane. Second, the 3D volume is rotated about a central axis through sets of user-defined steps ranging from 6 degrees to 30 degrees. It therefore takes from 6 to 30 planes, depending on the rotating pattern chosen for completing a full 180-degree rotation. Finally, upon completion of a full 180-degree rotation, volume acquisition is automatically generated and its characteristics are calculated, leading to more reliable and accurate volume measurements (Fig. 33-9A to C). Experimental calculations indicated that precision of the volume measured increased with the number of rotation steps, from 30 degrees, to 9 degrees, to 6 degrees.[109] Practically, however, the 9-degree[109] and 15-degree rotation steps[110] are preferred and are more commonly used.

From a first volume of reference (i.e., the endometrial volume), secondary volumes can be generated that extend to set distances of the primary reference, as for example 1-5 mm subendometrial extensions of the primary endometrial volume, using the *shelling* properties of the VOCAL system.

In a prospective trial, Raine-Fenning et al. scanned a population of 30 presumably fertile volunteers on alternate days until evidence of ovulation was obtained and collapse of the follicle was witnessed and every 4 days thereafter.[111] The 3D volumes of the uterus were acquired using a Voluson 530D ultrasound machine from an appropriate longitudinal scan of the uterus. Then 3D volume measurements were performed off-line using the VOCAL system with endometrium boundaries

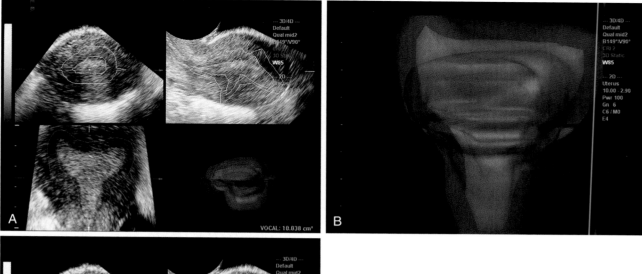

Figure 33-9. *Endometrial volume calculation using a virtual organ computer-aided analysis (VOCAL) imaging program together with the calculation of a secondary subendometrial volume extending at 5 mm (**A** and **B**) or 1 mm (**C**) outside the endometrial-myometrial interphase.*

identification conducted on the coronal C plane in successive manual 9-degree rotation steps. As illustrated in Figure 33-9B, the changes in endometrial thickness and volume throughout the menstrual cycle followed similar patterns with progressive increments during the follicular phase and stable values throughout the luteal phase. As expected from the diagram, the changes in endometrial thickness and volume were highly correlated ($R^2 = 0.767$; $P < 0.001$). Studies looking at correlations between endometrial volume and ART outcome revealed the same kind of relationship already described for endometrial thickness. Like their endometrial thickness counterparts, 3D endometrial volume studies revealed poor pregnancy rates in cases of marginal endometrial volume. Specifically, pregnancy rates were directly related to endometrial volume for values from 2 to 4 mL, significantly reduced when the endometrium was less than 2 mL, with no pregnancy if the volume was less than 1 mL. Conversely, however, further an increase in endometrial volume above 4 mL was not associated with better outcome, as compared to 2 to 4 mL.[12] In a study of 47 women, Schild et al. showed no correlation between endometrial volume and pregnancy rates,[108] a finding in agreement with that of Yaman et al.[112]

UTERINE DOPPLER

Principles and Applications

The Doppler effect (named after the German physicist Christian Doppler) refers to the phenomenon whereby a change in frequency is perceived when relative motion exists between the wave source (in our case, the reflected ultrasound waves) and the receiver. Yet, the frequency of the emitted wave (here, ultrasound waves bouncing back toward the receiver) does not physically change, as the Doppler phenomenon only affects the perception of the received wave (ultrasound), not the wave itself. If ultrasound waves are emitted (or reflected) from a source that moves toward the receiver, an increase in frequency will be perceived. The reverse will take place if the target on which ultrasound waves are reflected moves away from the receiver. In either case, the perceived frequency change (i.e., the intensity of Doppler effect) is proportional to the speed of displacement of the target on which ultrasound waves are reflected. The actual frequency of the reflected ultrasound waves remains constant, however.

In medical ultrasound studies, the primary practical application of the Doppler effect has been for analyzing the movement of blood particles on which ultrasound waves are reflected in order to study flow parameters and the vascularization status of a given area. Using distinct methodologic approaches, Doppler-based analyses may either look at individual vessels or measure perfusion in a whole tissue area. Flow analyses of specific vessels (i.e., the uterine artery) are conducted with the *pulsed* Doppler technique, which consists of sending sound signals at timed intervals in a given volume or *sampling gate* and studying the perceived frequency changes in the return signal or Doppler *waveform*.

Blood flow analyses based on studying Doppler effect in vessels of various territories of the body stem from the formidable advancements that this technology made in cardiology, which set the methodologic groundwork for all Doppler analyses performed today.[113] Pulse Doppler (Fig. 33-10) involves first physically locating the vessel to be studied in order to properly position the Doppler *sampling gate*. This can be done with a duplex system providing concomitant gray-scale imaging or more easily with *color Doppler*, which directly identifies vessels (see later discussion). Once the emitting signal is targeted at the designated vessel, calculation of actual blood flow and resistance in that vessel results from analyzing the frequency changes that are perceived in the received signal or *Doppler waveform*. The recorded changes in the return signal (i.e., the intensity of the Doppler effect) reflect the speed of displacement of the moving blood particles toward or away from the probe on which the pulsed ultrasound signal is reflected. An exact computation of flow and resistance in that vessel requires that we know the angle made between the ultrasound wave and the great axis of the studied vessel in order to determine the true speed of displacement of blood in the vessel. This calculation is unfortunately impossible in the gynecologic organs because uterine and ovarian vessels are far too tortuous.

For drawing practical advantages from pulsed Doppler technology in gynecology we must therefore approximate the global resulting effect or *impedance* to flow, as the accurate determination of blood flow and resistance are impossible.[10,11,114,115] Practically, the impedance to flow is assessed by descriptive analyses of how the *Doppler flow wave* is modulated throughout the systolic and diastolic phases of the cardiac cycle. For this semiquantitative measurement, different indices have been proposed that compute ratios of maximum systolic and minimum diastolic Doppler signals. The most common indices, the resistance index (RI) and pulsatility index (PI), are directly calculated on the flow wave either manually or using semi- or fully automated methods. Both RI (values, 0-1) and PI (values, ≥0) are therefore directly related to vascular resistance with higher values corresponding to lower flow.

An alternate approach for Doppler analysis is based on using various ever more complex electronic means for decoding and interpreting the Doppler effect directly on the return of the ultrasound signal used for constructing the gray-scale images. This approach applies color coding to voxels that are subjected to Doppler effect while the rest of the voxels serve for gray-scale imaging. The end result or *color Doppler* function and its variant angle-independent and highly sensitive *power Doppler* imaging directly depict (or map) vessels of various sizes live on ultrasound images. Color and power Doppler therefore

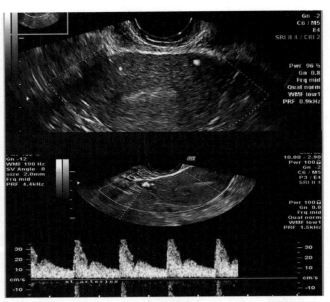

Figure 33-10. *Pulsed Doppler waveform analyzed by computation of the semiquantitative pulsatility index (PI), which directly reflects the impedance to flow in the territory downstream from the area of measurement.*

offer a novel way of easily identifying vessels in a given organ or territory. This can serve for identifying vessels on which pulsed Doppler studies are going to be conducted. Color and power Doppler studies also permit global assessments of vascularization in a given area by direct visual or computer-based analysis of the colored voxels present in a territory using computer-assisted systems, a principle called *power* Doppler *angiography* (PDA).[116] Contrary to PI and RI, PDA values are directly related to local flow, with higher values indicating higher flow. Various technologic systems have been developed for filtrating nonspecific color Doppler signals or "flash" artifacts that are triggered by nonspecific displacements of the targeted tissue as a result of bowel or respiration linked movements.

More recently, power Doppler assessments have been associated with 3D volume reconstruction (3D-PDA)[117] (Fig. 33-11A and B). This approach offers improved reproducibility because measurements are conducted in a defined anatomic territory, as for example, the endometrium or ovary, rather than in an area that is arbitrarily selected.[13] Practically speaking, 3D-PDA is measured in a given volume of interest, using a VOCAL imaging program for volume measurement, as described in detail in the next section of this chapter.[13] 3D-PDA results are displayed on a histogram from which three indices, VI, FI and VFI, are derived. The vascular index (VI, %) represents the proportion of lighted voxels over all voxels, thus reflecting the degree of vascularity of the studied volume. The flow index (FI, 0-100) represents the mean power Doppler intensity of the lighted voxels, a parameter meant to reflect the vascularization flow rate (VFI, 0-100), which is a product of the VI and FI (Fig. 33-12).

Generally speaking, pulsed and color Doppler functions have become refinements of ultrasound techniques that

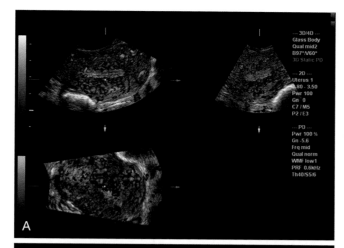

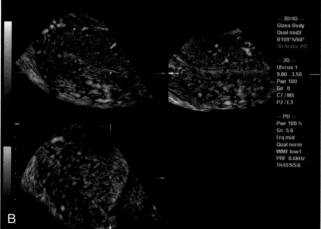

Figure 33-11. Computation of color Doppler finding in a given area by computation power Doppler angiography (PDA) in a 3D-defined territory, as for example, the endometrium and subendometrial volume using the virtual organ computer-aided analysis (VOCAL) and shelling functions. PDA score is directly related to flow. Three primary indexes are computed, the vascularization (VI), flow (FI), and vascularization-flow indexes (VFI). VI reflects the number of vessels in a given area, whereas FI is porportional to blood flow in these vessels and VFI constitutes a product of VI and FI. **A,** In normal conditions, color Doppler shows no to minimal vascular entries in the endometrium. **B,** In case of endometrial polyps vessels are shown entering a given territory of the endometrium (right cornua).

over time have become readily available in all but strictly entry-level ultrasound equipment. Hence, the Doppler function extends the diagnostic usefulness of ultrasound imaging by providing pertinent data related to the vascular status of a given organ or area. From a practical standpoint, Doppler data have been used for two main purposes:

1. For refining cancer detection by identifying or excluding characteristic increases in vascularity in relation to specific findings on gray-scale imaging (i.e., detecting an ovarian cyst)
2. For assessing the effects of hormones (endogenous or exogenous) on blood flow

Most commonly but not exclusively, the intent is to infer information pertinent to reproductive physiology and pathophysiology, such as endometrial receptivity that may be linked to infertility or its treatment.

Vascular Changes Related to the Menstrual Cycle and Hormonal Effects

From the early days of Doppler availability in gynecology, investigators have tried to identify the changes in uterine vascularization that take place during the menstrual cycle. Early studies using pulsed Doppler looked at changes in Doppler waveforms recorded from the uterine artery[10,118] and its major branches.[114,119,120]

In a prospective trial Raine-Fenning et al. used the novel technology 3D-PDA to quantify changes in blood flow recorded in the endometrium and subendometrium territories during the menstrual cycle.[121] These authors observed that both endometrial and subendometrial blood flow as measured by the 3D-PDA based calculation of VI, FI, and VFI increased during the follicular phase, peaking 3 days prior to ovulation and decreasing to a nadir 5 days after ovulation (Fig. 33-13). This pattern differs from prior findings made with pulsed Doppler showing a steady increase of blood flow throughout the menstrual cycle.[114,121-125] Smoking was associated with significantly lower VI and VFI throughout the menstrual cycle, whereas parous women had higher values than their nulliparous counterparts.[121]

Exogenous hormones administered to women suffering from premature[11,120] or normally occurring menopause[119] induced a prompt and profound decrease in uterine PI and RI indices, thereby reflecting vasodilatory effects of E_2. Menopausal[126] and donor egg IVF regimens[11] provided similar vasodilation of uterine arteries, suggesting that maximal vasodilation effects are achieved at subphysiologic levels of E_2 with no further increase in flow with higher exposure to E_2. In these studies, the vasodilation of uterine arteries induced by E_2 administration was partially antagonized by synthetic progestins[126] but not by progesterone administration.[11]

Vascular changes observed in the uterus during COH do not parallel those that would be anticipated from the mere increase in exposure to E_2. These data, therefore, indicate that the stimulated ovaries, which interfere with endometrial and subendometrial blood flow, produce vasoactive factors other than E_2. In a prospective trial, Ng et al.[68] compared endometrial and subendometrial blood flow measured using the 3D-PDA approach in the menstrual and COH cycles of the same women. Their findings showed a significant decrease of endometrial and subendometrial blood flow during the stimulated cycle,[68] with excessive responders having further reduction in endometrial blood flow as compared to moderate responders.[127] These findings suggest that vasoconstrictive substances stimulated by exogenous gonadotropins are released during ovarian stimulation that antagonize the vasodilative properties of E_2, causing the decreased blood flow observed during COH.[75,128] Among the putative factors possibly responsible for the decrease in uterine flow during COH are ovarian androgens, which are produced in increased amounts under the influence of exogenous follicle-stimulating hormone (FSH).[129,130]

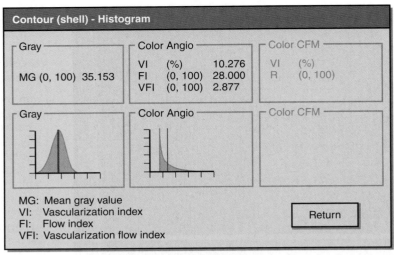

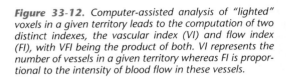

Figure 33-12. *Computer-assisted analysis of "lighted" voxels in a given territory leads to the computation of two distinct indexes, the vascular index (VI) and flow index (FI), with VFI being the product of both. VI represents the number of vessels in a given territory whereas FI is proportional to the intensity of blood flow in these vessels.*

Supporting the concept that ovarian androgens interfere with the vasodilative properties of E_2 is the observation of increased uterine artery resistance in case of polycystic ovary syndrome (PCOS),[131] a finding not shared by others, however.[132] Further supporting the vasoconstrictive role of androgens or of a substance released in conjunction with androgens is the report of an improvement of uterine flow in PCOS following administration of the anti-androgen flutamide.[131] In a different study Ng et al.[133] observed a negative correlation between E_2 levels and blood flow, suggesting that the putative vasoactive factor produced during COH is triggered by FSH administration in a proportional manner to that of E_2. This is further supported by the observation that the decrease in endometrial flow is more pronounced in women whose response to COH is excessive as compared to moderate responders.[133]

The promising findings of early Doppler studies that proposed Doppler landmarks that defined endometrial receptivity[134] have not been confirmed by recent 3D-PDA data on either fresh[135] or frozen embryo transfers,[65] although increased vascularitiy may be predictive of lesser risk of miscarriage.[127] The complex relationship between Doppler data and endometrial receptivity are discussed later in this chapter.

DYSFUNCTIONAL UTERINE BLEEDING: BENIGN AND MALIGNANT ENDOMETRIAL DISEASE

Investigations for a suspected endometrial disease such as polyp or submucosal fibroid is either driven by the cardinal symptom of endometrial dysfunction, dysfunctional uterine bleeding (DUB), or as part of a workup for infertility. On uterine imaging, a thickened endometrium with irregular echogenicity is cause to suspect endometrial disease. Three-dimensional endometrial volume reconstruction and 3D-PDA analyses may prove to be most valuable for investigating DUB, but not at predicting endometrial receptivity. Odeh et al. prospectively evaluated 89 perimenopausal women and 56 menopausal women with dysfunctional bleeding.[136] Although endometrial thickness is simpler to measure, Odeh et al. found that endometrial

volume was more accurate in identifying endometrial hyperplasia and carcinoma according to the receiver-operating characteristic (ROC) curves. According to ROC curve analysis, a sensitivity of 100% implied a cut-off value of 1.45 mL, which resulted in an unrealistic low sensitivity of 0.08%. A more reasonable cut-off value for the endometrial volume of 3.56 mL had a sensitivity of 93% and a specificity of 36%. With this value, two carcinomas would have been missed in the patient cohort; one had alarming 3D-PDA data and the other had negative 3D-PDA results. In our opinion, adopting more sophisticated tools, such as 3D-based endometrial volume measurement, should not preclude careful analysis of heterogeneous echogenicity, which warrant histologic exploration.

When endometrial polyps are suspected based on irregularly thickened endometrium on plain vaginal ultrasound scans, direct power Doppler often but not always will help in identifying the feeding vessel that enters the polyp from its base. Conversely, vessels identified on power Doppler normally stop in the subendometrial layers of the endometrium, with none seen entering the endometrium.[137] As discussed in a later section, suspicious findings on plain ultrasound examinations today justify SIS, which normally sorts out the issue of whether there is an intrauterine structure (or not) that would need to be surgically removed.

As reviewed by Montgomery et al., the primary suspicion of a cancerous lesion of the endometrium comes from identifying an abnormally thick endometrium.[138,139] The cardinal sign of endometrial carcinoma remains a thick endometrium with irregular and erratic echogenicity.[140] In 339 women with postmenopausal DUB, no women with an endometrial thickness of 4 mm or less developed endometrial carcinoma over a 10-year follow–up period.[141] Doppler has been claimed to differentiate between cancer and noncancerous lesions. Although noncancerous lesions tend to have lower impedance indices, there is an overlap between the PI and RI of benign and malignant lesions.[142] Based on these findings, Tabor et al. conclude at the end of their meta-analysis on the value of endometrial thickness for detecting endometrial cancer among postmenopausal bleeders that a thin endometrium still requires histologic

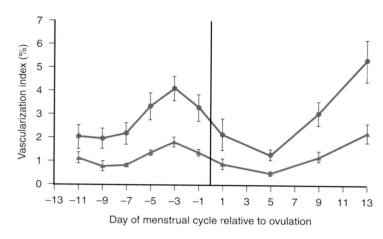

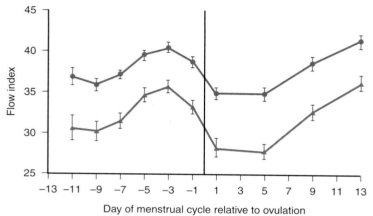

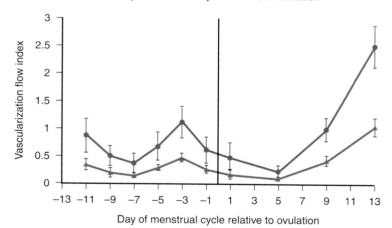

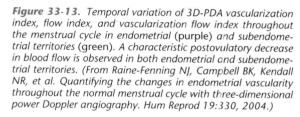

Figure 33-13. Temporal variation of 3D-PDA vascularization index, flow index, and vascularization flow index throughout the menstrual cycle in endometrial (purple) and subendometrial territories (green). A characteristic postovulatory decrease in blood flow is observed in both endometrial and subendometrial territories. (From Raine-Fenning NJ, Campbell BK, Kendall NR, et al. Quantifying the changes in endometrial vascularity throughout the normal menstrual cycle with three-dimensional power Doppler angiography. Hum Reprod 19:330, 2004.)

exploration for endometrial hyperplasia or cancer.[143] Finally, in cases of cancer, vaginal ultrasound and MRI were found to be equivalent for determining the depth of myometrial invasion.[144]

THE MYOMETRIUM: PHYSIOLOGY AND PATHOLOGIC FINDINGS

Uterine leiomyomas or fibroids are the most common solid tumor, occurring in 20% to 40% of women in their reproductive life.[145] Fibroids are well-circumscribed lesions, often with a pseudocapsule containing feeding vessels

running at the surface of the fibroid from which they penetrate into the fibroid in a radiating manner (Fig. 33-14). In contrast, adenomyosis contains vessels that are sparse and scattered with usually indistinct borders. Fibroids originate from the middle layer of the myometrium from which they tend to extend either inward toward the cavity to become submucosal or outward toward the serosa possibly to the point of becoming pedunculated.

The possibility that fibroids may cause infertility and the extent to which this may take place and constitute a predisposing factor for miscarriages remains a matter of debate. First, fibroids may alter fertility by interfering with

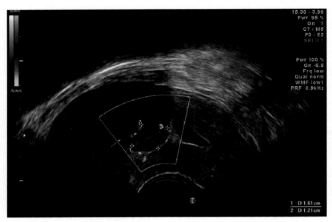

Figure 33-14. Uterine fibroid. Characteristically, vessels run around the surface of the fibroid from which radiating branches penetrate vertically.

sperm transport and embryo implantation, a possibility that has long been entertained.[146] This detrimental effect of fibroids on sperm transport has recently been further supported by MRI-based studies of uterine contractility.[147,148] Kido et al. observed that submucosal fibroids were more prone to affect uterine peristalsis than their intramural counterparts. Second, the possibility that fibroids alter endometrial receptivity has been entertained for many years. Fibroids may hamper embryo implantation, in part by physical effects when present in a subendometrial location, and in part by focal endometrial disturbances[149] and local inflammation and release of various vasoactive and other substances.[150]

The possibility that fibroids cause miscarriages remains a topic of debate. In a recent study, recurrent miscarriages were more frequent in a population that experienced fibroids than in their unaffected counterparts.[151] There are other studies, however, that failed to find such an association.[152]

CONTRAST-ENHANCED IMAGING OF THE UTERINE CAVITY

Hysterosonography

Early in the use of vaginal ultrasound, it became apparent that uterine exploration in early pregnancy offered images of the developing embryo of outstanding quality.[153,154] The remarkable definition of fetal images obtained in early pregnancy using vaginal ultrasound has been instrumental in the formidable forward leap that ultrasound-based prenatal diagnosis of fetal malformation has made in the past 20 years. Contrasting with this, however, ultrasound images of the nonpregnant uterine cavity remain of notoriously lower quality. This hampered the reliability with which intrauterine diseases, such as fibroids or polyps, can be identified. This led to a new diagnostic procedure aimed at improving the quality of uterine images on ultrasound; the procedure received different designations over time, including hysterosalpingo-contrast-sonography (Hy-Co-Sy), SIS, and hysterosonography (HySo)[14-16] (Fig. 33-15).

Over the years, the practice of SIS has been streamlined while its clinical soundness became validated in studies providing mounting evidence for the superiority of its images as compared to simple ultrasound studies. Two types of contrast products have been proposed that offer sono-transparent or sono-opaque properties. These products provide negative (black) or positive (white) contrast enhancement of the uterine cavity by comparison to the uterine tissue depicted on gray-scale imaging.[155] Negative contrast solutions have the acoustic properties of water (sono-transparent) with normal saline being most commonly used. Positive contrast solutions consist of preparations that gain sono-refracting properties from air entrapped in various microparticle systems from which it is progressively released over time.[156-158] This is achieved through albumin (Albumex) or saccharide microparticles (Echovist, later replaced by Levovist, BR1, EchoGen, etc.). These positive ultrasound contrast products are injectable solutions, which are available for various medical indications but are used within the uterus for gynecologic imaging.[159]

Positive contrast solutions instilled in the uterine cavity provide *white* contrast enhancement of the uterine cavity. Yet, in these images the far side of the uterine wall may at times be partially obscured by shadowing effects of the contrast product present in the uterine cavity. On the contrary, negative contrast solutions such as normal saline provide *black* contrast enhancement of the uterine cavity. This leaves the vision of the far side of the uterus totally unobstructed and offers a marked improvement in the identification of intracavitary lesions while retaining an unabated view of all aspects of the uterine tissue.[158,160,161] From these findings, it became universally recognized that negative contrast solution (NaCl) is the preferred option for exploring the uterine cavity, whereas positive contrast solutions serve for visualizing the fallopian tubes, organs that otherwise evade scrutiny on ultrasound examination.[162,163] Therefore, positive contrast ultrasound will be described in the section of this chapter dedicated to the fallopian tube. Positive echographic contrast solutions have also served for enhancing the Doppler signal and improving the assessment of tissue perfusion when administered systematically.[164] Yet, Doppler enhancement that requires IV administration of these contrast products has not yet provided clinically relevant advantages that would justify their use for diagnostic purposes. Lastly, a variety of harmonic imaging techniques with and without pulse sequencing methods has been developed for improving the signal-to-noise relationship.[165] The approaches currently in development may yield practical applications in gynecologic assessment some time in the future.

Practical issues are limiting factors for HySo. Particularly, the relative complexity of the procedure requiring the help of an assistant, which limits use that would likely be much greater if the procedure could be simplified. Two options exist for assuring the proper distention of the uterine cavity during the HySo procedure:

1. A simple catheter of the type used for intrauterine insemination (IUI) or one equipped with a specially designed cone-shaped stopper for better fitting against the external os of the cervix[9]

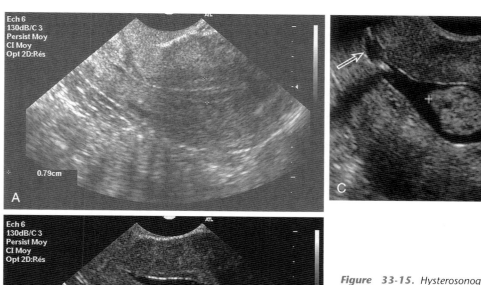

Figure 33-15. Hysterosonography (HySo): Intrauterine infusion of a contrast solution improves vision of the uterine cavity over that provided by plain ultrasound image (**A**). Providing an interphase that enhances contrast (**B**) facilitates the detection of intrauterine diseases such as polyps and fibroids (**C**).

2. A balloon-equipped catheter, which is inflated after positioning in the uterine cavity in order to prevent displacement

In the first scenario, the speculum needs to be removed very carefully after placement of the catheter so as not to displace it from its proper intrauterine position. This most often justifies using speculums that are articulated on one side only, although this facilitates extraction that are notoriously more uncomfortable. In the second option, the balloon catheter creates some degree of discomfort when it expands in the lower uterine segment. Moreover, the balloon may hinder proper visualization of the lower uterine segment. In short, albeit providing images of remarkable resolution, HySo is a three-hand procedure (one for holding the probe, one for instilling medium, and the third hand for making image adjustments and measurements). Recently, an innovative option has been proposed in which a phase-shifting medium is used.[166] This medium has a gel consistency at room temperature and the acoustic characteristics of water. Intrauterine instillation of 1 to 3 mL creates a slight distention of the cavity, thus offering negative or *black* contrast vision during the time necessary for ultrasound examination, which is conducted in the absence of any instrument present in the uterus. The medium later liquefies and is expelled naturally. In a pilot trial, this novel technique provided classic HySo-like images while performing an ultrasound exploration in regular ultrasound-like conditions with no catheter present in the uterine cavity during the examination.[166]

Hysterosonography for Visualizing Endometrial Polyps and Fibroids

HySo, designed for visualizing intrauterine disease, has been primarily indicated in women suffering from DUB. In these women, HySo aims at identifying a possible anatomic cause, such as a polyp or a subendometrial fibroid, in order to determine the need for surgical exploration. Thus, HySo is in direct competition with other noninvasive diagnostic procedures, primarily with regular vaginal ultrasound and office diagnostic hysteroscopy.

In a prospective trial, de Kroon et al.[167] reported that HySo provided conclusive information in 84% of 180 consecutive women presenting with DUB. In all these cases, the positive and negative findings of HySo were confirmed in women undergoing surgery, showing a sensitivity and specificity of 100%. In 5.6% of cases, however, HySo could not be performed because of cervical stenosis; its results were judged inconclusive in a further 10.3% because of constant leaking of saline solution resulting in inadequate distention of the cavity, a finding that might have been reduced by the use of a balloon catheter instead of the catheter with the Goldstein cone-stopper used by these authors.[167] A recent meta-analysis of trials looking at the value of HySo in women presenting with DUB confirmed de Kroon's original findings, reporting pooled sensitivity and specificity in the 24 retained trials of 0.95 (95% CI, 0.93, 0.97) and 0.88 (95% CI, 0.85, 0.92), respectively.[168] The results of this analysis are in general agreement with those of other meta-analyses.[169] In a study of 48 women presenting with DUB, Leone et al. showed that when strict methods for assessing SIS findings are used this noninvasive exploration is as effective as hysteroscopy,[170] a finding in agreement with others.[171]

The recent advent of 3D reconstruction appears to further enhance the clinical value of HySo.[16,172] If 2D or 3D HySo is negative, invasive procedures such as surgical hysteroscopy can be avoided. Practically speaking, 3D volume acquisitions limit the duration of the uterine distention to the time strictly necessary for carrying out the electronic acquisition of a 3D volume. Subsequently it is possible to review 3D images after the uterine distention subsides (Fig. 33-16).

Similarly HySo can benefit from the added information provided by Doppler, showing for example a vessel entering a polyp or circling around the surface of a submucosal fibroid.[173] Unusual use of Doppler in conjunction with SIS includes identification of a uteroperitoneal fistula[174] and intrauterine vascular malformation.[175]

Besides DUB, other indications for HySo include the evaluation of women receiving tamoxifen[176,177] and, according to certain authors, asymptomatic women entering menopause and considering initiating hormonal therapy.[178] HySo in preparation for ART is discussed in a separate section later in the chapter.

Discomfort generated by HySo examination is usually mild to minimal. In a prospective trial Dessole et al.[179] looked at the side effects and complications of 1153 intended HySo procedures. In 93% of cases, HySo was conducted appropriately. No usable data were available in only 7% of women for various reasons (mainly leaks of the contrast solution). Side effects of moderate to severe pain, vaginal reactions, and nausea and vomiting occurred in 102 (8.8%) cases. Severe complications such as fever and clinical signs of peritonitis were encountered in 0.95% of cases. This group does not routinely perform cervical cultures or use routine antibiotics. The reported low incidence of infectious complications does not constitute an absolute indication for routine measures of prophylaxis, a recommendation shared by the American College of Obstetricians and Gynecologists.[180] These recommendations, however, could be proposed in selected cases who stand at higher risk because of their past history or the existence of pelvic tenderness. Further expanding their study of the safety of HySo, Dessole et al. looked at the specific risk of propagating cancer cells in the cases of endometrial cancer.[181] In this trial fluid spilling from the fallopian tube was collected while HySo was conducted preoperatively in 32 women diagnosed with endometrial cancer. Malignant and suspicious cells were recovered from tubal spill in 2 (6.25%) and 6 (18.8%), respectively, for a total of 8 findings of suspicious or malignant cells recovered from 32 (25%) women undergoing HySo while suffering from endometrial carcinoma. These authors strongly recommended that HySo not be performed in cases of proven or suspected endometrial cancer.[181] The practical value of operating to remove polyps smaller than 1.5 cm in women prior to IVF has been a matter of debate. In a retrospective trial, Isikoglu et al.[182] observed that even if small endometrial polyps might not affect pregnancy rates they bore a negative toll on fecundity by causing an increase in miscarriages, a finding in agreement with those of others.[183] The corollary of this is that HySo should be part of the regular workup in cases of repeated miscarriages.[184] Interestingly, some investigators recommend surgical removal of

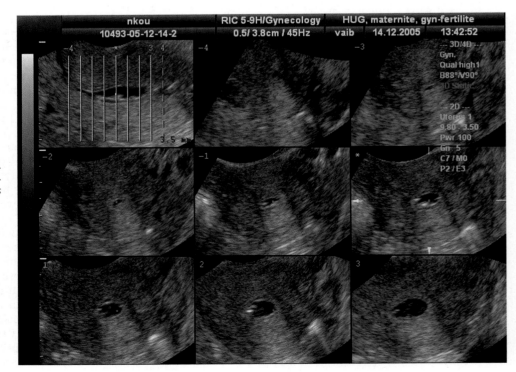

Figure 33-16. *3D-hysterosonography (HySo) allows secondary reviews of images for detailed analysis of intrauterine content.*

the polyp upon starting IVF without cycle cancellation.[185] In our own program in which women are synchronized with a short 7- to 14-day use of oral contraceptive (OC) pills during which routine SIS is performed, we commonly perform the surgical removal of incidental polyps while the patient is still on the OC pill. Performing HySo while the patient is on the pill offers the further advantage of having an atrophic mucosa, which precludes confusing a mucosal fold for a polyp.

Ultimately, it is important to underscore that a comparison between HySo and office hysteroscopy goes beyond the sheer ability that these diagnostic techniques offer for detecting intrauterine diseases such as polyps and fibroids, a difference that is now reduced to a draw. Besides detecting intrauterine disease, each technique offers other specific advantages that will drive the preferences for one or the other technique. On the one side, office hysteroscopy provides information about possible chronic inflammation/infection of the endometrium, a condition not totally clarified yet, but otherwise not identifiable.[186] On the other hand, pelvic ultrasound and its possible refinements (Doppler, 3D reconstruction and HySo) offer information about organs other than the uterus, namely, the ovaries, that may be pertinent for sorting out the cause of DUB. Hence, the choice between SIS and office hysteroscopy should result from a global clinical process that takes into account all the issues pertinent to each clinical situation. When DUB is encountered in the perimenopause, ultrasound will offer the added advantage of checking for the possible presence of ovarian cysts. In preparation for ART, however, office hysteroscopy offers added information about the inflammation status of the endometrium, which might call for specific treatments.

Hysterosonography in ART

In an unselected population of 500 consecutive infertile women submitted to routine HySo, Hamilton et al.[187] reported that HySo could be performed in 96.8% of the women with interpretable observations in all but one of these women. Twenty of these women underwent surgical hysteroscopy based on their HySo findings, with false positive HySo findings disclosed in 6 (30%) women. In a different study, Ragni et al.[188] compared data from routine pre-ART vaginal ultrasound, HySo, and diagnostic hysteroscopy in 98 infertile patients with a mean age of 33.9 years. Compared to hysteroscopy, vaginal ultrasound and HySo had false positive and negative rates of 9.2% and 5.1% and 2% and 1%, respectively, HySo is more accurate than vaginal ultrasound. This finding is similar to that reported by Tur-Kaspa et al. of 13% as identified by HySo, but not by standard ultrasound.[189] Together, these findings support prior reports[183,190,191] that recommend systematic prospective use of contrast imaging to verify the functionality of the uterine cavity prior to undertaking costly assisted reproductive treatments. Considering that including systematic HySo in all infertility workups may lead to false positive findings generated by mucosal folds, we recommend that HySo be done either in the first 10 days of the follicular phase or while women are on the OC pill. At our institution, all IVF participants undergo routine evaluation of the uterine cavity with HySo while taking a 7- to 14-day course of OC pills routinely used for synchronizing ovarian follicles and cycles. This protocol has revealed otherwise unsuspected intrauterine polyps in 5% to 10% of cases.

Müllerian Anomalies and Recurrent Pregnancy Losses

Uterine anomalies have a reported incidence ranging from 16% to 10%,[192] mainly based on interpretation of hysterosalpingographic (HSG) studies. However, a selection of better structured studies reported a similar incidence of approximately 1% in infertile or presumably fertile women.[193-195] A higher incidence approximating 3% was found in women having a history of recurrent pregnancy losses.[196-198]

Early in development (approximately 9-10 weeks), the paramesonephrotic ducts fuse caudally while the uterine septum starts regressing in an unidirectional manner from the lower part of the uterocervical canal upward.[199] An alternate bidirectional regression theory exists, however.[200]

In a recent study Mazouni et al. undertook a full evaluation of 110 women suspected of bearing a müllerian anomaly, using vaginal ultrasound, HSG, computed tomography (CT) scan, and in cases diagnosed in the later years MRI.[201] Müllerian duct anomalies were reported according to American Fertility Society (AFS) classification[202] (Fig. 33-17). Of the 110 patients referred for müllerian anomalies, 73 women had a septate uterus, 20 a bicornuate uterus, 10 a uterine hypoplasia, 4 a unicornuate uterus, and 3 Rokitansky-Hauser syndrome. In 33% of the cases, the diagnosis was made as part of infertility workup, in 18.2% because of repeat early abortion, and in 12.7% on the occasion of ultrasound performed during pregnancy. In case of septate vagina, dyspareunia was a presenting symptom accounting for 8.2% of all müllerian anomalies diagnosed in this series.

The issue of how müllerian anomalies are best diagnosed has not yet been resolved. HSG was the traditional approach and remains a useful if not indispensable examination in many cases. MRI, although helpful, should not be looked at as the primary means for diagnosing müllerian malformations, but rather used secondarily for further defining certain cases too complex or atypical for definitive diagnosis on ultrasound.[201] 3D ultrasound with contrast enhancing solution stands as the diagnostic tool of choice for first-line screening for uterine malformation. Yet, admittedly, this novel approach has not been sufficiently challenged in certain low-prevalence populations. Woelfer et al. prospectively studied 1089 women with no history of infertility or recurrent early fetal losses using 3D ultrasound.[203] The scanned uteri were analyzed in reconstructed coronal plans, looking at a series of parallel transverse sections and analyzed according to AFS classification (see Fig. 33-17). Briefly, normal and arcuate uteri were recognized by their uniformly convex external contour with indentation less than 10 mm. The fundal contour, which was straight or convex in the normal uterus, was concave in the case of an arcuate uterus (indentation at obtuse angle) and showed the presence of a septum, with the central point of the septum at an acute angle. In the bicornuate uterus, the external contour showed an indentation greater than 10 mm, dividing the two cornua with a convex fundal contour in each. Of the original 1289 women recruited into the study, 200 were not suitable for analysis because of poorly visualized uteri, primarily because of fibroids distorting the cavity. Of the remaining 1089 women, 983 had a normally shaped uterine cavity. Of the 106 (9.7%) uterine anomalies, there were 72 (68%) arcuate, 29 (27%) septate, and 5 (4.7%) bicornuate uteri.[211]

Extending their research on uterine malformations, this team looked at uterine anomalies in 509 women with a history of unexplained recurrent miscarriages and 1976 asymptomatic women in whom a uterine anomaly had been diagnosed fortuitously on ultrasound.[204] There was no difference in relative frequency of various müllerian anomalies or depth of fundal distortion between the two groups. However, in the case of both arcuate and septate uteri, the length of the remaining undisturbed uterine cavity was significantly shorter with more pronounced distortion in the recurrent miscarriage group. This observation is clinically important. It indicates that it is the degree of the müllerian malformation that bears the most important consequences on reproductive outcome rather than the type of malformation encountered.

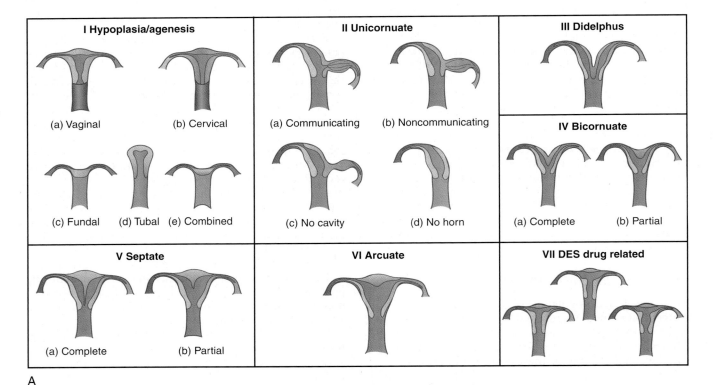

A

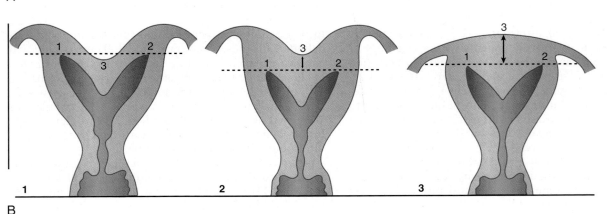

B

Figure 33-17. Müllerian anomalies: **A,** American Fertility Society classification of müllerian anomalies. **B,** Differentiation of septate from bicornuate uteri. The uterus is bicornuate when apex of the fundal external contour occurs below (1) or within 5 mm above (2) a straight line between the tubal ostia. The uterus is septate when the apex is more than 5 mm above the line between the tubal ostia (3). DES, diethylstilbestrol.

UTERINE CONTRACTILITY: DIRECT VISUALIZATION ON ULTRASOUND

Contractility of the Nonpregnant Uterus

The advent of high-resolution vaginal probes has offered the possibility of directly visualizing contractions in the nonpregnant uterus, a physiologic parameter that previously required the invasive measure of intrauterine pressure (IUP). Therefore, the possibility of studying uterine contractility noninvasively has revived interest in this facet of uterine physiology, leading to numerous studies aimed at understanding the role of contractility in reproductive physiology. As in the case of all forms of contractile events, uterine contractions (UCs) are characterized by three primary parameters: frequency, amplitude, and direction of contraction. Also pertinent to the contractile status of the uterus is the IUP value that prevails between UCs or *resting tone.*

Identifying UCs on ultrasound scans has benefited from various forms of image management, which were necessary because of the relatively slow frequency of UCs (maximum of 5 UCs per minute in late follicular phase), making direct UC identification difficult. Most commonly, uterine scans have been accelerated by 5 to 10 times for UC identification, using fast plays of VHS recordings[205,206] or digitized image sequences.[207] Some investigators have used custom computer-assisted systems for UC recognition and computation of UC frequency. Fanchin et al.[208] used an offline 3D reconstruction system providing time mode image sequences depicting time-related changes of the myometrial to endometrial interphase (Fig. 33-18). On these sequences, UCs appear as successive waves created by the periodic displacement of the myometrial to endometrial interphase, which facilitated direct UC recognition. Yet, in spite of our personal technical interest in 3D-based systems of UC recognition, we demonstrated in a prospective trial that the 3D-based approach and direct identification of UC on fast plays of digitized image sequences provide identical UC frequency results.[207] More recently, Pierzynski et al. used a system based on image distortion recognition for UC identification.[209] In a prospective trial conducted in estrogenized women, Bulletti et al. reported perfect concordance between UC frequency measurements made by IUP analysis and UC recognition on ultrasound scans using a 3D-based approach for UC identification.[210] This study provided definitive validation of the noninvasive ultrasound-based approach for UC frequency measurement.

Based on direct UC visualization, various types of contractions have been described, ultimately leading to recognition of two primary types that show either retrograde (cervix to fundus) or antegrade (fundus to cervix) displacement of the contractile process. It is of note, however, that ultrasound-based analyses of UC displacement have never been validated by comparing ultrasound findings against the actual propagation of the pressure wave, as measured by multiple IUP recorders[211] or true displacement of the uterine content.[212,213] Hence, to this date, UC displacement data remain unvalidated and of descriptive value only. UC amplitude and uterine resting tone also evade ultrasound-based analyses. Attempts have been made of using noninvasive methods for studying the actual involvement of uterine muscle cells that participate in the contractile event, which in theory could reflect the contractile event and, therefore, correlate with actual changes in IUP. Such data, which could potentially provide information about UC physiology, are still at the research stage. Attempts in this direction using MRI must be recognized, however.[214,215]

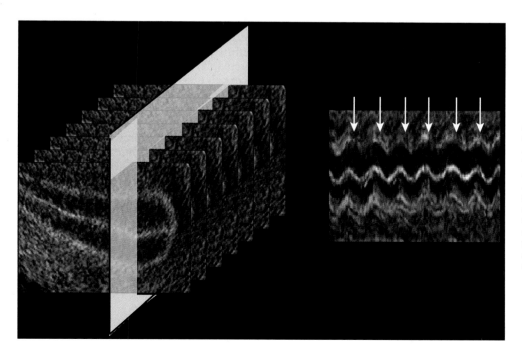

Figure 33-18. *3D-based approach of uterine contraction assessment. 2D images are recorded over time without sweeping through a given territory. Hence, the z-axis represents time. On these electronically reconstructed time mode scans, displacements of the myometrial-endometrial interphase take the appearance of periodic waves (arrows), with each wave individually representing an actual contraction of the uterus.*

Uterine Contractility during the Menstrual Cycle

Typically, three patterns of uterine contractility are recognized during the menstrual cycle. These are emblematic of the late follicular phase, luteal phase, and intercycle interval (i.e., during menses).[216,217] Each of these patterns is defined by sets of UC characteristics such as frequency, amplitude, and direction of contractions and, moreover, response to specific hormonal stimuli.

Follicular Phase. *During the follicular phase*, there is a progressive increase in UC frequency under the influence of rising E_2 levels,[218-220] which culminates at approximately 5 UC per minute just prior to ovulation.[63] Characteristically, only the subendometrial layers of the myometrium are involved in the contractile events encountered in the preovulatory period. They are never perceived by women despite UC frequency being higher at that time than at any other time in the menstrual cycle.[19]

An overwhelming majority of investigators,[207,218,221] but not all,[222] have reported a clear predominance of UCs displaying retrograde cervix-to-fundus displacement during the late follicular phase. In these studies UC displacement was judged on fast plays of ultrasound sequences or by analyzing the propagation of the increase in IUP signal.[212] Yet determining the UC direction and its physiologic relevance is complicated by the presence two distinct unknowns:

1. Although the contractile structure that is actually responsible for UCs is the subendometrial part of the myometrium, the visualized phenomenon on sequences of ultrasound images is the resulting effect, the displacement of the endometrium. Hence, the parameter that is analyzed is an indirect reflection of the contractile process rather than the true phenomenon itself.

2. Ultrasound scans identify the apparent retrograde displacement of contractile waves recording on the endometrium by the myometrium without actually indicating whether this does or does not result in a true displacement of the uterine content. In the case of sperm, for example, retrograde transport will also depend on whether an appropriate opening takes place or does not at the uterotubal junction when the contractile event reaches there.

Retrograde UCs identified during the late follicular phase have been viewed as being instrumental in the rapid transport of sperm that takes place from the vagina to the pelvic cavity following intercourse in the late follicular phase.[212,223,224] UCs or possible disruptions of their functionality may therefore play a key role in the reproductive process and in certain forms of infertility. Yet, as stated above, echographic analyses of UC direction have never been challenged to determine whether a correlation exists with the actual displacement of uterine content.

Using ^{99}Tc-labeled macroalbumin aggregates (MAA), Leyendecker's team showed that contractions with retrograde displacement of uterine content predominate during the late follicular phase.[220] Interestingly, these authors also observed that an elective transport takes place toward the tube facing the developing follicle.[225,226] In various intervention trials, Leyendecker's team showed evidence for the involvement of oxytocin (OT) in the retrograde contractions encountered during the late follicular phase.[213,227] That OT and possibly vasopressin (AVP) actually play a physiologic role in late follicular phase UCs and are instrumental in the control of sperm transport remain to be determined, however. As discussed later in this chapter, retrograde displacement of uterine content triggered by late follicular phase UCs appears to be seriously disrupted in women suffering from endometriosis[226] or intramural uterine fibroids.[147]

Retrograde contractions that prevail during the late follicular phase and partake in sperm transport are decreased in cases of endometriosis and uterine fibroids.[148] This disruption of uterine contractility elegantly identified by Kido's group is likely to bear some responsibility for the infertility that accompanies both conditions associated with decreased uterine contractility, particularly, endometriosis.[148]

Luteal Phase. *During the luteal phase*, the UC pattern is characterized by a state of uterine quiescence brought on by the uterorelaxing properties of progesterone. In a prospective trial, Wilcox et al.[228] showed that pregnancies never occurred when a single instance of unprotected intercourse took place after the day of ovulation. This finding may be explained in part by the uterorelaxing properties of progesterone and the resulting decrease in uterine contractility, particularly the retrograde UCs that are involved in sperm transport. In experimental trials, exogenous E_2 and progesterone reproduce the UC patterns encountered in the follicular and luteal phases, respectively (Fig. 33-19). Ayoubi et al. observed that physiologic E_2 replacement administered to young women suffering from premature ovarian failure (POF) resulted in UC frequency patterns that were similar to those encountered in the menstrual cycle, particularly during the follicular-luteal transition.[207] In these authors' hands, transvaginal administration of 45, 90, and 180 mg of progesterone per day using the sustained release vaginal gel (Crinone) resulted in a prompt decrease in UC frequency with no dose-related differences. This indicates that following physiologic estrogen exposure minimal amounts of progesterone suffice to induce full uteroquiescence, as seen in the luteal phase of the menstrual cycle.[207]

Intercycle Interval. *During the intercycle interval* (menses), uterine contractility increases sharply in response to withdrawal from the uterorelaxing properties of progesterone upon demise of the corpus luteum or discontinuation of exogenous progesterone or progestin administration. The role of concomitant withdrawal from E_2 also produced by the corpus luteum and supplied by most oral contraception (OC) preparations remains a matter for debate. Contrary to the late follicular phase situation, all layers of myometrium are involved in UC experienced by women at the time of menses. Moreover, UCs are commonly perceived by women at that stage of the cycle. At times, UCs occurring during the intercycle interval are painful enough to cause a true medical condition, dysmenorrhea, characterized by painful uterine cramping to the point of requiring specific treatment. Contrasting with the late follicular phase, however, UC frequency is markedly lower during the intercycle interval when it usually does not exceed 2.5 UCs per minute. Moreover, UC amplitude and resting tone, which are markedly higher during menses than at any other time during the menstrual cycle,[211,217,229] are the two parameters that are most significantly increased in cases of dysmenorrhea.[229] Using MRI analyses, Kataoka et al. showed an enlargement of the subendometrial sonolucent layer of the myometrium in dysmenorrheic women on cycle day 1, at a time when these women experienced strong cramping. Conversely, uterine images returned to normal on day 3 of the cycle when cramping had subsided[214] (Fig. 33-20). In a prospective trial, Kido et al. compared the characteristics of MRI of the endometrium and subendometrial sonolucent layer of the myometrium in 25 women on OC pills and 23 others having regular menstrual cycles.[215] This trial revealed that endometrial distortion was significantly less prominent and the subendometrial low-intensity area significantly thinner in the OC group who also presented a lesser degree of cramping as compared to their cycling counterparts.[215] To this day, therefore, MRI is the only approach that provided noninvasive UC parameters that parallel clinical symptoms in cases of dysmenorrhea. However, the relative complexity of the technique precluded any form of large-scale use and, consequently, the practical verification of the pilot trials. Hence, this MRI-based approach, albeit promising, awaits experimental verification.

Effects of Uterine Contractility on ART Outcome

Fanchin et al.[208] were first to report an inverse correlation between UC frequency at the time of embryo transfer (ET) and IVF outcome (Fig. 33-21), a finding that supported data from other.[230] but not all teams.[231] From Fanchin's results, high UCs had negative consequences on implantation and pregnancy rates. As UCs were measured prior to conducting ETs, the study reflected the state of contractility prevailing prior to ET, not the impact of the ET procedure itself on contractility. In further trials, the same team also observed that an inverse correlation existed between progesterone levels on the day of ET and UC frequency.[232] Furthermore, an earlier onset of progesterone treatment on the day of oocyte retrieval rather than after ET resulted in an abrupt decrease in UC frequency on the day of ET with a trend toward better pregnancy rates.[233] Similarly, delaying ET to the fifth day after oocyte retrieval resulted in a profound reduction in UC frequency, thus permitting the transfer of blastocysts under better conditions.[234]

Following extensive analyses of UC displacement patterns as observed on ultrasound, IJland et al.[222] reported that women in whom predominantly retrograde UCs persisted until the day of oocyte retrieval had higher pregnancy rates than those in whom a shift in UC direction took place prior to the retrieval. In spite of these early studies, no definitive answer was ever provided regarding the role of direction of contraction on fecundity in general and IVF outcome in particular, in part because ultrasound is not a validated method of measuring UC direction.

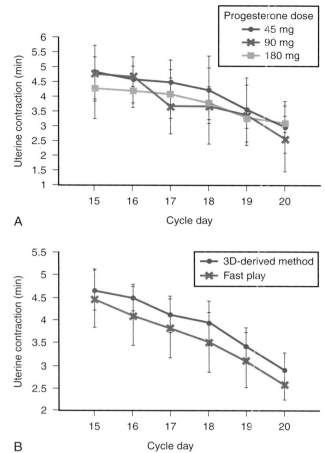

Figure 33-19. Effects of exogenous progesterone on uterine contractility. **A,** In estrogenized women, exogenous administration of 45, 90, and 180 mg of progesterone per day resulted in a prompt decrease in uterine contraction frequency without dose-related differences. **B,** Direct measurements from fast plays of ultrasound sequences or using the 3D-derived method gave similar results. (From Ayoubi JM, Fanchin R, Kaddouz D, et al. Uterorelaxing effects of vaginal progesterone: comparison of two methodologies for assessing uterine contraction frequency on ultrasound scans. Fertil Steril 76:736, 2001.)

The observation that many IVF patients have an increase in UC frequency at the time of ET raises puzzling questions about the mechanism(s) responsible for this phenomenon. In a prospective trial, we studied UC frequency in the same patients during the menstrual cycle that preceded IVF and the IVF cycle itself.[63] In these women, UC frequency reached a similar maximum on the day of LH surge and hCG administration despite E_2 levels being markedly higher in IVF as compared to the menstrual cycle. This indicates that E_2 levels encountered in the menstrual cycle already exert a maximal effect on UC frequency.[63] As illustrated in Figure 33-22, the UC frequency patterns observed in the same women after the LH surge and hCG administration were markedly different in the midluteal phase. In the menstrual cycle, the state of uterine quiescence induced by progesterone is observed as early as day 4 after the LH surge when mean UC frequency was 1.1 per minute. In contrast, UC frequency was 3.6 per minute on the fourth day after hCG administration. In IVF,

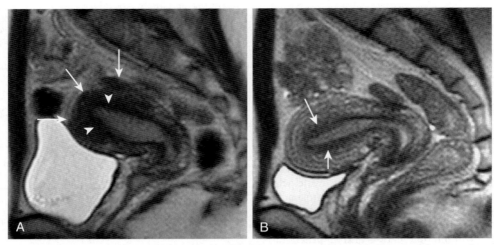

Figure 33-20. *Using MRI, differences were observed in the junctional zone between women experiencing severe dysmenorrhea on day 1 of the menstrual cycle (A) and the same women assessed on day 3 when cramping had subsided (B). On day 1 a characteristic distortion of the endometrium (arrows) and a thickened junctional area (arrowheads) was noticed, a finding that paralleled the intensity of perceived pain. On day 3 when pain had subsided the endometrium and junctional area had returned to normal (arrows). (From Kataoka M, Togashi K, Kido A, et al. Dysmenorrhea: evaluation with cine-mode-display MR imaging—initial experience. Radiology 235:124, 2005.)*

UC frequency dropped to reach a state of uterine quiescence on the sixth day after hCG administration. Note, however, that these women started to receive exogenous progesterone administration on the fourth day after hCG administration (after the UC measurement). Exogenous progesterone therefore may have been instrumental in the decrease in UC frequency observed on the sixth day after hCG administration in IVF. Taken together, these findings suggest that some degree of resistance to the uterorelaxing properties of progesterone exists in IVF. This resistance is likely to result from the effect of the high levels of E_2 encountered in IVF, which can be countered by exogenous progesterone administration.

Pierzynski et al.[209] provided pilot data suggesting that exogenous administration of the OT antagonist, atosiban, resulted in decreased UC frequency prior to ET. This finding is interesting in view of the fact that all other uterorelaxing substances, such as beta mimetics used for

decreasing UC frequency at the time of ET, failed to significantly increase pregnancy rate.[235] Non-ultrasound methods for studying uterine contractility and particularly, MRI approaches have been developed but for studying the impact of endometriosis on contractility not the correlations between contractility and ART outcome. Therefore, this issue will is addressed in the section on endometriosis in which a large place is given to the MRI and its various applications such as cineloop analysis.

IMAGING MARKERS OF ENDOMETRIAL RECEPTIVITY

The endometrial parameters assessed by uterine imaging that have been proposed as markers of endometrial receptivity are endometrial thickness and volume, echogenicity, Doppler perfusion parameters, and contractile patterns. The issue of endometrial thickness and endometrial receptivity can be summarized by saying that the endometrium should be sufficiently thick to forecast an appropriate response to progesterone and in turn a proper deployment of the sequence of changes that lead to endometrial receptivity. Rashidi et al.[236] reported no correlation between endometrial thickness on the day of hCG administration and pregnancy rate by receiver-operating characteristic (ROC) curve and multiple logistic regression analysis. These authors concluded that the echographic characteristics of the endometrium (thickness and pattern) on the day of hCG administration did not differ between pregnant and nonpregnant patients with thickness of 10.1 and 10.2 in pregnant and nonpregnant patients. De Geyter et al. comparing endometrial thickness in COH-IUI and IVF cycles, predictably found the endometrium was thicker in IVF as compared to COH-IUI.[77] In this comparison of endometrial thickness in COH-IUI and IVF, a correlation between thinner endometrium and poor outcome existed in COH-IUI but not in IVF. In our opinion, this suggests that a thin endometrium in COH-IUI primarily reflects a

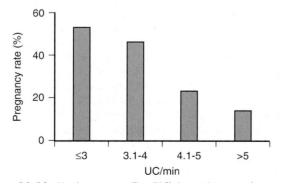

Figure 33-21. *Uterine contractility (UC) just prior to embryo transfer and pregnancy rates. In women who all had three good embryos available for transfer, an inverse correlation was observed between UC frequency and pregnancy rates. (From Fanchin R, Righini C, Olivennes F, et al. Uterine contractions at the time of embryo transfer alter pregnancy rates after in-vitro fertilization. Hum Reprod 13:1968, 1998.)*

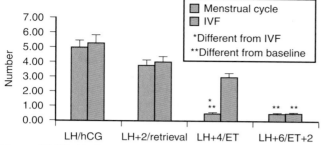

Figure 33-22. *Uterine contraction (UC) frequency was measured in the same patients, in menstrual and IVF cycles. UC frequency was similar on the day of LH surge and hCG administration, indicating that the supraphysiologic levels of E_2 encountered in assisted reproductive technology (ART) do not further stimulate UC frequency over what is encountered in the menstrual cycle. Following ovulation, UC frequency decreased earlier in the menstrual cycle (on LH + 4 day) than it did in ART (on ET+2 or hCG+6 day), indicating that a relative degree of resistance to the uterorelaxing properties of progesterone exists in ART, most likely as a result of elevated E_2 levels. E_2, estradiol; ET, embryo transfer; hCG, human chorionic gonadotropin; IVF, in vitro fertilization; LH, luteinizing hormone; LH +2, +4, +6: days after LH surge. (From Ayoubi JM, Fanchin R, Kaddouz D, et al. Uterorelaxing effects of vaginal progesterone: comparison of two methodologies for assessing uterine contraction frequency on ultrasound scans. Fertil Steril 76:736, 2001.)*

weak response to the milder stimulation used outside IVF rather than a true endometrial parameter reflective of poor receptivity.

In spite of not finding a correlation between endometrial thickness and ART outcome, Rashidi's data[236] showed that pregnancy rates declined when endometrial thickness was either less than 7 mm or had uncommonly high values (>12 mm). Studying 139 IVF cycles, Oliveira et al. made a similar observation yet with thinner endometrial measurements across the board of 8 and 8.6 mm in pregnant and nonpregnant patients as compared to Rashidi's finding of 10.1 and 10.2 mm, respectively.[99] Along these lines, Isaacs et al. report that endometrial thickness is a valid predictor of pregnancy with a 91% pregnancy rate seen in women whose endometrial thickness is greater than 10 mm and no pregnancies when it is less than 7 mm.[237] In a retrospective study of 1294 patients, Richter et al. found a clear correlation between endometrial thickness and pregnancy rates.[76] These authors also failed to find any negative impact of very high endometrial thickness on pregnancy rates as previously reported by Casper's team.[85]

The possibility of a positive bias between thicker endometrium and heftier responses to COH, a parameter of better IVF outcome, is reported by Zohav et al.[238] a phenomenon which could easily suggest that thicker endometrium is inherently more receptive. By extension, this observation indicates the possibility of further biases between Doppler findings of higher perfusion and stronger ovarian responses to human menopausal gonadotropin (hMG)/FSH and consequently better oocyte quality when in fact endometrial perfusion may not be directly related to endometrial receptivity. The possibility that different ovarian stimulation protocols had different impacts on endometrial thickness was examined by Imoedemhe et al.[239] These authors compared the effects of regimens using

clomiphene citrate (CC) alone (regimen I) or in combination with 75 IU (regimen II) or 150 IU of hMG (regimen III) and found no differences in endometrial thickness.

Raga et al. looked at the predictive value of 3D endometrial volume calculation for the development of pregnancy in ART.[12] In a study on 72 IVF cycles, pregnancy rates were significantly lower when endometrial volume was less than 2 mL as compared to 2 to 4 mL or greater than 4 mL. Consonant findings were reported by Zohav et al. who found no differences in endometrial volume in 60 pregnant IVF women depending on pregnancy outcome but observed that endometrial volume less than 2 mL was associated with a significant increase in pregnancy loss.[238] Martins et al. reported on endometrial volume values measured 1 week after embryo transfer.[240] A significant difference was found between the endometrial volume of pregnant (6.49 ± 1.97mL) and nonpregnant women (3.4 ± 1.1mL), and to a lesser extent, endometrial thickness. This latter observation of a difference in endometrial volume by a factor of nearly 2 between pregnant and nonpregnant women appears to reflect a direct early effect of the developing pregnancy on the endometrium rather than preexisting differences. This finding is in agreement with the report of an early increase in E_2 production that even precedes that of hCG in the late luteal phase of conception cycles.[241]

Endometrial echogenicity has been proposed as a marker of endometrial receptivity. In early work, Casper's team, who observed no differences in endometrial thickness between pregnant and nonpregnant women, reported three different patterns of endometrial echogenicity on the day after hCG administration.[92] In these investigators' hands a hypoechoic endometrium was associated with a good prognosis whereas pregnancy rates were lower in the case of a hyperechogenic, intermediate pattern. Numerous publications support the concept that a hypoechoic endometrium with a full three-line aspect is associated with good ART outcome.[93-98] Other articles failed to find good predictive value to endometrial echogenicity, however.[99,100]

According to Rosenwaks' team, hyperechoic endometrium is a particularly ominous sign in women exposed to DES.[242] The objective of this study was to compare prospectively pregnancy outcome as it is related to ultrasonic endometrial echo pattern in women exposed to DES in utero by their mother's consumption with women not exposed to DES, all of whom were undergoing IVF. Pregnancy outcome relative to endometrial thickness and pattern was evaluated in 540 cycles of IVF including DES-exposed (n = 50) and non-DES-exposed (n = 490) women. Endometrial patterns were designated as p1 (solid); p2 (ring); and p3 (intermediate). DES patients exhibited p1 more often than the majority of the non-DES-exposed group. There was no significant difference in endometrial thickness among the cycles where p1 was noted when comparing the DES-exposed (10.3 mm) with the non-DES-exposed (10.7 mm) groups. Notably, within the group exhibiting p1, no pregnancies occurred in the 18 cycles of DES-exposed women compared with a 39.2% clinical pregnancy and 36.5% delivery rate in the non-DES-exposed control subjects ($P < 0.0001$ and $P = 0.008$, respectively). Pregnancy rates were not significantly different in the cycles in which the other endometrial patterns were found when comparing the two groups. The impact of uterine shape on pregnancy outcome was also investigated. A T-shaped uterine configuration was noted in 11 of 18 (61.1%) cycles of DES-exposed women with pattern p1 compared with 9 of 23 (39.1%) with pattern p2. Of cycles in which a T-shaped uterus was demonstrated, none of 11 (0%) with pattern p1 compared with 4 out of 9 (44.4%) with pattern p2 resulted in pregnancy (P = 0.026). These data suggest that the endometrial pattern is one of the most significant variables for pregnancy outcome in DES-exposed women undergoing IVF.

The two last parameters proposed as markers of endometrial receptivity are Doppler data on endometrial and subendometrial vascularization and uterine contractility. Early Doppler studies that claimed to identify flow parameters that precluded the possibility of embryo implantation, thus recommending freezing all the embryos for a different transfer, were never verified. Instead, all available studies that used either pulsed Doppler data or the more sophisticated and operator independent 3D-PDA failed to find differences between conception and nonconception cycles.[135] Hence, Doppler data cannot be considered any more a marker of endometrial receptivity. Finally, in our hands, increased uterine contractility bore an ominous prediction on embryo implantation,[200] a finding confirmed by others[209] but challenged by one study that failed to confirm these findings.[231]

EMBRYO TRANSFERS

Embryo transfers should be performed with utmost care. Conversely, sloppy practice or simply suboptimal care, let alone imprecise placement of the transferred embryos in the uterine cavity, will undermine the good clinical and biologic work that came together to obtain these embryos. Interestingly, the very person who first achieved oocyte retrieval under ultrasound guidance[1] was also the first to advocate using ultrasound for directing embryo transfers.[243] In both cases, however, the route proposed by this pioneer team turned out to not be the one that proved itself best in the end and that remains in use today. The visionary value of these original propositions remains, however.

In 1991, J. Leeton's team[244] first provided objective evidence in favor of ultrasound-guided transcervical transfers, as we know them today. In a prospective trial, pregnancy rates were higher in 94 women who had an ultrasound-guided transfer as compared to 246 control subjects who underwent the classical or *clinical touch* approach. Similar benefit was found in donor egg recipients. In a retrospective comparison of 137 embryo transfers, Lindheim et al. showed that pregnancy and embryo implantation rates were higher in women whose transfers were ultrasound guided as compared to their counterparts in whom ultrasound was not used,[245] a finding confirmed by Coroleu et al. with even more drastic differences.[246] These pioneer studies were later supported by a wealth of others, including sets of meta-analyses,[247-250] although some noticeable reports failed to document the superiority of ultrasound-guided transfers.[251-253] In a letter to the editor, Ata and Urman

argued with the conclusions drawn by Kosmas et al.[253] based on findings of non-superiority.[254] These authors' contention was that, although the superiority of ultrasound-guided transfers was not universally recognized, none of the trials had reported lower results when compared to the classical alternate "clinical touch" method. After alluding to the possible independent benefit from a full bladder condition, Ata and Urman also underscored that not all ultrasound-guided trials placed the embryos where their implanting chances are optimal, halfway down the uterine cavity (or possibly lower).[254] Lastly, we ourselves endorse these authors' ultimate pledge in support of routinely conducting embryo transfers *with a view*, because it does not harm and may help (possibly very much so) if the embryos are placed lower in the uterine cavity. Supporting the same line of thought, Flisser and Griffo, whose own study showed no improvement in pregnancy rates with ultrasound-guided transfers, nonetheless recommended its systematic use in a recent review article.[255] Their stand is rooted on the grounds that it is clinically impossible to preemptively determine who is likely to truly benefit from ultrasound-guided embryo transfers. Ata and Urman remind us that ultrasound-guided transfer is reassuring to the patient, constitutes an excellent teaching experience for shortening the learning curves of trainees, and is likely to help in certain circumstances.[254]

As alluded to above, there is a question that looms large today: Where is the most optimal and efficacious location for placing transferred embryos within the uterine cavity? As this issue evaded our scrutiny before the current interest in ultrasound-guided embryo transfers, our answers to these questions are still fragmentary and subject to further refinements before becoming definitive. To date, data from prospective trials unveiled a counterintuitive scenario: Embryo transfers are more successful when performed low rather than high in the uterine cavity. As early as 2002, Coroleu et al. reported a prospective trial in which embryos were transferred in 180 consecutive IVF patients at 1, 1.5, and 2 cm from the fundus.[256] Unequivocally, embryo transfers performed 2 mm and 1.5 mm from the fundus resulted in higher pregnancy rates than when embryos were placed 1 mm from the fundus. In agreement with these findings, Pope et al. observed in a retrospective analysis that the further away the tip of the catheter was from the fundus, the higher the pregnancy rate.[257] A regression analysis in this trial indicated that each millimeter in excess of 1 cm from the fundus translated in a whopping 11% increase in pregnancy rate, a trend later confirmed by others.[258]

As the clinical interest for ultrasound-guided transfers gained momentum, industry designed catheters specially equipped with echogenic tips that facilitated their recognition on ultrasound to more accurately follow how far the catheter is moved inside the uterine cavity. These new catheters have been evaluated for the ease of use and efficacy at optimizing embryo placement. In a prospective randomized trial, a standard catheter (n = 95) and a new echogenic soft Wallace catheter (n = 98) were compared. The results showed a trend, albeit not statistically significant (P = 0.08), for higher pregnancy rates at 54.1% with the echogenic as compared to 41% with the regular catheter,[259] a finding confirmed by others.[260] It appears, therefore, that although new echogenic catheters are more agreeable to use, they do not bring higher pregnancy rates, at least in the hands of these investigators. Wishing to err on the safe side, we contend that results may be different in real-life conditions. The easier vision provided by the echogenic ring placed at the tip of these catheters will facilitate a more precise and reliable placement of the transferred embryos at the exact location selected in the uterine cavity. Notably, these catheters are likely to safely protect against the risk of *following* the second instead of the first air bubble present in the catheter and consequently transferring the embryos too high in the cavity. We believe, therefore, that the use of echogenic catheters constitutes a sound measure for securing more reliable and predictable pregnancy rates.

Taken together, these data indicate that embryo transfers should be routinely performed under vision, aiming at placing embryos lower in the uterine cavity than intuitively thought and previously done. In our opinion, this unexpected and surprising information about the benefit of lower embryo placement further supports the choice of routinely performing all embryo transfers under ultrasound guidance in order to optimize embryo placement. These findings, we believe, should direct the objectives of future trials, which rather than persisting in proving the benefit of ultrasound-guided transfers, which are sufficiently self-evident today, should aim at precisely determining the most optimal way of placing embryos at the time of transfer. New trials should, therefore, validate the current belief about the value of lower transfers, not just in normal uteri, but also in the case of fibroids and other anomalies of the uterus, such as when a uterine septum is present or in DES-exposed women.

OVARIES

Contrary to the uterus, which reaches a definitive and stable size at the time of puberty (short of developing tumors like fibroids), the ovaries change size and aspect throughout the different phases of their functional life. Hence, morphologic analyses of the ovaries as they appear on ultrasound and other imaging techniques need to be repeated because their normal appearance will be affected by the various facets and stages of ovarian function. Therefore, ovarian imaging will be reviewed in parallel with the functional changes encountered during the transition of puberty, throughout the menstrual cycle, and in relation to aging and the menopause.

Ultrasound, in the modern era high-resolution vaginal probes, provides an unrestricted view of the ovaries even in case of obesity. For this reason ultrasound is the first-choice imaging approach for exploring the ovaries. Specifically, ovarian ultrasound studies identify the two constituents of the organ, the ovarian cortex and stroma.[261] Following a description by Pache et al.[262] all follicles 2 to 10 mm are counted in each ovary, the sum of which constitutes the total antral follicle count (AFC). As granulosa cells of antral follicles are freshly endowed with FSH receptors, these follicles constitute the cohort of follicles capable of responding to rising FSH levels, called recruitable follicles.

Recruitment by FSH takes place either through the physiologic intercycle FSH signal or with exogenous FSH/hMG treatments administered in the context of ART. Therefore, the size of this cohort of recruitable follicles (AFC) is inherently linked to the magnitude of the ovarian response to COH. Hence, AFC is expected to predict the magnitude of the ovarian response to COH as well as its outcome.

The cohort of antral follicles identified on ultrasound—expressed by the total AFC score—represents a constant fraction of the pool of primordial follicles remaining in the ovary at any given time.[263,264] Therefore, the AFC can serve to determine the number of remaining follicles and thus the ovarian reserve. These considerations explain the two primary grounds on which AFC constitutes an important parameter of ovarian function. Specifically, AFC aims at (i) predicting the amplitude of the ovarian response to exogenous FSH/hMG (for singling out excessive and poor responses and therefore adjusting the doses of FSH/hMG accordingly) and (ii), as AFC assesses the ovarian reserve based on the number of recruitable follicles available, it can predict ART outcome based on the number of primordial follicles remaining. The latter point begs a question about whether a link exists between the quantity of remaining follicles and quality of these follicles and the chances of conceiving. As discussed in the following paragraph, the nature of this link between quantity and quality of remaining follicles differs based on the circumstances that pertain to the reduction in the AFC score.

The joint ESHRE/ASRM Rotterdam consensus conference[265] included the echographic characteristics of the ovaries (volume and AFC) as criteria for making the diagnosis of PCOS. Ovarian volume and AFC represents now one of the 2 out of 3 criteria that are necessary for making the diagnosis of PCOS. The echographic criteria of PCOS will be addressed in a later section of this chapter.

The ovaries are the sites of tremendous changes in blood flow that take place at various stages of physiologic (from follicular maturation to corpus luteum formation)[266] and pathologic functioning (ovarian stromal flow in PCOS)[267,268] or in the context of specific diseases, such as cancer.[269,270] A separate section discusses ovarian flow assessments using the various methodologies available.

OVARIAN ANATOMY AND FUNCTIONAL CHANGES

The Ovary Before and After Puberty

Ovarian growth in infants and children reflects functional changes rather than chronological ages. In a prospective trial, Buzi et al. examined 117 normal girls between the ages of 1.1 and 15.6 years and 87 girls presenting with premature sexual maturation.[271] In girls showing no signs of abnormal sexual maturation, ovarian volume was 1.1, 2.3, and 5.3 mL in prepubertal, pubertal, and postmenarchial girls, respectively. These changes correlated better with Tanner stages of sexual development than with chronological age.[272]

In infancy and childhood, follicles begin their maturation to rapidly become atretic in the absence of gonadotropin stimulation, giving the ovary a microcystic pattern.[273] Upon increasing gonadotropin cyclicity,[274] but before secondary sexual characters become visible, the promise of puberty is evident, with the ovaries showing changes in morphologic pattern characterized by the presence of several follicles 4 to 9 mm in diameter. This aspect, sometimes referred to as *megalocystic* or *multicystic*,[275,276] needs to be distinguished from the *polycystic* ovary,[277-279] as the morphologic and clinical expressions of this constitutional disorder classically begin at the time of puberty.

The Ovary in the Menstrual Cycle

The intercycle interval constitutes the *baseline* state of the ovaries during their functioning in the menstrual cycle. Therefore, efforts have focused on timing ovarian scans at this reference point, notably for measuring parameters such as AFC that are used for predicting the ovarian reserve and in order to select the optimal COH regimen and adjust the doses of gonadotropin used (Fig. 33-23). During the intercycle interval, the number of small ovarian follicles 2 to 9 mm in diameter computed in the AFC score constitutes the cohort of recruitable follicles endowed with FSH receptors. They are the follicles capable of responding to FSH elevation whether naturally occurring as part of the intercycle FSH signal or resulting from exogenous FSH administered in COH treatments.

From the extensive work of Gougeon and colleagues, we know that a correlation exists between the size of the cohort of recruitable follicles and the remaining endowment in primordial follicles at any given time of the reproductive life[263,264] (Fig. 33-24). As discussed in the section on AFC, correlations have been sought between AFC and COH responses and outcome and with ovarian reserve at large in search for a predictor of future reproductive outcome whether spontaneously occurring or through ART.

Through daily evaluations of individual ovarian follicles on repeated transvaginal scans, Pierson's team identified bursts of synchronous growth in a cohort of follicles, or *waves* of follicle development. In their analysis of the menstrual cycle, these authors identified two to three of these waves. A distinction is made between *minor* waves of follicular growth leading to all the follicles ultimately undergoing atresia and *major* waves leading to further follicular growth and single follicular dominance.[280] The nature of the mechanisms controlling these successive minor waves (2-3) of follicular growth encountered during the menstrual cycle is unknown and cannot be explained simply by the gonadotropin profile.

Follicular growth leading to follicular dominance can be ascertained by witnessing follicles of more than 10 mm. From repeated measurements, it was determined that follicles reach the 12- to 13-mm mark by day 9 of the menstrual cycle on average.[281] At this stage, granulosa cells acquire LH receptors with evidence that follicular maturation can be pursued with LH only[282] or minidoses of hCG.[283] Follicular growth rate appears fairly constant in the menstrual cycle once follicles are more than 13 mm with a daily mean increment in diameter of 1.4 to 1.5 mm/day. Follicular growth is accelerated in COH, however, during which it reaches 1.6 to 1.8 mm/day.[284]

The side of ovulation in the menstrual cycle and whether this regularly alternates from one cycle to the next has been

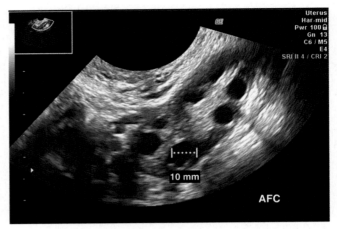

Figure 33-23. *Antral follicles are best assessed and counted for computing the antral follicle count (AFC) at baseline of the menstrual cycles (i.e., during the intercycle interval). Classically, all follicles of 2 to 9 or 10 mm are counted.*

the matter of enduring debate. Some reports based on histologic evidence support the concept that alternate sides of ovulation is the rule,[285] but others claim that it is not more frequent than expected by chance alone.[286] Finally, some propose that the side of follicular growth and ovulation alternates in the case of short cycles,[287] but that ovulation side is randomly determined in the case of long cycles. Reassessing this latter paradigm, Fukuda et al. studied 410 natural cycles of 123 infertile women undergoing 267 IUI and 143 IVF natural-cycle treatments, respectively.[288] In this population, ovulation occurred contralaterally by reference to the preceding cycle in 57% of the 410 cycles but in 72% of women whose follicular phase was 13 days or less. Conversely, ovulation occurred randomly on either side when the follicular phase was more than 14 days, thereby giving credence to the concept that the side of ovulation only alternates in short cycles. From these authors' observation, ovulation appeared of better quality when occurring on the contralateral side with reference to the previous ovulation, with better outcomes of both IUI and IVF cycles in these cases. This observation supports the concept that ovulation is of better quality when the dominant follicle is contralateral to the prior ovulation rather than ipsilateral. Moreover, significantly higher estradiol-to-androstenedione and estradiol-to-testosterone ratios and lower androstenedione levels were observed in *contralateral* as compared to *ipsilateral* ovulation cycles. Practically speaking, therefore, the chance of conceiving during a natural cycle may be affected by the site of ovulation in the preceding cycle. The side of ovulation, however, did not influence Doppler blood flow of the ovarian stroma or follicular and uterine arteries.[289]

Pierson's team prospectively assessed imaging characteristics of the corpus luteum (CL) with daily ultrasound scans in 50 normo-ovulatory women.[290] A CL was detectable on ultrasound scans in 100% of women during the luteal phase with persistent image found in 90% of women during the subsequent follicular phase. Two days after ovulation, a central fluid-filled cavity (CFFC) was present in 88% of the cases, down to 34% after 13 days and 2% after

Early reproductive life   **Late reproductive life**

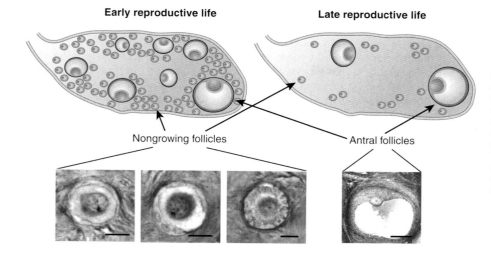

Nongrowing follicles   Antral follicles

Figure 33-24. *Nongrowing and antral follicles in early and late reproductive life. In early and late reproductive life, antral follicles as identified by computing the total antral follicle count (AFC) score, which reflects the total number of follicles remaining, or ovarian reserve. (From Hansen KR, Knowlton NS, Thyer AC, et al. A new model of reproductive aging: the decline in ovarian non-growing follicle number from birth to menopause. Hum Reprod 23:699, 2008.)*

27 days. It is possible to measure the CL volume excluding the CFFC. This volume is correlated with serum progesterone levels over time.[286]

The Resting Ovary during Hormonal Contraception

The impact of OC treatment on ovarian follicles depends on the size of the follicles when OC treatment is initiated. In a prospective trial, Baerwald et al. determined that no follicular growth took place when all the follicles were 10 mm or smaller at the time of starting OC.[291] Conversely, approximately 30% of follicles that were larger than 14 mm at the onset of OC treatment went on to ovulate while the rest regressed and became atretic. In parallel work, this group of investigators determined that follicular development takes place during the 1-week hormone-free interval of classical OC regimens.[292] In a trial looking at normal volunteers on OC pills, these investigators determined that nearly half (47%) of the women grew follicles larger than 10 mm with 53% of them having follicles reaching 14 mm in diameter with, in the latter case, an increase in E_2 production. Contrasting with these findings, echographic assessments showed similar rates of follicular growth in women using progestin-only or barrier contraception in the postpartum period. Endometrial thickness was markedly reduced in the progesterone-only contraception group, indicating that this form of contraception acts on the uterus and cervix, rather than by blocking ovulation.[293]

Hormonal contraception induces a significant reduction in ovarian volume in normally cycling women[294] and in women suffering from PCOS.[295,296] In cycling women, the effect of hormonal contraception on ovarian volume was more profound during continuous rather than cyclic administration of hormonal contraception.[297] Remarkably, however, AFC and anti-müllerian hormone (AMH) values remained unaltered in PCOS women receiving hormonal contraception, in spite of the reduction in ovarian volume observed.[296]

The Ovary through Functional Aging and Menopausal Changes

Ovarian volume decreases with age. Early in the high-resolution ultrasound era, optimistic views prevailed about the predictive value of ovarian volume for future reproductive performance. Surveys of published data indicated that ovarian volume represented a good and easily obtainable index of the primordial follicle population based on comparisons with Faddy's data.[298] Pavlik et al. retrospectively reviewed data from 58,673 ovarian scans obtained from 13,963 women 25 to 91 years of age who underwent annual scanning as part of an ovarian cancer screening program in the context of a familial risk. Ovarian volume was calculated using the prolate ellipsoid formula (L × H × W × 0.523).[107] Mean ovarian volume was 6.6 ± 0.19 cm³ in women younger than 30 years with a decrease that reached statistical significance in women between the ages of 30 and 39. Yet the practicality of ovarian volume data for predicting ovarian reserve on an individual basis is somewhat limited, as clinically meaningful changes only materialize when women are at the edges of their entrance into the naturally infertile period of life. In Pavlik's analyses, in the group of women between the ages of 40 and 49 ovarian volume was found to be markedly reduced at 4.8 ± 0.3 cm³. Ovarian volume decreased to 2.6 ± 0.01 cm³ in postmenopausal women aged 50 to 59 with further decreases observed during the sixth and seventh decades of life.[107] In their extensive study, these authors also looked at relationships between height and ovarian volume. Their findings showed no steady increase with height but a statistical break showed higher volumes in women over 5 feet 8 inches tall. There was a statistically significant reduction in ovarian volume in women younger than 50 years taking estrogens but not in postmenopausal women. In a retrospective chart review, Syrop et al. looked at possible different predictive values of the volume of the smallest and largest ovaries.[299] Their results indicated that the volume of the smallest ovary was a better predictor of peak E_2 levels and numbers of oocytes and embryos and clinical pregnancy in IVF.

In the strict sense of the definition, premature ovarian failure (POF) occurs when ovarian function fails before the age of 40 years. More commonly encountered in everyday ART practice are the cases of premature ovarian dysfunction (not failure) or occult POF (oPOF), which is obscured by seemingly normal ovulatory cycles. These cases of POF classically associate various alterations of the markers of ovarian function. We commonly encounter increases in day 3 FSH/E$_2$ and deceases in AMH and AFC, or poor-insufficient or even lack of ovarian response to ART treatments. Taken together, these findings constitute the clinical characteristics of oPOF. In oPOF, the menstrual cycle is commonly maintained and seemingly ovulatory with no visible anomaly except may be a slight shortening of the cycle and a characteristic early ovulation. Hence oPOF may at times be suspected based on a thorough assessment of ovarian reserve and menstrual history. Conversely, oPOF may be revealed unexpectedly in the course of exploring poor responses to ART cycles prescribed after milder treatments have failed.

Embedded among cases of classical POF and oPOF, which constitute an early expression of ovarian aging, there are sporadic cases of a variant disorder, the state of insensitive ovaries. This complex diagnosis results not from a true advancement of the ovarian aging process but rather from some form of masking of FSH receptor that impedes the biologic activity of this hormone on the ovaries with the net result of inducing an insufficient or absent ovarian response to FSH. Assessing ovarian volume in cases of POF or oPOF may identify a subgroup of women suffering from insensitive ovaries rather than true aging and for whom certain treatments may be undertaken with reasonable chances of success. In a prospective trial Mehta et al. looked at 17 women with fully expressed POF.[300] Based on the ecographic appearance of their ovaries, these authors sorted POF women into two groups, with ($n = 7$) and without ovarian follicles ($n = 10$). Hormonal parameters (FSH and E$_2$) and endometrial thickness were identical in the two groups, whereas ovarian volume was markedly larger in the group with follicles (at 2.8 ± 0.4 mL) than in the group without (1.4 ± 0.2 mL). On average, two follicles were identified in the follicle group, whereas by definition, none were identified in the other group. These authors contend that ultrasound imaging of the ovaries allows identification of a subgroup of women presenting with hypergonadotropic hypogonadism who suffer from insensitive ovaries rather than POF. Practically speaking, pregnancies are more likely to occur in women with insensitive ovaries than in women with POF. The putative diagnosis of insensitive ovaries based on ultrasound images showing preserved ovarian size with follicles supports efforts for possibly attempting various techniques for re-sensitizing ovaries to FSH. These techniques are based on 2- to 3-month treatment periods with E$_2$ and progesterone for lowering FSH levels followed by FSH administration. In a different series Falsetti et al. observed normal ovarian volumes (3.1 ± 0.3 mL) in 14 of 40 women (35%) with frank POF, whereas it was significantly smaller in the remaining 26 women (65%).[301]

In all forms of POF and, more importantly, oPOF, we believe that women must be screened for possible premutations of the FMR1 gene. Ignored, these may transform to the full mutation stage at the next generation, possibly causing fragile X syndrome.[302] Unfortunately, there are no imaging or other characteristics that have been identified as specific to oPOF syndromes associated with FMR1 mutations. Hence, we believe that at the current state of knowledge, all forms of oPOF must be screened for premutations in the FMR1 gene.

In Turner syndrome the number of primordial follicles has been estimated to be normal until at least the 18th week of fetal life with uncertainties as to when atresia starts to accelerate beyond the normal progression.[303] The recent possibility of transplanting cryopreserved ovaries,[304] including the report of live birth successes,[305] sparked interest for contemplating cryopreserving ovaries from Turner syndrome patients before follicle depletion is completed. In a prospective trial, Hreinsson et al. reported ovarian follicles present in 8 of 9 adolescent girls diagnosed with Turner syndrome but who all underwent spontaneous onset of puberty.[306] In these adolescent girls, the density of primordial follicles in ovarian samples studied surgically showed an inverse correlation with plasma FSH levels. It would probably be more useful to cryopreserve ovaries in infanthood or childhood, when the pool of primordial follicles remaining is likely to be much larger, provided that the diagnosis of Turner syndrome can be made that early. However, landmarks on infant and child ovaries imaging (transvesical) have not been delineated yet that determine the limits (ovarian volume, follicles, etc.) above which the cryopreservation of ovaries is worthwhile, and thus, justifies the laparoscopic exploration. We anticipate, however, that these parameters will be determined in the near future so that the decision about surgical exploration can be made from ovarian imaging data at the time of diagnosing Turner syndrome.

Assessing ovarian volume, and particularly differences in size between the two ovaries, is useful for screening for ovarian cancer. Based on their echographic analyses of postmenopausal ovaries, Campbell et al. concluded that the percentage mean difference between the two ovaries was 42.88% ± 32.05%.[307] Based on their observation, these authors concluded that any finding showing an ovary with a volume that is more than twice the size of the other ovary should be considered as suspicious of ovarian cancer until proved otherwise.

ANTRAL FOLLICLE COUNT: A VIEW OF THE OVARIAN RESERVE

In each woman, the endowment of primary oocytes is a finite value established during intrauterine life. From then on, it progressively decreases to reach approximately 2 million at birth and 400,000 at puberty. Drawing their views from extensive histologic reviews of ovaries from women of all ages, Faddy et al. described a progressive decay of primordial follicles over time that follows a bimodal pattern[263] (Fig. 33-25). These authors first identify a slow depletion rate that prevails until the age of approximately 37. If it remained unchanged until final exhaustion of all ovarian follicles, this decay process would lead to complete follicular exhaustion, and therefore menopause, at the age of

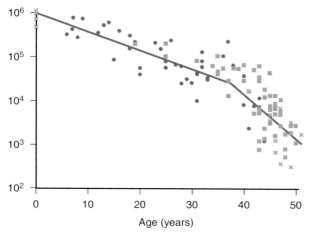

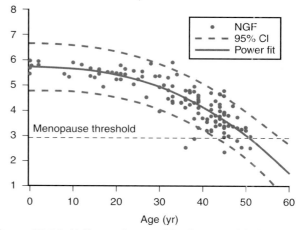

Figure 33-25. *Depletion of primordial follicles over time. In their global analysis, Faddy et al. observed that the number of primordial follicles declines bi-exponentially rather than as a simple exponential function of age, with a first exponential rate parameter of –0.097 and a second of –0.237. The change occurred when numbers had fallen to the critical figure of 25,000 at age 37.5 years. Data were obtained from studies by Block (blue), Richardson (purple), and Goujon (gold). (From Faddy MJ, Gosden RG, Gougeon A, et al. Accelerated disappearance of ovarian follicles in mid-life: implications for forecasting menopause. Hum Reprod 7:1342, 1992.)*

Figure 33-26. *Unlike previous models of ovarian follicle depletion, Hansen et al describe a model predicting no sudden change in decay rate, but rather a constantly increasing rate. NGF, nongrowing follicles. (From Hansen KR, Knowlton NS, Thyer AC, et al. A new model of reproductive aging: the decline in ovarian non-growing follicle number from birth to menopause. Hum Reprod 23:699, 2008.)*

71 years. Yet, Faddy's data indicate that when the number of oocytes remaining reaches a critical value of 25,000, an abrupt increase in oocyte depletion rate takes place, which constitutes the second or fast depletion rate of the bimodal curve of follicular depletion over time. The change from the first *slow* to the second *fast* depletion rate of primordial follicles takes place at approximately the age of 37 years. However, these authors stress that it is reaching the absolute number of remaining oocytes (i.e., the reference mark of 25,000 remaining primordial follicles) that triggers the acceleration in the depletion rate, not age per se. In circumstances of increased follicular losses, as might be encountered following repeated ovarian surgery, it is the moment when the number of remaining oocytes reaches the critical value of 25,000 that will precipitate entrance into the rapid depletion stage. Likewise, the practical impact of single oophorectomy on future reproductive life will depend on whether the abrupt loss of 50% of the remaining oocytes leads to reaching the critical number of 25,000 primordial follicles or not. From arithmetical calculations based on Gougeon's extensive studies of ovarian morphology, it can be calculated that an oophorectomy performed at the age of 20 preserves a number of remaining oocytes well above 25,000. This is no longer the case when oophorectomy takes place at the age of 27 years, when single oophorectomy will accelerate follicular depletion.

Gougeon's claim that follicular depletion over time follows a bimodal pattern has been recently challenged by Hansen et al.[308] who contend that follicular depletion over time follows a progressive acceleration pattern instead of Gougeon's classical bimodal model (Fig. 33-26).

From their morphologic observations, Gougeon's team confirmed that a correlation exists between the number of

primordial and antral follicles.[264] Primordial follicles can only be identified on histologic preparations whereas antral follicles represent the cohort of 2- to 9-mm follicles identified on ultrasound and constitute the AFC score. As stated earlier, antral follicles are endowed with FSH receptors. Hence, they constitute the cohort of recruitable follicles from which the dominant follicle is selected in the menstrual cycle. The whole cohort will be stimulated in case of exogenous gonadotropin (recombinant FSH, urinary FSH, or hMG) administration as prescribed in COH. Therefore, an inherent link exists between AFC and the ovarian response to COH. Clinicians have tried to see how AFC can predict two primary shortcomings of COH: (1) the excessive responses leading to OHSS and (2) the insufficient ones leading to too few oocytes and ultimately ART failure. Practically, the questions are:

1. Can AFC predict ovarian responses to COH in terms of number of follicles and oocytes retrieved?
2. Can AFC be used to single out poor and excessive responses at risk of OHSS?
3. Can AFC predict ART outcome, therefore reflecting oocyte quality not just quantity?
4. Can AFC be used to assess the ovarian reserve and future reproductive potential?

The methodology of AFC measurement has been the source of debate. Using either 2D or 3D approaches for AFC measurements showed good overall inter- and intraobserver reliability.[309] Recently, a novel method of AFC assessment was developed based on automatically isolating volumes of low echogenicity that reflect the antral follicles, the *3D inversion mode rendering method*[310] (Fig. 33-27). Reviewing the methodology of AFC measurement, Jayaprakasan et al. determined that the variability of AFC scoring was significantly lower with inversion mode while it was equivalent when measured with the 3D multiplanar and 2D equivalent method. Yet the authors determined that interobserver reliability was affected by image quality when using the 3D-rendered inversion method. Moreover, mean time for measurement varied greatly with the methods used, ranging from 34, to 50, to 216 seconds for the three methods.[311]

In various trials, AFC was found to correlate to the number of oocytes retrieved in COH[312-314] and the risk of developing OHSS.[315] In a prospective trial, AFC was found superior to basal FSH for predicting ovarian response to COH.[316] In a different trial, Ng et al[317] compared AFC to serum FSH measured at baseline and after clomiphene citrate challenge test (CCCT) for their predictive values regarding ART outcome. These authors found that AFC that remained unchanged after stimulation (CCCT) or after gonadotropin-releasing hormone (GnRH) down-regulation had the best predictive value of the quantitative outcome of COH expressed by the number of oocytes retrieved. This was followed by combined baseline and post-CCCT FSH concentration and age of the woman. Baseline and post-CCCT FSH concentration was a slightly better predictor of E_2 values.

In a prospective trial, Jayaprakasan et al. looked at the predictive value of AFC assessed from 3D ovarian data and compared their data to baseline FSH levels. One of three methods of measurement was used, including the new 3D-rendered inversion mode.[318] These authors' results indicated that total AFC was the best predictor of the number of oocytes retrieved in ART, followed by baseline FSH. Moreover, AFC was significantly lower in the nonpregnant group. AFC less than 7 (<6 using 3D-rendered inversion mode) predicted poor ovarian response leading to cycle cancellation with sensitivity of 100% and specificity

ranging from 93% to 96%, depending on the method used. Prediction of nonconception was low for all methods of AFC measurement. Based on linear regression analysis, the actual number of oocytes retrieved was 40%, 53%, and 72% of total AFC calculated using the 3D-derived three methods. Data obtained from 3D-rendered inversion mode were the closest to the actual number of oocytes retrieved.

Haadsma et al. proposed that among the cohort of 2- to 10-mm follicles retained for AFC computation, the subgroups of smaller and larger antral follicles had different predictive values.[319] In a cohort of 474 women, the number of very small follicles (2-6 mm) declined with age, while that of larger follicles (7-10 mm) remained fairly constant over time. Independent of age, the number of small follicles was related to the results of ovarian reserve tests. These authors claimed that the number of small antral follicle represents the functional ovarian reserve. Following along these lines, Scheffer et al. observed a steeper yearly decline in the number of small antral follicles (2-5 mm) as compared to that seen for larger follicles (6-10 mm).[320]

As stated earlier, a direct correlation has been established between the size of the antral follicle cohort and the number of remaining primordial follicles.[264] Interest has focused on determining the rate of depletion of antral follicles over time. In a prospective trial, Ng et al. determined that the rate of AFC decrease was 0.35 follicle per year (95% CI, 0.26-0.45).[321] These findings are of similar magnitude as the rate of decline of 0.52 follicle per year (95% CI, 0.26-0.45) observed by the same group in a subsequent study conducted in a different cohort of women.[322] Yet, both results were obtained in Chinese women, and other publications reported faster AFC decays in white women in whom an annual loss of 0.95 follicle (8.2%) was

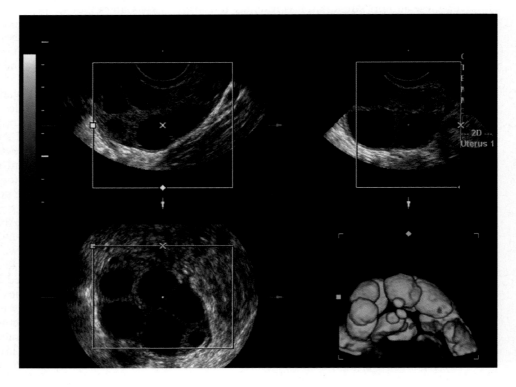

Figure 33-27. Method of antral follicle count (AFC) measurement in predicting poor response. The AFC score can be computed from 2D or 3D images. In the latter case, antral follicles can be counted using the multiplanar approach, scanning through the ovarian volume either instantaneously or at a later stage, or using the 3D inversion mode rendering method.

observed.[323,324] There is no easy explanation for the lower AFC losses observed in Chinese women as compared to their white counterparts.

Hendriks et al. conducted a meta-analysis looking at the respective values of ovarian volume versus AFC for predicting IVF outcome.[325] A total of 17 studies, 11 from a prior meta-analysis[316] and 6 new ones, were included for examining the predictive value of AFC. Comparison of ROC curves showed that the prediction of poor response was significantly better for AFC than for ovarian volume ($P < 0.005$) (Fig. 33-28). The prediction of nonpregnancy was poor for both tests, but the performance of AFC was slightly better than that of ovarian volume.

In recent years, sensitive assays for AMH, also known as müllerian inhibiting substance, have revealed that AMH is not just produced by fetal gonads of male fetuses but also by gonads of male and female adults. In women, AMH is produced by in-growth small ovarian follicles, often referred to as preantral follicles, and a smaller fraction of antral follicles.[326] The follicles producing AMH are, therefore, at a slightly earlier stage of development than the antral follicles identified in the AFC score. Yet, the two cohorts of follicles are inherently linked together because follicles identified on pelvic imaging by the AFC score evolve from the other group of earlier follicles reflected by AMH levels.

The cohort of antral follicles is believed to remain constant throughout the menstrual cycle, thus providing constant AFC scores throughout the menstrual cycle and limited intercycle variability as compared to day 3 FSH levels.[327,328] Likewise, AMH levels show a high degree of correlation with AFC[329] and remain essentially constant throughout the menstrual cycle[330-332] with limited intercycle variability.[333-335] AMH levels are not affected by prolonged treatment with OC[332] in spite of the profound decrease observed in ovarian volume[295] and remain constant in pregnancy and post-partum[336] and following FSH administration in regularly ovulating women[337] and women suffering from PCOS.[338] Recently, a question has been raised about possible postovulatory fluctuation.[339] Reviewing this issue, we concluded that this discrepancy did not result from methodologic differences and that if a slight postovulation decrease truly exists, it is of lesser magnitude than intercycle variability of AMH measurements and can therefore be ignored clinically.[340]

Some studies have questioned whether AMH measurements add any value over simple AFC determination.[341,342] It is important to stress that AMH also offers the practical advantages of identifying PCOS and rating the degree of PCOS expression among women whose AFC scores are so elevated that follicles are too numerous to count.

In conclusion, AFC appears as the best available predictor of ovarian response to COH with good predictive value of excessive and insufficient ovarian responses but poor prediction of overall ART outcome. Recently serum determination of AMH has provided an easily available biologic marker of a cohort of ovarian follicles that are at a slightly earlier stage of maturation than antral follicles identified by the AFC score. As both AFC and AMH levels reflect the remaining endowment of primordial follicles at any given time, their use serves fairly similar purposes. AMH

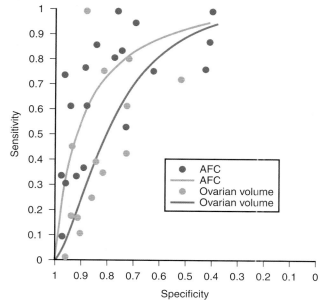

Figure 33-28. *Relative predictive value toward poor ovarian response of ovarian volume and antral follicle count (AFC). The results of a meta-analysis of 17 studies clearly show the superiority of AFC over ovarian volume toward the prediction of poor ovarian response in assisted reproductive techniques (ART). From each study, all cutoff points are plotted. Summary ROC (receiver-operating characteristic) curves for both ovarian volume and AFC are given: the* green line *represents the summary of the ROC curve for ovarian volume, and the* purple line *represents the summary ROC curve for AFC. In conclusion, the predictive performance of ovarian volume toward poor response is clearly inferior compared with that of AFC. (From Hendriks DJ, Kwee J, Mol BW, et al. Ultrasonography as a tool for the prediction of outcome in IVF patients: a comparative meta-analysis of ovarian volume and antral follicle count. Fertil Steril 87:764, 2007.)*

certainly offers a practical edge in certain cases of extreme PCOS ovaries, when the number of antral follicles is too high to count. AFC and AMH are both reflectors of the quantity of follicles, but neither reflects follicular quality. In the normal ovarian aging process, the decrease in the number of oocytes is paralleled by a decrease in oocyte quality. In this context a correlation exists between lower AMH and AFC and lower oocyte quality. Yet, this link is not an inherent one, with all indications that it does not exist when the decrease in oocyte quantity results from mechanisms other than age, as for example, after successive ovarian surgery or endometriosis.

OVARIAN PERFUSION

Perfusion in the Maturing Follicle and Corpus Luteum

Power Doppler has revealed the development of vessels in the follicular wall of the dominant follicles in the later stages of the follicular phase[343] and in COH[344-346] and suggests a link with oocyte quality and reproductive outcome. Characteristically, this vascular development gives an colored annular ring that circles the maturing follicle. Typically this ring is observed around certain but not all follicles developing in COH, starting on average 1 to 2 days prior to the time when hCG is commonly administered in

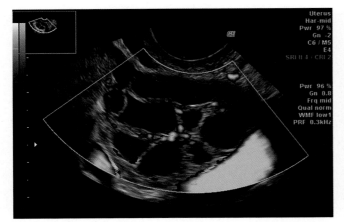

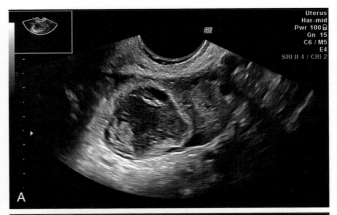

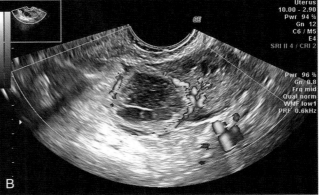

Figure 33-29. Vascularization of maturing ovarian follicles in controlled ovarian hyperstimulation (COH). Starting 1 to 2 days prior to follicular maturity and human chorionic gonadotropin (hCG) administration in COH cycles, color Doppler mode identifies the development of follicular vascularization. Characteristically some but not all follicles display the development of end-follicular phase vascularization.

Figure 33-30. Corpus luteum appearance in gray scale imaging **(A)** and color Doppler mode **(B).** On color Doppler mode, the characteristic intense vascularization of the corpus luteum confers the typical "ring-of-fire" appearance.

COH[347] (Fig. 33-29). We have observed that an educated eye can identify the development of a shining reflection in the contour of the follicle on gray-scale images that signal the presence of the vessels that identified the follicular wall on power Doppler.

Claims have been made that oocytes originating from well-vascularized follicles yield better reproductive outcome than their counterparts originating from less vascularized follicles.[348-350] In line with this, a decrease in follicular flow in aging ovaries has been reported.[351] In 2007, however, these results were challenged by Ragni et al.[352] In a prospective trial on 318 women, these authors found that vascularity of the developing follicle did not appear to predict the chance of pregnancy in women undergoing mild COS and IUI cycles. Pregnancy rates in the low-, medium-, and high-grade vascularity groups were 14.1, 10, and 11.8%, respectively.

Lozano et al. used the natural cycle IVF model in order to assess how follicular vascularization correlates with oocyte quality.[353] In this study, 61 normally ovulating women were prospectively examined. Their treatment consisted of daily GnRH antagonist (Cetrotide 0.5 mg/day) and 150 IU of hMG, starting when a growing follicle larger than 12 mm was observed. Ovulation was triggered as soon as the single dominant follicle reached 16 mm in diameter. Follicular vascularization was assessed just prior to oocyte retrieval, 34 to 36 hours after hCG (5000 IU) administration. Using 3D-based methodology, the vascularization index (VI) and flow index (FI) were taken as quantitative and qualitative reflectors, respectively, of follicular vascularization. In these authors' hands, VI had no predictive value for IVF outcome, but FI strongly predicted clinical pregnancies. These authors concluded that a qualitative rather than quantitative relationship exists between follicular vascularization and oocyte quality.

After ovulation, the developing CL is the site of intense neovascularization and rapidly becomes the most vascularized organ of the body (based on blood flow per tissue volume). Ultimately, on color and power Doppler images, the CL acquires the characteristic "ring of fire" appearance described in all textbooks (Fig. 33-30). In a longitudinal study throughout the luteal phase and early pregnancy, Tamura et al. showed that the resistance index in the CL (luteal RI) was associated with CL function.[354]

Claims have been made that correlations exist between CL Doppler data and quality of the luteal phase,[355] leading to the proposal that Doppler data could be used to assess the luteal phase[356] and predict pregnancy outcome.[357] In spontaneously occurring singleton pregnancies, Frates et al. failed to find a correlation between the echographic characteristics of the CL and first trimester pregnancy outcome.[357]

On gray-scale images, we believe that an educated eye can easily identify the fine dual contours of vessels that run around the CL, an impression supported by the finding of a correlation between Doppler data and vascular density.[358] Yet, it is noteworthy that the increased vascularity of the CL may at times be confused with the vascular ring that characterizes certain ectopic pregnancies.[359]

Perfusion of the Ovarian Stroma

Color Doppler has revealed the presence of ovarian stromal vascularization. From the outset it was suspected that a difference in the degree of vascularization exists between normally ovulating and PCOS women. According to Battaglia et al. ovarian stromal vascularization is identified in 50% and 88% of normally cycling and PCOS women, respectively.[360,361]

In ART, a link has been claimed between the degree of stromal vascularization and the responsiveness to gonadotropin stimulation.[362,363] According to Popovic et al. ovarian power Doppler together with AFC are the two most significant predictors of ovarian response of the 12 possible predictive factors investigated in normally cycling women.[364] The observation of significantly lower 3D power Doppler indexes of ovarian stromal blood flow in poor responders as compared to normoresponders[365] was taken as supporting evidence of this claim. Studying the effect of age on ovarian stromal blood flow, Ng et al. observed that an age-related decrease was observed only in women aged 41 years or older.[322]

Numerous papers have suggested that the link between ovarian stroma perfusion and the number of oocytes retrieved in ART is the result of confounding factors, not an independent one. Using a 3D-based approach, Merce et al. indeed found a correlation between ovarian VI and FI and the number of oocytes recovered.[366] Vascular parameters, however, were not independent predictors of the number of developed follicles and oocytes retrieved, but ovarian volume and AFC were, a finding consonant with other reports.[367]

Ng et al. observed that AFC, ovarian volume, and ovarian 3D power Doppler flow indices did not significantly change after a short-term treatment with GnRH agonist (GnRHa) for pituitary down-regulation.[368] In a prospective study, Jarvela et al. examined the power Doppler signal in the ovaries after pituitary suppression by GnRHa. They observed that Doppler data did not provide any additional information beyond those of ovarian volume and AFC with respect to predicting the subsequent response to gonadotropin stimulation during IVF.[369]

Ovarian stromal vascularization as assessed by power Doppler data was used to compare ovarian function following salpingectomy. The concern was that this procedure, which is indicated to prevent the backflow of fluid in cases of hydrosalpinx, might interfere with vascular supply to the ovary and in turn its proper functioning. In their trial, Chan et al. found that differences in ovarian blood flow actually existed, depending on the surgical technique used. Ovarian volume, AFC, and 3D power Doppler indices were comparable between the operated and the nonoperated sides when salpingectomy was done by laparotomy, but they were significantly reduced on the operated side when salpingectomy was done by laparoscopy.[110] These authors concluded that ovarian function seems to be impaired after laparoscopic unilateral salpingectomy at short-term assessment.

THE OVARY IN POLYCYSTIC OVARY SYNDROME

Echographic Characteristics of PCOS Ovary

In its original description by Stein and Leventhal, the diagnosis of PCOS implied verification of characteristic histologic findings that included prominent theca, thickening of the tunica albuginea, and multiple cystic follicles.[370] Later, this clinical feature of PCOS became part of the diagnostic criteria.[371] In 2003, the ovarian characteristics again officially returned as part of the diagnostic criteria of PCOS when the joint ESHRE/ASRM consensus or Rotterdam conference retained echographic criteria of the ovary for making the diagnosis of PCOS. Thus, the Rotterdam conference departed from the prior criteria required for diagnosing PCOS, from the National Institutes of Health Conference held in Bethesda, MD, in 1990.[372] According to the Rotterdam conference,[265] the diagnosis of PCOS is made when two of the following three clinicopathologic features are present: (i) oligo-anovulation, (ii) clinical or biochemical hyperandrogenism, and (iii) PCOS ovaries on ultrasound. The latter is defined by the presence of either more than 12 follicles 2 to 9 mm in diameter (AFC) in each ovary or a volume of 10 cm³ or more. Hence, the total ovarian volume is considered as being an acceptable surrogate marker for AFC and increased stromal volume, the latter criteria being what is specific to PCOS in terms of ovarian volume.[373]

Making the ovarian volume one criterion that suffices for qualifying the ovaries as being of PCOS type raises several issues. First among these is the reliability of ovarian volume measurement. In PCOS, the primary modification is an increased stromal volume,[374] which in turn translates to an overall increase in ovarian volume.[373] A possible exception to the rule that ovarian volume is increased in PCOS concerns women who are on the OC pill because of increased ovarian volume; the OC pill has been found to result in reduced ovarian volume in these cases,[294] but this finding is not shared by everyone.[375] Interestingly, however, in spite of the profound reduction in ovarian volume observed by Wachs et al. in PCOS women after they had been on the OC pill for 6 months, AFC and AMH levels remained unchanged.[338]

Calculating AFC and determining whether the score exceeds 12 in each ovary in order to qualify for the Rotterdam criteria also poses methodologic issues of its own. Originally, 2D measurements of ovarian volume used the simplified formula for the prolate ellipsoid (0.5 × width × length × thickness), which assumes a regular ovoid shape of the ovary.[376,377] Methodologically speaking, direct 3D measurements, particularly when using the VOCAL-based rotation approach,[13,378] surpass volume values calculated from three diameters using the ellipse formula.[379] In this latter study, the investigators based their conclusion on a comparison of 2D and 3D approaches for measuring ovarian follicle volume, taking the actual volume of follicular fluid collected at the time of IVF as reference.

The novelty of the Rotterdam criteria stands out in having introduced echographic criteria for the definition of PCOS, which are integrated, however, with rich data on the echographic appearance of PCOS ovaries in cases of PCOS.[380,381] More important in our view from a reproductive endocrine imaging standpoint, the Rotterdam criteria have implicitly defined a new category of women who do not qualify for PCOS diagnosis but have PCOS-like ovaries, yet without androgen excess, and who ovulate regularly.[261] Practically speaking, these women need to be identified because women with "PCOS ovaries" tend to behave like PCOS women in terms of ovarian response to exogenous gonadotropins administered in ART and risk for frank ovarian hyperstimulating syndrome (OHSS).[317] Moreover, women with PCOS ovaries have AMH levels lower than encountered in full blown PCOS, but nonetheless higher than in cycling control subjects whose ovaries do not meet PCOS criteria.[382]

The Rotterdam criteria for making the diagnosis of PCOS have been challenged by certain investigators. Stephen Franks objects that the consensus reached by the Rotterdam conference participants did not truly settle the controversy concerning the diagnosis of PCOS.[383] This author contends that the association of hyperandrogenism and anovulation are the mainstay of the definition of PCOS, and yet the Rotterdam criteria include women with androgen excess without anovulation and women with anovulation without hyperandrogenism. Further elaborating along the same line of thinking, Ricardo Azziz stresses the fact that little is known about the degree of insulin resistance and long-term metabolic risk of oligoanovulatory women with PCOS ovaries but no sign of hyperandrogenism.[384] Based on uncertain phenotypes included under the diagnosis of PCOS by the Rotterdam criteria, Azziz considers the new definition of PCOS premature. From an imaging standpoint, we hold the position that the clarification brought by the Rotterdam conference was actually long overdue and most likely warranted in view of the increasingly important role played by ultrasound imaging of the ovaries.

Recently, Allemand et al.[385] challenged the number of small follicles that had been included in the Rotterdam criteria for diagnosing PCOS. In his communication, he suggested a higher number of follicles or ovarian volume as cutoff criteria for PCOS. Using receiver operating characteristic (ROC) curves, these authors concluded that a diagnosis cutoff point set at AFC greater than 20 follicles per ovary resulted in positive predictive value of 100% and negative predictive value of 91%. Similar values were obtained if the cutoff value for the ovarian volume was raised from 10 to 13 cm^3.

Dewailly et al. stressed the fact that some of the small 2- to 5-mm follicles found in PCOS are actually atretic follicles, reflecting follicular arrest.[386] The latter is believed to result from an exaggerated physiologic inhibitory effect from the pool of small 2- to 5-mm follicles on terminal follicle growth.[387]

In PCOS, as in normally ovulating women, a strong correlation exists between AFC scores and AMH levels. Chen et al. observed that a significant correlation existed between the number of antral follicles and the ovarian volume on the one hand and AMH on the other. AMH levels also correlated with total testosterone and the free androgen index.[388] AMH, however, was inversely correlated with body mass index (BMI), fueling the argument that the ovarian expression of PCOS was more profound in lean as well as hirsute individuals.[389] All findings indicate, therefore, that AMH levels constitute an accurate marker of the ovarian early antral follicle endowment with good prospect for helping the diagnosis of PCOS. Yet, at this stage, the precise cutoffs between AMH levels

encountered in normally ovulating women and women with PCOS has not yet been established. AMH measurements are likely to help when accurate ultrasonographic data are not available, as for example, in virgin girls.[390] In the future it is likely that AMH will become part of the diagnostic criteria for PCOS, being a surrogate for AFC, as an extension of the current Rotterdam consensus criteria.

The Ovarian Stroma in PCOS

The description of the echographic characteristics of PCOS goes way beyond what originally stood as the cardinal feature of PCOS, an increase in size and number of small 2- to 10-mm follicles arranged like a necklace of pearls identified prior to vaginal ultrasound studies.[391] A cardinal echographic criterion often put forth, yet rarely objectively studied, in case of PCOS is a putative increase in ovarian stromal echogenicity.[392,393] In a prospective trial Bucket et al.[374] looked at the echographic appearance of 67 women on no medication who were scheduled to undergo IVF. Using a 7.5-MHz vaginal probe these authors measured total and stromal ovarian echogenicity, computing the stromal index as the ratio of stromal echogenicity over total echogenicity. Criteria for PCOS, including AFC greater than 12, were found in 37% of the cases. Total ovarian volume and stromal volume were higher in PCOS ovaries, but contrary to expectation, there was no significant difference in the mean stromal echogenicity between women with PCOS and their normally cycling counterparts. There was, however, a reduction in mean echogenicity resulting from the increase in ovarian follicles, which accounted for a significant increase in stromal index in spite of the lack of change in stromal echogenicity. These results were confirmed with the most recent VOCAL volume measurements. Kyei-Mensah[394] calculated the ovarian stromal volume by subtracting the follicular volume from total ovarian volume. Using a less operator-dependent approach, Lam et al. used the VOCAL rotational approach (15-degree rotation steps) to measure ovarian and stromal volumes, applying an arbitrary 6-mm inner shell beneath the ovarian capsule for stromal volume measurement.[395] In a prospective trial, these authors compared 40 white women identified to have PCOS as per Rotterdam criteria and 40 cycling control subjects having normal non-PCOS ovaries on ultrasound.[395] Ovarian and stromal volumes were markedly larger in the PCOS group (12.56 and 10.79 mL) as compared to control subjects (5.66 and 4.69 mL). There was no difference, however, in stromal echogenicity between PCOS and control groups at 32.3 and 30.4 (not significant), respectively. Likewise, Jarvela et al.[396] failed to find a difference in echogenicity when measured by 3D calculation in 14 women with PCOS as compared to 28 women with echographically normal ovaries. In a subgroup analysis, Lam et al. observed that hirsute PCOS patients had larger stromal volume than the nonhirsute counterparts[395] but did not find differences in ovarian stroma echogenicity between these subgroups of PCOS patients either. It can reasonably be concluded that the overall impression of denser ovarian stroma in PCOS results from a visual illusion linked to the increase in stromal volume component of total ovarian volume but not from a true increase in stromal echogenicity.

Interestingly, AFC remains constant in PCOS women taking OC pills in spite of the profound decrease in ovarian volume.[295] This finding indicates that the effect of hormonal contraception is on ovaran stroma, not follicles, as suggested by the profound effect observed on androgens in the majority of patients.[397]

The advent of pulsed and color Doppler function on vaginal ultrasound probes led to study of intraovarian stromal flow as a distinct phenomenon from changes in flow taking place in the follicular walls[398] and after ovulation in the CL.[343,399,400] Stromal flow was found to be increased in women suffering from PCOS,[362] as compared to findings made in cycling control subjects.[124,401] Zaidi et al. compared ovarian stromal flow status as by Doppler (peak systolic blood flow velocity) to ovarian responsiveness to FSH/hMG in ART cycles. A positive correlation was found between blood flow at baseline measured by Doppler and ovarian response to COH, with higher values in 13 POCS patients and compared to 63 cycling control subjects.[402] Conversely, ovarian blood flow was decreased at baseline in women bound to have a poor response as compared to normal responders.[362]

In 2D studies, Balen et al. reported an increase in ovarian blood flow in PCOS,[261] a finding shared by some[268] but not other investigators who, using 3D-PDA, failed to find an increase in stromal vascularitiy in 14 women with PCOS as compared to 28 control women.[396] In a recent prospective trial, Lam et al.[395] compared ovarian flow assessed by 3D ultrasound in 40 women fulfilling the Rotterdam criteria for PCOS with those of 40 age-matched cycling control women whose ovaries were not of PCOS type. Ultrasound data were obtained on days 3 to 5 of spontaneous or induced bleeding. A 3D data set was acquired using a sweep angle set to 90 degrees and a slow-sweep mode. AFC was significantly higher in the PCOS group (median, 16.3; range, 9-35) as compared to control subjects (5.5; 2-10). The results showed an increase in ovarian blood flow by some (VI) but not all 3D-PDA indices (FI). Interestingly, differences were observed among various phenotypes of PCOS. Ovarian blood flow was frankly increased in a subgroup of 30 (of 40) hirsute PCOS women as compared to their 10 nonhirsute PCOS counterparts. Likewise, blood flow was also higher in 14 lean PCOS women as compared to their overweight counterparts. Yet there were no differences in AFC between lean and obese PCOS and hirsute and nonhirsute women. In a different protocol, Ng et al. confirmed the differences in ovarian blood flow between different PCOS phenotypes. This team also found a significant increase in ovarian blood flow in women whose BMI was less than 25 as compared to their overweight counterparts, with a significant negative correlation between total ovarian indices (VI, FI, and VFI) and BMI.[389] There was also a strong trend toward higher LH levels in lean women with PCOS. Hirsute women with PCOS had increased stromal volume (median, 11.5 mL; range, 6.8-17.1) compared to nonhirsute women with PCOS (9.8 mL; 5.7-136). Globally, this supports the concept that the source of excessive androgens in these women is the thecal cells in the ovarian stroma that undergo hypertrophy.

Early Diagnosis of PCOS in Adolescent and Prepubertal Girls

Chang and Coffler stress the importance of diagnosing PCOS early in adolescent girls in order to offer treatment for the hormonal (hyperandrogenism and hirsutism) and metabolic expression of the disease.[279] Based on studying AMH levels through the pubertal process, Crisosto et al. observed that the increase in follicular mass is established during early development and persists during puberty.[403] First among individuals in whom an early diagnosis of PCOS is important are daughters of PCOS women. Indeed, Sir-Petermann et al. determined that daughters of women with PCOS are at increased risk of suffering from PCOS.[404] These authors compared 14 female infants (2-3 months old) and 25 prepubertal girls (4-7 years old) born to PCOS mothers to a control group of 21 female infants and 24 prepubertal girls born to mothers with regular menses and without hyperandrogenism. Serum concentrations of AMH were significantly higher in the PCOS group compared with the control group during early infancy (20.4 ± 15.6 versus 9.16 ± 8.6 pmol/L; $P = 0.024$) and during childhood (14.8 ± 7.7 versus 9.61 ± 4.4 pmol/L; $P = 0.007$). Yet, gonadotropin and serum sex steroid concentrations were similar in both groups during the two study periods, except for FSH, which was lower during childhood in girls born to PCOS mothers. The discrepancy between the alteration of the follicular cohort, as expressed by the increase in AMH levels, and the lack of hormonal alteration in these infants and prepubertal girls suggests that the ovarian facet of PCOS precedes the altered gonadotropin pattern. Evidence of altered follicular development during infancy and childhood opens opportunities for early screening either directly by ultrasound or in the future through the surrogate for the follicular cohort, AMH levels. This should be considered when PCOS is suspected, notably because of metabolic alterations or because of an increased risk, as in daughters of PCOS mothers.

ADNEXAL CYSTS AND TUMORS

Ovarian versus Extraovarian Disease

Through the marked improvement in image resolution that stemmed from using high-frequency, high-resolution vaginal probes, vaginal ultrasound has now become the primary approach used for investigating adnexal masses. As stressed in a review by Brown,[270] the primary question that pelvic imaging needs to answer is whether the adnexal mass is of ovarian or extraovarian origin. Most adnexal masses arise from the ovary, but not always. When the mass is of ovarian origin, the issue of cancer is a real one. Once established that the mass is of extraovarian origin, it can be ascertained that, short of rare cases of tubal cancer,[405] the mass is not cancerous. The primary clinical presentation of tubal cancer actually is most commonly pelvic pain rather than an asymptomatic pelvic mass.[406] When suspected at the time of laparoscopy the principle of Hu should prevail, according to which if the ovary and the tube are both involved with tumor, the bulk of the tumor should be in the tube.[407]

Identifying ovarian tissue with small antral follicles helps in determining whether a mass is of ovarian origin or not. Likewise, recognizing an ipsilateral ovary independent from the adnexal mass suggests the nonovarian nature of the mass. In postmenopausal women, the lack of visible ovarian follicles may render the process more complex. Helpful tips for determining the ovarian or nonovarian nature of the mass include the possibility of mobilizing the structure that is being investigated by pressure applied with the vaginal probe with or without the help of external pressure applied manually. In case of a cystic mass, the impact of the pressure applied with the probe on the cystic dilatation can be carefully followed. In case of ovarian cyst, the pressure applied on the probe bounces against the nondeformable nature of the cyst. Conversely, when the cystic structure is caused by a hydrosalpinx, pressure of the probe will modify the shape of the cystic dilatation as fluid pushed by the probe will move elsewhere along the length of the tube, allowing for a change in shape of the visualized structure.

The vascular supply of the lesion may also help in delineating its ovarian or extraovarian origin. In case of pedunculated fibroids, one might identify vessels bridging with the uterus. The peripheral developments of vessels can also help in recognizing the fibroid nature of an adnexal mass.

Extraovarian Cysts

Paraovarian (or paratubal) cysts appear as simple cysts indistinguishable from ovarian cyst if it were not for their nonovarian nature, which can normally be determined in premenopausal women because ovarian tissue can easily be identified,[408,409] including identifying an ipsilateral ovary.[410]

Hydrosalpinges are the most important paraovarian structures encountered in clinical reproductive endocrinology. Typically they appear as an elongated cystic mass with characteristic incomplete stations, although the reliability of this echographic sign has been challenged.[411] Other typical findings of hydrosalpinges include the waist sign and the findings evoking *beads on a string*. In a review of 67 cystic adnexal masses, Patel et al. observed 26 (39%) hydrosalpinges. These authors concluded that the association of an elongated aspect together with the identification of the waist sign carried the highest probability for hydrosalpinx.[412] Ultrasound scans aimed at excluding the presence hydrosalpinges in ART need to be performed at midcycle because fluid tends to accumulate during the follicular phase or after ovarian stimulation,[413] including in women with PCOS.[414]

Peritoneal inclusion or pseudocysts are believed to result from fluid trapped within pelvic adhesions, giving the impression that the ovary lies within the cyst itself.[270,415]

Ovarian Cysts and Tumors

In his extensive review, Brown lists five primary findings for ovarian masses, each having their echographic characteristics, which most often permit a positive diagnosis.[270]

Simple Cysts. In premenopausal ovaries, a cyst is a structure less than 3 cm in diameter with a thin anechoic wall free of protrusion and showing characteristic distal enhancement. Structures of lesser diameter are best described as follicles, which may have stopped developing or failed to regress because of isolated or recurrent ovarian dysfunction. Simple cysts most often disappear spontaneously, a process that may be hastened by suppressing ovarian function with OC pills. The majority of persisting cysts treated surgically turned out to be serous cystadenomas.

The Corpus Luteum. The CL is not a pathologic finding, but rather constitutes a normal occurrence on one ovary during the luteal phase. Yet imaging characteristics of the CL may be so dramatic that they can easily be mistaken for cancer because of the intense low impedance blood flow if not properly recognized. In a prospective trial, Baerwald et al. followed luteal images and serum E_2 and progesterone in 50 women daily from one ovulatory episode to the next.[290] The day of ovulation was defined as the day of follicular disappearance. The CL was detected on the day of ovulation and later in 100% of women and during the subsequent follicular phase in 90% of them. Some CL presented a central fluid-filled cavity (identified in 88%) and some without (12%). A progressive decrease in echogenicity was observed throughout the luteal phase. The CL is intensely vascularized with annular arrangements of vessels, which can be recognized on gray scale images by a circular dual contour line.[266]

Hemorrhagic Cyst. Hemorrhagic cyst is a common occurrence in premenopausal women. It can be associated with acute pain or may be a fortuitous finding in routine scans, such as scans done prior to ART. The internal echo pattern varies depending on the stage of the hemorrhage and the amount of fluid present. The acutely hemorrhagic cyst is typically more echogenic than the surrounding ovarian tissue. Characteristically, findings will evolve from a sponge-like appearance, followed by the development of irregular internal echos after the clot starts to retract after a few days, leaving a mesh-like maze of intertwined fine structures that are the echographic expression of fibrin strands.[416,417] These strands rarely run totally across the cyst, being therefore fairly easily distinguished cyst septa. A gentle yet brisk pressure stroke applied with the vaginal probe may generate a disruption wave that propagates through the mesh-like network of internal echos with a characteristic jello-like effect where the wave rebounds backward when hitting the cyst wall.

The retracted blood clot may mimic a mural nodule. The sharp angles of the retracting clot are different from solid tumors that do not tend to have acute angles.[417] To distinguish the clot from more ominous internal echos it is most helpful to document the absence of vessels entering the solid area. MRI is classically of little help for diagnosing hemorrhagic cysts, as its features are atypical and variable.[418] Most commonly, hemorrhagic cysts rapidly change their echographic appearance and ultimately disappear, a process that may be hastened by suppressing ovarian function with the OC pill.[419,420] The pill is commonly started on day 2 of the menstrual cycle or arbitrarily, provided that endogenous progesterone is low (<1.5 ng/mL), which precludes the possibility of pregnancy. The differential diagnosis includes endometrioma and dermoid cysts. Typically, the former has a homogeneous mixed echogenic (gray) appearance, whereas the latter may add to that grayish appearance the finding of brightly echogenic calcifications and, on occasion, a denser mesh image when the dermoid cyst contains an accumulation of hair. A hemorrhagic CL may accompany a clinical course suggestive of ectopic pregnancy. The hemorrhagic process linked to a cyst is characteristically embedded within the ovary, whereas it lies outside the ovary in ectopic pregnancy.

Endometrioma. Contrary to other localizations of endometriosis, which can be difficult to positively identify, ultrasound studies are efficient for diagnosing the paramount expression of ovarian endometriosis, the endometriotic cyst, or endometrioma. Out of a cohort of 1170 scans yielding 252 adnexal masses the diagnosis of endometrioma was made in 40 cases (prevalence 16%).[421] Taken in isolation, low-level internal echos have a sensitivity of 93% and a specificity of 83%. At the other end of the spectrum, identifying all characteristic findings of endometriomas, namely, low-level internal echos, no neoplastic features, and hyperechoic wall foci or multilocularity, led to a specificity of 99%, whereas sensitivity dropped to 45%. These data demonstrate that gray-scale vaginal ultrasound can achieve a high degree of accuracy in diagnosing endometriomas. Hence, an adnexal mass with diffuse low-level internal echos and no neoplastic features is most likely to be an endometrioma.

Mature Cystic Teratoma or Dermoid Cyst. Typical features of dermoid cysts include shadowing echodensity, regional diffuse bright hyperechoic area with an attenuating effect, hyperechoic lines and dots, and fat-fluid levels.[422] Yet great variability in the appearance of cystic teratomas has been emphasized. Practically, this led to needing further data from MRI in order to rule out the possibility of ovarian cancer except in the most typical echographic presentations. Suspecting that echographic findings were often specific enough, Patel et al. demonstrated in a prospective study that 55 of 74 cystic teratomas diagnosed among 252 adnexal masses had two or more sonographic features associated with dermoids.[423] These authors observed a positive predictive value of 80% for shadowing echogenicity, 75% for regionally bright echos, 50% for hyperechoic lines and dots, and 20% for fat-fluid level. Taking these signs together, each reviewer had 98% positive predictive value, which reached 100% when an adnexal mass had two or more sonographic findings associated with dermoids.

Most ovarian cancers are epithelial neoplasms, which include serous, mucinous, endometrioid, and clear cell neoplasms. Additionally there are borderline tumors, or tumors of low malignant potential of all epithelial cell types, with the mucinous and serous cell types being by far the most common. The presence of a solid component is the most common feature that reveals the cancerous nature of an ovarian tumor. In spite of the initial wide interest in color and power Doppler, there is a consensus today that Doppler indices do not provide much more information than gray-scale morphologic assessment.

Contrast Imaging of the Fallopian Tubes

In normal physiologic conditions, the fallopian tubes are not identified on pelvic ultrasound nor with other imaging approaches such as MRI and CT scans. Dilated tubes in case of hydrosalpinges are easily seen, however, by the contrast effect generated by fluid contained in the tubes.

Exploring the fallopian tubes therefore requires the use of some sort of contrast material. Classically, the fallopian tubes are being visualized on x-ray images by transcervical infusion of an opaque dye (HSG). Newer approaches use positive (*white*) ultrasound dyes (SIS or HySO).

HYSTEROSALPINGOGRAPHY

Indications

HSG is the preeminent ancestor of the imaging tools used for investigating infertility.[424] Its modern development, including the description of methodology and interpretation of images, dates back from pre-IVF time but remains valid today and nearly unchanged.[425]

The ability of HSG to explore the uterine cavity is challenged by transvaginal ultrasound and HySO on one hand, and hysteroscopy on the other. The former offers the advantage of depicting both the cavity itself and the myometrial contour. This made HySO the undisputed primary imaging tool for investigating uterine malformations. The miniaturization of endoscopic instruments has permitted diagnostic hysteroscopy to be an office procedure, thereby leading to marked increases in its use. For intrauterine disease, diagnostic hysteroscopy offers the advantage of permitting direct visualization of the pathologic structures causing the problem under investigation and determining the surgical procedure, if surgery is needed.

Tubal exploration by HSG is sometimes compared to HySO using positive contrast products that delineate the tubal lumen, which appears in white on gray-scale images. Positive (white) contrast agents include Echovist, Levovist, and Albumex, none of which are approved for use as fallopian tube contrast medium by the Food and Drug Administration (FDA).[426]

The need for HSG, classically included in all infertility workups, has been recently challenged in women whose serology for chlamydiae is negative. In these women, it has been claimed that the practice of HSG has a yield of tubal pathologic findings so low that it makes the routine use of HSG not cost effective.[427,428]

Technical Considerations

Traditionally, HSG is performed during a relatively short interval between cycle day 5 and day 12 to 14. This time limit achieves two objectives: (i) menses must be finished in order to minimize the risk of enhancing retrograde bleeding by the procedure; and (ii) the x-ray procedure is performed before ovulation in order to minimize the risk of irradiating a developing pregnancy. For practical purposes, it may be handy at times to place the patient on a short course of OC pills for better programming.

Several recent and thorough reviews on HSG have covered the details about the many practical aspects of this procedure.[429-431] Many groups routinely prescribe 600 mg of ibuprofen or other nonsteroidal anti-inflammatory drugs (NSAIDs) 30 minutes to 1 hour before the procedure in a effort to ease the uterine cramping that may be generated by the procedure.[430] Frishman et al. randomly compared the effects of intrauterine instillation of 2% lidocaine solution or saline before performing HSG.[432] Lidocaine, unfortunately, failed to alleviate pain generated by HSG. The issue of routine antibiotic prophylaxis has been much debated because infectious complications have occurred but represent a risk of less than 1%.

With the patient in the dorsal lithotomy position and a speculum in place, the instillation device is positioned in order to provide a sealed connection with the cervix. The instillation instrument is either the Jarcho cannula,[433] which is held to the cervix with tenaculums, or modern plastic catheters equipped with inflatable balloons, such as the 5-F HSG catheter (Cooper Surgical, Trumbull, CT). The balloon is inflated once it has passed the internal os of the cervix. The balloon must be filled with the same contrast material as used for the examination. Although these catheters are probably easier to handle, they may create pain because of the balloon and in certain circumstances may hinder the vision of the cervical canal. The speculum needs to be removed once the instillation instruments are in place. Air needs to be meticulously expelled from the instilling device so that only the contrast medium is being pushed inside the uterine cavity. Failing to do so could lead to false diagnoses of filling defects.

Prior to instilling contrast medium and after a mark identifies the sides, a scout x-ray of the pelvic cavity is examined, looking for possible calcifications. Water-soluble contrast material is slowly instilled under intermittent control on fluoroscopic vision. A minimum of four spot radiographs is commonly recommended.[431] The first image is obtained during early filling of the uterine cavity in search of filling defects, which may later stop being visualized when the uterus is totally opacified. The second image is obtained when the uterus appears fully distended. The third image aims at depicting the fallopian tubes. Finally a fourth image is obtained to depict free spillage of dye in the pelvic cavity and proper mixing. Additional spot radiographs are obtained as necessary, including oblique views when it is necessary to avoid the superimposition of images.

Choice of Contrast Medium: Oil-Based or Water Soluble?

The original contrast medium used in HSG was lipid-based, with Lipiodol being used since it became available in the early 1920s.[434] In a pre-IVF era study, Mackey et al. compared the occurrence of spontaneous pregnancies in women who had HSG and those who did not, sorting out results for when the oil-based ethiodol or a water-soluble contrast medium was used.[435] In their study population of 460, the spontaneous pregnancy rate over 1 year following oil-based dye HSG was 58%, whereas it was 38% in women in whom a water-soluble dye was used. These puzzling results, speaking in favor of a fertility-enhancing effect of HSG using lipid-based dye as compared to findings observed following HSG using water-soluble dyes, were confirmed by other studies.[436-438] However, the use of oil-based contrast media incurs the risk of developing granulomas[436] or the serious complication of a pulmonary or cerebral oil embolism.[439] A sequential combination of water-soluble dye for documenting tubal patency followed later by instillation of the oil-based dye ethiodol has been proposed in order to benefit from the fertility-enhancing effects of HSG using oil-based dye while avoiding its risk. Alternatively, the use of the oil-based dye has been proposed in women whose tubal patency had been demonstrated by laparoscopy.[440] Furthermore, water-soluble dyes offer better visualization of the distal sections of the fallopian tube.[441]

Attempting to provide an explanation for the pregnancy-promoting properties of oil-based dye HSGs, Goodman et al. proposed that the lipid dye inhibited the activity of peritoneal lymphocytes and macrophages.[442] That HSG was found to enhance fecundity in women whose infertility was of unknown cause[436] suggests that it might be in these patients that the inhibiting effect of the lipid dye on macrophages is most valuable.[443]

The Uterine Cavity

Filling defects constitute a common finding in HSG. Once artifacts such as air bubbles and endometrial folds have been excluded, the differential diagnosis is synechiae as a result of post-traumatic or infectious endometrial scarring. Full-fledged development of endometrial scarring suggests the Asherman syndrome, which is classically associated with multiple scarring of the endometrium and, clinically, amenorrhea.

Myomas may indent the uterine cavity. For practical purposes, the degree of distortion must be assessed for determining whether surgery is indicated in the absence of symptoms and whether an intracavitary approach is feasible. For this, however, more complete information is obtained by transvaginal ultrasound and its refinement for exploring the uterine cavity, SIS. This latter procedure allows simultaneous visualization of the whole fibroid and the part that extends into the uterine cavity. SIS offers crucial clues, therefore, for deciding the most appropriate surgical approach by assessing the extent of intracavitary extension of the fibroid to determine the ease of endocavitary excision of the fibroid.

Assessment of the uterine cavity includes a search for congenital malformation of the organ. HySO offers simultaneous vision of the uterine cavity dilated by saline and of the organ itself identified on gray-scale imaging. The 3D reconstruction of the uterus in the frontal plane is of great practical help.[444] HSG may uncover uterine malformations (Fig. 33-31). Finally, the assessment of the uterus must include the cervical canal, notably to rule out cervical incompetence.

Clues about the possibility of adenomyosis may arise from HSG images. The characteristic image is one of diverticula filled with contrast medium that extend into the myometrium. This may exist in the context of an overall

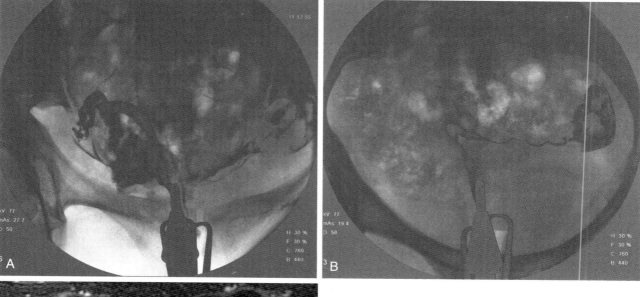

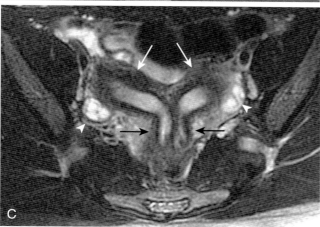

Figure 33-31. Hysterosalpingography (HSG) showing a completely unfused uterus with two cervices and two corpora uteri. Note right (**A**) and left (**B**) uterus and tube. **C**, Similar findings seen on magnetic resonance imaging. White arrows *point at the two corpora uteri;* black arrows *indicate the two cervices. (From Imaoka I, Wada A, Matsuo M, et al. MR imaging of disorders associated with female infertility: use in diagnosis, treatment, and management. RadioGraphics 23:1401, 2003.)*

irregular contour with multiple outpouching. The ultimate expression of this pattern is referred to as the classical honeycomb pattern.[445,446] This finding, however classical, that has been held as diagnostic of adenomyosis is now recognized as not really specific,[447] being at times encountered in lymphatic extravasation.

For large adenomyomas, the image may be one of a mass-like filling defect, with contrast material filling the mass itself and delineating it entirely. Adenomyosis is more accurately diagnosed by MRI, in which it is characterized by a thickening of the junctional zone. This is the only feature that has been formally validated against histologic identification of adenomyosis in women undergoing hysterectomy.

The Fallopian Tubes

In spite of emerging new approaches based on positive contrast-enhanced ultrasound imaging, HSG remains today the best method for visualizing and evaluating the fallopian tubes. Normal tubes appear thin, with smooth outlines and a characteristic distention in the ampullary area. Proximal disease that prevents the visualization of

the tubes may be the reflection of salpingitis isthmica nodosa (SIN) or the expression of a simple spasm. In case of SIN, a characteristic penetration of the contrast medium within the thickness of the fallopian tube wall may result in the typical honeycomb appearance (Fig. 33-32). Classically, SIN is the result of PID that leads to fibrosis of the proximal tubal section with stricture of the lumen and tubal occlusion.[448] We now know that SIN may also result from a tubal form of endometriosis.[448] In this latter case, temporary treatment with a GnRHa has been documented to be effective,[449] a significant departure from the classical surgical approach for SIN.[450] Our experience showed that 3 months of treatment with GnRHa resulted in reopening 15 of 18 women who had bilateral proximal occlusion and in whom a laparoscopy showed some expression of endometriosis and no evidence of distal tubal disease.[451] Spastic contriction of the tube may result in complete tubal occlusion, thereby opening the door to the possible erroneous diagnosis of proximal disease of the fallopian tube. Timely use of glucagon can result in uterine muscle relaxation.[452] We believe that medical treatment of SIN should be considered each time endometriosis is present and there is no evidence of distal tubal disease.

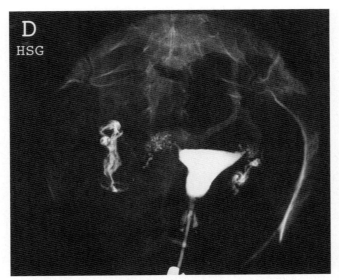

Figure 33-32. *Characteristic honeycomb appearance in the proximal segment of the fallopian tube seen in salpingitis isthmica nodosa as a result of penetration of contrast medium within the fallopian tube wall.*

Distal disease is classically expressed by dilatation of the tube to form hydrosalpinges or the incomplete form, sactosalpinges. PID is the most common cause of distal tubal disease, but such disease may at times result from endometriosis.[453,454]

Visualizing dilated tubes on HSG does not mean that there are hydrosalpinges present at times other than when the HSG is performed. Hence, we believe that the diagnosis of hydrosalpinx is made on visualizing dilated tubes on ultrasound at midcycle. This nuance is important, as today it is commonly held that hydrosalpinges must be removed (salpingectomy) to optimize IVF outcome.[455] From clinical trials that exist, there is now a consensus that pregnancy rates in IVF are approximately halved when a hydrosalpinx is visible on ultrasound.[456,457] From their analyses, Taylor's group suggested that hydrosalpinges probably, by the release of fluid into the uterine cavity, interfered with *HOXA10*,[455] thus providing an explanation for the fact that their removal is justified.[458-460]

Complications

Minor complications of HSG include pain and cramping, which is usually mild to moderate and subsides within hours of the procedure.

The most serious complication is a pelvic infection. Albeit rare (<1%), the risk exists, particularly if there is a history of PID.[461] In view of this, some have advocated antibiotic prophylaxis, either systematically or in selected cases felt to be at higher risk of infection.[462] The most common regimen has been doxycycline 100 mg twice a day, administered for 1.5 to 5 days. We commonly administer 100 mg immediately prior to the procedure, on the evening of the procedure, and on the morning after the procedure in women at higher risk of infection as per history or findings on HSG.

Other complications, fortunately extremely rare, include allergic reaction to iodine-based contrast agents. In this case, gadolinium can be used as a replacement.[463] Perforation of the uterus or fallopian tube has been reported to occur during HSG, but is extremely rare.

HYSTEROSONOGRAPHY

Numerous publications have described the possibility of documenting tubal patency by infusion sonography.[464] In the numerous attempts that have been made to perfect the methodology, a consensus has been established over the fact that positive contrast solutions providing a white visualization offer better and easier visualization of the tubes, particularly of the proximal tubal sections.[426,465] Solutions such as Echovist or Levovist, although offering unquestionable interest for assessing tubal patency, have the disadvantages of (i) not offering an anatomic depiction of the fallopian tubes that matches that of HSG, particularly of the distal segment, and (ii) adding the not-insignificant cost (>$100) of the insemination product. 3D reconstruction capability is likely to facilitate tubal assessment by sonography but without inherent changes the image capabilities.[466] It is our impression that even though the proximal section of the fallopian tube can easily be identified, HSG images remain largely superior for assessing the distal ends of the tubes.

We foresee that in the future, HySO is likely to have a role for assessing tubal physiology rather than being limited, as it is today, to assessing tubal anatomy (patency). For the latter purpose, sonography is in direct competition with the remarkable images obtained with HSG. Conversely, the issue at stake when attempting to assess tubal physiology is to determine whether the retrograde transport of sperm takes place normally during the late follicular phase. Using ^{99}Tc-labeled macroalbumin aggregates in a procedure referred as hysterosalpingoscintigraphy, Kissler et al. reported evidence of retrograde sperm transport alteration in endometriosis,[467] and even more so in adenomyosis.[468] This approach based on studying ^{99}Tc-labeled macroalbumin aggregates is cumbersome, however, and does not lend itself to repeat measurements nor to studies conducted in mock reproductive conditions.

A clear advantage of HySO over x-ray-based methods for assessing tubal function is its noninvasiveness and the possibility of repeating examinations. The ideal infusion preparation for assessing tubal function is still lacking, though. An ideal preparation capable of fulfilling the expectations of infertility specialists would be a product that would have the following characteristics: (i) positive contrast imaging for best identification of the fallopian tubes, (ii) a consistency that permits lasting contrast properties for a duration sufficient for studying whether an actual transport takes place through the tubes, and (iii) nontoxicity to gametes. This latter characteristic would be helpful for studying retrograde tubal transport in actual intercourse-like conditions when the uterotubal unit is exposed to prostaglandins and other constituents of sperm. This is necessary because constituents of sperm may exert clinically relevant effects on retrograde contractility[469] or other uterine functions.[470] Uterine and tubal influences exerted by sperm constituents are likely to result from a direct vagina-to-uterus transport through a true functional portal system, or *first uterine pass effect*.[471]

From the perspective of studying the contractility of the uterotubal unit in intercourse-like conditions, we found the work of Mansour et al. of particular interest.[472] These authors used a sperm preparation that was visible by ultrasound. The injected sperm preparation (5 mL) could be identified in all 45 (100%) women who participated in the study.[472] According to their study paradigm, women in whom the speculum was *closed* at the time of the IUI in an effort to prevent expulsion from the uterus (in an ET-like manner) had a longer retention of sperm in the upper segment of the uterus as compared to control subjects in whom the speculum was kept open. If these data are validated, they might serve for assessing retrograde transport of sperm in infertile individuals as a function of the underlying cause of their infertility.

Endometriosis

Endometriosis is the *preeminent* disease of the pelvis. It can affect all the territories of the pelvic cavity in an isolated or combined manner, touching numerous pelvic organs and areas in the latter scenario. The clinical expression of endometriosis is either infertility or pain or any combination of both symptoms. Classically, one distinguishes the manifestations of endometriosis that are identifiable on ultrasound from the others that usually evaded conventional vaginal ultrasound scrutiny. Typically, the endometriotic cysts of the ovary are easily identified on ultrasound, and the other localizations of endometriosis are classically considered as nonvisible to ultrasound, a situation that is in the process of changing.

Identifying and staging endometriosis and its possible deep pelvic infiltration have formed the primary basis for reverting to MRI in benign gynecology. In certain circumstances, rectal ultrasound or special procedures such as sono-vaginography[473] have been proposed for judging the presence and extension of deep infiltrating endometriosis. Preoperative staging, which aims at determining the nature and extent of surgery to be performed, is an even more challenging step and requires exploring all the various possible localizations of endometriosis.

It is widely accepted that the ovary constitutes the most common site for the development of endometriosis when endometriotic cysts or endometrioma are formed. In general, peritoneal lesions are classified as either superficial or deep, depending on whether penetration exceeds 5 mm or not. Anterior endometriosis includes invasion of the bladder and particularly its detrusor muscle.[474] Posterior endometriosis includes the extension of the disease to the uterosacral ligament, the upper and posterior portions of the cervix (torus), and finally, vaginal, bowel, and ureteral sites.[475,476]

ENDOMETRIOTIC CYSTS (ENDOMETRIOMA)

Edometriomas are best diagnosed and described on ultrasound, where they present as isolated or multiple cystic structures filled with homogeneous low-level echos.[416]

This appearance gives what is commonly referred to as a grayish, fairly homogeneous appearance to the cystic structure. The vast majority of endometriomas range from 30 to 60 mm. Color Doppler helps in identifying clues to the endometriotic nature of the cyst and notably documents the absence of blood vessels within the walls of the cyst or penetrating inside the cyst.[475] Differential diagnosis consists of benign teratomas[423] and hemorrhagic cysts, particularly CL cysts.[477] The teratoma, by its frequent sebum content, which has the thickness and general consistency of the old blood found in endometriomas, can provide echographic characteristics that are fairly similar to those of endometriomas. The presence of echos of hairballs or shadowing effects from calcified structures (bones) strongly speaks for a dermoid cyst.[478]

Hemorrhagic CL cysts vary in size (2.5-10 cm) and are known to have a variable wall thickness. They differ from endometriomas by the presence of complex internal architecture that reflects the presence of a retracted clot and its fibrin content.[417] Moreover, a sponge-like reticular pattern is often identified within the cyst. Characteristically, these two findings are not encountered in endometriomas. Retracted clot often identified on the inner aspect of the cyst wall may have an ominous appearance at first glance because it is likely to mimic mural nodules of cancerous nature. Typically, however, the retracting clot presents with sharp angles, whereas this finding is not seen in tumors. Moreover, Doppler scans confirm the absence of blood vessels within the clot,[417] possibly with improved predictability when taking advantage of 3D Doppler analysis.[269] Likewise, it is helpful at times to identify the typical intense circular vascularity, or *ring of fire*, that characterizes the intense vascularization of the CL that is often still visible when hemorrhagic CL cysts are commonly encountered.[357] We found that the fibrin nature of the reticular pattern identified within an hemorrhagic cyst can be confirmed by applying a pressure smack with the tip of the probe and watching it propagate through the inner echo-positive stucture like shock waves traveling through gelatin. On rare occasions, central fibrin present in a hemorrhagic cyst may mimic a yolk sac, leading to the erroneous diagnosis of an ectopic pregnancy. That the suspect image arises from the ovary and not the tube is an argument against the diagnosis of ectopic pregnancy.[479] The ultimate hemorrhagic nature of cysts is confirmed by witnessing their disappearance (or profound change) on repeat ultrasound studies performed 2 to 4 weeks later, a measure that we believe is recommended whenever practical when evaluating an ovarian cyst, even when the suspicion of endometrioma is high.[480]

Endometriomas are often multiple. They characteristically have hyperchoic wall foci that are clearly identified in nearly a third of the cases.[421] In a recent study conducted in 65 women suspected of having an endometrioma, Alcazar et al. observed that peripheral vascularization of the endometrioma's wall was more important when pelvic pain was present than when it was not.[481] It is generally admitted that ultrasound is the diagnostic tool of choice for exploring endometriomas. Yet in certain circumstances, MRI may prove to be more helpful, let alone necessary when ultrasound findings are indefinite or their interpretation is hampered by the presence of other disorders, such as uterine fibroids. In all these and other difficult cases, MRI may add information and increase the diagnostic performance.[482,483]

ENDOMETRIOSIS OF PELVIC AREAS OTHER THAN THE OVARY

As stated earlier, deep endometriosis, which relates to lesions that extend 5 mm or more beneath the surface of the endometrium, is a specific entity.[484] Chapron et al. observed that pelvic examination does not suffice for reliably diagnosing and locating deep endometriosis.[485] These authors recommended relying on MRI for diagnosing deep penetrating endometriosis,[486] using previously described diagnostic criteria.[487,488] Although the superiority of MRI for diagnosing deep penetrating endometriosis remains an established fact today, ultrasound data are becoming ever more efficient. Notably, promising results have been reported with transvaginal ultrasound, which was found to be equivalent or superior to rectal ultrasound.[489] These authors describe deep endometriosis lesions as hypoechoic linear thickening or nodules/masses with and without regular contour in the cul-de-sac, retrocervical region, and rectovaginal septum, involving the vaginal wall or not. In a recent prospective study, Abrao et al., benefiting from improvements in ultrasound equipment, found that transvaginal ultrasound offered better sensitivity and specificity for identifying deep endometriosis than pelvic examination and even MRI.[490] That all patients were submitted to a Fleet enema prior to the ultrasound examination might have been instrumental in Abrao's positive findings with this technique. Bowel preparation may have been particularly helpful for visualizing bowel. Further improving the discriminating capacity of transvaginal ultrasound and its value as a *functional* diagnostic tool, Guerriero et al. proposed a fusion of ultrasound and pelvic examination in a *tenderness-guided* approach.[491] These authors also added 12 mL of ultrasound gel meant to improve visualization of near-field area. This approach proved to be as effective at identifying posterior and rectovaginal lesions as sonovaginography, a procedure in which saline is placed in the vagina for improving near vision and hence visualization of the vaginal wall as described by Dessole et al.[473]

Anterior and bladder involvement of endometriosis is an extension that is found in a little under 10% of cases. Most commonly bladder endometriosis translates into localized bladder wall thickening seen on ultrasound.[492] At times infiltration may be recognized by witnessing the presence of deep irregular hypoechogenic infiltration of the bladder wall, particularly in the area of uterobladder flap, with a protrusion that extends inside the bladder itself.[493] On MRI, bladder lesions are identified as heterogeneous T_2 isointense thickening of the bladder wall,[475] with lesions varying from 10 to 40 mm.[488] In a trial on 195 patients, MRI had a sensitivity and specificity of 88% and 99%, respectively, for the diagnosis of bladder endometriosis.[494] Extension of endometriosis to the ureter can be identified on T_2-weighted sequences.[475,495]

Endometriosis of the uterosacral ligament and posterior aspect of the cervix (an area defined as the "torus uteri") could be positively assessed by transvaginal ultrasound in 64% of cases, a diagnosis confirmed surgically in 88% of cases (specificity).[496] MRI provides higher sensitivity, however, with reported values ranging from 76% to 86%.[488,494] Retrocervical endometriosis is identified when thick irregular nodular formations of hypoechoic nature are found in this area (torus uteri) with possible extension to one or both uterosacral ligaments. Signs of adhesion are looked for by sliding loops of bowel along the uterosacral ligament and retrocervical area. The sensitivity of ultrasound is notoriously weak, however, reaching 64% in Bazot's hands[496] for diagnosing retrocervical endometriosis. Conversely, MRI offers an improved sensitivity for diagnosing deep endometriosis of the retrocervix (torus uteri).[488] An elegant MRI study demonstrated that deep infiltrating endometriosis does not originate from the rectovaginal septum but rather from the posterior of the cervix at the height of insertion of the uterosacral ligaments (torus uteri).[486]

Endometriosis of the bowel most often but not exclusively affects the rectosigmoid colon. It is characterized by long, nodular, predominantly solid hypoechogenic lesions with varying degrees of infiltration from the serosal layer down to the muscularis propria identified as two hypoechoic lines separated by a fine hyperechoic line.[490,497] On MRI, the reported sensitivity and specificity is 84% and 99%, respectively, in 60 women with documented intestinal involvement.[494] Diagnostic criteria of rectal invasion include rectal wall thickening and a characteristic triangular attraction of the rectum toward the posterior aspect of the cervix or torus uteri.[475,494,498,499]

ADENOMYOSIS

A variant of endometriosis, adenomyosis, is characterized by the heterotopic development of glands and stroma in the subendometrial myometrium with various degrees of hyperplasia present among adjacent smooth muscle cells. Adenomyosis can be either diffuse or focal. In the diffuse form, glandular and stromal constituents of the endometrium extend throughout the subendometrial layers of the myometrium, resulting in an overall enlargement of the whole uterus. In the localized variant, the affected area is isolated in the frontal or posterior wall of the uterus taking an appearance that may be difficult to distinguish from a fibroid.[500] Various modern transvaginal ultrasound approaches are being tested and developed for their ability to identify and delineate the territorial extension of adenomyosis. The most commonly identified marker of diffuse adenomyosis on ultrasound is a poorly marginated hypoechoic extension in the subendometrial layers of the myometrium.[501] According to Devlieger et al. localized adenomyosis can be distinguished from fibroids based on the following most typical criteria: (i) absence of circular vascularization at the border of the lesion, which may be replaced by vessels actually penetrating into the lesion, and (ii) presence of a shaggy limit between the lesion and the outer myometrium that typically lacks the characteristic edgy shell common to fibroids with its acoustic shadowing effect[500] (Fig. 33-33).

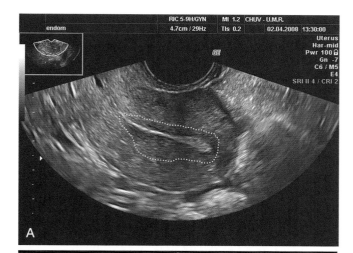

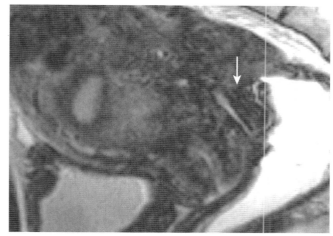

Figure 33-34. Endometriotic lesion: Sagittal T$_2$-weighted fast spin-echo magnetic resonance image of the pelvis showing infiltrative and retractile lesion (typical fibromuscular lesion of endometriosis, arrow) extending to the anterior rectal wall and posterior wall of the uterus.

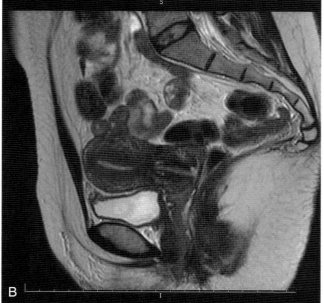

Figure 33-33. Diffuse adenomyosis. *A,* The ultrasound appearance is characterized by a thickened subendometrial sonolucent area. *B,* Magnetic resonance imaging is characterized by a diffuse and fairly regular thickened subendometrial transitional zone.

In spite of ever more sophisticated developments and accomplishments in the field of ultrasound, their efficacy at identifying diffuse or focal adenomyosis remains to this date largely surpassed by MRI, which still stands as the diagnostic tool of choice.[447] MRI, especially through T$_2$-weighted images, has been able to provide excellent soft tissue differentiation. In the uterus, MRI delineates a subendometrial band of low signal referred to as the junctional zone (JZ). Histologic analyses have demonstrated that the JZ corresponds to the subendometrial layer of the myometrium.[502,503] Yet these studies failed to provide clues as to the nature of the histologic basis that accounts for the low signal on MRI. Contrary to the outer layers of the myometrium, the subendometrial layer of the myometrium is of müllerian origin and the site of changes in E$_2$ and progesterone receptors that follows the pattern of changes encountered in the menstrual cycle.[20] Considerable varia-

tion in JZ thickness has been reported, with values ranging from 2 to 8 mm.[504,505] In one report, transvaginal ultrasound was as effective as MRI for delineating the subendometrial layer of the myometrium.[506] Excessive local or diffuse thickening of the low-signal JZ with ill-defined boundaries has been the hallmark of adenomyosis, with many authors proposing 8 mm as the cutoff value between normal and overt diffuse adenomyosis.[507] In a prospective trial of 119 patients undergoing hysterectomy, the JZ was 7.7 mm (mean) in 91 women without adenomyosis and 15 mm (mean) in 28 women with adenomyosis.[506] In women whose JZ was between 8 and 12 mm, associated findings, such as focal further thickening of the JZ or high-signal foci within areas of low signal on T$_2$-weighted sequences, may represent islands of ectopic endometrium.

Focal adenomyosis consists of an area of low signal intensity on T$_2$-weighted images consisting of smooth muscle hyperplasia associated with heterotopic endometrial tissue[447,508] (Fig. 33-34). Practically, it is most important to distinguish focal adenomyosis from leiomyomas. In 21 women clinically suspected to have focal adenomyosis, MRI adequately diagnosed signs of focal adenomyosis in 12 women. In 10 of these women, the diagnosis was ultimately confirmed by histologic analysis of the pathologic specimen.[509] According to Reinhold et al.[447] features in favor of the diagnosis of adenomyosis on MRI include (i) lesion with poorly defined borders, (ii) lesion that extends along the endometrium, (iii) minimal mass effect on the endometrium relative to the size of the lesion, (iv) linear striation radiating out of the endometrium into the myometrium, and (v) absence of large vessels at the margins of lesions contrary to the typical findings of leiomyomas. Furthermore, these authors stress the possibility that uterine contractions and the resulting deformation of the endometrial-myometrial interphase may generate images evocative of focal adenomyosis.[447] There is consensus regarding the high sensitivity of MRI at detecting focal adenomyosis, with sensitivity reported at 88% and 86% in prospective trials by Ascher et al.[507] and Reinhold et al.[506] respectively. These authors disagreed, however, about the ability of endovaginal ultrasound to detect focal adenomyosis with the former and the latter groups reporting 53% and 89%, respectively.

ENDOMETRIOSIS AND UTERINE CONTRACTILITY

In a provocative series of publications Leyendecker's team spearheaded the concept that endometriosis is associated with a hyperkinetic-dyskinetic condition of the uterus[468,510] as a result of structural abnormalities of the uterine wall.[511] This impairs the retrograde transport of sperm during the follicular phase[212,225,512] and the proper antegrade emptying of uterine contents at the time of menses.[221] Following these authors' vision, endometriosis causes a state of local intrauterine hyperestrogenism that increases as well as it disorganizes uterine contraction. From their studies using the uterine displacement of ^{99}Tc-labeled MAA, these authors observed two pathologic findings in endometriosis: (i) a pathologic increase in retrograde transport at the time of menses and (ii) the loss of the elective retrograde transport characteristically targeted toward the tube that faces the developing follicle during the late follicular phase of natural cycles.[226,227] Both phenomena are likely to contribute to the existence of the disease, with the latter participating in the infertility that accompanies even the milder forms of endometriosis. The original report of activation of the aromatase gene in the eutopic endometrium in cases of endometriosis,[513] which has been amply confirmed,[514] offers an explanation for the local state of hyperestrogenism purported as the likely cause for the relative progesterone resistance[515] and the dyskinetic alterations encountered in case of endometriosis.[229,516] That COH-IUI cycles have markedly lower pregnancy rates in case of endometriosis as compared to unaffected control subjects[517-519] further supports the concept that endometriosis is accompanied by a sperm transport problem stemming from uterine dyskinetic alterations.

Conclusions

The advent of transvaginal ultrasound and its ever wider applications in diagnostic gynecology have laid the foundation for the development of functional imaging in reproductive endocrinology. Medical imaging seen in this perspective provides not just anatomic data about pelvic organs but also information about their functional status and the hormonal environment at large. This, therefore, goes well beyond the realm of static images. Specifically, pelvic imaging with transvaginal ultrasound tells us about the state of ovarian function, providing the most reliable reflector of the ovarian reserve, the AFC score. Uterine imaging on transvaginal ultrasound tells us about the hormonal environment at large by analyzing endometrial thickness, volume, and echogenicity. Endometrial thickness and volume inform us about estrogenic exposure, whereas endometrial echogenicity is a marker for progesterone effects, although not only those effects. Yet vaginal ultrasound tells us whether the minimum prerequisite for proper endometrial development, minimal endometrial thickness and volume, are satisfied or not. Expanding in an unexpected direction, however, vaginal ultrasound studies have offered a new direct approach for prying into uterine contractility and its possible impact on uterine receptivity to embryo implantation. Although not all has been unveiled yet and more work is ongoing for assessing UC amplitude and direction, vaginal ultrasound has become a validated tool for measuring UC frequency. Finally, aided by contrast-enhanced imaging (HySO) and possibly 3D volume reconstruction, vaginal ultrasound has become the first line, if not the definitive diagnostic tool, for identifying intrauterine disease (polyps and submucosal fibroids) and assessing uterine malformations.

The advent of 3D facilities, which are now offered on an ever larger segment of new ultrasound equipment, has offered emerging new possibilities for conducting quality control. This stems from the possibility of reconstructing and rereading pertinent new ultrasound *cuts* generated from saved 3D volumes in order to reassess and possibly reconsider original diagnoses. Saved 3D volumes constitute objective data that lend themselves to reassessment, whereas saved 2D images, the only record that existed until now, were essentially subjective.

Contrast-enhanced hysterosonography has become the diagnostic measure of choice for investigating uterine malformations because it offers a simultaneous vision of the uterine cavity(ies) and core uterine muscle. Doppler facilities widely available today and provided on nearly all new ultrasound equipment sold today failed, however, to live up to the original hopes sparked by early reports that alluded to the possibility that Doppler data reliably predicted endometrial receptivity. On the contrary, a consensus exists today to indicate that Doppler has no independent predictive value of endometrial receptivity in ART. Whether Doppler might predict endometrial receptivity in certain contexts, for example in DES-exposed women, remains to be demonstrated as current practices in this field stem from isolated unreproduced case reports. Doppler in its various applications remains useful, however, as a handy complement of gray-scale imaging in various circumstances, as for example, the exploration of ovarian cysts and building confidence about their benign nature or for assessing the vascular status of a uterine septum.

Although MRI stood until now as the primary diagnostic tool for exploring nonovarian endometriosis, the improvements made by vaginal ultrasound are closing the gap to the point that we predict that ultrasound will soon be the first-line tool for diagnosing and staging endometriosis.

The complete reference list can be found on the companion Expert Consult Web site at www.expertconsultbook.com.

Suggested Readings

Chapron C, et al. Magnetic resonance imaging and endometriosis: deeply infiltrating endometriosis does not originate from the rectovaginal septum. Gynecol Obstet Invest 53:204-208, 2002.

Chapron C, et al. Presurgical diagnosis of posterior deep infiltrating endometriosis based on a standardized questionnaire. Hum Reprod 20:507-513, 2005.

de Kroon CD, et al. Saline contrast hysterosonography in abnormal uterine bleeding: a systematic review and meta-analysis. BJOG 110:938-947, 2003.

de Ziegler D, et al. Contractility of the nonpregnant uterus: the follicular phase. Ann N Y Acad Sci 943:172-184, 2001.

Fanchin R, et al. New look at endometrial echogenicity: objective computer-assisted measurements predict endometrial receptivity in in vitro fertilization-embryo transfer. Fertil Steril 74:274-281, 2000.

Hamilton JA, et al. Routine use of saline hysterosonography in 500 consecutive, unselected, infertile women. Hum Reprod 13:2463-2473, 1998.

Herter LD, et al. Ovarian and uterine sonography in healthy girls between 1 and 13 years old: correlation of findings with age and pubertal status. AJR Am J Roentgenol 178:1531-1536, 2002.

Holm K, et al. Pubertal maturation of the internal genitalia: an ultrasound evaluation of 166 healthy girls. Ultrasound Obstet Gynecol 6:175-181, 1995.

Kaufman RH, et al. Upper genital tract changes associated with exposure in utero to diethylstilbestrol. Am J Obstet Gynecol 128:51-59, 1977.

Kunz G, et al. Sonographic evidence for the involvement of the utero-ovarian counter-current system in the ovarian control of directed uterine sperm transport. Hum Reprod Update 4:667-672, 1998.

Leyendecker G, et al. Endometriosis: a dysfunction and disease of the archimetra. Hum Reprod Update 4:752-762, 1998.

Lindheim SR, et al. Ultrasound guided embryo transfer significantly improves pregnancy rates in women undergoing oocyte donation. Int J Gynaecol Obstet 66:281-284, 1999.

Ng EH, et al. The role of endometrial and subendometrial blood flows measured by three-dimensional power Doppler ultrasound in the prediction of pregnancy during IVF treatment. Hum Reprod 21:164-170, 2006.

Raine-Fenning N, et al. The reproducibility of endometrial volume acquisition and measurement with the VOCAL-imaging program. Ultrasound Obstet Gynecol 19:69-75, 2002.

Tur-Kaspa I, et al. A prospective evaluation of uterine abnormalities by saline infusion sonohysterography in 1,009 women with infertility or abnormal uterine bleeding. Fertil Steril 86:1731-1735, 2006.

CHAPTER 34

Contraception

Courtney A. Schreiber and Kurt Barnhart

The last decade has hosted the advent of many new contraceptive technologies—short-acting, long-acting, and permanent methods of contraception are now available in many varieties and delivery systems. Such a breadth of possibilities provides an opportunity for clinicians to tailor their contraceptive counseling to women based on the patient's co-morbidities, future plans for childbearing, and lifestyle needs.

Contraceptive Use in the United States

According to the U.S. census bureau, 62 million American women are in the childbearing years (15-44 years). The vast majority (7 out of 10) of women age 18 to 44 are sexually active and trying to avoid pregnancy. Without effective contraception, this population of women is at risk for unintended pregnancy. The typical American woman must use contraceptives for roughly three decades of her life.[1] Sixty-two percent of the 62 million women of reproductive age in the United States are using a contraceptive method. Seven percent of women are at risk of an unintended pregnancy and not using contraceptives. The majority of American women use the oral contraceptive pill or tubal sterilization for contraception. Eighteen percent of couples use the male condom.

Table 34-1 demonstrates the subtle changes over time in American contraceptive use and underscores that although long-term effective contraceptive methods are increasing in use, these methods still make up a slim minority of contraceptive technologies utilized by American couples. The oral contraceptive pill is the most widely used method by women in their teens and 20s, women who have never been married, and women who have at least a college degree. Poor and low income women are twice as likely as higher income women to use the 3-month injectable

method, with depo-medroxyprogesterone acetate. Fifty percent of all women age 40 to 44 who practice contraception have been sterilized. The proportion of women who use a contraceptive method at first intercourse has doubled in recent times to 79% at present.[2] The majority of these couples use condoms at first intercourse. Teenagers who do not use a contraceptive at first intercourse are twice as likely to become teen mothers as teenagers who do use a contraceptive method. As demonstrated by Table 34-1, contraceptive use has increased overall among American women. Despite this, the unintended pregnancy rate remains approximately 49% in the United States. Unintended pregnancies are associated with poor social, health, and economic outcomes for women and children alike.[3]

Contraceptive Effectiveness and Efficacy

Contraceptive clinical trials typically report their failure rates either by the Pearl Index or Life Table Analysis. The Pearl Index is defined as the number of contraceptive failures per 100 women-years of exposure, and uses as the denominator the total months or cycles of exposure from the initiation of the product to the end of the study or the discontinuation of the product. Life Table Analysis, on the other hand, provides the contraceptive failure rate for each month of use and can provide a cumulative failure rate for any specific length of exposure. A recent Food and Drug Administration (FDA) briefing reviewed the actual utility of the Pearl Index, noting that it does not take into account the effect of failures over time (www.fda.gov/ohrms/dockets/ac/07/briefing/2007-4274b1-01-FDA.pdf). The Life Table Analysis method of reporting effectiveness is considered an actuarial method. Effectiveness can be difficult to compute because there are many factors that influence contraceptive use. The term "effectiveness" is defined as

TABLE 34-1

Percentage Distribution and Number (in Thousands) of Contraceptive Users Aged 15 to 44 in the United States, by Current Method, 1982-1995

Method	1982 %	1982 No.	1988 %	1988 No.	1995 %	1995 No.
Sterilization	34.1	10,295	39.2	13,686	38.6	14,942
Female	23.2	6998	27.5	9614	27.7	10,727
Male	10.9	3298	11.7	4069	10.9	4215
Pill	28.0	8431	30.7	10,734	26.9	10,410
Implant	NA	NA	NA	NA	1.3	515
Injectable	NA	NA	NA	NA	3.0	1146
Intrauterine device	7.1	2153	2.0	703	0.8	310
Diaphragm	8.1	2436	5.7	2000	1.9	720
Male condom	12.0	3608	14.6	5093	20.4	7889
Foam	2.4	711	1.1	371	0.4	161
Periodic abstinence	3.9	1166	2.3	806	2.3	883
Withdrawal	2.0	588	2.2	778	3.0	1178
Other[*]	2.5	754	2.1	733	1.3	508
Total	100.0	30,142	100.0	34,912	100.0	38,663
Sample n	NA	4242	NA	5176	NA	7145

[*]Other consists of douche, sponge, jelly or cream alone, and other methods.
From Piccinini LJ, Mosher WD. trends in contraception use in the United States 1982-1995. Fam Plann Perspect 30:4-10 and 46, 1998. With permission of the Alan Guttmacher Institute.

the ability of a contraceptive to prevent pregnancy in a clinical trial setting, meaning a failure or success that occurs when a product is used perfectly in accordance with the recommended dose regimen. "Efficacy" is a term used to define the ability of a contraceptive to prevent pregnancy in typical use, for example, when the subject does not completely follow the recommended dosing regimen. The terms "typical use failure rate" and "perfect use failure rate" are also used to describe these differences. Table 34-2 demonstrates the differences in the typical use failure rate from the perfect use failure rate in the different contraceptive methods. It is critical to note that typical use applies to the population in general whereas perfect use refers to the clinical trial setting.

Spermicides and Barrier Methods

Spermicides are a nonprescription barrier method of reversible contraception. All spermicidal agents contain a surfactant, usually 1000 mg nonoxynol-9 (N-9), that immobilizes or kills sperm on contact. They also provide a mechanical barrier and can be used with other barrier methods of contraception, such as condoms; therefore, they need to be placed into the vagina before each coital act. Spermicides used alone are 75% to 85% effective in preventing pregnancy.[4] The effectiveness of these agents increases with increasing age of the woman and is similar to that of the diaphragm in all age and income groups.

There was a great deal of hope invested in the possibility that N-9 might act as an anti-infective agent as well as a spermicide, and prevent against HIV and other sexually transmitted infections. While initial in vitro studies were promising, clinical trials have demonstrated that N-9-containing spermicides do not provide protection

against HIV or sexually transmitted infections (STIs). According to a recent study by the World Health Organization (WHO), such compounds appear to increase the incidence of these infections in sex workers, perhaps by causing lesions and ulcerations in the genital mucosa of the female, leading to increased risk of transmission of infective agents. These effects were also found to be dose related, so at lower doses, the gel did not have a protective or promotive effect on HIV transmission or disruptions in the vaginal ecology.[5]

Microbicides

Microbicides are products in development designed to protect against HIV and STIs. Many of the candidate microbicides will also be effective contraceptives. The development of microbicides is urgent because the incidence of transmission of HIV and STIs is greatest in women of reproductive age,[6] and the only proven way to protect against the sexual transmission of HIV is with the male condom (not a viable option for all women because it requires male cooperation). Many microbicidal compounds are currently under development, and they will provide additional protection when used with condoms, but may be used as primary protection for those who are unable or unwilling to use condoms consistently.

The pharmacologic action of microbicides is based on several different mechanisms: either killing or immobilizing pathogens by forming a barrier between pathogen and vaginal tissues; preventing the infective agent from entering target cells; preventing a pathogen from replicating once it has entered cells; boosting the vagina's or rectum's own defense system; or by acting like invisible condoms. The focus is on developing such products that can be

TABLE 34-2

Percentage of Women Experiencing an Unintended Pregnancy During the First Year of Typical Use and the First Year of Perfect Use of Contraception and the Percentage Continuing Use at the End of the First Year: United States

Method	Women Experiencing an Unintended Pregnancy within the First Year of Use (%)		Women Continuing Use at One Year[3] (%)
	Typical Use[1]	Perfect Use[2]	
No method[4]	85	85	42
Spermicides[5]	29	15	43
Withdrawal	27	4	51
Periodic abstinence	25	—	—
Calendar	—	9	—
Ovulation method	—	3	—
Sympto-thermal[6]	—	2	—
Postovulation	—	1	—
Cap[7]			
Parous women	32	26	46
Nulliparous women	16	9	57
Sponge			
Parous women	32	20	46
Nulliparous women	16	9	57
Diaphragm[7]	16	6	57
Condom[8]			
Female (reality)	21	5	49
Male	15	2	53
Combined pill and minipill	8	0.3	68
Evra patch	8	0.3	68
NuvaRing	8	0.3	68
Depo-Provera	3	0.3	56
Lunelle	3	0.05	56
Intrauterine device (IUD)			
Progestasert (progesterone T)	2	1.5	81
ParaGard (copper T)	0.8	0.6	78
Mirena (LNG-IUS)	0.1	0.1	81
Norplant and Norplant-2	0.05	0.05	84
Female sterilization	0.5	0.5	100
Male sterilization	0.15	0.1	100

Emergency contraceptive pills: Treatment initiated within 72 hours after unprotected intercourse reduces the risk of pregnancy by at least 75%.[9] Lactational amenorrhea method (LAM) is a highly effective, *temporary* method of contraception.[10]

[1]Among *typical* couples who initiate use of a method (not necessarily for the first time), the percentage who experience an accidental pregnancy during the first year if they do not stop use for any other reason.

[2]Among couples who initiate use of a method (not necessarily for the first time) and who use it *perfectly* (both consistently and correctly), the percentage who experience an accidental pregnancy during the first year if they do not stop use for any other reason.

[3]Among couples attempting to avoid pregnancy, the percentage who continue to use a method for 1 year.

[4]The percentages becoming pregnant in columns 2 and 3 are based on data from populations where contraception is not used and from women who cease using contraception in order to become pregnant. Among such populations, about 89% become pregnant within 1 year. This estimate was lowered slightly (to 85%) to represent the percentage who would become pregnant within 1 year among women now relying on reversible methods of contraception if they abandoned contraception altogether.

[5]Foams, creams, gels, vaginal suppositories, and vaginal film.

[6]Cervical mucus (ovulation) method supplemented by calendar in the preovulatory phase and basal body temperature in the postovulatory phase.

[7]With spermicidal cream or jelly.

[8]Without spermicides.

[9]The treatment schedule is one dose within 120 hours after unprotected intercourse, and a second dose 12 hours after the first dose. Both doses of Plan B can be taken at the same time. Plan B (1 dose is 1 white pill) and Preven (1 dose is 2 blue pills) are the only dedicated products specifically marketed for emergency contraception. The Food and Drug Administration has in addition declared the following 17 brands of oral contraceptives to be safe and effective for emergency contraception: Ogestrel or Ovral (1 dose is 2 white pills), Alesse, Lessina, or Levlite (1 dose is 5 pink pills), Levlen or Nordette (1 dose is 4 light-orange pills), Cryselle, Levora, Low-Ogestrel, or Lo/Ovral (1 dose is 4 white pills), Tri-Levlen or Triphasil (1 dose is 4 yellow pills), Portia or Trivora (1 dose is 4 pink pills), Aviane (1 dose is 5 orange pills), and Empresse (1 dose is 4 orange pills).

[10]However, to maintain effective protection against pregnancy, another method of contraception must be used as soon as menstruation resumes, the frequency or duration of breastfeeding is reduced, bottle feeds are introduced, or the baby reaches 6 months of age.

From Trussell J. Chapter 13. *In* Hatcher RA, Trussell J, Stewart F, et al (eds). Contraceptive Technology, 18th rev. New York, Ardent Media, 2004.

TABLE 34-3

Microbicide Compounds Under Development

Microbicide Group	Mode of Action	Examples
Surface active agents (detergents)	Penetrate cervical mucus, disrupt viral envelopes, cover the surface of viral STDs	Nonoxynol 9, octoxynol 9, benzalkonium chloride, menfegol, and *n*-docosanol
Sulfated compounds	Bind to virus or host cell receptors and block viral uptake	Dextrin sulfate, Dextran 2 sulfate, carageenan, polystyrene sulfonate, heparin sulfate: cholic acid, cellulose sulfate, PC-515, and naphthalene sulfonate (PRO 2000)
Anti-HIV compounds	Antiretroviral agents that prevent virus replication	X-2371 (low-molecular-weight, nonpeptide oligospecific integrin modulator), PMPA (adenine antiretroviral drug), serine proteinase inhibitor, novel aryl phosphate derivatives of AZT, nevirapine gel/cream, and cyanovirn N
Natural defense compounds	Increase host natural defenses against STIs by maintaining the normal acidic pH of the vagina in the presence of semen, contain lactobacillis which produces hydrogen peroxide killing HIV and STDs	Lactobacillus suppositories, buffer gel, and acid gel (ACIDFORM)

applied in advance before sexual intercourse, and spread evenly over the vagina and cervix or rectum.

Many potential microbicides are in various phases of development; but most of them are in early phases of clinical trial or in preclinical stages. Other drugs undergoing trials are those that were previously approved for antiretroviral therapy because they are effective against herpes simplex, bacteria, yeast, fungi, viruses, and potentially effective against other STIs as well.

Some of the groups of compounds that are being developed as microbicides are noted in Table 34-3.

Barrier Techniques

DIAPHRAGM

Diaphragms are soft latex or silicone barriers that cover the cervix. They provide contraception by blocking the entrance to the uterus and preventing the sperm from fertilizing the egg. They may also be used in conjunction with spermicides that immobilize the sperm, and therefore, lead to better contraception. Diaphragms provide no protection against HIV or sexually transmitted infections.

A diaphragm must be fitted by the health care provider. The largest size that does not cause discomfort or undue pressure on the vaginal epithelium should be used. After the fitting, the woman should remove the diaphragm and reinsert it herself. She should then be examined to make sure the diaphragm is covering the cervix. The diaphragm should be used with a spermicide and be left in place for at least 8 hours after the last coital act. If repeated intercourse takes place or coitus occurs more than 8 hours after insertion of the diaphragm, additional spermicide should be used. Although spermicide use with the diaphragm is advised, it has not been conclusively demonstrated that pregnancy rates are lower when a spermicide is used with a diaphragm than when the diaphragm is used alone.[11] The number of urinary tract infections in women who use diaphragms is significantly higher than in nonusers, probably because of the mechanical obstruction of the outflow of urine by the diaphragm.[12] A one-size-fits-most nonlatex diaphragm is currently being studied and, if approved for use, has the potential to simplify this method of contraception significantly.

Advantages

The diaphragm has several advantages:

- Safe to use during breastfeeding
- Not easily felt by either partner (reasonably discreet)
- Immediately effective
- Immediately reversible
- Nonhormonal

Disadvantages

Disadvantages of the diaphragm are as follows:

- Requires personalized fitting by health care professional
- Difficulty in insertion may be experienced
- May need to be refitted after full-term pregnancy or pelvic or abdominal surgery
- Must be used with every coital act
- Moderately effective

CERVICAL CAP

The *cervical cap* is a cup-shaped plastic or rubber device that fits around the cervix. It may be either a cavity rim cap (Prentif and Oves), a cap that fits the vaginal walls around the cervix (FemCap, Dumas, Vimule), or a large cap-like device (Lea's shield). Prentif, Femcap and Lea's shield are approved for use in the United States. These barrier methods can be left in place longer than the diaphragm.

The various types of caps are manufactured in different sizes and should be fitted to the cervix by a health care provider.

The cap should be left on the cervix for no more than 48 hours, and a spermicide should always be placed inside the cap before use.[13] The *cavity rim cervical cap* is manufactured in four sizes and requires more training than the diaphragm, both for the provider to fit it and for the user to place it correctly. Failure rates with the cervical cap for nulliparous women are similar to those observed with the diaphragm, but for parous women they are twice as high.

Constraints of Fitting of a Cervical Cap

- Fitting is to be done by a health care professional.
- Vaginal delivery may lead to a scarred or irregularly shaped cervix.
- Antiflexed uterus requires cavity rim caps.
- Not all sizes are available.
- Refitting may be needed after childbirth.

MALE CONDOM

The male condom is the only method of contraception that has been shown to prevent transmission of sexually transmitted infections, so its use by individuals at risk for infection should be encouraged. The male condom should not be applied tightly against the tip of the penis, but rather the condom tip should extend beyond the end of the penis by about half an inch to collect the ejaculate. Care must be taken on withdrawal not to spill the ejaculate. When used by strongly motivated couples, the male condom is very effective. The male condom has a "typical use" failure rate of 14%. Recent studies have shown that teens were most likely to use condoms for birth control and that 66% used a condom when they became sexually active.[7] The male condoms provide a physical barrier that prevents sperm and egg interaction. They are intended for one-time use only. Condoms also provide protection against HIV and STI.

FEMALE CONDOM

A female condom was approved for marketing in the United States in 1994. It consists of a soft, loose-fitting sheath and two flexible polyurethane rings. One ring lies inside the vagina at the closed end of the sheath and serves as an insertion mechanism and internal anchor.

The outer ring forms the external edge of the device and remains outside the vagina after insertion, thus providing protection to the labia and the base of the penis during intercourse. The condom is prelubricated and is intended for one-time use only. Fitting by a health professional is not required.[8] In comparison to the male condom, the female condom has the advantage of being able to be inserted before beginning sexual activity and to be left in place for a longer time after ejaculation occurs. Because the female condom also covers the external genitalia, it should offer greater protection against the transfer of certain sexually transmitted organisms, particularly genital herpes. Because polyurethane is stronger than the latex used in male condoms, the female condom is less likely to rupture.

In a multicenter clinical trial in U.S. centers, the cumulative pregnancy rate for this device at 6 months was 12.4%. The 6-month pregnancy rate with perfect use was 2.6%, indicating that the probable 1-year pregnancy rate with perfect use would be slightly more than 5%.[9] At the end of 6 months in the U.S. study, about one third of the women had discontinued this method. Clinical trials with the female condom have not directly compared its use with other barrier techniques. Trussel and colleagues,[9] using the data of other studies, concluded that the efficacy rate of the female condom with perfect use would be similar to that of the diaphragm and cervical cap, but the failure rate of the female condom with typical use would be higher than that of the diaphragm. Because of the lack of prospective clinical trials with the male condom, no statistical comparison of the effectiveness of the two types of condoms can be made. Moreover, the effectiveness of the female condom for reducing sexual infection transmission has not been evaluated. However, because polyurethane does not allow virus transmission, it should reduce a woman's risk of acquiring HIV infection.

INVISIBLE CONDOMS

Thermoreversible gel prevents infection by forming a protective barrier after being inserted into the vagina or rectum. It is a liquid at room temperature and quickly turns into an impermeable gel inside the rectal/vaginal canal.

Steroid Contraceptives

Hormonal contraception was initially marketed in the United States in pill form in 1960. The original formulation included 50 µg of estrogen. Such dosing is rarely used today, and the majority of hormonal contraceptives on the U.S. and European markets include doses of 35 µg of estrogen or less, all of which qualify as "low-dose" hormonal contraceptives. The oral contraceptive pill is still the most widely used hormonal contraceptive delivery system. However, steroid contraceptives also take the form of a transdermal patch, a combined hormonal vaginal ring, and progestin-only methods include a 3-month injectable, a subdermal implant, and an intrauterine contraceptive. The oral contraceptive pill is perhaps the most widely studied medication in history. Although it is biologically plausible that other delivery systems, such as the transdermal patch and the vaginal ring, carry with them similar contraceptive benefits, side effects, and contraindications as the combined contraceptive pill, verification of this biologic plausibility has not yet been done in large clinical trials. For this reason, we will focus on the combined hormonal contraceptive pill when discussing the details of the mechanism of action, the side effects, the noncontraceptive benefits, and the contraindications to combined hormonal contraceptive use. The specific issues related to the other delivery systems will be addressed in the respective sections.

HORMONAL CONTRACEPTION

The history of hormonal contraception dates back into the early 1900s when it was observed that ovulation is linked to pregnancy and the presence of a corpus luteum. The history of hormonal contraception is not glamorous, but instead exemplifies the dedicated, multidisciplinary efforts required to make scientific advances that may be politically challenging. The chemist Russell Marker purified progesterone from both animal and plant sources. Carl Djerassi, another chemist at the company Syntax, found that the progestational activity of yam-derived progesterone could be enhanced by removing the 19-carbon from this plant progesterone. A reproductive health activist named Margaret Sanger brought the scientist Gregory Pincus together with the philanthropist Catherine McCormick in the 1950s. Pincus, together with other scientists from Boston, worked with the funding supplied by Catherine McCormick to develop a progestational agent in pill form to act as a contraceptive. The clinical trials of the early oral contraceptive pill were conducted in Puerto Rico. The initial compound consisted of 10 to 40 mg of synthetic progestin. The initial products, however, were contaminated with 1% mestranol, a synthetic estrogen. When the mestranol was removed from the compound for a more pure progestational agent, clinical trial results demonstrated more breakthrough bleeding and the decision was made to retain the estrogen for cycle control. This is the history behind the combined hormonal contraceptive as we know it today.

Pharmacology

There are three main formulations for combined hormonal contraception delivered orally. These include monophasic combination pills, multiphasic combination pills, and progestin-only pills. The progestin component of the combined hormonal contraceptive is most commonly a 19-nortestosterone progestin. These progestins more closely resemble testosterone than their alternative, the 21-carbon

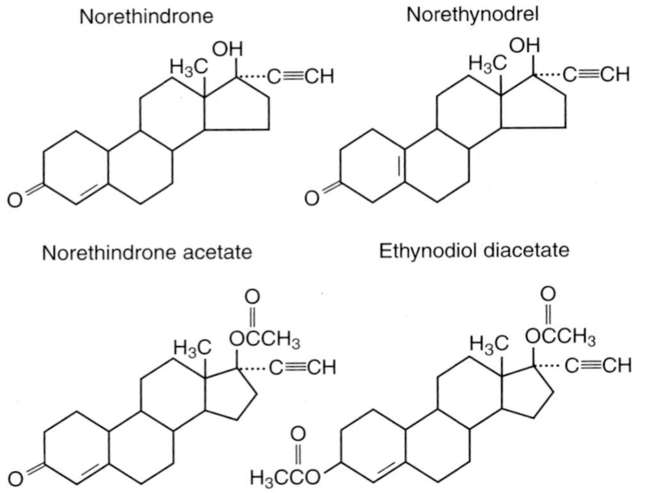

Figure 34-1. *Chemical structures of the estrane progestins used in oral contraceptives.*

acetoxyprogesterone derivative. Medroxyprogesterone acetate and megestrol acetate are 21-carbon progestins. The two classes most commonly used are the estranes and gonanes. Those derived from 17α-acetoxyprogesterone are referred to as the pregnanes. 19-Nortestosterone derivatives are orally active, but they do carry some androgenic and progestational effects. The estrane family of progestin, norethindrone derivatives (Fig. 34-1), include norethindrone, norethynodrel, norethindrone acetate, ethynodiol diacetate, lynestrenol, norgestrel, norgestimate, desogestrel, and desogen. Regardless of the nomenclature, most estrane progestins are converted to norethindrone when they are metabolized. The norgestrel family of progestins, the gonane progestins (Fig. 34-2), include desogestrel, gestodene, norgestimate, and etonogestrel, and are utilized in the combination vaginal ring. Drospirenone is one progestin that is used in oral combination hormonal contraception but is not a member of the estrane or gonane families. Drospirenone is considered to have less androgenicity than the 19-nortestosterone-derived progestins. Drospirenone is derived from spironolactone and it has

Figure 34-2. *Chemical structure of the gonane progestins used in oral contraceptives.*

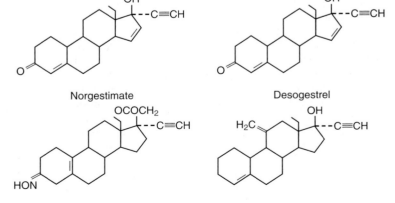

anti-androgenic and anti-mineralcorticoid activity. This formulation has not been shown to have decreased progestin associated side effects in randomized control trials at a population based level. However, it is an option for women using combined hormonal contraception today. Because the progestin component of combined hormonal contraception is what is responsible for the contraceptive efficacy, most dosages of oral contraceptive pills are dependent upon the amount of progestin required to achieve contraceptive efficacy. The gonane class has greater progestational activity per unit weight than the estrane class, which accounts for the smaller amount required in these oral contraceptive formulations.

Combination hormonal contraceptive pills by definition combine the progestin with one of two types of estrogens, most commonly ethinyl estradiol and less commonly ethinyl estradiol 3-methyl ether, which is otherwise known as mestranol (Fig. 34-3). The original oral contraceptive formulations contain mestranol, which was utilized in the 50-µg formulation. These 50-µg formulations are termed first-generation combined hormonal contraceptives. These forms are rarely utilized today, and most oral contraceptives contain estrogen doses of 35 µg or less and are referred to as low-dose estrogen oral contraceptives. Oral contraceptive pills with 20 to 35 µg of ethinyl estradiol are termed second-generation products. The third-generation formulation refers to those with the newer versions of the levonorgestrel derivatives, the newer versions of the gonane progestins, and they include desogestryl, norgestimate and gestodene. Combination oral contraceptives are given continuously for 3 weeks, and the traditional formulation allows for a placebo, medication-free week, in the fourth week. The withdrawal of the estrogen in the combined hormonal contraceptives results in endometrial sloughing. This sloughing results in a withdrawal bleed that usually lasts 3 to 4 days. Uterine blood loss is about 25 mL and this is less than the average 35 mL that is lost with menses in an ovulatory cycle.

Mechanism of Action

The traditional contraceptive pills are given for 3 out of 4 weeks in the month. Newer formulations have focused on diminishing or eliminating the pill-free week in order to allow for a decreased number of bleeding days or elimination of bleeding days entirely. The progestin component of the combination pills prevents ovulation by inhibiting gonadotropin secretion. This effect comes directly from the progestational agent's suppression of luteinizing hormone (LH) secretion, thereby preventing ovulation. The estrogenic agent suppresses follicle-stimulating hormone

(FSH). However, it is important to note that even if follicles do develop, which is commonly seen with combination pills of 20 µg or less, these follicles do not develop sufficiently and the progestational component still inhibits the luteinizing hormone surge that is necessary for ovulation. The progestin component also works by thickening the cervical mucus and altering the endometrium such that it is not receptive to implantation. The endometrium in a progestin-dominant milieu is decidualized and atrophic. These lower genital tract effects are sufficient in and of themselves to afford good contraception. In fact, many progestin-only methods work primarily by cervical mucus thickening and endometrial lining decidualization.

The FDA has approved three new contraceptive formulations for continuous use. These methods are called Lybrel, Seasonale, and Seasonique. The efficacy of these regimens appears to be similar to the 21/7-day efficacy period. The clinical trials that were done initially for the approval of these formulations demonstrate that continuous use of hormonal contraception suppresses folliculogenesis at improved rates over the traditional 21/7-day regimens. This choice should be considered in the clinical scenario when patients may have ovarian cysts and are looking for suppression of follicle growth as a noncontraceptive benefit of their hormonal contraceptive. Studies have demonstrated that these new formulations are acceptable to women of reproductive age. They are highly convenient with fewer bleeding days over time. Noncontraceptive benefits include decreased dysmenorrhea, decreased endometriosis pain, and fewer instances of headaches, bloating, and mood swings. Good candidates for continuous hormonal contraceptives are all women but specifically women who have symptoms in their pill-free week. Breakthrough bleeding is, however, more common than during the first 3 months of use in the conventional 21/7-day regimen. Over time, this breakthrough bleeding reaches the usual rate.

Long-term safety data have not yet been amassed with continuous hormonal contraceptives, but markers of safety and pregnancy after discontinuation appear to be similar to the traditional 21/7-day oral contraceptive pill. Lybrel is a 20-µg ethinyl estradiol pill with 0.09 mg of levonorgestrel. It can be taken 365 days per year. There is no placebo or pill-free interval. The Pearl Index for efficacy is 1.55 per 100 user-years.[10] There appear to be no differences in pregnancy rates between Lybrel and a 20-µg ethinyl estradiol/0.1 mg levonorgestrel pill.[11] Sixty percent of women are amenorrheic by the year's end.[11] Breakthrough bleeding is common, with 40% of women complaining of breakthrough bleeding at the third pack, decreasing over time to 21% at pack 13.[10] So, a large percentage of women on Lybrel are

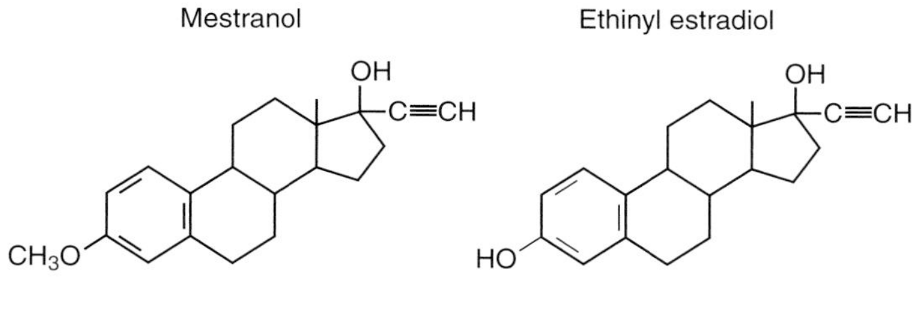

Mestranol   Ethinyl estradiol

Figure 34-3. Structures of the two estrogens used in combination oral contraceptives.

amenorrheic, and those who are not will likely have unscheduled bleeding. Once Lybrel is discontinued, 99% of women will resume regular menses within 90 days.

Seasonale was FDA approved in 2003 as a 30-μg ethinyl estradiol and 0.15 mg levonorgestrel 84-day pill regimen with 7 days of placebo every 3 months. Patients have four withdrawal bleeds per year with 91-day cycles. A randomized control trial[12] comparing Nordette, which is the same hormonal dosing but in a traditional 21/7-day regimen, to Seasonale showed that Nordette had a higher continuation rate at 1 year, and an improved acceptability of bleeding patterns. Both have high compliance, however, and the Pearl Index is 0.6 for Seasonale and 1.78 for Nordette, rendering Seasonale a more effective contraceptive. Total number of bleeding days is decreased with Seasonale but there is increased breakthrough bleeding in the first 3 months. Its safety profile approximates that of other hormonal contraceptive pills with no unexpected laboratory changes, no lipid changes, and no thromboembolic events in greater than 1000 cycles of Seasonale use. Seasonique[13] is a 30-μg ethinyl estradiol pill with 0.15 mg of levonorgestrel for 84 days, followed by 7 days of 10 μg of ethinyl estradiol. This pill allows for four withdrawal bleeds per year and has a Pearl Index of 0.78. Unscheduled bleeding decreased with time in clinical trials, and scheduled bleeding occurs for about 2 to 3 days in duration. The reasoning behind these newer formulations is to increase efficacy and theoretically decrease side effects associated with the pill-free period. Shorter hormone-free intervals suppress the hypothalamic-pituitary axis more consistently.[14] Studies have demonstrated less folliculogenesis in the extended cycle regimen.[15] A randomized control trial[16] was done to compare a 21/7-day pill consisting of 20 μg of ethinyl estradiol and 100 μg of levonorgestrel versus a 20-μg ethinyl estradiol/150-μg desogestrel regimen, followed by two placebo pills, followed by five pills of 20 μg of ethinyl estradiol versus 28 solid days of 20 μg ethinyl estradiol and 150 μg desogestrel. This trial had three arms and examined the traditional pill-free interval versus estrogen alone in place of a pill-free interval and demonstrated a statistically significant decrease in folliculogenesis on ultrasound and lower FSH and LH levels during the pill-free interval. A Cochrane review[17,18] of traditional 21/7-day administration versus continuous administration showed no difference in efficacy, no difference in safety profiles, high compliance rate, and high satisfaction rate. Continuous administration was in this review associated with a decrease in headaches, genital irritation, feelings of fatigue, bloating, and menstrual pain. Mood, headache, and pelvic pain scores improved with continuous hormonal contraception. In women who had undergone ablation for endometriosis and then failed traditional 21/7-day low-dose monophasic contraception for suppression of pain, there was significantly reduced frequency and severity of pain on continuous low-dose monophasic contraceptives for up to 24 months. Continuous oral contraceptive pills (OCPs) suppress both the ovary and the endometrium to a greater extent than cyclic OCPs and have been shown to have beneficial effects on both pain and mood symptoms related to menstruation.[19] It is important to note that although the FDA has approved these three formulations for extended use, many physicians have been using extended cycle regimens for their patients for years. Most monophasic hormonal contraceptive pills will produce acceptable results when used continuously.

Adverse Effects of Continuous Cycle Oral Contraceptives

There are limited long-term data to answer the question of adverse outcomes in continuous hormonal contraception. The longest study is a 2-year study on Seasonale.[20] What these data do show are that unexpected bleeding and spotting decrease with length of use: this is an important counseling point for any woman considering use of extended cycle OCPs. The incidence of thromboembolism is not well known. There has only been one reported case.[12] No endometrial hyperplasia or cancers were reported in these clinical trials.[12,20] In terms of lipid profiles, triglycerides and low-density lipoproteins (LDLs) were similar in range for women on continuous hormonal contraception as those who were cycling.[12,13] In one study. there were five cases of women with cholecystitis or cholelithiasis, but it is unclear if this was due to other risk factors.[13] Return to fertility appears to be fairly prompt after continuous hormonal oral contraception is discontinued.[11,15,20] The study of Lybrel[11] demonstrated that 99% of women were ovulating within 90 days of discontinuing the 365-day per year pill. Ninety-two percent ovulated within 60 days, and 38.5% ovulated within 30 days of discontinuing the oral contraceptive.

Metabolic Effects

The use of synthetic steroids and combination hormonal contraceptive formulations has multiple metabolic effects. The vast majority of these effects, including effects on lipids, carbohydrate metabolism, and other hormonally responsive organs, such as the breasts, are generally transient and self-limited and minor. Rarely, however, these other effects can result in serious consequences. The majority of the serious side effects associated with hormonal contraception are cardiovascular events that are related to the effects that estrogen has on the coagulation system.

Cardiovascular Events

The increased cardiovascular events including venous thromboembolism and arterial thromboembolism appear to be due to coagulation-mediated effects, not atherosclerosis. Epidemiologic data have shown us that the risk of venous thromboembolism (VTE) is dose-dependent with the amount of estrogen in the oral contraceptive formulation.[21] The background rate of venous thromboembolism in women of reproductive age is thought to be about 0.8 per 10,000 women-years. Recent data,[22] however, have demonstrated that the true prevalence of VTE in the population of women is difficult to elucidate. Deep venous thromboembolism (DVT) in particular is often silent and self-limited. Given that symptomatic venous thromboembolism is clearly a rare event, but potentially also asymptomatic and therefore underreported, background risk is hard to discern. This should be kept in mind at all times given the reporting bias that may be present when venous thromboembolism is attributed to the use of oral contraceptives.

Several observational studies have been performed to determine the occurrence of VTE in users of oral contraceptive containing formulations with less than 50 μg of estrogen.[23-25] These studies were consistent and showed that the risk of DVT was increased approximately three- to fourfold among women using oral contraceptives compared with women not using oral contraceptives. Thus, the use of oral contraceptives with less than 50 μg of estrogen is still associated with about a threefold to fourfold increased risk of VTE compared with a nonpregnant population who are not taking oral contraceptives, but about a 50% reduction in risk of VTE compared with a pregnant or recently postpartum population.[25]

In 1995, the U.K. Committee on Safety of Medication sent a letter to all physicians and pharmacists in the United Kingdom stating that women taking oral contraceptives containing desogestrel or gestodene should discontinue utilizing these specific formulations because of an apparent risk in venous thromboembolism in women using these formulations compared with other progestins, which was mostly levonorgestrel. This letter was prompted by epidemiologic data that retrospectively suggested an association between desogestrel- or gestodene-containing hormonal contraceptives and an increased risk of 1.5 to 2 of VTE.[26] This event was unfortunately associated with an increase in unintended pregnancy and induced abortions in the United Kingdom and given the nature and design of these studies, the differences that were found in risk of thromboembolism could be, in fact, due to an increased risk with these progestins or just as easily could be due to bias of study design—for example, the common biases associated with pharmacoepidemiologic studies, including selection bias, reporting bias, and referral bias. Women taking OCs containing drospirenone have a similar risk of VTE to those taking levonogestrol-containing OCs.[27]

The use of 50-μg oral contraceptive pills did appear to have an impact on the coagulation system. This was due to an increase in clotting factors, such as factors V, VIII, X, and fibrinogen. Studies that addressed this question in the group taking OCPs of 35 μg and less have not demonstrated clearly increased risk of clotting related events in women using pills at this dose.[28,29] The incidence of a cardiovascular event is not associated with duration of OC use.[30] There is no increased risk of cardiovascular morbidity among past-users of OCs.[31] Most of the studies that have shown an increased risk of myocardial infarction have been observational studies in which the women at risk for myocardial infarction (MI) also had other risk factors that cause arterial narrowing, such as preexisting hypercholesterolemia, hypertension, diabetes mellitus, or smoking more than 15 cigarettes per day. Smoking is clearly thrombogenic in and of itself,[32] and smoking is an independent risk factor for MI.[28] It appears, however, that the use of low-does oral contraceptives by heavy cigarette smokers significantly enhances their risk of experiencing an MI because these two factors act synergistically.[28] Prior oral contraceptive use in a smoker and prior smoking in an oral contraceptive user does not seem to be associated with an increased risk of MI. Both the Royal College and the WHO studies report that the risk of MI in oral contraceptive users was severalfold greater if they had hypertension than if they did not. Two large case control studies in the United States have shown no significantly increased risk of MI in oral contraceptive users.[29,33] A recent WHO technical report stated that women who do not smoke and have their blood pressure checked and who do not have hypertension or diabetes have no increased risk of MI if they use combined oral contraceptives, regardless of their age.[34]

Exogenous estrogen does increase the synthesis of several coagulation factors that promote thrombosis in a dose-dependent manner. The small increased risk of VTE exists in all women using combined oral contraceptives (COCs). The risk of MI or stroke in nonsmoking, normotensive women is not increased with COC users. However, in women with preexisting medical problems, the risk of thrombosis may be further increased by simultaneous use of combined hormonal contraceptives. The potential risk of stroke with combined hormonal contraceptives is even more difficult to assess than the risk of MI or DVT. Early studies in the 1970s of higher dose (50 μg) combined hormonal contraceptives did suggest a potential relationship between this dose of pill and stroke. However, even these data were conflicting. Data on early formulations of pills do not apply to the contemporary pills. Women without other risk factors do not appear to have an increased risk of stroke while on oral contraceptive pills.[35,36] The safety of pills with doses under 35 μg of estrogen in women who smoke or have other thrombogenic medical problems, such as hypertension, is not known because women with these risk factors are rarely on combined hormonal contraceptives today.

Other Metabolic Effects

Although combined hormonal contraceptives do have metabolic effects that are detected at the laboratory level, such effects are very rarely associated with statistically significant or concerning outcomes. Table 34-4 shows the chemical and clinical effects that estrogens and progestins have on the human metabolic system.

Mood Changes

The 19-nortestosterone derivatives do have central nervous system effects and estrogen does as well. It was postulated that high doses of synthetic estrogens would replace changes in luteal depression. No study to date has demonstrated an increase in depression due to estrogen at the dosing currently used in combined oral contraceptives.[37,38] However, the progestin component may be associated with an increase in irritability, fatigue, and depression.

Hepatic Proteins

Synthetic estrogens in oral contraceptives cause an increase in hepatic production of several proteins and these include sex hormone–binding globulin (SHBG) and

TABLE 34-4

Metabolic Effect of Contraceptive Steroids

Steroid	Chemical Effects	Clinical Effects
Estrogen: Ethinyl Estradiol		
Proteins		
Albumin	↓	None
Amino acids	↓	None
Globulins	↑	
Angiotensinogen		↑ Blood pressure
Clotting factors		Hypercoagulability
Carrier proteins (CBG, SHBG, TBG, transferrin, ceruloplasmin)		None
Carbohydrate		
Plasma insulin	↑	None
Glucose tolerance	↓	None
Lipids		
Cholesterol	↑	None
Triglyceride	↑	None
HDL cholesterol	↑	? ↓ Cardiovascular disease
LDL cholesterol	↓	? ↓ Cardiovascular disease
Electrolytes		
Sodium excretion	↓	Fluid retention
		Edema
Vitamins		
Vitamin B complex	↓	None
Ascorbic acid (vitamin C)	↓	None
Vitamin A	↑	None
Other		
Breast	↑	Breast tenderness
Endometrial steroid receptors	↑	Endometrial hyperplasia
Skin	↓	↓ Sebum production
		↑ Facial pigmentation
Progestins: 19-Nortestosterone Derivatives		
Proteins (SHBG)	↓	None
Carbohydrate		
Plasma insulin	↑	None
Glucose tolerance	↓	None
Lipids		
Cholesterol	↓	None
Triglyceride	↓	None
HDL cholesterol	↓	? ↑ Cardiovascular disease
LDL cholesterol	↑	? ↑ Cardiovascular disease
Other		
Nitrogen retention	↑	↑ Body weight
Skin—sebum production	↑	↑ Acne
CNS effects	↑	Nervousness, fatigue, depression
Endometrial steroid receptors	↓	No withdrawal bleeding

↑, increases; ↓, decreases; ?, questionable; CBG, corticosteroid-binding globulin; CNS, central nervous system; HDL, high-density lipoprotein; LDL, low density lipoprotein; SHBG, sex hormone–binding globulin; TBG, thyroid-binding globulin.

globulins that are part of the coagulation cascade, such as factors V, VIII, and X and fibrinogen.[39] Progesterone and progestins decrease the synthesis of SHBG. The balance between these effects make one pill more appropriate for, for example, a woman with hyperandrogenicity due to polycystic ovary syndrome over another.

Increased angiotensin may be the mechanism by which blood pressure can become elevated.[40] This seems to be an estrogen-driven effect, because there an increase in mean blood pressure in women who ingest oral contraceptive pills levels, but this is lower in women who ingest formulations with 30 to 35 μg of ethinyl estradiol. Women who use oral contraceptive pills are slightly more likely to develop hypertension and about 0.4% of current low-dose oral contraceptive users became hypertensive in one study. Women who receive progestins without an estrogen component do not have an increase in blood pressure over time.[40]

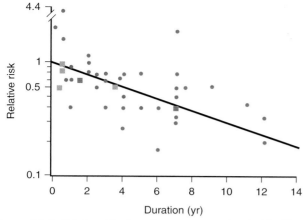

Figure 34-4. Relative risk of ovarian cancer associated with different durations of oral contraceptive use: Findings of 15 studies. Study categories, indicating category weights ranging from smallest (weight in bottom 25% of range) to largest (weight in top 25% of range): tan squares, 1 (smallest); blue squares, 2; purple dots, 3; green dots, 4 (largest). (From Hankinson SE, Colditz CA, Hunter DJ, et al. A quantitative assessment of oral contraceptive use and risk of ovarian cancer. Obstet Gynecol 80:708-714, 1992.)

Oral Contraceptives and Malignancies

Given the extensive history now of oral contraceptive pills and our ability to follow populations of women who used these pharmaceuticals in their reproductive years, both prospective cohort and retrospective case control designs have been used to assess the relationship between OCs and cancer risk. In general, hormones are considered promoters but not initiators of cancer, so the oncologic effects, if any, of steroids should be seen as a dose response and may or may not be related to duration of use.

A study examining cancer incidence in relation to OC use in the Oxford Family Planning Association contraceptive study included 17,032 women recruited at family planning clinics at ages 25 to 39 years between 1968 and 1974, who were using OCs, a diaphragm, or an intrauterine device. Breast cancer findings (844 cases) were very reassuring (relative risk ratio [RR] comparing women ever using OCs with those never doing so 1.0, 95% confidence interval [CI] 0.8-1.1). There was a strong positive relationship between cervical cancer incidence (59 cases) and duration of OC use (RR comparing users for 97+ months with nonusers 6.1, 95% CI 2.5-17.9). Uterine body cancer (77 cases) and ovarian cancer (106 cases) showed strong negative associations with duration of OC use: RRs for 97+ months of use were 0.1 (95% CI 0-0.4) and 0.3 (95% CI 0.1-0.5), respectively. This apparent protective effect for both cancers persisted more than 20 years after stopping OCs.[41]

Ovarian Cancer and Benign Ovarian Neoplasms

Over 20 reports of oral contraceptives and the subsequent evolvement of ovarian cancer have been published. Eighteen of these have found a reduction in risk in the most common of epithelial ovarian cancers (Fig. 34-4).

The magnitude of the risk reduction appears to be linked to the duration of time of use of the oral contraceptive pill.[42] A large case control study has demonstrated that not only is the duration of oral contraceptive use related to the protective effect, but that this risk reduction lasts for years after the cessation of oral contraceptive use.[41] Oral contraceptives appear to also significantly reduce the incidence of benign ovarian neoplasms, including serous and mucinous cystadenomas, benign cystic teratomas, fibromas, and endometriomas.[43] Endometrial cancer has similarly been well studied in relation to oral contraceptive use. Twelve retrospective studies have suggested an association between oral contraceptive use and endometrial cancer risk reduction.[44] One study has shown that oral contraceptive users have one third the risk of endometrial cancers as nonusers and this likewise persists after cessation of use, and the duration of oral contraceptive use seems to correlate with the amount of risk reduction found.

Cervical Cancer

To date, epidemiologic data is conflicting with regard to a correlation between oral contraceptive use and invasive cervical cancer. There are multiple important confounding factors that include the use, for example, of barrier contraceptives for women who do not use oral contraceptive pills and the fact that barrier contraceptives are protective against sexually transmitted infections including the human papillomavirus (HPV). It is also possible that women who are oral contraceptive users obtain more frequent Pap tests (cervical cancer screening) than do women who are not oral contraceptive pill users. There have been studies of women who use oral contraceptives that demonstrate an increased risk of cervical cancer.[45] Long-term oral contraceptive use may have a promotional effect upon the carcinogenic action of HPV. In one study, OCs increased the risk of cervical cancer only in women infected with HPV, not women without HPV.[46] However, it is well known that HPV is necessary but not sufficient for the development of cervical cancer. Case-control studies have reported that there is an increased risk of adenocarcinoma of the cervix among OC users when compared to nonusers. This risk appears to increase with duration of use.[47]

Breast Cancer

Multiple studies have tried to address the concern that estrogen might stimulate the growth of neoplastic breast tissue. One study of over 53,000[48] women did show that there is a slightly increased risk (RR 1.24, 95% CI 1.15-1.3) of women who are actively using oral contraceptives developing breast cancer. This association appears to decline after stopping OCs and was no longer present after 10 years of use. These cancers appear to be less advanced clinically than the cancers that occur in non-OC users. It is possible that breast cancer is diagnosed earlier in OC users than in nonusers, but this could also be due to a biologic effect of the OCs in terms of tumor promotion. New data demonstrate that OCs do not further increase risk for women with a family history of breast cancer and may be associated with a reduction in risk of breast cancer.[49,50]

Novel Delivery Systems

Newer delivery systems have been developed in attempt to address some of the compliance issues associated with daily pill taking. The systems include the transdermal patch, contraceptive vaginal rings, injectables, and intra-uterine contraception.

TRANSDERMAL CONTRACEPTIVE SYSTEM

Approved for use in the United States in 2001, the trans-dermal contraceptive system (TCS) consists of a 20-cm², beige-colored, three-layered matrix patch that releases 150 µg of norelgestromin (the active metabolite of norgesti-mate) and 20 µg of ethinyl estradiol at a constant rate each day into the systemic circulation.[51] The three layers of the thin matrix consist of an outer protective layer of polyester, a medicated adhesive middle layer, and a polyester inner liner that is removed just prior to application to the skin.

Circulating blood levels of each steroid remain relatively constant during the 7 days the patch is scheduled to be in place, as well as for an additional 2 days, in contrast to the peaks and troughs that occur after ingestion of an oral contraceptive pill[52] (Figs. 34-5 and 34-6). In a pharma-cokinetic study,[51] steady-state conditions of each steroid were achieved in the serum of women using the patch for three cycles. Steady-state serum concentrations increased only slightly from the first week of the first treatment cy-cle until the third week of the third treatment cycle, in-dicating minimal accumulation. The circulating levels of norelgestromin are sufficient to inhibit ovulation while the patch is in place.

The patches are applied to the skin of either the abdo-men, buttocks, upper arm, or upper torso (except for the breasts) for 1 week and then removed. A patch is applied to a different site for 3 consecutive weeks; no patch is ap-plied during the fourth week to allow withdrawal bleeding to occur. Withdrawal bleeding similar in duration to that which occurs with OC use usually begins 2 to 3 days after the last patch is removed.

Contraceptive effectiveness of the TCS is similar to that for OCs. In a pooled analysis from three large clinical studies, the overall pregnancy rate from more than 22,000 treatment cycles was 0.88 pregnancies per 100 woman-years.[53] In these studies the pregnancies were uniformly distributed among the 3236 subjects with body weight less than 198 pounds, but five pregnancies occurred among the 83 subjects weighing 198 pounds or more. Thus, the TCS appears to have a lower level of effectiveness in women with body weight of 198 pounds or more.

A randomized trial demonstrated that the incidence of perfect compliance with the TCS, 88.2% of cycles, was significantly better than with the OC, 77.7% of cycles.[54] The convenient dosing schedule of the patch likely en-hances compliance and may result in greater effectiveness than the OC in actual use. In the clinical trials during which 70,552 patches were worn, the rate of replacement for complete detachment of the patch was 1.8%, and for partial detachment was 2.9%.[55] Various conditions of exercise, heat, and humidity did not increase the inci-dence of detachment or the force required to remove the patch.[56]

Adverse effects were analyzed in the comparative study with the OC. The patch had a higher incidence of inter-menstrual spotting and breast tenderness than the OC in the first two cycles of use but not thereafter.[54] About 20% of women using the TCS noted intermenstrual spotting and breast discomfort in the first cycle of use. Applica-tion site reaction also occurred in 20% of the subjects us-ing the TCS. Other adverse effects, such as headache and

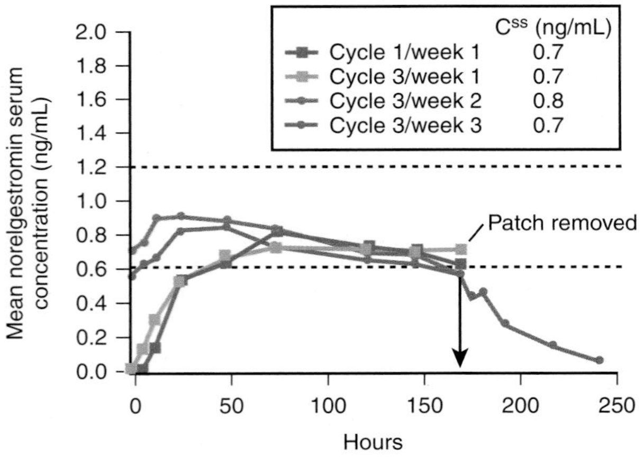

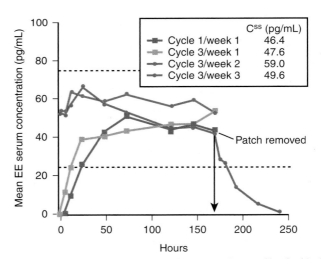

Figure 34-5. *Mean serum concentration-versus-time profile of norel-gestromin after patch application on the buttock for three consecutive cycles. Dashed horizontal lines indicate the reference range. C^{ss}, steady-state concentrations. (From Abrams LS, Skee DM, Natarajan J, et al. Multiple-dose pharmacokinetics of a contraceptive patch in healthy women participants. Contraception 64:287-294, 2001.)*

Figure 34-6. *Mean serum concentration-versus-time profile of ethinyl estradiol (EE) after patch application on the buttock for three consecutive cycles. Dashed horizontal lines indicate the reference range. C^{ss}, steady-state concentrations. (From Abrams LS, Skee DM, Natarajan J, et al. Multiple-dose pharmacokinetics of a contraceptive patch in healthy women participants. Contraception 64:287-294, 2001.)*

nausea, were similar with these two methods of steroid contraception.[54] Thus, the TCS is an effective reversible alternative method of steroid contraceptive.

Venous Thromboembolism Risk

In 2006 the U.S. product labeling for the TCS was revised to include a warning that the TCS provides a higher steady-state concentration of ethinyl estradiol than OCs and lower peak concentrations. Pharmacokinetic studies reveal that steady-state levels are approximately 60% higher than an OC containing 35 μg of ethinyl estradiol while the peak concentration on the TCS is 25% less than that in women taking OCs (Ortho Evra [norelgestromin/ethinyl estradiol transdermal system], Raritan, NJ; Ortho-McNeil Pharmaceuticals, Inc, 2006).

It is not clear whether this difference in pharmacokinetics translates to a change in the risk of serious adverse events, such as venous thromboembolism. Two studies on this subject have been reported to date. The first was a case-control study with data abstracted from a managed-care database; 68 new cases of idiopathic VTE in TCS users were identified, and when compared to control subjects, the odds ratio (OR) was 0.9 (95% CI 0.5-1.6), demonstrating a similar risk for both methods.[57] A second study performed from insurance claim outcomes from a major national health insurer reported a more than twofold increase in the VTE rate (adjusted incidence rate ratio 2.2, 95% CI 1.3-3.8) among TCS users compared to norgestimate-containing OC users. Acute myocardial infarction and ischemic stroke were also investigated in this study, but each had too few outcomes to provide conclusive results.[58] Although the two studies are discrepant, until more definitive data is known, the possible increased risk of VTE on TCS needs to be considered when counseling individual patients regarding their contraceptive options. The counselor should keep in mind that the risk of VTE on either TCS or OCs remains lower than the risk of VTE during pregnancy, and if the patient and health care provider believe that the TCS is the best way to prevent pregnancy, it use is certainly warranted.

Continuous Regimens/Extended Use

The TCS had also been studied to evaluate for extended use to delay or prevent menses. A study performed to evaluate the bleeding profile and satisfaction on a continuous regimen compared 158 women using an extended regimen (weekly application for 12 weeks, followed by 1 week off, then 3 more weeks) to 81 women using the usual cyclic regimen (weekly application for 3 weeks followed by 1 week off, continued for four cycles). Extended use resulted in fewer bleeding days overall, with delayed median time to bleeding of 54 days. Women were equally satisfied with both regimens.[59]

CONTRACEPTIVE VAGINAL RING

The vaginal contraceptive ring contains ethinyl vinyl acetate that releases ethinyl estradiol and the third-generation progestin, etonorgestrel. The ring currently on the market has an outer diameter of 54 mm and a cross-sectional diameter of 4 mm. It was approved by the FDA in 2001. The vaginal contraceptive ring is highly efficacious with a Pearl Index of 1.18 and an efficacy of 99.1%. The vaginal ring is a flexible, soft device and is available in one size only and does not need to be fitted. If desired, the ring can be removed for up to 3 hours without altering the contraceptive effectiveness. In a review of 12 randomized controlled trials comparing the contraceptive vaginal ring and combined oral contraceptives, both forms achieved the same contraceptive efficacy and adequate ovarian suppression with comparable incidence of adverse effects, such as breast tenderness, headache, and nausea. Vaginal administration was associated with higher local adverse events such as leukorrhea, vaginal discomfort, vaginitis, foreign body sensation, expulsions, and coital problems, leading to higher discontinuation rates. Overall, both contraceptives improved overall sexual function and were highly acceptable. Advantages to the ring included lower systemic estradiol exposure (50% compared to a 30-μg ethinyl estradiol pill) with a lower incidence of irregular bleeding and spotting.[60]

INJECTABLE CONTRACEPTIVES

Injectable contraceptives are used throughout the world. These include depo-medroxyprogesterone acetate (DMPA), norethisterone enanthate (NET-EN), and combined injectable contraceptives of different combinations of estrogens and progestins that are given monthly. DMPA is the only currently available injectable contraceptive in the United States. It is used by approximately 3% of women of reproductive age.

Medroxyprogesterone Acetate

Medroxyprogesterone acetate (MPA) is a 17-acetoxyprogesterone compound. Unlike most other synthetic progestins, MPA is structurally most closely related to progesterone, instead of testosterone, and possesses less androgenic activity. MPA is rapidly metabolized in humans to progesterone. The 3-month injectable dosage is 150 mg. The drug is delivered by intramuscular injection into the deltoid or gluteus muscle and is released slowly into the circulation.

MPA is an extremely effective contraceptive with a 1-year pregnancy rate of 0.1% and a 2-year accumulative pregnancy rate of 0.4%. Its primary mechanism of contraceptive action is ovulation inhibition, but it works by increasing the cervical mucus viscosity and creating progestational changes in the endometrium as well.

Mechanisms of Action

With consistent use, DMPA is highly effective, with a failure rate of approximately 0.4% per WHO clinical trial.[61] DMPA requires re-dosing every 3 months intramuscularly. The contraceptive levels are maintained for at least 14 weeks and may be metabolized differently in different women. There is a margin of safety built into the dosing regimen of intramuscular DMPA. Unlike other lower dose progestin-only methods, DMPA works primarily by blocking the LH surge and ovulation. FSH is not systematically suppressed with progestin-only methods. In addition to LH blockade, the progestin-dominant hormonal milieu results in thickening of the cervical mucus and alteration of the endometrium. Estrogen levels are comparable to those in early follicular phase of noncontracepting women. Because of this, symptoms of estrogen deficiency, such as vasomotor symptoms or vaginal atrophy, are not present with this method of contraception. In order to obtain suppression of ovulation in the initial injection cycle, DMPA must be administered within several days after the onset of menses.[62] Studies show that if DMPA is administered as late as 9 days after the onset of menses, 2 out of 13 women showed evidence of ovulation.[63] It is recommended in the package labeling that the first dose be given within the first 5 days of the onset of menses and evidence supports giving DMPA no later than 7 days after the onset of menses.

Pharmacokinetics

DMPA is effective within 20 minutes of IM injection.[64] Effective blood levels are found at greater than 0.5 ng/mL and this occurs within 24 hours after injection. MPA appears to be cleared slightly differently depending on the assay used in the study. MPA levels plateau at about 1 to 1.5 ng/mL and remain at that level for approximately 3 months, after which they begin to decline. In some subjects it appears that MPA levels remain detectable in the circulation for 7 to 9 months after initial injection. Estradiol levels in these subjects are found to be in the range of the early follicular phase during these times. However, other studies demonstrated that MPA levels decreased to less than 0.5 ng/mL after 4 to 6 months of use and one study demonstrated a decrease in circulating levels at 13 weeks of use.[65]

The pharmacodynamics of MPA may be variable based on individual metabolism or based on the study assay used, and further studies are needed to improve our understanding of this. However, no study has shown metabolic clearance of therapeutic levels of the drug before 12 weeks after the initial dose, and this supports the current product labeling.

Return to Fertility

The lag time in the clearing of MPA from the circulation results in delayed resumption of ovulation for women in the population.[66] This quality is a by-product of the injectable delivery system. Women who use MPA should be counseled that there will be a delay in the resumption of fertility. This, however, is not a permanent effect. Ninety percent of MPA users become pregnant by 18 months after the last injection.

Disadvantages of MPA Use

Women who use MPA will experience unscheduled bleeding during the early months of use. Perhaps most important, women who experience breakthrough bleeding on MPA should be reassured that this is a well-understood side effect of use of MPA. Weight changes are another disadvantage of MPA use. Other studies have shown longitudinally

that MPA users may gain between 1.5 and 4 kg in the first year of use.[67] The weight gain associated with MPA may also have some individual risk factors such as tendency to gain weight and ethnic background. One study demonstrated a statistically significant increase in weight gain among Navajo women randomized to MPA versus combined hormonal contraceptives. The metabolic effects of MPA on body weight are unclear, and weight and exercise should be evaluated in all women who are concerned about weight gain on MPA before the method is discontinued.

There have been no randomized control trials to assess the effects of DMPA on mood. There have, however, been several observational studies that demonstrate that the clinically significant difference in mood is rare with MPA.[68]

Headaches are the most common reason cited for discontinuation of MPA in the first year. However, only 2.3% of MPA users discontinue in the first year due to headaches.[69] There is no conclusive evidence to suggest that the use of DMPA increases the severity of tension of migraine headaches and the presence of headaches is not a contraindication to initiation or continuation of MPA use. However, if women find that their headache incidence increases while on this method, counseling regarding the benefits of perhaps changing to another method should be initiated.

Metabolic Effects of DMPA

DMPA does not increase liver production of proteins as the estrogen component of combined hormonal contraception does. Therefore, there is no evidence to suggest that clotting factors are increased with DMPA use. A WHO study also reported that blood pressure measurements are unchanged with DMPA users over 2 years.[69] Injectable progestins do not appear to be associated with increased risk of VTE, MI, or stroke. This makes DMPA a very desirable method of contraception in women with co-morbidities, in an aging cohort, or in potentially obese women because these women may all have other risk factors for venous or arterial thromboembolic events.

Bone Mineral Density

The FDA recently placed a black box warning on MPA labeling which stated that MPA has been shown to be associated with a decrease in bone mineral density in women with long-term use. Many studies have demonstrated that bone mineral density is decreased in women on MPA.[70-72] No studies, however, demonstrated that MPA users are at increased risk of fracture.[71,73] Furthermore, the use of a DEXA (dual energy x-ray absorptiometry) scan, the test used to asses bone mineral density, may not be a valid test in the premenopausal population. Studies also suggest that the loss in bone density is likely to be entirely reversible with discontinuation of MPA. This biologic effect of a progestin-dominant hormonal milieu on bone mineral density can be likened to that of a breastfeeding woman, who also will experience a transient loss in bone mineral density while breastfeeding which appears to be reversible after breastfeeding is discontinued. For women who do well on MPA as their long-term contraceptive method, we encourage continued use for the duration of time that contraception is required.

We do not recommend discontinuing the use of MPA based on concerns of bone mineral density alone. Women and adolescents who use MPA for contraception or control of menorrhagia should be encouraged to have a calcium-rich diet, or perhaps to supplement with calcium if necessary during this time. DEXA scan should not be used routinely in women who are using DMPA for contraception.

Recommendations for Initiating MPA Use

Women should be counseled about the importance of repeat dosing every 3 months of MPA, as well as about the primary side effect experience: abnormal bleeding for the first one to two injections followed by a high likelihood of amenorrhea. If these bleeding patterns are acceptable to the patient, then MPA is a reasonable method. Women who are cycling can be dosed within the first 5 days of the onset of their menses and do not require backup contraception after this point. Women can also receive MPA within the first 5 days postpartum. MPA can be used immediately after abortion or miscarriage. Women who are using lactational amenorrhea as their contraceptive method can institute MPA at any time so long as hCG value is negative. For a woman seeking a repeat dose of DMPA beyond the 13–week period, if she is still amenorrheic and her hCG value is negative, it is appropriate to redose at this time. Concerns about new pregnancy should always be balanced with the understanding that pregnancies that have occurred with DMPA during DMPA use have not demonstrated any evidence of increase risk of teratogenicity in this population or on adverse pregnancy outcomes.

Injectable progestin-only contraceptives inhibit the secretion of gonadotropins and thereby suppress ovarian estrogens. There are several recent studies that show trends toward decreased bone mineral density with the use of DMPA, but it is unclear if this decrease is associated with fracture risk. Two recent meta-analyses highlight the need for further research on the long-term consequences of DMPA. Recent studies reveal that bone loss during progestin-only contraceptive use is completely recovered several years after the cessation of use.[74,75]

COMBINED ESTROGEN-PROGESTIN INJECTABLE CONTRACEPTION

A combined method of injectable contraception is no longer on the U.S. market. However, in other parts of the world this method is available and it is a highly discreet method of contraception. Because of the combined estrogen and progestin in the injectable formulation, the bleeding irregularities that are associated with progestin-only injection (DMPA) are not experienced with this combined method. Progestin and estrogen combined injectables contain a low dose of a long-acting progestin and a low dose of an estradiol. The most widely used method contains 17α-hydroxyprogesterone caproate (250 mg) and estradiol valerate (5 mg). This is a commonly used method in Asia and in Latin America. Previously in the United States, a combined injection of medroxyprogesterone acetate, 25 mg, and estradiol cypionate (E_2C), 5 mg, was available under the name Lunelle, but this is not currently the case.

MPA-E_2C is a well-tolerated method of contraception with a reasonable side effect profile.[76] The amount of pregnancy data is sparse owing to the short amount of time that it was on the market. However, in clinical trials, no pregnancies occurred in 782 women over 8008 cycles.[77] Side effects and clinical effects of the injectable combined hormonal contraceptive are similar to those of oral contraceptive pills.

PROGESTIN-ONLY IMPLANT SYSTEM

Norplant is a sustained release progestin-only system that consists of six capsules, each measuring 34 mm in length, with a 2.4 mm outer diameter. Each capsule contains 36 mg of levonorgestrel for a total of 216 mg of steroid hormone that remains unchanged within capsules over 9 years of use. Norplant is no longer available on the U.S. market. However, it is widely used in other parts of the world. Implanon is a new progestin-only method that contains 68 mg of 3-ketodesogestrel (etonogestrel) within a single 4-cm flexible rod. Subdermal implants were approved by the FDA in 1990. The major mechanism of action of subdermal implants is ovulation inhibition via inhibition of luteinizing hormone.[67,78] Insertion is accomplished in the outpatient setting. The capsules are implanted in the subcutaneous tissue through a trocar that is enclosed in the contraceptive implant kit. Local anesthetic is sufficient and the entire procedure takes approximately 5 minutes. As with all progestin-only methods, the cervical mucus is thickened and the endometrial lining becomes decidualized. The effects on the endometrial lining produce the clinical symptoms of initial irregular unscheduled bleeding, followed by scant bleeding or amenorrhea.[78,79]

Amenorrhea rates with Implanon in clinical trials run about 50% of women. Frequent and prolonged bleeding occurred in 20%.[78,79] In one multicenter study in Europe and Canada, the discontinuation of this method for abnormal bleeding reached a rate of 23% within the first 2 years of use.[80] However, in a comparative study of the single implant (Implanon) with the six capsules of levonorgestrel (Norplant), there were fewer bleeding episodes and less blood loss per episode with the single implant. The most common adverse effects with the implant were acne, breast pain, headache, and weight gain.[79] The etonogestrel implant (Implanon) lasts for 3 years. It releases 60 to 70 mg of etonogestrel per day and this gradually decreases over time.[81] Levels of etonogestrel in the serum are therapeutic within 8 hours of insertion. In clinical use, etonogestrel implant (Implanon) can be inserted within 5 days of the onset of the menstrual cycle in a cycling woman and in the setting of a negative hCG in a noncycling woman. Etonogestrel implant has not yet been FDA approved for postpartum use; however, it is approved for use immediately after miscarriage and after abortion.

POSTCOITAL CONTRACEPTION

Postcoital contraception, also known as emergency contraception or the morning-after pill, is the use of a contraceptive method after a single unprotected act of intercourse. For women who have had known unprotected intercourse, meaning they were not using a primary method of contraception or in whom a barrier method may have failed, postcoital contraception provides a second opportunity to decrease the risk of pregnancy from a midcycle act of intercourse. Both the ParaGard IUD and hormonal methods can be used to effect postcoital contraception. The original methods of emergency or postcoital contraception were developed by using high doses of estrogen compounds. Examples of such compounds include diethylstilbestrol 25 to 50 mg/day, ethinyl estradiol 5 mg/day, on conjugated estrogens 30 mg/day. With these compounds, treatment was continued for 5 days. If treatment was initiated within 72 hours of an isolated midcycle act of intercourse, the efficacy is estimated at 75%.[82] If more than one act of intercourse has occurred, or if the treatment is delayed, the efficacy is decreased.

The side effects associated with these high doses of estrogenic compounds led to the development of the first alternative approach, tested in Canada in the 1970s, known as the Yuzpe method. This is a combination oral contraceptive method of postcoital contraception that initially consists of using the Ovral oral contraceptive pill, four tablets of ethanyl estradiol (0.05 mg) and DL-norgestrel (0.5 mg). These are given in two doses, 12 hours apart. Studies[83,84] demonstrated that this regimen had a similar degree of efficacy and decreased adverse side effects when compared with the 5-day estrogen regimens. The FDA approved a dedicated product that is a combined method of estrogen and progestins called Preven. This method, however, is no longer on the American market. In recent times, progestin-only methods of postcoital contraception have been developed and one is now available in the dedicated product called Plan B. Plan B consists of two tablets of 0.75 mg of levonorgestrel. The product labeling indicates that the pills should be taken at time zero (the first) and 12 hours later (the second). Pooled data from studies on the Yuzpe method from 1977 until 1993, that include 5226 women treated with the Yuzpe method, demonstrated a failure rate of about 1.5%.[82] Demographers estimated that the Yuzpe regimen prevents about 75% of expected pregnancies when used within 72 hours of unprotected intercourse.

The use of levonorgestrel alone has been compared directly to levonorgestrel plus estradiol in a randomized control trial.[83] Failure rates (about 2%) were similar when these two regimens were ingested within 48 hours of unprotected intercourse. Substantially less nausea and vomiting was noted with the levonorgestrel-alone method.[84,85] Because of the comparable efficacy and improved side effect profile, when available, progestin-only methods of postcoital contraception are now preferable. A randomized control trial performed by the WHO[84] that included 2000 women in 21 centers evaluated the efficacy of levonorgestrel alone within 72 hours after a single act of unprotected intercourse. In this trial, there was a 1.1% pregnancy rate and this was actually more effective than the Yuzpe method it was compared to, which had a 3.2% pregnancy rate. The calculated estimates by the authors demonstrated that 85% of pregnancies were prevented compared to 57% of pregnancies prevented with the combined regimen. Again, less nausea and vomiting were demonstrated with levonorgestrel alone. Effectiveness is greatest with any method of

postcoital contraception when it is given within 24 hours of sexual intercourse than in the subsequent 48 hours.

Randomized trials have shown that taking both the 0.75 mg tablets of levonorgestrel at once offers the same efficacy as taking them 12 hours apart without increasing side effects.[86,87] In addition, original studies all tested the efficacy of emergency contraceptive regimens within 72 hours of unprotected intercourse. More recent studies have demonstrated efficacy up to 120 hours after intercourse.[86,88] The efficacy does, however, decline with increasing time from the unprotected intercourse event. Patients should thus be counseled that emergency contraception can be taken within 120 hours of unprotected intercourse but that it is a time-sensitive drug and the maximum efficacy is yielded when the method is used as early as possible.

Advance prescription or advance supply of Plan B has been shown to increase use among various populations including adolescents and has not been shown to decrease use of the primary method of contraception, either condoms or hormonal contraception.[89] Advance prescription of Plan B should be the standard of care given its potential to help prevent unintended pregnancy as a backup method. No adverse effects in terms of increased risk taking or decreased contraceptive use have been noted in multiple studies. In the United States, Plan B was recently made available over the counter for women above the age of 18. There is no reason to suspect that levonorgestrel is unsafe for woman younger than the age of 18, and because of the increased difficulty for teens, who are at particularly high risk of unintended pregnancy, advance prescription of this should be encouraged for all young women using barrier method contraception or daily methods of contraception. Reproductive health care providers should discuss the availability of postcoital contraception with all their patients who are seeking pregnancy prevention. Its use may be necessary in women who are not using long-term methods of contraception, such as an intrauterine device (IUD), an implant, or sterilization.

The exact mode of action of emergency contraception has not yet been established. Initially it was thought that the estrogen and progestin combination alter the endometrium to prevent implantation of the fertilized egg.[90,91] More recent studies, however, have suggested that emergency contraception may work through delaying ovulation, or, if taken post ovulation, through the interference of egg or transport or through impairment of corpus luteum function.[92,93] However, the type of data to support any single mechanism of action with postcoital contraception is poor at this point, and it may be a combination of effects that lead to the efficacy of this method.

Several studies have found that the insertion of a copper IUD within 5 to 10 days of midcycle unprotected intercourse is an effective method to prevent pregnancy.[94,95] One study included nine different trials involving almost 900 women who had received an IUD in the postcoital midcycle. Only one pregnancy occurred in this population, giving a pregnancy rate of 0.1%. Thus, based on studies to date, the insertion of a copper IUD is the most effective method of postcoital contraception. This method can be effective up to 10 days after unprotected midcycle intercourse safely. It is a good option for women who also desire an IUD for long-term contraception after this initial unprotected intercourse event.

Intrauterine Contraception

Intrauterine contraception is the most widely used method of reversible birth control globally. Benefits of IUDs include a high level of effectiveness, lack of associated systemic metabolic effects, and the need for only a single act of motivation for long-term use, as well as its ability to be used over several years. Although IUDs are a prevalent contraceptive method globally, less than 1% of married couples of reproductive age use IUDs in the United States.

TYPES OF INTRAUTERINE CONTRACEPTION

Currently there are two intrauterine contraceptives available on the United States market: The copper ParaGard IUD and the levonorgestrel-containing Mirena intrauterine system. Over the past 35 years, however, many intrauterine contraceptives have been designed and used clinically throughout the world. The design of IUDs has evolved since their original use in the 1960s. IUDs were initially developed in the 1980s as T-shaped plastic devices covered with copper wire. The amount of copper in the IUD accounts for the length of time of efficacy. Each IUD does have a certain rate of copper dissolution, which accounts for its need to be replaced over time. In the United States, the T380A IUD is the only copper-bearing IUD. The multi-load CU375 is widely used in Europe. The T380A has a frame of polyethylene with a vertical length of 36 mm and a horizontal length of 32 mm. The exposed surface area of copper is 380 mm², hence its name. The amount of copper dissolution daily amounts to less than what the ingested amount of copper is in the normal diet. The copper T380A is currently approved in the United States for 10 years, but evidence has shown that it is effective for up to at least 12 years.[96] All copper-containing IUDs have a number as a part of their name and this indicates the surface area of copper that the IUD provides.

Copper Intrauterine Devices

Copper T IUDs have failure rates of less than 1% per year and cumulative 10-year failure rates of approximately 2% to 6%. A large WHO trial[96] reported a cumulative 12-year failure rate of 2.2% for the T380A (ParaGard). This is an average of 0.18% per year over 12 years of use. This failure rate is equivalent to the failure rate seen with female sterilization methods. The mechanism of action is not fully understood for the copper IUD. The presence of in intrauterine device has been shown to prompt the release of leukocytes and prostaglandins by the endometrium.[97] This creates a hostile milieu to both sperm and eggs. The presence of copper increases the spermicidal effect.

Hormonal Intrauterine Devices

A reservoir of progestin in the vertical arm of the T-shaped IUD increases its efficacy. The progestin-releasing IUD was marketed initially as a 1-year device but is no longer manufactured. Currently, a T-shaped IUD containing a levonorgestrel in the vertical arm has been developed and has undergone extensive clinical testing. It is available in the United States and other countries as the levonorgestrel intrauterine system (LNG-IUS), or Mirena. A large comparative trial of the copper T380A and the levonorgestrel-releasing IUD found that the efficacy of the two methods is similar, as are the continuation rates. The LNG-IUS measures 32 mm both horizontally and vertically. It is made with a silicone reservoir containing 52 mg of levonorgestrel in the vertical stem. There is an initial burst release of levonorgestrel of 20 μg/day, resulting in plasma levels of 150 to 200 pg/mL.[98] The plasma concentrations of levonorgestrel decrease over the number of years it is used. There is sufficient levonorgestrel in the intrauterine system to last for the estimated duration of 5 years.[99] The levonorgestrel-releasing intrauterine system produces high concentrations of progestins in the endometrium. The progestin-dominant effect allows the endometrium to remain thin and not proliferate. In addition to the contraceptive efficacy that is obtained, bleeding patterns change. Approximately 20% of women who use this device become amenorrheic at 1 year.[99]

The mechanism of action of the levonorgestrel intrauterine system is slightly better understood than is that of the copper intrauterine device. The LNG-IUS works primarily by changing the endometrial lining and thickening the cervical mucus. This thick cervical mucus obstructs the passage of sperm through the cervix. The foreign body reaction also makes the environment hostile to sperm and eggs. The frequency of ovulation is reduced with the LNG-IUS overall. However, this is not the primary mechanism of action. Women may ovulate variably with the LNG-IUS in place. All the effects that render both intrauterine contraceptives effective are reversed promptly upon their removal.

Resumption of fertility seems to occur at the same rate as discontinuation of barrier methods of contraception. The incidence of varied pregnancy outcomes including term delivery, spontaneous abortion, and ectopic pregnancies after IUD removal is unchanged from the baseline incidence of these events in the population.

CONSIDERATIONS FOR IUD PLACEMENT

Considerations that should be reviewed with patients before IUD placement include the appropriateness of the patient's candidacy, the timing of insertion, the bleeding patterns to be expected, the adverse effects of the method, and the expected interval of use. Appropriate candidates for the IUD include all women who desire long-term contraception. This is one of the primary benefits of this method. There are few contraindications to IUD placement. It is important to assess on physical examination the woman's uterus for the possibility of distorting anatomy due to fibroids or any anatomic defects. IUDs are appropriate for nulliparous women as they are for any woman who is seeking long-term contraception. It has been widely considered that menses is the best time during which to insert an IUD. The insertion of an IUD during the menstrual period does lend some benefits which include lubrication and slight opening of the cervical os from the menstrual flow, a decrease in bleeding symptoms after IUD placement due to the pre-existing bleeding from the menses, and the assurance that the patient is not pregnant. However, IUDs may be inserted at any time during the cycle so long as pregnancy has been excluded.

Bleeding patterns may change with both intrauterine contraceptive methods. The copper-T 380A is associated with approximately a 55% increase in menstrual blood loss.[100] In contrast, the amount of blood loss is significantly reduced to about 5 mL per cycle with the LNG-IUS.[101] The bleeding patterns with the T380A IUD may be most increased during the first few months of use, and some patients may require supplemental iron and prostaglandin synthetase inhibitors during menses to help counteract these effects. Bleeding patterns with the LNG-IUS are variable. The general picture of bleeding patterns is unscheduled bleeding during the first few months of use due to the erratic thinning of the endometrium. Over time, bleeding days decrease and approximately 20% of women are amenorrheic at 1 year of use. Women who do experience menstrual periods with the LNG-IUS in place generally have light periods or perhaps even spotting as opposed to longer and full menstrual flow.

Potential complications of IUD insertion include infection and perforation. There has been a documented transient increase in the risk of pelvic inflammatory disease (PID) within the first 20 days of intrauterine device placement.[102] This is likely due to the introduction of bacteria into the upper genital tract with the placement of the IUD or with the sounding of the uterus. However, over time PID prevalence is the same with IUD users as in the general population. One study has shown a decreased risk of PID among LNG-IUS users when compared to those who use the T380A. For this reason, some have advocated the levonorgestrel intrauterine system as an optimal method for younger women who may be at a baseline increased risk of PID. As with all nonbarrier methods of contraception, patients should be counseled that the intrauterine system does not protect against sexually transmitted infections, and if such a risk is present, condoms should be used.

Perforation is another uncommon risk of IUD insertion, but it is potentially serious. Perforation occurs at the time of insertion, and perforation rates are approximately 1 in 3000 insertions.[216] This risk is due to the blind introduction of the device into the uterus. At any time, if an IUD is found to be outside the uterus, even in asymptomatic patients, it should be removed from the peritoneal cavity. The presence of the copper IUD in the peritoneal cavity has been associated with complications, including severe adhesions and bowel obstruction. Such data are not available for the levonorgestrel intrauterine system, but until there is reason to believe otherwise, this IUD should also be removed, usually via laparoscopy.

RISKS OF IUD USE IN THE SETTING OF PREGNANCY

Pregnancies are rare with an IUD in place given their efficacy. However, if a woman conceives while using an IUD and the device is not subsequently removed, the incidence of spontaneous abortion is about 55%, about three times greater than would occur in pregnancies without an IUD. There has been concern over the risk of septic abortion due to an apparent increased risk in this adverse outcome with a historically used intrauterine device. There is no evidence that the IUDs that are currently on the market cause sepsis during pregnancy. There is a study that has demonstrated a decreased risk of a spontaneous abortion in women who have a copper IUD removed after pregnancy is diagnosed.[103] Since this percentage is similar to the baseline incidence of spontaneous abortion and significantly less than the reported incidence of abortion if the IUD remains in situ, the current recommendations include removal of an IUD should a woman conceive with the IUD in place and wishes to continue the pregnancy. There is difficulty with removal of the IUD at the time of pregnancy diagnosis. Ultrasound guidance may improve the ability to safely remove the IUD without repeated prodding.[104,105] There is evidence that IUD users may have increased rates of colonization with *Actinomyces* in the upper genital tract. Certain laboratories will report *Actinomyces* on Pap smear and this is often increased in women who have an IUD in place. The relationship of *Actinomyces* to PID is unclear because many women without intrauterine devices have *Actinomyces* in their vagina and are asymptomatic.[106] If *Actinomyces* organisms are identified on routine cervical cytologic examination and the woman is symptomatic, she may be treated with the appropriate antimicrobial therapy or expectant management as appropriate as well. The IUD need not be removed in an asymptomatic woman who is colonized with but not infected with actinomycosis.

The overall safety of intrauterine contraceptives demonstrate that they are not associated with an increased risk of endometrial or cervical carcinoma and may actually be associated with a reduced risk in these neoplasms during use and after removal.[107,108] The IUD is a very useful method of contraception for women who have completed their families and do not wish to have permanent sterilization. The LNG-IUS has many noncontraceptive benefits such as a decrease in menstrual symptoms and bleeding, and it is also a treatment for endometrial hyperplasia. Studies have also shown that the LNG-IUS is useful for treatment of women with adenomyosis and endometriosis. Women in the United States who use an IUD have a higher level of satisfaction with their method of contraception than do women using any other method of reversible contraception. IUD use is very common among female gynecologists but is underutilized by a large proportion of candidate women in the United States.

Noncontraceptive Benefits of Hormonal Contraception

The noncontraceptive health benefits of hormonal contraception are derived from a variety of epidemiologic studies that have been conducted since combined hormonal contraceptive pills were initially marketed in the 1960s. A study of combined hormonal contraceptive pills containing less than 35 µg of ethinyl estradiol (those that are routinely in clinical use today) estimate that use of these oral contraceptive pills allows for a 70% reduction in ovarian cancer (see Fig. 34-4), 50% reduction in endometrial cancer, 45% reduction in uterine blood loss, 50% reduction in dysmenorrhea, 65% reduction in premenstrual symptoms, 50% reduction in acne, 20% reduction in benign ovarian tumors, and 80% reduction in ectopic pregnancy.[109] Twelve case-control studies and three cohort studies have examined the relation between OCs and endometrial cancer, and all but two of these studies have indicated that the use of these agents has a protective effect against endometrial cancer, the third most common cancer among U.S. women.[110,111] Women who use OCs for at least 1 year have an age-adjusted relative risk of 0.5 for diagnosis of endometrial cancer between the ages of 40 and 55 years compared with nonusers. This protective effect is related to duration of use, increasing from a 20% risk reduction with 1 year of use to a 40% reduction within 2 years of use, to about a 60% reduction with 4 years of use. A prospective study of almost 30 years showed that OC users had one third the risk of endometrial cancer as nonusers (RR, 0.34; CI, 0.17-0.66) and one third the risk of dying of uterine cancer (RR, 0.3), compared with age-matched non-OC users.[112,113]

Eighteen studies on ovarian cancer and oral contraceptives have found a reduction in risk[42] (see Fig. 34-4). The relative risk of ovarian cancer among ever-users of OCs was 0.64, a 36% reduction. The magnitude of the decrease in risk is directly related to the duration of OC use, increasing from about a 40% reduction with 4 years of use to a 53% reduction with 8 years of use and a 60% reduction with 12 years of use. Beyond 1 year, there is about an 11% reduction in ovarian cancer risk for each of the first 5 years of use. The protective effect begins within 10 years of first use and continues for at least 20 years after the use of OCs ends. In the 1968-1995 analyses of the RCGP data,[113] OC users were half as likely to develop ovarian cancer as nonusers (RR, 0.49; CI, 0.3-0.8) and had a 40% decreased risk of death due to ovarian cancer (RR, 0.5). In a large case-control study, OC users had a 40% decrease in risk of ovarian cancer that increased to 70% reduction with 10 or more years of use.[114]

With the advent of the ability to test for hereditary predispositions to breast and ovarian cancer, the potential value for chemoprophylaxis with hormonal contraceptive regimens has become more important. Results from three studies indicate that women with *BRCA1* and *BRCA2* mutations who use combined hormonal contraceptive pills have a decreased risk for developing ovarian cancer.[50] It is important to counsel women who are at increased risk for ovarian cancer due to hereditary reasons that chemoprophylaxis can offer a safe and effective way to reduce their risk of developing ovarian cancer. Furthermore, the use of combined hormonal contraception does not increase a woman's risk of developing breast cancer.[41,48] In a large study by the Centers for Disease Control, current or past use of combined hormonal contraceptive pills did not increase the risk for developing breast cancer in women who were 35 to 64 years of age.[115] Women who are at increased risk of breast cancer due to genetic or family history were not at increased risk if they used combined hormonal contraceptives. Most studies show a similar pattern of risk

with hormonal contraceptive use regardless of a woman's reproductive history or her family history of breast cancer when it comes to her personal risk for breast cancer development.

Recent studies have shown that OCP use is not associated with an increase in breast cancer incidence, even in those who carry the *BRCA1* and *BRCA2* mutations.[50] The odds ratio for developing breast cancer with COC use was 0.74 (CI 0.55-0.99) for women with neither mutation; 0.18 (CI 0.08-0.42) for women with *BRCA1* mutation; and 0.92 (CI 0.3-2.84) with the *BRCA2* mutation. Therefore, it is evident that the use of the low-dose hormonal contraceptive pills that are currently in clinical practice today do not increase the risk for breast cancer in women who are genetically predisposed to developing this disease and afford a risk reduction for ovarian cancer in this same population.[49,50]

Contraception in Women of Special Subpopulations

Given the overall safety of hormonal contraception, especially in young healthy women, and when compared to the risk that pregnancy conveys, there are few instances when the risks of providing contraception outweigh the benefits. Overall mortality rate in the general population is not increased by OC use.[116] However, there are occasions when special consideration to contraceptive method must be given due to a woman's co-morbidities or health circumstances.

OBESITY

Obesity and its accompanying co-morbidities is becoming an increasing concern in both developed and underdeveloped countries. Although obesity does impair fertility it does not the eliminate risk of unintended pregnancy. Furthermore, pregnancy in obese women increases risks for obstetric and neonatal complications. For this reason, appropriate contraception is important in the obese population in order to help this population reduce unnecessary risk of stillbirth neonatal death, cesarean delivery, endometritis, and thromboembolism—all of which appear to be increased in pregnancy in obese women. Several epidemiologic studies conducted in the United States have demonstrated an increased risk of pregnancy in women using combined hormonal contraceptive pills. The reason for this is not understood, whether it be due to metabolism or other mechanisms. Health care providers and patients alike should be aware of the possible reduction in efficacy in this population. Authors analyzed the National Survey for Family Growth Data and identified women who had a BMI of 30 kg/m^2 or more and demonstrated that these women had an 80% increased risk of pregnancy compared to women who had a BMI of 20 to 24.9 kg/m^2.[117] The adjusted relative risk resulted in a 51% increased risk of pregnancy.

A case-control study of 454 patients with a first episode of thrombosis revealed that, among women aged 15 to 45 years, there is a combined effect of obesity with hormonal contraceptives on the risk of thrombosis leading to a 10-fold increased risk among women with a BMI greater than 25 kg/m². This risk increase was 2 to 4.6 times greater than in patients with one risk factor alone. On these data, some organizations, specifically the Royal College of Obstetricians and Gynecologists, advised that the risk for oral contraceptives generally outweighs the benefits for women with BMI of 35 to 39 kg/m² and that oral contraceptive pills that are combined should not be used in women with a BMI of 40 kg/M² or more.[118,119]

HORMONAL CONTRACEPTIVE IMPLANTS

The current etonogestrel implant now available cannot be assessed yet for differential efficacy in obese and nonobese populations. The number of pregnancies thus far has been too low for such conclusions to be drawn. However, the previously used six rod levonorgestrel implant was associated with a fivefold increase in risk of pregnancy in women who weighed more than 70 kg. These women are also at increased risk for endometrial cancer; progestin-only methods, specifically the progestin-only intrauterine contraceptive device, may be an appropriate choice in obese women because efficacy does not appear to be decreased in this population and it provides protection against endometrial hyperplasia.

WOMEN WITH CARDIOVASCULAR DISEASE

A meta-analysis of 10 studies found the odds ratio (OR) for myocardial infarction (MI) and ischemic stroke in OC users versus nonusers was 2.01 (95% CI 1.63-2.48). Second-generation OCs were associated with a significant increased risk of both MI and ischemic stroke events (OR 1.85, 95% CI 1.03-3.32; and 2.54, 95% CI 1.96-3.28, respectively) and third-generation OCs, for ischemic stroke outcome only (OR 2.03, 95% CI 1.15, 3.57).[120] Another meta-analysis found that current OC users have an overall adjusted OR for MI of 2.48 (95% CI 1.91-3.22) compared to never-users. The risk of MI for past OC users is not significantly different from that for never-users, overall OR 1.15 (95% CI 0.98-1.35; $P = 0.096$).[121]

There is an emerging population of women who are adult survivors of congenital heart disease. This population represents a challenge as pregnancy may either be contraindicated or certainly impose increased risk. Careful assessment of the independent risk of thrombosis in these women, based on the specific heart defect and the degree of correction, must be made when evaluating such patients for appropriate contraception. In general, using progestin-only methods or intrauterine devices is probably the safest mode in these patients. Barrier methods will likely not give sufficient efficacy, and although estrogen-containing methods may be appropriate in some subsets of this population, this choice may require careful attention and thought. Progestin-only methods, however, are safe in women who are at increased risk of MI or thrombosis and therefore can be used in this population.

HEREDITARY THROMBOPHILIA

In a retrospective family cohort study, women with hereditary deficiencies of protein S, protein C, or antithrombin who were taking an oral contraceptive had an annual incidence of venous thromboembolism of 3.5%, increasing to 12% in women with more than one type of hereditary thrombophilia.[122] A systematic review found a total of 10 studies together that provided "good" evidence of a greater risk of VTE (risk ratios of 1.3-25.1) and cerebral vein or cerebral sinus thrombosis among COC users with factor V Leiden mutation when compared with nonusers who have the mutation.[123] The evidence for prothrombin and other thrombogenic mutations was not as strong as for factor V Leiden mutation. It is unclear whether the type of COC or duration of use modifies the risk of VTE among women with thrombogenic mutations.[21] However, one study found that women with factor V Leiden polymorphisms may remain asymptomatic after prolonged use of OCs. Some authors support the use of SHBG levels and activated protein C resistance as markers of thromboembolic risk with OCPs.[116] The WHO discourages use of OCs in women with either an underlying thrombophilia or a history of a previous VTE.[23] These women are good candidates for progestin-only contraceptives or intrauterine contraceptives.

The complete reference list can be found on the companion Expert Consult Web site at www.expertconsultbook.com.

Suggested Readings

Collaborative Group on Hormonal Factors in Breast Cancer. Breast cancer and hormonal contraceptives: collaborative reanalysis of individual data on 53 297 women with breast cancer and 100 239 women without breast cancer from 54 epidemiological studies. Lancet 347:1713-1727, 1996.

Frost JJ, Singh S, Finer LB. Factors associated with contraceptive use and nonuse, United States, 2004. Perspect Sex Reprod Health 39:90-99, 2007.

Gray RH, Parker RA, Diethelm P. Vaginal bleeding disturbances associated with the discontinuation of long-acting injectable contraceptives. From the World Health Organization Special Programme for Research, Development, and Research Training in Human Reproduction; Task Force on Long-acting Systemic Agents for the Regulation of Fertility. Br J Obstet Gynaecol 88:317-321, 1981.

Hannaford PC, Kay CR. The risk of serious illness among oral contraceptive users: evidence from the RCGP's oral contraceptive study. Br J Gen Pract 48:1657-1662, 1998.

Jensen JT, Speroff L. Health benefits of oral contraceptives. Obstet Gynecol Clin North Am 27:705-721, 2000.

Rosenberg L, Zhang Y, Constant D, et al. Bone status after cessation of use of injectable progestin contraceptives. Contraception 76:425-431, 2007.

Schlaff WD, Lynch AM, Hughes HD, et al. Manipulation of the pill-free interval in oral contraceptive pill users: the effect on follicular suppression. Am J Obstet Gynecol 190:943-951, 2004.

Schlesselman JJ. Net effect of oral contraceptive use on the risk of cancer in women in the United States. Obstet Gynecol 85:793-801, 1995.

von Hertzen H, Piaggio G, Van Look PF, Task Force on Postovulatory Methods of Fertility Regulation. Emergency contraception with levonorgestrel or the Yuzpe regimen. Lancet 352:1998, 1939.

World Health Organization Collaborative Study of Cardiovascular Disease and Steroid Hormone Contraception. Effect of different progestagens in low oestrogen oral contraceptives on venous thromboembolic disease. Lancet 346:1582-1588, 1995.

Index

Note: Page numbers followed by f indicate figures; those followed by t indicate tables; and those followed by b indicate boxed material.